Principles of
Neurological
Surgery Third Edition

Principles of Neurological Surgery

Third Edition

Richard G. Ellenbogen, MD, FACS

Professor and Chairman
Theodore S. Roberts Endowed Chair
Department of Neurological Surgery
University of Washington
Seattle, Washington
USA

Saleem I. Abdulrauf, MD, FAANS FACS

Professor and Chairman
Department of Neurological Surgery
Saint Louis University School of Medicine
Director, Saint Louis University Center
    for Cerebrovascular and Skull Base Surgery
Neurosurgeon-in-Chief
Saint Louis University Hospital
St. Louis, Missouri
USA

Laligam N. Sekhar, MD, FACS

Vice Chairman
William Joseph Leedom and Bennett Bigelow Professor
Director, Cerebrovascular Surgery and Skull Base Surgery
Department of Neurological Surgery
University of Washington
Seattle, Washington
USA

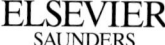

ELSEVIER
SAUNDERS

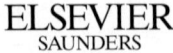

1600 John F. Kennedy Blvd.
Ste 1800
Philadelphia, PA 19103-2899

Notices

Knowledge and best practice in this field are constantly changing. As new research and experience
broaden our understanding, changes in research methods, professional practices, or medical treatment may become necessary.

Practitioners and researchers must always rely on their own experience and knowledge in evaluating and using any information, methods, compounds, or experiments described herein. In using such
information or methods they should be mindful of their own safety and the safety of others, including
parties for whom they have a professional responsibility.

With respect to any drug or pharmaceutical products identified, readers are advised to check the
most current information provided (i) on procedures featured or (ii) by the manufacturer of each
product to be administered, to verify the recommended dose or formula, the method and duration of
administration, and contraindications. It is the responsibility of practitioners, relying on their own
experience and knowledge of their patients, to make diagnoses, to determine dosages and the best
treatment for each individual patient, and to take all appropriate safety precautions.

To the fullest extent of the law, neither the Publisher nor the authors, contributors, or editors,
assume any liability for any injury and/or damage to persons or property as a matter of products
liability, negligence or otherwise, or from any use or operation of any methods, products, instructions, or ideas contained in the material herein.

Library of Congress Cataloging-in-Publication Data

Principles of neurological surgery / editors, Richard G. Ellenbogen, Saleem I. Abdulrauf;
associate editor, Laligam N. Sekhar. -- 3rd ed.
      p. ; cm.
   Rev. ed. of: Principles of neurosurgery / edited by Setti S. Rengachary, Richard G. Ellenbogen.
2nd ed. 2005.
   Includes bibliographical references and index.
   ISBN 978-1-4377-0701-4 (hardcover : alk. paper)
   I. Ellenbogen, Richard G. II. Abdulrauf, Saleem I. III. Sekhar, Laligam N.
IV. Principles of neurosurgery.
   [DNLM: 1. Neurosurgical Procedures. 2. Nervous System Diseases—surgery. WL 368]
   LC classification not assigned
   617.4'8–dc23   2011046359

Associate Content Strategist: Julie Goolsby
Content Development Specialist: Julia Bartz
Publishing Services Manager: Patricia Tannian
Senior Project Manager: Sharon Corell
Senior Book Designer: Louis Forgione

Working together to grow
libraries in developing countries

www.elsevier.com | www.bookaid.org | www.sabre.org

ELSEVIER   BOOK AID International   Sabre Foundation

Printed in the United States of America

Last digit is the print number: 9 8 7 6 5 4 3 2 1

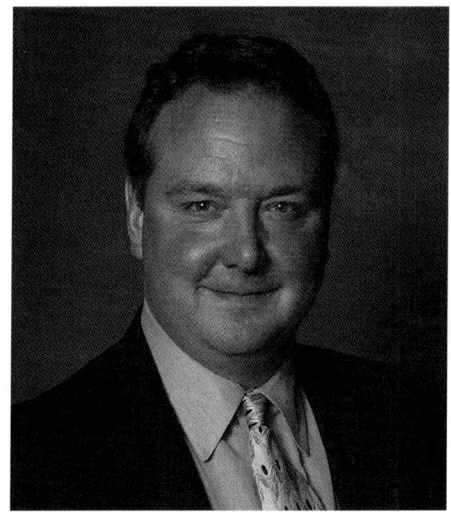
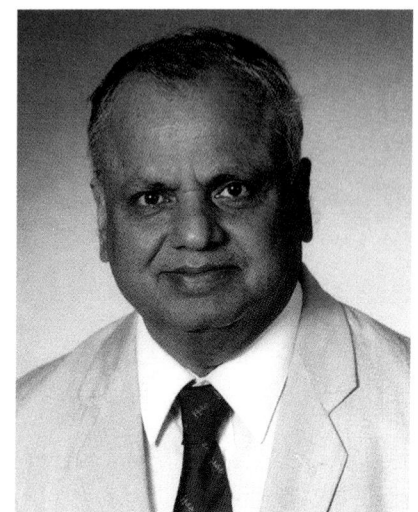

IN MEMORIUM

CHRISTOPHER C. GETCH, MD (1961-2012)

SETTI S. RENGACHARY, MD (1937-2008)

They floated through our lives for far too short a time. Professors Getch and Rengachary were renowned neurological surgeons, husbands, fathers, and mentors. These leaders taught using the tools of inspiration and patience. They operated with skill and compassion. And they brought happiness to all whose lives they touched. They remain heroes to their patients and role models to their students. They were forces of light and kindness in our field, and as our friends, made us better. We shall miss their intellect, humor, and gentle spirits. They shall forever remain as beacons of what the best of our field can bring to those we serve. We dedicate this edition to them.

"Concern for man and his fate must always form the chief interest of all technical endeavors. Never forget this in the midst of your diagrams and equations." Albert Einstein

To the loves of my life: Sandy, Rachel, Paul, and Zachary…thank you for my happiness and your great humor!

Richard G. Ellenbogen, MD, FACS

I dedicate this book to my patients for placing their deepest trust in us, as there is no higher trust than to place their lives in the hands of others. This trust represents our most seminal obligation.

I dedicate this book to my students, residents, and fellows, as there is no higher achievement than to see those whom we mentor go on to become compassionate and technically exceptional neurosurgeons.

Saleem I. Abdulrauf, MD, FAANS, FACS

I dedicate the book to my wife, Gordana, and my children, Raja, Daniela, and Krishna.

Laligam N. Sekhar, MD, FACS

Contributors

Saleem I. Abdulrauf, MD, FAANS, FACS
Professor and Chairman
Department of Neurological Surgery
Saint Louis University School of Medicine
Director, Saint Louis University Center for Cerebrovascular
   and Skull Base Surgery
Neurosurgeon-in-Chief
Saint Louis University Hospital
St. Louis, Missouri, USA

Francesco Acerbi, MD, PhD
Department of Neurosurgery Fondazione IRCCS Istituto
Neurologico Carlo Besta
Milan, Italy

Geoffrey Appelboom, MD
Department of Neurological Surgery
Columbia University College of Physicians and Surgeons
New York, New York, USA

Col. Rocco A. Armonda, MD
Director, Cerebrovascular Surgery and Interventional
   Neuroradiology
National Capital Neurosurgery Service
Walter Reed Military Medical Center
Director, Department of Neurosurgery
Uniformed Services University of the Health Sciences
Bethesda, Maryland, USA

Danielle Balériaux, MD
Emeritus Professor and Senior Consultant
Department of Neuroradiology
Erasme Hospital
Université Libre de Bruxelles
Brussels, Belgium

Nicholas C. Bambakidis, MD
Department of Neurological Surgery
University Hospitals Case Medical Center
Cleveland, Ohio, USA

H. Hunt Batjer, MD
Professor and Chair
Northwestern University Feinberg School of Medicine
Chairman
Department of Neurological Surgery
Northwestern Memorial Hospital
Chicago, Illinois, USA

Joel A. Bauman, MD
Resident
Department of Neurosurgery
University of Pennsylvania
Philadelphia, Pennsylvania, USA

LCDR Randy S. Bell, MD
Assistant Professor
Uniformed Services University of Health Sciences
Attending Neurosurgeon
National Capital Neurosurgery Service
Walter Reed National Military Medical Center
Bethesda, Maryland, USA

Shawn A. Belverud, DO, LCDR, MC, USN
Staff Neurosurgeon
Naval Medical Center San Diego
San Diego, California, USA

Bernard R. Bendok, MD, FACS
Associate Professor of Neurosurgery
Department of Neurosurgery
Northwestern University Feinberg School of Medicine
Northwestern Memorial Hospital
Chicago, Illinois, USA

Edward C. Benzel, MD
Chairman
Department of Neurosurgery
Neurological Institute
Cleveland Clinic
Cleveland, Ohio, USA

Mitchel S. Berger, MD
Professor and Chairman
Department of Neurological Surgery
University of California, San Francisco
San Francisco, California, USA

Sandeep S. Bhangoo, MD, MS
Chief Resident
Department of Neurosurgery
Henry Ford Hospital
Detroit, Michigan, USA

William Bingaman, MD
Vice Chairman
Neurological Institute
Head
Department of Epilepsy Surgery
Cleveland Clinic
Cleveland, Ohio, USA

Peter Black, MD, PhD
Professor of Neurosurgery
Harvard Medical School
Founding Chair
Department of Neurosurgery
Brigham and Women's Hospital
Boston, Massachusetts, USA
President of the World Federation of Neurosurgical Societies

Benjamin Blondel, MD
Spine Division
Hospital for Joint Diseases
New York University
New York, New York, USA

Giovanni Broggi, MD
Professor of Neurosurgery
Department of Neurosurgery
Fondazione IRCCS Istituto Neurologico Carlo Besta
Milan, Italy

Morgan Broggi, MD
Department of Neurosurgery
Fondazione IRCCS Istituto Neurologico Carlo Besta
Milan, Italy

Jacques Brotchi, MD, PhD, FACS
Emeritus Professor and Honorary Chairman
Department of Neurosurgery
Erasme Hospital
Brussels, Belgium

Samuel R. Browd, MD, PhD
Assistant Professor of Neurological Surgery
Associate Residency Director
Department of Neurological Surgery
University of Washington
Attending Pediatric Neurosurgeon
Director, Hydrocephalus Program
Seattle Children's Hospital
Seattle, Washington, USA

Michaël Bruneau, MD, PhD
Associate Professor
Department of Neurosurgery
Erasme Hospital
Brussels, Belgium

David W. Cadotte, MSc, MD
Neurosurgical Resident
Division of Neurosurgery
University of Toronto
Toronto, Ontario, Canada

Paolo Cappabianca, MD
Professor and Chairman of Neurosurgery
Department of Neurological Sciences
Division of Neurosurgery
Università degli Studi de Napoli Federico II
Naples, Italy

Ricardo L. Carrau, MD, FACS
Professor
Department of Otolaryngology–Head and Neck Surgery
Director of the Comprehensive Skull Base Surgery Program
The Ohio State University Medical Center
Columbus, Ohio, USA

Luigi Maria Cavallo, MD, PhD
Neurosurgery Instructor
Department of Neurological Sciences
Division of Neurosurgery
Università degli Studi de Napoli Federico II
Naples, Italy

Juanita M. Celix, MD
Resident
Department of Neurological Surgery
University of Washington
Seattle, Washington, USA

Chris Cifarelli, MD, PhD
Chief Resident
Department of Neurological Surgery
University of Virginia
Charlottesville, Virginia, USA

Lt. Michael Cirivello, MD
Neurosurgery Resident
National Capital Neurosurgery Consortium
Walter Reed National Military Medical Center
Bethesda, Maryland, USA

Alan R. Cohen, MD, FACS, FAAP
Reinberger Professor of Neurological Surgery
Chief of Pediatric Neurosurgery
Surgeon-in-Chief
Rainbow Babies and Children's Hospital
Case Western Reserve University School of Medicine
The Neurological Institute
University Hospitals Case Medical Center
Cleveland, Ohio, USA

E. Sander Connolly Jr., MD
Bennett M. Stein Professor and Vice-Chair
Department of Neurological Surgery
Department of Neurological Intensive Care
Columbia University College of Physicians and Surgeons
New York, New York, USA

Victor Correa-Correa, MD
Research Fellow
Harborview Medical Center
National Institute of Neurology and Neurosurgery in Mexico
Tlalpan, Mexico

Aneela Darbar, MD
Assistant Professor
Department of Neurological Surgery
Saint Louis University School of Medicine
St. Louis, Missouri, USA

Salvatore Di Maio, MDCM, FRCS(C)
Fellow
Department of Neurological Surgery
University of Washington
Harborview Medical Center
Seattle, Washington, USA

Christopher S. Eddleman, MD, PhD
Department of Neurosurgical Surgery and Radiology
UT Southwestern Medical Center
Dallas, Texas, USA

Richard G. Ellenbogen, MD, FACS
Professor and Chairman
Theodore S. Roberts Endowed Chair
Department of Neurological Surgery
University of Washington
Seattle, Washington, USA

Jorge L. Eller, MD
Assistant Professor
Department of Neurological Surgery
Saint Louis University School of Medicine
St. Louis, Missouri, USA

Felice Esposito, MD, PhD
Neurosurgery Instructor
Department of Neurological Sciences
Division of Neurosurgery
Università degli Studi de Napoli Federico II
Naples, Italy

Isabella Esposito, MD
Neurosurgery Instructor
Department of Neurological Sciences
Division of Neurosurgery
Università degli Studi de Napoli Federico II
Naples, Italy

Aria Fallah, MD
Resident
Division of Neurosurgery
University of Toronto
Toronto, Ontario, Canada

Michael G. Fehlings, MD, PhD, FRCSC, FACS
Professor and Krembil Chair in Neural Repair and Regeneration
University of Toronto
Toronto, Ontario, Canada

Manuel Ferreira, Jr., MD, PhD
Assistant Professor
Department of Neurological Surgery
University of Washington
Seattle, Washington, USA

Aristotelis S. Filippidis, MD
Division of Neurological Surgery
Barrow Neurological Institute
St. Joseph's Hospital and Medical Center
Phoenix, Arizona, USA

James R. Fink, MD
Assistant Professor
Department of Radiology
University of Washington
Seattle, Washington, USA

Kathleen R. Tozer Fink, MD
Assistant Professor
Department of Radiology
University of Washington
Seattle, Washington, USA

John C. Flickinger, MD, FACR
Department of Radiation Oncology
University of Pittsburgh Medical Center
Pittsburgh, Pennsylvania, USA

Rabindranath Garcia, MD
Research Fellow
Department of Neurological Surgery
University of Washington
Seattle, Washington, USA

Fred H. Geisler, MD, PhD
Founder
Illinois Neuro-Spine Center at Rush-Copley Medical Center
Aurora, Illinois, USA

Mikhail Gelfenbeyn, MD, PhD
Assistant Professor
Department of Neurological Surgery
University of Washington
Puget Sound Health Care System
Veterans Administration Medical Center
Seattle, Washington, USA

Venelin M. Gerganov, MD
Associate Neurosurgeon
Department of Neurosurgery
International Neuroscience Institute
Hannover, Germany

Christopher C. Getch, MD
Professor
Department of Neurological Surgery
Northwestern University Feinberg School of Medicine
Chicago, Illinois, USA

George M. Ghobrial, MD
Neurosurgery Resident
Department of Neurological Surgery
Thomas Jefferson University Hospital
Philadelphia, Pennsylvania, USA

Carlo Giussani, MD, PhD
Division of Neurosurgery
University of Milano-Bicocca
Monza, Italy;
Department of Neurological Surgery
University of Washington School of Medicine
Seattle, Washington, USA

Atul Goel, MD
Department of Neurosurgery
K.E.M. Hospital
Parel, Mumbai, India

Ziya L. Gokaslan, MD, FACS
Donlin M. Long Professor
Professor of Neurosurgery, Oncology and Orthopaedic Surgery
Vice-Chair
Director of Neurosurgical Spine Program
Department of Neurosurgery
Johns Hopkins University School of Medicine
Johns Hopkins Hospital
Baltimore, Maryland, USA

James Tait Goodrich, MD, PhD, DSci (Hon)
Director, Division of Pediatric Neurosurgery
Department of Neurosurgery
Montefiore Medical Center
Professor of Clinical Neurosurgery, Pediatrics, Plastic
  and Reconstructive Surgery
Albert Einstein College of Medicine
Bronx, New York, USA

Gerald A. Grant, MD
Associate Professor of Neurosurgery and Pediatrics
Duke University
Durham, North Carolina, USA

Murat Gunel, MD
Nixdoff-German Professor of Neurosurgery
Chief, Yale Neurovascular Surgery Program
Co-Director, Yale Program on Neurogenetics
Yale University School of Medicine
New Haven, Connecticut, USA

Todd C. Hankinson, MD, MBA
Assistant Professor of Neurosurgery
Children's Hospital Colorado
University of Colorado Denver
Aurora, Colorado, USA

James S. Harrop, MD
Associate Professor of Neurologic and Orthopedic Surgery
Jefferson Medical College
Philadelphia, Pennsylvania, USA

Alia Hdeib, MD
Neurosurgery Resident
Department of Neurological Surgery
Neurological Institute
University Hospitals Case Medical Center
Cleveland, Ohio, USA

Alan Hoffer, MD
Director of Neurotrauma Program
Assistant Professor
Department of Neurological Surgery
University Hospitals Case Medical Center
Cleveland, Ohio, USA

L. Nelson Hopkins, MD, FACS
Professor and Chairman
Departments of Neurosurgery and Radiology and
Toshiba Stroke Research Center, School of Medicine and
  Biomedical Sciences
University at Buffalo, State University of New York
Department of Neurosurgery
Millard Fillmore Gates Hospital
Kaleida Health
Buffalo, New York, USA

Clifford M. Houseman, DO
Resident
Department of Neurological Surgery
Cushing Neuroscience Institute
Hofstra North Shore-LIJ School of Medicine
Manhasset, New York, USA

Gwyneth Hughes, MD
Resident
Neurological Surgery
Cleveland Clinic Foundation
Cleveland, Ohio, USA

David F. Jimenez, MD, FACS
Professor and Chairman
Department of Neurosurgery
University of Texas Health Sciences Center, San Antonio
San Antonio, Texas, USA

M. Yashar S. Kalani, MD, PhD
Resident
Division of Neurological Surgery
Barrow Neurological Institute
St. Joseph's Hospital and Medical Center
Phoenix, Arizona, USA

Amin B. Kassam, MD, FRCS(C)
Professor and Chief of Neurosurgery
University of Ottawa
Ottawa, Ontario, Canada

Robert F. Keating, MD
Professor and Chief
Division of Neurosurgery
Children's National Medical Center
George Washington University School of Medicine
Washington, DC, USA

Daniel Kelly, MD
Director, Brain Tumor Center
John Wayne Cancer Institute at Saint John's Health Center
Santa Monica, California, USA

Joanna Kemp, MD
Department of Neurosurgery
Saint Louis University School of Medicine
St. Louis, Missouri, USA

Melin Khandekar, MD, PhD
Instructor
Department of Radiation Oncology
Harvard Medical School
Assistant in Radiation Oncology
Massachusetts General Hospital
Boston, Massachusetts, USA

Louis J. Kim, MD
Assistant Professor
Department of Neurological Surgery
University of Washington
Seattle, Washington, USA

Douglas Kondziolka, MD, MSc, FRCSC
Peter J. Jannetta Professor of Neurological Surgery
University of Pittsburgh
Pittsburgh, Pennsylvania, USA

Virginie Lafage, PhD
Director, Spine Research
Spine Division
Hospital for Joint Diseases
New York University
New York, New York, USA

Federico Landriel, MD
Neurosurgery Chief Resident
Fellow of the WFNS at Harvard University/
    Brigham and Women's Hospital
Department of Neurological Surgery
Hospital Italiano de Buenos Aires
Buenos Aires, Argentina

Geneviève Lapointe, MD, FRCSC
Department of Neurological Surgery
Saint Louis University School of Medicine
St. Louis, Missouri, USA

A. Noelle Larson, MD
Assistant Professor
Department of Orthopedic Surgery
Mayo Clinic
Rochester, Minnesota, USA

Ilya Laufer, MD
Assistant Attending
Department of Neurosurgery
Memorial Sloan-Kettering Cancer Center
New York, New York, USA

Jonathon J. Lebovitz, MD, MS
Department of Neurological Surgery
Saint Louis University School of Medicine
St. Louis, Missouri, USA

Florence Lefranc, MD, PhD
Department of Neurosurgery
Erasme Hospital
Université Libre de Bruxelles
Brussels, Belgium

Michael R. Levitt, MD
Resident
Department of Neurological Surgery
University of Washington
Seattle, Washington, USA

Elad I. Levy, MD, FACS, FAHA
Professor
Departments of Neurosurgery and Radiology and
Toshiba Stroke Research Center
School of Medicine and Biomedical Sciences,
University at Buffalo, State University of New York
Department of Neurosurgery
Millard Fillmore Gates Circle Hospital
Kaleida Health
Buffalo, New York, USA

James K.C. Liu, MD
Resident
Department of Neurological Surgery
Neurological Institute
Cleveland Clinic
Cleveland, Ohio, USA

Jay Loeffler, MD
Chief
Radiation Oncology
Massachusetts General Hospital
Boston, Massachusetts, USA

John Loeser, MD
Professor Emeritus
Departments of Neurological Surgery and
Anesthesiology and Pain Medicine
University of Washington
Seattle, Washington, USA

Ramón López López, MD
Research Fellow
Department of Neurological Surgery
University of Washinigton
Seattle, Washington, USA

Timothy H. Lucas, II, MD, PhD
Assistant Professor
Department of Neurological Surgery
University of Pennsylvania
Philadelphia, Pennsylvania, USA

L. Dade Lunsford, MD
Lars Leksell Professor and Distinguished Professor
Professor of Neurological Surgery and Radiology Oncology
Director, Center for Image-Guided Neurosurgery
Director, Residency Training Program
University of Pittsburgh Medical Center
Pittsburgh, Pennsylvania, USA

Luke J. Macyszyn, MD
Resident
Department of Neurosurgery
University of Pennsylvania
Philadelphia, Pennsylvania, USA

Marcella A. Madera, MD
Neurosurgeon
Austin Brain and Spine
Seton Brain and Spine Institute
Austin, Texas, USA

Suresh N. Magge, MD
Assistant Professor of Neurosurgery and Pediatrics
George Washington University
Division of Pediatric Neurosurgery
Children's National Medical Center
Washington, DC, USA

Ghaus M. Malik, MD
John R. Davis Chair in Neurosurgery
Vice-Chairman
Department of Neurosurgery
Henry Ford Health System, Detroit
Chief of Neurosurgery
Henry Ford West Bloomfield Hospital
Detroit, Michigan, USA

Paul N. Manson, MD
Professor of Surgery
University of Maryland Shock Trauma Unit
Professor of Surgery
Johns Hopkins Hospital
Baltimore, Maryland, USA

Edward M. Marchan, MD
Resident Physician
Department of Neurosurgery
Thomas Jefferson University
Philadelphia, Pennsylvania, USA

Carlo Marras, MD
Center for Epilepsy Surgery and Neuro-Oncology
Division of Neurosurgery
Ospedale Pediatrico Bambino Gesù
Roma, Italy

Henry Marsh, CBE, MA, MD, FRCS
Consultant Neurosurgeon
Atkinson Morley's/St. George's Hospital
London Professor
Department of Neurological Surgery
University of Washington
Seattle, Washington, USA

Christian Matula, MD, PhD
Professor of Neurosurgery
Neurosurgical Department
Medical University of Vienna
Vienna, Austria

Nancy McLaughlin, MD, PhD, FRCSC
Neuroscience Institute and Brain Tumor Center
John Wayne Cancer Institute at Saint John's Health Center
Santa Monica, California, USA

Giuseppe Messina, MD
Department of Neurosurgery
Fondazione IRCCS Istituto Neurologico Carlo Besta
Milan, Italy

Alessandra Mantovani, MD
Research Fellow
Department of Neurological Surgery
University of Washington
Seattle, Washington, USA

Ryan Morton, MD
Resident
Department of Neurological Surgery
University of Washington
Seattle, Washington, USA

Carrie R. Muh, MD, MS
Assistant Professor of Neurosurgery and Pediatrics
Division of Neurosurgery
Duke University Medical Center
Durham, North Carolina, USA

Raj K. Narayan, MD
Professor and Chairman
Department of Neurosurgery
Director
Cushing Neuroscience Institute
Hofstra North Shore-LIJ School of Medicine
Manhasset, New York, USA

Sabareesh K. Natarajan, MD, MS
Clinical Assistant Instructor
Department of Neurosurgery and
Toshiba Stroke Research Center,
School of Medicine and Biomedical Sciences
University at Buffalo, State University of New York
Department of Neurosurgery
Millard Fillmore Gates Circle Hospital, Kaleida Health
Buffalo, New York, USA

Ajay Niranjan, MD, MBA
Associate Professor of Neurological Surgery
Director of Radiosurgery Research
University of Pittsburgh Medical Center
Pittsburgh, Pennsylvania, USA

Jeffrey G. Ojemann, MD
Professor
Department of Neurological Surgery
University of Washington
Richard G. Ellenbogen Chair in Pediatric Neurological
  Surgery
Center for Integrative Brain Research, Seattle Children's
  Research Institute
Chief
Division of Neurological Surgery
Seattle Children's Hospital
Seattle, Washington, USA

Chima O. Oluigbo, MD, FRCSC
Assistant Professor of Neurological Surgery
Department of Neurological Surgery
The Ohio State University Medical Center
Columbus, Ohio, USA

Nelson M. Oyesiku, MD, PhD, FACS
Al Lerner Chair and Vice-Chairman
Department of Neurosurgery
Professor of Neurosurgery and Medicine (Endocrinology)
Emory University School of Medicine
Director
Neurosurgery Residency Program
Editor-in-Chief, NEUROSURGERY
Atlanta, Georgia, USA

Ali K. Ozturk, MD
Resident Physician
Department of Neurosurgery
Yale University School of Medicine
New Haven, Connecticut, USA

Sheri K. Palejwala, MD
Department of Neurological Surgery
Saint Louis University School of Medicine
St. Louis, Missouri, USA

Matthew Piazza
Clinical Research Fellow
Department of Neurological Surgery
Columbia University College of Physicians and Surgeons
New York, New York, USA

David W. Polly, Jr., MD
Professor and Chief of Spine Surgery
Spine Division
University of Minnesota
Minneapolis, Minnesota, USA

Daniel M. Prevedello, MD
Assistant Professor
Department of Neurological Surgery
Director of Minimally Invasive Cranial Surgery Program
The Ohio State University Medical Center
Columbus, Ohio, USA

Anja-Maria Radon
Department of Neurological Surgery
Saint Louis University School of Medicine
St. Louis, Missouri, USA

Govind Rajan, MBBS
Associate Professor of Anesthesiology, Surgery, and Critical Care
Director of Clinical Anesthesiology and Operating Room Affairs
Director, Liver Transplant Anesthesia
Saint Louis University School of Medicine
St. Louis, Missouri, USA

Ali R. Rezai, MD
Julius F. Stone Chair
Professor of Neurosurgery
Director
Ohio State University Center for Neuromodulation
Vice Chair, Clinical Research
Department of Neurological Surgery
The Ohio State University Medical Center
Columbus, Ohio, USA

Eduardo Rodriguez, MD, DDS
Chief of Plastic Surgery
Associate Professor
University of Maryland Shock Trauma Unit
Associate Professor
Johns Hopkins Hospital
Baltimore, Maryland, USA

James T. Rutka, MD, PhD, FRCSC
Professor and Chair
Department of Surgery
University of Toronto
Toronto, Ontario, Canada

Madjid Samii, MD, PhD
President of the International Neuroscience Institute
Hannover, Germany
President of the China International Neuroscience Institute
  at the Capital University of Medical Sciences
Beijing, China

Mical Samuelson, MD
Neurosurgery Resident
Department of Neurosurgery
University of Texas Health Science Center, San Antonio
San Antonio, Texas, USA

Nader Sanai, MD
Director
Division of Neurosurgical Oncology
Director, Barrow Brain Tumor Research Center
Barrow Neurological Institute
Phoenix, Arizona, USA

Deanna Sasaki-Adams, MD
Assistant Professor
Department of Neurological Surgery
Saint Louis University School of Medicine
St. Louis, Missouri, USA

Jennifer Gentry Savage, MD
Neurosurgery Chief Resident
Department of Neurosurgery
University of Texas Health Science Center, San Antonio
San Antonio, Texas, USA

David Schlesinger, PhD
Assistant Professor of Radiation Oncology and Neurological
  Surgery
University of Virginia
Charlottesville, Virginia, USA

Frank Schwab, MD
Clinical Professor
Chief of the Spinal Deformity Service
Spine Division
Hospital for Joint Diseases
New York University
New York, New York, USA

Daniel Sciubba, MD
Assistant Professor
Department of Neurosurgery
Johns Hopkins Hospital
Baltimore, Maryland, USA

R. Michael Scott, MD
Professor of Surgery
Department of Surgery (Neurosurgery)
Harvard Medical School
Neurosurgeon-in-Chief
Children's Hospital Boston
Boston, Massachusetts, USA

Laligam N. Sekhar, MD, FACS
Vice Chairman
William Joseph Leedom and Bennett Bigelow Professor
Director, Cerebrovascular Surgery and Skull Base Surgery
Department of Neurological Surgery
University of Washington
Seattle, Washington, USA

Warren Selman, MD
The Harvey Huntington Brown, Jr., Professor and Chair
Department of Neurological Surgery
Case Western Reserve University
Director
The Neurological Institute
University Hospitals
Cleveland, Ohio, USA

Mitchel Seruya, MD
Resident
Plastic Surgery
Georgetown University Hospital
Washington, DC, USA

Spyros Sgouros, MD, FRCS(SN)
Assistant Professor of Neurosurgery
University of Athens
Director
Department of Pediatric Neurosurgery
"Mitera" Childrens Hospital
Athens, Greece

Jason P. Sheehan, MD, PhD
Alumni Professor of Neurological Surgery and Radiation
  Oncology
Director of Lars Leksell Gamma Knife Center
Vice Chair of Academic Affairs
University of Virginia
Charlottesville, Virginia, USA

Helen Shih, MD, MS, MPH
Assistant Professor of Radiation Oncology
Harvard Medical School
Chief, Central Nervous System and Eye Services
Department of Radiation Oncology
Massachusetts General Hospital
Boston, Massachusetts, USA

Adnan H. Siddiqui, MD, PhD
Associate Professor
Departments of Neurosurgery and Radiology and
  Toshiba Stroke Research Center,
School of Medicine and Biomedical Sciences
University at Buffalo, State University of New York
Department of Neurosurgery
Millard Fillmore Gates Circle Hospital, Kaleida Health
Buffalo, New York, USA

Daniel L. Silbergeld, MD, FACS
Arthur A. Ward, Jr., Professor
Department of Neurological Surgery
University of Washington
Seattle, Washington, USA

Justin Singer, MD
Resident
Department of Neurological Surgery
University Hospitals Case Medical Center
Cleveland, Ohio, USA

Edward R. Smith, MD
Director, Pediatric Cerebrovascular Surgery
Department of Neurosurgery
Children's Hospital Boston
Associate Professor of Surgery
Harvard Medical School
Boston, Massachusetts, USA

Vita Stagno, MD
Resident
Department of Neurological Sciences
Division of Neurosurgery
Università degli Studi de Napoli Federico II
Naples, Italy

Juraj Šteňo, Prof, MD, PhD
Professor
Head of the Department of Neurosurgery
Comenius University Medical Faculty
Bratislava, Slovakia

Leslie N. Sutton, MD
Professor
University of Pennsylvania School of Medicine
Chief Neurosurgery
Children's Hospital of Philadelphia
Philadelphia, Pennsylvania, USA

Justin M. Sweeney, MD
Department of Neurological Surgery
Saint Louis University School of Medicine
St. Louis, Missouri, USA

Alexander S. Taghva, MD
Department of Neurological Surgery
University of Southern California, Keck School of Medicine
Los Angeles, California, USA

Farzana Tariq, MD
Senior Fellow
Department of Neurological Surgery
University of Washington
Seattle, Washington, USA

Charles Teo, MD
Associate Professor and Chairman
Prince of Wales Private Hospital
University of New South Wales
Director
Centre for Minimally Invasive Neurosurgery
Sydney, Australia

Nicholas Theodore, MD, FACS
Professor
Chief, Spine Section
Division of Neurological Surgery
Director, Neurotrauma Program
Barrow Neurological Institute
St. Joseph's Hospital and Medical Center
Phoenix, Arizona, USA

R. Shane Tubbs, MS, PA-C, PhD
Anatomist/Research
Children's Hospital
Birmingham, Alabama, USA

Aimee Two, MD
Resident Physician
Department of Neurological Surgery
University of Southern California, Keck School of Medicine
Los Angeles, California, USA

Scott D. Wait, MD
Pediatric Neurosurgery Fellow
LeBonheur Children's Hospital/St. Jude's Children's Research Hospital
Memphis, Tennessee, USA

Grace Elisabeth Walter
Central Michigan University
Mount Pleasant, Michigan, USA

Adrienne Weeks, PhD
Department of Neurosurgery
University of Toronto
Toronto, Ontario, Canada

John C. Wellons, III, MD
Professor of Surgery and Pediatrics
Section of Pediatric Neurosurgery
University of Alabama–Birmingham
Children's Hospital of Alabama
Birmingham, Alabama, USA

Lynda J-S Yang, MD, PhD
Associate Professor
Department of Neurosurgery
University of Michigan Health System
Ann Arbor, Michigan, USA

Chun Po Yen, MD
Clinical Instructor
Department of Neurological Surgery
University of Virginia
Charlottesville, Virginia, USA

Preface

Concern for man and his fate must always form the chief interest of all technical endeavors...Never forget this in the midst of your diagrams and equations.

Albert Einstein

Principles of Neurological Surgery is in its third edition because of the popular demand of our students. As I walk through the hospital and operating room, I am thrilled to see the previous editions being read by medical students, house officers, nurses, and practicing neurosurgeons. It is for these treasured students, young and old, novice and experienced, that this book is intended. It is to be used to guide both those learning and those teaching. We are indebted to our students for inspiring us to perform at our best every day, for in the operating room our best is required by our patients all the time. At the end of the day, we hope this edition contributes to the modest goal of shaping more effective clinicians, ultimately for the benefit of our patients.

The world of medical education has evolved rapidly, and our students do not necessarily learn in the same manner we once learned. We have listened carefully to their constructive comments and re-created a book that addresses their individual approach to learning basic neurological surgery principles. Scientific information is growing at an exponential rate. Thus, mastering the wide spectrum of neurological surgery is arguably even more challenging for the current generation of students than it was for our generation. A host of excellent encyclopedic neurological surgery reference texts currently are available. Our work is intended to be comprehensive without being encyclopedic. We hope it could be the sort of tool that students can use every day of their training and then carry into practice. We realize that the internet and searchable peer-reviewed literature have often supplanted multivolume collections. So we took a different approach with this text. It is our goal to make the complex and broad spectrum of neurological surgery more comprehensible by reviewing the surgical principles in a concisely written, template-oriented,

and visually attractive format. The text is purposely designed to fit in a single volume so that the information is digestible and can be successfully reinforced with subsequent review. The chapter topics represent both basic core areas and novel subject matter in our rapidly evolving field. The authors have added CLINICAL PEARLS to their chapters that sum up the critical bullet points of the chapters. The chapters are further supplemented with five SELECTED KEY REFERENCES from the bibliography, which the authors believe are worthy of in-depth investigation. Furthermore, we have listened to our students' desire for visual reinforcement and simulation to master psychomotor skills in the operating room. For that reason, we have added video clips for key operations in this textbook. They can be downloaded from the Elsevier website and reviewed at any time from any location by those who desire to augment their understanding of the material.

In the third edition, I was fortunate to be joined by two exceptional neurological surgery talents: Professors Sekhar and Abdulrauf. These two professors possess a keen eye for the critical elements of our field. They are internationally recognized as master educators, as well as technical virtuosos. Of course, the success of this book truly rests upon a team of world class contributing scholars, known for their specific expertise. Therefore the third edition enlisted new contributions from these internationally renowned neurosurgeons. The text by these authors was then combined with the work of highly skilled artists employing cutting-edge art technology. The entire project was then overseen by a patient and experienced Elsevier editing team.

I am deeply grateful to the authors, artists, and editors for the precious time and hard work invested in this third edition. They created a book with extraordinary visual appeal, containing accurate, evidence-based explanations, beautiful color illustrations, simple tables, illustrative photographs, and video highlights. It is our hope that this approach will be substantive, long lived, and enjoyable for our readers and beneficial to our patients.

Richard G. Ellenbogen

Contents

Part 6. Tumors

Part 7. Radiosurgery

Part 8. Functional/Pain

ONLINE ONLY

Online Video Contents

- Video 13: Clipping of a large right ophthalmic aneurysm through a right transylvian approach
- Video 14: Clipping of a basilar tip aneurysm 1
- Video 15: Clipping of a basilar tip aneurysm 2
- Video 16: Clipping of a giant carotid wall aneurysm

AVM Surgeries
Saleem I. Abdulrauf

- Video 1: Resection of a previously ruptured temporal-frontal AVM; stepwise approach
- Video 2: Obliteration of tentorial dural AVM
- Video 3: A stepwise technique on how to resect an arterial-venous malformation (AVM) and resection of an AVM
- Video 4: Demonstration of the interior petrosal trans-tentorial approach for an AVM of the tentorial surface of the cerebellum

Approaches for Brainstem and Thalamic Legions
Saleem I. Abdulrauf

- Video 1: Interior hemispheric petrosal approach for a midbrain cavernoma
- Video 2: Resection of a midbrain cavernoma through a right interior petrosal approach
- Video 3: Resection of a pulvinar cavernoma through a right-sided posterior inter-hemispheric transcingulate approach
- Video 4: Resection of a midbrain cavernoma through a right-sided interior petrosal approach
- Video 5: Teloe-velar approach to the floor of the fourth ventricle for a pontine cavernoma

Operative Approaches to the Supra-Sellar and Third Ventricular Regions
Saleem I. Abdulrauf

- Video 1: Resection of an interior third ventricular craniophyarngioma through a right-sided transylvian translamina-terminalis approach
- Video 2: Resection of a retro-chiasmatic craniophyarngioma going through the optical-carotid and oculomotor-carotid triangles

- Video 3: Resection of a craniophyarngioma through a right transylvian approach; demonstration of how to dissect the capsule of the tumor off the ICA
- Video 4: Demonstration of the resection of a craniophyarngioma away from the basilar artery
- Video 5: Resection of a colloid cyst using the interhemipsheric transcallosal approach
- Video 6: Tuberculum sellae menengioma resection through a left cranial orbital approach
- Video 7: Resection of a hypothalamic tumor
- Video 8: Demonstration of hypothalamic-chiasmatic glioma

EC/ IC Bypass Surgeries
Saleem I. Abdulrauf

- Video 1: Demonstration of the proximal anastomosis for a high flow bypass
- Video 2: Demonstration of STA-MCA bypass
- Video 3: Preparation for a high flow radial artery ECIC bypass
- Video 4: Demonstration of an intracranial anastomosis of the radial artery graft to M2
- Video 5: Intercranial anastomosis of radial artery to the middle cerebral artery
- Video 6: Preparation of the radial artery graft for anastomosis
- Video 7: Demonstration of the intracranial anastomosis (M2) using a radial artery graft

Special Technical Nuances
Saleem I. Abdulrauf

- Video 1: Resection of a posterior fossa epidermoid using the far lateral approach
- Video 2: A dissection of an adherent meningioma away from optic nerve (left cranial-orbital approach)
- Video 3: Resection of an upper clival meningioma through a right-sided cranial-orbital-zygomatic approach
- Video 4: Demonstration on how to split the sylvian fissure
- Video 5: Demonstration of the reconstruction of the orbital roof following cranial-orbital approach using porex implant

Online Cases Studies Contents

(University of Washington)

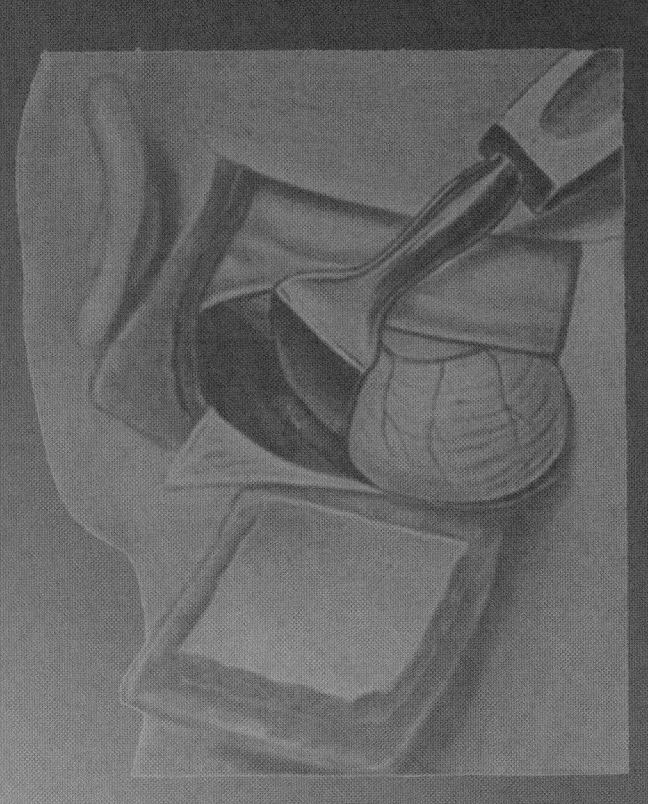

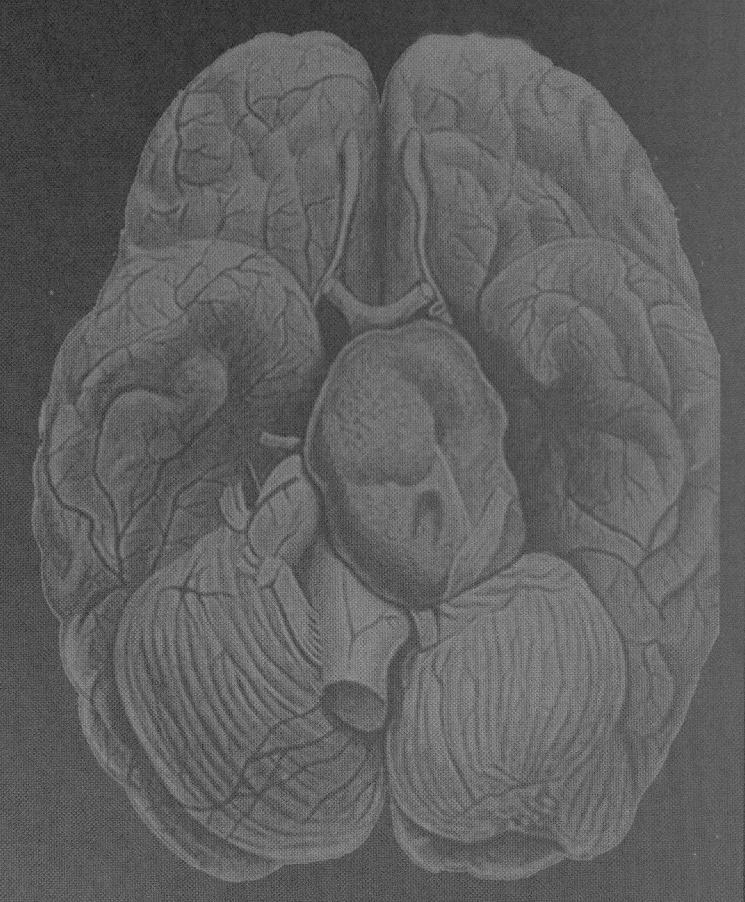

PART 1
General Overview

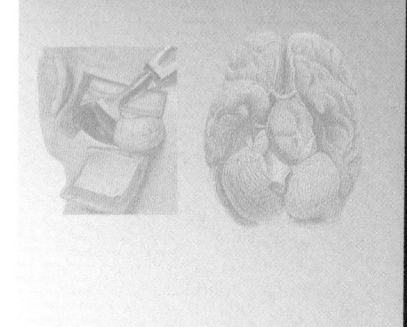

CHAPTER 1

Landmarks in the History of Neurosurgery

James Tait Goodrich

If a physician makes a wound and cures a freeman, he shall receive ten pieces of silver, but only five if the patient is the son of a plebeian or two if he is a slave. However it is decreed that if a physician treats a patient with a metal knife for a severe wound and has caused the man to die—his hands shall be cut off.
—Code of Hammurabi (1792-1750 BC)

In the history of neurosurgery there have occurred a number of events and landmarks and these will be the focus of this chapter. In understanding the history of our profession perhaps the neurosurgeon will be able explore more carefully the subsequent chapters in this volume to avoid having his or her "hands cut off."

To identify major trends and events in neurosurgery this chapter has been organized into a series of rather arbitrary historical time periods. In each period the key themes, personalities, and neurosurgical techniques developed and used are discussed.

PREHISTORIC PERIOD: THE DEVELOPMENT OF TREPHINATION

Neurosurgeons are often considered the second oldest profession, the first being prostitution. Early man (and woman) recognized that to take down a foe or an animal a direct injury to the head was the quickest means. Having said that, prehistoric surgery, compared with its modern successor, lacked several essentials in its early development: an understanding of anatomy, recognition of the concept of disease, and comprehension of the origin of illness in an organic system. Failure to grasp these vital principles retarded the practice of both medicine and surgery. The "modern" art of surgery, and in particular that of neurosurgery, was not recognized as a discrete specialty until the early twentieth century. Neurosurgeons have now advanced from mere "hole drillers" to sophisticated computer nerds running complex twenty-first century stereotaxic frameless guided systems.

In many museum and academic collections around the world are examples of the earliest form of neurosurgery—skull trephination.[1-4] A number of arguments and interpretations have been advanced by scholars as to the origin and surgical reasons for this early operation—to date no satisfactory answers have been found. Issues of religion, treatment of head injuries, release of demons, and treatment of headaches have all been offered. Unfortunately, no adequate

archaeological materials have surfaced to provide us with an answer. In reviewing some of the early skulls the skills of these early surgeons were quite remarkable. Many of the trephined skulls show evidence of healing, proving that these early patients survived the surgery. Figure 1.1 shows examples of two early (Peru circa AD 800) skulls that have been trephined and show evidence of premorbid bone healing. In the Americas the tumi was the most common surgical instrument used to perform a trephination and some examples of these tumis are shown in Figure 1.1. In Figure 1.2 is a fine example of a well-healed gold inlay cranioplasty done by an early South American surgeon.

Included in many museum and private collections are examples of terra cotta and stone figures and other carvings that clearly depicted several common neurological disorders. Commonly depicted by contemporary artisans were images of hydrocephalus, cranial deformation, spina bifida, and various forms of external injuries and scarring. We have added two examples from the Olmec and Mayan civilizations, where we see demonstrated a young adult with achondroplasia and a young adult with severe kyphoscolosis likely due to a myelomeningocele[5] (Fig. 1-3).

EGYPTIAN AND BABYLONIAN MEDICINE: EMBRYONIC PERIOD

The Egyptian period, covering some 30 successive dynasties, gave us the earliest known practicing physician—Imhotep (I-em-herep) (3000 BC). Imhotep ("he whom cometh in peace") is considered the first medical demigod, one likely more skilled in magic and being a sage. From this period came three important medical and surgical documents that give us a contemporary view of the practice of surgery. These collections are the Ebers, Hearst, and Edwin Smith papyri, two of which are considered here.[6,7]

The Egyptians are well remembered for their skills developed in mummification. Historians have now shown that anatomical dissection was also performed in this period. An examination of the existing Egyptian papyri shows that the practice of medicine was based largely on magic and superstition. Therapeutic measures depended on simple principles, most of which allowed nature to provide restoration of health with little intervention. In treating skeletal injury the Egyptians realized that immobilization was important and they prescribed splints for that purpose. Their materia medica was impressive, as their substantial pharmacopeias attest.

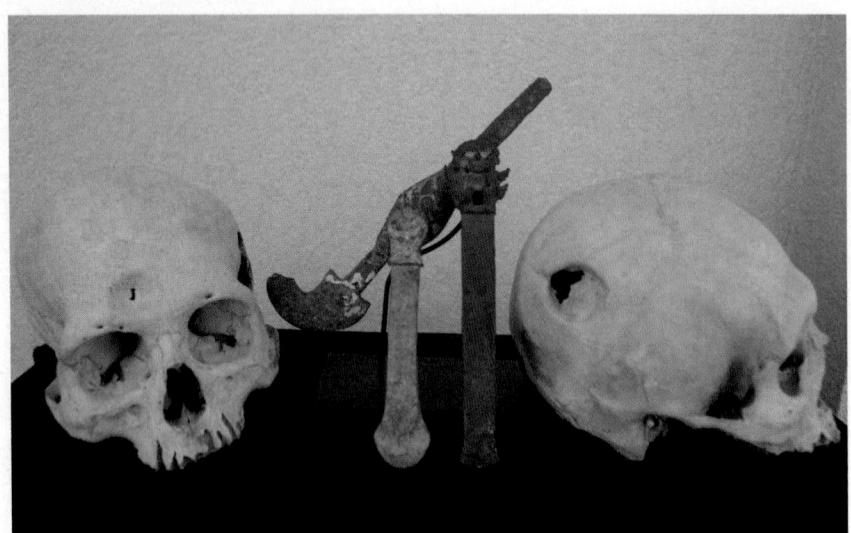

FIGURE 1.1 Two Peruvian skulls that date from about AD 600 showing a well-healed occipital trephination (*right skull*) and a well-healed frontal trephination (*left skull*). Three typical bronze/copper "tumis" used to make the trephination are illustrated between the skulls. *(From the author's collection.)*

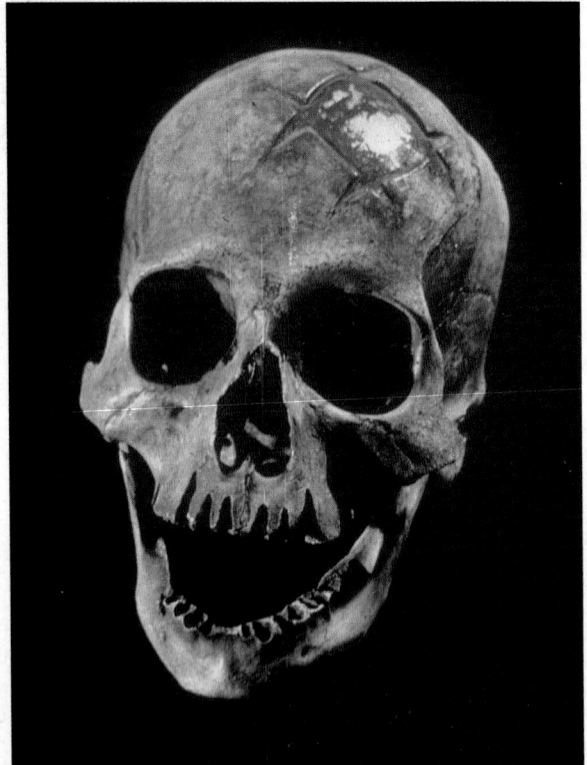

FIGURE 1.2 An early cranioplasty done with a gold inlay which is well healed. *(From the Museum of Gold, Lima, Peru.)*

Written some 500 years after Hammurabi (1792-1750 BC), and the oldest medical text believed to exist (including about 107 pages of hieratic writing), the Ebers papyrus is of interest for its discussion of contemporary surgical practice.[7] The text discusses the removal of tumors, and recommends surgical drainage of abscesses.

The Edwin Smith papyrus, written after 1700 BC is considered to be the oldest book on surgery per se and is a papyrus scroll 15 feet in length and 1 foot in width (4.5 m by 0.3 m; Fig. 1.4).[6] The text contains a total of 48 cases including those with injuries involving the spine and cranium. Each case is considered with a diagnosis followed by a formulated prognosis. Owing to the scholarly work of James Breasted this papyrus has been translated from the original Egyptian to English. The original document remains in the possession of the New York Academy of Medicine.[6]

Other than the isolated cases found in these papyrus fragments, little can be gleaned on the actual practice of neurosurgery. However, it is clearly evident from these papyri that the Egyptian physician could classify a head and spine injury and would even elevate a skull fracture if necessary. In the Edwin Smith papyrus (ca. 1700 BC) are the first descriptions of the skull sutures, the presence of intracranial pulsations, and the presence of cerebrospinal fluid (CSF). The use of sutures in closing wounds and the applications of specifically designed head dressings for cranial injury appear here for the first time. The Egyptian physician's understanding of the consequences of a cervical spine injury is clear from case 31, in which the injured individual is described with quadriplegia, urinary incontinence, priapism, and ejaculation in a cervical spine subluxation. The understanding of head and spine injury was further developed in the Greek schools of medicine; here we see the first treatment principles being offered on the management and codification of head injury.

GREEK AND EARLY BYZANTINE PERIOD: THE ORIGINS OF NEUROSURGERY

The first formal development of neurosurgery occurred with the golden age of Greece. During the ancient period there were no surgeons who restricted themselves *in stricto sensu* to "neurosurgery." Head injuries were plentiful then as the result of wars and internecine conflicts, as recorded by Herodotus and Thucydides as well as by Homer. The Greeks' love of gladiator sports also led to serious head injuries. So sports and war were then, as now, a principal source of material for the study and treatment of head injury.

The earliest medical writings from this period are those attributed to Hippocrates (460-370 BC), that most celebrated of the Asclepiadae, and his schools (Fig. 1.5).[8] To Hippocrates we owe the description of a number of neurological conditions,

FIGURE 1.3 A, A Jadeite figure from the Olmec culture of Pre-Conquest Mexico dating from about 1500 BC showing a figure of an achondroplastic dwarf with likely arrested hydrocephalus. Individuals with some deformations such as achondroplasia were highly prized in the noble courts. **B**, A west Mexico figure from the Pre-Conquest Nayarit area showing a severe kyphoscolosis in a young adult with likely a primary problem of a myelomeningocele. *(from the author's collection.)*

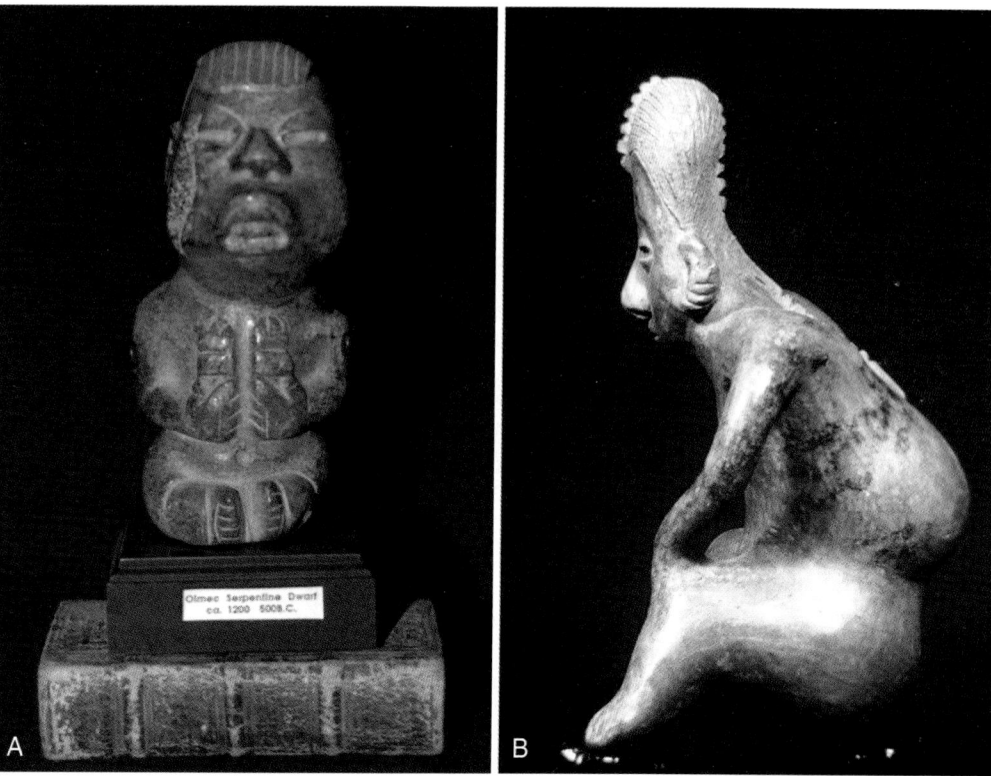

FIGURE 1.4 A manuscript leaf from the Breasted translation of the Hearst papyrus discussing a head injury. *(From Breasted JH. The Edwin Smith Papyrus. Published in Facsimile and Hieroglyphic Transliteration with Translation and Commentary. Chicago: University of Chicago Press; 1930; from the author's collection.)*

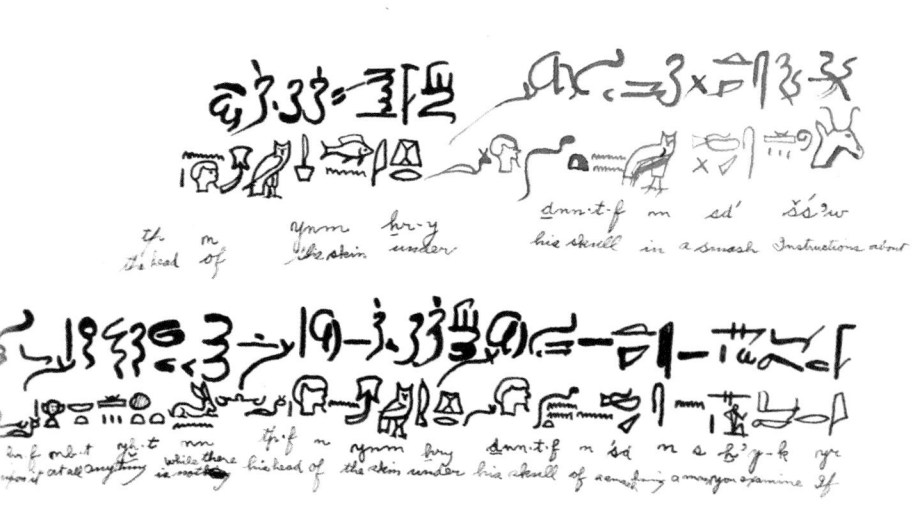

many of them resulting from battlefield and sport injuries. Hippocrates was the first to develop the concept that the location of the injury to the skull was important in any surgical decision. The vulnerability of the brain to injury was categorized from lesser to greater by location, with injury to the bregma representing a greater risk than injury to the temporal region, which in turn was more dangerous than injury to the occipital region.[9]

Hippocrates wrote on a number of neurological conditions. From his *Aphorisms* is one of the earliest descriptions of subarachnoid hemorrhage: "When persons in good health are suddenly seized with pains in the head, and straightway are laid down speechless, and breathe with stertor, they die in seven days, unless fever comes on."[10]

Hippocrates provides the first written detailed use of the trephine. Insightful, he argued for trephination in brain contusions but not in depressed skull fractures (the prognosis was too grave) and cautioned that a trephination should never be performed over a skull suture because of the risk of injury to the underlying dura. Hippocrates demonstrated good surgical technique when he recommended "watering" the trephine bit while drilling to prevent overheating and injury to the dura.

Hippocrates had great respect for head injury. In the section on "Wounds of the Head," Hippocrates warned against incising the brain, as convulsions can occur on the opposite side. He also warned against making a skin incision over the temporal artery, as this could lead to contralateral convulsions (or perhaps severe hemorrhage from the skin). Hippocrates had a simple understanding of cerebral localization and appreciated serious prognosis in head injury.

Herophilus of Chalcedon (fl. 335-280 BC) was an important early neuroanatomist who came from the region of the Bosporus and later attended the schools of Alexandria. Unlike his predecessors, Herophilus dissected human bodies in addition to those of animals—more than 100 by his own account. Herophilus was among the first to develop an anatomical nomenclature and form a language of anatomy. Among his contributions was tracing the origin of nerves to the spinal cord. He then divided these nerves into motor and sensory tracts. He made the important differentiation of nerves from tendons, which were often confused at that time. In his anatomical writings are the first anatomical descriptions of the ventricles and venous sinuses of the brain. From him comes the description of confluens sinuum or *torcular Herophili*. The first description of the choroid plexus occurs here, so named for its resemblance to the vascular membrane of the fetus. Herophilus described in detail the fourth ventricle and noted the peculiar arrangement at its base, which he called the "calamus scriptorius" because it "resembles the groove of a pen for writing." Among his many other contributions was his recognition of the brain as the central organ of the nervous system and the seat of intelligence, in contrast to Aristotle's cardiocentric view.[11]

All was not perfect with this anatomist as Herophilus is also remembered for introducing one of the longest standing errors in anatomical physiology: the rete mirabile (Fig. 1.6),[12] a structure present in artiodactyls but not in humans. This structure acts as an anastomotic network at the base of the brain. This inaccurately described structure later became dogma and important in early physiological theories of human brain function. The rete mirabile was later erroneously described in detail by Galen of Pergamon and further canonized by later Arabic and medieval scholars. Scholarship did not erase this anatomical error until the sixteenth century, when the new anatomical accounts of Andreas Vesalius and Berengario da Carpi clearly showed it did not exist in humans.

Entering the Roman era and schools of medicine, we come to Aulus Cornelius Celsus (25 BC to AD 50). Celsus was neither a physician nor a surgeon; rather, he can best be described as a medical encyclopedist who had an important influence on surgery. His writings reviewed, fairly and with moderation, the rival medical schools of his time—dogmatic, methodic, and empiric. As counsel to the emperors Tiberius and Gaius (Caligula), he was held in great esteem. His book, *De re Medicina*,[13] is one of the earliest extant medical documents after the Hippocratic writings. His writings had an enormous influence on early physicians. So important were his writings that when

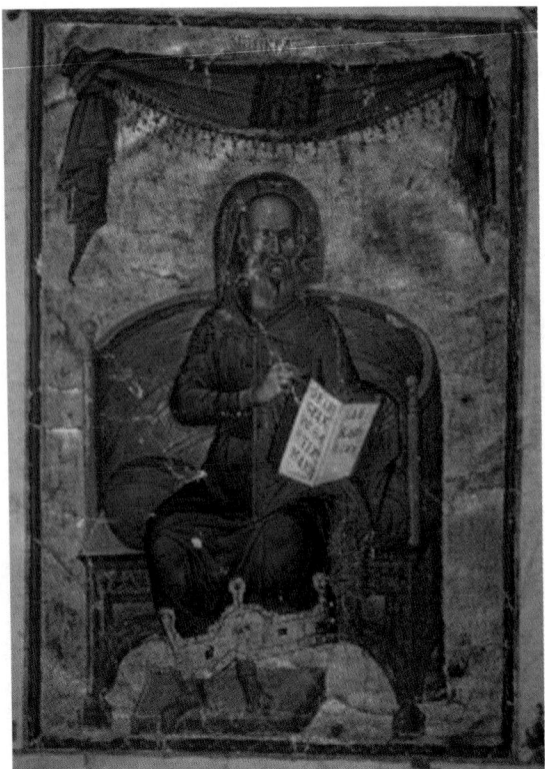

FIGURE 1.5 One of the earliest known paintings of Hippocrates, Father of Medicine, dating from about the eighth century BC. *(Courtesy of the Bibliothèque Nationale, Paris, France.)*

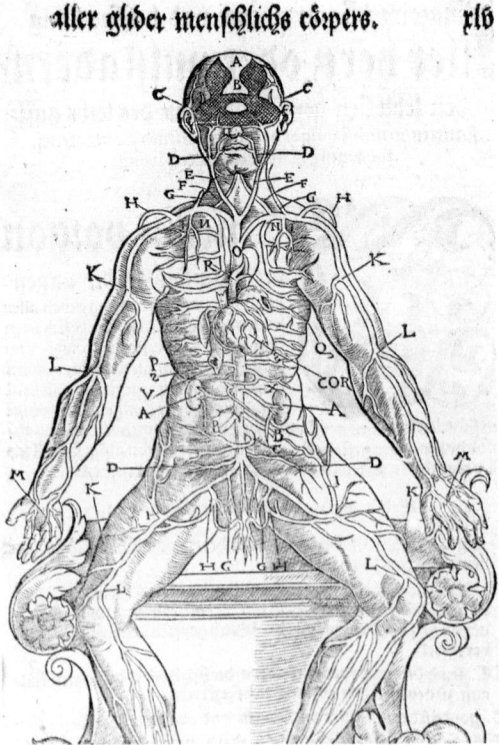

FIGURE 1.6 Introduced in antiquity was the rete mirabile, an erroneous anatomical structure first discussed by Herophilus. This anatomical error was carried further in the writings of Galen and others and not corrected until the Renaissance. A nice example of this structure is illustrated here, from the Ryff 1541 book on anatomy. *(From Ryff W. Des Aller Furtefflichsten ... Erschaffen. Das is des Menchen ... Warhafftige Beschreibund oder Anatomi. Strasbourg: Balthassar Beck; 1541.)*

printing was introduced in the fifteenth century, Celsus' works were printed before those of Hippocrates and Galen.

Celsus made a number of interesting neurosurgical observations. *De re Medicina* contains an accurate description of an epidural hematoma resulting from a bleeding middle meningeal artery.[8] Celsus comments that a surgeon should always operate on the side of greater pain and place the trephine where the pain is best localized. Considering the pain sensitivity of dura and its sensitivity to pressure, this has proved to be good clinical acumen. Celsus provided accurate descriptions of hydrocephalus and facial neuralgia. Celsus was aware that a fracture of the cervical spine can cause vomiting and difficulty in breathing, whereas injury of the lower spine can cause weakness or paralysis of the legs, as well as urinary retention or incontinence.

Rufus of Ephesus (fl. AD 100) lived during the reign of Trajan (AD 98-117) in the coastal city of Ephesus. Many of Rufus' manuscripts survived and became a heavy influence on the Byzantine and medieval compilers. As a result of his great skill as a surgeon, many of his surgical writings were still being transcribed well into the sixteenth century.[14] Rufus' description of the membranes covering the brain remains a classic. Rufus clearly distinguished between the cerebrum and cerebellum, and gives a credible description of the corpus callosum. He had a good understanding of the anatomy of the ventricular system with clear details of the lateral ventricle; he also described the third and fourth ventricles, as well as the aqueduct of Sylvius. Rufus also provided early anatomical descriptions of the pineal gland and hypophysis, and his accounts of the fornix and the quadrigeminal plate are accurate and elegant. He was among the first to describe the optic chiasm and recognized that it was related to vision. The singular accuracy of Rufus' studies must be credited to his use

of dissection (mostly monkeys) in an era when the Roman schools were avoiding hands-on anatomical dissection.

An individual of enormous influence was Galen of Pergamon (Claudius Galenus, AD 129-200). Galen was skilled as an original investigator, compiler, and codifier, as well as a leading advocate of the doctrines of Hippocrates and the Alexandrian school. As physician to the gladiators of Pergamon he had access to many human traumatic injuries.

His experience as a physician and his scientific studies enabled Galen to make a variety of contributions to neuroanatomy. Galen was the first to differentiate the pia mater and the dura mater. Among his contributions were descriptions of the corpus callosum, the ventricular system, the pineal and pituitary glands, and the infundibulum. Long before Alexander Monro's *Secundus* (1733-1817) eighteenth century anatomical description, Galen clearly described the structure now called the *foramen of Monro*. He also gave an accurate description of the aqueduct of Sylvius. He performed a number of interesting anatomical experiments, such as transection of the spinal cord, leading him to describe the resultant loss of function below the level of the cut. In a classic study on the pig he sectioned the recurrent laryngeal nerve and clearly described that hoarseness was a consequence (Fig. 1.7). Galen provides the first recorded attempt at identifying and numbering the cranial nerves. He described 11 of the 12 nerves, but by combining several, he arrived at a total of only seven. He regarded the olfactory nerve as merely a prolongation of the brain and hence did not count it.[15]

In viewing brain function Galen offered some original concepts. He believed the brain controlled intelligence, fantasy, memory, and judgment. This was an important departure from the teaching of earlier schools, for example, Aristotle's cardiocentric view. Galen discarded Hippocrates' notion that

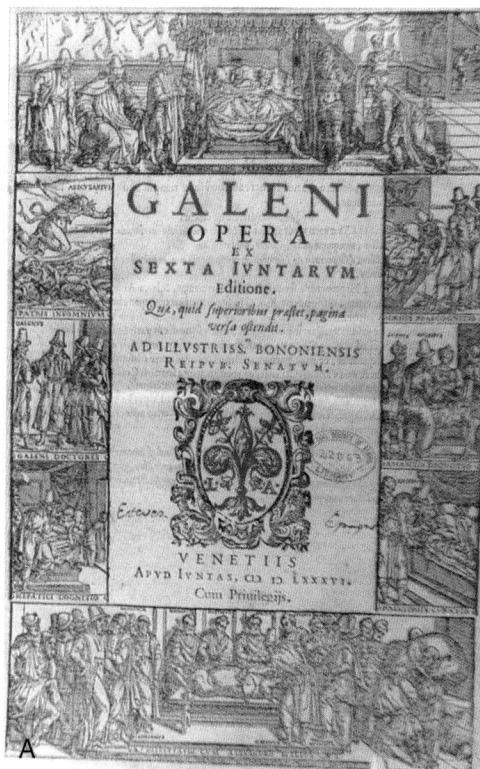
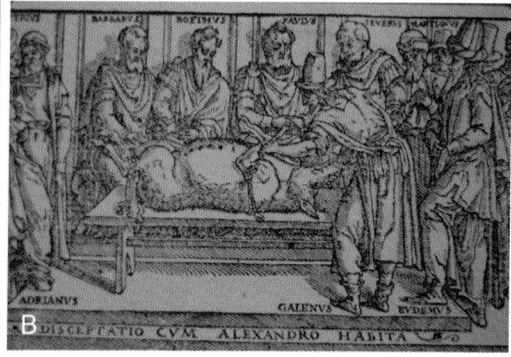

FIGURE 1.7 A, Title page from Galen's *Opera Omnia*, Juntine edition, Venice. The border contains a number of allegorical scenes showing the early practice of medicine. **B,** The bottom middle panel is shown here enlarged in which Galen is performing his classic study on the section of the recurrent laryngeal nerve and resulting hoarseness in the pig. *(From Galen. Omnia Quae Extant Opera in Latinum Sermonem Conversa, 5th ed. Venice: Juntas; 1576-1577.)*

the brain is only a gland and attributed to it the powers of voluntary action and sensation.

With animal experimentation Galen recognized that cervical injury can cause disturbance in arm function. In a study of spinal cord injury, Galen detailed a classic case of what is today known as *Brown-Séquard syndrome*—i.e., a hemiplegia with contralateral sensory loss in a subject with a hemisection of the cord.[16] Galen's description of the symptoms and signs of hydrocephalus is classic. This understanding of the disease enabled him to predict which patients with hydrocephalus had a poorer prognosis. Galen was much more liberal in the treatment of head injury than Hippocrates, arguing for more aggressive elevation of depressed skull fractures, fractures with hematomas, and comminuted fractures. Galen recommended removing the bone fragments, particularly those pressing into the brain. Galen was also more optimistic than Hippocrates about the outcome of brain injuries, commenting that "we have seen a severely wounded brain healed."

Paul of Aegina (AD 625-690), trained in the Alexandrian school, is considered the last of the great Byzantine physicians. He was a popular writer who compiled works from both the Latin and Greek schools. His writings remained extremely popular, being consulted well into the seventeenth century. Beside his medical skills Paul was also a skilled surgeon to whom patients came from far and wide. He venerated the teachings of the ancients as tradition required, but also introduced his own techniques with good results. This author is best remembered for his classic work, *The Seven Books of Paul of Aegina*, within which are excellent sections on head injury and the use of the trephine.[17,18] Paul classified skull fractures in several categories: fissure, incision, expression, depression, arched fracture, and, in infants, dent. In skull fractures he developed an interesting skin incision which involved two incisions intersecting one another at right angles, giving the Greek letter X. One leg of the incision incorporated the scalp wound. To provide comfort for the patient the ear was stuffed with wool so that the noise of the trephine would not cause undue distress. In offering better wound care he dressed it with a broad bandage soaked in oil of roses and wine, with care taken to avoid compressing the brain.[18]

Paul of Aegina had some interesting views on hydrocephalus, which he felt was sometimes a result of a man handling midwife. He was the first to suggest the possibility that an intraventricular hemorrhage might cause hydrocephalus:

> The hydrocephalic affection ... occurs in infants, owing to their heads being improperly squeezed by midwives during parturition, or from some other obscure cause; or from the rupture of a vessel or vessels, and the extravasated blood being converted into an inert fluid ... (Paulus Aeginetes).[18]

An innovative personality, he designed a number of surgical instruments for neurosurgical procedures. Illustrated in his early manuscripts are a number of tools including elevators, raspatories, and bone-biters. An innovation for his trephine bits was a conical design to prevent plunging, and different biting edges were made for ease of cutting. Reviewing his wound management reveals some sophisticated insights—he used wine (helpful in antisepsis, although this concept was then unknown) and stressed that dressings should be applied with no compression to the brain. Paul of Aegina was later to have an enormous influence on Arabic medicine and in particular on Albucasis, the patriarch of Arabic/Islamic surgery.[19]

ARABIC AND MEDIEVAL MEDICINE: SCHOLARSHIP WITH INTELLECTUAL SOMNOLENCE

From approximately AD 750 to AD 1200 the major intellectual centers of medicine were with the Arabic/Islamic and Byzantine cultures. As Western Europe revived after AD 1000, a renewed study of surgery and medicine developed there as well.

Arabic/Islamic Scholarship

As we move out of the Byzantine period the Arabic/Islamic schools became paramount in the development of medicine and surgery. Thriving Arabic/Islamic schools undertook an enormous effort to translate and systematize the surviving Greek and Roman medical texts. Thanks to their incredible zeal, the best of Greek and Roman medicine was made available to Arabic readers by the end of the ninth century, an enormous contribution. Although a rigid scholastic dogmatism became the educational trend, original concepts and surgical techniques were clearly introduced during this period. In anatomical studies some of the more prominent figures actually challenged Galen and some of his clear anatomical errors.

Islamic medicine flourished from the tenth century through the twelfth century. Among the most illustrious scholars/writers/physicians were Avicenna, Rhazes, Avenzoar, Albucasis, and Averroes. In the interpretative writings of these great physicians one sees an extraordinary effort to canonize the writings of their Greek and Roman predecessors. Islamic scholars and physicians served as guardians and academics of what now became Hippocratic and Galenic dogma. But having said this, there is clear evidence that these scholars and physicians continued original research and performed anatomical studies, a procedure not forbidden in either the Koran or Shareeh, a common Western view.

In reviewing this period, one finds that physicians rarely performed surgery. Rather, it was expected that the physician would write learnedly and speak *ex cathedra* from earlier but more "scholarly" writings. The menial task of surgery was assigned to an individual of a lower class, that is, to a surgeon. Despite this trend several powerful and innovative personalities did arise and we will review their contributions.

In this era of Islamic medicine we see introduced a now common medical tradition—bedside medicine with didactic teaching. Surgeons, with rare exceptions, remained in a class of low stature. One unfortunate practice was the reintroduction of the Egyptian technique of using a red-hot cautery iron, applied to a wound, to control bleeding. In some cases hot cautery was used instead of the scalpel to create surgical incisions, and this practice clearly led to a burned and subsequent poorly healed wound (Fig. 1.8).

An important Islamic scholar of this period, as reflected in his writings, was Rhazes (Abu Bakr Muhammad ibn Zakariya' al-Razi, AD 845–925). Reviewing his works one sees clearly a scholarly physician, loyal to Hippocratic teachings, and

FIGURE 1.8 A, Ottoman empire physician applying cautery to the back. B, Manuscript leaf showing Avicenna reducing and stabilizing a spinal column injury. *(From Sabuncuoglu S. Cerrahiyyetü'l-Haniyye [Imperial Surgery] [translated from Arabic]. Ottoman Empire circa fifteenth century. From a later copied manuscript in the author's collection, circa 1725.)*

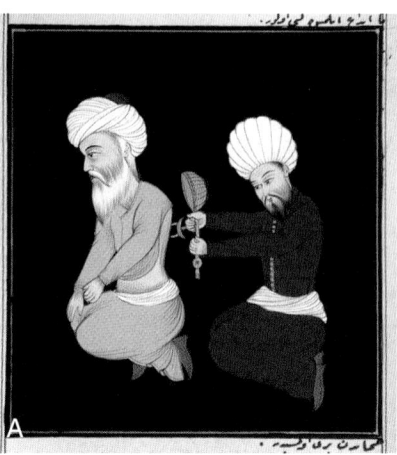
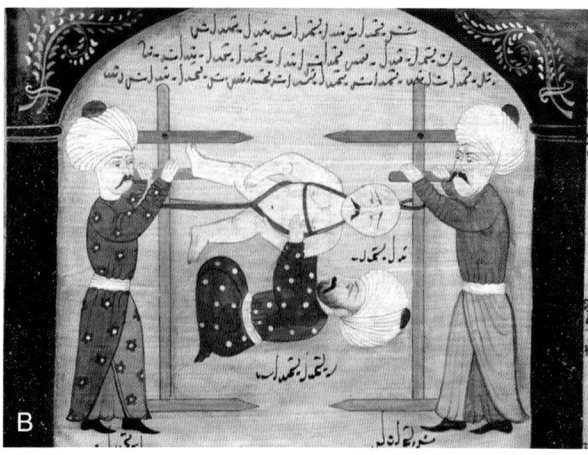

learned in diagnosis. Although primarily a court physician and not a surgeon, he provided writings on surgical topics that remained influential through the eighteenth century.[20] Rhazes was one of the first to discuss and outline the concept of cerebral concussion. Head injury, he wrote, is among the most devastating of all injuries. Reflecting some insight he advocated surgery only for penetrating injuries of the skull as the outcome was almost always fatal. Rhazes recognized that a skull fracture causes compression of the brain and thereby requires elevation to prevent lasting injury. Rhazes also understood that cranial and peripheral nerves have both a motor and sensory component. In designing a surgical scalp flap one needed to know the anatomy and pathways of the nerves so as to prevent a facial or ocular palsy.

Avicenna (Abu 'Ali al-Husayn ibn 'Abdallah ibn Sina, AD 980-1037), the famous Persian physician and philosopher of Baghdad, was known as the "second doctor" (the first being Aristotle). During the Middle Ages his works were translated into Latin and became dominant teachings in the major European universities until well into the eighteenth century. With the introduction of the printed book it has been commented that his *Canon (Q'anun)* was the second most commonly printed book after the Bible. Avicenna disseminated the Greek teachings so persuasively that their influence remains an undercurrent to this day. In his major work, *Canon Medicinae (Q'anun)*, an encyclopedic effort founded on the writings of Galen and Hippocrates, the observations reported are mostly clinical, bearing primarily on materia medica (Fig. 1.9).[21] Avicenna's medical philosophy primarily followed the humoral theories of Hippocrates along with the biological concepts of Aristotle. Within Avicenna's *Canon (Q'anun)* are a number of interesting neurological findings, such as the first accurate clinical explanation of epilepsy, for which treatment consisted of various medications and herbals along with the shock of the electric eel. He describes meningitis and recognized it was an infection and inflammation of the meninges. It appears that Avicenna might have conducted anatomical studies inasmuch as he gives a correct anatomical discussion of the vermis of the cerebellum and the "tailed nucleus," now known as the *caudate nucleus*. Avicenna introduced the concept of a tracheostomy using a gold or silver tube placed into the trachea and provided a number of innovative techniques for treating spine injuries and included some devices for stabilizing the injured spine. Avicenna also had some insightful thoughts on

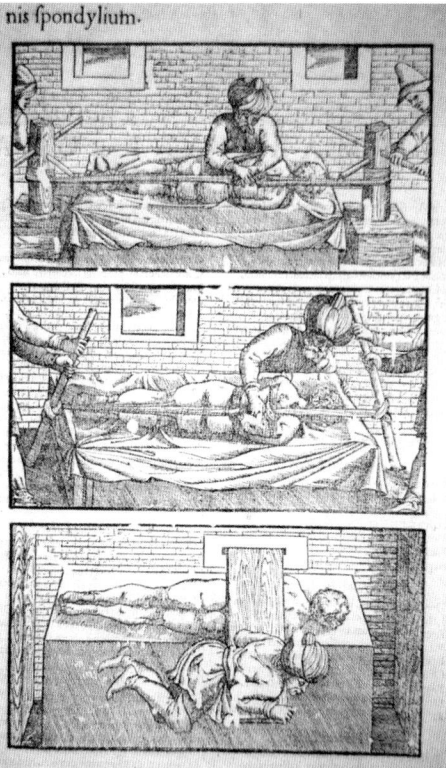

FIGURE 1.9 Avicenna developed a number of different devices to deal with spinal injury and spinal stabilization. Illustrated here is a "rack" system using a series of winches and stretching devices to realign the spine. *(From Avicenna. Liber Canonis, de Medicinis Cordialibus, et Cantica. Basel: Joannes Heruagios; 1556.)*

the treatment of hydrocephalus. He recognized that external hydrocephalus (fluid between the brain and dura) could be drained with low morbidity risk. However, true internal hydrocephalus was more dangerous to treat and best left alone or treated with herbals and medications.[22] The *Canon (Q'anun)* was clearly his greatest contribution, along with his collation and translation of Galen's collected works, a book that remained a dominant influence until well into the eighteenth century.

A personality often overlooked in neurosurgical history was a prominent Persian/Islamic physician by the name

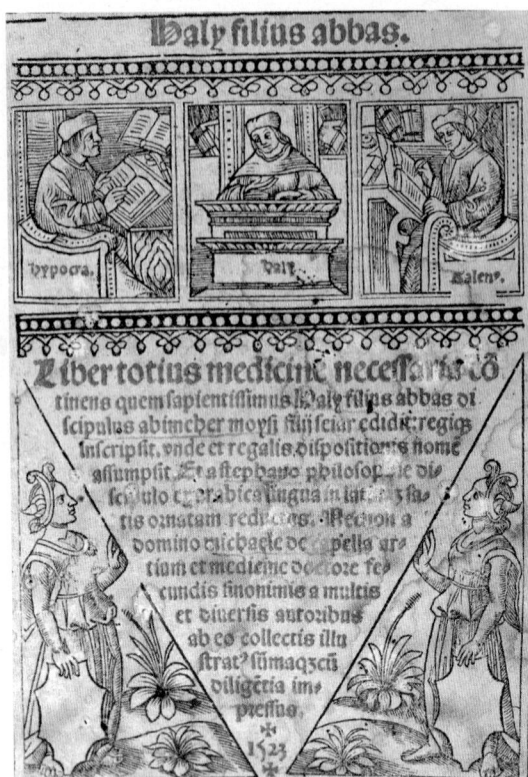

FIGURE 1.10 Title page from the second printed edition of Haly Abbas' writings on medicine and surgery. In this allegorical title page we see Haly Abbas in the center and Galen and Hippocrates to each side. *(From Haly Abbas [Abdul-Hasan Ali Ibn Abbas Al Majusi]. Liber Totius Medicine necessaria continens quem sapientissimus Haly filius Abbas discipulus Abimeher Muysi filii Sejar editit: regique inscripsit unde et regalis depositionis nomen assumpsit. Et a Stephano philosophie discipulo ex Arabica lingua in Latinam . . . reductus. Necnon a domino Michaele de Capella. . . Lugduni. Lyons: Jacobi Myt; 1523.)*

of Haly Abbas (Abdul-Hasan Ali Ibn Abbas Al Majusi) (?AD 930-944). This writer from the Golden Age of Islamic medicine produced a work called *The Perfect Book of the Art of Medicine*,[23] also known as the *Royal Book* (Fig. 1.10). Born and educated in Persia, a place he never left, it was here he produced his important writings on medicine. In his book he dedicated 110 chapters to surgical practice. A review of his work shows that his writings on spine injuries were essentially copied from the earlier Greek writers, in particular Paul of Aegina, and consisted mostly of external stabilization of spinal column injuries. Surgical intervention via a scalpel was rarely advocated. In his nineteenth discourse, Chapters 84 and 85 is clearly presented his management of depressed skull fractures. He also described the different types of fractures that can occur along with potential mechanisms of injury. He clearly appreciated that the dura should be left intact and not violated, the exception being those fractures where the skull bone had penetrated through the dural membrane, in which case these fragments needed to be removed. His technique of elevating a bone flap involved drilling a series of closely placed holes and then connecting them with a chisel. He showed some interesting consideration for the patient by advocating placing a ball of wool into the ears so as to block the sounds from the drilling. The head wound was then dressed with a wine-soaked dressing, the wine likely providing a form of antisepsis. In these chapters are also an interesting discussion about intraoperative brain swelling and edema, in which case the surgeon should look further for possible retained bone fragments and remove them. If later swelling occurred from too tight a head dressing, then it should be loosened. Unfortunately, Haly Abbas also advocated cephalic vein bleeding and inducing diarrhea for those who did not respond well; such primitive techniques were not to be abandoned until the mid-nineteenth century.

In the Islamic tradition Albucasis (Abu al-Qasim Khalaf ibn al-Abbas Al-Zahrawi, AD 936-1013) was both a great compiler as well as a serious scholar, whose writings (some 30 volumes!) were focused mainly on surgery, dietetics, and materia medica. In the introduction to his *Compendium*[24] there is an interesting discussion of why the Islamic physician had made such little progress in surgery—he attributed this failure to a lack of anatomical study and inadequate knowledge of the classics. One unfortunate medical practice that he popularized was the frequent use of emetics as prophylaxis against disease, a debilitating medical practice that survived, as "purging," into the nineteenth century.

The final section of the *Compendium* is the most important part for surgeons and includes a lengthy summary of surgical practice at that time.[24-26] This work was used extensively in the schools of Salerno and Montpellier and hence was an important influence in medieval Europe. A unique feature of this text was the illustrations of surgical instruments along with descriptions of their use, which Albucasis detailed in the text. Albucasis designed many of the instruments, and some were based on those described earlier by Paul of Aegina. His design of a "nonsinking" trephine is classic (he placed a collar on the trephine to prevent plunging) and was to become the template of many later trepan/trephine designs (Fig. 1.11).

Albucasis' treatise on surgery is an extraordinary work—a rational, comprehensive, and well-illustrated text designed to teach the surgeon the details of each treatment, including the types of wound dressings to be used. Yet one can only wonder how patients tolerated some of the surgical techniques. For chronic headache a hot cautery was applied to the occiput, burning through the skin but not the bone. Another headache treatment described required hooking the temporal artery, twisting it, placing ligatures, and then in essence ripping it out! Albucasis recognized the implications of spinal column injury, particularly dislocation of the vertebrae: in total subluxation, with the patient showing involuntary activity (passing urine and stool) and flaccid limbs, he appreciated that death was almost certain. Some of the methods he advocated for reduction of lesser spinal injuries, using a combination of spars and winches, were rather dangerous. With good insight he argued that bone fragments in the spinal canal should be removed. To provide comfort for the patient undergoing surgery he developed an "anesthesia" sponge in which active ingredients included opium and hashish; the sponge would be applied to the lips of the patient until the patient became unconscious.

For hydrocephalus (following the teachings of Paul of Aegina, he associated the disorder with the midwife grasping the head too roughly) Albucasis recommended drainage, although he noted that the outcome was almost always fatal. He attributed these poor results to "paralysis" of the

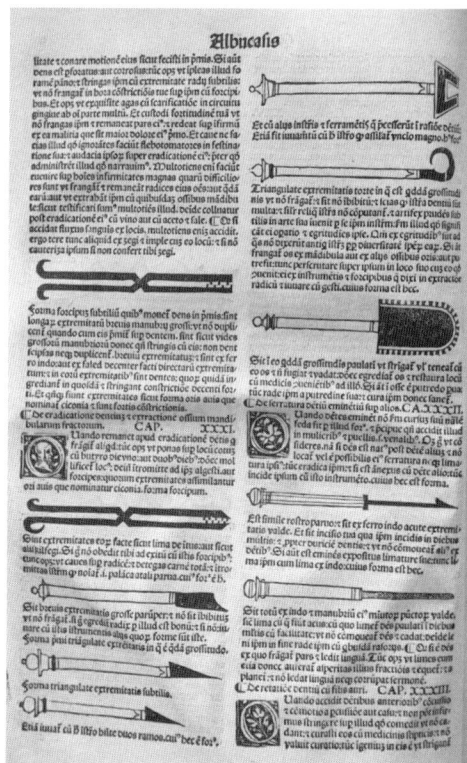

FIGURE 1.11 Illustrated here are some of Albucasis' instrument designs including a couple of cephalotomes for dealing with hydrocephalus in the infant. *(From Albucasis. Liber Theoricae Necnon Practicae Alsaharavii. Augsburg: Sigismundus Grimm & Marcus Vuirsung; 1519.)*

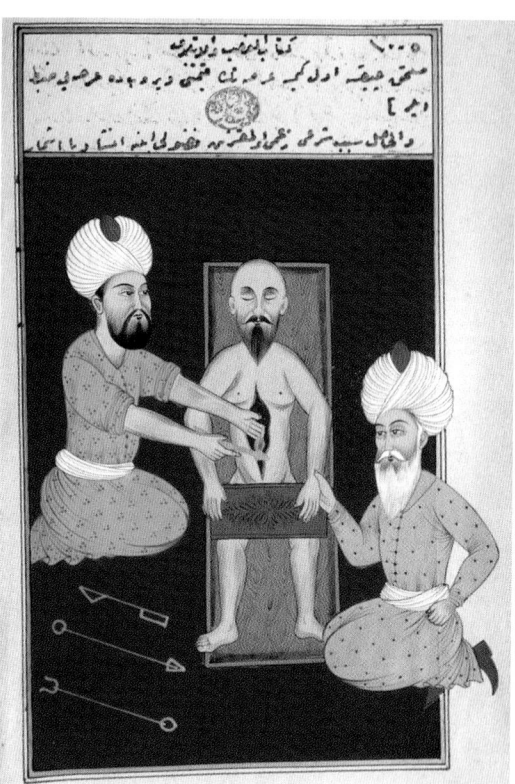

FIGURE 1.12 An unusual colored illustration of an anatomical dissection being done by Arabic/Islamic physicians. Often thought to have been forbidden by the Koran, anatomical dissections were done in the Byzantine and Medieval periods by this group of physicians and anatomists. *(From the author's personal collection.)*

brain from relaxation. With regard to the site for drainage, Albucasis noted that the surgeon must never cut over an artery, as hemorrhage could lead to death. In the child with hydrocephalus he would "bind" the head with a tight constricting head wrap and then put the child on a "dry diet" with little fluid—in retrospect a progressive treatment plan for hydrocephalus.[25,26]

An important figure in the history of surgery, and one who bridged the Islamic and medieval schools, was Serefeddin Sabuncuoglu (1385-1468). Sabuncuoglu was a prominent Ottoman surgeon who lived in Amasya, a small city in the northern region of Asia Minor, part of present-day Turkey. This was a glorious period for the Ottoman Empire and Amasya was a major center of commerce, culture, and art. While working as a physician at Amasya Hospital, and at the age of 83, he wrote a medical book entitled *Cerrahiyyetü'l-Haniyye* [*Imperial Surgery*], which is considered the first colored illustrated textbook of Turkish medical literature.[27-30] There are only three known copies of this original manuscript, two are in Istanbul and the third at the Bibliothèque Nationale in Paris.[27] First written in 1465 the book consists of three chapters dealing with 191 topics, all dealing with surgery. Each topic consists of a single, poetical sentence in which the diagnosis, classification, and surgical technique of a particular disease are described in detail. This book is unique for this period in that virtually all the surgical procedures and illustrations were drawn in color, even though drawings of this type were prohibited in the Islamic religion (Fig. 1.12).

Medieval Europe

Constantinus Africanus (Constantine the African) (1020-1087) introduced Islamic medicine to the school of Salerno and thus to Europe (Fig. 1.13). Constantine had studied in Baghdad, where he came under the influence of the Islamic/Arabic scholars. Later, he retired to the monastery at Monte Cassino and there translated Arabic manuscripts into Latin, some scholars say rather inaccurately. Thus began a new wave of translation and transliteration of medical texts, this time from Arabic back into Latin.[31] His work allows one to gauge how much medical and surgical knowledge was lost or distorted by multiple translations, particularly of anatomical works. It is also notable that Constantine reintroduced anatomical dissection with an annual dissection of a pig. Unfortunately the anatomical observations that did not match those recorded in the early classical writings were ignored! As had been the theme for the previous 400 years surgical education and practice continued to slumber.

Roger of Salerno (fl. 1170) was a surgical leader in the Salernitan tradition, the first writer on surgery in Italy. His work on surgery was to have a tremendous influence during the medieval period (Fig. 1.14). His *Practica Chirurgiae* offered some interesting surgical techniques.[32] Roger introduced an unusual technique of checking for a tear of the dura, i.e., cerebrospinal fluid (CSF) leakage, in a patient with a skull fracture by having the patient hold his breath (Valsalva maneuver) and then watching for a CSF leak or air bubbles.

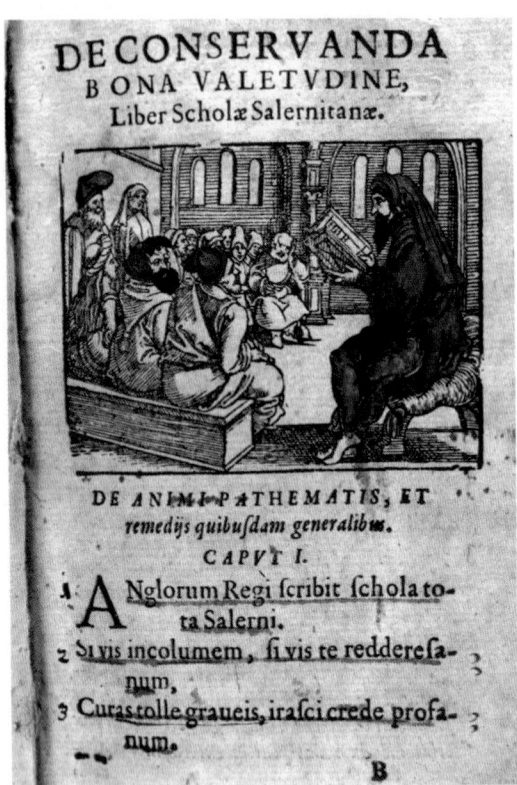

FIGURE 1.13 Constantine the African lecturing at the great School of Salerno. In the typical fashion of the day, the professor is giving an "ex cathedra" lecture to the students on medicine reading from the codices of Hippocrates and Galen. *(A 17th-century leaf from the author's collection.)*

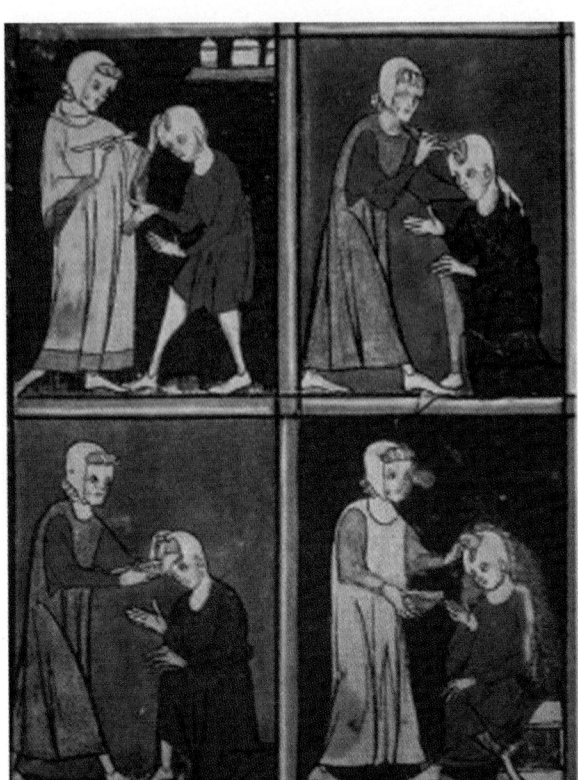

FIGURE 1.14 This early medieval manuscript illustrates a craniotomy being performed by Roger of Salerno. *(From Bodleian Library, Oxford, UK.)*

A pioneer in the techniques of managing nerve injury, he argued for reanastomosis of severed nerves. During the repair he paid particular attention to alignment of the nerve fasicles. Several chapters of his text are devoted to the treatment of skull fractures. The following is a discussion of a skull fracture:

> When a fracture occurs it is accompanied by various wounds and contusions. If the contusion of the flesh is small but that of the bone great, the flesh should be divided by a cruciate incision down to the bone and everywhere elevated from the bone. Then a piece of light, old cloth is inserted for a day, and if there are fragments of the bone present, they are to be thoroughly removed. If the bone is unbroken on one side, it is left in place, and if necessary elevated with a flat sound (spatumile) and the bone is perforated by chipping with the spatumile so that clotted blood may be soaked up with a wad of wool and feathers. When it has consolidated, we apply lint and then, if it is necessary (but not until after the whole wound has become level with the skin), the patient may be bathed. After he leaves the bath, we apply a thin cooling plaster made of wormwood with rose water and egg.[32]

In reviewing the writings of Roger of Salerno we see little offered that is new in the field of anatomy. He contented himself with recapitulating earlier treatises, in particular those of Albucasis and Paul of Aegina. He strongly favored therapeutic plasters and salves; fortunately he was not a strong advocate of the application of grease to dural injuries. Citing the writings of *The Bamberg Surgery*,[33] he advocated trephination in the treatment of epilepsy.

An unusually inventive medieval surgeon, Theodoric Borgognoni of Cervia (1205-1298) is remembered as a

pioneer in the use of aseptic technique—not the "clean" aseptic technique of today but rather a method based on avoidance of "laudable pus." He made a number of attempts to discover the ideal conditions for good wound healing; he concluded that they comprised control of bleeding, removal of contaminated or necrotic material, avoidance of dead space, and careful application of a wound dressing bathed in wine—views that are remarkably modern for the times (Fig. 1.15).

Theodoric's surgical work, written in 1267, provides a unique view of medieval surgery.[34] He argued for meticulous (almost Halstedian!) surgical techniques. The aspiring surgeon was to train under competent surgeons and be well read in the field of head injury. Interestingly, he argued that parts of the brain could be removed through a wound with little effect on the patient. He appreciated the importance of skull fractures, especially depressed ones, recognizing that they should be elevated. He believed that punctures or tears of the dura mater could lead to abscess formation and seizures. To provide comfort for the patient about to undergo surgery, he developed his own "soporific sponge," which contained opium, mandragora, hemlock, and other ingredients. It was applied to the nostrils until the patient fell asleep. He describes results in improved comfort that were better for both patient and surgeon (Figs. 1.16, 1.17).

William of Saliceto (1210-1277) might be considered the ablest surgeon of the thirteenth century. A professor at the University of Bologna, William of Saliceto wrote his *Chirurgia*,[35] which many consider to be highly original, though it does carry the strong influence of Galen and Avicenna. To his credit William replaced the Arabic technique of incision by cautery with the surgical knife. He also devised techniques for nerve

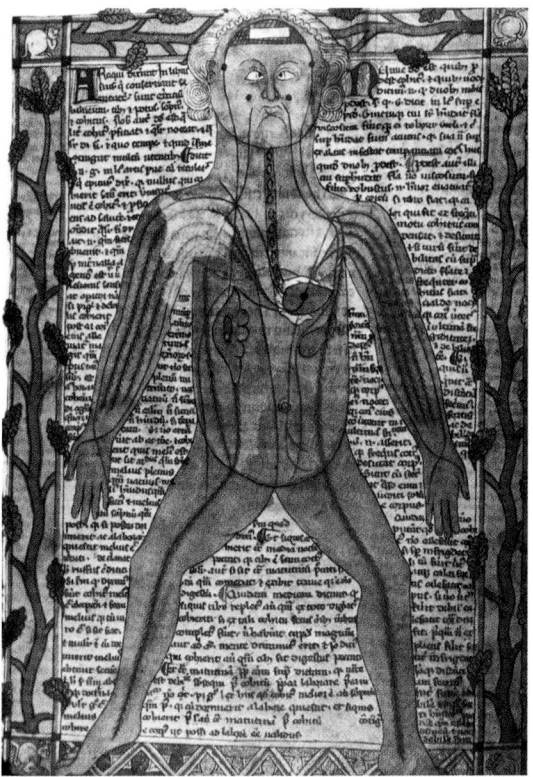

FIGURE 1.15 From the "five-figure series," this illustration reveals the Middle Ages understanding of the circulatory and nervous system of man with the Galenic anatomical error of the rete mirabile clearly illustrated. *(From Bodleian Library Collection, Oxford, England.)*

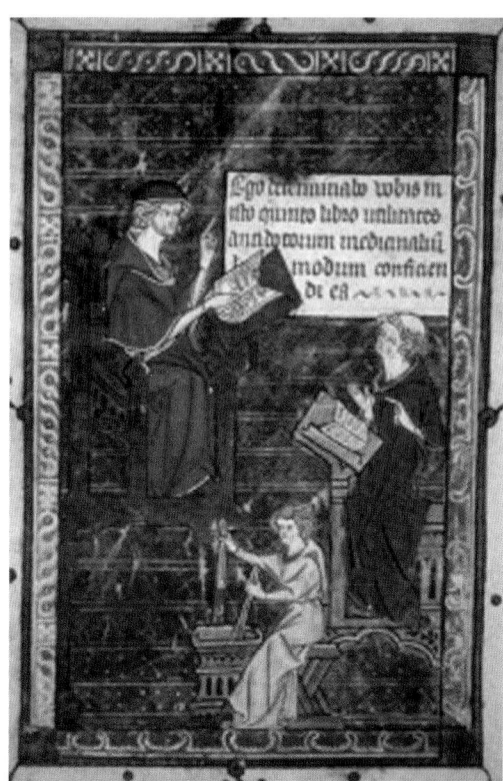

FIGURE 1.16 A medieval image of the "typical" lecture of the period with the professor speaking "ex cathedra" to the student reading from classic texts from Hippocrates, Galen, and other classical writers. *(Attributed to Gerard of Cromona, a translator of Avicenna Canon Medicinae, Paris circa 1320. Bibliotheca Nationale, Paris, France.)*

suture. In neurology, he recognized that the cerebrum governs voluntary motion and the cerebellum involuntary function.

Leonard of Bertapalia (1380?–1460) was a prominent figure in medieval surgery. Leonard came from a small town near Padua and established an extensive and lucrative practice there and in nearby Venice. He was among the earliest proponents of anatomical research—in fact, he gave a course of surgery in 1429 that included the dissection of an executed criminal. Leonard had a strong interest in head injury—he ended up devoting a third of his book to surgery of the nervous system.[36,37] He considered the brain the most precious organ, regarding it as the source of voluntary and involuntary functions. He provided some interesting and accurate insights into the management of skull fracture. He argued that the surgeon should always avoid materials that might cause pus, always avoid the use a compressive dressing that might drive bone into the brain, and if a piece of bone pierces the brain, remove it!

Lanfranchi of Milan (c. 1250-1306), a pupil of William of Saliceto, continued his teacher's practice of using a knife instead of cautery. In his *Cyrurgia Parva* he pioneered the use of suture for wound repair.[38] His guidelines for performing trephination in skull fractures and "release of irritation" of dura are classic. He even developed a technique of esophageal intubation for surgery, a technique not commonly practiced until the late nineteenth century.

Guy de Chauliac (1298-1368) was the most influential surgeon of the fourteenth and fifteenth centuries and a writer of rare learning and fine historical sense. So important to surgical practice did Guy de Chauliac's *Ars Chirurgica* become,

it was copied and translated into the seventeenth century, a span of nearly 400 years. Most historians consider this surgical manual to be the principal didactic surgical text of this era.[39,40]

The discussion of head injuries in his *Ars Chirurgica* reveals the breadth of his knowledge and intellect. He recommended that prior to doing cranial surgery the head should be shaved to prevent hair from getting into the wound and interfering with primary healing. When dealing with depressed skull fractures he advocated putting wine into the depression to assist healing—an interesting early form of antisepsis. He categorized head wounds into seven types and described the management of each in detail. Surgical management of a scalp wound requires only cleaning and débridement, whereas a compound depressed skull fracture must be treated by trephination and bone elevation. For wound repairs he advocated a primary suture closure and described good results. For hemostasis he introduced the use of egg albumin, thereby helping the surgeon to deal with a common and difficult problem.

SIXTEENTH CENTURY: ANATOMICAL EXPLORATION

With the beginnings of the Renaissance profound changes began to occur in surgical practices. To resolve medical and surgical practice issues, both physicians and surgeons reintroduced basic hands-on investigative techniques. Of profound

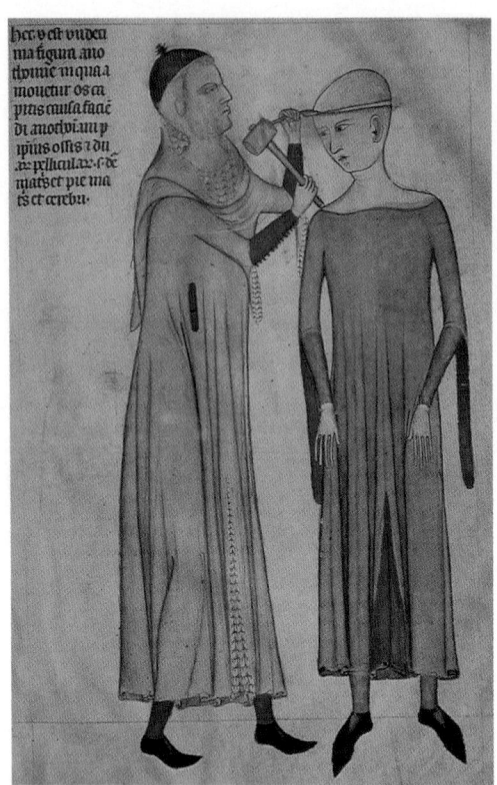

FIGURE 1.17 Medieval anatomist performing a dissection of the head. *(From Guido de Papia (Papaya), Anatomia circa 1325. Musèe Condé, Chantilly, France.)*

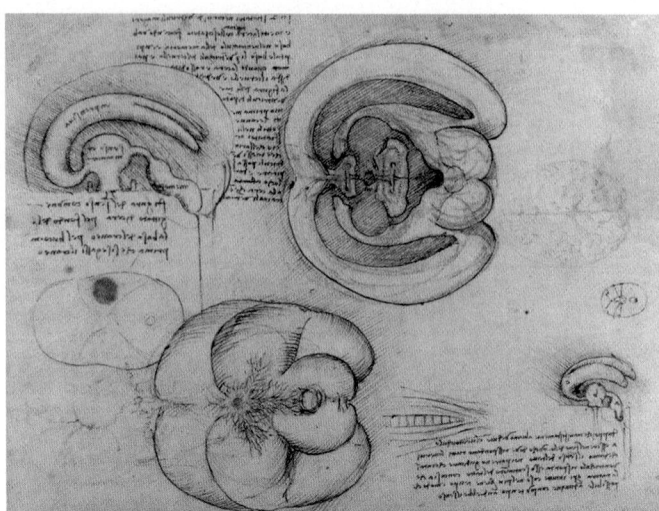

FIGURE 1.18 From Leonardo's anatomic codices: using a wax casting design of his own Leonardo was able to outline the ventricular system. The technique involved filling the ventricles with a warm wax and an egress tube to allow the air out. *(From Leonardo da Vinci. Quaderni d'Anatomia. Christiania: Jacob Dybwad; 1911-1916.)*

influence was the now routine practice of anatomical dissection of humans. A series of prominent figures including Leonardo da Vinci, Berengario da Carpi, Johannes Dryander, Andreas Vesalius, and others led the movement. Anatomical errors, many ensconced since the Greco-Roman era, were corrected, and a greater interest in surgery developed. This radically inventive period and its personalities laid the foundations of modern neuroanatomy and neurosurgery.

Leonardo da Vinci (1452-1519) was the quintessential Renaissance man. Multitalented, recognized as an artist, an anatomist, and a scientist, Leonardo went to the dissection table so as to better understand surface anatomy and its bearing on his artistic creations. On the basis of these studies he founded iconographic and physiological anatomy.[41-43] Leonardo, being a well-read man, was familiar with the writings of Galen, Avicenna, Mondino, and others. From his knowledge of these writings he developed an understanding of their anatomical errors.

To Leonardo's studies we owe a number of anatomical firsts. Leonardo provided the first crude diagrams of the cranial nerves, the optic chiasm, and the brachial and lumbar plexuses. Leonardo made the first wax casting of the ventricular system and in so doing provided the earliest accurate view of this anatomy. His wax casting technique involved removing the brain from the calvarium and injecting melted wax through the fourth ventricle. Tubes were placed in the lateral ventricles to allow air to escape. When the wax hardened he removed the brain, leaving a cast behind—simple but elegant (Fig. 1.18).

In connection with his art studies he developed the concept of "antagonism" in muscle control. His experimental studies

included sectioning a digital nerve and noting that the affected finger no longer had sensation, even when placed in a fire. Leonardo had great plans for publishing a stupendous opus on anatomy, which was to be issued in 20 volumes. The work did not appear owing to the early death of his collaborator, Marcantonio della Tore, who died in 1509.[44] From 1519, the year of Leonardo's death, until the middle of the sixteenth century, his anatomical manuscripts circulated among Italian artists through the guidance of Francesco da Melzi, Leonardo's associate. Sometime in the mid- to late sixteenth century the anatomical manuscripts were lost, and were rediscovered only in the eighteenth century, by William Hunter.

Ambroise Paré (1510-1590), a poorly educated and humble Huguenot, remains one of the greatest figures in surgical history; indeed, many considered him to be the father of modern surgery. Using the surgical material from a long military experience he was able to incorporate a great deal of practical knowledge into his writings. Paré did a very unusual thing in that he published his books in the vernacular, in this case French rather than Latin. His using French, rather than Latin, allowed a much wider dissemination of his writings. Owing to his surgical prowess and good results, Paré became a popular surgeon with royalty. The fatal injury sustained by Henri II of France was an important case, from which some insight into Paré's understanding of head injury can be obtained. Paré attended Henri II at the time of the injury and was also present at the autopsy. Paré's clinical observations of this case included headache, blurred vision, vomiting, lethargy, and decreased respiration. At autopsy the king was found to have developed a subdural hematoma. Using the clinical observations and the history, Paré postulated that the injury was due to a tear in one of the bridging cortical veins, and the autopsy confirmed his observations.

In reviewing Paré's surgical works,[45,46] the part on the brain best reflects a contemporary surgical practice. Book X is devoted to skull fractures. Paré reintroduced the earlier technique of elevating a depressed skull fracture by using the Valsalva maneuver: "... for a breath driven forth of the chest

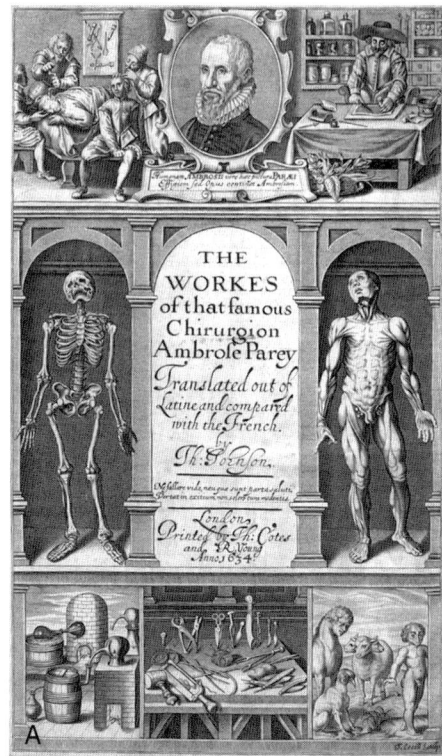
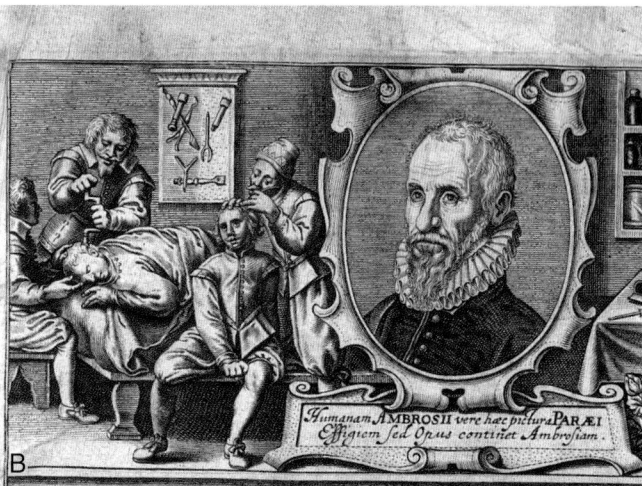

FIGURE 1.19 **A,** Title page from the English translation of Ambroise Paré's great surgical treatise. Paré is illustrated in the top middle panel, and a trephination scene is in the top left panel, which is enlarged in the next figure. **B,** Trephination scene from the title of Paré's work enlarged. As a military surgeon Paré performed numerous treatments of head injuries and skull fractures. *(From Paré A. [Johnson T, translator] The Workes of That Famous Chirurgion Ambroise Parey. London: Richard Coates; 1649.)*

and prohibited passage forth, swells and lifts the substance of the brain and meninges where upon the frothing humidity and sanies sweat forth."[36] This maneuver also assisted in the expulsion of blood and pus (Fig. 1.19).

In reviewing Paré's surgical techniques we find a remarkable advance over previous writers. Paré provides extensive discussions on the use of trephines, shavers, and scrapers. He advocates removing any osteomyelitic bone, incising the dura and evacuating blood clots and pus—procedures previously carried out with great trepidation by less well-trained surgeons. Paré strongly advocated wound débridement, emphasizing that all foreign bodies must be removed. An important advance in surgery by Paré was the serendipitous discovery that boiling oil should not be poured into wounds, particularly gunshot wounds. While in battle he ran out of the boiling oil and instead he made a dressing of egg yolk, rose oil, and turpentine. With this new formulation he found greatly improved wound healing and dramatically reduced morbidity and mortality. He also discarded the use of hot cautery to control bleeding, substituting the use of ligatures, which enhanced healing and significantly reduced blood loss, particularly in amputations.

In 1518 a remarkable book by Giacomo Berengario da Carpi (1460-1530) appeared.[47] This book came about because of Berengario's success in treating Lorenzo de' Medici, Duke of Urbino, who had received a serious cranial injury and survived. In a dream that occurred shortly after this episode Berengario was visited by the god Hermes Trismegistus (Thrice-Great Mercury), who encouraged him to a write a treatise on head injuries. As a result of this dream Berengario's

Tractatus appeared and was the first printed work devoted solely to treating injuries of the head. Not only are original surgical techniques discussed but also illustrations of the cranial instruments for dealing with skull fractures are provided (Fig. 1.20). Berengario introduced the use of interchangeable cranial drill bits for trephination. Included in the text are a number of case histories with descriptions of the patients, methods of treatment, and clinical outcomes. This work remains our best sixteenth century account of brain surgery.

Berengario, besides being a skilled surgeon, was also an excellent anatomist. Through Berengario we are provided with one of the earliest and most complete discussions of the cerebral ventricles. From his anatomical studies Berengario developed descriptions of the pineal gland, choroid plexus, and lateral ventricles. His anatomical illustrations are believed to be the first published from actual anatomical dissections rather than historical caricatures. Of enormous significant for this period were his anatomical writings, which were among the earliest to challenge the dogmatic beliefs in the writings of Galen and others.

An important book, *Anatomiae*, is most likely the earliest to deal with "accurate" neuroanatomy and appeared in 1536 (with an expanded version in 1537). The book was written by a professor of medicine from Marburg, Johannes Dryander (Johann Eichmann, 1500-1560).[48,49] This work contains a series of full-page plates showing successive Galenic dissections of the brain (Fig. 1.21). Dryander starts with a scalp dissection in layers. He continues a series of "layers," removing the skull cap. He next illustrates the meninges, brain, and posterior fossa. The first illustration of the metopic suture appears in one of the skull

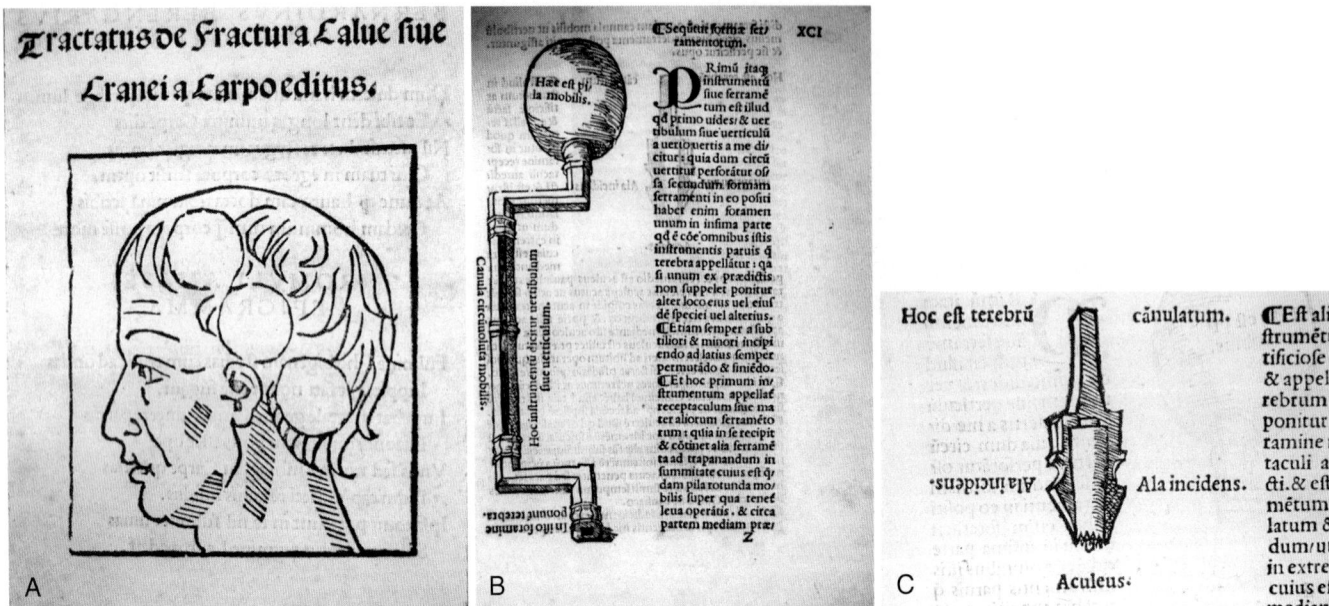

FIGURE 1.20 A, Woodcut device from the title page of Berengario da Carpi's *Tractatus de Fractura Calvae.* **B,** Berengario's design for a trephine brace. **C,** Berengario's trephines reveal a number of sophisticated designs for bone cutting and angles to avoid plunging into the brain. *(From Berengario da Carpi J. Tractatus de Fractura Calvae Sive Cranei. Bologna: Hieronymus de Benedictus; 1518.)*

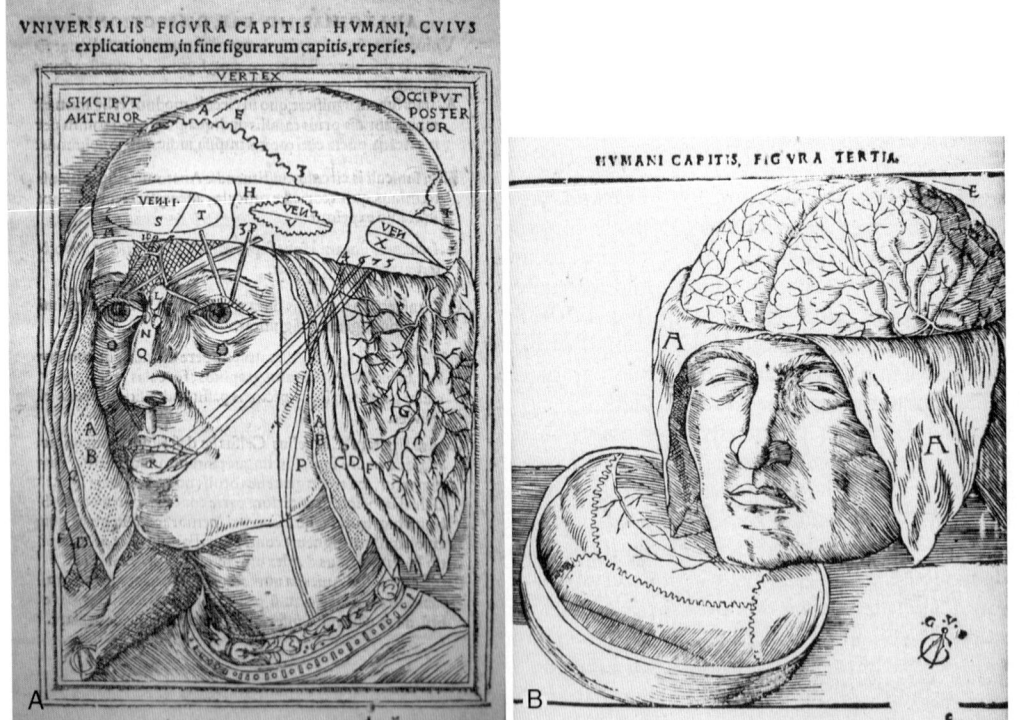

FIGURE 1.21 A, Illustration from Dryander's *Anatomiae* showing his layered dissection of the scalp and head. Also illustrated is the cell doctrine theory in which function of the brain rested in the ventricular system, not in the brain. **B,** Illustration from Dryander's *Anatomiae* showing a dissection of the scalp, skull, and brain plus the skull sutures seen in the skull cap. *(From Dryander J. Anatomiae. Marburg: Eucharius Ceruicornus; 1537.)*

figures. Important to Dryander's studies was the performance of public dissections of the skull, dura, and brain, the results of which he details in this monograph. In one image is depicted the ventricular system and the cell doctrine theory in which imagination, common sense, and memory are placed within the ventricles. There are a number of inaccuracies in the work, reflecting medieval scholasticism, but despite these errors this book should be considered the first textbook of neuroanatomy.

Volcher Coiter (1534-1576) was an army surgeon and city physician at Nuremberg who had the good fortune to study under Fallopius, Eustachius, and Aldrovandi. These scholars provided the impetus for Coiter's original anatomical and physiological investigations. He described the anterior and posterior spinal roots and distinguished gray from white matter in the spinal cord. His interest in the spine led him to conduct anatomical and pathological studies of the spinal cord, including a study on the decerebrate model. He performed a number of experiments on living subjects including work that predated William Harvey on the beating heart. He trephined the skulls of birds, lambs, goats, and dogs, and was the first to associate the

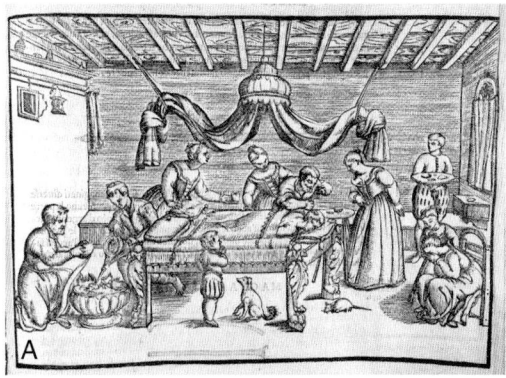
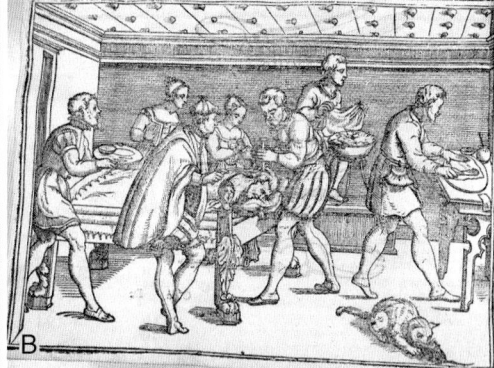

FIGURE 1.22 A, A classic scene of a sixteenth century Renaissance trephination being performed in a noble's elegantly furnished bedroom, complete with pet dog and child at bedside, from Croce's classic monograph on surgery. **B,** An Italian surgeon performing a burr hole with his assistants and instruments surrounding him. *(From Croce GA della. Chirurgiae Libri Septem. Venice: Jordanus Zilettus; 1573.)*

pulsation of the brain with the arterial pulse. He even opened the brain and removed parts of it, reporting no ill effects—an early, surprising attempt at cerebral localization.[50] Because of his enthusiastic anatomical studies via human dissection he ran afoul of the Inquisition and ended up being jailed by the Counter-Reformation, who held great distrust of physicians and anatomists who were challenging already accepted studies.

Using a combination of surgical skill and a Renaissance flair for design, Giovanni Andrea della Croce (1509?–1580)[51] produced some very early engraved scenes of neurosurgical operations. The scenes are impressive to view as the surgeries were performed in family homes, and typically in the bedrooms. Most of the neurosurgical procedures illustrated were trephinations (Fig. 1.22). Croce also provides a series of newly designed trephines with safety features to prevent plunging. An unusual innovation involved his trephine drill, which was rotated by means of an attached bow, copying the style of a carpenter's drill. Various trephine bits with conical designs are proposed and illustrated. Included in his armentarium are illustrations of surgical instruments that include some cleverly designed elevators for lifting depressed bone. In reviewing Croce's book we find it is mainly a compilation of earlier authorities from Hippocrates to Albucasis, but his recommendations for treatment and his instrumentation are surprisingly modern.

A discussion of surgery in the sixteenth century would not be complete without mention of the great anatomist and surgeon Andreas Vesalius (1514-1564). Clearly a brilliant mind, he early on rejected the anatomical views of his Galenic teachers. Vesalius studied in Paris under Johann Günther (Guenther) of Andernach, an educator of traditional Galenic anatomy. Günther quickly recognized Vesalius' skills and described him as a gifted dissector, one with extraordinary medical knowledge, and a person of great promise. Despite the laudatory praise Vesalius quickly came to the conclusion, from his Paris medical studies, that many errors in basic anatomy existed. Following the theme of earlier sixteenth century anatomists such as Berengario da Carpi, Vesalius strongly argued that anatomical dissection must be performed by the professor, not by prosectors. The common practice was to have a prosector, typically an uneducated surgeon, probe the body under the direction of the professor, who read from a Galenic anatomical text. Errors of text that did not agree with the dissection findings were merely overlooked. Vesalius' anatomical descriptions came from his own observations rather than an

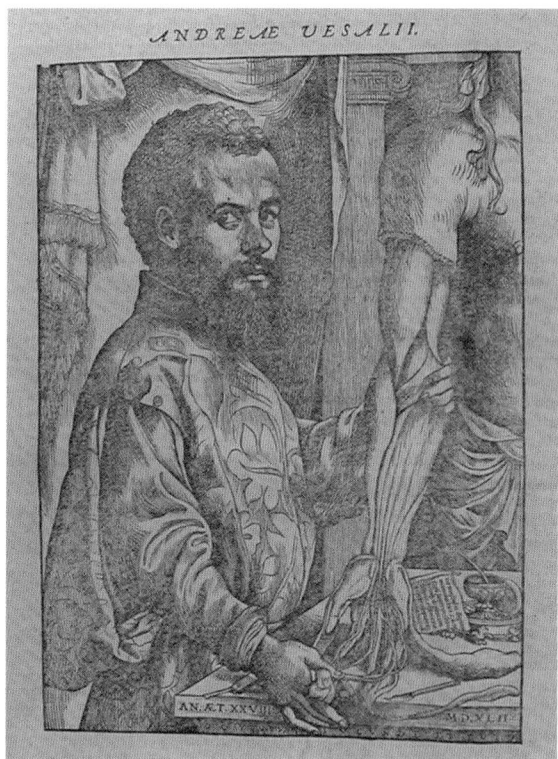

FIGURE 1.23 Portrait of the great anatomist Andreas Vesalius demonstrating a dissection of the arm from his *magnum opus. (From Vesalius A. De Humani Corporis Fabrica Libri Septem. Basel: Joannes Oporinus; 1543.)*

interpretation of the writings of Galen and others. Considering the staunch orthodox Galenic teaching of the time, he clearly faced some serious opposition from his teachers.

Vesalius's anatomical studies culminated in a masterpiece, *De Humani Corporis Fabrica*, published in 1543.[52] In Book VII is the section on the anatomy of the brain that presents detailed anatomical discussions along with excellent engravings (Fig. 1.23). Vesalius noted that "heads of beheaded men are the most suitable [for study] since they can be obtained immediately after execution with the friendly help of judges and prefects."[53]

Vesalius was primarily a surgeon and the section of text on the brain and the dural coverings discusses mechanisms of injury and how the various membranes and bone have been designed to protect the brain.[53] Interestingly, close examination of several of the illustrated initial letters in the text shows little cherubs performing trephinations! For neurosurgeons Vesalius made an interesting early contribution to the understanding of hydrocephalus: In Book 1 is a discussion of "Heads of other shape" wherein he provides the following early description of a child with hydrocephalus:

> ... at Genoa a small boy is carried from door to door by a beggar woman, and was put on display by actors in noble Brabant in Belgium, whose head, without any exaggeration, is larger than two normal human heads and swells out on either side.[52]

In the second edition (1555) of his work,[54] Vesalius describes a second case, that of hydrocephalus in a young girl whom he noted to have a head "larger than any man's," and at autopsy he describes the removal of 9 lb of water. As a result of these studies Vesalius made the important observation that fluid (i.e., cerebrospinal fluid) collects in the ventricles and not between the dura and skull, an earlier Hippocratic error. Vesalius made a number of interesting clinical observations but offered no insight into any effective treatment, either surgical or medical.

A remarkable work on anatomy by Charles Estienne (1504-1564) appeared in Paris in 1546.[55] This book was the fifth in a series of books on anatomy to be published in Europe, following Berengario da Carpi (two books), Dryander, and Vesalius. Although published 3 years after Andreas Vesalius' work, the book had actually been completed in 1539, but legal problems delayed publication. This work contains a wealth of beautiful but bizarre anatomical plates with the subjects posed against sumptuous, imaginative Renaissance backgrounds (Fig. 1.24). The anatomical detail clearly lacks the details of Vesalius and the book repeats many of the errors of Galen. The plates on the nervous system are quite graphic but flawed in the anatomical details. A typical plate shows a full anatomical figure with the skull cut to show the brain. Although gross structures like the ventricle and cerebrum are recognizable they do lack solid anatomical details.

With the end of the sixteenth century anatomy has come full circle, rejecting earlier doctrines flawed with numerous errors. In works by Vesalius and Berengario hands-on dissection by the professor clearly corrects many of the anatomical errors long ensconced in the literature. Without these fundamental changes in both thought and concept the development of neuroanatomy would not have been possible. Without accurate neuroanatomy how can one practice neurosurgery? As we will see, nearly 300 more years of surgical art, skill, and anatomy are needed to let that happen.

SEVENTEENTH CENTURY: ORIGINS OF NEUROLOGY

In the sixteenth century anatomy was the main theme, and with the seventeenth century we see the development of a period of spectacular growth in science and medicine. Individuals such as Isaac Newton, Francis Bacon, William Harvey, and Robert Boyle made important contributions in physics, experimental design, the discovery of the circulation of blood, and physiological chemistry. For the first time open public communication of scientific ideas came with the advent of scientific societies

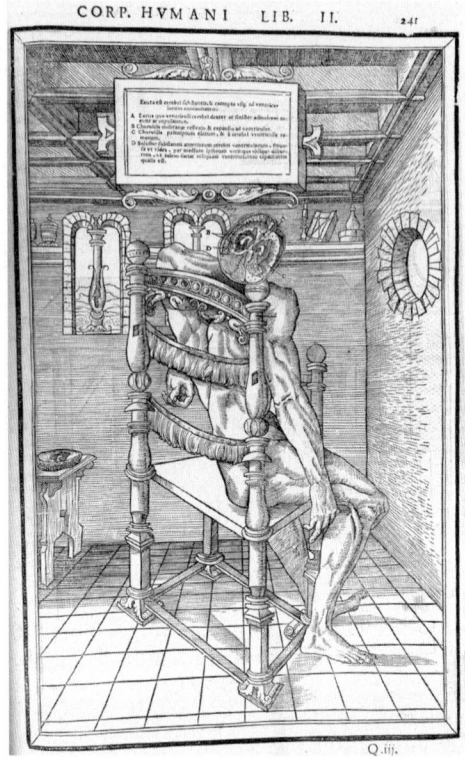

FIGURE 1.24 A neuroanatomical plate from Estienne's *De Dissectione* showing an axial dissection of the brain of a man seated in a sumptuous room in a villa. *(From Estienne C, De Dissectione Partium Corporis Humani Libri Tres. Paris: Simon Colinaeus; 1546.)*

(e.g., the Royal Society of London, the Académie des Sciences in Paris, and the Gesellschaft Naturforschenden Ärzte in Germany). These societies and the individuals associated with them dramatically improved scientific design and education along with unparalleled exchanges of scientific information.

Within this century came the first intense exploration of the human brain. Leading the many investigators was Thomas Willis (1621-1675), after whom the circle of Willis is named (Fig. 1.25). A fashionable London practitioner, educated at Oxford, Willis published his *Cerebri Anatome* in London in 1664 (Fig. 1.26).[56] With its publication we have now the first accurate anatomical study of the human brain. Willis was assisted in this work by Richard Lower (1631-1691). In Chapter VII Lower demonstrates by laboratory experimentation that when parts of the "circle" were tied off, the anastomotic network still provided blood to the brain. Lower noted, "if by chance one or two [of its arteries] should be stopt, there might easily be found another passage instead of them . . ." (see Figure 1a, p. 27).[56] The striking brain engravings were drawn and engraved by the prominent London personality, Sir Christopher Wren (1632-1723), who was often present at Willis' dissections. Most surgeons are not aware that the eponym was not applied to the circle until Albrecht Haller used it in his eighteenth century bibliography on anatomy.[57,58]

To Thomas Willis we owe the introduction of the concept of "neurology," or the doctrine of neurons, here using the term in a purely anatomical sense. The word *neurology* did not enter general use until Samuel Johnson defined it in his dictionary of 1765, in which the word *neurology* now

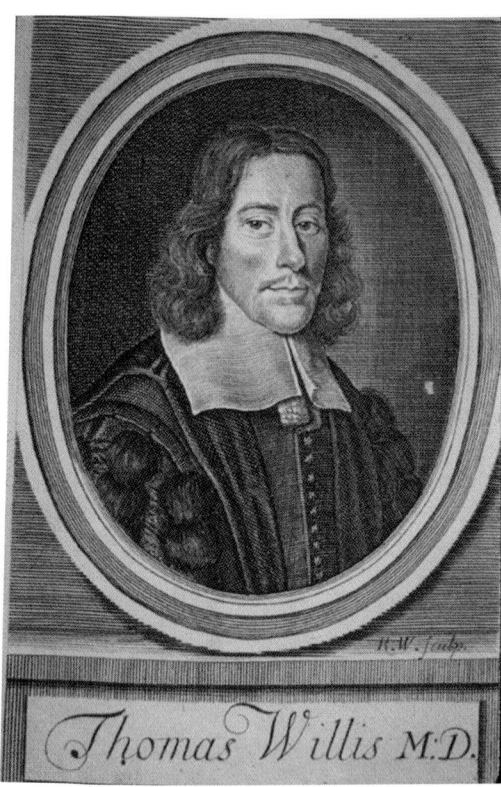

FIGURE 1.25 Thomas Willis (1621-1675).

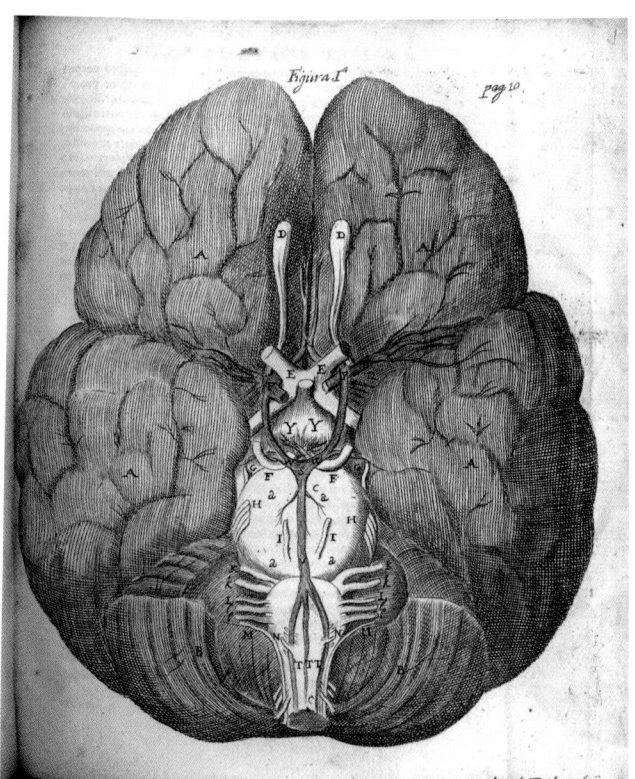

FIGURE 1.26 Thomas Willis' *Cerebri Anatome*, published in 1664, showing his depiction of what is now called the *circle of Willis*. The eponym for the circle of Willis did not appear until the eighteenth century when Albrecht Haller assigned it in his anatomical bibliography.[57] *(From Willis T. Cerebri Anatome: Cui Accessit Nervorum Descriptio et Usus. London: J. Flesher; 1664.)*

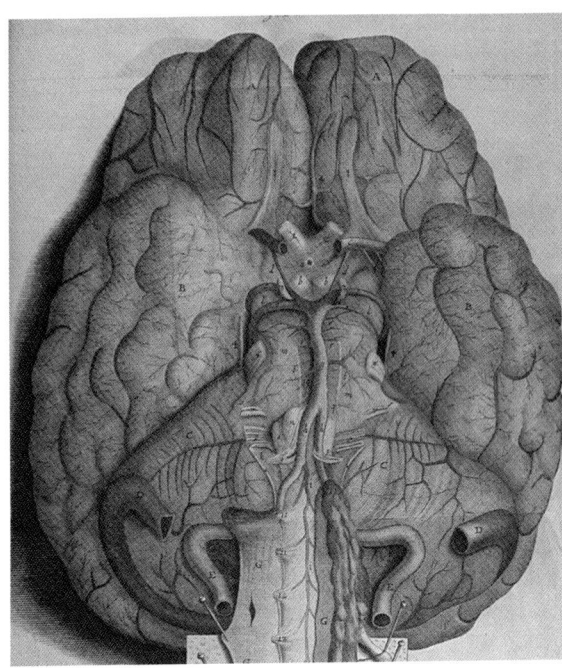

FIGURE 1.27 Circle of Willis as detailed by Ridley in an anatomically more correct rendition than that of Willis. *(From Ridley H. The Anatomy of the Brain, Containing its Mechanisms and Physiology: Together With Some New Discoveries and Corrections of Ancient and Modern Authors Upon That Subject. London: Samuel Smith; 1695.)*

encompassed the entire field of anatomy, function, and physiology. The circle of Willis was also detailed in other anatomical works of this period by Vesling,[59] Casserius,[60] Fallopius,[61] and Humphrey Ridley.[62]

Another important work on the anatomy of the brain appeared under the authorship of Humphrey Ridley (1653-1708). The book was unique in that it was written in the vernacular (English), not the usual academic Latin, and became widely circulated (Fig. 1.27).[62] Ridley was educated at Merton College, Oxford, and at the University of Leiden, where he received his doctorate in medicine in 1679. At the time his work on the brain appeared, many ancient theories of the brain were still prevalent. Shifting away from the earlier cell doctrine theory, seventeenth century anatomists came to recognize the brain as a distinct anatomical entity. Cerebral function, instead of residing within the ventricles, was now known to be a property of the brain parenchyma.

Ridley described a number of original observations in this volume on brain anatomy. He ingeniously conducted anatomical studies on freshly executed criminals, most of whom had been hanged. Ridley realized that hanging caused vascular engorgement of the brain and hence allowed easier identification of the anatomy. In reviewing his description of the circle of Willis we find an even more accurate view than Willis'. Ridley added a more complete account of both the posterior cerebral artery and the superior cerebellar artery. The anastomotic principle of this network was even further elucidated with his injection studies of the vessels. His understanding of the deep nuclei and, in particular, the anatomy of the posterior fossa, was superior to that of previous writers including Thomas Willis. The first accurate description of the fornix and its pathways appears in this monograph. Ridley provided an early and accurate description of the arachnoid membrane. Ridley's book was not totally without error as he argues here in favor of the belief that the rete mirabile exists.

Although Wilhelm Fabricius von Hilden (1560-1634) had received a classical education in his youth, family misfortune did not allow him a formal medical education. Following the apprenticeship system then prevalent, he studied the lesser field of surgery. Fortunately, the teachers he selected were among the finest wound surgeons of the day. With this education, he had a distinguished career in surgery, during which he made a number of advances.

His large work, *Observationum et Curationum,* included over 600 surgical cases and a number of important and original observations on the brain.[63] Congenital malformations, skull fractures, techniques for bullet extraction, and field surgical instruments are all clearly described. He performed operations for intracranial hemorrhage (with cure of insanity), vertebral displacement, congenital hydrocephalus, and occipital tumor (i.e., encephalocele) of the newborn; he also carried out trephinations for abscess and claimed a cure of an old aphasia. To remove a splinter of metal from the eye he used a magnet, a cure that enhanced his reputation.

Johann Schultes (Scultetus) of Ulm (1595-1645) provided in his *Armamentarium Chirurgicum XLIII* the first descriptive details of neurosurgical instruments to appear since those published by Berengario in 1518.[64] His book was translated into many languages, influencing surgery throughout Europe. Its importance lies in the exact detail of surgical instrument design and in the presentation of tools from antiquity to the present. Interestingly a number of the instruments illustrated by Scultetus are still in use today. Scultetus details a variety of surgical procedures dealing with injuries of the skull and brain. The text is further enhanced by some of the best seventeenth century illustrations detailing surgical technique (Fig. 1.28).

James Yonge (1646-1721) was among the first since Galen to argue emphatically that "wounds of the brain are curable." Appropriately enough, Yonge's remarkable little monograph was entitled *Wounds of the Brain Proved Curable.*[65] Yonge was a Plymouth naval surgeon, remembered mostly for his flap amputation technique. In his monograph Yonge gives a detailed account of a brain operation on a child aged 4 years with extensive compound fractures of the skull from which brain tissue issued forth. The surgery was a success and the child lived. Yonge also included reports on more than 60 cases of brain wounds that he found in the literature, beginning with Galen, which had been cured.

EIGHTEENTH CENTURY: ADVENTUROUS SURGEONS

The eighteenth century was a period of intense activity in the medical and scientific world. Chemistry as a true science was propelled forward by the work of Priestley, Lavoisier, Volta, Watt, and many others. Thomas Sydenham, William Cullen, and Herman Boerhaave reintroduced clinical bedside medicine, a practice essentially lost since the Byzantine era. Diagnostic examination of the patient advanced in this period; especially notable is Auenbrugger's introduction of percussion of the chest. Withering introduced the use of digitalis for cardiac problems. Edward Jenner provided the world with

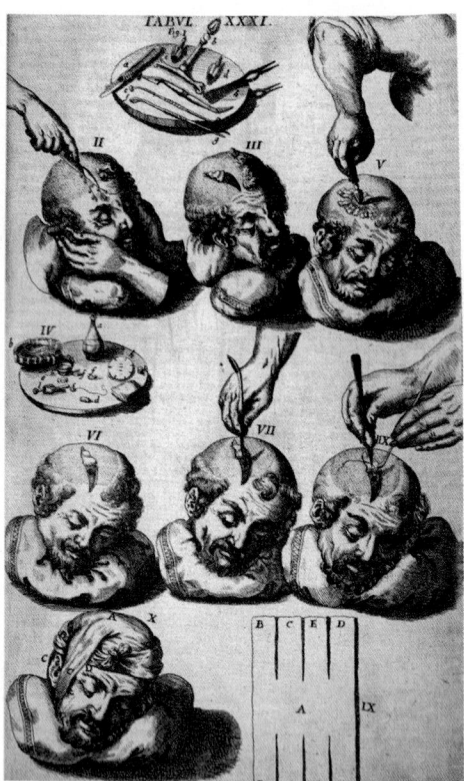

FIGURE 1.28 Seventeenth century neurosurgical trephination techniques as detailed by Scultetus. *(From Scultetus J. Armamentarium Chirurgicum XLIII. Ulm: Balthasar Kühnen; 1655.)*

cowpox inoculation for smallpox, beginning the elimination of the terror of this scourge.

The eighteenth century produced some quite clever and adventurous surgeons. Percival Pott (1714-1788) was the greatest English surgeon of the eighteenth century. His list of contributions, several of which apply to neurosurgery, is enormous. His work *Remarks on That Kind of Palsy of the Lower Limbs Found to Accompany a Curvature of the Spine* describes the condition now known as *Pott's disease.*[66] His clinical descriptions are excellent, with the gibbous and tuberculous condition of the spine well outlined. Interestingly, he failed to associate the spinal deformity with the paralysis. He also described an osteomyelitic condition of the skull with a collection of pus under the pericranium, now called *Pott's puffy tumor.* Pott felt strongly that these lesions should be trephined to remove the pus and decompress the brain.

In the ongoing argument over whether to trephine, Pott was a strong proponent of intervention (Figs. 1.29, 1.30). In his classic work on head injury,[67] Pott appreciated that symptoms of head injury were the result of injury of the brain and not of the skull. He made an attempt to differentiate between "compression" and "concussion" injury of the brain.

The reasons for trepanning in these cases are, first, the immediate relief of present symptoms arising from pressure of extravasated fluid; or second, the discharge of matter formed between the skull and dura mater, in consequence of inflammation; or third, the prevention of such mischief, as experience has shown may most probably be expected from such kind of violence offered to the last mentioned membrane. …

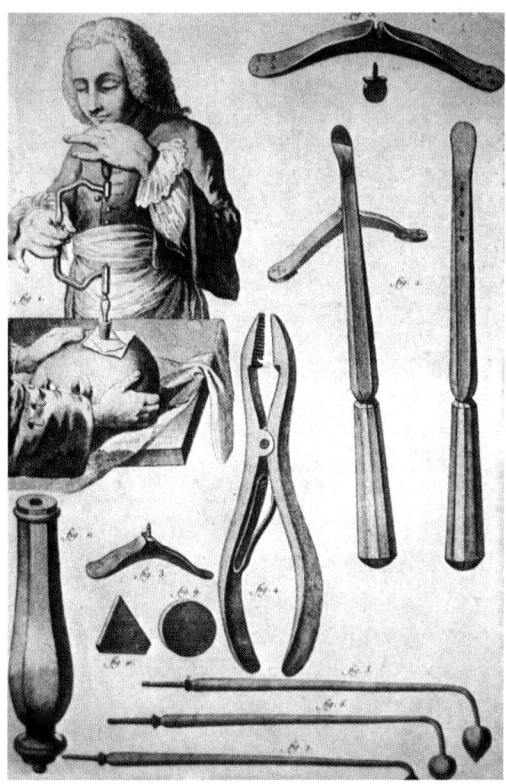

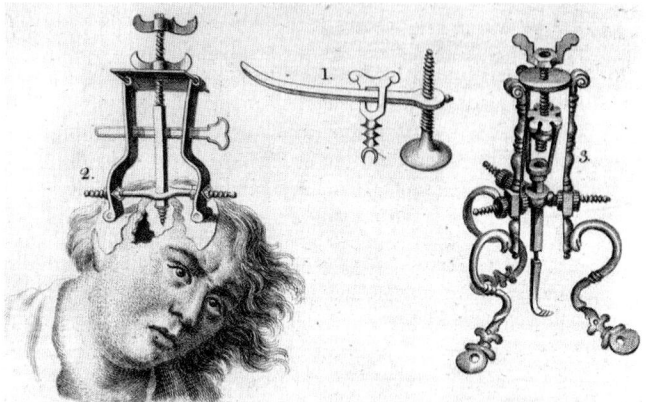

FIGURE 1.30 A trephination set designed by Percival Pott that includes a tripod-type system. To elevate a depressed skull fracture he designed a trephine screw that was driven into the fracture and then used a lever action to elevate the fracture. *(From Pott P. Observations on the Nature and Consequences of Wounds and Contusions of the Head, Fractures of the Skull, Concussions of the Brain. London: C. Hitch and L. Hawes; 1760.)*

FIGURE 1.29 An eighteenth century trephination illustrated in Diderot's *Encyclopédie.* In this case the surgeon can rest his chin on the trephination handle and thereby is able to apply additional pressure to the trephine bit. The surrounding instruments are various bone elevators, bone rongeur, and cautery applicators. *(From Diderot D. Encyclopedie ou Dictionnaire Raisonnes Des Sciences Des Arts et Des Metiers. Paris: 1751-1752.)*

In the ... mere fracture without depression of bone, or the appearance of such symptoms as indicate commotion, extravasation, or inflammation, it is used as a preventative, and therefore is a matter of choice, more than immediate necessity.[67]

Pott's astute clinical observations, bedside treatment, and aggressive management of head injuries made him the first modern neurosurgeon. His caveats, presented in the preface to his work on head injury, still hold today.

John Hunter (1728-1793) was one of the most remarkable and talented figures in English surgery and anatomy. His knowledge and skills in anatomy, pathology, and surgery and his dedication to his work allowed him to make a number of important contributions. Hunter received minimal formal education, though Percival Pott was an early teacher and mentor. In his book *A Treatise on the Blood, Inflammation, and Gun-Shot Wounds,*[68] Hunter drew on his years of military experience (he served as a surgeon with the British forces during the Spanish campaign of 1761-1763). Unfortunately, the section on skull fractures took up only one paragraph and offered nothing original. However, his discussion of vascular disorders was quite advanced, with an appreciation of the concept of collateral circulation. His views on this subject grew out of his surgical experimentation on a buck whose carotid artery he tied off; he noted the response to be development of collateral circulation.[69]

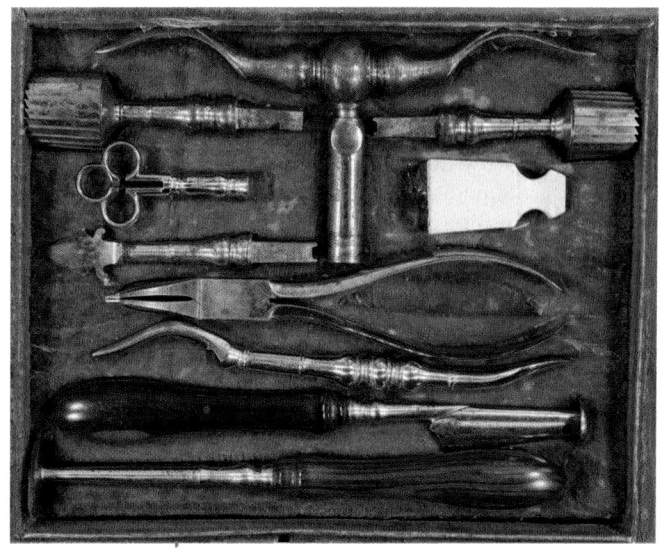

FIGURE 1.31 An eighteenth century traveling trephine set with the tools and elevators necessary for a trephination and elevating a skull fracture. In the preantisepsis era these instruments were often encrusted with bone dust and debris from the previous surgery. *(From the author's personal collection.)*

Benjamin Bell (1749-1806) was among the most prominent and successful surgeons in Edinburgh. He was one of the first to emphasize the importance of reducing pain during surgery. His text, *A System of Surgery,*[70] is written with extraordinary clarity and precision, qualities that made it one of the most popular surgical texts in the eighteenth and nineteenth centuries. In the section on head injury there is an interesting and important discussion of the differences between concussion, compression, and inflammation of the brain—each requiring different modes of treatment.[70] Bell stressed the importance of relieving compression of the brain, whether it be caused by a depressed skull fracture or pressure caused by pus or blood—a remarkably aggressive approach for this period (Fig. 1.31). Bell was among the first to note that hydrocephalus is often associated with spina bifida. His treatment of a myelomeningocele involved placing a ligature around the base of the myelomeningocele sac and tying it down. The concept of an epidural hematoma and its symptoms were detailed by Bell; he argued for a rapid and prompt evacuation. His discussion of the symptoms of brain compression caused by external trauma is classic:

A great variety of symptoms … indicating a compressed state of the brain [among which] … the most frequent, as well as the most remarkable, are the following: Giddiness; dimness of sight; stupefaction; loss of voluntary motion; vomiting; an apoplectic stertor in the breathing; convulsive tremors in different muscles; a dilated state of the pupils, even when the eyes are exposed to a clear light; paralysis of different parts, especially of the side of the body opposite to the injured part of the head; involuntary evacuation of the urine and faeces; an oppressed, and in many case an irregular pulse … (volume 3, chapter 10, section 3).[70]

Lorenz Heister (1683-1758) produced another of the most popular surgical textbooks of the eighteenth century. A German surgeon and anatomist (a common combination at the time), he published his *Chirurgie* in 1718. It was subsequently translated into a number of languages and circulated widely.[71] The book's popularity was due to the wide range of surgical knowledge it communicated and its many valuable surgical illustrations. In the treatment of head injury Heister remained conservative with regard to trephination (Fig. 1.32). In wounds involving only concussion and contusion, he felt trephination to be too dangerous. In this preantiseptic era considering the additional risk of infection and injury to the brain, this was not too far off the mark:

XXVII. But when the Cranium is so depressed, whether in Adults or Infants, as to suffer a Fracture, or Division of its Parts, it must instantly be relieved: the Part depressed, which adheres, after cleaning the Wound, must be restored to its Place, what is separated must be removed, and the extravasated Blood be drawn off through the Aperture … (p. 100).[71]

Heister introduced a number of techniques that proved most useful. To control scalp hemorrhage he used a "crooked needle and thread" that when placed and drawn tight reduced bleeding from the wound edges. He also pointed out that when the assistant applied pressure to the skin, edge bleeding could also be reduced. In spinal injuries Heister was quite aggressive, advocating exposure of the fractured vertebrae and removing fragments that damaged the spinal marrow, even though he recognized that grave outcomes of such attempts were not uncommon.

Francois-Sauveur Morand (1697-1773) describes one of the earliest operations for abscess of the brain. Morand had a patient, a monk, who developed an otitis media and subsequently mastoiditis with temporal abscess.[72] He trephined over the carious bone and discovered pus. He placed a catgut wick within the wound, but it continued to drain. He reopened the wound and this time opened the dura (a very adventurous maneuver for this period) with a cross-shaped incision and found a brain abscess. He explored the abscess with his finger, removing as much of the contents as he could, and then instilled balsam and turpentine into the cavity. He placed a silver tube for drainage, and as the wound healed he slowly withdrew the tube. The abscess healed, and the patient survived.

Domenico Cotugno (1736-1822) was a Neapolitan physician and was the first to provide descriptions of cerebrospinal fluid (CSF) and sciatica[73] (Fig. 1.33). He performed a number of experiments on the bodies of some 20 adults. Using the technique of lumbar puncture, he was able to demonstrate the

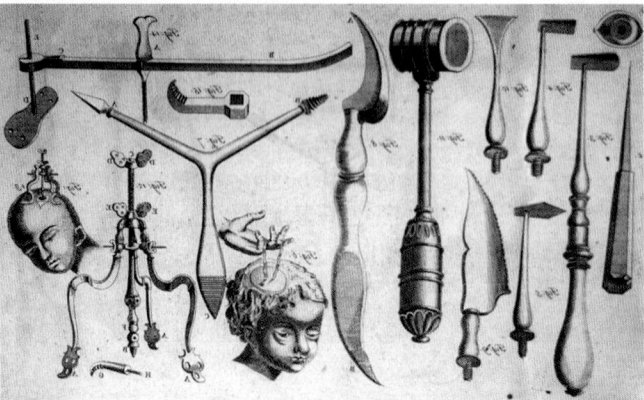

FIGURE 1.32 Lorenz Heister, an ingenious eighteenth century German surgeon, designed his own trephination set, which included a number of interesting surgical designs. Heister illustrated an unusual technique to elevate a depressed fracture in a child. Heister made two small holes in the depressed fracture, a leather string was placed through the holes, and then the fracture was elevated outward with string. *(From Heister L. A General System of Surgery in Three Parts. London: W. Innys; 1743.)*

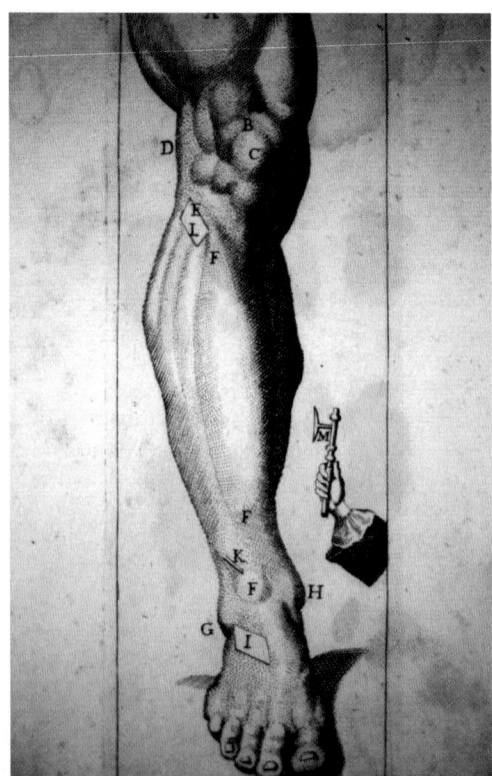

FIGURE 1.33 Cotugno was the first to ascribe sciatica to the sciatic nerve and not rheumatism, the then prevalent concept. *(From Cotugno D. De Ischiade Nervosa Commentarius. Napoli: Fratres Simonii; 1764.)*

characteristics of CSF. In *De Ischiade Nervosa Commentarius* he demonstrated the "nervous" origin of sciatica, differentiating it from arthritis, with which it was generally equated at that time. Cotugno discovered the pathways of CSF, showing that it circulates in the pia-arachnoid interstices and flows through the brain and spinal cord via the aqueduct and convexities. He also described the hydrocephalus *ex vacuo* seen in cerebral atrophy.

In 1709, a small, and now very rare, monograph by Daniel Turner (1667-1741) appeared.[74] The book was entitled *A Remarkable Case in Surgery: Wherein an Account is given of an uncommon Fracture and Depression of the Skull, in a Child about Six Years old; accompanied with a large Abscess or Aposteme upon the Brain* ... (Fig. 1.34). This rather poignant piece of writing is perhaps our best view of the treatment of brain injuries in the early eighteenth century.

The case is most disturbing to read, written in the frank and somewhat verbose style of this period. Turner was "... called in much hast, to a Child about the Age of Six Years ... wounded by a Catstick ... He was taken up for dead and continued speechless for some time." Turner examined the head, found a considerable depression, and arrived at the prognosis that the child was in great danger. He sent for the barber to shave the head; while waiting for the barber he opened a vein in the arm to bleed the child, taking about 6 ounces. The patient regained consciousness, vomiting and complaining of a headache. Turner chose to delay surgery. But finding the child the next day still vomiting, restless, and hot, he decided on an exploration. Through a typical X incision he found "the Bones were beat thro' both meninges into the substance of the brain." He elevated the bone and found "... a cavity sufficient

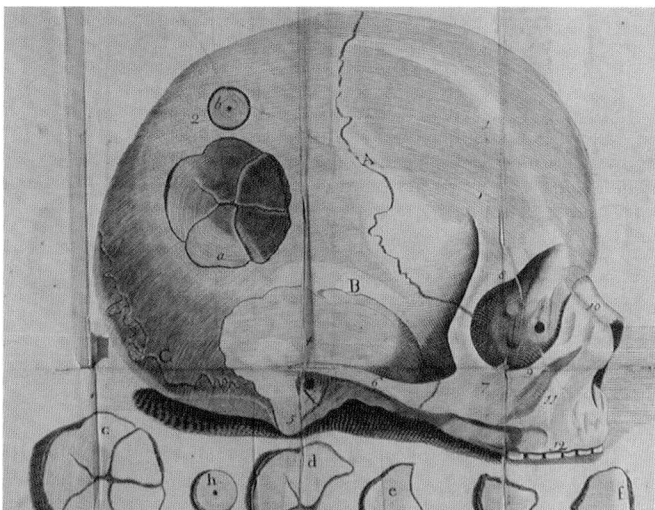

FIGURE 1.34 A child with a severe skull fracture who survived his injury. Illustrated here are the various trephinations done and bone fractures removed along the lower margin. *(From Turner D. A Remarkable Case in Surgery: Wherein an Account is Given of an Uncommon Fracture and Depression of the Skull, in a Child About Six Years Old; Accompanied With a Large Abscess or Aposteme Upon the Brain. With Other Practical Observations and Useful Reflections Thereupon. Also an Exact Draught of the Case, Annex'd. And for the Entertainment of the Senior, but Instruction of the Junior Practitioners, Communicated. London: R. Parker; 1709.)*

to contain near two Ounces of Liquor." Postoperatively the patient was awake with "... a quick pulse, thirst and headache ... but no vomiting. He was very sensible." He visited the child the next day and found him still feverish but without other symptoms. He removed the dressings and realized the extent of the fracture, which had been only partially elevated. He now took a trephine, removed what bone he thought it was safe to remove, and applied a clyster.

A careful report of the operation follows, including a description of a piece of bone that flew across the room upon elevation. Four pieces of bone were removed. The dura now pulsated nicely. The wound was cleaned out with soft sponges soaked in claret. The patient was carried to bed and refreshed with "two or three Spoonfulls of his Cephalic Julep." Despite all this effort and although the patient was doing well, upon removing the dressings "an offensive smell" and fetid matter were noted. A consultant's advice was to redress the wound. Instead, Turner opened the right jugular vein and bled 6 ounces. A vesicatory was also applied to the neck and an emollient clyster given in the evening. The next day Turner was still not satisfied with what was happening, and so he re-explored the wound, venting a great deal of purulent matter.

This patient was to have several additional explorations for removal and drainage of pus. Cannulas were placed for drainage and the wound carefully tended, but despite all this the patient died after 12 weeks.

Louis Sebastian (also listed as Nicolas) Saucerotte (1741-1814) was first surgeon to the King of Poland and later a surgeon in the French Army. As has often been the case in the history of neurosurgery, war provided Saucerotte with training and multiple opportunities to deal with head injury. He reintroduced the concept of the contre-coup injury. In a review of head injury, he described in detail a series of intracranial injuries and their symptoms, including compression of the brain due to blood clot.[75] Saucerotte described a classic case of incoordination, including opisthotonos and rolling of the eyes, as a result of a cerebellar lesion. He divided the brain into "areas" of injury, pointing out that areas of severe injury are at the base of the brain, while injuries of the forebrain are the best tolerated.

During the eighteenth century there was a remarkable change in the approach to surgery of the brain. Surgeons became much more aggressive in their management of head injuries and the clinical symptoms associated with brain injury were better recognized. Unfortunately in many cases the outcomes remained poor because of infection and a lack of understanding on how to control this morbidity. As anesthesia was not yet well developed the best surgeons were the "fastest" and most adroit with their hands.

NINETEENTH AND TWENTIETH CENTURIES: ANESTHESIA, ANTISEPSIS, AND CEREBRAL LOCALIZATION

During the nineteenth century three major innovations made possible great advances in surgery. Anesthesia allowed patients freedom from pain during surgery, antisepsis and aseptic technique enabled the surgeon to operate with a greatly reduced risk of postoperative complications caused by infection, and

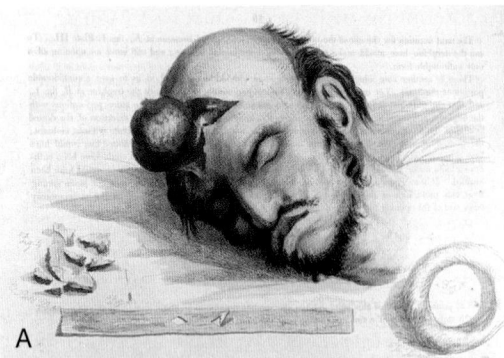
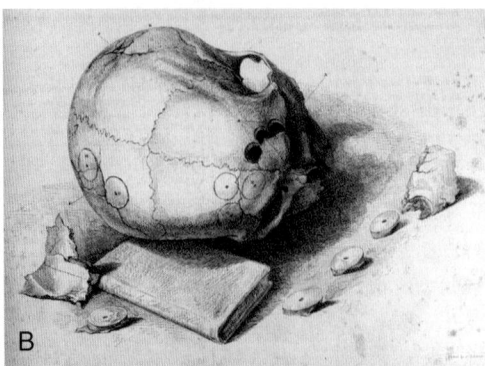

FIGURE 1.35 A, Charles Bell, both a surgeon and a skilled artist, illustrates his surgical technique for exploration and repair of an open skull fracture with herniating brain; the bone fragments removed are shown at the lower left of the illustration. **B,** From Bell's surgical atlas is a clinical sketch from a skull localizing the various areas where it would be safe to perform trephinations. *(From Bell C. Illustrations of the Great Operations of Surgery. London: Longman, Rees, Orme, Brown, and Greene; 1821.)*

the concept of cerebral localization helped the surgeon make the diagnosis and plan the operative approach.

In the first half of the century, improvements in surgical technique and neuropathology helped prepare the way for these innovations. John Abernethy (1764-1831) succeeded John Hunter at St. Bartholomew's Hospital and followed his tradition of experimentation and observation. Abernethy's surgical technique did not differ from that of his predecessors; what is remarkable in his *Surgical Observations*[76] is the thoughtful, very thorough discussion of all the mechanisms of injury to the brain and spinal cord. He performed one of the earliest known procedures for removal of a painful neuroma. The neuroma was resected and the nerve reanastomosed; the pain resolved and sensation returned, proving the efficacy of the anastomosis.

Sir Charles Bell (1774-1842), a Scottish surgeon and anatomist, was a prolific writer. He was educated at the University of Edinburgh and spent most of his professional career in London. He is remembered for many contributions to the neurosciences, including the differentiation of the motor and sensory components of the spinal root. He wrote a number of works on surgery, many of which were beautifully illustrated with his own drawings. These hand-colored illustrations were unrivaled at the time in detail, accuracy, and beauty (Fig. 1.35). In describing a trephination Bell details the technique as he practiced in 1821:

> Let the bed or couch on which the patient is lying be turned to the light—have the head shaved—put a wax-cloth on the pillow—let the pillow be firm, to support the patient's head. Put tow or sponge by the side of the head—let there be a stout assistant to hold the patient's head firmly, and let others put their hands on his arms and knees.

> The surgeon will expect the instruments to be handed to him in this succession—the scalpel; the rasparatory; the trephine; the brush, the quill, and probe, from time to time; the elevator, the forceps, the lenticular (p. 6).[77]

Also in the first half of the nineteenth century, a number of industrious individuals provided the basis for study of neuropathological lesions. Several excellent atlases appeared, beautifully colored and pathologically correct. Among the best known are those of Robert Hooper, Jean Cruveilhier, Robert Carswell, and Richard Bright (Fig. 1.36). Cruveilhier's atlas

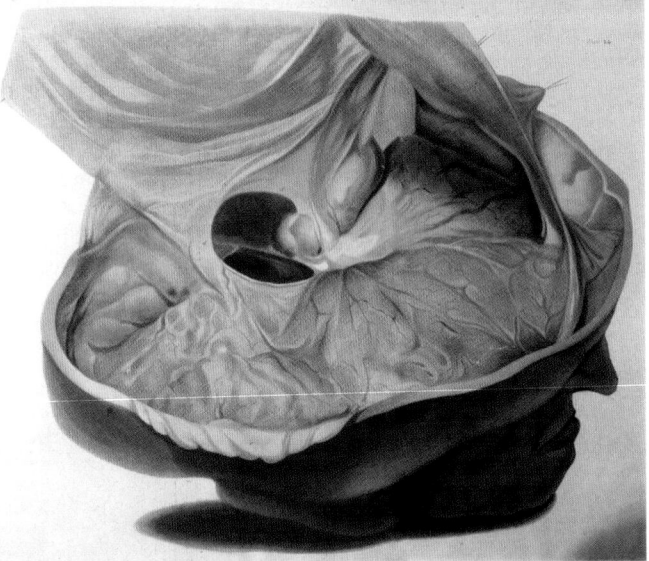

FIGURE 1.36 In one of the great nineteenth century neuropathological atlases Richard Bright illustrated a classic case of a young adult with severe hydrocephalus who died in his 20s. The autopsy findings in hydrocephalus are beautifully illustrated in this hand-colored lithograph. *(From Bright R. Report of Medical Cases. London: Longman, Rees, Orme, Brown, and Greene; 1827.)*

is the most dramatic in appearance with illustrations of the brain and spine that were unparalleled for the period.[78]

Jean Cruveilhier (1791-1874) was the first occupant of a new chair of pathology at the University of Paris. He had at his disposal an enormous collection of autopsy material provided by the dead house at the Salpêtrière and the Musée Dupuytren. Using material from these sources he made a number of original descriptions of pathologies of the nervous system, including spina bifida (Fig. 1.37), spinal cord hemorrhage, cerebellopontine angle tumor, disseminated sclerosis, muscular atrophy, and perhaps the best early description of meningioma. This work was published in a series of fascicles issued over 13 years.[79] The detailed descriptions by Cruveilhier and others provided the basis for the later cerebral localization studies. An understanding of tumors and

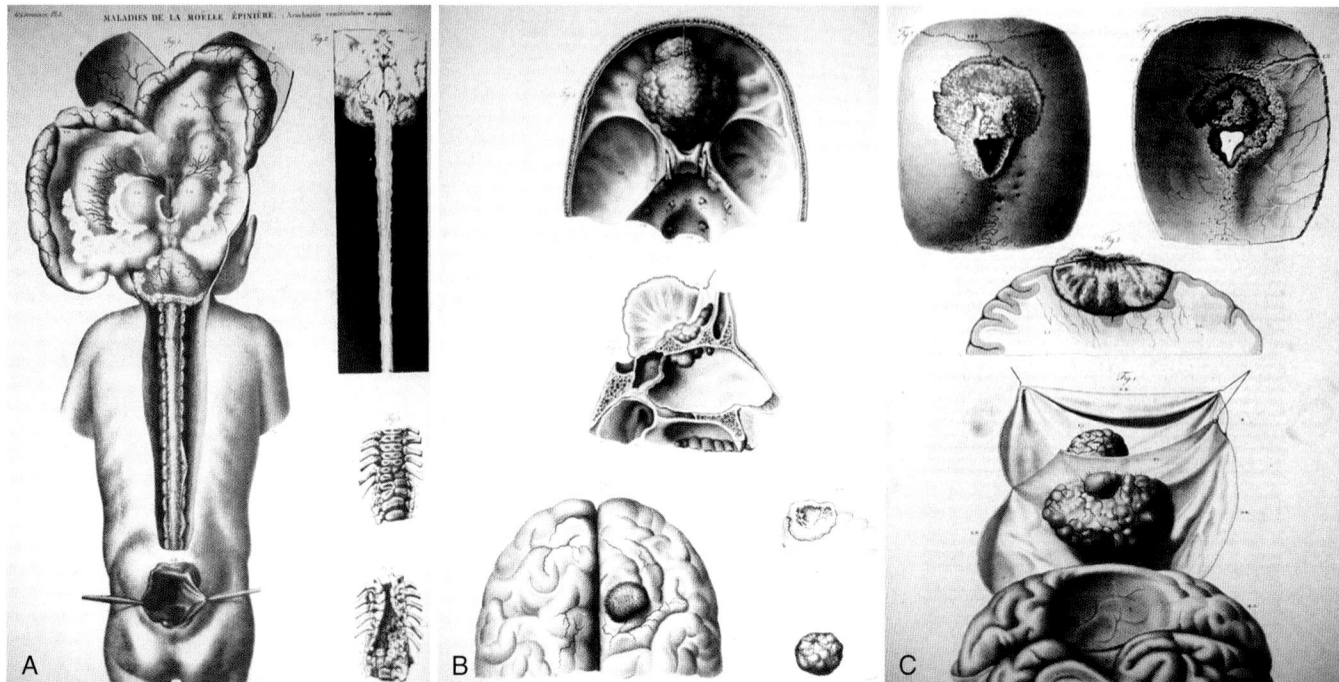

FIGURE 1.37 A, A fine graphic illustration by Cruveilhier showing a child with spina bifida and associated hydrocephalus: an excellent example of the developing quality of pathological illustrations in the first half of the nineteenth century. **B,** A fine example of various meningiomas involving the skull base, olfactory region, and convexity. **C,** A nice example of convexity dural meningioma with destructive bone invasion and loss. *(From Cruveilhier J. Anatomie Pathologique du Corps Humain. Paris: J.-B. Baillière; 1829-1842.)*

their clinicopathological effects on the brain was critical for the later development of neurosurgery and the neurological examination. Harvey Cushing was the first to call attention to Cruveilhier's accuracy in pathology and clinical correlation. He used portions of Cruveilhier's works in his treatise on acoustic neuromas and his classic meningioma monograph.[79-81]

Anesthesia

Surgeons have tried various methods of reducing sensibility to pain over the centuries. Mandrake, cannabis, opium and other narcotics, the "soporific sponge" (saturated with opium), and alcohol had all been tried. In 1844, Horace Wells, a dentist in Hartford, Connecticut, introduced the use of nitrous oxide in dental procedures; however, the death of one of his patients stopped him from investigating further. At the urging of W.T.O. Morton, J.C. Warren used ether on October 16, 1846, to induce a state of insensibility in a patient, during which a vascular tumor of the submaxillary region was removed. James Y. Simpson, who preferred chloroform, introduced in 1847, as an anesthetic agent, undertook similar efforts in the United Kingdom. There were many arguments about which was the best agent. However, the end result was that the surgeon did not need to restrain the patient or operate at breakneck speed, and patients were free of pain during the procedure.

Antisepsis

Even with the best surgical technique, 3-minute (!) trephinations, the patient often died postoperatively of suppuration and infection. Fever, purulent material, brain abscess, and draining wounds all defeated the best surgeons. For many

centuries surgeons dreaded opening the dura mater for fear of inviting disaster from infection. Until the issue of infection could be dramatically reduced no surgeon comfortably approached surgery of the head or spine.

Utilizing the recent bacterial concepts developed by Louis Pasteur, Joseph Lister introduced antisepsis in the operating room (Fig. 1.38). For the first time a surgeon, using aseptic technique and a clean operating theater, could operate on the brain with a reasonably small likelihood of infection. The steam sterilizer, the carbolic sprayer, the scrub brush, and Halsted's rubber gloves truly heralded a revolution in surgery.

Cerebral Localization

To make a diagnosis of a brain lesion or brain injury was not meaningful until the concept of localization was formulated (Fig. 1.39). During the 1860s several investigators, including G.T. Fritsch and E. Hitzig[82] as well as Paul Broca, introduced the concept of cerebral localization, that each part of the brain was responsible for a particular function (Fig. 1.40).

Paul Broca (1824-1880) conceived the idea of speech localization in 1861.[83] His studies were based on the work by Ernest Auburtin (1825-1893?), who had as a patient a gentleman who attempted suicide by shooting himself through the frontal region. He survived, but was left with a defect in the left frontal bone. Through this defect Auburtin was able to apply a spatula to the anterior frontal lobe and with pressure abolish speech, which returned when the spatula was removed. Auburtin immediately recognized the clinical implications. Broca further localized speech in an epileptic patient who was aphasic and could only emit the utterance "tan," for which the patient became named. At autopsy, Broca found

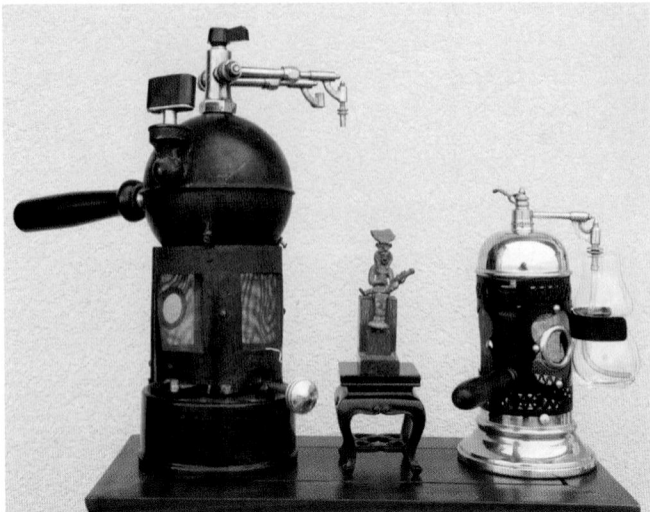

FIGURE 1.38 One of the great nineteenth century advances for surgeons was the introduction of the surgical antisepsis technique. Illustrated here are two early examples of carbolic acid sprayers. The surgeon or his associate would spray the room and the patient prior to the start of the surgery. Despite early promising results it was nearly 25 years before all surgeons adopted the principles of the Listerian antiseptic technique. *(From the author's personal collection.)*

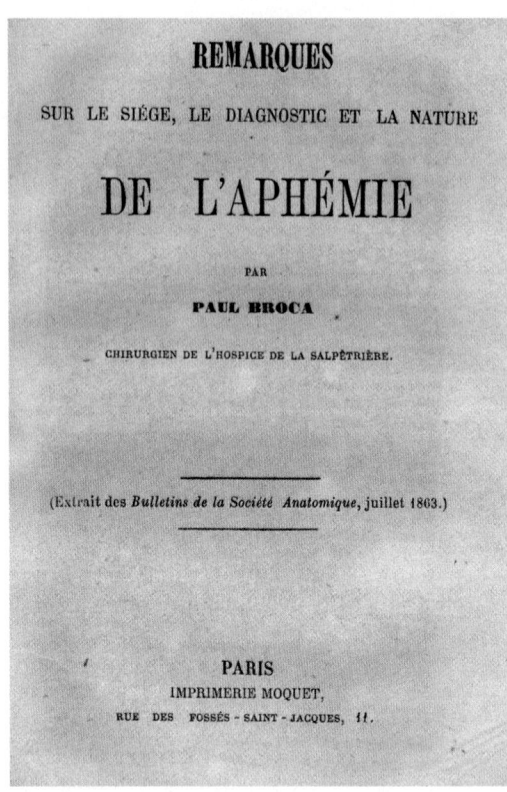

FIGURE 1.40 Paul Broca (1824-1880), a pioneer in cerebral localization studies, presenting here one of his classic studies on aphasia and cerebral localization, in this case a patient with a left inferior frontal lobe injury who developed an expressive aphasia. *(From Broca P. Remarques sur le siège de la faculté du language articulé suivie d'une observation d'aphémie (perte de la parole). Bull Soc Anat Paris 1861;36:330-357.)*

softening of the third left frontal convolution, and from this he postulated the cerebral localization of speech.[83,84] Later, Karl Wernicke (1848-1904) identified a different area of the brain where speech was associated with conduction defects.[85]

These studies led to an explosion of research on the localization of brain function, such as the ablation studies by David Ferrier (1843-1928).[86] John Hughlings Jackson (1835-1911), the founder of modern neurology, demonstrated important areas of function by means of electrical studies and developed the concept of epilepsy.[87] Robert Bartholow (1831-1904), working in Ohio, published a series of three cases of brain tumors in which he correlated the clinical observations with the anatomical findings.[88]

Bartholow later performed an amazing clinical study correlating these types of pathological findings. In 1874 he took under his care a lady named Mary Rafferty who had developed a large cranial defect from infection, which had in turn exposed portions of each cerebral hemisphere. Through these defects he electrically stimulated the brain; unfortunately she subsequently died of meningitis. Bartholow records that "two needles insulated were introduced into left side until their points were well engaged in the dura mater. When the circuit was closed, distinct muscular contractions occurred in the right arm and leg."[89] Bartholow stimulated a number of different areas, carefully recording his observations. These clinical observations supported his postulated functional localizations in the brain. The ethics of his studies would be called into question today!

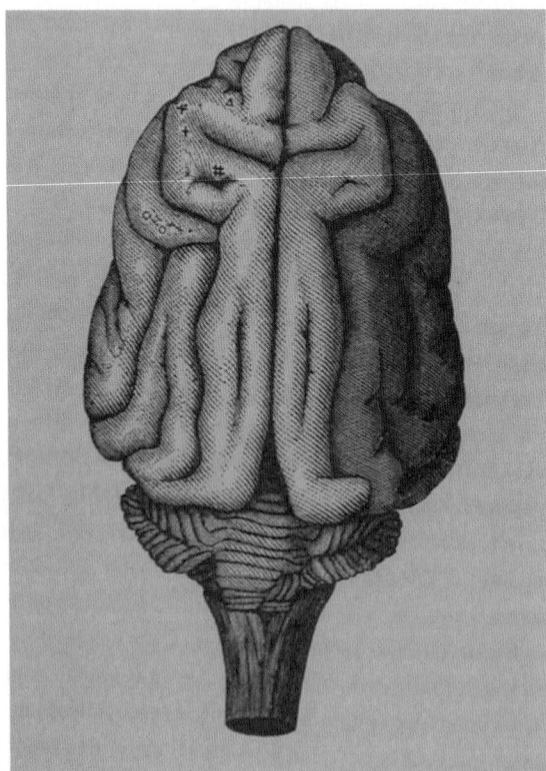

FIGURE 1.39 The 1870s opened the dawn of the concept of cerebral localization. Two German investigators by the name of Fritsch and Hitzig accomplished one of the earliest localization studies using electrical stimulation of the cortex and noting motor movement. This illustration of the exposed cortex of a dog's brain demonstrates the sites of cortical stimulation. *(From Fritsch GT, Hitzig E. Über die elektrische Erregbarkeit des Grosshirns. Arch Anat Physiol Wiss Med 1870:300-332.)*

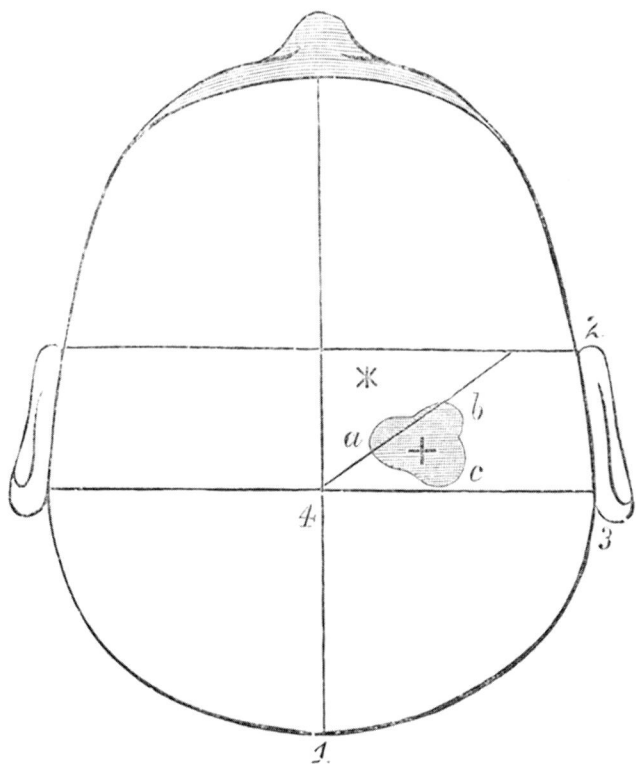

FIGURE 1.41 Illustration from Bennett and Godlee's classic paper of 1884 on an early operation for brain tumor in which a neurologist (Bennett) localized the tumor (seen in this drawing) and a surgeon (Godlee) removed it successfully. *(From Bennett AH, Godlee RJ. Excision of a tumour from the brain. Lancet 1884;2:1090-1091.)*

Advances in Surgical Techniques

Some prominent surgical personalities of the nineteenth century led to some major advances in surgical technology, particularly in neurosurgery. Until the end of the nineteenth century, neurosurgery was not a subspecialty; general surgeons, typically with a large black top hat, bewhiskered, and always pontifical, performed brain surgery!

Sir Rickman Godlee (1859-1925) (Fig. 1.41) removed one of the most celebrated brain tumors, the first to be successfully diagnosed by cerebral localization, in 1884.[90] The patient, a man by the name of Henderson, had suffered for 3 years from focal motor seizures. They started as focal seizures of the face and proceeded to involve the arm and then the leg. In the 3 months prior to surgery the patient also developed weakness and eventually had to give up his work. A neurologist, Alexander Hughes Bennett (1848-1901), basing his conclusions on the findings of a neurological examination, localized a brain tumor and recommended removal to the surgeon. Godlee made an incision over the rolandic area and removed the tumor through a small cortical incision. The patient survived the surgery with some mild weakness and did well, only to die a month later from infection. Bennett, the physician who had made the diagnosis and localization, along with J. Hughlings Jackson and David Ferrier, two prominent British neurologists, observed this landmark operation. All of these physicians were extremely interested in whether the cerebral localization studies would provide necessary results

in the operating theater. The results were good; this operation remains a landmark in the progress of neurosurgery.

Sir William Gowers (1845-1915) was one of an extraordinary group of English neurologists. Using some of the recently developed techniques in physiology and pathology, he made great strides in refining the concept of cerebral localization. Gowers was noted for the clarity and organization of his writing; his neurological writings remain classics.[91-93] These investigative studies allowed surgeons to operate on the brain and spine for other than desperate conditions.

Sir Victor Alexander Haden Horsley (1857-1916) was an English general surgeon who furthered the development of neurosurgery during its embryonic period. Horsley began his experimental studies on the brain in the early 1880s, during the height of the cerebral localization controversies. Horsley worked with Sharpey-Schäfer in using faradic stimulation to analyze and localize motor functions in the cerebral cortex, internal capsule, and spinal cord of primates.[94-96] In a classic study with Gotch, done in 1891, using a string galvanometer, he showed that electrical currents originate in the brain.[97] These experimental studies showed Horsley that cerebral localization was possible and that operations on the brain could be conducted safely using techniques adapted from general surgery. In 1887, working with William Gowers, Horsley performed a laminectomy on Gowers' patient, Captain Golby, a 45-year-old army officer. Golby was slowly losing function in his legs from a spinal cord tumor. Gowers localized the tumor by examination and indicated to Horsley where to operate; the tumor, a benign "fibromyxoma" of the fourth thoracic root, was successfully removed.[98]

Horsley made a number of technical contributions to neurosurgery, including the use of beeswax to stop bone bleeding. He performed one of the earliest craniectomies for craniostenosis and relief of increased intracranial pressure. For patients with inoperable tumors he developed the decompressive craniectomy. For treatment of trigeminal neuralgia Horsley advocated sectioning the posterior root of the trigeminal nerve for facial pain relief. Using his technical gifts he helped Clarke design the first useful stereotactic unit for brain surgery (Fig. 1.42). Although never used in human surgery, the Horsley-Clarke stereotactic frame inspired all subsequent designs.[99]

Sir Charles A. Ballance (1856-1936) was an English surgeon who received his medical education at University College, London. Ballance was an early pioneer in neurosurgery, performing the first mastoidectomy with ligation of the jugular vein. Ballance was one of the first to graft and repair the facial nerve. In his monograph on brain surgery Ballance sets forth many ideas that were quite modern.[100] The book came from a series of Lettsomian Lectures given in 1906 in which are contained a series of three lectures on cerebral membranes, tumors, and abscesses. Ballance's treatise recognized and described chronic subdural hematoma with great accuracy and detailed an operative success. Additional successful operations included one for subdural hygroma. Ballance routinely used the recently introduced lumbar puncture for cases of head injury and suppurative meningitis. An interesting and apparent cure of congenital hydrocephalus was recorded by Ballance using a technique that included ligation of both common carotid arteries. In his treatment of brain abscesses Ballance urged evacuation of the abscess with drainage recommended; in some cases he felt that complete enucleation of an abscess was advisable. Ballance devoted 243 pages of his monograph to a discussion of brain tumors and noted a wide operative experience with 400 such lesions. One of his most important cases, and one only recently recognized in the literature, involved a patient who was reported well in 1906 from whom he removed "a fibrosarcoma from the right cerebellar fossa" (i.e., an acoustic neuroma) in 1894; this would appear to be one of the earliest surgeries for an angle tumor[100,101] (Fig. 1.43). In a profound comment on surgical operations for tumors Ballance had a hopeful outlook: "... I am convinced that the dawn of a happier day for these terrible cases has come."

William Macewen (1848-1924), a Scottish surgeon, successfully accomplished a brain operation for tumor on July 29, 1879 (Fig. 1.44). Using meticulous technique and the

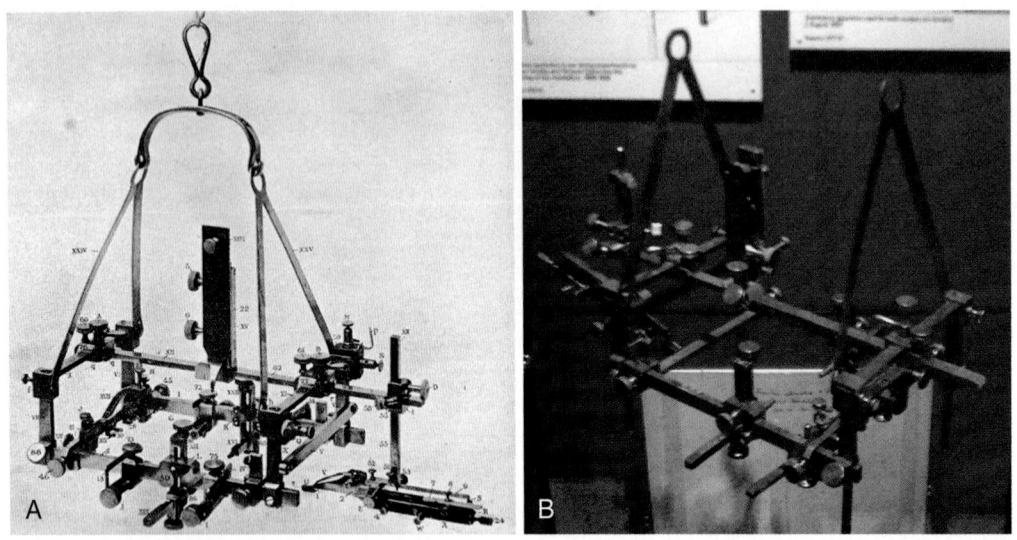

FIGURE 1.42 A, The Horsley-Clarke stereotactic frame was designed for animal studies but never used on humans; nevertheless, it became the precursor for the modern human stereotactic frame. **B,** An original Horsley-Clarke stereotactic frame on display at the Science Museum, London, England. Very few of these original frames now exist. (**A,** *from the author's personal collection;* **B,** *photograph taken by the author October 13, 2009. From Horsley VAH , Clarke RH. The structure and functions of the cerebellum examined by a new method. Brain. 1908;31:45-124.)*

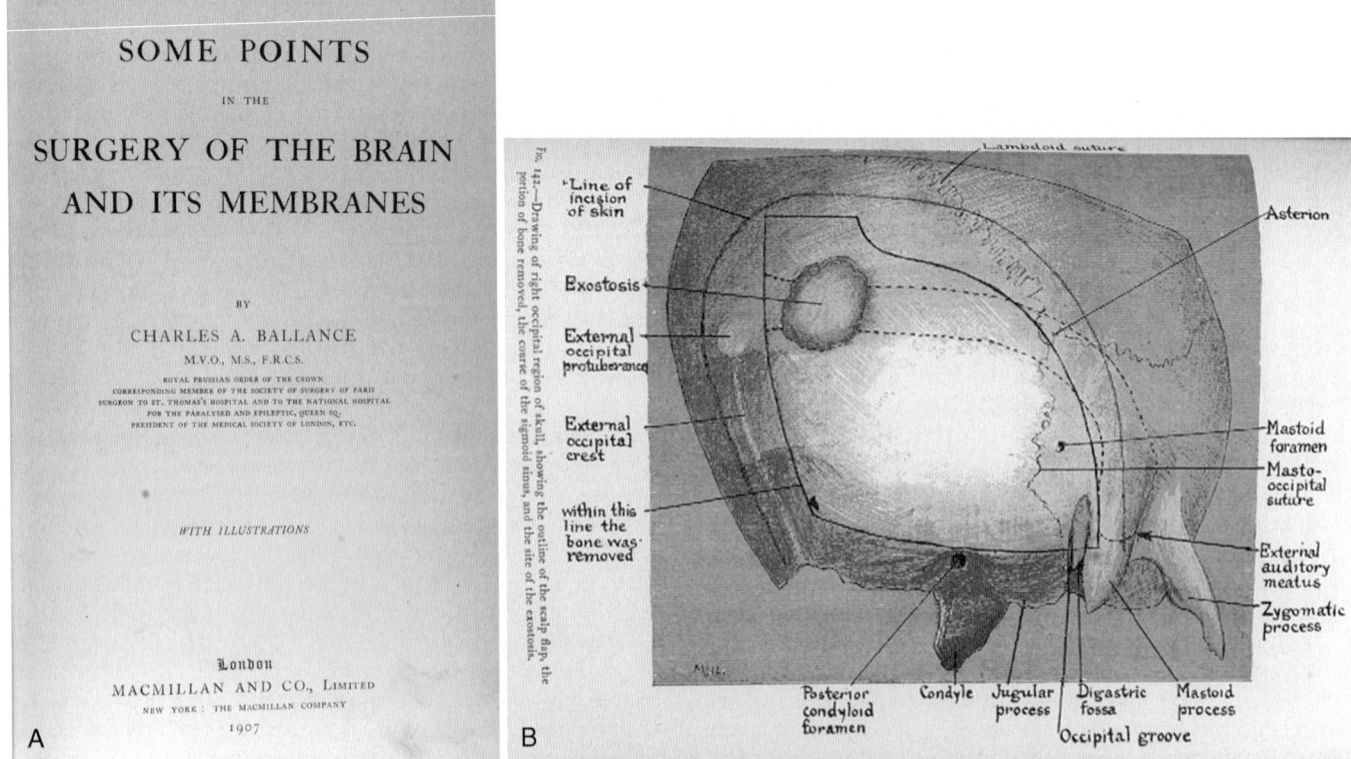

FIGURE 1.43 A, Title page from Ballance's nineteenth century monograph on brain surgery. **B,** An anatomical diagram outlining the anatomy of Ballance's posterior fossa approach for what is thought to be the first successful removal of an acoustic neuroma. *(From Ballance CA. Some Points in the Surgery of the Brain and Its Membranes. London: Macmillan; 1907.)*

recently developed neurological examination, he localized and removed a periosteal tumor from over the right eye of a 14-year-old. The patient went on to live for 8 more years, only to die of Bright's disease; at autopsy no tumor was detected. By 1888, Macewen had operated on 21 neurosurgical cases with only three deaths and 18 successful recoveries, a remarkable change from earlier series. Macewen considered his success to be the result of excellent cerebral localization and good aseptic techniques. Macewen's monograph on pyogenic infections of the brain and their surgical treatment, published in 1893,[102] was the earliest to deal with the successful treatment of brain abscess. His morbidity and mortality statistics are as good as those in any series reported today.

Joseph Pancoast (1805-1882) produced one of the most remarkable nineteenth century American monographs on surgery in the era just before the introduction of antisepsis and anesthesia[103] (Fig. 1.45). Pancoast spent his academic career in Philadelphia, Pennsylvania, where he was physician and visiting surgeon to the Philadelphia Hospital. He later became professor of surgery and anatomy at Jefferson's Medical College in 1838. Pancoast's *Treatise* has 80 quarto plates comprising 486 lithographs with striking surgical details. These plates remain some of the most well-executed and graphical illustrations of different surgical techniques. The lithographs are exceedingly graphic, so much so that religious purists often removed numbers 69 and 70 because of their depiction of the female genitalia. The section on head injury and trauma clearly demonstrates the techniques of trephination and the elevation of depressed fractures. Pancoast was one of the first to devise an operation for transecting the fifth cranial nerve for trigeminal neuralgia.

Fedor Krause (1857-1937) was a general surgeon whose keen interest in neurosurgery made him the father of German neurosurgery. His three-volume atlas on neurosurgery, *Surgery of the Brain and Spinal Cord*, published in 1909-1912, was one of the first to detail the techniques of modern neurosurgery; it has since been through some 60 editions[104] (Fig. 1.46). Krause, like William Macewen, was a major proponent of aseptic technique in neurosurgery. His atlas describes a number of interesting techniques. The "digital" extirpation of a meningioma is graphically illustrated. A number of original neurosurgical techniques are reviewed, including resection of scar tissue for treatment of epilepsy. Krause was a pioneer in the extradural approach to the gasserian ganglion for treatment of trigeminal neuralgia. He pioneered the transfrontal craniotomy in addition to transection of the eighth cranial nerve for severe tinnitus. To deal with tumors of the pineal region and posterior third ventricle he pioneered the supracerebellar-infratentorial approach. Krause was the first to suggest that tumors of the cerebellopontine angle (e.g., acoustic neuromas) could be operated on safely. Interestingly, Krause retired to Rome, where he gave up neurosurgery and continued his greatest love, playing the piano. When asked what he would most like to be remembered for, it was not as a neurosurgeon but rather as a classical pianist.

Antony (Antoine) Chipault (1866-1920) has remained an obscure historical figure in neurosurgery yet nevertheless he was one of the pioneers and was once considered the potential father of French neurosurgery. Chipault was named at

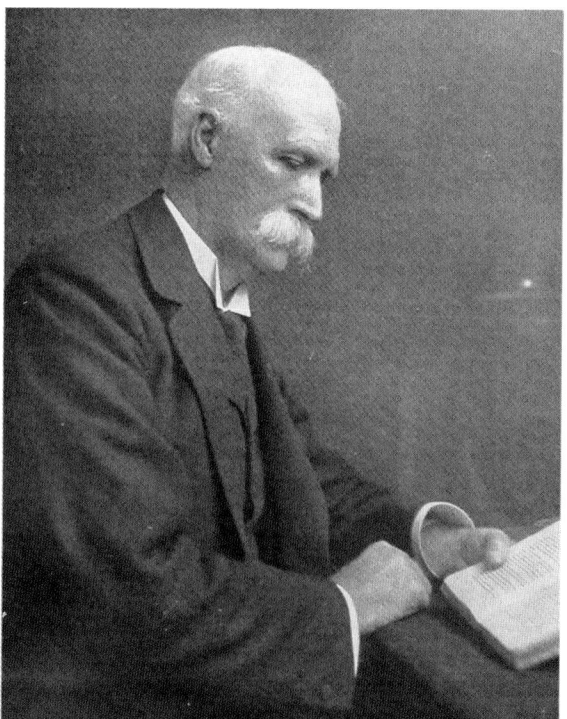

FIGURE 1.44 William Macewen (1848-1924), a pioneering Scottish surgeon who specialized in brain surgery starting in the 1880s.

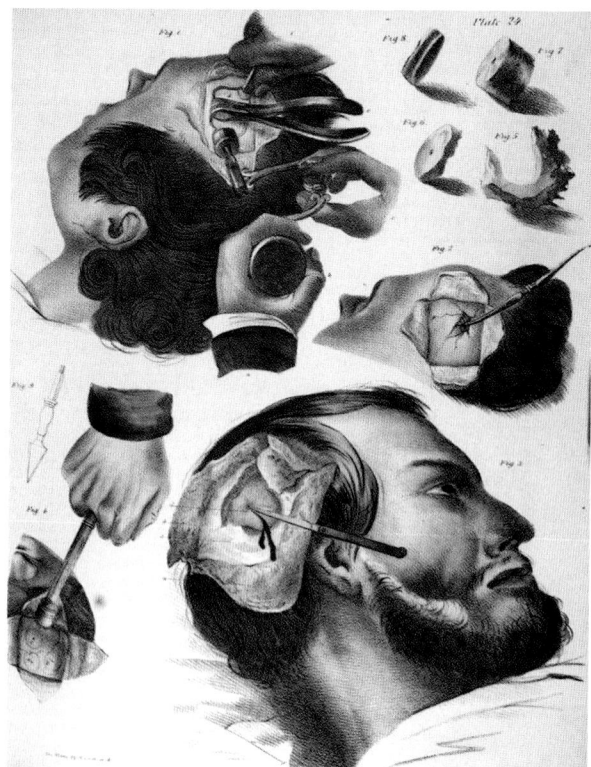

FIGURE 1.45 In the preantisepsis Listerian period we find Joseph Pancoast, with ungloved hands and street dress, performing a craniectomy for a depressed skull fracture. *(From Pancoast J. A Treatise on Operative Surgery; Comprising a Description of the Various Processes of the Art, Including all the New Operations; Exhibiting the State of Surgical Science in its Present Advanced Condition. Philadelphia: Carey and Hart; 1844.)*

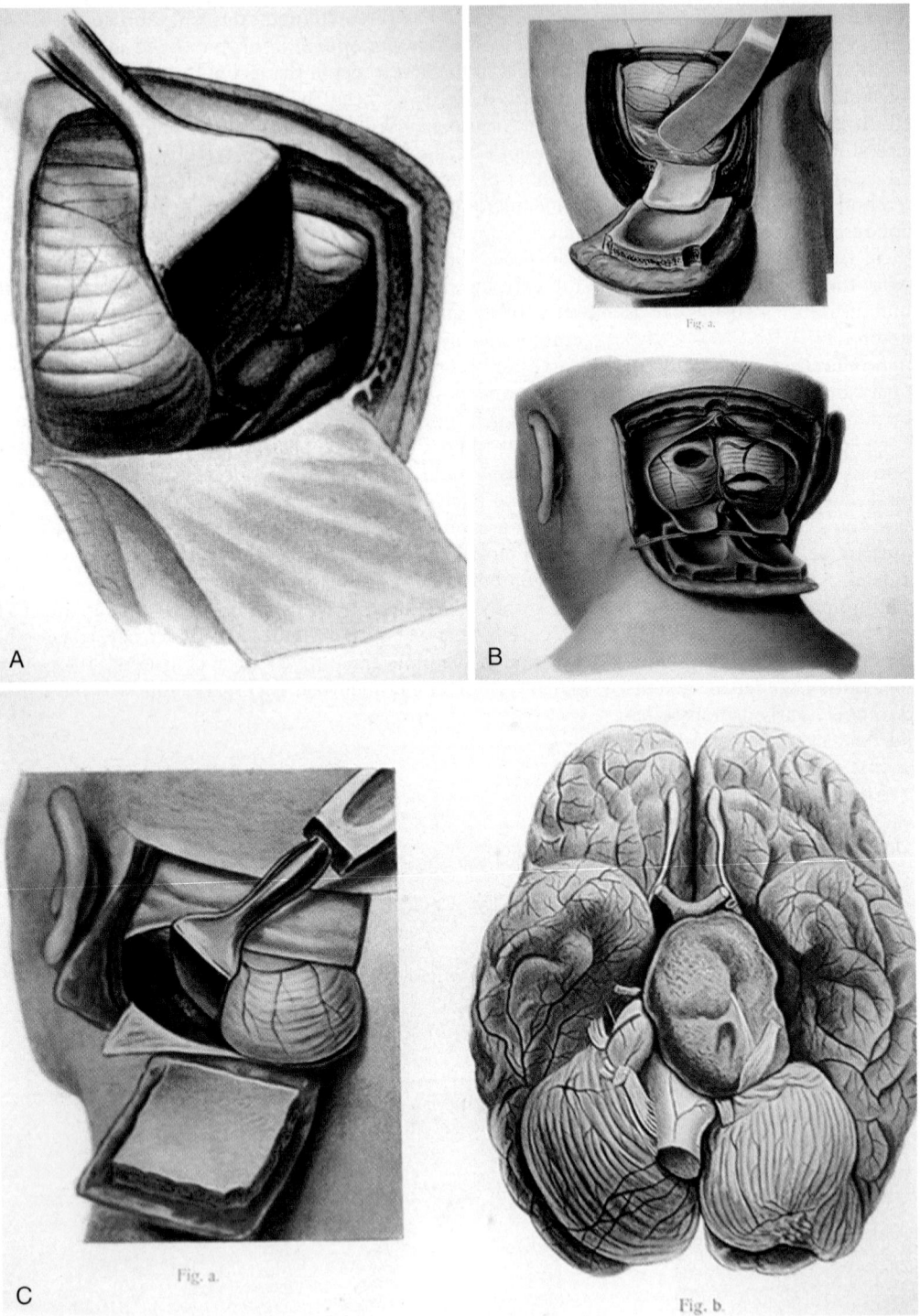

FIGURE 1.46 A, By the beginning of the twentieth century we find several talented general surgeons doing neurosurgery. Illustrated here is Fedor Krause's exposure for a cerebellopontine exposure. **B,** Krause's technique for an osteoplastic flap in a posterior fossa craniotomy. **C,** Krause illustrating his approach for a cerebellopontine tumor. The image on the right clearly outlines the anatomy of an acoustic neuroma and its relationship to the facial nerve. *(From Krause F, Haubold H, Thorek M, translators. Surgery of the Brain and Spinal Cord Based on Personal Experiences. New York: Rebman Co.; 1909-1912.)*

birth Antonie Maxime Nicolas Chipault on July 16, 1866, in the town of Orleans, France. His father was a surgeon and he began his medical studies in Paris at the age of 18. He initially qualified as a gynecologist but later became interested in neurology. He became initially interested in the anatomy of the spine and published a now rare seminal monograph *Etudes de Chirurgie Médullaires.*[105] In 1891 he began working with Professor Duplay at the Hotel Dieu under whom he became interested in craniocerebral pathology. In 1894 he published his classic work on surgery of the spine and spinal cord. Chipault published a series of papers on the brain and spinal cord including writings on Pott's disease, osteoplastic craniotomy, spinal trauma, posterior root section for pain, and surgical treatment of brain tumors and hemorrhage, among other subjects. He made a number of technical innovations in neurosurgery, including introducing the removal of the underlying dura in meningiomas, a new laminectomy technique, plus development of small clamps for closing a scalp incision. He treated hydrocephalus by tapping the ventricles through a burr hole, and proposed a

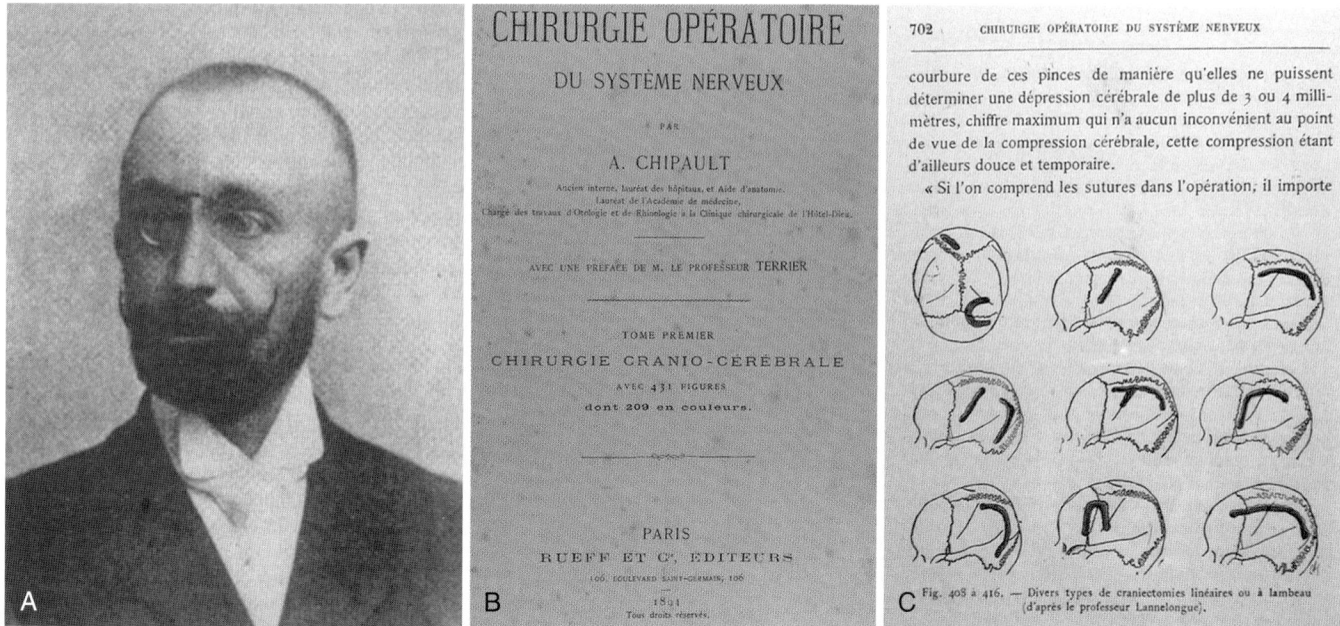

FIGURE 1.47 A, Antoine Chipault, one of France's pioneers in neurosurgery. **B,** Title page from Chipault's monograph on surgery of the nervous system. **C,** Chipault's schema of craniectomies for treating craniosynostosis. *(From Chipault A. Chirurgie Opératoire du Systéme Nerveus. Paris: Rueff et Cie; 1894-1895.)*

scheme of craniectomies for treatment of craniosynostosis (Fig. 1.47). He pioneered the use of wires and steel splints in the stabilization of the spine in trauma and deformities. In 1894 his surgical masterpiece appeared *Chirurgie Opératoire du Systéme Nerveux*, an extremely popular work that was translated into English, Spanish, Italian, German, Romanian, and Serbo-Croatian.[106] He also introduced one of the first journals devoted to surgery of the spine and brain—*Les Travaux de Neurologie Chirurgicale*. Despite this illustrious career he dropped out of sight in 1905 ceasing all writing and works in neurosurgery. The cause is thought to be the onset of paraplegia, the etiology of which remains unknown. Chipault moved with his family to the Jura mountains near Orchamps. He died in 1920 at the age of 54 in total obscurity, a state in which he remains.

William W. Keen (1837-1932), professor of surgery at Jefferson Medical College in Philadelphia, was one of the strongest American advocates for the use of listerian antiseptic techniques in surgery. A description of Keen's surgical setup provides a contemporary view of this innovative surgeon's approach to antisepsis:

All carpets and unnecessary furniture were removed from the patient's room. The walls and ceiling were carefully cleaned the day before operation, and the woodwork, floors, and remaining furniture were scrubbed with carbolic solution. This solution was also sprayed in the room on the morning preceding but not during the operation. On the day before operation, the patient's head was shaved, scrubbed with soap, water, and ether, and covered with a wet corrosive sublimate dressing until the operation, then ether and mercuric chloride washings were repeated. The surgical instruments were boiled in water for 2 hours, and new deep-sea sponges (elephant ears) were treated with carbolic and sublimate solutions before usage. The surgeon's hands were cleaned and disinfected using soap and water, alcohol, and sublimate solution (pp. 1001-1002).[107]

One of the earliest American monographs on neurosurgery, *Linear Craniotomy*, was prepared by Keen.[108] He described the difficult differentiation between microcephalus and craniosynostosis. He then performed, in 1890, one of the first operations for craniostenosis in America. He developed a technique for treatment of spastic torticollis by division of the spinal accessory nerve and the posterior roots of the first, second, and third spinal nerves.[109] He was also responsible for introducing the Gigli saw, first described in Europe in 1897, into American surgery in 1898.[110,111]

The first American monograph devoted to brain surgery was written not by a neurosurgeon but by the New York neurologist Allen Starr (1854-1932) (Fig. 1.48).[112,113] Starr was Professor of Nervous Diseases at Columbia University and an American leader in neurology. He trained in Europe, working in the laboratories of Erb, Schultze, Meynert, and Nothnagle, experiences that gave him a strong foundation in neurological diagnosis. Working closely with Charles McBurney (1845-1913), a general surgeon, he came to the realization that brain surgery not only could be done safely but was necessary in the treatment of certain neurological problems (Fig. 1.49).[114] He summarized his views in the preface:

Brain surgery is at present a subject both novel and interesting. It is within the past five years only that operations for the relief of epilepsy and of imbecility, for the removal of clots from the brain, for the opening of abscesses, for the excision of tumors, and the relief of intra-cranial pressure have been generally attempted ... It is the object of this book to state clearly those facts regarding the essential features of brain disease which will enable the reader to determine in any case both the nature and situation of the pathological process in progress, to settle the question whether the disease can be removed by surgical interference, and to estimate the safety and probability of success by operation.[112]

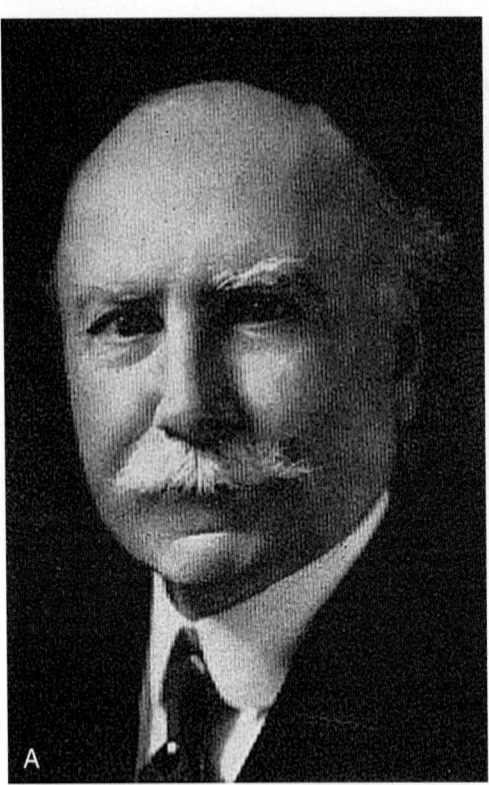

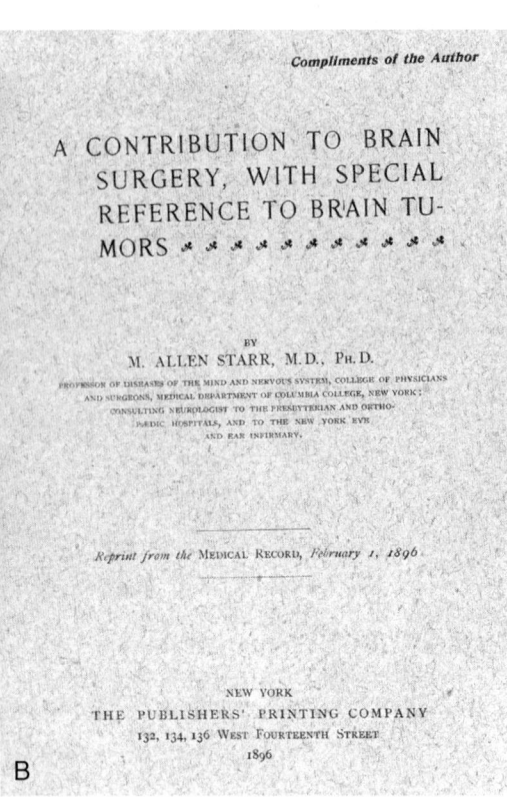

Compliments of the Author

A CONTRIBUTION TO BRAIN SURGERY, WITH SPECIAL REFERENCE TO BRAIN TUMORS

BY
M. ALLEN STARR, M.D., Ph.D.
PROFESSOR OF DISEASES OF THE MIND AND NERVOUS SYSTEM, COLLEGE OF PHYSICIANS
AND SURGEONS, MEDICAL DEPARTMENT OF COLUMBIA COLLEGE, NEW YORK;
CONSULTING NEUROLOGIST TO THE PRESBYTERIAN AND ORTHO-
PÆDIC HOSPITALS, AND TO THE NEW YORK EYE
AND EAR INFIRMARY.

Reprint from the MEDICAL RECORD, *February 1, 1896.*

NEW YORK
THE PUBLISHERS' PRINTING COMPANY
132, 134, 136 WEST FOURTEENTH STREET
1896

FIGURE 1.48 A, Allen Starr (1854-1932), a prominent New York City neurologist who wrote one of the first American monographs devoted to surgery of the brain. **B,** In one of Allen Starr's early papers he advocated that cranial surgery could be done and done safely for brain tumors. *(From Starr MA. Discussion on the present status of the surgery of the brain, 2: a contribution to brain surgery, with special reference to brain tumors. Trans Med Soc NY 1896;119-134.)*

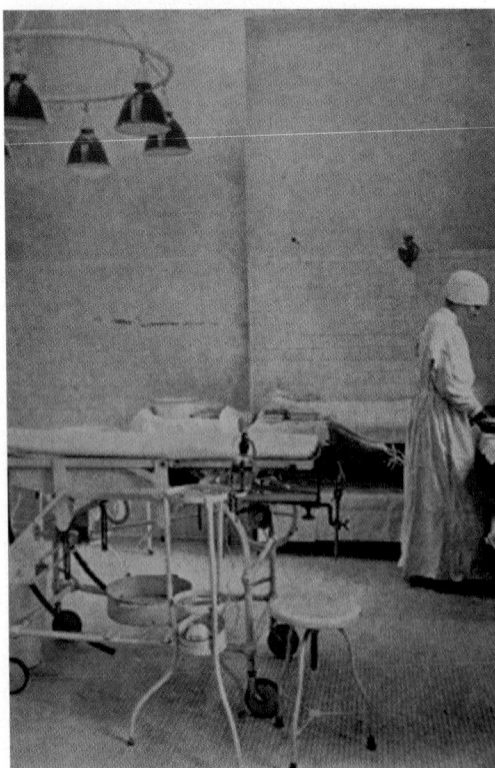

FIGURE 1.49 An aged early albumin print showing the operating room at the New York Neurological Institute, circa 1910. The New York Neurological Institute was the first institute in the United States devoted solely to both neurological and neurosurgical treatment. This early operating room is clearly far sparser in technical equipment than the "modern" operating room of the twenty-first century.

In 1923 Harvey Cushing, reviewing one of his own cases, commented about Allen Starr:

> I am confident that if Allen Starr, in view of his position in neurology and his interest in surgical matters, had taken to the scalpel rather than the pen we would now be thirty years ahead in these matters, and I am sure his fingers must many times have itched when he stood alongside an operating table and saw the operator he was coaching hopelessly fumble with the brain.[115]

Harvey William Cushing (1869-1939) is considered the father of American neurosurgery (see Fig. 1.49). Educated at Johns Hopkins under one of the premier general surgeons, William Halsted (1852-1922), Cushing learned meticulous surgical technique from his mentor. As was standard then, Cushing spent time in Europe; he worked in the laboratories of Theodore Kocher in Bern, investigating the physiology of CSF. These studies led to his important monograph in 1926 on the third circulation.[116] It was during this period of experimentation that the cerebral phenomenon of increased intracranial pressure in association with hypertension and bradycardia was defined; it is now called the "Cushing phenomenon." While traveling through Europe he met several important surgical personalities involved in neurosurgery, including Macewen and Horsley. They provided the impetus for him to consider neurosurgery as a full-time endeavor (Fig. 1.50).

Cushing's contributions to the literature of neurosurgery are too extensive to be listed in this brief chapter. Among his most significant work is a monograph on pituitary surgery published in 1912.[117] This monograph inaugurated a prolific career in pituitary studies. Cushing syndrome was defined in his final monograph on the pituitary published in 1932.[118] In a classic monograph, written with Percival Bailey in 1926, Cushing brought a rational approach to the classification of

FIGURE 1.50 A, Harvey Cushing as a dapper young man in training at the Johns Hopkins University, circa 1900. This image comes from an album put together for the Johns Hopkins University faculty that was never published. **B,** Harvey Cushing was one of the early pioneers in the transsphenoidal approach to the pituitary and sella regions. It was rumored that Cushing used the hot headlight to effectively keep annoying or nonattentive residents out of the field. (From the author's personal collection.)

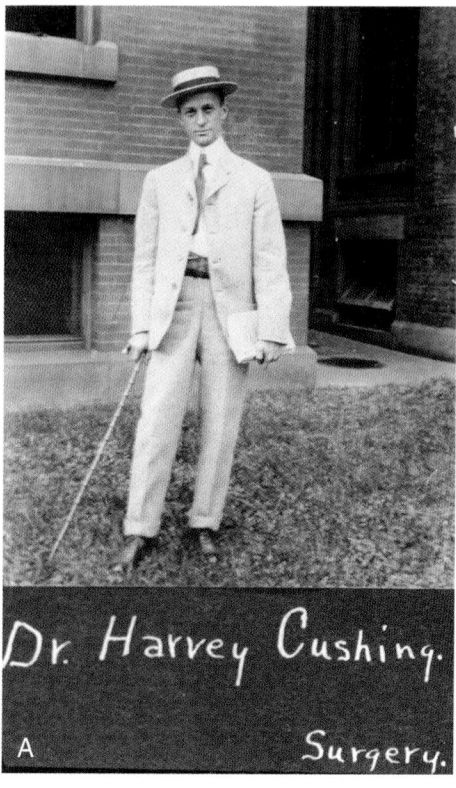

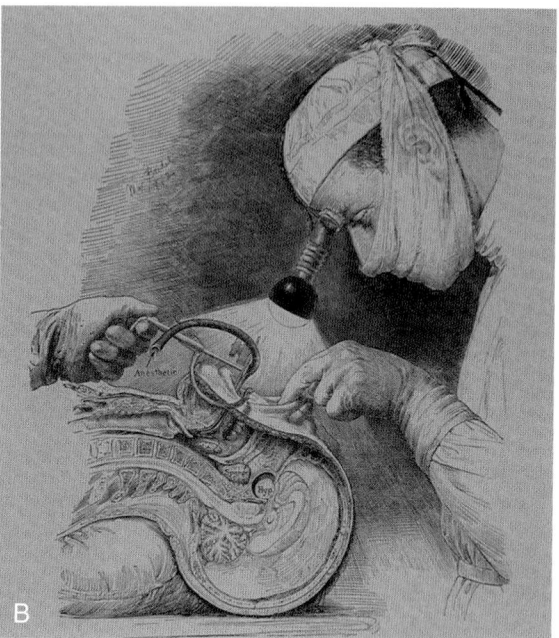

brain tumors.[119] His monograph on meningiomas, written with Louise Eisenhardt in 1938, remains a classic.[120]

Cushing retired as Moseley Professor of Surgery at Harvard in 1932. By the time he completed his 2000th brain tumor operation,[121] he had unquestionably made some preeminent contributions to neurosurgery, based on meticulous, innovative surgical techniques and the effort to understand brain function from both physiological and pathological perspectives. An ardent bibliophile, Cushing spent his final years in retirement as Stirling Professor of Neurology at Yale, where he put together his extraordinary monograph on the writings of Andreas Vesalius.[122] Cushing's life has been faithfully recorded by his close friend and colleague John F. Fulton.[123]

Walter Dandy (1886-1946), who trained under Cushing at Johns Hopkins, made a number of important contributions to neurosurgery. Based on Luckett's serendipitous finding of air in the ventricles after a skull fracture,[124] Dandy developed the technique of pneumoencephalography (Fig. 1.51).[125-127] This technique provided the neurosurgeon with the opportunity to localize the tumor by analyzing the displacement of air in the ventricles.[127] A Philadelphia neurosurgeon, Charles Frazier, commented in 1935 on the importance of pneumoencephalography and the difference it made in the practice of neurosurgery:

Only too often, after the most careful evaluation of the available neurologic evidence, no tumor would be revealed by exploration, the extreme intracranial tension would result in cerebral herniation to such an extent that sacrifice of the bone flap became necessary, and subsequently the skin sutures would give way before the persistent pressure, with cerebral fungus and meningitis as inevitable consequences. But injection of air has done away with all these horrors. The neurologist has been forced to recognize its important place in correct intracranial localization and frequently demands its use by the neurosurgeon.[128]

Dandy was an innovative neurosurgeon, far more aggressive in style and technique than Cushing. He was the first to show that acoustic neuromas could be totally removed.[129,130] He devoted a great deal of effort to the treatment of hydrocephalus.[131-133] He introduced the endoscopic technique of removing the choroid plexus to reduce the production of CSF.[134] He was among the first to treat cerebral aneurysms by obliterating them using snare ligatures or metal clips.[135] His monograph on the third ventricle and its anatomy remains a standard to this day, with anatomical illustrations that are among the best ever produced.[136]

In the field of spinal surgery, two important American figures appeared in the first quarter of the twentieth century: Charles Elsberg (1871-1948), Professor of Neurosurgery at the New York Neurological Institute, and Charles Frazier (1870-1936), Professor of Surgery at the University of Pennsylvania. Toward the end of the nineteenth century studies on the spine had been initiated by J. L. Corning, who had shown that lumbar puncture could be performed safely for diagnosis.[137] H. Quincke went on to popularize this procedure; these early studies encouraged the development of spinal surgery.[138,139]

From a surgical experience developed during World War I Charles Frazier decided on a career in neurosurgery. Charles Frazier's 1918 textbook on spinal surgery was the most comprehensive work on the subject available[140]; he summarized much of the existing literature and established that spinal surgery could be performed safely.

From New York City came Charles Elsberg, another pioneer in spinal surgery. Elsberg's techniques were impeccable and led to excellent results. By 1912 he had reported on a series of 43 laminectomies and by 1916 he had published the first of what were to be three monographs on surgery of the

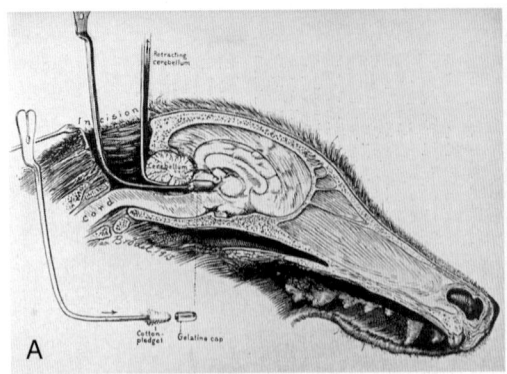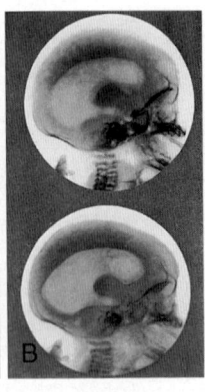

FIGURE 1.51 **A,** One of Walter Dandy's greatest contributions to neurosurgery was his work on experimental hydrocephalus. In this drawing he shows his experimental model for developing hydrocephalus in the dog model. **B,** These x-ray studies for showing brain lesions were produced in Walter Dandy's classic studies on ventriculography. A technique whereby cerebrospinal fluid was removed and replaced with air, thereby outlining the ventricles on x-ray. *(From Dandy WE. Experimental hydrocephalus. Trans Am Surgical Assoc 1919;37:397-428; Dandy WE. Ventriculography following the injection of air into the cerebral ventricles. Ann Surg 1918;68:5-11.)*

spine.[141,142] In the treatment of intramedullary spinal tumors Elsberg introduced the technique of a first-stage myelotomy. By waiting some time afterward, this allowed the intramedullary tumor to deliver itself, so then, at a second-stage procedure, the tumor was resected[143] (Fig. 1.52). He worked with a fierce intensity and was always looking for new techniques. Working with Cornelius Dyke, a neuroradiologist at the New York Neurological Institute, he treated spinal glioblastomas with directed radiation in the operating room after the tumor had been exposed! These procedures were performed with the patients receiving only local anesthesia. During the half-hour therapy, while the radiation was being delivered, the surgeon and assistants stood off in the distance behind a glass shield.[144]

Leo Davidoff (1898-1975) was one of the prodigies of twentieth century neurosurgery (Fig. 1.53). Starting from humble origins in Lithuania, the son of a cobbler, he immigrated to the United States with his eight siblings. As a teen Davidoff worked in a factory to support his family; the factory's manager admired his skill and dedication and sponsored his education, leading to his graduation from Harvard University in 1916. He completed his medical degree at Harvard in 1922 as an AOA (the national honor society for graduating medical students) member. Davidoff trained under Harvey Cushing and became one of his most popular students, not always an easy achievement with Cushing's personality. When Cushing was once asked who he would allow to operate on him for a brain tumor his response was "Well I guess I would have Davey [Davidoff] do it." Davidoff initially joined the staff of the New York Neurological Institute with Charles Elsberg in 1929. Here he began his seminal studies on the normal anatomy seen in pneumoencephalograms utilizing the hundreds of pneumoencephalograms performed at the Neurological Institute. In 1937 he issued a classic monograph with Cornelius Dyke (1900-1943), *The Normal Encephalogram*.[145] This work, and a later publication with Bernard Epstein (1908-1978), *The Abnormal Encephalogram* (1950),[146] became two of the most important neuroradiological texts, remaining influential for over 30 years. Davidoff's meticulous and detailed studies led him to be called the father of neuroradiology. He left the Neurological Institute in 1937 when Bryon Stookey became chief, moving on to Brooklyn to the Jewish Hospital. Davidoff became chief of neurosurgery at Montefiore Hospital in 1945, working with two contemporary giants, Houston Merritt in neurology and Harry Zimmerman in neuropathology. Davidoff later became instrumental in the founding of the Albert Einstein College

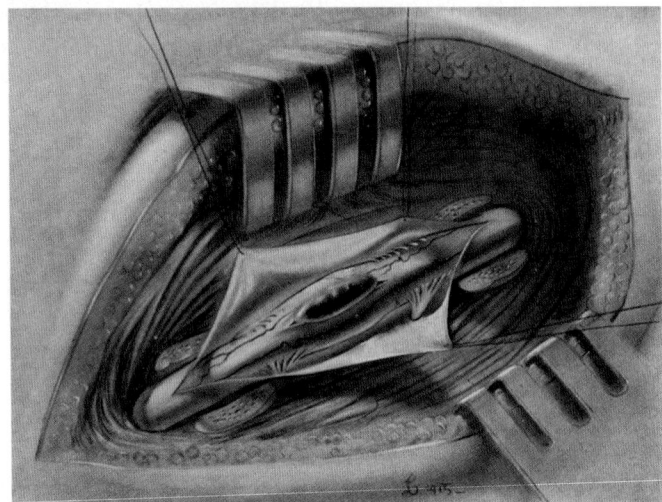

FIGURE 1.52 Elsberg's two-stage procedure for removing an intramedullary spinal tumor. Elsberg's technique involved a laminectomy and then a myelotomy over the tumor. The pressure of the tumor causes its extrusion; then in a later second operation the surgeon removes the "extruded" tumor safely. *(From Elsberg CA. Tumors of the Spinal Cord. New York: Hoeber; 1925:381.)*

of Medicine, becoming the first chairman of neurosurgery in 1955. Davidoff was a charter member of the Harvey Cushing Society and served as president of the American Association of Neurological Surgeons from 1956 to 1957. Davidoff was described by his staff as a hard taskmaster, punctual, demanding, and critical. His operating room was meticulous and organized, with no unnecessary sound or speech allowed. Never one to raise his voice, a mere look, even behind a surgical mask, could be a chilling experience for the new house officer or scrub nurse. His legacy remains in over 200 scientific publications, his pioneering work in neuroradiology, and his total commitment to the highest standards in patient care and resident training.

Besides the pioneering techniques of Dandy, Cushing, and others, a number of diagnostic techniques were introduced whereby the neurosurgeon could localize lesions less haphazardly, thereby shifting the emphasis from the neurologist to the neurosurgeon. One such technique, myelography using opaque substances, was brought forward by Jean Athanase Sicard (1872-1929).[147] With the use of a radiopaque iodized oil, the spinal cord and its elements could be outlined on

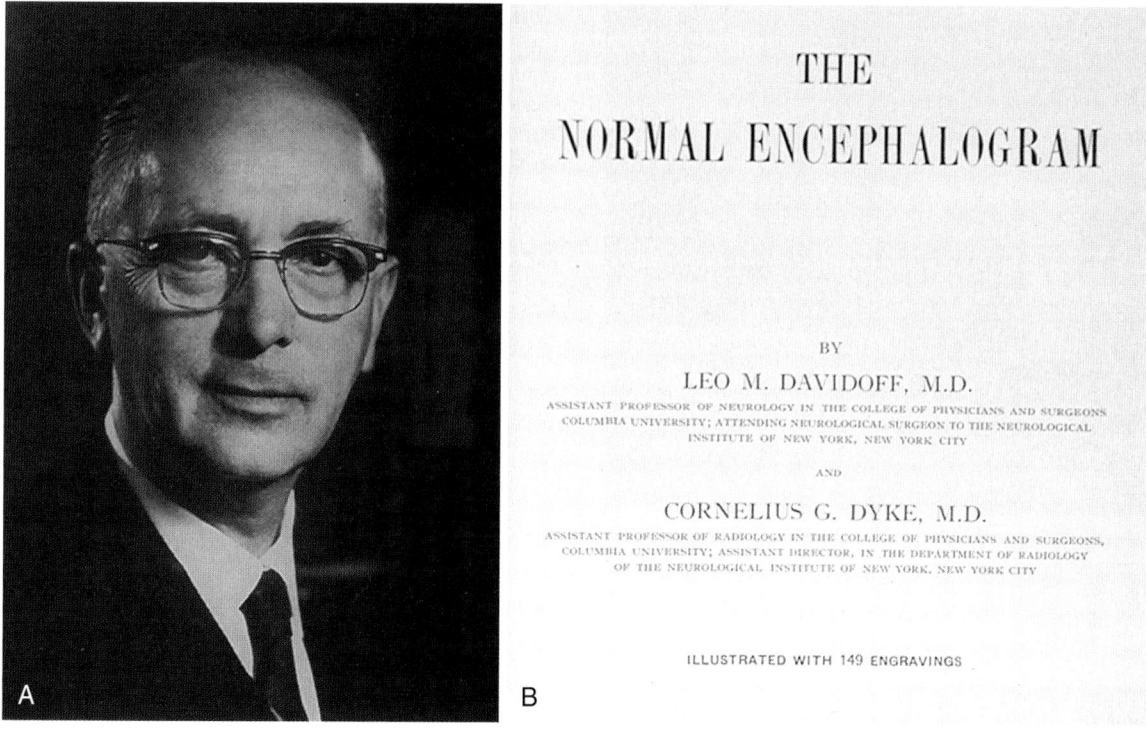

THE

NORMAL ENCEPHALOGRAM

BY

LEO M. DAVIDOFF, M.D.

ASSISTANT PROFESSOR OF NEUROLOGY IN THE COLLEGE OF PHYSICIANS AND SURGEONS
COLUMBIA UNIVERSITY; ATTENDING NEUROLOGICAL SURGEON TO THE NEUROLOGICAL
INSTITUTE OF NEW YORK, NEW YORK CITY

AND

CORNELIUS G. DYKE, M.D.

ASSISTANT PROFESSOR OF RADIOLOGY IN THE COLLEGE OF PHYSICIANS AND SURGEONS,
COLUMBIA UNIVERSITY; ASSISTANT DIRECTOR, IN THE DEPARTMENT OF RADIOLOGY
OF THE NEUROLOGICAL INSTITUTE OF NEW YORK, NEW YORK CITY

ILLUSTRATED WITH 149 ENGRAVINGS

FIGURE 1.53 A, Leo Davidoff trained with Harvey Cushing and later became the first chairman of neurosurgery at the Albert Einstein College of Medicine, New York. **B,** Title page from Davidoff's monograph on the normal encephalogram, a seminal work that followed up on Dandy's early work on the ventriculogram. *(From Davidoff L, Dyke C. The Normal Pneumoencephalogram. Philadelphia: Lea & Febiger; 1937.)*

x-ray. Antonio Caetano de Egas Moniz (1874-1955), Professor of Neurology at Lisbon, perfected arterial catheterization techniques and the cerebral angiogram in animal studies. This work required that a number of iodine compounds be studied, many of which caused convulsions and paralysis in laboratory animals. However, his ideas were sound and by 1927 angiography, used in combination with pneumoencephalography, offered the neurosurgeon the first detailed view of the intracranial contents.[148,149] Ironically Moniz was later awarded the Nobel Prize in medicine in 1949 for his work in psychosurgery and not for his work in cerebral angiography.

In 1929, Alexander Fleming (1881-1955) published a report on the first observation of a substance that appeared to block the growth of a bacterium. This substance, identified as penicillin, heralded a new era of medicine and surgery.[150] With World War II, antibiotics were perfected in the treatment of bacterial infection, reducing even further the risk of infection during craniotomy.

One area of neurosurgery in which developments in the twentieth century clearly outlined the disease, the pathology, and surgical treatment was in hydrocephalus. Walter Dandy and his team researched the etiology of the disorder and in the 1952 Nulsen and Spitz developed a unidirectional valve for the treatment of hydrocephalus. Key to the design was the prevention of reflux and maintaining a unidirectional flow. John Holter (1956) took advantage of the recently introduced silicone rubber to design a valve and a tube system to take CSF from the brain to the heart; in the 1960s literally thousands of these systems were placed. The technology has continued to improve with better valve designs, better implantable materials, and lower morbidity rate for our patients.

A defining moment in operative neurosurgery came with the Nobel Prize–winning work of an engineer by the name of Sir Godfrey Newbold Hounsfield and his design of the computer-assisted tomography (CAT).[151] For the first time a neurosurgeon was able to visualize intracranial pathology by a noninvasive technique. The original images were poor quality grainy images on Polaroid film, whereas in a mere 40 some years the neurosurgeon now has elegant, high-resolution three-dimensional images with multimodality grids being easily obtained. This pioneer work led to an engineer (not a physician) receiving the first Nobel Prize in medicine in 1979, only 6 years after the publication of his seminal paper in 1973 (Fig. 1.54).

CONCLUSION

The first half of the twentieth century brought the formalization of the field of neurosurgery. In the 1920s, Elsberg, Cushing, and Frazier persuaded the American College of Surgeons to designate neurosurgery as a separate specialty. It has taken some 5000 years of constant study and the experience of generations to make neurosurgery what it is today (Fig. 1.55).

In just under 160 years the patient entering a neurosurgical operating room can have a painless operation with minimal risk of infection, and surgery will rarely be in the wrong location. Thanks to magnetic resonance imaging and computed tomography, the localization of neurological problems is hardly an issue. Intraoperative computerized localization of brain pathology is rapidly becoming the standard throughout the world. Some provocative forward thinkers feel that the

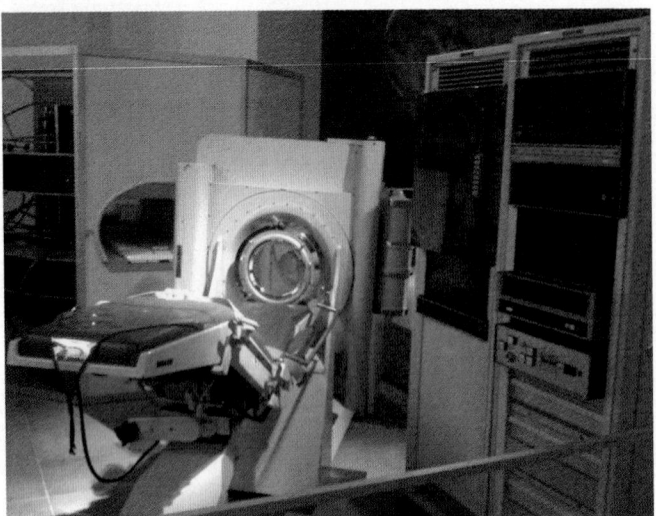

FIGURE 1.54 An early model of Godfrey Hounsfield's EMI computer-assisted tomography (CAT) scanner, now housed at the Science Museum, London, England. *(Picture taken by author October 13, 2009.)*

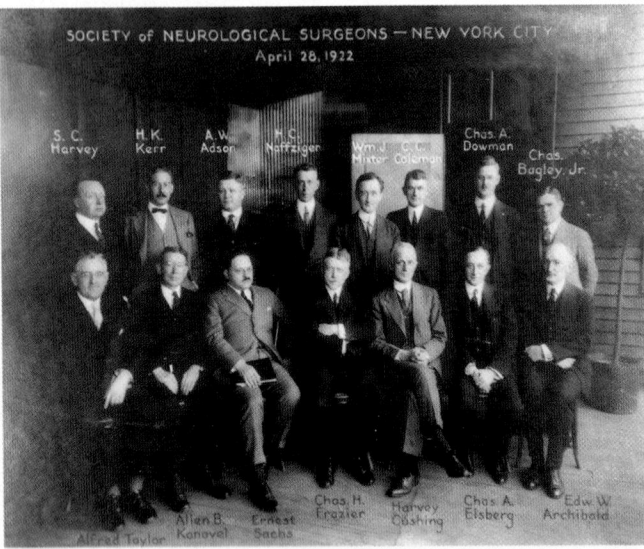

FIGURE 1.55 The Society of Neurological Surgeons, later the American Association of Neurological Surgeons, meeting in New York City on April 28, 1922. The figures portrayed here were early founders of American neurosurgery as an independent surgical specialty. *(Photograph from the estate of Leo Davidoff, acquired by the author in 2007.)*

neurosurgeon of the 2020s will be mere data engineers inputting into a computerized operation room with robots and in-place scanners. This scenario is a far cry from our Asclepiad fathers, who could only whisper secret incantations, lay on the hands, and provide herbal medicaments that only occasionally worked.

SELECTED KEY REFERENCES

Cushing H. *The Pituitary Body and Its Disorders: Clinical States Produced by Disorders of the Hypophysis Cerebri.* Philadelphia: JB Lippincott; 1912.

Dandy WE. Localization or elimination of cerebral tumors by ventriculography. *Surg Gynecol Obstet.* 1920;30:329-342.

Fulton JF. *Harvey Cushing: A Biography.* Springfield, IL: Charles C Thomas; 1946.

Goodrich JT. Sixteenth century Renaissance art and anatomy: Andreas Vesalius and his great book—a new view. *Med Heritage.* 1985;1:280-288.

Leonardo da Vinci. Corpus of the Anatomical Studies in the Collection of Her Majesty the Queen at Windsor Castle. In: Keele KD, Pedretti C, eds. New York: Harcourt Brace Jovanovich; 1979.

Moniz CE. L'encéphalographie artérielle: son importance dans la localisation des tumeurs cérébrales. *Rev Neurol.* 1927;2:72-90.

Please go to expertconsult.com to view the complete list of references.

Clinical Evaluation of the Nervous System

Gerald A. Grant, Richard G. Ellenbogen

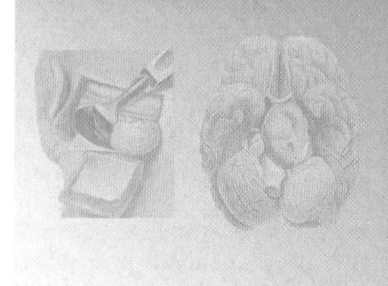

CLINICAL PEARLS

- Step back and observe the patient walking, reading, or moving in bed before beginning the clinical examination. If you focus on an obvious deficit, you may miss many important details. The examiner must master the skill of observing and listening to the patient. A thorough and artfully elicited history and examination are still essential and constitute the cornerstone of what we do and should be used in conjunction with the imaging studies to help direct therapy.

- Signs of pyramidal tract dysfunction include spasticity, weakness, slowing of rapid alternating movements, hyperreflexia, and a Babinski sign. Pyramidal lesions often cause rapid alternating movements to become slowed, but accuracy is preserved, in contrast with cerebellar lesions, which can result in fast but inaccurate, sloppy movements.

- A basal ganglion tremor often is present at rest but disappears with movement, in contrast with a cerebellar tremor, which is minimal at rest and exaggerated with movement (intention tremor).

- Use caution investigating the cause of the dilated pupil on one side, because the larger pupil is always the more impressive, even though the patient actually has a constricted pupil on the opposite side because of Horner syndrome.

- A compressive lesion, such as an aneurysm, may produce a dilated pupil with ptosis and *painful* ophthalmoplegia, in contrast with a pupil-sparing, *painless* ophthalmoplegia due to diabetes.

- The presence of optokinetic nystagmus can be used to confirm cortical vision and rule out hysterical blindness; its absence, however, is inconclusive.

- A fourth cranial nerve lesion causes weakness of the superior oblique muscle and results in a compensatory head tilt away from the side of the affected eye to compensate for the diplopia. Patients with a fourth nerve paresis have difficulty walking down steps or looking down when they walk.

- Note any asymmetry or marked preference for one hand or the other in a young child; the presence of definite hand preference before 24 months may raise the suspicion of central nervous system or peripheral nerve impairment.

- Asymmetry of the Babinski response is abnormal at any age and may reflect an upper motor neuron lesion.

- The open fontanelle in a child under 15 months of age provides good access for checking intracranial pressure. If it is bulging in a quiet child in an upright posture, you can assume that the intracranial pressure is high.

There are only two sorts of doctors; those who practice with their brains and those who practice with their tongues.
—Sir William Osler

The analytical approach required to bring a patient with a neurological problem from diagnosis to surgery is much akin to the work a detective must perform to solve a mystery. The evolution of magnetic resonance imaging (MRI) and other sophisticated imaging techniques may cause the student to view history-taking skills or those of the neurological clinical examination as superfluous, but this idea is simply not an accurate reflection of the neurosurgeon's intellectual responsibility. Thus, neurosurgeons around the world are still trained to hone their analytical and interpersonal skills so that they may elicit a history and an examination to provide a context for the radiological examination.

The history and neurological examination is still the centerpiece in the evaluation of a patient with a surgically correctable neurological disease. The neurosurgeon's job requires basic investigative work, a thorough knowledge of neuroanatomy, appropriate utilization of the currently available diagnostic tools, and last, substantial interpersonal skills. Correctly identifying the neurological problem is one of the most satisfying parts of a neurosurgeon's job, for it is a mandatory skill that must precede a successful surgical outcome for the patient. It is what everything we do is built upon.

NEUROLOGICAL HISTORY

It is a common medical school teaching that acquiring an accurate medical history can help the clinician secure the correct diagnosis in approximately 90% of all patients. Historical information obtained by a skilled clinician, more often than not, will uncover a patient's entire anatomical and etiological illness. The history is followed by the neurological examination, which should simply confirm dysfunction of the organ system one has already decided is abnormal, prior to reliance on sophisticated neuroimaging. It is paramount that the astute clinician masters the skill of anatomical localization in the nervous system. This complex but beautiful system is composed of *ten subsystems* (from a practical standpoint): cortex, pyramidal tracts, basal ganglia, brainstem, cranial nerves, cerebellum, spinal cord, nerve roots, peripheral nerves, and muscle. Understanding each subsystem of the nervous system is equivalent to mastering the anatomy of one entire internal organ. Many of the subsystems stretch over long distances either vertically (i.e., pyramidal tracts, posterior columns) or horizontally (i.e., cortex, cranial nerves, brainstem), which can complicate accurate anatomical localization. To evaluate the functional state of the nervous system, the neurosurgeon requires a basic knowledge of the pertinent anatomy as well as an understanding of the role of ancillary imaging and laboratory tests. Apart from the optic nerve head, which can be evaluated by a funduscopic examination, the rest of the nervous system is hidden from direct observation, and therefore, at the clinical level, disease usually must be inferred from a disorder of normal function.

FOCAL CORTICAL SIGNS

We will begin this tour at the top with the cerebral cortex and then continue down the line. In general, conversation with the patient during the course of the examination will elicit the cortical deficits that are obvious. The ability to talk and respond to questions in a sensible and coherent fashion reveals a great deal about the cerebral cortices. Asking a patient to perform a simple task such as reading a newspaper to the examiner requires activation of an incredibly complex set of neural circuits. In so doing, the examiner is able to test the visual system, cranial nerves, and the motor and sensory systems as well as higher cortical function. This seemingly straightforward, everyday task helps the examiner quickly close down on a wide spectrum of neurological functions that may be affected by the patient's disease. More subtle cortical deficits require meticulous testing, often by neuropsychological examinations, the interpretation of which requires specific training. Neuropsychological examinations are performed more commonly in the pre- and postoperative stages of modern neurosurgical intervention.[1] It is simply not sufficient to know if the patient did "OK" after complex intracranial surgery. It is important to understand what subtle deficits existed preoperatively and how well the deficits improved postoperatively, or which new deficits will require active rehabilitative intervention to improve after surgery.

In broad strokes, the examiner must understand two major types of pathognomonic cortical signs: focal and bihemispheric. Focal cortical signs direct the examiner to a specific area of cortex in one hemisphere, or if bihemispheric, in both hemispheres. Certain portions of the cerebral hemispheres are also termed "silent" areas, because the localizing evidence for lesions here may be absent.[2,3]

Left occipital lobe dysfunction produces a right homonomous hemianopia (loss of the right half of a visual field), although loss of this field can theoretically result from a lesion of the left optic tract or left thalamic lateral geniculate body. A right or left hemianopia can therefore result from any retrochiasmal lesion (behind the chiasm). Color dysnomia (inability to name colors) is the result of an interruption of fibers streaming from the occipital lobe to Wernicke's area, the comprehension center in the left temporal lobe. In 98% of right-handed people, Wernicke's area is located in the left temporal lobe. In most left-handed people, Wernicke's area is still located in either the left temporal lobe alone or in both temporal lobes.[4,5] In only a minority of left-handed people is Wernicke's area confined to the right temporal lobe.[6] A lesion in Wernicke's area results in a sensory or receptive aphasia characterized by fluent speech filled with gibberish words. Written words come from the occipital cortex, while spoken words may come from both temporal lobes. A mistake in naming results in a paraphasia and is often the result of a lesion in the posterosuperior temporal lobe, but can have quite variable localization. Adjacent to Wernicke's area in the temporal lobe is another area called the "dysnomia center," which shows variable localization from person to person. Another pathognomonic sign of temporal lobe dysfunction is a focal, temporal lobe seizure, described as fits consisting of a sense of fear, smell, pleasure, or déjà vu. Another common manifestation of temporal lobe seizures is the automatism, a brief episode of automatic behavior during which the patient is unaware of his or her surroundings and is unable to communicate with others. Patients with complex partial seizures may experience sudden unpleasant smells (e.g., burning rubber) of brief duration which constitute olfactory auras. Temporal lobe dysfunction may also cause a superior quadrantopia (loss of a quarter of the visual field), described as a "pie in the sky," as a result of a disruption of the optic radiations, called *Meyer's loop*, which dip into the temporal lobe.

Pathognomonic signs of left parietal dysfunction include right-sided cortical sensory loss, right-sided sensory-motor seizures, or a Gerstmann syndrome, characterized by finger agnosia (inability to recognize one's fingers), acalculia (inability to calculate numbers), right/left confusion, and agraphia without alexia (an ability to read but not write). Another sign of left parietal cortical dysfunction is cortical sensory loss and results in agraphesthesia (inability to identify numbers written on his/her skin). Sensory seizures may spread up or down the sensory strip and have been described as the *jacksonian march*. The movement, usually clonic, begins in one portion of the body, for example, the thumb or fingers, and spreads to involve the wrist, arm, face, and leg on the same side along the stereotypical pattern of cortical organization termed the *homunculus* (Fig. 2.1). A Todd's paralysis may then occur following the attack, with the same distribution.

Left frontal lobe dysfunction can result in Broca's aphasia, also known as motor or expressive aphasia, and is characterized by halting, slow, and nonfluent speech.[7] Speech lesions in the arcuate fasciculus, a dense bundle of fibers connecting Wernicke's area to Broca's, prevent patients from repeating phrases but does not impair comprehension (Table 2.1).

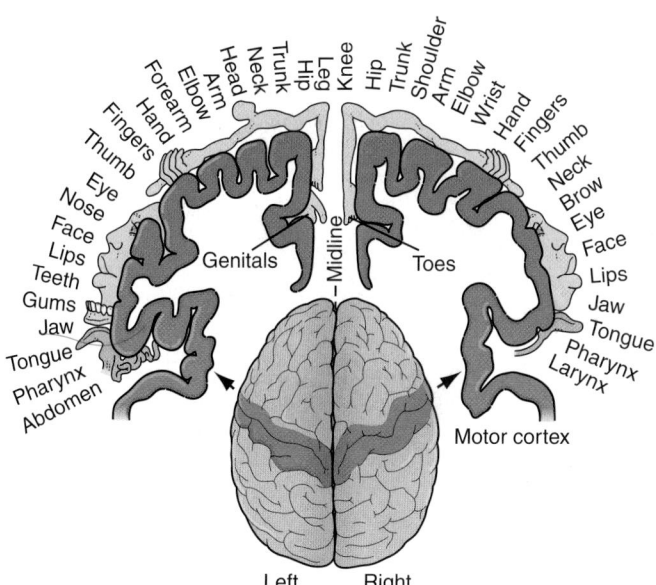

FIGURE 2.1 Somatosensory and motor homunculi.

Left   Right

Motor cortex

TABLE 2.2 MRC Scale for Muscle Strength Grading

Grade	Strength
0	No muscle contraction
1	Flicker or trace of contraction
2	Active movement with gravity eliminated
3	Active movement against gravity
4	Active movement against gravity and resistance
5	Normal power

bihemispheric dysfunction and are not derived from a simple focal cortical lesion.[2]

PYRAMIDAL TRACT

The pyramidal tract begins in the motor strip of the cortex and courses downward through the brain and into the spinal cord. In the hemispheres it is called the *coronal radiata* and then becomes the internal capsule, cerebral peduncle, and pyramidal tract, which crosses at the medulla–spinal cord junction, and finally in the spinal cord becomes the corticospinal tract. Functionally, a lesion anywhere along this tract can produce the same long tract signs. Signs of pyramidal tract dysfunction include spasticity, weakness, slowing of rapid alternating movements, hyperreflexia, and a Babinski sign.[8] Muscle tone is examined by manipulating the major joints and determining the degree of resistance. Spasticity is one type of increased tone (resistance of a relaxed limb to flexion and extension). Muscle strength is commonly graded from 0 to 5 using the grading system shown in Table 2.2.

Acute lesions anywhere along the pyramidal tract may also produce flaccid hemiparesis, at least initially, with spasticity developing later. If the whole area of cortex supplying a limb is damaged, the extrapyramidal pathways may be unable to take over and an acute global flaccid weakness of the limb can occur. Intraoperative monitoring has been used to mitigate injury to the corticospinal tract.[3] Pyramidal tract lesions typically produce weakness of an arm and leg, or face and arm, or all three together.[9] Facial weakness may manifest with a slight flattening of the nasolabial fold; however, the forehead will not be weak (frontalis muscle) because the muscles on each side of the forehead have dual innervation by both cerebral hemispheres (corticopontine fibers). The less affected muscles are the antigravity muscles (wrist flexors, biceps, gluteus maximus, quadriceps, and gastrocnemius). Specific tests of grouped muscle strength can also be quite useful (Table 2.3): pronator drift (arms outstretched with the palms up), standing on each foot, hopping on one foot, walking on toes (gastrocnemius), walking on heels (tibialis anterior), and deep knee bend (proximal hip muscles). Typically, pyramidal lesions often cause rapid alternating movements to become slowed but accuracy is preserved. This is in contrast to cerebellar lesions (see later discussion), which can result in fast but inaccurate, sloppy movements.

Reflexes can also be quite important in detecting subtle pyramidal tract lesions, especially if asymmetrical. Reflexes are graded by a numerical system: 0 indicates an absent reflex, trace describes a reflex that is palpable but not visible,

TABLE 2.1 Classification of Dysphasias

Lesion	Deficit	Aphasia Type
Temporal	Retained repetition and fluency, no comprehension, no naming	Transcortical sensory
Wernicke's	Retained fluency, no comprehension, repetition, or naming	Wernicke's
Parietal	Retained comprehension and fluency, no repetition	Conduction
Broca's	Retained comprehension, no fluency, repetition, or naming	Broca's
Frontal	Retained comprehension and repetition, no fluency or naming	Transcortical motor

Lesions of the corpus callosum prevent the interhemispheric transfer of information, so a patient cannot follow instructions with his or her left hand but retains the ability to perform these same instructions with the right hand. Another syndrome of the corpus callosum is *alexia without agraphia* (inability to read but retained ability to write) and is caused by a lesion extending from the left occipital lobe and into the splenium of the corpus callosum.

The right frontal lobe, despite its size, is a relatively silent lobe, other than loss of speech intonation (inflection and emotion in speech). The areas of major clinical importance are the motor strip (area 4), the supplementary motor area (area 6), the frontal eye fields (area 8), and the cortical center for micturition (medial surface of the frontal lobe). Frontal lobes play a major role in personality and acquired social behavior. Frontal lobe dysfunction may result in loss of drive, apathy, loss of personal hygiene, inability to manage one's family affairs or business, and disinhibition. The right parietal lesions cause a characteristic disturbance of space perception and left-side neglect.

Signs such as lethargy, stupor, coma, disorientation, confusion, amnesia, dementia, and delirium often result from

TABLE 2.3 Deep Tendon Reflexes

Reflex	Segmental Level*	Peripheral Nerve
Biceps	**C5**-C6	Musculocutaneous
Triceps	C6, **C7**, C8	Radial
Brachioradialis	C5-C7	Radial
Quadriceps	L2, **L3**, L4	Femoral
Achilles	L4, L5, **S1**, S2	Sciatic

*Roots in bold type indicate spinal segment with greatest contribution.

1+ is hypoactive but present, 2+ is normal, 3+ is hyperactive, 4+ implies unsustained clonus, and 5+ is sustained clonus. *Clonus* is a series of rhythmic involuntary muscle contractions induced by sudden stretching of a spastic muscle such as at the ankle. The cutaneous reflex (abdominal twitch obtained when you gently stroke someone's abdomen) and the cremasteric reflex (L1, L2 innervation; retraction of the testicle upward with a brush along the inner thigh) may also be lost in pyramidal tract lesions. The *abdominal cutaneous reflexes* in the upper quadrant of the abdomen are mediated by segments T8 and T9; the lower by T10 to T12. If, for example, the lower abdominal reflexes are absent but the upper are preserved, the lesion may be between T9 and L1. The *Hoffmann reflex* is reflective of hyperreflexia and spasticity on that side and suggests pyramidal tract involvement. It is elicited by snapping the distal phalanx of the middle finger; a pathological response consists of thumb flexion. The Babinski reflex is the best-known sign of disturbed pyramidal tract function. The *Babinski reflex* is an important sign of upper motor neuron disease, but should not be confused with a more delayed voluntary knee and toe withdrawal due to oversensitive soles of the feet.[10] The Babinski reflex is sought by stroking the lateral border of the sole of the foot, beginning at the heel and moving toward the toes. The stimulus should be firm but not painful. The abnormal response, referred to as the *Babinski sign*, consists of immediate dorsiflexion of the big toe and subsequent separation (fanning) of the other toes. The Babinski sign is present in infancy but usually disappears at about 10 months of age (range 6-12 months). When planar responses produce equivocal results, a related reflex may be tested by stroking the lateral aspect of the dorsum of the foot, and is known as the *Chaddock sign*.

In general, the more spasticity is present, the more likely the pyramidal tract lesion is in the spinal cord, especially if the spasticity is bilateral.[11] Conversely, it is unusual for a pyramidal tract lesion in the spinal cord to produce a hemiparesis or monoparesis. A hemiparesis that involves the face places the lesion somewhere above the facial nucleus, although if the hemiparesis spares the face, the lesion need not be below the facial nucleus. Mild or more chronic hydrocephalus may also cause impressive pyramidal tract dysfunction in the legs more than in the arm fibers. Bladder axons also become stretched by the dilated ventricles associated with hydrocephalus and cause urinary urgency and incontinence. Finally, it should be remembered that the spinal cord terminates normally at the level of the L1-L2 vertebral body, and therefore, neurologically L5 is anatomically in the lower thoracic region.

THE EXTRAPYRAMIDAL SYSTEM

Unlike the pyramidal tracts, which govern strength and fine dexterity, the basal ganglia govern the speed and spontaneity of movements. Two basic patterns emerge with basal ganglia dysfunction: either too much or not enough movement. The number one characteristic of a *basal ganglia tremor* is its presence at rest and disappearance with movement, in contrast to a *cerebellar tremor* which is minimal at rest and exaggerated with movement (intention tremor). The strength and deep tendon reflexes are normal in extrapyramidal diseases and there is no Babinski sign. However, the tone is either hypotonic, as occurs in choreiform disorders, or increased (rigid), as in the bradykinetic (slowness of movements) varieties with rachety rigidity appropriately called *cogwheeling*. Choreiform movements are involuntary random jerky movements of small muscles of the hands, feet, or face and may be proximal enough to cause the whole arm to jerk gently. If instead of the small distal muscles, the larger more proximal muscles involuntarily flinch, the patient may have ballismus. Ballismus can be unilateral, but chorea is almost always bilateral. Athetoid movements are slower, more continuous, and sustained, and may involve the head, neck, limb girdles, and distal extremities. Dystonic movements resemble a fixation of athetoid movements involving larger portions of the body. Torticollis, or torsion of the neck, is an example of a neck dystonia that is the result of the continuous contraction of the sternocleidomastoid muscle on one side. Postural and gait abnormalities of extrapyramidal disease are most diagnostic in patients with Parkinson's disease (tremor, bradykinesia, and rigidity).[12] A blank expression and infrequent blinking, walking with a leaning forward posture, and a festinating gait (running, shuffling feet) are typical findings of a Parkinson's patient. Once in gear, the initially bradykinetic patient may have difficulty stopping. At the same time, the patient's hand is coarsely shaking at three times a second and the patient's speech is also devoid of normal changes in pitch and cadence.

CRANIAL NERVES

There are 12 cranial nerves but only nerves III to XII enter the brainstem (I and II do not). Diagnosing a cranial neuropathy is only the beginning, because the lesion may lie anywhere along the course of the cranial nerve.

Cranial Nerve I

Cranial nerve I, the olfactory nerve, begins at the cribriform plate and travels back underneath the frontal lobe to the temporal lobe without relaying in the thalamus. To test olfaction, test each nostril independently and avoid using a caustic substance such as ammonia, which tests the trigeminal nerve (V) in addition to the olfactory nerve due to irritation of the nasal mucosa. An olfactory groove tumor may present with unilateral anosmia (loss of smell), although the most likely explanation is local nasal obstruction. *Foster-Kennedy syndrome* is characterized by ipsilateral anosmia, ipsilateral scotoma with optic atrophy (direct pressure on the optic nerve), and contralateral papilledema (elevated intracranial pressure) and is classically due to an olfactory groove or medial sphenoid wing meningioma. Loss of smell can also complicate up to 30% of head injuries as a result of shearing of the nerves as they pass through the cribriform plate.

Cranial Nerve II

The second cranial nerve, the optic nerve, is the most complex. Visual acuity, color vision, Marcus Gunn pupil, visual fields, and direct ophthalmoscopic observation must all be assessed. Visual acuity is affected early in optic neuropathies, because 20% to 25% of all optic fibers come from the macula and travel in the center of the nerve. If the patient's visual acuity is not 20/20 and cannot be improved by refraction (looking through a pinhole in a piece of cardboard is a good bedside test), then the visual impairment is most likely neurological. The size, shape, and symmetry of the pupils in moderate lighting conditions should be noted. If the pupils are unequal it is important to decide which pupil is the abnormal one. One frequent mistake is to investigate for the cause of the dilated pupil on one side, because the larger pupil is always the more impressive, even though the patient actually has a constricted pupil on the opposite side because of *Horner syndrome.* If there is ptosis of the eyelid on the side of the small pupil, the patient may have Horner syndrome, although if the ptosis is on the side of the large pupil, the patient may have an ipsilateral partial third cranial nerve lesion. Furthermore, the light and accommodation reflexes will be normal in a Horner syndrome and impaired in a partial third nerve lesion. Whenever a patient is found to have a widely dilated pupil that is fixed to light and accommodation without accompanying ptosis, there is a possibility of a pharmacological pupil (e.g., atropine drops instilled into the eye). A *Marcus Gunn pupil* (afferent pupillary defect), a form of optic nerve dysfunction, is elicited by the swinging flashlight test: shine a dim light into the right eye, and note how small the right pupil constricts (left pupil also constricts). Swing the light over to the left eye and carefully note the left pupil. If the very first reaction of that pupil is dilation instead of maintaining its previous small size, then there may be left optic nerve dysfunction, i.e., an afferent papillary defect (Fig. 2.2). The examiner must ignore "hippus," which is a normal phasic instability of the pupil with waves of alternating constriction and dilatation. An optic nerve lesion can be corroborated with visual field testing and direct funduscopy, both of which will be discussed later in this chapter in the neuro-ophthalmology section. The approach to patients with diplopia also requires a systematic approach because double vision may arise from ocular, neurological, or extraocular muscle disorders (i.e., thyrotoxicosis). The *Cover test* can be useful in the evaluation of a patient with binocular diplopia. The test is based on the fact that the separation of two images becomes greatest as the eyes attempt to look in the direction of the action of the weak muscle. By determining which eye must be covered to obliterate the outer image, the affected eye is identified, because the false image is always projected as the outer image.

Cranial Nerves III, IV, and VI

The third cranial nerve, or oculomotor nerve, is one of the three nerves that move the eye, the others being the fourth (trochlear) and the sixth (abducens) cranial nerves. Defective

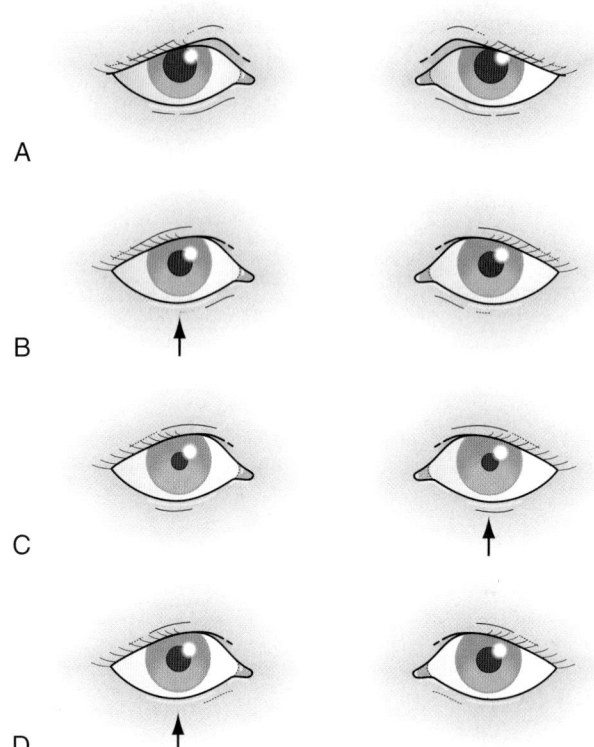

FIGURE 2.2 Marcus Gunn pupil paradoxically dilates with direct light (↑).

adduction and elevation with outward and downward displacement of the eye suggests a third cranial nerve palsy. The third cranial nerve also innervates the levator palpebrae superioris, the muscle that opens the eyelid. Parasympathetic fibers travel within the superior and medial perimeter of the third cranial nerve to constrict the iris and stimulate the ciliary body to round up the lens. As a general rule, if the pupil is affected, the cause is more likely to be surgical (compressive) and if spared, the cause is more likely to be medical (diabetes, cranial arteritis, arteriosclerosis, syphilis, migraine). A compressive lesion, such as an aneurysm, selectively injures these superficially situated parasympathetic fibers, producing a dilated pupil with ptosis and painful ophthalmoplegia. In contrast, diabetes more often causes a pupil-sparing, painless ophthalmoplegia by damaging the interior motor axons through arterial thrombosis.[13] The sympathetic nerves supply Müller's muscle, which also slightly elevates the eyelid and when injured causes the upper eyelid to droop and results in ptosis and miosis (eyelid droop and a dilated pupil), or Horner syndrome. If the sympathetic nerves to the eye are interrupted prior to the carotid bifurcation, ipsilateral facial anhidrosis (no sweating) may also result. Some of the sympathetic nerves also ascend the common carotid and follow the external carotid onto the face to stimulate the facial sweat glands.

If the pupils do not react to light, the anatomical differential diagnosis includes the afferent limb (retina, optic nerves, optic tracts) and the efferent limb (pretectum, Edinger-Westphal nucleus, parasympathetic fibers in the oculomotor nerves, and the pupillary constrictor muscle in the iris). A pupil able to accommodate to near vision but not react to light is referred to as an *Argyll Robertson pupil* and has been classically seen in patients with tertiary syphilis. This, of course, is a rare

TABLE 2.4 Classification of Nystagmus

Nystagmus Type	Characteristic(s)	Location of Pathology	Possible Etiological Disorder(s)
Upbeat	Upbeating nystagmus	Cerebellar vermis	Cerebellar or medullary lesion, Wernicke's encephalopathy
Downbeat	Downbeating	Cervicomedullary junction	Chiari I malformation, basilar invagination, syringobulbia, foramen magnum lesion, multiple sclerosis, Wernicke's encephalopathy
Convergence-retraction	Convergence motions and simultaneous retraction of globes into orbits	Rostral midbrain, pretectum, posterior third ventricle	Pineal tumors
Ocular bobbing	Downward jerk with slow drift back into primary position	Pons	Pontine tegmentum hemorrhage or stroke
Ocular flutter	Rapid back and forth saccades, associated with ocular dysmetria	Cerebellum	Neuroblastoma, occult lung or breast carcinoma
Opsoclonus	Continuous, involuntary, random chaotic saccades (dancing eyes), continues during sleep	Cerebellum, dentate nucleus	Neuroblastoma, occult lung or breast carcinoma
Ocular dysmetria	Overshoot or undershoot on rapid refixation, side to side oscillation, fast component toward the side of lesion	Cerebellum	Multiple sclerosis
Monocular nystagmus	Vertical	Eye	Acquired blindness
Congenital nystagmus	Horizontal jerk, remains horizontal even in upgaze and downgaze	Eye	Congenital
Spasmus nutans	Torticollis, head nodding, and pendular nystagmus	Unknown	Developmental, 6 months to 3 years

finding because of the decrease in this disease over the past century. Light-near dissociation is also seen in *Adie's pupil*, which is usually unilateral and is caused by parasympathetic dysfunction. When parasympathetic innervation is first lost in Adie syndrome, the pupil is relatively large, but with time and reinnervation the pupil constricts. This is a curious but benign disorder of unknown cause, usually affecting one eye, and results from injury or illness to the ciliary ganglion, usually inflammatory in nature. Pineal region tumors can also damage the midbrain pretectum and cause light-near dissociation. Pineal region tumors more classically damage the midbrain upgaze center and cause a constellation of dorsal midbrain signs called Parinaud syndrome: (1) impaired upward or downward gaze; (2) bilateral light-near dissociation; (3) pupillary dilatation; and (4) retraction of the eyelids.

In general, nystagmus can be due to labyrinthine or brainstem/cerebellar pathology, may be central or peripheral, and is defined in the direction of the fast movement (Table 2.4). *Upbeat or downbeat nystagmus* is almost always of central origin, and represents disrupted connections between the cerebellum and brainstem (Chiari malformations, basilar invagination, platybasia, or a midline cerebellar lesion such as medulloblastoma in children). *Horizontal nystagmus* is more commonly peripheral in origin, especially if the patient can stop the nystagmus by fixating on a target. Two axes of nystagmus, as seen in rotary nystagmus, suggest a disturbance of two semicircular canals. *Opsoclonus* is another form of nystagmus and is characterized by chaotic, repetitive, saccadic movements in all directions, preventing fixation, and has also been termed *dancing eyes*.[14] In an adult, opsoclonus is associated with postinfectious encephalopathy as well as with carcinomas of the lung or breast, although in younger children

it has been described in association with neuroblastoma. The presence of optokinetic nystagmus can be used to confirm cortical vision; its absence, however, is inconclusive.[15] When the optokinetic tape (a series of vertical black lines on a white background) is pulled from the patient's left to his or her right, the right parieto-occipital lobe tracks the target to the right (smooth pursuit, slow phase). The eyes saccade left to track each newly arriving target (fast phase). In right parieto-occipital lesions, a smooth pursuit (slow phase) to the right is lost. However, occipital stroke due to a posterior cerebral artery infarct do not usually impair optokinetic nystagmus. A tumor, in contrast, may cross vascular boundaries and interrupt a smooth pursuit generators.

Looking left involves two cranial nerves: the left sixth (left lateral rectus) and the right third (right medial rectus) (Fig. 2.3). There are three classic signs of a pontine medial longitudinal fasciculus (MLF) lesion, or *internuclear ophthalmoplegia* (INO): (1) weakness of the contralateral medial rectus muscle causing paralysis of adduction on lateral gaze, because the MLF cannot transmit its message to the third cranial nerve to pull the eye medially; (2) nystagmus in the abducting eye; and (3) the retained ability to converge, demonstrating that the reason for medial rectus weakness on adduction is not in the third cranial nerve or muscle itself. In the setting of a third nerve lesion, the eye will be deviated downward (secondary depressant action of superior oblique) and outward (lateral rectus action) and the diplopia would improve when testing lateral gaze in the affected eye.

A fourth or trochlear nerve lesion causes weakness of the superior oblique muscle and diplopia. This weakness results in a compensatory head tilt away from the side of the affected eye to compensate and is called the *Bielschowsky sign*. Patients

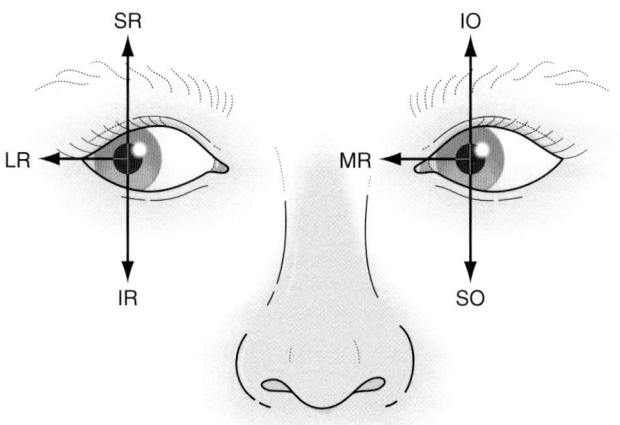

FIGURE 2.3 Simplified scheme for testing the major pulling actions of extraocular muscles. IO, inferior oblique; IR, inferior rectus; LR, lateral rectus; MR, medial rectus; SO, superior oblique; SR, superior rectus.

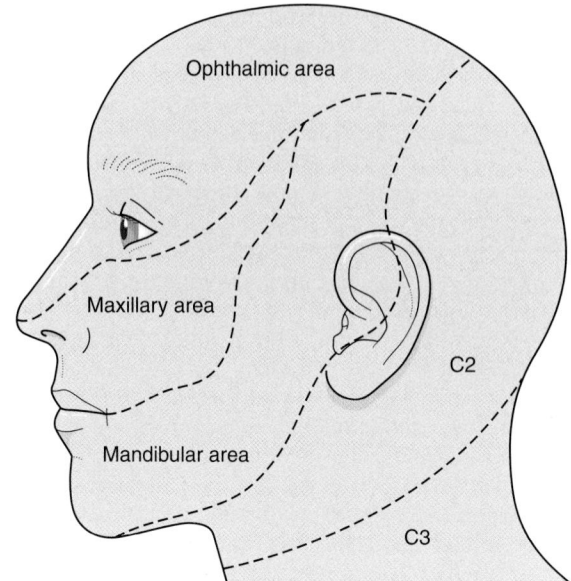

FIGURE 2.4 Diagrammatic representation of the cutaneous nerve supply of the head.

with a fourth cranial nerve palsy can lessen or extinguish their double vision by tilting their head toward the unaffected side. Tilting their head toward the shoulder on the affected side makes the diplopia worse. The diplopia is particularly troublesome on looking downward and thus especially problematic when the patient is attempting to walk down a set of stairs. In some patients, this head tilt may be misdiagnosed as torticollis. A sixth or abducens nerve palsy is the most disabling eye movement abnormality because the diplopia persists in nearly all directions of gaze. At rest, the affected eye is pulled medially by the unopposed action of the medial rectus muscle. Multiple sclerosis is the most common cause of an isolated sixth cranial nerve palsy due to a plaque in the brainstem. The sixth nerve takes a ventral course from the pontine tegmentum over the petrous ridge to the dorsum sellae and into the cavernous sinus lateral to the carotid nerve and medial to cranial nerves III, IV, V_1, and V_2. A posterior fossa tumor can cause hydrocephalus, which can also stretch the sixth nerve over the petrous tip and cause diplopia. As the sixth nerve has a rather long course, it is the most vulnerable cranial nerve to closed head injury. Benign transient sixth nerve palsies can also occur in children following mild infections. More severe cases of mastoiditis (*Gradenigo syndrome*) can cause ear pain and a combination of sixth, seventh, eighth, and occasionally fifth cranial nerve lesions. These symptoms must be differentiated from *Ramsay Hunt syndrome* (geniculate herpes zoster), in which there is vesicular eruption in the ear and a seventh cranial nerve palsy.

Cranial Nerve V

The fifth cranial nerve, the trigeminal, controls both sensory and motor function: sensation of the forehead and face (including inside the mouth) and strength of chewing muscles (temporalis, masseter, pterygoids). The three branches of the trigeminal nerve are denoted as V1, V2, and V3. It is important to recognize that there is a large area over the angle of the jaw supplied by nerve roots C2 and C3 and that patients with nonorganic sensory loss over the face usually claim anesthesia extending to the line of

the jaw and the hairline (Fig. 2.4). When testing for a corneal reflex, a wisp of cotton wool should not be allowed to cross in front of the pupil or the patient will see it and blink (false positive). In addition, both eyes should shut simultaneously if the corneal reflex is present. A depressed or absent corneal reflex can be an early physical sign of an acoustic neuroma in the cerebellopontine angle. Intracavernous lesions (i.e., aneurysms, meningiomas, carotid-cavernous fistulas, and pituitary tumors) can all cause facial numbness. However, jaw numbness does not typically occur with cavernous sinus lesions because nerve V_3 does not enter the cavernous sinus like nerves III, IV, VI, V_1, and V_2. Patients suffering from lightning jabs of terrible facial and jaw pain, often precipitated by a trigger point along the gums or lips, may have trigeminal neuralgia.[16] The cardinal feature of trigeminal neuralgia is pain without any objective neurological abnormality (i.e., sensory or motor dysfunction). The cause is thought to be an arterial or venous loop that pulsates against the trigeminal nerve at the pontine root entry zone or sometimes a small plaque of brainstem demyelination as in multiple sclerosis, although attacks of trigeminal pain may occur with any tumor of the cerebellopontine angle or petrous apex. Although herpes zoster can affect any nerve in the body, the thoracic roots are usually affected in younger age groups, although in the elderly, the virus has a predilection for nerve V_1.

Cranial Nerve VII

The seventh cranial nerve, the facial, controls all the facial and forehead muscles. The seventh nerve does not contribute to normal eye opening but instead contributes to forced eye opening. Paralysis of facial movement including both the cheek and forehead on one side of the face, both volitional and emotional, indicates a lesion in the seventh cranial nerve (peripheral) somewhere between the pontine facial nerve nucleus and the facial muscles. In general, if the forehead is spared, then the facial paralysis is "central" and is the result of a lesion in the descending corticopontine upper motor neuron. Eye closure and forehead movement will remain relatively intact because the intact hemisphere pathways provide adequate cross-innervation. Recent evidence also suggests that upper facial motor neurons receive little direct cortical input, whereas lower facial neurons do and are therefore more affected.[17] As the facial nerve leaves its nucleus in the brainstem, other nerves piggyback it on their way to the lacrimal gland, stapedius muscle (dampens loud noises in the ear), and the taste buds along the anterior two thirds of the tongue. Ipsilateral loss of taste and tear production, and the presence of hyperacusis (noises sound too loud) confirm that the patient's facial weakness is the result of lower motor neuron dysfunction. Most often, an acute peripheral facial weakness without associated sensory loss is the result of *Bell's palsy*, a poorly understood acute inflammatory attack on the facial nerve within the facial canal. This disorder has an excellent prognosis for recovery within weeks or months. Blepharospasm is a recurrent involuntary spasm of forceful eye closure (both eyes) with some spread into other facial muscles. Hemifacial spasm is characterized by recurrent spasms of one side of the face and is most likely the result of an irritation of the facial nerve as it leaves the brainstem by a pulsating arterial loop.[17,18]

Cranial Nerve VIII

The eighth cranial nerve, or acoustic nerve, relays hearing to the brainstem from the cochlea as well as balance information from the labyrinth. The early loss of speech discrimination amid background noise raises the suspicion to a diagnosis of an acoustic neuroma. The closest nerve to the eighth cranial nerve is the facial nerve; however, after the acoustic nerve, the most common nerve to be affected is the trigeminal nerve. There is a relative loss of higher tones in nerve deafness whereas lower tones are lost in middle ear deafness. A tuning fork is also helpful to distinguish between nerve deafness hearing loss due to middle ear disease (conductive deafness) and that due to eighth nerve damage (sensorineural deafness). For the Rinne test, a tuning fork is held on the mastoid while the opposite ear is masked. A *Rinne positive test* test result occurs when the tuning fork can still be heard in front of the ear but is no longer heard on the mastoid and is the normal situation (air conduction > bone conduction). For the *Weber test*, a tuning fork is placed on the vertex, and if heard equally in both ears, then hearing is normal. In conductive deafness, the fork will be heard more loudly in the affected ear, and in sensorineural hearing loss the fork will not be heard in the affected ear. It is also important to recognize that unilateral temporal lobe lesions do not produce hearing loss. After the eighth cranial nerve enters the brainstem, spoken words are directed to both sides of the brainstem and ascend to both temporal lobes. Disturbances in the vestibular system may occur in the labyrinth (i.e., Meniere's disease) or in the nerve (acoustic neuroma, petrous temporal bone fracture), or in the temporal lobe of the brain (epilepsy). Meniere's disease is characterized by a triad of recurring attacks of vertigo associated with tinnitus and progressive deafness.

Cranial Nerves IX, X, and XI

The ninth cranial nerve, or glossopharyngeal nerve, controls primarily sensation of the posterior tongue and pharynx. The only muscle supplied by the nerve is the stylopharyngeus muscle, which cannot be easily tested clinically, although there is much overlap of the vagal and glossopharyngeal sensory supply to the pharynx. The tenth or vagus nerve is the longest of the cranial nerves. It is primarily motor and when weak can cause ipsilateral vocal cord paralysis. Paralysis of one vocal cord can lead to hoarseness, loss of voice volume, and an inability to cough explosively. Unilateral palatal or pharyngeal palsies may even be asymptomatic. The eleventh cranial nerve, the spinal accessory, has two parts: the spinal part exits the upper cervical spinal cord and tracks up through the foramen magnum into the posterior fossa where it joins the accessory part of nerve XI exiting the medulla. The spinal accessory then does a U-turn back through the jugular foramen to innervate the ipsilateral sternocleidomastoid (SCM) and trapezius muscles. To test the left SCM muscle, ask the patient to put the chin on the right shoulder. Try to pull the face back over to the left and feel the left SCM muscle. The left SCM muscle therefore pulls the head to the right and the trapezius muscle helps shrug the shoulders and elevate the arm above the horizontal. Torticollis is caused in part by intermittent contractions of the SCM muscle on the opposite side.

Cranial Nerve XII

The twelfth cranial nerve, the hypoglossal, supplies the tongue muscle and damage results in ipsilateral tongue atrophy. On attempted tongue protrusion, the tongue deviates toward the weak side, due to the unopposed genioglossus muscle. Bilateral weakness or paralysis of the tongue is more common than unilateral paralysis and may be caused by amyotrophic lateral sclerosis or myasthenia gravis, although in the latter, no wasting or fasciculations accompany the weakness. Tongue fasciculations may be present normally when the tongue is resting quietly on the floor of the mouth.

CEREBELLUM

The smooth and efficient performance of volitional movements depends on the coordination of agonist and antagonist muscles, acting in synergy. A failure of a group of muscles to act harmoniously is a sign of cerebellar dysfunction. Dysdiadochokinesis is characterized by difficulty in performing rapid alternating movements. Dysmetria is the difficulty in reaching a target accurately or past-pointing. The rate, rhythm, amplitude, and smoothness of movement may all be affected in cerebellar disease. A relatively common cerebellar tremor, called *titubation,* affects elderly people with a rapid, fine, bobbing motion of the head. The side-to-side imbalance of cerebellar ataxia is in contrast to the front-to-back imbalance of parkinsonian patients. However, unlike the crossed pyramidal and extrapyramidal systems, the right cerebellar hemisphere controls the right arm and right leg and vice versa. Often a cerebellar tremor is present with the arms outstretched (postural tremor), but the tremor almost always worsens with intention (intention tremor). Speech is also affected in cerebellar disorders, causing ataxia of speech called *scanning speech.* In addition, the inability to perform finger-to-nose movements or to tandem walk is characteristic of cerebellar dysfunction. Postural instability can be best evaluated by the Romberg test, which is a nonspecific test of vestibular function and often used to demonstrate loss of joint position sense. A positive test results when the patient falls with his or her eyes closed when standing with the feet together. In unilateral vestibular or cerebellar disease, the patient sways toward the damaged side.

Saccades are tested by having a patient glance back and forth between two targets about a foot apart. A patient with ocular dysmetria who consistently overshoots the target is likely to be suffering from cerebellar dysfunction. Lesions of one cerebellar hemisphere may cause coarse nystagmus when the patient gazes toward the side of the lesion. The most extreme example of fixation instability is opsoclonus, which is most likely of cerebellar origin. Opsoclonus classically occurs in infants with neuroblastoma and is described as lightning-fast random eye movements often called *dancing eyes.*

SPINAL CORD, NERVE ROOTS, AND MUSCLES

The last neural circuits to consider are the spinal cord, nerve roots, and muscles. However, before distinguishing between a root and peripheral nerve lesion it is important to discriminate an upper motor neuron from a lower motor neuron lesion. As discussed earlier, *upper motor neuron* signs include spasticity, weakness, slowing of rapid alternating movements, hyperreflexia, and a Babinski sign. *Lower motor neuron* lesions (root or peripheral nerve) can cause muscular atrophy, fasciculations, hypotonia, or weakness in a particular root or peripheral nerve distribution, and diminished reflexes. To diagnose a myelopathy, the long tract signs need to be combined with root or segmental signs (Fig. 2.5). Fasciculations are spontaneous, random contractions of muscle, usually too small to move a joint but visible when the skin over the affected muscle is inspected. However, in order to call a spontaneous muscular twitch a fasciculation, the muscle must be fully at rest. The presence of fasciculations implies a lower motor neuron dysfunction; however, the abnormality may be in the spinal cord (ventral horn) or anywhere along the peripheral nerve up to the point of muscle insertion. Fibrillations are the smallest potentials obtainable from individual muscle fibers and occur in denervated muscle fibers after 3 weeks when the motor neurons supplying a muscle are damaged, either in their cell bodies, the ventral roots, or the peripheral nerve itself.

A *Brown-Sequard syndrome* affects the left or right half of the spinal cord and is characterized by ipsilateral weakness, contralateral pain and temperature loss, and ipsilateral vibration and proprioception loss below the lesion (Fig. 2.6). *Anterior spinal artery syndrome* is characterized by flaccidity followed by spasticity, weakness, slowing of rapid alternating movements, hyperreflexia, and a Babinski sign, as well as bilateral pain and temperature loss below the lesion but no vibratory or proprioceptive loss (dissociated sensory loss).[19] *Syringomyelia* (slowly expanding cyst of the spinal cord) or a centrally located spinal cord tumor can also cause dissociated sensory loss. A constellation of lower motor neuron signs and upper extremity dissociated sensory loss is virtually pathognomonic of syringomyelia in the cervical spinal cord. A syrinx can be congenital, developmental, or even post-traumatic and can present in a delayed fashion following a spinal cord injury. Occasionally, the syrinx extends up into the medulla (called *syringobulbia*) and causes atrophy, fasciculations, and

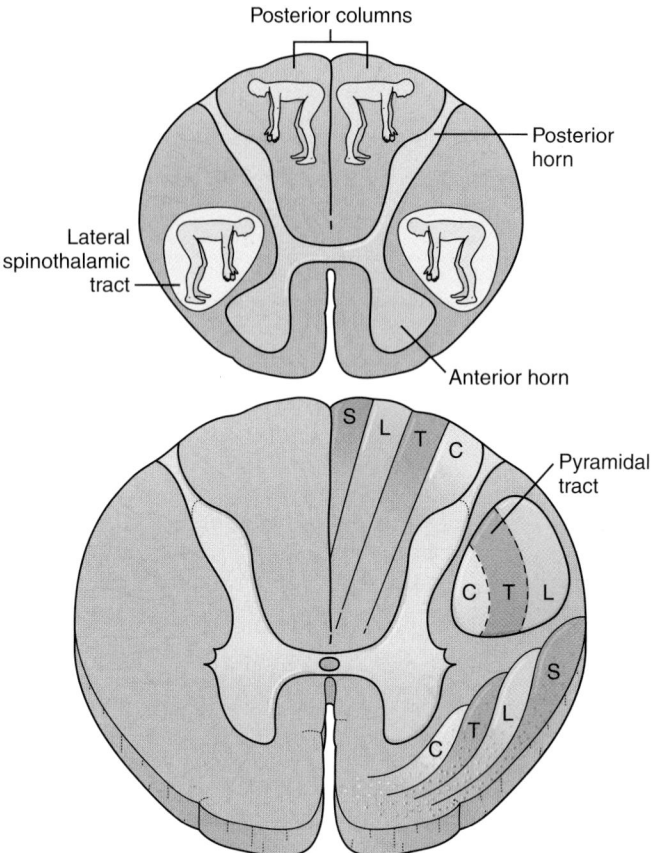

FIGURE 2.5 The posterior columns and lateral spinothalamic tracts are both somatotopically organized, but the lamination scheme is opposite in the two systems. In the posterior columns, the sacral fibers are mostly medial; in the spinothalamic tracts, the sacral fibers are mostly lateral.

weakness of the tongue and pharynx.[20,21] Vitamin B_{12} deficiency causes another type of dissociated sensory loss called *combined systems disease.* In this disease, vibration and proprioception are lost but pain and temperature sensation are spared. Lower motor neuron signs may also be present from the peripheral neuropathy due to vitamin B_{12} deficiency. *Central cord syndrome* is another spinal cord syndrome characterized by post-traumatic quadriparesis (worse in the arms) without sensory loss following a hyperextension cervical injury and usually occurs in the elderly with preexisting cervical canal stenosis. Injury to the ventral horns can cause the lower motor signs in the arms and hands, and injury to the corticospinal tracts results in a spastic quadriparesis.[22] The center of the spinal cord is a vascular watershed zone, which renders it more vulnerable to injury from edema, and furthermore, the cervical fibers are located more medially than lumbar fibers for the lower extremity. A *cruciate paralysis* due to a foramen magnum lesion may also result in hand weakness that will start in one hand and then go to the ipsilateral leg and the contralateral side.

There are a few pitfalls to consider when examining a patient with a potential myelopathy.[3] First, remember that the pyramidal tracts to the legs terminate neurologically at about L4 (Babinski is extensor hallucis longus: L5) and anatomically at around the T12 vertebral body (Fig. 2.7). Therefore,

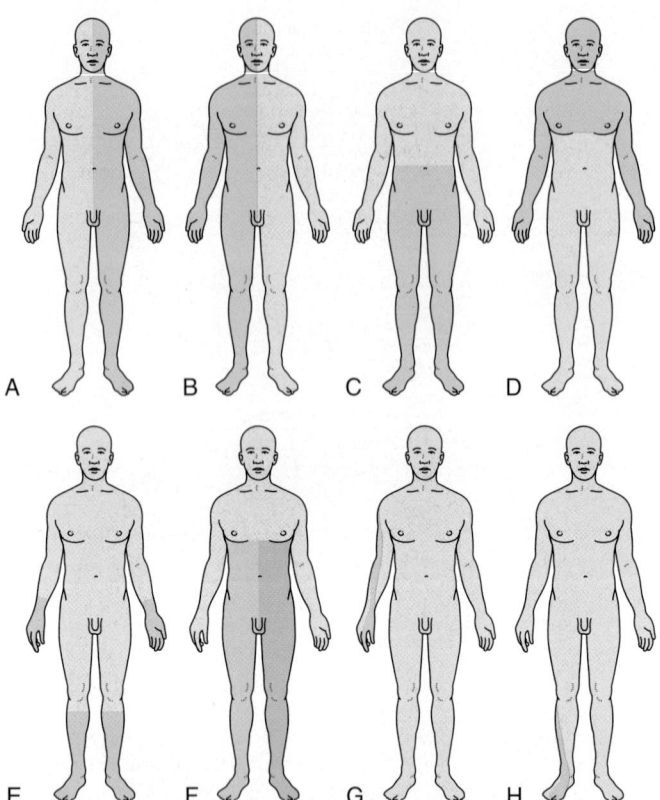

FIGURE 2.6 Common patterns of organic sensory loss. **A,** Hemisensory loss as a result of a hemispheric lesion. **B,** Crossed sensory loss to pain and temperature because of a lateral medullary lesion. **C,** Midthoracic spinal sensory level. **D,** Dissociated sensory loss to pain and temperature as a result of syringomyelia. **E,** Distal, symmetrical sensory loss because of peripheral neuropathy. **F,** Crossed spinothalamic loss on one side with posterior column loss on the opposite side because of Brown-Séquard syndrome. **G,** Dermatomal sensory loss because of cervical radiculopathy. **H,** Dermatomal sensory loss due to lumbosacral radiculopathy.

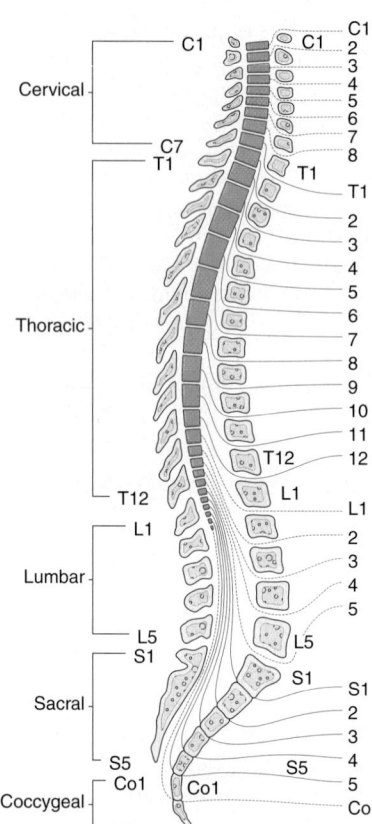

FIGURE 2.7 Relationship of the spinal cord segments and spinal nerves to the vertebral bodies and spinous processes.

a spastic paraparesis warrants a cervical or thoracic MRI and not a lumbar MRI. A spastic paraparesis does not automatically place the lesion between the thoracic and lumbar regions, because compressive lesions of the upper cervical cord can damage the cord's blood supply, and in addition, the descending leg fibers in the corticospinal tracts are more vulnerable to ischemia than the arm fibers. Second, a hemiparesis sparing the face is not necessarily the result of a cervical myelopathy because a pyramidal tract lesion in the internal capsule can also spare the face. Myelopathies, however, rarely result in a hemiparesis. Third, atrophy of the hands and arms may be the result of a high cervical extramedullary mass at the foramen magnum. An *extramedullary mass* is one that lies outside the spinal cord, either intradurally or extradurally. It is difficult by history and examination to distinguish an intramedullary from an extramedullary spinal cord lesion. In general, extramedullary lesions stretch nerve roots and can be more painful than intramedullary lesions and can cause compression of the spinal cord and nerve roots at the affected segment. Also, extramedullary lesions cause more pain in the supine position, which is the opposite of a herniated disk, in which lying flat can relieve the pain. Palpation of the spinous

processes and straight leg raising will often elicit pain from an extramedullary lesion but not an intramedullary lesion. *Intramedullary lesions*, in contrast, are more likely to produce atrophy, dissociated sensory loss, and early bowel and bladder problems. Sacral sparing can also be helpful, since the sacral sensory fibers are lateral in the spinothalamic tracts and may not be affected in a patient suffering from an intramedullary lesion. The cauda equina and conus medullaris syndromes are also important to distinguish from peripheral root symptoms. Lesions at either location interrupt multiple motor and sensory roots to the legs, producing bilateral lower extremity atrophy and weakness, depressed reflexes, down-pointing toes, and often a sensory level.

The peripheral nervous system is the final common pathway, whatever the movement involved. There are three classes of peripheral nerve lesions—those affecting a single peripheral nerve (mononeuropathy: carpal tunnel), multiple random individual nerves (mononeuropathy multiplex), and all peripheral nerves (polyneuropathy). A diagnosis of mononeuropathy is made by finding mixed motor/sensory loss in the distribution of individual peripheral nerves. A polyneuropathy is diagnosed by the constellation of distal, symmetrical stocking/glove sensory loss or lower motor neuron signs, and absent distal deep tendon reflexes. Electrical studies may also be of value in the diagnosis and prognosis of certain disorders and may help to distinguish between lesions of the motor neuron and the muscle and between spinal and peripheral nerve lesions.

Proximal weakness alone is the most common sign of a myopathy. Patients with proximal weakness waddle, because the weak gluteus medius muscles allow the pelvis to tilt from side to side. A patient may also have to lean forward and push off with both hands to get up from a chair, signifying pelvic girdle weakness. When trying to get up off the floor, children also adapt to pelvic girdle weakness and from the all-fours position, lock both their knees and push their trunk back over their legs by bracing their hands on their thighs (*Gower's sign*). *Myotonia* is a myopathic sign resulting from delayed relaxation after the muscle contracts and occurs in myotonia congenita, myotonic dystrophy, and paramyotonia congenita. As a rule, a myotonic patient shakes your hand and does not let go. In patients with widespread symmetrical weakness, pay attention to any sensory loss so that myopathic weakness is not confused with *Guillain-Barré syndrome*, an acute peripheral neuropathy with some distal vibratory loss and areflexia. Muscles above the shoulders are particularly susceptible to myasthenia gravis and botulism, two illnesses that attack the neuromuscular junction. Patients may present with a pure motor syndrome dominated by ophthalmoplegia, ptosis, weakness of chewing, difficulty sucking through a straw, dysphagia, and tongue weakness, but without pyramidal signs in the arms and legs. Almost any external ophthalmoplegia can be mimicked by myasthenia gravis[23]: internuclear ophthalmoplegia, up- or down-gaze palsy, sixth cranial nerve palsy, and a pupil-sparing third cranial nerve palsy. Neuromuscular blockade produces "fatigable" weakness that worsens with each contraction.

THE PEDIATRIC PATIENT

The neurological evaluation of the infant or child begins with the birth history, social history, developmental history, family history, and physical examination. The general appearance of the child should be noted, particularly the presence of any dysmorphic features or neurocutaneous abnormalities such as café au lait spots, neurofibromas,[24] facial port-wine stain in Sturge-Weber disease, depigmented lesion nevi in tuberous sclerosis, as well as a craniofacial dysmorphism seen with craniosynostosis. It is important to inspect the midline of the neck, back, and pilonidal area for any defects, particularly for small dimples above the level of the gluteal fold in the midline that might indicate the presence of occult spinal dysraphism or a dermal sinus tract. The head should be examined by inspection, palpation, and auscultation. The shape, size, and asymmetry may point to microcephaly, hydrocephalus, craniosynostosis (premature cranial suture fusion), or cerebral atrophy. Maximum head circumference should be recorded on a standard chart according to the patient's age and sex. The charting of the head circumference by the primary care provider and the neurosurgeon examining that plotted curve are essential parts of the examination and may indicate an intracranial pathology before it becomes symptomatic. The general appearance of the skull, prominence of venous pattern, and palpation of the anterior fontanelle may suggest increased intracranial pressure. The palpation of the anterior fontanelle is another essential part of the neurological examination. In the sitting position the fontanelle should be concave or sunken; in the supine position it may be more full (Fig. 2.8). Intracranial pressure can be estimated within several millimeters of water by palpating the anterior fontanelle. The baby

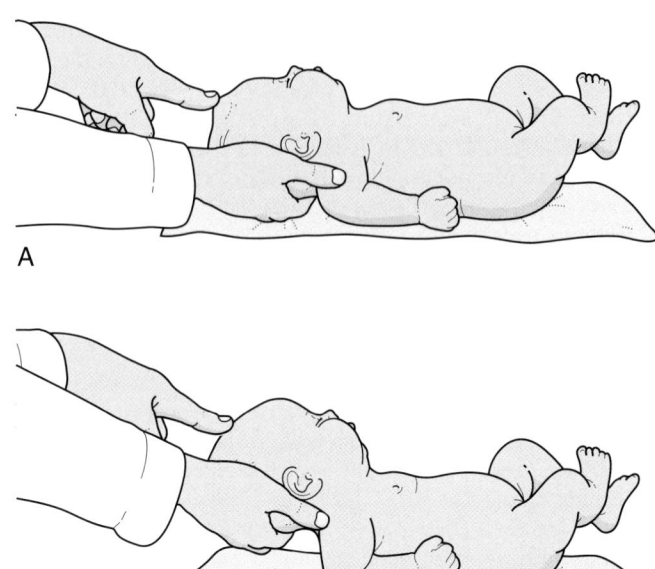

A

B

FIGURE 2.8 Positional changes in appearance of the fontanelle can be used to assess changes in intracranial pressure in children. In **B**, as this child's head is raised to 5 cm above the level of the right atrium of the heart (arbitrary physiological "zero" point), the fontanelle goes from bulging (**A**) to flat. The flat fontanelle means that the intracranial pressure equals the extracranial pressure. Because the height of the head is about 5 cm above the heart, the intracranial pressure is approximately 5 cm H_2O. This method can be used for estimating the intracranial pressure in a child with an open fontanelle (younger than 15 months). If the fontanelle is still bulging in the upright position in a quiet baby, this denotes raised intracranial pressure.

should be laid flat and the head should be gently raised off the examining table. At the point the fontanelle becomes flat, the intracranial pressure equals the extracranial pressure. If one measures the height the head has been raised in millimeters above a horizontal line drawn through the child's heart (the physiological zero point), then one has a fairly good estimate of the child's intracranial pressure. If the patent's anterior fontanelle consistently remains bulging and full when a quiet child is fully erect or sitting, then that denotes increased intracranial pressure. An imaging study such as a computed tomography (CT) or MRI of the head is a reasonable option. The anterior fontanelle is often closed by 18 to 24 months of age, although the posterior fontanelle closes after 2 to 3 months. Transillumination of the head with a flashlight in absolute darkness up to the age of approximately 9 months is an old-fashioned but useful way to detect severe hydrocephalus, arachnoid cysts, or subdural effusions at the bedside. However, it has become a lost art and cranial ultrasound has replaced this once important historical diagnostic modality. Percussion of the head, also of historical note, may produce a hollow or "cracked pot" resonance in patients with severe hydrocephalus (*Macewen's sign*). Cranial nerve examination can be more reliably tested beyond 30 weeks' gestation since prior to that time, the pupillary response to light is not predictably present, and the gag reflex is also not easily elicited.[4] The "blink reflex" is often used to determine the presence of functional vision in small infants but is absent in the newborn.[25] A slight degree of anisocoria is not unusual, particularly in infants and small children. The funduscopic examination is an essential part of the neurological examination (see discussion under neuro-ophthalmology). True papilledema with early obliteration of the disk margins and absent pulsations of the central veins is rare in patients under the age of 2 years because of the ability of the expansile skull to dissipate a rise in intracranial pressure. Medulloblastoma, a midline cerebellar tumor that can infiltrate the superior medullary velum, may produce bilateral fourth nerve palsies. A *setting sun sign* is the forced downward deviation of the eyes at rest with associated upward gaze palsy. *Parinaud syndrome* is an upward gaze palsy that can also be seen in any patient as a result of pressure on the upward gaze eye center in the region of the suprapineal recess and quadrigeminal plate due to hydrocephalus or a pineal region mass lesion.

Muscle tone is examined by passive movement of the joints and extremities, and both sides should be compared. During the first few months of life, normal hypertonia of the flexors of the elbows, hips, and knees occurs. Fine motor development is indicated by the appearance of a pincer grip at the age of 9 months. Careful note should be made of asymmetry or marked preference for one hand or the other in a young child, since the presence of definite hand preference before 24 months may raise suspicions of central nervous system or peripheral nerve impairment. Crawling is normally seen at 9 to 12 months on average, and at 12 to 15 months the infant begins to walk, although the gait is broad-based and unsteady.

Small, choreiform-like movements are common in healthy infants and are transient, emerging at approximately 6 weeks of age and tapering off between 14 and 20 weeks of age. Extremity tone can also be assessed by a number of reflexes. The "grasp reflex" is modulated by the frontal lobes and is present at birth but should disappear between 4 and 6 months. The Moro reflex is a primitive startle response and consists of extension of the arms followed by their flexion with simultaneous spreading of the fingers and is elicited by rapidly changing the infant's head position. The Moro reflex is present from birth to 4 months of age. The rooting reflex is elicited with gentle stimulation around the mouth, which produces turning of the head in the direction of the stimulus. The Landau reflex is evaluated by holding the infant in a prone position by supporting his or her abdomen. Normally the head extends and hips flex. If there is weakness of the lower extremities, hip flexion may not occur. Generalized reflexes of the extremities can be elicited beyond 33 weeks' gestation. The Babinski response is a nociceptive reflex elicited by noxious stroking of the lateral aspect of the plantar surface from the heel toward the toes. This response is normal in newborns until the age of 2 years. However, asymmetry of the Babinski response is abnormal at any age and may reflect an upper motor neuron lesion. Unsustained clonus can also be normal if symmetrical, although sustained clonus is suspect at any age.

NEURO-OPHTHALMOLOGY

No neurological examination is complete without a detailed study of the visual system. Because of the extent of the visual system and its intimate relations with other areas of the brain,

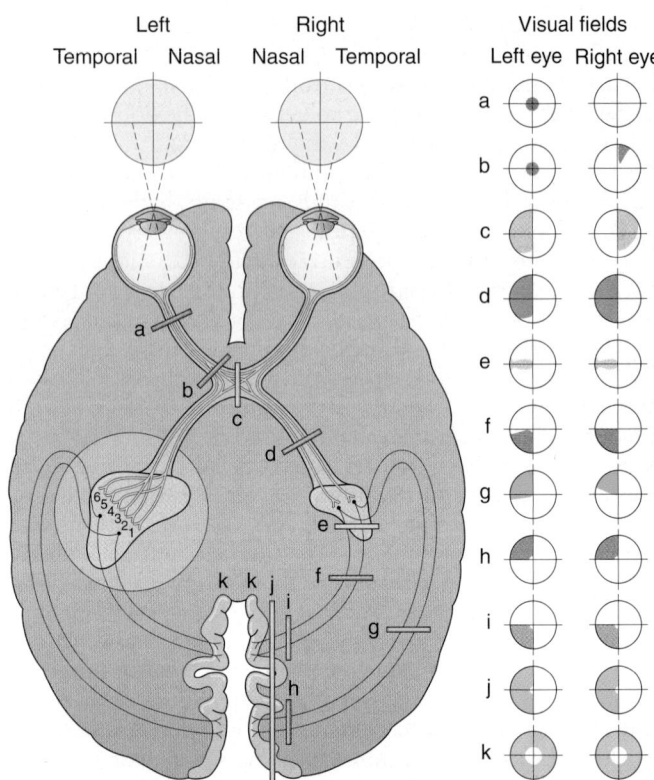

FIGURE 2.9 Characteristic defects of the visual field produced by lesions at various points along the visual pathways.

much valuable information can be obtained. Color vision is especially important in neuro-ophthalmology in the detection of pregeniculate pathway lesions. The visual field to a red object is interestingly more affected by damage in these areas. Similarly an optic tract lesion may produce an incongruous hemianopic defect of color vision. The results of confrontation testing are conventionally recorded as seen by the patient, which means reversing the defect as seen by the examiner during confrontation testing. The nature of the field defect should be carefully documented: left central scotoma (optic nerve lesion), bitemporal hemianopia (chiasmatic lesion), right upper quadrantic hemianopia (left temporal), macula-sparing hemianopia (lesions of the optic tract), and right homonomous hemianopia's scotoma lesion (tip of occipital pole) (Fig. 2.9). The areas of calcarine cortex subserving the peripheral fields lie anteriorly and those subserving macular vision are concentrated at the extreme tip: the upper fields are represented in the lower half below the calcarine sulcus and the lower fields in the upper half of the cortex. Special attention should be paid to whether the defect crosses the horizontal meridian, because retinal lesions due to vascular occlusion cannot do so. The defect may extend to the blind spot, and defects due to vitamin B_{12} deficiency, toxins, or glaucoma usually extend into it. Lastly, the defect may cross the vertical meridian because organic visual field defects have a sharp vertical edge at the midline. The macula of the retina responsible for central vision is situated to the temporal side of the optic nerve head, which then moves centrally into the optic nerve as it joins the chiasm. This papillomacular bundle conveying central vision in the optic nerve is very vulnerable to extrinsic compression

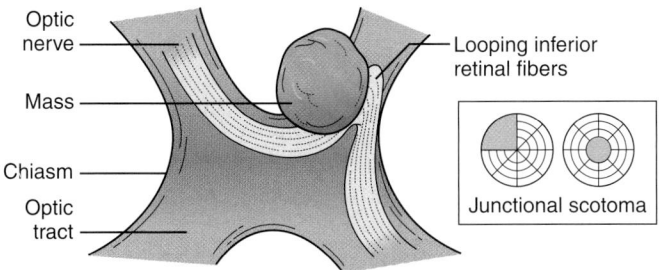

FIGURE 2.10 A junctional scotoma may result from a mass impinging on the optic nerve at its junction with the chiasm.

by mass lesions. It is equally important to check for an early temporal field cut (contralateral junctional scotoma) in the opposite eye due to damage to the decussating nasal fibers (anterior chiasmatic syndrome of Traquair) (Fig. 2.10).

The importance of papilledema is that it is usually associated with raised intracranial pressure, of which it may be the only objective sign. Papilledema (swelling of the optic nerve head) may cause field defects in several ways: enlargement of the blind spot, exudate into the macula, chronic papilledema causing gliosis, papilledema due to hydrocephalus, and a binasal hemianopia, a stretched posterior cerebral artery with cerebral herniation causing a macular-sparing hemianopia. Raised intracranial pressure due to any mass lesion in the brain has to be included in the differential diagnosis, although conditions interfering with cerebrospinal fluid (CSF) circulation or resorption should also be considered. Papilledema develops within a day or two after intracranial pressure begins to rise, but will not often be found in the first few hours of such a rise. Papilledema may also persist for several weeks upon normalization of the intracranial pressure. A similar ophthalmoscopic picture can result from acute retrobulbar neuritis, which is a response of the optic nerve to a variety of toxic and metabolic insults and is commonly seen with an attack of multiple sclerosis (Devic's disease). The classic field defect is a central scotoma, and symptomatically, the patient complains that central vision is impaired by a "fluffy ball" or a "steamed-up window" associated with some eye discomfort.

Diplopia may not always be due to extraocular nerve palsies. For example, thyrotoxicosis is characterized by weakness of the superior rectus and lateral rectus muscles as a result of an inflammatory myopathic process. Myasthenia gravis is characterized by diplopia and ptosis of the eyelid which is fatiguable. Diplopia under conditions of fatigue may also be due to lateral strabismus and unmasking of a lifelong squint. The acuity of onset of the diplopia must be determined as well as if there is any variability or remission to help differentiate the preceding diagnoses. A painful onset may suggest a compressive lesion due to aneurysmal dilatation causing a third cranial nerve palsy. Associated congestion of the eye may raise the possibility of a granulomatous lesion in the orbit, either pseudotumor or Tolosa-Hunt syndrome (recurrent unilateral orbital pain accompanied by transient extraocular nerve palsies and a high erythrocyte sedimentation rate with a dramatic response to steroids). A caroticocavernous fistula can also cause a painful and red eye that is proptotic and can be associated with rapidly deteriorating visual acuity.

ANCILLARY DIAGNOSTIC TESTS

If a definite diagnosis is not reached either on clinical grounds alone or with the aid of ancillary neurodiagnostic tests, sometimes the best test is said to be a second examination. However, the rapidly increasing sophistication and diagnostic accuracy of neurodiagnostic procedures have challenged the continued need for a detailed and systematic neurological examination.

CT and MRI have revolutionized the diagnostic evaluation of neurological patients and have eliminated the need for invasive pneumoencephalography and ventriculography. Almost uniformly, an unenhanced (i.e., noncontrast) CT of the brain suffices for patients seen in the emergency room presenting after trauma or with a new neurological deficit. CT is the best test to rule out the presence of hemorrhage and is more sensitive than MRI for detecting acute blood loss. CT with three-dimensional (3D) reconstruction is also preferable to MRI for the detection of intracranial calcifications and craniosynostosis. CT angiography (CTA) is obtained by administering a rapid bolus intravenous contrast agent that allows the selective imaging of vascular structures, and can be quite useful in the evaluation of subarachnoid hemorrhage to localize aneurysm pathology, carotid stenosis in a patient with transient ischemic attacks, or a traumatic carotid or vertebral dissection. CT is also the study of choice in the evaluation of the skull base and cranial vault (i.e., craniofacial disorders) because of the potential for exquisite bony detail.

MRI is noninvasive and has a number of diverse clinical uses in the evaluation of neurological disorders without exposure to ionizing radiation. However, as a result of the longer acquisition time and less access to the patient during the study, it is not routinely used for acute trauma or unstable patients. MRI offers superb anatomical detail in the detection of structural causes for neurological dysfunction such as tumors, arteriovenous malformations, demyelinating disease, or stroke. Generally, T1-weighted images provide a better view of structural anatomy, whereas T2-weighted images are exquisitely sensitive to water (hydrocephalus) and cerebral edema and are preferred for the detection of pathology. MRI has been shown to be superior to CT for the detection and characterization of posterior fossa lesions. MRI has been used to define the anatomy in epilepsy patients with mesial temporal sclerosis or with anomalies of cortical architecture, depict the compression of the trigeminal nerve by a vascular loop, and evaluate CSF flow in patients with Chiari malformation and syringomyelia or normal-pressure hydrocephalus. Diffusion-weighted MRI is extremely sensitive to the brownian motion of water protons and is used in the early evaluation of stroke in evolution. MRA (arteriography or venography) is an excellent way to evaluate the vascular structures and avoids invasive cerebral angiography. MR perfusion techniques have evolved to quantify blood flow to areas of ischemia or hyperemia and have been used in patients with brain tumors, stroke, and subarachnoid hemorrhage. MRI can be combined with high-resolution MR spectroscopy to evaluate the spectral peaks obtained that reflect the concentrations of the metabolites and some neurotransmitters in the voxel area under investigation. Spinal MRI is the most efficient way to screen for spinal disease and can be combined with a gadolinium contrast agent in the setting of neoplasia or infection. Functional MRI is useful in the preoperative localization of the motor and somatosensory cortex based on the identification of cortical activation by detecting changes in venous oxygen.

Following funduscopic and CT or MRI examinations, CSF analysis is indicated in patients suspected of having central nervous system bacterial, fungal, or viral infection as well as subarachnoid hemorrhage. Lumbar CSF pressure recordings are also useful in the diagnosis of pseudotumor cerebri and normal-pressure hydrocephalus, although it is important to recognize that falsely high pressures result when the knees are pressed against the abdomen and when the patient holds his breath. The chief danger of a lumbar puncture (spinal tap) is uncal herniation in patients with raised intracranial pressure because of focal disease. The spinal fluid is normally clear and colorless. Turbidity can result from the presence of leukocytes or bacteria, and hemorrhage can result from a "bloody tap" or a subarachnoid hemorrhage. In normal adult CSF, there are 0 to 4 lymphocytes or mononuclear cells per mm^3, and no polymorphonuclear lymphocytes or red blood cells. Polymorphonuclear lymphocytes can be present in the newborn, but they are not normally found in CSF taken from healthy children older than 1 year of age. In general, 1 white blood cell can be subtracted for every 700 red blood cells in the CSF. The CSF/plasma ratio for glucose is normally 0.60 to 0.80. Low protein content suggests its relative exclusion by the blood-brain or blood-CSF barriers, although high protein levels are found in patients with blood (1000 red blood cells raise the total protein level by 1.5 mg/dL) or intraspinal tumors. Among spinal cord tumors, intradural extramedullary tumors such as meningiomas or neurofibromas often have elevated CSF protein values greater than 100 mg/dL (Table 2.5).

Angiography now plays a supplementary role in defining the vascularity except in the setting of subarachnoid hemorrhage, a suspected carotid-cavernous fistula, trauma, or in the preoperative planning stages for the treatment of an arteriovenous malformation or for adjuvant preoperative embolization of a tumor. MRA or CT angiography may one day replace the diagnostic capabilities of cerebral angiography if their sensitivity or specificity prove equal to those of angiography, the gold standard.

A positron emission tomography (PET) scan combined with fluorodeoxyglucose, or FDG ([^{18}F]fluoro-2-deoxy-D-glucose 6-phosphate) is used clinically in the evaluation of patients with dementia, brain tumors, and epilepsy. FDG is transported into the cell and is not a substrate for further degradation after conversion to glucose 6-phosphate and therefore is an excellent marker of brain metabolism. Patients with dementia often have abnormal PET scans with reduced metabolism in the frontal and parietal regions. FDG-PET techniques have been used to evaluate patients with temporal lobe epilepsy, both ictal and interictal. In general, hypometabolism in the temporal lobe is lateralized to the side of seizure onset interictally, but may be hypermetabolic during the ictal state. Finally, FDG-PET studies have been used in patients with brain tumors to characterize the most malignant component (i.e., hypermetabolic) of a tumor, assess prognosis, and differentiate recurrent tumor from radiation necrosis.

Single-photon emission computed tomography (SPECT) often uses gamma-emitting isotopes, such as technetium (^{99m}Tc), to assess brain perfusion and cerebrovascular reserve. Using HMPAO (hexamethyl-propylene amine oxime) as a marker for cerebral blood flow, cerebrovascular reserve can be determined with or without Diamox, a cerebral vasodilator. HMPAO is lipophilic and crosses the blood-brain barrier and is then rapidly converted to a hydrophilic form and trapped in the brain. SPECT has also proved useful in localizing abnormalities in patients with temporal lobe epilepsy.

Transcranial Doppler ultrasound has been used to record flow velocities from extra- and intracranial arteries. The recorded velocity is not a direct measurement of flow, but proportionality does exist between velocity and flow when the arterial diameter remains constant. Transcranial Doppler ultrasound has been invaluable in its capacity to determine noninvasively the degree of vasospasm after subarachnoid hemorrhage, to evaluate the hemodynamic significance of intracranial stenosis, to monitor changes in autoregulation following closed head injury and microemboli in the circulation, and to assess changes in cerebral blood flow during a carotid endarterectomy or arteriovenous malformation resection.

Electromyography and nerve conduction studies can often aid in the evaluation of neuromuscular disorders or spinal disease, such as herniated disks or spondylosis. A needle electrode is inserted into the muscle and action potentials are generated by muscle activity. Normal resting muscle is electrically silent except for the insertion potential produced by

TABLE 2.5 Typical Cerebrospinal Fluid Findings in Various Disorders

Condition	Pressure	Red Blood Cells/mm³	White Blood Cells/mm³	Differential	Glucose (mg/dL)	Protein (mg/dL)
Normal	Normal	0	0-5	Mononuclear	45-80	15-45
Bacterial meningitis	↑	0	500-100,000	Neutrophils	Low	↑
Tuberculous meningitis	↑	0	50-500	Mononuclear	Low	↑
Viral meningitis	Normal to ↑	0	5-500	Mononuclear	Normal	15-100
Subarachnoid hemorrhage	Normal to ↑	10,000-500,000	↑ in proportion to red blood cells	Mononuclear and neutrophils	Normal	↑
Multiple sclerosis	Normal	0	0-50	Mononuclear	Normal	20-100
Guillain-Barré syndrome	Normal	0	0-50	Mononuclear	Normal	20-500
Brain tumors	Normal to ↑	0	0-100	Mononuclear	Normal	Variable (↑ in acoustic schwannoma)

needle insertion. After denervation of the muscle, fibrillation potentials appear. Nerve conduction velocities can be used to differentiate demyelination and axonal degeneration from muscular disorders. Conduction rates of motor nerves can be measured by stimulating the nerve at two points and recording the latency between each stimulus and the muscle contraction. Somatosensory evoked potentials are recorded after stimulation of peripheral nerves and are sensitive to compare side to side.

DIAGNOSIS AND INVESTIGATION OF CEREBRAL TUMORS

History and physical examination remain the gold standard for the initial assessment of any patient suspected of suffering from a primary or secondary cerebral neoplasm. However, the advent of CT and MRI has transformed the investigation.[26] The cardinal symptoms and signs of a cerebral tumor are headache, vomiting, malaise, cognitive decline, and papilledema. These are most commonly seen with posterior fossa tumors or those which have blocked the flow of CSF. However, in general, less than 0.1% of patients referred to the hospital for headaches have a cerebral tumor. Thus lies the diagnostic dilemma for the primary care physician. A first (nonfebrile, nonmetabolic-induced, nontraumatic) epileptic seizure occurring in an adult patient warrants an electroencephalogram (EEG) or an imaging study such as an MRI or CT scan. An EEG is of value in the assessment of patients who have presented with an epileptic fit, although it may be misleadingly normal. The EEG does not exclude the presence of epilepsy or organic disease and a single normal EEG is of little value. The basic rhythm observed in an adult is called the *alpha rhythm* (frequency of 8-13 Hz) and is present when the patient is relaxed with his or her eyes closed and suppressed when the patient opens his or her eyes or concentrates.

Angiography still retains a role in the investigation of tumors, particularly in demonstrating and embolizing (occluding) the blood supply of highly vascular tumors such as meningioma, choroid plexus neoplasms, or hemangioblastoma. Adult supratentorial tumors account for 90% of cerebral neoplasms and occur in the lobes in a frequency roughly proportional to the size of the lobe. Unlike in children, 20% to 30% of cerebral tumors in adults prove to be metastases. Therefore a chest radiograph and careful physical examination are essential.

HEADACHE

Luckily not all bad headaches are the result of brain tumors or aneurysms and the seriousness of a headache does not uniformly correlate with its pathological severity. However, a careful headache history is essential in deciding on a further workup, especially is acute situations. We often suggest a headache log for a patient whose headaches are problematic. All the extracranial structures, including the arteries and muscles, are pain sensitive. Intracranially the dura and dura-based vessels are pain sensitive, although the brain itself, cortical vessels, and pia-arachnoid are pain insensitive. Pain can also be referred to the head from other structures sharing its innervation such as the eye, ear, sinuses, and

teeth.[6,7,27] The temporal pattern of the headache; its site and radiation; precipitating, aggravating, and mitigating factors; accompanying symptoms; and family history should all be considered.[28]

Headaches occur in about 97% of all subarachnoid hemorrhages from aneurysms. They are often severe, described as "the worst headache of my life." They are sudden and may be associated with vomiting, photophobia, syncope (apoplexy), meningismus, and loss of consciousness. Classic migraine is frontotemporal in site, pulsatile, and often unilateral and may be accompanied by a prodrome of visual phenomena, nausea, and mood changes. A cluster headache is of very rapid onset, short-lived, and characterized by pain in and around the eye with associated lacrimation and nasal watering. Nocturnal attacks are more frequent and the attacks are often clustered together for 6 to 12 weeks. Benign thunderclap headaches will reach maximum intensity in less than a minute and are sudden, severe global headaches associated with vomiting in 50% of patients. It is not always trivial to distinguish a severe migraine or thunderclap headache from a subarchnoid hemorrhage headache. It often requires a lumbar puncture or CT scan, which are the most sensitive screening tests. Cerebral angiography remains the gold standard for aneurysm diagnosis but CT angiography in many institutions is being used in a parallel fashion.

A typical tension headache is characterized by a tight feeling in the suboccipital muscles which spreads over the top of the head and is exacerbated by stress. A typical pressure headache is one that occurs on waking or at the end of the day, is aggravated by bending or movement, and may be responsive to analgesics.[29] A patient with a Chiari I malformation–related headache often complains of "tussive" symptoms that are felt in the back of the head or neck and are worse with coughing, laughing, bending, or any Valsalva-related action. They are better at rest. Analgesics often do not work for these headaches. A headache starting after the age of 60 with pain and tenderness over the temporal region may represent temporal arteritis and is associated with a high erythrocyte sedimentation rate, visual impairment, and generalized malaise.

VASCULAR DISEASES

To make the clinical differentiation between a neoplastic or other space-occupying lesion and a stroke one must substantially rely on the temporal history. Following a stroke, it is unusual to find a vessel actually occluded because most occlusions are the result of temporary embolic blockage with rapid subsequent recanalization. Stroke or "brain attack" emphasizes the abrupt onset of symptoms, the single characteristic feature of a vascular accident. It is important to recognize a stuttering onset of symptoms, characterized by repeated identical brief episodes of hemiparesis with full recovery, known as *transient ischemic attacks*. There are three main types of hemorrhagic strokes: (1) classic hypertensive intracerebral hemorrhage as a result of rupture of one of the peripheral lenticulostriate arteries; (2) hemorrhage associated with a cerebral arteriovenous malformation; and (3) subarachnoid hemorrhage as a result of aneurysms arising from the vessels traversing the subarachnoid space. Thunderclap headache, acute nausea, vomiting, and neck stiffness are the hallmarks of both subarachnoid hemorrhage and meningitis. Three considerations should be applied to working up a patient with cerebrovascular disease. (1) Is the extent of the lesion typical of occlusion of an identifiable vessel? (2) Is there any hematological disorder that could have predisposed to or mimicked a cerebrovascular accident? (3) Are there any causative factors or comorbidity such as hypertension, atrial fibrillation, vessel stenosis, or myocardial infarction? If the clinical suspicion is high for a subarachnoid hemorrhage and the CT scan is normal, a lumbar puncture should be performed. Normally the CSF is clear and colorless, and therefore, if the CSF is pink or bloody, differentiation between a traumatic lumbar puncture and a subarachnoid hemorrhage must be made by performing cell counts on three sequential samples of CSF. Classically, a small amount of CSF is centrifuged and the supernatant is inspected. If the supernatant is xanthochromic, there is a high likelihood that a subarachnoid hemorrhage has occurred. However, an ultra-early lumbar puncture (<2 hours) may precede the window to establish whether or not a subarachnoid hemorrhage has occurred. On occasion, an ophthalmological examination may reveal retinal or vitreous hemorrhage thought secondary to the subarachnoid hemorrhage.[8,30] This syndrome of retinal hemorrhage in association with subarachnoid hemorrhage is known as *Terson's syndrome.*

HYSTERIA AND MALINGERING

A single disease can often explain all the symptoms and signs; however, a patient may have a variety of diseases, old and new, organic and functional.[3] Although the accuracy of neurodiagnostic tests is superb, it is the additional duty of the neurosurgeon to identify the malingering patient, for hysterical signs present more often in the nervous system than in any other organ system.[3]

Beginning in the cortex, functional signs manifest as seizures, stuttering, amnesia, and coma. The most definitive test for psychogenic seizures is a normal EEG during the ictus or seizure. A postictal EEG should also be abnormal with slowing. If the physician happens to witness a motor seizure, concentrate on the jerking, which should have a quick and slow phase (a true jerk) and not simply a tremor. Amnesia that includes the patient's own name is often hysterical. Hysterical coma can most easily be diagnosed by performing cold calorics. The presence of nystagmus indicates retained physiological connections between the brainstem and cortex.

Reactive pupils do not necessarily indicate hysterical blindness, because there may still be a lesion behind the midbrain, damaging the optic radiations or occipital cortex. Normal optokinetic nystagmus in the face of blindness does indicate hysteria or malingering, because optokinetic nystagmus requires intact connections from the retina to the occipital cortex. A constricted visual field should also be cone-shaped. Each time the examiner doubles the distance between him and the patient, the intact field should double in diameter and not leave only a central core of retained tunnel vision. Some patients can mimic a sixth cranial nerve palsy by converging the eyes while looking to the side. The tip-off is that convergence also constricts the pupil. Diplopia should often disappear when one covers one eye; however, monocular diplopia does occur in rare cases such as a retinal detachment or lens dislocation.[31]

Eliciting collapsing or ratchety weakness versus true weakness when the muscle gradually gives way can be a challenge.

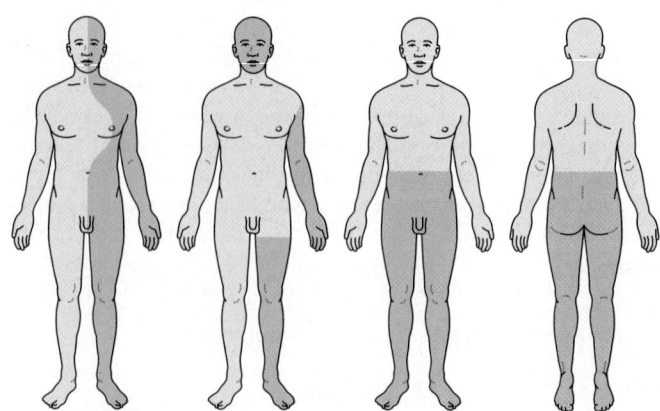

FIGURE 2.11 Common patterns of nonorganic sensory loss.

While vigorously testing the strength of an individual muscle, the examiner suddenly lets go. If the muscle fails to spring back to its contracted position, hysterical weakness may be present. When testing grip strength, watch the thumb; if the flexor pollicis longus does not flex the distal interphalangeal joint, the patient was not really giving maximal effort. The Hoover maneuver is another method of detecting insufficient effort by the patient. After placing one palm under the patient's heel, the examiner asks the patient to lift the other leg against the examiner's other hand. If the examiner does not feel the heel digging into his palm, the patient is not really trying to lift his leg. Hysterically hemiparetic patients also forget that pyramidal lesions selectively weaken the tibialis anterior. Although they drag the leg, there's no circumduction; in fact, they purposely elevate the toe to keep it from scraping the floor. Withdrawal of a limb to pain also belies another common hysterical complaint: marked sensory loss. Hysterical hemihypesthesia may be uncovered by demonstrating nonorganic splitting of vibration at the midline (Fig. 2.11). Several nonorganic physical signs have also been described by Waddel, such as pain with gently tapping the lower back or with toe dorsiflexion,[32] and are collectively referred as *Waddel signs.*

We hope this review has provided a comprehensive and systematic approach to the evaluation of a patient with a neurological disorder.

SELECTED KEY REFERENCES

Damasio AR. *Aphasia. N Engl J Med.* 1992;326:531-539.
Ojemann GA. Cortical organization of language. *J Neurosci.* 1991;11:2281-2287.
Strub RL, Black FW. *The Mental Status Examination in Neurology.* Philadelphia: FA Davis; 1985.
Schneider RC, Crosby EC, Russo RH, Gosch HH. Traumatic spinal cord syndromes and their management. *Clin Neurosurg.* 1973;20:424-492.
Shareef AH, Dafer RM, Jay WM. Neuro-ophthalmologic manifestations of primary headache disorders. *Semin Ophthalmol.* 2008;23(3):169-177.
Waddel G. Nonorganic physical signs in low-back pain. *Spine.* 1980;5:117.

Please go to expertconsult.com to view complete list of references.

3 Principles of Modern Neuroimaging

Kathleen R. Tozer Fink, Michael R. Levitt, James R. Fink

CLINICAL PEARLS

- Noncontrast head computed tomography (CT) is the imaging test of choice in the evaluation of acute neurological disease such as head trauma, hemorrhage, and acute hydrocephalus.

- Noncontrast head CT can also detect early signs of ischemic stroke, including sulcal effacement, and insular ribbon and dense MCA (middle cerebral artery) signs.

- In CT perfusion (CTP) of acute stroke, areas of ischemic penumbra show prolonged mean transit times (MTTs) and normal cerebral blood volume (CBV). These areas are potentially salvageable with neurointerventional therapies.

- Intravenous contrast agent is useful in the detailed evaluation of vascular structures, as well as for identification of blood-brain barrier breakdown, such as occurs with mass lesions and infection.

- Vascular flow-voids are best seen on T2-weighted magnetic resonance imaging (MRI), and edema is best assessed with fluid attenuated inversion recovery (FLAIR) imaging.

- Gradient echo (GRE) sequences highlight blood products in assessment of subtle hemorrhage or small cavernous malformations.

- Functional MRI detects changes in blood oxygenation in areas of the brain involved in specific tasks such as speech, vision, or movement.

- Areas of restricted diffusion (such as acute stroke) appear bright on diffusion sequences and dark on ADC (apparent diffusion coefficient) maps. These sequences also distinguish between ring-enhancing lesions; central areas of abscess and lymphoma are bright on diffusion, but those of glioma and metastasis are not.

- Diffusion tensor imaging (DTI) measures organized fluid movement along white matter tracts and can aid in the surgical resection of lesions in eloquent cortex.

- Seizure foci show ictal hyperperfusion and interictal hypoperfusion in single-photon emission computed tomography (SPECT) imaging.

Neuroimaging is vital to the practice of neurosurgery, and an understanding of the strengths and limitations of available imaging modalities is important for the practicing neurosurgeon. As the number of imaging studies performed worldwide has increased, issues of patient safety, including the risks of ionizing radiation and contrast use, and rising health care costs have become increasingly important.

Even though the number of randomized controlled studies and cost effectiveness analyses regarding the use of imaging in neurosurgical practice remains small, this is changing. In an effort to provide clinicians with easy access to the latest data on the most effective imaging modalities for a particular clinical question, the American College of Radiology has established a set of criteria to evaluate the use of imaging in patient care, called the ACR Appropriateness Criteria.[1] These criteria are composed by consensus among a panel of experts in radiology with input from nonradiology experts based on critical reviews of the literature. The criteria are available online through a searchable database based on patient symptom and imaging modality using a free search engine (http://acsearch.acr.org/).[2]

This chapter aims to describe the fundamentals of currently used imaging techniques and to highlight the advantages of different techniques in neurosurgical illness. Important considerations of radiation exposure and risks of contrast agents are discussed briefly. Next, a survey of key general imaging findings pertinent to neurosurgeons are described in detail in the sections on computed tomography (CT). The section on magnetic resonance imaging (MRI) approaches the topic from a different angle, highlighting advantages of specific imaging sequences. Angiographic modalities of CT and MRI are then addressed. Advanced imaging techniques including diffusion tensor imaging (DTI), spectroscopy, and functional MRI are also briefly discussed.

PRINCIPLES

Radiography

Discovered by Wilhelm Roentgen in 1895, x-rays are photons carrying electromagnetic energy which are created by an anode-cathode system within a vacuum.[3] These photons are of higher energy and shorter wavelength than visible light. When photons collide with atoms of varying sizes, they either pass through or are absorbed. Larger (heavier, radiopaque) atoms, such as calcium or metals, are more likely to absorb the energy of the photons than smaller (lighter, radiolucent) atoms and small molecules, such as water or air. When a patient is positioned in a beam of x-rays, the x-rays will be differentially absorbed based on the tissue components (bone, soft tissue, aerated sinuses). Photons that pass through the patient strike a detector and create an x-ray image, producing a two-dimensional projected image of the different attenuation properties of body tissue.

Fluoroscopy is a variation of radiography in which images are obtained in rapid succession and displayed in real time on a screen. In angiography, intravenous contrast material is injected into vessels during continuous fluoroscopy. Digital subtraction angiography (DSA) is a technique in which a baseline or mask image is initially obtained of the area of interest. This baseline image is subtracted from subsequent images obtained during intravascular contrast injection, optimizing visualization of the contrast agent itself within opacified vessels. With modern angiography systems, images can be acquired from multiple different projections during a single contrast injection by rapidly rotating the fluoroscopy unit around the patient, allowing reconstruction of a three-dimensional image of the vascular structures.

Computed Tomography

Sir Godfrey Hounsfield and Dr. Allan Cormack invented the first computed axial tomographic scanner in 1972, which earned them the Nobel Prize for Medicine in 1979.[4] Computed tomography (CT) scanners have advanced significantly since that time, rapidly increasing in speed and resolution. Modern scanners use a rotating x-ray tube and detector array that revolve around the body, obtaining tissue attenuation information from beams or rays of tissues within a slab. Standard axial images are obtained by applying a reconstruction algorithm, typically filtered back projection, to reconstruct the two-dimensional image.[5] Sagittal, coronal, or oblique imaging planes can be reconstructed from the axial sequences by computer reformatting. Radiodense contrast material administered intravenously or parenterally can outline hollow structures such as blood vessels or the digestive system.

CT density is quantitatively measured in Hounsfield units (HU).[5] Hounsfield units describe a linear scale of attenuation that is constant across scanner platforms, with water and air given arbitrary values of 0 and –1000, respectively. Materials with increased x-ray attenuation with respect to water have a positive HU value, and those with less x-ray attenuation than water have a negative HU value (Table 3.1).[4,6]

CT images can be viewed in different ways to accentuate different tissues. Window level describes the center point of the gray scale, and window width describes the range of CT

TABLE 3.1 Computed Tomography Hounsfield Unit Values	
Tissue	**Hounsfield Units**
Air	–1000
Fat	–(60-100)
Water	0
White matter	35
Gray matter	45
Blood—acute hemorrhage	50-70
Calcium	>150
Dense bone	1000
Metal	>>1000

values displayed.[6] For example, gray matter has an attenuation of approximately 35 HU, and white matter attenuation is approximately 45 HU. In order to differentiate gray matter from white matter, a narrow window is needed to highlight small changes in HU values. On the other hand, if detailed evaluation of dense material such as bone is desired, a wide window better delineates the margins. Window level and width are easily manipulated using most imaging viewing software.

In addition to window width and level, CT scans are generally processed using different reconstruction filters, frequently referred to as *bone* and *standard algorithms*.[5] Both filters can be applied to a single acquisition of data, allowing accentuation of different structures. Standard algorithm is a method of averaging adjacent pixels to accentuate soft tissue detail. Standard algorithm images are useful for evaluating gray-white matter differentiation and for detecting blood. Bone algorithm images are processed to maximize edges, thus accentuating high-density materials such as calcium and metal. Bone algorithm images are also useful for evaluating lung parenchyma due to the differences in attenuation between aerated lung and small soft tissue attenuation structures such as blood vessels and pulmonary nodules.

Issues with Computed Tomography

Radiation Exposure

There is increasing awareness among health care providers and the general public of radiation exposure from medical imaging and the carcinogenic potential of x-rays. This is in part related to the dramatic increase in the utilization of CT over the past few decades. According to the American College of Radiology White Paper on Radiation Dose in Medicine[7] approximately 3 million CT studies were performed in 1980, compared to approximately 60 million in 2005. Although CT has undoubtedly contributed positively to the care of patients, the cumulative radiation dose may have increased the risk of cancer in exposed patients, and up to 1% of U.S. cancers may be related to medical exposures. Based on studies of Japanese atomic bomb survivors, cancer risk increases with exposures as low as 50 mSv (millisieverts). Millisieverts are a measure of effective radiation dose, which is weighted for tissue sensitivity to the negative effects of radiation.[8]

Cancer risk depends on tissue type, and neural tissue is relatively resistant. Exposure to more radiosensitive tissues may also occur with neuroimaging. For example, exposure of the cornea may lead to cataracts in a dose-dependent fashion.

The lens of the eye receives a dose of 40 to 50 mGy (milliGray, a measure of absorbed dose) per head CT,[9,10] which can be reduced by eye shielding. Lens opacities have been seen with as little exposure as 500 mGy (10 CT scan equivalents), with vision-limiting cataracts forming at doses greater than 4 Gy (approximately 80 CT scan equivalents). Children are more susceptible than adults.

The ALARA principle (As Low As Reasonably Achievable) of keeping exposure to a minimum is an important guideline to follow when imaging patients, particularly when ionizing radiation will be used. This principle aims to balance the clinical benefit of the imaging study with the risks, however low they may be. Additionally, physicians should take care to protect themselves when using fluoroscopy for angiography and during implant and spine procedures. Specific questions about radiation exposure and protection can be addressed to the local staff radiologist or medical physicist.

Iodinated Contrast Agents

Iodinated contrast material may be associated with contrast-induced nephropathy (CIN) in patients with renal failure, particularly those with diabetes mellitus. Strategies to reduce the risk of CIN include volume expansion through intravenous or oral fluids. Sodium bicarbonate infusion and prophylactic *N*-acetylcysteine have also shown efficacy compared to normal saline infusion.[11] In patients with diminished renal function, reduced doses of contrast agent or iso-osmolar nonionic contrast agent can be considered. Of course, the best prevention of CIN is the avoidance of intravenous contrast material altogether, although this is not always feasible.

Another potential complication of iodinated contrast agent is contrast reaction. The incidence of contrast reaction after CT contrast scan is 0.2% to 0.7% (approximately 1/225).[12,13] Contrast reactions may be mild or severe. Most reactions are mild, including nausea, vomiting, or rash. Severe reactions occur infrequently, with an incidence of approximately 0.05% (1/2000) for low osmolar iodinated contrast agent.[12,13] Severe contrast reactions include bronchospasm, laryngeal edema, and cardiovascular collapse.

In patients with a history of moderate or severe contrast allergy, premedication strategies decrease, but do not eliminate, the risk of recurrent contrast reaction. Premedication strategies include prednisone (50 mg by mouth at 13, 7, and 1 hour prior to contrast injection) or methylprednisolone (32 mg by mouth at 12 and 2 hours before contrast injection), along with diphenhydramine (50 mg 1 hour prior to injection).[14]

Magnetic Resonance Imaging

Magnetic resonance imaging (MRI) was developed by a host of innovative scientists over multiple decades of development from a scientific tool to a medical imaging necessity. MRI is based on the principles of nuclear magnetic resonance (NMR), first discovered by Felix Bloch and Edward Purcell, for which they were awarded the Nobel Prize in physics in 1952. NMR can be utilized to characterize and differentiate tissues based on their intrinsic NMR signal. Using NMR techniques, chemist Paul C. Lauterbur and physicist Sir Peter Mansfield developed the gradients and mathematical formulations required for rapid 2-dimensional MR images, publishing the first images in 1973[15] and 1974.[16] Drs. Raymond

Damadian, Larry Minkoff, and Michael Goldsmith were also instrumental in the development and refining of this technology for use in humans.[17] For their pioneering work in MRI development, Drs. Lauterbur and Mansfield shared the Nobel Prize in physiology or medicine in 2003.

The detailed physics principles underlying MRI are highly complex and beyond the scope of this chapter. In brief,[18] a powerful electromagnetic field is created within the bore of an MRI machine, typically along the cranial-caudal (z) axis. Protons that are present in the human body predominantly as hydrogen atoms in water molecules reach equilibrium aligned along the direction of this magnetic field (longitudinal magnetization). A radiofrequency (RF) pulse is applied at a resonance frequency specific to the protons within the main magnetic field (B-zero), causing them to absorb energy and change their alignment toward the horizontal/vertical plane (x-y axes), called *transverse magnetization.* When the RF pulse ends, the protons first dephase in the x-y direction (free-induction decay, the basis of T2 signal) at a rate dependent on the molecular structure of the sample. The protons then realign along the z-axis (spin-lattice relaxation, the basis of T1 signal) at a slower rate, which is dependent on the molecular structure surrounding the proton. As the protons realign toward equilibrium, they emit RF energy that is detected by antennas (receiver coil) surrounding the patient in the scanner. By inducing small changes in frequency and phase of the proton resonance frequency that vary as a function of proton position, the MRI system reconstructs the precise location of each signal within the patient. The MRI system thus produces cross-sectional images through the patient where each pixel (corresponding to a defined volume of tissue, or voxel) depends upon the magnetic microenvironment of the corresponding tissue.

From this general principle, a variety of pulse sequences have been developed to emphasize different tissue characteristics.[18] A pulse sequence refers to a specific pattern of RF pulses that may vary in timing, order, repetition, and direction. Basic pulse sequences include spin echo, inversion recovery including short tau inversion recovery (STIR) and fluid attenuated inversion recovery (FLAIR), and gradient echo imaging. The clinical applications of those sequences most pertinent to neuroradiology are described in this chapter.

MR angiography (MRA) can be performed by several techniques, including time-of-flight, phase-contrast, and gadolinium-enhanced MRA. In time-of-flight angiography, protons in moving blood are tagged in one tissue slab by applying an RF pulse to change their longitudinal magnetization.[18] Tagged protons are subsequently detected in a different tissue slab that has not experienced the RF pulse. The direction of blood flow can be selected by applying a saturation pulse to null the longitudinal magnetization from protons traveling in the opposite direction. For example, to selectively visualize tagged blood protons moving superiorly within the cervical arteries, a saturation pulse is applied superior to the scan volume (e.g., within the head) to neutralize the longitudinal magnetization of the tagged protons within the intracranial compartment before they travel inferiorly in the cervical veins.

Phase contrast angiography is another method to detect moving protons such as those in blood or CSF.[18] Phase contrast imaging depends on applying bipolar gradients to protons, so that stationary protons experience both positive and negative gradients, with no net phase change. Moving protons experience only one gradient before moving out of the field, resulting in positive or negative excitation.

Contrast-enhanced angiography uses gadolinium-based contrast agents to highlight blood vessels. Gadolinium is strongly paramagnetic, resulting in significant T1 shortening (high signal on T1-weighted sequences). After intravenous administration of gadolinium, T1-weighted sequences can be obtained during the arterial or venous phase to highlight vascular anatomy. Three-dimensional reformatted sequences can be constructed after any of the angiographic techniques.

Issues with Magnetic Resonance Imaging

MRI offers many advantages over CT. MRI provides excellent soft tissue detail and does not use ionizing radiation, but it does have several drawbacks. Study times for MRI are significantly longer than those for CT. MR images are significantly degraded by motion artifact, which coupled with the longer scan times becomes problematic in acutely ill patients and children. MRI coils must be in close approximation to the body area being imaged, and the bore of the MRI scanner is generally both smaller and more enclosed than CT. This can be a significant problem for patients with claustrophobia or those with a large body habitus.

Because of the strong magnetic fields used for MRI, it is not safe to scan patients with certain metal implants or ferromagnetic foreign bodies. Some metal implants or foreign bodies can move because of the influence of the external magnetic field, with potentially devastating consequences depending on the nature of the object (e.g., older ferromagnetic aneurysm clips). Certain metallic objects can heat during scanning, which can be uncomfortable to the patient or cause tissue damage. These effects of the magnetic field are more pronounced at higher field strength magnets (that is, 3-tesla compared to 1.5-tesla scanners). In addition, certain implants, such as vagal nerve stimulators, deep brain stimulators, and cardiac pacemakers, can malfunction during exposure to strong magnetic fields. It is worth remembering that implanted devices or other foreign bodies do not need to lie within the area of interest (scan volume) in order to be affected by the magnetic fields of the MR scanner, and that in most modern scanners the main magnetic field is always present.

There are several resources available to determine whether a particular implant is compatible or considered safe to scan with MRI, including a website maintained by the Institute for Magnetic Resonance Safety, Education, and Research (http://mrisafety.com).[19] This website includes a free searchable database of the safety profile of many different implants and devices. The radiologist or MRI technologist can also provide valuable advice on MR safety.

Gadolinium Contrast Agents

Gadolinium-based contrast agents used in MRI have associated risks. The risk of contrast reaction after gadolinium-based contrast agent injection is lower than for iodinated contrast, with a reported incidence of 0.04% to 0.07% (approximately 1/2000).[12,13] In one large series of contrast reactions after gadolinium-based contrast agent, 88% were considered mild. The overall incidence of severe reactions (those requiring epinephrine for treatment) was 0.001% to 0.01% of injections (approximately 1/20,000).

A relatively recent development in the use of gadolinium-based contrast agents has been the recognition of the link between contrast administration and nephrogenic systemic fibrosis (NSF) in patients with renal failure. NSF is a progressive fibrosing disease affecting the skin and soft tissues, often of the extremities. NSF may also affect striated muscle and the diaphragm.[20,21] There is no clearly effective treatment. This entity is believed to be associated with gadolinium deposition in tissues and is not prevented by dialysis.[22] The risk of NSF may vary depending on the particular contrast agent, but this is still under investigation.

NSF is rare, with an incidence of 1% to 7% in patients with renal dysfunction[12,21] who receive gadolinium. It is associated with severe acute renal failure or chronic renal failure with an estimated glomerular filtration rate (GFR) of less than 15 to 30 mL/minute. It is also associated with renal or liver transplantation.[20] Because of this association, gadolinium agents should be used with caution in patients with compromised renal function and should be avoided if possible in patients with GFR less than 30 mL/minute. As research in this area continues to evolve, discussion of these cases with the local radiologist is recommended.

CLINICAL IMAGING

Radiography

Once the mainstay of neuroradiology, skull radiography and its permutations have been largely replaced by cross-sectional imaging modalities such as CT and MRI. Radiography is still used in the evaluation of shunts and other neurosurgical implants such as intrathecal pumps and deep brain stimulators.

Shunt series are the most commonly encountered of these studies and include radiographs of the shunt components in two planes. Shunt series are used to evaluate the nature of the shunt, including the location of the ventricular and distal catheters, drainage location (e.g., atrial, peritoneal, pleural), and the type and setting of the shunt valve, as well as to identify causes of shunt dysfunction.[23] Shunt catheters, valves, and tubing can be quickly examined for kinks or disruption, without the cost or radiation exposure of CT or the time and cost of MRI. The type and setting of most implanted shunt valves can also be determined based on radiographic appearance.

Radiography is also sometimes used in the evaluation of the bony calvarium. Although CT has largely replaced radiography for evaluation of facial fractures or sinusitis, skull films are occasionally obtained for these purposes. Linear nondisplaced skull fractures that may be missed on axial CT can at times be detected by radiography. Such occult fractures can sometimes be visualized by either examining the scout tomographic view obtained as part of a routine CT scan, or by constructing surface rendered reformats of CT images. In addition, skull films are sometimes obtained to evaluate for radiolucent bone lesions prior to the placement of stereotactic frames for gamma knife treatment or stereotactic biopsy.

Computed Tomography

The nonenhanced head CT has become the workhorse of acute neuroimaging, due to its wide availability, speed, and relatively low cost. CT provides rapid imaging of many intracranial processes and is excellent for the detection of intracranial hemorrhage, mass lesions, and evaluation of the ventricular system. CT is highly sensitive for calcifications, fat, and air, as well as metallic foreign bodies. In addition, CT allows rapid evaluation of the sequelae of intracranial pathology, including mass effect and brain herniation. Potential drawbacks of head CTs include radiation exposure and cost. In addition, MRI is more sensitive at detecting many parenchymal processes such as stroke, subtle enhancement, and small masses.

Noncontrast Imaging

Because of the importance of the noncontrast head CT to the practice of neurosurgery, clinically relevant findings commonly found on head CT are described here.

Mass Effect and Herniation

Space-occupying lesions within the intracranial compartment distort normal cranial anatomy and can cause mass effect and brain herniation. Mass effect can affect local structures, distorting the ventricles or narrowing the cerebral sulci. Focal mass effect can also result in herniation of brain across fixed structures such as the falx cerebri and tentorium. Brain herniation is an important predictor of severe neurological injury.

There are several types of brain herniation, including subfalcine, uncal, transtentorial (upward and downward), and tonsillar herniation (Fig. 3.1). Brain can also herniate extracranially through a skull defect. CT is excellent at detecting all types of brain herniation.

Subfalcine herniation occurs from a space-occupying lesion in the cerebral hemisphere causing the cingulate gyrus to be pushed under the rigid falx cerebri into the contralateral cranial vault[24] (Fig. 3.1G). Subfalcine herniation commonly occurs with frontal lobe and parietal lesions. If midline shift is severe, the anterior cerebral arteries may be compressed, potentially leading to infarction. Subfalcine herniation is often measured as midline shift at either the level of the septum pellucidum, foramen of Monro, or third ventricle. It is important to measure midline shift at the same location to assess for changes between scans.

Uncal herniation is a type of unilateral descending transtentorial herniation involving the uncus, a component of the mesial temporal lobe that appears as a focal convexity at the anterior margin of the parahippocampal gyrus (Fig. 3.1B). Uncal herniation occurs when the mesial temporal lobe herniates medially and inferiorly, usually because of a temporal lobe or middle cranial fossa mass (Fig. 3.1F). To diagnose uncal herniation, find the suprasellar cistern and look for medial displacement of the uncus with compression of the ipsilateral perimesencephalic cistern. In severe cases, the herniated uncus will compress the ipsilateral cerebral peduncle[24] and the brainstem may be shifted to the opposite side. There may be entrapment of the contralateral temporal horn of the lateral ventricle as CSF outflow is compressed. Recognizing and alleviating uncal herniation before progression to brainstem compression are important to minimize severe neurological consequences.

Transtentorial herniation is assessed by evaluating the basilar cisterns around the midbrain, including perimesencephalic cistern, ambient cistern, and quadrigeminal plate cistern.[24] In the case of severely increased intracranial pressure or focal mass effect, the brain herniates downward through the tentorial incisura, first resulting in narrowing, then effacement of the basilar cisterns. If intracranial pressure continues to increase, the herniated brain will compress the brainstem (Fig. 3.1D and E), with narrowing of the transverse diameter of the midbrain. Transtentorial herniation may lead to compression of branches of the posterior cerebral artery against the tentorium with temporal or occipital infarction. Hydrocephalus may occur if the cerebral aqueduct is compressed. Severe transtentorial herniation may result in hemorrhages within the brainstem (Duret's hemorrhages), which are a sign of grave prognosis.

If intracranial mass effect arises in the posterior fossa, cerebellar contents can herniate upward through the tentorial incisura.[24] This displacement is usually accompanied by tonsillar herniation, the downward herniation of the cerebellar tonsils through the foramen magnum. Upward tentorial herniation appears similar to downward tentorial herniation on axial images at the level of the incisura, but a mass lesion in the posterior fossa will be present. Tonsillar herniation appears on axial CT as crowding of the contents at the foramen magnum with effacement of the perimedullary cistern. Sagittal reconstructions may be particularly helpful in delineating upward transtentorial herniation and cerebellar tonsillar herniation.

Hemorrhage

CT is highly sensitive for detecting intracranial hemorrhage. In general, acute hemorrhage (within hours of injury) is hyperdense to brain, with Hounsfield units in the range of 50 to 70[25] (Fig. 3.2A). As the blood products break down and are reabsorbed, the density of the hematoma decreases. Subacute blood products (1-6 weeks) may appear isodense to brain (Fig. 3.2B). As the hematoma becomes chronic, the density approaches that of CSF. In the case of chronic subdural hematoma, there may be blood products of different density or fluid-fluid levels due to hemorrhages of different ages (Fig. 3.2C).

Hyperacute blood (ongoing bleeding or imaging immediately after hemorrhage) is heterogeneous in appearance (see Fig. 3.2A). If contrast agent is given as part of the study, active hemorrhage is evident as contrast extravasation. Acute hemorrhage may occasionally appear isodense in the setting of anemia or coagulopathy.

CT is also excellent for determining the location of hemorrhage (Fig. 3.3). In general, different compartments within the cranium include the epidural space, between the dura and inner table of the calvarium; the subdural space, between the dura and arachnoid membranes; the subarachnoid space, between the arachnoid membrane and brain surface; within the brain parenchyma; and within the ventricles. The location and pattern of bleeding can yield vital clues to the underlying cause of hemorrhage.

Trauma can result in hemorrhage in any of the above-named compartments. Epidural and subdural hemorrhages commonly occur after trauma. Epidural hemorrhage is associated with arterial bleeding, classically related to a skull fracture and often temporal in location. Epidural hemorrhage can also be present in the setting of venous sinus injury. Subdural hemorrhage can result even from minor trauma, and classically results from tearing of the subdural veins, especially in the elderly who have experienced cerebral atrophy.

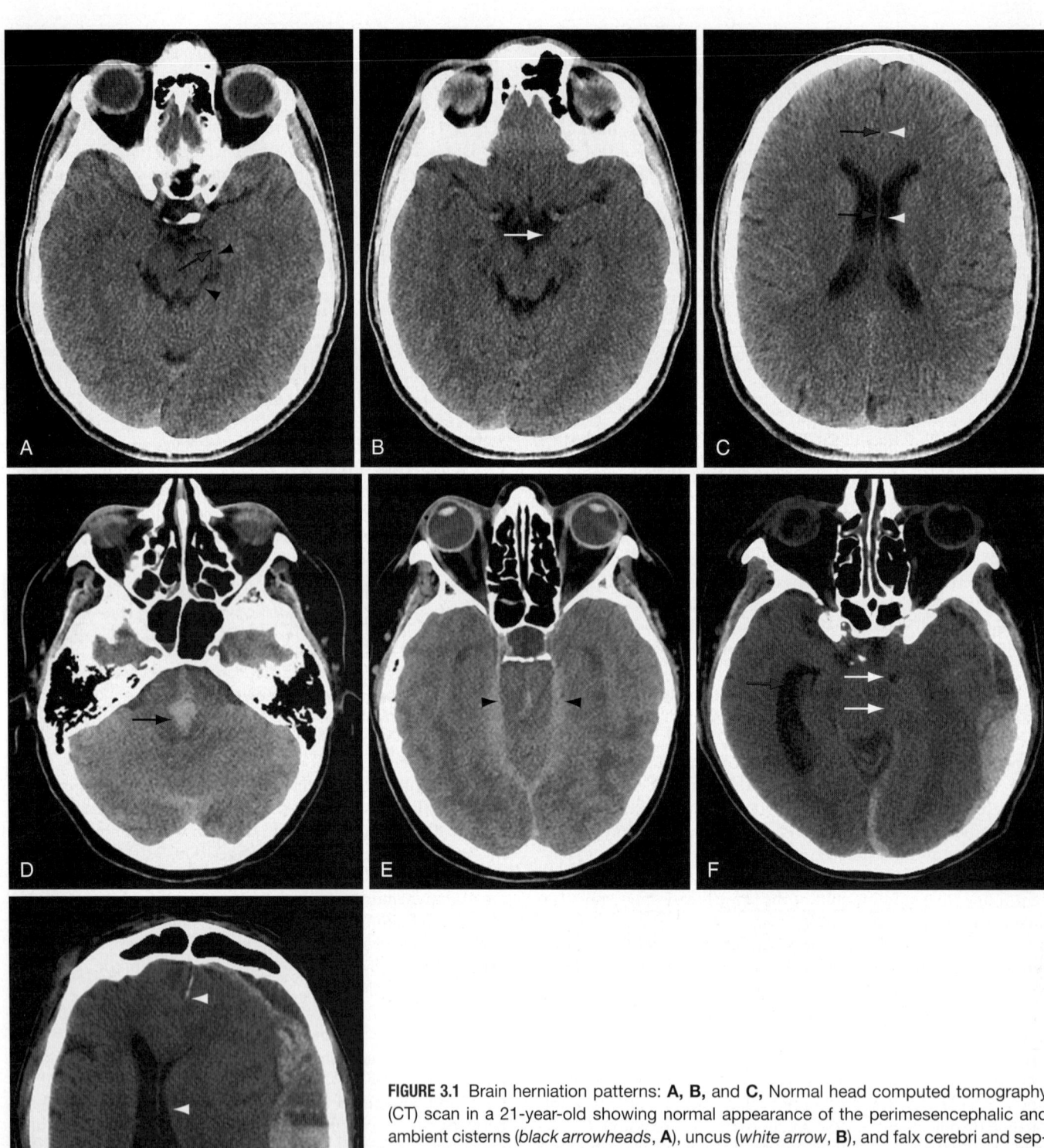

FIGURE 3.1 Brain herniation patterns: **A, B,** and **C,** Normal head computed tomography (CT) scan in a 21-year-old showing normal appearance of the perimesencephalic and ambient cisterns (*black arrowheads*, **A**), uncus (*white arrow*, **B**), and falx cerebri and septum pellucidum (*white arrowheads*, **C**). **D** and **E,** Downward transtentorial herniation in a 50-year-old woman with rapid neurological decline. There is complete effacement of the perimesencephalic and ambient cisterns (*black arrowheads*, **E**) with a Duret hemorrhage in the pons (*black arrow*, **D**). **F** and **G,** Uncal and subfalcine herniation in a 71-year-old confused man with an acute subdural hemorrhage (SDH). Note the medial placement of the uncus and parahippocampal gyrus (*white arrows*, **F**), enlarged temporal horn of the right lateral ventricle (*red arrows*), and rightward shift of the septum pellucidum under the falx cerebri (*white arrowheads*, **G**).

FIGURE 3.2 Blood of various ages: A 67-year-old woman on heparin with acute decline in mental status: **A,** Noncontrast head computed tomography (CT) scan shows hyperdense acute hemorrhage within the pons (*black arrows*). Note hypodense areas with fluid-fluid levels reflecting hyperacute hemorrhage. **B,** Postcontrast CT image in the same patient shows layering contrast material (*arrowhead*) within the hemorrhage, indicating active extravasation. **C,** A 50-year-old with 2 weeks of severe headaches. Noncontrast CT image shows isodense subdural hemorrhage (SDH) (*black arrows*). Hyperdense focus in the SDH (*arrowhead*) indicates more recent hemorrhage. **D,** A 72-year-old who fell. Noncontrast CT image shows hypodense chronic SDH (*black arrows*). Layering isodense component on the right and fluid-fluid level on the left (*arrowheads*) represent more recent blood products.

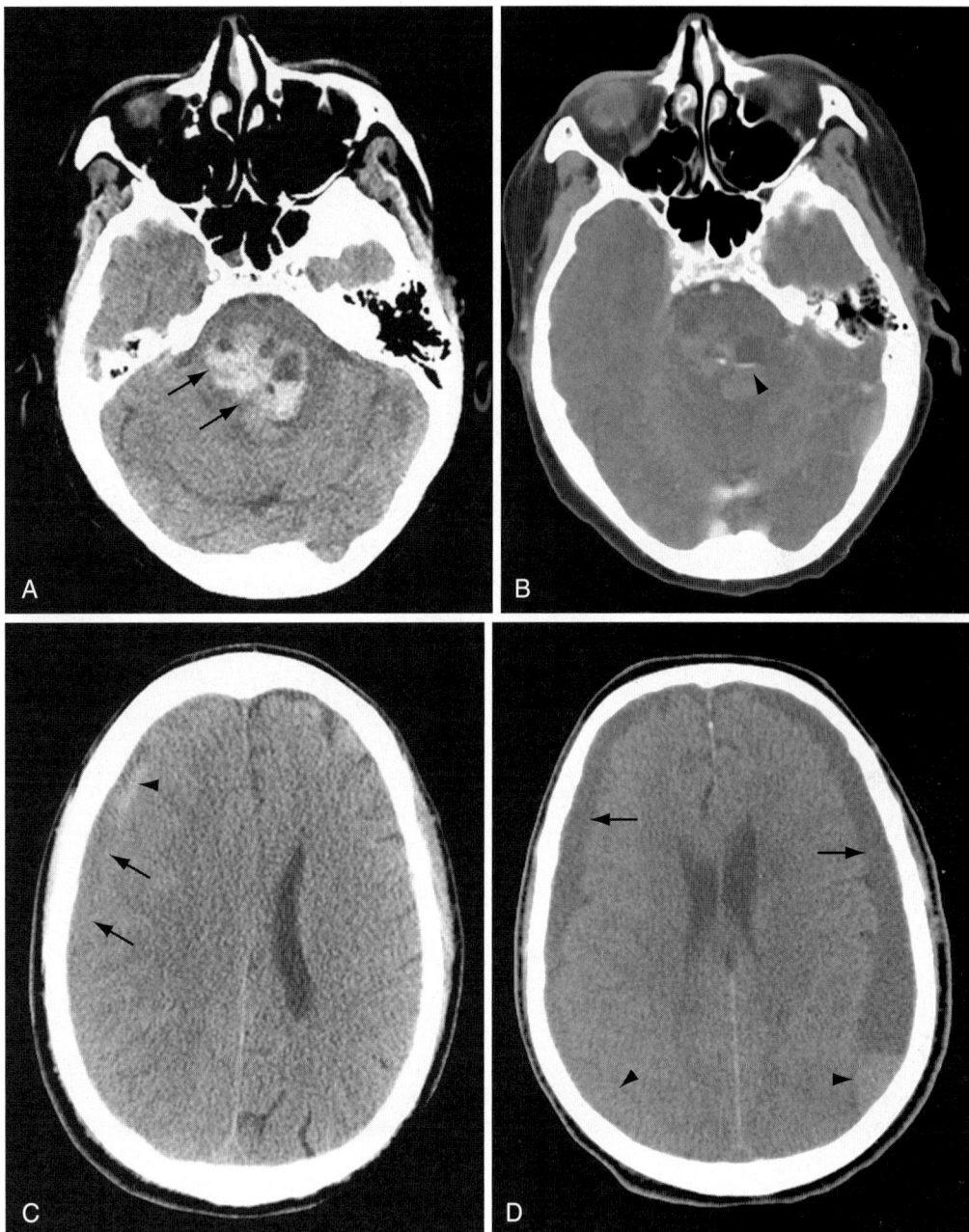

Subarachnoid hemorrhage (SAH) can result from trauma or cerebrovascular disease. Classically, subarachnoid hemorrhage is associated with rupture of intracranial aneurysm, and in the absence of trauma or in the setting of a suspicious pattern of SAH, vascular imaging (CTA or MRA) should be pursued. SAH can also result from venous abnormalities including cortical venous infarction.

Intraventricular hemorrhage often results from extension of a parenchymal hematoma. In rare cases, isolated intraventricular hemorrhage can result from a ruptured aneurysm, arteriovenous malformation, choroid plexus lesion, or metastasis.

Parenchymal hemorrhage has a variety of causes other than trauma. Parenchymal hemorrhage can be the result of hypertensive vasculopathy, vasculitis, amyloid angiopathy, or

bleeding from arteriovenous malformations. Mass lesions such as tumors or cavernous hemangiomas can also bleed. Patients who experience ischemic infarctions can hemorrhage into the infarcted brain. Because of the wide variety of underlying causes of parenchymal hemorrhage, correlation with clinical history is vital, and further studies such as contrast-enhanced studies, vascular evaluation, or MRI are often needed.

Edema

Edema manifests on CT as decreased brain parenchymal attenuation due to increased water content. Vasogenic edema appears as low attenuation areas of the white matter with accompanying gyral enlargement and sulcal effacement. The cortical ribbon is preserved, and gray-white matter differentiation is accentuated. Vasogenic edema is associated with mass

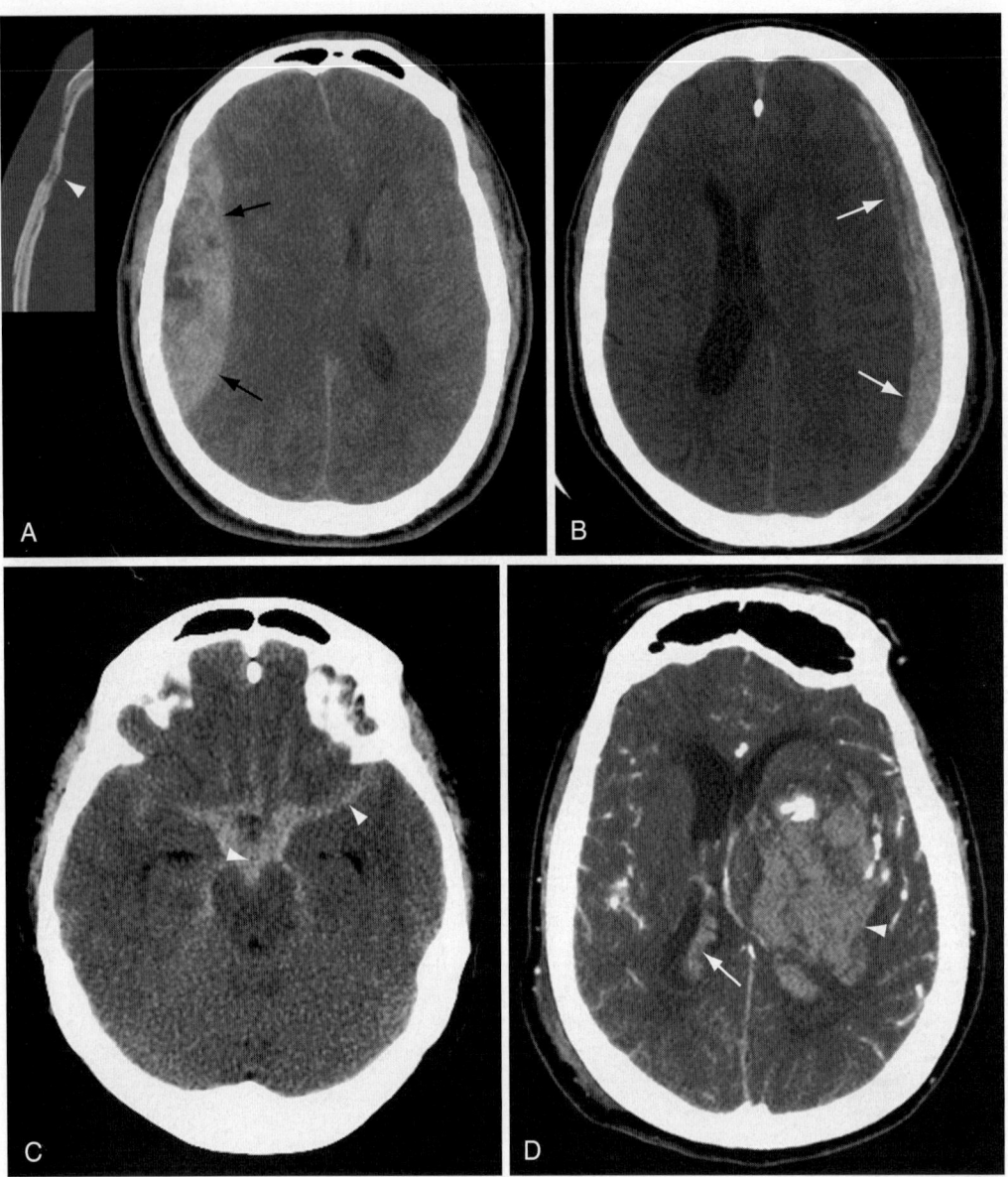

FIGURE 3.3 Acute hemorrhage in different compartments: **A,** Acute epidural hemorrhage (EDH) with hyperacute (low attenuation) components (*black arrows*) in a 38-year-old who fell 20 ft. Inset shows associated linear nondisplaced skull fracture (*arrowhead*). **B,** Acute hemispheric subdural hematoma (*white arrows*) in a 50-year-old who fell. Note subfalcine herniation in A and B. **C,** Extensive basilar and sylvian subarachnoid hemorrhage (SAH) (*arrowheads*) from a ruptured aneurysm in a 45-year-old with thunderclap headache. **D,** In a 55-year-old who was found unresponsive, postcontrast computed tomography (CT) scan shows large basal ganglia parenchymal hemorrhage (*white arrowhead*) with intraventricular extension (*white arrow*). Note focus of bright contrast extravasation within the parenchymal hemorrhage indicating active bleeding.

lesions, venous congestion, and hemorrhage, among other things. Cytotoxic edema is manifested as gyral enlargement with loss of gray-white differentiation. Cytotoxic edema is associated with ischemia, infarction, and anoxic brain injury. Diffuse cerebral edema is manifested by diffuse sulcal and cisternal effacement with loss of gray-white matter differentiation. Diffuse cerebral edema may result from acute traumatic brain injury or severe, widespread anoxic injury.

Infarction

CT is relatively insensitive for acute stroke. Nevertheless, CT is important in the evaluation of acute stroke, primarily to identify or exclude other causes of neurological deficit such as hemorrhage or mass lesion.[26] Early signs of ischemia by CT include sulcal effacement, indicating focal cerebral edema in the ischemic tissue, and loss of gray-white differentiation (Fig. 3.4). Careful examination of the gray-white junction on CT using a narrow window width to accentuate the difference in attenuation between gray and white matter is vital

for early detection of ischemia/infarction. In early ischemia, this gray-white differentiation is obscured owing to cytotoxic edema. A second look at the CT in the brain area corresponding to symptoms may also increase sensitivity. Post-contrast-enhanced CT is generally not indicated in the evaluation of stroke, as the enhancement seen in subacute strokes may confound early diagnosis.

Classic signs of a middle cerebral artery (MCA) territory stroke include the insular ribbon sign and the dense MCA sign. The insular ribbon sign refers to loss of gray-white differentiation of the insular cortex. Similarly, effacement of the lateral margin of the putamen or caudate head may provide early indication of an MCA infarction (see Fig. 3.4).

The dense MCA sign is seen with an acute thrombus in the middle cerebral artery. Because calcified atherosclerotic plaque is also dense, care should be taken to compare the affected MCA to the contralateral MCA to increase the specificity of this sign. A similar sign indicating basilar artery occlusion is also described but is less sensitive. Ultimately, if

FIGURE 3.4 MCA infarction: 44-year-old with profound left hemiplegia and sensory loss. **A,** Dense MCA sign: linear hyperdensity in the expected location of the right M1 segment of the MCA (*white arrowhead*). **B,** Loss of gray-white differentiation around the right caudate and lentiform nucleus (*white arrowhead*). Left side is preserved (*white arrow*). **C** and **D,** CTA in the same patient demonstrates nonopacification of the right cavernous ICA (**C**) and MCA (**D**) (*white arrowheads*), compared to the normal left side (*white arrows*). CTA, computed tomography angiogram; ICA, inferior cerebral artery; MCA, middle cerebral artery.

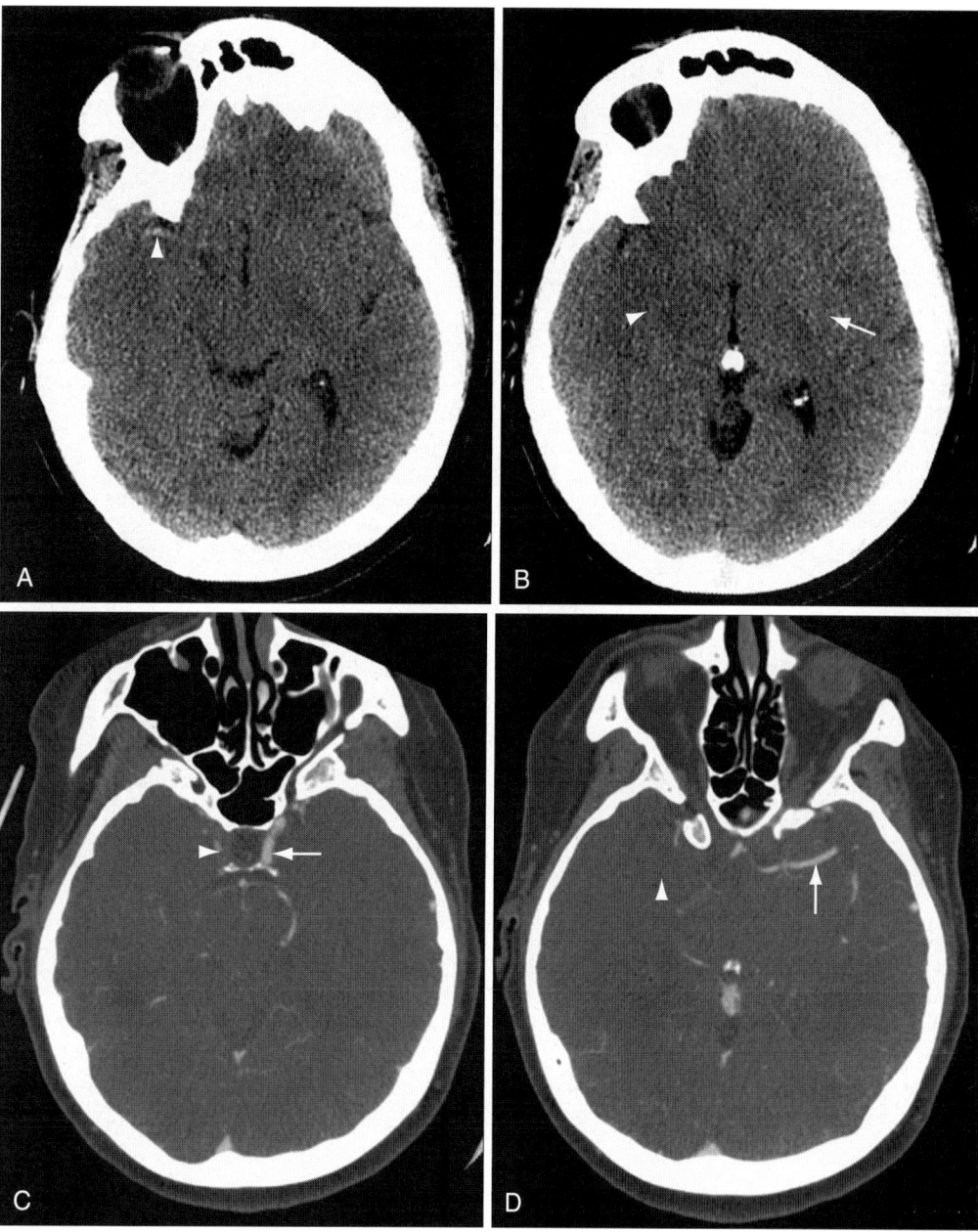

there is a question of a branch occlusion of the circle of Willis, vascular evaluation such as CTA or MRA should be pursued.

Hydrocephalus

The ventricular system is seen well on noncontrast CT. Ventricular size depends in part on the age of the patient and the extent of cerebral parenchymal volume loss. It is important to evaluate ventricular size in relation to sulcal size. Enlarged ventricles with preserved sulci and widely patent basilar cisterns may simply reflect cerebral volume loss. Even slightly increased ventricular size in a young person with effaced sulci and cisterns is much more concerning for hydrocephalus (Fig. 3.5). Secondary signs of hydrocephalus include transependymal CSF flow, where pressurized CSF collects in the parenchymal interstitial space, particularly around the frontal horns.

Hydrocephalus can either be communicating, due to compromised CSF reabsorption, or noncommunicating, due to obstruction of CSF outflow. Communicating hydrocephalus involves the entire ventricular system, including the fourth ventricle, but noncommunicating hydrocephalus results in dilatation of only the ventricles proximal to the obstruction. If obstructive hydrocephalus is suspected, a search for underlying cause should be undertaken. CT may be helpful in some cases, but MRI is more sensitive for subtle lesions and can provide multiplanar anatomical evaluation.

Contrast-Enhanced Computed Tomography

Iodinated contrast agent may be useful in some situations. For example, in patients with a suspected mass lesion such as tumor or abscess, contrast enhancement will better demonstrate the

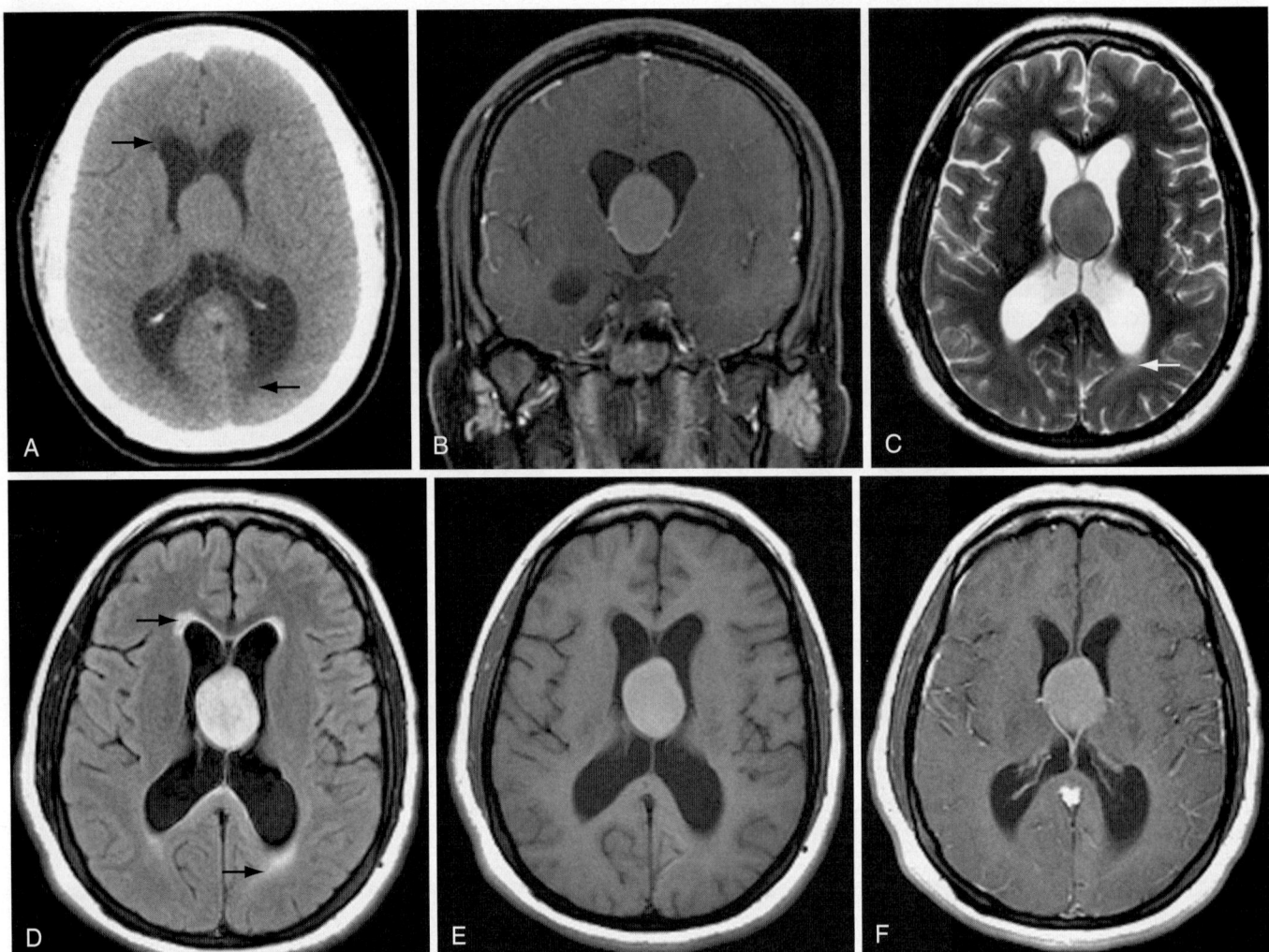

FIGURE 3.5 Hydrocephalus due to a colloid cyst in a 32-year-old. **A,** Noncontrast head computed tomography (CT) scan demonstrates enlarged lateral ventricles with low-density areas extending from the corners of the lateral ventricles (*black arrows*), indicating hydrocephalus. Postcontrast coronal T1 (**B**), T2 (**C**), and FLAIR (**D**) images, along with precontrast (**E**) and postcontrast (**F**) T1-weighted images, demonstrate a homogeneous nonenhancing mass centered at the foramen magnum, a classic colloid cyst. Note the periventricular transependymal cerebrospinal fluid displacement on T2 and FLAIR sequences (**C, D,** *arrows*). FLAIR, fluid attenuated inversion recovery.

lesion. Contrast also increases the sensitivity of CT for small masses. Contrast can be helpful in the evaluation of infection after craniotomy by highlighting peripheral enhancement of fluid collections. In general, MRI is more sensitive than CT for mass lesions. The advantages of contrast-enhanced CT over MR include availability and rapidity of the examination, ability to perform CT in unstable patients or patients with contraindications to MR (e.g., metal implants), and the ability to perform CT in larger patients than many MRI scanners can accommodate.

Computed Tomographic Angiography

Arterial phase CT of the head or neck (CTA) is useful in the evaluation of cerebrovascular diseases, including atherosclerosis/stroke, aneurysms, and arteriovenous malformations. CTA is often the initial study in the evaluation of subarachnoid hemorrhage and is useful in the workup of intracranial hemorrhage of unknown etiology. The arterial phase of the study will evaluate for the presence of a vascular lesion.

A postcontrast head CT scan obtained at the same sitting can reveal mass lesions and active contrast extravasation. Venous phase CT (CTV) can be used to evaluate the dural venous sinuses and cerebral veins for occlusion or injury.

CTA offers the advantages of wide availability, speed of acquisition, and avoidance of many of the potential complications of conventional angiography such as stroke and vascular dissection. Angiography does provide useful physiological information that CTA does not, such as blood flow dynamics. For example, angiography can detect delayed flow through a vascular stenosis, or arteriovenous shunting in arteriovenous malformations and dural arteriovenous fistulas (Fig. 3.6). Angiography also exquisitely reveals the arterial supply and venous drainage pattern in these cases.

In many centers, CTA is replacing conventional angiography in the evaluation of subarachnoid hemorrhage. CTA is not as sensitive as conventional angiography for the detection of small aneurysms,[27] but newer multislice scanners with three-dimensional reformation may increase the sensitivity

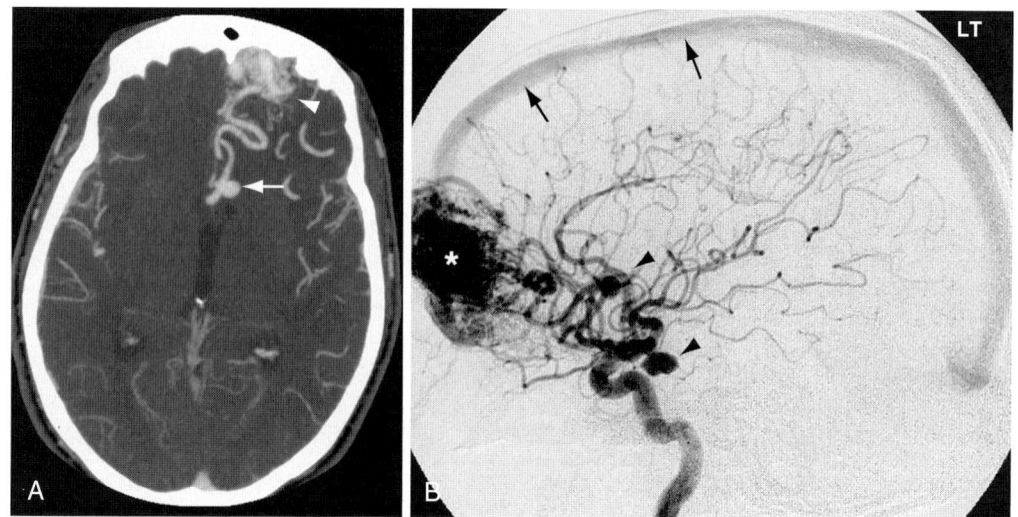

FIGURE 3.6 Computed tomography angiogram (CTA) and conventional angiogram in a 26-year-old with an arteriovenous malformation. **A,** CTA shows an aneurysm arising from a dilated anterior cerebral artery feeder (*white arrow*). Left frontal lobe nidus (*arrowhead*) is well visualized. **B,** Conventional angiography again shows the nidus (*) as well as arteriovenous shunting with early filling of the superior sagittal sinus (*black arrows*). Black arrowheads highlight aneurysms.

of CTA.[28] In addition, CTA provides additional anatomical information, such as the relationship of an aneurysm to the bony skull base and presence of a thrombosed component (Fig. 3.7).

Computed Tomography Perfusion

Perfusion CT (CTP) is a type of contrast-enhanced CT study in which serial images are obtained through a section of brain parenchyma during the administration of intravenous contrast agent. Maps of cerebral blood flow (CBF, measured in mL/100 g tissue/minute), mean transit time (MTT, measured in seconds), and cerebral blood volume (CBV, measured in mL/100 g tissue) can be derived using the central volume principle.[29] Briefly, the tissue residual function, based on parenchymal contrast enhancement per pixel as a function of time, and the arterial input function, based on arterial contrast enhancement (typically an anterior cerebral artery), can be deconvolved using a singular value decomposition method to derive CBV and MTT. CBF can then be calculated from the equation:

$$CBF = CBV / MTT.$$

Qualitative analysis of colorized perfusion maps reveal areas of the brain with altered perfusion. Quantitative analysis of perfusion parameters can also be performed to obtain numerical values of CBF, CBV, and MTT.[30] Table 3.2 contains normal values for each parameter.[31]

A common clinical application of perfusion CT is to assess for potentially salvageable tissue (penumbra) in acute stroke patients. With ischemia, cerebral blood flow decreases. Tissue is considered ischemic when CBF is less than 20 mL/100 g/minute. As CBF falls below 10 mL/100 g/minute, the ischemic threshold is passed and the tissue suffers irrevocable damage.[32] When evaluating a stroke patient, comparison of the CBV and either TTP or MTT maps is most helpful for detecting infarct penumbra.[33]

The CBV map best correlates with the size of subsequent core infarction.[33,34] There is a correlation between the infarct core determined by CBV map and the area of restricted diffusion by MRI. The MTT map is the most accurate for detecting regions of decreased perfusion.[33] The infarct penumbra is the brain parenchyma with prolonged MTT (>6 seconds)[32] but relatively normal CBV (i.e., MTT abnormality minus the infarct core). Patients with a large infarct penumbra may benefit from intra-arterial thrombolysis or other aggressive therapies.

Perfusion CT is also used in assessing cerebrovascular reserve.[32] Similar to xenon-CT with acetazolamide challenge, patients can undergo perfusion CT at baseline and following either acetazolamide or CO_2 challenge. Administration of either agent results in cerebrovascular dilatation. In a person with impaired perfusion to a portion of brain parenchyma, the physiological mechanism of cerebral autoregulation compensates by dilating cerebral vasculature, lowering cerebrovascular resistance and maximizing CBF to the region of ischemic tissue. Cerebrovascular reserve refers to how much capacity the cerebrovasculature has for additional vasodilatation. In a person with no cerebrovascular reserve, no additional vasodilatation is possible. When given vasodilating agents, normally perfused brain will experience vasodilatation and increased CBF. Areas without cerebrovascular reserve already are at maximal cerebrovascular dilatation and will experience relatively decreased CBF compared to the normal areas (Fig. 3.8). Steal phenomenon may occur when areas without cerebrovascular reserve experience a decrease in CBF due to the increased perfusion to normal areas. Patients without cerebrovascular reserve may benefit from further therapies aimed at revascularization.

Magnetic Resonance Imaging

MRI is a sensitive method for detecting many abnormalities of the brain. MRI provides excellent soft tissue contrast and is sensitive for infarction, hemorrhage, and small masses, among other things. Because MRI is used for such a variety of pathologies, this chapter focuses on the strengths of different MRI

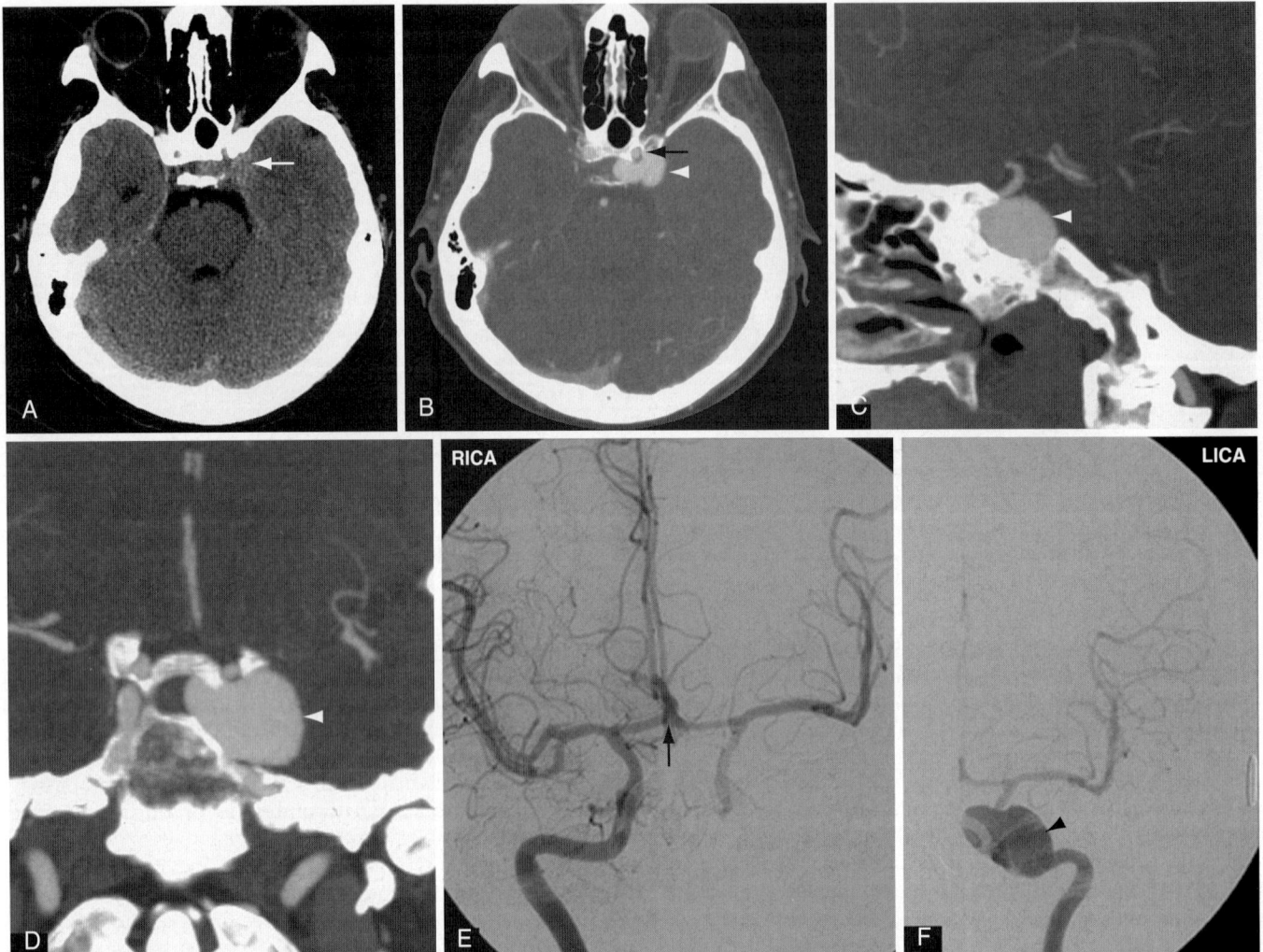

FIGURE 3.7 A 66-year-old woman with diplopia. **A,** Noncontrast head computed tomography (CT) image demonstrates hyperdense lesion in the region of the right cavernous sinus extending into the sella (*arrow*). Computed tomography angiograms (CTA) in the axial (**B**), sagittal (**C**), and coronal (**D**) planes better show the saccular left cavernous carotid aneurysm (*arrowheads*) herniating into the sella. Note the relationship to the paraclinoid carotid artery (*black arrow*, **B**). Conventional angiogram shows robust cross-filling of the left anterior circulation through the anterior communicating artery on right inferior cerebral artery (ICA) injection (**E**). Left ICA injection again demonstrates the aneurysm (**F**, *arrowhead*).

TABLE 3.2 Perfusion Computed Tomography Values		
Parameter	**Value**	**Units**
CBF	30-70	mL/100 g/min
CBV	2.2-4.2	mL/100 g
MTT	3-6	sec

CBF, cerebral blood flow; CBV, cerebral blood volume; MTT, mean transit time.

sequences for diagnosis. MRI research continues to advance, with the development of new and faster pulse sequences. The basics of MR physics are very briefly described.

T1-Weighted Imaging

T1-weighted images are commonly used to assess anatomy. On T1 sequences, gray matter is darker (hypointense) than white matter. Certain substances demonstrate inherent T1 shortening, meaning they appear brighter (hyperintense) relative to other structures (Fig. 3.9). Substances that appear bright on T1 sequences include fat, methemoglobin, some calcifications, melanin (as can be seen in melanoma metastases), proteinaceous fluid, and gadolinium contrast agents. In some cases, blood flow can cause T1 signal hyperintensity even in the absence of contrast administration, particularly at the skull base. This flow-related enhancement or flow artifact is caused by unsaturated protons moving into the imaging plane.[35]

T1-weighted images are also used to evaluate enhancement after intravenous gadolinium contrast administration. Breakdown of the blood-brain barrier allows intravenous gadolinium contrast to accumulate in the extravascular space within tissue, resulting in contrast enhancement on MRI (Fig. 3.10). Detection of tumors is a common reason to use contrast material, but abscesses, hematomas, demyelinating lesions, and subacute infarcts may all have areas of blood-brain barrier disruption, and therefore may also enhance. If the area of concern is within the bone marrow,

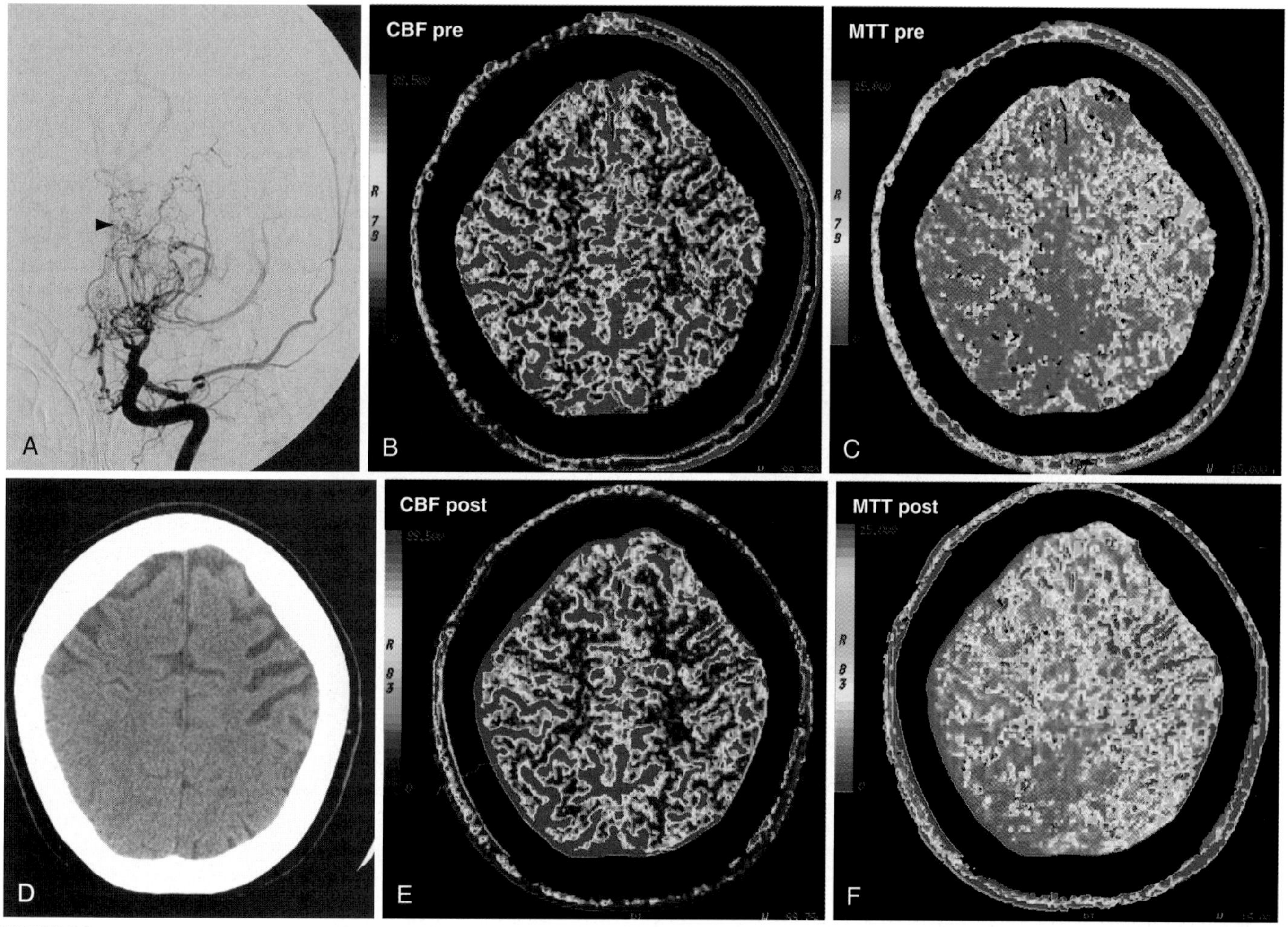

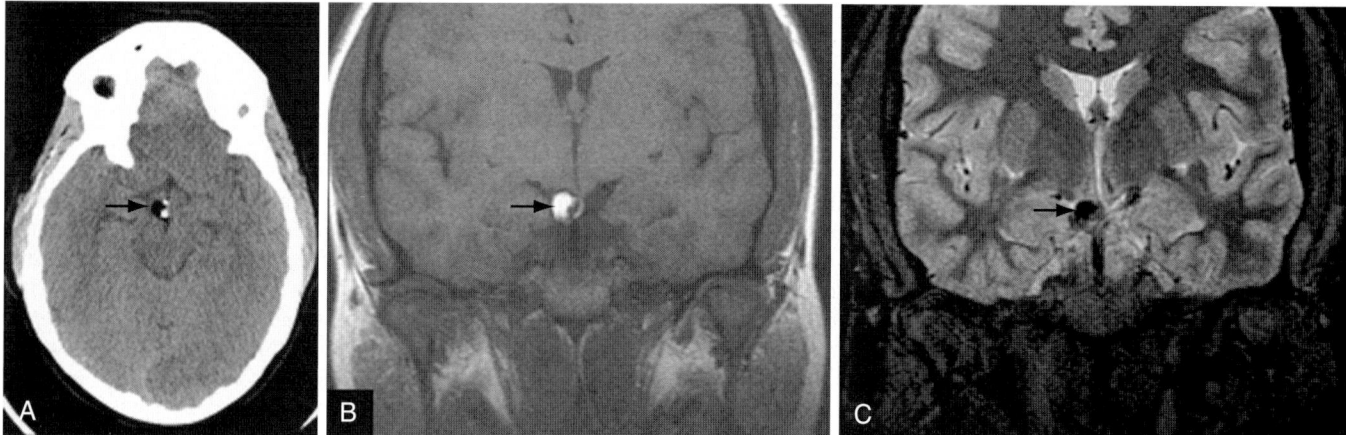

FIGURE 3.8 A 26-year-old with moyamoya disease. **A,** Angiogram showing characteristic puff-of-smoke vessels. **B** and **C,** Cerebral blood flow (CBF) and mean transit time (MTT) maps at baseline showing mildly decreased CBF and prolonged MTT within the affected left hemisphere. **D,** Noncontrast CT shows parenchymal volume loss in the left hemisphere but no focal encephalomalacia to indicate prior cortical infarct.**E** and **F,** CBF and MTT maps after vasodilatation with CO_2 inhalation show worsened asymmetry, indicating impaired cerebrovascular reserve.

FIGURE 3.9 A 35-year-old man with suprasellar dermoid. Computed tomography (CT) image shows fat density lesion with peripheral calcifications (**A,** *arrow*). Coronal T1 (**B**) shows inherent bright signal of the fat-containing lesion, with signal loss on fat-suppressed T2-weighted image (**C**).

including the calvarium, skull base, and spine, postcontrast fat suppression is helpful to null the inherent T1 signal hyperintensity due to bone marrow fat content, allowing optimal visualization of gadolinium enhancement.

T2-Weighted Imaging

T2-weighted images and the closely related FLAIR sequence are commonly used to assess for fluid and edema. Many pathological

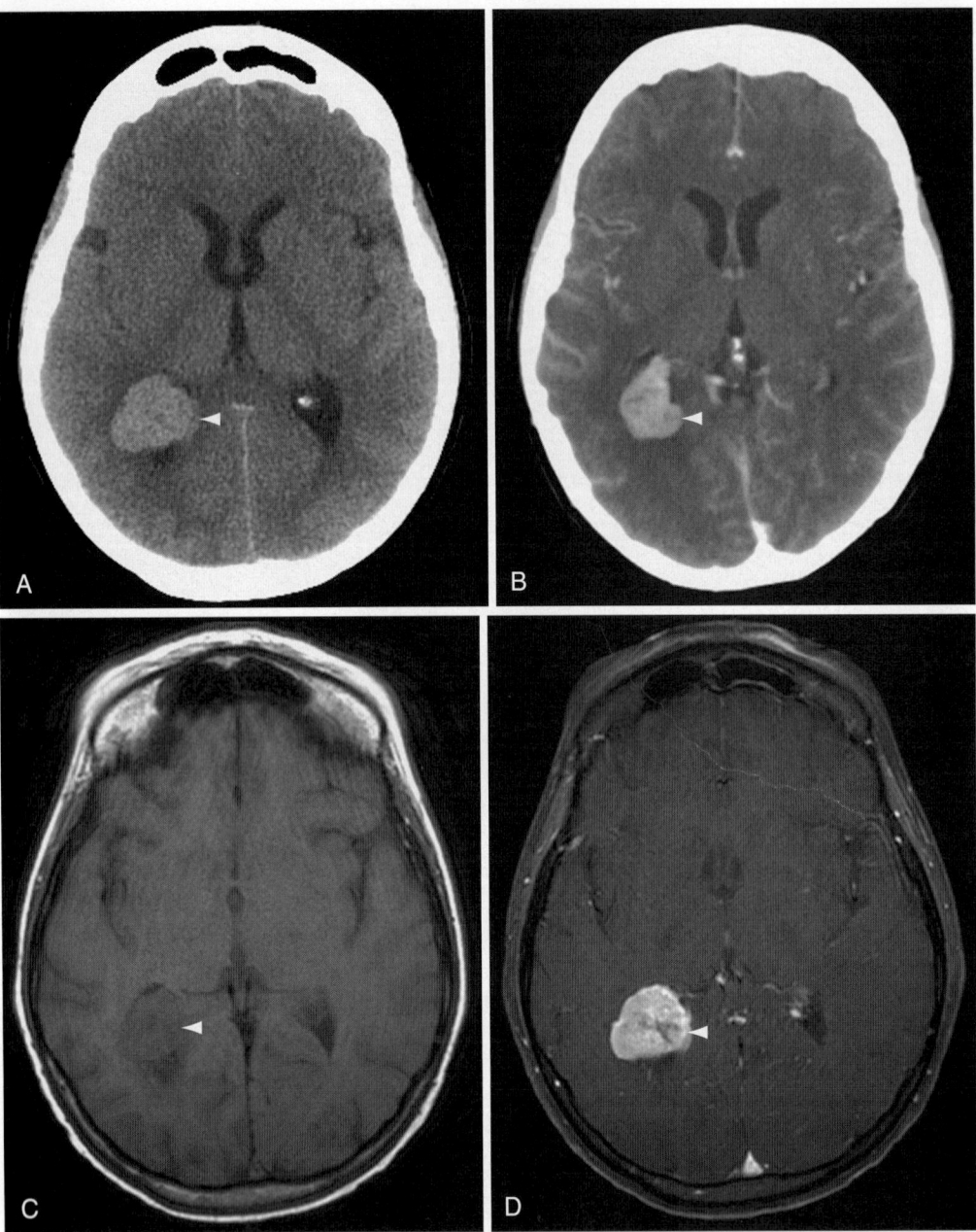

FIGURE 3.10 A 30-year-old who underwent cranial radiation as a child. Computed tomography (CT) scans without (**A**) and with (**B**) contrast agent show an enhancing lesion in the atrium of the right lateral ventricle. T1 precontrast (**C**) and T1 post-contrast (**D**) fat-suppressed sequences again show the enhancing lesion, an intraventricular meningioma.

processes in the brain are bright on T2 and FLAIR sequences, including edema, neoplasms, gliosis, and demyelinating lesions, among other entities. The FLAIR sequence is essentially a T2-weighted sequence in which simple fluid signal from CSF, for example, has been nulled and appears dark rather than bright as on T2. Proteinaceous fluid incompletely nulls and therefore appears brighter than CSF on FLAIR, allowing for differentiation of a CSF-filled space from a space containing proteinaceous fluid. However, FLAIR imaging is susceptible to CSF flow-related artifacts, particularly in the posterior fossa where T2 is often most useful for finding small posterior fossa and brainstem lesions.

High-resolution, heavily T2-weighted sequences can be helpful for looking closely at small structures in the basilar cisterns, such as the cranial nerves. These sequences are helpful in diagnosing very small vestibular schwannomas or neurovascular compression disorders such as trigeminal neuralgia.

These sequences can also be used to evaluate CSF spaces such as the third ventricle in preparation for a third ventriculostomy, or the cerebral aqueduct to assess for aqueductal stenosis as a cause of hydrocephalus. The names of these specific pulse sequences vary among vendors.

T2-weighted images are also useful for evaluating vascular flow voids. Flow voids of the circle of Willis are often seen on T2 sequences, as are the carotid, vertebral, and basilar artery flow voids. Dural venous sinuses flow voids may also be evaluated for patency on T2. Pathological flow voids from arteriovenous malformations are also readily assessed on T2 imaging.

T2*-Weighted Imaging

T2*-weighted gradient echo sequence highlights areas of magnetic field inhomogeneity that cause magnetic susceptibility artifacts. Areas of field inhomogeneity result in signal dropout and appear dark black. These areas may be caused by imperfections in the magnet, but also can be caused by certain ferromagnetic or paramagnetic material such as metal and blood products. Calcium causes susceptibility artifacts as well, but these areas of susceptibility are less intense than metal and blood products. T2* sequences are highly sensitive for small areas of hemorrhage, and are useful for detecting subtle or old microhemorrhages from hypertension, cerebral amyloid angiopathy, diffuse axonal injury, and cavernous malformations (Fig. 3.11).

Susceptibility-weighted imaging is a newer sequence that provides high-resolution images highlighting areas of altered magnetic susceptibility such as hemorrhage, calcium, and blood vessels.[36] The advantages of this sequence include the ability to reformat in multiple planes and high sensitivity. In fact, susceptibility-weighted imaging is more sensitive than standard T2* sequences in detecting small microhemorrhages[37] and can also detect a variety of vascular malformations.[38] The high sensitivity of susceptibility-weighted imaging may also be a disadvantage, because there are many potentially distracting areas of signal dropout that do not represent hemorrhage.

Diffusion-Weighted Imaging

Diffusion-weighted imaging (DWI) is inherently a series of T2-weighted sequences that detect movement of protons in water molecules by applying opposite gradient pulses in each of three orthogonal directions. If there is no net movement of water molecules, their underlying T2 signal intensity is preserved, resulting in hyperintense DWI signal. Conversely, net movement of water molecules along the direction of the applied gradients[39] causes dephasing with underlying T2 signal loss, resulting in hypointense DWI signal. In regions in which brownian movement of water molecules is constrained, DWI signal is increased (called *restricted diffusion*) owing to lack of net movement. However, because DWI sequences contain T2-weighting, areas within the brain with high inherent T2 signal intensity can also show increased signal on DWI sequence, so-called T2 shine-through. To distinguish T2 shine-through from true restricted diffusion, consult the apparent diffusion coefficient (ADC) map. Areas of T2 shine-through will be bright on both DWI and its corresponding ADC map, whereas areas of restricted diffusion appear bright on DWI and dark on ADC.

The most important cause of restricted diffusion on DWI is acute ischemia. Although commonly thought to reflect areas of infarct core, a recent systematic review found reversible DWI lesions in 24% of patients in reviewed studies,[40] half of whom had received thrombolytic therapy. This finding suggests that DWI hyperintense lesions in acute stroke may reflect both ischemic core and some reversibly ischemic tissue.

Restricted diffusion can also be present in cerebral abscesses, diffuse axonal injury, active demyelination, and highly cellular tumors such as CNS lymphoma. DWI is particularly helpful in two classic cases. The differential diagnosis for a ring-enhancing parenchymal mass frequently includes intracranial neoplasm such as metastasis or high-grade astrocytoma as well as cerebral abscess. The central nonenhancing component of a pyogenic abscess classically demonstrates markedly restricted diffusion, with decreased ADC values (Fig. 3.12). This differentiates abscess from neoplasm, in which DWI signal is usually, but not always, normal or elevated.

Another classic situation in which DWI is particularly helpful is in differentiating an epidermoid cyst from arachnoid cyst, for example, in the cerebellopontine angle cistern. Epidermoid cysts exhibit bright DWI signal (Fig. 3.13).[41] Arachnoid cysts follow CSF on all sequences, and will therefore have low DWI signal.

Blood Degradation on Magnetic Resonance Imaging

Parenchymal hematomas can have a confusing MR appearance because of the changes in imaging appearance over time.[25,42] The state of hemoglobin affects the magnetic properties of iron by changes in the oxidation state, resulting in changes in T1 and T2 signal properties. Knowledge of the pattern of changes can be helpful for establishing the time course of hemorrhage evolution as well as preventing misdiagnosis of hemorrhage as a different mass lesion (Table 3.3).

Hyperacute hemorrhage is liquid and predominantly contains intracellular oxygenated hemoglobin. At this stage, the hemorrhage is isointense on T1 and bright on T2. During the acute phase (approximately 12 hours to 2 days), the hemoglobin becomes progressively deoxygenated, and the hematoma becomes dark on T2 while remaining isointense on T1. As the hematoma continues to break down in the early subacute phase (2 to 7 days), the hemoglobin is denatured to methemoglobin, which initially remains in the intracellular compartment. Methemoglobin appears hyperintense on T1 but remains dark on T2. As the red blood cells lyse in the late subacute phase (approximately 8 days to 1 month), the extracellular methemoglobin becomes bright on T2 and remains bright on T1. Finally, as the hematoma further evolves into the chronic stage (months to years), the iron from degraded hemoglobin is stored within hemosiderin and ferritin, and becomes dark on both T1 and T2.[42]

Magnetic Resonance Angiography

MR angiography can be performed without or with intravenous contrast agent. Noncontrast MR angiography depends on tagging moving protons, and thus relies on inherent inflow for visualizing vessels. Contrast-enhanced MRA is similar to CTA in that vascular visualization relies on contrast opacification. Contrast-enhanced MRA is thus dependent on accurate contrast bolus timing for the acquisition of high-quality imaging. The basic physics of these techniques has been described earlier.

Time-of-flight (TOF) MRA of the intracranial circulation is performed using three directions, because blood flows in the anteroposterior, superoinferior, and transverse directions in the circle of Willis. Three-dimensional TOF MRA provides excellent, high-resolution images of the major intracranial vessels without the risks of contrast agent or radiation, as long as the patient remains still during the acquisition. Contrast-enhanced MRA of the brain may be helpful in certain situations, such as in the evaluation of arteriovenous malformations, in which there might be slow flow or in which flow in small vessels is important.

Noncontrast MRA of the neck uses a two-dimensional TOF technique, because flow in the neck occurs primarily

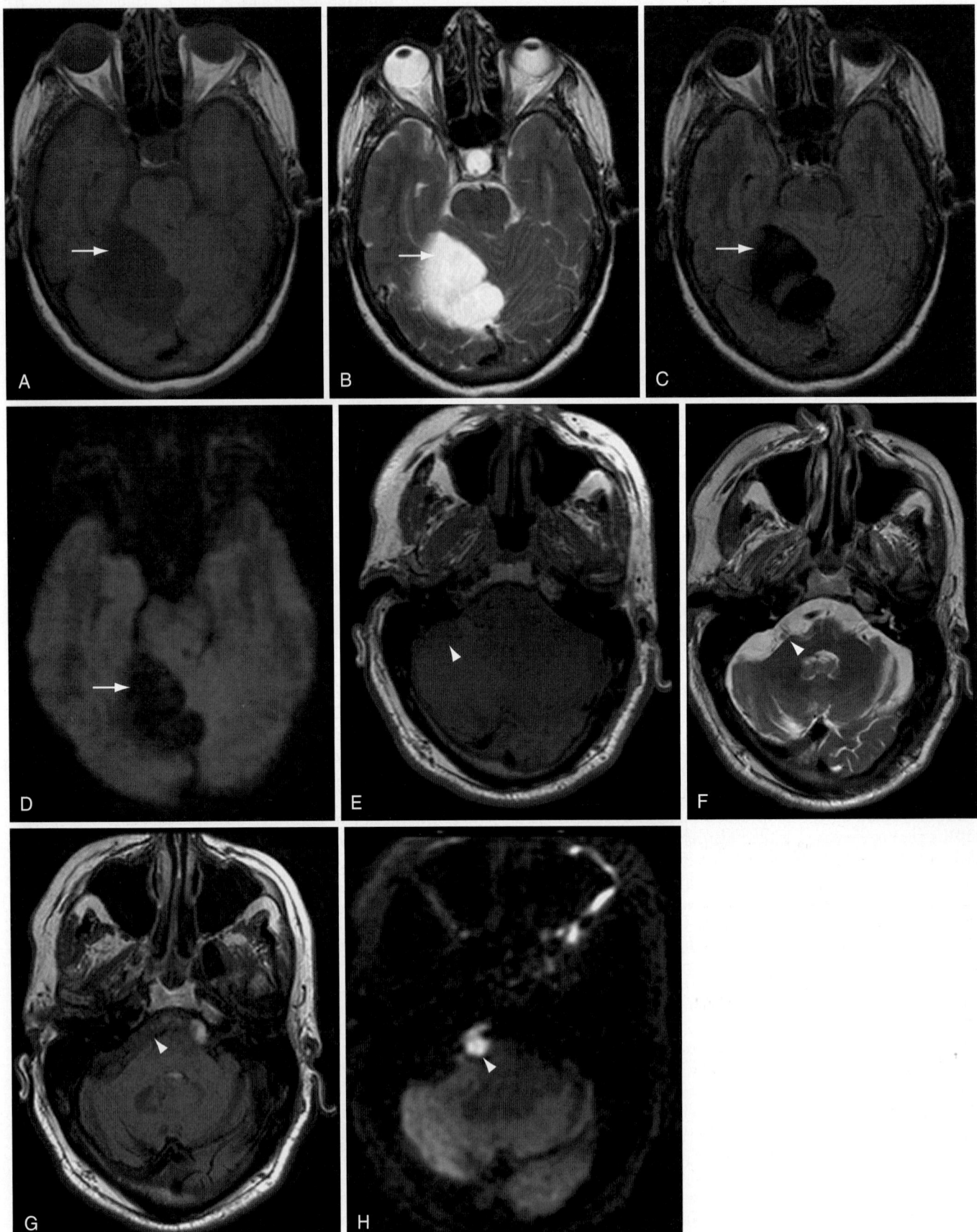

FIGURE 3.11 Two patients with posterior fossa lesions. T1 (**A**), T2 (**B**), FLAIR (**C**), and diffusion-weighted (**D**) images from a 77-year-old woman with an incidental posterior fossa arachnoid cyst. Note the cystic structure follows cerebrospinal fluid (CSF) signal on all sequences, a hall-mark of an arachnoid cyst. T1 (**E**), T2 (**F**), FLAIR (**G**), and diffusion-weighted (**H**) images from a 37-year-old with an epidermoid cyst in the right cerebellopontine angle (CPA) cistern. Note that this lesion appears similar to CSF on T1 and T2, but does not suppress completely (as would simple fluid) on FLAIR. Note flow artifact in the left CPA cistern, appearing as increased FLAIR signal. The epidermoid is bright on DWI sequence, a classic finding. FLAIR, fluid attenuated inversion recovery.

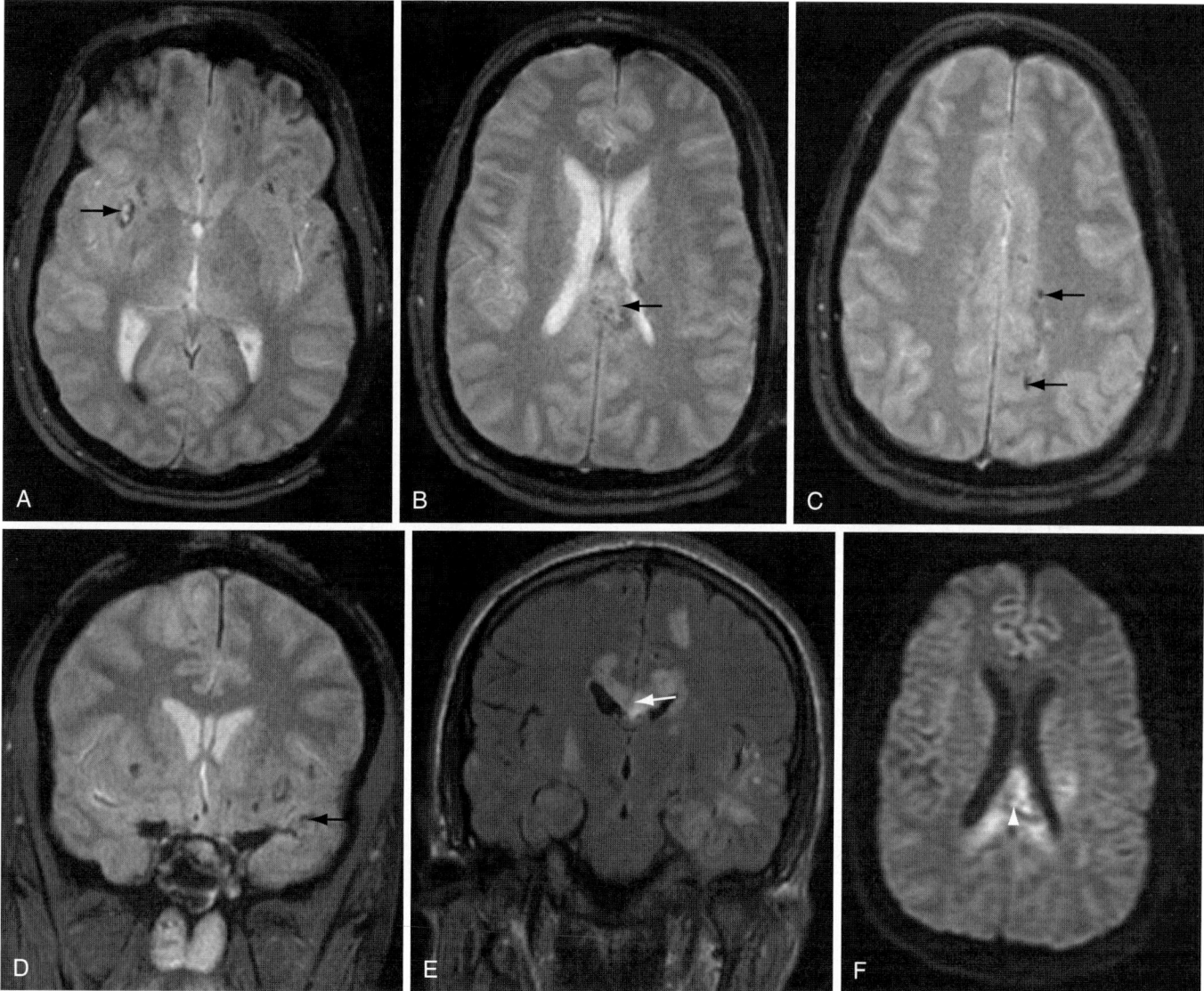

FIGURE 3.12 Hemorrhage on T2* gradient echo (GRE) sequence. A 34-year-old in a high-speed motor vehicle crash. Axial (**A, B, C**) and coronal (**D**) T2* GRE-weighted images demonstrate multiple areas of signal dropout corresponding to microhemorrhages (*black arrows*). FLAIR (**E**) and diffusion-weighted (**F**) images demonstrate extensive involvement of the splenium of the corpus callosum. Findings are consistent with diffuse axonal injury. FLAIR, fluid attenuated inversion recovery.

in the superoinferior direction. The larger region of interest requires acquisition of images in multiple slabs. If there is movement between the acquisitions of adjacent slabs, there will be stair-step artifact along the course of the vessel that can limit interpretation. One way to avoid this artifact is to perform gadolinium bolus MRA of the neck. In this case, direct coronal acquisition through the cervical vessels during peak arterial enhancement phase of the contrast bolus can be performed. Images from either MRA technique are reformatted to provide three-dimensional images with maximum intensity projections (MIP reformatted images).

The differences in contrast and noncontrast MRA of the neck can be illustrated by comparing vessel occlusion with subclavian steal syndrome (Fig. 3.14). In the case of vessel occlusion, there will be no flow-related signal on TOF sequence because there are no tagged protons traveling through the occluded vessel. In addition, there will be no

contrast opacification of the occluded vessel (see Fig. 3.14, carotid artery).

Conversely, in the case of subclavian steal there is reversal of flow in the affected vertebral artery. In this case, a two-dimensional TOF sequence through the vessel will not detect flow-related signal, because flow in the vessel runs superior to inferior. A saturation pulse superior to the cervical vessels is applied to remove flow-related signal in the cervical veins, which may overlap and thereby obscure the cervical arteries. Because the flow in the left vertebral artery also runs superior to inferior in the case of subclavian steal, the tagged protons in this flow-reversed vertebral artery are also suppressed on two-dimensional TOF MRA. However, the flow-reversed vertebral artery continues to opacify with contrast on gadolinium-bolus MRA, because the vessel remains patent (see Fig. 3.14).

Noncontrast TOF or phase contrast sequences through the dural venous sinuses can also be performed to evaluate

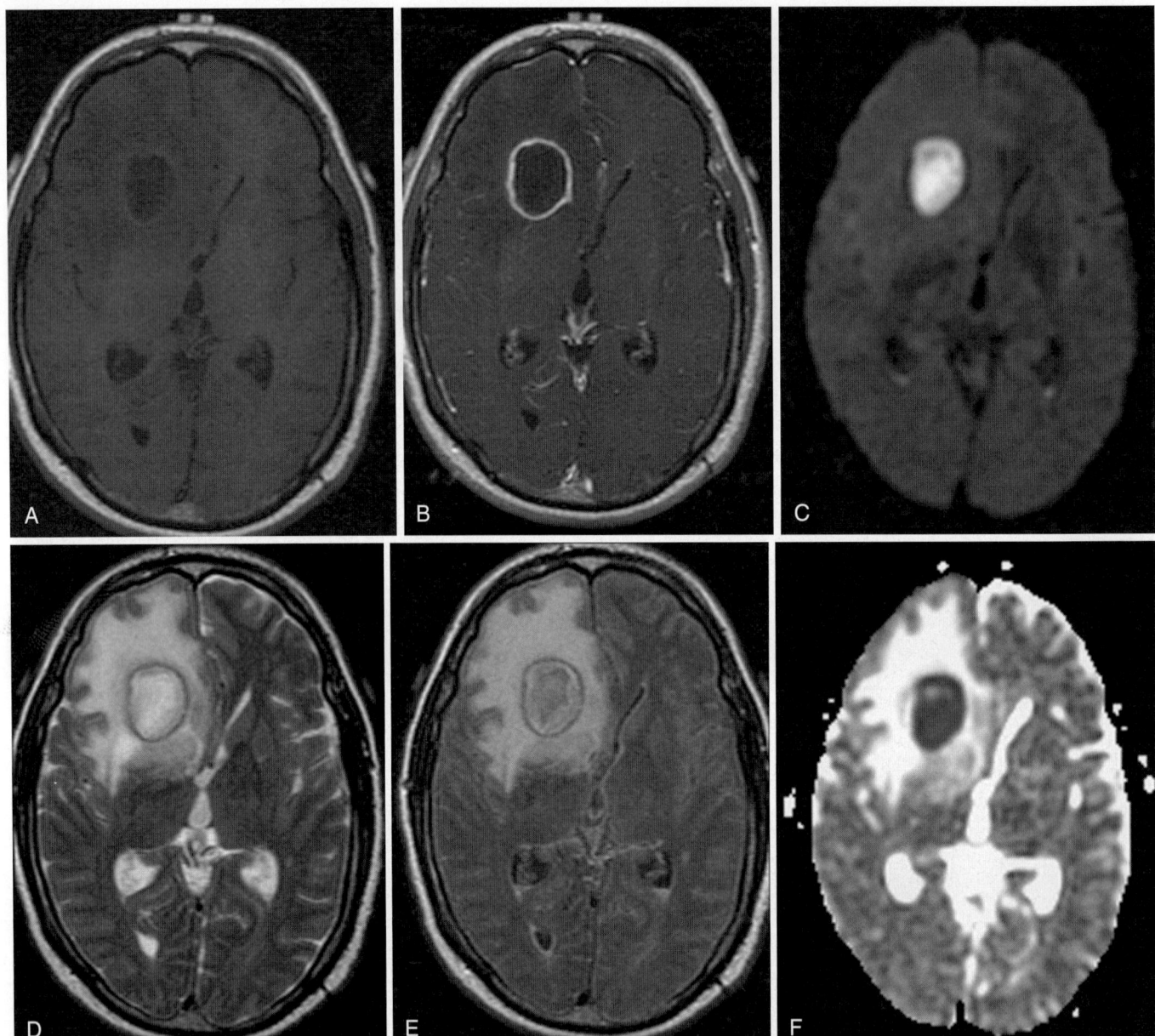

FIGURE 3.13 Restricted diffusion. A 45-year-old man with headache. T1 (**A**), T1 postcontrast (**B**), diffusion-weighted (**C**), T2 (**D**), and FLAIR (**E**) images, as well as ADC map (**F**), show a ring-enhancing left frontal lesion. Findings typical of abscess include restricted diffusion (bright on DWI, **C**; dark on ADC, **F**) and a low T2 ring (**D**) around the lesion. Note layering debris in the ventricles on DWI (**C**) and FLAIR (**E**), indicating intraventricular extension. ADC, apparent diffusion coefficient; DWI, diffusion-weighted imaging; FLAIR, fluid attenuated inversion recovery.

intracranial venous structures (MR venography, MRV). In general, imaging in both the axial and coronal planes is recommended to detect flow in the superior sagittal sinus as well as the transverse sinuses.

Magnetic Resonance Perfusion

A complementary perfusion technique to CT perfusion is MR perfusion. MR perfusion is performed by one of two methods, either with intravenous contrast agent or by using arterial spin labeling. In contrast-enhanced MR perfusion, images are acquired during rapid contrast bolus transit through the entire brain. The dynamic susceptibility contrast (DSC) technique uses a T2*-sensitive pulse sequence to image the contrast agent over time as it passes through the brain parenchyma. Gadolinium causes signal loss on T2*-sensitive sequences due to the paramagnetic effects of gadolinium. This signal loss is plotted against time to reveal a signal intensity curve. The negative enhancement integral is the calculated area under this curve, which corresponds to the cerebral blood volume.[43] From this graph, perfusion maps equivalent to CBV, CBF, and MTT can be derived.[43] If the perfusion images are acquired using a T1-based pulse sequence, the technique is called *dynamic contrast-enhanced* (DCE) MR perfusion. In this technique, perfusion maps are derived in a similar fashion to perfusion CT, as described previously.[40]

TABLE 3.3 Appearance of Hemorrhage on Magnetic Resonance Imaging

Stage	Age of Bleed	Composition	T1	T2
Hyperacute	<12 hours	Intracellular oxyhemoglobin	Isointense	Hyperintense
Acute	12 hours to 2 days	Intracellular deoxyhemoglobin	Isointense	Hypointense
Early subacute	2-7 days	Intracellular methemoglobin	Hyperintense	Hypointense
Late subacute	8 days to 1 month	Extracellular methemoglobin	Hyperintense	Hyperintense
Chronic	Months to years	Hemosiderin	Hypointense	Hypointense

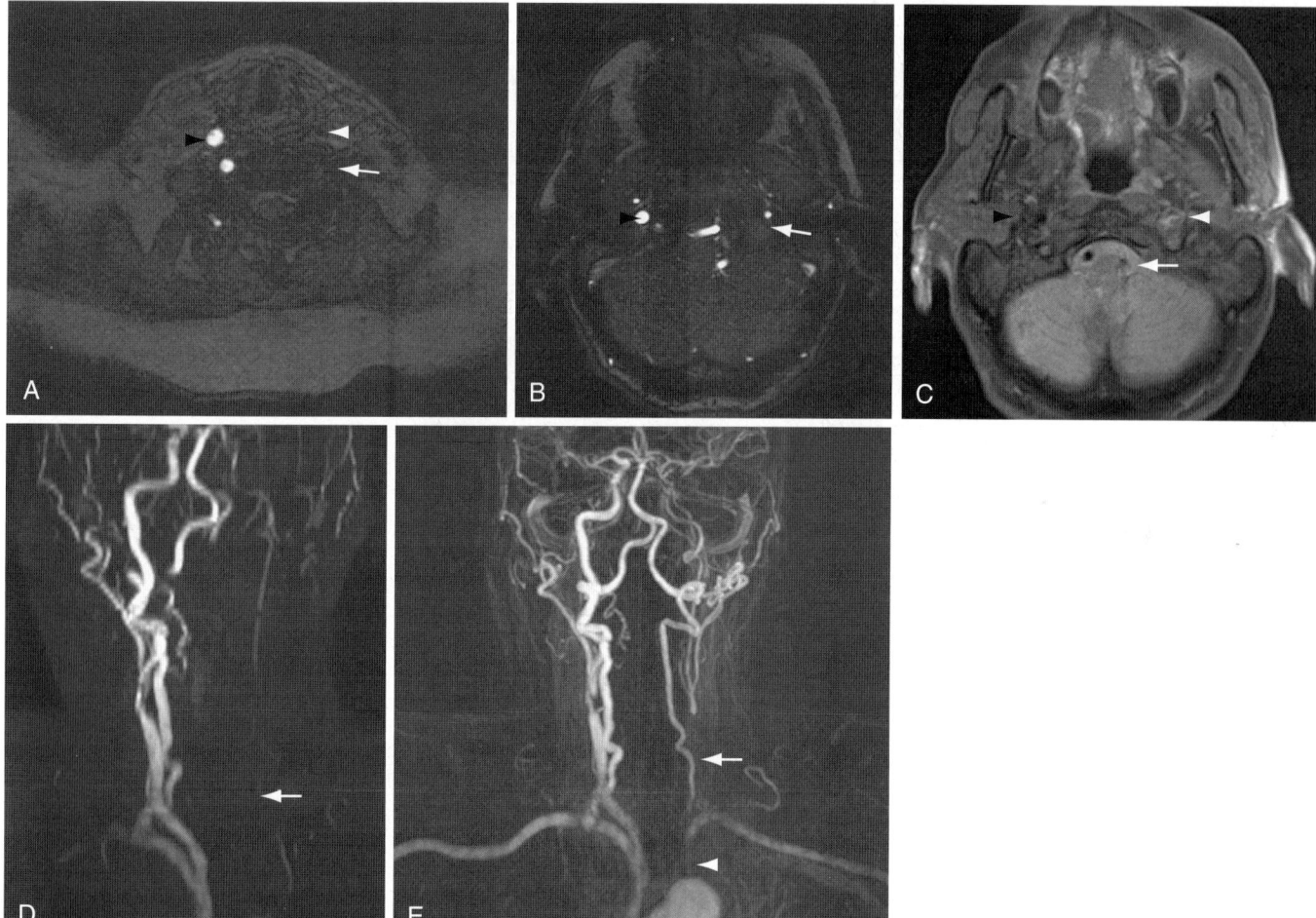

FIGURE 3.14 Magnetic resonance angiography (MRA). A 70-year-old woman who has had multiple falls. Unenhanced two-dimensional (2D) time-of-flight (TOF) MRA (**A, B, D**) shows normal right carotid and vertebral arteries (*black arrowheads* in **A, B**). No flow-related signal in the left vertebral (*white arrow*) or left carotid artery (*white arrowhead*). Axial proton density fat-saturated image (**C**) shows abnormal left carotid artery flow void (*white arrowhead*), compared to normal appearance of the right carotid (*black arrowhead*) and vertebral artery (*white arrow*) flow voids. **E,** Gadolinium-enhanced MRA shows contrast opacification of the left vertebral artery (*white arrow*), but nonfilling of the left carotid artery. Note stenosis of the left subclavian origin (*arrowhead*). Angiogram confirmed subclavian steal syndrome with reversal of flow in the left vertebral artery (thus, no flow-related signal on the 2D TOF) and occlusion of the left carotid artery (no flow on either TOF or gadolinium-bolus MRA).

Both dynamic susceptibility contrast and dynamic contrast-enhanced MR perfusion have been used in a variety of clinical settings, including stroke and the evaluation of unknown brain lesions. In acute stroke imaging, a mismatch between perfusion and diffusion abnormalities on MRI is thought to represent ischemic penumbra; that is, brain tissue that is ischemic but not yet infarcted. The perfusion abnormality has been defined in many ways, most commonly as delayed time to peak (TTP),[44] but also as an area of prolonged MTT. The infarct core is generally defined as the area of restricted diffusion. Patients in whom there exists a large ischemic penumbra may benefit from intra-arterial thrombolysis or other therapies intended to salvage the at-risk tissue defined by the penumbra (Fig. 3.15).

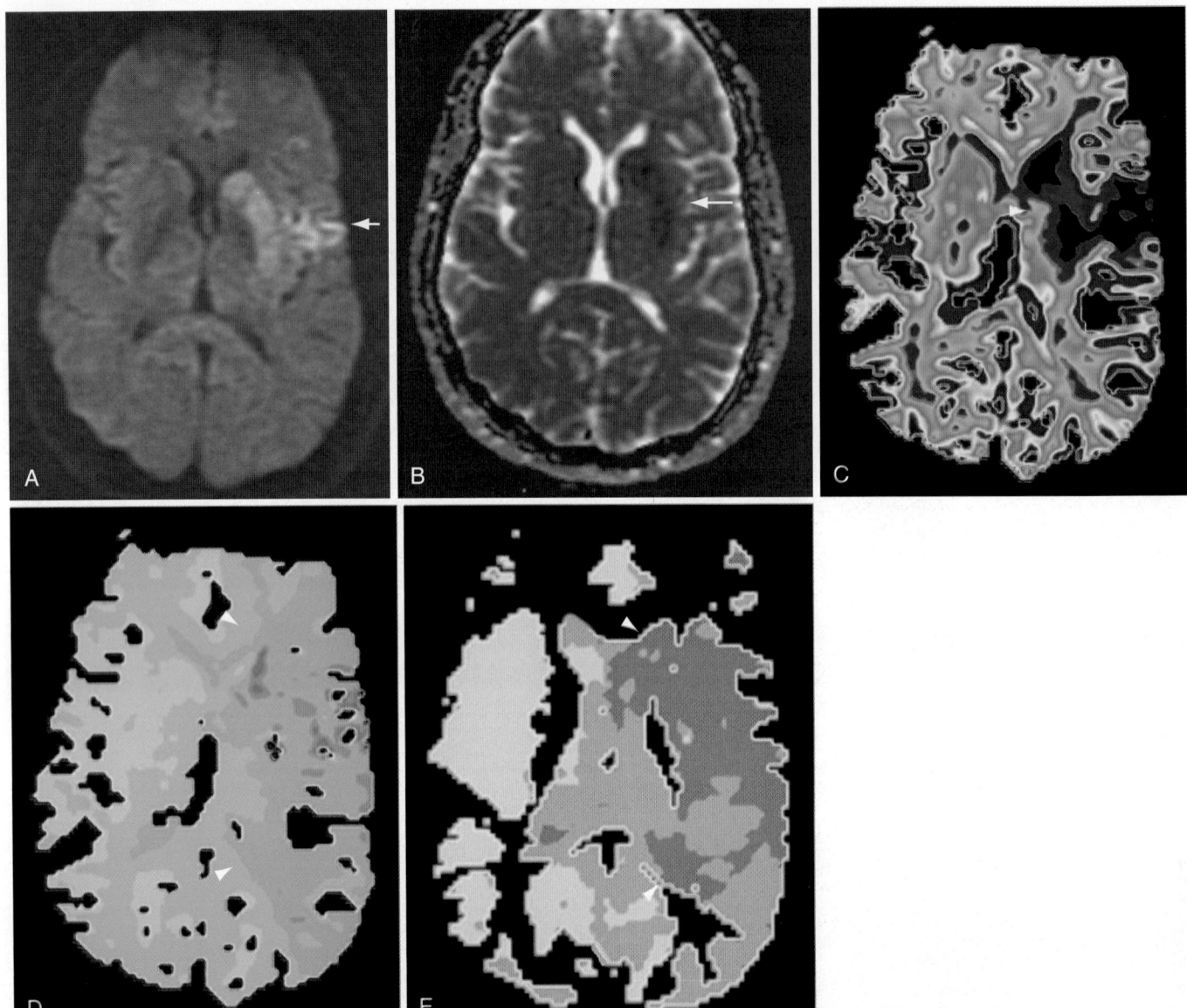

FIGURE 3.15 A 56-year-old man with acute right hemiplegia. Diffusion-weighted image (**A**) and ADC map (**B**) show an area of restricted diffusion in the left basal ganglia and insula, consistent with acute infarction. Cerebral blood volume map (**C**) is similar to the area of restricted diffusion, indicating infarct core. Mean transit time (MTT) (**D**) and time to peak (TTP) (**E**) maps show a much larger area of perfusion abnormality, demarcated by white arrowheads. The tissue within the region of the perfusion abnormality that does *not* show restricted diffusion is thought to represent the ischemic penumbra.

Arterial spin labeling perfusion MR is a different technique in which contrast material is not given, but arterial water is tagged by an inverted pulse applied proximal to the imaging plane.[45] As these magnetically tagged protons flow into the imaging slabs covering the brain, they equilibrate with tissues, acting as a diffusible tracer. Images acquired with and without spin labeling are subtracted, resulting in a map of relative concentration of arterial water, corresponding to a cerebral blood flow map. Quantitative values of CBF in mL/100 g tissue/minute can be calculated.

Arterial spin labeling (ASL) perfusion MR has been used for many applications, including stroke. Comparing CBF maps either visually or by quantitative analysis of CBF values to DWI maps can also demonstrate areas of perfusion-diffusion mismatch, thought to correlate to ischemic penumbra.[46] Other

indications for ASL perfusion MR reported in the literature include assessing chronic ischemia, epilepsy, neoplasms, vascular malformations, and luxury perfusion.[47,48]

Functional Magnetic Resonance Imaging

Functional MRI (fMRI) is a technique in which serial images of the brain are obtained while a patient performs a functional task. Pulse sequences are maximized for the detection of increased blood oxygenation level, felt to represent activation of a brain area.[49] The signal changes detected are extremely small, and repetitive performance of the task with accumulation of the imaging data is required to achieve adequate signal-to-noise for analysis.

Functional MRI has been used in a variety of clinical settings.[49] fMRI has been used to lateralize language and memory in patients with epilepsy in whom surgical treatment is planned. Functional cortex can be mapped prior to surgery in cases of planned tumor resection when the tumor lies within or near eloquent areas. This technique is also widely used in research studies to evaluate and localize different brain functions. Undoubtedly, new uses of fMRI will continue to be developed as research in this field progresses.

Diffusion Tensor Imaging

Diffusion tensor imaging is a sophisticated version of diffusion-weighted imaging in which detection of the movement of water molecules is performed in six or more directions rather than the standard three dimensions, as with DWI.[50] In the brain, water molecules tend to exhibit motion preferentially in certain directions over others according to the underlying cellular architecture, a property termed *anisotropy* that is mapped according to fractional anisotropy (FA mapping). Areas with high fractional anisotropy (relatively closer to an FA value of 1.0) show a strong directionality of water molecular movement, whereas areas with low fractional anisotropy (closer to an FA value of zero) show relatively less directionality of water motion. Most often, water molecular motion appears to be organized along known white matter tracts. By analyzing the movement of water molecules throughout the brain, a map of these fiber tracts can be constructed (DTI tractography).

DTI has been used in neurosurgical practice to map important fiber tracts in patients with tumors in eloquent areas. The technique of isolating important fiber tracts by selecting key anatomical areas and mapping pathways of anisotropic water movement between them can help to identify the location of important white matter fiber tracts with respect to the mass lesion. Using techniques such as these may facilitate safe maximal resection.[51] However, it must be emphasized that the fiber tracts revealed by diffusion tractography are not the actual white matter tracts themselves, but instead a representation of white matter tracts based on the analysis of anisotropic water movement.

DTI has also been studies in a variety of research setting to assess white matter integrity. Important areas of research include evaluating loss of axonal pathways in multiple sclerosis, head trauma, and aging/dementia.

Magnetic Resonance Spectroscopy

MR spectroscopy (MRS) is a method of sampling a volume of brain tissue for known metabolites. In clinical MRS, proton (^{1}H) MRS is most commonly used because of the abundance of protons in tissue. MR spectroscopy can be acquired in several different fashions. In single voxel MRS, a single volume of tissue is selected for study. This tissue can be sampled at different echo times (TE) to highlight different metabolites. The echo times used in short TE studies are approximately 35 msec, whereas long TE studies frequently use either 144 msec or 288 msec. MRS at any of these echo times shows metabolite peaks corresponding to *N*-acetyl aspartate (NAA), creatine (Cr), choline (Cho), lactate (Lac), and lipid (Lip) if present. At 144 msec, the lactate peak often projects (inverts) below the baseline rather than above, and it frequently displays a doublet peak pattern, helping to differentiate it from the broader, adjacent lipid peak. Short TE studies also reveal the peaks of additional metabolites including glutamine and glutamate (Glx) and myoinositol (mI), among others.

Multivoxel MRS differs from the single voxel technique in that a slab of tissue is sampled, comprising many smaller voxels within the slab. When processing the spectra after acquisition, individual voxels within the slab can be interrogated and adjacent voxels can be summed, allowing greater flexibility in selecting a region of interest. The multivoxel slab can also be positioned at the time of acquisition to include adjacent normal brain for comparison.

Different metabolites are felt to represent different physiological processes.[52] Creatine is generally used as an internal reference peak for cellular metabolism and, as a first approximation, is assumed to be relatively stable in concentration throughout the parenchyma. NAA is often used as a marker of neuronal integrity, whereas choline is frequently used as a marker for cellular membrane turnover reflecting cellular proliferation. Lactate indicates the presence of anaerobic glycolysis. Myoinositol is a marker of myelin degradation. Lipids may indicate necrosis or disruption of myelin.

The pattern of the spectral peaks can help determine whether a lesion is neoplastic in nature, for example.[53] Elevated Cho:Cr peak height ratio, depressed NAA, and presence of lactate are all findings associated with neoplasia (Fig. 3.16). However, one of the diagnostic challenges with MRS is that changes in relative metabolic peak height for the various metabolites may be nonspecific as to etiology, and in such cases MRS spectra should always be interpreted in the context of other available imaging data.

Nuclear Medicine Studies

Neurosurgeons may also encounter nuclear medicine studies in clinical practice. Nuclear medicine refers to a type of imaging study in which radiolabeled compounds are administered to a patient and the distribution of that agent within the body is then evaluated with specialized detectors. The many types of nuclear medicine studies include positron emission tomography (PET) and single-photon emission computed tomography (SPECT), but only the latter will be discussed here.

SPECT is a nuclear medicine imaging modality that can be used to detect changes in brain perfusion,[54] among other things. For brain SPECT, a tracer agent is tagged with a radionuclide and inhaled or intravenously injected. The agent accumulates in brain parenchyma proportionate to cerebral blood flow in a given region of brain tissue. As the radionuclide decays, photons are emitted. Areas with relatively higher cerebral blood flow such as gray matter accumulate more radiotracer and therefore emit more photons than relatively lower flow areas such as white matter. These photons are detected by gamma cameras positioned around the head, and the information is reconstructed into tomographic slices. The intensity of each voxel in SPECT imaging represents the relative uptake of the radiotracer. Because voxels are compared to each other, actual blood flow is not directly measured, and brain SPECT in its usual clinical form is a qualitative test (with the exception of inhaled xenon gas; see later discussion).

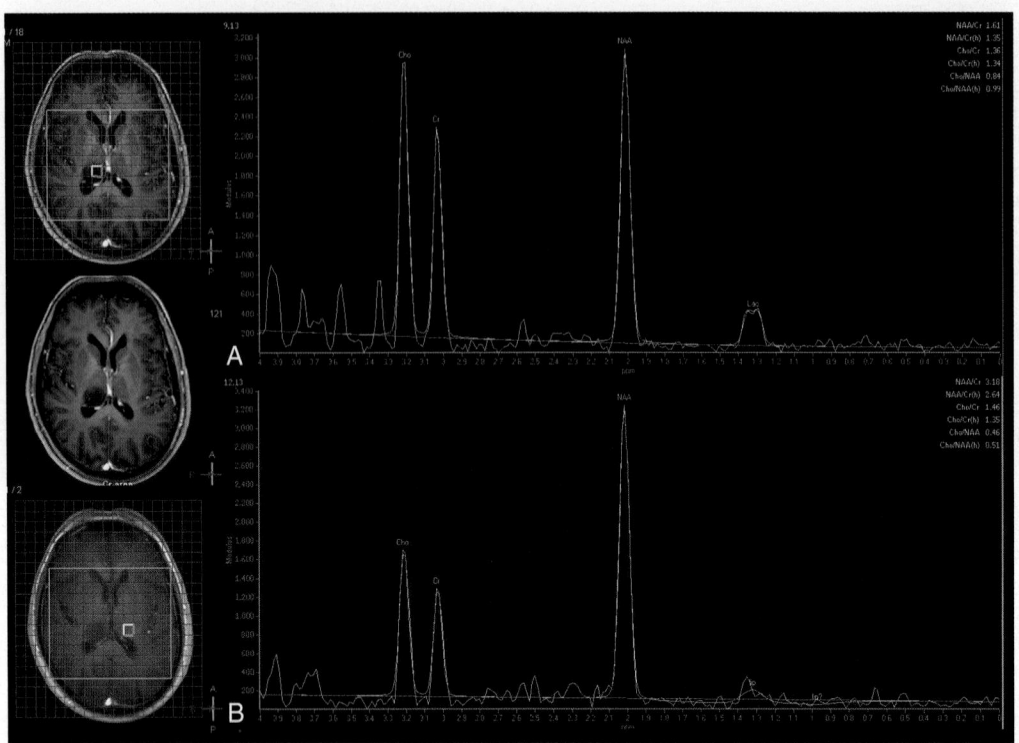

FIGURE 3.16 A 42-year-old man with thalamic tumor who underwent multivoxel long echo time (TE) magnetic resonance spectroscopy of a right thalamic lesion compared to the contralateral normal side (center inset, T1 postcontrast image). **A,** Voxel chosen within the right thalamic lesion shows decreased *N*-acetyl aspartate (NAA) and elevated choline compared to the creatine peak, with presence of lactate. **B,** Voxel chosen within the normal left thalamus showing normal spectral pattern. Surgical pathological findings revealed anaplastic astrocytoma (WHO III).

Tracer agents must be lipid soluble to pass through the blood-brain barrier. The most commonly used radiotracer agents for brain SPECT are intravenous technetium-99m (^{99}Tc) labeled compounds and inhaled radiolabeled xenon gas (^{133}Xe). Intravenous tracers are taken up within minutes and remain fixed for many hours, allowing the characterization of perfusion at a specific time point, the time of injection. Brain SPECT with inhaled ^{133}Xe can yield quantitative measurements of cerebral blood flow, but this technique requires specific and expensive equipment and is seldom clinically used.

In addition to the detection of cerebral perfusion, the SPECT technique can be applied to other compounds and other areas of the body. For instance, the density of radiolabeled leukocytes in a lesion suspicious for abscess can support that diagnosis.[55] Brain SPECT can also be used for molecular imaging. For example, a radiolabeled receptor ligand, such as a neurotransmitter, can be used to localize receptor activity.[56]

In clinical practice, brain SPECT is most often used in cases of epilepsy, cerebrovascular disease, and the evaluation of dementia. Seizures can significantly increase focal cerebral blood flow in epileptogenic tissue[57] (Fig. 3.17). Because ^{99}Tc tracers are rapidly taken up by brain tissue and remain there for up to 6 hours, the radionuclide can be injected within a minute of seizure onset, and SPECT imaging can then subsequently be performed when the seizure is over and the patient is stable. The perfusion during a seizure (ictal SPECT) is compared to perfusion between seizures (interictal SPECT). Seizure foci show ictal hyperperfusion and interictal hypoperfusion, which can be useful when electroencephalography (EEG) or clinical data are conflicting or nonspecific, or to highlight the epileptic focus in secondary generalized seizure disorders. In addition, lack of perfusion changes in a patient with clinical seizure-like activity may imply pseudoseizure or other nonepileptogenic phenomena. Combined with MRI and EEG, SPECT is a useful adjunct in the presurgical evaluation of epilepsy patients.[58]

Cerebrovascular disease and stroke can also be evaluated with brain SPECT.[59] SPECT can be used to define ischemic penumbra in an ongoing stroke, although CT and MR perfusion are more commonly used for this purpose owing to their relatively wider availability, more rapid acquisition times, and higher spatial resolution.[60] Brain SPECT can also be used to evaluate cerebrovascular reserve in a patient with chronic cerebral ischemia. Such tests require the introduction of a vasodilatory agent (acetazolamide or inhaled 5% CO_2), followed by the injection of radionuclide tracer. In normally perfused tissue, administration of a vasodilator causes hyperperfusion. In areas supplied by diseased vasculature, hyperperfusion does not occur, as the affected vessels are either unable to dilate, or are already maximally dilated, and in fact hypoperfusion induced by the steal phenomenon may be observed. Revascularization procedures may be considered in such patients.[61]

Cerebral vasospasm has also been studied using SPECT. Vasospasm is a well-known complication of subarachnoid hemorrhage, and can cause ischemia or infarction.[62,63] Cerebral angiography is the gold standard for the diagnosis of cerebral vasospasm, but SPECT has also been used to evaluate hypoperfusion in the setting of suspected vasospasm.[64] A recent study of SPECT obtained within 24 hours of angiographically confirmed vasospasm failed to confirm the predictive utility of SPECT, however, thus potentially limiting the role of brain SPECT imaging in vasospasm.[65]

Finally, nuclear medicine studies including SPECT can be used as a noninvasive corroborative test in the evaluation of brain death.[66] In brain death there is absent cerebral perfusion manifesting as an intracranial compartment devoid of any radiotracer uptake. The majority of head and neck blood flow is routed to the external carotid circulation, resulting

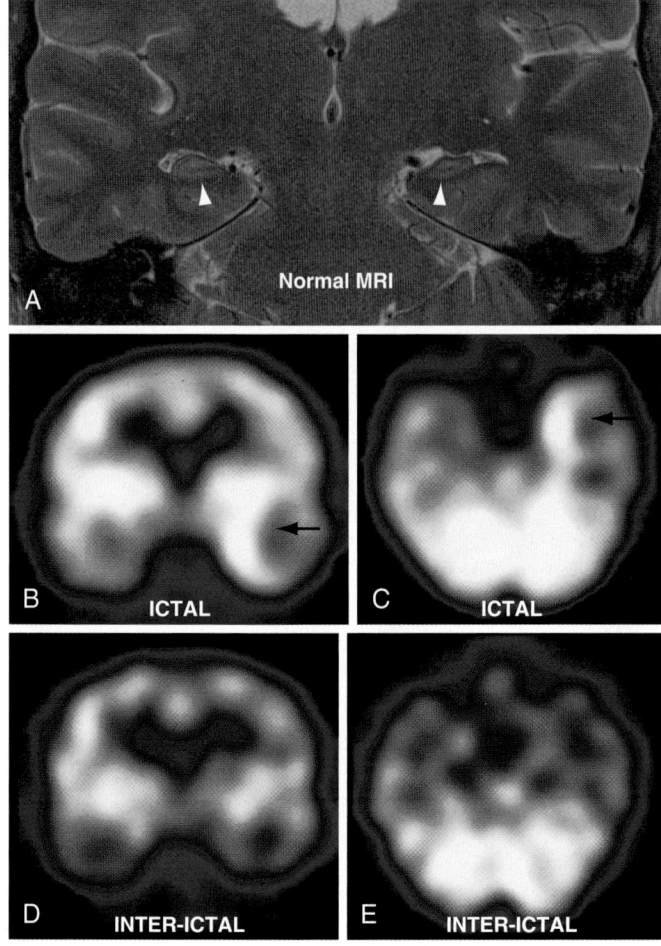

FIGURE 3.17 A 39-year-old woman with medically intractable seizures. **A,** Coronal high resolution T2-weighted magnetic resonance image through the temporal lobes showing normal hippocampi (*arrowheads*). Technetium-99m ethylcysteinate dimer (ECD) brain single-photon emission computed tomography (SPECT) obtained during (**B, C**) and between (**D, E**) seizures. Coronal (**B, D**) and axial images (**C, E**) demonstrate increased radiotracer uptake in the left mesial temporal lobe during ictus (*black arrows*) compared to the resting state.

in the characteristic "hot nose" sign. This test must be interpreted in conjunction with high clinical suspicion of brain death, as brain SPECT alone is not sufficient to diagnose brain death.[67]

SUMMARY

Neuroimaging plays an important role in the practice of clinical neurosurgery. An understanding of the imaging findings of basic neurosurgical processes such as mass effect, brain herniation, edema and ischemia is the first step to rapidly diagnosing neurosurgical emergencies. MRI is a useful adjunct for the diagnosis of many diseases in the brain, and different MR sequences provide unique information to aid in the differential diagnosis. Neuroimaging is an exciting field, with advances being made in many areas, particularly perfusion imaging, DTI, and fMRI. An understanding of the basic concepts underlying these newer modalities will allow incorporation of these techniques into clinical practice as their utility in clinical practice continues to emerge.

SELECTED KEY REFERENCES

ACR Appropriateness Criteria: Neurologic Imaging. American College of Radiology; 2010. Accessed March 1, 2010, at http://www.acr.org/SecondaryMainMenuCategories/quality_safety/app_criteria.aspx2010.

de Lucas EM, Sanchez E, Gutierrez A, et al. CT protocol for acute stroke: tips and tricks for general radiologists. *Radiographics*. 2008;28:1673-1687.

Kidwell CS, Wintermark M. Imaging of intracranial haemorrhage. *Lancet Neurol*. 2008;7:256-267.

Laine FJ, Shedden AI, Dunn MM, Ghatak NR. Acquired intracranial herniations: MR imaging findings. *AJR Am J Roentgenol*. 1995;165:967-973.

Shih LC, Saver JL, Alger JR, et al. Perfusion-weighted magnetic resonance imaging thresholds identifying core, irreversibly infarcted tissue. *Stroke*. 2003;34:1425-1430.

Please go to expertconsult.com to view complete list of references.

4 Principles of Surgical Positioning

Geneviève Lapointe, Joanna Kemp, Govind Rajan,
Grace Elisabeth Walter, Saleem I. Abdulrauf

CLINICAL PEARLS

- Surgical positioning is a critical step of every operation that needs to be planned and executed carefully in order to avoid any significant potential complications.

- It is crucial to avoid traction on the patient's extremities and to ensure proper padding of all bony prominences, as these steps will prevent the occurrence of easily avoidable complications.

- Venous air embolism (VAE) can occur in any surgery where the wound is above the heart but is seen more frequently

with the sitting position. Less favored these days, this position still offers great advantages but requires adequate preoperative investigation and intraoperative monitoring to decrease the risks for the patient.

- Surgeons must play a leading role in ensuring the safety and comfort of the patient, for themselves, and for every other personnel member in the operating room.

Surgical positioning is one of the first obligatory steps in adequate surgical planning. Proper patient positioning is a critical part of every operation: it allows the surgeon the ability to comfortably gain access to the surgical site while avoiding potential complications. Positioning is particularly important in neurosurgery because procedures are often lengthy and many different trajectories can be used to access a single lesion. Neurosurgical positioning can vary greatly depending on the indication for surgery, the patient's body habitus, and the surgeon's preference. Several general principles of patient positioning must be understood in order to avoid potentially devastating complications. In this chapter the main neurosurgical positions, potential complications related to each position, and important considerations to decrease morbidity associated with each position are discussed in detail.

GENERAL PRINCIPLES OF PATIENT POSITIONING

Positioning the neurosurgical patient is a critical part of the procedure, perhaps more so than in any other surgical subspecialty. Appropriate patient positioning is not only important for the safety of the patient, but it also plays a key role in optimizing surgical exposure, ensuring adequate and safe anesthesia, and allowing the surgeon to comfortably operate during long procedures.

A thorough preoperative assessment by the anesthesia and nursing staff is necessary, as is a general understanding of the

indications, advantages, disadvantages, and potential complications that may arise from commonly utilized neurosurgical patient positions. The final position of the patient should be conveyed to the entire team as early as possible by the surgeon so that appropriate equipment is readily available and to ensure optimal selection and placement of the endotracheal tube, intravenous and arterial lines, noninvasive equipment, and monitors.[1-4]

Typically, patient positioning occurs subsequent to the induction of general anesthesia, intubation, acquisition of vascular access, and bladder catheterization. Neurophysiological monitoring leads are placed at various stages throughout the perioperative period. Unlike other surgical subspecialties, the planar rotation of the operative table varies depending on the planned surgical approach. The table can be neutral, turned 90 degrees, or often positioned at 180 degrees to allow adequate space and optimal placement of equipment required during complex neurosurgical procedures. This equipment may include the operating microscope, image guidance equipment, C-arm, endoscope tower, headlight sources, and occasionally intraoperative magnetic resonance imaging (MRI) or computed tomography (CT).[1]

During table rotation and patient positioning, it is often necessary to disconnect the ventilator and monitors temporarily. All members of the team should pay special attention to the duration of this period in order to avoid hypoxic insult to the patient. Eye protection with lubrication and tape provides a barrier that prevents corneal abrasion and introduction of caustic material into the eyes during positioning, intubation, and patient preparation and draping.[2]

Preoperative Assessment
- When judged appropriate, it is helpful to ascertain that patients can comfortably tolerate the anticipated operative position.

Upper Extremity Positioning
- Arm abduction should be limited to 90 degrees in supine patients; patients who are positioned prone may comfortably tolerate arm abduction greater than 90 degrees.
- Arms should be positioned to decrease pressure on the postcondylar groove of the humerus (ulnar groove). When arms are tucked at the side, a neutral forearm position is recommended. When arms are abducted on armboards, either supination or a neutral forearm position is acceptable.
- Prolonged pressure on the radial nerve in the spiral groove of the humerus should be avoided.
- Extension of the elbow beyond a comfortable range may stretch the median nerve.

Lower Extremity Positioning
- Lithotomy positions that stretch the hamstring muscle group beyond a comfortable range may stretch the sciatic nerve. Prolonged pressure on the peroneal nerve at the fibular head should be avoided.
- Neither extension nor flexion of the hip increases the risk of femoral neuropathy.

Protective Padding
- Padded armboards may decrease the risk of upper extremity neuropathy. The use of chest rolls in laterally positioned patients may decrease the risk of upper extremity neuropathies.
- Padding at the elbow and at the fibular head may decrease the risk of upper and lower extremity neuropathies, respectively.

Equipment
- Properly functioning automated blood pressure cuffs on the upper arms do not affect the risk of upper extremity neuropathies.
- Shoulder braces in steep head-down positions may increase the risk of brachial plexus neuropathies.

Postoperative Assessment
- A simple postoperative assessment of extremity nerve function may lead to early recognition of peripheral neuropathies.

Documentation
- Charting specific positioning actions during the care of patients may result in improvements of care by (1) helping practitioners focus attention on relevant aspects of patient positioning; and (2) providing information that continuous improvement processes can use to lead to refinements in patient care.

From American Society of Anesthesiologists Task Force on the Prevention of Perioperative Peripheral Neuropathies: Practice Advisory for the Prevention of Perioperative Peripheral Neuropathies. Anesthesiology 2000;92:1168-1182.

Principles of padding, taping, and positioning of the patient's extremities are based on the Summary of Task Force Consensus on the Prevention of Perioperative Peripheral Neuropathies Relevant to Positioning for Neurosurgery (Box 4.1).[5] In general, maintaining the patient's arms and legs in an anatomically neutral and relaxed position with soft protective barriers over areas with associated bony prominences helps prevent neurovascular compression, muscle damage, and cutaneous pressure injuries. A combination of gel pads, foam cushions, pillows, and padded arm rests are used for these purposes. For thoracoabdominal and pelvic protection and positioning, large gel rolls or specially designed frames and operative tables provide padding while simultaneously allowing relaxation of this region, aiding in both ventilation and venous return (Fig. 4.1). Such devices include but are not limited to the Wilson frame, Relton-Hall frame, Andrews frame, and Jackson table and frame.[3,4,5]

Cranial surgeries and occasionally posterior cervical surgeries require rigid skull fixation. Historically the use of stereotactic navigation universally required skull fixation; however, the development of electromagnetic systems has allowed the head to be mobile during a stereotactic procedure, obviating the need for pins. If rigid fixation is not required, the head may be placed on a gel or foam doughnut (Fig. 4.2) or in a padded horseshoe. The Mayfield frame (Fig. 4.3) is a three-pin device that is typically used for rigid skull fixation.[1,2] Both radiolucent and metal versions exist depending on the need for intraoperative x-ray. In cases in which spinal distraction and reduction may be necessary, Gardner-Wells tongs or a halo ring with attached weights are used. For prone positioning the head can be maintained in the Mayfield frame or placed on a foam pillow that is usually precut with openings for the eyes, nose, and endotracheal tube (Fig. 4.4).[1] Lateral positioning requires the use of specially positioned arm rests and usually an axillary roll to prevent brachial plexus compression.[5] More detailed requirements for the various positions are discussed in the respective sections later in this chapter.

In positions other than prone, placement of the Mayfield frame is carried out on the operative table prior to patient positioning. In the prone position, the pins are usually inserted on the hospital bed prior to transferring the patient to the operative table. In adults pins are placed under 60 pounds per square inch (psi) of pressure.[1] Inserting and tightening the pins has a profoundly stimulating effect on the patient that usually leads to an increase in heart rate and blood pressure. This hemodynamic change may incur potential complications, for example, in patients with unsecured

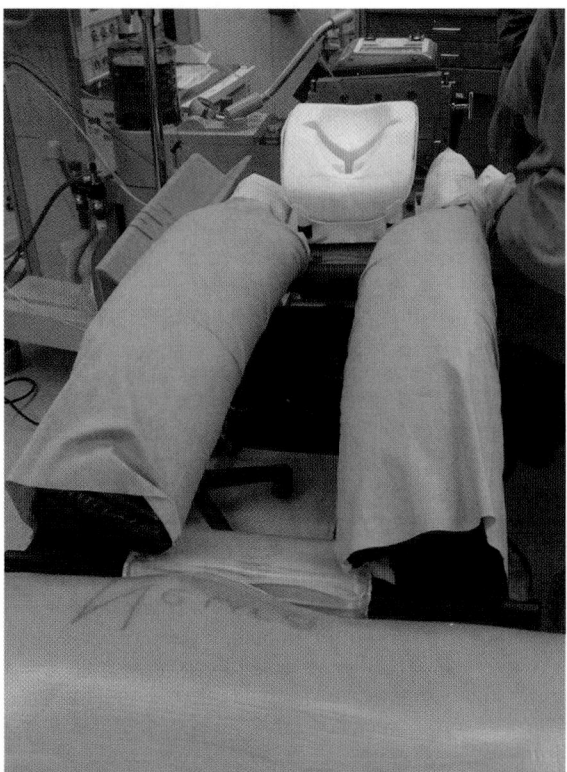

FIGURE 4.1 Table preparation for prone position.

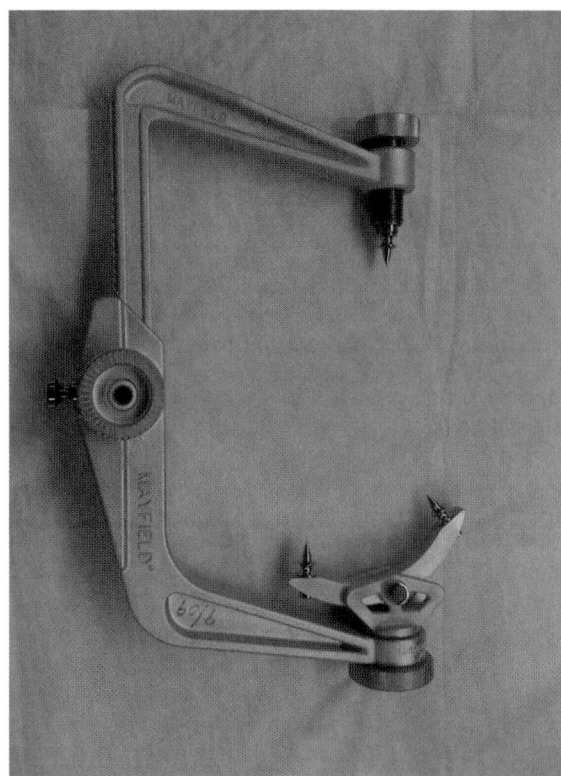

FIGURE 4.3 Mayfield head holder.

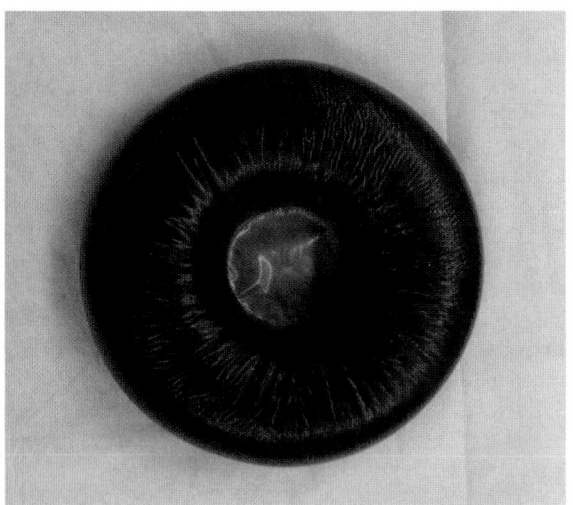

FIGURE 4.2 Gel doughnut.

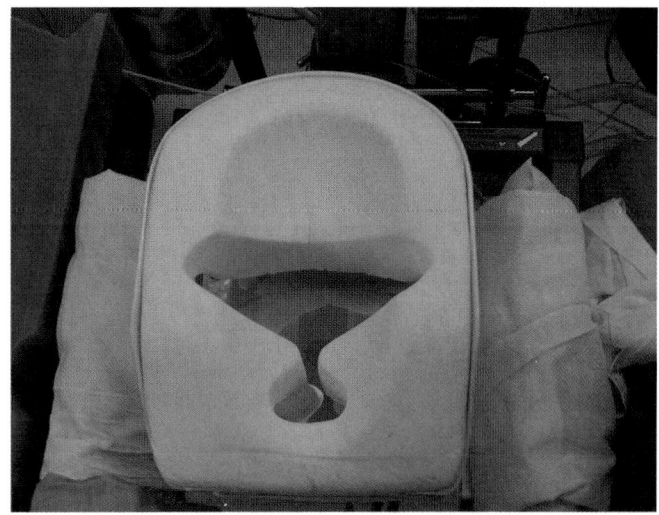

FIGURE 4.4 Foam pillow.

aneurysms or intracerebral hemorrhage. The timing of pin insertion should be clearly communicated between the surgeon and anesthesiologist so that the depth of anesthesia can be increased with additional bolus administration of an agent such as propofol (Diprivan). The patient's vital signs should be closely monitored during this time. This assumes that appropriate invasive and noninvasive forms of monitoring are in place and functioning prior to this step. Additionally, antibiotic ointment should be applied to each of the pins prior to their percutaneous insertion as a bacterial barrier and to avert air embolism, particularly in the sitting position.[2,6]

Head and neck configuration is perhaps the most important aspect of neurosurgical patient positioning. Final orientation of the head and neck is based on the planned surgical approach and exposure. There are several basic cranial approaches that determine head and neck positioning. The head can be safely rotated approximately 45 degrees in the supine position in healthy individuals. Access to the skull beyond 45 degrees requires manipulation and rotation of the patient's body into any of the specific positions described later in the chapter.[2] Various degrees of anteroposterior and lateral flexion and extension of the neck provide additional modification to the surgical trajectory.[1]

Avoidance of neurovascular complications during head and neck positioning requires vigilance on the part of the surgeon and the anesthesiologist. Hyperflexion beyond approximately 2 to 3 fingerbreadths between the mandibular protuberance and the manubrium is considered the upper limit of safe neck flexion. Hyperflexion of the neck in both the anteroposterior and lateral planes may lead to a series of complications. These complications include decreased cranial venous return and lymphatic outflow leading to facial swelling, macroglossia, and raised intracranial pressure, compression of the vertebral arteries leading to ischemia, and increased airway pressures affecting ventilation and oxygenation. Awareness of the distance between the patient's chin and the edge of the operative table is also important. In the prone position if the patient shifts downward on the table, the chin can press against the edge, leading to skin necrosis.[1,2,7]

The same basic principles and guidelines of patient positioning in general surgery also apply to the neurosurgical patient. However, a number of important considerations should be given to this subset of patients. Each patient position has its own indication and benefit but also carries a set of unique risks and potential complications that can be avoided with a thorough understanding of the use of the position.

SUPINE POSITION

The supine position (Fig. 4.5) is perhaps the most commonly used patient position in neurosurgery and across all surgical specialties. Because it is a familiar position, it is arguably the safest with the fewest number of associated complications. As an additional advantage, no special equipment is required.

In the supine position, the patient's head can be free on a padded doughnut or horseshoe, rigidly fixed in the Mayfield clamp, or in traction with Gardner-Wells tongs or a halo ring. The elbows, wrists, and heels are appropriately padded with gel or foam cushions. The knees are maintained in a slightly flexed position over a pillow. The arms are generally maintained at the patient's side on padded arm rests.[3] The head can safely be turned 45 degrees, as previously mentioned. Additional rotation can be achieved by placing a roll or bolster under the shoulder ipsilateral to the surgical side. If pins are not used and the head is turned, the ear and contralateral

scalp should be protected with a gel doughnut or foam pad to avoid compressive injury to the pinna and to prevent pressure alopecia.[2] If a shoulder roll is used, the contralateral or dependent arm is often placed in a slightly abducted position on an arm rest. The ipsilateral arm is either placed in a flexed position across the abdomen or maintained at the side on an arm rest, depending on the degree of patient rotation and whether access to the abdomen is desired (e.g., for ventriculoperitoneal shunt or if abdominal fat graft is desired).[1] Arms should not be abducted more than 90 degrees at the shoulder and supination of the forearm is recommended in order to minimize ulnar nerve injury.[5]

In addition to patient position, bed configuration plays an important role in the supine patient. In anterior spinal procedures and endarterectomies, the bed is maintained in the horizontal position. In cranial procedures in which both venous drainage from the brain and venous return from the legs are desired, the lawn chair position is preferable. Maximal venous drainage from the head is achieved with either the Fowler or reverse Trendelenburg position, both of which help to minimize venous bleeding and to reduce cerebral swelling.[1,2]

The supine position is a familiar position that is commonly used, is easily achieved, and requires no special equipment. The very few complications that are associated with this position can be avoided by using basic principles of patient positioning.

PRONE POSITION

The prone position refers to three primary patient configurations: straight prone, Concorde, and kneeling (Figs. 4.6 to 4.8). In general, the prone position is used for access to the suboccipital region and the posterior spine. For prone procedures the patient is placed under general anesthesia and intubated on the hospital bed in the supine state. Vascular access is also obtained and a bladder catheterization occurs prior to placing the patient into the final position on the operative table.[3]

Extreme caution should be used when rotating the patient from the hospital bed to the prone position on the operative table, particularly in cases of presumed or known spinal instability. The surgeon, not the anesthesiologist, should be

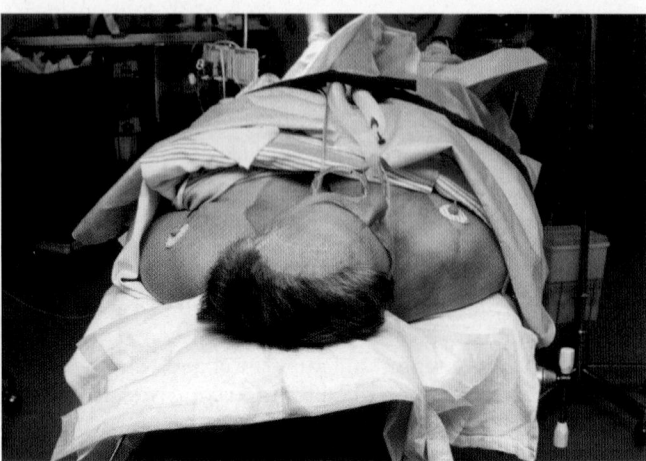

FIGURE 4.5 Patient in supine position.

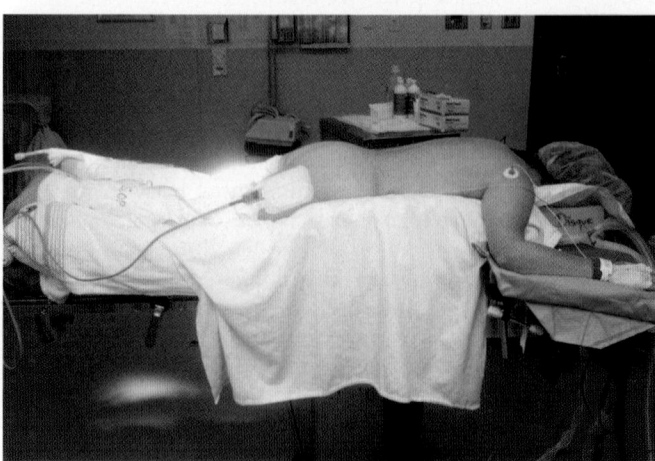

FIGURE 4.6 Patient in prone position.

responsible for control of the cervical spine and skull during this maneuver. Gripping the Mayfield clamp during this step does not provide optimal craniocervical stabilization. Instead, the Mayfield clamp should be locked in place, the surgeon's receiving hand should be placed directly onto the patient's face with the endotracheal tube stabilized between two fingers on the same hand, and the surgeon's other hand should be placed on the occiput. This configuration offers maximal airway protection and control of the patient's cervical spine and skull simultaneously. All members of the team should monitor intravenous/arterial lines, catheters, and tubing during this transition. Many of the circuits are intentionally disconnected prior to this maneuver.[1,2,7]

The use of large gel pads for the chest or special padded frames or tables allows for appropriate cushioning while preventing excessive thoracoabdominal compression. Female breasts and nipples should be positioned medially and male genitalia should hang freely.[3] The patient's knees are padded and usually flexed. The wrists and elbows are also appropriately padded.[5] The neck is maintained in either a neutral or flexed position, the degree of which is determined by the surgeon and the indication for surgery. The head may or may not be fixed and can be tilted up to 30 degrees to one side and rotated up to 45 degrees, also depending on the precise location of the pathology being treated and surgeon preference.[2]

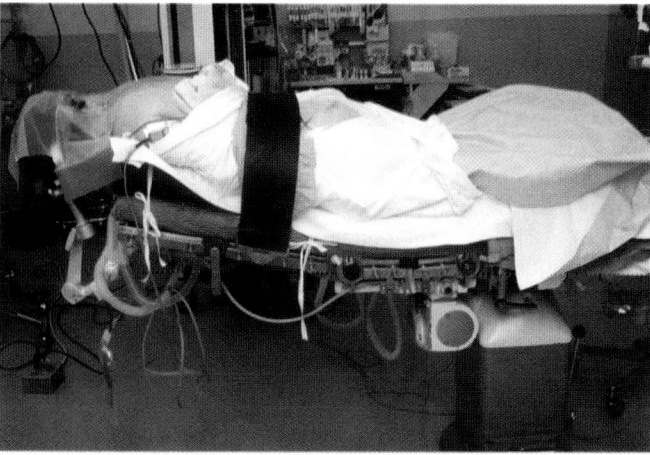

FIGURE 4.7 Patient in Concorde position.

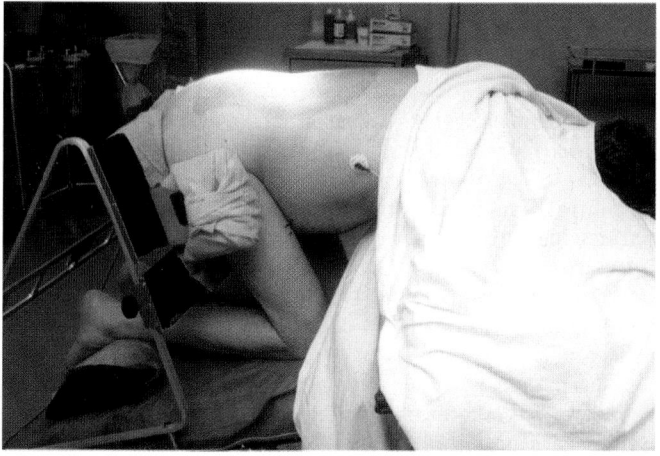

FIGURE 4.8 Patient in kneeling position.

Posterior cervical surgeries may be performed with the patient in a three-point headholder, halo ring, or traction tongs, or with the face on a padded pillow with cutouts for the endotracheal tube and eyes. Special consideration should be given to corneal lubrication, lid taping, and eye positioning so as to avoid ocular pressure that may lead to blindness.[2,8] The neck is often maintained in a neutral position, particularly if fusion is desired. For thoracolumbar surgeries, the patient is often placed on a Jackson table or Wilson frame, and the head is placed on a padded pillow with cutouts as mentioned earlier.[2] For spinal procedures in which intraoperative x-rays are planned, it is important to consider the placement of the patient's arms. For thoracolumbar procedures the arms are maintained in abduction at approximately 90 degrees at the shoulder and elbow ("airplaned") on arm rests. For cervical and cervicothoracic junction procedures, the arms are often padded and wrapped at the patient's side. To enhance radiographic visualization of the cervicothoracic junction, traction applied toward the feet by using either tape on the shoulders or soft wrist restraints anchored to the foot of the bed is often necessary. However, excessive traction should be avoided because it can lead to neuromuscular and vascular injuries, cutaneous burns, and very rarely joint dislocation.[3,5]

For cranial approaches, especially the occipital transtentorial and supracerebellar infratentorial approaches, the Concorde position is advocated. In this position, the skull is fixed in pins, the patient's neck and knees are flexed, the arms are maintained in the neutral position at the side with thumbs pointing downward, and the thoracolumbar region is extended so that the head is elevated slightly above the level of the heart. The Concorde position is commonly used for suboccipital approaches and has a relative benefit over the sitting position (used for similar surgical approaches) in that it is associated with a significantly lower incidence of venous air embolism.[1,9]

Finally, the kneeling prone position is rarely used. In this position, the patient is placed on an operative table that approximates the outline of the letter Z. Historically patients were placed in the kneeling position to minimize the amount of intraoperative blood loss. Although this was demonstrated clinically and experimentally, the disadvantages of the kneeling position are well documented and include increased potential for neurovascular and muscular pressure injuries,[5] hypotension from pooling of blood in the dependent lower extremities, a concomitant increase in the incidence of venous thrombosis and pulmonary embolism, and muscle necrosis and rhabdomyolysis that can lead to renal failure. For these reasons, placing the patient in the kneeling configuration is rarely justified.[2]

LATERAL POSITION

The lateral position (Figs. 4.9 to 4.11) allows the best access to the temporal lobe, the lateral skull base, and the lateral suboccipital area. From a spine perspective, the lateral position is utilized for transthoracic and retroperitoneal approaches to the thoracolumbar spine as well as posterior approaches to the lumbar spine for unilateral decompressive procedures. Specific uses of the lateral position also include lumboperitoneal and syringoperitoneal shunts, intrathecal baclofen pumps, pain

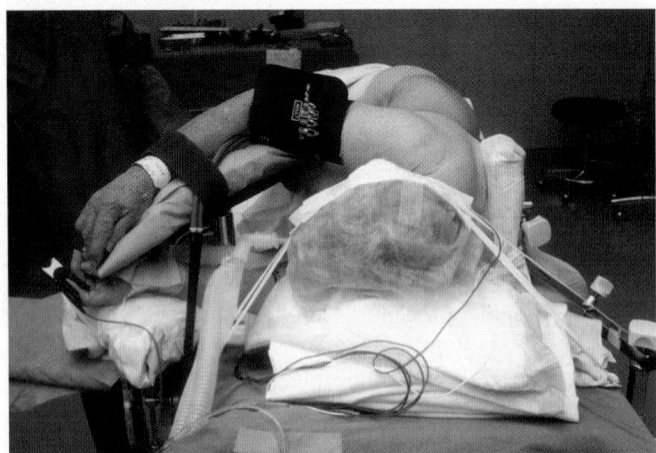

FIGURE 4.9 Patient in lateral position.

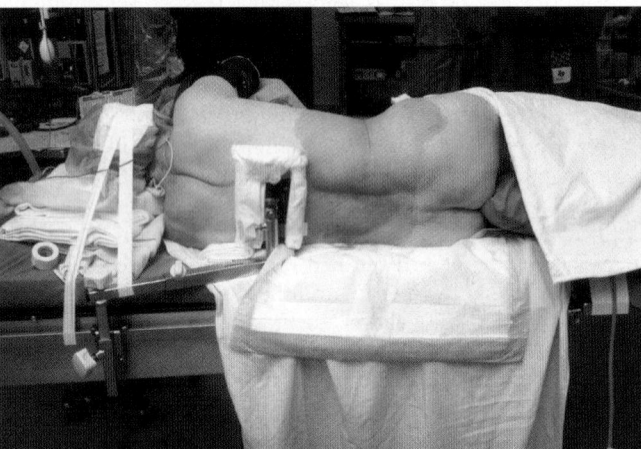

FIGURE 4.10 Patient in lateral position.

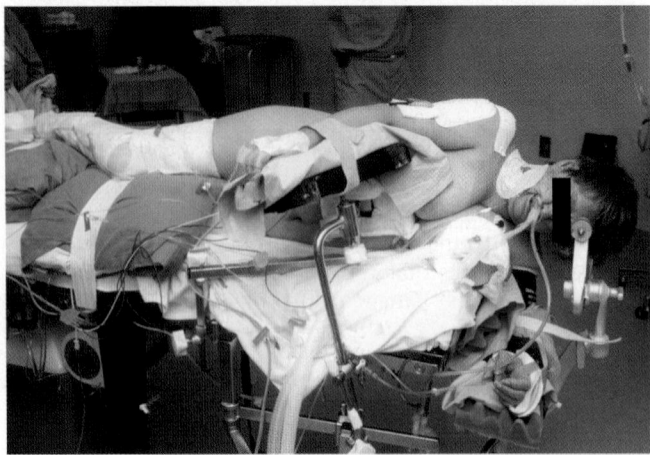

FIGURE 4.11 Patient in park bench position.

pumps, and dorsal sympathectomies. From a cranial standpoint, the lateral position can be approximated from supine position by using a shoulder bolster. However, the true lateral position usually requires that the patient's hips be perpendicular to the floor.[1]

This position is achieved by first placing the patient supine on the operative table. A bean bag is often used to secure the patient in the lateral position and is placed on the table prior to the patient.[3] The patient is then rotated laterally, and an axillary roll the diameter of the upper arm is inserted approximately 4 cm below the dependent armpit to avoid injury to the long thoracic nerve and the C5-C6 roots.[5] Finally the bean bag is compressed against the patient's torso and deflated. For cranial procedures the skull is pinned, secured to the table, and the dependent arm is then placed in a hanging position on a padded arm rest. This arm rest is placed between the Mayfield clamp and the edge of the operative table. The shoulder is slightly abducted with the elbow minimally flexed, and the entire extremity is positioned outstretched in front of the patient. A modification in the lateral position, the park bench position (see Fig. 4.11), has the nondependent arm taped in a slightly flexed position at the elbow over the patient's side, the neck flexed toward the floor, and the head rotated contralaterally in order to allow access to the posterior fossa.[1,2]

For spinal procedures, a similar configuration is achieved with the head resting on a padded doughnut and the table flexed at the level of the lumbar spine or with the kidney rest elevated. This maneuver theoretically opens the interlaminar space on the nondependent side of the vertebral column (i.e., the side of the pathology).[1]

In all lateral configurations, the lower extremities are positioned with a pillow between the legs and the dependent knee flexed to avoid compressive injury to the peroneal nerve over the fibular head. Care should be taken not to hyperflex the knee as this position is often associated with excess hip flexion that can lead to undue traction on the lateral femoral cutaneous nerve.[5]

The lateral position is frequently used. It is most often associated with compressive neuropathies and brachial plexus injuries. Additional equipment is usually necessary to prevent these complications. With a thorough understanding of how the lateral position is achieved, its indications, and its potential complications, this position can be safely and effectively implemented.

THREE-QUARTER PRONE POSITION

The three-quarter prone position (Fig. 4.12) resembles the lateral position in many ways. Indications for this position include approaches to the parieto-occipital region, the posterior fossa, and the pineal region. Although it is not the most popular position for spinal surgeries, reports of its use have been documented for thoracic extracavitary approaches. Compared to the sitting position, the three-quarter prone position leads to lower risks of air embolism.[9] It also allows less retraction of the parietal and occipital lobes during a parafalcine approach performed on the hemisphere positioned inferiorly.[1] Another important advantage of this position is that, in comparison to the sitting position, it provides more comfort to the surgeon and decreases fatigue imposed on the arms and shoulders.[10]

The patient is placed on the table supine and undergoes general anesthesia, intubation, and placement of invasive and noninvasive monitors. Although not an obligatory step, the skull is generally fixed in pins at this stage. The patient's body

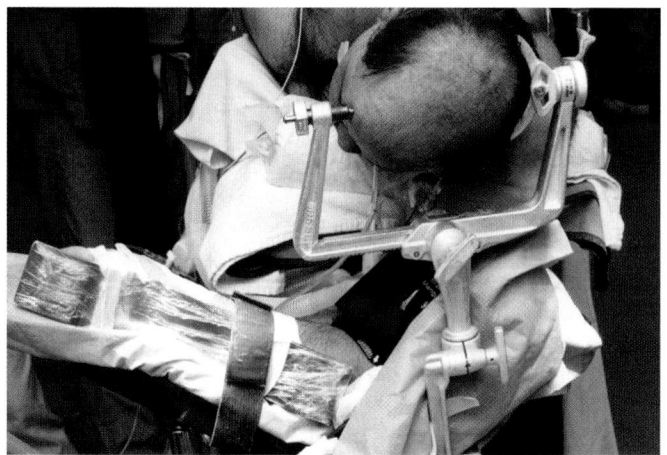

FIGURE 4.12 Patient in three-quarter prone position.

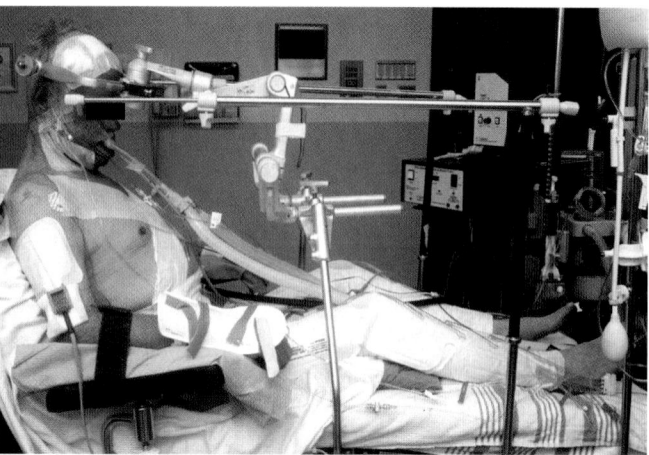

FIGURE 4.13 Patient in sitting position.

is then rotated approximately 130 degrees while keeping the head and torso centered on the table. As previously stated the surgeon should be in charge of mobilizing and positioning the head. Careful avoidance of excessive neck movement is important because the patient is under the effects of general anesthesia and muscle relaxant. The dependent arm is then positioned either next to the body or, as in the lateral position, dependent on a padded arm rest at the head of the table. In order to decrease the risk of injury to the brachial plexus and the rib cage, an axillary roll is inserted in the same manner as described for the lateral position. The superior nondependent arm is then flexed and placed on a soft barrier over the chest. Gentle traction toward the feet can be applied on the superior shoulder. This traction can be achieved by applying tape from the lateral aspect of the shoulder to the foot of the bed. However, care should be taken to avoid traction or direct compression of the brachial plexus. The lower extremities are positioned with the dependent leg straight, underneath, and the superior leg slightly flexed to allow for greater stability and to decrease the risk of stretch neuropathy. Both legs are separated by pillows. The head can finally be secured to the table in the desired position with varying degrees of rotation and flexion in the direction of the floor to allow for maximal exposure of the surgical site. The importance of making sure that all bony prominences are padded and that there is no stretch on any extremity cannot be emphasized enough because these complications are easily avoidable.[1-3,5]

As in any other position, because the surgical site is above the heart, there is an increased risk of air embolism, but this risk is significantly less than that for the sitting position. If the Mayfield frame is not used and the patient's head is placed on a horseshoe or doughnut, potential ocular complications such as blindness can occur. The risk of injury to the brachial plexus or other peripheral nerves is decreased by appropriately padding the extremities and avoiding excessive traction on the arms as delineated earlier.[2,5,8]

The three-quarter prone position is indicated for parieto-occipital and posterior fossa surgeries. It offers a comfortable position for the surgeon and allows a significantly lower risk of air embolism than the sitting position. Although a relatively safe position, risks can be encountered, and complication avoidance still relies on the same general principles described earlier in this chapter.

SITTING POSITION

Traditionally, the sitting position (Fig. 4.13) has been the preferred position for posterior fossa and posterior cervical spine surgeries. Over time this position has fallen out of favor because of a higher risk of complications associated with it such as quadriplegia, pneumocephalus, and venous air embolism (VAE). However, the sitting position can still offer significant advantages, and many surgeons continue to use this position for posterior fossa disease, pineal region lesions, and posterior cervical spine approaches. Today the sitting position and its variations are used most commonly during deep-brain stimulation (DBS) procedures. In certain scenarios the benefits of this position outweigh the associated risks, and it is preferred by many surgeons. Specifically, the position offers excellent anatomical exposure, lowers intracranial pressure and venous pressure, allows drainage of cerebrospinal fluid and blood to gravity, reduces the need for cerebellar retraction during the supracerebellar infratentorial approach, and provides direct access to the face for control of the airway and for cranial nerve monitoring. Careful preoperative planning, perioperative monitoring, as well as close collaboration with an experienced anesthesia team are required in order to minimize and avoid complications.[1,2]

Relative contraindications should be determined and evaluated before a patient is deemed a suitable candidate for the sitting position. There are several key considerations that are unique to this position and should be assessed during the preoperative period. Although the effects of gravity may have advantages on the technical aspects of surgery, they contribute to the majority of the serious complications that arise in this configuration. These effects are compounded by general anesthesia and muscle relaxation. Hypotension is one such risk that requires careful consideration. Relative contraindications to the sitting position in the context of hypotension include a patient history of orthostasis, cardiac atherosclerotic disease, and long-standing antihypertensive therapy. Slow verticalization during table positioning and the use of vasopressors can minimize the likelihood of hypotension. The use of trunk and lower extremity compressive bandages, elastic leg stockings, and sequential compression devices decreases the extent of venous pooling. However, these measures may be inadequate in obese patients.[2]

Cases of cervical spinal cord injury resulting in quadriparesis or quadriplegia are well documented in the literature. Although this complication occurs more frequently in patients with a history of cervical stenosis, this devastating outcome can occur in healthy patients. In the latter case, the injury is thought to be secondary to hemodynamic changes induced in the spinal cord vasculature during neck flexion. The most commonly reported level of injury is C5. In order to reduce the risk of postoperative position-induced myelopathy, a simple preoperative evaluation can be performed by asking the patient to simulate the surgical position and to hold the head flexed for at least 5 minutes. If the patient complains of any neck pain or other neurological symptom, additional preoperative investigation should be performed or another surgical position should be considered. Unfortunately this simple bedside test cannot completely eliminate the risk of neurological complications, but by allowing early identification of high-risk patients, it may reduce the occurrence of complications. Additionally, the use of intraoperative monitoring can be helpful in detecting and preventing spinal cord injury in this setting.[2,7,11-14]

Finally, well-documented cases of fatal VAE occurring in the sitting position have been reported. Although VAE is most commonly discussed in the context of the sitting position, any surgical position that maintains the patient's wound above the heart carries a theoretical and actual risk of this complication. However, in the sitting position this distance is greatest and is therefore seen more commonly. In the context of VAE, an absolute contraindication arises in patients with a patent foramen ovale (PFO) or other type of right-to-left shunt. In these patients paradoxical air emboli can cross into the systemic arterial circulation with devastating consequences. This topic has been a popular subject in the literature.[6,8,9,15-22] A recent review published by Fathi and associates concluded that, when considering the sitting position, routine preoperative investigation with transesophageal echocardiography or contrast-enhanced transcranial Doppler to rule out PFO is necessary because its incidence in the general population is as high as 20% to 25%.[20] If the sitting position appears to be the only suitable position, patients with a PFO can undergo a low-risk percutaneous procedure to achieve closure of the foramen and reduce the risk of paradoxical air embolism.[23]

Upon completion of the preoperative assessment, the patient is brought to the operating room, positioned supine on the operative table, placed under general anesthesia, and intubated. Standard noninvasive cardiopulmonary monitoring is used with or without the use of additional invasive monitors, depending on surgeon preference. An arterial line and a central venous catheter are almost universally advocated in this position. Central access to the venous system allows the patient's volume status to be continuously monitored while also providing a means to treat VAE should it occur. Although it remains controversial, the central line can be used to aspirate air directly from the superior vena cava and the right atrium. To achieve proper monitoring for VAE, Mirski and colleagues suggested using different combinations of end-tidal nitrogen and carbon dioxide monitoring as well as esophageal stethoscope, precordial Doppler, transcranial Doppler, or transesophageal echocardiography.[9] According to an editorial published by Leonard and Cunningham, at least three of these monitoring modalities should be used.[24]

Unfortunately, intraoperative interpretation of transesophageal echocardiography and transcranial Doppler by an anesthesiologist require expertise that is not widely available at every center. The use of precordial Doppler offers excellent sensitivity, allowing detection of air embolus of about 0.05 mL/kg, which is well below the estimated lethal 3 to 5 mL/kg volume. Because hypotension can have deadly consequences, continuous knowledge of the patient's fluid status is also crucial. Although the use of a Swan-Ganz catheter is not advised for every patient, it may be indicated in certain high-risk patients with tenuous cardiovascular and cardiopulmonary conditions.[9,16,19,20,22] Intermittent compression devices or compressive elastic stockings and bandages are typically applied as a way to reduce venous pooling in the lower extremities and the lower part of the trunk. Using a G-suit or military antishock trouser, although proved to increase right atrial pressure while the patient is in the sitting position, is not advocated because the potential complications outweigh the benefits. These complications include lower extremity compartment syndrome, abdominal organ hypoperfusion, and lower vital capacity.[2,9,19,20,22]

Once the various forms of invasive and noninvasive monitors are in place, the Mayfield head clamp is applied, and the operative table is flexed in the middle. The head and the thighs are slowly elevated and pillows are placed underneath the knees. The foot of the table is slightly lowered, thereby flexing the knees and minimizing pressure on the sciatic nerve. The entire table is then tilted backward and the head slowly elevated to the sitting position, which varies from 45 to 90 degrees. At this stage careful observation of the blood pressure is necessary. The next step involves flexing the head in a manner that avoids compression of the cervical spinal cord and allows proper venous drainage. A distance of 2 to 3 fingerbreadths between the chin and the sternum is generally acceptable. The head is then fixed to the table using the Mayfield clamp, which is secured anteriorly to the foot of the bed. The table and its remote control are then locked to avoid any alteration in the general position and prevent serious injury to the cervical spine. The table can still be tilted during the surgery to accommodate the surgical team's needs as long as the general position remains the same. After the desired position is achieved, the arms are cautiously placed either on arm boards or directly on the patient. Standard measures should be undertaken to prevent traction on the brachial plexus and avoid pressure on neurovascular structures and bony prominences.[1-3,5]

Because the most common complication cited by surgeons as a reason to avoid the sitting position is the risk of VAE, additional consideration should be given to this topic. Only a 5-cm gravitational gradient between the wound and the heart is necessary for air to enter the venous system. Although VAE is most commonly discussed in the context of the sitting position, this short distance is also present in many of the more standard positions described here. In fact, a retrospective analysis published by Black and associates compared posterior fossa surgeries in the sitting position with surgeries performed in the horizontal position. The occurrence of VAE was 45% in the first group versus 12% in the latter. However, when the patient is sitting, the incidence of VAE can range from as low as 7% to as high as 60%, depending on the means used for its detection. Clinically significant VAE still remains rare with reported morbidity rates ranging from 0.5% to 2% in different published series. Other factors that contribute to the development of VAE include traversing noncompressible large venous structures such as dural sinuses or intraosseous emissary veins.[6,12,16]

Important preoperative and perioperative steps discussed earlier must be taken to prevent the occurrence of VAE. Both anesthesia and the surgical teams play important roles in recognizing and treating the condition at the onset of systemic symptoms. VAE can affect the cardiovascular, pulmonary, and neurological systems. For a patient under general anesthesia, these symptoms may range from early cardiac arrhythmia and electrocardiogram changes to complete vascular collapse secondary to right-sided heart failure. The respiratory alterations can include bronchoconstriction, a decrease in oxygen saturation and end-tidal CO_2, and an increase end-tidal N_2 and systemic CO_2. Neurological symptoms associated with VAE occur from hypoperfusion secondary to vascular collapse or direct occlusion of the cerebral vasculature by paradoxical emboli. Postoperative neurological consequences vary from simple mental status alteration to focal neurological deficit to coma. The presence and degree of such symptoms will depend on two main factors: the volume and rate of air accumulation. In humans, the acute lethal volume is estimated to be approximately 200 to 300 mL.[11,14,25] The rate of accumulation can be significant as demonstrated by Flanagan and co-workers, who proved that a 5-cm gravity gradient applied to a 14-gauge needle could lead to entrapment of air as quickly as 100 mL/second.[26] At this rate rapid actions need to be taken to prevent dramatic consequences from occurring. The first step involves actively irrigating the wound and covering with sponges. The operating table can be tilted backward to reduce the gravity gradient. Prompt identification of the origin of the air embolus is necessary. Waxing of all exposed bony surfaces and repairing or coagulating open veins and dural sinuses are obligatory actions to prevent further entry of air into the circulation. While the surgical team is attempting to identify and eliminate the source, the anesthesiology team must maintain hemodynamic stability. Strategies include increasing the inspiratory oxygen, discontinuing nitrous oxide, and using vasopressors as necessary to keep the blood pressure within a normal range.[9,11,14,25] If a central line is in place, an attempt at aspirating the entrapped air should be made and has been successful according to many published reports independent of the volume of air removed. However, there is no indication to proceed with emergent line placement if one was not previously placed. In the case of refractory vascular collapse, chest compression can be performed, facilitating mobilization and dispersion of the air embolus. Hyperbaric oxygen therapy has also been used postoperatively as long as the patient remains hemodynamically stable. These patients should be monitored closely in the intensive care unit for the delayed development of pulmonary edema.[15,20,26]

Although less frequently mentioned, other potential complications have been reported with the sitting position. According to a recent study published by Sloan, postoperative supratentorial pneumocephalus related to decreased intracranial pressure was seen in more than 40% of the patients. Simple pneumocephalus occurs more often when the patient has a ventriculostomy catheter and if the surgery is prolonged. Simple pneumocephalus tends to resolve spontaneously over the course of 2 to 3 postoperative days. More severe complications include tension pneumocephalus as well as supratentorial hematoma, both of which have been reported after surgery in the sitting position. Very little can be done to prevent these adverse events, but fortunately they rarely occur.[27]

Excellent visualization of posterior fossa and cervical spine anatomy, decreased cerebellar retraction, drainage of CSF and blood to gravity, and reduced intracranial pressure are strong arguments for instituting the sitting position. Specific measures can be employed to reduce the risk of VAE, which is clearly highest in the sitting position. With experienced surgical and anesthesia teams, the sitting position can be relatively safe and effectively used with minimal complications.

SURGICAL ERGONOMICS

The importance of patient positioning has been thoroughly described in previous sections. However, the ergonomics of the operating room and its impact on the surgical team cannot be underestimated. Neurosurgical operations can be long and strenuous both mentally and physically. They often require a high degree of concentration, repetitive movements of the upper extremities over long periods of time, and very fine motor control. The presence of various types of equipment such as the operating microscope, C-arm, intraoperative CT or MRI, image guidance systems, and two- and three-dimensional displays all leads to crowded operating rooms and a more restricted corridor to access the surgical field (Fig. 4.14). It is known from laparoscopic experience that the strategic placement of devices such as these has been shown to reduce fatigue and improve concentration. Although this issue has not been specifically studied in the neurosurgical literature, many would argue that these principles are universal across surgical specialties. Simple maneuvers such as providing rests for the arms and hands, keeping the elbows flexed at 90 degrees, sitting for prolonged operations that require fine

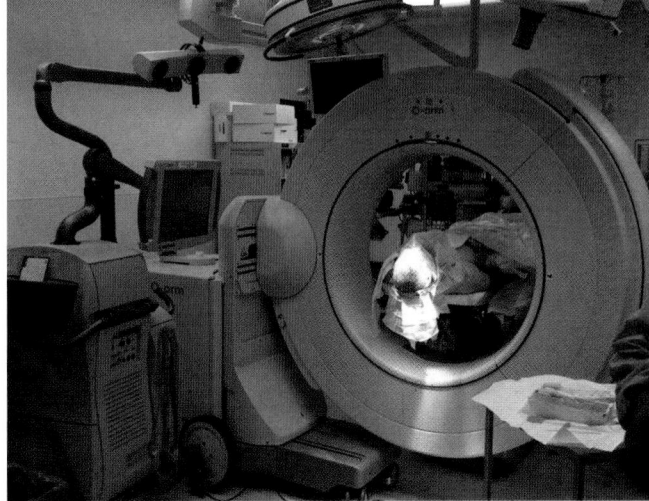

FIGURE 4.14 Crowded operating room with C-arm and neuronavigation system.

repetitive movements, avoiding excessive neck flexion for the surgeon, maintaining the operating scope perpendicular to the surgical trajectory, altering the bed position to allow additional anatomical visualization, and placing displays and navigation equipment in the surgeon's line of site will all aid in reducing discomfort, fatigue, and injury. Surgical ergonomics encompasses all aspects of patient, surgeon, and equipment placement and position. It impacts each member of the operating room team, but its effective implementation is ultimately the responsibility of the operating surgeon.[10]

ACKNOWLEDGMENT

We would like to thank Dr. Martin Côté and the staff of the Département audio-visuel, Centre hospitalier *affilié*-Hôpital Enfant-Jésus Université Laval for their contribution from their image library.

SELECTED KEY REFERENCES

Mirski MA, Lele AV, Fitzsimmons L, Toung TJ. Diagnosis and treatment of vascular air embolism. *Anesthesiology.* 2007;106(1):164-177.

Practice advisory for the prevention of perioperative peripheral neuropathies: a report by the American Society of Anesthesiologists Task Force on Prevention of Perioperative Peripheral Neuropathies. *Anesthesiology.* 2000;92(4):1168-1182.

Rozet I, Vavilala MS. Risks and benefits of patient positioning during neurosurgical care. *Anesthesiol Clin.* 2007;25(3):631-653.

St. Arnaud D, Paquin MJ. Safe positioning for neurosurgical patients. *AORN J.* 2008;87(6):1156-1168:quiz 1169–1172.

Winn HR, ed. *Youmans Neurological Surgery.* 5th ed. Philadelphia: WB Saunders; 2004:4vols., 38 pp plates.

Please go to expertconsult.com to view the complete list of references.

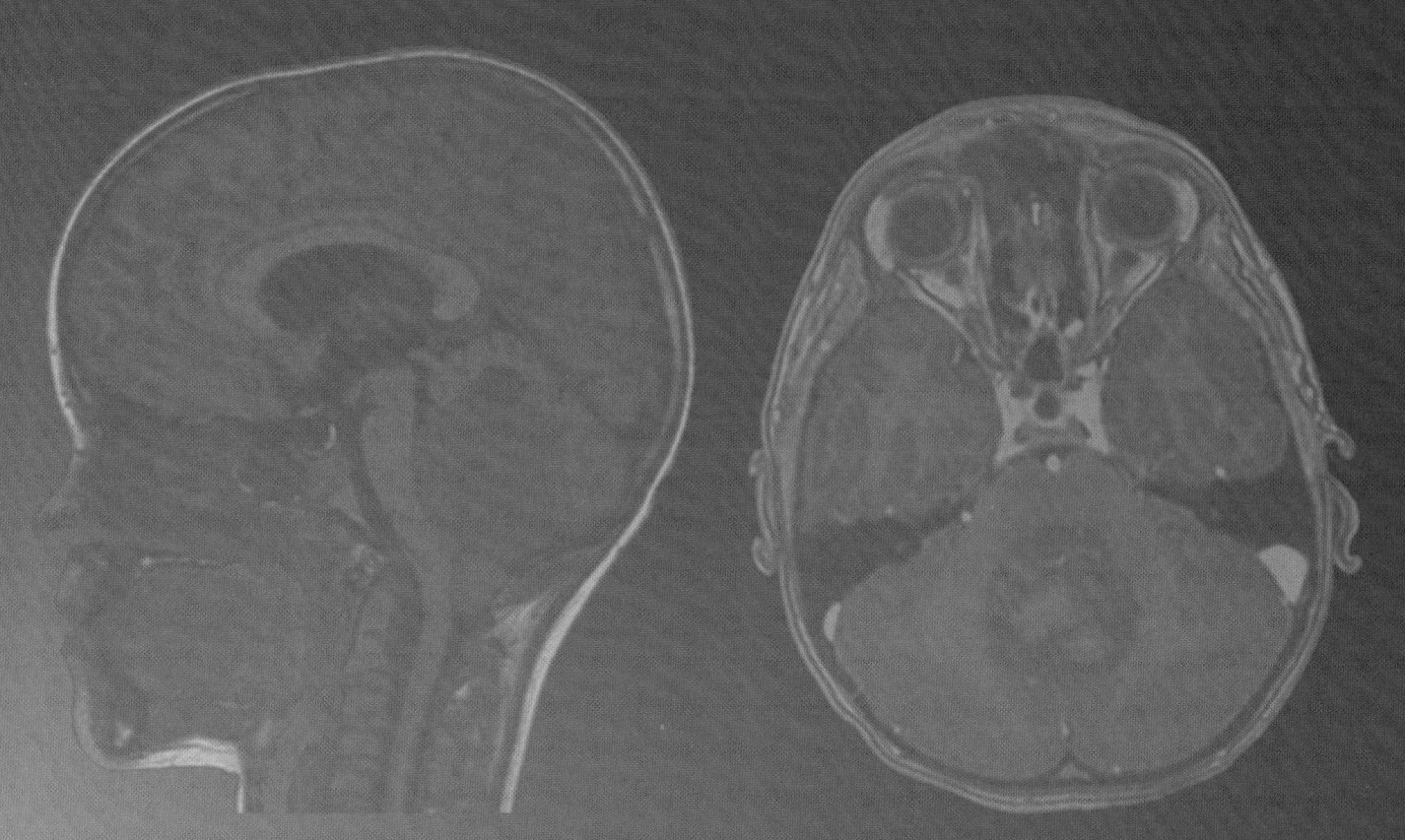

PART 2
Pediatric
Neurosurgery

Spinal Dysraphism and Tethered Spinal Cord

Leslie N. Sutton, Joel A. Bauman, Luke J. Macyszyn

CLINICAL PEARLS

- Spinal dysraphism refers to anomalies of the spine in which the midline structures do not fuse. Myelomeningocele is the most common significant birth defect involving the spine.

- The prevalence of spina bifida in industrialized countries has been decreasing because of the steadily increasing proportion of affected fetuses that are detected prenatally and electively terminated. In addition, there is strong scientific evidence that the use of preconception folate appears to decrease the risk of developing a neural tube defect such as myelomeningocele.

- Embryologically, the abnormality manifests between 3 and 4 weeks of gestation, during the period called *neurulation.* The abnormality represents the failure of the posterior neuropore to close properly. Patients with myelomeningocele usually have hydrocephalus and a Chiari II malformation. Surgical closure of the dorsal defect is performed shortly after birth.

- In utero closure of myelomeningocele is a promising surgical technique that has been pioneered at several medical centers. The goal is to decrease the incidence of hydrocephalus and hindbrain abnormalities found in this population. A randomized clinical trial demonstrated efficacy

of this treatment option in reducing shunt placement and improving motor function.

- Developmental anomalies involving the caudal portion of the neural tube are increasingly important in clinical practice. This is the result of advances in radiological diagnostic techniques and a consequent change in the philosophy of treatment, which includes prophylactic cord untethering to prevent neurological deficits. Greater awareness of the conditions of lipomyelomeningocele, tethered cord, diastematomyelia, and sinus tracts, by pediatricians, orthopedists, pediatric surgeons, and urologists, in concert with the widespread application of magnetic resonance imaging in addition to the clinical examination, have led to earlier recognition of these congenital surgically correctable problems. Recognition of the cutaneous, orthopedic, neurological, and urological stigmata of "occult" spinal anomalies has been helpful for early diagnosis.

- Patients with sacral agenesis, cloacal extrophy, and other caudal regressions syndromes may require magnetic resonance imaging after initial pediatric surgery intervention to identify potential tethered cord anatomy.

The term *spinal dysraphism* refers to a group of congenital anomalies of the spine in which the midline structures fail to fuse. If the lesion is confined to the bony posterior arches at one or more levels, it is termed *spina bifida.* Simple spina bifida of the lower lumbar spine is a common radiological finding, especially in children, and by itself carries no significance; in contrast, bony spina bifida may accompany any of several complex anomalies involving the spinal cord, nerve roots, dura, and even the pelvic visceral structures. In these cases, spinal dysraphism constitutes a major source of disability among children and adults.

There are two distinct syndromes of spinal dysraphism: (1) *spina bifida cystica,* which includes the familiar myelomeningocele, is characterized by herniation of elements through the skin as well as the bony defect and is obvious at birth; and (2) *spina bifida occulta,* in which the underlying neural

defect is masked by intact overlying skin. The external signs are often subtle; symptoms may not develop until late childhood, or even adulthood, as the result of spinal cord tethering. Included in the latter group are diastematomyelia, lipomyelomeningocele, tethered filum terminale, anterior sacral meningocele, myelocystocele, and the caudal regression syndromes. Early recognition of these entities is important, because neurological function may be preserved only by early (prophylactic) and appropriate surgical intervention.

MYELOMENINGOCELE

Myelomeningocele is the most common significant birth defect involving the spine. Since the early 1980s the prevalence of spina bifida in industrialized countries has been decreasing because of the steadily increasing proportion of affected fetuses that are detected prenatally and electively terminated. The incidence of the condition ranges from less than 1 case per 1000 live births in the United States to almost 9 cases per 1000 in areas of Ireland. The etiology is unknown, but evidence exists for both environmental and genetic influences. A role for genetic risk factors is supported by numerous studies documenting familial aggregation of this condition. In addition, several lines of evidence point to the potential importance of maternal nutritional status as a determinant of the risk for having a child with spina bifida. Indirect evidence for this association is provided by studies indicating that the season of conception, socioeconomic status, and degree of urbanization may be related to the risk of spina bifida. In August 1991, the Centers for Disease Control and Prevention (CDC) advised that women with a history of an affected pregnancy should take 4 mg of folic acid daily, starting at the time they planned to become pregnant, after publication of the Medical Research Council in Britain Vitamin Study Group report.[1] This recommendation was based on a randomized, double-blind, multicenter study performed in Europe that clearly showed the protective effect of periconception folate in reducing the recurrence of spina bifida when ingested by the mothers who had previous births of children with spina bifida. A second randomized, double-blind study was performed in Hungary and demonstrated conclusively the beneficial effects of periconception folic acid intake by mothers on decreasing the incidence of first occurrence of spina bifida.[2] It was anticipated that these recommendations would have a substantial impact on reducing the risk of neural tube defects in the offspring of such women. Although it is hoped that this benefit will be the case, it should be noted that the vast majority of affected pregnancies (approximately 95%) occur in women with no history of a prior affected fetus or child.[3] Currently the recommended daily dose of folic acid is 0.4 mg for all women of childbearing age who are capable of becoming pregnant. Fortification of the food supply may be a more effective strategy at preventing neural tube defects, rather than individual supplementation.

Embryologically, the abnormality manifests between 3 and 4 weeks of gestation. At this point in development, the neural plate folds into the neural tube, a process termed *neurulation*. Neurulation begins in the dorsal midline and progresses cephalad and caudad simultaneously. The last portion of the tube to close is the posterior end (neuropore) at 28 days. Myelomeningocele presumably occurs when the posterior neuropore fails to close, or if it reopens as the result of distention of the spinal cord's central canal with cerebrospinal fluid (CSF). The spinal abnormality is only part of a more widespread complex of central nervous system abnormalities, which also include hydrocephalus, gyral anomalies, and the Chiari II malformation of the hindbrain.

Recent developments in the prenatal diagnosis of fetal anomalies have made antenatal recognition of myelomeningocele commonplace. Families at risk are routinely offered amniocentesis for amniotic alpha fetoprotein and acetylcholinesterase, which are important in separating open lesions from skin-covered masses, such as myelocystocele. Amniocentesis along with ultrasound screening has a combined accuracy of more than 90%. Prenatal magnetic resonance imaging (MRI), using ultrafast T2-weighted sequences, may also be used to characterize the Chiari II malformation and other associated anomalies.[4] Furthermore, fetal MRI may augment ultrasound by detecting spinal cord abnormalities underlying bony abnormalities.[5] Recent studies indicate that such prenatal imaging studies can help to determine prognosis. Specifically, lesion level determined by prenatal imaging studies appears to predict neurological deficit and ambulatory potential, but not the degree of fetal ventriculomegaly or the extent of hindbrain deformity.[6] Families can be professionally counseled regarding the expected prognosis and decisions about abortion or the new option of fetal closure.

The majority of fetuses with spina bifida that are not electively terminated receive no specific treatment until after birth. In the United States, these babies are generally delivered by cesarean section.[7] However, the benefit of this approach relative to vaginal delivery has not been clearly demonstrated. Data suggest that if broad-spectrum antibiotics are administered, closure of the myelomeningocele can be safely delayed for up to a week to allow time for discussion with the parents. In most instances, however, the closure is performed within 48 to 72 hours of birth. The parents should be told the infant's prognosis based on the functional spinal level, and it should be emphasized that closure of the defect is a life-saving measure but will not alter the preexisting neurological deficits. Pending plans for definitive care, the infant is nursed in the prone position with a sterile, saline-soaked gauze dressing loosely applied over the sac or neural placode.

The initial step in managing the newborn with myelomeningocele is a careful physical examination by a pediatrician and neurosurgeon. A thorough evaluation should reveal associated anomalies, including cardiac and renal defects that might contraindicate surgical closure of the spine defect. Approximately 85% of myelomeningocele patients either present with hydrocephalus or develop it during the newborn period.[8] A large head or bulging fontanelle suggests active hydrocephalus and indicates the need for a head ultrasound or computed tomography (CT) scan. Stridor, apnea, or bradycardia in the absence of overt intracranial hypertension suggests a symptomatic Chiari II malformation, which carries a poor prognosis. The myelomeningocele is inspected; the red, granular neural placode is surrounded by a pearly "zona epitheliosa" that must be entirely excised to prevent the appearance of a dermoid inclusion cyst. Most myelomeningoceles are slightly oval with the long axis oriented vertically. If the lesion is oriented more horizontally, a horizontal skin closure may be preferable. Neurological examination is difficult in a newborn infant, and it is hard to separate voluntary leg motion from reflex movement. It must be assumed that any leg movement in response to a painful stimulus to that limb is reflexive. Contractures and foot deformity denote paralysis at that segmental level. Virtually all affected neonates have abnormal bladder function, but this is difficult to assess in the newborn. A patulous anus lacking in sensation confirms sacral denervation.

Generally, the back is closed first, and a CSF shunting procedure is deferred unless necessary. In cases with overt hydrocephalus, the back closure and the shunt can be performed at the same time to protect the back closure from CSF leakage. The goal of back closure is to seal the spinal cord with multiple tissue layers to inhibit the entrance of bacteria from the skin and to prevent CSF leakage while preserving neurological function and preventing tethering of the spinal cord.

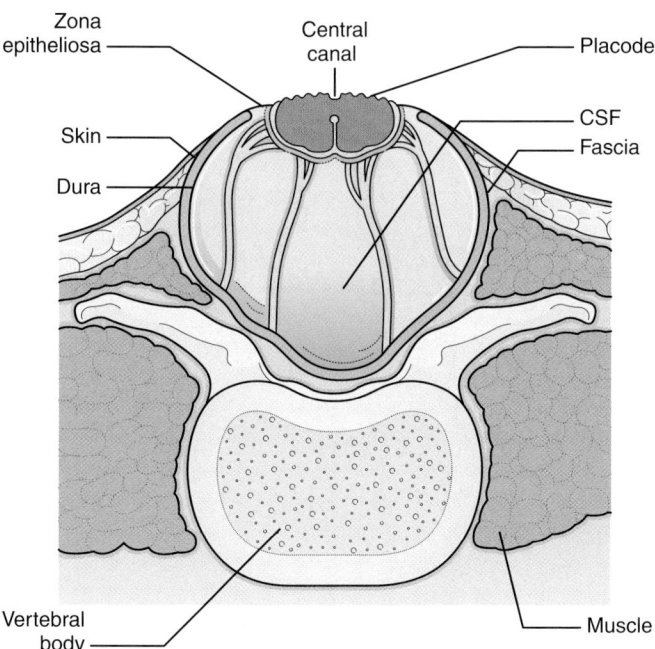

FIGURE 5.1 Cross-sectional anatomy of a myelomeningocele. The neural placode is visible on the back, usually at the center of the sac. It is separated from the full-thickness skin by a fringe of pearly tissue, the "zone epitheliosa." The neural tissue herniates through a defect in the skin, fascia, muscle, and bone. The dorsal dura and zona epitheliosa converge to attach laterally to the placode, forming the roof of the sac.

Accomplishing this goal requires a thorough understanding of the three-dimensional anatomy of the tissue layers involved (Fig. 5.1).

Surgical Technique

General anesthesia is used, and the patient is placed in the prone position, with rolls under the chest and hips to allow the abdomen to hang freely (Fig. 5.2). If the sac remains intact, fluid is aspirated and sent for culture. The surgeon gently attempts to approximate the base of the sac or defect vertically, then horizontally, to determine which direction of closure will produce the smallest skin defect. An elliptical incision is made, oriented along that axis, just outside the junction of the normal, full-thickness skin and the thin, pearly zona epitheliosa. Full-thickness skin forming the base of the sac is viable and should not be excised. The incision is carried through the subcutaneous tissue until the glistening layer of everted dura or fascia is encountered. The base of the sac is mobilized medially until it is seen to enter the fascial defect (Fig. 5.3A). The sac is entered by radially incising the cuff of skin surrounding the neural placode. This skin is sharply excised circumferentially around the placode with scissors and discarded (Fig. 5.3B). It is important to excise all of the zona epitheliosa to prevent later formation of an epidermoid cyst. At this point, the neural placode is lying freely above the everted dura (Fig. 5.4).

In some instances it is appropriate to "reconstruct" the neural placode so that it fits better within the dural canal and a pial surface is in contact with the dural closure to

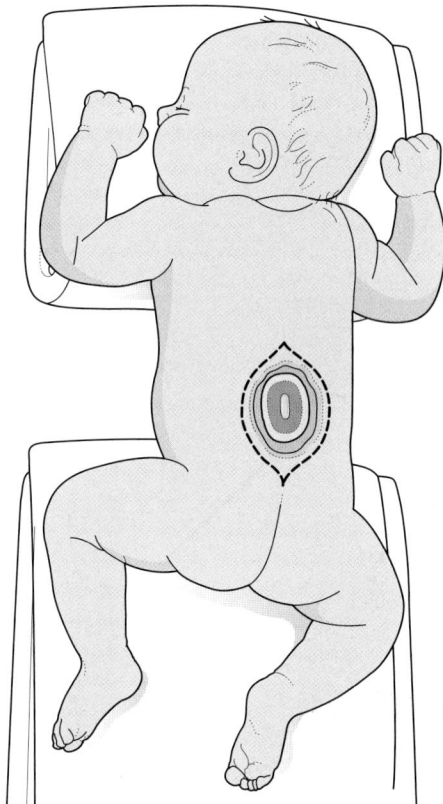

FIGURE 5.2 Positioning the patient for myelomeningocele closure. The infant is placed in the prone position, with rolls beneath the chest and iliac crests to minimize epidural bleeding. The skin incision is outlined circumferentially on the outside of the zona epitheliosa. A vertical orientation of the elliptical incision is appropriate for most closures.

prevent tethering. Interrupted 6-0 sutures approximate the pia-arachnoid-neural junction of one side of the placode with the other, folding the placode into a tube. The central canal is closed along its entire length.

Attention is then directed to the dura, which is everted and loosely attached to the underlying fascia. The dura is undermined bluntly and reflected medially on each side until enough has been mobilized to enable a closure (see Fig. 5.4). The dura is closed in a watertight fashion using a running suture of 4-0 neurilon. If possible, the fascia is closed as a separate layer by incising it laterally in a semicircle on both sides, elevating it from the underlying muscle, and reflecting it medially. Like the dura, the fascia is closed with a continuous stitch of 4-0 suture material (Fig. 5.5). The fascia is poor at the caudal end of a lumbar myelomeningocele as well as with most sacral lesions; thus, closure at this level may be incomplete.

The skin is mobilized by blunt dissection with dissecting scissors or a finger. It may be necessary to free up the skin ventrally all the way to the abdomen (see Fig. 5.5). In most instances, midsagittal (vertical) plane closure is easiest, but occasionally horizontal closure results in less tension. A two-layer closure using vertical interrupted mattress skin sutures is preferred.

Very large lesions require special techniques. Various types of "Z-plasties" and relaxation incisions have been described and may be necessary in very large or difficult lesions. Large

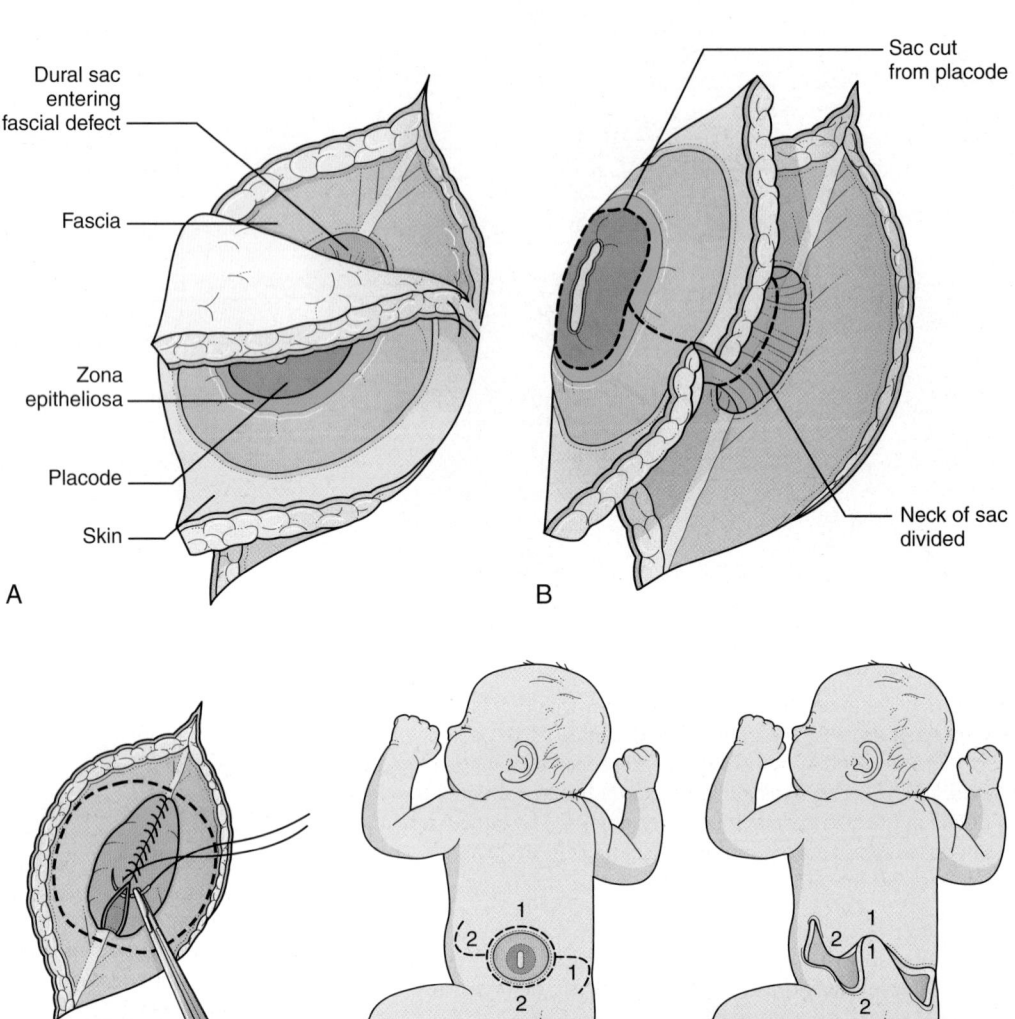

FIGURE 5.3 A, Mobilizing the sac. The skin is undermined medially until the dural sac is seen to enter the fascial defect. **B,** Excising the fringe of skin surrounding the placode. A radial cut is used to enter the sac, and it is continued around the placode to excise the skin. A separate circumferential cut amputates the base of the sac.

Dural sac entering fascial defect

Fascia

Zona epitheliosa

Placode

Skin

Sac cut from placode

Neck of sac divided

A

B

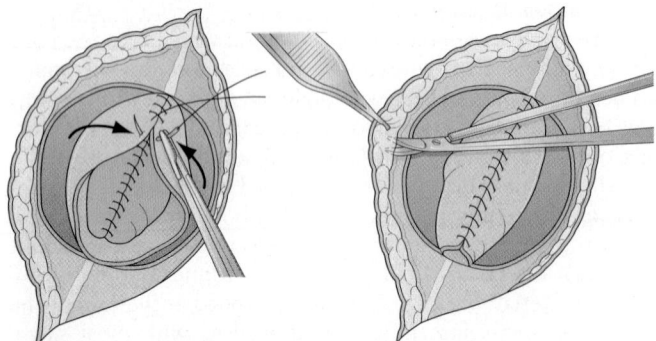

FIGURE 5.4 Mobilizing and closing the dura. The dura is undermined and closed using a continuous 4-0 nonabsorbable suture.

FIGURE 5.5 The fascial closure. The fascia is closed with a continuous stitch. The caudal end of the repair may be incomplete. Skin is mobilized by blunt dissection with scissors or a finger.

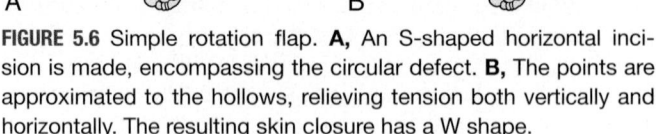

A

B

FIGURE 5.6 Simple rotation flap. **A,** An S-shaped horizontal incision is made, encompassing the circular defect. **B,** The points are approximated to the hollows, relieving tension both vertically and horizontally. The resulting skin closure has a W shape.

circular defects can be closed using a simple rotation flap (Fig. 5.6). Alternative techniques such as allogeneic skin grafts and tissue expansion may be used in rare circumstances.[9,10]

Care of the child with a myelomeningocele is life-long; it only begins with the surgical closure. Any deterioration in neurological function signals a progressive process such as shunt malfunction, hydromyelia, tethered cord, or symptomatic Chiari II malformation. Significant advancements have been made in the treatment of these children over the past two decades, particularly in the widespread use of multidisciplinary teams of specialists to manage their urological, orthopedic, and other needs. Among those who undergo early back closure, 92% will survive to 1 year.[11] From prospective outcome cohort data, it is known that the survival rate until age 17 is 78%,[12] but it drops to 46% by the fourth decade of life.[13] Death is the result of problems associated with the Chiari II malformation, restrictive lung disease secondary to chest deformity, shunt malfunction, or urinary sepsis. A sensory level higher than T11 is associated with increased risk of mortality,[13] likely due to increased risk of urosepsis.[14] Approximately 75% of children with myelomeningocele are ambulatory, although most require braces and crutches. Approximately 75% of surviving infants will have normal intelligence (defined as IQ > 80), although only 60% of those requiring shunts for hydrocephalus will have normal intelligence.[15] Normal intelligence drops to 70% in surviving adults.[16]

In a few centers, the fetus with spina bifida may be a candidate for in utero treatment, because this condition is routinely detected before 20 weeks of gestation. There is evidence that neurological deterioration occurs during gestation.[17] Normal lower extremity movement can be seen on sonograms of affected fetuses before 17 to 20 weeks of gestation, but most late-gestation fetuses and newborns have some degree of deformity and paralysis. Such deterioration could be the result of exposure of neural tissue to amniotic fluid and meconium or direct trauma as the exposed neural placode impacts against the uterine wall. In theory, such deterioration could be reduced or eliminated by in utero closure of the lesion. Animal studies (in which a model for spina bifida is created by laminectomy and exposure of the fetal spinal cord to the amniotic fluid) have demonstrated improved leg function if the lesion is closed before birth.[18] There is also evidence that the Chiari II malformation, which occurs in the vast majority of individuals with spina bifida, is acquired and could potentially be prevented by in utero closure.[19]

The first cases of in utero spina bifida repair were performed in 1994 using an endoscopic technique. This technique proved unsatisfactory and was quickly abandoned. In 1997, in utero repair of spina bifida was performed by hysterotomy at Vanderbilt University and at the Children's Hospital of Philadelphia.[20,21] Fetuses treated in utero are delivered by cesarean section because the forces of labor are likely to produce a uterine dehiscence. The early experience at both institutions suggested that relative to babies treated postnatally, those treated in utero had a decreased incidence of hindbrain herniation, and possibly a decreased need for shunting.[22,23] The combined experience at the Children's Hospital of Philadelphia and Vanderbilt, indicates that the incidence of hydrocephalus requiring shunting in patients treated in utero is less than in historical control subjects stratified by spinal level who received standard postnatal care.[24,25] It is hypothesized that fetal closure of the spinal lesion reduces the need for shunting by eliminating the leakage of spinal fluid which puts back-pressure on the hindbrain. This allows reduction of the hindbrain hernia and relieves the obstruction of the outflow from the fourth ventricle.[26]

In utero spina bifida closure appears to be generally well tolerated by the expectant mothers. Approximately 5% of fetuses have died from complications associated with uncontrollable labor and premature birth. An analysis of leg function in children treated prenatally revealed no significant difference from a set of historical control subjects who were treated with conventional postnatal repair.[27] However, many of the children evaluated in this series had lower limb paralysis at the time of the surgery, which may have diluted any possible benefit. In contrast, a series from the Children's Hospital of Philadelphia suggested potentially improved leg function in patients with prenatally confirmed intact leg movement on ultrasound prior to fetal surgery.[28] Problems with delayed development of dermoid inclusion cysts and tethered cord may adversely affect outcome in the long term.[29] The preliminary experience suggests that children treated in utero have the same urodynamic abnormalities that are seen in conventionally treated

children with spina bifida.[30,31] The incidence of the Chiari II malformation, and the need for shunting may be decreased,[23] but there are currently no long-term data.

Prior to the Management of Myelomeningocele Study (MOMS) trial,[32] outcomes for spina bifida babies treated in utero were assessed relative to outcomes in conventionally treated, historical control subjects.[8] Such comparisons are, however, prone to substantial biases because fetuses that undergo in utero closures represent a highly selected subset of cases. In addition, the medical management of spina bifida is continuously improving, making comparisons with historical control subjects particularly problematic.

A consortium of three institutions (Children's Hospital of Philadelphia, Vanderbilt, and University of California San Francisco) performed an unblinded, randomized, controlled trial of in utero treatment of spina bifida ([MOMS] to obtain definitive answers regarding the benefits of fetal myelomeningocele closure.[32]). Pregnant women who receive a prenatal diagnosis of spina bifida between 16 and 25 weeks of gestation were randomized to either in utero repair at 19 to 25 weeks' gestation or cesarean delivery after demonstration of lung maturity. The primary study end points were the need for a shunt procedure at 12 months, and fetal/infant death. Secondary end points included neurological function, cognitive outcome, and maternal morbidity. The intent to treat analysis demonstrated a significant risk reduction with regard to the primary endpoint, and the study was closed early due to efficacy of prenatal surgery. The prenatal surgery group benefited from decreased shunt requirement (40% versus 82%) and a higher proportion of normal hindbrain anatomy, and it was more likely to ambulate independently at 30 months compared to the postnatal group. There were no maternal deaths, and adverse neonatal outcomes were similar between groups; however, prenatal surgery was associated with more pregnancy complications, increased frequency of pre-term delivery, and a higher rate of respiratory distress syndrome in the neonate. To date, this is the only randomized study that demonstrates clear benefits of in utero treatment of spina bifida. These benefits were realized at experienced centers with strict inclusion criteria and must be carefully weighted against the higher rates of prematurity and maternal morbidity. Longer follow up is required to determine the longevity of these benefits as well as the effect on urinary function.

OCCULT SPINA BIFIDA AND THE TETHERED CORD SYNDROME

Developmental anomalies involving the caudal portion of the neural tube are increasingly important in clinical practice, largely as a result of advances in diagnostic techniques and the consequent change in the philosophy of treatment. Greater awareness of these conditions by pediatricians, orthopedists, and urologists, and the development of MRI have led to earlier recognition of these relatively rare problems.

The term *occult spinal dysraphism* actually encompasses several separate, possibly coexisting, entities. Most of these entities are localized to the lower spine segments and hidden by full-thickness skin. Embryologically, they arise from abnormal retrogressive differentiation of the caudal cell mass, a process by which the previously formed tail structures undergo a precise, ordered necrosis, leaving only the filum terminale, the coccygeal ligament, and the terminal ventricle of the conus as remnants by 11 weeks of gestation. Failure of regression presumably gives rise to the hypertrophied filum terminale; abnormal and incomplete regression result in lipomyelomeningocele. The embryology of diastematomyelia remains poorly understood,[33] but it may involve persistence of the fetal neurenteric canal between the yolk sac and the amniotic cavity, allowing herniation of endodermal elements through a split notochord, and causing migrating mesenchymal elements to form the bony "spike."

TABLE 5.1 Presenting Symptoms and Signs of Occult Spinal Dysraphism

Symptoms/Signs	Frequency
Foot deformity	39%
Scoliosis	14%
Gait abnormality	16%
Leg weakness	48%
Sensory abnormality	32%
Urinary incontinence	36%
Recurrent urinary tract infections	20%
Fecal incontinence	32%
Cutaneous abnormality	48%

Adapted from Pang D: Sacral agenesis and caudal spinal cord malformations. Neurosurgery 1993;32:755-758.

Symptoms may have several causes. Abnormal formation of the spinal cord and roots during embryogenesis can result in permanent neurological deficits, as seen in myelomeningocele. Local masses growing within the spinal canal (lipomas or neurenteric cysts) can cause compression. Tethered cord syndrome, the result of traction on the spinal cord, occurs with any of the entities associated with occult spinal dysraphism. It can also occur in the adult in whom the conus has already completed its ascent.

To recognize occult dysraphic states, one must appreciate the significance of the various syndromes that occur in association with the various entities (Table 5.1). The *cutaneous syndrome* refers to any midline skin anomaly overlying the lower spine. This anomaly often signals a dysraphic state, and its recognition is especially important in the infant, in whom urological or orthopedic complaints are not yet manifest. Dimples may be significant if they are at the level of the upper sacral or lumbar spine above the gluteal fold, but the common coccygeal pit overlying the lowest point of the coccyx in or below the gluteal fold has no particular significance.[34,35] The cutaneous abnormality may include the striking "faun's tail" of hair (Fig. 5.7), dermal sinus tract, hemangioma (Fig. 5.8), or skin-covered fatty mass (Fig. 5.9). The *orthopedic syndrome* is apparent at birth or develops progressively in childhood. Common components include high arched feet, claw toes, unequal leg length, and scoliosis. The *urological syndrome* should be considered in any infant or small child who has an abnormal voiding pattern,

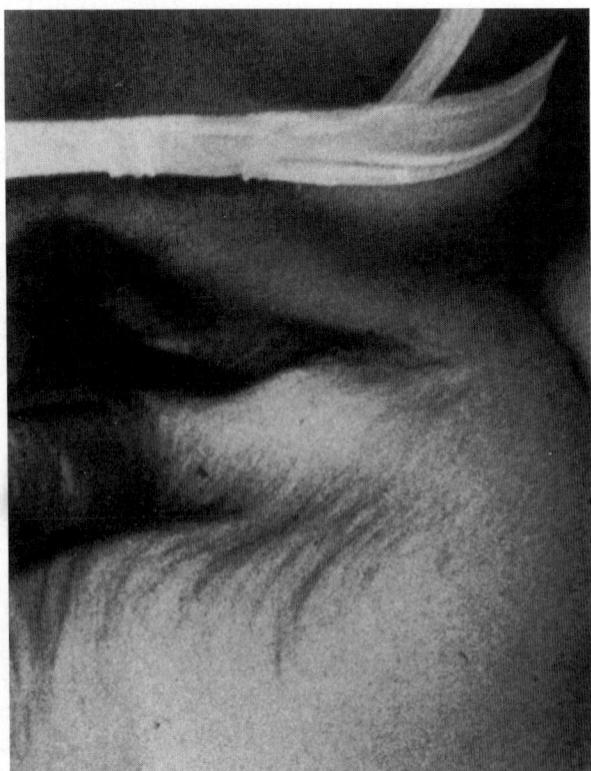

FIGURE 5.7 Faun's tail. This patch of hair in the midline overlying the lower spine is highly suggestive of a dysraphic state. It is not associated with any particular entity, and it may occur in lipomyelomeningocele, diastematomyelia, or hypertrophied filum terminale. *(Reprinted with permission from Rothman RH, Simeone FA. The Spine, 3rd ed. Philadelphia: WB Saunders; 1992.)*

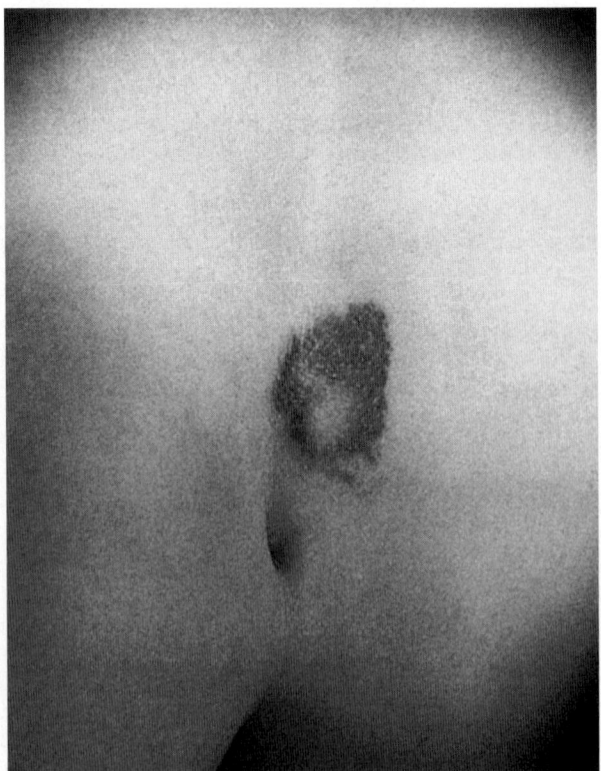

FIGURE 5.8 Hemangioma and dermal sinus. Dermal sinus tracts overlying the distal sacrum or coccyx are common in normal infants and do not generally represent dysraphic states. Any midline hemangioma or sinus tract over the lumbar spine warrants an investigation. *(Reprinted with permission from Rothman RH, Simeone FA. The Spine, 3rd ed. Philadelphia: WB Saunders; 1992.)*

a child with a new onset of incontinence after toilet training, or with urinary tract infection in a child of any age. The *neurological syndrome* presents as leg muscle atrophy or weakness, numbness of the feet, or radicular lower extremity pain and can occur at any age. In summary, patients may present with any of the abovementioned syndromes, but in general, infants primarily present with skin manifestations, older children present with

urological, neurological, or orthopedic syndromes, and adults often complain of pain (see Table 5.1).[36]

The current method of choice for a suspected occult spinal dysraphic lesion is MRI scanning, which is usually definitive. In newborn infants the image quality can be suboptimal because of their small size, and if the clinical suspicion is high, a repeat scan at 6 months is indicated. The scan is examined for the level of the conus, which should not be below the L2-L3 interspace, and for the presence of fatty masses, a split cord, or a thickened filum. A large distended urinary bladder suggests sacral root dysfunction. In some cases of hypertrophied filum terminale the MRI scan may be equivocal, and if the clinical suspicion is high, surgical exploration may be warranted.[37,38] Fat in the filum is a frequent incidental MRI finding, and if the conus is at a normal level and there are no clinical indications of a tethered cord, surgery is usually not indicated. Fat that occurs near the conus may represent a different clinical situation and may be more likely to cause tethering.[39]

LIPOMYELOMENINGOCELE

Lipomyelomeningocele is one of the more common forms of occult spinal dysraphism seen in pediatric neurosurgical practice. The term is actually a misnomer, because it suggests herniation of neural elements through a spina bifida defect into a meningeal sac, which is not the case. In fact, the lipomatous tissue inserts into the conus, and it is fat that herniates through the bony defect dorsally to attach to a subcutaneous mass. Nonetheless, the term has gained wide acceptance and is likely to stay. The distinction between lipomyelomeningoceles that insert caudally into the conus and those that attach to the dorsal surface of the spinal cord is of considerable value in planning the operative approach.[40] If the lipoma inserts into the dorsal surface of the conus there is usually a substantial subcutaneous mass (Fig. 5.10). Along the lateral interface of the attachment of the lipoma to the spinal cord, the dura and pia are also

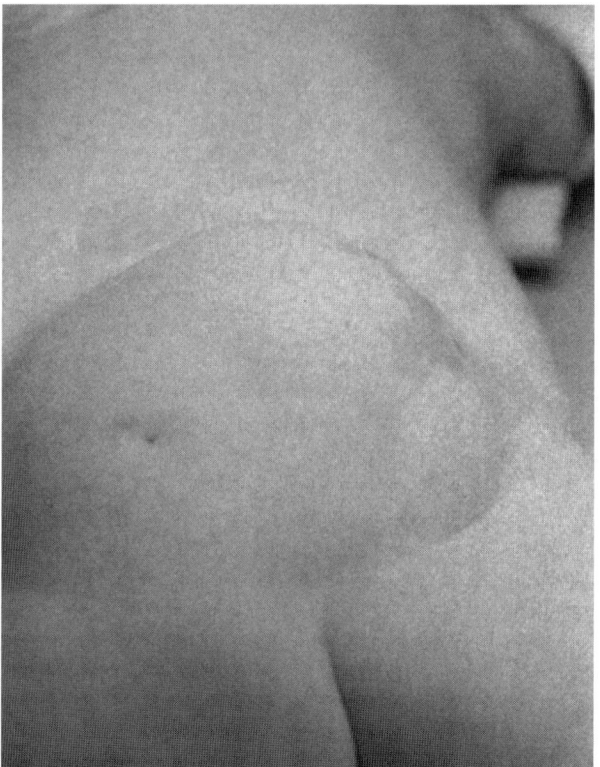

FIGURE 5.9 Lipomyelomeningocele in an infant. The skin-covered fatty mass in the lumbosacral region is typical.

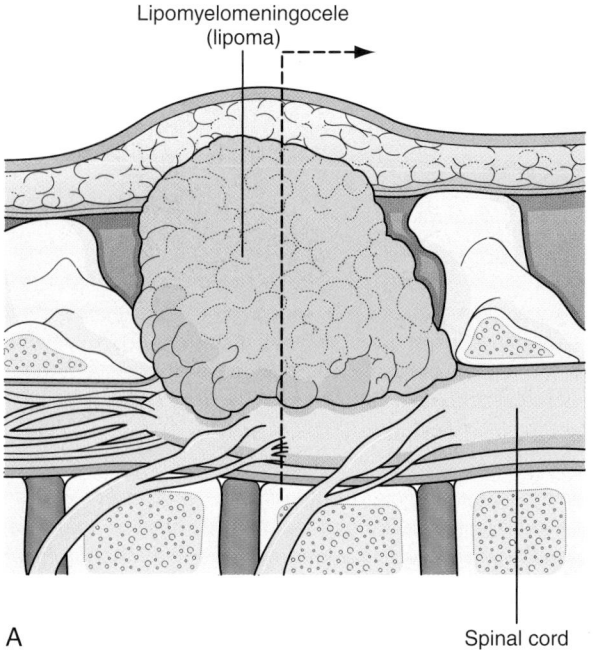

Lipomyelomeningocele (lipoma)

A

Spinal cord

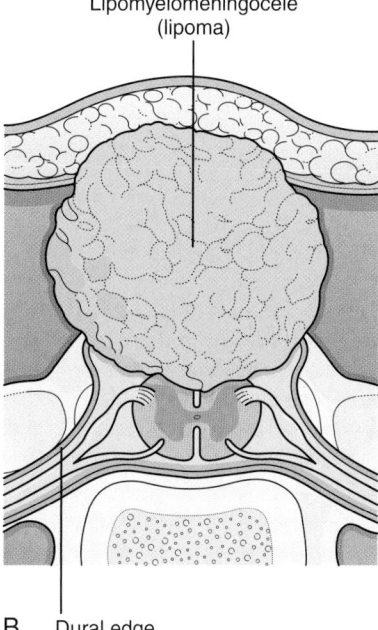

Lipomyelomeningocele (lipoma)

B Dural edge

FIGURE 5.10 A, Dorsally inserting lipomyelomeningocele. The mass of the lipoma attaches broadly on the dorsal surface of the conus, extending through a dural and bony defect to be continuous with the subcutaneous mass. The nerve roots are ventral to the lipoma. **B,** Cross-sectional view of a dorsal lipoma. The lateral lines of attachment are formed by the lipoma and the dural edge, and must be divided to release the tether. Note that the nerve roots are ventral to this line.

FIGURE 5.11 Cross-sectional view of a caudal lipoma. The roots run anteriorly and may attach to the ventral wall of the lipoma.

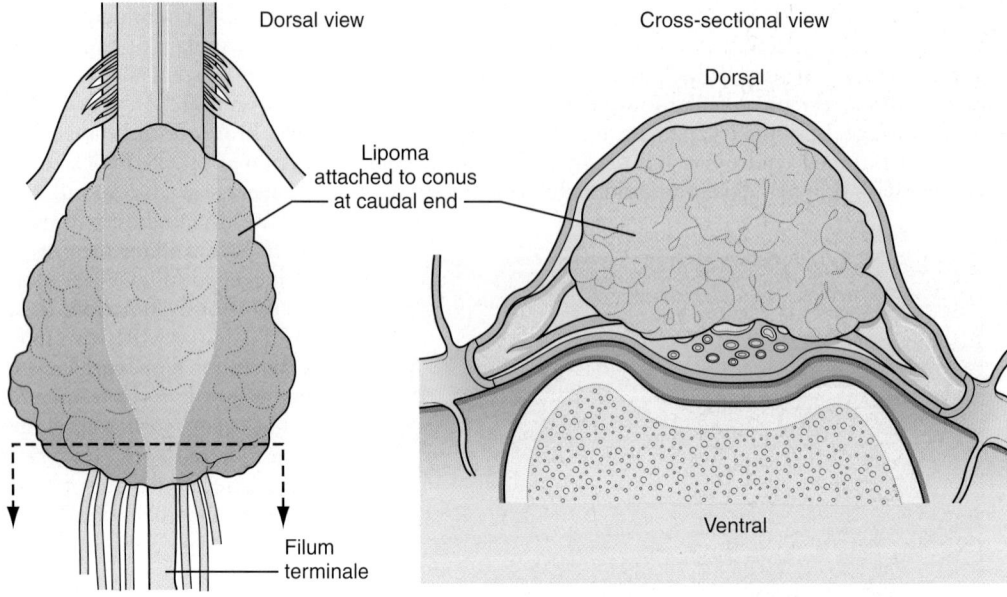

fused. Sensory roots emerge just anterior to this "lateral line of fusion," and as a result, neither the sensory nor the motor roots lie within the actual substance of the lipoma. Alternatively, the lipoma joins the conus at its caudal end, almost as a continuation of the cord itself. The remaining lipomatous mass then lies entirely within the spinal canal or extends dorsally through a spina bifida defect. The fatty tumor either replaces the filum terminale, or a separate filum lies anteriorly. The nerve roots usually lie anterior to the lipoma, although they can lie within the fibrous anterior portion of the mass itself (Fig. 5.11). A third, least common, type is the chaotic lipomyelomeningocele, which has a prominent ventral component, as described by Pang and associates.[41] Transitional forms of these types may occur, but this schema is extremely useful in planning surgery.

The surgical indications for lipomyelomeningocele have changed over the past 20 years. Although some neurosurgeons have questioned the value of prophylactic surgery,[42] almost all modern authorities strongly favor it, preferably in the first 6 months of life.[43-45] The rationale is that once a significant neurological deficit occurs, due to natural history in a lipomyelomeningocele patient, the chance of reversing this deficit is not uniformly assured. The risks of creating a new neurological deficit in an experienced neurosurgeon's hands are low albeit not negligible. Thus, the goals of prophylactic surgery are to untether the spinal cord, remove as much of the lipomatous mass as possible, and reconstruct the dura to avoid leakage of CSF and to discourage retethering. This seems to provide a better outcome than the natural history of this condition in which neurological deficits can occur during periods of rapid growth and activity in which the spinal cord can become stretched and compromised. Surgical planning begins with review of the MRI scan. The lipoma can usually be determined to fit either the dorsal group (Fig. 5.12) or the caudal group (Fig. 5.13).

Surgical Technique

General anesthesia is used, and the patient is positioned prone with rolls under the hips and chest so the abdomen hangs free. If electrophysiological monitoring with electromyography (EMG)

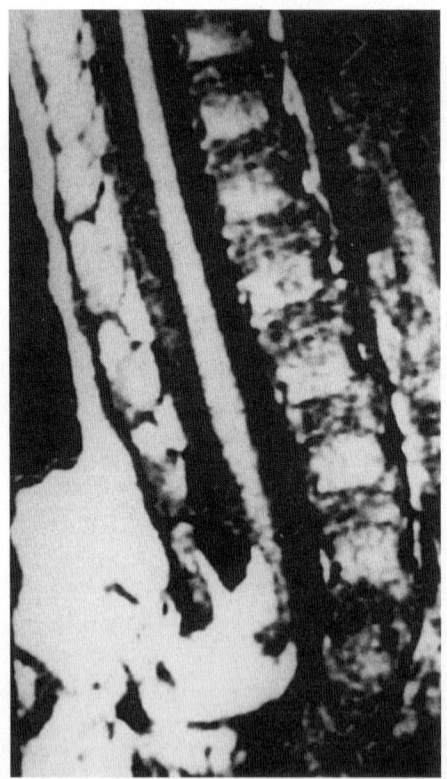

FIGURE 5.12 Magnetic resonance image of a dorsally inserting lipoma. The mass inserts dorsally within the conus. It extends through a spina bifida defect to be continuous with the subcutaneous mass. *(Reprinted with permission from Rothman RH, Simeone FA. The Spine, 3rd ed. Philadelphia: WB Saunders; 1992.)*

or continuous motor evoked potentials is to be used, muscle relaxants must be discontinued before the dura is exposed. An elliptical skin incision surrounding the subcutaneous mass is made along a vertical axis. The subcutaneous tissue is then incised circumferentially down to the lumbodorsal fascia (Fig. 5.14). The lipoma is undermined and separated bluntly from

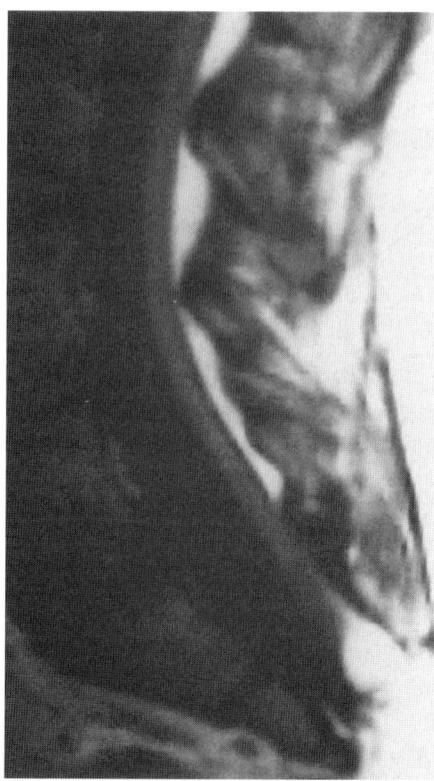

FIGURE 5.13 Magnetic resonance image of caudal lipoma. The lipoma is entirely within the caudal spinal canal, and the cord is tethered to the caudal portion of the thecal sac. *(Reprinted with permission from Rothman RH, Simeone FA. The Spine, 3rd ed. Philadelphia: WB Saunders; 1992.)*

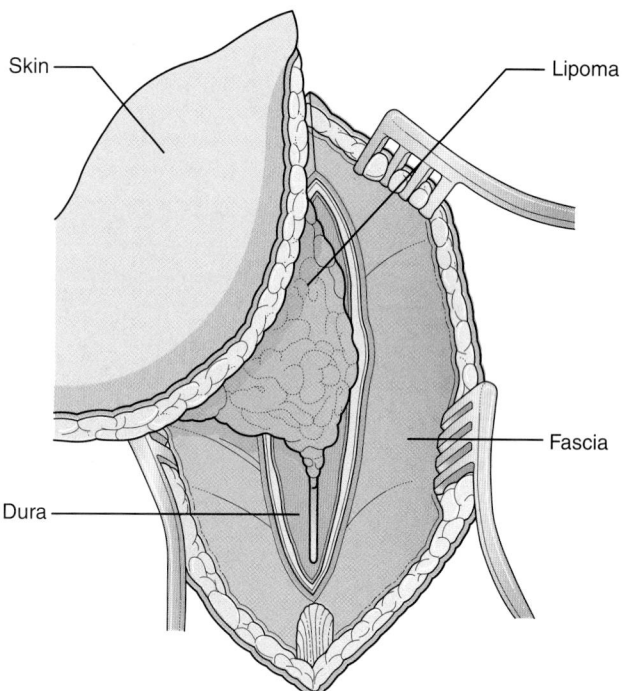

FIGURE 5.15 Surgery for spinal lipoma (*continued*). A laminectomy of the lowest intact neural arch has been performed and the dura has been opened at this level. The dural incision is extended caudally until the lipoma is encountered.

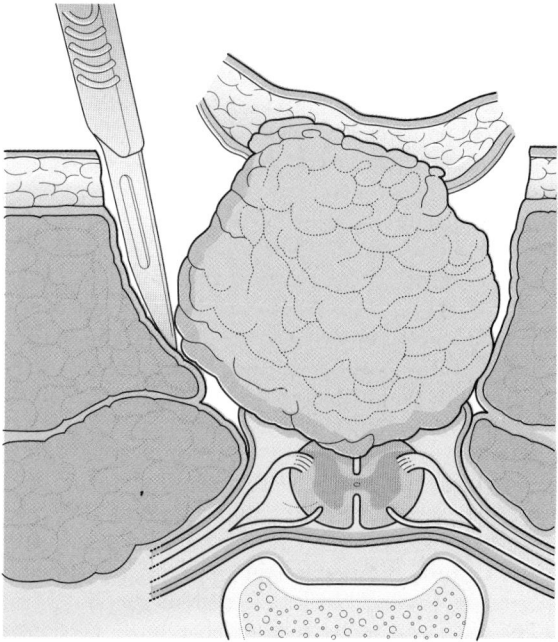

FIGURE 5.14 Initial exposure of a spinal lipoma. The skin has been elliptically incised around the subcutaneous mass and the incision has been carried to the lumbodorsal fascia. Dissection has proceeded medially, until the stalk of the lipoma is seen entering the spinal canal through the spinal bifida and the dural defect.

the underlying fascia, until it can be seen to enter the fascial defect medially. A self-retaining retractor is inserted, and the lowest intact laminar arch is palpated. The fascia overlying this spinous process and lamina is opened in the midline, and a laminectomy of this segment is performed, exposing the underlying normal dura. At this point it can help to amputate the large fatty mass with its island of skin attached at the level of its stalk.

Starting at the level of normal dura cephalad to the mass, the epidural fat is melted with a bipolar cautery until the dural defect with fatty tissue extruding through it is encountered. A midline dural opening is made above the defect, exposing the spinal cord. As the dural opening is carried inferiorly toward the defect, a transverse band of thick, fibrous tissue, which kinks the spinal cord, is noted at the rostral end of the lipoma stalk. This is opened widely along with the dura. The dural opening is extended caudally on either side of the exiting lipoma circumferentially (Fig. 5.15).

At this point, the lipoma will usually be found to correspond to one of the two types previously described. Lipomas that insert into the conus dorsally can be removed from the dorsal aspect of the cord in a plane superficial to the lateral lines of fusion, with the nerve roots emerging anteriorly (Fig. 5.16). These lines of fusion are divided laterally, first on one side and then the other, with a bipolar cautery and microscissors or a knife blade over a dissector. A CO_2 laser may be of help to shave down the mass of the lipoma. The filum is identified and divided. After the lipoma has been largely removed from the spinal cord, it is sometimes possible to reapproximate the pial edges of the cord to reconstitute the normal tubular configuration (Fig. 5.17), which discourages retethering.

Lipomas that insert caudally into the conus must be sectioned distally to the take-off of any functional roots. It is

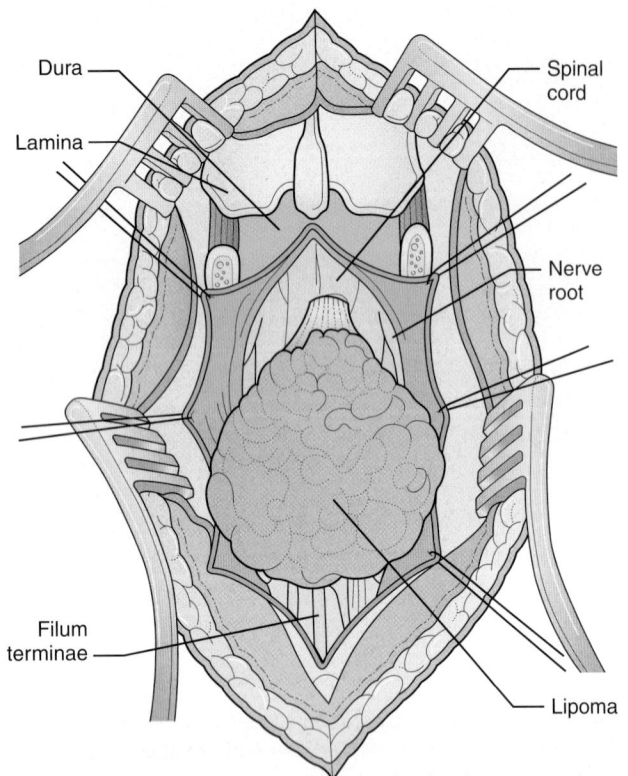

FIGURE 5.16 Lateral dissection of the lines of fusion. The lateral lines of fusion are sharply incised on either side of the lipoma. A tunnel can usually be formed between the lateral lines of fusion and the nerve roots beneath.

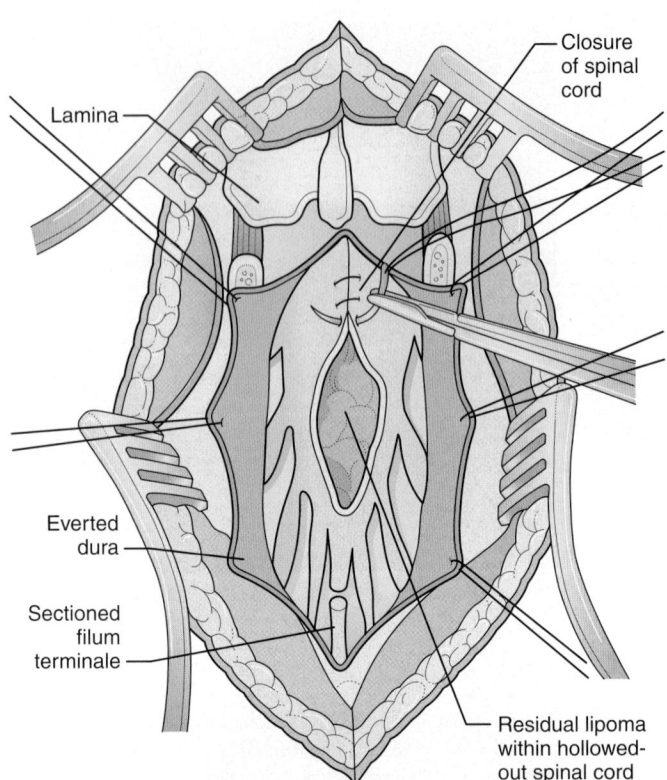

FIGURE 5.17 Reconstruction of the spinal cord. The lipoma has been largely removed with a CO_2 laser, creating a cavity within the conus. This may be closed with interrupted sutures to prevent retethering.

unnecessary to remove all of the gross lipoma; attempting this can cause damage to the conus and roots. Simple sectioning of the lipoma releases the point of tethering and typically fulfills the goal of the operation. However, Pang and colleagues have reported that a more aggressive sharp excision of the lipoma can decrease the rate of retethering.[46]

When the cord is free of adhesions, the dura is closed. In some cases, the dura is approximated and closed with a running suture directly. In most cases, however, a graft is required to prevent stricture of the canal. The muscle and fascia are closed as much as possible, and the skin is closed in the usual fashion.

Surgery is relatively safe. The major problems are post-operative CSF leaks and pseudomeningoceles, which require re-exploration. Most series report a small number of patients whose condition is made worse by the procedure; however, when the outcome of the procedure is compared with that of untreated cases, which are characterized by progressive worsening and disability, the benefits outweigh the risks. The major late problem is retethering, which is suggested by clinical deterioration, and requires re-exploration.[47]

DIASTEMATOMYELIA AND THE SPLIT CORD MALFORMATIONS

The term *diastematomyelia*, which derives from the Greek word *diastema*, meaning cleft, refers to a congenital splitting of the spinal cord. The term is used to describe the split, not the bony spike that often accompanies the abnormality.

Clinically, it presents as tethered cord syndrome.[48] It occurs predominantly in females and most often in the lower thoracic or upper lumbar spine. Most patients have a midline cutaneous abnormality, but it does not necessarily correspond to the level of the cleft. The most common finding is a hairy patch, but a variety of other cutaneous abnormalities are seen. The spinal deformity (kyphoscoliosis), which eventually develops in virtually all patients, is thought to be primarily the result of the bony structure abnormalities, rather than of neurological involvement.

Pang has suggested a useful classification scheme.[33,48] It is proposed that the term *diastematomyelia* be replaced by the more general term *"split cord malformation"* (SCM), which may occur as one of two types: The type I SCM consists of two hemicords separated by a bony or cartilaginous median septum, with each housed in its own dural sheath. The type II SCM consists of two hemicords enveloped in the same dural sheath, and separated by a fibrous septum. Both are associated with tethering.

Neurological symptoms are the result of spinal cord tethering and may not occur until adulthood, if at all. Symptoms can include back pain, gait disturbance, muscular atrophy, spasticity, or urological complaints. These abnormalities are not specific, and other conditions, such as spinal cord tumor, Friedreich's ataxia, and syringomyelia, must be considered in the differential diagnosis. Neurological deterioration can occur following corrective surgery for scoliosis, if spinal cord tethering is not recognized beforehand.

The classic appearance of the SCM on plain spine roentgenograph is a fusiform interpedicular widening of the

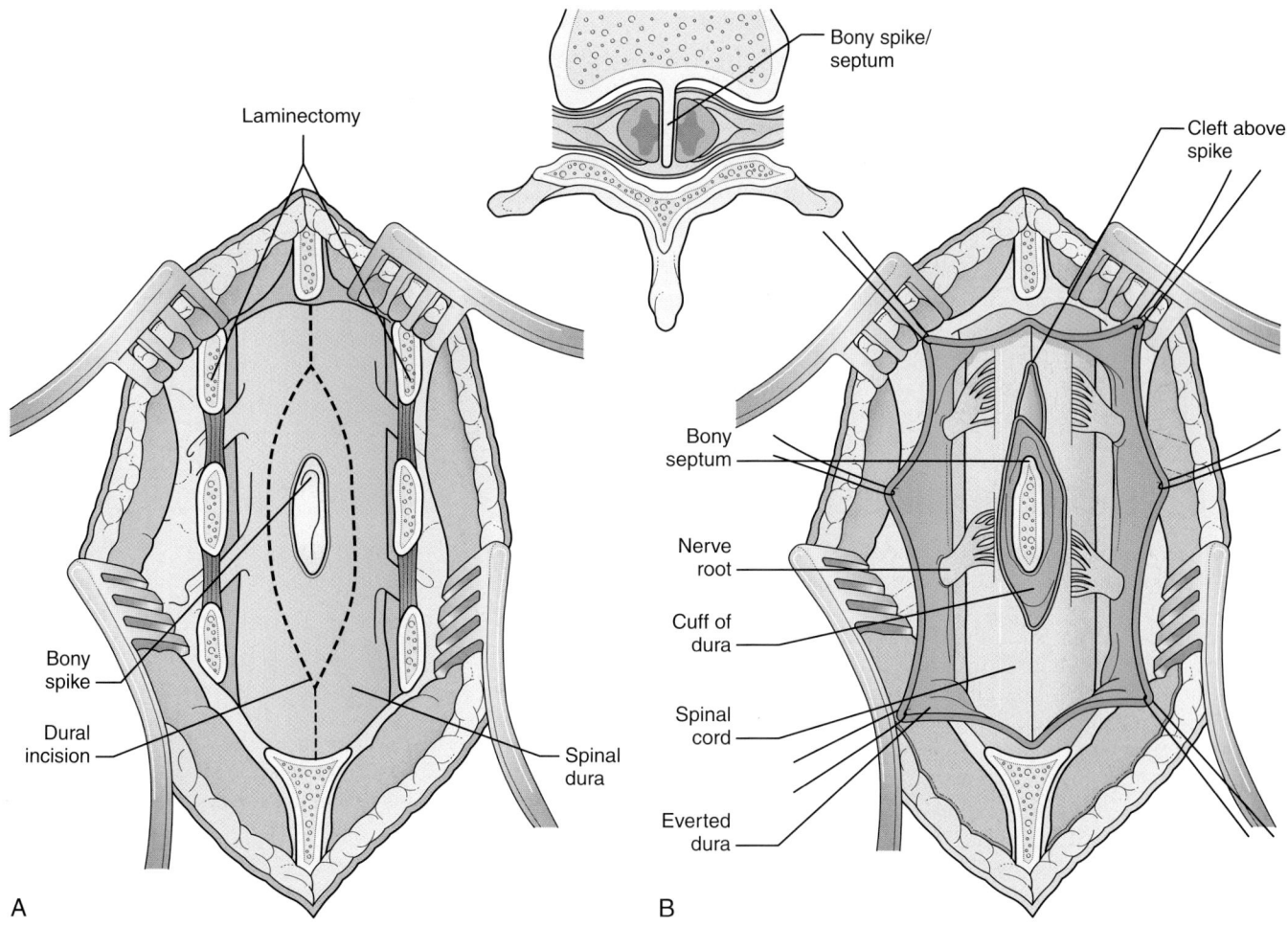

FIGURE 5.18 A, Diastematomyelia. Full laminectomy has been performed above and below the bony septum and the bone has been removed laterally to expose the dural cleft. The proposed dural incision is shown. **B,** Diastematomyelia, dura open. The cuff of dura is used to protect the spinal cord as the bony septum is drilled to the level of the vertebral body below. Note that the caudal end of the split cord tightly hugs the inferior surface of the bony spike, suggesting tethering.

spinal canal on the anteroposterior view with a midline oval bony mass projecting posteriorly from the vertebral body. The spur is usually not visible on lateral views. CT myelography will clarify the diagnosis, but MRI is currently the primary diagnostic test. The coronal study shows the split nicely, but severe kyphoscoliosis can make the study difficult to interpret. Newer imaging sequences, in which the scan is obtained along the curve of the spine, will probably solve this problem. It is important to evaluate the entire spine so that secondary lesions such as lipomas or hypertrophied fila are not missed.

Clear indications for surgery include progressive neurological deficit and scoliosis. When performing surgery to untether the cord for scoliosis, it is usually advisable to operate on the SCM first as a separate procedure; removal of the bony spike most often results in the temporary loss of evoked potential signals, which can reduce the safety of the orthopedic procedure. In select cases, however, the two procedures can be performed together.[49] The management of the asymptomatic patient remains controversial. Historically, some authors have favored a more conservative approach because of the potential risks of surgery and the significant number of patients

who remain asymptomatic (or with stable deficits) throughout growth.[50] However, more recently, other authors have advocated for prophylactic surgery within the first 2 years in asymptomatic children.[51,52] Risk of postsurgical neurological decline is likely highest in SCM subtypes in which the bony septum maximally overlaps the region of cord split.[52]

Surgical Technique

The patient is positioned as for a standard laminectomy. The paraspinal muscles on either side of the midline are freed and retracted laterally as in any standard laminectomy, but vigorous blunt dissection with a periosteal elevator and sponges is avoided, because spina bifida can coexist with the bony septum. The laminectomy is initiated at least one full segment above and below the septum, and it is carried out around the bony spike itself, exposing the dural cleft (Fig. 5.18A). The cleft will usually extend cephalad to the spur but hug it tightly caudally, which indicates tethering. A septal elevator frees the septum from the surrounding dura. The superficial portion of the septum is removed by a rongeur or a high-speed drill that has a diamond burr within the investing dural sheath, which protects the spinal cord. Once the cleft is decompressed, the dura is opened around the cleft, and all intradural adhesions at the cleft are divided (Fig. 5.18B). The dural cuff and the deeper portions of the septum are removed to the level of the anterior spinal canal. It is not necessary or appropriate to close the anterior dura. The posterior dura is closed in a watertight fashion, using a graft if necessary. If an associated hypertrophied filum is suspected, it is divided, using a separate laminectomy if needed.

The procedure should be considered largely prophylactic, although some patients may show neurological improvement. Complications include worsening of neurological status and CSF leak. Late deterioration after surgery can be the result of failure to remove the spike completely, failure to address associated lesions, or rarely, of regrowth of the septum.

ANTERIOR SACRAL MENINGOCELE

Anterior sacral meningocele is a relatively rare condition in which there is herniation of the dural sac through a defect in the anterior surface of the spine, usually in the sacrum. The sac is composed of an outer dural membrane and an inner arachnoid membrane. It contains CSF and, occasionally, neural elements. If the sac is large, it may present as a pelvic mass. Most anterior meningoceles are congenital, as evidenced by their appearance in children. Unlike the typical posterior myelomeningocele, there is no association with hydrocephalus or Chiari malformation. The embryology of these lesions is incompletely understood; most likely, the primary problem is a defect in dural development, resulting in a defect through which the arachnoid herniates, resulting in pulsations that erode the bone.

The lesion is more commonly detected in women, but this most likely reflects the gynecological presentation of a pelvic mass. Symptoms are usually produced by pressure of the presacral mass on adjacent pelvic structures, causing constipation, urinary urgency, dyspareunia, or low back pain. Headache while defecating is occasionally described by children. The cardinal sign is a smooth, cystic mass detected on rectal or pelvic examination.

MRI scanning is the imaging study of choice. When communication between the pelvic cyst and the spinal subarachnoid space is not evident, a metrizamide CT-myelographic study may be indicated.

Surgical treatment of symptomatic lesions is advised because there is no possibility of spontaneous regression, and untreated female patients have a significant risk of pelvic obstruction at the time of labor. Asymptomatic lesions may be followed without operation, if there is no possibility of pregnancy and the lesion does not enlarge on repeated rectal examinations.

Aspiration of the cyst through the rectum or vagina may result in meningitis and should not be performed. If the meningocele is discovered at laparotomy for other reasons, the operation should be terminated and further workup carried out. Surgical treatment via laparotomy has been described historically and recently.[53,54] Nevertheless, most authors prefer the sacral laminectomy approach because it allows visualization of the intraspinal contents of the cyst, resection of adhesions, and sectioning of the filum terminale.[55] The goal of surgery is

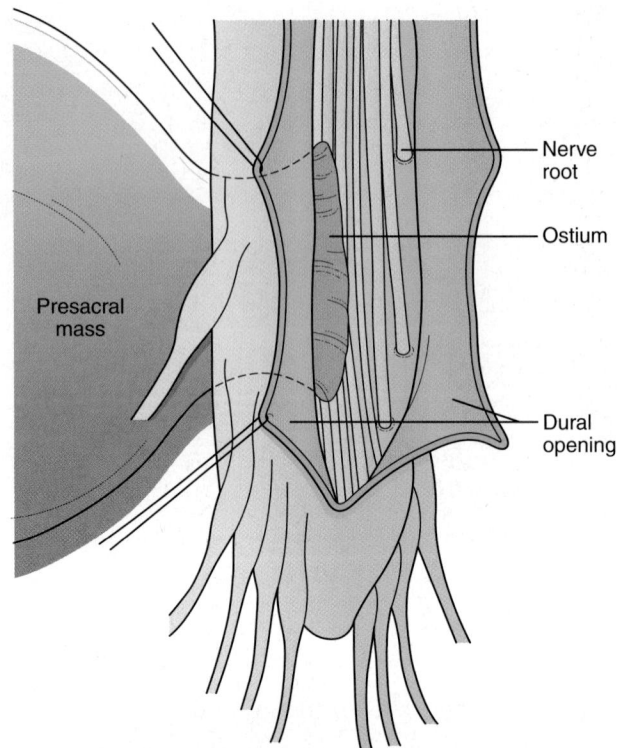

FIGURE 5.19 Approach to anterior sacral meningocele by sacral laminectomy. The posterior dura is opened longitudinally, exposing the sacral nerve roots and the ostium to the pelvic mass.

to untether the spinal cord, decompress the pelvic mass, and obliterate the CSF fistula.

Surgical Technique

The surgical technique has been reviewed.[56] Antibiotic coverage and a bowel preparation are begun 48 hours prior to surgery in case bowel perforation occurs. Under general anesthesia the patient is positioned for laminectomy. A lumbosacral laminectomy is performed from L5 to S4, and the posterior dura is opened longitudinally (Fig. 5.19). Nerve roots within the dural canal are carefully retracted, and the filum terminale is divided to expose the dural ostium leading to the pelvic sac. If no roots enter the sac and the neck is narrow, the anterior dura is simply oversewn (Fig. 5.20). If the sac arises as a caudal extension of the dural sac, and the sacral roots have exited above, the dural sleeve may simply be ligated. If the anterior defect is wide and cannot be mobilized into the field sufficiently for primary closure, digital collapse of the sac through the rectum can be helpful or a fascial graft can be sewn to the edges of the defect. If roots exit through the defect, the dura or graft will have to be plicated around the roots as they exit. The posterior dura is closed. Postoperatively, stool softeners are given to prevent straining. In difficult cases, a second pelvic procedure is required.

The results of surgery described in the literature have been generally good.[54] Complications include meningitis, CSF leak, and neurological problems when nerve roots enter the meningocele sac.

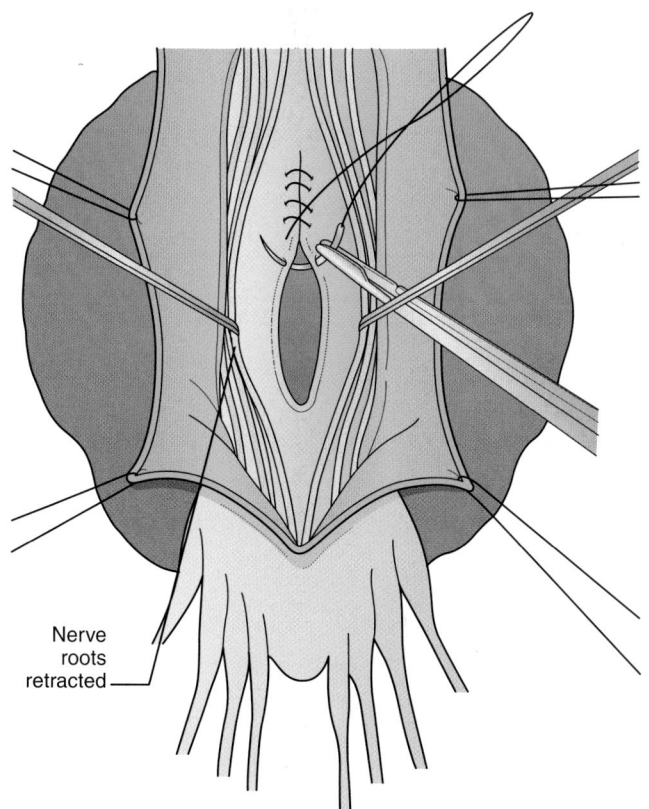

FIGURE 5.20 Anterior sacral meningocele. The nerve roots are retracted, and the ostium is oversewn using a continuous suture. No attempt is made to resect the pelvic mass.

CONGENITAL DERMAL SINUS AND HYPERTROPHIED FILUM TERMINALE

The term *congenital dermal sinus* refers to a group of congenital malformations in which a tubular tract lined with squamous epithelium extends from the skin overlying the spine inward to varying depths. The sinus terminates in the subcutaneous tissue, bone, dura, subarachnoid space, filum terminale, or within an intradural dermoid cyst or neuroglial mass within the spinal cord itself. They occur at all levels within the spine but are most commonly seen in the lower lumbosacral area, where they are frequently confused with simple pilonidal sinuses or coccygeal pits. Pilonidal sinuses are acquired lesions in adults, believed to be secondary to trauma or chronic inflammation, that have no connection with the subarachnoid space or neural elements. Coccygeal pits represent a minor embryonic defect in which the sacrococcygeal ligament produces a dimple in the overlying skin as the spine begins to elongate. There is no connection with the spinal canal, and the coccyx can be palpated directly beneath. In contrast, a congenital dermal sinus is a significant lesion because it enables skin flora to enter the spinal fluid pathways, resulting in repeated bouts of meningitis. It also causes spinal cord tethering, which leads to progressive neurological problems. The hallmark of the lesion is a midline cutaneous dimple overlying the lumbosacral spine above the gluteal fold. There can be other associated cutaneous abnormalities (see Fig. 5.10), such as hemangiomas or hairy patches.

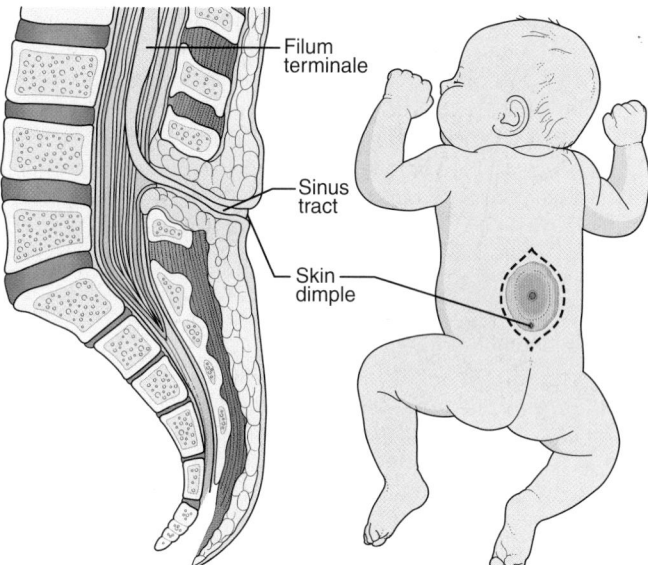

FIGURE 5.21 Cross-sectional anatomy of typical congenital dermal sinus tract. The tract may extend to any depth but it often continues in a cephalad direction, enters the dura, and becomes continuous with the filum terminale.

A somewhat related condition is the so-called meningocele manqué, which is believed to represent an incomplete form of open dysraphism in which bands of meninges, fibrous tissue, and some neural tissue tether the cord to a small area of atretic skin on the back. The radiographic hallmark is a tract extending from the low-lying conus to the cutaneous abnormality. However, it is now recognized that the spinal cord may be tethered even with the conus at a normal level.[57] This condition may be suspected only if there are clear clinical symptoms.

Prophylactic surgery is performed as early as possible, even in newborns, to excise the entire tract.[58,59] When there is clinical evidence of spinal cord compression, MRI scanning is indicated to determine the extent of abscesses or dermoid cysts. In asymptomatic cases, the lesions can simply be explored and the tract followed to its termination. The surgeon undertaking such an operation must be prepared to carry out an extensive intradural dissection, because the tract can extend for a considerable distance. In typical cases, the sinus tract begins at the skin dimple and proceeds cephalad through the soft tissues overlying the spine to traverse the dorsal dura. Once intradural, the tract often becomes continuous with the filum terminale, which is thickened and may contain dermoid elements (Fig. 5.21).

Surgical Technique

The operation begins with an elliptical skin incision that surrounds the sinus opening and encompasses any abnormal skin surrounding it. The tract is sharply dissected and followed through the defect in the fascia. If the tract appears to continue through the dura, a laminectomy is performed above the level of the tract. If the tract attaches to the dura, the dura is opened above the attachment in the midline and incised inferiorly around the point of entry. Any intradural tract must be followed to its termination, even if this involves an extensive laminectomy, because remaining tissue has the capacity to grow into a dermoid inclusion cyst. Intradural dermoids are completely removed, if possible without violating the capsule. If the cyst has ruptured or has been infected, a dense arachnoiditis with scarred nerve roots will prevent complete excision. In this case, judicious intracapsular removal of purulent material and dermoid material is performed, and no attempt is made to remove the scarred capsular wall from the nerve roots. A watertight dural closure is accomplished, except when closure would compress residual infected dermoid cyst material, in which case the dura is left open and the muscle and fascia are closed.

The syndrome of the hypertrophied filum terminale may occur without a cutaneous dimple or sinus tract. If a patient presents with the typical picture of the tethered cord syndrome, an MRI scan is indicated. The scan will demonstrate the low-lying conus, but it may not demonstrate the thickened filum. In these cases, a metrizamide CT-myelogram can demonstrate the pathology, although surgical exploration may be more expeditious.

SACRAL AGENESIS, MYELOCYSTOCELE, AND CLOACAL EXTROPHY

A number of complex anomalies involving the caudal spine have been described, some of which may come to the attention of the neurosurgeon.[61,62] These may involve multiple organ systems, and include imperforate anus, the VACTERL syndrome (*v*ertebral anomalies, *a*nal atresia, *c*ardiac anomalies, *t*racheoesophageal fistula, *e*sophageal atresia, *r*enal and *l*imb anomalies), the OEIS complex (*o*mphalocele, cloacal *e*xtrophy, *i*mperforate anus, *s*pinal deformities), and sacral agenesis. Any of these conditions may be associated with the tethered cord syndrome.

Some consider these caudal regression syndromes to be a continuum, while others feel that they are distinct entities. The severity of the anomaly determines the likely spinal pathology and the management. Simple imperforate anus is associated with hypertrophy of the filum terminale, and there may be no cutaneous stigmata of this condition. Screening with MRI is often recommended. Sacral agenesis is suspected by flattening of the buttocks, shortening of the intergluteal cleft, and prominence of the iliac crest. The newborn with an omphalocele, ambiguous genitalia, and cloacal extrophy may have an associated skin-covered lumbosacral mass, which may represent a myelocystocele or a lipomyelomeningocele. Myelocystocele may occur in association with these complex syndromes, or in isolation. It is generally considered to be an extreme form of the common *ventriculus terminalis*, which is a normal anatomical variant seen often on MRI scans performed for unrelated indications. The central canal of the terminal spinal cord is massively dilated to form a huge cystic structure, which presents as a skin-covered lumbosacral mass. Fetal ultrasound may confuse a myelocystocele with a cystic myelomeningocele. The spinal cord is invariably tethered. Sacral agenesis is associated with maternal diabetes. Pang has divided these cases into five types, based on the appearance of the sacrum.[61] As a practical matter, one can divide these anomalies into those with a high conus and those with a low conus. High symmetrical sacral agenesis is correlated with a truncated,

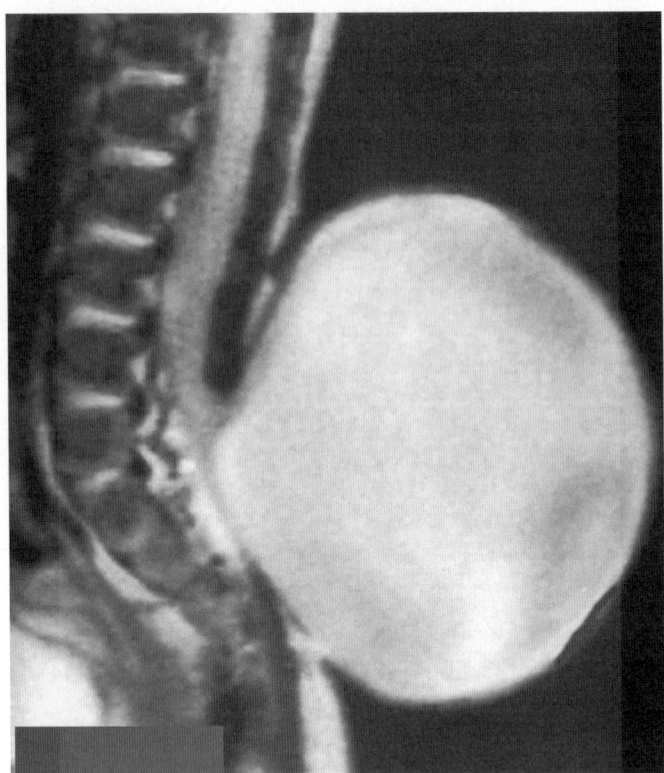

FIGURE 5.22 Lateral magnetic resonance image of a terminal myelocystocele. A large, skin-covered lumbosacral mass is seen clinically. The radiographic finding is a cystic mass, which is a massively dilated terminal central canal of the spinal cord.

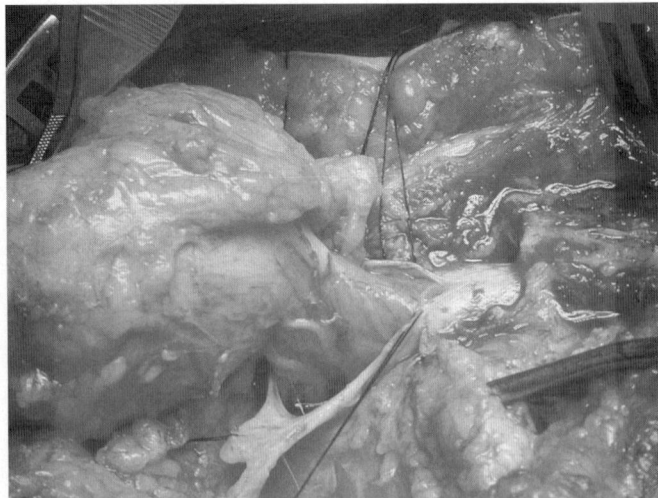

FIGURE 5.23 Operative photograph of a terminal myelocystocele. The terminal end of the spinal cord protrudes through the dural defect. The surgery consists of amputating this tissue while preserving the anterior roots, which remain within the spinal canal.

club-shaped conus ending around T11 or T12. Tethering is not present, although dural canal stenosis has been reported as the cause of delayed deterioration. The lower asymmetrical forms of sacral dysgenesis are more likely to have a low-lying tethered cord. Altogether, tethering is reported in 24% of children with anorectal malformations and as frequently

TABLE 5.2 Evidence-Based Medicine

Statement	Reference*	LOE
Periconceptional folate results in a 72% relative risk reduction in the recurrence of spina bifida when taken by mothers with previous birth of a child with spina bifida.	1	I
Periconceptional folic acid intake results in a 42% relative risk reduction in the incidence of first occurrence of spina bifida.	2	I
In utero spina bifida repair is associated with a 52% relative risk reduction in the need for shunt placement at 12 months and twice the likelihood of independent ambulation at 30 months. (Reference 32, LOE I.) For the fetus with uncomplicated myelomeningocele, cesarean delivery before the onset of labor results in an average postnatal motor functional level 2.2 segments lower (better) than that noted for vaginal delivery.	7	II
In patients with lumbosacral dimples, ultrasound examination is more cost-effective than MRI in screening for occult spinal dysraphism. MRI becomes more effective for higher-risk patients, such as those with anorectal malformations.	35	II/III
Patients requiring revision spinal lipoma surgery are 2.2 times more likely to have an enlarged neural tube–to–canal ratio than those initially presenting for spinal lipoma surgery.	41	III
Patients with symptomatic retethering after lipomyelomeningocele repair are 6.6 times more likely to have a transitional lipomyelomeningocele than those who do not experience retethering.	47	III
Patients with skin stigmata of occult spinal dysraphism who present with neurological deficit are 11 times more likely to be older than 1 year of age than those presenting without neurological deficit.	58	III

*See numbered list of references.
LOE, level of evidence.

as 43% in those with complex malformations.[63] Mechanisms of tethering include myelocystocele, lipomyelomeningocele, or simple hypertrophy of the filum.

Initial management of infants with multisystem anomalies is usually non-neurosurgical, and consists of colostomy, closure of an omphalocele, urinary diversion, and reconstruction for tracheoesophageal fistula. An MRI of the spine is obtained electively, when the infant is stable (Fig. 5.22). Fetal MRI can also make the diagnosis.[64] When the conus is at a normal level, neurosurgical intervention is usually not required. Those cases in which the conus is low-lying should undergo tethered cord release at about 3 months of age, or when the systemic condition permits. It is useful to perform the tethered cord release prior to reversing the colostomy, because the wound is protected from fecal contamination. Even infants with high motor levels should undergo prophylactic untethering, because improvement is possible.

Surgery is similar to that for other tethered cord syndromes. Surgery for myelocystocele consists of defining normal anatomy above the sac, and amputating the sac and all of the tissue below the level of the last intact nerve roots with untethering (Fig. 5.23). The dural reconstruction may require a graft.

Patients who do not have tethering, or who have undergone successful untethering procedures, should remain with stable deficits. If new signs or symptoms appear, a repeat MRI should be performed to define retethering, syrinx formation, or dural constriction. Patients may require long-term management by neurosurgeons, pediatric general surgeons, urologists, and orthopedists.

CONCLUSIONS

The treatment of spinal dysraphism is still evolving. Little in the way of randomized controlled studies is available to support current practice (Table 5.2), However, the recently completed MOMS trial may provide the impetus for further work in this area.

SELECTED KEY REFERENCES

Adzick NS, Thom EA, Spong CY, et al. A randomized trial of prenatal versus postnatal repair of myelomeningocele. *N Engl J Med*. 2011;364:993-1004.

Chapman P. Congenital intraspinal lipomas. Anatomic considerations and surgical treatment. *Childs Brain*. 1982;9:37-47.

Pang D, Dias M, Ahab-Barmada M. Split cord malformation: Part I: a unified theory of embryogenesis for double cord malformations. *Neurosurgery*. 1992;31(3):451-480.

Pang D. Split cord malformation: Part II: clinical syndrome. *Neurosurgery*. 1992;31(3):481-500.

Warder D, Oakes W. Tethered cord syndrome and the conus in a normal position. *Neurosurgery*. 1993;33(3):374-378.

Please go to expertconsult.com to view the complete list of references.

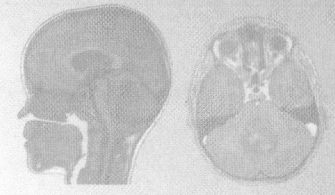

Alia Hdeib, Alan R. Cohen

CLINICAL PEARLS

- Hydrocephalus is one of the most challenging and common conditions that a neurosurgeon encounters.

- This condition can be due to intraventricular hemorrhage in the preterm infant, and its many other causes include trauma, intracranial hemorrhage, tumor, infection, aqueductal stenosis, and idiopathic origin in both the infant or adult.

- For 50 years, the mainstay of hydrocephalus treatment for patient survival and improved quality of life has been cerebrospinal fluid (CSF) diversion by shunting the ventricle or lumbar subarachnoid space to the peritoneum or atrium.

- However, the long-term complications of placement of a CSF shunt apparatus include infection, overshunting, and failure from obstruction.

- A more recent advance or alternative to shunting in a selected population of patients with hydrocephalus is endoscopic third ventriculostomy (ETV), in which CSF diversion is achieved via minimally invasive endoscopic fenestration of the floor of the third ventricle. It appears safe and is most effective for children over 1 month of age, those with aqueductal stenosis, and those who have not had a shunt previously.

Although it is one of the most commonly encountered clinical diagnoses in neurosurgical practice, hydrocephalus across the age spectrum is a humbling entity with a long history. Hydrocephalus (from the Greek words *hydro* ["water"] and *kefale* ["head"]) has been recognized for over 2000 years. Despite great strides in diagnosis and treatment, hydrocephalus remains a challenge for the clinician.

Hydrocephalus refers to the buildup of cerebrospinal fluid (CSF) within the intracranial compartments usually associated with clinical sequelae from an increase in intracranial pressure (ICP). It can develop at any time, from the fetal period into adulthood, and it can have a myriad of causes including, but not limited to, congenital defects, perinatal insults, acquired conditions such as infection, tumor, traumatic and nontraumatic hemorrhage, and rarely CSF overproduction (Fig. 6.1).

Hydrocephalus is one of the most commonly encountered conditions in neurosurgery. One recent study by Sipek and colleagues analyzed data from the Czech national registry from 1961 to 2000 retrospectively and found the mean incidence of congenital hydrocephalus diagnosed both pre- and postnatally to be 6.35 per 10,000 liveborn infants.[1] Another series by Fernell and Hagberg from Sweden found that the prevalence of infantile hydrocephalus was 6.99 per 1000 in the 1970s, increasing to 25.37 in the 1980s.[2] The increase was thought to be due to the increased survival of very preterm infants. In the 1990s the prevalence of infantile hydrocephalus in the Swedish population decreased to 13.69. Despite changes in prevalence rates, outcome in surviving children with hydrocephalus remained similar. Other studies have looked at the prevalence of hydrocephalus in the adult population. A recent Norwegian study by Brean and Eide found the prevalence of idiopathic normal-pressure hydrocephalus (NPH) to be 21.9 per 100,000 and the incidence to be 5.5 per 100,000, reflecting minimum prevalence/incidence rate estimates.[3] The incidence of hydrocephalus in developing countries is unknown but may be higher.

HISTORY

The recognition of hydrocephalus as a clinical entity dates back to antiquity. In the fifth century BC Hippocrates described the clinical presentation of hydrocephalus secondary to water accumulation within the head.[4,5] Later, Galen described the choroid plexus and the relationship of CSF to the brain, though his understanding of CSF physiology was lacking.[4] In the seventeenth century, Willis proposed the secretion of CSF by the choroid plexus and its absorption into the venous system, although the pathways he described were less than accurate.[4] In 1701 Pacchioni described the arachnoid granulations, though he misidentified their function as the site of CSF production rather than absorption, and it was not until the late nineteenth century that the current accepted physiology of CSF production and absorption was clarified.[4,6,7]

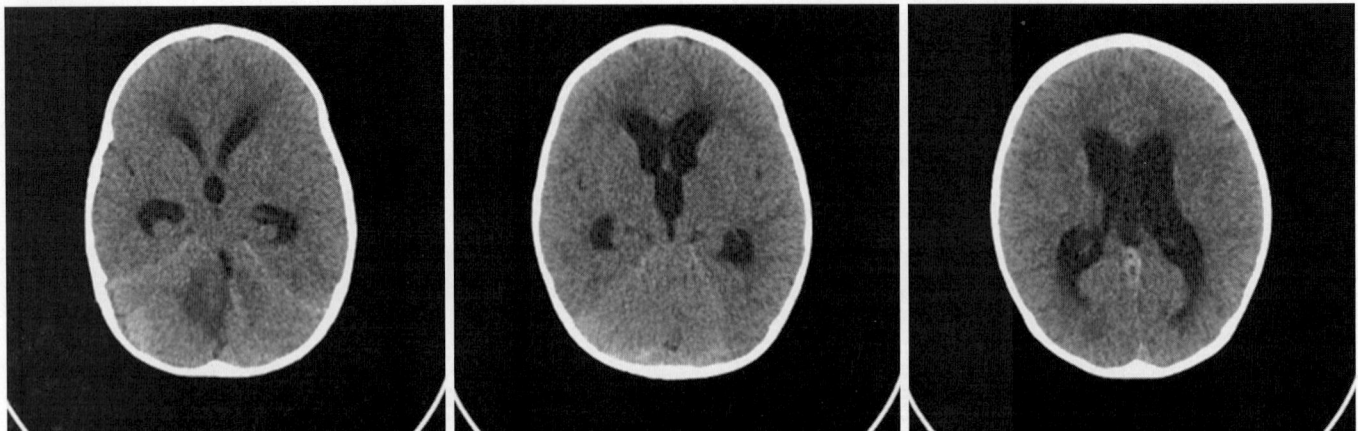

FIGURE 6.1 Axial noncontrast computed tomography (CT) scan of a 2-year-old child with hydrocephalus due to a posterior fossa chloroma.

The evolution of the treatment of hydrocephalus can be described by three stages.[7] The first stage, up to the Renaissance, was characterized by poor medical understanding of CSF dynamics and pathology; therefore, nonsurgical and surgical treatment was largely useless. The second stage encompasses the period between the nineteenth and mid-twentieth centuries, when CSF physiology and pathology were elucidated but treatment options were in their infancy. In 1891 Quincke described lumbar puncture as a diagnostic modality and a means of treating hydrocephalus. Keen drained the cerebral ventricles through a temporal approach.[4] Various lumbar and ventricular cannulation attempts were described, some more successful than others. Cushing reported treating hydrocephalus by a lumbar peritoneal connection, which was encouraging. Lespinasse in 1910 was the first to describe choroid plexus coagulation and the use of an endoscope (cystoscope) for the cannulation of the cerebral ventricles.[4,7] In 1922 Dandy was the first to perform a third ventriculostomy through a subfrontal approach, and a year later Mixter performed the first endoscopic third ventriculostomy for noncommunicating hydrocephalus using a urethroscope.[4] In 1939 Torkildsen described the use of a valveless rubber catheter to connect the lateral ventricles with the cisterna magna for noncommunicating hydrocephalus.[4]

The third stage of evolution in the treatment of hydrocephalus started with the development of silicone shunts with unidirectional valves in the 1950s. Nulsen and Spitz used a stainless steel unidirectional ball valve connected to a rubber catheter to divert CSF from the ventricles to the jugular vein in a hydrocephalic child.[8] This was a landmark operation that marked the beginning of a new and powerful way of treating hydrocephalus. Variations and improvements on the valve used by Nulsen and Spitz ensued. Eventually, ventriculoperitoneal shunting became the standard surgical treatment for hydrocephalus, although both historically and in current clinical practice various sites for CSF diversion have been, and are still, used. However, shunt systems represent the introduction of a foreign material in the body, and complications related to infection and plugging of the shunt system are often encountered in clinical practice. Currently advances in technology and endoscopy have prompted resurgence in the use of third ventriculostomy for treating noncommunicating hydrocephalus as a means of obviating the inherent complications associated with shunts.

TABLE 6.1 Sites of Cerebrospinal Fluid Production

Compartment	Site
Intracranial	Choroid plexus of the lateral, third, and fourth ventricles
	Ependymal lining
	Interstitial space
Spinal	Dura of the nerve root sleeves

CEREBROSPINAL FLUID AND PATHOPHYSIOLOGY OF HYDROCEPHALUS

CSF is a clear colorless fluid produced mostly by the choroid plexus of the lateral, third, and fourth ventricles, and to a lesser degree (<20%) by the interstitial space and ependymal lining of the ventricles. In the spinal compartments, the nerve sleeve dura is responsible for CSF production[9] (Table 6.1). Ninety-five percent of CSF produced by the ventricular choroid plexus occurs at the level of the lateral ventricles. CSF is found within the ventricles and cisterns of the brain and subarachnoid space, and surrounds both the brain and spinal cord. The infant has an approximate total volume of about 50 mL of CSF, and adults average 150 mL, half in the cranial compartment and half in the spinal compartment. Newborns produce CSF at a rate of 25 mL/day, which increases to about 500 mL/day in the adult (0.3-0.35 mL/minute).[9] Intracranial pressure ranges from 9 to 12 cm H_2O in the newborn to less than 18 to 20 cm H_2O in the adult population. Generally, the rate of CSF formation is not dependent on intracranial pressure (ICP); however, CSF absorption is pressure dependent, and it occurs at the level of the arachnoid villi that are found in proximity to the dural venous sinuses.

The circulation and physiology of CSF and its circulation can be quite complex. More than 2 centuries ago Alexander Monro applied principles of physics to the relationship of intracranial contents.[10] This was supported by experiments conducted by Kellie.[10] Today their work is known as the Monro-Kellie doctrine (Table 6.2), which states that within the rigid container of the skull, the sum of intracranial contents, including CSF, blood, and brain, is constant.[10,11] Therefore, a change in one component (e.g., increase in CSF)

TABLE 6.2 The Monro-Kellie Doctrine

The sum of intracranial contents to include blood, CSF, and brain should remain constant in a fixed container, such as the skull.

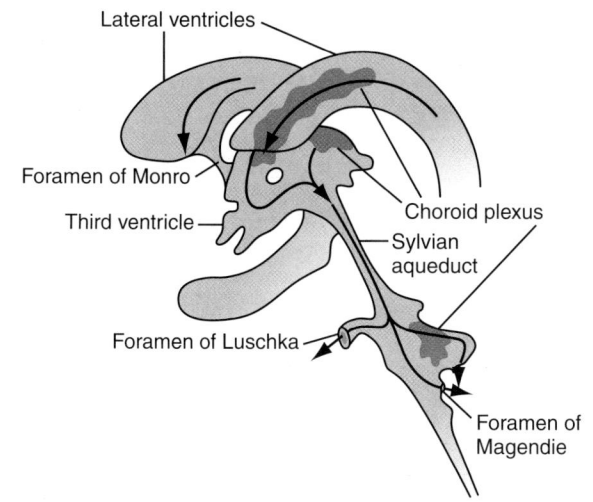

FIGURE 6.2 Cerebrospinal fluid flow through the ventricular system.

requires a compensatory change in one or both of the other components. However, in very young children, usually less than 2 to 3 years of age, the fontanelles are still open and the system is no longer closed; in this scenario the hypothesis does not apply.

CSF flow through the ventricular system occurs in a progressive manner, from the lateral ventricles through the foramina of Monro to the third ventricle, through the sylvian aqueduct to the fourth ventricle, then through the foramina of Luschka and Magendie to the subarachnoid spaces (Fig. 6.2). From the subarachnoid spaces, CSF is absorbed into the venous circulation through the arachnoid granulations. A dysregulation in production, absorption, or circulation of CSF can lead to symptomatic hydrocephalus.

Rarely hydrocephalus can be associated with CSF overproduction, as in the case of choroid plexus tumors. However, in most instances hydrocephalus is due to an obstruction along the pathway of CSF flow. Tumors of the lateral ventricles can cause hydrocephalus by mass effect or CSF overproduction in the case of tumors derived from the choroid plexus. Common tumors of the lateral ventricles include meningiomas, gliomas, and choroid plexus tumors. Choroid plexus tumors are rare, seen more commonly in children younger than 2 years of age, and account for less than 1% of all intracranial tumors[12] (Fig. 6.3). Even with complete surgical tumor resection, hydrocephalus may still persist and require treatment. This is thought to be due to more distal obstruction (i.e., aqueduct, arachnoid villi) either from preoperative microhemorrhages or scarring after surgery. Rarely choroid plexus villous hypertrophy can lead to CSF overproduction, which can be treated by choroid plexus coagulation.[13] Obstruction at the foramina of Monro can also be caused by congenital atresia, membranes, or gliosis after hemorrhage, and can lead to unilateral ventriculomegaly.[14]

In the third ventricle, cysts and tumors can cause hydrocephalus by CSF obstruction. Colloid cysts, found at the anterior superior part of the third ventricle, generally represent less than 2% of intracranial tumors and are more commonly symptomatic in the adult population, with clinical presentations ranging from acute to chronic hydrocephalus due to obstruction of the foramina of Monro[15] (Fig. 6.4). Treatment is aimed at stereotactic aspiration, endoscopic resection, or open microsurgery.[16] Other cystic lesions include arachnoid and ependymal cysts, and rarely dermoid cysts. Third ventricular neoplasms include craniopharyngiomas and gliomas, including hypothalamic astrocytomas and subependymal giant cell astrocytomas (in association with tuberous sclerosis). Hydrocephalus may persist after glioma resection, necessitating shunt placement.

Obstruction may be seen at the level of the sylvian aqueduct, especially in neonates in whom the small diamter (0.2-0.5 mm) of the aqueduct puts it at risk for obstruction from congenital and acquired causes (Fig. 6.5). This leads to enlargement of the third and lateral ventricles. Congenital aqueductal malformations include stenosis, forking, septum formation, and subependymal gliosis due to in utero infections. True luminal stenosis is not as common. In addition, lesions such as arteriovenous malformations and periaqueductal tumors such as tectal gliomas and pineal region tumors can cause obstruction at or near the sylvian aqueduct, leading to triventricular obstructive hydrocephalus (Fig. 6.6). Often, resection of the lesion is sufficient to treat the hydrocephalus. Newer methods of endoscopic aqueductoplasty and stenting are showing promise.[16]

The fourth ventricle and basal foramina can also be sites of obstruction leading to hydrocephalus. Dandy-Walker malformations present in infants with a large posterior fossa cyst in the setting of cerebellar vermian hypoplasia and cerebellar atrophy, commonly associated with hydrocephalus as well as other congenital abnormalities (Fig. 6.7). Tumors of the posterior fossa and fourth ventricular region can present with acute or chronic hydrocephalus in addition to other associated posterior fossa symptoms. In the adult population common tumors include metastases, gliomas, meningiomas, neuromas, and hemangioblastomas. In the pediatric population, infratentorial tumors are common causes of hydrocephalus and common offenders include medulloblastomas, ependymomas, cerebellar astrocytomas, and brainstem gliomas. Across the age spectrum, infections and subarachnoid hemorrhage can lead to arachnoid scarring and hydrocephalus (Fig. 6.8). Congenital conditions such as Chiari malformations may cause hydrocephalus by obstruction of CSF flow around the base of the skull. Obstruction of CSF flow can also occur at the level of the arachnoid granulations with impairment of CSF absorption. This may be idiopathic or may be seen after infection, subarachnoid hemorrhage, trauma, or tumors and can lead to enlargement of CSF spaces over the convexities.

In models of adult hydrocephalus, conditions leading to scarring distal to the ventricular system (e.g., subarachnoid hemorrhage or infection) cause a resistance to normal CSF outflow. However, the pathophysiology of CSF circulation is quite complex. CSF pulsation variability and cerebral blood flow dynamics have been implicated in both idiopathic and secondary hydrocephalus, though their exact role is still a topic of investigation.[17,18] In addition, the properties of the surrounding parenchyma, particularly its compressibility,

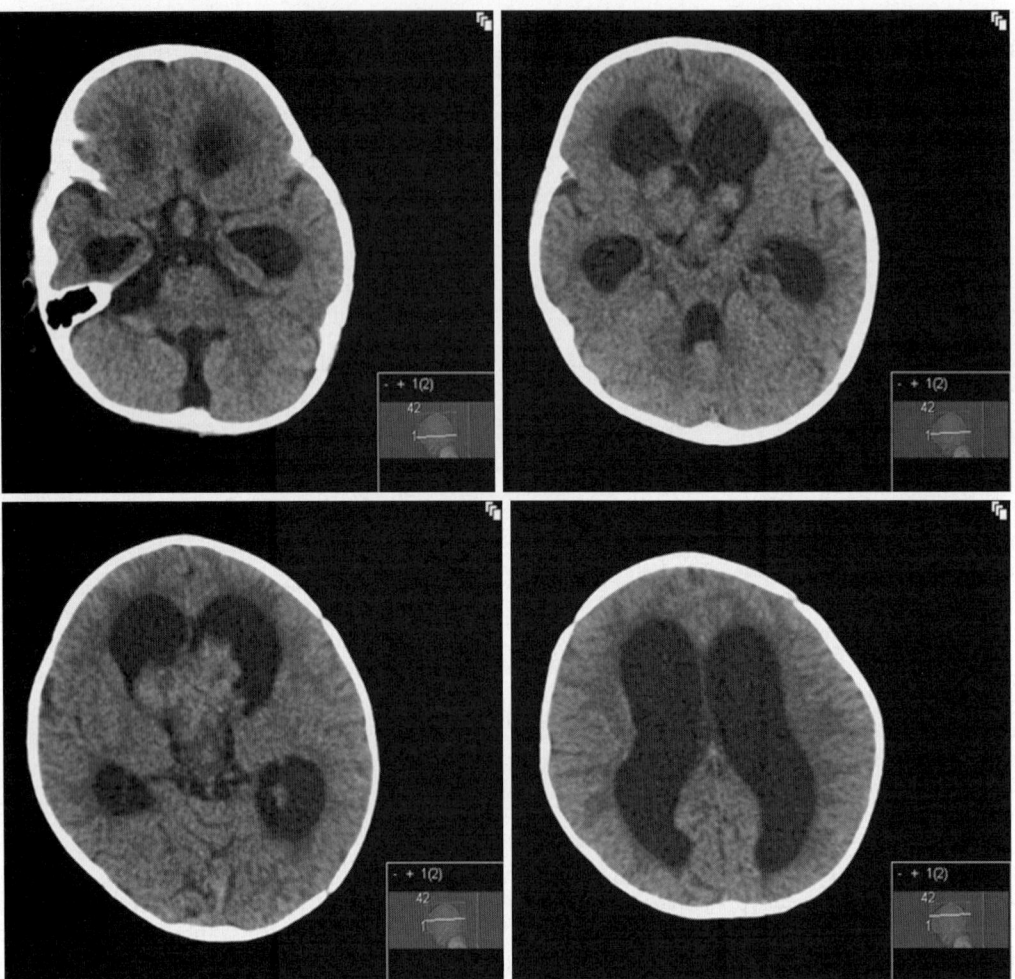

FIGURE 6.3 Axial noncontrast computed tomography (CT) scan of a 7-month-old with a choroid plexus papilloma and hydrocephalus.

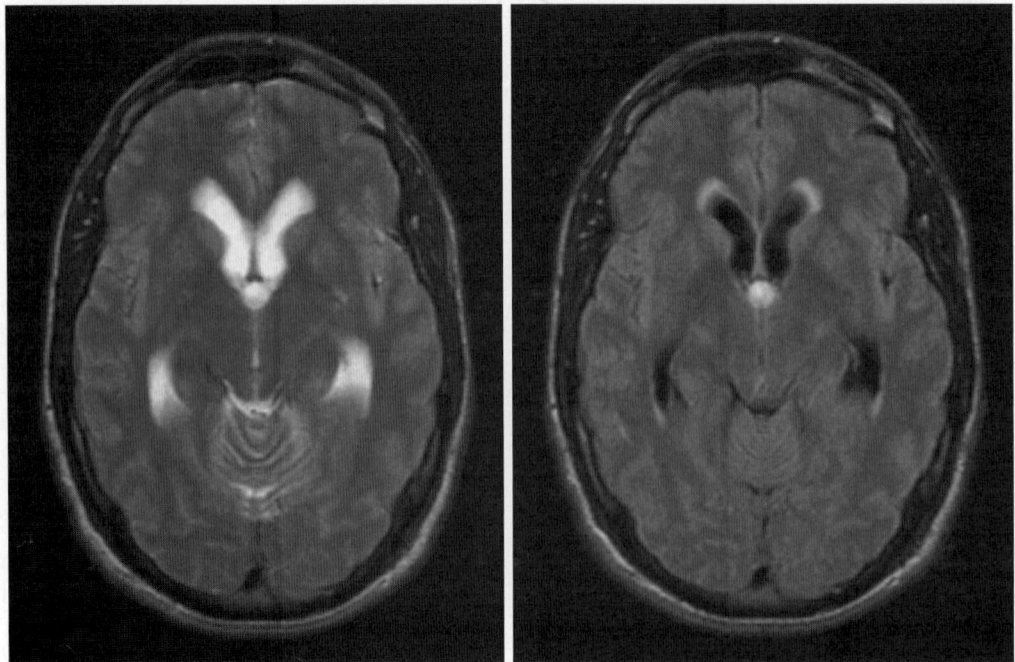

FIGURE 6.4 A 39-year-old patient with hydrocephalus from obstruction at the foramen of Monro from a colloid cyst. T2-weighted axial image (*left*) and fluid attenuated inversion recovery (FLAIR) sequence (*right*) showing the colloid cyst and enlarged lateral ventricles.

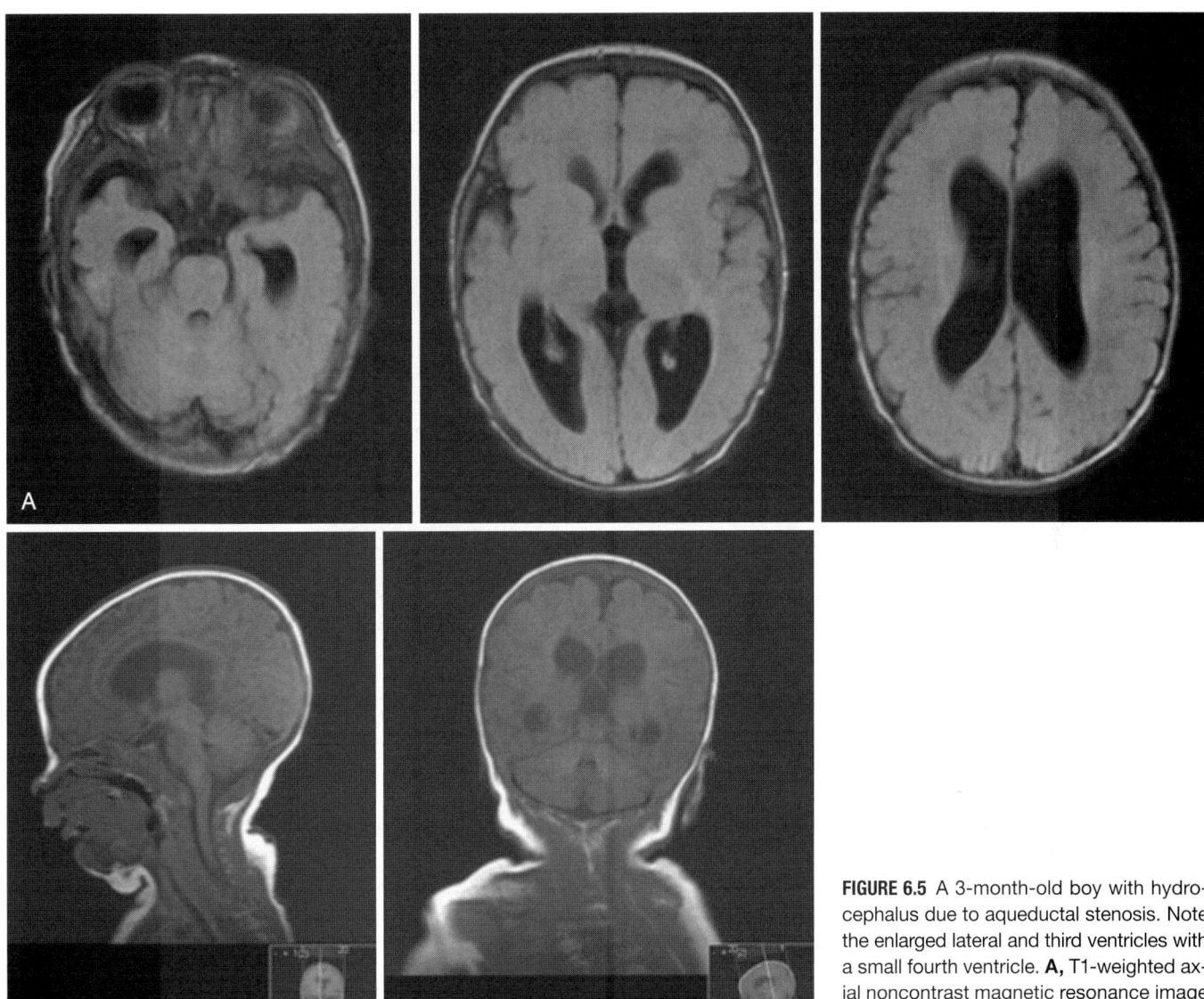

FIGURE 6.5 A 3-month-old boy with hydrocephalus due to aqueductal stenosis. Note the enlarged lateral and third ventricles with a small fourth ventricle. **A,** T1-weighted axial noncontrast magnetic resonance image (MRI). **B,** T1-weighted sagittal and coronal noncontrast MRI.

has been proposed as a means of explaining the observation of hydrocephalic symptoms in the settings of lower ventricular pressures.[19] For example, if the brain parenchyma is able to attenuate increases in intraventricular pressure, the overall intracranial pressure does not need to rise above normal levels in the setting of abnormal transventricular pressure gradients, leading to the entity commonly called *normal-pressure hydrocephalus* (NPH).[19] It is not clear if parenchymal damage plays a primary or secondary role in the development of NPH.

CLASSIFICATION OF HYDROCEPHALUS

There are different classifications and means of describing hydrocephalus. Often different schemes are employed for hydrocephalus in infants and children versus adults, delineating the difference in pathophysiology and clinical presentation across the age spectrum. In general, hydrocephalus can be defined as nonobstructive, associated with ventricular system enlargement (e.g., hydrocephalus ex vacuo), or obstructive, associated with defective CSF circulation or absorption (Table 6.3). A more clinically useful scheme divides obstructive hydrocephalus into communicating and noncommunicating types. Generally, communicating hydrocephalus refers to an obstruction outside the ventricular system, often at the level of the subarachnoid space or the arachnoid villi. Noncommunicating hydrocephalus refers to an impedance of CSF flow within the ventricular system, such as blockage at the aqueduct of Sylvius or the basal foramina of Luschka and Magendie. Less clinically useful schemes describe hydrocephalus as physiological (secondary to CSF overproduction) or nonphysiological, external or internal (obstruction outside or within the ventricular system, respectively).

A system proposed by Gowers in 1888, still useful today, divides hydrocephalus as either acute or chronic, primary or

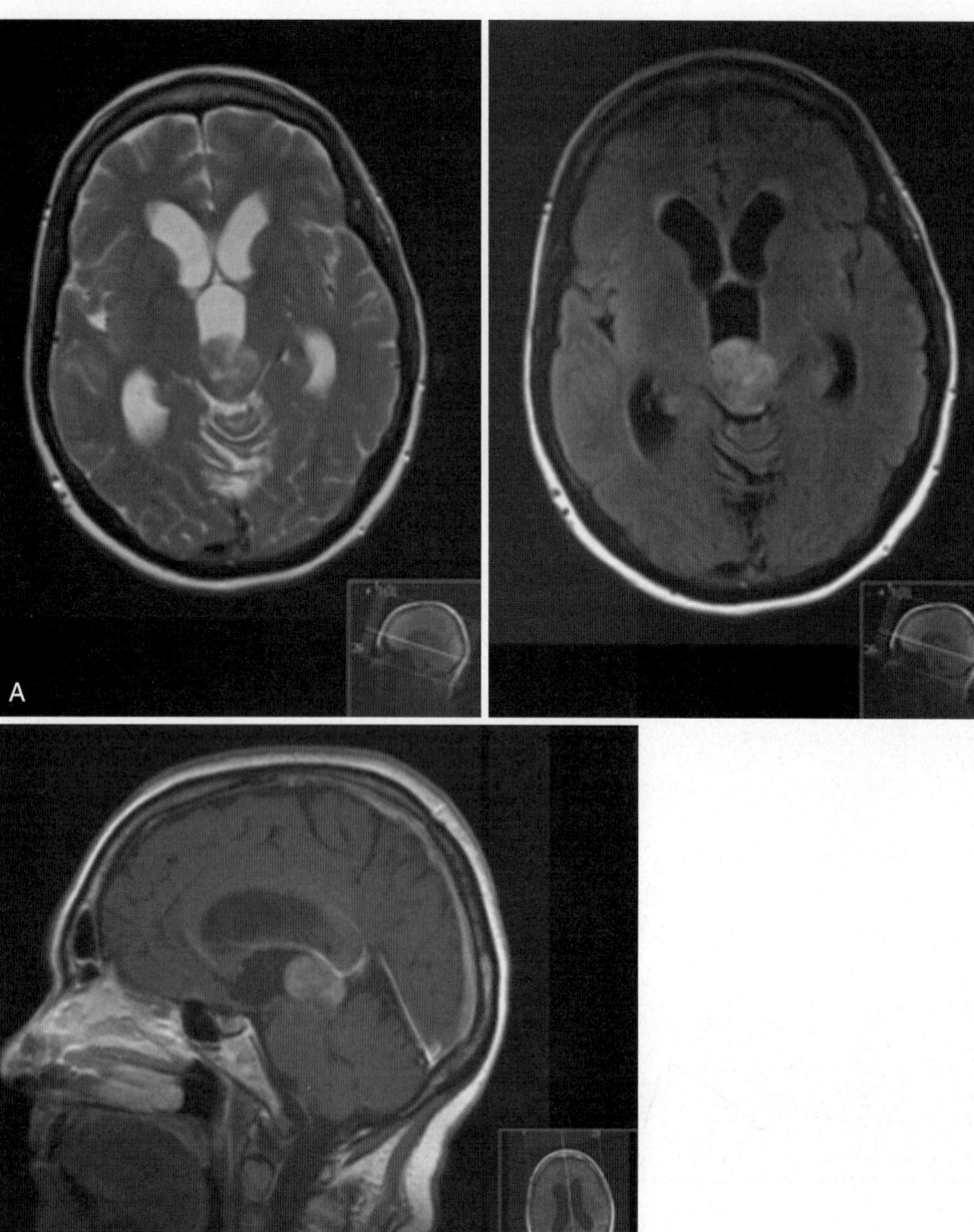

FIGURE 6.6 Magnetic resonance imaging (MRI) scan of a patient with a pinealocytoma. **A,** Axial T2-weighted and fluid attenuated inversion recovery (FLAIR) MRI. **B,** Sagittal T1-weighted enhanced MRI scan.

secondary.[20] Generally, acute hydrocephalus implies a rapid decompensation usually associated with an underlying condition and presents with elevated intracranial pressure. Chronic hydrocephalus may be either idiopathic or secondary to a known pathological condition, and generally is associated with lower or normal intracranial pressures. Secondary hydrocephalus can be due to a number of clinical conditions, including but not limited to tumors, hemorrhage, trauma, and infection.

ETIOLOGY AND CLINICAL PRESENTATION

There are different etiologies for hydrocephalus depending on the age group of patients (Table 6.4). In infants, numerous causes are clinically identified. Particularly in premature infants, posthemorrhagic hydrocephalus (PHH) is often seen as a sequela of intraventicular or germinal matrix hemorrhage (Table 6.5). The intraventricular blood leads to fibrosing arachnoiditis, meningeal fibrosis, and subependymal gliosis, altering the physiology of CSF flow.[21] In full-term infants hydrocephalus can be ascribed to a different etiological set, including but not limited to aqueductal stenosis, Dandy-Walker malformations, tumors, arachnoid cysts, vein of Galen malformations, Chiari malformations, and so on.[22] Intrauterine infections can also lead to congenital hydrocephalus. In older children, common causes include various tumors that obstruct CSF flow along its ventricular path, as well as trauma and infection (e.g., meningitis).

Several studies have looked at trends in causes of hydrocephalus in specific groups. A retrospective review by Green and co-workers of 253 infants and children with hydrocephalus treated at a British tertiary care center over a 10-year

FIGURE 6.7 Child with a Dandy-Walker malformation and shunted hydrocephalus. Note the right occipital ventricular shunt catheter.

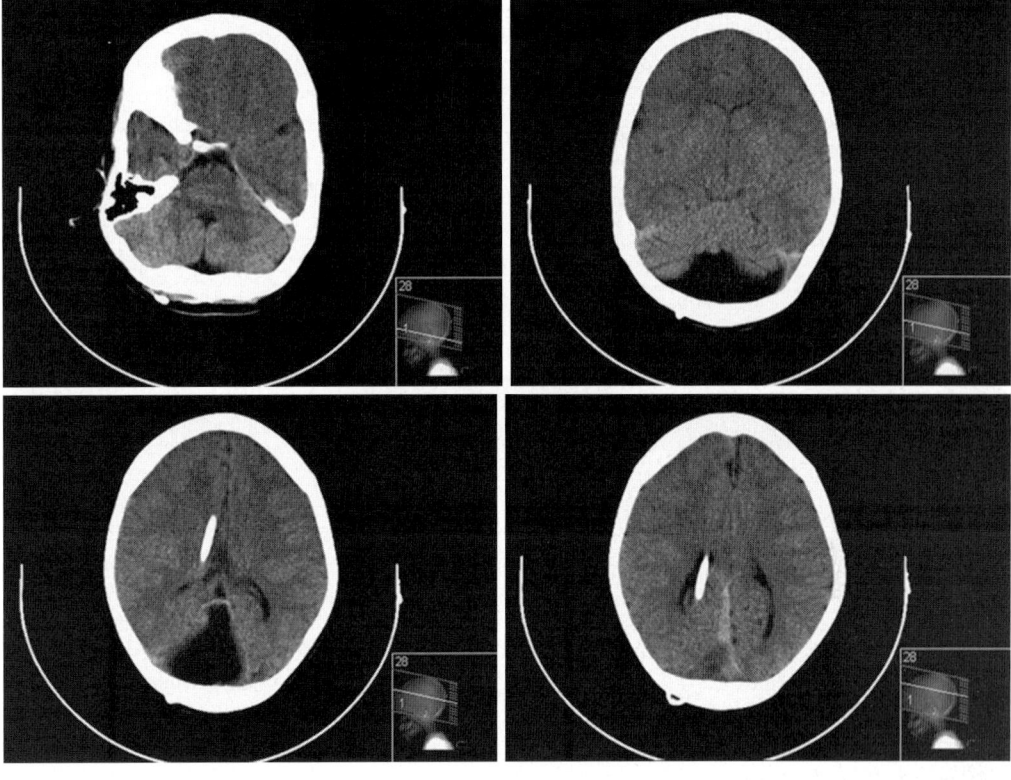

FIGURE 6.8 Axial computed tomography (CT) scan of a patient with hydrocephalus from aneurysmal subarachnoid hemorrhage who underwent a right frontal external ventricular drain placement.

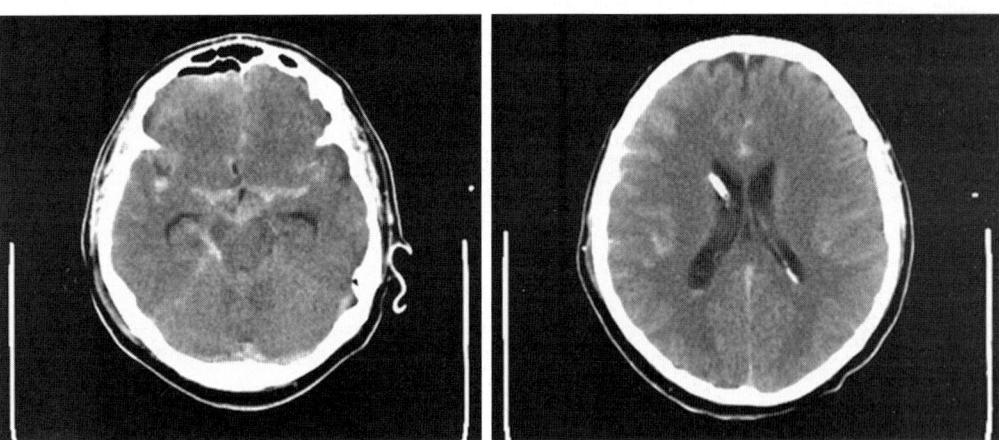

period revealed interesting trends in the causes of this condition.[23] In the first half of the decade, the predominant causes were posthemorrhagic hydrocephalus and hydrocephalus due to brain tumors, which decreased from over half of the children to one third by the end of the decade; the rate of neonatal intraventricular hemorrhage decreased by 45%.[23]

Infants with hydrocephalus can present with various symptoms. Apnea and bradycardia may be noted. As ventriculomegaly and intracranial pressure increase, the anterior fontanelle becomes more convex and tense. The head circumference is also seen to increase, generally by 0.5 cm to 2 cm per week in premature infants with posthemorrhagic hydrocephalus. In older infants and children, as the skull becomes less distensible, presenting signs can include lateral rectus palsies and vertical gaze palsies (e.g., Parinaud's sign). Full-term infants with hydrocephalus can also present with poor feeding, vomiting, irritability, macrocephaly, bulging fontanelle,

splaying of cranial sutures, and frontal bossing. Normal head circumference for full-term infants ranges from 33 to 36 cm, and rapid increases that cross percentile lines are more concerning for hydrocephalus than head circumferences that are above the 95% percentile but that parallel the normal head growth curve.

In older children, hydrocephalus may occur secondary to neoplasms or trauma (Fig. 6.9). Children can present with headaches (dull, typically upon awakening), vision changes (blurry or double vision), lethargy, vomiting, decreased food intake, behavioral disturbances, poor school performance, and endocrinopathies (e.g., short stature, precocious puberty). On examination, papilledema and lateral rectus palsies can be seen, as well as hyperreflexia and clonus. If progressive lethargy is noted, diagnosis and treatment become urgent. In severe cases of increased intracranial pressure and severe hydrocephalus, Cushing's triad can be seen. Cushing's triad

TABLE 6.3 Hydrocephalus Classification

Type	Features
Nonobstructive	Ventricular enlargement (e.g., hydrocephalus ex vacuo)
Obstructive	
Communicating	Obstruction outside the ventricular system (e.g., subarachnoid space or arachnoid villi)
Noncommunicating	Obstruction within the ventricular system (e.g., aqueduct or basal foramina)

TABLE 6.4 Pathologic Conditions Associated With Hydrocephalus

Congenital	Acquired
Chiari I malformation	Postinfectious
Chiari II malformation (associated with myelomeningocele)	Posthemorrhagic (including subarachnoid and intraventricular hemorrhage)
Primary aqueductal stenosis (or gliosis secondary to intrauterine infection or germinal matrix hemorrhage)	Post-traumatic
Dandy-Walker malformation	Secondary to mass lesions (e.g., tumors, vascular malformations, cysts)
Hydranencephaly	Postoperative (e.g., after tumor resection including posterior fossa tumors)

TABLE 6.5 Grading of Germinal Matrix Hemorrhage

Grade	Description
I	Subependymal hemorrhage
II	Intraventricular hemorrhage with no ventricular dilatation
III	Intraventricular hemorrhage with ventricular dilatation
IV	Intraventricular hemorrhage with intracerebral hemorrhage

consists of bradycardia, hypertension, and irregular breathing, and requires emergent evaluation and treatment.

In the adult population the causes and clinical presentations of hydrocephalus are varied. Therefore, it is easier to describe hydrocephalus as acute (generally high pressure) or chronic (normal or low pressure). Various pathological processes can be associated with acute hydrocephalus (e.g., tumors, posterior fossa infarcts, subarachnoid hemorrhage, infection), which generally closely follows the causative disease. Common signs and symptoms include generalized headaches, usually worse when lying down (ICP is maximal), nausea, vomiting, vision changes (blurring or diplopia), papilledema, lateral rectus palsies, ataxia, and changes in mental status.

The presentation of chronic hydrocephalus is different from that of acute hydrocephalus. Symptoms are often more

insidious, and become apparent over weeks, months, or years. Chronic hydrocephalus may be secondary to a known pathological process or may be idiopathic. Patients present with cognitive dysfunction including dementia or intellectual and behavioral changes, urinary incontinence, motor difficulties, vision changes, and skull changes such as thinning and widening of the suture line. Hydrocephalus can be seen in the setting of brain tumors that obstruct CSF pathways. Sometimes the signs of hydrocephalus can be obscured by the symptoms of the primary process. The chronicity of symptoms depends on the rate of growth and location of the tumor. Post-traumatic hydrocephalus usually presents as chronic hydrocephalus. Because encephalomalacia often occurs in post-traumatic patients, the diagnosis of hydrocephalus can be difficult, especially because the cognitive effects of traumatic brain injury can confound the clinical picture.

NPH is a common diagnosis encountered by neurosurgeons in the adult population (Fig. 6.10). Patients with NPH present with the clinical triad of gait disturbances, dementia, and urinary incontinence, usually in the sixth to eight decades of life[24] (Table 6.6). Generally, gait disturbances, described as apraxic or magnetic, are the first symptoms noted. Patients develop a slow, wide-based shuffling walking pattern. Urinary incontinence is a common presentation of NPH. Early in the course patients develop urinary frequency and urgency, which progress to incontinence owing to bladder hyperactivity.[24] The cognitive decline must be differentiated from other causes of dementia (vascular, Alzheimer's disease, dementia with Lewy bodies, etc.). Generally, the dementia associated with NPH is subcortical in nature. Often patients show apathy, psychomotor retardation, difficulty with executive function, and inattention; apraxia, aphasia, and agnosia are not seen.[24] In the elderly, the symptoms associated with NPH must be distinguished from other common causes seen in this patient population, including vascular and neurodegenerative disorders.

A nonhydrocephalic clinical entity presenting with increased intracranial pressure, seen in both the pediatric and adult populations, is the syndrome of idiopathic intracranial hypertension, also commonly known as *pseudotumor cerebri*. The ventricles are not enlarged and are usually small. Patients are generally overweight women who develop increased intracranial pressure without an identifiable source, and it remains a diagnosis of exclusion. The pathophysiology of this syndrome is still unclear, though venous stenosis and effects of the hormone leptin have been implicated.[25] Symptoms include headaches and papilledema, and up to 25% of patients develop visual deterioration from optic nerve atrophy.

DIAGNOSIS

Neuroimaging studies are the mainstay for visualizing and understanding ventricular anatomy and diagnosing hydrocephalus in symptomatic cases. In utero diagnosis of hydrocephalus is often accomplished via ultrasound studies, though fetal MRIs are gaining popularity as diagnostic adjuncts.[26] In infants with intraventricular hemmorrhage (IVH) and suspected hydrocephalus, sonography is often used to evaluate the ventricles because the anterior fontanelle provides a good window for ventricular visualization.[27] Diagnosis of mono-,

FIGURE 6.9 Magnetic resonance imaging (MRI) scan of a 2-year-old child with hydrocephalus due to a posterior fossa tumor. Axial fluid attenuated inversion recovery (FLAIR), sagittal T2-weighted, and coronal T1-enhanced sequences. Note the transependymal edema seen on the axial FLAIR images.

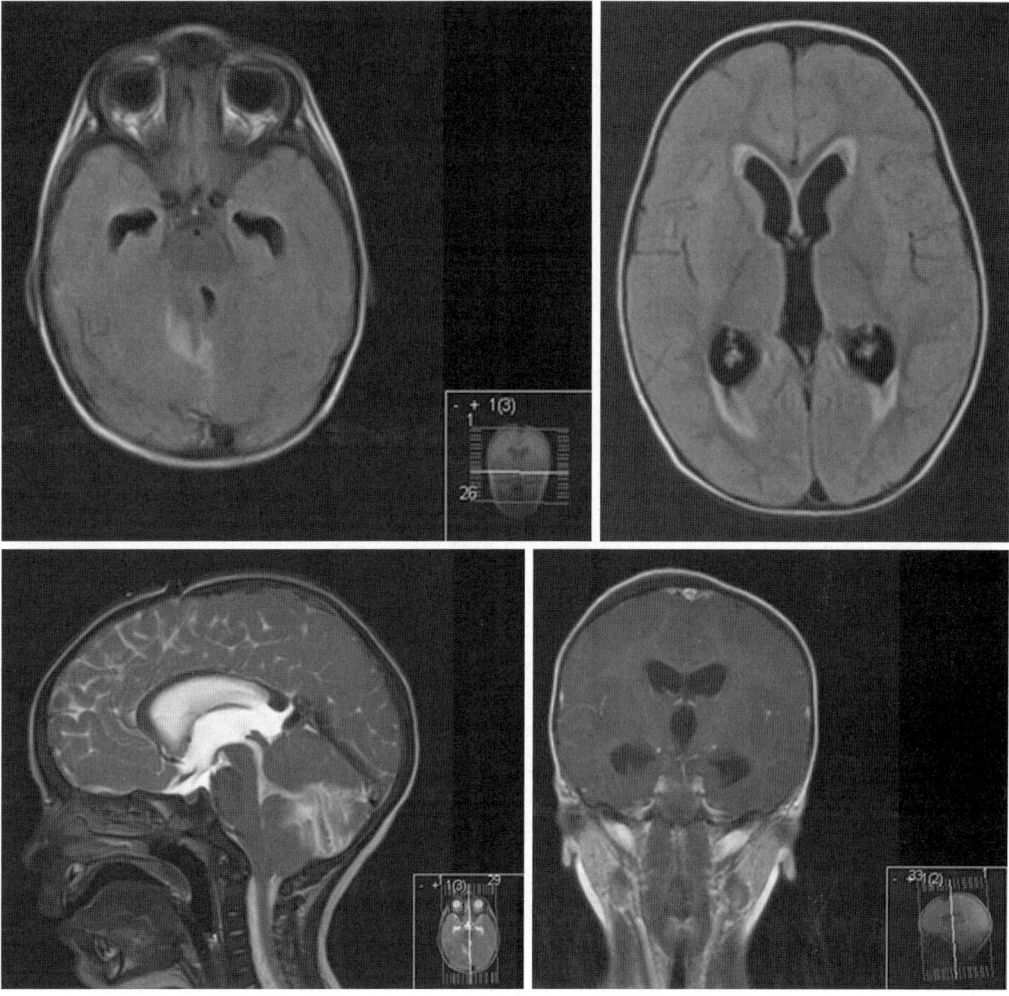

bi-, or triventricular hydrocephalus can be made by using ultrasound evaluation of the lateral and third ventricles; however, posterior fossa imaging is limited (Fig. 6.11).

The current standard imaging method in the diagnosis of hydrocephalus is CT scanning. CT scans provide an effective way of visualizing ventricular morphology, blood products complicating the picture of hydrocephalus, transependymal edema, and signs of increased intracranial pressure such as sulcal/gyral effacement and obliteration of subarachnoid spaces. The Evans ratio describes the ratio of the lateral ventricular frontal horn width to the maximal biparietal diameter, and is abnormal and indicative of ventriculomegaly if it is greater than 0.3.[28] Occasionally, in select cases, cisternography or ventriculography can be performed. This often entails the administration of a radiopaque contrast agent into the ventricular system to evaluate the compartmentalization of cysts and determine whether communication of CSF is present (i.e., posterior fossa cysts in Dandy-Walker malformations, or a trapped fourth ventricle).[29] MRI studies are particularly useful in delineating disease responsible for CSF pathway obstruction, such as tumors compressing the ventricular system, and provide a better evaluation of the posterior fossa and foramen magnum. MRIs allow for the evaluation of ventricular anatomy in coronal, sagittal, and axial planes (Fig. 6.12). In addition, MRI CSF flow studies (e.g., cine flow

studies) timed to the cardiac cycle can provide useful information in selected cases.

Though CT and MRI studies have made it significantly easier to evaluate ventricular morphology, it is important to note that morphology and symptomatology do not always correlate.[30,31] Therefore, these studies have to be interpreted in the context of the appropriate clinical setting. Occasionally, in the setting of altered ventricular compliance, ventricular size may not change despite increases in intracranial pressure and clinical symptoms.[30,31] Invasive intracranial pressure monitoring can be used in certain settings when symptoms and imaging do not correlate.

Several studies have examined ICP monitoring for chronic NPH as a means of understanding responders to CSF shunting, though results are often inconclusive and not widely accepted at all institutions. The Dutch NPH study by Boon and associates concluded that positive predictors of outcome from shunting were observed with patients whose resistance to outflow of CSF was about 18 mm Hg/mL/minute; at lower levels outcomes became dependent on clinical and imaging findings to support shunting.[32] Some studies, such as the one by Eide and Stanisic from Norway, suggest that CSF pulsatility, determined by ICP wave amplitude, can help identify clinical responders to shunting versus nonresponders.[33] Another study by Eide and Sorteberg showed that in patients shunted

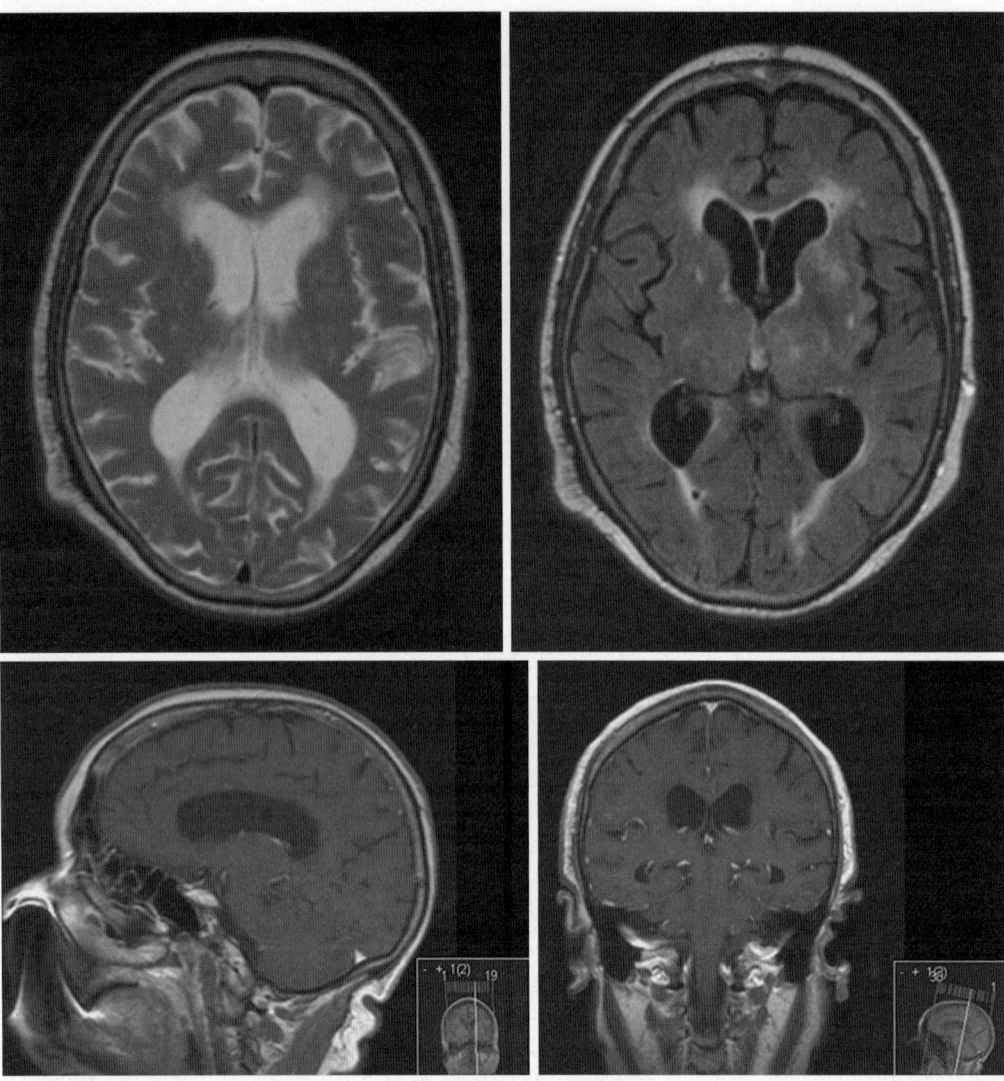

FIGURE 6.10 Magnetic resonance imaging (MRI) scans of an 81-year-old patient with normal-pressure hydrocephalus. Prominent ventricular system noted on axial T2-weighted, fluid attenuated inversion recovery (FLAIR), sagittal, and coronal noncontrast T1-sequences.

TABLE 6.6 Symptomatic Triad of Normal-Pressure Hydrocephalus (NPH)
■ Gait disturbance
■ Dementia
■ Urinary incontinence

for NPH whose intracranial pressure and waveforms were monitored invasively, 93% of those with increased CSF pulsatility (ICP waveform of >4 mm Hg amplitude on average) showed response to shunting as opposed to 10% of those without increased pulsatility.[34]

Normal-Pressure Hydrocephalus

The diagnosis of acute hydrocephalus can often be made effectively through a combination of clinical signs and imaging findings indicating increased intracranial pressure. However, the diagnosis of chronic hydrocephalus, particularly idiopathic NPH, has been a much studied and debated topic in the literature since the initial seminal work from the Massachusetts General Hospital in 1964. The true incidence is unknown

and it is likely an underreported condition because it can be challenging to diagnoses in the patients who most commonly suffer from this condition, and are typically 60 to 80 years of age. In 2009, the incidence reported in Norway was estimated to be 1.09 per 100,000 per year.[35] Currently several criteria are used for diagnosis and include history and clinical presentation, including the classic triad of gait disturbance, urinary incontinence, and dementia. These clinical findings are usually described in the setting of CT and MRI imaging showing ventriculomegaly with no evidence of extrinsic obstruction to CSF flow. Although not common, transependymal CSF flow occasionally can be seen in a patient's MRI with NPH. Recent published idiopathic NPH consensus guidelines classify this entity as probable, possible, or unlikely based on the constellation of history, physical examination, and clinical findings.[24,36] In addition, adjunctive prognostic tests can be used to help in diagnosis. Large volume lumbar punctures, in which 40 to 50 mL of CSF are withdrawn, are performed in conjunction with detailed examination before and after the procedure to document clinical response to the CSF removal[24] in terms of intellectual function, memory, gait, and continence. Symptomatic improvement is correlated with response to shunting, with a positive predictive value of 73% to 100%.[24] However,

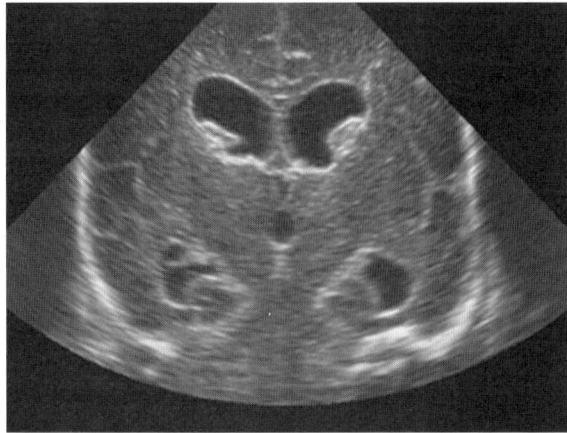

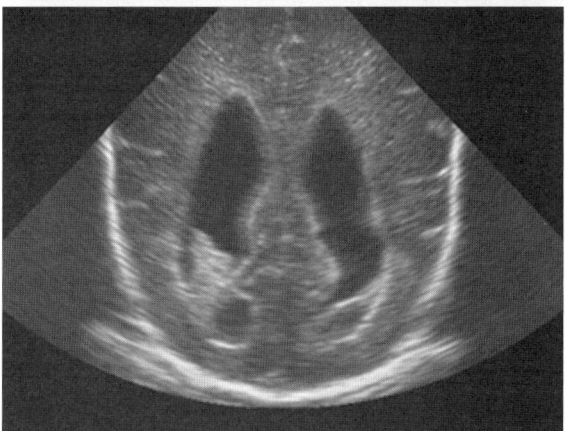

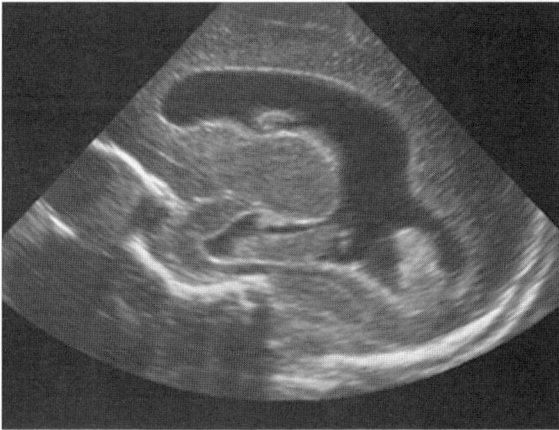

FIGURE 6.11 Transfontanelle ultrasound of 28-week-old premature infant with hydrocephalus due to germinal matrix hemorrhage.

this test has a low sensitivity (26-61%).[37] Prolonged external CSF drainage of 300 mL of CSF has a higher sensitivity (50-100%) and a high positive predictive value (80-100%), though it is a more invasive test with higher complication rates.[37] However, many centers prefer to place a temporary indwelling lumbar catheter and drain CSF over the space of 24 to 72 hours, as part of their screening paradigm because improvements in gait, cognition, and continence can be more carefully compared to pretest analyses and carefully quantified during the hospital stay. The higher predictive value of this test also makes the need for placement of an unnecessary permanent CSF diversion device in an older, often more fragile patient less likely.

TREATMENT OF HYDROCEPHALUS

The treatment of hydrocephalus includes both nonsurgical and surgical interventions. Though surgical treatment is more definitive, nonsurgical treatment has been used with variable success.

Nonsurgical Approaches

Nonsurgical management, historically mostly used in infants, was aimed at preventing shunt placement by controlling intracranial pressure and ventricular dilatation until the cranial sutures fused, at which point there would be an establishment of pressures sufficient to promote a balance between CSF production and absorption. Conservative measures work with variable success, and often these measures serve only to temporize hydrocephalus until shunt placement.

Pharmacological treatment is aimed at decreasing CSF production and increasing CSF absorption. The medications commonly used to decrease CSF production include acetazolamide and furosemide. Acetazolamide is a carbonic anhydrase inhibitor and furosemide is a loop diuretic. Their effect on hydrocephalus has been especially studied in infants with posthemorrhagic hydrocephalus. In a large randomized controlled trial, the International Posthaemorrhagic Ventricular Dilation Trial Group enrolled 177 patients to either standard therapy alone or treatment with acetazolamide (100 mg/kg/day) and furosemide (1 mg/kg/day) to determine if there is an advantage in preventing shunt dependence in infants with posthemorrhagic hydrocephalus.[38] The study was stopped prematurely when the data showed increased neurological sequelae and increased shunt placement rate in the group receiving the medications.[38] This emphasizes the conclusion that these drugs are not without side effects, including but not limited to metabolic acidosis, lethargy, poor feeding, electrolyte imbalances, tachypnea, and diarrhea. Other drugs have been used in the treatment of hydrocephalus with mixed success. Hyaluronidase promotes increase CSF absorption; however, its efficacy as a means of obviating shunting has not been shown.[39] Medications used to decrease intracranial pressure include osmotic diuretics such as mannitol, urea, and glycerol.[4] Usually these provide temporizing measures until definitive treatment is initiated.

Other nonsurgical means of treatment historically and currently used include head wrapping and intermittent CSF removal. Head wrapping has been used in the past to treat hydrocephalus, thought to be effective by creating a constant force high enough to promote increased CSF absorption in infants with unfused skulls.[40] This is not a common practice, particularly due to complications including increased intracranial pressure. Intermittent CSF removal through lumbar or ventricular puncture has been used as a means of temporizing hydrocephalus until a more definitive treatment is undertaken. It has been particularly studied in infants with posthemorrhagic hydrocephalus, and has been used as a means of treatment until the infants' CSF profiles and body weight increase permit shunt placement.[41] Several studies looked at the efficacy of intermittent CSF removal and concluded that it is not effective in preventing hydrocephalus.[42]

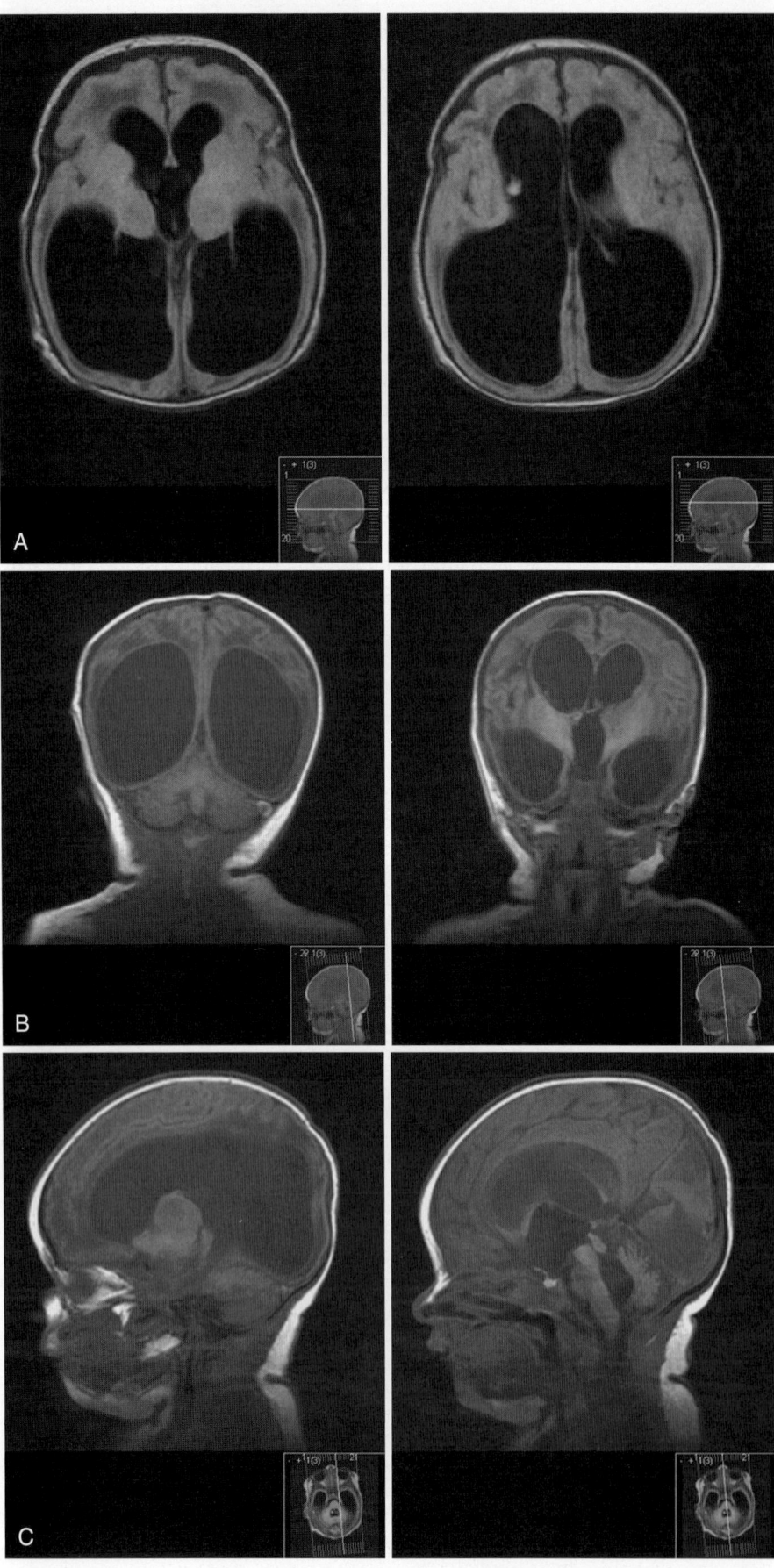

FIGURE 6.12 Noncontrast magnetic resonance imaging (MRI) scan of a newborn with hydrocephalus. **A,** Axial fluid attenuated inversion recovery (FLAIR) scans. **B,** Coronal sequences. **C,** Sagittal sequences.

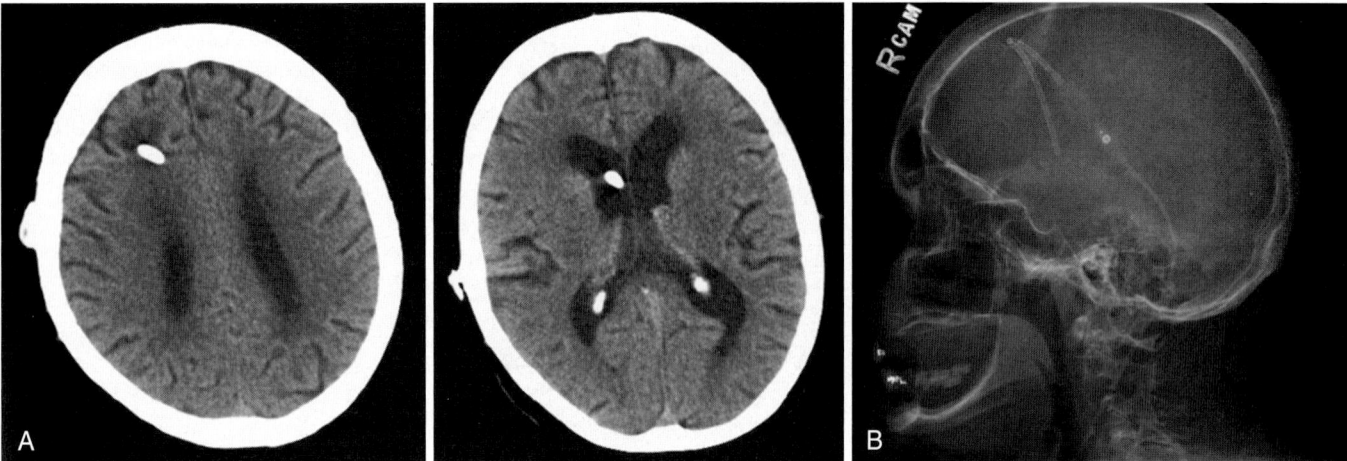

FIGURE 6.13 A 76-year-old patient with shunted hydrocephalus. **A,** Axial computed tomography (CT) scan showing a right frontal ventricular shunt catheter. **B,** Lateral skull radiograph showing ventricular and extracranial portions of the shunt, and a programmable valve.

Surgical Management

Surgical management of hydrocephalus has a long history, though ancient methods for treatment were not effective.[43] Today surgical management of hydrocephalus can be divided into nonshunting versus CSF shunting options. Nonshunting options include endoscopic third ventriculostomy, resection of an obstructing lesion causing the hydrocephalus, when possible, and choroid plexus ablation. The success of choroid plexus coagulation has been mixed. Dandy described the procedure in 1918 with high morbidity and mortality rates.[44] In the past it has been useful in temporarily decreasing the rate of CSF production, but does not completely halt hydrocephalus, because a portion of CSF is still produced by the ependymal lining. With the advent of neuroendoscopy there has been a recent resurgence in endoscopic choroid plexus ablation for hydrocephalus treatment.[45]

The mainstay of surgical management of hydrocephalus involves CSF diversion through shunting procedures. Since the time of Nulsen and Spitz, a number of shunt equipment and techniques have been developed. CSF shunts entail using silicone polymer silastic tubes to divert CSF from the ventricles to body cavities where it can be reabsorbed (i.e., the peritoneum, cardiac atrium, pleura). Shunting systems generally have three components: a proximal catheter that drains the intracranial ventricles, a one-way valve system, and distal tubing that diverts the CSF to its final body cavity destination. Occasionally antisiphoning devices are also included in tandem with the valve to prevent overdraining effects when the patient is upright.

There are different types of valves currently in use. In general, the most commonly used system is a pressure-dependent valve, which allows CSF flow across the valve when the pressure differential exceeds its preset opening pressure. Flow-controlled valves, on the other hand, allow a constant flow of CSF across different pressure gradients with different patient positions. The choice of valve does not generally affect shunt failure rates. This was shown in a randomized study by Drake and colleagues in which 344 patients were shunted with one of three valve systems (a standard differential pressure valve, a valve with an antisiphon component, and a valve with a flow-limiting component).[46] The study found no difference in shunt failure-free interval among the different kinds of valves. Newer advances in technology have introduced the variable pressure programmable valves. These are pressure-differential valves that can have their preset pressure changed by extrinsic devices without requiring surgery to change the valve itself. Studies show that both programmable and conventional valves have similar safety and efficacy profiles.[47] Of note, since most programming devices work through a magnetic field interaction, exposing patients to MRIs may inadvertently change the valve setting.[48] Therefore, patients with programmable valves should have their valve settings evaluated and reprogrammed appropriately after routine MRIs.

The most common type of CSF shunt currently performed is a ventriculoperitoneal shunt (Fig. 6.13). This procedure involves ventricular cannulation and tunneling of a distal subcutaneous catheter to the peritoneal cavity (Fig. 6.14). Cannulating the ventricle can be performed in several ways, which includes placing either a frontal, occipital or parietal catheter (Table 6.7). The frontal horn can be accessed at Kocher's point, the occipital horn through Frazier's point, and the trigone can less commonly be entered through a parietal approach at Keen's point.[9] Some surgeons prefer the parietal approach because it provides an easier pass from the scalp to the abdomen. Some choose the frontal approach both because of easier landmarks and because of migration of the catheter away from the choroid plexus with patient growth. Some studies suggest that regardless of the surgical approach, the most important factor in shunt failure is the final relationship of the ventricular catheter to the choroid plexus.[49] Preoperative imaging can be used to optimize catheter length at insertion into the ventricle, though often infants outgrow their ventricular catheters and require revision to replace the ventricular catheter that tends to pull out of the ventricle with patient growth. In addition, frameless stereotactic guidance and endoscope-assisted ventricular catheter placement are gaining popularity when ventricular systems are difficult to cannulate.[50,51]

The proximal catheter is connected to a one-way valve and then to a distal catheter that is passed subcutaneously through

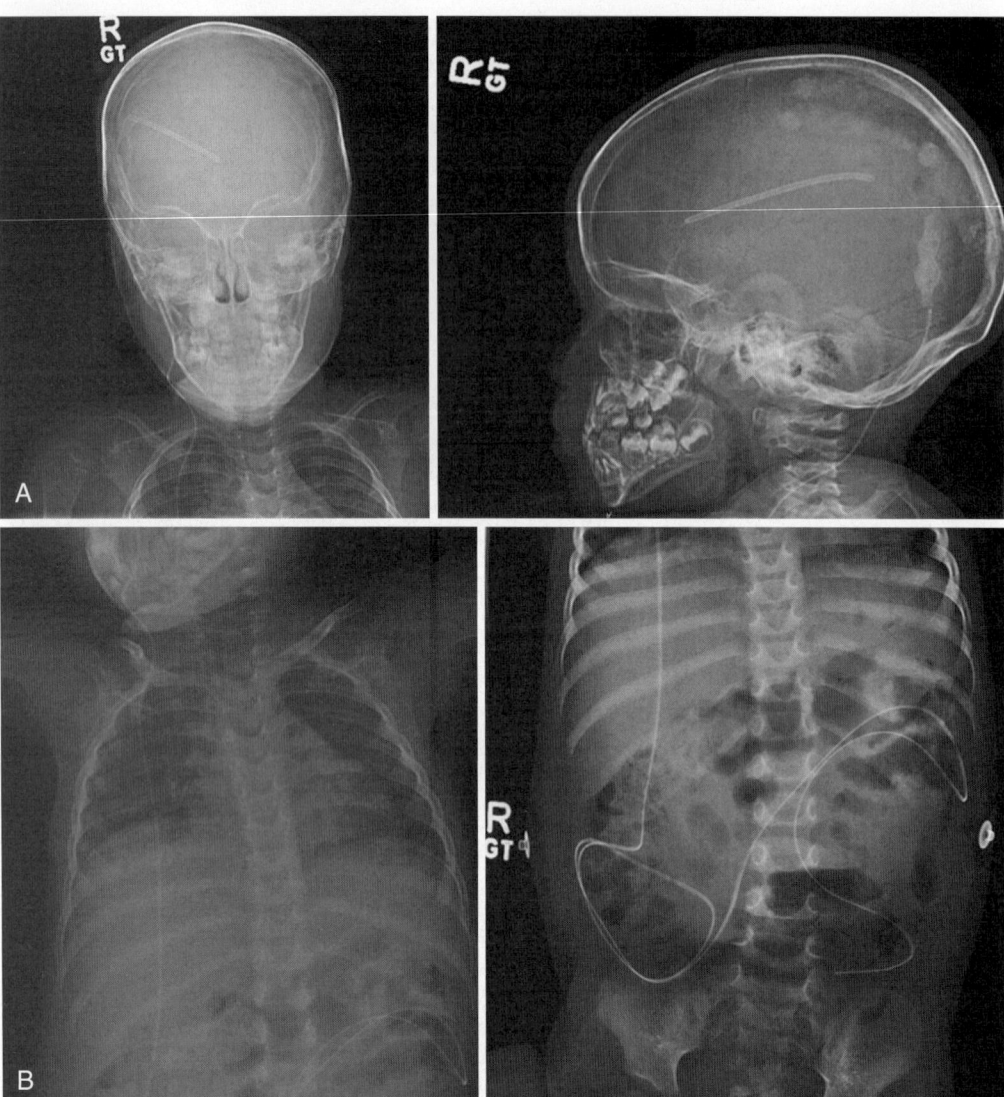

FIGURE 6.14 Ventriculoperitoneal shunt. Radiographs show the course of a ventriculoperitoneal shunt catheter. **A,** Anteroposterior and lateral skull films. **B,** Chest and abdominal radiographs.

TABLE 6.7 Sites for Ventricular Cannulation

Site	Entry	Trajectory and Course
Frontal (Kocher's point)	Frontal horn, 2-3 cm from midline, midpupillary line, 1 cm anterior to coronal suture	Perpendicular to skull, medial canthus in the coronal plane, external auditory meatus in the sagittal plane
Parietal (Keen's point)	Trigone, 2.5-3 cm posterior and superior to pinna	Perpendicular to skull
Occipital (Frazier's point)	Occipital horn, 6-7 cm above inion, 3-4 cm from midline	Parallel to skull base, aiming for middle of forehead

a tunneling device to the final destination. Generally, patients are placed supine, with the head turned sharply to the opposite side (Fig. 6.15). A shoulder roll is placed to facilitate the passing of the distal catheter from the head, across the neck and clavicle, to the abdomen. The senior author performs a small ipsilateral paraumbilical incision, incises the anterior rectus sheath, bluntly dissects the rectus muscle, incises the posterior rectus sheath and the peritoneum, and uses a small dissector to verify peritoneal location. The catheter is then passed into the peritoneal cavity. Some surgeons prefer to use minimally invasive laparoscopic means of distal catheter placement into the abdomen.[52] In infants, care must be taken to place sufficient distal catheter into the abdomen (generally

>30-40 cm) to avoid the catheter's pulling out of the abdomen with patient growth.

If the peritoneum is not a physiological option for shunting CSF (i.e., in the presence of peritonitis), an alternative site is the cardiac atrium or the pleura (Fig. 6.16). Techniques for placement of a ventriculoatrial shunt include an open cervical approach to cannulate the internal jugular vein or common facial vein, or a more commonly used modified Seldinger technique for percutaneous insertion of the distal tube through the subclavian vein, via a peel-away catheter, into the right atrium.[53] Complications of ventriculoatrial shunts include migration out of the atrium, cardiac embolism, and immune-mediated glomerulonephritis. For ventriculopleural shunts,

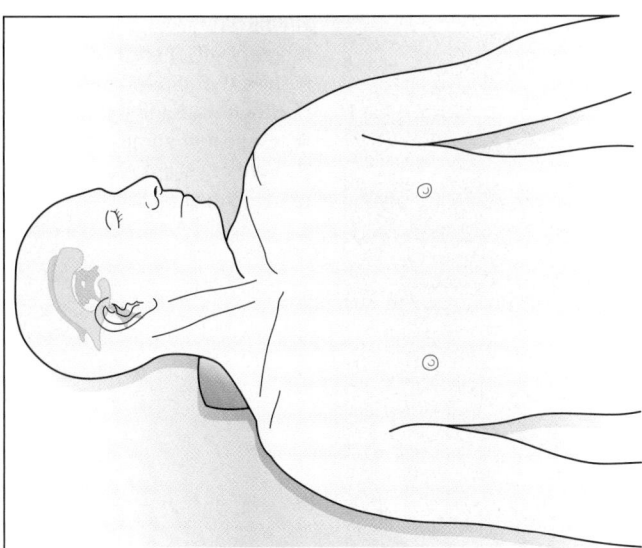

FIGURE 6.15 Positioning for ventriculoperitoneal shunt. The patient is supine with a roll between the shoulder blades and the head turned to the contralateral side.

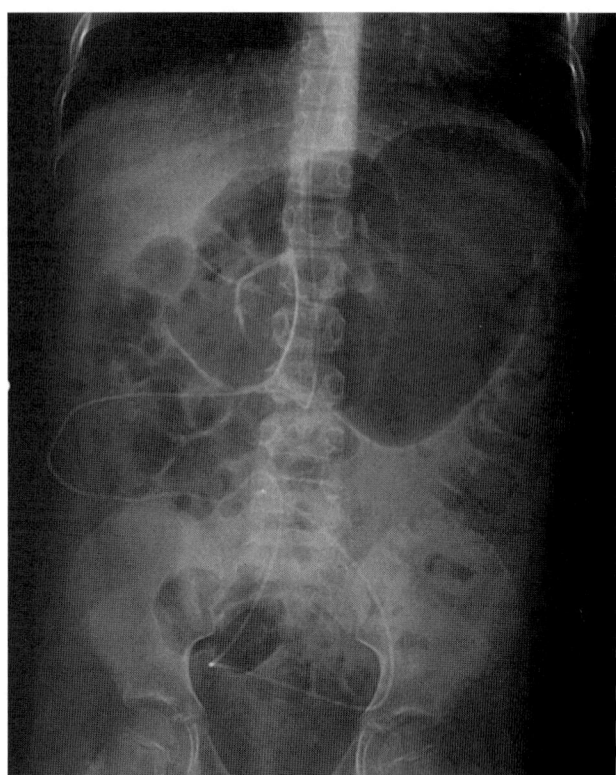

FIGURE 6.17 Radiographs showing catheter tubing in a patient with a lumbar peritoneal shunt.

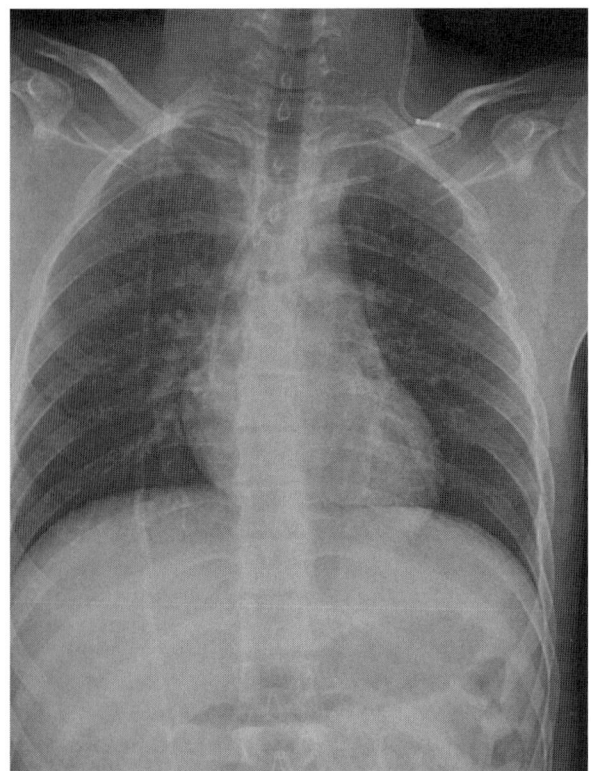

FIGURE 6.16 Chest radiograph showing a left ventriculoatrial shunt in place. The distal tubing terminates in the right cardiac atrium. Of note there is a retained subcutaneous catheter on the right from a previous failed ventriculoperitoneal shunt.

the second intercostal space is accessed on the superior aspect of the rib to prevent injury to the neurovascular bundle.[4] The pleura is opened at end expiration, the catheter is inserted under direct visualization, and the wound is irrigated while the patient is ventilated.[4] In children younger than 4 years of age pleural shunts may not be practical because of their association with pleural effusions and respiratory compromise.

Lumboperitoneal shunts (Fig. 6.17) can also be placed in cases of communicating hydrocephalus, especially in instances when the ventricles cannot be easily accessed (e.g., slit-ventricle syndrome)[54] (Fig. 6.18). The technique entails accessing the L4-L5 interspace, cannulating the subarachnoid space with a Tuohy needle, passing the catheter into the subarachnoid space, tunneling it to the peritoneal cavity, and securing it to the lumbar fascia with an anchor.[4] Complications include sequelae of overdrainage, which are more difficult to assess and control, difficulties in pressure regulation, lumbar nerve root irritation, progressive cerebellar tonsillar herniation, arachnoiditis, and arachnoid adhesions.[55] Other distal sites of CSF drainage that can be used if there are specific problems with diverting to the common locations (i.e., peritonitis, subacute bacterial endocarditis, pleural adhesions/effusions) include the gallbladder and the ureter or urinary bladder.

After shunt placement, patients are followed closely. An initial postoperative CT scan is obtained as a baseline evaluation of the ventricular system and catheter position after shunting. For programmable valves, radiographs can be obtained to confirm the valve setting. With ventriculoatrial shunts, radiographs postoperatively show the catheter's position and evaluate for pneumothorax, which can occur after placement. In the first 1 to 2 years, there is more frequent radiographic surveillance, which may be performed less frequently afterward if no clinical or radiographic problems are noted.

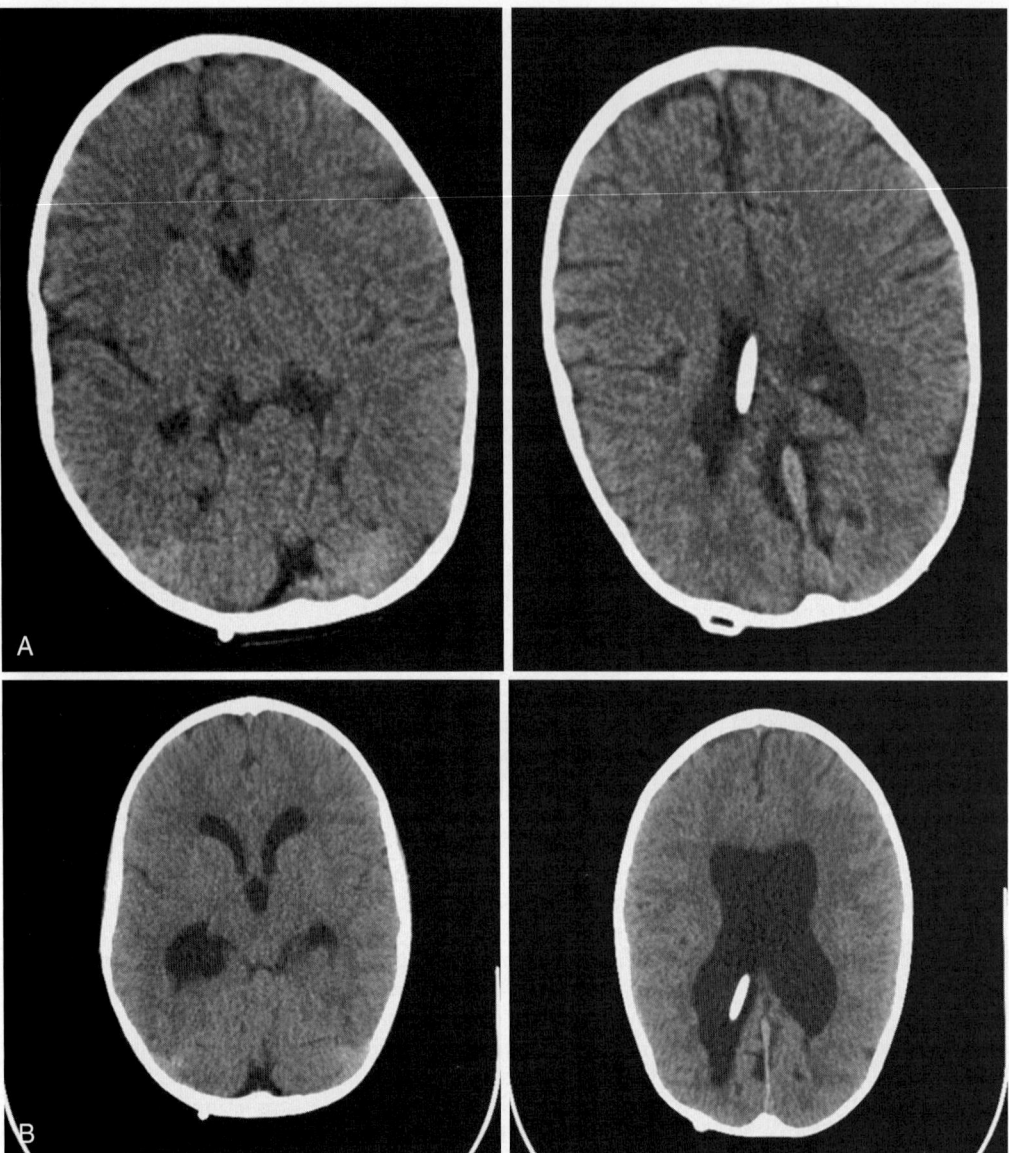

FIGURE 6.18 Axial computed tomography (CT) scan of a patient with an occipital ventriculoperitoneal shunt malfunction. **A,** Baseline small ventricles. **B,** Ventricles are enlarged due to shunt malfunction.

TABLE 6.8 Common Shunt Complications

- Underdrainage of CSF (from obstruction or disconnection)
- Overdrainage of CSF
- Infection

CSF, cerebrospinal fluid.

COMPLICATIONS OF HYDROCEPHALUS TREATMENT

CSF shunts have become a powerful way to treat hydrocephalus. With the advent of CSF shunts, hydrocephalus and the sequelae of increased intracranial pressure can be successfully managed. However, shunting systems are troublesome devices. Common complications include shunt malfunction including underdrainage of CSF (usually from shunt system obstruction), overdrainge of CSF, or infection of the shunt system or of the CSF (Table 6.8).

Shunt Infections

Shunt infection is unfortunately still seen after shunt insertion, despite the best precautions taken at the time of surgery. Generally, shunt infection rates are in the 5% to 15% range, with more than 70% developing within 1 month of surgery, and 90% within 6 months.[56] In some centers, the shunt infection rates are significantly lower or higher. Patients commonly present with low-grade fevers, headaches, malaise, elevation of inflammatory markers (e.g., erythrocyte sedimentation rate, C-reactive protein), erythema along the shunt tract, and symptoms of shunt malfunction if the shunt system becomes obstructed. In severe cases bacteremia, peritonitis, ventriculitis, bacterial endocarditis, and pleural empyema can occur. Peritoneal pseudocysts may be associated with CSF shunt infections. They may be diagnosed by ultrasound or CT evaluation of the abdomen.

CSF shunt catheters are foreign bodies that can be prone to bacterial infection. The most common organisms are coagulase-negative staphylococci followed by *Staphylococcus*

FIGURE 6.19 Shunt disconnection. **A,** Skull lateral radiograph showing a disconnection of the shunt catheter tubing (*arrow*). **B,** Chest radiograph showing shunt tubing disconnection in the chest (*arrow*).

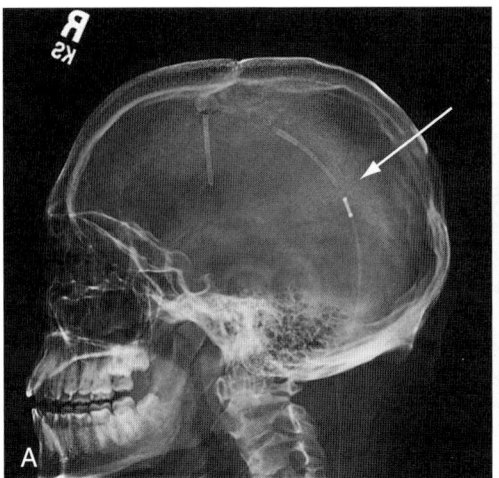
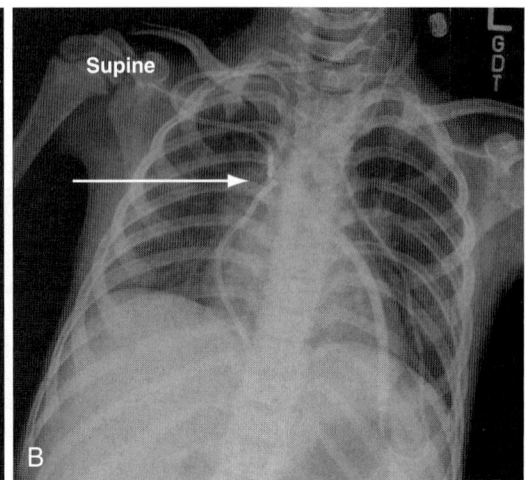

aureus.[57] Other organisms less commonly seen include other gram-positive (streptococci, enterococci), gram-negative, and anaerobic bacteria (*Propionibacterium acnes*).

Treatment of shunt infections always includes antibiotic therapy. Broad-spectrum antibiotics are started initially and tailored to the specific offending organism once it is isolated in culture. Some advocate administration of intrathecal antibiotics in addition to systemic treatment, though this is not routine practice in most centers.[58] In addition, either externalization or removal of the shunt and external drainage are performed in suspected cases of infection. The management of infected CSF shunts varies greatly among clinicians. A recent study surveyed all active members of the American Society of Pediatric Neurosurgeons (ASPN) about their clinical practices.[59] Most of the neurosurgeons who responded reported that they remove the infected shunt system and place an external ventricular drain.[59] Another reported method involved distal externalization of the shunt system and drainage. There was considerable variation in the practices of the surveyed neurosurgeons as far as the duration of antibiotic therapy. In addition there is also substantial variation in how long to continue external ventricular drainage and how long to evaluate cultures before reinternalization of the shunt system.[60] The senior author advocates waiting until the CSF cultures have been sterile for at least 72 hours before replacing the ventricular shunt.

In an attempt to improve shunt infection rates, antibiotic impregnated shunt catheters were introduced. Several series looked at the effectiveness of these catheters. One recent retrospective study of 353 shunt placements found a 2.4-fold decrease in infection rate with the use of antibiotic impregnated catheters.[61] Other series show more modest effects.[62,63] Most studies reported in the literature are retrospective, and large randomized controlled prospective studies comparing antibiotic impregnated versus standard shunt catheters are lacking.

Shunt Malfunction

A common complication of CSF shunting is malfunction from underdrainage of CSF (see Fig. 6.18). Generally, this is due to an obstruction or disconnection causing impedance of CSF drainage anywhere along the course of the shunt system.[64]

Patients present with symptoms of increased intracranial pressure, which differ depending on the age group. Often the presentation can be with symptoms similar to a previous malfunction, though patients can develop a different constellation of symptoms with subsequent obstructions, and such complaints should not be dismissed.

Shunt malfunctions can be proximal, from obstruction of the ventricular catheter, or distal, from a blockage in the extracranial components. Ventricular catheters that migrate toward the choroid plexus are more prone to occlusion. Disconnections can be seen along the distal tubing in areas with increased movement, generally occurring in children undergoing growth spurts in areas with increased movement. The presence of multiple tubing connectors puts the shunt at risk for disconnection (Fig. 6.19). With time distal tubing can calcify, predisposing the shunt system to fracture.

Shunt catheters can migrate and dislodge. Proximal catheters can malfunction from migration into the brain parenchyma or subependymal space, either because of initial misplacement or because of continued head growth in children or ventricular collapse. Sometimes catheters can even migrate outside the cranial vault. Ventricular catheters connected to reservoirs are felt to be less likely to migrate. Particularly in children undergoing growth spurts, catheters can dislodge from the peritoneum, especially if not enough tubing was initially placed in the abdomen.

If a shunt obstruction is suspected, the initial evaluation includes imaging studies. A CT of the head allows for evaluation of the ventricles, especially when compared to previous scans. Though many shunted patients present with some degree of ventricular enlargement if the shunt becomes obstructed, those with altered ventricular compliance (e.g., slit-ventricle syndrome) may not show any change in ventricular size on imaging studies with a malfunction.[30] A shunt series is also obtained, which includes radiographs of the skull and the body along the peripheral shunt tract, which allows for evaluation of the continuity of the distal tubing. Other adjunctive studies include radionuclide scans, which require injection of a tracer into the reservoir, which travels into the ventricle and then through the distal tubing.[65] Failure of visualization of the tracer into the peritoneum indicates a shunt failure.

The valve can be examined at the bedside. The valve can be compressed against the skull. If the valve depresses but does not refill, it may indicate a shunt system obstruction. The shunt reservoir can also be accessed percutaneously with a small-gauge needle (23-25 gauge butterfly needle). Good flow of CSF indicates that the proximal part of the shunt is patent; in addition, ICP can be measured. In patients with symptoms concerning for shunt malfunction, but with imaging studies that are equivocal, CSF pressure can be measured by performing a lumbar puncture and checking the opening pressure, if there are no contraindications (e.g., mass lesion, history of myelomeningocele).

CSF shunt malfunctions require prompt operative revision. Most shunt malfunctions are secondary to occlusion of the ventricular catheter. When possible, a new ventricular catheter can be inserted before removing the old obstructed catheter. If there is resistance to removing the obstructed catheter, a stylet can be inserted into the catheter and monopolar cautery can be used along the stylet to free it from tethering tissue (e.g., choroid plexus adhesions). Sometimes the new catheter can be inserted without a stylet along the trajectory of the malfunctioning catheter, but sometimes such a catheter may again become obstructed by scar tissue.

Shunt malfunction can also be observed from shunt overdrainage.[66] This is can be seen with a variety of shunt valves, and is particularly augmented by the negative hydrostatic pressures generated when a patient is upright. Common symptoms include low-pressure headaches more pronounced in the upright position. A review of the literature by Pudenz and Foltz revealed that complications of overdrainage occur in at least 10% to 12% of patients with shunted hydrocephalus, usually within 6.5 years from the time of initial shunt placement.[67] Overdrainage complication includes the formation of subdural hematomas, intracranial hypotension, craniosynostosis and microcephaly, and slit-ventricle syndrome.[67] Valve pressure upgrades and the addition of antisiphoning devices may help with overdrainage symptoms.

Occasionally patients with known shunted hydrocephalus can present with concerning symptoms in the setting of small ventricles on imaging studies. Slit-ventricle syndrome refers to headaches lasting 10 to 90 minutes in the setting of imaging studies showing small ventricles and slow refill of pumping devices.[68] However, consensus is still lacking as far as the exact definition of the condition, and evaluation and treatment paradigms. Overdrainage symptoms are treated accordingly, while patients with increased ICP without ventriculomegaly are treated with shunting procedures such as lumboperitoneal shunt placement.

Subdural hematoma (SDH), acute or chronic, may occur from brain collapse due to ventricular overshunting, with resultant tearing of bridging veins. SDH can be ipsilateral to the side of the shunt (more common), contralateral (less common), or bilateral. Symptomatic SDHs should be removed, and the shunt valve pressure may need to be upgraded or a siphoning control device may need to be added.

Uncommon Complications

Less commonly encountered complications from CSF shunt placements include hemorrhage along the shunt tract or at the site of insertion, seizures, and shunt metastasis (Table 6.9). Although very uncommon, systemic metastasis of intracranial

TABLE 6.9 Uncommon Complications of Cerebrospinal Fluid Shunts	
Cranial	**Peripheral**
Subdural hygroma	Shunt tube migration
Hemorrhage (subdural or	Shunt tube disconnection/fracture
intraparenchymal)	Abdominal pseudocyst formation
Seizure	Bowel perforation
Hemiparesis/new	Peritonitis
neurological deficits (due	Abdominal hernia
to misplaced catheters)	Endocarditis (VA shunts)
	Immune-mediated glomerulonephritis (VA shunts)

VA, ventriculoatrial.

tumors in shunted patients has been described, particularly in patients with medulloblastoma and other types of malignant tumors.[69,70]

TREATMENT OUTCOMES AND SPECIFIC PROBLEMS ASSOCIATED WITH HYDROCEPHALUS

Clinical long-term outcomes after hydrocephalus treatment are largely dependent on the underlying pathology, response to shunting, and overall neurological comorbid factors. Despite frequency of ventricular shunting, data on long-term outcomes, particularly in the pediatric population, are scarce. Often the overall prognosis is dependent on the underlying congenital malformations. A study by Casey and co-workers followed a cohort of 155 children shunted for hydrocephalus over a 10-year period.[71] Outcome measures were surgical morbidity and mortality rates, and academic achievement records. Fifty-nine percent of children attended public school; however, those shunted secondary to IVH more often required special schooling. Forty-four percent did not require shunt revision. The most common complications of shunting included obstruction and infection, most presenting within the first year after placement. An 11% mortality rate during the 10-year follow-up was noted. Another study by Billard and associates looking at IQ in shunted children found that 75% of patients had an IQ greater than 70. However, many children had a marked decrease in visual spatial skills.[72] There was a trend toward lower IQ values in patients with hydrocephalus due to infection as opposed to other causes.

Hydrocephalus can be diagnosed in utero and can be detected often on prenatal ultrasonography and further evaluated with prenatal MRI (Fig. 6.20). In the 1980s fetal surgery for hydrocephalus was undertaken in an attempt to improve postnatal outcome in infants with hydrocephalus.[73] However, outcomes were so poor that in utero treatment was largely abandoned.[73]

Premature infants weighing less than 1.5 kg are at risk for developing germinal matrix hemorrhages, leading to CSF obstruction and hydrocephalus (see Fig. 6.20). Generally these hemorrhages are thought to be due to fragility of the germinal matrix vasculature in the setting of dysautoregulation of cerebral blood flow.[74] Prognosis depends on the extent of

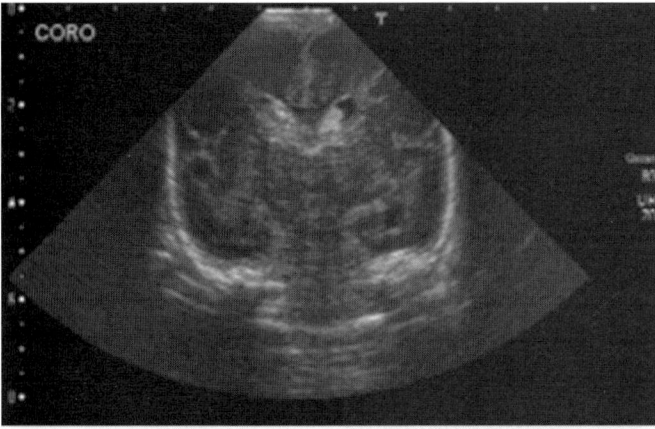

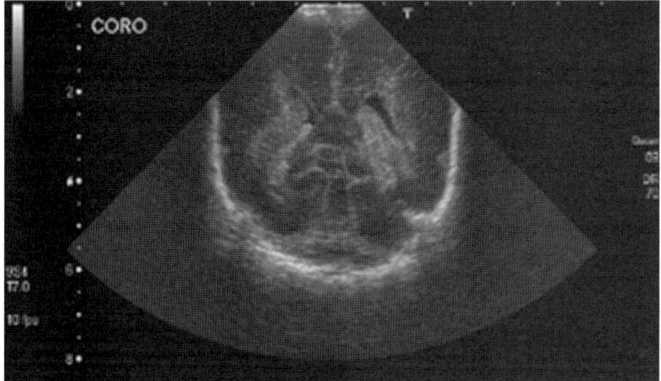

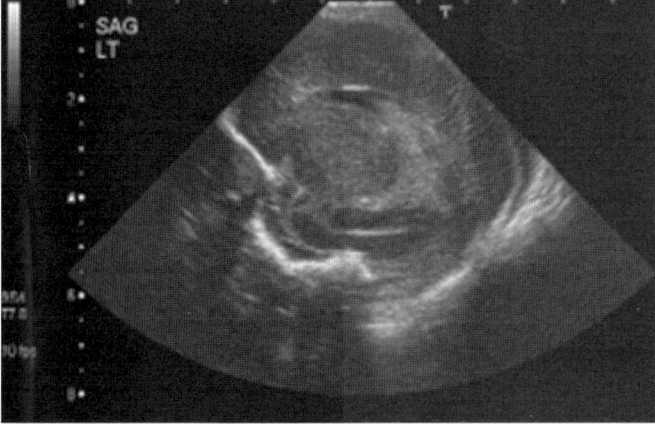

FIGURE 6.20 Transfontanelle sonogram of a premature infant with germinal matrix hemorrhage, coronal and sagittal views.

hemorrhage, which is described by four clinical grades (see Table 6.5). Several studies describe higher morbidity and mortality rates for higher grades, associated with more extensive hemorrhage.[75] Treatment centers on a multimodal evaluation of all medical problems of the preterm infant. The infant is monitored closely with daily head circumferences, fontanelle evaluations, and serial transfontanelle ultrasound examinations. If hydrocephalus develops, CSF removal can be done by lumbar puncture, ventriculosubgaleal shunt, ventricular catheter and reservoir placement with percutaneous taps, or external ventricular drain placement. A ventriculoperitoneal shunt can be inserted at any point when necessary, although delaying shunt placement until the infant weighs more than 1.5 kg may reduce the chance of infection.

Other congenital conditions are associated with hydrocephalus. The Dandy-Walker malformation refers to a fourth ventricular cyst associated with cerebellar vermian hypoplasia, with a large posterior fossa, and associated hydrocephalus and systemic problems.[76,77] Initial management is aimed at determining if there is communication of the cyst with the ventricular system. An infratentorial cystoperitoneal shunt can be used to decompress the cyst, and an additional ventricular shunt may or may not be needed as well.[76] If both supra- and infratentorial shunts are placed, a Y-connector can be used to allow drainage from both compartments through the shunt.[76] Alternatively, two separate shunt systems can be used, but if separate valves are used, they should have the same pressure settings. A high incidence of lower IQ scores has been observed in Dandy-Walker patients, thought to be due to associated congenital intracranial anomalies rather than initial hydrocephalus.[77] Hydrocephalus associated with myelomeningocele is generally treated with ventriculoperitoneal shunting. The timing of shunt placement has been debated, but current literature suggests that shunt complications are not necessarily associated with the timing of surgery, and many practitioners advocate concurrent shunt placement at the time of myelomeningocele repair if there is significant hydrocephalus.[78]

Posterior fossa tumors can be associated with postresection hydrocephalus in up to 40% of patients (Fig. 6.21). Shunting is required for persistent ventricular dilatation and symptoms. Recently endoscopic third ventriculostomy has been described as an option to avoid the need for a shunt.[79,80]

Hydranencephaly is a developmental abnormality in which there is absence of the cerebral hemispheres (Fig. 6.22). Although life expectancy is markedly reduced, occasionally patients can survive into the teen or adult years.[81] Shunt placement does not improve function. Patients with hydranencephaly and severe macrocephaly may benefit from ventricular shunt placement or endoscopic coagulation of the choroid plexus as palliative procedures.

Occasionally, compartmentalization of the ventricular system can be noted after CSF shunting. For instance, after shunt placement in the lateral ventricles there may be persistent and progressive dilatation of the fourth ventricle with associated brainstem and cerebellar dysfunction. This can be due to an obstruction at the aqueduct or at the basal foramina, either from prior hemorrhage or meningitis. Endoscopic fenestration of cyst membranes can help to simplify shunt systems in the management of complex hydrocephalus.

For normal-pressure hydrocephalus there remains debate about the optimal valve pressure settings, the use of antisiphon devices, and whether to use ventriculoperitoneal or lumboperitoneal shunts. One study by Hebb and Cusimano reviewing the Medline literature found that 29% of patients had significant symptom improvement, with a complication rate of 6% after shunting.[82] Some studies have also shown that patients who respond to intermittent CSF drainage and undergo shunt placement for NPH tend to show significant improvement in executive function and cognition on neuropsychological testing.[83,84] A retrospective study by McGirt and colleagues of 132 patients undergoing 179 shunt placements showed that up to 75% had objective improvement in symptoms up to 24 months after shunting.[85] Gait dysfunction was the first symptom to improve in 93% of patients,

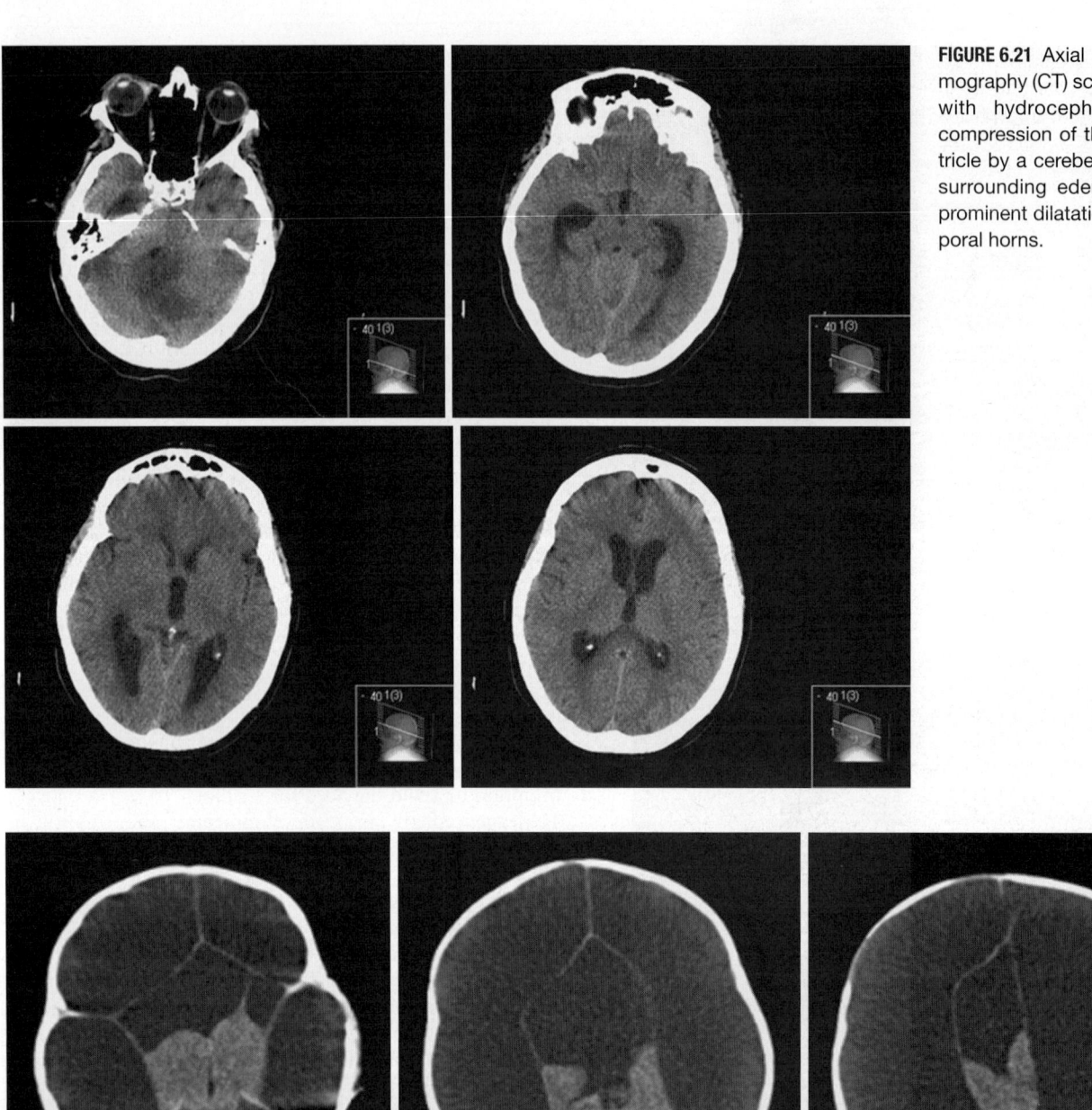

FIGURE 6.21 Axial computed tomography (CT) scan of a patient with hydrocephalus due to compression of the fourth ventricle by a cerebellar mass with surrounding edema. Note the prominent dilatation of the temporal horns.

FIGURE 6.22 Axial computed tomography (CT) scan of an infant with hydranencephaly.

but dementia and urinary incontinence did not improve as dramatically as gait dysfunction.[85]

ENDOSCOPIC TREATMENT OF HYDROCEPHALUS

With advances in optics and computer technology, neuroendoscopic treatment of hydrocephalus has regained popularity since its introduction in the early 1900s. Endoscopic third ventriculostomy (ETV) is a particularly attractive option in

selected patients with noncommunicating hydrocephalus, with aqueductal or fourth ventricular obstruction.[86] It provides a means of bypassing a downstream obstruction and when successful, it obviates the need for extracranial CSF shunting and the long-term complications associated with this procedure.

To determine which patients with hydrocephalus are good candidates for ETV, MRI findings become helpful in patient selection.[4,86] In particular, careful consideration is given to the anatomy of the floor of the third ventricle, and generally the procedure becomes more challenging if the floor is thicker (Fig. 6.23). The relationship of the basilar artery to the floor

FIGURE 6.23 Preoperative magnetic resonance imaging (MRI) of a patient with hydrocephalus due to stenosis of the caudal sylvian aqueduct.

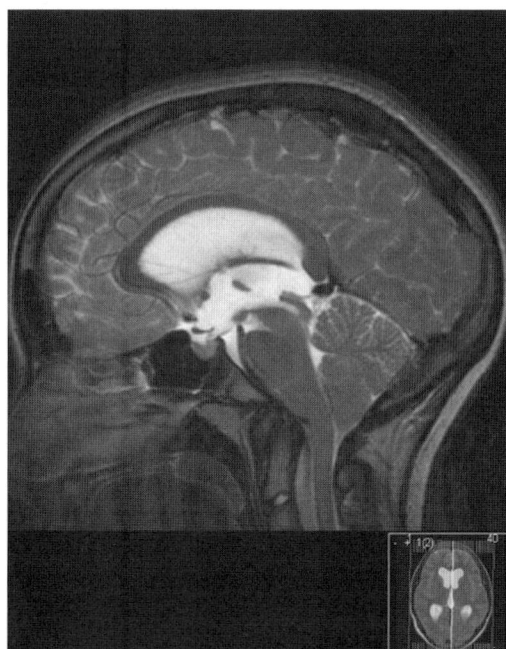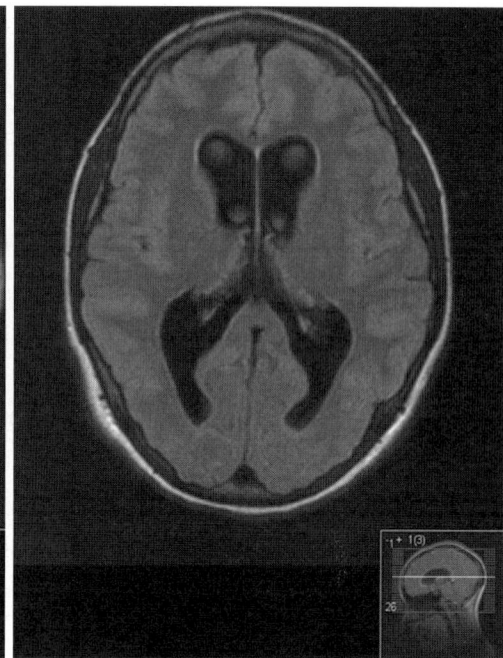

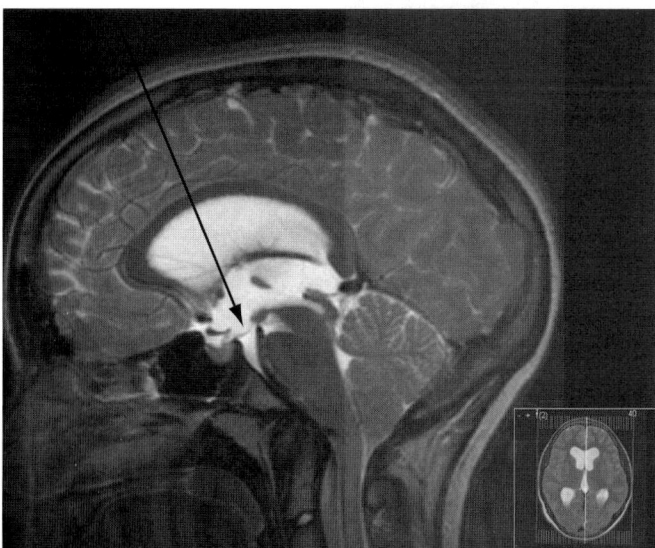

FIGURE 6.24 Trajectory for endoscopic third ventriculostomy. The arrow points to the site of fenestration along the floor of the third ventricle, anterior to the mammillary bodies.

of the third ventricle needs to be evaluated carefully. ETV is more likely to be successful in patients with acquired or late occlusion of the sylvian aqueduct, as well as patients with posterior fossa tumors causing ventricular obstruction.[87] The results of ETV in young children are not as good as those in older children or adults.

The technique for performing ETV is well established.[4,88,89] The patient is positioned supine with the brow up. A coronal burr hole is placed just medial to the midpupillary line. The lateral ventricle is entered and then the endoscope is passed through the foramen of Monro into the third ventricle (Fig. 6.24). The fenestration is performed anterior to the mammillary bodies and posterior to the infundibular

recess, through the thinned tuber cinereum using a blunt probe. The fenestration is then enlarged using a balloon catheter (Fig. 6.25). Image guidance can be used to facilitate the trajectory.

The outcome following ETV is good in properly selected cases. In a recent study by Sacko and co-workers from France evaluating 368 ETVs, the overall success rate was 68.5%.[90] Factors related to increased failure of the ventriculostomy were age younger than 6 months, and hemorrhage-related or idiopathic chronic hydrocephalus. The associated morbidity rate was 10%, and 97% of failures occurred within 2 months. Another series by Gangemi and associates reported results in 125 patients who had undergone ETV, with an overall success rate of 86.4%.[91] Amini and Schmidt reported their experience with 36 ETVs performed selectively in an adult population, with a success rate of 72%.[92] Of those patients, 22% demonstrated delayed failure of the ventriculostomy at a mean of 3.75 years, emphasizing the need for longer follow-up of patients undergoing this procedure.[92]

In 2009, a very important paper by Kulkarni and colleagues from the Canadian Pediatric Neurosurgery Study Group elucidated which children did best from an ETV. The researchers analyzed 618 patients undergoing an ETV at 12 international centers and followed up at 6 months.[93] An ETV Success Score was validated and hovered around 64% at the time of follow-up, which is when most ETV failures become evident. The three most important parameters for ETV success appeared to be patient age at the time of ETV, etiology of hydrocephalus, and whether or not the patient was previously shunted. Table 6.10 shows the ETV success score, which approximates the percentage success of performing a successful ETV in a particular patient. The patients whose ETV was most successful were those over 10 years of age, those with aqueductal stenosis, and those who did not have a previous shunt. Those patients whose ETV fared the worst were patients under 1 month of age, those with postinfectious hydrocephalus, and those with a previous shunt.

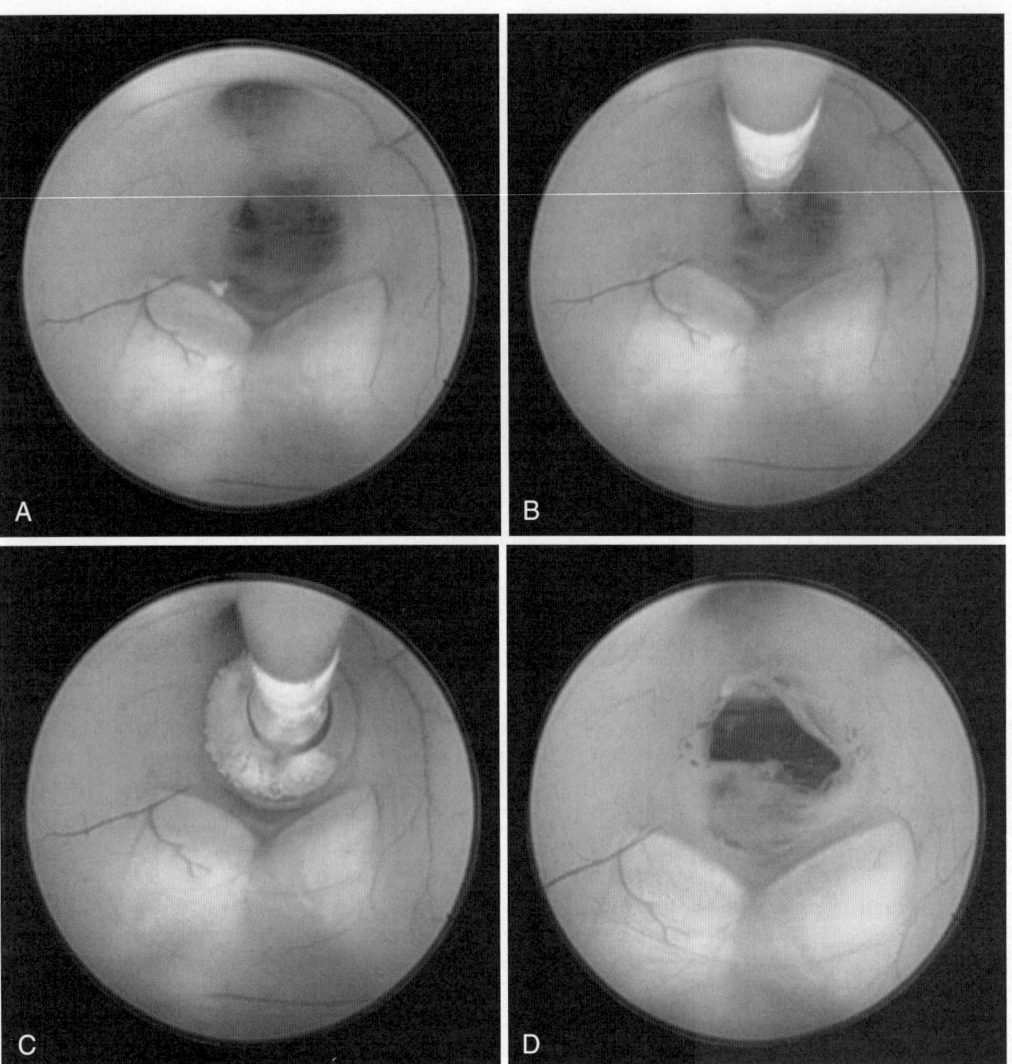

FIGURE 6.25 Intraoperative photographs showing the steps of endoscopic third ventriculostomy in a hydrocephalic patient. **A,** View of a thinned floor of the third ventricle between the infundibular recess and the mammillary bodies. **B,** Perforation of the floor of the third ventricle using a Fogarty balloon catheter. **C,** Inflation of the balloon catheter. **D,** Fenestration in the floor of the third ventricle.

It is unclear whether or not the success of an ETV is more sustainable than a shunt. Based on a 2010 paper from the same Canadian/International group, the relative risk of failure of an ETV is initially higher than that of a shunt but drops below the failure of a shunt after 3 months, and the long-term benefit of ETV may be realized in several years.[94]

Neuroendoscopic treatment of multiloculated hydrocephalus, including endoscopic cyst fenestration and fenestration of the septum pellucidum, is yet another effective alternative to multiple CSF shunt placements in selected patients.[95-97] Recent studies have suggested a role for ETV for communicating hydrocephalus as well.[98]

TABLE 6.10 ETV Success Score*			
Component Score	Age +	Etiology +	Previous Shunt
	↓	↓	↓
0	<1 month	Postinfectious	Previous shunt
10	1 month– <6 months		No previous shunt
20		Myelomeningocele Intraventricular hemorrhage Nontectal brain tumor	
30	6 months– <1 year	Aqueductal stenosis Tectal tumor Other etiology	
40	1–<10 years		
50	≥10 years		

ETV, endoscopic third ventriculostomy.

*As calculated using the given equation with values from the table, the **ETV Success Score approximates the percent success of performing a successful ETV:**
ETV Success Score = Age score + Etiology score + Previous shunt score ≈ percent probability of ETV success
The higher the score, the higher the chance of a successful ETV.
From Kulkarni AV, Drake JM, Mallucci CL, et al. Endoscopic third ventriculostomy in the treatment of childhood hydrocephalus. J Pediatr 2009;155(2):254-259. ee1. Epub 2009 May 15.

SUMMARY

Although hydrocephalus is a commonly encountered entity in clinical practice, its diagnosis and optimal treatment remain complex. The past century has seen great strides in the treatment of hydrocephalus with the introduction of CSF shunting systems. Although lifesaving, CSF shunts are still associated with significant complications. Clinicians and investigators are continuing to develop better shunt systems and novel techniques to treat this condition.

ACKNOWLEDGMENTS

This chapter contains material from the second edition, and we are grateful to Paul P. Wang, Anthony M. Avellino, and Sherman C. Stein for their contributions.

SELECTED KEY REFERENCES

Aronyk KE. The history and classification of hydrocephalus. *Neurosurg Clin North Am.* 1993;4(4):599-609.

Aschoff A, Kremer P, Hashemi B, et al. The scientific history of hydrocephalus and its treatment. *Neurosurg Rev.* 1999;22(2-3):67-93.

Greitz D. Paradigm shift in hydrocephalus research in legacy of Dandy's pioneering work: rationale for third ventriculostomy in communicating hydrocephalus. *Childs Nerv Syst.* 2007;23(5): 487-489.

Kulkarni AV, Drake JM, Mallucci CL, et al. Endoscopic third ventriculostomy in the treatment of childhood hydrocephalus. *J. Pediatr.* 2009;155(2):254-259.

Whitehead WE, Kestle JR. The treatment of cerebrospinal fluid shunt infections. Results from a practice survey of the American Society of Pediatric Neurosurgeons. *Pediatr Neurosurg.* 2001;35(4):205-210.

Please go to expertconsult.com to view the complete list of references.

CHAPTER 7

Developmental Anomalies: Arachnoid Cysts, Dermoids, and Epidermoids

David F. Jimenez, Jennifer Gentry Savage, Mical Samuelson

CLINICAL PEARLS

- Treatment for arachnoid cysts is indicated only if the cyst is associated with clinical symptoms.

- When treating arachnoid cysts the choices include
  - Cystoperitoneal shunt
  - Craniotomy and fenestration
  - Endoscopic minimally invasive fenestration

- When resecting dermoids associated with dermal sinus tracts, the entire cyst and sinus tract must be removed in order to prevent recurrence.

- When removing intracranial epidermoids, meticulous care must be undertaken to prevent spillage of the contents into the subarachnoid spaces in order to prevent postoperative chemical meningitis.

ARACHNOID CYSTS

Arachnoid cysts contain cerebrospinal fluid (CSF) and are most typically enclosed in arachnoid or arachnoid-like membranes and can be located anywhere within the craniospinal axis. With the advent and widespread use of magnetic resonance imaging (MRI), these lesions have been encountered with significant frequency. However, despite being well described throughout the literature, arachnoid cysts are actually rare, accounting for around 1% of intracranial space-occupying lesions. They exhibit a male predominance, at approximately a 3:1 ratio,[1,2] and a predilection for the sylvian region. Although these cysts are occasionally bilateral and multiloculated, they are usually unilateral and single.[3]

Diagnosis of arachnoid cyst can be made easily with currently available imaging modalities. Computed tomography (CT) and MRI are the gold standard for visualizing and making the diagnosis. Arachnoid cysts will appear markedly hypodense on CT scan (Fig. 7.1) and show low signal on T1 MRI and high signal intensity on T2 MRI (Fig. 7.2), as they are generally isointense with CSF. Diffusion MRI reveals a low signal secondary to high water diffusibility and high apparent diffusion coefficient (ADC). Arachnoid cysts display a smooth, well-demarcated surface and are heterogeneous and nonenhancing, distinguishing them from other cystic lesions such as epidermoids.[4] In utero, arachnoid cysts may be visible via ultrasound.[5]

The embryogenesis of arachnoid cysts remains controversial. Some authors report the arachnoid layer originating strictly from neural crest cells, but others propose the arachnoid originating from two layers: neural crest ectoderm and mesoderm. The primitive mesenchyme, or mesoderm, surrounding the neural tube separates into an endomeninx, which forms the pia-arachnoid membrane, and an ectomeninx.[6]

The subarachnoid space is then formed by the rupture of the rhombic roof and dissection of the ecto- and endomeninges by CSF pulse pressure from the choroid plexus. Any disruption of this separation is thought to be the initiating event in arachnoid cyst formation.[7,8] This disruption can occur anywhere along the neuraxis as evidenced by reports of spinal intradural and extradural arachnoid cysts.[9] Congenital spinal arachnoid cysts have been mostly described in patients with neural tube defects.[10] Posterior fossa arachnoid cysts have been specifically discussed in the literature along with Chiari malformations and Dandy-Walker syndrome as a possible result of embryonal atresia of the fourth ventricle.[4] Two theories predominate in the literature with respect to the pathogenesis of middle fossa arachnoid cysts. Robinson's theory proposes primary temporal lobe agenesis as the main factor in middle fossa arachnoid cyst formation. Starkman and co-workers propose the arachnoid cyst as the primary abnormality leading to eventual temporal lobe hypoplasia secondary to cyst expansion.[11] Both theories are supported equally well throughout the literature.

In 1831, Bright submitted what is considered the first pathological description of arachnoid cysts. He reported the cysts as malformations caused by a splitting of the arachnoid membrane.[12] More recently, Rengachary and Watanabe described the structural features of arachnoid cysts after review of several hundred cases: (1) splitting of the arachnoid membrane at the margin of the cyst; (2) thickened collagen layer in the cyst wall; (3) absence of normal arachnoid trabeculations within the cyst; and (4) hyperplastic arachnoid cells in the cyst wall.[6,13] On pathological review of optic nerve arachnoid cysts, authors report three common features of the cyst wall: meningothelial cell proliferation, thickened dura, and psammoma bodies.[14-16]

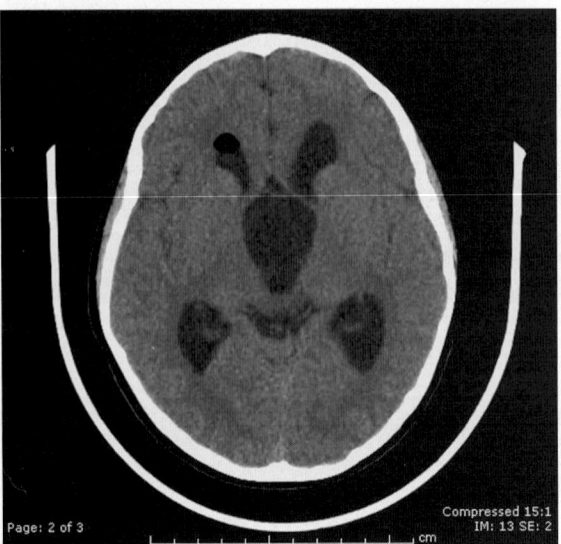

FIGURE 7.1 Computed tomography (CT) scan of a patent with a large suprasellar arachnoid cyst extending into the third ventricle and causing headaches, declining school performance, and progressively impaired memory. The patient underwent an endoscopic fenestration into the ventricles (Video 1) which led to complete symptom resolution.

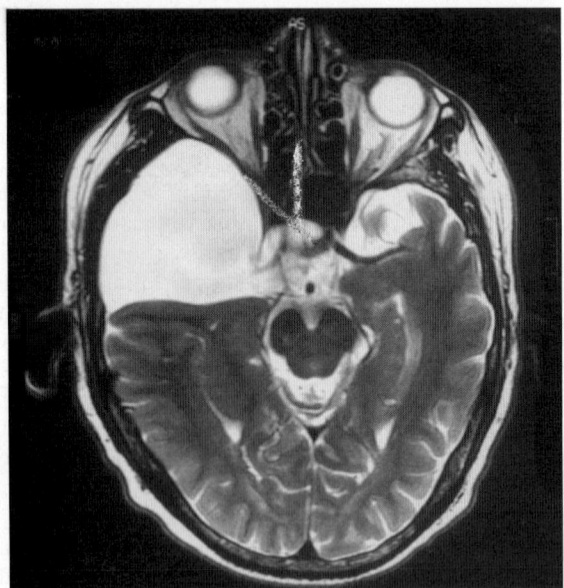

FIGURE 7.2 T2-weighted magnetic resonance image showing an area of high signal intensity on the right temporal fossa and marked compression of the temporal lobe. Lesion is consistent with an arachnoid cyst.

Galassi and associates introduced a classification scheme for arachnoid cysts based on their communication with the adjacent cisterns. In this classification scheme, type I arachnoid cysts freely communicate with the cisterns. Type II cysts are intermediate and may or may not communicate with the cisterns but it is likely they communicated with the subarachnoid space at one time, before sealing off their communication.[17] Type III cysts do not communicate with any region of the subarachnoid space and cause local mass effect.[2,18] This classification scheme also hints at a possible treatment guide, with type I cysts rarely needing surgical intervention, owing to the free communication with the subarachnoid space, and type III cysts more frequently requiring surgical intervention secondary to mass effect.

The most common location for arachnoid cysts is the middle fossa or sylvian fissure, usually behind the greater wing of the sphenoid bone[19] accounting for nearly 50% of arachnoid cysts in one study. Posterior fossa cysts including cerebellopontine angle and the cerebellar vermis comprise 20% to 30% of lesions,[20] and supracellar cysts, 9%. Other documented locations include interventricular, optic nerve, cerebral convexity, and clival interpeduncular area arachnoid cysts.[12,21] Intraspinal arachnoid cysts are rare and mostly traumatic except in the cases of intramedullary cysts, which have been reported as truly congenital. Most intradural spinal arachnoid cysts occur in the thoracic region (80%) followed by the cervical (15%) and lumbar regions (5%).[22]

Macrocephaly is one of the most common presenting signs of an arachnoid cyst in infants and can be diagnosed in utero. In older patients, cyst location correlates with presenting symptoms. Headache, secondary to increased intracranial pressure from mass effect, is usually the most common presenting symptom, frequently seen with middle fossa cysts. Middle fossa cysts are also often associated with post-traumatic subdural hemorrhages and may present with signs of mass effect from the hemorrhage.[19] Suprasellar, pineal, and posterior fossa region arachnoid cysts present with signs of obstructive hydrocephalus. Suprasellar cysts in particular may present with precocious puberty, hyperinsulinism, and even visual loss.[23,24] These cysts are frequently symptomatic and rarely respond to surgical treatment, requiring initiation of long-term hormonal therapy regimens. In cases of optic nerve arachnoid cysts, patients may present with a childhood history of blindness in the affected eye with progressive complaints of proptosis, erythema, and pain.[8] There are also several reports of patients presenting with cranial nerve palsies of the occulomotor, trigeminal, abducens, facial, vestibulocochlear, and hypoglossal nerves.[25-29] Patients with spinal arachnoid cysts may present with a constellation of symptoms if associated with a congenital syndrome. Others may present with back pain or, rarely, with progressive spastic paraparesis.[30]

The natural history of arachnoid cysts is not yet clearly delineated given that most are found incidentally and remain static in size over time. Patients are frequently asymptomatic throughout their lives and many are found at autopsy. However, arachnoid cysts are often associated with other congenital disorders and in these cases the natural history may be related to the associated disorder. Glutaric aciduria type I (GAT1) is an inborn metabolic disorder that appears to have a strong association with bitemporal intracranial arachnoid cysts, the most consistent reported finding on all imaging modalities.[7] Patients with these findings in combination with macrocephaly, psychomotor development, and dystonic cerebral palsy warrant a detailed metabolic workup. Recently, a case of bitemporal arachnoid cysts was also reported in a patient with tuberous sclerosis. Short-rib polydactyly syndromes and their variants, including Beemer-Langer syndrome, have been associated with arachnoid cysts, along with other genetic syndromes including cri-du-chat, autosomal dominant polycystic kidney disease, Aicardi syndrome, neurofibromatosis, and proteus syndrome. Further supporting a genetic basis of arachnoid cyst formation are reports of familial cysts. Familial arachnoid cysts usually occur in the same location in affected family members and have even been documented as mirror-image cerebellopontine-angle arachnoid cysts in monozygotic twins. An association with behavioral and cognitive disabilities has been recently documented and centers largely around attention-deficit hyperactivity disorder (ADHD), epileptic aphasia (Landau-Kleffner syndrome), and other developmental language disorders. Some authors report positron emission tomography (PET) studies revealing hypometabolism in cortical regions surrounding the cyst. After surgical decompression of the cysts, repeat PET studies demonstrated improvement in cortical metabolism and clinical performance on language testing.[19,31]

Another area of controversy surrounds arachnoid cysts in middle fossa locations of epileptic patients. Many studies suggest only an incidental association, yet others report improvement in seizures following surgical treatment. There are several reports of epileptic foci over the region of the arachnoid cyst as confirmed by electroencephalography.[3] However, other reports describe epileptic patients with temporal lobe arachnoid cysts and seizure onset localization far from the cyst,[32-34] varying treatment decisions on among cases. With regard to spinal arachnoid cysts, associations with congenital spinal malformations including caudal regression syndrome and acquired anomalies such as syringomyelia have been documented.[35]

In incidental cases of arachnoid cysts, and those unrelated to other congenital anomalies, the size and dynamic status of the cyst appear to play a role in the natural history. Several theories have been proposed to explain the mechanism of arachnoid cyst expansion, the most common being the ball-valve theory. In this theory, an anatomical communication exists between the cyst and the subarachnoid space which acts as a unidirectional valve. Multiple reports of MRI studies have demonstrated this effect through cine-mode studies. However, this mechanism has not been observed in all arachnoid cysts and cannot explain the spontaneous resolution of cysts reported in the literature.[36-38] Another proposed mechanism is an osmotic gradient between the cyst and the surrounding CSF. This theory is not widely accepted in cases of congenital arachnoid cysts given that the cystic content is quite similar to the composition of CSF. This theory could be plausible in cases of traumatic arachnoid cyst formation, especially in the presence of hemorrhagic or inflammatory foci. A third theory, backed by clinical evidence, is that of fluid production by the cells of the cyst wall. There are many reports of isolated or closed compartment cysts that expand over time and, as discussed previously, the cyst wall is physiologically similar to the subdural and arachnoid granulation neurothelium.[13]

Another factor affecting the natural history of arachnoid cysts is related to location of the cyst and susceptibility to hemorrhage. Middle fossa arachnoid cysts can be complicated by post-traumatic subdural hemorrhages, regardless of the age of the patient.[39] The mechanism of the hemorrhage is likely secondary to the displacement at stretching of the bridging veins by the cyst as they extend from the cortical surface to the dura. As they stretch, and tear, hemorrhage accumulates mostly in the subdural space, and occasionally in the cyst itself.[19,40] Some authors cite annual increases in the risk of

subdural hemorrhage by 20- to 40-fold in patients with arachnoid cysts.[19,41,42]

The lack of evidence-based data or studies has led to significant controversies regarding the appropriate treatment protocol for patients presenting with arachnoid cysts. No significant controversy is present when the patient is found to have a small asymptomatic cyst. Even with larger cysts, if the patient has no clinical symptoms, no intervention is necessary. In patients with more dynamic cysts without signs of increased intracranial pressure or focal neurological deficit, nonoperative management may also be considered in conjunction with close follow-up and serial imaging.[43]

Perhaps the most challenging treatment decision concerns when to treat patients who present with a medium-size arachnoid cyst and have mild symptoms (headaches, dizziness, mild ataxia, etc.) and it is not clear if the symptoms are causally related to the presence of the cyst. Assessment of the patient, looking for signs of elevated intracranial pressure, and clinical judgment play a crucial role in the decision-making process. The easiest clinical scenario is one in which the patient presents with marked symptoms and large cysts producing significant mass effect, midline shift, or obstructive hydrocephalus, as in the case of large suprasellar cysts (Fig. 7.3). Moreover, in these cases controversy exists as to which surgical approach is the best to treat the patient.

Open craniotomy with cyst fenestration has been reported in cases of well-circumscribed cysts without hydrocephalus. This procedure allows for total or subtotal (as is most commonly the case) resection of the cyst wall and pathological diagnosis. Some authors even report arachnoidoplasty via an open craniotomy. The surgeons incised the cyst microsurgically to initially enter the cyst and then again to allow communication with the cisterns followed by subsequent closure of the outermost membrane to prevent CSF leakage.[44] Cyst fenestration may also be accomplished via an endoscopic approach with possible marsupialization of the cyst and even varying degrees of resection of the cyst wall. This technique is favored by many, especially in the management of symptomatic suprasellar arachnoid cysts.[43,45,46] Shunting of the cyst, most commonly to the peritoneum, allows for appropriate diversion of the CSF and is favored by some for middle fossa cysts and recurrent cysts in the setting of increased intracranial pressure. This technique allows for a gradual decompression of the cyst and concomitant gradual expansion of the brain. Neuronavigation techniques have been combined with most types of surgical treatments for arachnoid cysts yielding a minimally invasive approach and higher precision, particularly with suprasellar and multiloculated cysts.[43] With regard to spinal arachnoid cysts, surgical interventions are again usually reserved for symptomatic patients. In the cases of extradural cysts, some authors favor amputation at the stalk near the dural cleft from which the cyst protrudes.[47] In other cases, a decompressive laminectomy may be warranted.

DERMOID CYSTS

Dermoid cysts are by definition inclusion cysts, which mean that they are made up of implanted epithelial tissue into an area that should not contain it. As such, these cysts can be found in many parts of the body to include the face, nose,

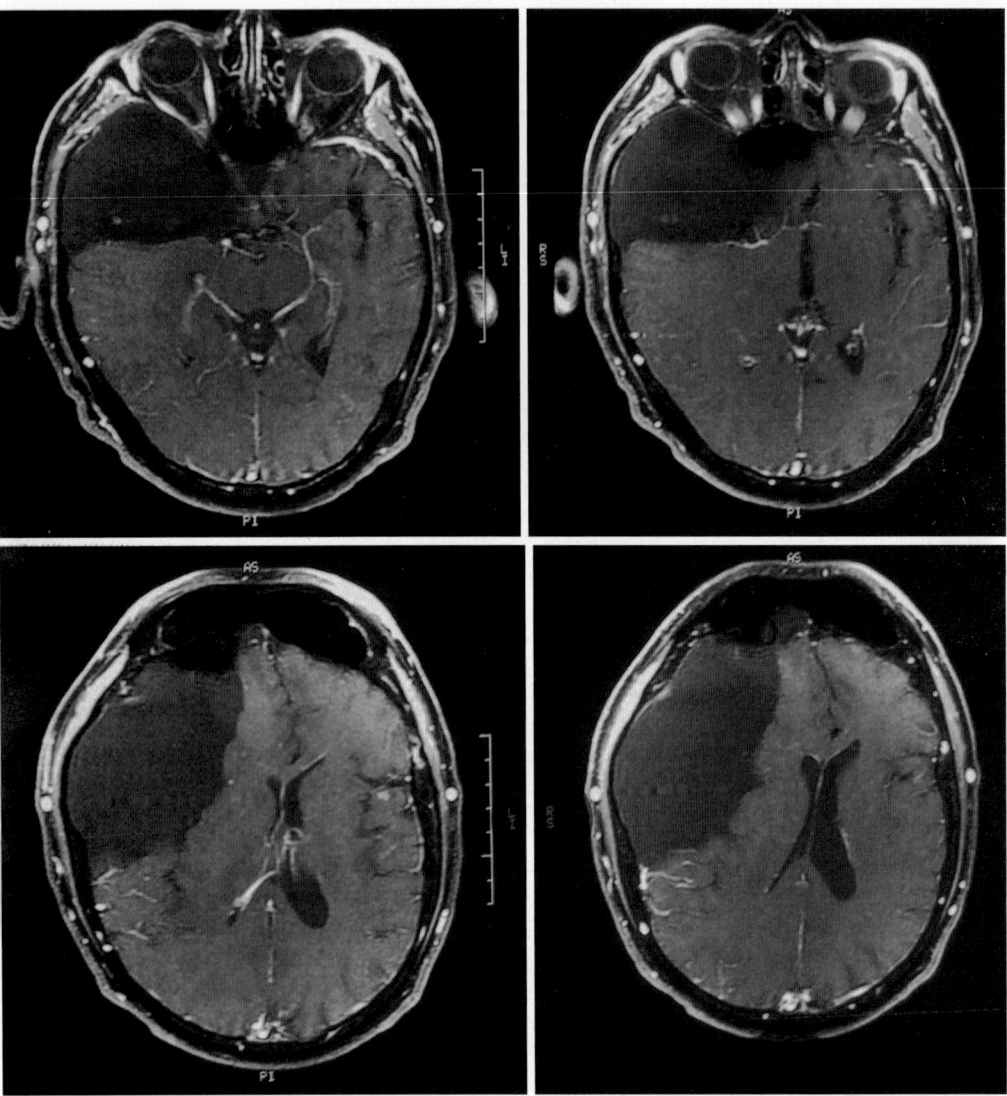

FIGURE 7.3 Magnetic resonance imaging of an 18-year-old male patient who presented with seizures, severe headaches, and papilledema. There is a large temporal arachnoid cyst causing midline shift and expansion of the temporal bone secondary to large standing pressure within the cyst.

scalp, skull, brain, spinal cord, orbits, neck, and oral and nasal cavities. These congenital lesions are thought to arise from misplaced ectodermal elements during the third to fifth week of embryonic life due to failure of the neural tube closure at the midline. They are more commonly associated with dermal sinus tracts (Fig. 7.4) and spinal abnormalities than are epidermoid tumors. Dermoid inclusion cysts account for approximately 0.3% of all brain tumors. The tumors are usually benign slow-growing lesions that rarely undergo malignant transformation, and can occur anywhere along the spinal axis. Histologically, dermoid tumors usually contain desquamated epithelial keratin and some lipid material, which gives its external surface a smooth, lobulated, pearly appearance. These tumors have an outer connective tissue capsule and are lined with stratified squamous epithelium that also contains hair follicles, sebaceous glands, and sweat glands. Because they contain mature tissues, these cysts are almost universally benign (Figs. 7.5, 7.6).

On CT scans, dermoids are usually rounded, well-circumscribed, extremely hypodense lesions with a Hounsfield unit of 220 to 2140, in keeping with their lipid content (Fig. 7.7). Peripheral capsular calcification is frequent. Enhancement

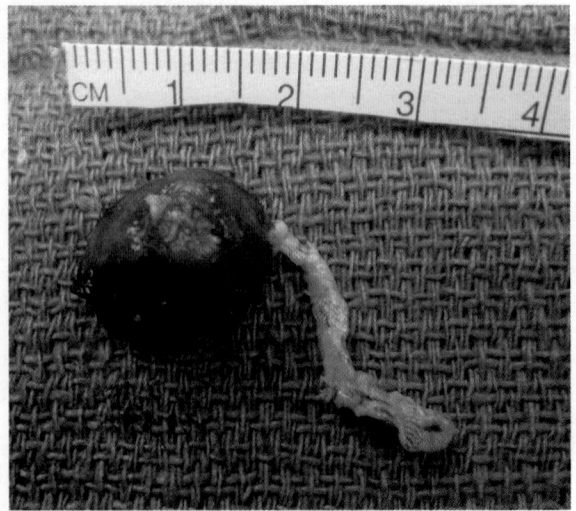

FIGURE 7.4 Surgical specimen of an intracranial dermoid cyst and its associated dermal sinus tract. Care must be taken to remove the cyst along with the capsule to ensure that no recurrence takes place.

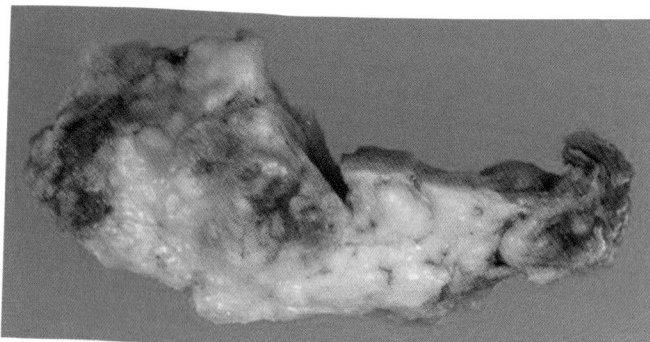

FIGURE 7.5 Gross specimen of dermoid seen in Figure 7.4. Keratinized material is seen along with an outer capsule. Care should be taken to avoid spillage of this material in the subarachnoid spaces.

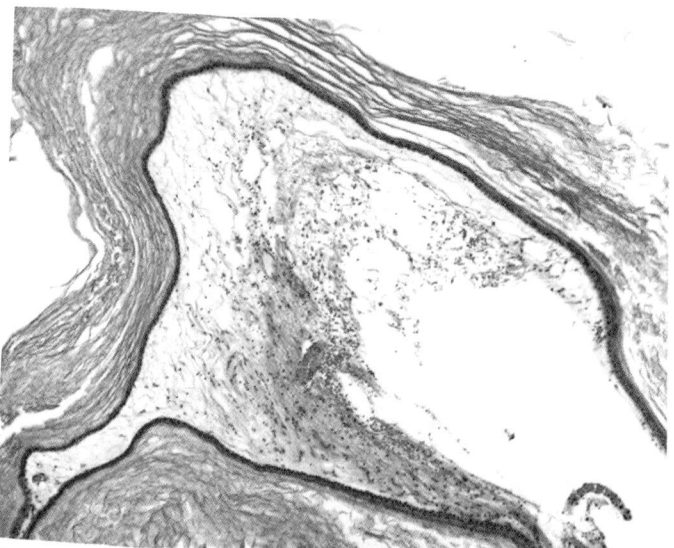

FIGURE 7.6 Histological slide of the same intracranial dermoid shown in Figures 7.4 and 7.5, showing multiple layers of attenuated epithelium that shed the anucleated squames that make up most of the mass.

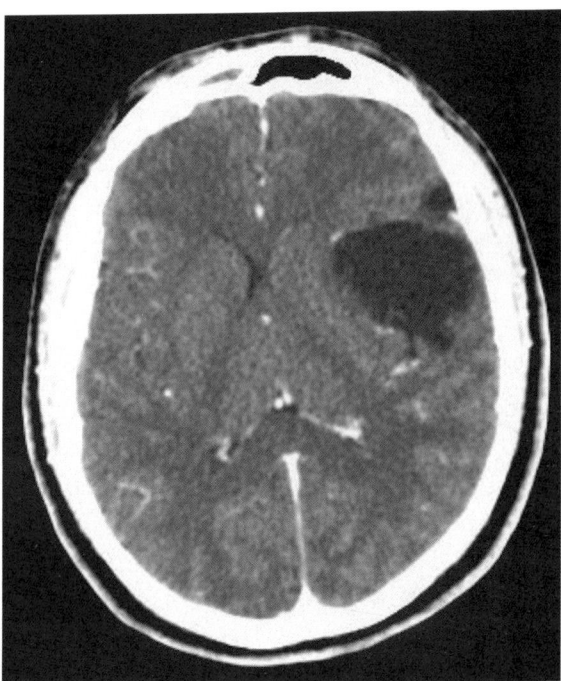

FIGURE 7.7 Axial computed tomography scan of a 32-year-old male patient who presented with progressively increasing left-sided headaches. Scan shows an area of hypodensity located on the left temporal fossa and causing mass effect on the ipsilateral ventricular system. Contrast enhancement shows no evidence of contrast uptake by the lesion.

after contrast agent administration is rare but has been reported. On MR images, dermoids are typically hyperintense on T1-weighted images but vary from hypo- to hyperintense on T2-weighted studies (Figs. 7.8, 7.9). There is usually no associated vasogenic edema or contrast enhancement. Serpiginous hypointense elements may be seen if the lesion contains hair. Mural calcification can sometimes be identified. Orakcioglu and colleagues noted that diffusion-weighted imaging (DWI) hyperintensity in dermoid cysts is related to a decrease of water proton diffusion and should be used for both the diagnosis and follow-up of these lesions.[48] Imaging findings vary, depending on whether the cyst has ruptured. On both CT and MR images, fat-density droplets may be seen throughout the subarachnoid space and in the ventricular system if rupture of the cyst has occurred. Extensive pial enhancement can be seen from chemical meningitis caused by ruptured cysts.

Intracranial dermoid tumors are seen most frequently in patients up to 20 years of age and show a slight male predominance. They are usually solitary and commonly occur in posterior fossa (within the fourth ventricle or cerebellar region. Symptoms and signs

are associated with the location of the tumor and the mass/ pressure effect on adjacent tissues. Suprasellar tumors can cause visual abnormalities from compression of the optic chiasm. Diabetes insipidus and hypopituitarism may occur. Parasellar tumors may be associated with seizures from mass effect or extension to the temporal lobe and sylvian fissure. Intraventricular dermoid tumors are most frequently located in the fourth ventricle and sometimes cause hydrocephalus. It has been suggested that the CSF flow may occur through interstices on the surface of the tumor. Spinal dermoid tumors are most commonly situated near the thoracolumbar junction and tend to involve the conus medullaris and cauda equina. About 50% are intradural intramedullary, and 50% are intradural extramedullary. Extradural location is least common. Less common sites of dermoid tumors include the scalp, skull, orbit, nasal and oral cavities, and neck. Dermoid tumors in the spinal canal may cause back or leg pain due to mass effect. Headache and meningitis may occur if an associated dermal sinus tract becomes infected. Vertebral abnormalities, such as diastematomyelia, hemivertebra, and scoliosis, are frequently associated with dermal sinuses, dermoid tumors, or epidermoid tumors.

Morbidity depends on the location of the tumor and on the involvement of adjacent structures. Dermoid tumors can rupture, releasing lipid contents into the ventricular or subarachnoid spaces (Fig 7.5). This causes a chemical meningitis that can lead to recurrent symptoms, most commonly headache. The subsequent meningeal inflammation may result in arterial vasospasm, possible stroke, and death. Orakcioglu and colleagues reviewed the charts of five men and two women

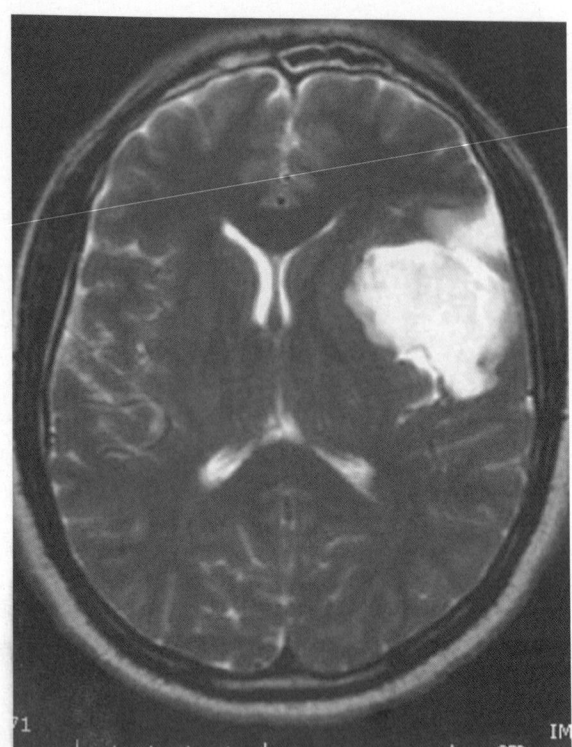

FIGURE 7.8 Axial T2-weighted magnetic resonance image demonstrates a high signal intensity lesion expanding the left sylvian fissure and placing mass effect on the left frontal horn.

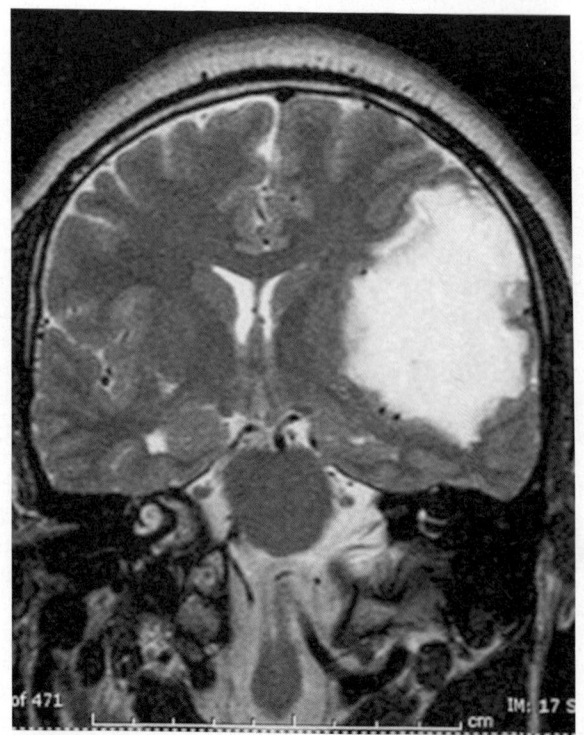

FIGURE 7.9 Coronal T2-weighted magnetic resonance image of same patient in Figure 7.8 demonstrates a high signal intensity lesion displacing the surrounding frontal and temporal lobes. The lesion was found to be a dermoid cyst at surgery.

with intracranial dermoid cysts and found that clinical presentations included focal neurological deficits, epileptic seizures, persistent headache, mental changes, and psycho-organic syndromes. One patient underwent delayed ventriculoperitoneal shunting after ruptured fatty particles caused obstructive hydrocephalus. In three patients, despite dermoid rupture into the subarachnoid space, hydrocephalus did not develop. In one patient, diffuse vascular supratentorial lesions occurred as a result of aseptic meningitis. In addition, they noted that although rupture does not necessarily cause hydrocephalus, radical removal of the tumor and close monitoring of ventricular size are necessary.

Surgical treatment is indicated when the patient presents with symptoms related to mass effect. Craniotomy with careful resection of the lesions is recommended. Utmost care should be taken to avoid spillage of the keratinized contents into the subarachnoid space. Perioperative steroids help decrease the incidence of postoperative meningitis.

EPIDERMOID CYSTS

Epidermoid cysts (sebaceous cysts) are benign congenital lesions of ectodermal origin. Intracerebral epidermoid cysts are rare and possibly account for approximately 1.5% of all intracranial epidermoids and approximately 1% of all intracranial tumors. Epidermoids usually present around 20 to 40 years of age and occur with equal frequency in men and women. They can be congenital or acquired. They can be both intradural and extradural. They most commonly present within the cerebellopontine (CP) angle, parasellar region, and middle cranial fossa. There have also been case reports within the ventricular system, brain parenchyma, and spinal cord. Congenital epidermoids are thought to arise from ectodermal inclusions during neural tube closure in the third to fifth weeks of embryogenesis. Ectodermal inclusions occurring at the third week of embryogenesis could account for intracerebral and intraventricular epidermoids. Most epidermoid cysts in the cerebellopontine angle cistern and the parasellar region are thought to occur during neural tube closure between the third to fifth weeks of gestation when the optic and otic vessels are being formed. In a review of 39 cases described in the literature, these lesions were noted to occur most commonly in the frontal and temporal lobes. Less frequent locations include the corpus callosum, pineal gland, parietal lobe, and occipital lobe. Acquired epidermoid tumors are believed to form as a result of trauma when epithelial cells are deposited within the lumbar spinal canal. Sites of epithelial deposition can occur anywhere between the neural tube and the overlying skin surface. The clinical presentation and symptoms depend on the location of the mass. Presentations for cerebellopontine angle masses include headache, diplopia, trigeminal hypoacusia, and gait ataxia.

Epidermoids are well-circumscribed, smooth, lobulated, encapsulated lesions. Histologically, their internal layer is composed of stratified squamous epithelium with a fibrous capsule. They tend to slowly enlarge as epithelial cells desquamate, with the formation of keratin and cholesterol crystals in the center of the lesion. Handu and co-wo̶r̶k̶e̶r̶s̶ the aspirates of epidermal i̶n̶c̶l̶u̶s̶i̶o̶n̶ cytological features.[49] The aspirates showed a clear background with high cellularity, along with nucleate and anucleate squames. In some cases, keratinous material was present but less than the cellular elements. In 31 cases, a diagnosis of infected EIC was made on the basis of dense inflammatory infiltrate in addition to the squames. Of 56 cases for which histopathological data were available, 45 cases of EIC were diagnosed, 5 cases of dermoid cyst, 2 cases of branchial cyst, 2 cases of pilomatricoma, 1 case of sebaceous cyst, and 1 case of thyroglossal cyst.

Typical imaging findings on CT include a round/lobulated mass with a density resembling CSF; the mass may have a crenated margin,which, when present, could be characteristic. Calcification is reported to be present in approximately 10% of all intracranial epidermoids,[50] which may be due to saponification of the desquamated debris. In their review of reported intracerebral epidermoids, Kaido and associates found high density in 2 out of 13 patients with a CT description[51] and Watanabe and colleagues[52] described a right frontal lobe epidermoid with nodular peripheral calcification. On MRI epidermoid cysts appear hypointense on T1-weighted images and hyperintense on T2-weighted images. There is usually some internal heterogeneity, which is best seen in the proton-density and fluid attenuated inversion recovery (FLAIR) images, and this finding could help distinguish these cysts from arachnoid cysts. In a review of the MRI appearance of epidermoids, signal heterogeneity was observed on T1 and proton-density weighted images in 65% of cases. MRI may also show insinuating margins of the cyst, extending into the adjacent cisterns or fissures, features that are not usually associated with arachnoid cysts. Lesions typically do not enhance. When present, contrast enhancement is minimal and peripheral; it has been seen in up to 35% of cases.[53] DWI is the most helpful imaging sequence in diagnosing an epidermoid cyst. Because of a combination of T2 and diffusion effects, epidermoid tumors appear markedly hyperintense compared with CSF and brain tissue on diffusion-weighted images. Epidermoid tumors demonstrate an ADC that is similar to that of gray matter and lower than that of CSF. In contrast, arachnoid cysts or other cystic intracranial lesions do not show restricted diffusion and follow the CSF signal on DWI and ADC maps.

Epidermoid cysts are benign, slowly but ineluctably growing tumors that require surgical treatment. Similar to dermoid cysts, morbidity of epidermoids depends on the location of the tumor and on the involvement of adjacent structures. Lopes and co-workers reviewed the postoperative morbidity and mortality rates in 44 patients (22 men and 22 women) between 1980 and 2000. Their postoperative morbidity rate was 13.6% and the mortality rate was 8.9%, with a median follow-up period of 8 years and a recurrence rate of 4.5%. Morbidity and mortality rates for epidermoid cysts seem to be unrelated to classical aseptic meningitis (22.7% in their series) or hydrocephalus (10%). They concluded prolonged cerebral retraction could be one of the responsible factors for increased morbidity and mortality rates.[54]

Other common locations for epidermoids include the scalp and skull. These slow-growing lesions commonly present in infancy or childhood and grow unabated until adulthood. They may be located anywhere in the scalp and may be multicentric (Fig. 7.10). As opposed to dermoids which may also contain hair, teeth, and skin glands, epidermoids

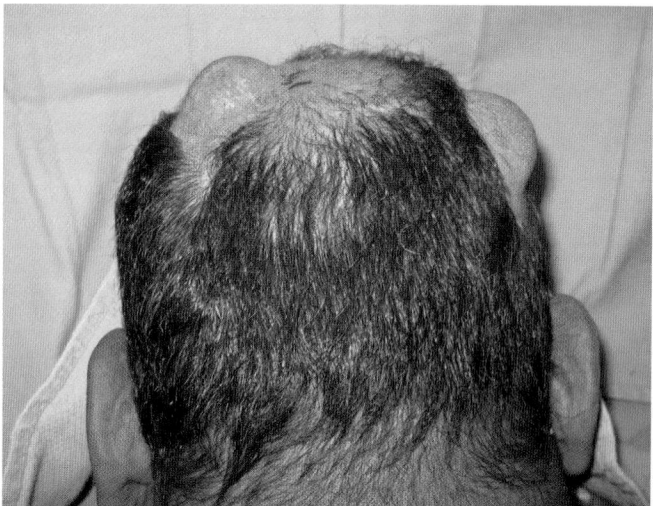

FIGURE 7.10 This 50-year-old male patient presented with painful enlarging scalp masses. These masses were present since childhood and only became symptomatic 1 year prior to presentation.

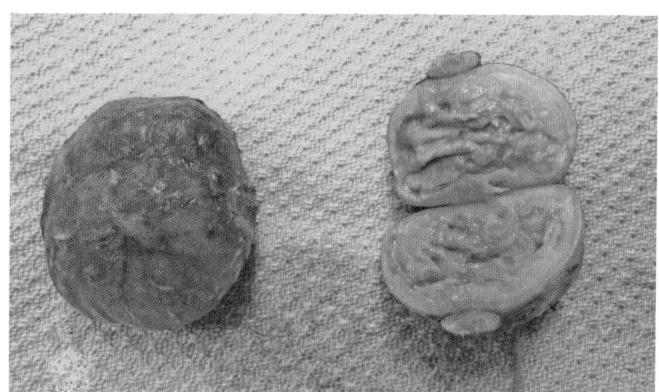

FIGURE 7.11 Cystic lesions removed from patient shown in Figure 7.10. Note thick capsule with green-yellowish keratinized material inside dissected lesion.

typically only contain epidermal tissue and keratin debris (Fig. 7.11). Gross total resection is curative and provides excellent results.

SELECTED KEY REFERENCES

Akor CA, Wojno TH, Newman NJ, Grossniklaus HE. Arachnoid cysts of the optic nerve. *Ophthal Plast Reconstr Surg.* 2003;19:466-469.

Cincu R, Agrawal A, Eiras J. Intracranial arachnoid cysts: current concepts and treatment alternatives. *Clin Neurol Neurosurg.* 2007;109:837-843.

Peraud A, Ryan G, Drake JM. Rapid formation of a multicompartment neonatal arachnoid cyst. *Pediatr Neurosurg.* 2003;39:139-143.

Piatt Jr JH. Unexpected findings on brain and spine imaging in children. *Pediatr Clin North Am.* 2004;51:507-527.

Tatli M, Guzel A. Bitemporal arachnoid cysts associated with tuberous sclerosis complex. *J Child Neurol.* 2007;22:775-779.

Please go to expertconsult.com to view complete list of references.

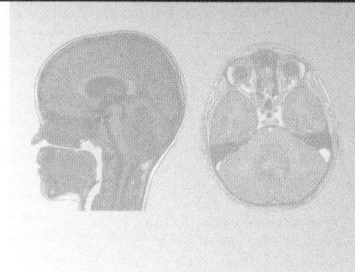

CHAPTER

8 Diagnosis and Surgical Options for Craniosynostosis

Mitchel Seruya, Suresh N. Magge, Robert F. Keating

CLINICAL PEARLS

- In craniosynostosis, skull growth is arrested in the direction perpendicular to the fused suture and expanded at the sites of unaffected sutures (Virchow's law), leading to characteristic calvarial deformations. In addition, the skull base and calvarial development are interrelated and changes at one location may affect the growth parameters at the other location.

- Intracranial hypertension can accompany craniosynostosis and is a function of the number of affected sutures, ranging from approximately 14% for single-suture synostosis to roughly 47% in multisuture synostosis. Children suspected of having elevated intracranial pressure may present with irritability, feeding difficulties, failure to thrive, headache, developmental delays, visual changes, calvarial towering, supraorbital recession, or lack of circumferential skull growth. Computed tomography (CT) scan changes may include "beaten copper" appearance of the inner table of the skull and compression of the ventricles and cisterns. Hydrocephalus and Chiari malformation can be associated

- with children with syndromic craniosynostosis (e.g., Crouzon, Apert, Pfeiffer syndromes).

- An increasing number of growth factor receptors (FGFR, TGF-βR), growth factors (FGF2, TGF-β, BMP), as well as transcription factors (MSX-2 and Twist), have been implicated in the pathogenesis of craniosynostosis and this list will undoubtedly grow in the future.

- The optimal timing of craniosynostosis surgery remains controversial even today, although the majority of craniofacial surgeons operate when patients are between 3 and 12 months of age. Because the normal brain and skull grow most rapidly in the first 2 years of life, early surgery takes advantage of this rapid period of growth and facilitates cranial volume expansion.

- Posterior deformational plagiocephaly, secondary to a supine sleeping position, will generally resolve with positional changes, physiotherapy, or helmet therapy and is only rarely a surgical condition.

Craniosynostosis is defined as the premature closure of a cranial suture which causes abnormal calvarial growth. Skull growth is arrested in the direction perpendicular to the fused suture and expanded at the sites of unaffected sutures, leading to characteristic calvarial deformations (Virchow's law).[1] In addition to the morphological changes accompanying craniosynostosis, functional problems related to brain development and possible intracranial hypertension are major considerations. Although the likelihood of elevated intracranial pressure remains low for patients with single-suture craniosynostosis, children with multiple-suture involvement or delayed presentation of single-suture synostosis are at significantly higher risk.[2-4] A broad range of surgical options exist in the armamentarium of contemporary craniofacial surgical reconstruction, all with the primary objective of releasing the affected suture to permit normalization of skull growth in the setting of accelerated cerebral growth. Over time, progressively earlier recognition of craniosynostosis and its subsequent treatment have led to improved surgical results with correspondingly decreased

perioperative morbidity. With a greater understanding of technologies relying on dynamic cranial vault alteration, including endoscopic sutural release, spring-assisted cranioplasty, and distraction osteogenesis, new horizons will inevitably unfold.

HISTORY

Craniosynostosis has long been recognized as an abnormal process originating at the calvarial suture. Early recognition of the importance of the skull sutures and their relationship to head shape was first made by investigators such as Hippocrates, Galen, and Celsus. In 1791, Sommerring noted that calvarial growth occurred at the suture line and that premature suture closure led to restriction of growth perpendicular to the affected suture.[5] In addition to confirming Sommerring's findings, Virchow was the first to describe the compensatory calvarial growth that occurred at the sites of unaffected sutures and associate a characteristic head shape

137

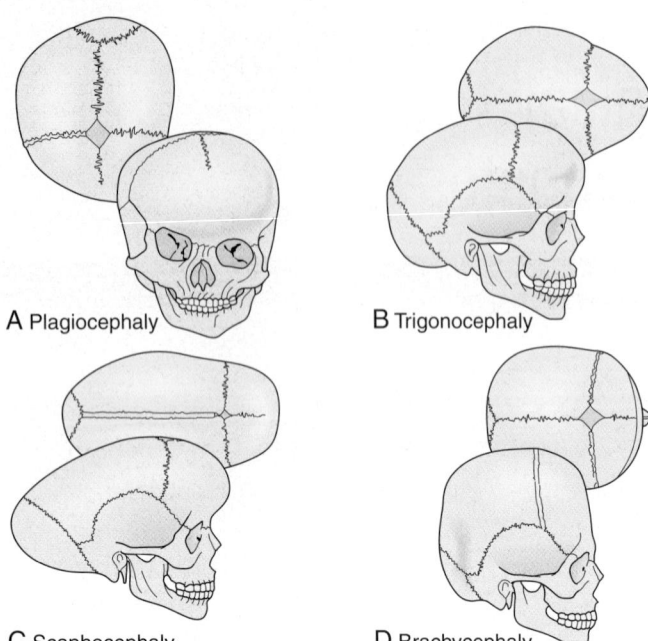

A Plagiocephaly   B Trigonocephaly

C Scaphocephaly   D Brachycephaly

FIGURE 8.1 Restriction of growth at particular sutures will lead to characteristically abnormal head shapes. Unicoronal synostosis is associated with ipsilateral flattening of the supraorbital and frontal regions with contralateral compensatory frontal bossing (anterior plagiocephaly). Premature closure of the metopic suture may lead to the formation of a triangular-shaped head (trigonocephaly). Sagittal synostosis is marked by an elongated and narrowed head (scaphocephaly). Bilateral coronal synostosis leads to a short, wide head with frontal towering (brachycephaly).

with its corresponding abnormal suture (Fig. 8.1).[1] These observations served as principal tenets directing craniosynostosis surgery over the subsequent century.

Over time, the relationship between calvarial growth and the skull base became better appreciated. In 1959, Moss pointed out the importance of the skull base in the promotion and development of the calvarial vault.[6] His contributions included the observation that the cranial base developed prior to the calvarial vault and that characteristic abnormalities in the cranial base were associated with classic sutural abnormalities. Nevertheless, subsequent experimental work in animal models demonstrated that restriction of growth at specific sutures resulted in characteristic skull deformities that mimicked shapes seen in simple (nonsyndromic) craniosynostosis.[7-9] As a result, the pathogenesis of craniosynostosis is currently thought to be a combination of skull base and calvarial growth disturbances.

EPIDEMIOLOGY

Craniosynostosis occurs in approximately 1 in 2000 to 1 in 2500 live births.[10] This condition can be classified into simple (single-suture) versus complex (multiple sutures) or nonsyndromic versus syndromic (Table 8.1). Single-suture synostosis represents the majority of patients, with multiple-suture synostoses comprising approximately 5% to 15% of cases.[10] As reported by large craniofacial centers, syndromic patients

TABLE 8.1 Classification of Synostosis

Affected Suture	Phenotypic Presentation
Sagittal	Dolichocephaly, scaphocephaly
Coronal (unilateral)	Anterior plagiocephaly
Coronal (bilateral)	Brachycephaly
Metopic	Trigonocephaly
Lambdoid	Posterior plagiocephaly
Multiple sutures	Cloverleaf (Kleeblattschädel), acrocephaly, oxycephaly

account for 15% to 20% of cases, whereas nonsyndromic patients constitute 80% to 85%.[11]

Single-suture synostosis most frequently occurs sporadically, with familial aggregation accounting for 7% to 8% of sagittal and metopic synostosis.[11] An equal frequency is found for all ethnic populations; however, gender predilection will vary depending on the type of suture pathology. The most commonly involved location is the sagittal suture, which accounts for 45% to 68% of all individuals[12,13] and is marked by a male/female ratio ranging from 3.5:1 to 7:1.[14] An autosomal dominant inheritance pattern with 38% penetrance was reported for sagittal synostosis.[15] Metopic synostosis is now the second most common form of craniosynostosis (23.7-27.3% of cases), an observation that currently evades definitive etiopathogenesis, and shows a male predominance of 75%.[11-13] Unicoronal synostosis, also known as *anterior plagiocephaly*, accounts for approximately 18% of patients with craniosynostosis,[12] with girls outnumbering boys by a 3:2 ratio.[16] Lambdoid suture synostosis, referred to as *posterior plagiocephaly*, is a relatively rare event in children with an observed incidence ranging from 0.9% to 4%.[17-19] True lambdoid synostosis must be distinguished from posterior deformational plagiocephaly, also known as positional molding, in which there is occipital flattening on the affected side without associated suture fusion. This epiphenomenon is possibly related to the supine sleeping position in young children, instituted in 1992 to address sudden infant death syndrome (SIDS).[20]

Although the sporadic nature of simple craniosynostosis makes an accurate prediction of risk difficult to ascertain, it appears that the risk doubles for future siblings if there are no other family members involved. When one parent and child are affected, the subsequent risk rises to 50%. Conversely, if both parents are unaffected and two siblings are affected, the risk for additional sibling involvement approaches 25%.[21]

More than a hundred syndromes have been associated with craniosynostosis, often marked by an autosomal dominant mode of transmission.[22] Among them, Crouzon, Apert, and Pfeiffer (Fig. 8.2) syndromes are the most frequently occurring. Syndromic synostosis is commonly associated with multiple suture closure (coronal, sagittal, etc.) combined with other systemic manifestations (Table 8.2).

GENETIC AND ETIOLOGICAL FACTORS

The etiology of craniosynostosis remains elusive because of its heterogeneous nature. Nevertheless, numerous factors are now known to promote or have been implicated in the

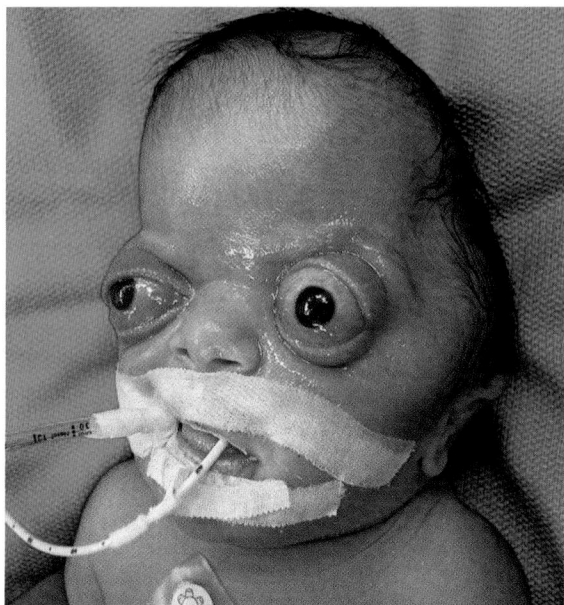

FIGURE 8.2 Newborn infant with Pfeiffer syndrome presenting with a cloverleaf skull (Kleeblattschädel) deformity. This is characterized by frontal towering, bitemporal expansion, bilateral supraorbital recession and proptosis, and midfacial hypoplasia.

TABLE 8.3 Recognized Causes of Craniosynostosis

Hematologic disorders	Thalassemias
	Sickle cell anemia
	Polycythemia vera
Teratogens	Valproic acid
	Retinoic acid
	Aminopterin
	Diphenylhydantoin
Genetic conditions	
Metabolic disorders	Rickets
	Hyperthyroidism
Mucopolysaccharidoses	Hurler syndrome
	Morquio syndrome
	Mucolipidosis III
β-Glucuronidase deficiency	
Malformations	Holoprosencephaly
	Encephalocele
	Microcephaly
	Hydrocephalus (shunted)

TABLE 8.2 Craniofacial Dysostosis Syndromes

Syndrome	Involved Suture	Morphological Presentation
Crouzon	Coronal, sagittal	Midface hypoplasia, shallow orbits, proptosis, hypertelorism
Apert	Coronal, sagittal, lambdoid, others	Midface hypoplasia, shallow orbits, proptosis, hypertelorism, *symmetrical syndactyly of hands and feet,* choanal atresia, ventriculomegaly, genitourinary/cardiovascular anomalies
Pfeiffer	Coronal, sagittal	Midface hypoplasia, proptosis, hypertelorism, *broad great toe/thumb*

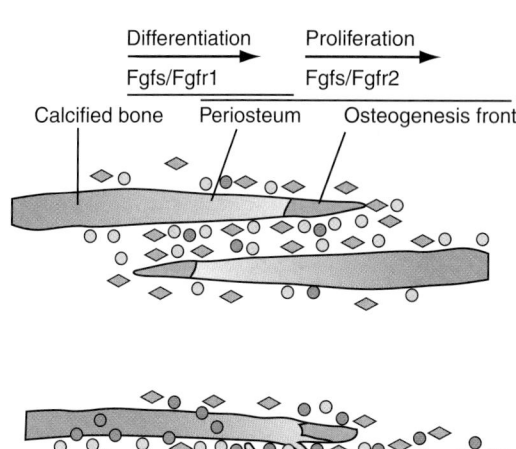

FIGURE 8.3 Normal suture growth and morphogenesis is dependent upon a delicate balance between the proliferation of osteoprogenitors within the suture mesenchyme and differentiation to osteoblasts at the osteogenic fronts. *(Adapted from Lin C, Li D, Li C, et al. A Ser250Trp substitution in mouse fibroblast growth factor receptor 2 (Fgfr2) results in craniosynostosis. Bone 2003;33:169-178, used with permission from Elsevier.)*

development of premature closure of the calvarial sutures. Multiple teratogens, genetic mutations, metabolic disorders, and blood dyscrasias have been associated with craniosynostosis (Table 8.3). Interestingly, maternal smoking has been associated with isolated craniosynostosis[23] and advanced paternal age has been found to trend with a higher frequency of metopic synostosis.[12]

With advances in molecular genetics, candidate gene mutations as well as the molecular interactions underlying cranial deformities have been elucidated.[24,25] Normal suture growth and morphogenesis is dependent upon a delicate balance between the proliferation of osteoprogenitors within the suture mesenchyme and differentiation to osteoblasts at the osteogenic fronts (Fig. 8.3).[26] It is now known that the majority of syndromic craniosynostoses are caused by mutations in genes encoding fibroblast growth factor receptors (FGFR-1, FGFR-2, and FGFR-3) and the transcription factors Twist and

MSX-2.[27-33] Moreover, these same genes are responsible for approximately 25% of all cases of craniosynostosis.[34] In general, gain-of-function mutations are associated with the *MSX2* and *FGFR* genes, while loss of function or haplo-insufficiency abnormalities are found in *TWIST* gene mutations.[35]

Genetic alterations in FGFR-1 and FGFR-2 have been implicated in Crouzon, Apert, Pfeiffer, and Jackson-Weiss syndromes.[30,36-39] FGFR-1 has been found to regulate osteoblast differentiation; therefore, a gain-of-function mutation may precipitate premature suture fusion through promotion of osteoblast differentiation and bone formation.[40] Moreover, FGFR-2 has been linked to activation of osteogenic cell apoptosis. As shown by Chen and co-workers, a gain-in-function mutation leads to increased apoptosis and results in decreased cell numbers and distance between two overlapping bones. Ultimately, this develops into physical contact of two opposing bones, eventually leading to premature closure.[41]

Alterations in growth factor receptors have also been observed in nonsyndromic craniosynostoses. FGFR-3-associated coronal synostosis, also known as Muenke-type craniosynostosis, has been identified in up to 52% of patients with nonsyndromic bicoronal synostosis,[42] either as a result of de novo mutations or associated with an autosomal dominant inheritance pattern.[43] Gripp and colleagues observed that 10.8% of patients with unilateral coronal synostosis were positive for an FGFR-3 mutation and subsequently recommended testing of all patients with unilateral coronal synostosis to assess the risk of recurrence.[44] These guidelines stem from the observation that Muenke-type craniosynostosis has been associated with a reoperation rate of at least 43%.[45]

Studies have implicated transforming growth factor-beta receptors (TGF-βR) in syndromic and intrauterine head constraint-related craniosynostosis. Loeys and co-workers have discovered a link between mutations of TGF-βR1 and TGF-βR2 and a syndrome of altered cardiovascular, craniofacial, neurocognitive, and skeletal development.[46] Hunenko and colleagues demonstrated upregulation of TGF-βR1 and TGF-βR2 in mice undergoing intrauterine constraint leading to coronal suture synostosis.[47] Such data points to the ability of mechanical forces to alter growth factor–mediated signaling during craniofacial growth and development.

In addition to the aforementioned growth factor receptors, their corresponding ligands have been found to be an integral component of calvarial osteoblast proliferation and subsequent sutural fusion. FGF2 has been shown to enhance proliferation rates in rat fetal osteoblasts, promote premature fusion of frontal sutures in calvarial organ cultures, and correlate with intrauterine constraint-related coronal suture synostosis.[47,48] Inverse patterns of TGF-β isoform expression between fusing and patent sutures have been demonstrated in animal and human models. Opperman and colleagues demonstrated declining levels of TGF-β3 but continued expression of TGF-β1 and TGF-β2 posterior frontal suture fusion.[49] Bone morphogenetic proteins (BMPs), members of the TGF-β superfamily, are involved in a broad range of developmental roles, including bone formation, skeletal patterning, and limb development. Several investigators have demonstrated the critical role of BMPs and their antagonists in dictating cranial suture biology. In particular, in situ hybridization of mouse cranial sutures localized expression of BMP-2 and BMP-4 to the osteogenic fronts and BMP-4 to suture mesenchyme and dura mater in the sagittal and posterior frontal sutures.[50] Nacamuli and co-workers found BMP-3, a bone morphogenic protein antagonist, to be decreased in normally fusing posterior frontal sutures and increased in normally patent sagittal sutures.[51]

Mutations of transcription factors have also been implicated in causing syndromic forms of craniosynostosis. Liu and co-workers linked a gain-of-function mutation in the MSX-2 transcription factor with Boston-type craniosynostosis.[52] Loss-of-function mutations in Twist proteins, transcription factors activating osteoblast differentiation, have been found to cause Saethre-Chotzen syndrome.[28] Woods and colleagues have recommended *TWIST1* mutation screening of all patients with either bicoronal or unicoronal synostosis, given that this genetic alteration confers a greater risk of recurrent intracranial hypertension and subsequent reoperation than nonsyndromic synostosis of the same sutures.[53]

ANATOMICAL AND PATHOLOGICAL CONSIDERATIONS

Skull development can be divided into neurocranium and viscerocranium formation, a process starting between 23 and 26 days of gestation. Neurocranium growth leads to cranial vault development via membranous ossification, while viscerocranium expansion leads to facial bone formation by endochondral ossification. Cranial sutures form by 16 weeks' gestation at the junction of numerous osteogenic fronts and are particularly active areas of bone formation and deposition, directly affected by underlying tension forces of brain growth and dural reflections as well as local growth factors.

The calvarium grows most rapidly during the first 12 months, with the brain doubling in volume in the first 6 months and again by the second birthday. While calvarial expansion is most pronounced during the first 2 years, growth continues in a linear fashion until the age of 6 to 7 years, at which time the cranium is 90% of the adult size. Most of this cranial growth takes place in the sutures between the bone plates. Within the center of the sutural area, a population of proliferating osteoprogenitor cells is maintained. A portion of these cells enters the pathway of osteogenic differentiation, forming bone-matrix-secreting osteoblasts at the bone edges and contributing to skull expansion.[54] Normal cranial suture closure occurs from front to back and from lateral to medial, with the metopic suture usually closing between 9 and 11 months of age[55] and the remaining sutures fusing in adulthood.

A disturbance in the balance between proliferation, differentiation, and apoptosis causes premature ossification within the suture and its synostosis.[56] Factors disturbing this balance include genetic or acquired changes in growth factor receptor/ligand profiles, loss of direct contact between dural and sutural cells, and increased external mechanical forces. As mentioned previously, many of the syndromic forms of craniosynostosis are attributed to alterations in the FGF/FGFR, TGF-β/TGF-βR, and BMP cascades. Both cerebral hypoplasia and overshunted hydrocephalus have been associated with secondary craniosynostosis, phenomena likely attributed to loss of dural contact.[55,57] Both breach positioning and twin pregnancies have been associated with intrauterine constraint-related craniosynostosis, stemming from mechanical force signal transduction.[58]

DIAGNOSTIC EVALUATION AND IMAGING

Preoperative assessment for craniosynostosis includes a detailed medical history, physical examination, and radiographic imaging. Medical history should elicit for asymmetrical calvarial deformities noted by friends or other family members, family history of calvarial deformities, and symptoms of intracranial hypertension (headache/vomiting, developmental changes, irritability, and oculomotor paresis). Physical examination should evaluate for characteristic calvarial shapes and asymmetries, premature closure of the anterior fontanelle (normally open until 12-18 months of age), perisutural ridging (calcification), and signs of intracranial hypertension (papilledema, supraorbital retrusion, severe towering, and severe frontal/occipital bossing). Routine funduscopic examination for papilledema is an accurate predictor of raised pressure in the older child but may not be 100% sensitive for the younger child (<8 years old).[59] Craniofacial asymmetries should be documented in the form of head circumferences, cranial indices, and anthropometric measurements. The history combined with the examination is often confirmatory in an experienced primary care physician/nurse or craniofacial surgeon's initial evaluation.

The role of radiological workup for craniosynostosis varies among clinicians. Currently, it is not uncommon for prenatal ultrasound to document craniosynostosis in utero.[60-63] In addition to the ultrasound evaluation, fetal magnetic resonance imaging (MRI) (Fig. 8.4) at some centers has offered significant prenatal definition.[64] Radiological investigation may be necessary to corroborate the diagnosis and rule out any associated intracranial abnormalities in the postnatal consultation period. Computed tomography (CT) studies remain the most sensitive barometer of bony fusion, as skull plain films suffer from poor sensitivity and a high false positive rate. The recent advent of three-dimensional CT (3D CT) has provided an excellent view of affected suture(s) as well as overall head shape, thereby simplifying the diagnosis and helping with surgical planning.[60,65,66] This modality is not mandatory, but rather is reserved for multiple/complicated suture pathology, confirmation of diagnosis, or demonstration of skull base pathology.

CT scans may also provide radiological evidence for raised intracranial pressure. The presence of intracranial hypertension is dependent on the number of affected sutures, ranging from approximately 14% for single-suture synostosis to approximately 47% in multiple-suture synostosis, as well as

on patient age.[2,3] Although few children will manifest clinical symptoms of increased intracranial pressure, it is not uncommon to visualize erosion of the inner calvarial table (beaten copper appearance) on CT scan. A diffuse beaten copper appearance has been associated with greater intracranial pressure, as reported by Tuite and co-workers.[67] Though it is common to see expanded subarachnoid spaces in all types of craniosynostoses, these spaces usually spontaneously resolve and are not felt to represent an increase in intracranial pressure.[68] If there is any evidence for elevated pressure, surgical consideration should be expedited. This is especially vital in patients with syndromic synostosis (e.g., Crouzon, Apert, Pfeiffer syndrome), who are at a greater risk for hydrocephalus and Chiari malformations with associated intracranial hypertension.

CT and MRI studies are also helpful in evaluating the underlying brain for any structural or functional abnormalities. Unrecognized intracranial abnormalities may exist in a small number of patients and may include hydrocephalus (more common in patients with Crouzon syndrome), partial agenesis of the corpus callosum, holoprosencephaly (seen in patients with trigonocephaly), or focal cortical dysplasias. Indeed, as reported by Boop and colleagues, up to 5% of their patients with sagittal synostoses had unappreciated underlying intracranial pathology.[69]

THERAPEUTIC CONSIDERATIONS

Surgical Indications

Correction of calvarial contour deformities and prevention of psychosocial dysfunction, intracranial hypertension, and mental retardation are the thrusts for surgical intervention in craniosynostosis. In the past, surgical intervention for simple craniosynostosis was undertaken primarily because of cosmetic and psychosocial considerations.[70,71] Recently, sutural release in simple craniosynostosis has been advised owing to the concerns regarding raised intracranial pressure as well as mild but significant developmental delay in the aging child with uncorrected single-suture synostosis.[2,3,72-74] In contrast to simple craniosynostosis, patients with complex or syndromic synostoses present with increased severity in neurological and cosmetic symptoms;[3,75-77] therefore, surgical intervention in these infants is even more imperative.

Timing of Surgery

The optimal timing for reconstructive surgery in craniosynostosis remains controversial, as the age at surgery has different effects on intraoperative hemodynamics, postoperative cranial growth, and subsequent mental development. With regard to intraoperative hemodynamics, Meyer and co-workers demonstrated that older patient age (>6 months) was associated with decreased blood loss.[78] In addition to benefiting from decreased blood loss, older infants can tolerate extensive blood loss better than younger infants. From the perspective of long-term skull growth, data are conflicting. In 1987, Whitaker demonstrated that as surgical age increased, the likelihood of secondary surgery also elevated.[79] On the other hand, Fearon and colleagues recently found that older patient

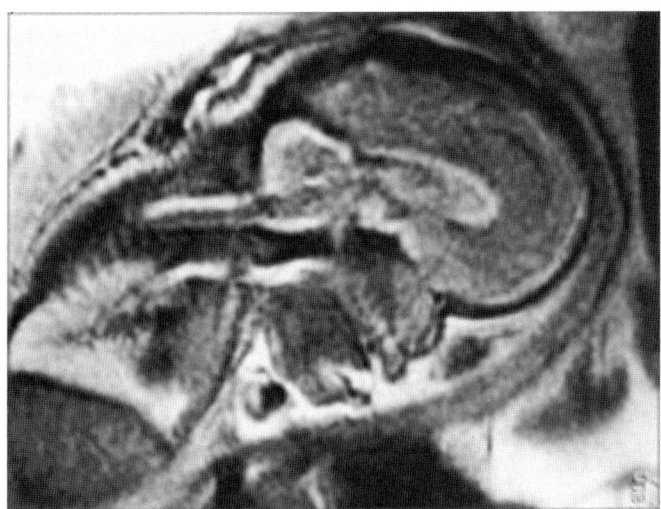

FIGURE 8.4 Sagittal MRI of a 30-week fetus with Pfeiffer syndrome depicting a cloverleaf skull, which required a near-total calvarectomy within the first week of life.

age (≥12 months) was associated with less diminished cranial growth following correction of all types of single sutural craniosynostosis.[80] These findings must be weighed against the need to fully reconstruct any advanced postoperative skull defects in children over 12 months of age, because dura will not regenerate bone as readily. From the standpoint of mental development, Arnaud and co-workers reported that postoperative mental outcome was significantly better when surgery was performed before the patient reached 12 months of age.[42]

Although the literature is inconclusive regarding the appropriate timing for correction of craniosynostosis, the majority of craniofacial surgeons operate between 3 and 12 months of age. The specific time period is dependent on the type of surgical approach used. In general, endoscopic corrections are done at an earlier age, namely, by 3 to 4 months of age. Open surgical corrections are often done later. Fearon and colleagues perform treatment at 4 months of age for sagittal synostosis and 9 months of age for all other single-suture synostoses (metopic, coronal, and lambdoid).[80] Marchac and associates reviewed their craniofacial experience with 983 patients operated on over 20 years, discussing their timing of surgical operations.[81] Children with brachycephaly underwent a floating forehead procedure between 2 and 4 months of age, infants with sagittal synostosis underwent parasagittal craniectomies between 2 and 4 months of age or a frontocranial remodeling procedure if presenting between 6 and 9 months of age, and infants with either metopic or unicoronal synostoses had a frontocranial remodeling procedure between 6 and 9 months of age.

Type of Surgery

There is a growing debate in the literature regarding the optimal type of operation for correction of craniosynostosis. An open craniofacial approach was proposed as early as 1890, with Lannelogue advocating early open surgical release of a fused suture to prevent intracranial hypertension.[82] Building on the principles of Lannelogue, a number of centers have reported their large-volume experience with open cranial vault remodeling procedures for all types of craniosynostoses.[79,80,83-87] In 421 intracranial operations with movement of one or both orbits, Whitaker and co-workers in 1979 reported a 2.2% rate of mortality, 6.2% rate of infection, and 2.2% frequency of CSF leak.[85] With increased experience and refinement in technique, Whitaker and colleagues reported a 0% mortality rate, 3.7% infection rate, and 1.2% CSF leak rate in a 1987 report of 164 open craniofacial procedures for craniosynostosis.[79] Regarding longevity of the open craniofacial procedure, McCarthy and associates identified a 13.5% rate of reoperation for simple craniosynostoses and 36.8% revision rate for complex craniosynostoses during a 20-year experience.[86,87] Reoperation rates have also decreased with experience and refinement of open surgical technique, with Sloan and co-workers reporting a 7.2% overall rate of reoperation in 250 patients and Fearon and associates noting a 2% rate of revision in 248 cases of simple craniosynostosis.[80,84]

To address concerns regarding the extent of incision length, operative blood loss, and length of stay for open craniofacial procedures, minimally invasive techniques that rely on dynamic cranial vault alteration have been proposed. Techniques include endoscopic sutural release, spring-assisted

cranioplasty, and distraction osteogenesis. A brief overview of each of these evolving techniques follows.

Endoscopic Craniosynostosis Correction

Jimenez and Barone pioneered endoscopic sutural release in the mid-1990s,[88-94] and it has been used by increasing numbers of surgeons who treat craniosynostosis. In general, the idea is to perform a minimally invasive strip craniectomy of the fused suture at an early age. The child then wears a cranial molding helmet, which slowly corrects the deformity over several months.

For coronal (Fig. 8.5) or metopic craniosynostosis, the child is positioned supine. One small incision is used to access the fused suture. A burr hole is drilled, and an endoscope is used to separate the dura from the overlying bone. Bone-cutting scissors are then used to cut out the fused suture. Irrigation and Gelfoam are used for hemostasis, and the incision is closed.

For sagittal craniosynostosis, the child is positioned prone. Two small incisions are used on either side of the fused suture in the midline. A burr hole is drilled through each suture, and an endoscope is used to separate the dura of the superior sagittal sinus from the overlying bone. Bone-cutting scissors are then used to remove the fused sagittal suture. Gelfoam is placed over the superior sagittal sinus, and both incisions are closed.

Postoperatively, patients are placed in orthotic helmets for 7 to 12 months to facilitate dynamic cranial vault alteration. Summarizing the data from studies by Jimenez and Barone,[88-94] average age at operation is between 3 and 4 months, mean operating time centers around 60 minutes, average estimated blood loss is approximately 30 mL or approximately 5% estimated blood volume (EBV), transfusion rate hovers around 10%, average length of stay is generally 1 day, and complication rates range from 0% to 6%. These numbers are far lower than the blood loss of 25% to 500% of EBV, blood transfusion volume of 25% to 500% of EBV, and 4- to 7-day length of stay associated with open craniofacial techniques.[93] MacKinnon and co-workers also found that children treated with endoscopic repair of unicoronal craniosynostosis may have less severe eye findings, such as V-pattern strabismus, than children treated with fronto-orbital advancement at a later age.[95]

There has been a lot of enthusiasm for this technique in recent years, and many parents prefer the less invasive approach to the traditional open surgical approaches. Because this technique is relatively new, many centers are still compiling their results. Although early data look promising, more long-term data will be needed.

Spring-Assisted Cranioplasty

Spring-assisted cranioplasty was first undertaken on human subjects by Lauritzen in 1997, based upon success in the rabbit model by Persing and co-workers.[96,97] This technique relies on a standard open access incision, osteotomies at the sites of stenosed sutures, placement of omega-shaped tension springs across the osteotomy sites, and possible placement of compressive springs along areas of compensatory growth (Fig. 8.6). Implantable springs are typically removed 4 to 7 months

FIGURE 8.5 Endoscopic sutural release for right unicoronal synostosis. **A,** Placement of a small incision behind the hairline, over the stenosed coronal suture. **B,** Subgaleal dissection aided with the use of a lighted retractor and fine needle electrocautery. **C,** Use of a pediatric burr to create a cranial opening for passage of an endoscope, allowing dissection of the stenosed suture away from the underlying dura. **D,** Bone-cutting scissors are used to facilitate the osteotomy, extending from the incision toward the pterion. *(Reprinted from Barone CM, Jimenez DF. Endoscopic approach to coronal craniosynostosis. Clin Plast Surg 2004;31:415-222, used with permission from Elsevier.)*

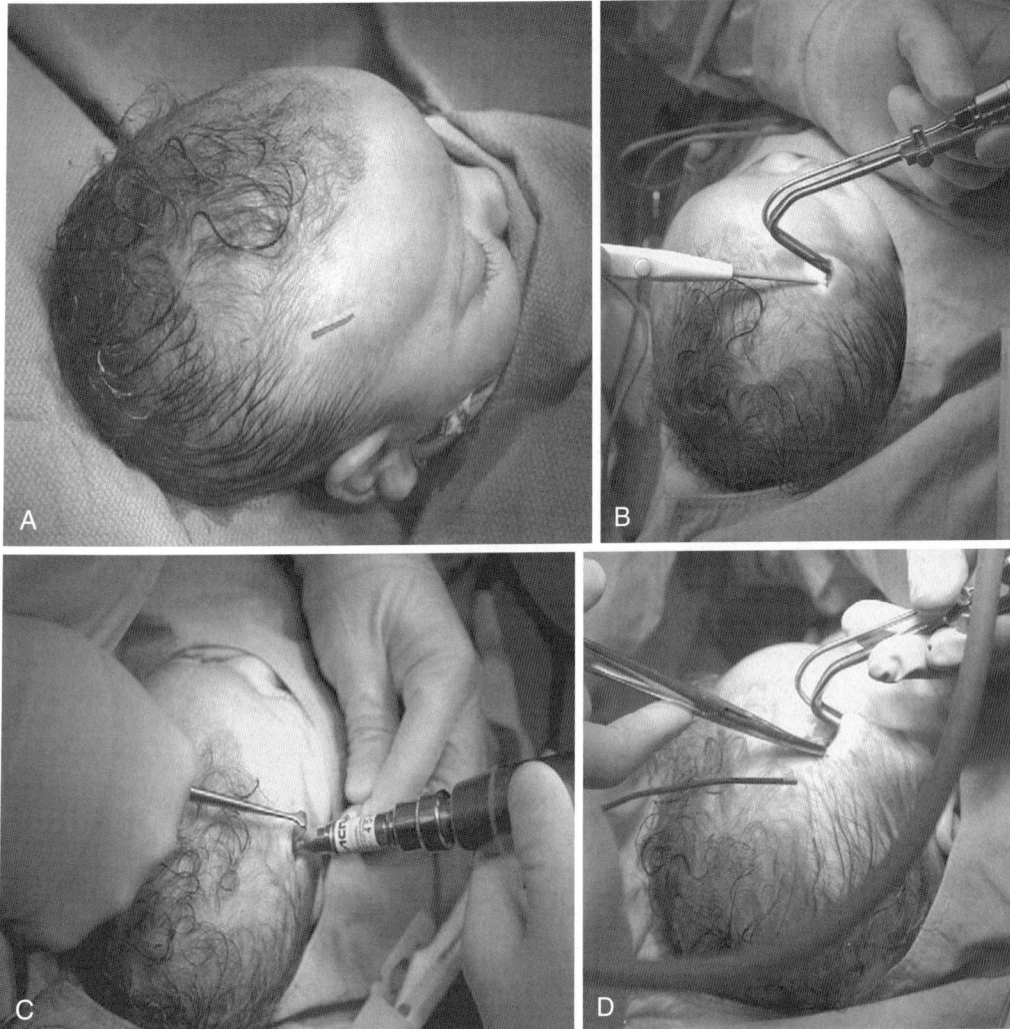

postoperatively. In 2008, Lauritzen and co-workers reported their large-volume experience with spring-assisted cranioplasty for all forms of craniofacial surgery.[98] Results included an average operative time of 97 to 215 minutes, mean blood loss ranging from 143 to 503 mL, average length of stay between 5 and 6 days, mean cephalic index of 74 in scaphocephalic infants 6 months following cranioplasty, 6% reoperation rate, 3% rate of intracranial hypertension secondary to compressive springs, and a 0% mortality rate. On the heels of this study, David and co-workers reported their experience with the first 75 spring-assisted surgeries for scaphocephaly.[99] With a mean follow-up period of 46 months, mean cephalic index was 75.4, which is comparable to patients with open cranial vault reconstruction and was maintained at 3- and 5-year follow-ups. Optimism with this emerging modality must be balanced against the need for a second operation for spring removal as well as the lack of control of spring action.

Distraction Osteogenesis

Along the lines of spring-assisted cranioplasty, distraction osteogenesis has been investigated for the treatment of craniosynostosis. This method entails a standard open access incision, osteotomies at the sites of stenosed sutures, and placement of internal versus external distraction devices (Fig. 8.7). After a latency period of 3 to 5 days, the devices are activated for a number of weeks until desired expansion and then followed by a 2- to 3-week consolidation period. Given that appraisal of this technique has been limited to the setting of small case reports,[100-112] its safety and efficacy cannot be commented upon at this time.

Given the senior author's extensive experience with open craniofacial reconstruction for craniosynostosis, operative steps and surgical outcomes shall be described for this type of surgery in the accompanying sections on different types of craniosynostoses.

CLINICAL PRESENTATION/ THERAPEUTIC CONSIDERATIONS

Metopic Synostosis (Trigonocephaly)

Clinical Features

Metopic synostosis is often accompanied with a variable degree of phenotypic severity. Patients may present with mild ridging of the metopic suture, unaccompanied by other

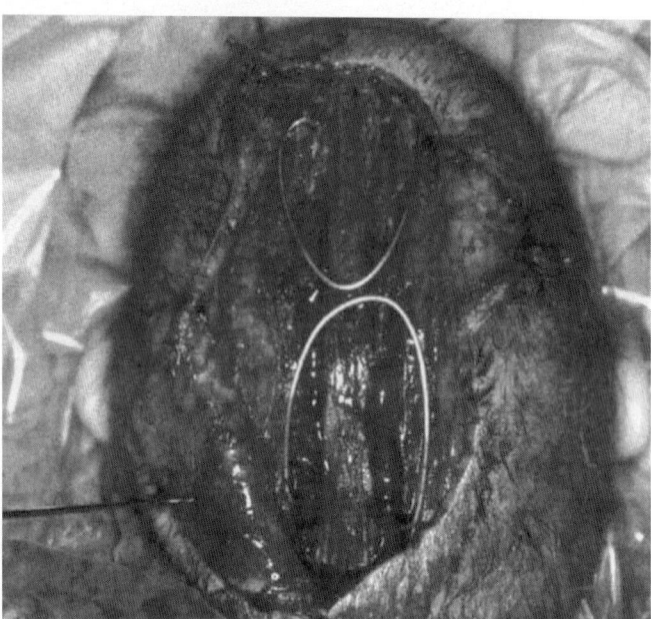

FIGURE 8.6 Spring-assisted cranioplasty for sagittal synostosis. Note the placement of two omega-shaped tension springs across the sagittal synostectomy defect. (*Reprinted from Guimaraes-Ferreira J, Gewalli F, David L, et al. Spring-mediated cranioplasty compared with the modified pi-plasty for sagittal synostosis. Scand J Plast Reconstr Surg Hand Surg 2003;37:208-215, used with permission from Taylor & Francis Group.*)

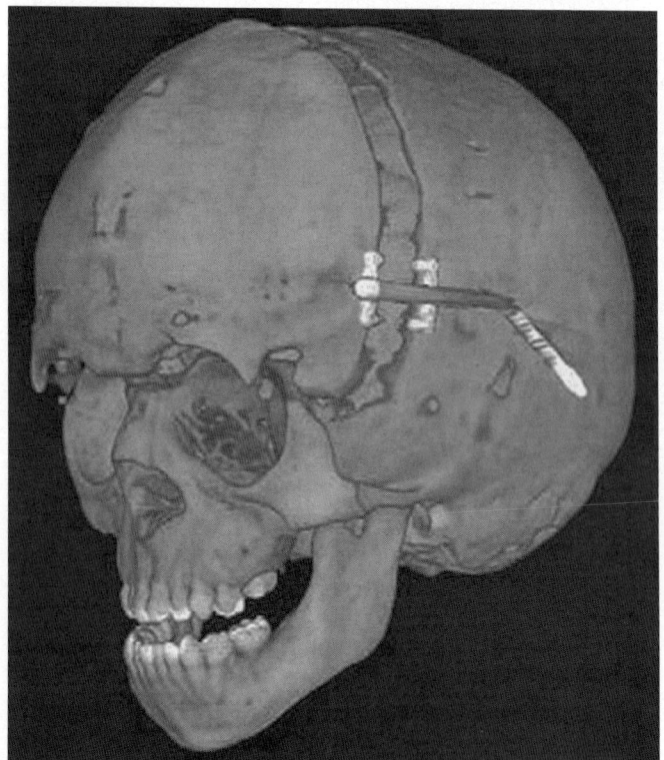

FIGURE 8.7 Three-dimensional computed tomography image showing placement of single-vector, internal distraction devices across a one-piece fronto-orbital osteotomy. (*Reprinted from Choi JW, Koh KS, Hong JP, et al. One-piece frontoorbital advancement with distraction but without a supraorbital bar for coronal craniosynostosis, J Plast Reconstr Aesthet Surg 2009;62:1166-1173, used with permission from Elsevier.*)

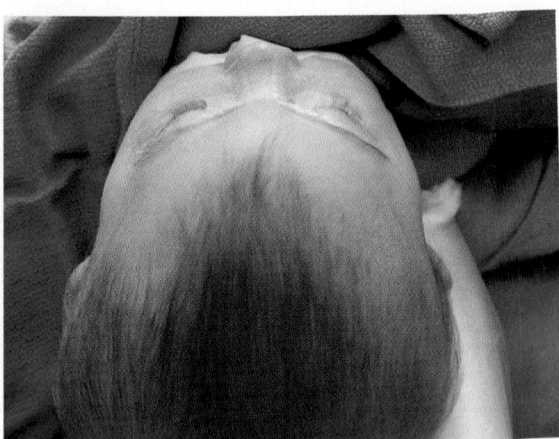

FIGURE 8.8 Aerial view of a 6-month-old infant with trigonocephaly, manifesting significant ridging over the midline (metopic suture) as well as supraorbital recession and hypotelorism.

manifestations. Premature closure of the metopic suture may also lead to the formation of a triangular head, otherwise known as *trigonocephaly*. On the severe end of the spectrum, patients may present with a prominent "keel" forehead accompanied by recession of the lateral orbital rims, hypotelorism, and constriction of the anterior frontal fossa (Fig. 8.8).

Among the nonsyndromic craniosynostoses, metopic synostosis is most associated with chromosomal abnormalities, other brain malformations, and cognitive/behavioral dysfunction. Mild variants of metopic synostosis have been recently associated with abnormalities of chromosomes 3, 9, and 11.[113-115] In addition, Tubbs and co-workers found a 30% incidence of type I Chiari malformations in the evaluation of patients with simple metopic ridges and postulated that these children were at greater risk secondary to the diminished anterior cranial volume.[116] At the other end of the spectrum, severe cases of metopic synostosis have been associated with underlying frontal brain dysmorphology as well as other congenital anomalies.[117]

Metopic synostosis has also been associated with neurodevelopmental delay, with reported deficits ranging from modest to severe. Historically, metopic synostosis had been considered the form of single-suture synostosis with the highest degree of neuropsychological morbidity.[118] Although Becker and co-workers confirmed a high prevalence of speech, cognitive, and behavioral abnormalities in patients with metopic synostosis, reported as 57%, they observed no differences in the degree of neuropsychological morbidity between different forms of single-suture synostoses.[119] More recently, however, studies have concluded a modest to no delay in neurodevelopment.[120,121] Da Costa and co-workers found that children with nonsyndromic craniosynostoses did not display obvious evidence of intellectual dysfunction, with mean intelligence quotients within the normal range. In 2007, Speltz and colleagues demonstrated a modest but reliable neurodevelopmental delay in children with all forms of single-suture synostoses in comparison to case-matched control subjects.[121] Similar to Becker's study, they found no difference in the extent of neuropsychological morbidity between different types of single-suture synostoses.[119,121]

FIGURE 8.9 A, Axial computed tomography (CT) scan depicting increased bone thickness over the midline at the region of the metopic suture as well as a narrowed interorbital distance, consistent with hypotelorism. **B,** Three-dimensional view clearly demonstrates the fusion of the metopic suture as well as trigonocephaly.

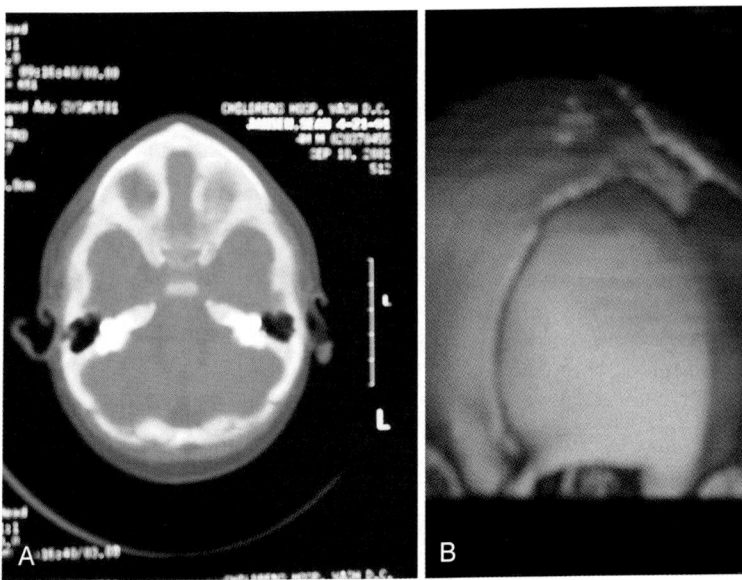

Radiological Evaluation

Radiographic imaging by plain skull radiographs may demonstrate a hyperostotic, midline metopic suture in addition to hypoteloric orbits in severe examples of trigonocephaly. Nevertheless, definitive diagnosis is best made by CT, which will offer better bone definition while also evaluating the cerebral parenchyma (Fig. 8.9). Frontal dysmorphology is most commonly seen in this type of craniosynostosis and may consist of corpus callosum dysgenesis, holoprosencephaly, and other frontal dysembryogeneses. Patients suspected of harboring a Chiari malformation are best served by an MRI, although CT scans with low cuts through the posterior fossa may also demonstrate a crowded foramen magnum as a result of tonsillar herniation.

Surgical Therapeutics

Delashaw and colleagues proposed that metopic synostosis and trigonocephaly represent an embryological continuum, directing their surgical approach based on the severity of the frontal calvarial deformities.[122] In general, the goals of surgery are the normalization of the forehead with reconstitution of a normal supraorbital rim if necessary.[123-129] Individuals presenting solely with a prominent midline keel may be best served by simple contouring of the frontal bone or by removal of the frontal bone flap followed by reconfiguration. These children otherwise demonstrate normal orbital and supraorbital anatomy. Conversely, patients with significant trigonocephaly and hypotelorism will require a fronto-orbital reconstruction, recontouring the frontal bone and laterally expanding the orbits at the same time. Evolution of surgical technique has included more radical treatment of the involved sphenoid bone with simultaneous correction of the hypotelorism.[130-132]

The essentials of fronto-orbital reconstruction involve a standard bicoronal incision, which will provide adequate exposure of the fronto-orbital region while minimizing any postoperative scar. Perioperative antibiotics (cefazolin 10-20 mg/kg loading dose, 8 mg/kg intravenously every 8 hours for 48 hours) [...] mg/kg intravenous every

6 hours for 48 hours) are given. Prior to the start of surgery, bilateral tarsorrhaphies are undertaken. The incision is infiltrated with 0.5% lidocaine and 1:400,000 parts epinephrine to minimize intraoperative bleeding. The frontal and temporal regions are dissected in the subgaleal plane leaving the periosteum intact on the surface of the bone which also helps to minimize bleeding (Fig. 8.10A). The dissection is taken down to the level of the periorbital tissues, taking care to avoid any injury to the underlying globes. Following exposure of the frontal and orbital regions, the frontal bone is removed, providing access to the intracranial compartment (Fig. 8.10B). The supraorbital rim is then removed in one piece to facilitate reconstruction of the previously triangular supraorbital bar. Care is taken to remove sufficient bone in the region of the sphenoid bone to allow for growth at the midface and orbits (Fig. 8.10C). If the orbits require correction of hypotelorism, it will be necessary to displace the lateral walls of the orbit as well as to split the midline and interpose a calvarial bone graft. Reconfiguration of the supraorbital bar often requires a midline osteotomy to facilitate a flattened forehead with additional partial-thickness bone cuts at the lateral (pterional) angle to promote normalization of the lateral supraorbital angle (Fig. 8.10D and E). The supraorbital reconfiguration is maintained by the utilization of intervening bone grafts as well as absorbable hardware (Fig. 8.10F). Following placement of the supraorbital bar as a foundation (Fig. 8.10G), the frontal bone is reconstructed using the remaining portions of bone. It is often possible to reverse the original frontal bone flap (posterior portion now in an anterior position) to obtain an adequate width and contour with the new frontal bone flap. It is important to provide an adequate enhancement at the pterional region to avoid long-term supratemporal hollowing or recession. Reconstruction is facilitated with absorbable hardware, as permanent hardware has been associated with transcranial migration (Fig. 8.10H).

Outcome and Complications

Following fronto-orbital reconstruction for metopic synostosis, the long-term outcome is generally excellent for more than 90% of patients unless there are manifestations of syndromic overlay.[80,83,123,133-137] Recently, Pearson and co-workers reported a 7% rate of reoperation and Fearon and colleagues reported a 2.5% rate of revision in infants treated for metopic synostoses.[80,83] Additional surgery may be needed in children who initially do well but subsequently develop new metopic ridging, progressive frontal towering, or continued laterosuperior fronto-orbital restriction.[138] It has also been the author's experience to witness the subsequent development of additional sutural stenosis (sites other than the metopic suture) despite the lack of suture fusion or sclerosis at the time of the initial CT scan.

Surgical morbidity rate remains low for patients undergoing fronto-orbital reconstruction with wound infections, CSF leaks, post-traumatic encephaloceles (Fig. 8.11), and orbital/neural injuries being relatively uncommon events. Intraoperative blood loss and transfusion requirements, leading to hemodynamic instability, constitute greater dangers to the patient and should never be underestimated. Studies have reported blood loss ranging from 19% to 58% of EBV and blood transfusion volumes of approximately 34% of EBV.[139-142] It is imperative to accurately gauge the extent of blood loss and match accordingly with packed red blood cells.

Sagittal Synostosis (Scaphocephaly, Dolichocephaly)

Clinical Features

Children with sagittal synostosis will present with a narrow, elongated skull (*dolichocephaly*—long-headedness, *scaphocephaly*—boat-shaped). Perisutural ridging is often observed in addition to

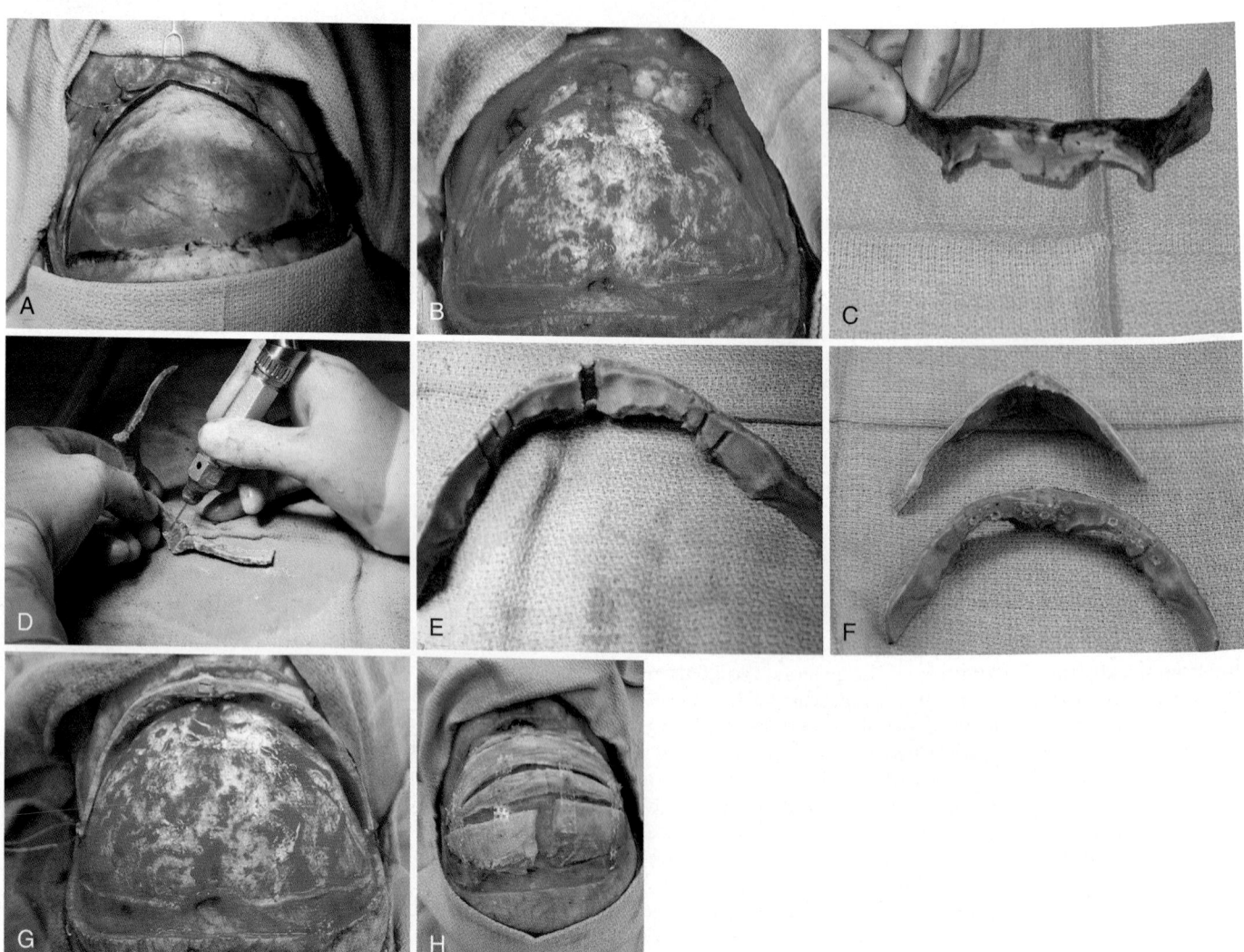

FIGURE 8.10 **A,** Subgaleal dissection exposing a triangular-shaped frontal bone with synostosis of the metopic suture. **B,** Removal of the frontal bone flap demonstrating significant hypotelorism and restricted frontal development. **C,** Removal of the supraorbital bandeau. **D,** Partial osteotomies in the midline and at the lateral wings to facilitate reconfiguration. **E,** Midline placement of a small bone graft coupled with lateral partial osteotomies for correction of hypotelorism and supraorbital recession, respectively. **F,** Resorbable hardware placed on the internal surface to maintain the final configuration. **G,** Securing the orbital bandeau in the midline and lateral regions with resorbable hardware. Note the degree of supraorbital advancement at the frontolateral dural margins. **H,** Filling the remaining defects with reconfigured frontal bone and calvarial bone grafts to ensure a satisfactory frontal contour while avoiding increased towering. Frontal recon... facilitated by the utilization of resorbable hardware.

premature or occasionally delayed closure of the anterior fontanelle. Depending upon the region of greatest premature fusion of the sagittal suture, the child may manifest frontal or occipital bossing, or a combination of both (Fig. 8.12). Some children will also demonstrate a "towering" skull, also known as *turricephaly,* which may be a harbinger of intracranial hypertension (see earlier section on Diagnostic Evaluation and Imaging).

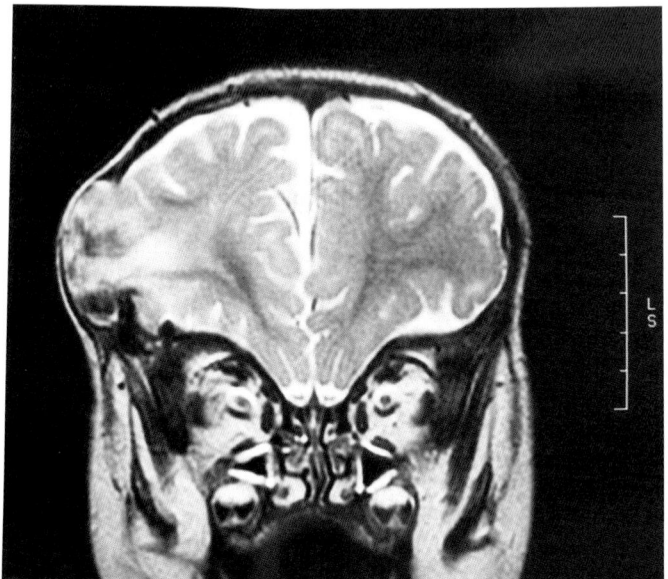

FIGURE 8.11 Coronal magnetic resonance imaging (MRI) scan demonstrating the presence of a right leptomeningeal cyst in a 26-month-old male presenting with right frontal swelling and seizures. Patient had undergone a subtotal calvarial reconfiguration, which was complicated by numerous postoperative episodes of head banging. The cyst was corrected with a dural repair and split-calvarial graft.

The presence of neurodevelopmental delay in children with sagittal synostosis remains debated. In a critical review of 17 historical studies, Speltz and co-workers concluded that isolated craniosynostosis was associated with a three- to five-fold increase in risk for cognitive deficits or learning/language disabilities.[143] Becker and colleagues reported a 39% rate of speech, cognitive, and behavioral abnormalities in patients with sagittal synostosis, which trended as the lowest rate of neuropsychological morbidity for single-suture synostoses.[119] More recently, however, studies have concluded a modest to no delay in neurodevelopment for all forms of single-suture synostoses.[120,121]

Radiological Evaluation

Although radiological workup often starts in the office of the pediatrician with skull plain films, the physical examination is frequently sufficient. The yield on plain films may be poor, although good-quality films will demonstrate fusion or ridging of the sagittal suture. Occasionally, concurrent premature fusion of the coronal or lambdoid suture or manifestations of increased intracranial pressure (e.g., digital markings) will be seen.

All patients identified as requiring surgical correction benefit from a preoperative CT scan. A subset of patients may demonstrate scaphocephaly, with an otherwise normal radiographic workup. It has been postulated that these children have "sticky sutures" secondary to microspicules of bone in the involved suture, inhibiting normal growth and development of the calvarium.[144] Nevertheless, these children exhibit similar morphological characteristics to those with clear-cut fusion and may benefit from calvarial reconfiguration in severe examples.

Three-dimensional CT may offer a more accurate depiction of the state of sutural fusion. Unanticipated intracranial pathology is seen in 5% or more of patients with sagittal synostosis,[145] including hydrocephalus, agenesis of the corpus

FIGURE 8.12 A, Lateral view of a 4-month-old male infant demonstrating frontal bossing in the setting of scaphocephaly. **B,** Aerial view highlighting the elongated skull shape as well as the marked frontal and occipital bossing.

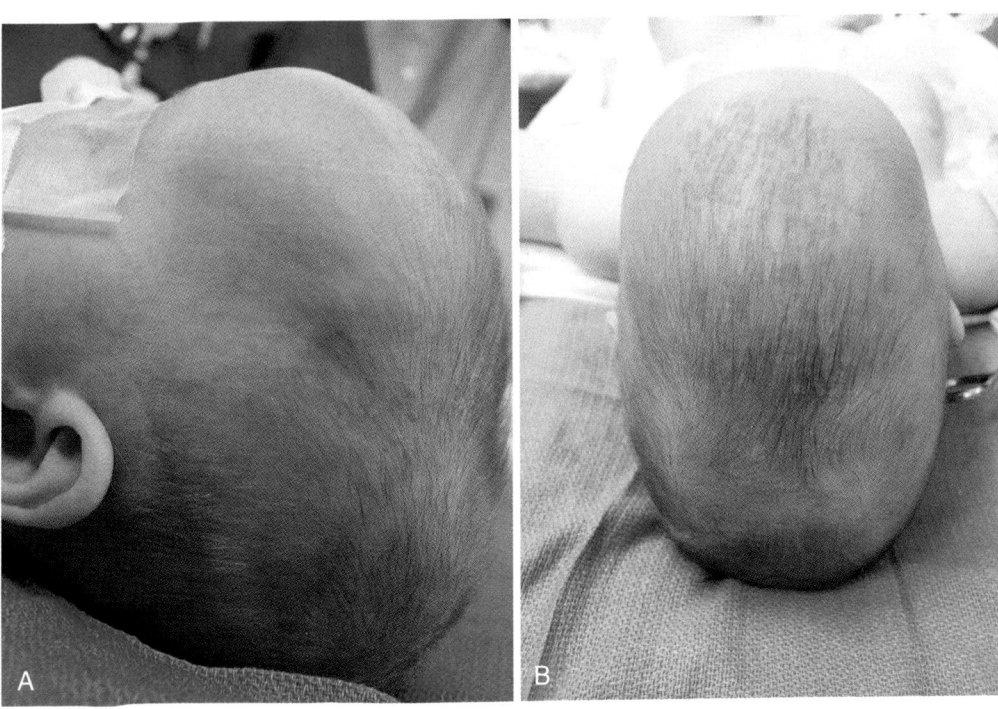

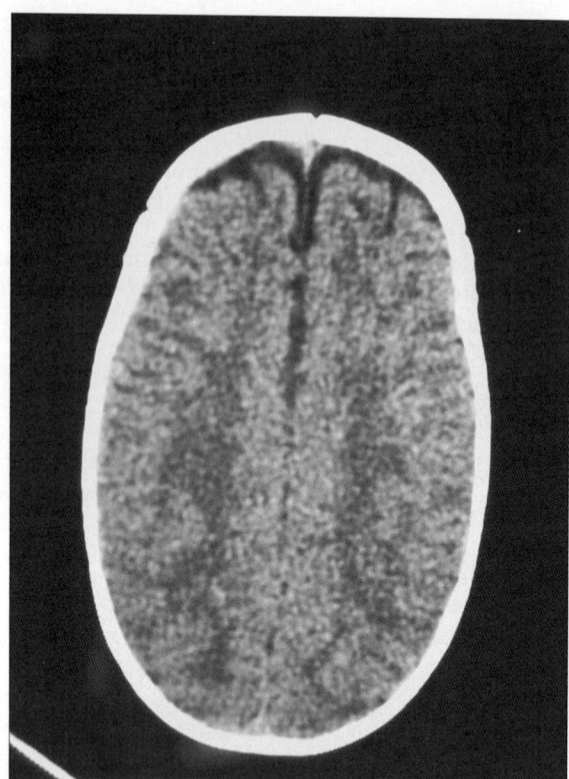

FIGURE 8.13 Axial computed tomography (CT) scan of a 6-month-old male infant with sagittal synostosis, demonstrating skull elongation and expansion of bifrontal subarachnoid spaces.

callosum, and focal cortical dysplasia. In addition, expanded subarachnoid spaces, often bifrontal, are commonly seen in patients with sagittal synostosis (Fig. 8.13).[67,140] Typically, this will resolve spontaneously and does not reflect increased intracranial pressure.

Surgical Therapeutics

The treatment for sagittal synostosis has changed considerably over the past century, with surgical approaches evolving from minimal removal of involved suture and bone[82,146] to extensive total calvarectomy.[147-151] Despite relative long-term experience and numerous publications, the optimal timing for surgery as well as the extent of bony resection and need for extensive reconstruction remain contested. These issues are especially difficult to answer, given that the extent of calvarial resection and reconfiguration can sometimes be a function of the age at presentation.

A minimalist approach was taken early in the history of reconstructive surgery for sagittal synostosis. In 1892, Lane advocated the simple removal of the pathological sagittal suture, referred to as *simple synostectomy* or *single strip craniectomy*.[146] Shillito and Matson in 1968 and Hunter and Rudd in 1976 revisited the idea of single strip craniectomy for this deformity.[118,152] The general conclusions were that the technique is safe and well tolerated, providing adequate cosmetic results in select patients with mild deformities under the age of 2 to 3 months. Simple synostectomy, however, has several disadvantages stemming from the fact that it strictly addresses the fused suture and not the compensatory changes in skull shape. Specifically, it does not provide immediate or long-term cosmetic improvement in the majority of patients, by failing to shorten the anteroposterior dimension of the skull or address frontal bossing. It also leaves a large unprotected area over the vertex of the skull, an area with a high rate of restenosis and renewed growth restriction.[153-156]

In an effort to provide more immediate restoration of normal skull contour, extended strip craniectomy procedures were proposed.[69,156-160] Venes and Sayers[160] and Albright[157] described occipitoparietal extension craniectomies as a means of shortening the anteroposterior dimension, expanding the biparietal dimension, and addressing the frontal and occipital prominences.[155,156] Immediate cosmetic improvement was secured at the expense of large calvarial defects.

Striving to maintain the advantages of other extended strip craniectomies while simultaneously eliminating the disadvantage of postoperative calvarial defects, Jane and associates reported an extended strip craniectomy in the design of the Greek letter pi (π).[158] The pi procedure has become a widely utilized approach for older infants (3-12 months of age) with scaphocephaly. Although multiple modifications with this approach have been proposed, including 12 different variations suggested by Jane depending upon the patient's clinical presentation,[161] the essential steps involve removal of bone along both sides of the sagittal suture as well as over the coronal suture (or lambdoid for the reverse pi) (Fig. 8.14). Cranial bone overlying the sagittal sinus is left intact to minimize bleeding.

To address older infants (>9-12 months of age) as well as those children with significant frontal or occipital prominence, procedures with more aggressive craniectomies and reconstruction have been proposed. In children beyond the period of maximal cerebral growth (>12-18 months of age), correction of the cephalic index will require substantial realignment of the calvarium and skull base. In the setting of significant pathology at the skull base, as proposed by Moss,[162,163] many believe that a larger procedure should be undertaken to provide optimal surgical correction as well as avoiding potential recurrence. To accomplish these goals, a number of different approaches have been reported, ranging from variations of the pi procedure with wider or additional craniectomies over the lambdoid or coronal suture to total calvarial reconfiguration.

Total calvarectomy and reconstruction in the setting of severe or late presentation scaphocephaly has been proposed to offer superior cosmetic results with a minimal increase in morbidity.[147-151,164,165] This may be accomplished by removal of the frontal, occipital, and both parietal bones. Subsequently, reconfiguration is carried out and aimed at providing a shortened anteroposterior dimension in addition to a widened biparietal diameter (Fig. 8.15). The use of rigid fixation is indispensable in these cases, providing greater three-dimensional conformational stability and decreased intraoperative time, bleeding, and postoperative infection. Although questions regarding transcranial migration of permanent titanium hardware have been raised in the developing infant, there is less controversy in the older patients undergoing total calvarial reconstruction. In addition, the introduction and increasing use of absorbable plates and screws has mitigated concerns regarding transcranial migration and inhibition of calvarial growth.

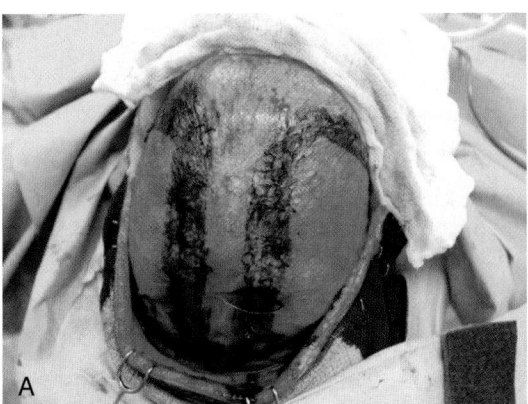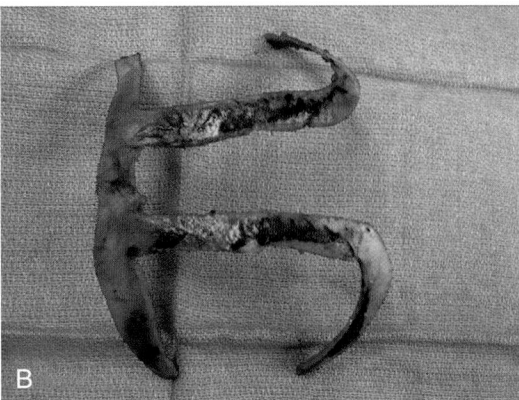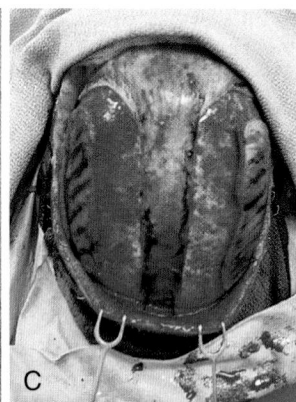

FIGURE 8.14 A 4-month-old infant undergoing a modified pi procedure. **A,** Methylene blue marks out the extended strip craniectomy, which begins posterior to the coronal sutures, runs along both sides of the sagittal suture, and ends anterior to the lambdoid sutures. **B,** The removed bone has the appearance of the Greek symbol pi, hence the name of the procedure. **C,** The remaining bone in the midline is then brought forward with two sutures, effectively shortening the anteroposterior length, widening the biparietal diameter, and thus improving the cephalic index.

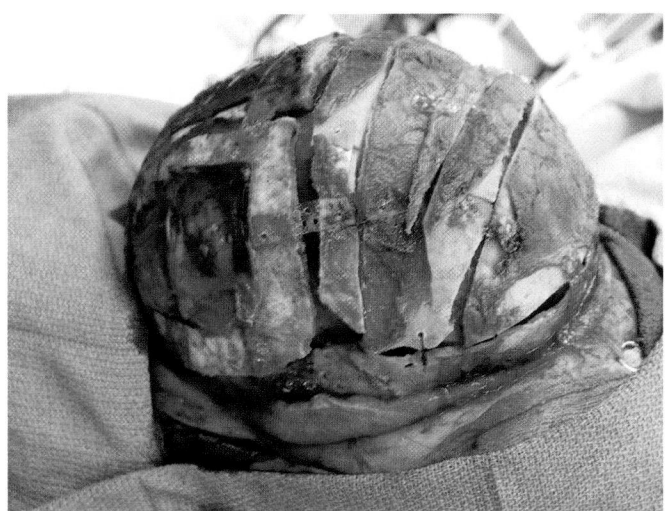

FIGURE 8.15 Lateral view of a subtotal calvarial reconfiguration in an older child with scaphocephaly. Surgical objectives include widening of the biparietal diameter and correction of frontal/occipital bossing, which is stabilized with resorbable hardware.

The patient presenting in a delayed fashion (after the age of 18-24 months) merits special consideration. Despite the lack of initial concern over the head shape, the significant calvarial deformity may become readily apparent as the child encounters greater social interaction through preschool, day care, or even later in kindergarten[71,73,166] In addition to the myriad number of psychosocial issues, a subset of individuals may also harbor elevated intracranial pressure.[3,59,167-170] Older children with significant scaphocephaly, often accompanied by both frontal and occipital bossing in association with midvertex depression, should be evaluated closely for any evidence of intracranial hypertension (see earlier section on Diagnostic Evaluation and Imaging).

The absence of any of the aforementioned signs or symptoms of intracranial hypertension does not preclude the possibility of intracranial hypertension. It has been the senior author's experience to observe significant elevations in intracranial pressure in patients with a paucity of clinical findings. Therefore, the senior author currently monitors older children undergoing repair of their scaphocephaly if there is any evidence (even subtle) for elevated intracranial pressure. Intracranial pressure is monitored via a ventriculostomy and CSF is actively drained during calvarial reconfiguration to protect the brain from transient elevations in pressure. At the surgical conclusion, if intracranial pressures are normal (or have returned to a normal baseline), the ventriculostomy is removed prior to closure. In the event of uncertainty regarding persistently elevated intracranial pressure or when the diagnosis of hydrocephalus remains unclear, the ventricular drain may be left in place for postoperative monitoring.

Outcome and Complications

Studies have compared outcomes following different types of open craniofacial surgery for sagittal synostosis, with the consensus being improved quantitative and qualitative morphological results with the more extensive procedures.[154,164,171,172] Reported cranial indices have been in the range of 71 to 73 for simple strip craniectomy,[11,164] 71 to 79 for extended strip craniectomy,[164,171] and 74 to 78.5 for subtotal/total calvarial remodeling.[148,149,164,171] Qualitatively, Kaiser found that extended strip craniectomy had an 83% rate of correction of cranial index, whereas simple strip craniectomy only has a 43% correction rate.[171] Maugans and co-workers found the cosmetic outcomes of total calvarial reconstruction to be superior to strip craniectomy, with 79% in the calvarial remodeling group rated as excellent as opposed to 41% in the strip craniectomy group. Additionally, they commented that two patients required a second operation for poor cosmetic results with the strip craniectomy.[172]

Concerns regarding increased morbidity and mortality rates for more extensive procedures have been alleviated by the favorable outcomes data from several large series. Boop and co-workers reported three simple dural lacerations following 85 cases of the pi procedure,[69] and Kanev and Lo described 65 cases without incident.[159] Greensmith and co-workers found a 3.3% rate of major complications (one air embolus) and 10% rate of minor complications (one hematoma and two prominent wires) following total cranial vault remodeling.[148] Nevertheless, the more extensive procedures do require larger blood transfusions and a longer hospital stay. Mean intraoperative blood transfusion volumes have been reported in the range of 85 to 120 mL for extended strip craniectomies,[153,173] 159 mL for subtotal calvarial reconfiguration,[174] and 460 to 485 mL for total cranial vault remodeling.[148,150] Contemporary average lengths of stay have included 3.7 to 5.6 days for extended strip craniectomies,[69] 2.8 to 8.9 days for subtotal calvarial reconfiguration[174,175] and 5 days for total cranial vault remodeling.[150]

Coronal Synostosis (Anterior Plagiocephaly/ Brachycephaly)

Clinical Features

Patients with unicoronal synostosis present with anterior, or frontal, plagiocephaly whereas those with bilateral coronal involvement display brachycephaly. Anterior plagiocephaly shows a predilection for right-sided pathology, with approximately a 3:2 ratio comparing right to left coronal involvement.[11] Phenotypic features of anterior plagiocephaly include ipsilateral perisutural ridging, forehead flattening, and orbital recession, coupled with contralateral compensatory frontal bossing (Fig. 8.16). Facial deformities are also common, including nasal root displacement toward the ipsilateral side, anterior displacement of the ipsilateral ear, and chin deviation toward the contralateral side. Pathognomonic for unicoronal synostosis, elevation of the ipsilateral orbit can be seen secondary to superior displacement of the greater wing of the sphenoid, also known as the "harlequin" appearance. The presence of strabismus is common (50-60%), stemming from superior oblique muscle dysfunction as a result of skull base shortening in the anteroposterior direction with concomitant displacement of the orbital roof and trochlea.[176,177] Although correction of the plagiocephaly occasionally improves the strabismus, surgery is frequently needed for ultimate correction. Interestingly, left-handedness recently has been shown to be three times more common in patients with anterior plagiocephaly than control subjects and four times more likely with left-sided fusion.[178]

Phenotypic features of brachycephaly include forehead retrusion and flattening, frontal towering, and biparietal widening. The nasal dorsum can be low and hypertelorism may be present. Temporal bulging may be prominent in Muenke-type bicoronal synostosis.[179] The presence of a named syndrome can be frequently seen, with an incidence reported as high as 57.1% by Sloan and co-workers.[84] Other features that may be associated with bicoronal synostosis include brachydactyly, sensorineural hearing loss, and developmental delay.

Neurodevelopmentally, children with unicoronal and bicoronal synostoses have been associated with varying degrees of functional delay, ranging from minimal to severe.[42,119,120,166,180] Becker and co-workers found 52% to 61% of patients with unicoronal and 55% of patients with bicoronal synostosis to demonstrate abnormalities in speech-language, cognitive, or behavioral function.[119] In contrast, Speltz and colleagues discovered only a modest neurodevelopmental delay in cognitive and motor skills in patients with unicoronal synostosis.[121] Along those lines, Arnaud and co-workers observed a mean preoperative intelligence quotient (IQ) of 95 and postoperative IQ of 97 in children with nonsyndromic brachycephaly, both scores falling within the "normal" range based on normative standards.[42]

Radiological Evaluation

Radiological imaging, such as CT scans and MRI, serve to confirm fusion of the affected sutures, identify coexisting abnormalities, and help visualize the extent of craniofacial bony disease. Associated abnormalities may include Arnold-Chiari malformations and hydrocephalus, more common in syndromic brachycephaly than in nonsyndromic anterior plagiocephaly. As for other synostoses, plain skull radiographs have high false positive and false negative rates and are of limited value.

Surgical Therapeutics

Surgical intervention in unicoronal and bicoronal synostoses aims to correct both the frontal and orbital asymmetries. With the current understanding that unilateral coronal synostosis presents with bilateral dysmorphic changes, bilateral correction is now believed to be the optimal approach.[87,181-183] For

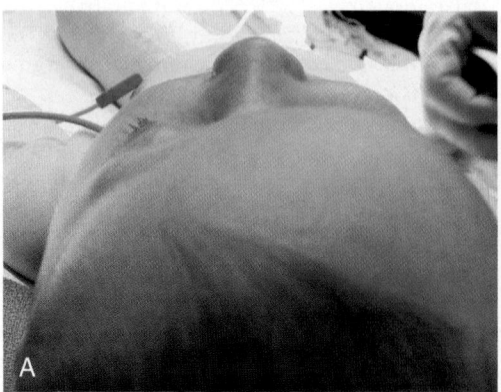
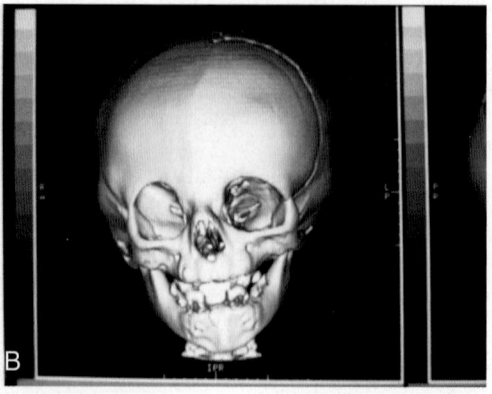

FIGURE 8.16 **A,** A 6-month-old infant with left coronal synostosis, manifested by significant left supraorbital retrusion, left forehead flattening, and compensatory right frontal bossing. **B,** Three-dimensional computed tomography (CT) image in a child with right coronal synostosis, depicting elevation of the right orbit as part of the "harlequin" deformity as well as nasal root deviation toward the right side.

anterior plagiocephaly, a bilateral fronto-orbital advancement procedure is employed for expansion of the affected forehead and orbit with concomitant recession of the contralateral orbit. Bilateral fronto-orbital advancement also serves in the correction of bicoronal synostosis, first proposed by Marchac and Renier in 1979 in the form of the "floating" forehead procedure.[184]

The timing of surgery remains a debated topic. However, an increasing number of surgeons have favored earlier surgery. Based on experience in 164 patients with craniosynostosis, Whitaker and co-workers proposed that the ideal age for treatment of both asymmetrical and less severe symmetrical synostoses was 4 to 12 months.[79] In a 1994 report, Marchac and co-workers recommended performing a frontocranial remodeling procedure between 6 and 9 months for anterior plagiocephaly and between 2 and 4 months for brachycephaly.[81] McCarthy and colleagues stated that patients with anterior plagiocephaly should undergo operations at approximately 6 months of age.[185] Recently, Whitaker's group has updated their recommendations and stated that surgery for unicoronal synostosis should be delayed until at least 6 months of age to avoid relapse.[186] In contrast to these opinions, Posnick recommended waiting until 10 to 12 months for patients with anterior plagiocephaly.[182]

The bilateral fronto-orbital advancement procedure involves the release of both coronal sutures while providing bilateral frontal and orbital correction. After performing bilateral tarsorrhaphies, a standard bicoronal skin incision is made. A bifrontal bone flap is removed typically in one piece, leaving a 1- to 2-cm-wide supraorbital bandeau. Extending the osteotomy posterior to the coronal suture will often provide adequate width and a satisfactory new frontal reconstruction when this bone flap segment is inverted. The sphenoid wing is removed down to the level of the clinoid process and the coronal sutures are opened to the level of the skull base (Fig. 8.17), serving to prevent continued growth restriction and resultant postoperative hollowing of the pterional regions. Care must be taken when performing the osteotomy across the sphenoid wing on the affected side, as its superior displacement may cause technical difficulty upon frontal bone flap removal and lead to dural laceration if caution is not exercised. After removal of the frontal bone flap, the orbital bandeau is freed with osteotomies taken across the lateral orbit at the frontozygomatic suture, the orbital roof, and nasion just above the nasofrontal suture. Care is taken to protect the underlying brain as well as orbital contents with judicious placement of retractors. The bandeau is then reconfigured via partial osteotomies at the midline while utilizing absorbable hardware on the interior surface to maintain the newly contoured shape. The newly configured supraorbital bar is replaced, its lateral aspects and midline fixed to the calvarial foundation with rigid fixation (absorbable hardware) for improved healing and postoperative maintenance of the surgical construct (Fig. 8.18A). It is frequently necessary to overcorrect the expansion of the affected side by 5% to 10%, while also providing a convex shape at the lateral border for a satisfactory reconstruction (Fig. 8.18B). Often, the unaffected orbit is mildly set back to correct for preoperative compensatory overgrowth. The frontal bone flap is then attached to the supraorbital bar, taking care to match it to the previously overbuilt (5-10%) orbital bandeau on the affected side (Fig. 8.18C). Remaining portions of bone are fixed with absorbable plates or suture, and closure is performed in a routine fashion with subgaleal drains.

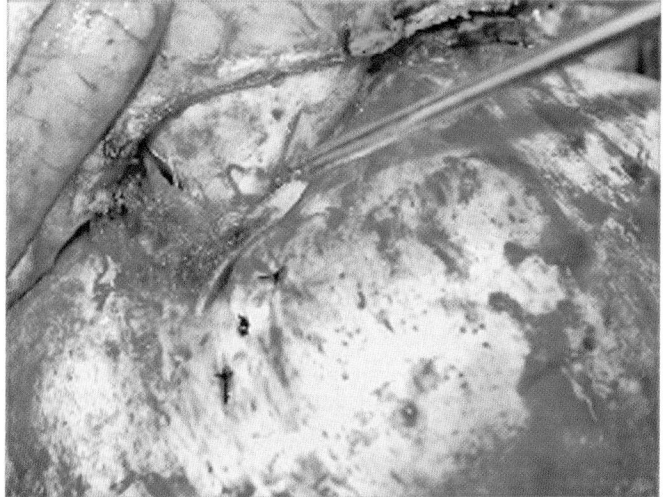

FIGURE 8.17 Removal of the sphenoid wing down to the level of the clinoid process on the affected side, serving to prevent continued growth restriction and resultant postoperative hollowing of the pterional.

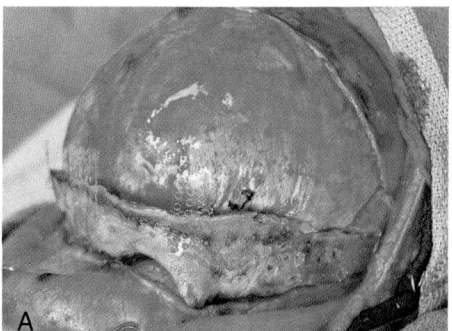
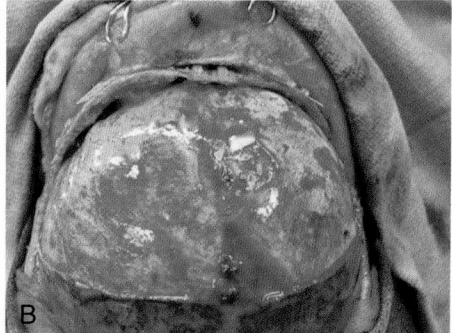
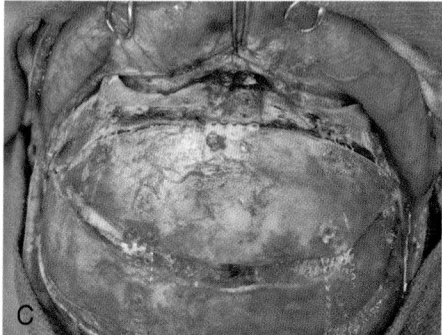

FIGURE 8.18 A, Three-quarter oblique view showing placement of the newly reconfigured orbital bandeau. **B,** Aerial view of the orbital bandeau, demonstrating asymmetrical inset with slight overcorrection on the previously affected side and slight recession on the unaffected side. **C,** Inversion of the frontal bone to provide adequate width and contour to match the newly constructed supraorbital region, followed by resorbable hardware fixation.

Outcome and Complications

A number of studies have addressed outcomes and complications following correction of unicoronal and bicoronal synostoses.[79,80,83,84,87,186-188] Reported reoperation rates have ranged from 3.1% to 29% for unicoronal synostosis[79,80,83,84,87,186] and 20% to 50% for bicoronal synostosis.[83,84,87,187,188] Interestingly, two recent studies have focused on the impact of surgical age on postoperative outcome in unicoronal synostosis.[80,186] Selber and co-workers determined that patients with unicoronal synostosis treated at 6 to 12 months had the lowest rate of secondary surgery (7%), which was statistically significant as compared to patients operated on less than 6 months of age or those receiving surgery at greater than 12 months of age.[186] Looking at outcomes from a different perspective, Fearon and colleagues investigated the impact of surgical age on postoperative growth in patients with unicoronal synostosis. Head circumferences in 21 patients with unicoronal synostosis were measured, demonstrating that growth was more than twice as impaired in the early treatment group (mean = 5 months) versus the late treatment group (mean = 14 months).[80]

A broad range of numbers has been reported for postoperative complications and mortality rate.[79,80,84,87,186-188] Complication rates have ranged from 0% to 27% for unicoronal synostosis[79,84,87,186] and 20% to 50% for bicoronal synostosis.[84,87,187,188] Perioperative morbidity may include wound infection, dural laceration, superficial brain injury, cerebrospinal fluid leak, encephalocele formation, subgaleal hematoma, and ocular injury including corneal abrasion. More serious perioperative complications can involve ischemic brain injury, epidural and subdural hemorrhage, and severe transfusion reactions. Long-term postoperative concerns include recurrent calvarial deformities, cranial bone defects that fail to fill in over time, and hardware-related problems. Defects greater than 2 cm in patients older than 18 to 24 months will often persist and may need eventual correction. Persistent hardware may also be problematic, particularly in patients in whom absorbable hardware was utilized. It is not uncommon for the polylactic/polyglycolic constructs to remain in place for 12 to 18 months before eventual resorption. In rare individuals, sterile abscesses may develop at sites of hardware resorption and subsequently require exploration for débridement. Postoperative mortality rates are near 0% for unicoronal synostosis[83,84,186] and range from 0% to 10% for bicoronal synostosis.[83,84,87,187]

Lambdoid Synostosis and Posterior Deformational Plagiocephaly

Clinical Features

Posterior plagiocephaly due to lambdoid suture synostosis is a rare event today, with the majority of observed posterior plagiocephaly secondary to positional molding. Understanding the phenotypic differences between lambdoid synostosis and posterior deformational plagiocephaly is critical toward making the appropriate diagnosis and designing the proper course of treatment. Children with lambdoid synostosis characteristically have a trapezoid-shaped head in association with posterior displacement of the ipsilateral ear, contralateral occipital bossing, and frequent ridging of the affected lambdoid suture.

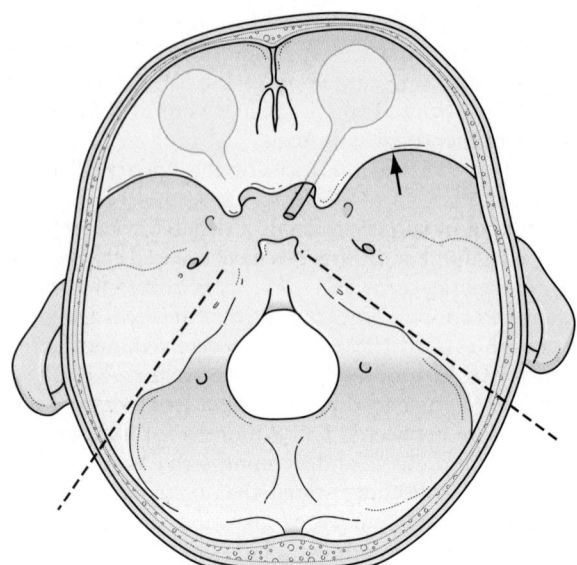

FIGURE 8.19 Skull base changes in the setting of right posterior deformational plagiocephaly, or positional molding. Note the parallelogram-shaped head, anterior displacement of the right ear, and right frontal bossing. This is in contrast to unilateral lambdoid synostosis, which is marked by a trapezoid-shaped skull, posterior displacement of the ipsilateral ear, and contralateral occipital bossing.

In contrast, posterior deformational plagiocephaly is marked by a parallelogram-shaped head, anterior displacement of the ipsilateral ear, and ipsilateral frontal bossing in the absence of palpable ridging along the lambdoid sutures (Fig. 8.19).

An increasing number of studies have focused on uncovering the etiological pathogenesis and associated clinical features of positional deformational plagiocephaly. In 2004, Littlefield and co-workers reported an incidence of 1 in 68 infants.[189] A prospective cohort study identified male gender, supine position, limited head rotation, lower activity levels, and first-born status as risk factors.[190] Indeed, one of the unforeseen consequences of the "back to sleep" campaign was a nearly exponential rise in asymmetrical and symmetrical occipital flattening.[20,191-193] Furthermore, about 30% of cases are associated with torticollis, or a tight sternocleidomastoid muscle.[11]

Radiological Evaluation

Routinely, radiographs are unnecessary in differentiating lambdoid synostosis from posterior deformational plagiocephaly, given that significant morphological differences exist to help separate the two entities on clinical grounds. In situations in which the diagnosis is unclear, skull plain films or facial CT scans can be employed. Lambdoid synostosis is consistent with fusion of the affected lambdoid suture, and posterior deformational plagiocephaly can be associated with sclerosis along a patent lambdoid suture.[194]

Surgical Therapeutics

Infants with true lambdoid synostosis may benefit from a variety of surgical approaches,[195-204] aiming to release the affected suture(s) and normalize the posterior calvarial vault contour.

Options include simple synostectomy, unilateral reconfiguration of the affected occipital region, and bilateral occipital reconstruction with or without the use of an occipital bandeau. The majority of lambdoid surgical candidates have significant parietal and frontal compensatory changes in addition to their occipital deformation; therefore, they are best served by a more extended calvarectomy and reconstruction.

For an extended calvarial reconfiguration, the globes are protected with bilateral tarsorrhaphies and patients are placed in a prone position. Perioperative antibiotics and steroids are administered. Intraoperative bleeding is minimized with the use of local anesthetic mixed with epinephrine as well as controlled hypotensive anesthesia. A bicoronal incision is then undertaken followed by subgaleal dissection to expose the occipitoparietal regions. Both parietal bone flaps are subsequently removed with osteotomies taken posterior to the coronal and anterior to the lambdoid sutures. A midline strip of bone is then left to protect the underlying sagittal sinus. After removal of the parietal bone flaps, dissection is carried out at the level of the lambdoid suture under direct visualization, taking great caution at the level of the transverse, sagittal, and sigmoid sinuses. Osteotomies are brought to within 1 cm on either side of the midline, with the final cut made after the underlying dura and sinus have been clearly dissected free under direct vision. Inadvertent entry into the sinus, particularly at the region of the asterion, may lead to significant blood loss over a short period and constitutes the greatest risk encountered for this approach. Nevertheless, with appropriate care and attention, this complication may be avoided in the majority of individuals. The removed calvarial plates are reconfigured to provide adequate normalization of the occipital contour and stabilized with resorbable hardware, deliberately leaving open the region of the prior lambdoid suture (Fig. 8.20). Subgaleal drains are then placed and closure is carried out in routine fashion.

Treatment of posterior deformational plagiocephaly is a function of both the age and severity at presentation. When presenting before the age of 6 months, therapy consists of positional modifications combined with physiotherapy in the case of constrained neck movements or asymmetric neurological development.[205] In cases of no improvement or progression of the deformity despite repositioning after 2 to 3 months, cranial orthotic (helmet) therapy (Fig. 8.21) is indicated.[11] Additionally, Graham and co-workers recommended helmet therapy if the cephalic index is larger than 90 or if the diagonal diameter difference is more than 1 cm at the age of 6 months.[206] Despite conservative management, a small subset of patients (<7%) may require surgical correction for excellent long-term results.[195,207]

Outcome and Complications

Given the infrequency of unilateral and bilateral lambdoid synostoses, only a handful of studies have large enough patient numbers to glean accurate outcomes data.[80,83,84,196,197,199] Reoperation rates range from 0% to 10% and complication rates fall between 5.4% and 13.6%. In addition to improvement of the posterior vault, studies have noted correction of the majority of facial asymmetries with surgeries performed at less than 1 year of age.[196,199] Complications can consist of wound infections, transfusion-related problems, hemorrhage, dural injury, and rare intracerebral injury.

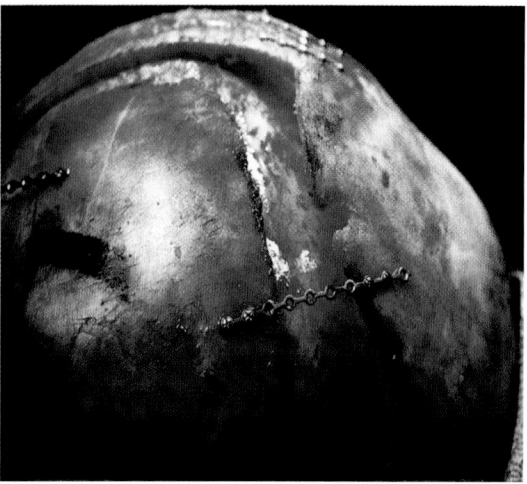

FIGURE 8.20 Extended calvarial reconfiguration for unilateral lambdoid synostosis. Note the newly reconfigured parietal and occipital bones, with the region of the prior lambdoid suture left open via rigid fixation.

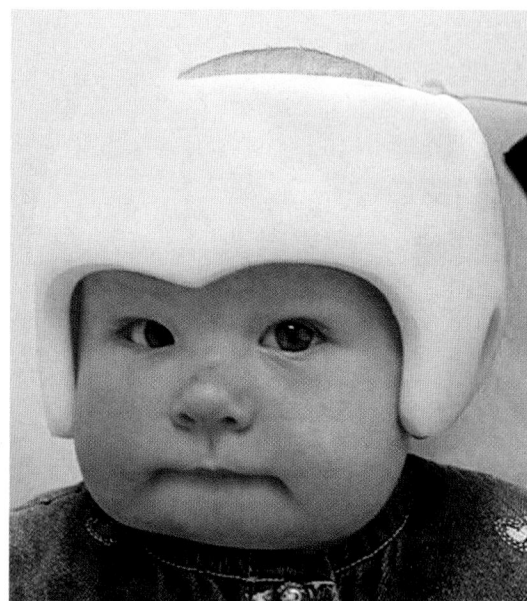

FIGURE 8.21 Cranial orthotic (helmet) therapy serves to redirect calvarial growth in children with positional molding or posterior deformational plagiocephaly.

Outcome studies have also demonstrated conservative therapy to be beneficial in the reduction of calvarial deformities secondary to positional molding.[19,208-215] Postural changes and helmet therapy are most effective between 4 and 12 months of age, during the period of rapid brain growth.[205] Approximately 95% of infants can be expected to have satisfactory cosmetic improvement with conservative management. Following a recent systematic review of 16 studies, it was concluded that counterpositioning with or without physiotherapy or helmet therapy may reduce skull deformity; however, it was not possible to draw conclusions regarding the relative effectiveness of these interventions.[209] On the issue of duration of therapy, Thompson noted an improvement in head shape after 4 months of helmet therapy, observing better results with increased compliance.[211]

TABLE 8.4 Evidence-Based Medicine on Craniosynostosis

Year	First Author*	Study Type	Level†	Conclusions
1993	Prevot[216]	Case-control study; comparing characteristics of patients with lack of calvarial ossification with those of patients with no calvarial defects	III	5% rate of lack of ossification; risk factors include infection, forehead advancement with resorbable hardware, and brachycephaly
1996	Gosain[177]	Prospective cohort study; determining relationship between strabismus and head posture in frontal plagiocephaly	II	Extraocular motor paresis is a major cause of abnormal head posture in frontal plagiocephaly
1996	Renier[77]	Retrospective cohort study; comparison of IQ scores in children with Apert syndrome operated on before the age of 1 year and in those undergoing surgery after 1 year	III	Age at surgery significantly associated with mental development; IQ > 70 in 50% of patients operated on before 1 year of age versus 7% of those operated on after 1 year
1996	Tuite[67]	Case-control study; comparing radiographs of patients with craniosynostosis and age/sex-matched control subjects	III	Presence of beaten copper appearance (BCA) no more common in synostosis, but severity significantly increased; x-ray studies not recommended for ICP screening
1997	Hansen[217]	Retrospective cohort study; comparison of three surgical techniques for anterior plagiocephaly	III	Data support bilateral repositioning of forehead/orbit and nasal root correction
2002	Kan[218]	Prospective cohort study; assessing presence of FGFR2 mutation in syndromic synostoses	III	9.8% of patients with syndromic craniosynostoses possess FGFR2 mutation
2003	Boltshauser[219]	Case-control study; assessed neuropsychological function in uncorrected scaphocephalic children versus their unaffected siblings	III	No statistical significance between mean IQ scores
2006	Da Costa[120]	Cross-sectional case series; comparing IQ scores in nonsyndromic and syndromic craniosynostoses (ages 7-12) and in norms	III	Both nonsyndromic and syndromic craniosynostoses with normal intelligence; average IQ scores lower in syndromic
2006	Kelleher[220]	Case-control study; comparing neurodevelopment in operated with that in unoperated trigonocephaly	III	No difference between patients with/without surgical correction
2006	Mathijssen[221]	Prospective cohort study; comparing cognitive development of unmatched control subjects (UCS) in early (<1 yr) versus late (>1 yr) correction	II	Cognitive development not related to age at surgery, FGFR3 P250R status, or presence of high ICP
2007	Agrawal[222]	Case-control study, relationship of BCA on postoperative films to ICP symptoms	III	45% of children with BCA on postoperative films develop symptoms of raised ICP
2007	Rasmussen[223]	Case-control study; comparison of maternal factors in craniosynostosis and in control subjects	III	Maternal thyroid disease significantly associated with craniosynostosis (OR, 2.47)
2007	Speltz[121]	Case-control study; assessing neurodevelopment in single-suture synostoses presurgery versus that in case-matched control subjects	III	Modest but reliable delay in neurodevelopment (cognitive, motor) in single-suture synostoses, unaffected by location of synostosis
2008	Windh[224]	Retrospective cohort study; comparing spring-mediated cranioplasty with modified pi-plasty for sagittal synostosis	III	Pi-plasty associated with cephalic index marginally closer to normal range at 3 years; spring-mediated cranioplasty, with less blood loss, transfusion requirements, operative time, ICU and recovery times, and total hospital stay
2009	Fearon[80]	Retrospective cohort study; comparing anthropometric measurements for early and late corrected single-suture synostosis	III	Earlier surgery for metopic sutures (4 months) associated with more growth inhibition than with later surgery (12 months); similar tendencies for other synostoses
2009	MacKinnon[95]	Retrospective cohort study; comparing ophthalmological outcomes for endoscopic strip craniectomy with those for fronto-orbital advancement (FOA) in unicoronal synostosis	III	Less severe subsequent V-pattern strabismus, excyclotorsion, and range of aniso-astigmatism in endoscopically treated patients than in those treated by FOA
2009	White[225]	Prospective cohort study; determining predictors of blood loss in FOA	II	Increased bleeding with syndromic, pansynostosis, operating room time >5 hr, and age <18 mo

*Numbers refer to references listed for this chapter online.
†ASPS scales for rating levels of evidence.
ICP, intracranial pressure; ICU, intensive care unit; IQ, intelligence quotient; OR, odds ratio.

FUTURE DIRECTIONS

Significant advances over the past decade have contributed to the improvement in diagnosis and treatment of craniosynostosis while concurrently reducing the risks involved in its surgical treatment. A summary of the available evidence-based medicine can be found in Table 8.4.[216-225] An understanding of the genetic underpinnings has provided investigators with an in-depth view of the potential mechanisms involved in the pathogenesis of sutural fusion and may eventually lead to new approaches in future treatment. New surgical treatment methods continue to refine the operative arena, with enhanced cosmetic outcomes and decreasing rates of recurrence. Minimally invasive techniques that rely on dynamic cranial vault alteration, including endoscopic sutural release, spring-assisted cranioplasty, and distraction osteogenesis, will undoubtedly play a greater role in the surgical correction of craniosynostosis. In time, answers will be forthcoming with respect to the appropriate surgical approaches for each type of craniosynostosis in addition to the optimal timing for correction. The value of orthotic devices in the setting of positional plagiocephaly will be eventually clarified by objective prospective data. The future will help clarify some of the current issues facing the craniofacial surgeon and no doubt will also bring new challenges to the forefront.

SELECTED KEY REFERENCES

Bellus GA, Gaudenz K, Zackai EH, et al. Identical mutations in three different fibroblast growth factor receptor genes in autosomal dominant craniosynostosis syndromes. *Nat Genet.* 1996;14(2):174-176.

Bialocerkowski AE, Vladusic SL, Howell SM. Conservative interventions for positional plagiocephaly: a systematic review. *Dev Med Child Neurol.* 2005;47(8):563-570.

Kapp-Simon KA, Speltz ML, Cunningham ML, et al. Neurodevelopment of children with single suture craniosynostosis: a review. *Childs Nerv Syst.* 2007;23(3):269-281.

Lannelongue M. De la craniectomie dans la microcéphalie. *Compt Rend Seances Acad Sci.* 1890;50:1382-1385.

Renier D, Sainte-Rose C, Marchac D, et al. Intracranial pressure in craniostenosis. *J Neurosurg.* 1982;57(3):370-377.

Please go to expertconsult.com to view complete list of references.

CHAPTER 9

The Chiari Malformations and Syringohydromyelia

R. Shane Tubbs, Todd C. Hankinson, John C. Wellons, III

CLINICAL PEARLS

- Chiari malformations are pathological herniations of the hindbrain through the foramen magnum and into the cervical spinal canal. Chiari malformations are being recognized with increasing frequency because of the increased availability of magnetic resonance imaging (MRI).

- Chiari I malformation (CIM) represents downward herniation of the cerebellar tonsils into the cervical canal at least 3 to 5 mm on sagittal MRI. The impaction of the tonsils in the foramen magnum causes an anatomical and physiological block of cerebrospinal fluid (CSF), which normally flows from the posterior fossa into the cervical subarachnoid space. The symptoms of CIM commonly include headache or neck pain worsened by activity or Valsalva maneuver, or signs of brainstem compression. Syringomyelia may be associated with CIM, and those patients often present with signs of spinal cord dysfunction.

- The most widely accepted treatment of CIM is a posterior fossa decompression with removal of the posterior arch of C1 and dural augmentation graft. The goal of surgery is to enlarge the posterior fossa and permit normal flow of CSF from the posterior fossa to the cervical subarachnoid space. In the majority of patients, the symptoms of headache resolve and there is a concomitant collapse of

the associated syrinx. Only rarely does the surgeon have to treat directly the associated syringomyelia.

- Chiari II malformation (CIIM), which is a downward migration of the cerebellar vermis and brainstem through the foramen magnum, is most commonly seen in patients with myelomeningocele. It is associated with hydrocephalus in 90% of the patients. Syringomyelia is also very common. In addition, on MRI, patients often have low-lying tentorium, tectal beaking, cervicomedullary kinks, agenesis of the corpus callosum, and other brain abnormalities. A small, but significant, number of patients will present with acute brainstem, cerebellar, or progressive spinal cord dysfunction. The initial step in this treatment should be the surgical establishment of a functioning shunt. If the symptoms progress or do not resolve in this setting, then a formal decompressive procedure may be required.

- Syringomyelia, or cavitation of the spinal cord, has many causes in addition to hindbrain herniation. Signs and symptoms of a syrinx include pain and temperature loss, reflex changes, or motor weakness. Treatment of the syrinx, when not the result of hindbrain herniation, often includes shunting of the syrinx into the peritoneum or pleura. The goal is to drain the syrinx and to reestablish a patent subarachnoid space.

In the early 1890s, the pathologist Hans Chiari[1] described four congenital malformations that would later become known as the *Chiari malformations*. The four traditional varieties of Chiari malformations represent varying degrees of involvement of rhombencephalic derivatives. Three of these (types I to III) have progressively more severe herniation of these structures outside the posterior fossa as a common feature. These three also have in common a pathogenesis that involves a loss of free movement of cerebral spinal fluid (CSF) out of the normal outlet channels of the fourth ventricle. Pathological differences between Chiari I malformations (CIMs) and Chiari II malformations (CIIMs) can be explained with knowledge of the differences in the timing of the development of the hindbrain herniation.[2]

Although a large majority of hindbrain hernias are congenital, acquired CIMs occur and are not rare. Not considered

further in this chapter are the patients who have movement of their cerebellar tonsils into the cervical spine as a result of an intracranial tumor, or other mass lesion, especially within the posterior fossa. Technically, these patients have a CIM but treatment of the cause of their hindbrain hernia usually allows resolution of their secondary CIM.

Within the large group of patients with hindbrain hernias due to some problem with equilibrating CSF across the craniocervical junction, several subclassifications have been developed and are included with the following brief descriptions of the traditional forms of Chiari malformations:

Chiari 0—These patients do not appear to have significant hindbrain hernias, although the posterior fossa may appear "crowded"; they have large syringes that resolve with posterior fossa decompression and have a unique position in our thinking about this subject.[3,4] These malformations have been informally termed *Chiari 0* because they behave as though they have fourth ventricular outlet obstruction, and at surgery they frequently do have physical barriers to CSF movement but do not have caudal displacement of the cerebellar tonsils beyond a point that could be considered pathological.

Chiari I—This common group of patients has been found to have caudal displacement of the cerebellar tonsils more than 5 mm below the foramen magnum. The brainstem is in a normal position and they may or may not have a syrinx. The 5 mm "rule" concerning the definition of pathological extent of caudal migration of the tonsils is arbitrary. Numerous patients have tonsils well below this point and are asymptomatic, especially young infants and children. When followed over time they frequently remain asymptomatic if their initial evaluation was performed for an unrelated reason. The extent of their caudal migration may progressively improve with time and become less impressive. This, however, is not assured and the patient should be followed for the development of symptoms. Syringomyelia is often associated with the CIM.

Chiari I.5—Although somewhat confusing, this term is applied to patients who bridge the gap between the CIM and CIIM. They have characteristics of both groups and are best considered separately. They are unassociated with neural tube defects and have caudal displacement of the cerebellar tonsils similar to that seen in the CIM patient. However, their brainstem and fourth ventricle are displaced inferiorly like CIIM patients. In our series of patients with a hindbrain hernia but without a neural tube defect, 17% had significant caudal displacement of the brainstem.[5,6]

Chiari II—This lesion almost always occurs in patients with neural tube defects (myelomeningoceles and encephaloceles). It consists of caudal migration of the cerebellar vermis, brainstem, and fourth ventricle. Syringomyelia is common in this group.

Chiari III—The Chiari III malformation is a rare and extreme form of hindbrain hernia that may be confused with an occipital encephalocele. It comprises less than 1% of all patients in this category. Patients have low occipital or high cervical sacs containing significant portions of the cerebellum and brainstem.[7] Other intracranial anomalies such as are found with CIIM patients may be seen with this group. Hydrocephalus is common and severe neurological and developmental problems are almost always present.

Chiari IV—Type IV Chiari malformation patients have cerebellar hypoplasia or aplasia; this malformation is not a form of hindbrain hernia. For this reason, inclusion in a discussion of hindbrain hernias is debatable and will not be considered further.

CHIARI I MALFORMATION

Many theories have been put forth to explain the development of Chiari malformations in the absence of hydrocephalus (Figs. 9.1 to 9.3). Currently, the most appealing theory emphasizes the difficulty in rapidly equilibrating the CSF

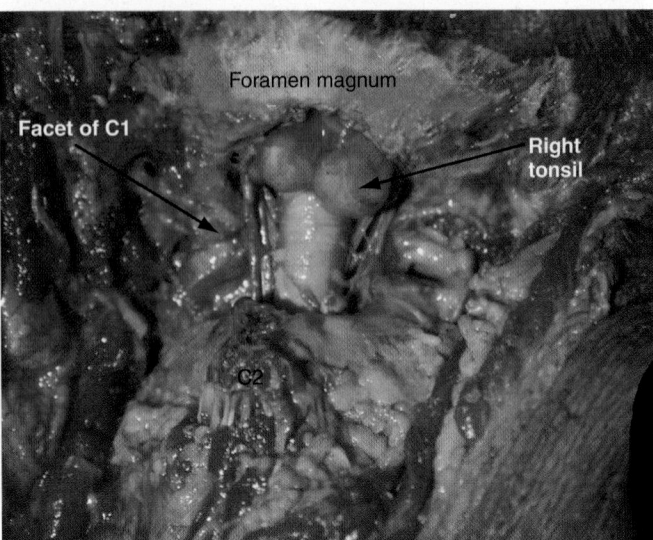

FIGURE 9.1 Postmortem view of the Chiari I malformation from an adult male cadaver. Note the right tonsil that is descended more inferiorly.

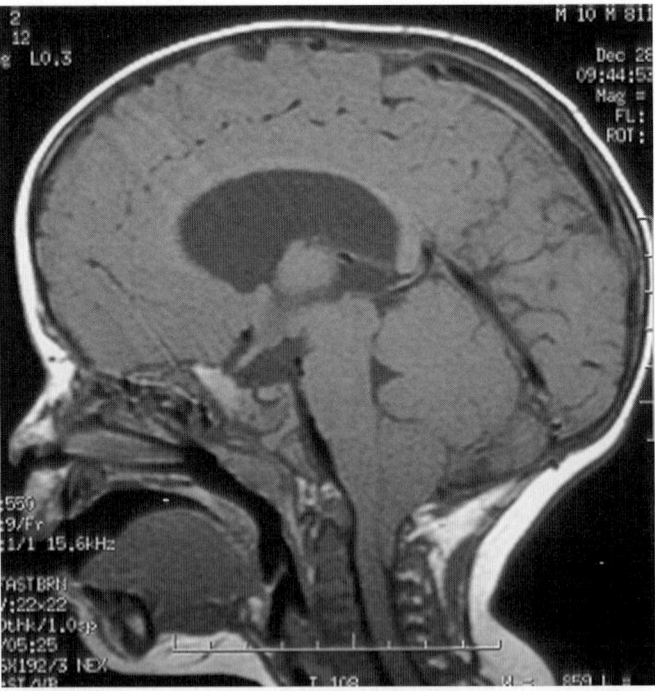

FIGURE 9.2 Sagittal T1-weighted magnetic resonance image of a child with swallowing difficulty and Chiari I malformation. Note the dilated ventricular system.

pressure wave seen during the Valsalva maneuver.[8-10] During this delay in achieving equilibrium, there is a vector of force out of the intracranial cavity (Fig. 9.4). The prolonged intracranial hypertension relative to the intraspinal compartment may result in the downward migration of the cerebellar tonsils, resulting in obstruction of normal CSF flow between the posterior cranial fossa and the cervical subarachnoid space. Conditions that impede the physiological flow of CSF at the foramen of Magendie enhance the formation of the malformation. These could include arachnoid veils or septations in this

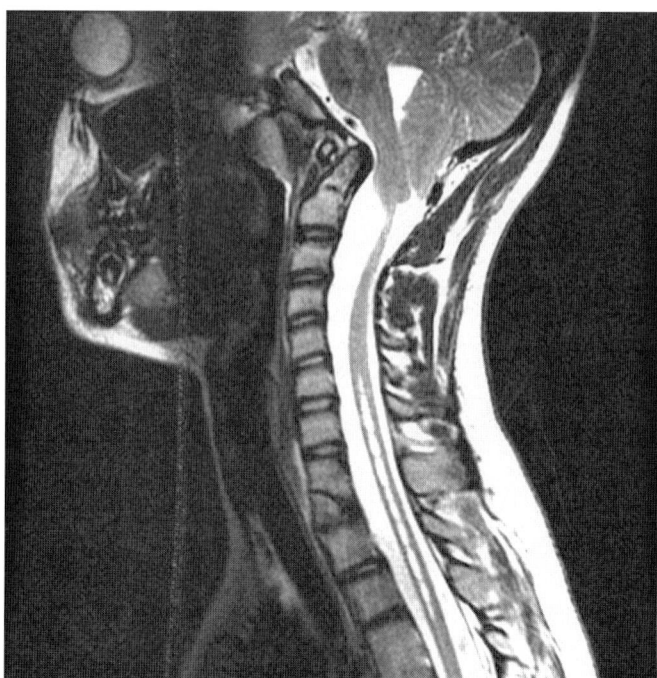

FIGURE 9.3 Sagittal magnetic resonance image noting a Chiari I malformation in an adolescent girl with Valsalva-induced headaches. Also, note the retroversion of the odontoid process resulting in simultaneous ventral compression.

region as well as adhesions.[11] Alternatively, conditions that artificially lower the intraspinal pressure relative to the intracranial pressure (lumboperitoneal shunts) have been observed to "cause" the CIM with the subsequent development of syringomyelia. Parenthetically, there is some evidence that the CIM may result from derailment on chromosomes 9 and 15.[12]

Initially considered an "adult" disease, the CIM is reported more frequently now in the pediatric population as a result of the widespread availability of detailed MRI. The clinical presentation of CIM essentially falls into three categories (Fig. 9.5):

1. Signs or symptoms related to brainstem compression
2. Signs or symptoms associated with cerebellar compression
3. Spinal cord dysfunction secondary to syringomyelia

Most commonly, patients present with occipital or cervical pain that is nonradicular but frequently associated with dysesthesias in the C2 dermatome.[13] The neck pain or headache is frequently brought on by exertion or by coughing or sneezing (Valsalva-induced). Nonverbal children may relate their pain via irritability, crying, failure to thrive, or the presence of opisthotonos.

The diagnosis of CIM can easily be confirmed with MRI. The presence and extent of syringomyelia, seen in 50% to 75% of patients,[5,14-16] should be determined with an MRI of the entire spinal cord. Computed tomography (CT) may further elucidate the bony abnormalities and plain films may assist in the evaluation of stability issues. Dynamic MRI (cine-MRI) has been used to evaluate CSF flow around the craniocervical junction. In a review of 800 MRI examinations, one study noted that "normal" or "asymptomatic" patients may have cerebellar tonsils that extend 3 mm below the foramen magnum.[17] The tonsillar herniation was noted to be clearly

pathological when it exceeded 5 mm. Similarly, Barkovich and associates[18] studied 200 normal patients and 25 patients with a "firm" diagnosis of CIM. Tonsils 2 mm below the foramen magnum were considered as the lowest extent of the tonsils in normal patients (specificity of 98.5% [three false positive results] and a sensitivity of 100%). Tonsils 3 mm below the foramen magnum were considered the lowest extent in normal patients (sensitivity 96% and specificity 99.5%). An additional study has documented ascent of the tonsils with increasing age in some patients.[19]

No medical treatment exists for the Chiari malformations. Numerous therapeutic paradigms exist (Fig. 9.6). The first decision that must be made is whether the lesion is truly symptomatic. Observation is warranted in asymptomatic patients without an associated syrinx. In symptomatic patients or asymptomatic patients with syringomyelia, surgical intervention is recommended. The degree of brainstem compression and tonsillar herniation is taken into account as well. In about 10% of patients hydrocephalus is associated with the CIM, in which case a CSF diversionary shunt or endoscopic third ventriculostomy should be the initial form of therapy. Similarly, symptomatic ventral compression out of proportion to dorsal compression may require a ventral decompression (i.e., transoral odontoid resection), especially in cases of myelopathy. The most common surgical procedure for the treatment of CIM is posterior fossa decompression. The goal of the operation is to enlarge the posterior fossa and to re-create the cisterna magna, thereby permitting normal flow of CSF from the posterior fossa to the cervical subarachnoid space. In the majority of CIM patients with a syrinx, the syrinx decreases in size and does not require direct treatment because the posterior fossa decompression treats the underlying pathological process causing the syringomyelia.

For decompression, the patient should be prone and the neck flexed (Fig. 9.7). The incision extends from a point just below the inion to the spinous process of C2. An avascular plane (nuchal ligament) between the paraspinous muscles is followed down to bone, and a subperiosteal dissection is then performed. A moderate suboccipital craniectomy, the width of the foramen magnum, is followed by the removal of the posterior arch of C1. Some techniques advocate either stopping here or opening the outer layer of the dura and then closing.[20,21] We open all layers of the dura and clip the opened arachnoid to the dural edge. Any arachnoid adhesions potentially obstructing the outflow of CSF from the foramen of Magendie are removed and the floor of the fourth ventricle is examined (Fig. 9.8). A portion of the occipital pericranium is harvested through a separate incision and duraplasty performed. The wound is closed in anatomical layers.

The results of craniocervical decompression are encouraging in long-term follow-up. Postoperative outcome is not age-based and early treatment tends toward better outcomes. Nearly 85% of patients will have relief of their head and neck pain, especially if it was Valsalva-induced.[5,20] Associated syringes decrease in size or collapse in the majority, albeit not all, of the patients who undergo a well-performed posterior fossa decompression. If decompression fails to improve the symptoms or decrease the size of the syrinx in a 6-month period, consideration should be given to either a reexploration of the posterior fossa with coagulation or resection of a cerebellar tonsil. Placement of a syringosubarachnoid shunt may

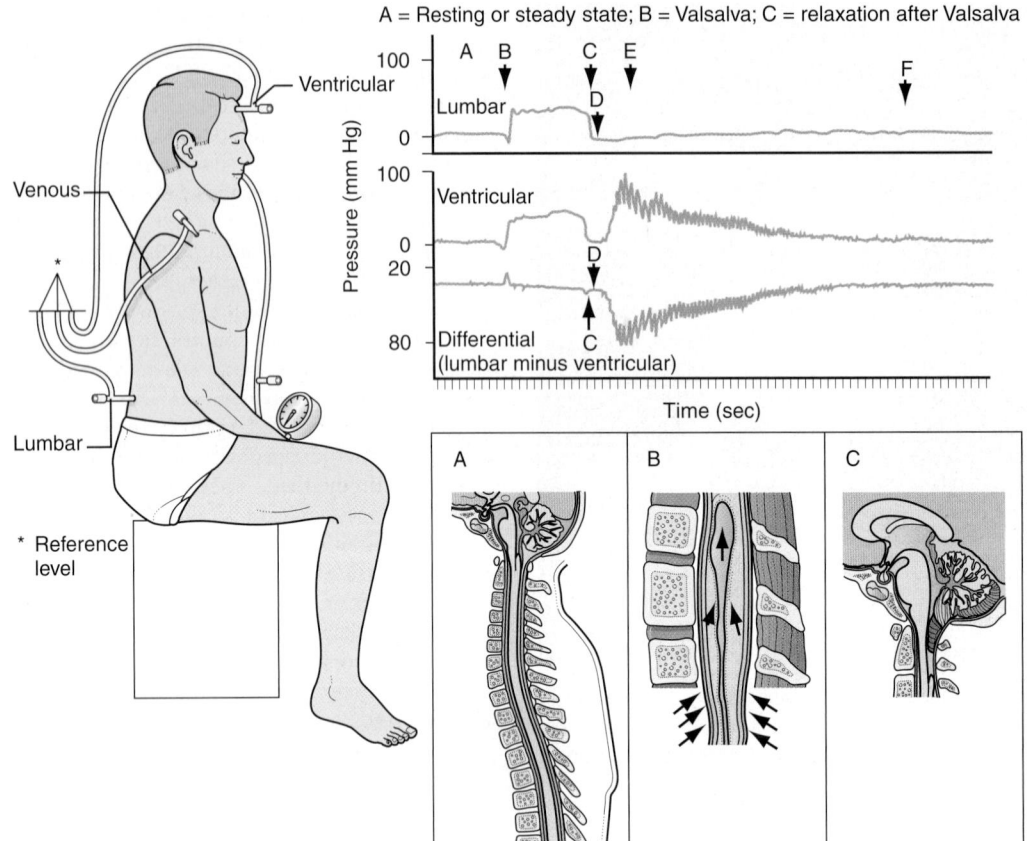

FIGURE 9.4 A, When ventricular and lumbar subarachnoid pressures are simultaneously monitored in a patient with a Chiari I malformation the pressures are the same in the resting state when calibrated against a reference. **B,** With the Valsalva maneuver there is an abrupt rise of lumbar pressure exceeding that seen in the ventricular system. **C,** With relaxation the lumbar space has its pressure rapidly fall and return to the baseline. The ventricular pressure, on the other hand, cannot equilibrate, and sustained intracranial hypertension relative to the intraspinal compartment is maintained for several seconds to a few minutes. This vector of force is the pathophysiological mechanism for the development of progressive displacement of the cerebellar tonsils into the cervical spine and the development of syringomyelia. (*From Williams B. Cerebrospinal fluid pressure-gradients in spina bifida cystica, with special reference to the Arnold-Chiari malformation and aqueductal stenosis. Dev Med Child Neurol Suppl. 1975;17:138-150.*)

Brainstem
- Neck pain/headache
- Downbeat nystagmus
- Hoarse voice
- Palatal dysfunction
- Tongue atrophy/ fasciculations
- Dysphagia
- Hiccups
- Severe snoring
- Respiratory dysrhythmias
- Facial numbness
- Drop attacks
- Dysarthria

Spinal cord (Syringomyelia)
- Scoliosis
- Suspended dissociated sensory loss (pain/ temperature)
- Trunk/extremity dysesthesia
- Wasting of hands or arms
- Spasticity of legs
- Charcot joint destruction
- Urinary incontinence
- Arm/hand weakness

Cerebellum
- Ataxia
- Nystagmus

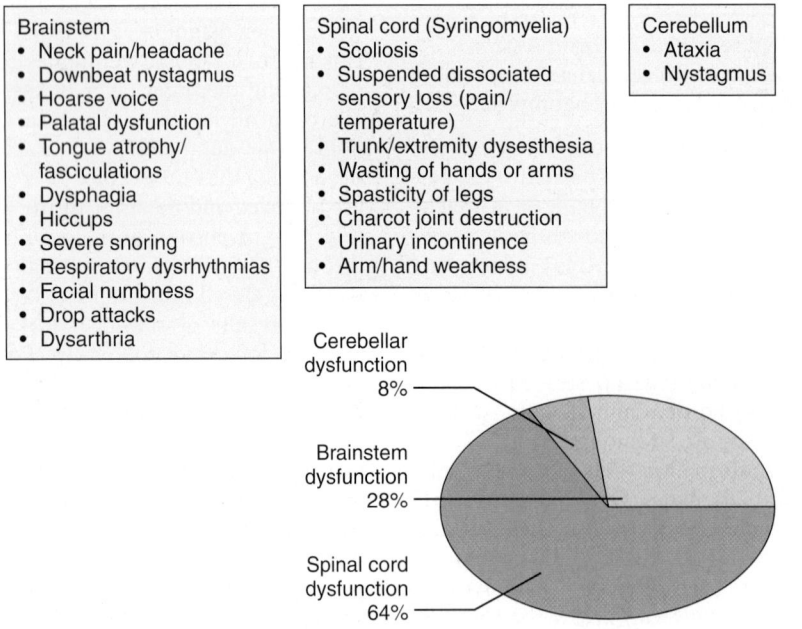

FIGURE 9.5 Symptoms and signs of patients with Chiari I malformation.

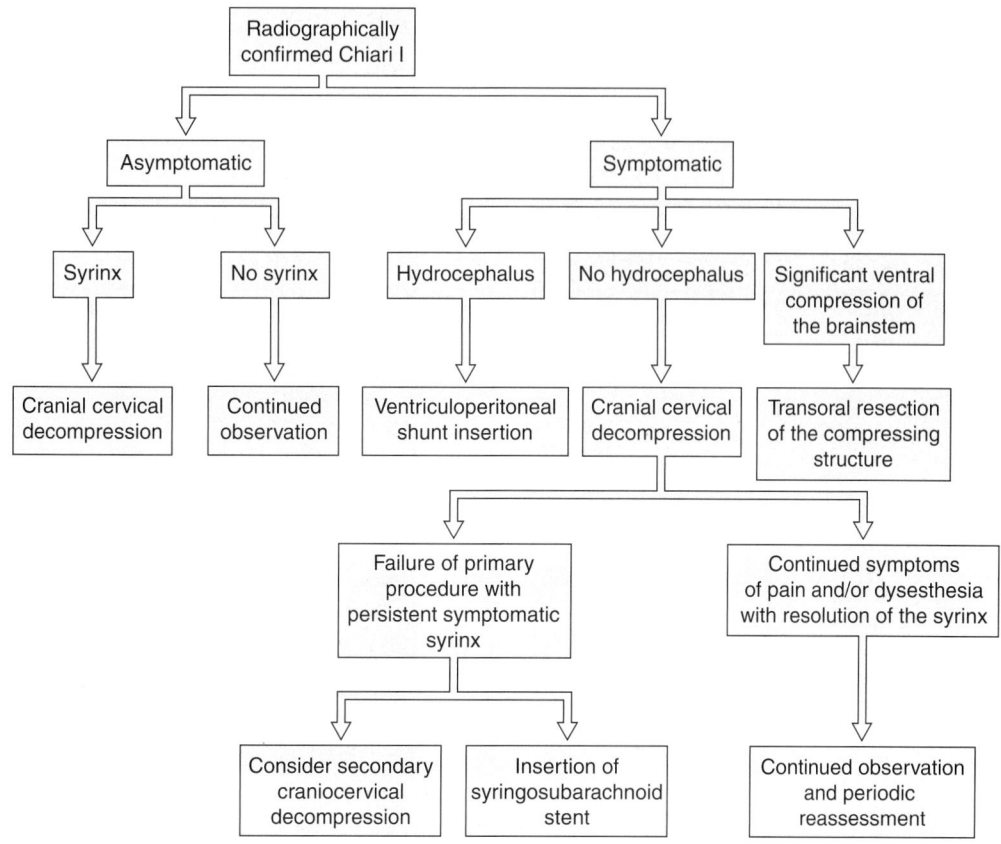

FIGURE 9.6 Therapeutic options for treating Chiari I malformation.

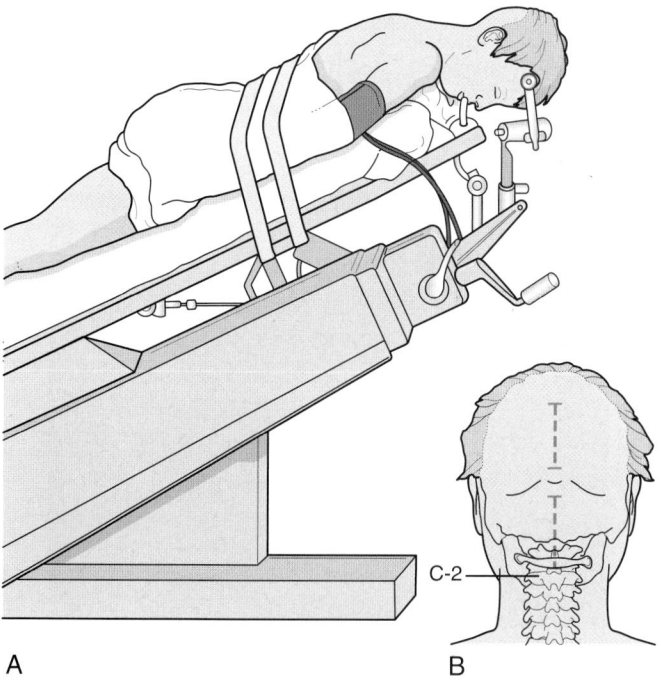

A   B

FIGURE 9.7 Operative position for posterior fossa decompression. **A,** The operative field is maintained horizontally with the head flexed and held in a pin fixation device. **B,** Preparation is made for a midline linear incision 2 cm below the external occipital protuberance and extending to the spinous process of C2. A 3-cm incision is made above the inion to harvest pericranium for grafting material.

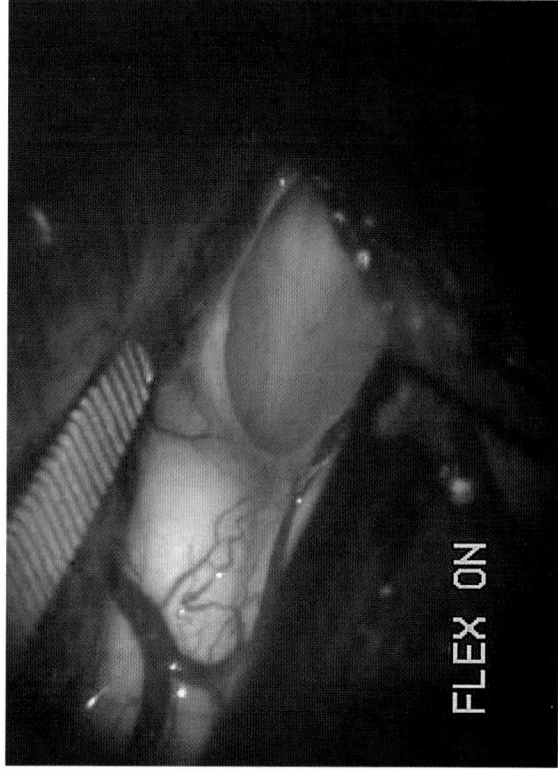

FIGURE 9.8 Intraoperative view following decompression of a Chiari I malformation. The left and right cerebellar tonsils are spread with forceps to observe the floor of the fourth ventricle.

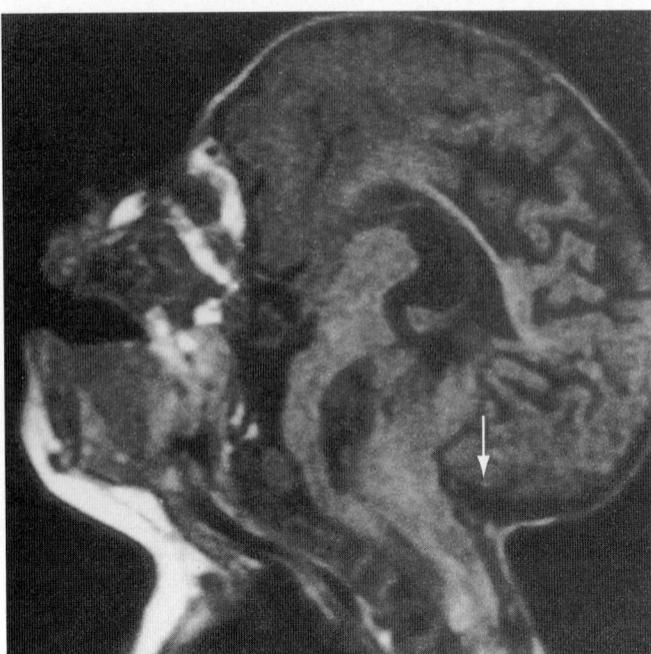

FIGURE 9.9 Sagittal T1-weighted magnetic resonance image of a child with the Chiari II malformation. Note the large massa intermedia, thin corpus callosum, beaked tectum, and cortical dysplasia.

be indicated in recalcitrant cases of syringomyelia that do not respond to an adequate posterior fossa decompression, although this lack of response is rare. Advanced symptoms of medullary dysfunction, muscle wasting, or dysesthesias in the trunk or extremities are unlikely to resolve but should not progress. Mild to moderate scoliosis has a high likelihood of improvement.

CHIARI II MALFORMATION

The caudal displacement of the cerebellar vermis, lower brainstem, and fourth ventricle is seen almost exclusively in patients with myelomeningoceles (Fig. 9.9). Numerous other anomalies of the nervous system and its support structure are seen in various combinations (Fig. 9.10). Of particular note is the vertical straight sinus resulting from the low-lying tentorium cerebelli, as well as the possibility of large venous lakes in the tentorium. Fenestrations may also be seen in the falx cerebri, which is often not well formed, and on occasion allow the gyri of the left and right cerebral hemispheres to interdigitate, giving the appearance of "Chinese lettering" on axial MRI (Fig. 9.11). Hydrocephalus occurs in approximately 90% of patients with CIIM.[22] Split cord malformation is seen in up to 6% of patients with CIIM and syringomyelia has been reported to occur in between 20% and 95% of patients.[2] Other associated anomalies include tectal beaking secondary to partial or complete fusion of the colliculi into a single backward pointed peak and kinking at the level of the cervicomedullary junction. The latter anomaly is caused by caudal displacement of a portion of the medulla in conjunction with a spinal cord that is held in relative immobility by the dentate ligaments. The tracts of the spinal cord then double back on themselves for a short distance. The cerebellum is smaller than usual; in addition, the

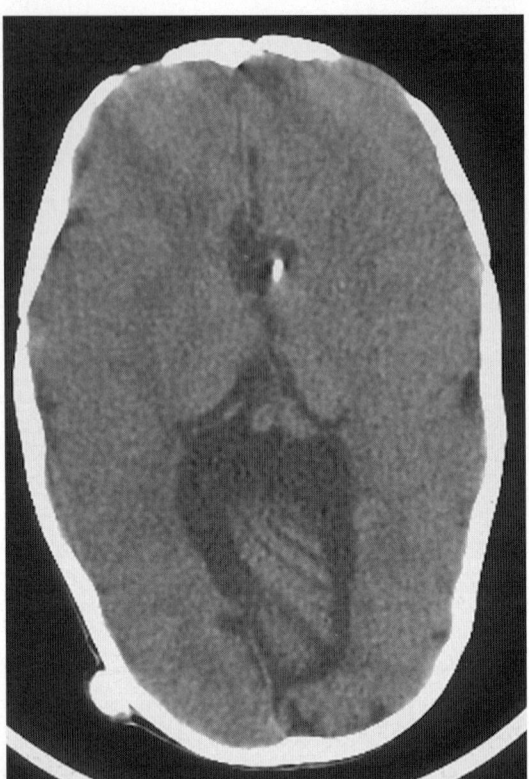

FIGURE 9.10 Axial CT image noting the towering cerebellum seen in patients with Chiari II malformation.

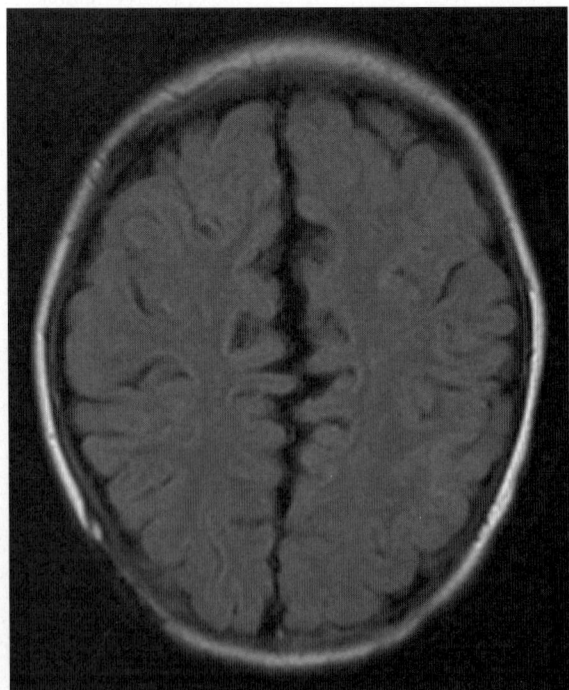

FIGURE 9.11 Axial CT image demonstrating the Chinese lettering that occurs in the Chiari II malformation and the absence of the falx cerebri.

vermis and adjacent medial cerebellar hemispheres are poorly differentiated from each other. The extent of the medial cerebellar protrusion and the character of tissues involved vary considerably from case to case. Abnormalities of the cerebral cortical pattern have frequently been described in Chiari II

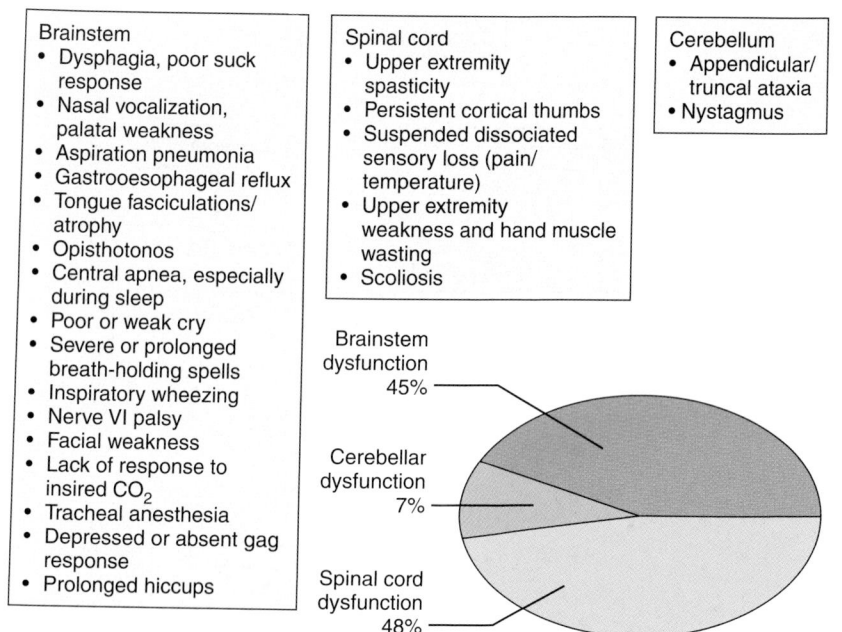

FIGURE 9.12 Symptoms and signs of patients with Chiari II malformation.

patients. Radiographic signs of CIIM evident on CT scans include lückenschädel (85% of cases), scalloping of the posterior surface of the petrous pyramid (80%), tentorial hypoplasia (95%) with a wide incisura and a small posterior fossa, enlargement of the foramen magnum (73%), and inversion (or transtentorial upward herniation) of the cerebellum. Most of these abnormalities may be observed with other conditions; however, their combination is highly suggestive of CIIM. In addition to hydrocephalus, the ventricular system displays multiple abnormalities: the third ventricle may be only mildly dilated and contains a large massa intermedia (75%); the fourth ventricle is typically small or nonvisualized (70%); it is often flattened and elongated, extending into the cervical canal; the lateral ventricles may be asymmetrically dilated, with prominence of the atria and occipital horns (colpocephaly), and the septum pellucidum is frequently absent. The frontal horns and the anterior portion of the third ventricle are frequently pointed and acutely angulated. This sharpness of the frontal horn (lemon sign) and the caudal displacement of the fourth ventricle (banana sign) are relatively easily seen on in utero ultrasound examinations. The upper cervical canal also displays several bony and spinal cord anomalies in association with the CMII. The C1 arch may be incomplete in up to 70% of these patients, with the missing bone being replaced by a fibrous band corresponding to the periosteal envelope. The dorsal arch of C2 is almost always intact. Klippel-Feil fusion anomalies of the cervical spine are present in a small group of patients.[23] Basilar impression and C1 assimilation are quite uncommon in CIIM as opposed to CIM. Significant shortening and scalloping of the clivus can be seen.

The pathophysiology of the malformation has been postulated to be similar to that of the CIM, that is, a difficulty in equilibrating the dynamic CSF pulse pressure induced by Valsalva.[10,24] In the case of CIIM, the presence of CSF pooling in or leaking from the myelomeningocele sac lowers the intraspinal pressure and the result is the ectopia of not only ... but the abovementioned portions of

the brainstem. In support of this theory is the observation of reduced hindbrain herniation observed in some children who undergo fetal myelomeningocele closure.[25]

Similarly grouped as in the earlier section, the symptoms of CIIM are best considered according to the area demonstrating disturbed function: brainstem, cerebellar, or spinal cord dysfunction (Fig. 9.12). Approximately 33% of these patients will develop some symptom of hindbrain herniation prior to the age of 5 years and outcome significantly worsens for presentation of these symptoms before 3 months of age.[26,27] Symptoms that may result in death if left untreated include stridor, apnea, and dysphagia resulting in aspiration, and are the leading cause of death in myelodysplastic patients. Nystagmus may be the earliest sign of cerebellar dysfunction and the initial spinal cord symptoms (weakness, bowel and bladder dysfunction) are secondary to the inadequate formation of the lower spinal cord. It is important to note that spinal cord function can worsen during development and that CSF diversionary shunt malfunction, syringomyelia formation, or spinal cord tethering must be ruled out and surgically dealt with if present. Scoliosis may also be present in this population and may be related to syringomyelia.

MRI continues to be the imaging procedure of choice in these patients. Indeed, the advent of MRI technology enabled the identification of the associated developmental abnormalities mentioned previously. Plain dynamic cervical spine radiographs may assist with any question of instability, just as plain thoracic and lumbar radiographs would help to follow the degree of scoliosis. Spinal cord syringes are best identified and followed with spinal MRI.

It is important to stress that adequate shunt function must be established prior to pursuing decompression of a symptomatic CIIM (Fig. 9.13).[28] This examination includes surgical inspection of the shunt because the ventricular system may not change size in this group. The number of CIIM decompressions at our institution has decreased significantly following the establishment of this paradigm. Symptoms warranting

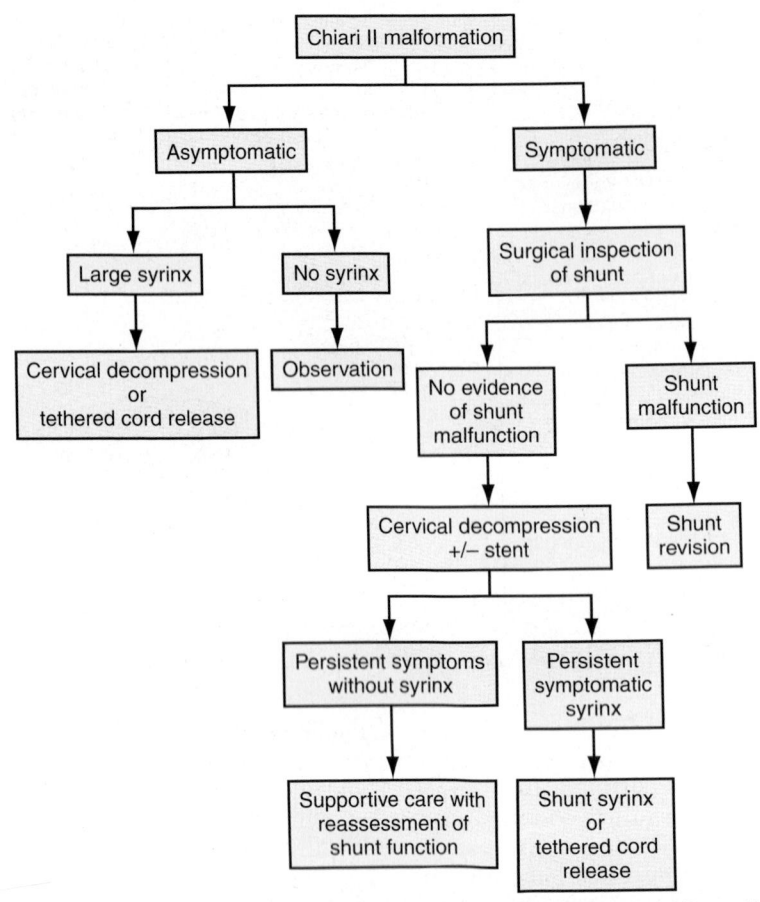

FIGURE 9.13 Therapeutic options for treating patients with Chiari II malformation.

intervention include inspiratory stridor, sleep apnea, recurrent aspiration pneumonia, opisthotonos, and progressive spasticity or ataxia.

When surgical decompression is elected, patients are positioned prone with the neck flexed. Unlike surgical decompression of a CIM, decompression of a CIIM rarely includes removal of the foramen magnum. Removal of the posterior elements of the vertebrae overlying the displaced cerebellar vermis must be performed (Figs. 9.14 and 9.15). The dura is opened widely and the fourth ventricle is identified. The choroid plexus is often in its embryonic extraventricular position. Following this frequently ectopically placed choroid plexus through the dense arachnoidal scarring will usually lead to the foramen of Magendie and the fourth ventricle. This is the crucial goal of the procedure. If any question exists as to the patency of the foramen, then a stent should be placed. The medullary kink, if present, must not be mistaken for the vermis, or the surgeon will end up dissecting into the brainstem. An expansion duraplasty is performed and the remainder of the wound is closed in anatomical layers.

Outcome following surgery is dependent on the severity of symptoms prior to intervention. Infants presenting with brainstem symptoms are less likely to have a significant improvement in their symptoms following decompression. Few studies exist regarding outcome; however, earlier intervention and fewer symptoms are thought to predict success.[27]

SYRINGOHYDROMYELIA

Syringohydromyelia is a secondary process with many causes. The term *syringomyelia* has been used to describe any longitudinal fluid collection within the spinal cord. This term, however, refers to fluid collections outside the central canal. *Hydromyelia* refers to fluid collections enlarging the central canal. A combination of these two words, *syringohydromyelia* better connotes this disease process. However, for the purposes of simplicity we have used the term *syringomyelia* or *syrinx* throughout this chapter to denote any fluid collection within the spinal cord. Known pathological situations in which a syrinx may form include post-traumatic circumstances or in association with Chiari malformations (Figs. 9.16 to 9.18), neoplasms, arteriovenous malformations, arachnoiditis, or occult spinal dysraphism. Idiopathic syringomyelia also exists. The mechanism by which the fluid accumulates varies significantly and a useful informal system to classify syringes divides them into either communicating (Chiari, occult spinal dysraphism) or noncommunicating (neoplasm, arteriovenous malformations, arachnoiditis, traumatic). A terminal syrinx (lower one third of the spinal cord) is normally not a result of hindbrain herniation.

Fluid collections that begin in the ependyma-lined central canal (hydromyelia) may cause an outpouching in weak areas that can grow into the white matter of the cord (Fig. 9.19). The absence of ependyma then enables the syrinx to enlarge with less constraint. Of note are the

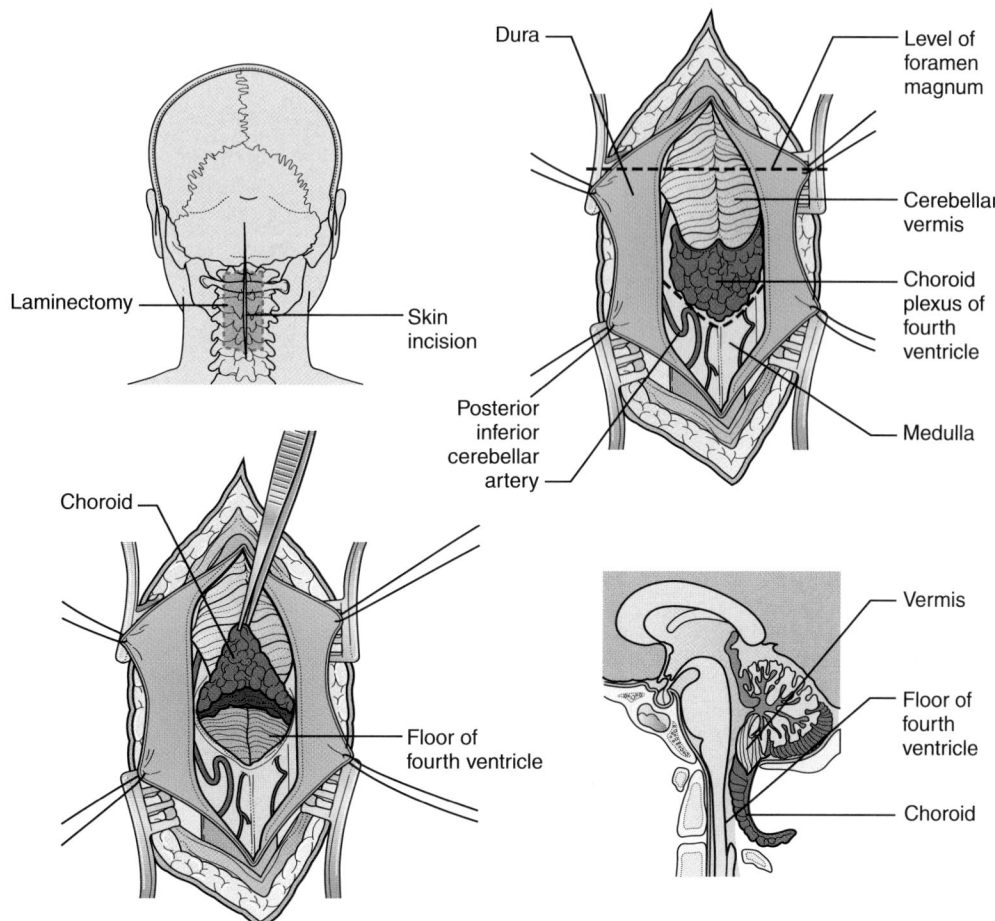

FIGURE 9.14 Operative exposure of the Chiari II malformation.

spinothalamic tract in the ventral white commissure that are particularly vulnerable to syrinx expansion.

Symptoms include loss of pain and temperature sensation in the arm or chest, diminished or absent deep tendon reflexes, and spasticity of the lower extremities. Longer-term findings include wasting of the intrinsic muscles of the hand and scoliosis. Dysesthetic pain over the thorax and arms is a particularly poor prognostic indicator for postoperative relief of symptoms. Acute loss of neurological function may occur with coughing or straining. When the Valsalva maneuver causes the epidural venous complex to expand, the cavity may be forced to dissect through white matter within the cord (Fig. 9.20). This may result in symptomatic or asymptomatic enlargement of the syrinx.

MRI is the diagnostic procedure of choice for syringohydromyelia. Up to 75% of patients with CIM will have an associated syrinx identified on MRI, and between 20% and 95% of patients with CIIM will have a syrinx seen on imaging.[2] An extreme form of syringomyelia, which has ruptured through the pia mater of the spinal cord and expanded, may be seen in this group and is referred to as an *exophytic syrinx*. These syringes may be confused with spinal arachnoid cysts in this population.

If symptoms are functionally significant (Fig. 9.21) or progressive, intervention should be considered, with the recommended procedure varying widely depending on the underlying condition (Fig. 9.22). No medical therapy exists for syringomyelia. If no alternative explanation for a surgically

significant syrinx is identified, exploration of the craniocervical junction should be considered. Follow-up MRI can readily evaluate residual or recurrent fluid. In the setting of a residual syrinx following a decompressed CIM, the patient should return to the operating room and the posterior fossa should be explored for readhesion of the arachnoid at the outlet of the fourth ventricle.[29-31] There is no consensus as to how long to wait and at our institution, we wait at least 6 months in asymptomatic patients. It is common for a cerebellar tonsil to be either partially coagulated or resected subpially during the secondary procedure. When operative therapy turns to stenting or shunting the syrinx, note that the arachnoid flow tends to be compromised in certain pathological states (i.e., arachnoiditis, post-traumatic) and therefore the distal end of the shunt should be placed either in the pleural space or the peritoneum. If the distal end of a syrinx stent is placed in the intrathecal space, it is imperative that it be placed in the subarachnoid space for absorption to take place properly. Reestablishment of a patent spinal canal and subarachnoid space may be undertaken in the setting of traumatic disruption through removal of bone fragments or bony realignment. This is made more difficult in the setting of a previous surgical fusion. Occasionally, syringes are multicompartmental and will require drainage at multiple sites. If the syrinx is the result of either arteriovenous malformations or tumor, primary treatment is directed at the appropriate pathology. Outcome

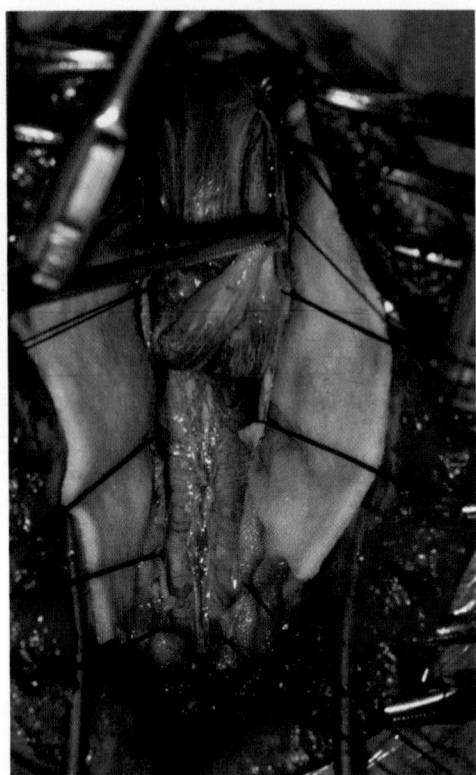

FIGURE 9.15 Operative view of the Chiari II malformation.

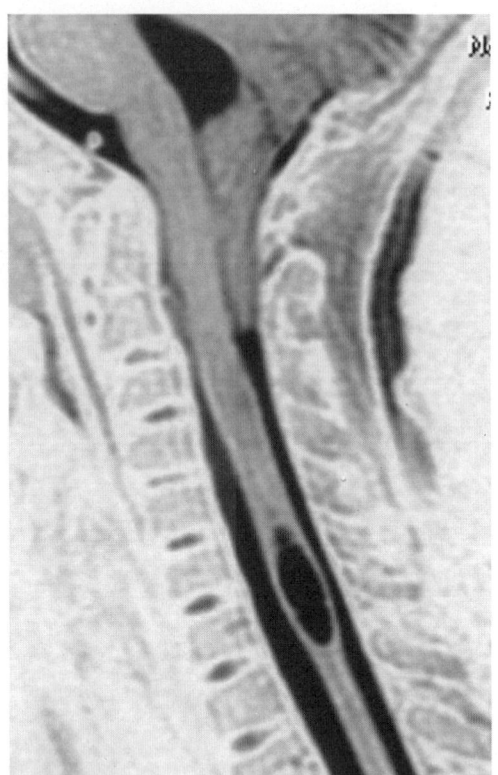

FIGURE 9.16 Sagittal magnetic resonance imaging demonstrating small syringes.

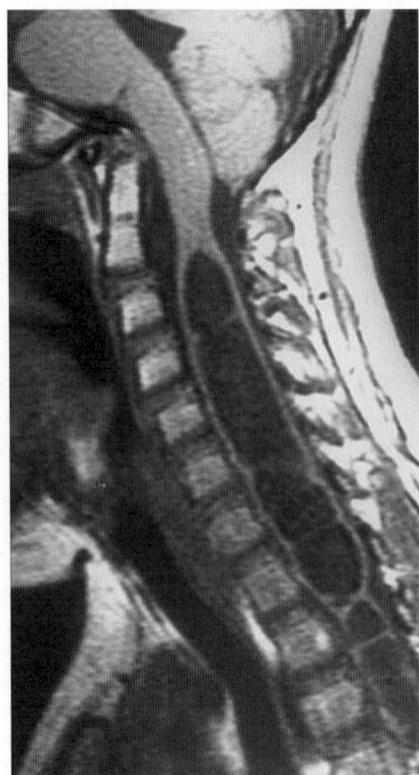

FIGURE 9.17 Sagittal magnetic resonance imaging demonstrating large syringes.

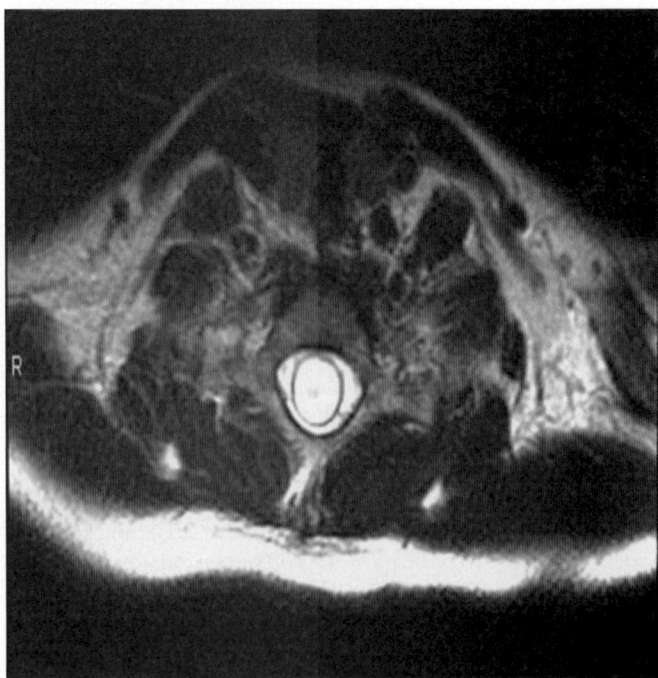

FIGURE 9.18 Axial view of Figure 9.17 noting the distended syrinx.

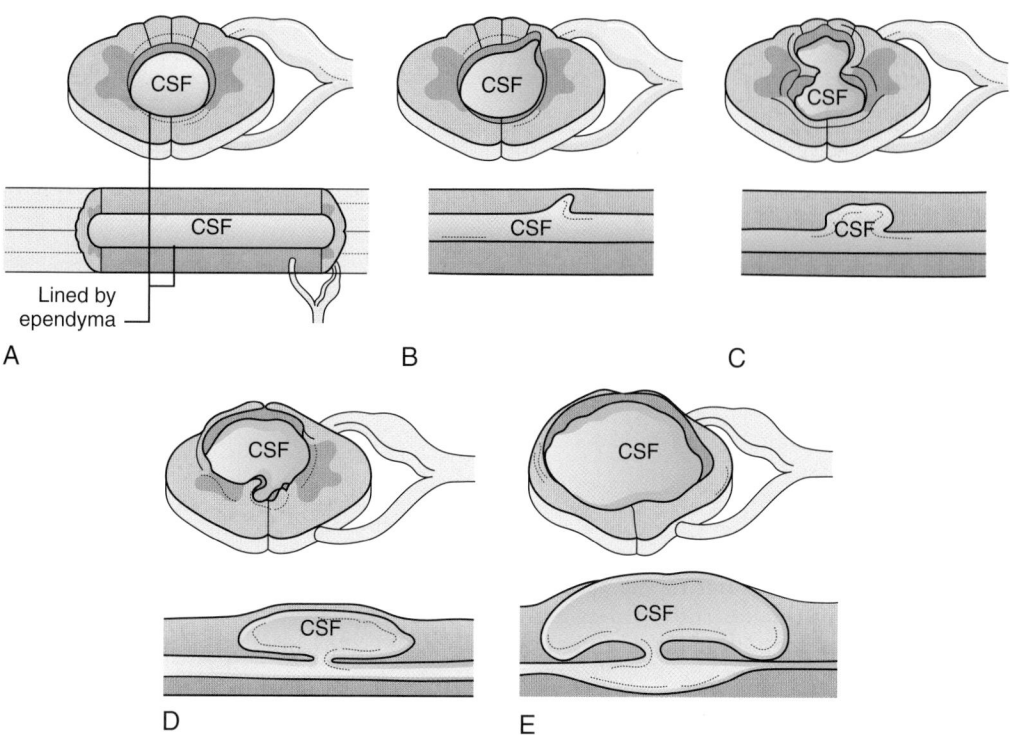

FIGURE 9.19 Stages in the progressive expansion of an ependyma-lined hydromyelia to a larger cavity compressing the central canal. This large cavity has no ependymal lining and so could be termed a syrinx.

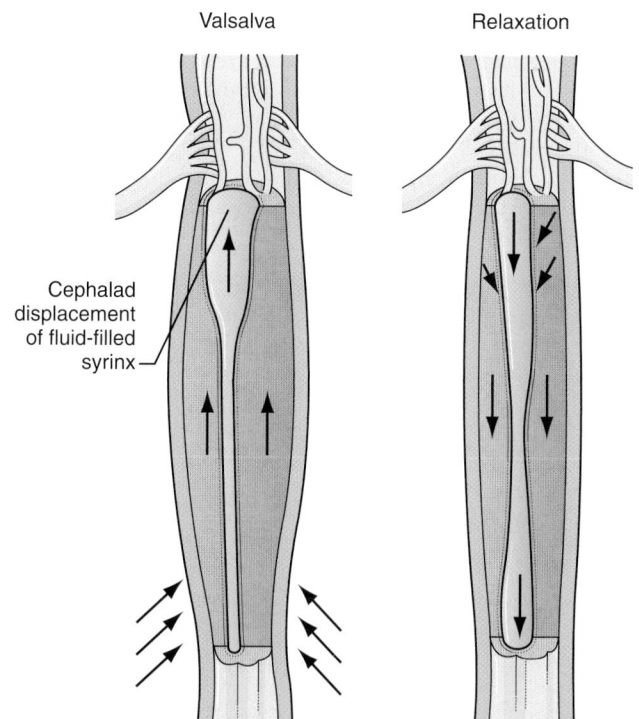

FIGURE 9.20 Increased intra-abdominal pressure caused by the Valsalva maneuver forces blood into the epidural venous complex. When the epidural veins are forcefully expanded against the enlarged cystic cord they may force the cyst to be displaced (usually cephalad). This sudden displacement with forceful coughing or sneezing may actually be associated with a significant worsening of the patient's neurological condition.

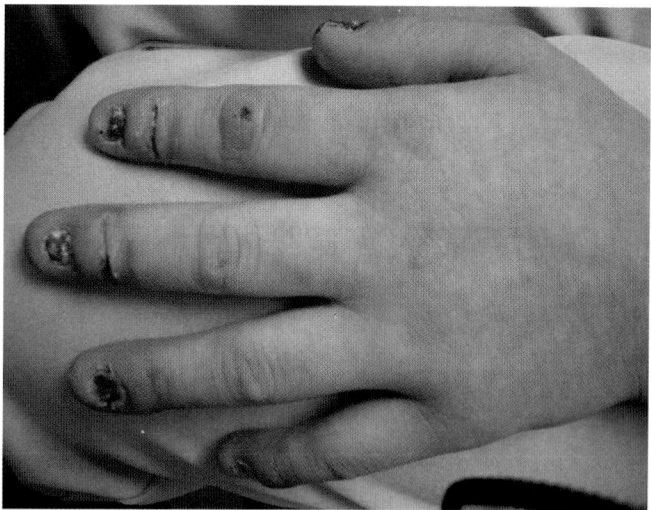

FIGURE 9.21 Left hand from a patient with a large cervicothoracic syringomyelia and dysesthetic pain that resulted in her biting the nails off her fingers.

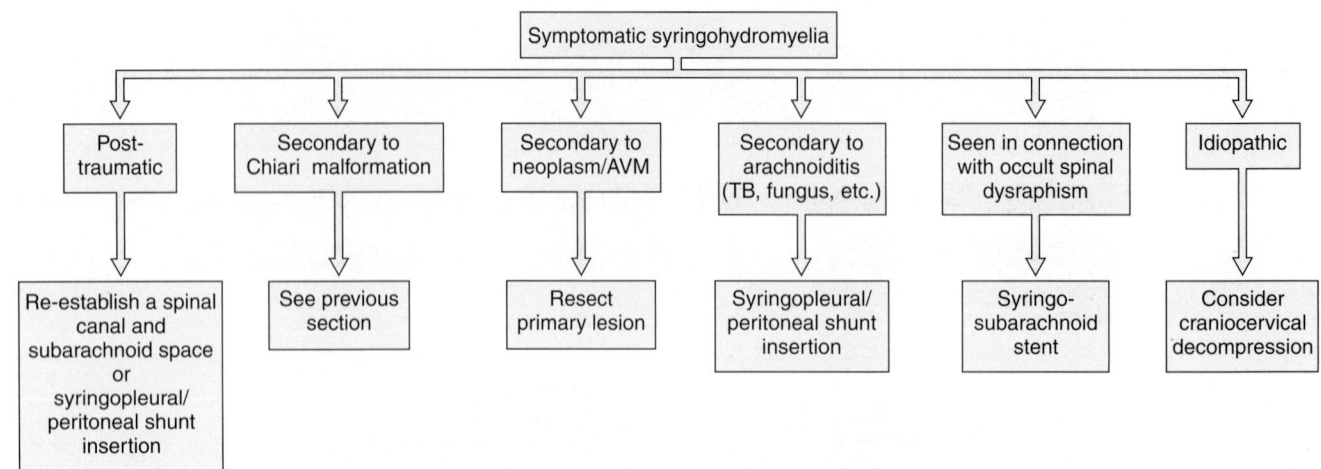

FIGURE 9.22 Therapeutic options for patients with symptomatic syringomyelia.

is dependent on the degree of disability prior to intervention and the cause of the syrinx. Evaluation for any tethering elements (e.g., fatty filum terminale) should be made in patients with terminal syringes. If tethering is found, the offending element is addressed. If no tethering pathology is found, these patients can be watched unless there is unequivocal evidence for neurological decline (e.g., bladder function).

SUMMARY

Time and, when necessary, surgical intervention are needed to better elucidate the natural history of the hindbrain herniation syndromes known as the Chiari malformations. Numerous abnormalities of the nervous system may also be associated with them, and a unified theory has yet to be fully discerned. To date, all studies aimed at the Chiari malformations are classified as levels II and III. Syringomyelia is most often due to these abnormalities at the craniocervical junction but also occurs in response to other pathological processes of the spinal cord.

SELECTED KEY REFERENCES

Hayhurst C, Richards O, Zaki H, et al. Hindbrain decompression for Chiari-syringomyelia complex: an outcome analysis comparing surgical techniques. *Br J Neurosurg.* 2008;22:86-91.

Milhorat TH, Chou MW, Trinidad EM, et al. Chiari I malformation redefined: clinical and radiographic findings for 364 symptomatic patients. *Neurosurgery.* 1999;44:1005-1017.

Oakes WJ, Tubbs RS. Chiari malformations. In: Winn HR, ed. *Youmans Neurological Surgery: A Comprehensive Guide to the Diagnosis and Management of Neurosurgical Problems.* 5th ed. Philadelphia: WB Saunders; 1993.

Tubbs RS, McGirt MJ, Oakes WJ. Surgical experience in 130 pediatric patients with Chiari I malformation. *J Neurosurg.* 2003;99:291-296.

Tubbs RS, Shoja MM, Ardalan MR, et al. Hindbrain herniation: a review of embryological theories. *Ital J Anat Embryol.* 2008;113:37-46.

Please go to expertconsult.com to view the complete list of references.

Posterior Fossa and Brainstem Tumors in Children

Adrienne Weeks, Aria Fallah, James T. Rutka

CLINICAL PEARLS

- Presentation and Investigation
- Presentation of posterior fossa lesions is dictated by location, and aggressiveness of the lesion involved. The most common presenting symptom of a posterior fossa mass is headache related to mass effect, or obstruction of cerebrospinal fluid (CSF) pathways.

- Seizures from a posterior fossa mass are rare. If a patient with a posterior fossa tumor presents with seizures, consider the possibility of leptomeningeal spread.

- Magnetic resonance imaging (MRI) of the brain and spinal cord should be obtained to rule out disseminated disease. Occasionally lumbar puncture may be required for cytological examination.

- Pilocytic Astrocytoma
- Pilocytic astrocytomas are the most common pediatric cerebellar neoplasm.

- The degree of mitotic activity, cellular atypia, and microvascular proliferation do not affect grade of pilocytic astrocytomas.

- Gross total resection of a pilocytic astrocytoma is considered curative. If the cyst wall enhances, it should be removed by the neurosurgeon.

- Medulloblastoma
- Desmoplastic medulloblastomas have a more favorable prognosis than classical medulloblastoma. Anaplastic/large cell histological finding has a poor prognosis and qualifies as high-risk medulloblastoma.

- The most common genetic anomaly in medulloblastoma is isochromosome 17q. In the near future, prognostic and risk stratification of medulloblastoma will be based on molecular profiling.

- "Second look" surgery should be considered when significant residual disease is evident on postoperative imaging.

- The current standard of care for average-risk medulloblastoma, age above 3 years, is gross total

resection, postoperative craniospinal radiation of 23.4 Gy with a posterior fossa boost of 54 Gy, followed by 12 months of chemotherapy. Postoperative intensive chemotherapy can be used to delay radiation in children younger than 3 years of age.

- Ependymoma
- The 5-year survival rate for ependymoma is 60%.

- Classic histological features include ependymal rosettes and pseudorosettes.

- Ependymoma of the cerebellopontine (CP) angle can encase vital neurovascular structures.

- Extent of surgical resection is the only factor with significant prognostic value.

- Atypical Teratoid/Rhabdoid Tumor
- Loss of INI1 is found in 90% of atypical teratoid/rhabdoid tumors (AT/RTs).

- Owing to intermixed histopathological features, AT/RT can be confused with medulloblastoma or primitive neuroectodermal tumors (PNETs) if only small areas are biopsied.

- Gross total resection predicts for improved survival. Radiation therapy should not be used for children under 3 years of age. Intrathecal chemotherapy is being tested in recent clinical trials.

- Choroid Plexus Tumors
- Histologically, choroid plexus papillomas are difficult to distinguish from normal choroid epithelium.

- Choroid plexus tumors are more common in the very young.

- Choroid plexus tumors are extremely vascular and intraoperative blood loss can lead to morbidity and fatal outcome.

- Dermoid/Epidermoid Cysts
- Dermoids typically present in midline locations in association with a dermal sinus tract. The sinus tract should be completely excised to prevent recurrence.

- Epidermoid cysts occur laterally and are commonly found in the CP angle.

- High signal on diffusion-weighted imaging aids in differentiating an epidermoid from an arachnoid cyst.

- Treatment of Hydrocephalus
- A third ventriculostomy prior to tumor resection in children over age 3 can be effective in eliminating CSF shunt requirements postoperatively.

- Brainstem Gliomas
- Not all brainstem tumors have an unfavorable prognosis. Subsets of focal brainstem gliomas are associated with long-term survival. Diffuse intrinsic pontine gliomas account for 60% to 80% of brainstem gliomas, with an average survival of 9 months. NF1 patients have brainstem tumors with a more favorable survival time.

- The use of neuronavigation and neurophysiological mapping and monitoring is essential for maximizing resection while minimizing harm to patients.

- Diffuse Intrinsic Pontine Glioma
- There is no current role for biopsy or surgical excision of these tumors.

- Palliative radiation will provide transient symptom relief in 75% of patients.

- Focal Tectal Gliomas
- More than 80% of these lesions have an indolent course.

- Large size (>2 cm), enhancement, and invasion of adjacent structures are signs of more aggressive tectal lesions.

- Benign tectal lesions in children older than 3 years can be managed with a third ventriculostomy and serial follow-up.

- Surgical Approaches to the Posterior Fossa
- The telovelar approach to the fourth ventricle offers an alternative to the midline approach in which the cerebellar vermis is split.

- Intraoperative mapping/monitoring helps the surgeon in identifying and preserving lower cranial nerves and the brainstem nuclei during surgery.

- Use corridors created by the lesion such as cysts, or presentation to the pial surface, as landmarks to begin the resection of posterior fossa tumors. Do not transgress the floor of the fourth ventricle when resecting brainstem tumors.

Pediatric brain tumors are the leading cause of solid cancer–related death in children. Approximately 60% of these tumors occur below the tentorium, including the brainstem, cerebellum, fourth ventricle, and cerebellopontine angle. In contrast, in the adult population the majority of these neoplasms occurs in the supratentorial compartment. The pathological features of these tumors are diverse, and prognosis ranges from excellent to dismal, depending on histopathological findings, extent of surgical resection, and use of adjunctive therapies (Table 10.1). Great technological strides have been made in regard to improving and understanding tumor biology, imaging, surgical techniques, and chemotherapeutic/radiation protocols, leading to increased survival time in these patients. For example, survival time for medulloblastoma in Cushing's day in the 1920s averaged 17 months. The addition of craniospinal radiation in the 1950s yielded 3-year survival rates of 65% and in the modern era with combined surgery, radiation, and chemotherapy average-risk medulloblastoma patients can achieve a 5-year survival rate of 80% to 85%.[1] However, these treatments can lead to significant morbidity to the developing brain and thus we still have more to learn from these complex and challenging tumors.

CLINICAL PRESENTATION

Presentation is dictated by both location in the posterior fossa and aggressiveness of the lesion involved. The more malignant the lesion is, the shorter the time from symptom onset to diagnosis. The most common presenting sign of a posterior fossa lesion is hydrocephalus, and symptoms related to intracranial hypertension include headache, macrocephaly (in small children), vomiting, blurred vision (papilledema), strabismus (sixth nerve palsies), lethargy, and failure to thrive.

Focal compression of the brainstem may result in cranial nerve deficits from injury to the nuclei or tracts. The most commonly involved cranial nerves are the third, fourth, and sixth. However, long tract findings of hemiparesis and sensory disturbances can also occur as a result of brainstem compression. Compression of the midline cerebellum can cause truncal ataxia and unsteady gait. More lateral compression of the cerebellar hemispheres may result in appendicular ataxia and dysmetria.

Children with lesions in the cerebellopontine angle (CPA) can present with brainstem compression or any number of cranial nerve deficits from direct compression or involvement of the nerve. In addition, patients with leptomeningeal spread may present with signs and symptoms related to the site of metastasis. Supratentorial spread may result in seizures or communicating hydrocephalus, whereas metastasis to the spinal cord may result in spinal cord or nerve compression.

GENERAL DIAGNOSTIC IMAGING FEATURES

Once stabilized, patients with a posterior fossa lesion require magnetic resonance imaging (MRI) of both the brain and spinal cord to rule out leptomeningeal spread.

TABLE 10.1 Survival Data for Pediatric Posterior Fossa Tumors With Current Best Management	
Tumor Subtype	Survival with Current Best Management
Pilocytic astrocytoma	EFS > 90% at 5 years[28]
Medulloblastoma	*Average risk*: EFS 80% at 5 years[67]
	High risk: EFS 60% at 4 years[71]
Ependymoma	GTR: 70-80% 5-year survival rate[101]
	STR: 20-40% 5-year survival rate
AT/RT	3-year EFS 50-78% with radiation[122,123]
	3-year EFS 11% in young children with no radiation[123]
Choroid plexus papilloma	OS 100% at 2 years[132]
	Atypical tumor: OS 89% at 2 years[132]
Choroid plexus carcinoma	OS 36% at 2 years[132]
Diffuse pontine glioma	9-month survival[207, 228]
Focal brainstem glioma	5-year survival rates 50-100%[194, 226-228, 239]

AT/RT, atypical teratoid/rhabdoid tumor; CPP, choroid plexus papilloma; EFS, event-free survival rate; GTR, gross total resection; OS, overall survival rate; STR, subtotal resection.

Cerebrospinal fluid (CSF) may be acquired by lumbar puncture if deemed safe prior to surgery to look for malignant cells. If a metastatic workup cannot be performed prior to surgery, then a waiting period of 10 to 14 days prior to imaging or obtaining lumbar CSF should elapse after surgery to avoid false positive results from surgical intervention.[2] MRI can also alert the surgeon to instances when the brainstem or floor of the fourth ventricle has been compromised by an invading tumor.

Despite the classic imaging of each tumor type, it can be very difficult to differentiate these tumors based on MRI or CT alone. Classically, medulloblastoma has a higher cellularity than either pilocytic astrocytoma or ependymoma and as such has a higher density on CT or is hypointense on T1 MRI. The solid portion of a pilocytic astrocytoma is hyperintense to CSF on T2 sequences in 50% of cases.[3] Ependymoma can typically be seen exiting laterally or inferiorly from the foramen of Luschka or Magendie, respectively. However, imaging characteristics often overlap or are atypical, and diagnosis based on traditional imaging alone is not reliable. Recently, studies have utilized diffusion-weighted imaging (DWI) and magnetic resonance spectroscopy (MRS) to enhance predictive values. DWI measures the microscopic diffusion of water in tissues. Highly cellular tumors such as medulloblastoma have restricted diffusion and higher signals on apparent diffusion coefficient (ADC) maps. Proton MRS analyzes the metabolic composition from tissues such as choline (high in tumors), N-acetylaspartate (reduced in tumors), lactate, taurine (high in medulloblastoma), glutamine, myoinositol, and alanine. Utilizing these two methods in conjunction may help increase predictive values of imaging for pediatric posterior fossa tumors or help distinguish relapse from radiation necrosis.[4]

INDIVIDUAL POSTERIOR FOSSA TUMOR TYPES

Pilocytic Astrocytoma

Cerebellar astrocytomas were first described in a series of 76 tumors by Harvey Cushing.[5,6] Pilocytic astrocytomas (PAs) are the most common pediatric cerebellar neoplasm and occur at a mean age of 7 to 8 years.[7,8] There is no gender predilection. Pilocytic astrocytomas are WHO (World Health Organization) grade I lesions, indicating their slow growth, indolent behavior, and high survival rate. They can occur in any location of the neuraxis, but the cerebellar hemispheres (~50%), optic pathways, thalamus, and hypothalamus are the most common sites.[7] There are case reports of pilocytic tumors occurring within the CPA.[9,10] The vast majority of cerebellar astrocytomas are pilocytic (WHO I), as was found in 88% of patients in the Hospital for Sick Children series.[11] However, distinctions between fibrillary and pilocytic tumors of the cerebellum have not been useful in predicting prognosis.

Imaging

Typically, cerebellar pilocytic astrocytomas appear as well-circumscribed cystic lesions with a solid enhancing nodule (Fig. 10.1). Computed tomography (CT) imaging reveals a well-demarcated lesion with cystlike features, very occasional calcifications, and intense enhancement of the solid component with contrast agent administration.[12,13] A pilocytic astrocytoma can present on imaging in four patterns: (1) An enhancing mural nodule or mass accompanied by a nonenhancing cyst; (2) an enhancing mural nodule with an intensely enhancing cyst; (3) a predominantly solid mass with no cyst component; and (4) a necrotic mass with a central nonenhancing zone.[14] Pilocytic tumors typically arise from the vermis and the cerebellar hemispheres but can extend into the ventricular system.[15] Pilocytic astrocytomas are isointense to hypointense relative to normal brain on T1 images and hyperintense to normal brain in T2 images.[7] However, diagnosing pilocytic astrocytomas, medulloblastomas, and ependymomas with complete accuracy is not possible based on traditional imaging. Next-generation MRS and DWI techniques (described earlier) may be helpful in the future.

Dissemination or leptomeningeal spread of pilocytic astrocytoma is rare and is more common in tumors arising from the hypothalamus, partially resected tumors, and tumors of the very young.[16] In contrast with other more aggressive tumors, leptomeningeal dissemination of a pilocytic astrocytoma is not incompatible with long-term survival.[17]

Histology

Histologically, pilocytic astrocytomas are characterized by a classic biphasic pattern of loose glial tissue and compacted piloid tissue (see Fig. 10.1). The piloid component comprises dense sheets of bipolar cells with fibrillary process containing Rosenthal fibers. The loose glial component contains protoplasmic astrocytes and eosinophilic granular bodies.[18] Macroscopically pilocytic tumors appear well circumscribed; however, on the microscopic level 64% show

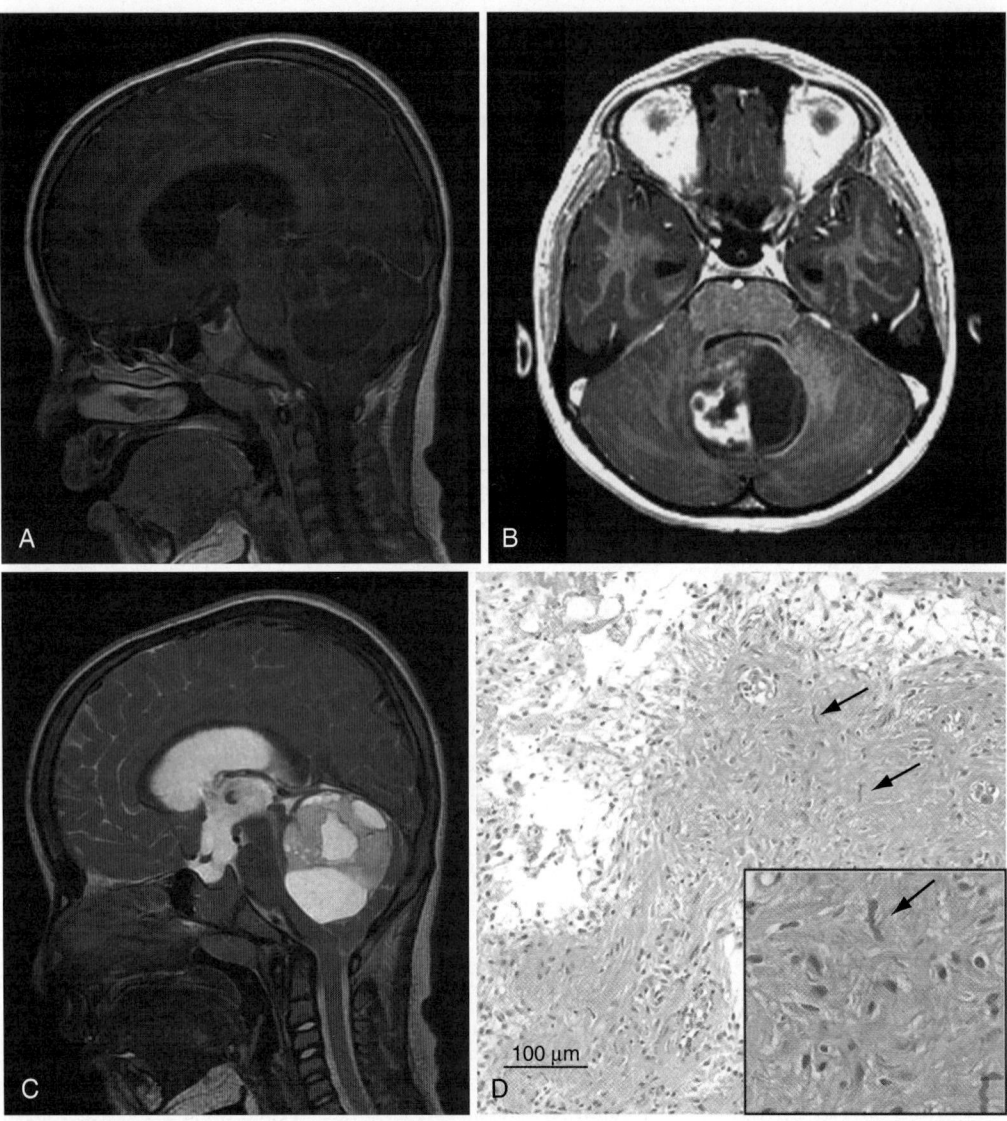

FIGURE 10.1 Magnetic resonance imaging (MRI) scan of a 7-year-old boy with a pilocytic astrocytoma presenting with a long-standing history of headache. **A to C,** Midsagittal T1-weighted image with gadolinium contrast enhancement, axial T2-weighted image, and midsagittal T2-weighted image showing a mainly cystic posterior fossa lesion with an enhancing solid component and associated hydrocephalus. The highly cystic nature and high T2 signal intensity suggest the diagnosis of pilocytic astrocytoma. **D,** Hematoxylin and eosin (H&E) staining of a pilocytic astrocytoma. Arrows are pointing at Rosenthal fibers, which are characteristic of this tumor. Inset is a higher magnification of the image.

infiltration of the surrounding brain, making surgical extirpation difficult.[13] In the cerebellar pilocytic astrocytoma, invasion of the leptomeninges is common.[18] However, this invasion does not correlate with a poor prognosis. Interestingly, the degree of mitotic index, cellular atypia, and microvascular proliferation has no effect on event-free survival. However, histopathological evidence of vascular hyalinization, calcification, necrosis, or oligodendroglioma-like features may predict a poorer clinical outcome.[19] Very rarely, pilocytic astrocytomas undergo malignant transformation to an anaplastic pilocytic astrocytoma.[7] The majority of malignant transformation has occurred after administration of radiotherapy.[20,21]

Contrary to the supratentorial and brainstem pilocytic tumors, cerebellar pilocytic astrocytomas are rare in the neurofibromatosis type 1 (NF1) population. Recently, genetic investigations have revealed gains at 7q34 resulting in the discovery of two important fusion proteins: KIA1546-BRAF and SRGAP3-RAF1. These fusion proteins lead to constitutive activation of the ERK/MAP kinase pathway.[22-25]

Management

Gross total resection of a pilocytic astrocytoma is considered curative.[8,15,16,26,27] Resection of the mural nodule is key in the surgical extirpation of pilocytic astrocytomas. Surgeons debate the need for removal of the cystic wall, but no statistical difference in survival has been noted between patients with cyst wall removal and those without.[14] Postoperative MRI is imperative to evaluate degree of resection because direct neurosurgical evaluation is unreliable. With gross total resection 10-year survival rates are in excess of 90%.[28] Subtotal resection increases rate of recurrence (7% vs. 27%) but not overall survival.[7,28] Spontaneous regression after partial resection as measured by MRI occurs more frequently than growth. Thus, a good argument can be made for observation of residual tumor in cases in which reoperation for total resection carries a high morbidity rate, such as when the tumor invades the fourth ventricle (~10%).[28,29] No adjunctive therapy is required for the treatment of pilocytic astrocytoma unless leptomeningeal spread is evident. Leptomeningeal dissemination

FIGURE 10.2 Magnetic resonance imaging (MRI) scan of a 7-year-old boy with an anaplastic medulloblastoma presenting with a short history of nausea, vomiting, and headache. **A** to **C,** Midsagittal T1-weighted, axial T1-weighted with gadolinium contrast, and coronal T2-weighted images showing a predominantly solid posterior fossa lesion with T1 hypointensity and heterogeneous enhancement; note the obstructive hydrocephalus. The hypointense T1 signal and predominantly solid nature of this lesion suggest medulloblastoma. **D,** Hematoxylin and eosin (H&E) staining showing a highly cellular small blue cell tumor. Note the numerous mitotic figures present in the magnified inset (*arrows*).

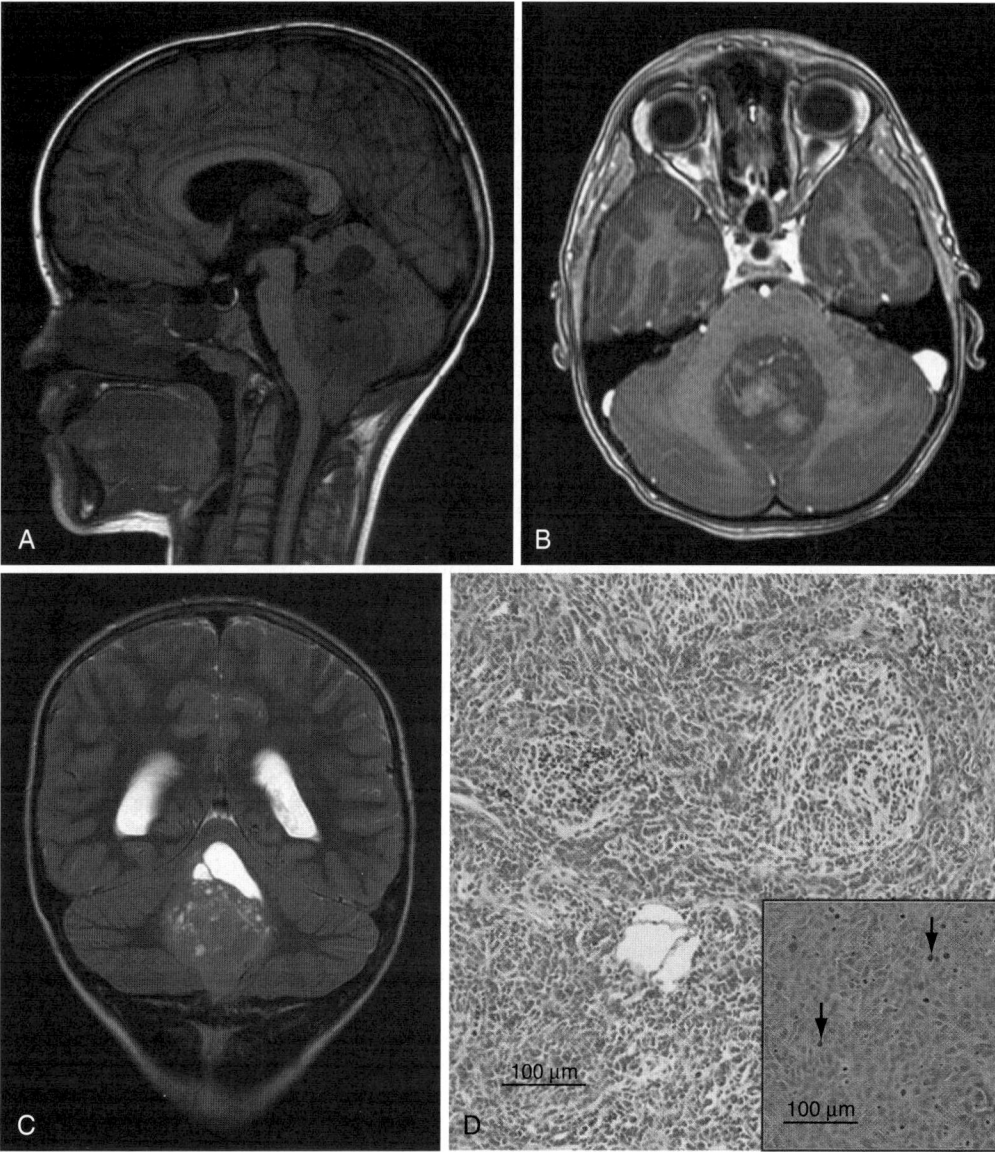

can then be treated with chemotherapy or radiation, although no standard protocol exists.[16,17,30,31]

Medulloblastoma

Medulloblastoma is the most common malignant solid neoplasm of childhood. Medulloblastomas are related to primitive neuroectodermal tumors (PNETs) and occur exclusively in the posterior fossa. The median age at presentation is 9 years in the entire population and 7.3 years in the pediatric population.[32] There is a slight male predominance of 1.6:1.[32]

Histology and Genetics

The WHO classifies medulloblastoma as a grade IV lesion and recognizes five subtypes: classic, desmoplastic/nodular, medulloblastoma with extreme nodularity, anaplastic, and large cell.[33] Desmoplastic/nodular lesions have a more favorable prognosis as opposed to large cell and anaplastic lesions, which have a poorer prognosis when compared to classic

medulloblastoma.[34-36] Classic medulloblastoma appears as a small blue cell tumor, composed of densely packed undifferentiated oval cells with hyperchromatic nuclei and scant cytoplasm (Fig. 10.2). As with other malignant lesions, there is marked nuclear pleomorphism and brisk mitotic activity.[37] Homer-Wright rosettes composed of neoplastic cells concentrically arranged around fibrillary processes are a common histological feature. The desmoplastic type of medulloblastoma contains "pale islands" of reticulin fibers surrounding a nodular reticulin-free zone.[37] The large cell and anaplastic subtypes are characterized by large nuclei with prominent nucleoli, and a lower nuclear-to-cytoplasmic ratio than classic medulloblastoma.[38,39]

Genetic insights into medulloblastoma were gained by studying the familial tumor predisposition syndromes: Gorlin's syndrome (a mutation in the *PTCH* gene in the sonic hedgehog signaling pathway), Turcot's syndrome (a mutation in the *APC* gene affecting the beta-catenin/Wnt signaling pathway, and Li-Fraumeni syndrome (a mutation in *p53* tumor suppressor gene).[40] However, these familial syndromes account for only a small percentage of medulloblastomas.

The largest genetic analysis on sporadic medulloblastoma comes from a study by Northcott and associates in which they analyzed 212 medulloblastomas with high-resolution SNP (single nucleotide polymorphism) genotyping. Isochromosome 17q was confirmed as the most common genetic alteration in medulloblastomas, found in 28% of specimens.[41] This large data set corroborated other genes associated with medulloblastoma such as amplification of *MYC* oncogenes, *OTX2*, *TERT*, *PDGFRA*, and *CDK*.[41] Interestingly, this paper identified a novel pathway of medulloblastoma pathogenesis including histone lysine methylation genes, which regulate gene expression during development.[41]

The cell of origin in medulloblastoma remains elusive. Some groups have proposed medulloblastoma to arise from the external granule layer of the developing cerebellum and others have proposed that the cell of origin arises from a subventricular progenitor zone. Recent genetic subgroup analysis has classified medulloblastoma into one of four or five distinct genetic groups.[42,43] In a series of over 400 patients which was linked to patient prognostic data, medulloblastomas could be segregated into one of four subgroups: group A (characterized by defects in WNT pathway signaling), group B (characterized by defects in SHH signaling), group C, and group D. Prognosis was correlated with subgroup and revealed that patients with group B medulloblastoma were at the extremes of age (infant or adult), have a desmoplastic phenotype, and have a more favorable prognosis. Group A medulloblastoma behaved in a similar fashion to classic medulloblastoma, whereas group C and D tumors had a poorer prognosis, and presented with disseminated disease. Of greatest interest, however, was the ability to predict genetic subgroup based on immunohistochemistry alone (Table 10.2). These distinct genetic and prognostic subgroups argue for a multiple cell of origin for medulloblastoma, but what is more important, they may change the way we risk stratify and treat patients with medulloblastoma in the future.

Imaging

Medulloblastomas are typically midline cerebellar lesions arising from the vermis; however, in older children and adults they can arise from the cerebellar hemispheres.[44] Classic CT imaging of medulloblastoma is a hyperdense lesion in the cerebellar vermis with surrounding vasogenic edema.[45,46] Calcification (22%) and cyst formation (59%) may be observed in some cases.[47] There is a high degree of variability of MR appearances of medulloblastoma. T1 sequences are usually iso-hypointense to white matter and hyperintense on T2 sequences (see Fig. 10.2). Tumor enhancement can be both homogeneous or heterogeneous.[46] Similar to ependymoma, approximately 14% of medulloblastomas may show foraminal extension.[48] Leptomeningeal seeding on MRI is found in approximately 33% of patients. The spinal canal is the most common location of seeding; however, the supratentorial compartment may also be involved. Nodular or diffuse enhancement along the leptomeninges, nerve roots in the spinal canal, or cranial nerves in the CPA are common findings of CSF seeding (Fig. 10.3).[46,49-51] Interestingly only 15% to 60% of patients with evidence of metastasis by MRI have positive CSF by cytological examination and only 70%

TABLE 10.2 Novel Stratification of Medulloblastoma Based on Genetic Subgroup Analysis

Subtype	Genetic Background	Immunohisto-chemical Stain
A	WNT tumors	DKK1
B	Sonic Hedgehog (SHH) tumors	SFRP1
C		NPR3
D		KCNA1

Data from Northcott PA, Korshunov A, Witt H, et al. Medulloblastoma comprises four distinct molecular variants. J Clin Oncol 2011;29(11): 1408-1414.

of patients with positive cytological findings have evidence of metastasis by MRI. This highlights the importance of CSF cytological examination, especially in cases in which the MRI imaging is negative.[52,53] Rare cases of extraneural spread have been reported to bone, lymph nodes, liver, and lung.[54]

Management

With combined surgical resection, radiation, and high-dose chemotherapy, 5-year progression-free survival rate in average-risk medulloblastoma is approximately 80%. Currently risk stratification is based on age (less than 3 years of age), presence of disseminated disease, and extent of surgical resection (Table 10.3). However, this stratification system fails to take into consideration the biology of medulloblastoma tumors, and a system based on molecular markers and genetic subgroup analysis may provide a better way of categorizing patients in the future. Current treatment studies are including favorable molecular markers such as nuclear beta-catenin and TrkC expression and unfavorable markers such as *Myc* genes and *ERBB2* in their stratification paradigms.[55]

Surgery for Medulloblastoma

The goal of surgery in medulloblastoma is complete resection without causing neurological injuries. Several clinical trials have shown that extent of surgical resection correlates with recurrence-free survival.[56-59] Postoperative imaging should be obtained 24 to 48 hours after surgery and compared to preoperative scans to determine extent of resection. In cases in which there is greater than 1.5 cm^2 of residual tumor, a repeat procedure should be considered, if safe and anatomically feasible, to place the patient in the best prognostic category.

Treatment of Children Over Age 3 with Average-Risk Medulloblastoma

Management of medulloblastoma has evolved over time as new clinical trials are published on risk stratification and treatment paradigms. Medulloblastoma is a radiosensitive tumor and incorporation of radiotherapy has become a standard of care in treatment of children older than 3 years of age. The original radiation dose of 36 Gy to the neuroaxis and 54 Gy to the posterior fossa resulted in numerous detrimental side effects including cognitive decline, endocrine insufficiency, hearing loss, vascular complications, and secondary malignancies.[60-65] Because of these detrimental effects of craniospinal

FIGURE 10.3 Metastatic spread of medulloblastoma. **A,** Fluid-attenuated inversion recovery (FLAIR) sequence showing thickening of the leptomeninges in the left sylvian fissure indicative of leptomeningeal spread (arrow). **B,** Midsagittal lumbar spine T1-weighted image showing a drop metastasis behind the sacrum.

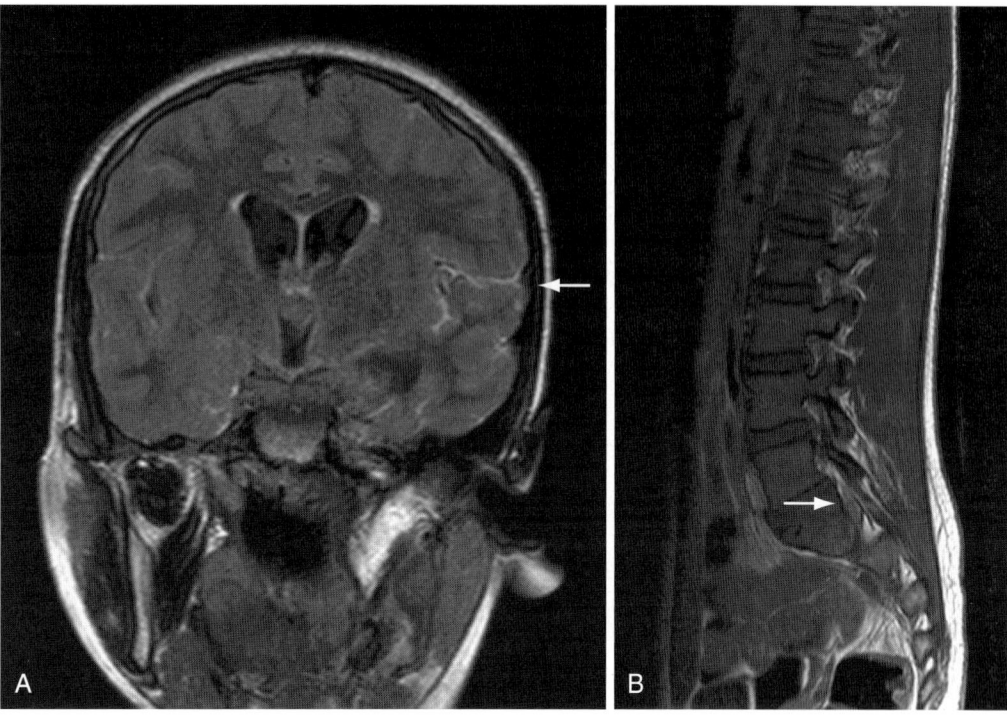

TABLE 10.3 Risk Stratification of Medulloblastoma	
Average-Risk Medulloblastoma	**High-Risk Medulloblastoma**
Age < 3 years	Age □ 3 years
□1.5 cm² residual disease	>1.5 cm² residual disease
M₀—no dissemination of tumor	M₁—positive lumbar CSF cytological findings, negative MRI of brain and spine
	M₂—macroscopic dissemination on MRI of brain and negative MRI of spine
	M₃—macroscopic spinal dissemination on MRI
	M₄—extraneural spread
	Anaplastic histological pattern

CSF, cerebrospinal fluid; M₀-M₄, distant metastasis (staging); MRI, magnetic resonance imaging.

radiation, efforts began to reduce the degree of craniospinal radiation in average-risk patients aimed at preserving neurological function. This was accomplished by increasing the intensity of chemotherapy. Chemotherapy had already proved an effective adjunct to radiation and surgery in earlier studies.[66,67] Packer and colleagues reduced the degree of cranial spinal radiation to 23.4 Gy by adding chemotherapy during and after radiotherapy and still maintained excellent control with event-free-survival (EFS) of greater than 80% in nondisseminated medulloblastoma.[68] Typical chemotherapeutics used in medulloblastoma include cisplatin, CCNU, vincristine, cyclophosphamide, and etoposide. There is some evidence to support a further reduction of craniospinal radiation to 18 Gy and the Children's Oncology Group is currently examining this possibility.[69] The current standard of care for average-risk medulloblastoma is gross total resection, postoperative craniospinal radiation of 23.4 Gy with a posterior fossa boost of 54 Gy, followed by 12 months of chemotherapy.

Treatment of Children Over Age 3 with High-Risk Medulloblastoma

The 5-year event-free survival rate across studies in high-risk medulloblastoma ranges from 30% to 70%.[70] The best outcomes to date involve surgery, craniospinal radiation with 36 to 39.6 Gy, with a posterior fossa boost followed by intense cyclophosphamide, vincristine, cisplatin, and peripheral stem cell rescue. This regimen yielded a 5-year EFS rate of 70%.[71] A 4-year EFS rate of 66% was reached by the Children's Oncology Group (COG 99701) with surgery, concomitant daily vincristine/carboplatin and craniospinal radiation (36 Gy), and a posterior fossa boost followed by monthly cyclophosphamide and vincristine.[72] These studies highlight the intensive regimens required to treat high-risk medulloblastoma. The adverse effects associated with these intensive treatments must be taken into consideration when one considers the enhanced survival rates for these patients.

Treatment of Infants and Young Children with Medulloblastoma

Treating infants and young children with medulloblastoma remains challenging and suboptimal. The developing brain is particularly susceptible to the toxicity of treatment regimes. These patients suffer from severe neurocognitive decline secondary to craniospinal irradiation. Thus, recent neuro-oncology clinical trials have promoted the use of chemotherapeutic strategies to delay or avoid craniospinal radiation. The Pediatric Oncology Group (POG) initiated a trial in the 1980s (the Baby POG study) treating infants with prolonged postoperative chemotherapy in an attempt to delay radiation until 3 years of age. The overall 5-year progression-free survival (PFS) rate was 31.8% but increased to 69% in those children with gross total resection.[73] This study showed that craniospinal radiation could be delayed.[73] The best results, to date, come from the Head Start 1 and 2 trials using induction chemotherapy of cisplatin, vincristine, etoposide, and cyclophosphamide followed by myeloablative chemotherapy and autologous stem cell rescue (methotrexate was added for disseminated disease). The 5-year PFS rates for infants was 64% in those with localized disease and 45% for disseminated disease. Interestingly, 50% of survivors never received radiation.[74]

Salvage Strategies

There are no defined standards of care to salvage children after relapse from medulloblastoma. In infants in whom irradiation was avoided, radiation therapy can be initiated. Other treatments usually include further resection, myeloablative chemotherapy with autologous stem cell rescue, and intrathecal chemotherapy.

Novel Therapeutics

As we begin to understand the molecular biology of medulloblastoma we have come to recognize and identify possible therapeutic targets. One such example is the use of a sonic hedgehog (SHH) pathway inhibitor GDC-0449. A 26-year-old man with recurrent resistant medulloblastoma with aberrant activation of SHH signaling was treated with the inhibitor and showed rapid (albeit transient) response.[75]

Proton beam therapy is a type of radiation therapy that utilizes charged beams that have a finite range in tissues and potentially allows sparing of normal tissues compared to conventional types of radiotherapy. To date, only a few patients with medulloblastoma have been treated with proton beam therapy; however, there is currently a phase II trial being undertaken at this time.[76]

Intrathecal (IT) chemotherapy to delay radiation threapy, salvage recurrent disease, or treat leptomeningeal seeding is being used now in several trials. IT chemotherapeutic regimens have been successfully used to avoid craniospinal radiation in the pediatric leukemia population.[77] Case reports have shown moderate success and phase I and II trials for pediatric medulloblastoma are currently ongoing.[78,79]

Ependymoma

Ependymomas are the third most frequent brain tumor in the pediatric population. First described in 1926 by Cushing and Bailey, they account for 6.4% of primary brain tumors in children aged 0 to 14 years and for 30% of tumors in children less than 3 years of age.[80] The mean age of presentation is 3.7 years.[11] Unlike medulloblastoma, 5-year survival rates for ependymoma are approximately 60%.[81]

Ependymoma can occur throughout the neuraxis. Posterior fossa ependymoma (fourth ventricle, CPA) is more frequent in infants and young children (70%) whereas supratentorial lesions occur more commonly in older children and adults. Ependymomas of the spinal cord and, in particular, the filum terminale occur in both age groups.

Imaging

The classic infratentorial ependymoma fills the fourth ventricle and extends laterally through the foramina of Luschka (15%) and inferiorly through the foramen of Magendie (60%). Typically, ependymoma demonstrates low T1, high T2, and intermediate to high fluid attenuated inversion recovery (FLAIR) signal intensity (Fig. 10.4).[82] However, the lesions can be heterogeneous owing to cystic areas, calcifications (50%), and hemorrhage. Postcontrast imaging shows a heterogeneous enhancing tumor with areas of avid enhancement mixed with poorly enhancing regions. Diffusion-weighted imaging (DWI) is intermediate between pilocytic astrocytomas (low) and primitive neuroectodermal tumors (PNETs) (high).[83] Ependymomas often encase neurovascular structures in the CPA, thus making surgical removal difficult without causing cranial nerve or vascular injury. Ikezaki and co-workers, classified posterior fossa ependymomas into three groups based on location: (1) the lateral type presenting in the CPA characterized by a poor prognosis secondary to involvement of cranial nerves and brainstem; (2) ependymomas localized to the floor of the fourth ventricle with an intermediate prognosis; and (3) those localized to the roof of the fourth ventricle with the most favorable outcome.[84] Leptomeningeal dissemination occurs in 8% to 12% of patients by CSF cytological findings and occurs more frequently with anaplastic grades.[85] Leptomeningeal disease with drop metastasis is most common in the lumbosacral region.

Histology

The WHO recognizes three grades of ependymoma and four histological variants (Table 10.4).[33,80] The classic histological features of ependymoma are perivascular and ependymal rosettes. The former corresponds to ependymal cell processes radially arranged around a cell-free perivascular zone. The latter, ependymal rosettes, comprise tumor cells concentrically arranged to form a lumen.[80] Ependymomas are given an anaplastic grade when there is evidence of (1) brisk mitotic activity; (2) increased cellularity; (3) microvascular proliferation; or (4) pseuodopalisading necrosis. However, there is debate in the literature as to the precise definition of anaplastic criteria. In part, this controversy has called into question whether or not histological grade predicts for survival.[86-95]

The most common genetic alteration in ependymoma is loss of chromosome 22; however, in posterior fossa ependymoma the putative tumor suppressor at this locus remains elusive.[96] Other genetic events common in posterior fossa ependymomas are 9q and 1q gain, loss of 6q, and monosomy 17p.[96] Interestingly, DNA identical to portions of the SV40 virus has been isolated from ependymoma, and SV40 is capable of inducing ependymoma in rodents.

Surgical Management

The key to treatment of ependymoma remains complete macroscopic surgical resection, as it is known that the degree of resection is the most significant predictor of survival. The goals of surgery are tissue diagnosis, management of hydrocephalus, and cyotoreduction. Complete surgical resection leads to 5-year survival rates ranging around 70% to 80%,[80] whereas patients with subtotal resection have significantly poorer outcomes with 5-year survival rates around 20% to 40%.[91,97] Given the predictive value of resection on survival, patients should undergo a postoperative MRI within 48 hours

FIGURE 10.4 Magnetic resonance imaging (MRI) appearance of ependymoma. **A** and **B**, Midsagittal T2- and contrast-enhanced T1-weighted images showing a posterior fossa lesion extending through the foramen of Magendie in a 6-year-old boy. **C**, FLAIR (fluid-attenuated inversion recovery) sequence MRI showing an ependymoma extending through the foramen of Luschka. A third ventriculostomy has been performed and the floor of the third ventricle is bowed upward (*white arrow*). **D**, Hematoxylin and eosin (H&E) photomicrograph staining showing typical perivascular rosettes (*black arrows*).

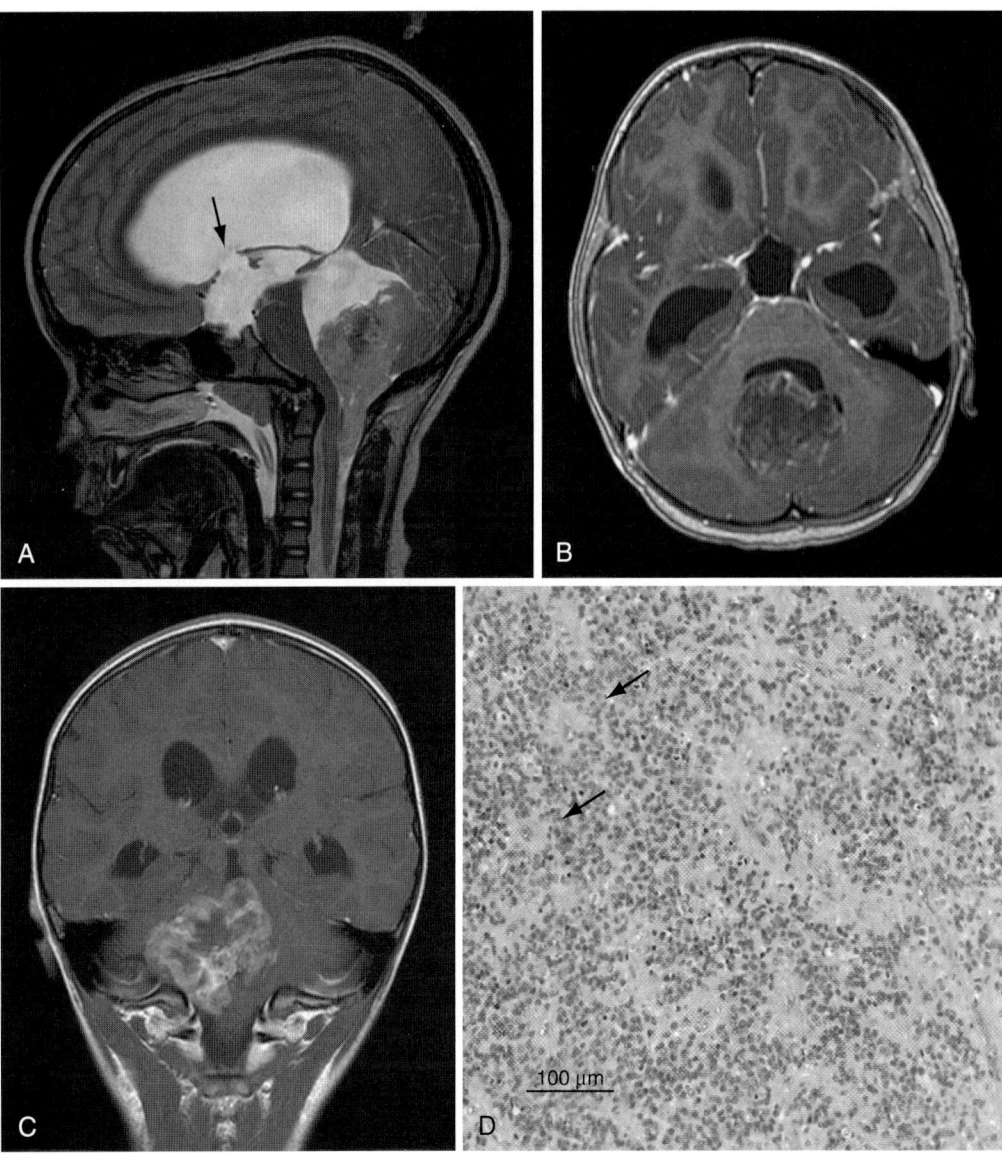

TABLE 10.4 WHO and Histological Grading of Ependymoma

WHO Grade	Histological Subtype(s)
Grade I (subependymoma and myxopapillary)	Cellular ependymoma (grade II)
Grade II (ependymoma)	Papillary ependymoma (grade II or III)
Grade III (anaplastic ependymoma)	Clear cell ependymoma (grade II or III)
	Tanycytic ependymoma (grade II or III)

WHO, World Health Organization.

to ensure macroscopic resection. "Second look" surgery is warranted in cases in which bulky residual disease is found after initial surgery.[91,98-100] It should be stressed here that gross total resection can be made difficult with large ependymomas extending into the CPA encasing cranial nerves and vascular structures or when invasion of the floor of the fourth ventricle occurs. The morbidity of complete resection in these cases may be high (10-30%).[101]

Adjunctive Therapies

Postoperative radiation treatment is an established standard of care for patients with ependymoma because it is a radiosensitive tumor. A recent study from St. Jude Children's Research Hospital showed a 7-year EFS rate and overall survival (OS) rate of 69% and 81%, respectively, with maximal surgical resection and local conformational radiation therapy. Craniospinal radiation was reserved for those cases with evidence of CSF dissemination by imaging or cytological appearance.[102] Interestingly, baseline and longitudinal testing of cognitive outcome demonstrate most survivors within normal range despite a large portion of patients being 3 years or less at treatment.[102]

Currently, there are no proven established protocols for chemotherapy in the treatment of ependymoma. There has been moderate success in using chemotherapy to delay radiation therapy in young children with ependymoma.[73,103,104] Current studies are being undertaken to evaluate molecularly targeted therapy such as the small molecule tyrosine kinase inhibitors (geftinib, erlotinib, baevacizumab).[105]

The rate of relapse following treatment ranges from 30% to 72%.[97,102,104,,106,107] The vast majority of relapses occurs locally, and median survival time after relapse varies from 8.4 to 24 months.[108] The literature supports reoperation for recurrence of ependymoma.[98,107] For children who have not received radiation therapy, radiation therapy should be given. Re-irradiation is an option for children previously treated with radiotherapy, but morbidity rate from radiation necrosis may be high.[109-111]

Atypical Teratoid/Rhabdoid Tumor

Malignant rhabdoid tumors (MRTs) were first described as a highly malignant subtype of Wilms' tumor.[112] It is now recognized that MRTs occur throughout the body. Biggs and associates first described an intracranial MRT in 1987.[113] These tumors were first termed *atypical teratoid/rhabdoid tumors* (AT/RTs) in a landmark paper in 1995 because of their histological characteristics, which showed neuroepithelial, peripheral epithelial, and mesenchymal elements.[114] The WHO first recognized AT/RT as a separate tumor entity in 2000. It is predominantly a tumor of infants and young children with a median age of diagnosis at 26 months with a slight male predominance.[114,115] Approximately 30% of AT/RTs occur infratentorially (CPA and cerebellum), and 22% have CSF dissemination at diagnosis.[115] The overall survival time is 18 months; however, in patients presenting with signs of metastasis the prognosis is significantly worse at 8 months.[115]

Histology

Pathologically, AT/RT is composed of nests or sheets of rhabdoid cells intermixed with areas indistinguishable from PNET or medulloblastoma.[114] The intermixed histological features of AT/RT underscores the issues with sampling errors in biopsies of the AT/RT. The histopathological diagnosis of AT/RT can be aided by staining for the loss of nuclear INI1.[116] *INI1* is a tumor suppressor gene found on chromosome 22q, and 60% to 90% of AT/RTs show monosomy or deletions of chromosome 22.[117]

Imaging

There are no distinguishing features on radiographic imaging that specifically distinguish AT/RTs from other fourth ventricular tumors. As with medulloblastomas, the solid portions of AT/RTs are hyperdense on CT, isointense on T1, and heterogeneous on T2, although the appearance can vary.[118-122] With contrast administration there is heterogeneous enhancement (Fig. 10.5).

Management

Given the overlap of AT/RT with other tumor subtypes of the posterior fossa, it is important to take into consideration the diagnostic tools used to classify AT/RT in each study cohort, specifically whether loss of INI1 by immunohistochemistry was utilized. The St. Jude Children's Research Hospital, Boston Children's Hospital, and the central registry in Cleveland have all published their series of patients with AT/RT. All studies showed that gross total resection correlated with OS and PFS rates.[123-125]

Radiation therapy, either craniospinal or focal, is important in the control of AT/RT. In a meta-analysis by Athale and colleagues, children receiving radiation in combination with chemotherapy versus children not treated with radiotherapy had an overall survival time of 18.4 versus 8.5 months.[116] The St. Jude group treated all patients with surgery and high-dose alkylator chemotherapy, and those over 3 years of age received craniospinal radiation. The 3-year EFS rate of those receiving chemotherapy was 78% versus 11% in children younger than 3 years who did not receive initial craniospinal radiation.[124] However, a large number of patients with AT/RT present before the age of 3 years, increasing the morbidity of radiation.

The variability of chemotherapeutic regimens and the small series of AT/RT cases render conclusions regarding specific chemotherapeutic regimens difficult. Investigators have used cisplatin, high-dose alkylators plus stem cell rescue, variations of the Intergroup Rhabdomyosarcoma Study, IRS III regimens, and temozolamide. In a meta-analysis of chemotherapeutic regimens, intrathecal (IT) chemotherapy increased the probability of survival at 2 years to 64%.[115] This survival benefit was maintained but was not as great in children younger than 3 years of age.[115,123] The Boston Children's Hospital recently published their prospective series of 25 children (mean 26 months) treated with intensive multi-modal therapy consisting of surgical resection, chemoradiation, consolidation therapy, and IT chemotherapy. Two-year EFS rate was 53% and OS rate reached 70%.[123] Whether IT therapy can substitute for craniospinal irradiation for CNS treatment or prophylaxis remains unclear.

Novel approaches to AT/RT treatment will be necessary to increase survival in this disease. A recent study on dendritic cell–based vaccinations was performed for three children with AT/RT (two at relapse and one at presentation with metastatic disease). The two patients who were treated with surgery, chemotherapy, radiation, and vaccination at relapse were still alive at 34- and 53-month follow-up. The patient with a metastatic presentation succumbed at 51 months.[126] In conclusion, AT/RT is an aggressive CNS tumor of young children that remains a therapeutic challenge.

Choroid Plexus Papilloma and Carcinoma

Choroid plexus tumors are rare primary brain tumors arising from choroid plexus epithelium. Guerard first described these neoplasms in 1833 and Bielschowsky performed the first operative procedure in 1906. Choroid plexus neoplasms represent 0.4% to 0.8% of all primary neoplasms of the brain. Although these tumors can occur in all age groups, a greater number of them occur in childhood, with 70% being diagnosed before the age of 2 years. Studies have shown a skewed distribution slightly in favor of the male gender 1-1.3:1.[127] The WHO recognizes three classes of choroid plexus neoplasms: the grade I choroid plexus papilloma (CPP), the grade II atypical CPP, and the grade III choroid plexus carcinoma (CPC).[33]

Anatomically, choroid plexus neoplasms occur more frequently in the lateral (50-70%), fourth (20-40%), and third (5-10%) ventricles.[128] They have also occurred in the CPA and in biventricular locations (5%).[128] However, the anatomical distribution differs markedly in relation to age. In young children, the vast majority of choroid plexus tumors present in the lateral ventricles, whereas fourth ventricular and CPA

FIGURE 10.5 Magnetic resonance imaging (MRI) appearance of atypical teratoid/rhabdoid tumor. **A** to **C,** Axial, coronal T2-weighted images and coronal T1-weighted image with gadolinium enhancement showing a heterogeneous posterior fossa lesion with associated hydrocephalus and a metastatic lesion in the right lateral ventricle in a 4-month-old girl presenting with rapid onset of nausea, vomiting, and decreased level of consciousness. **D,** Hematoxylin and eosin (H&E) histopathologic stain showing small blue cells intermixed with large spindle-shaped rhabdoid cells.

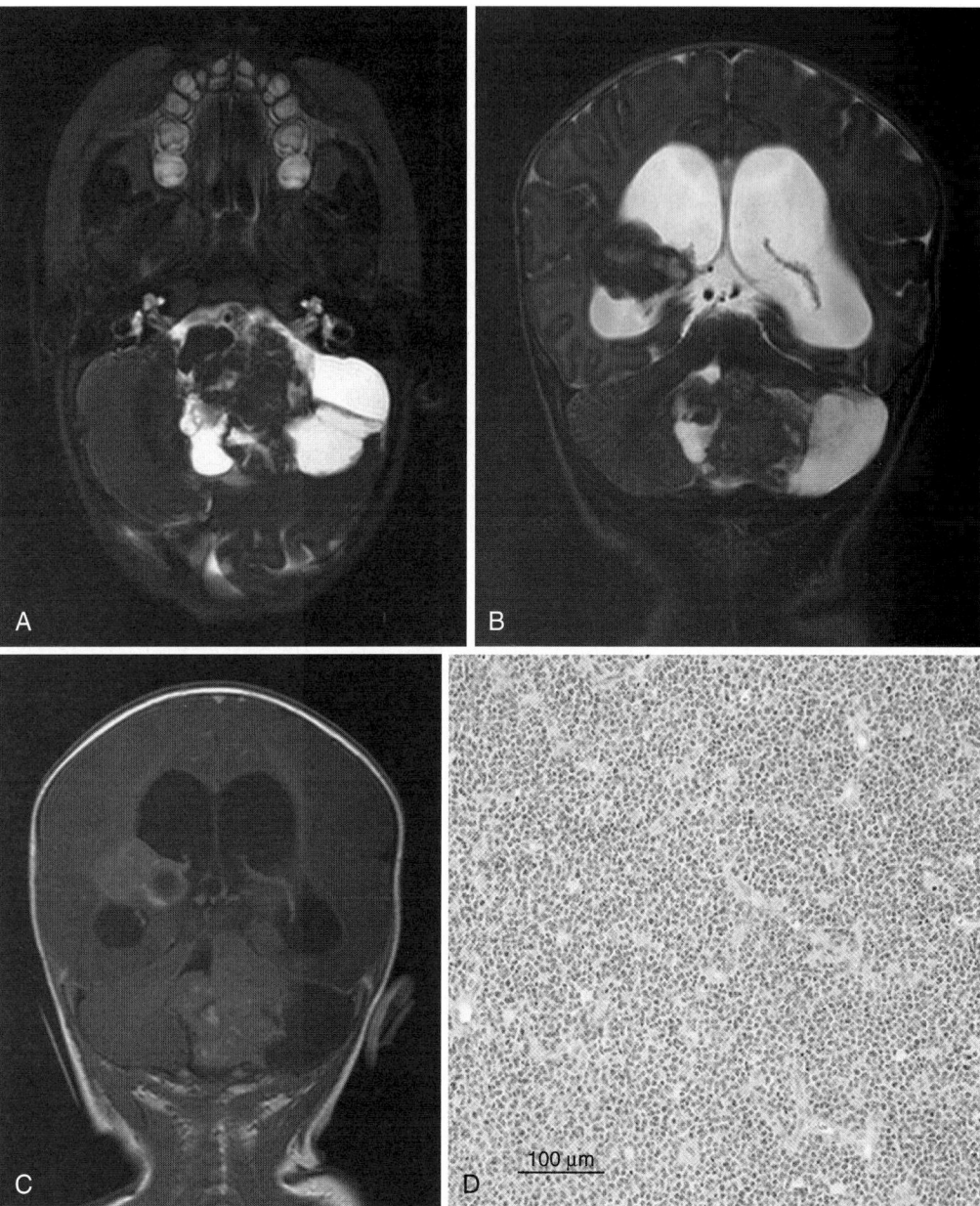

tumors are more common in older children and adults.[127] Metastatic disease from CPC has been documented anywhere along the neuraxis including the leptomeninges.

Histology and Genetics

Genetic syndromes predispose to the formation of CPP and CPC, such as Li-Fraumeni syndrome, neurofibromatosis type 2, Aicardi's syndrome, Down syndrome, and von Hippel-Lindau disease.[128] Germline mutations in *TP53* and *hSNF5/INI1* have been found in familial cases of choroid plexus tumors, and similar mutations have been found in tumors of sporadic cases of CPC and CPP.[129,130] Multiple chromosomal imbalances have been described in CPP and CPC.[131] The most clinically relevant cytogenetic abnormality was demonstrated in a small cohort of patients with a gain of 9p and loss of 10q, which provided a survival advantage.[132]

Histologically, CPPs are similar to normal choroid plexus in that they show many papillae covered by simple columnar or cuboidal epithelium, eosinophilic cytoplasm, round to oval nuclei situated basally, and papillary fronds consisting of vascular connective stroma.[127,128] CPPs do not have necrosis, brain invasion, or mitotic figures. As with other cancers, CPC can show marked cytological atypia, nuclear pleomorphism, loss of polarity, high cellular density, frequent mitosis, necrosis, vascular proliferation, hemorrhage, and brain infiltration.[127] Atypical CPPs show an intermediate degree of nuclear atypical and mitotic figures.[133]

Imaging

Imaging characteristics of CPPs often include a homogeneously enhancing tumor with vascular feeding pedicles along with a "frondlike" solid tumor and associated hydrocephalus. At times,

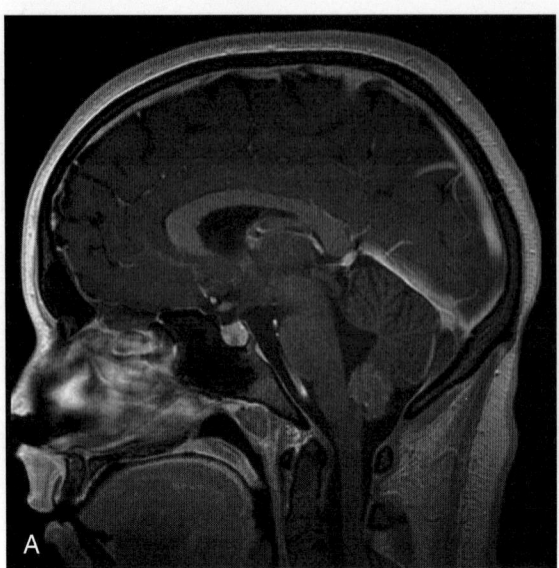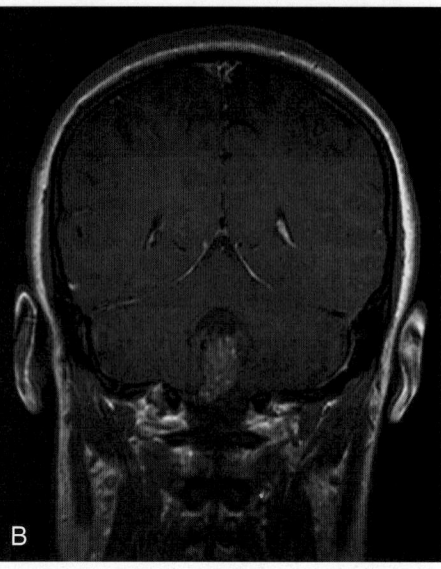

FIGURE 10.6 T1-weighted image with gadolinium enhancement of a fourth ventricular choroid plexus papilloma in an 11-year-old girl. Midsagittal and coronal T1-weighted images with gadolinium enhancement.

however, it is difficult to differentiate between CPP and CPC on imaging studies except that CPCs will often demonstrate parenchymal invasion and peritumoral edema whereas CPPs do not. Choroid plexus lesions are iso- to hyperdense on CT with 25% showing calcification. They are typically isointense on T1 and heterogeneous on T2 MRI sequences (Fig. 10.6).[127]

Management

Extent of surgical resection is a significant prognostic factor in choroid plexus tumors especially the CPC.[134-137] Choroid plexus tumors are highly vascular and perioperative blood loss may contribute to high perioperative morbidity.[138,139] Preresection chemotherapy has been successfully used by some groups to diminish tumor vacularity prior to surgery.[140] The CPT-SIOP-2000 trial recommends treating CPPs with gross total resection alone.[133] Atypical CPPs were treated with surgery alone unless evidence of metastasis or residual disease was present, and all patients with CPCs were treated with gross total resection where possible, chemotherapy, and craniospinal radiation (if >3 years of age). An early analysis of 106 patients and 2.2-year follow-up shows 100% overall survival in the CPP group (n = 39), 89% (n = 24) in atypical CPP, and 36% in CPC (n = 29).[133] Rates for complete surgical resection were 79%, 63%, and 47%, respectively; 9 of 24 patients with atypical CPP were treated with chemotherapy and 1 with radiation.[133]

Hemangioblastoma

Hemangioblastomas, WHO grade I, are highly vascular tumors seen in the cerebellum and spinal cord. They are the most common posterior fossa lesion in adults but are rarer in the pediatric population.[141,142] They can occur sporadically or as part of the von Hippel-Lindau (VHL) familial syndrome. Any patient diagnosed with a hemangioblastoma should be assessed for signs or symptoms of other manifestations of this rare syndrome. VHL is an autosomal dominant disorder characterized by CNS hemangioblastomas, retinal angionatosis, pancreatic cysts, renal cell carcinoma, pheochromocytoma,

and epididymal cysts.[143] VHL patients have a germline mutation in the *VHL* gene that normally acts as a sensor of hypoxia to induce vascular remodeling and increased levels of vascular endothelial growth factor (VEGF).[144] In VHL, this gene is constitutively active, leading to a highly vascular tumor. Sporadic hemangioblastomas are also found to have mutations to VHL.[145]

Hemangioblastomas are typically well-circumscribed cystic lesions with a small mural nodule abutting the pia; however, presentation can vary from a solid lesion to a lesion with a central cyst.[146,147] The cyst is hyperintense on both T1 and T2 MRI sequences, and the mural nodule is isointense on T1 and hyperintense on T2. There is strong contrast enhancement of the solid component.[146]

Surgical excision is the treatment of choice and can be curative with gross total resection.[148] In cases in which gross total resection cannot be achieved, gamma knife radiosurgery or fractionated radiotherapy can achieve tumor control.[149,150]

Dermoid/Epidermoid Cysts

Dermoid and epidermoid cysts are rare (<1%) intracranial congenital non-neoplastic lesions that arise from retained ectodermal cells and mesenchymal elements in dermoid cysts in the neural groove during embryonic neural tube closure.[151,152] They typically present in the third decade of life with a male predominance and are rare in the pediatric population.[153] In the adult population epidermoid cysts are significantly more common than dermoid cysts (4:1-10:1).[153] Interestingly, in children, dermoids may account for a higher percentage than epidermoids.[154] Dermoids and epidermoids are histologically benign but can present with mass effect, aseptic meningitis, infectious meningitis, or neurovascular compression.[155-157]

Dermoid cysts contain both dermal and epidermal elements, are typically midline in location, and are often associated with dermal sinus tracts.[154] The dermal sinus tract of posterior fossa dermoid cysts is typically located at the inion and is associated with the usual cutaneous stigmata of hair tufts, cutaneous angioma, and fluid leakage. There may be an association with Klippel-Feil syndrome.[158-162]

Epidermoid tumors contain epidermal elements and tend to occur in more lateral intracranial locations, commonly in the CPA. When in the CPA, epidermoids cause symptoms related to compression of adjacent cranial nerves or brainstem. They are often called *pearly white tumors* or *cholesteatomas* owing to their pearly appearance at surgery and characteristic cyst contents.

Generally, dermoid and epidermoid cysts appear as well-circumscribed lesions with no edema and moderate mass effect. The cysts appear as hypo- and hyperintense on T1- and T2-weighted MRI sequences, respectively.[154] Epidermoids commonly occur in the CPA and can mimic an arachnoid cyst on imaging with the exception that epidermoid cysts exhibit DWI changes on MRI sequences.[163]

Epidermoid and dermoid cysts are benign lesions for which surgical excision is curative.[153,154,164] A thick capsule adherent to vital neuroanatomical structures can complicate complete surgical removal.[165] In this case it is wise to perform a subtotal resection, and monitor for recurrence in the postoperative period. Malignant degeneration of dermoid or epidermoid cysts to squamous carcinoma has been reported but is extremely rare.[166] Care must be taken to avoid spillage of cyst contents into the subarachnoid space during surgical excision because this may result in aseptic meningitis.

SURGICAL MANAGEMENT OF POSTERIOR FOSSA TUMORS

Management of Hydrocephalus

A majority of patients (83%) with posterior fossa lesions in and around the fourth ventricle will present with hydrocephalus.[167-169] However, only about 30% of children will require postoperative shunting after tumor removal.[14,167,170-172] This number may be reduced to 6% if an endoscopic third ventriculostomy (ETV) is performed as the first CSF diversion technique or in combination with a ventriculostomy.[173] However, by performing an ETV in every child with hydrocephalus and a posterior fossa tumor, one would be exposing 70% of children to the morbidity of an extra surgical procedure. Riva-Cambrin and co-workers have developed a preoperative clinical grading system to aid in determining the need for postoperative CSF diversion.[174] This grading system scores children based on age (<2 years), initial degree of hydrocephalus, tumor histological features, and presence of metastasis to predict probability of hydrocephalus at 6 months.[174] This system can aid the surgeon in determining whether to perform CSF diversion (shunt or ETV) prior to surgical removal of tumor. Today there is an option to place an occipital or "Frazier" burr hole during the surgical procedure. This is for emergent decompression of the lateral ventricles should postoperative swelling result in obstruction of the fourth ventricle and acute hydrocephalus.

Surgical Approaches to Posterior Fossa Lesions

Patients are typically placed in the prone position for a cerebellar posterior fossa lesion; a slight head rotation can be employed if the lesion has lateral extension. Some surgeons favor the sitting position for cerebellar lesions, as blood does not pool in the operative field. However, the sitting position is associated with the risk of air embolism and thus must be done in close collaboration with the anesthesiologist. The park-bench position is often used for lesions mainly occupying the CPA.

The midline suboccipital craniotomy has been the workhorse for resection of fourth ventricular tumors. Classically, it involves splitting the inferior vermis for large tumors within the fourth ventricle. However, the process of splitting the vermis followed by lateral retraction of the dentate nuclei and affecting the dentatonucleocortical projection has raised concerns about cerebellar mutism (see later discussion). Thus, modifications of the midline approach, including the telovelar approach with dissection of the cerebellomedullary fissure to reach the fourth ventricle without splitting the vermis, have been developed.[175-177] In this procedure, after performing a standard suboccipital craniotomy, the cerebellomedullary fissure is opened by separating the tonsillo-uvular and tonsillomedullary spaces. The inferior roof of the fourth ventricle is exposed with retraction of the uvula superiorly and the tonsils laterally. The inferior medullary velum and the tela choroidea are then opened, exposing the fourth ventricle from aqueduct to obex. The opening of the tela can be continued laterally to expose the foramen of Luschka.[175,177,178] Proponents of the telovelar approach argue that with combined removal of the posterior arch of C1, one can obtain a larger working area and more lateral access to the foramen of Luschka, facilitating removal of large lesions.[179]

The suboccipital retrosigmoid approach can be used to reach lesions in the CPA. This approach allows for good visualization of the lower cranial nerves and preserves hearing. A curvilinear incision is made 1 to 2 cm behind the mastoid. The craniotomy is performed medial to the sigmoid sinus. Once the dura is opened, the arachnoid over the cisterna magna or the superolateral cerebellum is opened to allow for CSF drainage, thereby facilitating the retraction of the cerebellum medially to expose the CPA.[180,181] Care should be taken to monitor the seventh cranial nerve in these cases to aid in its preservation. Other more complex skull base approaches such as the posterior petrosal or far lateral approach can be utilized in conjunction or separately from the suboccipital retrosigmoid approach.[182]

Surgical Adjuncts

There are many tools available to the surgeon to assist in surgical removal of posterior fossa lesions. Image-guided surgery or neuronavigation based on presurgical MRI or CT scans can aid in planning craniotomy and identifying important surgical landmarks. These preoperative scans, however, can become less reliable as the surgical case proceeds, and thus the need for updated real-time imaging arises. This imaging may be more important in cases such as ependymoma and medulloblastoma in which degree of resection is critical. Many centers have reported on their case series of intraoperative MRI and have found it both helpful and safe.[157,165] When intraoperative MRI is not available, intraoperative ultrasound may aid the surgeon in understanding the degree of tumor resection and identifying surgical landmarks.[183,184]

Physiological mapping and monitoring during surgery can be invaluable to surgeons operating near the brainstem and cranial nerves. Mapping is the physical stimulation of a brain region of interest and awaiting a response. Mapping the floor of the fourth ventricle for the facial, glossopharyngeal, vagal, and hypoglossal nuclei has been performed to enhance surgical removal of posterior fossa tumors with promising results.[185,186] Monitoring is the ongoing activation and recording of neural circuits during surgery to provide "warnings" of a breach in pathway integrity. Electrodes can be placed in facial, pharyngeal, and tongue muscles, with sound-emitting electrodes in the ear, and stimulators of the gag reflex to monitor cranial nerves and their respective nuclei. Needle electrodes can be placed in the extremities to monitor the corticospinal tracts. Scalp electrodes can be placed in conjunction with stimulators to monitor evoked sensory potential activity from the extremities or auditory nerve.[187] A 50% drop in amplitude or an increased latency of 10% is thought to be indicative of pathway injury.[187] When this occurs, the neurosurgeon should stop operating until the potentials return to normal.

Complications of Therapy

Cerebellar mutism is one of the most feared complications following posterior fossa surgery and can complicate even the most anatomically successful of surgeries. Cerebellar mutism is defined as the complete absence of speech without impairment of consciousness. Other symptoms include hypotonia, ataxia, and emotional lability. Cerebellar mutism occurs in approximately 25% of cases and is more common after posterior fossa surgery for medulloblastoma.[188] Speech is typically intact immediately following surgery with abrupt cessation 1 to 5 days after surgery. Resolution occurs up to 6 months later but some form of speech impairment may persist thereafter.[189] The exact etiology of cerebellar mutism remains elusive; however, damage to the dentatothalamocortical outflow tracts is suggested by modern imaging modalities. Related to and perhaps an extension of cerebellar mutism is the cerebellar cognitive affective syndrome.[188] This syndrome is the chronic impairment of cognitive abilities from disruption of the cerebellum and its interconnections and manifests as speech, executive function, visual-spatial, and personality dysfunction. Cerebellar cognitive affective syndrome can occur in the absence of posterior fossa radiation.[188]

The long-term neurocognitive side effects of craniospinal radiation are well known. Craniospinal radiation (36 Gy) is associated with a 20- to 30-point decrease in IQ, and 23.4 Gy is associated with a 10- to 15-point decline.[190,191] These declines are more pronounced the younger the patient. Endocrine anomalies are strongly correlated with the degree of irradiation to the hypothalamus and commonly require hormone replacement therapy, such as growth hormone to increase stature in the pediatric population.[192] Neurovascular complications are present in up to 5% of patients.[193] Patients receiving cranial radiation are at risk for subsequent secondary malignancy. In a large cohort study of 1877 survivors of CNS tumors, 10.7% of patients had secondary tumors, most commonly nonmelanoma skin cancers and benign meningiomas. However, malignant neoplasms

occurred in 4.1% of patients including malignant glioma, malignant meningioma, and PNET.[194] Patients who have received radiation therapy have a significantly higher risk of mental health issues, unemployment, and remaining single.[194]

Conclusions

Posterior fossa lesions are a diverse group of neoplasms with varied prognosis and management. Great strides have been made in increasing survival in patients with malignant lesions such as medulloblastoma over the past few decades. With the advent of improvements in neurosurgical techniques, delivery of radiation therapy, and new chemotherapeutics, and with new molecular techniques which have helped us to better understand the genetic, epigenetic, and biological processes associated with these tumors, we expect to see improved survival and less treatment-related toxicity in the future.

BRAINSTEM GLIOMAS

Epidemiology and Classification

The brainstem is defined as the neural axis between the diencephalon and cervical spinal cord. Brainstem gliomas (BSGs) can occur anywhere in this neuraxis and account for 10% to 15% of primary pediatric intracranial neoplasms.[195] Two decades ago, tumors were considered inoperable owing to their anatomical location and therefore were frequently fatal. Experience over the last several decades has demonstrated that brainstem gliomas comprise a heterogeneous group of tumors, some of which are amenable to long-term survival.[196,197] BSGs are considered predominantly a pediatric entity with a mean age of presentation of 7 to 9 years.[196-199] The most commonly utilized classification system segregates brainstem tumors based on their radiological appearance into three major categories: (1) diffuse, (2) focal, or (3) exophytic.[196,200] In general, the focal and exophytic types are low-grade gliomas and carry a much better prognosis than the diffuse high-grade glioma. Diffuse intrinsic pontine gliomas (DIPGs) account for 60% to 80% of brainstem gliomas.[201]

Clinical Presentation

The specific signs and symptoms of brainstem tumors are dependent on their anatomical location. Patients with DIPGs typically have a rapidly progressive course of cranial neuropathies, with pyramidal tract and cerebellar signs. In contrast, the presentation of focal brainstem gliomas is more insidious with localizing signs such as isolated cranial nerve deficits and contralateral hemiparesis spanning months to years.[202] Tumors of the cervicomedullary junction commonly present with lower cranial nerve palsies, pyramidal tract signs, ataxia, spinal cord dysfunction, and nystagmus.[203-205] Signs and symptoms of hydrocephalus usually manifest later in the disease progression with the exception of tectal tumors to its location near the cerebral aqueduct.

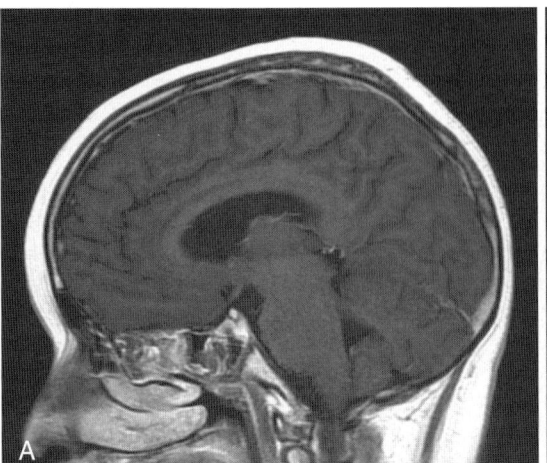
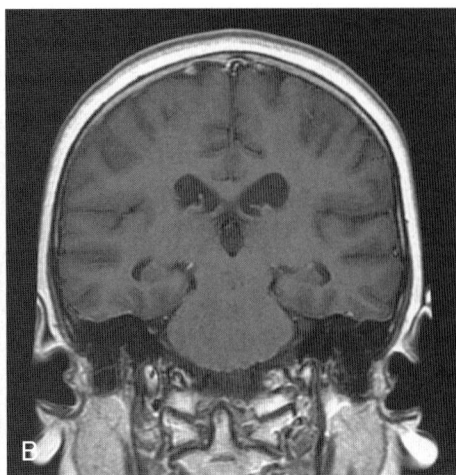
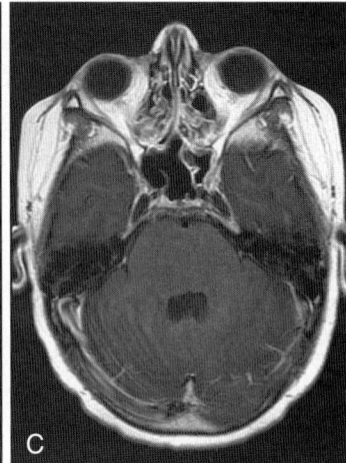

FIGURE 10.7 Sagittal, coronal, and axial T1-weighted magnetic resonance images with gadolinium contrast enhancement of a diffuse intrinsic pontine glioma (DIPG) in a 12-year-old boy. There is diffuse enlargement of the pons with little contrast enhancement. Note the lack of hydrocephalus, which is a late finding in DIPG.

Diffuse Intrinsic Pontine Glioma

DIPGs are the most common brainstem tumors, accounting for approximately 60% to 80% of lesions.[201] Unfortunately, DIPGs are the most devastating brainstem tumor with a median survival of 9 months despite treatment with multiple therapeutic modalities.[206-208] Children usually present with rapid onset and progression of a triad of symptoms (cranial nerve palsies, long tract and cerebellar signs).[209] Hydrocephalus occurs in the advanced stages of this disease.[210]

These lesions have a characteristic appearance on MRI. They appear hypointense on T1-weighted and hyperintense on T2-weighted images with indistinct margins, reflecting their infiltrative nature.[208] On midsagittal imaging, their confinement to the pons is better delineated (Fig. 10.7). Gadolinium enhancement is variable and provides no additional prognostic information.[211] Magnetic resonance spectroscopy (MRS) is an evolving imaging modality in brainstem tumors. DIPGs have increased metabolic ratios of choline to creatine and N-acetylaspartate, which is useful in delineating DIPG from demyelination, dysmyelination of NF1, encephalitis, and radionecrosis.[212,213]

Because the natural history and malignant course of DIPGs are well established, there is currently little clinical role for a diagnostic biopsy.[201,214-216] A biopsy is reserved for indeterminate lesions on MRI, an unusual presentation, or when mandated by a study protocol.[209] The rationale is that nearly all DIPGs are high-grade astrocytomas, outcomes are poor regardless of pathological grade, treatment strategies do not hinge on tumor grade, and biopsy is associated with significant morbidity and mortality rates. However, if we are to gain new insight into the biological and genetic behavior of these tumors, in the hopes of designing targeted therapies, biopsy may become an important strategy in the future.[198]

The mainstay of treatment for DIPGs is radiation therapy at a dose of 50 Gy. There is no role for surgical resection and very little long-term benefit from adjuvant chemotherapy.[217] Surgery may be required to treat hydrocephalus; however, the majority of these cases are mild and symptomatic relief may be achieved with steroid administration. Palliative radiation may provide temporarily relief of symptoms in 75% of children, but unfortunately, all patients eventually suffer recurrence.[218,219]

Focal Brainstem Tumors

Tectal Tumors

Tectal tumors are intrinsic lesions in the region of the mesencephalon representing 5% of brainstem lesions and are typically WHO grade I or II.[220] Given their close proximity to the cerebral aqueduct, tectal tumors cause hydrocephalus, rapid deterioration, and death at a small size.[221] Despite the vast majority of tectal gliomas exhibiting an indolent benign course (>85%) there is a second subtype that behaves more aggressively.[221] MRI may help distinguish this aggressive subtype, as they typically are greater than 2 cm; invade the adjacent tegmentum, thalamus, or pons; and demonstrate contrast enhancement (Fig. 10.8).

The more common benign intrinsic tectal region tumors generally follow an indolent course. These are typically low-grade astrocytomas that are well-circumscribed, nonenhancing lesions that present with signs and symptoms of hydrocephalus.[197] Other signs include gait disturbances, ataxia, Parinaud syndrome, and strabismus. Treating the underlying obstructive hydrocephalus and follow-up with serial MRI is a safe approach to nonsuspicious tectal lesions.[221] Some neurosurgeons favor a more aggressive surgical approach given that 18% to 30% of tectal tumors eventually progress.[220] Hydrocephalus can be treated with a ventriculoperitoneal shunt or endoscopic third ventriculostomy (ETV), which has demonstrated to be safe and effective.[220,222,223] It is important to continue to follow these patients because benign tectal gliomas may progress and ETVs can fail, leading to serious complications.[220,224] Gamma knife radiosurgery has been recently utilized on 13 patients with tectal tumors and result in tumor stabilization; however, it is uncertain whether this treatment provides an improvement over a more conservative approach.[225]

The aggressive tectal tumors are typically larger on presentation compared to the indolent variety. In addition, they

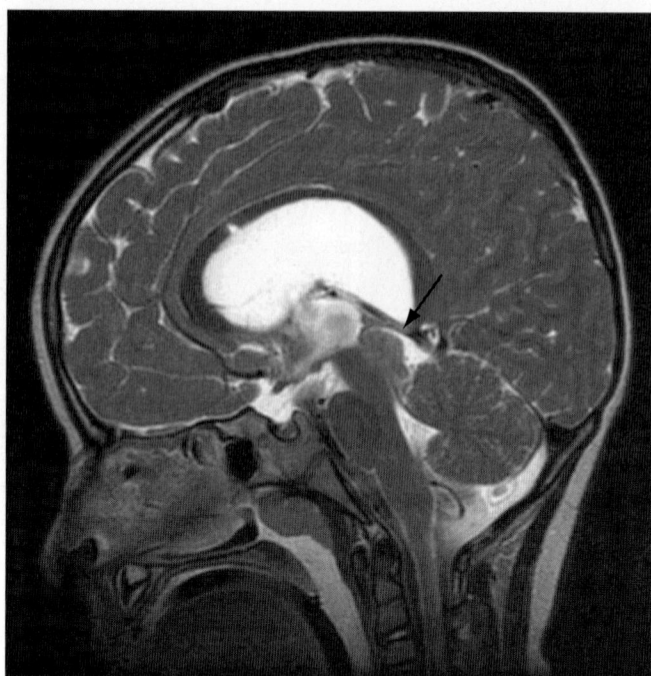

FIGURE 10.8 T2-weighted image of a tectal glioma in a 14-year-old boy. There is enlargement of the tectum with obstruction of the cerebral aqueduct resulting in hydrocephalus. This patient was treated successfully with a third ventriculostomy.

more frequently present with neurological symptoms, and may enhance and show evidence of invasion to adjacent neural structures on MRI. These aggressive lesions are rare and definitive management is debated in the literature with some authors supporting biopsy followed by radiotherapy and others supporting complete surgical resection followed by radiation therapy.[221,226]

Dorsally Exophytic Brainstem Tumors

The dorsally exophytic subtype accounts for approximately 10% to 20% of brainstem tumors.[227,228] Children usually present with an insidious history of headaches, vomiting, ataxia, and cranial nerve dysfunction (usually sixth and seventh).[227,228] Papilledema, torticollis, and long tract signs can be found on neurological examination.[227,228] By definition, these tumors protrude into the fourth ventricle, but occasionally they can be dorsolaterally exophytic, projecting into the CPA.[227] The hypointense signal on T1 and the hyperintense signal on T2 will generally display consistent tumor edges reflecting its less infiltrative nature. Contrast enhancement is typical. These tumors are predominantly pilocytic astrocytomas with occasional grade 2 and 3 astrocytomas and gangliogliomas, generally carrying a good prognosis.[227,229] Dorsally exophytic tumors are the most surgically accessible of all brainstem gliomas. Similar to pilocytic astrocytomas elsewhere in the neuraxis, the primary modality of treatment is surgical debulking followed by serial imaging. Radio- and chemotherapy is reserved for recurrence. Gross total resection is usually not possible owing to the critical nature of adjacent structures. Neuronavigation, diffusion tensor MRI, white matter tractography, and brainstem monitoring are aids to maximize tumor resection and minimize morbidity.

Cervicomedullary Tumors

Children with cervicomedullary tumors commonly present with slowly progressive lower cranial nerve palsies, pyramidal tract signs, ataxia, spinal cord dysfunction, or nystagmus. Lower cranial nerve deficits may include dysphagia, nasal speech, nausea, vomiting, palate deviation, facial nerve palsy, head tilt, apnea, or irregular breathing patterns. The gradual onset of these symptoms reflects the slowly growing, relatively benign histological picture that is most commonly found, namely, the pilocytic astrocytoma.[197]

MRI typically demonstrates a hypointense lesion on T1 and hyperintense lesion on T2-weighted images.[230] The craniocaudal extent can be best appreciated on the sagittal images. These tumors typically extend from the caudal two thirds of the medulla to the rostral portion of the cervical spinal cord. Some authors believe that cervicomedullary tumors may in fact be intramedullary tumors that expand rostrally.[231] There is some evidence that in the more benign pathological subtypes, the tumor is less likely to penetrate the "anatomical barrier" of the pyramidal decussating fibers, medial lemniscus, efferent fibers from the inferior olivary complex, and inferior cerebellar peduncle rostrally.[231]

The prognosis for these lesions is generally favorable following neurosurgical resection, given the low-grade nature of the majority of these lesions. An aggressive surgical resection is usually undertaken given that these tumors are more likely to possess a defined surgical plane compared to other brainstem tumors. However, surgery in this location carries significant risks including quadriparesis, sleep apnea, cranial nerve palsy, proprioceptive deficits, and spasticity.[232] Radiation therapy can be utilized after surgery, although most groups wait until evidence of recurrence.[205,233] The role of chemotherapy in cervicomedullary tumors is ill-defined. Some advocate its use as front-line therapy in children younger than 10 years and for older patients who have demonstrated tumor progression despite radiation; others recommend it only for patients who have failed surgery or as an adjuvant therapy.[230] Weiner and associates' retrospective study has shown that the 5-year progression-free survival rate was about 60%, with 89% of the patients being alive after 5 years.[205] Patients with good preoperative neurological status, early surgical intervention, and benign histological findings experience the longest progression-free survival.[205]

Other Focal Brainstem Tumors

Focal tumors in other location such as the medulla, midbrain tegmentum, or the pons are less common (<5%).[234] These lesion are typically low-grade; however, anaplastic astrocytoma and glioblastoma have been described. Non-neoplastic lesions such as vascular malformations, demyelination, and gangliosidoses need to be excluded by imaging or histological examination. If a biopsy is required, then surgical planning is crucial to minimize trajectories that will harm the patient; diffusion tensor imaging (DTI) or positron emission tomography (PET) may be useful in this situation. Surgical resection is the ideal treatment. However, owing to significant operative morbidity, conventional fractionated radiation therapy and radiosurgery have been tried with moderate results.[201,225] Chemotherapy may have a role in delaying radiation or treatment of refractory progressive low-grade gliomas.[197,235]

Brainstem Gliomas in Neurofibromatosis Type 1

Brainstem gliomas should not be confused with the "unidentified bright objects" seen in NF1 patients. These bright spots are common in the brainstem of children and disappear spontaneously.[236] Although less common than optic gliomas in the NF1 population, BSGs in NF1 may represent a distinct entity from non-NF1 brainstem gliomas. NF1 BSGs have a more favorable prognosis and survival rates of up to 90% at 5 years of age.[236]

Role of Surgery in Brainstem Gliomas

Biopsy of BSGs is reserved for lesions in which the diagnosis is indeterminate on MRI. Many authors have shown that biopsies can be accomplished with reasonable safety, with sufficient tissue for a histological diagnosis; complication rates range from 10% to 30%.[237-239] There is a concern with sampling errors when stereotactic biopsies are performed.

Surgical resection of the more common DIPG is currently futile.[208,229,232] The benefit of surgery is in the treatment of focal brainstem lesions. Sandri and colleagues reported their retrospective review of 17 focal BSGs treated with surgical excision and radiotherapy upon progression and achieved 4-year OS and EFS rates of 87% and 59%, respectively.[240] Gross total resection was achieved in only four patients and correlated with improved EFS.[240] Dorsal exophytic tumors have a good prognosis with long-term survival rates of 92% to 94%.[227,228] Intrinsic medullary tumors tend to have good survival rates and stable progression after surgery; however, the perioperative risk of ventilation, tracheostomy, and gastrostomy was 41% in a 41-patient series by Jallo and co-workers. Almost 80% of these patients had eventual complete recovery.[241] Patients with cervicomedullary BSGs can achieve favorable results with surgery, with 4- and 5-year survival rates of 72% to 100%.[205,230] In cervicomedullary tumors, the degree of preoperative morbidity predicts postoperative function.[197]

The prone position is used in most cases of focal BSGs in children with the exception of midbrain lesions. The goals of surgery are to debulk the lesion and avoid neurological sequelae.[229] Anterior focal pontine lesions can be accessed via the retrosigmoid approach, and dorsal focal intrinsic pontine lesions can be accessed via the midline suboccipital approach. "Safe" entry areas are regions of gliotic tissue presenting to the pial surface or in the zone around the facial colliculus when pial presentation does not occur.[242] Dorsal exophytic tumors can be reached via a suboccipital craniotomy with high cervical laminectomy and exposure of the fourth ventricle via a telovelar approach.[195] It is advisable not to follow the dorsal exophytic tumor into the brainstem as this will result in a high likelihood of cranial nerve nuclei injury. Cervicomedullary tumors can be approached via a laminectomy with or without suboccipital craniotomy for rostral extension. Intraoperative ultrasound can be utilized to define tumor margins.[195,232,234] A dorsal myelotomy is performed to preserve the posterior columns. The tumor is located and debulked. However, extension into the medulla may limit gross total resection to avoid injury to the lower cranial nerves. When operating near the medulla it is essential to identify normal anatomical structures and the lower cranial nerves to avoid injuring these structures.

The general principles for surgical debulking of BSGs include (1) identifying normal anatomy; (2) identifying the most direct route to the tumor, either by exploring tumor cysts or locating pial surfaces with discoloration for tumor bulge; and (3) debulking the center of the lesion prior to dissecting tumor margins. Neurophysiological monitoring such as brainstem auditory evoked responses, somatosensory evoked potentials, electromyography and motor evoked potentials, and neuronavigation are useful adjuncts in minimizing injury to the patient via damage to brainstem nuclei and tracts.

Conclusion

Despite improvements in understanding the biology and advances in treatment strategies (particularly radio- and chemotherapy), brainstem tumors continue to present a therapeutic challenge for neurosurgeons. Poor patient outcomes, especially for DIPGs, are still commonplace.[197] Surgical advancements in techniques, neurophysiological monitoring, and neuroimaging have allowed many patients with focal and dorsally exophytic brainstem tumors to experience a prolonged tumor-free survival.

Please go to expertconsult.com to view the the complete list of references.

Causes of Nontraumatic Hemorrhagic Stroke in Children: Pediatric Moyamoya Syndrome

Edward R. Smith, R. Michael Scott

CLINICAL PEARLS

- Ischemic stroke is relatively rare in children (approximately 2 to 3 per 100,000 children) compared to the adult population. In adults, 80% to 85% of strokes are ischemic, whereas the remaining 15% to 20% are hemorrhagic. In children, 55% of strokes are believed to be ischemic, and the remainder hemorrhagic.

- Early diagnosis of this condition is of paramount importance to minimize sequelae of potential strokes. The etiology of stroke in children covers a wide spectrum to include congenital heart disease, anemia, genetic causes, and moyamoya syndrome.

- The clinical status of the patient at the time of treatment is the most important predictor of long-term outcome. As such, any child with a stroke should have moyamoya syndrome considered in the differential diagnosis to minimize the risk of missing the presence of the disease. There is no medical treatment for moyamoya syndrome that can stop the progressive nature of this condition.

- Furthermore, the natural history of this condition is that of progressive narrowing of the cerebral vessels; therefore, referral of children with diagnosed moyamoya syndrome to a center experienced with the care of these complex patients is critical to providing optimal care.

- Optimal treatment of moyamoya syndrome appears to be operative, although class I data such as a randomized controlled trial between medical and surgical treatment does not exist. The surgical management of this condition is often successful in experienced centers and consists of cerebral revascularization through a variety of indirect means, such as pial synangiosis in which an extracranial vessel is laid on the cerebral cortex for vascular ingrowth or direct means in which an extracranial vessel is anastomosed to an intracranial vessel. Although direct methods afford immediate revascularization, it is not often technically possible in young children and indirect methods also offer success with revascularization in months.

Ischemic stroke in children is a relatively rare entity relative to the adult population. The World Health Organization's MONICA Project defines stroke as "rapidly developing clinical signs of focal (or global) disturbance of cerebral function, with symptoms lasting 24 hours or longer or leading to death with no apparent cause other than of vascular origin."[1] The definition includes ischemic and hemorrhagic infarction and intracerebral and subarachnoid hemorrhage. In adults, 80% to 85% of strokes are ischemic, whereas the remaining 15% to 20% are hemorrhagic. In children, 55% are believed to be ischemic, and the remainder hemorrhagic.[2,3]

PEDIATRIC ISCHEMIC STROKE

In this chapter, the major causes of ischemic stroke in children are reviewed with an emphasis on diseases with neurosurgical relevance, particularly moyamoya syndrome. Reference will be made to the recent American Heart Association (AHA) Scientific Statement on the Management of Stroke in Infants and Children as a resource for current management guidelines.[4] Causes of hemorrhagic stroke, including aneurysms and arteriovenous malformations (AVMs) are presented in other chapters in this text.

Incidence

It is difficult to ascertain the general incidence of ischemic stroke in children as there is limited information regarding pediatric stroke epidemiology. A population study from Rochester, Minnesota, of children under 15 years of age detected an incidence of cerebrovascular disease (including both ischemic and hemorrhagic stroke) of 2.5 per 100,000 population. In general, retrospective studies have reported stroke incidence of approximately 2.5 to 3.1 cases per 100,000 children per year.[5,6] In Japan, a series looking at ischemic cerebrovascular disease in children under 16 years of age (excluding moyamoya syndrome) identified a rate of 0.2 cases per 100,000 children. This reported rate may be low not only because of the exclusion of strokes caused by moyamoya disease (a leading cause of stroke in Japan) but also because of low rates of congenital heart disease.[6] The higher rate of approximately 13 cases of stroke per 100,000 children per year, in a prospective European study, probably reflects the increased availability of better imaging modalities, such as computed tomography (CT).[7] Hemorrhagic strokes account for approximately half of all strokes in the pediatric population. In a hospital autopsy series, 8.7% of patients died of complications related to cerebrovascular disease, but the most common cause of death was hemorrhage from an AVM, not ischemic stroke. The rate of recurrence is estimated to be 20% in these children.[8]

Causes

Strokes in adults are often caused by atherosclerosis; in contrast, the etiology of stroke in children can be diverse and determining the cause can be challenging. Although many different causes and potential risk factors for childhood stroke have been described, ischemic stroke in children frequently results from cardiac embolism, prothrombotic states, or vasculopathies, including the syndrome of moyamoya.[4]

Neonatal Stroke

The presentation of children with fixed neurological deficits during the perinatal period has been a topic of debate. Often grouped under the rubric of cerebral palsy, it appears that there may be multiple etiological factors in different children that account for the resultant neurological deficits. Perinatal hypoxia may result from birth-related trauma or asphyxia, and in utero arterial occlusions may occur secondary to embolic phenomena. Perinatal systemic disease may also contribute to ischemic brain injury, including disseminated intravascular coagulation (DIC), systemic infection, and congenital heart disease.

It may be difficult to dissect out cause versus effect of strokes in children who are hypotonic or have labile systemic vital signs (hypotension, apnea, bradycardia) at birth. Use of magnetic resonance imaging (MRI), ultrasound, and CT may be helpful in evaluation of parenchymal abnormalities in association with abnormal clinical presentation. Recent appreciation of the delayed risk of radiation use in children—especially the very young—has resulted in many institutions making efforts to minimize childhood exposure to CT when possible. In general, MRI can identify ischemic stroke earlier than CT or ultrasound, and offers better anatomical definition of the affected tissue. Although infarcted tissue cannot be repaired, knowledge of extent of infarct can be useful for prognostic purposes, including immediate risks from swelling, possibility of seizure with cortical injury, and overall prognosis with substantial stroke burden.

Genetic Disorders

Several heritable conditions have been implicated in pediatric ischemic stroke. These genetic conditions may be known from family history or may be newly diagnosed in a given patient.[9] Congenital metabolic derangements can contribute to premature arteriosclerosis and resultant ischemic stroke.

Dyslipoproteinemias, inborn errors in the metabolism of lipids and cholesterol, have been associated with increased stroke in children. Deficiencies of proteins C and S, antithrombin III deficiency, prothrombin G20210A mutant genotype, sickle cell disease, and activated protein C resistance are examples of inherited hematological abnormalities associated with ischemic stroke.[4,10,11] Homocystinuria is a genetic disorder in which endothelial cell injury occurs, with ensuing thrombotic and embolic infarcts. Other inherited metabolic disorders such as the syndrome of mitochondrial encephalomyopathy, lactic acidosis, and stroke-like episodes (MELAS), Fabry disease, Menkes disease, and Tangier disease may also be associated with strokes. Although direct correction of the underlying genetic defects of the aforementioned diseases is not yet available, treatment currently focuses on normalizing the metabolic abnormalities. Early knowledge of the predisposing condition can result in heightened vigilance in monitoring for neurological sequelae, and in some cases, stroke burden can be minimized through preventive measures.

Embolic Stroke: Congenital Heart Disease

Strokes may occur in children with either congenital or acquired heart disease. Congenital heart disease is reported to occur in approximately 5 to 10 per 1000 live births and has been implicated in up to one third of all ischemic strokes via embolic phenomena.[12,13] Emboli can result from a right-to-left shunt, valvular disease (including mitral valve prolapse), endocardial disease, thrombus/tumor in the left side of the heart, pulmonary arteriovenous fistula, or after cardiac surgery when bypass has been employed. Children with emboli from bacterial endocarditis are also at risk for mycotic aneurysms. The risk for stroke in patients with endocarditis is higher if the disease involves the left side of the heart.

Special note is made of the Fontan operation: essentially an anastomosis of the right atrium to the pulmonary artery. It is one of the most common cardiac operations for children over 1 year of age with congenital heart disease and the surgery is associated with a 2.6% risk of stroke. The risk period for stroke extends from the first postoperative day to 32 months following the Fontan procedure.[14]

Thrombotic Stroke: Sickle Cell Disease and Hypercoagulable Conditions

Thrombotic stroke is a phenomenon described in children, often in association with polycythemia, dehydration, and infection. One of the most common entities associated with thrombotic stroke in children is sickle cell disease.[4]

Sickle cell disease affects nearly 1 in 400 African Americans, with a nearly 10% lifetime risk of stroke.[15] Many strokes occur in children, with most strokes occurring before 10 years of age.[16] Cerebral infarction is often caused by progressive occlusion of the distal internal carotid artery, usually involving the anterior cerebral and middle cerebral artery distributions. Treatment includes hydration, transfusion, and in some cases bone marrow transplant to correct the underlying genetic disorder. Of particular note, recent literature—from our group and others—has highlighted the finding that a substantial number of children with sickle cell disease will fail medical therapy and develop moyamoya syndrome.[17,18] Importantly, there is evidence supporting the premise that this subset of children respond well to surgical treatment of their moyamoya disease and should thus be considered for referral to a neurosurgical center experienced in the management of this condition.[4,17,18]

Other conditions are also associated with prothrombotic disorders. In children who present with ischemic strokes, between 10% and 50% have been reported to have some type of prothrombotic state.[19-21] These prothrombotic processes can be genetic, such as factor V Leiden mutation, antiphospholipid antibodies, hyperhomocysteinemia, and elevated lipoprotein(a), or acquired, such as deficiencies in clotting pathways resulting from infection, medications, hepatic disease, or renal disease. Protein C, protein S, and antithrombin III deficiency may be either inherited or acquired. In all children who present with ischemic stroke, laboratory investigation of these hypercoagulable states should be undertaken.

Extracranial Arterial Dissection

Dissection of the carotid or vertebral arteries can occur in children spontaneously or may be secondary to trauma. Stroke can result from emboli from the site of dissection or from reduced blood flow from the narrowed vessel caliber. Of all patients (adult and pediatric) with dissections of these vessels, 6.8% were under the age of 18.[22] Presenting symptoms are usually pain (either headache or neck pain) and neurological signs referable to the site of injury. With carotid dissections, Horner syndrome may be present due to injury of the sympathetic plexus surrounding the artery, in addition to neurological deficits referable to the regions of the brain supplied by the carotid. In the posterior circulation, Horner syndrome can also be caused as a result of lateral medullary infarction.

The history may be notable for no injury or seemingly insignificant trauma and there may be an interval of several days between the presumed causative event and the presenting symptoms. Although the gold standard remains conventional six-vessel angiography, the diagnosis of craniocervical dissection is increasingly being made with noninvasive imaging modalities, such as computed tomographic angiography (CTA) and magnetic resonance angiography (MRA).[23] Because of technique constraints, MRA and CTA may miss some dissections, particularly those involving the posterior circulation. Particular attention should be paid to the C1-C2 region, as that is the most common site of vertebral artery dissection.[24]

Treatment is predicated on minimizing embolic events and allowing the injured vessel wall to heal. The risk for recurrent dissection is 12% and seems to be particularly high in the first several months immediately following presentation.[22] Optimal treatment remains controversial. At Children's Hospital Boston, we favor the use of anticoagulation, using heparin initially, followed by conversion to warfarin (Coumadin) for 6 months. Follow-up angiography often discloses healing of the dissection, after which anticoagulation is discontinued. If recurrent symptoms or radiographic progression occurs, endovascular therapy is considered.

Cerebral Vasculitis

Cerebral vasculitis is an uncommon cause of stroke in children. The vasculitis may be infectious or noninfectious. Infectious cases include sepsis of any type (particularly meningitis),

varicella, human immunodeficiency virus (HIV), and mycoplasma.[25-30] Noninfectious causes include a wide variety of autoimmune disorders, including Behçet disease, sarcoidosis, Sjögren syndrome, ulcerative colitis, Kawasaki disease, and Schönlein-Henoch purpura (SHP), among others.[4,31,32]

Cerebral vasculitis is often a difficult diagnosis to make. It should be considered when the stroke is associated with systemic manifestations such as fever, anorexia, myalgias, arthralgias, renal disease, and skin lesions. Presentation may be nonspecific, including both global (encephalopathy) and focal (often multiple) neurological deficits. Further complicating the diagnosis, stroke and other neurological symptoms might be the result of vasculitis or the result of a nonspecific disease process.

Previous work has demonstrated that only 4% of strokes in children were attributable to vasculitis.[33] Further study did not find any cause of vasculitis in children younger than 14 years of age with cerebrovascular disease.[5] Taken together, these findings suggest that the incidence of vasculitis, even in at-risk populations, is very low. These data are important, as the neurosurgeon will often be consulted for consideration of brain biopsy in an attempt to make the diagnosis of cerebral vasculitis.

Miscellaneous Causes

One increasingly common cause for stroke in children is the use of illicit drugs. Strokes have been reported in association with the use of amphetamines, cocaine, and phencyclidine (PCP) among others. Suggested mechanisms include transient cerebral vasoconstriction, unmasking of a preexisting cardiovascular disease, toxic vasculitis, and prothrombotic tendencies.[34]

Migraines are usually benign in children; however, there are reports of infarcts, usually in the vertebrobasilar distribution, associated with this disorder. Presumably these permanent deficits are the result of decreased vessel caliber during the migraine, leading to ischemia and infarction.[4]

Atherosclerotic cerebrovascular disease in children, although rare, has been implicated in stroke. Disorders of lipids may contribute to this process, as well as uncontrolled hypertension and diabetes.

Fibromuscular dysplasia has been associated with childhood stroke. Management of this disease is controversial, but many favor medical treatment with antiplatelet agents. Rarely, surgery or endovascular therapy may be utilized to bypass or dilate affected vessel segments.

Radiation-induced vasculopathy is a cause of stroke in patients involving either large or small vessels. Most commonly seen in patients treated for tumors, it may present in a delayed fashion. A recent study found that approximately 6% of children with central nervous system tumors treated with radiation had radiographic evidence of stroke.[35] One of the most important stroke syndromes associated with radiotherapy is moyamoya syndrome (see following section).[36,37]

MOYAMOYA SYNDROME

Moyamoya syndrome, a vasculopathy characterized by chronic progressive stenosis at the apices of the intracranial internal carotid arteries, is an increasingly recognized entity

TABLE 11.1 Frequency of Presenting Signs and Symptoms in Patients with Moyamoya Syndrome

Sign/Symptom	No. of Patients Affected (N = 143)*
Stroke	97 (67.8%)
TIAs (including drop attacks)	62 (43.4%)
Seizures	9 (6.3%)
Headache	9 (6.3%)
Choreiform movements	6 (4.2%)
Incidental finding	6 (4.2%)
Intraventricular or intracerebral bleed	4 (2.8%)

*Symptom totals are greater than patient total because some patients had multiple symptoms at presentation.
TIAs, transient ischemic attacks.

TABLE 11.2 Comorbid Conditions, Risk Factors, and Syndromes Associated with Moyamoya Syndrome

Condition/Risk Factor/Syndrome	No. of Patients Affected
No associated conditions (idiopathic)	66
Neurofibromatosis type I (NF 1)	16
Asian ethnicity	16
Cranial therapeutic irradiation for neoplasia	15
Hypothalamic-optic system glioma: 8	
Craniopharyngioma: 4	
Medulloblastoma, with Gorlin syndrome: 1	
Acute lymphocytic leukemia, intrathecal chemotherapy: 2	
Down syndrome	10
Congenital cardiac anomaly, previously operated	7
Renal artery stenosis	4
Hemoglobinopathy: 2 sickle cell, 1 Bryn Mawr (four African-American patients, two of whom were the individuals with sickel cell disears [see above])	3
Other hematological syndromes: 1 spherocytosis, 1 ITP	2
Giant cervicofacial hemangiomas	3
Shunted hydrocephalus	3
Idiopathic hypertension requiring medication	3
Hyperthyroidism (1 with Graves' disease)	2
Other conditions/syndromes	10
Reye (remote), Williams, Alagille syndromes; cloacal exstrophy; renal artery fibromuscular dysplasia; congenital cytomegalic inclusion virus infection (remote): 1 each	
Unclassified syndromic presentations: 2	
Among 4 African-American patients: 2 with sickle cell disease	

ITP, idiopathic thrombocytopenic purpura.

associated with cerebral ischemia.[38] This progressive stenosis occurs simultaneously as characteristic arterial collateral vessels develop at the base of the brain. These collateral vessels, when visualized on angiography, have been likened to the appearance of haze, a cloud, or a puff of smoke, which translates to "moyamoya" in Japanese.

This arteriopathy results in diminished blood supply to the brain, with resultant transient ischemic attacks (TIAs), seizures, headaches, hemorrhage, and strokes (Table 11.1). It has been associated with approximately 6% of childhood strokes.[39,40] There are few to no class I or II data on the treatment of pediatric moyamoya syndrome, and the evidence that serves as a basis for guidelines is aggregated class III data.[4] A recent meta-analysis of the literature of surgical treatment of pediatric moyamoya syndrome and a review article in the *New England Journal of Medicine* offer two sources for more comprehensive summaries of the literature.[38,41]

Epidemiology

First described in Japan, moyamoya syndrome has now been observed throughout the world and affects individuals of many ethnic backgrounds, with increasing detection of this disease in American and European populations.[42,43] In Japan, it is the most common pediatric cerebrovascular disease; affecting females almost twice as much as males with a prevalence of approximately 3 per 100,000.[39,44] In Europe, a recent study cited an incidence of 0.3 patients per center per year, which is approximately one tenth of the incidence in Japan.[45] A 2005 U.S. study suggests an incidence that was 0.086 per 100,000 persons. The ethnicity-specific incidence rate ratios compared to whites were 4.6 (95% confidence interval [CI]: 3.4 to 6.3) for Asian Americans, 2.2 (95% CI: 1.3 to 2.4) for African Americans, and 0.5 (95% CI: 0.3 to 0.8) for Hispanics.[46]

In the United States and Korea, reports corroborated historical claims of a bimodal age distribution of moyamoya syndrome, one group in the pediatric age range (around the first decade of life) and a second group of adults in the 30- to 40-year-old range. Adults—who still predominantly present with stroke—have a sevenfold increased likelihood of presenting with hemorrhage as compared to children.[38,47,48] In contrast, children usually present with TIAs or strokes, which may prove more difficult to diagnose because of the patient's age, leading to delayed recognition of the underlying moyamoya.[38,49]

Associated Conditions

A number of clinical conditions or predisposing factors have been associated with moyamoya syndrome.[18,50-52] Table 11.2 summarizes the clinical associations noted in a recently published series.[51]

Natural History and Prognosis

The prognosis of moyamoya syndrome is difficult to predict because the natural history of this disorder is not well known. The clinical progression of disease can be slow with rare, intermittent events or can be fulminant with rapid neurological decline.[50,51] However, regardless of the course, it seems clear that moyamoya syndrome, both in terms of arteriopathy and clinical symptoms, inevitably progresses in untreated patients.[53] It has been estimated that 50% to 66% of patients with moyamoya syndrome have progression of the neurological deficits with poor outcomes if left untreated.[54,55] This number contrasts strikingly to an estimated rate of only 2.6% of worsened neurological status in a recent meta-analysis of 1156 surgically treated pediatric patients.[41] Overall prognosis of patients with moyamoya syndrome depends heavily on the neurological status of the child at time of treatment, adding an imperative to early diagnosis and referral to an experienced center.[51,56]

Screening

There are no data to support indiscriminate screening for moyamoya syndrome and there is little evidence to justify screening first-degree relatives of patients with moyamoya syndrome when only a single family member is affected. However, a 2008 paper concerning patients with unilateral moyamoya syndrome documents decreased stroke burden and better clinical outcome when this specific population was imaged at intervals, providing evidence in support of selective screening.[57] Although widespread screening for moyamoya syndrome is not yet standard for any specific group, the diagnosis should be considered when patients with certain high-risk disorders such as neurofibromatosis type 1, Down syndrome, and sickle cell disease are undergoing routine examinations in order to uncover symptomatic patients and refer them for imaging.[58-61]

Diagnostic Investigations

Moyamoya syndrome should be considered and diagnostic evaluation begun in any child who presents with symptoms of cerebral ischemia (e.g., a TIA manifesting as episodes of hemiparesis, speech disturbance, sensory impairment, involuntary movement, or visual disturbance), especially if the symptoms are precipitated by physical exertion, hyperventilation, or crying. The diagnosis of moyamoya syndrome is made on radiographic studies that usually progress from CT scanning to MRI to formal arteriography.

Computed Tomography

The CT scan in a patient with moyamoya disease may demonstrate small areas of hypodensity suggestive of stroke in cortical watershed zones, basal ganglia, deep white matter, periventricular regions, or hemorrhage.[51] However, the CT scan can be normal, particularly in patients presenting solely with TIAs. The intracranial stenoses seen in moyamoya disease may be demonstrated by CTA. Thus, CTA should be considered when MRI is not readily available and a diagnosis of cerebral occlusive vasculopathy is being considered.

Magnetic Resonance Imaging

Widespread availability of MRI and MRA has led to increasing use of these modalities for primary imaging in patients experiencing symptoms suggestive of moyamoya syndrome.[62-64] An acute infarct is best seen using diffusion-weighted imaging (DWI), while a chronic infarct is better demonstrated with T_1 and T_2 imaging. Diminished cortical blood flow secondary to moyamoya syndrome can be inferred from so-called FLAIR (fluid attenuated inversion recovery) sequences, which demonstrate linear high signals that follow a sulcal pattern, which is called the *ivy sign*.[65] The finding most suggestive of moyamoya syndrome on MRI is reduced flow voids in the internal, middle, and anterior cerebral arteries coupled with prominent flow voids through the basal ganglia and thalamus from moyamoya collateral vessels. These imaging findings are virtually diagnostic of moyamoya syndrome.[66]

Angiography

Formal angiography should consist of a full six-vessel study that includes both external carotid arteries, both internal carotid arteries, and one or both vertebral arteries, depending on the collateral patterns visualized. In a study of 190 angiograms, complication rates in moyamoya patients were no higher than those in non-moyamoya patients with other forms of cerebrovascular disease.[67]

Definitive diagnosis is based on a distinct arteriographic appearance characterized by bilateral stenosis of the distal intracranial internal carotid artery extending to the proximal anterior and middle arteries. Disease severity is frequently classified into one of six progressive stages, originally defined by Suzuki.[53] Development of an extensive collateral network at the base of the brain along with the classic "puff of smoke" appearance on angiography is seen in the intermediate stages of the Suzuki grading system. External carotid imaging is essential to identify preexisting collateral vessels so that surgery, if performed, will not disrupt them. Aneurysms, and the rare arteriovenous malformation known to be associated with certain cases of moyamoya syndrome, can also be best detected by conventional angiography.

Other Diagnostic Techniques

Other diagnostic evaluations that may be useful in evaluating patients with moyamoya syndrome include electroencephalography (EEG) and cerebral blood flow studies. Specific alterations of EEG recordings are usually observed only in pediatric patients and include posterior or centrotemporal slowing, a hyperventilation-induced diffuse pattern of monophasic slow waves (called *build-up*), and a characteristic *rebuild-up* phenomenon,[68] which looks identical to the build-up slow waves seen in non-moyamoya patients, but differs in the timing of its presentation. Build-up occurs during hyperventilation while rebuild-up occurs after the hyperventilation is completed and indicates a diminished cerebral perfusion reserve.

Techniques such as transcranial Doppler (TCD), perfusion CT, xenon-enhanced CT, positron emission tomography (PET), MR perfusion imaging, and single-photon emission computed tomography (SPECT) with acetazolamide challenge have all been used in the evaluation of moyamoya syndrome. These studies may help to quantify blood flow, serve as a baseline prior to the institution of treatment, and occasionally aid in treatment decisions.

Treatment Considerations

There is no known treatment that will reverse the primary disease process of moyamoya syndrome, and current treatments are designed to prevent strokes by improving blood flow to the affected cerebral hemisphere. Improvement in cerebral blood flow may protect against future strokes, effect a concurrent reduction in moyamoya collaterals, and reduce symptom frequency.

The majority of data available supports the use of surgical revascularization as a first-line therapy for the treatment of moyamoya syndrome, particularly for patients with recurrent or progressive symptoms.[4,41] Abundant type III data, including two relatively large studies with long-term follow-up, have demonstrated a good safety profile for surgical treatment of moyamoya (4% risk of stroke within 30 days of surgery per hemisphere) with a 96% probability of remaining stroke-free over a 5-year follow-up period.[51,54] These type III data suggest that surgical therapy of moyamoya syndrome confers an effective, durable treatment for the disease and these findings are concordant with the recent AHA guidelines.[4]

Historically, there has been a paucity of data comparing the efficacy of medical versus surgical therapy for moyamoya syndrome. A large survey in 1994 from Japan noted that among 821 registered patients with moyamoya syndrome, there were no significant differences in outcome between medically and surgically treated patients.[69] However, a recent study indicated that 38.4% of 651 moyamoya patients who were not initially treated with surgery eventually came to surgery as a result of progressive symptoms.[70] Medical therapy is often used as treatment for moyamoya syndrome, particularly when the patient is a poor operative risk (severe cardiac disease, advanced debilitation from stroke burden, or other severe comorbid conditions) or has relatively mild moyamoya disease. Aspirin is a standard maintenance therapy for the syndrome without any published series demonstrating its long-term efficacy. A recent meta-analysis noted that medical therapy should not be employed for the treatment of patients with progressive neurological symptoms, stating that medical treatments (e.g., vasodilators, low-molecular-weight dextrans, and steroids) are ineffective.[41]

Indications for Surgery

Currently, there are no class I or II data to support specific determinants of indications for medical versus surgical therapy. The quality of evidence compiled in a recent meta-analysis of 1448 patients from 57 studies in the English language led to recommendations that were graded D (on a scale from A to D), meaning that they are based completely on class III data (non-analytic studies) and expert opinions.[41] Indications for surgery were noted in less than 15% of studies and varied between centers.[41] General indications and timing of surgery remain controversial.[71,72] Guidelines from Japan's Ministry of Health and Welfare regarding indications for surgical treatment of moyamoya syndrome state: "In the cases with (1) repeated clinical symptoms due to apparent cerebral ischemia, or (2) a decreased regional cerebral blood flow, vascular response and perfusion reserve, based on the findings of a cerebral circulation and metabolism study, surgery is indicated."[69] The 2008 AHA guidelines (Box 11.1) are concordant with those from Japan, stating, "Indications for revascularization surgery include progressive ischemic symptoms or evidence of inadequate blood flow or cerebral perfusion reserve in an individual without a contraindication to surgery."[4]

Medical Treatment

There is no known medical treatment capable of reversing the progression of moyamoya syndrome. However, there is support for the use of two classes of medications to slow the

---

BOX 11.1 AHA Guidelines for the Management of Children with Moyamoya Disease*

Class I Recommendations

1. Different revascularization techniques are useful to effectively reduce the risk of stroke resulting from moyamoya disease (Class I, Level of Evidence B).
2. Indirect revascularization techniques are generally preferable and should be used in younger children whose small-caliber vessels make direct anastomosis difficult, whereas direct bypass techniques are preferable in older individuals (Class I, Level of Evidence C).
3. Revascularization surgery is useful for moyamoya disease (Class I, Level of Evidence B). Indications for revascularization surgery include progressive ischemic symptoms or evidence of inadequate blood flow or cerebral perfusion reserve in an individual without a contraindication to surgery (Class I, Level of Evidence B).

Class II Recommendations

1. Transcranial Doppler may be useful in the evaluation and follow-up of individuals with moyamoya disease (Class IIb, Level of Evidence C).
2. Techniques to minimize anxiety and pain during hospitalizations may reduce the likelihood of stroke caused by hyperventilation-induced vasoconstriction in individuals with moyamoya disease (Class IIb, Level of Evidence C).

3. Management of systemic hypotension, hypovolemia, hyperthermia, and hypocarbia during the intraoperative and perioperative periods may reduce the risk of perioperative stroke in individuals with moyamoya disease (Class IIb, Level of Evidence C).
4. Aspirin may be considered in individuals with moyamoya disease after revascularization surgery or in asymptomatic individuals for whom surgery is not anticipated (Class IIb, Level of Evidence C).
5. Techniques to measure cerebral perfusion and blood flow reserve may assist in the evaluation and follow-up of individuals with moyamoya disease (Class IIb, Level of Evidence C).

Class III Recommendations

1. Except in selected individuals with frequent transient ischemic attacks or multiple infarctions despite antiplatelet therapy and surgery, anticoagulants are not recommended for most individuals with moyamoya disease because of the risk of hemorrhage and the difficulty of maintaining therapeutic levels in children (Class III, Level of Evidence C).
2. In the absence of a strong family history of moyamoya disease or medical conditions that predispose to moyamoya syndrome, there is insufficient evidence to justify screening studies for moyamoya disease in asymptomatic individuals or in relatives of patients with moyamoya syndrome (Class III, Level of Evidence C).

*Summarized from Roach ES, Golomb MR, Adams R, et al. Management of stroke in infants and children: a scientific statement from a Special Writing Group of the American Heart Association Stroke Council and the Council on Cardiovascular Disease in the Young. Stroke 2008;39:2644-2691.

progression of the disease: anticoagulants/antiplatelet agents and vasodilators.

The antiplatelet effect of aspirin is useful in moyamoya syndrome because some ischemic symptoms appear to occur as a consequence of emboli from microthrombus formation at sites of arterial stenoses.[50,51,72,73] Children with moyamoya syndrome typically receive lifelong aspirin therapy, with those younger than 6 years of age receiving 81 mg/day and older children receiving a variable dose depending on the presence or absence of symptoms.[51] Although anticoagulants such as warfarin are rarely used owing to the difficulty of maintaining therapeutic levels in children and the risk of hemorrhage from inadvertent trauma, low-dose low-molecular-weight heparin (Lovenox) has been used, at 0.5 mg/kg twice a day, particularly for those children who are neurologically unstable and need rapidly reversible anticoagulation prior to procedures such as surgery or angiography when ongoing aspirin therapy might be contraindicated.[74]

The other medication class that has been useful in the treatment of certain symptoms in moyamoya syndrome is calcium channel blockers.[73] These drugs may be particularly useful in ameliorating symptoms of intractable headaches or migraines, commonly seen in moyamoya patients, and may be effective in reducing both the frequency and severity of refractory TIA in certain patients.

Surgical Treatment

There are a number of studies in the literature that support a role for surgical management of moyamoya disease, and surgery is generally recommended for the treatment of patients with recurrent or progressive cerebral ischemic events and associated reduced cerebral perfusion reserve. Many different operative techniques have been described, all with the main goal of preventing further ischemic injury by increasing collateral blood flow to hypoperfused areas of cortex, using the external carotid circulation as a donor supply.[50,51]

The surgical procedures can generally be divided into direct and indirect revascularization techniques. Direct anastomosis procedures, most commonly superficial temporal artery (STA) to middle cerebral artery (MCA) anastomosis (STA-MCA bypass), may achieve instant improvement in focal cerebral perfusion, but these procedures are often technically difficult to perform because of small size of scalp donor vessels or middle cerebral artery recipient vessels. The small vessels limit the amount of additional collateral blood flow supplied to the brain by the procedure, and the basal moyamoya process itself tends to limit the amount of blood flow redistribution because of the proximal basal occlusive process. A variety of indirect revascularization procedures have been described: encephaloduroarteriosynangiosis (EDAS) whereby the STA is dissected free over a course of several inches and then sutured to the cut edges of the opened dura; encephalomyosynangiosis (EMS) in which the temporalis muscle is dissected and placed onto the surface of the brain to encourage collateral vessel development; and the combination of both, encephalomyoarteriosynangiosis (EMAS).[75-77] There are multiple variations of these procedures, including solely drilling burr holes, without vessel synangiosis,[78,79] and craniotomy with inversion of the dura in hopes of enhancing new dural revascularization of the brain.[80] Cervical sympathectomy and omental transposition or omental pedicle grafting have also been described, although

sympathectomy has largely been abandoned due to its ineffectiveness.[75,81-90] Finally, a number of groups have reported improved results in the use of combined direct and indirect anastomoses.[70,75,83,91] A modification of the EDAS procedure, termed *pial synangiosis*, employs a donor superficial temporal artery as the source of new collateral, a wide opening of the dura and arachnoid, and an attachment of the donor vessel directly to the brain surface by fine sutures.[51] The long-term efficacy of this variant of indirect revascularization has been validated by the largest surgical series of pediatric moyamoya patients reported in North America.[51]

One major consideration is the decision of which surgical technique to employ. In the United States, the AHA guidelines state that indirect procedures, such as pial synangiosis, are best suited to younger patients[4] (see Box 11.1).

Once the decision for surgical therapy has been made, several perioperative considerations need to be addressed. In addition to the general issues regarding surgery in children, moyamoya patients are at particular risk of ischemic events in the perioperative period. Crying and hyperventilation, common occurrences in children at times during hospitalization, can lower PCO_2 and induce ischemia secondary to cerebral vasoconstriction. Any techniques to reduce pain—including the use of perioperative sedation, painless wound dressing techniques, and absorbable wound suture closures—appear to reduce the incidence of strokes, TIAs, and length of hospital stay.[92] A further perioperative consideration is the use of specialized monitoring during surgery, such as EEG, which might identify and help prevent cerebral ischemia detected while the patient is under general anesthesia.

Perioperative and Intraoperative Considerations

The administration of general anesthesia can result in transient physiological changes that can affect cerebral blood flow. Blood pressure, blood volume, and $PaCO_2$ require careful monitoring because moyamoya patients have a diminished cerebral perfusion reserve and deviation from normal levels can result in stroke.[92] To reduce the risk of intraoperative and perioperative neurological morbidity, therefore, meticulous management of the patient is required to avoid hypotension, hypovolemia, hyperthermia, and hypocarbia both intraoperatively and perioperatively.[51] As noted previously, intraoperative EEG monitoring with a full array of scalp electrodes can be helpful in the neurological assessment of patients under general anesthesia. To help prevent hypovolemia during surgery, patients are often admitted the evening prior to surgery for aggressive intravenous hydration. Postoperatively, the patients are hydrated with intravenous fluids at 1.5 times the normal maintenance rate based on weight for 48 to 72 hours. Aspirin is given on the first postoperative day.

Potential complications associated with surgical treatment of moyamoya syndrome include postoperative stroke, subdural hematoma (both following trauma and spontaneous), and intracerebral hemorrhage.

Follow-up Considerations

Careful follow-up of patients with moyamoya syndrome is warranted.[41,69] Of patients treated conservatively or with medical management, 38.3% of unoperated patients required surgery eventually.[70] A study of patients initially diagnosed with unilateral moyamoya found that 27% (17 of 64) of those with unilateral disease progressed to bilateral involvement, with younger patients being most commonly affected, often within 1 to 5 years.[93] Other data further support the premise that younger children with unilateral disease commonly progress to bilateral involvement.[94] Of those patients who were treated operatively (for either bilateral or unilateral disease), the need for reoperation due to refractory disease ranged from 1.8% to 18%.[69] These data suggest that periodic clinical and radiographic examinations of patients with moyamoya disease, even if treated, should be performed on a regular basis.

Postoperative angiograms or MRI/MRA studies are usually obtained 12 months after surgery and typically demonstrate MCA collateralization from both the donor STA and the meningeal arteries.[51,70] A review of 143 children with moyamoya syndrome treated with pial synangiosis demonstrated marked reductions in their stroke frequency after surgery, especially after 1 month postoperatively: 67% had strokes preoperatively, 7.7% had strokes in the perioperative period, and only 3.2% had strokes after at least 1 year of follow-up. The long-term results are excellent, with a stroke rate of 4.3% (2 patients in a group of 46) in patients with a minimum of 5 years of follow-up.[51] This work supports the premise that surgical treatment of moyamoya syndrome provides a significant protective effect against new strokes in this patient population and is further supported by a recent meta-analysis of children treated surgically for moyamoya syndrome, which found that out of 1156 patients, 1003 (87%) derived symptomatic benefit from surgical revascularization (complete disappearance or reduction in symptomatic cerebral ischemia).[41]

CONCLUSIONS

Moyamoya syndrome is an increasingly recognized entity associated with cerebral ischemia. Diagnosis is made on the basis of clinical and radiographic findings, including a characteristic stenosis of the internal carotid arteries in conjunction with abundant collateral vessel development. Surgical revascularization is recommended for definitive treatment of children with moyamoya syndrome. Treatment is predicated on revascularization of the ischemic brain, which can occur following direct (STA-MCA bypass) or indirect (including pial synangiosis) procedures, both of which can be effective in children. Direct revascularization confers immediate protection, but often is not technically feasible in children. Indirect surgical revascularization can revascularize wide areas of the brain but is effective in preventing strokes in children only after the in-growth of new blood vessels from the donor vessel, usually a period of several months.

Patients with moyamoya syndrome should be referred to centers with experience with this disease, as demonstrated by annual volume and availability of the resources needed to treat them, including an appropriate team of physicians and an intensive care unit familiar with the issues related to moyamoya syndrome. Careful follow-up of these patients is warranted. Despite the compelling anecdotal evidence supporting the role for surgical treatment of moyamoya syndrome, there is a profound need for further research to validate these data. Future efforts should focus on organizing widespread consensus of diagnostic and therapeutic standards of care, supported by well-designed prospective studies. The genetic and metabolic bases for the disease remain fruitful areas of investigation and discoveries in these fields may lead to more directed metabolic therapy for the condition.

SELECTED KEY REFERENCES

Fung LW, Thompson D, Ganesan V. Revascularisation surgery for paediatric moyamoya: a review of the literature. *Childs Nerv Syst.* 2005;21:358-364.

Roach ES, Golomb MR, Adams R, et al. Management of stroke in infants and children: a scientific statement from a Special Writing Group of the American Heart Association Stroke Council and the Council on Cardiovascular Disease in the Young. *Stroke.* 2008;39:2644-2691.

Scott RM, Smith ER. Moyamoya disease and moyamoya syndrome. *N Engl J Med.* 2009;360:1226-1237.

Scott RM, Smith JL, Robertson RL, et al. Long-term outcome in children with moyamoya syndrome after cranial revascularization by pial synangiosis. *J Neurosurg Spine.* 2004;100:142-149.

Suzuki J, Takaku A. Cerebrovascular "moyamoya" disease: disease showing abnormal net-like vessels in base of brain. *Arch Neurol.* 1969;20:288-299.

Please go to expertconsult.com to view a complete list of references.

PART 3
Vascular Neurosurgery

Cerebrovascular Occlusive Disease and Carotid Surgery

Geoffrey Appelboom, Matthew Piazza, E. Sander Connolly, Jr.

CLINICAL PEARLS

- Atherosclerotic occlusive disease is the most commonly seen cervical common carotid bifurcation and involves the common, internal carotid arteries (ICAs). Other causes of ischemia are intracranial atherosclerotic narrowing or occlusion; extracranial or intracranial dissection of the internal carotid, vertebral, and other arteries; and moyamoya disease.

- Ischemic disease becomes symptomatic owing to distal thromboembolism or diminished flow. Symptoms may include stroke and transient ischemic attacks.

- Workup of a patient presenting with ischemic stroke may include magnetic resonance imaging (MRI; diffusion-weighted images and MR perfusion), magnetic resonance angiography (MRA), computed tomography angiography (CTA), carotid duplex ultrasonography, transcranial Doppler angiography, and digital subtraction angiography (DSA).

- Patients with symptomatic cervical ICA stenosis greater than 50% benefit from carotid endarterectomy at high-volume centers with low complication rates.

- Endovascular carotid artery stenting (CAS) has been evaluated as an alternative to carotid endarterectomy in two randomized international trials. The short-term results indicate higher complication rates with CAS. It may be performed in selected patients, especially with very high carotid lesions.

- Moyamoya disease is caused by progressive occlusion of the intracranial ICA, and adjacent major branches, with accompanying dilation of small collateral arteries. It may manifest in children with transient ischemic attack or strokes and in adults with ischemic symptoms or hemorrhage. Prevention of further ischemic episodes may be accomplished by indirect revascularization (encephalodural/glial/myosynangiosis) or direct revascularization (extracranial bypass, most commonly superficial temporal artery to middle cerebral artery anastomosis).

- At present, randomized trials do not support the use of external carotid/internal carotid (EC-IC) arterial bypass for chronic atherosclerotic ischemic disease.

The central nervous system is metabolically demanding, receiving approximately 20% of cardiac output despite comprising only 2% of body weight. Cerebral blood flow (CBF) is directly proportional to the difference between mean arterial pressure (MAP) and intracranial pressure (ICP) and inversely related to cerebrovascular resistance (CVR) as per Ohm's law. Alteration of cerebrovascular tone allows for maintenance of cerebral perfusion pressure over a wide range of mean arterial pressures. However, if cerebral perfusion pressure drops below 20 mm Hg, in the setting of arterial occlusion, for example, inadequate delivery of oxygen to brain tissue results in ischemia and subsequent infarction if CBF is not quickly returned to normal.[1]

Depending on the severity, location, and presentation of the occlusion a broad range of clinical symptoms may occur. For example, chronic occlusion leads to development of collateral vessels and neovascularization that will increase tolerance to the ischemia in cases of later acute occlusion. Moreover, a very proximal carotid occlusion, in the setting of weak anastomosis, could potentially lead to total hemiplegia. On the other end of the spectrum, patients may be asymptomatic with a distal occlusion of an artery. In cases in which a supra-aortic vessel becomes occluded, the collateral network afforded by the circle of Willis may provide blood flow to patients, although there is considerable anatomical variation among patients, which subsequently influences the degree of compensatory flow. Depending on the duration of the occlusion, neurological symptoms may be temporary (as in transient ischemic attacks or reversible ischemic neurological deficits) or permanent (ischemic stroke). Furthermore, brain tissue perfused by vessels with significant degrees of stenosis but not complete occlusion are vulnerable to ischemic insults with hemodynamic instability (i.e., shock); in these cases deficits may be specific to the stenotic vessel in addition to the classic watershed regions.

The differential diagnosis for arterial occlusion includes both acute and chronic disease processes that may affect either intracranial or extracranial vessels. This chapter focuses on cerebrovascular occlusive disease processes commonly encountered and treated by the neurosurgeon—atherosclerotic cerebrovascular occlusive disease (with a specific emphasis on carotid artery stenosis), moyamoya disease, and cerebral arterial dissection. Following a brief review of clinical anatomy, the pathophysiology, clinical presentation, diagnosis, and management of each of the aforementioned conditions will be discussed. The final section of this chapter will detail the neurosurgical technique for carotid endarterectomy and superficial temporal artery to middle cerebral artery bypass, important surgical treatments for cerebrovascular occlusive disease in the armamentarium of the neurovascular surgeon.

REVIEW OF CLINICAL ANATOMY

The anterior circulation consists of branches of the internal carotid artery, which originates at the bifurcation of the common carotid artery at the level of the thyroid cartilage in the neck. The extracranial portion of the artery passes into the carotid canal of the temporal bone. The intracranial segment of the artery consists of the petrosal, cavernous, and supraclinoid

portions. The latter segment gives rise to the ophthalmic artery, the anterior choroidal artery, and the middle cerebral artery. The right and left anterior circulations share flow via the anterior communicating artery, while the posterior communicating artery provides collateral flow to the middle cerebral artery from the respective posterior cerebral artery.

The posterior circulation is composed of the basilar artery formed at the pontomedullary junction by the confluence of both vertebral arteries. The vertebrobasilar system gives rise to numerous paramedian, short circumferential, and long circumferential branches that supply midline brainstem structures, lateral brainstem structures, and dorsolateral brainstem and cerebellar structures, respectively. Although the former two categories of arteries are unnamed, the three sets of long circumferential arteries (from most distal to proximal) are the posterior inferior cerebellar arteries, the anterior inferior cerebellar arteries, and the superior cerebellar arteries. The terminal branch of the basilar artery is the posterior cerebral artery (PCA); it supplies the midbrain, the thalamus, and the medial aspect of the temporal and occipital lobes.

Presenting symptoms of acute occlusion reflect the respective vascular territories (Fig. 12.1). Anterior circulation involvement may manifest as monocular blindness and an

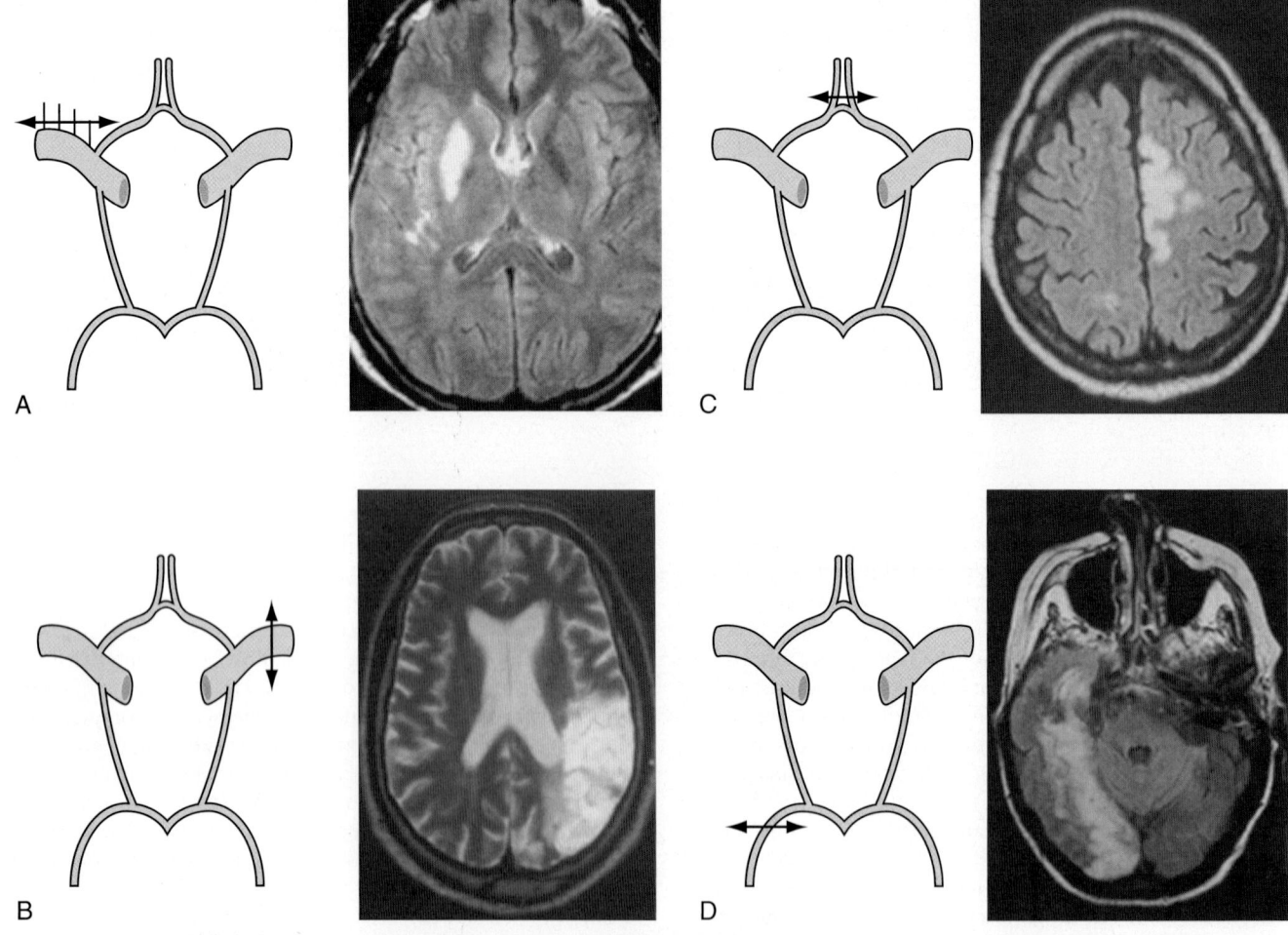

FIGURE 12.1 Expected ischemic lesion following intracranial occlusion. T1- and T2-weighted magnetic resonance imaging (MRI) of cerebral infarct with respective vascular territory. **A,** Proximal right middle cerebral arterial (MCA) occlusion. **B,** Distal left MCA occlusion. **C,** Left anterior cerebral arterial occlusion. **D,** Right posterior cerebral artery occlusion.

absent pupillary light response; hemispheric signs such as contralateral homonymous hemianopia, hemiparesis, and hemisensory loss; specific signs of dominant hemispheric ischemia including aphasia, alexia, agraphia, acalculia, and dysarthria; and nondominant hemispheric symptoms including visuospatial neglect, constructional apraxia, loss of prosody of speech, and anosognosia. Posterior circulation symptoms, aside from alteration in level of consciousness, include motor deficits such as hemiparesis, tetraparesis, and facial paresis from brainstem lesions, vertigo, vomiting, pupillary abnormalities, ataxia, oculomotor signs, and pseudobulbar manifestations.

ATHEROSCLEROTIC CEREBROVASCULAR OCCLUSIVE DISEASE

Pathophysiology

Arterial atherosclerotic plaques originate in regions of high permeability that are indistinguishable from surrounding tissue except on a microscopic level. Permeability is governed by the endothelial layer and appears to be the dysfunctional result of a combination of initial stressors that can include elevated or modified low-density lipoprotein (LDL) levels, flow-related mechanical stress, elevated serum cholesterol, elevated homocysteine levels, and potentially infection in some cases. The consequence of this excess permeability is that a higher than normal level of plasma components enters into the subendothelial layers and begins to aggregate.

The substance found to correlate highest with the generation of macroscopic plaques is unquestionably LDL, which initiates the fatty streak upon deposition in the subendothelial layers via focal activation and recruitment of monocytes. This inflammatory process is greatly exacerbated by the oxidation of LDL via lipoxygenases, nitric oxide, myeloperoxidase, and other mechanisms to the point of no longer being recognized by LDL receptors. Highly oxidized LDL thus becomes trapped in the subendothelial layers, promoting focal accumulations that stimulate local cells to secrete monocyte chemoattractants. Stimulation of scavenger receptors on local monocytes by oxidized LDL can also directly promote monocyte invasion into the subendothelial layer and subsequent differentiation into macrophages.

Macrophage uptake of LDL ultimately results in accumulation of LDL and cholesterol metabolites within these cells and the "foamy" histological appearance. The scavenger receptor pathway responsible for uptake is not down-regulated by this accumulation, which eventually results in unsustainable overload and cell death. The debris from early foamy cell death serves to promote more monocyte invasion fatty streak formation. An immunofibrotic plaque begins to form as foamy cells accumulate in subendothelial layers. Smooth muscle cells proliferate in the region of the growing fatty streak and begin to deposit collagen as a means of stabilizing the lesion, ultimately forming a fibrotic cap. The artery dilates to compensate for the thickening layer of smooth muscle and collagen, but years of plaque growth will ultimately surmount the maximum compensatory capacity of the vessel and a reduction in lumen volume occurs. This stenosis and the growing instability of the plaque due to size and inflammatory damage to its integrity

both contribute to potential cerebrovascular injury via the risk of ischemia and thromboembolic events.

Clinical Features

Given the chronic nature of cerebrovascular atherosclerosis, the cerebrovascular system can show a remarkable level of resilience prior to symptomatic presentation and often remains undiagnosed for many years. The remainder of the discussion will be focused on carotid disease given its responsiveness to neurosurgical intervention. Vertebrobasilar and intracranial atherosclerosis share a similar clinical presentation with carotid artery stenosis but specific neurological findings are localized to the vascular territories involved (Table 12.1).

Asymptomatic patients with carotid disease frequently are discovered because of the presence of a carotid bruit over the site of stenosis. Other signs in both asymptomatic and symptomatic patients include ocular bruits, pulsatile arteries arising from the external carotid artery. Nonetheless, the absence of signs does not exclude the presence of severe stenosis and subsequent complications, nor does the presence of these signs rule out other causes.

Symptomatic carotid disease is defined by the presence of neurological symptoms that are sudden in onset and referable to the appropriate carotid artery via its zone of dominant blood supply. Such disease often manifests in the form of a transient ischemic attack (TIA) or ischemic stroke. In most cases, carotid disease TIAs are less than 15 minutes in duration and present with either sensory, motor, or combined deficits of the contralateral side. Mechanistically, ischemic symptoms may result from embolism of platelet aggregates that form over the surface of the lesion leading to occlusion of a distal vessel or from hypoperfusion secondary to critical stenosis and hemodynamic alterations. In the former case, deficits may be quite specific (i.e., monocular blindness) and in the latter case, they are usually generalized to major vascular territories.

Diagnosis

The radiological evaluation of cerebrovascular atherosclerotic disease, specifically disease of the carotid arteries, consists of identifying the level and location of stenosis/occlusion, defining the etiology of these lesions, surgical planning, and patient follow-up. The four major modalities (most invasive to the least invasive techniques) are digital subtraction cerebral angiography (CA), computed tomographic angiography (CTA), magnetic resonance angiography (MRA), and duplex ultrasound (DUS).[2-4]

Cerebral angiography is the gold standard for imaging the carotid arteries (Fig. 12.2). Cerebral angiography has superior accuracy compared to noninvasive techniques, which may overestimate or underestimate the degree of stenosis, an important characteristic for accurately determining the extent of disease and for surgical planning. Moreover, more than one noninvasive modality is usually required to perform an accurate and comprehensive assessment of atherosclerotic disease. The advent of digital subtraction angiography (DSA) has reduced the size of catheter needed, the amount of contrast required, and the duration of this procedure. Although there is lower spatial resolution, DSA allows for dynamic visualization of blood flow at the site of stenosis as well as collateralization

TABLE 12.1 Clinical Syndromes with Cerebrovascular Occlusion

Site of Occlusion	Symptoms/Signs	Differential Diagnosis	Workup
Carotid circulation	Monocular blindness Unilateral somatosensory symptoms Unilateral leg/arm weakness Aphasia	Migraine with aura Seizure Transient amnesia Syncope Multiple sclerosis Subdural hematoma	MRI, MRA: diffusion- and perfusion-weighted CT angiography Duplex ultrasound Cerebral angiography General workup*
Vertebrobasilar circulation	Hemianopia/cortical blindness Bilateral face/leg/arm weakness Bilateral somatosensory symptoms Dizziness Dysphagia Dysarthria	Seizure Transient amnesia Syncope Multiple sclerosis Migraine with aura Cerebral amyloid angiopathy Subdural hematoma	MRI, MRA: diffusion- and perfusion-weighted CT angiography Duplex ultrasound Cerebral angiography General workup*
Intracranial circulation	Vertebrobasilar junction—see "Vertebrobasilar circulation" Internal carotid artery and the middle cerebral artery junction—see "Carotid circulation"	Vasculitis Seizure Multiple sclerosis Cerebral amyloid angiopathy Transient amnesia Syncope	Cerebral angiography: DSA Transcranial Doppler MRI, MRA: diffusion- and perfusion-weighted CT angiography General workup*

*General workup:
  Holter ECG, cardiac ultrasound (transthoracic, transesophageal)
  Blood workup: CBC, ESR, blood culture, ANA, PT, PTT
ANA, antinuclear antibody assay; CBC, complete blood count; CT, computed tomography; DSA, digital subtraction angiography; ECG, electrocardiogram; ESR, erythrocyte sedimentation rate; MRA, magnetic resonance angiography; MRI, magnetic resonance imaging; PT, prothrombin time; PT, partial thromboplastin time.

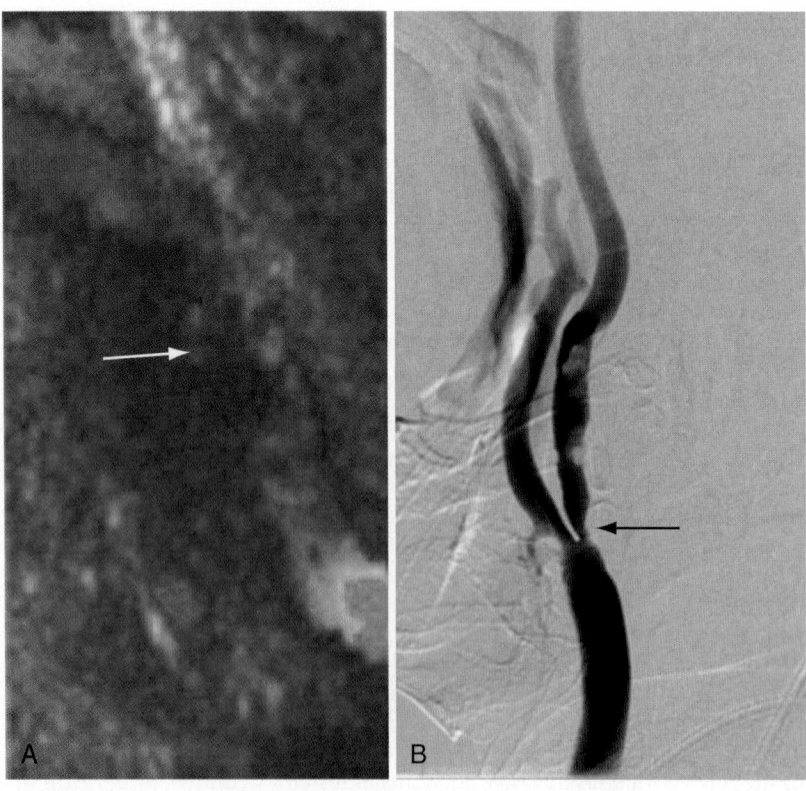

FIGURE 12.2 Diagnostic imaging of carotid artery stenosis. **A,** Color duplex sonography of the neck showing narrowing of the carotid artery and associated increase in flow velocity. **B,** Digital subtraction angiography of carotid artery demonstrating stenosis at the level of the carotid bifurcation and internal carotid artery.

and flow around the vascular lesion; this information provides an indication of the clinical impact of the stenosis. Patients should be screened for history of adverse reaction to contrast agent and renal disease, as contrast nephropathy and allergy are potential complications of cerebral angiography.

CTA combines CT technique with venous injection of contrast dye to visualize the supra-aortic vessels (both intracranially and extracranially). Unlike CA and DSA, CTA provides an anatomical description of the surrounding structures in addition to the vasculature, which is extremely useful in identifying nonatherosclerotic causes of stenosis. This technique is less invasive than DSA but requires contrast bolus comparable to angiography, and so contrast allergy and nephropathy are possible complications. Furthermore, as the quality and accuracy of the obtained image depends on both the timing of the injection and the scan itself, CTA often suffers from overestimation or underestimation of the degree of disease.

MRA uses intravenous injection of gadolinium and may be useful in evaluating extracranial carotid arteries. Alternative techniques are used without contrast enhancement, such as time-of-flight (TOF) measurement, which is often used for assessing intracranial lesions. MRA produces a reproducible three-dimensional image of the carotid bifurcation with good sensitivity for detecting high-grade carotid artery stenosis and is especially informative in the setting of symptomatic disease.

Carotid DUS is a relatively easy technique that can be performed at the bedside. It detects a focal increase in blood flow velocity, suggesting vessel stenosis. The peak systolic velocity is the most frequently used measurement to gauge the severity of the stenosis but the end-diastolic velocity, spectral configuration, and the carotid index or peak internal carotid artery velocity/common carotid artery velocity ratio provide additional information and allow accurate estimation of the lesion. Trancranial US is used to detect intracranial circulation as well and is very useful to assess intracranial atherosclerotic status. Although relatively inexpensive, portable, and easy to use at the bedside, this technique is still very physician and technician dependent.

Measurement of Carotid Artery Stenosis

Current indications for surgical intervention of carotid atherosclerotic disease require objective and reproducible methods to evaluate the degree of stenosis. Two major methods of measuring carotid stenosis were developed for use in the major clinical trials evaluating the efficacy of carotid endarterectomy: the North American Symptomatic Carotid Endarterectomy Trial (NASCET)[5] method and the European Carotid Surgery Trial (ESCT)[6] method. The primary difference in these methods lies in how the observer estimates the diameter of the reference vessel. The NASCET utilizes the normal carotid wall just distal to the stenotic lesion as the reference vessel, and ESCT defines the reference as the estimated diameter of the carotid bulb. Figure 12.3 diagrams each method of measurement and the mathematical relationship between these two methods. Note that the ECST and NASCET approximations are comparable with severe disease, but that their values diverge when the stenosis is not as pronounced. In contemporary practice, most patients are determined to have high-grade (>60-70%) stenosis on the basis of noninvasive color flow Doppler, CTA, or MRA. When two of these three modalities agree on the degree of stenosis and no other modality questions the result, the correlation with catheter angiography is excellent. Given the risk of catheter angiography, this is generally reserved for patients in whom the studies are not concordant.

Management

Medical Management

The mainstays of medical management for patients with carotid atherosclerosis are risk factor modification and antiplatelet therapy.

Traditional, modifiable cardiovascular risk factors, such as hypertension, diabetes mellitus, hyperlipidemia, and tobacco use, increase the risk of ischemic cerebrovascular events. Judicious use of antihypertensive agents to lower blood pressure in addition to antihyperlipidemic agents and proper glucose control, either through insulin or antihyperglycemic agents, are suitable options for slowing the progression of atherosclerotic disease and reducing the risk of ischemic events, but does not eliminate the risk of stroke in these patients. Patients should be counseled regarding the risks of smoking and its relationship to stroke and should be offered services to assist in smoking cessation.

Antiplatelet therapy has been shown to decrease the risk of ischemic stroke, although it does not eliminate this risk, presumably because of its multifactorial etiology. Antiplatelet therapy directly is thought to prevent the formation of

FIGURE 12.3 Methods of assessing carotid stenosis severity. **A,** Residual lumen diameter at most stenotic portion of vessel. **B,** Estimated diamater of carotid wall at the level of the lesion. **C,** Diameter of normal carotid artery just distal to stenosis.

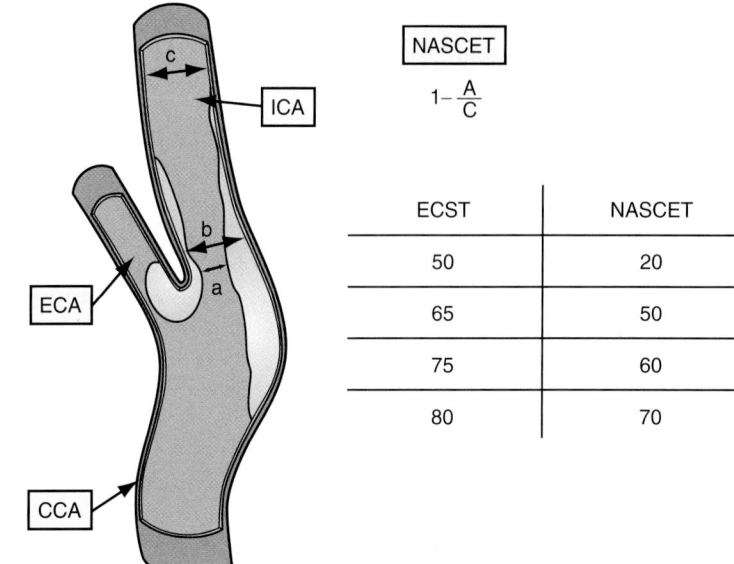

ECST	NASCET
50	20
65	50
75	60
80	70

mural-platelet aggregates that either lead to occlusion of large arteries or embolize to distal vessels. Aspirin (acetylsalicylic acid, ASA) is the typical agent used. The optimal dose prescribed remains controversial, although a daily dose of 325 mg has been shown to decrease the risk of stroke by 30% following a TIA. However, it should be noted that patients following carotid endarterectomy (CEA) have lower rates of morbidity and mortality with doses within the range of 81 mg to 325 mg when compared with patients using higher doses.[7] For patients who cannot tolerate ASA, thienopyridines may be used. Clopidogrel is preferred over ticlodipine owing to the greater risk of severe neutropenia in the latter.

Surgical Therapy

The efficacy of carotid endarterectomy at reducing the risk of stroke for both symptomatic and asymptomatic patients has been demonstrated in several large, randomized clinical trials, most notably the NASCET[5] and the Asymptomatic Carotid Artery Stenosis Trial (ACAST).[8]

The NASCET, which enrolled patients with transient ischemic attacks (TIAs) or mild stroke within 120 days of surgery, had an absolute risk reduction of ipsilateral stroke at 2 years of 17% when compared with best medical management (9% vs. 28%, respectively) for patients with severe stenosis defined as greater than 70%. A follow-up report found that patients with moderate stenosis (between 50% and 69%) demonstrated a modest risk reduction of 6.7% of any fatal or nonfatal stroke within the 5-year follow-up period for patients treated with surgery versus best medical management (15.7% vs. 22.2, respectively). The ACAST examined patients without symptomatic history and found that patients with greater than 60% stenosis had a 6.1% absolute reduction in risk of any ipsilateral stroke, perioperative stroke, or death at 5 years (5.1% vs. 11.0%, respectively).[9]

Contralateral stenosis is not uncommon, with one follow-up study of NASCET reporting approximately 8.6% with severe stenosis and 6.5% with complete occlusion of the contralateral carotid artery.[10] Although randomized controlled trials are needed to determine the efficacy of operating on patients with bilateral carotid stenosis/occlusion, subgroup analyses of NASCET suggest that patients with occluded contralateral carotid arteries have improved outcomes with surgery when compared with best medical management despite a greater risk of perioperative stroke or death.

Patients with concomitant intracranial atherosclerosis may especially benefit from carotid surgery as this subset of patients with carotid disease; a NASCET subgroup analysis of patients with intracranial atherosclerosis showed that patients who received medical management had a greater risk of stroke, but the surgically treated patients with and without intracranial atherosclerosis did not differ in rates of stroke.[11]

Alternatives to Carotid Endarterectomy

Carotid Stenting

The advent of endovascular surgery offers an alternative treatment for carotid atherosclerosis in patients who are at high risk for open surgery. Several large randomized trials have attempted to compare stenting versus CEA, but the results have largely been equivocal. Two recent trials are worth noting, the International Carotid Stenting Study (ICSS)[12] and the Carotid Revascularization Endarterectomy versus Stenting Trial (CREST).[13]

The ICSS examined outcome after carotid endarterectomy (CEA) and stenting in patients with recently symptomatic carotid artery stenosis. Short-term results (120 days) showed no significant difference in disabling stroke or death after CEA (3.2%) and stenting (4.0%). However, there was a significantly greater risk of stroke, death, or procedural myocardial infarction after stenting (8.5%) than with CEA (5.2%). Thirty-day results demonstrated that the incidence of any stroke, death, and fatal myocardial infarction in stenting patients exceeded twice the rate seen with CEA patients. CREST also studied outcomes after CEA and stenting in patients with both symptomatic and asymptomatic carotid artery stenosis. Preliminary results demonstrated no significant difference in the 30-day incidence of stroke, death, and myocardial infarction between the two treatment groups. However, the 4-year rate of stroke or death was significantly greater in the stenting versus surgery group with a hazard ratio of 1.5. Final, long-term results of both these trials are still pending, although it appears that carotid surgery remains the primary surgical intervention for both symptomatic and asymptomatic carotid stenosis but that carotid stenting may be used in select patients.[14]

External Carotid Artery/Internal Carotid Artery Bypass

External carotid/internal carotid (EC-IC) bypass surgery involves anastomosing a segment of the external carotid artery (most commonly, the superficial temporal artery, STA) to a segment of the internal carotid artery (usually the middle cerebral artery, MCA) using a venous graft and is an alternative surgical intervention for patients with atherosclerotic disease of the ICA (or MCA, for that matter). To date, the EC-IC Bypass Trial remains the only prospective randomized controlled trial evaluating the efficacy of bypass surgery in patients with atherosclerotic cerebrovascular disease compared with best medical management.[15] In this study, patients who experienced at least one TIA or stroke ipsilateral to the diseased vessel within 3 months were randomized to either STA-MCA bypass or best medical management. The trial demonstrated that surgery did not reduce the risks of major or fatal strokes, any ipsilateral stroke, major ipsilateral stroke, or all strokes and death. Moreover, operative patients had greater rates of perioperative stroke and death when compared to medically treated patients. As such, the authors concluded that EC-IC bypass was not effective in preventing ischemia or infarction in patients with atherosclerotic cerebrovascular disease. However, many critics of the study argue that the patient inclusion criteria were too broad and that additional prospective trials with better patient stratification, particularly with respect to cerebrovascular hemodynamic status, may demonstrate the utility of EC-IC bypass for a subset of patients.[16] The Carotid Occlusion Surgery Study (COSS) was a randomized trial that compared EC/IC bypass and best medical management in patients with hemispheric ischemia within the previous 120 days, and ipsilateral oxygen fraction (OEC) by positron emission tomography (PET). The trial was stopped early by the U.S. National

Institute of Health owing to a much better outcome than expected in the medically treated group.[17]

NONATHEROSCLEROTIC OCCLUSIVE DISEASE

Moyamoya Disease

Moyamoya disease is a relatively rare cause of cerebrovascular occlusive disease, with a typical reported incidence of less than 1 per 100,000 per year.[18] More common in females, moyamoya disease has a bimodal age distribution, with peak incidence in the first and fourth decades of life. Moyamoya disease manifests as chronic, progressive occlusion of the internal carotid artery at and distal to the carotid siphon that may also involve the proximal segments of the middle and anterior cerebral arteries. Over time, patients with moyamoya disease 3 develop networks of fragile, collateral vessels that resemble a "puff of smoke" on angiogram, hence its name.

The pathophysiology of moyamoya disease remains somewhat elusive. Cerebrospinal fluid (CSF) levels of cytokines, growth factors, and adhesion molecules are elevated in patients with moyamoya disease. Additionally, hepatocyte growth factor, which has increased expression in the media and thickened intima in moyamoya patients, has been implicated in the migration and proliferation of smooth muscle cells within the intima. Linkage studies also suggest that genetics may play a role in the development of moyamoya disease.

The clinical presentation depends on the age of the patient. Most pediatric patients present with ischemic symptoms (TIA or stroke), and adult patients can present with either ischemic or hemorrhagic symptoms. TIA or stroke in these patients usually involves the ICA distribution (usually centered around the frontal lobe) and results in focal neurological deficits. Pediatric patients, in particular, may present with intellectual impairments, and moyamoya disease can rarely masquerade as psychiatric illness. Crying spells in pediatric patients can precipitate ischemic events, as hyperventilation, with resulting hypocapnia and vasoconstriction, can lead to reduced blood flow to vulnerable and chronically poorly perfused tissues. Hemorrhage can result from ruptured fragile collateral vessels, commonly occurring in the basal ganglia, thalamus, or around the ventricles leading to intraventricular hemorrhage. Other causes of hemorrhage in these patients include rupture of intracranial aneurysm leading to subarachnoid hemorrhage. Atypical symptoms of moyamoya disease include migraine-like headaches, seizures, and involuntary movements.

Diagnosis

Cerebral angiography is the gold standard for diagnosing moyamoya disease. Hallmark features include narrowing of the C1 and C2 segments of the internal carotid artery and proximal involvement of the middle cerebral artery (MCA) and anterior cerebral artery (ACA) bilaterally. The pathognomonic, delicate collateral vessels typically are visualized near deep brain structures supplied by the thalamoperforating, lenticulostriate, and anterior choroidal vessels. The ethmoidal arteries may also be recruited to supply the ACA (ethmoidal moyamoya) and anastomoses between dural and pial vessels

(vault moyamoya). As collateral vessels disappear following revascularization, cerebral angiography may be used to assess success of bypass during follow-up. MRA is a noninvasive alternative, and angiography need not be performed if MRA/MRI shows the following bilaterally: (1) stenosis/occlusion of the terminal ICA and proximal ACA and MCA; (2) abnormal vascular network within the basal ganglia.[19]

Management

No interventions in the setting of acute ischemic stroke secondary to moyamoya disease have proved effective. Treatment is largely supportive and aimed at decreasing cerebral edema and increasing cerebral perfusion. Intravenous/intra-arterial thrombolysis is not typically performed in this patient population given the fragility of collateral vessels and the increased risk for intracerebral hemorrhage. Patients with intracerebral hemorrhage may benefit from surgical decompression and ventricular drainage.

Prevention of further ischemic or hemorrhagic events in moyamoya disease involves revascularization procedures.[20] Direct revascularization involves creating anastomoses between a branch of the external carotid artery and a branch of the internal carotid artery (typically the superficial temporal artery and M3 or M4 segment of the middle cerebral artery, respectively). This results in an immediate restoration of flow to previously poorly perfused areas of the brain. See later discussion for in-depth description of the operative technique for EC-IC bypass.

Indirect revascularization involves placement of vascularized tissue on the surface of ischemic brain, stimulation of angiogenesis, and formation of collateral networks between donor and recipient tissue. Vascularized donor tissue may consist of temporal muscle (encephalomyosynangiosis), galea (encephalogaleosynangiosis), superficial temporal artery (encephaloduroarteriosynangiosis), or combinations of these techniques (e.g., encephaloduroarteriomyosynangiosis). Although indirect bypass is not as technically challenging as direct revascularization and is a suitable alternative in moyamoya disease, angiogenesis may take months and patients remain at increased risk of ischemic stroke. A combination of direct and indirect revascularization techniques may be used to provide an immediate improvement of perfusion in addition to the progressive formation of collateral networks.

Dissection

Cerebral arterial dissection results from a tear in the arterial wall and extravasation of blood between the intima and media layers, with subsequent luminal narrowing or occlusion. The etiology of arterial dissection is multifactorial but can be grossly categorized as traumatic or spontaneous, although spontaneous dissections may be due to minor trauma to an already predisposed vessel. Conditions commonly associated with cerebral arterial dissections include fibromuscular dysplasia, Marfan syndrome, polycystic kidney disease, and vasculitides. The annual incidence of dissection is approximately 3.6 per 100,000, and vertebrobasilar dissections occur more frequently than carotid dissections.[21]

The clinical manifestations of cranial arterial dissection vary, but patients often present with either ischemic stroke (more common with carotid) or subarachnoid hemorrhage (more common with vertebrobasilar); however, patients may only have mild complaints, including headache, neck pain, incomplete Horner syndrome, transient deficits, or neck swelling. Ischemic symptoms represent occlusion of the cerebral arteries and can occur secondary to embolization of thrombus formed at the site of dissection, from intraluminal thrombosis, or from expansion of the false lumen with occlusion of the true lumen. As with atherosclerotic cerebrovascular disease, the clinical symptoms reflect the vascular territory involved.

Diagnosis

Cerebral angiography is the gold standard for diagnosis of cerebral arterial dissection.[21] Notable angiographic findings include a smooth, but irregular narrowing of the vessel, presence of a double lumen, or intimal flap, and arterial occlusion. The diagnosis may sometimes be confused with atherosclerosis or vasospasm in the setting of subarachnoid hemorrhage (SAH); the former can be distinguished by unusual location and relatively young age of the patient in dissection, and the latter occurs several days following the SAH. Angiography also has the advantage of allowing for immediate, endovascular intervention in select patients. However, there is a small, but real risk of ischemic stroke (<0.5%) as well as contrast nephropathy in patients with renal disease.[21] CTA has high sensitivity for both extracranial carotid and vertebral dissections. Additionally, this quick diagnostic allows for rapid diagnosis of dissection in patients, which is ideal for patients presenting acutely. However, as with angiography, patients are at risk of contrast-induced nephropathy and are exposed to significant levels of radiation. MRI/MRA is gaining favor and has particularly high sensitivity for detecting extracranial carotid dissection. Moreover, MRI allows for visualization of ischemic brain lesions. However, MRI/MRA has less utility in detecting vertebrobasilar dissections and may be associated with significant motion artifact in the restless patient. Finally, Doppler ultrasound can be used at the bedside to rapidly to diagnose extracranial carotid dissection the good sensitivity, but is not useful at identifying other dissecting vessels.

Management

Management of cerebral arterial dissection remains controversial given the absence of large, randomized clinical trials.[21] However, patients without evidence of hemorrhage and with extracranial disease (especially those with evidence of thromboembolic phenomena) may be treated with anticoagulation (intravenous heparin during the first week or so followed by several months of oral anticoagulation). Patients who do not respond to anticoagulation may benefit from endovascular or surgical intervention. Angioplasty, stenting, and intra-arterial thrombolysis are potential endovascular treatments. EC-IC bypass using high-flow conduit (either saphenous vein or radial artery grafts) with subsequent ligation of the ICA may be used in rare cases. Dissections that present with subarachnoid hemorrhage (usually intracranial cases involving the vertebral artery) usually require surgery. Options include sacrifice of the vertebral artery with or without vascular bypass, surgical clipping of dissection aneurysm, and endovascular coiling.

Surgical Management of Cerebrovascular Occlusive Disease

Carotid Endarterectomy

Choice of Anesthesia

Patients may undergo either local or general anesthesia per surgeon and patient preference, as previous studies have demonstrated that rates of poor short-term outcome following surgery are similar.[22] Choice of anesthesia determines intraoperative monitoring. Patients undergoing local anesthesia may be followed clinically throughout the procedure by frequently assessing neurological function. For patients receiving general anesthesia, EEG monitoring may be used to monitor for warning signs of intraoperative ischemia.

Operative Technique

Patients are placed in the supine position, with the neck extended and rotated gently contralateral from the side of the lesion of interest to maximize exposure of the internal carotid artery (the degree of neck rotation needed for optimal exposure may be ascertained by preoperative imaging) (Fig. 12.4). Care must be taken not to cause trauma to the lesion and subsequent thromboembolism to distal cerebral vessels when the operative region is prepped and draped.

The skin incision typically follows the anterior portion of the sternocleidomastoid; a transverse incision along the skinfold at the level of the carotid bulb may be more cosmetically pleasing but requires preoperative determination of the bulb location. Dissection of subcutaneous tissue and fascia, separation of the platysma muscle, and dissection of the neck to reveal the carotid sheath are performed. Meticulous hemostasis is maintained throughout. Medial retraction must be performed with care so as not to injure recurrent laryngeal nerves.

Once the carotid sheath is identified (Fig. 12.5), the jugular vein, which lies parallel and anteriorlateral to the carotid artery, is gently dissected from the carotid artery along its medial aspect. Division of the common facial vein enhances exposure of the carotid artery at the level of the bulb and the proximal common carotid, respectively. Following incision through the carotid sheath, the common, external, and internal segments of the carotid artery are identified and controlled using umbilical tape. Any hemodynamic instability noted during this time, principally bradycardia, can be treated with application of lidocaine to the carotid bulb. The patient is then heparinized and the internal, common, and external segments of the carotid artery are sequentially clamped. Cerebral shunting may be performed at this time, depending on surgeon preference; however, intraoperative neurological monitoring must be performed throughout the surgery and a shunt should be prepared and ready for insertion in the event that brain ischemia is suspected.

Longitudinal arterotomy of the common carotid near the bifurcation is made and extended proximally and distally through the internal segment. The atherosclerotic plaque (Fig. 12.6) must be carefully dissected away from the arterial wall; a smooth transition between normal and endarterectomized vessel should be made to avoid the creation of a false lumen of the artery.

Although primary closure of the arterotomy is preferred, a prosthetic or venous patch graft (usually harvested from the

FIGURE 12.4 Dissection of internal carotid artery. **A,** Anteroposterior view of magnetic resonance angiography demonstrating site of dissection. **B,** T1-weighted magnetic resonance imaging scan identifying false lumen of the dissected internal carotid artery imposing on the true lumen.

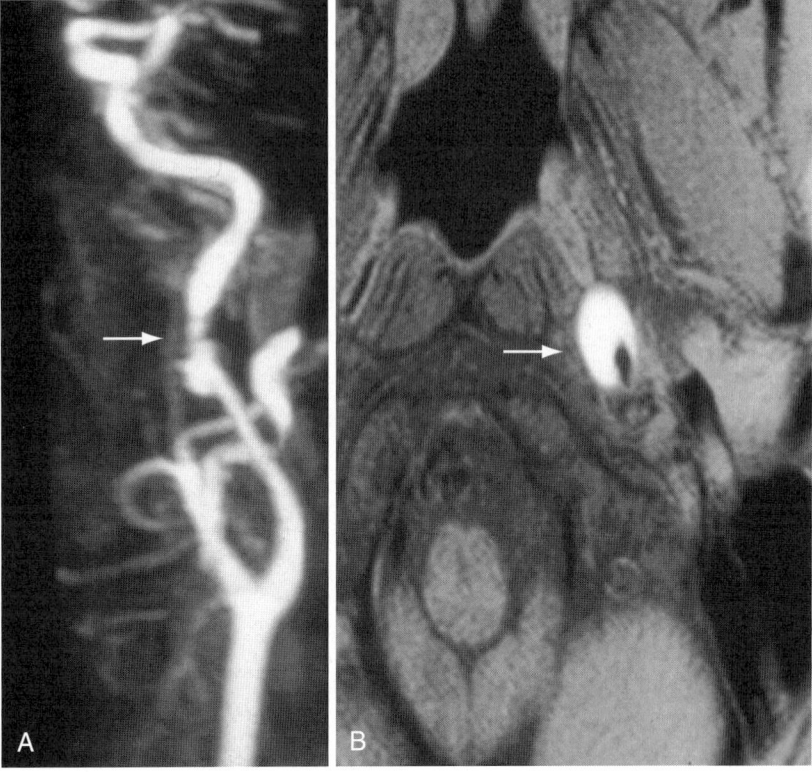

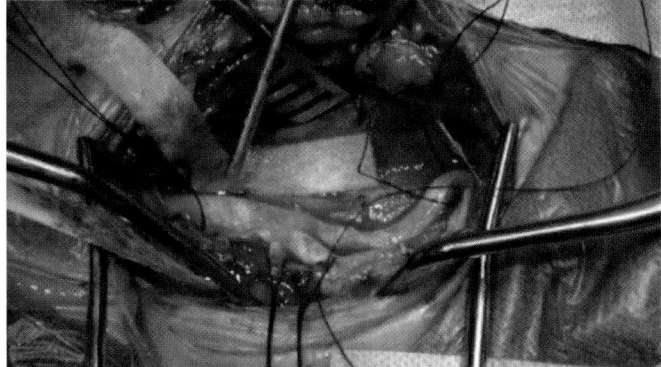

FIGURE 12.5 Intraoperative view of carotid endarterectomy. Prearterotomy view of carotid artery immediately prior to systemic heparinization and clamping the internal, common, and external carotid arteries in sequential fashion.

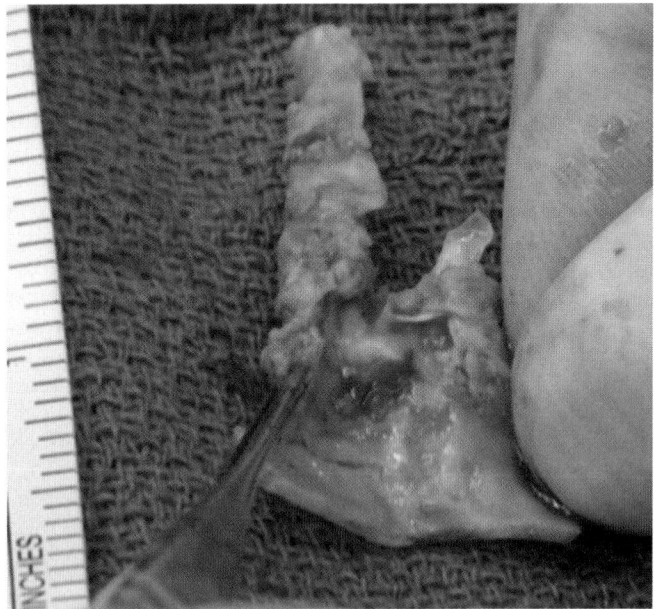

FIGURE 12.6 Postendarterectomy atherosclerotic plaque measuring approximately 1.8 inches in length.

saphenous vein) may be indicated in patients with repeat endarterectomy or with unusually small carotid arteries. In the latter case, a patch graft may be avoided by visualizing the artery under the microscope during closure. Unclamping for flushing before complete closure is routine. Carotid segments are unclamped following closure of the arterotomy beginning with the external carotid artery, and then the common carotid artery and internal carotid artery, in that order. Prior to final wound closure, meticulous hemostasis is performed and sufficient time is allowed to pass to guarantee its success. A Jackson-Pratt drain may be placed to avoid formation of neck hematomas, and the platysma, fascial layer, and skin are sutured.

Postoperative Care

Patients should be monitored in an intensive care unit with an arterial line in place. Blood pressure lability is common within the first 24 hours postoperatively and pressures should be kept within 110 mm Hg to 150 mm Hg, ideally with short-acting agents to avoid prolonged rebound hypotension or hypertension. Antiplatelet agents should be held for 24 to 48 hours after surgery but may be restarted as soon as 24 hours after surgery.

Frequent postoperative evaluations should focus on the identification of new neurological deficits, which may be due to iatrogenic nerve injury or postoperative stroke, evidence of hematoma development at surgical site, and cardiac abnormalities.

Postoperative Complications

Although CEA is an effective and durable treatment for carotid atherosclerosis, complications following CEA are common. The mortality rate of carotid endarterectomy varies between 0.5% and 2.5% depending on the experience and volume at individual institutions. Cardiac complications constitute the most common cause of death after CEA; patients should have the appropriate preoperative cardiac workup to assess risk and minimize postoperative cardiac complications.

Stroke is the second most common cause of death following CEA, occurring in approximately 5% of patients, and patients should have frequent neurological checks postoperatively to promptly identify those who are exhibiting signs of brain ischemia or infarction. Occlusion of the ICA is responsible for most cases of major stroke postoperatively, and thromboembolism originating at the endarterectomy site causes most minor strokes. The management of postoperative stroke varies depending on the surgeon and the institution. Bedside ultrasound may be used to assess for flow in the operated ICA, but many surgeons may prefer to reoperate and examine the surgical site visually. Although large randomized clinical trials are lacking, possible interventions include intravenous or intra-arterial alteplase administration or carotid stenting.

Nerve injury is not an uncommon complication of carotid surgery. The hypoglossal nerve is the most commonly affected and results in tongue deviation to the ipsilateral side. This injury usually results secondary to prolonged compression during retraction. Injury to this nerve can be minimized by early identification during neck dissection and gentle retraction. Common complaints include difficulty in speaking and swallowing, although bilateral injury from a contralateral endarterectomy can result in airway obstruction. Hence, in patients needing bilateral endarterectomy, hypoglossal nerve injury during the primary endarterectomy must resolve before proceeding to surgery on the contralateral side. Other commonly affected nerves include the recurrent laryngeal nerve, which may result in unilateral vocal cord paralysis, and the vagus nerve, which lies posteriorly within the carotid sheath.

Neck hematomas are not uncommon, especially in patients taking Plavix, but those requiring reintubation and evacuation are decidedly rare. In the advent of any sign of airway compromise, early elective intubation is usually best.

Hyperperfusion, which occurs in approximately 9% to 14% of patients postoperatively, is defined as more than 100% increase in cerebral blood flow over preoperative baseline. Cerebral hyperperfusion syndrome is a less common but serious complication of CEA characterized by ipsilateral headache, seizure, and focal neurological deficits in the absence of evidence of ischemia; symptoms usually occur secondary to ipsilateral hemorrhage or edema.[23] It occurs in approximately 0.75% to 3.0% of patients; it can occur at any time from hours to a month after surgery, but most commonly begins several days after surgery. Although the exact pathophysiology is unknown, a combination of ischemia-reperfusion injury, impaired cerebral autoregulation, and hypertension is thought to play a role. Hence, it is critical to maintain the systolic blood pressure less than 150 mm Hg following surgery to decrease the risk of developing this syndrome. Transcranial Doppler may be used to screen for patients at risk of developing hyperperfusion syndrome; urgent CT is warranted in suspected cases to rule out intracerebral hemorrhage.

External Carotid Artery/Internal Carotid Artery Bypass

Direct revascularization, which involves creating anastomotic connections between external and internal carotid branches, usually a superficial temporal artery/middle cerebral artery anastomosis, results in an immediate increase in perfusion of the affected portions of the brain. The choice of anastomotic arteries will depend on the ischemic territories and the surgeon's preference. Other possible combinations of vessel pairings include occipital artery to vessels of the posterior circulation (PICA or PCA). Interposed venous grafts may be utilized to create a high-flow conduit between donor and recipient vessels. The saphenous vein is commonly used for this purpose, but again, choice of graft varies depending on patient and surgeon. Because STA-MCA bypass is most commonly utilized, the remainder of the discussion will focus on this operative technique.

Anesthetic goals include induced hypothermia to 33° C for cerebral protection, maintenance of cerebral perfusion by keeping pressures in the normotensive to hypertensive range, and maintaining normocapnia to prevent dysregulation of cerebrovascular tone. Patients will also require continuous EEG monitoring intraoperatively to assess the degree of cerebral protection afforded by hypothermia and barbiturates.

Patients should undergo angiography of the external carotid artery preoperatively to assess candidate donor vessels. Doppler ultrasound may assist the surgeon in identifying the donor vessel in the operating room. Patients should be positioned supine on the operating table with the lateral aspect of the head turned parallel to the floor. The surgical site should be prepped and draped as usual.

Following incision, the STA is identified and dissected away; secondary branches are cauterized or ligated to ensure meticulous hemostasis and to prevent postoperative epidural hematoma formation, although cautery must be performed with care to avoid thermal injury to the donor artery. The temporalis muscle is incised down the skull, a burr hole is made just superior to the zygoma, and an approximately 3 cm craniotomy is performed. After meticulous hemostasis is ensured and the dura is opened, the cortical surface is examined for a suitable recipient vessel (typically an M3 or M4 branch); if such a vessel cannot be identified, continue with indirect revascularization (see later discussion).

Preparation of the donor involves proximally clipping, ligation of the artery distally, and performing an oblique cut just proximal to the point of ligation. The distal end is then washed in heparinized saline and excess adventitia at the anastomotic end is removed. Papaverine may be applied to the donor vessel to avoid arterial spasm.

The arachnoid should be incised to free the recipient vessel and small branches around the expected arterotomy site must be cauterized. A rubber dam is placed underneath the recipient vessel to isolate the vessel, define the operative field, and protect the underlying parenchyma. Continuous suction is applied to clear the operative field from excessive buildup of CSF.

Prior to trapping the recipient vessel, anesthesia should then induce pentobarbital burst suppression confirmed via continuous EEG for cerebral protection and systolic blood pressure should be within normal baseline values or slightly elevated to ensure sufficient cerebral perfusion. The recipient vessel is clipped proximally and distally to the site of anastomosis and an arterotomy is performed, with immediate washing with heparinized saline. The anastomosis is anchored at the proximal and distal ends, and a continuous stitch is applied, to the back wall first owing to difficult access, although interrupted suture may be used as well. The recipient vessel clips are removed first to assess for leakage; oozing usually resolves with heparin-free irrigation and Gelfoam, although significant or persistent leakage may be minimized with additional interrupted sutures. Patency may be assessed using intraoperative Doppler ultrasound or angiography.

For closure, Gelfoam is applied, the dura is loosely reapproximated and may be partially closed, and the bone is returned, with the appropriate remodeling performed to ensure adequate space for the donor vessel to pass. The temporalis fascia and muscle, galea, and skin are then closed in a manner to allow the graft to mature.

Indirect bypass is done in a similar manner but rather than divide the STA, the STA is mobilized anteriorly or posteriorly and the muscle incised and the bone removed on the more available side. The dura is opened and the graft sutured to the pia. The dura is laid directly on the brain and the bone replaced with openings for the vessel to enter and exit. All bypass patients are managed with perioperative low-dose aspirin (81 mg). Screening postoperative CT scanning is used to rule out subdural hematoma development.

Please go to expertconsult.com to view the complete list of references.

CHAPTER
13 Intracranial Aneurysms

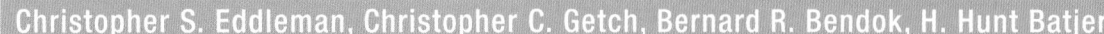

Christopher S. Eddleman, Christopher C. Getch, Bernard R. Bendok, H. Hunt Batjer

CLINICAL PEARLS

- The Incidence of intracranial aneurysms is variable throughout the world and is approximately 6% in the international population, with rates being higher in Asian/Finnish populations and those with a high-risk profile. In those patients without any risk factors, the incidence is approximately 2%. Once the aneurysm has ruptured, one third die and two thirds survive, with 50% of survivors leading independent lives.

- The majority of intracranial aneurysms arise at branching points of large arteries. Hemodynamic stress likely contributes to both the initial development and subsequent growth. Aneurysm formation can have many other associated conditions, including autosomal dominant polycystic kidney disease, Ehlers-Danlos syndrome, Loeys-Dietz syndrome, Marfan syndrome, tuberous sclerosis, fibromuscular dysplasia, and other genetic and structural predispositions.

- Approximately 25% to 50% of all patients will have warning symptoms that herald the onset of a major subarachnoid hemorrhage (SAH). The patient's description of the headache is very important, as most involve "thunderclap" onset or the "worst headache of my life." Computed tomography (CT) scans detect SAH with high sensitivity. If the scan is negative but suspicion remains high, a lumbar puncture may be performed. Although CT angiography is good for imaging aneurysms greater than 2 mm, cerebral

angiography remains the gold standard for intracranial vascular imaging.

- The risk of rebleeding after SAH is greatest on the first day (4.1%). By day 14, the cumulative rebleed incidence is 19%. Once an aneurysm is secure, the most significant cause of morbidity and death is cerebral vasospasm. The onset of cerebral vasospasm begins on day 3 and peaks between 7 and 14 days after SAH. Seventy percent of patients will develop radiographic signs of vasospasm and approximately 30% will develop clinical vasospasm requiring adjunctive therapy.

- The treatment goal of intracranial aneurysms is to exclude them from the parent circulation. In ruptured aneurysms, this must be done so early and safely so that maximum treatment of cerebral vasospasm can be administered if necessary. Symptomatic vasospasm can be treated with triple H therapy (involving hypertension, hypervolemia, and hemodilution) and endovascular means, namely intra-arterial injection of vasodilators or angioplasty.

- To achieve the goal of multidisciplinary cerebrovascular care, aneurysm patients are ideally treated at centers of excellence that employ expertise in all areas of neurovascular care, including endovascular, microvascular, and neurocritical care, and neuroanesthesia.

Intracranial aneurysms are potentially life threatening or disabling vascular lesions, which can pose formidable treatment challenges. Morphologically and pathologically they encompass diverse and occasionally overlapping entities including saccular, fusiform, and dissecting aneurysms with a wide variety of etiological origins, including hemodynamic, traumatic, infectious, and tumorogenic. Although intervention in most cases of ruptured intracranial aneurysms is indicated, the management of unruptured intracranial aneurysms remains controversial. On the other hand, as medicine shifts more toward prevention, greater interest has arisen in defining

screening and risk reduction strategies for high-risk populations. Over the last several decades, insight into the pathobiology and pathophysiology has significantly advanced, leading to improvements in the areas of natural history, epidemiology, biology, genetics, therapeutic intervention, and clinical outcomes. This chapter will provide an overview of intracranial aneurysms, clinical presentations, current therapeutic options, and technical aspects of surgical treatment. Although intracranial aneurysms encompass a diverse disease group, as stated earlier, this chapter will focus on the most common type, the so-called "saccular berry aneurysm."

EPIDEMIOLOGY

The incidence and prevalence of intracranial aneurysms in the general population are very difficult to estimate owing to clustering in various high-risk groups, large numbers of deaths without autopsy or neuroimaging, and the presence of asymptomatic lesions. Furthermore, autopsy studies have demonstrated disparate results that do not appear to link with the prevalence of subarachnoid hemorrhages (SAHs) and rupture risk incidence. Fox[1] reviewed the autopsy literature, which spanned from 1926 to 1973, and found the rate of occurrence to be 0.8% when studies included more than 5000 cases and 2% when studies included 2 to 5000 patients. Stehbens[2] conducted an autopsy study between 1952 and 1954 and found at least one aneurysm in 5.6% of cadavers. In his review of the pathological literature between 1890 and 1966, the prevalence of aneurysms at autopsy was found to be approximately 2.4% with a range of 0.2% to 9%.[3] Intracranial aneurysms in children are rare but are thought to occur in approximately 0.5% to 4.6%.[4] Currently, it is thought that approximately 6% of the international population harbor intracranial aneurysms with a higher prevalence in the Asian and Finnish populations (4-9%) and those who harbor significant risk factors, such as environmental, systemic, or genetic.[5] Risk factors associated with the presence and rupture of intracranial aneurysms have included high blood pressure, tobacco usage, and genetic- and ethnic-related factors; however, the prevalence of lesions is still thought to be approximately 2% in those without any known risk factors.[5] Although the most prevalent risk factors are those that are modifiable, the strongest risk factors are thought to occur through genetic and familial predisposition.

The risk of intracranial aneurysm rupture has also been a controversial topic. Although the annual risk of rupture has been reported to be between 0.1 and 8%,[5] depending on variable lesional characteristics, recent prospective data have challenged this view. The International Study of Unruptured Intracranial Aneurysms (ISUIA) reported in two recent publications[6,7] that the risk of aneurysm rupture was substantially lower than previously thought, that is, approximately 0% in anterior circulation aneurysms in those less than 7 mm, the most commonly encountered entities (Table 13.1). Although these studies represented the largest prospective collection of data regarding unruptured aneurysms, they have also been met with intense scrutiny and controversy, especially in light of a multitude of studies reporting an order of magnitude greater rupture risk.[8] Common problems with estimating the annual rupture risk are the inclusion of all patients with aneurysms, regardless of presentation, proper lesion classification and grouping, taking into account specific lesional characteristics, and proper classification of patients into various risk groups.[8] Given the broad spectrum of intracranial aneurysms, a balance of prospective data and clinical experience is necessary to properly and individually assess an individual patient's rupture risk.

Of those patients who experience (SAH) after aneurysmal rupture, approximately one third return to a functional life, one third live a dependent life, and the last third do not survive.[1,5,7,9] As advances in neurocritical care have increased survivability, neurological morbidity rate remains about the same. The greatest risk after the initial aneurysmal rupture is for re-rupture. Once the aneurysm is secure, the greatest risk is

TABLE 13.1 ISUIA 5-Year Cumulative Aneurysmal Rupture Rates According to Size and Location

Location	RUPTURE RATE BY ANEURYSM SIZE				
	<7 mm		7-12 mm	13-24 mm	>25 mm
	Group 1	Group 2			
Cavernous carotid artery	0	0	0	3.0%	6.4%
Anterior circulation*	0	1.5%	2.5%	14.5%	40%
Posterior circulation†	2.5%	3.4%	14.5%	18.4%	50%

*Includes anterior cerebral circulation, anterior communicating, middle cerebral artery, and internal carotid artery aneurysms.
†Includes posterior cerebral circulation, vertebrobasilar, and posterior communicating artery aneurysms.
ISUIA, International Study of Unruptured Intracranial Aneurysms.
Adapted from Wiebers DO, Whisnant JP, Huston J 3rd, et al. Unruptured intracranial aneurysms: natural history, clinical outcome, and risks of surgical and endovascular treatment. Lancet 2003;362(9378):103-110.

of cerebral vasospasm and ischemic complications from such events, thereby underlying the importance of early intervention and close monitoring in the postrupture period.

PATHOGENESIS

Intracranial arteries are unique to the systemic vascular system in that they lack the external elastic lamina present in extracranial vessels (Fig. 13.1). The pathogenesis of intracranial aneurysms has been thought to be due to a number of congenital factors such as vascular wall defects (i.e., media and elastic lamina), hemodynamic load on tortuous segments and bends with or without branch formation in the appropriate distribution, and discontinuity of the tunica media at origins of small vessels from larger parent vessels. Certainly, a multitude of systemic factors are thought to contribute to aneurysmal pathogenesis, such as degenerative changes, hypertension, atherosclerosis, connective tissue disease, and hemodynamic stress.

Genetic predisposition through various systemic and syndromic conditions has also been associated with the presence of intracranial aneurysms and is thought to represent approximately 10% to 12% of all aneurysms. Autosomal dominant polycystic kidney disease, Ehlers-Danlos syndrome, Loeys-Dietz syndrome, Marfan syndrome, tuberous sclerosis, and fibromuscular dysplasia have all been associated with the presence of intracranial aneurysms.[10-15] In recent years, many genetic loci have been proposed to be associated with familial linkage. Ruigrok and associates[14] recently reviewed the genetics of intracranial aneurysms and reported that probable loci included chromosomes 5q and 17cen, from which the strongest associations code for versican, an extracellular matrix protein, and TNFRSF13B, a transmembrane activator and a calcium modulator ligand interactor, respectively. Other suggestive loci are 1p34.3-p36.13, 7q11, 19q13.3, and Xp22.[9,14,16,17]

Despite the numerous factors likely to be related to intracranial aneurysm pathogenesis, it is most likely a complex,

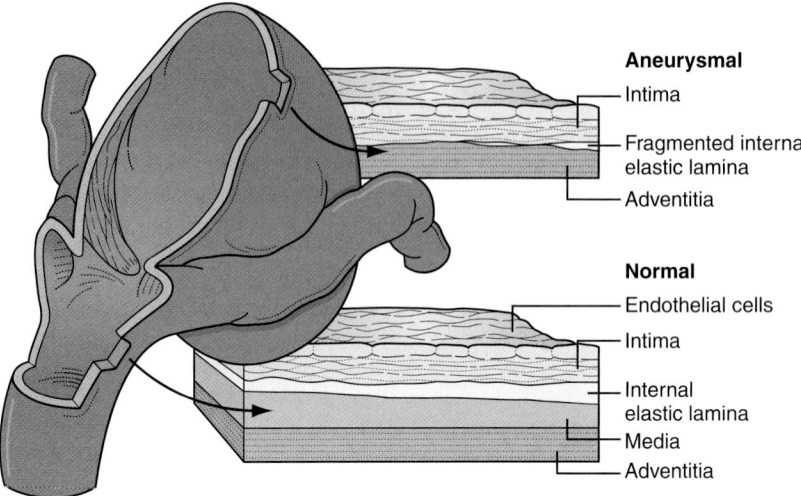

FIGURE 13.1 Histological layers of cerebral arteries. Note the absence of media in the aneurysmal wall and the fragmented internal elastic lamina. The wall may be quite sclerotic in some areas and extremely thin in others.

multifactorial set of circumstances involving anatomical, environmental, and genetic factors that lead to arterial wall weakening and aneurysm formation (Fig. 13.2). In fact, multiple aneurysms are present in up to 30% of patients. However, the majority of lesions are located at branching points along the proximal arterial tree, suggesting that hemodynamic factors play a significant role in aneurysm formation. In addition, formation of de novo aneurysms has been shown to occur at communicating arteries, and fatal rupture of aneurysms has occurred after recruitment of collateral blood flow through communicating arteries after the occlusion of carotid arteries. Furthermore, the incidence of aneurysms associated with high-flow states (e.g., arteriovenous malformations) is higher than in the general population, and some of these lesions regress after treatment of the vascular malformation. Finally, recurrent aneurysms can develop after incomplete treatment, whether by endovascular or microsurgical means.

Other factors related to aneurysm formation are trauma, infection, and tumor emboli. Traumatic aneurysms are more often fusiform and located near the skull base. Infectious aneurysms have a multitude of etiological factors but most commonly occur secondary to bacterial endocarditis. Finally, tumorigenic aneurysms are thought to form as a result of seeding of the arterial wall through hematogenous spread and are most often related to cardiac myxomas.

NATURAL HISTORY

The natural history of intracranial aneurysms can be conceptually separated into two general areas, namely, ruptured and unruptured. Of those patients who experience aneurysmal SAH, approximately one third will not survive 2 weeks after hemorrhage, one third will survive but have a dependent existence, and the last third will survive and be fully independent. The peak risk of re-hemorrhage is within the first 24 to 48 hours, with a 4% re-rupture risk within the first 24 hours, and 30% of patients rebleeding within 2 weeks if not treated.

For patients with unruptured intracranial aneurysms, the natural history is much more difficult to resolve. Prior to 1998, the estimated rupture rate for aneurysms was thought to be

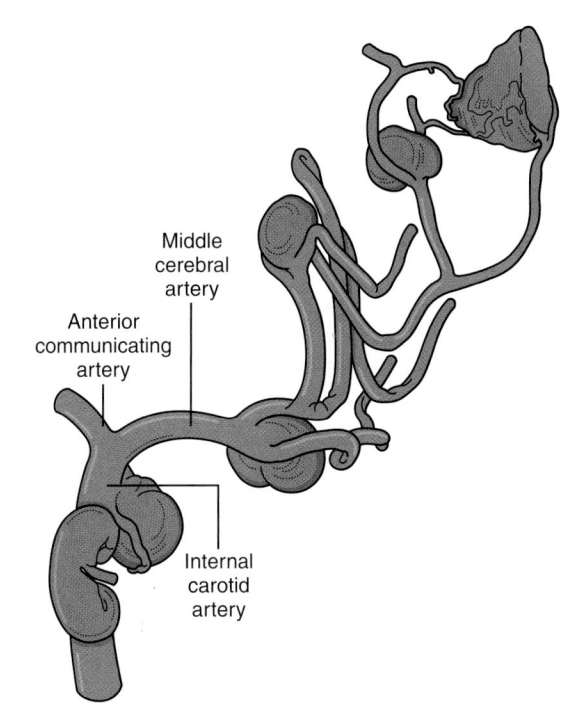

FIGURE 13.2 When high-flow situations complicate cerebral hemodynamics, such as an intracranial arteriovenous malformation, aneurysms are found with a relatively high frequency on feeding arteries and often in atypical distal sites.

1% to 2.5% per year cumulatively. For young patients, the data suggested that intracranial aneurysms should be treated, as the cumulative risk of rupture over many years is very significant. However, the largest and most debated prospective database on unruptured intracranial aneurysms was published in two parts by the International Study of Unruptured Intracranial Aneurysms (ISUIA) and suggested that the rupture risk of unruptured asymptomatic aneurysms was much more benign than once thought (see Table 13.1). The 5-year cumulative rupture rate without a prior history of SAH of anterior circulation aneurysms (not including cavernous carotid or posterior communicating artery aneurysms) was 0%, 2.6%, and 14.5% for aneurysms less than 7 mm, 7 to 12 mm, and 13 to 24 mm, respectively, and it was 2.5%, 14.5%, and 18.4%, respectively, for the same three size groups of aneurysms in the posterior circulation (including posterior communicating artery aneurysms). Patients with a history of SAH with aneurysms less than 7 mm had a 1.5% rupture rate over 5 years with further increases in rates with increasing aneurysmal size. Many limitations of the ISUIA study have been reported. Selection bias likely played a substantial role because patients with aneurysms that were thought to be at a high risk of rupture, namely, those with multiple lobulations, hemodynamic factors, and so on, were treated and therefore were not included as part of the study. Further, cavernous carotid aneurysms were included in these studies, but these aneurysmal lesions rarely result in SAH. Lastly, the annual incidence of SAH in the United States is approximately 30,000, which when calculated against the incidence of aneurysms, results in a rupture rate of at least 1% per year, significantly higher than that calculated in the ISUIA study.[18,19]

Other morphological factors of aneurysms, besides the size of the aneurysmal dome, have been thought to contribute to the annual rupture risk. More specifically, neck width, dome width, aneurysm shape, aspect ratio (height/neck width), and bottleneck factor (dome width/neck width) have been examined.[8] Among these, a higher aspect ratio (>1.6) is thought to be associated with an increased rupture risk. Other morphological characteristics, such as lobulations, daughter sacs, and surface irregularity, have long been associated with higher rupture

---

BOX 13.1   Morphological Factors That May Contribute to Aneurysmal Risk of Rupture

Neck width[52,53]
Aspect ratio (height/neck width)[20,54-56]
Bottleneck factor (dome width/neck width)[54]
Daughter sacs/blebs[57-60]
Surface irregularity[57,60,61]
Aneurysm angle to parent artery[58-60,62]
Aneurysm size to parent artery ratio[58-60,62]

Numbers refer to references listed for this chapter online.

---

risk[8] (Box 13.1). Finally, the hemodynamics of the surrounding vasculature to an unruptured aneurysm may put a particular lesion at a greater risk of rupture, for example, dominant A1 feeding into an anterior communicating artery aneurysm.[20]

CLINICAL PRESENTATION

The clinical presentation of patients who harbor intracranial aneurysms can be divided into several categories, namely, incidental (asymptomatic or unrelated symptoms), cranial nerve and other neurological deficits, sentinel events, or frank rupture (SAH).

For patients who present with frank aneurysm rupture, the most common clinical symptoms and signs are the sudden onset of the worst headache of their life, severe nausea and vomiting, altered mental status, nuchal rigidity, and loss of consciousness. Most emergency departments automatically order a head computed tomography (CT) scan without contrast to evaluate these patients for possible SAH, although misdiagnosis remains a major problem (Fig. 13.3). It is of paramount importance to identify these patients because aneurysmal re-rupture has devastating consequences. With the technological advancements of CT scanners, the sensitivity/specificity of SAH detection is greater than 98% in the first 2 days.[21] As such, lumbar puncture is not necessarily indicated unless the insinuating event happened at least 3 days prior or if head CT image is negative despite strong clinical suspicion. A lumbar puncture is used to detect evidence of red blood cells and xanthochromia. After confirmation of SAH on CT scan, a CT angiogram (CTA) is performed, especially if the clinical history is highly suggestive of aneurymal SAH. CTA detection of intracranial aneurysms is now on the order of 99% for aneurysms larger than 2 mm.[22,23] Digital subtraction angiography (DSA) is now often reserved at our center for the absence of or questionable intracranial lesions seen on CTA or when the clinical picture favors endovascular intervention.

Approximately 25% of patients who present with SAH have had sentinel headaches (same symptoms as those related

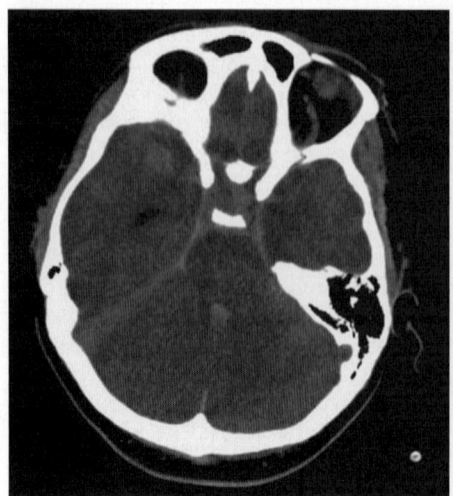 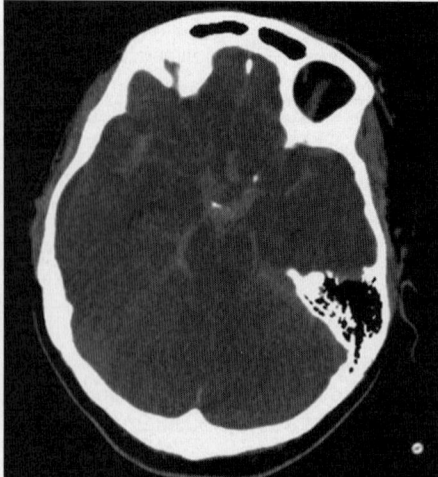 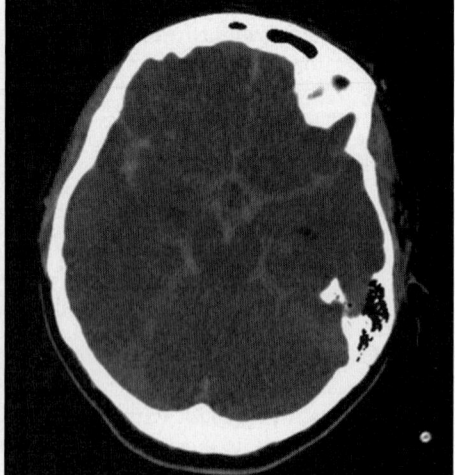

FIGURE 13.3 Noncontrasted computed tomography (CT) scan of the head showing diffuse subarachnoid hemorrhage (SAH) with mild enlargement of the ventricular temporal horns.

to SAH) in the weeks prior to presentation. The diagnosis of "sentinel headache" is only made in retrospect if the patient did not seek medical attention or was misdiagnosed recently when evaluated. These "sentinel headaches" are thought to be due to "minor leaks" or acute aneurysm expansion. Education of both the public and the medical community (especially physicians from primary care, neurology and emergency medicine) could go a long way to earlier diagnosis and improvement of outcomes. Any sudden onset thunderclap headache should be assumed related to an intracranial aneurysm until proved otherwise.

Various neurological deficits can be detected in aneurysm patients due to local mass effect, increased intracranial pressure, or thromboembolic complications from progressive thrombosis of a large or giant aneurysm. Common neurological findings include third cranial nerve palsy, visual loss (afferent pupillary defect), trigeminal symptoms, sixth cranial nerve palsy, nystagmus, vertigo, persistent nausea, and altered mental status (Fig. 13.4). These symptoms can occur from progressive enlargement of an unruptured aneurysm (Fig. 13.5). Focal neurological deficits can occur with embolization of clot from a thrombotic aneurysm. Magnetic resonance imaging (MRI) may be indicated in the workup of neurological findings but should not overlook the possibility of either aneurysms or the presence of subarachnoid blood.

Once aneurysmal SAH has been confirmed, the initial neurological examination is important in determining prognosis. A variety of grading scales have been developed, most commonly the World Federation of Neurosurgical Societies (WFNS) and Hunt-Hess grading scales (Table 13.2). Morbidity and mortality rates increase with a higher grade in each scale.

Initial treatment for SAH involves a complete medical evaluation. Some patients can present with acute mental status changes that are the result of hydrocephalus. In these cases, an extraventricular drain should be placed not only to relieve the hydrocephalus but also to monitor the intracranial pressure. Permanent cerebrospinal fluid (CSF) diversion is necessary in approximately 10% of patients, owing to the hematoma breakdown products affecting the functioning of the arachnoid granulations. However, the most common medical complication after SAH is cerebral ischemia secondary to cerebral vasospasm. Vasospasm usually starts by the fifth posthemorrhage day and can be a threat for up to 14 days after hemorrhage. Angiographic vasospasm has been shown in up to

70% of patients, whereas symptomatic clinical vasospasm occurs in only about 30% of patients.[24-26] Medications often administered to SAH patients, namely nimodipine, a calcium channel blocker, and pravachol, an HMG CoA (3-hydroxy-3-methylglutaryl coenzyme A) reductase inhibitor, are thought to limit, although not prevent, the onset of symptomatic vasospasm, thereby improving outcomes, not incidence.[27] However,

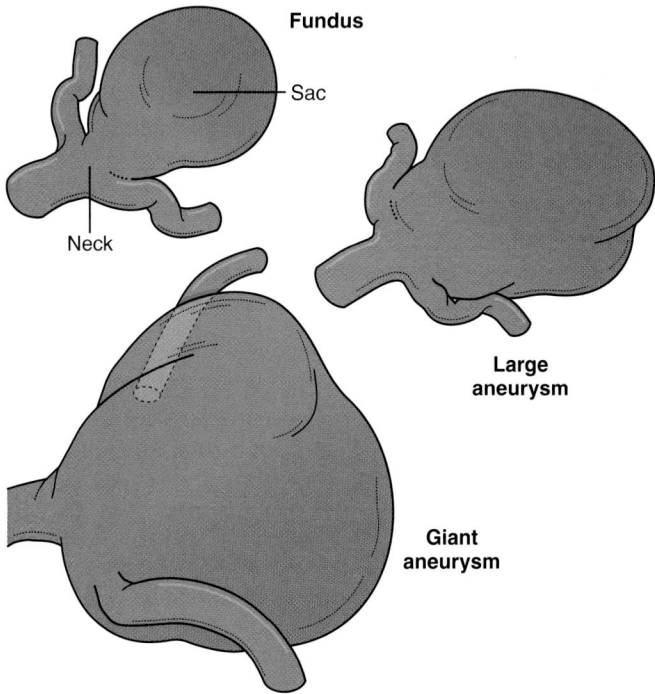

FIGURE 13.5 The potential evolution of a small aneurysm into a large and finally giant aneurysm. With each stage of enlargement, the efferent branches migrate farther out onto the sac itself.

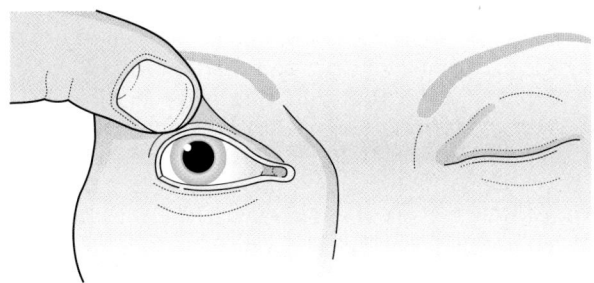

FIGURE 13.4 A patient with a third cranial nerve palsy will exhibit some or all of the following signs: ptosis, pupillary dilation, and inability to elevate, depress, or medially deviate (adduct) the eye. These findings (particularly pupillary dilation) strongly suggest focal mass effect.

Grade*	GCS Score	Motor Deficit	Clinical Description
I	15	Absent	Asymptomatic, mild headache or slight nuchal rigidity
II	13-14	Absent	Moderate to severe headache, nuchal rigidity, and no other neurological deficit except cranial nerve palsy
III	13-14	Present	Drowsiness, confusion, or mild focal deficit
IV	7-12	Present or absent	Stupor, moderate to severe hemiparesis, and possibly early decerebrate rigidity and vegetative disturbances
V	3-6	Present or absent	Deep coma, decerebrate rigidity, and moribund appearance

TABLE 13.2 Common Grading Scales for Patients with Subarachnoid Hemorrhage

*The World Federation of Neurosurgical Societies (WFNS) grade utilizes the combination of GCS score and motor deficit; the Hunt and Hess (H&H) grade utilizes only the clinical description.
GCS, Glasgow Coma Scale.

controversy still exists regarding the absolute effects of these medications.

SUBARACHNOID HEMORRHAGE

Medical Complications with Subarachnoid Hemorrhage

Subarachnoid hemorrhage has potentially devastating effects not only on the brain but also on the other organ systems of the body, both in the acute and chronic phases after aneurysmal rupture. Although it is beyond the scope of this chapter to detail every medical complication that can occur, brief mention will be made of the most commonly encountered medical complications (Box 13.2).

Soon after the event of SAH, a generalized sympathetic response is often encountered, which has profound effects on the cardiopulmonary system as well as the systemic vasculature. The massive surge of catecholamines after SAH likely induces various degrees of cardiac injury, as evidenced by increased serum troponin T levels, electrocardiogram (ECG) changes, and sometimes severe cardiac wall motion abnormalities.[28-31] Pulmonary complications are also anticipated after SAH. Pulmonary edema can occur after SAH and is usually secondary to cardiac failure from cardiogenic shock.[28,30] However, acute respiratory distress syndrome (ARDS) can result from primary pulmonary tissue damage from the initial sympathetic response. Further, in patients who lose consciousness after SAH, evidence of aspiration pneumonitis has been reported, which can develop into pneumonia or ARDS.[32] When patients are dependent on mechanical ventilators after SAH, an increased incidence of pneumonia occurs.[32]

Electrolyte disturbances are anticipated after aneurysmal SAH. The most common electrolyte abnormality after SAH is hyponatremia, which occurs in approximately one third of patients.[33] Owing to the endocrine disturbances of sodium and intravascular volume regulation, excessive renal excretion of sodium and dehydration lead to a condition known as *cerebral salt wasting*. In patients with lethal hemorrhages or aneurysms associated with hypothalamic tissue or vascular supply to such tissue, diabetes insipidus can occur, and leads to progressive hypernatremia and increasing urine output. In rare cases, SAH can lead to acute renal failure through posterior hypothalamic dysregulation, which may trigger renal vasoconstriction by activation of the renin-angiotensin system and thereby can reduce renal blood flow.[34]

Infectious complications also can accompany SAH patients in the chronic phases. Patients who are on mechanical ventilators, arterial and venous access lines, bladder catheters, and ventricular drains are always at an increased risk of infection. Appropriate changing of intravascular lines, tracheostomy procedures, timely removal of ventricular catheters, and changing of bladder catheters is thought to reduce the overall risk of infections.[35]

Finally, neurosurgical patients are known to experience a higher risk of developing deep venous thrombosis (DVT), potentially leading to an increased incidence of venous thrombosis and even thromboemboli.[36] Most medical centers currently use compression stockings and pneumatic compression devices to reduce the incidence of DVT and pulmonary

BOX 13.2	Major Medical and Neurological Complications of Subarachnoid Hemorrhage

Venous thromboembolism
Infection
Diabetes insipidus
Syndrome of inappropriate antidiuretic hormone secretion
Cardiac injury
Pulmonary failure
Hydrocephalus
Vasospasm
Rebleed
Direct brain injury

embolism (PE). In patients who develop DVTs and are not able to be anticoagulated due to recent SAH, vena cava filters are often placed. Early administration of prophylactic low-molecular-weight heparins is often used in SAH patients 48 to 72 hours after admission to decrease the risks of DVT/PEs (after aneurysm is secured).

Treatment of Subarachnoid Hemorrhage

Modern evaluation and treatment of intracranial aneurysms requires the participation of a multidisciplinary team, including neurosurgeons, neuroradiologists, endovascular practitioners, and neurocritical care specialists. Each patient has to be considered on an individual basis and the strategy for treatment is unique to each patient. In the current era, the options for treatment of intracranial aneurysms are observational, endovascular, microsurgical, or a combination of approaches.

The goal of treatment is to exclude the aneurysm from the circulation with minimal morbidity to the patient. Because the peak incidence of re-hemorrhage for ruptured aneurysms occurs within the first 48 hours, the most effective strategy to minimize this risk is to secure the ruptured aneurysm as soon as possible. However, if a patient presents at "off hours," the risks presented by suboptimal operating room and staff conditions may outweigh the risks of doing the procedure in the acute phase. It is therefore recommended to perform aneurysm surgery on the next elective surgical day, when an appropriate neurosurgical team can be assembled. Furthermore, each ruptured aneurysm is unique and may present technical challenges that may make surgery difficult, thereby necessitating endovascular therapy in the acute phase. However, a ruptured aneurysm should be secured before the onset of delayed cerebral ischemia so as to avoid the risk of re-hemorrhage with potential hypertensive and hypervolemic therapy for vasospasm. Despite this rationale, the issue of treatment timing remains somewhat controversial.

Systemic circumstances (e.g., cardiopulmonary instability) may prevent a patient from being ready for aneurysm treatment. Therefore, antifibrinolytic therapy has been suggested to aid in reducing the risk of re-bleeding. The Cooperative Aneurysm Study found that the re-bleeding rate at 14 days was 11.7% if antifibrinolytics were used and 19.4% if no antifibrinolytics were used.[37] However, in the face of vasospasm, the risk of ischemic events is higher in patients in whom antifibrinolytics were used, thus equalizing the mortality rates between the two groups. As such, we tend to use antifibrinolytics in patients who present in poor grade or who are medically

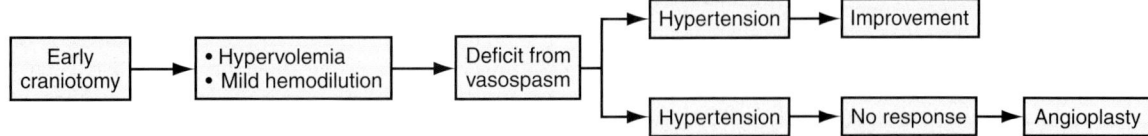

FIGURE 13.6 Prophylactic and therapeutic strategy for vasopasm at Northwestern University Medical School.

unstable for treatment with the knowledge that ischemic complications are possible and CSF diversion may be necessary.

Symptomatic vasospasm is the leading cause of morbidity and death following aneurysmal SAH.[25,26] Treatment for vasospasm has evolved over the past decade but still lacks definitive treatment (Fig. 13.6). Patients require diligent monitoring and treatment for up to 14 days after hemorrhage through invasive blood pressure monitoring, cerebral blood flow monitoring (transcranial ultrasound, CT/MRI perfusion studies), and often aggressive medical therapy including hypertensive and hypervolemic therapy and hemodilution (triple H therapy). In symptomatic patients, endovascular therapy can also be employed, which may involve intra-arterial injection of vasodilators or balloon angioplasty. In addition to spasm in the large conducting vessels, the phenomenon of SAH also triggers more complex events, which can lead to patchy infarcts in areas apparently unaffected by angiographically visible vasospasm.

Much study has been invested in pharmacological prevention of arterial narrowing but research has not demonstrated changes in the long-term outcome of patients treated with such agents. Calcium channel blockers (e.g., nimodipine) have been used since the 1980s but have produced modest results in the literature.[38-41] More specific pharmacological agents, namely, selective endothelin 1a receptor antagonists, have shown promise in effectively preventing and reducing arterial narrowing but failed to demonstrate any effect in long-term outcomes.[25,26] Lastly, it has been suggested that statin therapy in conjunction with calcium channel blockers may lower the incidence of delayed cerebral ischemic events and improve patient outcomes; this was demonstrated in a phase II study.[42] However, a recent meta-analysis of the literature claims that no statistical benefit could be gleaned from the literature. Nevertheless, many institutions now initiate acute therapy with both calcium channel blockers and statins.[43]

Approximately 70% of patients demonstrated some form of radiographic arterial narrowing, which does not necessarily warrant immediate treatment. However, up to 30% of these individuals will progress to have clinically symptomatic vasospasm, warranting immediate evaluation and treatment, medical or otherwise. Monitoring vasospasm in comatose patients becomes problematic because of the absence of a clinical examination to follow, thereby placing emphasis on indirect evidence such as transcranial Doppler or CT/MRI perfusion studies on progressively worsening cerebral blood flow changes to indicate time of potential treatment. Medical management of vasospasm has traditionally been through "triple H" therapy, involving hemodilution, hypertension, and hypervolemia.[26,30,38,41] Maximizing the rheological properties of blood (i.e., maintaining a hematocrit level from 30 to 34) improves tissue perfusion. Should a focal neurological deficit develop, we immediately raise the systolic blood pressure up to the 175 to 200 mm Hg range or until the deficit reverses. In addition, we will volume expand and raise the central venous pressure (CVP) of the patient to the 10 to 15 mm Hg range.

If these medical maneuvers do not result in an improvement of the patient's condition and a surveillance CT scan does not demonstrate any areas of obvious infarction, we then proceed immediately to the angiography suite for a diagnostic angiogram and potential intra-arterial therapy.

Hydrocephalus, either communicating or noncommunicating, frequently develops in the first few days after SAH and partly explains the appearance of a globally edematous brain. Upon recognition that symptomatic hydrocephalus exists, it is suggested that CSF diversion be performed, usually by placement of an extraventricular drain (EVD). Careful placement of an EVD and conservative drainage of CSF must be maintained to avoid the possibility of an acute increase in the transmural pressure across the aneurysm or ventricular shift leading to the destabilization of the tamponading aneurysmal clot. In about 10% of patients, permanent CSF diversion is necessary.[44] The risk of permanent hydrocephalus is higher in patients with ruptured upper basilar trunk aneurysms.

TREATMENT OF INTRACRANIAL ANEURYSMS

The treatment of intracranial aneurysms has undergone a paradigm shift such that endovascular therapy has emerged as a viable treatment regiment and is first-line therapy in several European countries. Aneurysm treatment in the United States is less standardized with both microsurgical and endovascular strategies employed depending on the individual lesion and surgeon/patient preference. However, endovascular therapy of intracranial aneurysms will not be discussed here as it is discussed elsewhere in this textbook. We will focus on the general problems caused by aneurysms in various locations such as anterior circulation artery aneurysm, proximal and posterior carotid artery wall aneurysm, caritid bifurcation, middle crerbral artery bifurcation, anterior communicating artery, distal basilar artery, vertebral artery and posterior inferior cerebellar artery, vertebral confluence, and lower basilar trunk, and illustrate the anatomical complexities and unique features found by neurosurgeons treating these various lesions. New developments over the past several years include advanced microscopic technology, intraoperative imaging techniques, neuromonitoring, and pharmacological agents utilized to aid clip reconstruction of complex aneurysms.

Adjunctive Techniques in Aneurysm Surgery

Several advancements have been made in adjunctive techniques and equipment that have significantly improved the surgical evaluation and management of aneurysms. Although the surgical microscope has been utilized in surgery for decades, its impact on aneurysm surgery continues to improve. With the reduction in the size of the microscope head as well as improvement in optics, neurosurgeons can work more comfortably and with improved visualization. The addition of using intraoperative fluorescence techniques such indocyanine green (ICG) video angiography allows the evaluation of aneurysm clip reconstruction in a fast and safe manner without the added risks of intraoperative catheter angiography.[45-47] This imaging modality can be repeated multiple times during the procedure. Although catheter angiography remains the gold standard of

intracranial vascular imaging, this new modality of intraoperative imaging allows quick and repeated evaluation of aneurysm clipping. Pharmacological agents have also been used more recently to aid in the clipping of complex intracranial aneurysms. Adenosine-induced cardiac arrest provides a safe method to reduce cerebral blood flow and softening of the aneurysmal dome, allowing manipulation and improved clip placement and reconstruction.[48-50] With adequate cerebral protection, adenosine obviates the need for temporary clip occlusion in carefully selected cases. However, in most cases, patients can tolerate temporary occlusion without issue (Fig. 13.7). These measures are only a few of the recent and important developments to aid in aneurysm surgery. With the ever-advancing technology of intraoperative navigation and imaging, aneurysm surgery will become safer and more efficient.

Surgical Management of Anterior Circulation Artery Aneurysms

Pterional "Frontotemporal" Craniotomy

The pterional craniotomy has been the workhorse surgical approach for a variety of anterior circulation artery aneurysms because of its versatility and many modifications. A key element of this approach is the patient's head position. Careful attention to this basic first step facilitates exposure and allows complex procedures to be carried out through small, tailored craniotomies, limited dural openings, and often without the need of brain retractors. The most frequent means of skull fixation in aneurysm surgery is the Mayfield-Keys three-point device, which provides almost absolute head stability (Fig. 13.8). Positioning of the three points varies for a pterional craniotomy and is at the discretion of the operating surgeon. Once the head is secured in the fixation device, the

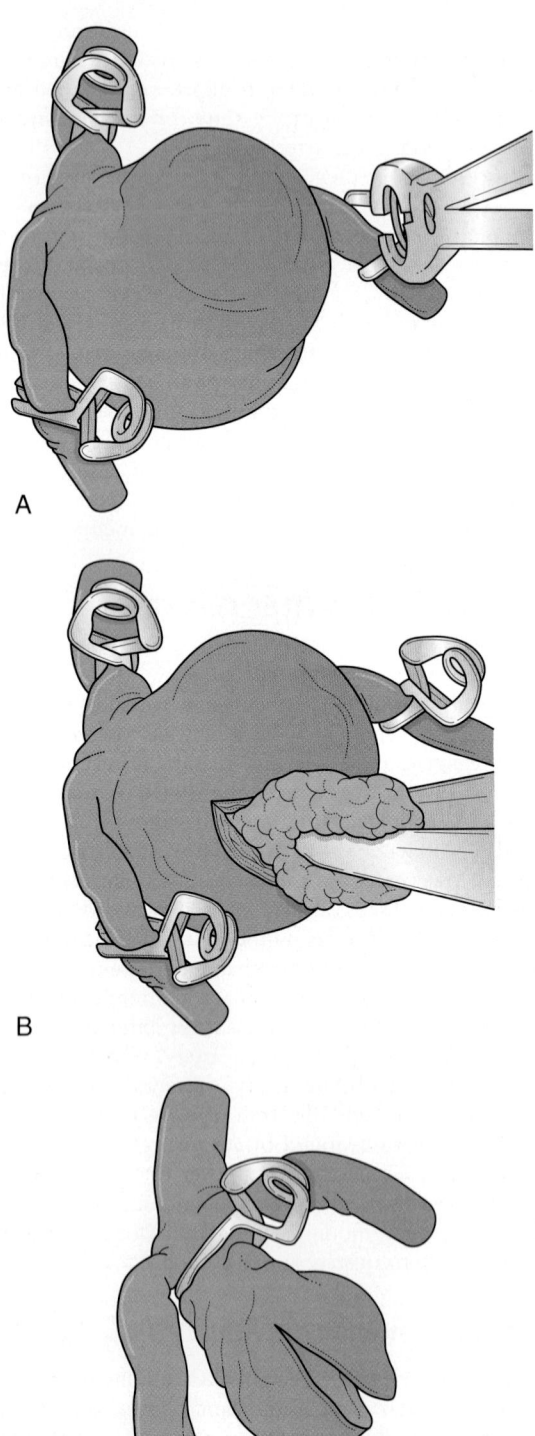

FIGURE 13.7 A to C, Temporary arterial occlusion is often necessary in repairing complex large or giant aneurysms. Not infrequently, the aneurysm must be widely opened to allow evacuation of debris and thrombus before definitive clip reconstruction can be performed.

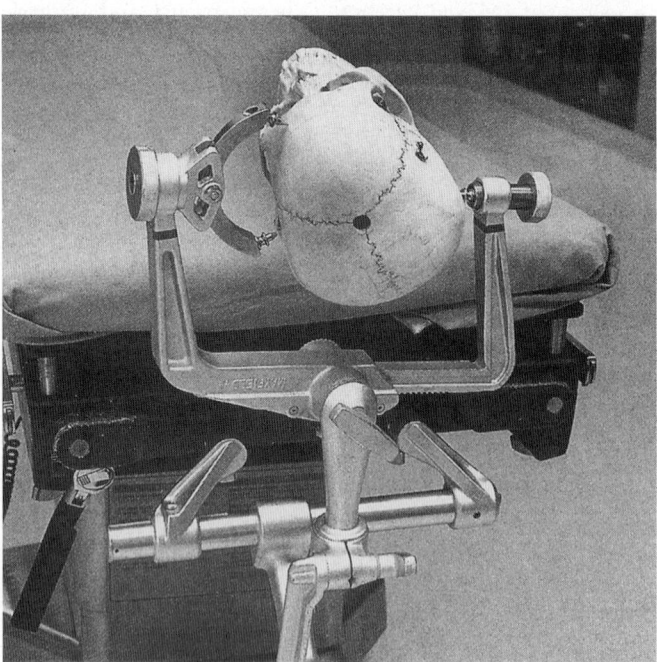

FIGURE 13.8 The Mayfield-Keys three-point skull fixation device provides optimal head stability so that inadvertent patient movement will not result in catastrophic injury to neural or vascular structures.

neurosurgeon performs three distinct maneuvers to position the head optimally for the necessary intracranial exposure.[51]

Rotation of the head is the first maneuver and is usually toward the contralateral or nonoperated side to an angle determined by the target anastomotic site (Fig. 13.9A). When the target site is the internal carotid or the distal basilar artery, minimal head rotation is required, usually approximately 20 degrees. Further angulation will allow the temporal lobe to migrate via gravity posteriorly and medially into the incisura and thus potentially obstructing the operative window. Aneurysms of the middle cerebral artery bifurcation require more angulation, approximately 40 to 45 degrees, to expose the sylvian fissure maximally, allowing both the temporal and frontal lobes to fall posteriorly once released from the fissure. For aneurysms of the anterior communicating artery, even more rotation is needed, approximately 45 to 60 degrees, to simplify the exposure of the medial gyrus rectus and interhemispheric fissure.

Flexion of the head is designed to maintain a perpendicular relationship between the floor of the anterior cranial fossa and the long axis of the patient's body (Fig. 13.9B). After positioning the head in the appropriate rotation, the neck is flexed gently, bringing the chin toward the contralateral clavicle without compromising cervical venous return. This maneuver brings the area of operation away from the ipsilateral shoulder.

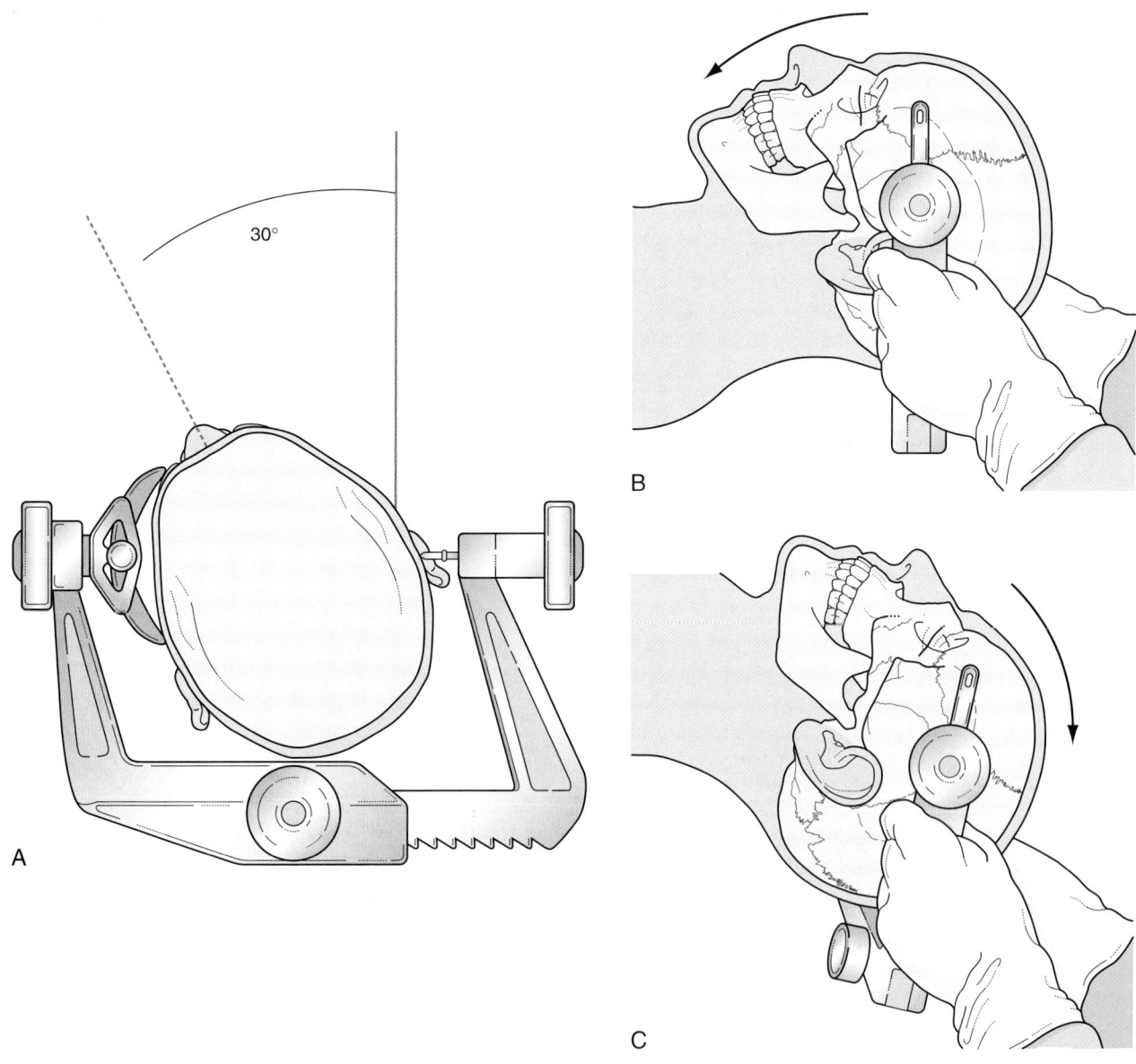

FIGURE 13.9 Patient positioning for pterional craniotomy. **A,** Rotation. The head is elevated slightly relative to the thorax and rotated contralaterally by an extent dictated by the specific operative target (less rotation for carotid and basilar bifurcation aneurysms and more rotation for aneurysm of the middle cerebral artery or anterior communicating region). **B,** Flexion. The neck should then be gently flexed, bringing the chin toward the contralateral clavicle. This subtle maneuver orients the floor of the anterior cranial fossa perpendicular to the long axis of the patient's body, maximizing the surgeon's access to the anatomical target without encroachment on the patient's ipsilateral shoulder. **C,** Extension (tilt). While maintaining the previous elements of rotation and flexion, the vertex is tilted inferiorly so that the maxillary eminence rises superior to the brow. The degree of extension will vary somewhat with the target aneurysm (less for paraclinoidal aneurysms and more with distal basilar aneurysms).

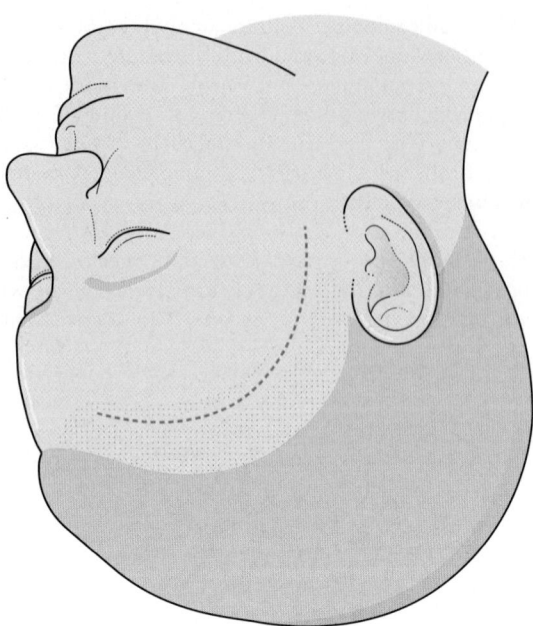

FIGURE 13.10 The skin incision for the pterional craniotomy extends from the zygoma to the midline, curving gently just posterior to the hairline.

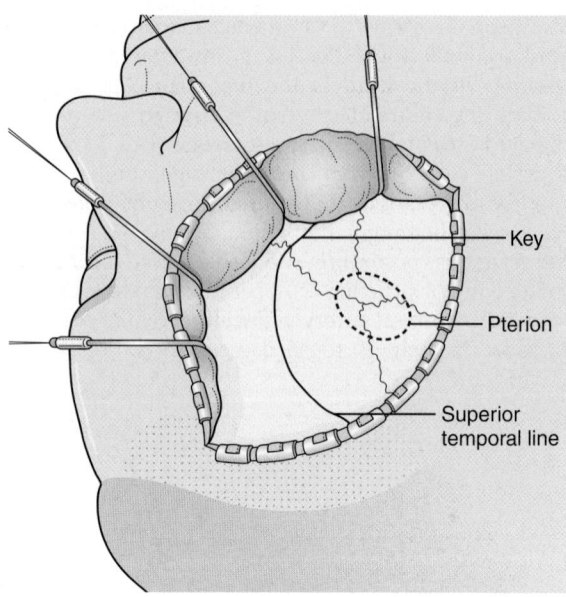

FIGURE 13.11 A commonly employed means of opening the scalp involves incision of the skin, galea, temporalis fascia, and muscle with reflection of the resultant flap in a single layer.

Extension or "tilting" of the head allows the frontal lobe to fall away from the floor of the anterior cranial fossa (Fig. 13.9C). To minimize retraction of the brain and to optimally display the vascular structures at the skull base, the vertex of the skull is tilted inferiorly so the maxillary eminence rises superior to the brow ridge.

Surgical Technique

The surgical incision is first drawn on the skin beginning at the level of the zygoma, 1 cm anterior to the tragus, and extends superiorly immediately behind the hairline and gently curves anteriorly to the midline (Fig. 13.10). A simple technique is to put the thenar eminence of the hand onto the brow ridge and rotate the hand starting at the zygoma. A curvilinear marking will result that just approaches the midline. Every attempt is made to keep the incision behind the hairline for cosmesis, although this can be difficult in a balding patient. Numerous options are available for reflecting the scalp. The most common scalp flap is the myocutaneous flap, which involves reflecting the scalp and temporalis muscle together anteriorly (Fig. 13.11). An alternative technique involves the interfacial dissection where the bulk of the temporalis muscle is reflected inferiorly and the intrafascial fat pad, containing the frontalis branch of the facial nerve, and the scalp are reflected anteriorly. When reflecting the scalp and temporalis muscle, the key target of exposure with respect to the skull is the anatomical keyhole. A variable amount of temporal squama is exposed as well, depending on the vascular target. Bur hole placement normally consists of one bur hole in the anatomical key, one at the floor of the middle fossa, and one just inferior to the superior temporal line posteriorly (Fig. 13.12). There are some aneurysmal lesions (e.g., carotid wall, anterior communicating, and basilar apex aneurysms) that may require additional bony removal in addition to the standard pterional craniotomy. The addition of an orbital or orbitozygomatic

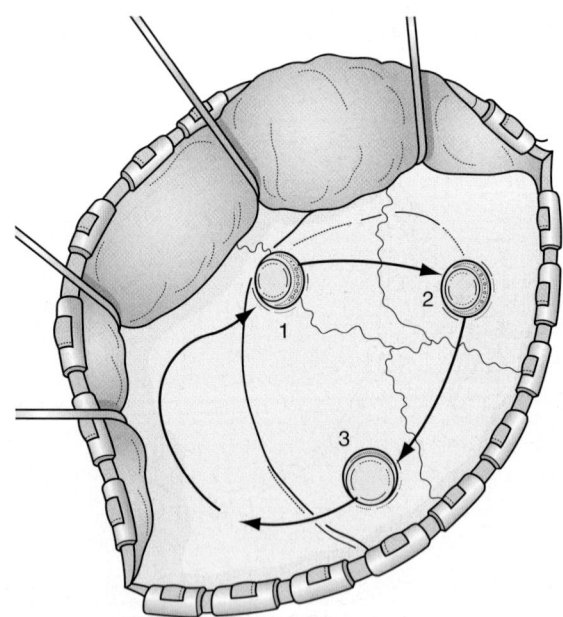

FIGURE 13.12 The pterional craniotomy is performed with power instruments so that three bur holes are placed: one at the anatomical key, one inferiorly on the temporal squama, and one posteriorly just inferior to the superior temporal line. The bone is cut as shown, exposing the frontal and temporal dura and the sphenoid ridge.

(OZ) osteotomy may add 10 to 15 degrees of exposure, which is especially helpful in situations in which a swollen, tense brain exists (Fig. 13.13). To prepare for the additional craniotomy, the dura overlying the orbital roof is stripped posteriorly toward the orbital apex, medial to the cribriform, and lateral to the dura of the superior orbital fissure. If exposed, the periorbita is stripped from the superior and lateral walls of the orbit to a depth of approximately 3 cm. If the zygomatic

FIGURE 13.13 Demonstration of orbital (**A**) and orbitozygomatic (**B**) osteotomies.

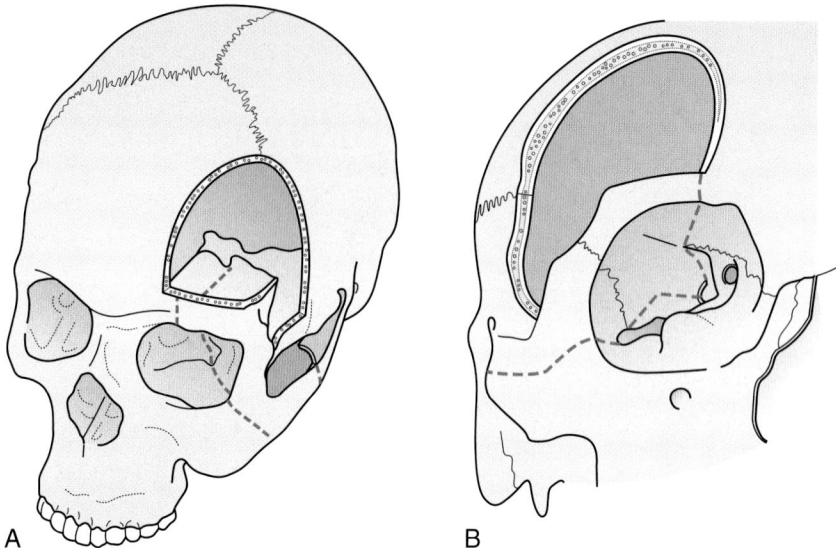

process is to be included in the osteotomy, the full extent of the zygomatic arch is exposed prior to the reflexion of the temporalis muscle. Resection of the orbital zygomatic segment is best accomplished with a combination of reciprocating saw and osteotomes. The initial bone cuts are made with a reciprocating saw through the supraorbital ridge and frontal zygomatic process with the former being just lateral to the supraorbital foramen. Narrow osteotomes complete the resection across the orbital roof and the greater and lesser wings of the sphenoid bone. Once the masseter has been released from the inferior surface of the zygomatic arch, the piece may be removed en bloc. It is important to preserve at least 3 cm of the orbital roof and lateral wall so as to minimize the possibility of a postoperative pulsatile enophthalmos.

Perhaps the most important element to the extended pterional is the resection of the proximal lesser and greater wings of the sphenoid bone inclusive of the anterior clinoid process. This bony resection is particularly useful for ophthalmic and superior hypophyseal aneurysms. The postclipping reconstruction is performed in a standard fashion with a microplating system and a hydroxyapatite compound or methylmethacrylate to fill in any bony defects.

Depending on the adherence of the dura or in older patients, a fourth bur hole may be placed in the frontal bone just superior to the midline of the superior temporal line. It is important to try to separate the dura from the bone flap through the bur holes with a Penfield 2 or 3. This maneuver will allow easier removal of the bone flap. A craniotome is used to make cuts between the bur holes. After the bone flap is removed, the anterior temporal bone is extracted with rongeurs, as is the lateral third of the sphenoid ridge. Often it is necessary to remove the deepest portion of the sphenoid ridge with a power drill (Fig. 13.14). The inner table of the frontal bone is also removed with careful drilling. This maneuver allows exposure of the parasellar region with minimal frontal retraction. The dural opening is centralized around the sylvian fissure and has a semilunar shape (Fig. 13.15).

After the surgical microscope is sterilely draped, it is positioned into place so that the parasylvian region can be easily visualized. Following the sphenoid ridge along the inferior frontal lobe will lead to the carotid cistern where the optic

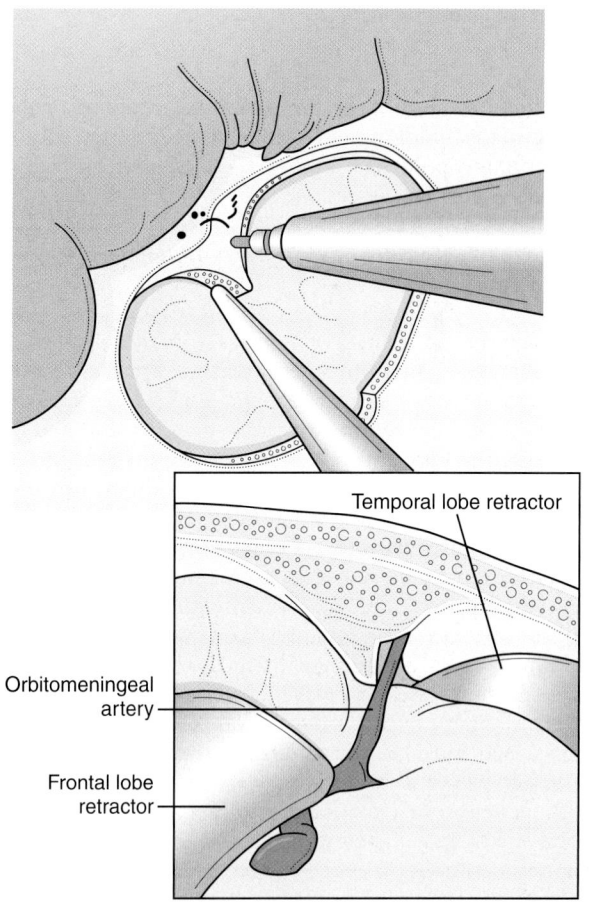

FIGURE 13.14 After removal of the bone flap, the sphenoid ridge is resected to the level of the orbitomeningeal artery. The inner table of the frontal bone can also be resected. This maneuver is particularly useful in exposing the anterior communicating region.

nerve and the carotid artery should be easily visualized. The surrounding arachnoid membranes, including the medial sylvian fissure, are opened sharply to separate the medial frontal and temporal lobes from the underlying carotid cisternal structures (Fig. 13.16). After this maneuver, the entire

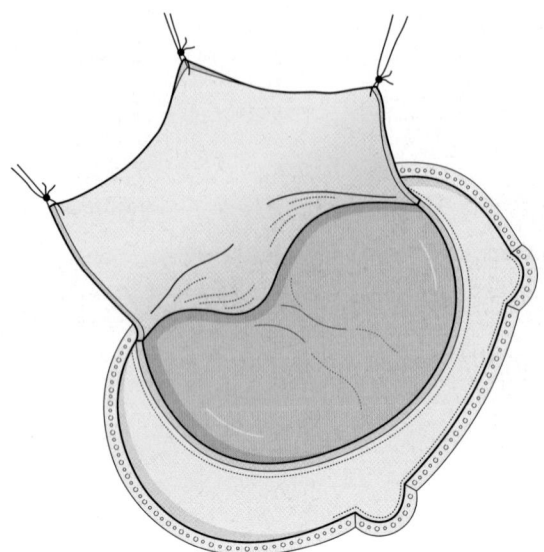

FIGURE 13.15 The dura is opened in a semilunar fashion and reflected with stay sutures.

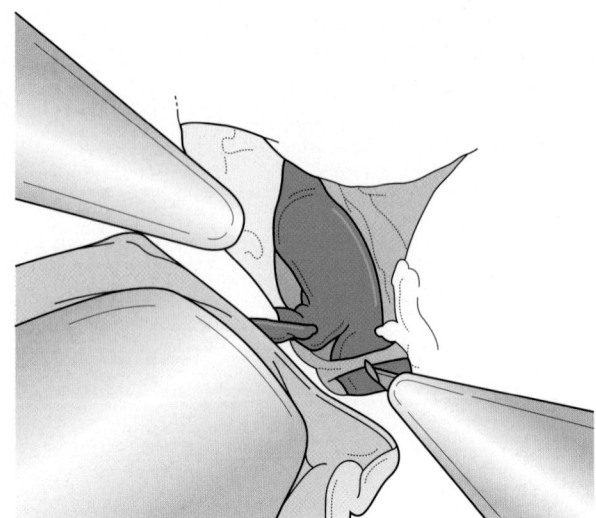

FIGURE 13.16 Sharp microinstruments are used to fully dissect the parasellar cisterns from the prechiasmatic cistern across the carotid cistern into the medial aspect of the sylvian fissure.

subarachnoid course of the carotid artery, including the bifurcation into the middle and anterior cerebral arteries, should be seen. From this point, the specific aneurysmal site governs the principles of further dissection.

Aneurysms of the Proximal (Paraclinoidal) and Posterior Carotid Artery Wall

This unique group of aneurysms arises from the most proximal intracranial segment of the internal carotid artery. Most of the aneurysms in this area can be separated into three subgroups, namely, carotid-ophthalmic, superior hypophyseal, and proximal posterior carotid wall. Each of these aneurysms presents several unique technical problems to the neurosurgeon. Although their proximity to the skull base was once a formidable problem in regard to obtaining any significant proximal vascular control, endovascular access and proximal control have reduced this difficulty. When these aneurysms reach a significant size, they can compress and distort the optic nerve, resulting in visual neurological deficits. The aneurysm must then be decompressed to relieve the mass effect. Further, large and giant aneurysms are often found to have thick, calcified walls, which must be refashioned with creativity, requiring multiple aneurysm clips because of the rigidity and differential wall thickness. The lateral aspect of paraclinoidal, especially carotid-ophthalmic, aneurysms can be partially covered by the anterior clinoid process as it emerges from the roof of the cavernous sinus (Fig. 13.17). The optic strut, the inferior bony aspect of the optic canal, can also obscure the proximal neck of the aneurysm. Our experience suggests that although large aneurysm domes can distort various neurovascular structures, the proximal portion of the normal carotid artery is *always* located at the lateral aspect of the optic canal. As such, this proximal portion of the carotid can normally be exposed via an incision in the falciform ligament, which will uncover the proximal carotid and ophthalmic artery origin, and the proximal neck of the aneurysm, particularly in carotid ophthalmic and superior hypophyseal variants. If the aneurysm

projects laterally or arises from within the carotid cave, then aggressive bony resection of the anterior clinoid process or the optic strut will be required to demonstrate the proximal neck. In ruptured proximal carotid aneurysms, it is important for proximal control to be established early either through an open cervical exposure to the internal carotid artery or through endovascular means with a proximal internal carotid balloon. Either way, it is important to guarantee early proximal control should difficulties arise and require temporary arterial occlusion, aneurysm decompression, and intraoperative angiography.

Posterior carotid wall aneurysms include lesions arising immediately distal to the posterior communicating artery as well as those arising immediately distal to the origin of the anterior choroidal artery (Fig. 13.18). These lesions are some of the most common aneurysmal lesions seen in neurosurgical practice, and intimate knowledge of the microanatomy is paramount in order to treat these lesions successfully. Neurological signs of an enlarging aneurysm in this area are pain, from compression of the tentorial incisura, and third cranial nerve deficits. The intimate association between the distal neck of the internal carotid–posterior communicating artery aneurysm to the fragile anterior choroidal artery place it at risk when treating these aneurysms. Injuring the anterior choroidal artery, which supplies the posterior limb of the internal capsule, the lentiform nucleus, the optic tract, the amygdala, and the choroid plexus of the temporal horn, can result in profound and devastating neurological deficits, including hemiplegia and hemianopia. Maneuvers that can result in injury include aggressive dissection of the aneurysm dome and the placement of Gelfoam or cotton to control minor intraoperative bleeding. It should be emphasized that the distal course of the anterior choroidal artery often runs close to the aneurysmal dome and should be carefully dissected away so that the distal clip blade does not compromise its blood flow or the vessel becomes "accordianed" by clip closure (Fig. 13.19). The posterior communicating artery usually arises just proximal to the aneurysmal neck, and every attempt should

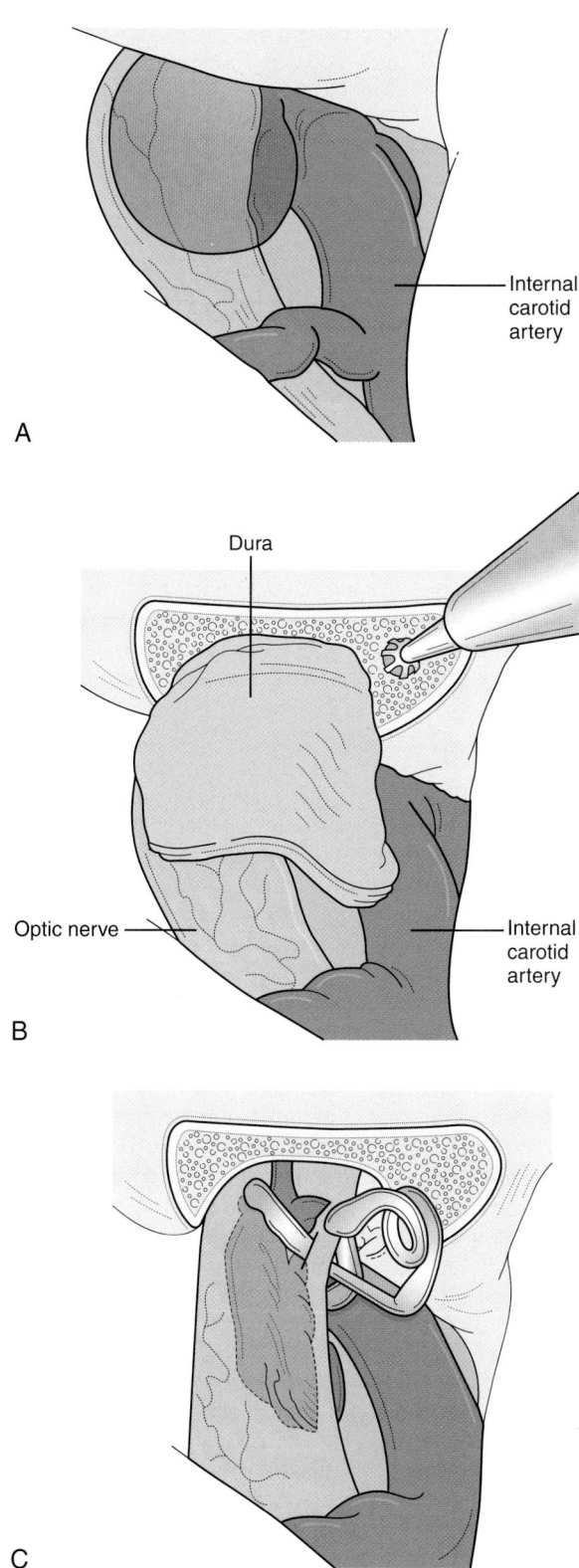

A

B

Dura

Optic nerve — Internal carotid artery

Internal carotid artery

C

FIGURE 13.17 Proximal carotid (paraclinoidal) aneurysm. **A,** These aneurysms often distort and attenuate the optic nerve and may have their proximal neck obscured by the dura covering the lateral aspect of the optic canal or by the bony anterior clinoidal process. Without securing proximal control in the neck or by endovascular means, it is obvious that true control of this aneurysm may be achieved intracranially only at some peril. **B,** To resect the anterior clinoid process, a dural flap is fashioned and reflected over the fundus of the aneurysm. A high-speed drill is then used to remove as much bone as is necessary to expose the proximal neck of the aneurysm. **C,** The specific clip placement chosen must not jeopardize the optic nerve or the patency of the internal carotid or the ophthalmic artery.

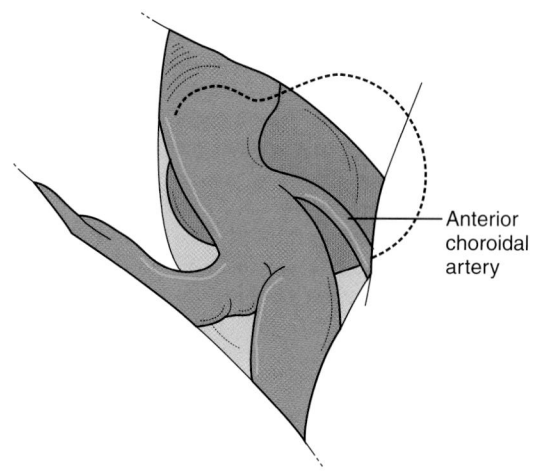

Anterior choroidal artery

FIGURE 13.18 Posterior carotid wall aneurysm. Despite their frequency and relative simplicity, especially the ease of achieving early proximal control intracranially, the neurosurgeon should not be nonchalant or complacent. The anterior choroidal artery is in intimate relationship with the distal neck, and simple retraction and mild compression can have devastating consequences.

be made to preserve this vessel because of important anterior thalamoperforating branches that ramify from its proximal portion. The neurosurgeon should also know if the posterior communicating artery is of fetal origin, therefore lacking an ipsilateral P1 segment. In this situation, it is paramount to

not sacrifice this artery. However, in patients with a normal circle of Willis, it is sometimes acceptable to include the posterior communicating artery in the clip, assuming the anterior thalamoperforators will fill from retrograde flow from the P1 segment off the basilar artery. This maneuver should be reserved for extreme situations because we have seen major deficits arise from it. Nevertheless, when possible, all components of the circle of Willis should be preserved, particularly in the setting of potential vasospasm after SAH and reliance on available collateral pathways. The most common clip arrangement for a posterior communicating artery aneurysm is perpendicular to the carotid artery. In smaller aneurysms, the carotid artery may narrow a bit after clipping but is usually trivial. In larger broad-based aneurysms, clipping perpendicular to the carotid artery can substantially narrow, even wrinkle, the carotid artery and impose shear forces on the fragile neck of the aneurysm during the closure of the clip. The angled fenestrated aneurysm clip allows clip placement

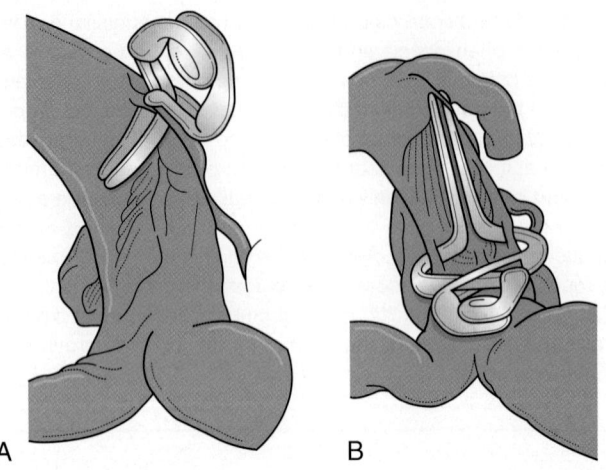

A   B

FIGURE 13.19 Alternatives for clipping posterior carotid wall aneurysms. **A,** For small aneurysms, a direct clip placement perpendicular to the carotid artery is often the best alternative. **B,** For larger aneurysms in this location, the degree of "gathering" of tissue by a perpendicular clip placement can jeopardize the carotid artery as well as apply serious shear stresses to the aneurysm neck during closure. The aperture clip allows blade closure parallel to the carotid artery, minimizing these deleterious events.

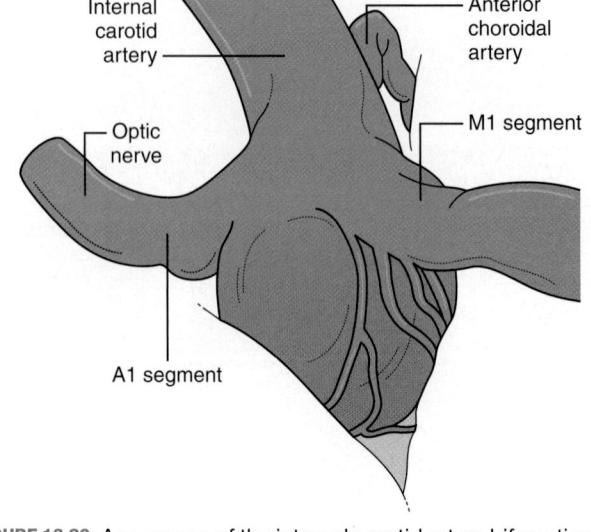

FIGURE 13.20 Aneurysms of the internal carotid artery bifurcation are frequently in intimate association with the distal course of the anterior choroidal artery as well as the medial lenticulostriate arteries arising from the middle and anterior cerebral arteries.

so that the blades close parallel to the carotid artery, minimizing the shear forces. Regardless of the clip chosen, it is critical to inspect the course of the anterior choroidal and the posterior communicating arteries to ensure that these vessels have not been compromised.

For patients presenting with third cranial nerve deficits, the aneurysm dome is not dissected away from the nerve. This maneuver can further damage the cranial nerve. Instead, the aneurysm is evacuated of its contents after clipping to eliminate the direct pulsations by the aneurysm on the nerve. Simple decompression will result in restoration of function in most patients within 6 months.

Aneurysms of the Carotid Bifurcation

Despite the fact that the carotid terminus/bifurcation is subject to continuous hemodynamic stress, it is a relatively rare site for aneurysm development. Aneurysms in this location typically project superiorly and occasionally superoposteriorly. Rupture of these aneurysms can often result in an intraparenchymal hematoma that mimics that of a putaminal hypertensive hemorrhage with little to no true subarachnoid blood. The diagnosis of aneurysmal rupture in these patients, especially without a history of hypertension, can be difficult.

Appropriate operative exposure of the carotid terminus/bifurcation requires judicious drilling of the sphenoid ridge and dissection of the opercular-insular cortex as well as the sphenoidal portions of the sylvian fissure. We prefer a lateral to medial approach followed by dissection of the carotid cistern to allow "unfolding" of the anatomy at the carotid terminus. The aneurysmal dome and neck can often be intimately associated with local vascular structures, namely, the anterior choroidal artery, anterior cerebral artery, the recurrent artery of Heubner, and sometimes medial lenticulostriate branches from the middle cerebral artery (Fig. 13.20). These vessels

typically hide posterior to the aneurysmal dome. It is paramount that the operating surgeon identify all of these important vessels so that the clip blades do not include them during closure of the aneurysm clip.

The two most important aspects of the exposure are gaining proximal control of the internal carotid artery and a wide opening of the carotid cistern. In addition, the sylvian fissure should be opened completely to expose the M1 segment, which can be followed proximally to the carotid terminus/bifurcation. Full exposure of the carotid terminus/bifurcation ensures both afferent and efferent circulation control. When treating difficult large and giant carotid terminus aneurysms, it is paramount for the neurosurgeon to know if there is a patent anterior communicating artery, which, if present, allows the potential sacrifice of the ipsilateral A1 segment in these cases and in the event of tears involving the medial aspect of the aneurysmal neck (Fig. 13.21).

Aneurysms of the Middle Cerebral Artery Bifurcation

Aneurysms of the middle cerebral artery, in particular at the site of the bifurcation, are quite common and hemorrhage from these lesions can produce several unique features. As such, diagnosis can be difficult in terms of the etiology of either an intraparenchymal or subdural hemorrhage in this location. Aneurysms at this location can also become very large or giant due to growth into the substance of the temporal lobe or invagination into the pia-arachnoid of the medial temporal lobe. When rupture occurs at the distal aspect of the aneurysmal dome, the resultant hematoma is in the temporal lobe parenchyma. Patients can present after a middle cerebral artery (MCA) aneurysm rupture with profound mass effect from the hematoma that necessitates surgical evacuation (Fig. 13.22). Modern CT angiography allows the immediate evaluation of the cerebral vasculature in cases such as these so that

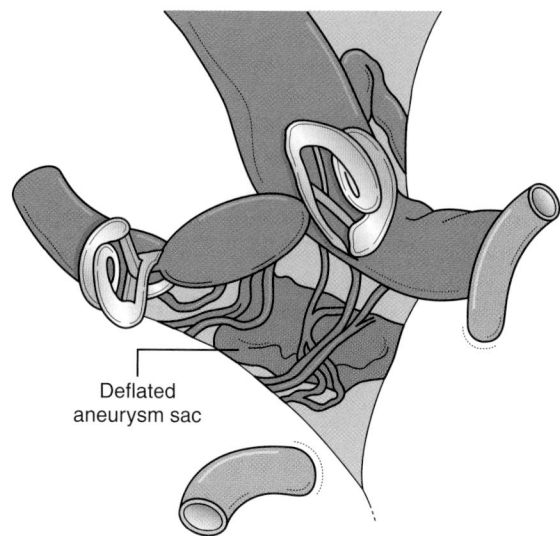

FIGURE 13.21 Carotid bifurcation aneurysm. If the anterior communicating artery is known to be patent, a valuable option for ceasing untimely intraoperative rupture is to incorporate the ipsilateral A1 segment into the definitive clipping, thus relying on the contralateral carotid to irrigate the anterior cerebral artery territory bilaterally.

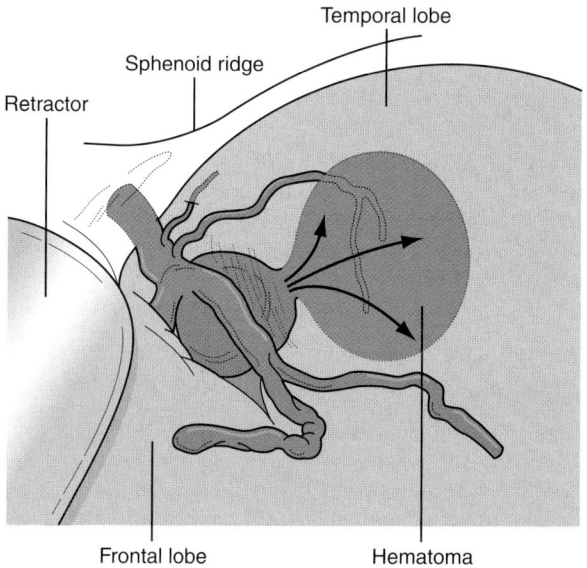

FIGURE 13.22 Aneurysms arising from the middle cerebral artery bifurcation often project into the medial aspect of the temporal lobe. Upon rupture, a hematoma may develop primarily within the temporal lobe itself and only minimally involve the subarachnoid space.

definitive treatment of the aneurysm can be considered during the evacuation of the hematoma.

The approach to MCA aneurysms is diverse and largely up to the experience and preference of the operating surgeon. One approach is to work medial to lateral from the carotids cistern, identifying the proximal M1 segment through the proximal sylvian fissure and dissecting distally until the bifurcation is reached. The serious disadvantage to this approach is the amount of frontal lobe retraction that is required to adequately expose the proximal M1 segment. Another approach is through the superior temporal gyrus, especially in cases in which there

is a temporal hematoma. Finally, the preferred approach to most MCA bifurcation lesions in most institutions is the direct transsylvian approach. The dissection is initiated in the lateral aspect of the sylvian fissure, approximately 2 to 3 cm from the sphenoid ridge. Frequently, an opening in the sylvian fissure can be made in the arachnoid membrane at this point. As the course of the distal sylvian veins is through this fissure, it is important to preserve all of the native vasculature. However, crossing sylvian veins may sometimes be sacrificed in order to open the fissure widely. Dissection via this route allows the surgeon to stay within the subarachnoid space from the outset, minimizing the degree of brain tissue retraction necessary and providing proximal control to be achieved safely. As the dissection deepens within the sylvian fissure, the small middle cerebral branches are followed down to the M2 segments, ultimately leading to the MCA bifurcation and M1 segment. Careful inspection of the aneurysm is important in this area because the M2 segments can often be intimately associated with or incorporated into the aneurysmal neck or dome. Dissection of these vessels must be carefully done to ensure continued distal blood flow after clipping. In cases of large or giant aneurysms that incorporate efferent vessels in the aneurysmal dome, these vessels may be either reimplanted into the distal vasculature or perfused with the aid of a revascularization strategy.

Aneurysms of the Anterior Communicating Artery

Aneurysms of the anterior communicating artery are perhaps the most common cause of SAH and represent approximately 30% of all cases of ruptured intracranial aneurysms. Furthermore, aneurysms in this location are thought to rupture at smaller diameters than those in other locations. The anterior communicating artery as well as the A1 segments of the anterior cerebral artery are some of the most variable components of the circle of Willis. The combination of hemodynamic factors with aberrant anatomy more often explains the propensity of aneurysm development in this location. Common anatomical anomalies are irregularities in size, asymmetrical dominance of A1 segments, and fenestration, duplication, or triplication of the anterior communicating artery. In fact, most anterior communicating artery aneurysms are thought to arise from the junction of the dominant A1 segment and the anterior communicating artery. Hemorrhagic presentation of ruptured aneurysms in this location can be highly varied and include diffuse SAH, interhemispheric SAH, intraventricular hemorrhage (by rupture through the lamina terminalis), and intraparenchymal hemorrhage (usually a flame-shaped frontal lobe hematoma). Unless they reach a large or giant size, aneurysms in this location rarely present with neurological deficits.

Treatment of anterior communicating artery aneurysms can present the surgeon with unique challenges. To adequately expose the surgical target, the bony craniotomy should be carried somewhat more medially and inferiorly than the craniotomy designed for other lesions because of the more anterior location of the anterior communicating artery complex. This is done by enlarging the craniotomy to the midpupillary line and carrying the bony incision as close to the brow as possible, without infiltrating the frontal sinuses. To augment this approach, a significant amount of bone, namely the sphenoid ridge to the superior orbital fissure and the inner tables of the anterior and middle fossa, must be removed. An alternative surgical

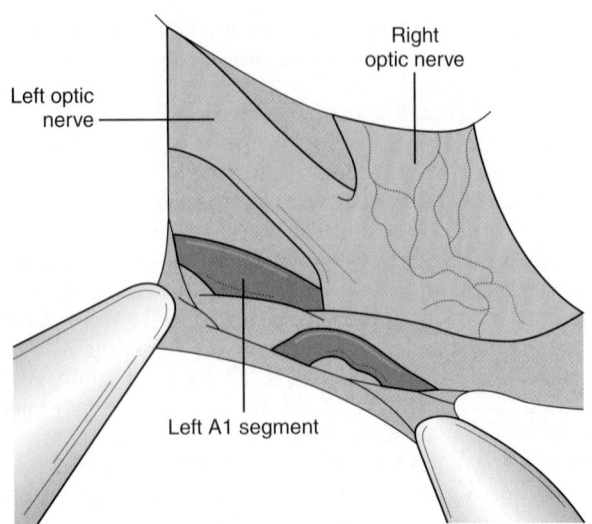

FIGURE 13.23 Isolation of the contralateral A1 segment completes acquisition of proximal control.

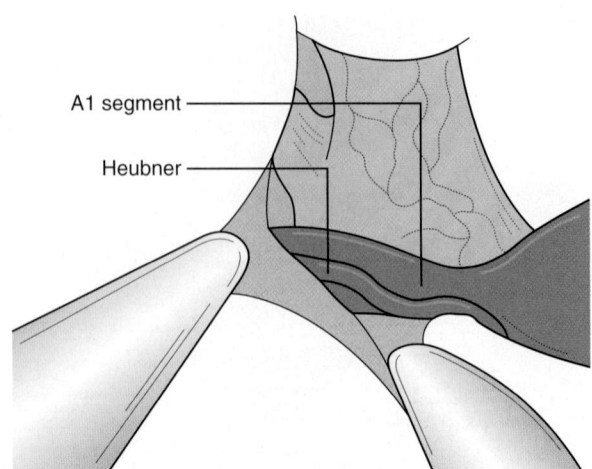

FIGURE 13.24 In approaching anterior communicating artery aneurysms, the additional brain retraction needed to isolate the origin of the A1 anterior cerebral segment at the carotid bifurcation can be avoided by dissecting the gyrus rectus from the optic nerve and tract. Deepening this plane will expose the A1 proximal to the anterior communicating artery.

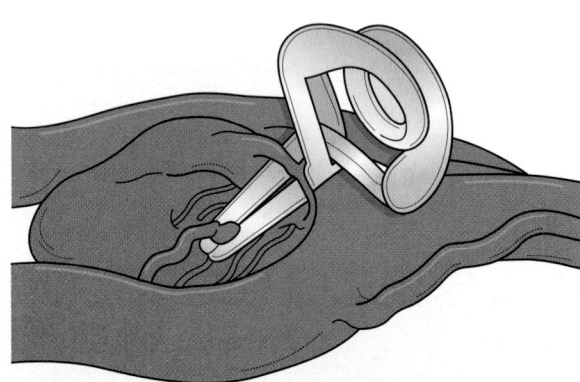

FIGURE 13.25 Multiple penetrating vessels arise from the posterior aspect of the anterior communicating artery. This schematic illustration shows that the use of excessive clip length and poor visibility behind the aneurysm can cause injury to these important vessels.

approach is the fronto-orbito-zygomatic, which involves the lateral superior and lateral orbital wall and zygomatic arch. Both of these approaches can lead to minimal visual obstruction by surrounding bone without significant cosmetic effects.

The microsurgical procedure for anterior communicating artery aneurysms focuses on the wide opening of the carotid cistern. One approach is to locate the proximal portion of the A1 segment at the carotid bifurcation and follow it to the anterior communicating complex. Alternatively, we advocate a direct dissection over the optic nerve toward the midline. The A1 segment swings anteriorly as it approaches the anterior communicating complex. The contralateral A1 segment should then be visualized by crossing the midline and working superior to the contralateral ophthalmic nerve (Fig. 13.23). This cistern may be filled with hematoma if done in a patient with SAH and, therefore, careful dissection in this area should be done to avoid inadvertently injuring the many important vessels traversing this region. The gyrus rectus, just inferior to the olfactory tract, can be aggressively resected with cautery and suction (Fig. 13.24). The overlying veil of pia can be manipulated to facilitate gyral resection. Once the gyrus resection is completed, the ipsilateral and contralateral A2 segments should be identified for distal control. Once both of the A1 and A2 segments are dissected and localized, the dissection can focus on the anterior communicating artery and the associated aneurysm. The relationship of the aneurysm to the surrounding vasculature as well as the proximal and distal aneurysmal necks needs to be understood completely before definite clipping can occur. It is paramount to identify the small perforating arteries that emanate from the posterior aspect of the anterior communicating artery (Fig. 13.25). Laceration or inclusion of these perforators in the clip blades can lead to serious and irreversible cognitive and hypothalamic sequelae.

Aneurysms of the Distal Basilar Artery

Aneurysms arising from the basilar apex or immediately distal to the origin of the superior cerebellar arteries are the most common form of posterior circulation aneurysms. Access to the distal basilar artery is complicated by the myriad of vital

perforating arteries arising from the posterior aspect of the distal basilar artery and both P1 segments (Fig. 13.26). As such, endovascular strategies are often employed as an initial treatment. However, some situations, such as efferent segments off the aneurysmal dome, acute angle of aneurysm neck from parent artery, or failed endovascular therapy make surgery more desirable. To ensure preservation of the vital perforating vessels, clear surgical strategies for clip placement must be made (Fig. 13.27). Pharmacological agents to induce systemic hypotension and asystole (i.e., adenosine) are especially helpful in the narrow surgical corridors through which these aneurysms are treated. Several surgical approaches are used to expose the distal basilar trunk, and the advantages, disadvantages, and limitations are discussed here.

Pterional Transsylvian Approach

The pterional approach, particularly with wide sylvian fissure dissection, is extremely versatile and used for many aneurysms of the distal basilar complex. Wide dissection of the parasellar

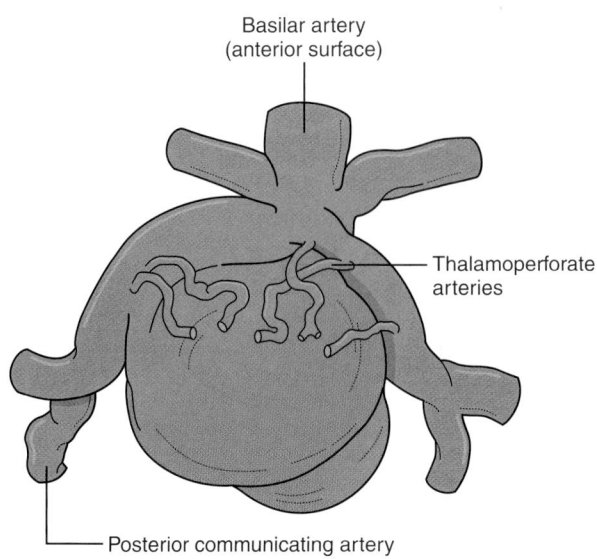

FIGURE 13.26 Aneurysms of the distal basilar artery must be treated with a precise awareness of the constant presence and infinite variability of the posterior thalamoperforating arteries supplying the mesencephalon and diencephalon.

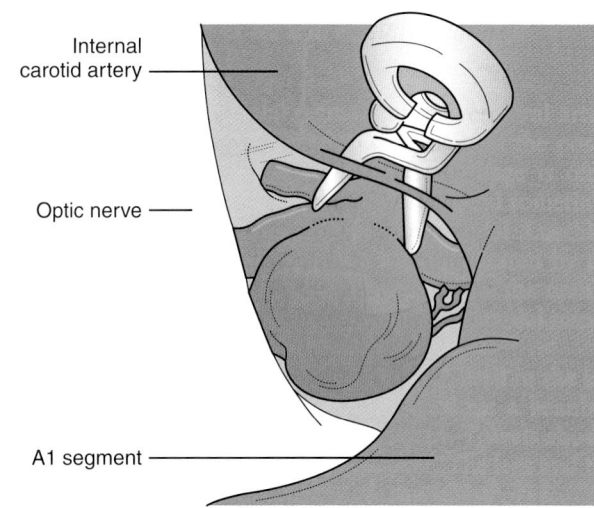

FIGURE 13.28 The surgeon can take advantage of the versatility of the pterional exposure by directing the microscope, and thus the line of sight, medial to the carotid artery and inserting the clip lateral and posterior to the carotid so the bulk of the clip and applier do not obscure the view.

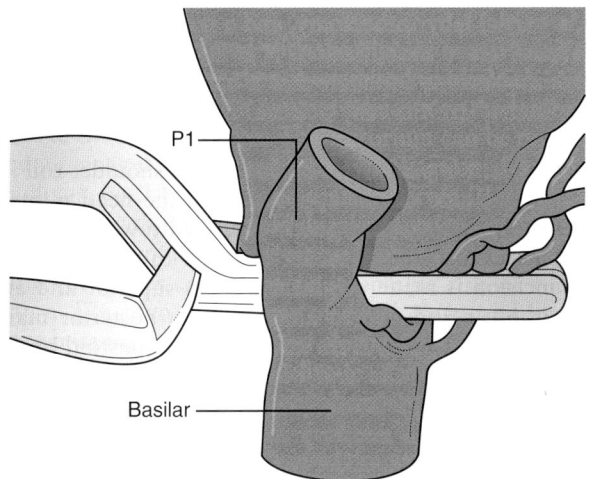

FIGURE 13.27 Clip applied to a basilar bifurcation aneurysm with inadvertent occlusion of thalamoperforating vessels. This error is almost always devastating to the patient.

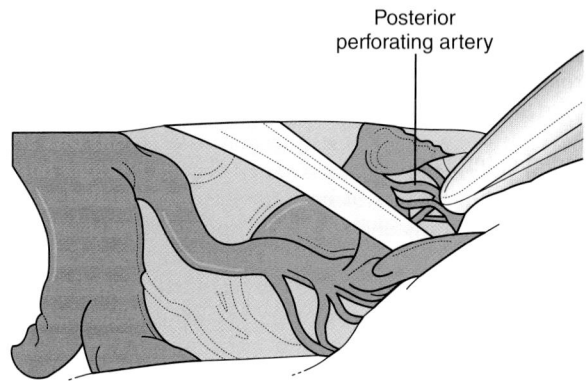

FIGURE 13.29 The subtemporal approach maximizes the surgical view of the thalamoperforating arteries while rendering the access to the contralateral posterior cerebral artery more difficult.

cisterns enables access to the interpeduncular cistern by one or multiple routes (Fig. 13.28). The dissection plane and the approach can be developed lateral to the internal carotid artery wherein the posterior communicating artery is followed to the junction of the P1 and P2 segments of the posterior cerebral artery. The P1 can be followed proximally to the basilar artery to gain proximal control. In a similar fashion, a dissection plane can be developed medial to the carotid artery that separates the small perforating arteries to the hypothalamic region and optic tract, opening the membrane of Liliequist, directly exposing the basilar trunk in the interpeduncular cistern. To achieve more superior exposure, the binding arachnoid fibers of the small lenticulostriate vessels can be divided to allow elevation of the optic tract opening up the interpeduncular cistern. To minimize the obstruction of this

limited surgical view, the clip applier is often passed lateral to the carotid artery toward the basilar apex. This exposure allows exquisite access to the proximal basilar trunk and both P1 segments for definitive temporary occlusion with aneurysmal decompression, adequate dissection space for large and giant lesions, and, if necessary, control of intraoperative bleeding.

Subtemporal Approach

The lateral view of the interpeduncular cistern offers the ideal view of the vital perforators posterior to the aneurysmal dome (Fig. 13.29). However, visualization of the contralateral P1 segment can be difficult. To improve visualization of the contralateral P1 segment; the space anterior to the aneurysmal neck can usually be gently retracted to expose the initial anterior course of this segment. The initial course of the P1 is superior and anterior. No vessels or neural structures obscure this route. When confusion arises as to whether the identified

tortuous, involves different calibers and lengths of vertebral arteries, and potentially involves fenestrations of the confluens and lower basilar trunk. As such, these configurations allow complex hemodynamics that predisposes this area to aneurysm development. Aneurysms of the lower basilar trunk are usually associated with the origin of the anterior inferior cerebellar artery (AICA) and the sixth cranial nerve.

The surgical exposure is normally done with the patient in the lateral position. The surgical approach is similar to the far lateral exposure explained previously except the initial dissection is carried out between the fibers of the ninth cranial nerve below and the seventh and eighth cranial nerves above. Exposure of lower basilar trunk usually involves a cranial base approach, either by sectioning the tentorium from a subtemporal approach or by an exposure anterior to or through the sigmoid sinus via a transpetrosal approach.

CONCLUSION

Intracranial aneurysms continue to provide significant rates of morbidity and mortality despite decades of advanced knowledge, technology, and research. The natural history of unruptured intracranial aneurysms is still controversial, especially with regard to aneurysms smaller than 7 mm. Other morphological factors have been associated with increased rupture risk but no one factor seems able to predict rupture, as would be expected from an entity that likely involves a multifactorial pathogenesis, pathobiology, and pathobehavior. Each individual unruptured aneurysm should be evaluated with all aspects taken into consideration, including lesional characteristics and patient comorbid conditions, as well as patients' risk aversion and expectations from the management plan.

Contemporary management strategies should involve all aspects of neurovascular care, including neuroendovascular physicians, neurocritical care, and neuroanesthesia. All of these specialties should be synergistic and complementary in their approach with the common goal of managing the obliteration of the aneurysm with minimal risk, both short-term and long-term, to the patient. It is now essential that all centers offering state-of-the-art cerebrovascular medicine have expertise in all specialized aspects of neurovascular care. Without such, we would be doing our patients a disservice.

SELECTED KEY REFERENCES

Bederson JB, Connolly Jr ES, Batjer HH, et al. Guidelines for the management of aneurysmal subarachnoid hemorrhage: a statement for healthcare professionals from a special writing group of the Stroke Council, American Heart Association. *Stroke*. 2009;40(3):994-1025.

Lall RR, Eddleman CS, Bendok BR, Batjer HH. Unruptured intracranial aneurysms and the assessment of rupture risk based on anatomical and morphological factors: sifting through the sands of data. *Neurosurg Focus*. 2009;26(5):E2.

Pluta RM, Hansen-Schwartz J, Dreier J, et al. Cerebral vasospasm following subarachnoid hemorrhage: time for a new world of thought. *Neurol Res*. 2009;31(2):151-158.

Rabinstein AA. The AHA guidelines for the management of SAH: what we know and so much we need to learn. *Neurocrit Care*. 2009;10(3):414-417.

Wiebers DO, Whisnant JP, Huston 3rd J, et al. Unruptured intracranial aneurysms: natural history, clinical outcome, and risks of surgical and endovascular treatment. *Lancet*. 2003;362(9378):103-110.

Please go to expertconsult.com to view complete list of references.

Vascular Malformations (Arteriovenous Malformations and Dural Arteriovenous Fistulas)

Ghaus M. Malik, Sandeep S. Bhangoo

CLINICAL PEARLS

- Arteriovenous malformations (AVMs) are congenital, high-flow, high-pressure lesions with the primary risk of devastating intracerebral hemorrhage.

- Important characteristics of any AVM include nidus size and location, number and locations of arterial feeders, and pattern of venous drainage.

- Only complete removal of the arteriovenous shunt has been shown to definitively reduce the risk of bleeding.

- Treatment modalities include surgical resection, radiosurgery, endovascular occlusion, or some combination of these approaches.

- Dural arteriovenous fistulas are a subset of AVMs that are thought to be acquired rather than congenital. Treatment focuses on the control of cortical venous drainage to reduce hemorrhage risk.

The arteriovenous malformation (AVM) and its cousin, the arteriovenous fistula (AVF), form a distinct subgroup of central nervous system disorders that have both fascinated and terrified neurosurgeons for decades. There are several reasons why such an otherwise rare disorder captures so much attention in the neurosurgical literature. Like an aneurysm, it is a vascular lesion is at risk of rupture, causing debilitating hemorrhage. Unlike aneurysms, they are not thought to develop de novo, yet the vast majority of them remains clinically silent for decades. Like a neoplasm, it is a pathological mass that has been seen to develop in every cranial structure. Unlike a neoplasm, it can grow along with the brain without necessarily displacing functional structures. Therefore, many never cause functional neurological compromise regardless of size. Like developmental anomalies, their early formation allows for considerable variability in presentation. Unlike most developmental anomalies, they have been notoriously difficult to classify because no two AVMs are alike.

Over the decades, the drive to understand these lesions has elucidated many concepts in cerebrovascular physiology, anatomy, and embryology. Despite all this, the most fascinating, yet terrifying, aspect of AVMs is their unpredictability. Other than epidemiological data, few tools can assist a neurosurgeon in helping patients understand the prognosis of this disease. Nevertheless, AVMs are one of the few disorders that can be definitively cured with surgical therapy. Modern imaging and multispecialty collaboration with interventional radiologists, neuro-intensivists, and radiation therapists give the practicing neurosurgeon the widest range of options in helping patients deal with this disease.

CLASSIFICATION AND DEFINITIONS

It is important to place AVMs and AVFs in the proper pathological classification given the multitude of names one may encounter in the literature.

First, a vascular malformation of the central nervous system is believed to be a dysplastic process, which should be distinguished from a neoplastic process (i.e., a hemangioma is defined as a neoplasm derived from the endothelial cells of a blood vessel). Some literature will, for example, refer to a cavernous malformation as a "cavernoma" or "cavernous angioma," with the suffix "oma" implying a neoplastic process. In a similar manner, one may also encounter the name "venous angioma" used to describe a developmental venous anomaly. In the category of dysplastic vascular malformations, there have traditionally been four pathological entities:[1-3] developmental venous anomalies, capillary telangiectasias, cavernous malformations, and AVMs. In addition, mixed malformations have been found, though they are thought to be rare.[4] What separates an AVM from the first three is the presence of an arteriovenous shunt, which is defined as oxygenated blood passing directly into the venous system without gas exchange occurring in a capillary bed. These shunts are characterized by high flow and high pressure, which distinguish them from other vascular malformations.

AVMs may be plexiform, fistulous, or both. A fistulous malformation may be an otherwise normal artery directly joining a vein. A plexiform malformation is defined as an artery connecting to a network of poorly differentiated, immature vessels before passing into a vein. This plexiform network

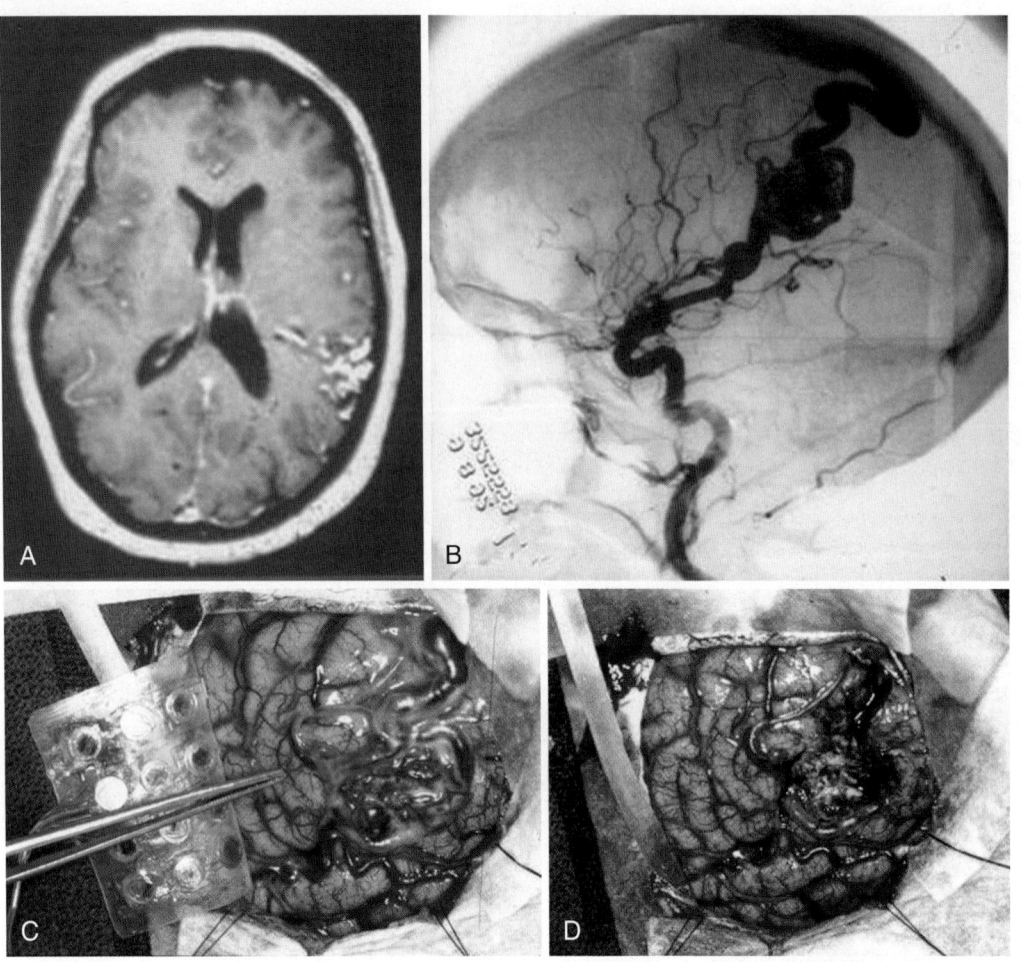

FIGURE 14.1 **A,** Axial magnetic resonance imaging with gadolinium shows an enhancing lesion in the left parietal cortex. **B,** Digital subtraction angiography (DSA) of the same patient shows an arteriovenous malformation (AVM) with a middle cerebral arterial feeder and a cortical draining vein to the superior sagittal sinus. **C,** Intraoperative image of the same AVM shows the nidus on the cortical surface. Note the large draining vein with oxygenated blood going superiorly. Here, intraoperative cortical stimulation was attempted because of the eloquent location of the nidus. **D,** Postresection image.

can be termed a *nidus* (Latin term for "nest"). Figure 14.1 shows a plexiform nidus on the cortical surface. AVMs with plexiform and fistulous components can be seen in any intracranial structure. Because of their developmental nature, they can span multiple structures that are otherwise anatomically distinct. Because they can occur anywhere in the brain, the term *brain AVM* (BAVM) is coming into wider use and becoming more accepted.[5] However, one may encounter multiple adjectives that attempt to describe the malformation (*true, cerebral, pial, parenchymal, cisternal, ventricular, medullary*) but do not necessarily imply a separate type of pathological entity. However, there is one exception: *Dural AVFs* (dAVFs) are a distinct pathological type in that their development is not thought to be strictly congenital but acquired. The dAVF will be treated as a separate pathological entity and will be discussed later.

DIAGNOSTIC RADIOLOGY

Cross-Sectional Imaging

Magnetic resonance imaging (MRI) is a useful tool in the diagnosis and management of AVMs. Its cross-sectional capability allows for geometric definition of complex structures such as the AVM nidus along with allowing the surgeon to better localize the lesion and adjacent structures. On T2-weighted

images, hypointense signals are indicative of flow voids representing the various feeding arteries, draining veins, or vessels of the nidus itself. Peripheral to the nidus, hypointense signals on T2 and gradient echo can also show hemosiderin deposition; this could be indicative of subclinical hemorrhage in the past. Magnetic resonance angiography (MRA) and magnetic resonance ventriculography (MRV) may be helpful in delineating the presence of flow in major vessels to and from the nidus and can be considered as a noninvasive method of determining the progress of obliteration after radiosurgical or embolic therapy.

A noncontrast head computed tomography (CT) scan is useful in the acute determination of intracranial hemorrhage. Because this is usually the first study acquired in patients with AVMs, it is important to recognize key features that could arouse suspicion of an AVM. First is that 25% to 30% of AVMs have calcium deposition[6] that may be apparent even in the presence of a mass-displacing hemorrhage. In addition, there may be evidence of iso- to hyperdense serpiginous vessels that might be located at some distance from the hemorrhage. Noncontrast CT has no role in ruling out an AVM because many cannot be visualized. A CT angiogram (CTA) may be helpful in an unruptured AVM to help delineate the nidus and associated vessels.

A weakness common to both CT and MR modalities is the lack of temporal sequencing of images to determine the dynamic aspect of the malformation. A good example of this

TABLE 14.1	Structures Visualized During Digital Subtraction Angiography				
	STRUCTURES SEEN IN STUDY PHASE (SECONDS ELAPSED)				
Feature	Early Arterial: 1–2 sec	Late Arterial: 2–3 sec	Capillary: 3–4 sec	Early Venous: 5–6 sec	Late Venous: 6–7 sec
Normal structures opacified	Main arteries	Arterial branches	Arterioles	Venules and veins	Veins and sinuses
AVM	Feeding arteries	Nidus	Draining veins and sinuses		
AVF	Feeding arteries	Draining veins and sinuses			

AVF, arteriovenous fistula; AVM, arteriovenous malformation.

for the MRA (or CTA) is that when all vessels are uniformly enhanced in any image one cannot distinguish between a nidus feeding artery or a draining vein without supplemental anatomical information which may be distorted in a malformation.

Angiography

No cerebral arteriovenous shunt can be completely understood without the aid of a selective cerebral angiogram. In fact, the history of the understanding of this pathology was dependent on the technological developments in the field of radiology. The modern equivalent is the digital subtraction angiogram (DSA), which can subtract out static components of the image (i.e., the skull) to allow the viewer a better visualization of the dynamic components. The main weakness of the angiography when compared to cross-sectional imaging is the lack of good geometric characterization and localization of the nidus. This is more evident as the size of the malformations increases. However, the primary utility of DSA is to establish the diagnosis of an arteriovenous shunt by locating early opacification of the nidus or draining veins in the routine arterial phase of the angiogram (Table 14.1).[7] The characterization of this shunting helps to determine not only the pathophysiology of a particular case but also provides a common communication platform upon which various treatment modalities can be discussed between specialists.

Radiological Findings

A judicious use of diagnostic imaging studies is warranted with these complex lesions. A Joint Writing Group publication, in 2001, was a multidisciplinary effort to provide guidelines in the standardized reporting of AVMs for the purposes of clinical research.[5] A summary of the important features is provided here. However, note that when AVMs are described, certain characteristics may have more clinical relevance.

Nidus

The size of an AVM usually refers to that of the nidus itself, though the presence of adjacent dilated veins may be confounding. Generally, cross-sectional imaging will provide a more accurate assessment using the same measurement techniques as those for any intracranial mass lesion. Location of the nidus is a second characteristic to note. One is particularly concerned about its proximity to eloquent brain structures.[8]

Both size and location, though better characterized on cross-sectional imaging, can be roughly estimated as well on angiography, as shown in Figure 14.2A. Additionally, one should characterize the shape for surgical or radiosurgical planning. Unusual geometries may be obscured in angiograms. In locating the nidus, the first step in microsurgical treatment would be consideration of the needed approach for any mass lesion in that location and the potential morbidity.

Arterial Supply

Arteries supplying the AVM should be noted for number, size, relative contribution to the nidus, and location. They can be characterized first by noting what vascular territory they arise from. Angiography from each intracranial vessel should be performed. The detailed description of the intracerebral anatomical vasculature is beyond the scope of this chapter. However, when describing the source of a feeding vessel it would be best to describe its course from the circle of Willis. For large AVMs, when there is concern for meningeal involvement, angiograms of the external carotid arteries should be done as well. Contribution from deep perforating arteries should be clearly noted as they are particularly difficult to deal with in surgery. Finally, one should note that large AVMs or even smaller ones in the temporal or occipital lobe may lie in the vascular border zone between the anterior and posterior circulations; they could, therefore, have vascular pedicles from both. In the era before digitized images, one could simply overlay the transparent films from multiple angiographic injections to get an idea of the complete nidus along with relative locations of erratic feeders. Modern, electronic PACS (picture archiving and communication system) software does not yet seem to have a simple equivalent (Fig. 14.2B).

There are three types of arterial feeders. *Direct feeders* are the simplest to conceptualize: they end directly and exclusively in the nidus, and they are also known as *terminal feeders*. *Transit arteries* are normal arteries that appear on angiogram to pass near or even through the nidus while going on to supply normal tissue. These normal arteries can be easily obscured during nidus opacification. At the same time, their distal territory may never get a sufficient supply of contrast to opacify. An example may be the pericallosal artery passing adjacent to a mesial frontal lobe nidus before proceeding posteriorly. The third type of feeding artery is the *indirect feeder* or artery *en passage*. This artery combines the previous two in that as it passes near the nidus it can contribute to the shunt before continuing on to supply normal brain.

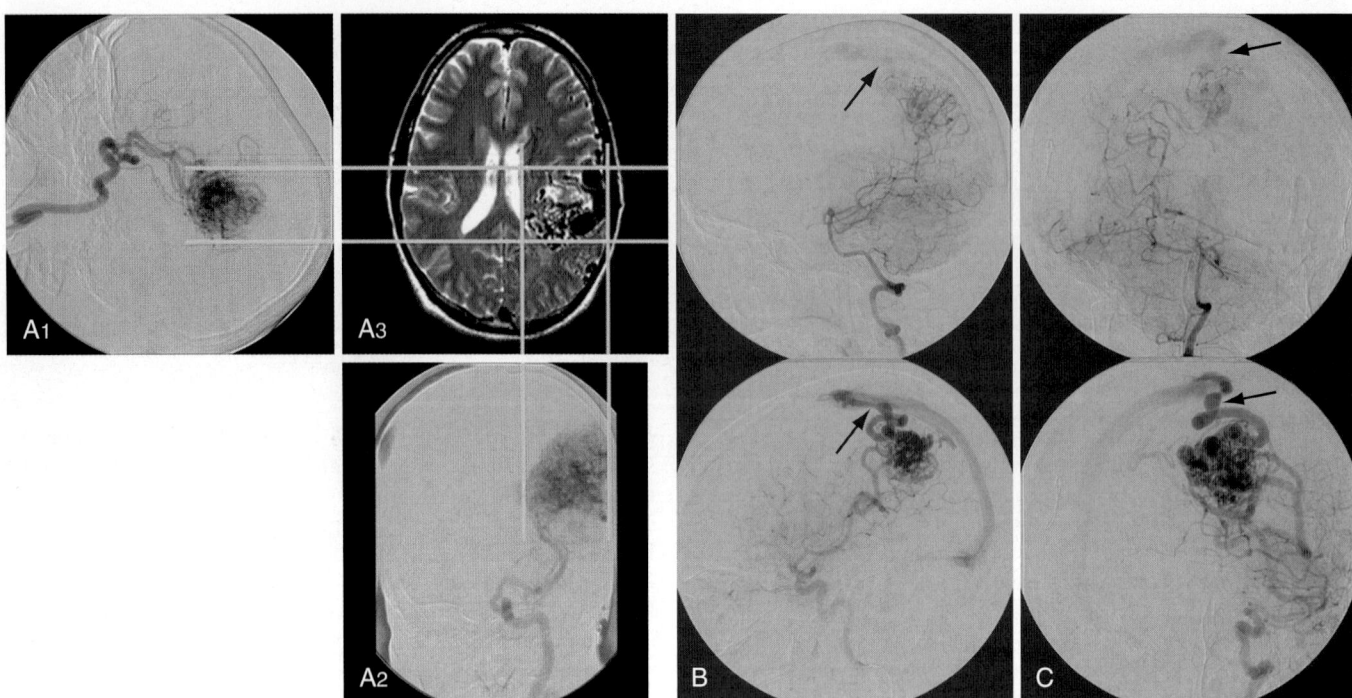

FIGURE 14.2 **A,** Use of digital subtraction angiography (DSA) in the early arterial phase lateral (I) and anteroposterior (II) projections to estimate the size and location of an arteriovenous malformation (AVM) nidus as seen on T2 axial magnetic resonance imaging (MRI) (III). Note that the conical shape of the nidus with the apex near the posterior lateral ventricle cannot be appreciated with DSA alone. Also note that the large flow void laterally on the MRI depicts a major draining vein that is not readily appreciated on this phase of the angiogram. **B,** An AVM with a 3-cm nidus in the parietal cortex as seen on lateral DSA vertebral injection (*above*) and left inferior cerebral artery (*below*). The arrows point to the same draining vein in order to help orient the reader to the same structures in each image. The primary arterial feeder is a middle cerebral artery branch from the carotid circulation. However, the early opacification of the same vein on the vertebral injection indicates a posterior circulation contribution as well. **C,** The same AVM seen on oblique views shows the posterior cerebral arterial feeders (*above*) are *en passage* arteries which likely supply normal brain tissue. The location of this nidus in a vascular border zone likely allowed the surrounding normal cerebral tissue to recruit additional arterial supply from the posterior circulation over time. During embolization or surgery, it is important to recognize the difference between these vessels to avoid a cerebral infarct. (*A from Hamm KD, Klisch J, Surber G, et al. Special aspects of diagnostic imaging for radiosurgery of arteriovenous malformations. Neurosurgery 2008;62(5):A44.*)

AVMs within the sylvian fissure usually harbor many *en passage* contributions from the distal middle cerebral arteries. Rotational angiography and three-dimensional reconstruction has now replaced the old-fashioned stereoangiography, which previously provided excellent tracking of the course of feeding arteries and draining veins.

Superselective angiography of a suspected vessel can show if it contributes to the nidus or not and help distinguish a transit artery. However, superselective catheterization of an artery *en passage* can have variable presentation on angiography depending on the hemodynamics of the vessel. Knowledge of normal cerebrovascular anatomy can help the neurosurgeon recognize where normal vessels should be expected. Also, a common theme among many, though not all, AVM feeders is that they do not seem to follow the traditional pattern of progressive luminal narrowing as they flow distally. Arterial feeders can even exhibit pathological stenosis or even aneurysms. Embolization or surgical ligation of an unrecognized *en passage* artery can lead to infarcts of normal tissue. The superselective angiography also helps identify any intranidal aneurysm as well as small prenidal aneurysms.

One other point of importance is the supply to AVM coming from pial collaterals. An AVM in the parietal area, for example, may have most of its supply from the middle cerebral artery, but it also gets its contribution from the posterior cerebral branches coursing over the hemisphere essentially supplying the distal territory of middle cerebral artery beyond the AVM (Fig. 14.2C). Even though these vessels are larger than normal, they are not suitable for endovascular occlusion. This fact also needs to be taken into consideration during microsurgery so that the supply to the normal brain is not affected.

Venous Drainage

The final feature to characterize in an AVM is the draining veins. In a similar manner to the arteries, one should note the number, size, and locations of the major veins.

The draining veins may be of unusual caliber with a tortuous course, ectasias, or stenosis.[9] Of particular importance to note is whether the veins drain superficially via the cortical surface or deeply to the vein of Galen. This is usually easy to identify with an angiogram as the first evidence of an arteriovenous shunt is early opacification of the veins by using anatomical recognition of the vein of Galen along with the major cerebral venous sinuses.

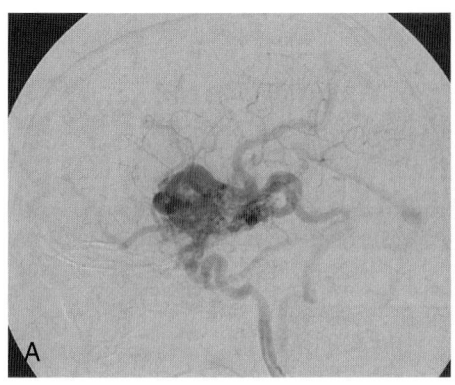
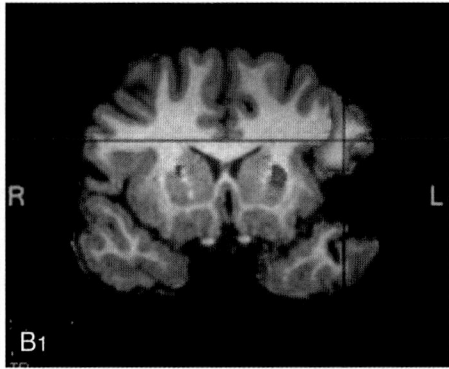
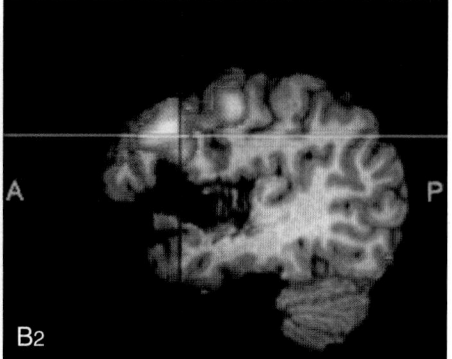

FIGURE 14.3 A, Digital subtraction angiography (DSA) left internal carotid artery injection shows perisylvian nidus in a 31-year-old female patient. **B,** Functional magnetic resonance imaging (fMRI) during verb generation showed activation of speech centers away from the nidus. Immediately postoperatively, however, the patient had aphasia. Though her speech eventually recovered, it is likely the fMRI results were inaccurate.

Like the transit arteries, it is important to recognize the possible existence of normal veins draining functional cerebral tissue that may be adjacent to the lesion. Again, careful study of the angiogram may show veins that opacify later than veins draining the nidus yet still in the same region. During surgical excision, it may be difficult to distinguish between them without knowing their locations relative to each other preoperatively.

Special Tests

Use of adjunctive diagnostic studies is helpful in selective cases. Functional MRI (fMRI) has helped assess the proximity of language and motor function in relation to AVM but has limitations (Fig. 14.3). Magnetic source imaging (MSI) can accurately localize sensory cortex and even visual and motor areas and the information can be overlaid on the MRI. Recently introduced, tractography should aid in assessing the relationship of deep white matter tracts to the AVM. The information derived from these studies is helpful in deciding the treatment and possibly assessing the neurological risk before intervention. Intraoperative functional mapping has limited value because one cannot do partial treatment in AVMs, in contrast to tumors.

GRADING SYSTEMS

Clinicians have been attempting to classify AVMs with the goal of helping patients understand the risks by comparison to historical outcomes. An ideal classification system would have the flexibility to cover many pathological variants, the simplicity to be used in a bedside fashion, and the utility to prognosticate. The variability and rarity of AVMs, however, have made this goal difficult to achieve in practice. Several classification schemes have been proposed.[10,11] Of these, the Spetzler-Martin system (Table 14.2)[12] has the most widespread use and should be known by the practicing neurosurgeon. Grades I and II AVM patients generally tolerated resection without morbidity while grade IV and V AVMs had higher risks of postoperative deficits. Retrospective and prospective studies have shown its utility for surgical decision making.[12,13] There are several weaknesses of this system, however. First, it lacks the ability to assess risks for interventions other than

TABLE 14.2 Spetzler-Martin Scale for Grading Arteriovenous Malformations

Lesion Characteristic	Points Assigned
Size	
Small: diameter <3 cm	1
Medium: diameter 3-6 cm	2
Large: diameter >6 cm	3
Location	
Noneloquent site	0
Eloquent site (sensorimotor, language, or visual cortex; hypothalamus or thalamus; internal capsule; brainstem; cerebellar peduncles; or cerebellar nuclei)	1
Pattern of venous drainage	
Superficial only	0
Any deep	1

*Total scores range from 0 to 5; high scores are associated with high risk of permanent neurological deficit after surgery.

exclusive microneurosurgery. Second, the studies were carried out by a highly experienced vascular team and may not necessarily be applicable to a general neurosurgeon's ability. Third, despite its simplicity, interobserver variability can still occur.[14] Finally, there is continuing concern that this system may oversimplify many AVMs. A more recent classification scheme attempts to add deep perforator supply and nidus diffuseness parameters to the Spetzler-Martin system[15] as predictors of higher surgical morbidity rates. The chief drawback is the difficultly applying the diffuseness parameter based on imaging (Fig. 14.4). These factors, however, have been recognized to make microsurgical resection more challenging.

In most of the grading schemes the size measurement is taken as a linear parameter, which when taken in the context of volume, has tremendous variation within the range of dimension. As an example, the spherical volume of a 5.54-cm-diameter AVM is approximately four times greater than an AVM measuring 3.5 cm, even though both of them are assigned 2 points in the Spetzler-Martin scale. Treatment with radiosurgery is volume dependent. In addition, several series have shown that volume is a better predictor of microsurgical risk and outcomes. The approximate volume can be determined by the formula: (length × width × height)/2.

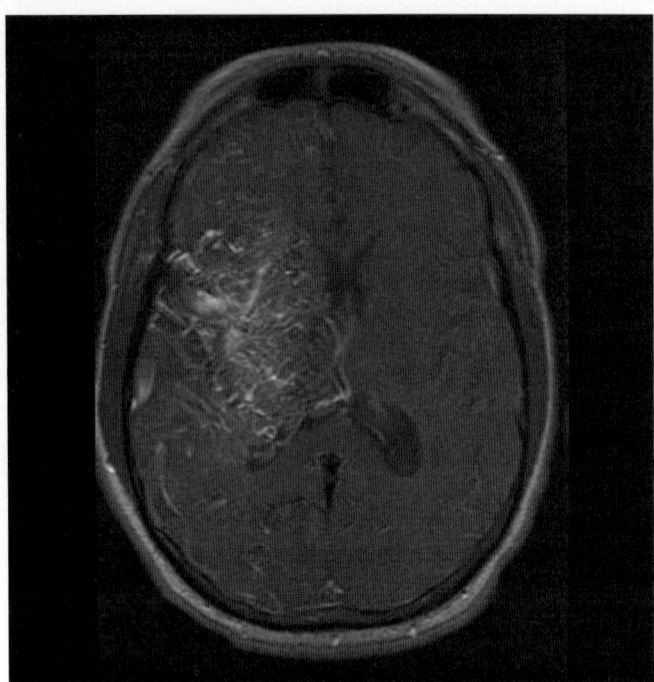

FIGURE 14.4 Axial magnetic resonance imaging (MRI) with gadolinium shows a large left frontal lobe nidus with a high level of diffuseness compared to the one seen in Figure 14.1. This characteristic, though not part of the Spetzler-Martin scale, may increase treatment morbidity. *(From Du R, Keyoung HM, Dowd CF, et al. The effects of diffuseness and deep perforating artery supply on outcomes after microsurgical resection of brain arteriovenous malformations. Neurosurgery 2007;60(4):638-646; discussion 646-648.)*

These measurements can be obtained from the anteroposterior (AP) and lateral views of the angiogram corrected for magnification.

Future attempts at classification may include more parameters, thus increasing the complexity beyond a simple bedside assessment. The ubiquity of computational devices even at the bedside, however, should allow for greater access to data-mining systems that can generate more granulated prognosis based on an ever greater number of parameters. Future studies, therefore, should focus on making classification schemes accurate rather than simple.

PATHOLOGICAL SEQUELAE

Hemorrhage

Over half of all AVMs are, unfortunately, discovered after an intracranial hemorrhage. The anatomical nature of the AVM often determines where the hemorrhage is seen. A small, deep AVM may hemorrhage exclusively intraparenchymally, but a cortical AVM may have a subarachnoid blood component. Intraventricular bleeds can occur from AVMs situated adjacent to the ventricles. Combinations of bleeding locations are also seen. dAVFs may present only with subarachnoid hemorrhage and should be considered in the differential diagnosis of a nonaneurysmal bleed. A six-vessel cerebral angiogram should be carried out in a subarachnoid hemorrhage patient

with no aneurysm seen on the intracranial vessels to rule out a dAVF.

The clinical sequelae of a hemorrhage depend upon the location and extent of intracranial mass effect; its initial medical management should be similar to a cerebral parenchymal hemorrhage. Headaches and seizures may also be associated with intracranial hemorrhage. In our own experience, a higher percentage of patients under the age of 20 and over the age of 60 present with hemorrhage, while seizure presentation is more likely between the ages of 20 and 60 years.

Seizures

Seizures are the second most common presenting symptom; they are associated with supratentorial AVMs. Approximately 15% to 30% of all patients with AVMs present with a focal or generalized seizure.[16-18] Angiographic characteristics of epileptogenic AVMs include cortical location of the nidus or feeding artery, feeding by the middle cerebral artery, absence of aneurysms, presence of varices in the venous drainage, and association of varix and absence of intranidal aneurysms. Other factors significantly associated with the onset of seizures include AVMs fed by the external carotid artery and a temporal or parietal cortical location.[19]

The causes of seizures are thought to be cortical irritation or remodeling from ischemia, altered hemodynamics, mass effect, or microhemorrhage. Despite this, most seizure disorders are well controlled with medical management alone. It is unclear whether AVM patients presenting with seizures, however, have similar risk profiles to those with hemorrhage. In the shorter term, hemorrhagic patients have higher risk for morbid rehemorrhage. However, the long-term risk for both presentations could converge.

An AVM patient presenting with epilepsy has a similar long-term risk profile for hemorrhage when compared to other presentations. That said, some patients may not wish to consider definitive treatment for reasons of age, comorbid conditions, or personal preference. Medical control of seizures with antiepileptic drugs (AEDs) is the first-line treatment. Consultation with neurological epileptologists for multidrug therapy is also indicated. There may, however, be a subset of patients harboring AVMs with medically refractory seizures. Neurological consultation can confirm location of the epileptic focus using clinical semiology or tools such as electroencephalography (EEG), magnetoencephalography (MEG), or single-photon emission computed tomography (SPECT). Given that most AVMs do not harbor functional tissue, the location of this epileptic focus with respect to the actual AVM nidus may help decide the best course of treatment, which may include radiosurgery.[20,21]

Headaches

Headaches are the presenting symptom in approximately 15% of patients without evidence of rupture.[16] They can be characterized as similar to migraines with lateralization to one side, but they may have a more permanent nature. This fact does not necessarily preclude migraines as an independent pathological entity, however, and patients should be informed that the goal of a successful AVM treatment is obliteration of

TABLE 14.3 Biological Processes Suspected in Arteriovenous Malformation Formation and Remodeling

	Vasculogenesis	Angiogenesis	Arteriogenesis
Definition	Formation of endothelium from progenitor cells	Formation and stabilization of capillary networks	Growth and formation of arterial collaterals
Stimulus	Preprogrammed molecular factors	Ischemia	Shear stress on vascular endothelium
Location	Embryonic cell bed	Post-vasculogenesis cell bed in embryo. Hypoxic cell bed in adult	Sprouting from existing arteries
Role in brain arteriovenous malformation	Dysplasia in initiation	Dyplasia in initiation. Later remodeling and recurrence	Growth, remodeling, and recurrence
Role in dural arteriovenous fistulas	Unlikely (noncongenital)	Ischemia or trauma may initiate dysplasia. Later remodeling and recurrence	Growth, remodeling, and recurrence

the nidus in order to mitigate risk of debilitating hemorrhage. Occipital AVMs may be a predisposing factor.

Neurological Deficit

A relatively rare presentation for an unruptured AVM is neurological deficit. Deficits may present as transient, progressive, or permanent and the spectrum of deficits varies with the morphological nature of the malformation. Deficits can arise through a number of mechanisms. First, the AVM itself may cause mass effect on adjacent neurovascular structures. Another possibility may be mass effect caused by arterial steal. The arteriovenous shunting may be disruptive to the vascular supply and regulation of surrounding normal brain structures by redirecting flow toward the shunt at a cost to normal vascular beds. This concept, if true, suggests that large AVMs with high flow should correlate with increased physiological evidence of steal. In fact, steal is thought to be relatively rare because the surrounding tissue does manage to adapt.[22,23]

DEVELOPMENT

There has been much speculation about how arteriovenous malformations are thought to develop. Traditionally it has been thought that they are congenital lesions that develop during the embryonic stage. This reasoning stems from histological examination of AVM structures that reveal characteristics that resemble the plexuses of developing vasculature in the embryo. There is also predisposition to develop AVMs in patients with genetic disorders such as Osler-Weber-Rendu and Wyburg-Mason syndromes.[24]

Against this theory, however, is the fact that AVMs have been known to recur after post-treatment angiographic evidence of obliteration by surgery or radiosurgery, although recurrence is very rare.[25] One must keep in consideration that the imaging resolution limit of an angiogram prohibits adequate visualization of the microcirculation. With this in mind, the question becomes whether these postnatal malformations arise de novo or develop into larger structures that can eventually be seen radiographically. In either case, the evidence supports the theory that AVMs are not static lesions but biologically dynamic and that they can develop and remodel over time.

The congenital theory of AVM development suggests that there is a failure of the development of a stable vascular and capillary plexus.[26] During embryological development of the nervous system, neuronal growth and migration help shape the vascular network that eventually will supply it. As an example, the population of neurons that develop in the germinal matrix near the ventricle and migrate radially outward toward the cortex can have vessels growing in tandem or, more commonly, migrating from the cortex inward in an antiparallel fashion.

Vascular development is believed to be a concerted mechanism that is a successive combination of three processes: vasculogenesis, angiogenesis, and arteriogenesis (Table 14.3).[26,27] Vasculogenesis is thought to occur exclusively in the embryonic period. It is defined as a process of differentiation of vascular progenitor cells into angioblastic cells which eventually form the endothelial layer of all vessels. The vasculogenesis process creates a haphazard network of immature cells that form angiocysts, which eventually fuse to form a primitive capillary plexus. The next process, angiogenesis, involves selective apoptosis along with the migration of supporting vascular smooth muscle cells to form a stable vascular bed. The interplay of these two processes during the embryonic stage requires multiple steps for cell proliferation, migration, differentiation, and programmed destruction. Any misstep during this stage could be the initiating factor in the formation of a congenital vascular malformation.

Although the interplay between vasculogenesis and angiogenesis during the embryological stage of development is thought to be the initiating factor in the formation of AVMs, arteriogenesis likely plays an important role in the later growth and remodeling of AVMs from the fetal stage onward. Both angiogenesis and arteriogenesis play a part in the maintenance and growth of AVMs into adulthood. Arteriogenesis, being mediated by vascular wall shear stress, is the likely mechanism by which an AVM with low resistance is able to recruit additional blood supply over time.

MOLECULAR BIOLOGY AND GENETICS

The study of the molecular changes with AVMs has revealed the altered expression of many factors that are known to have key roles in the developmental processes noted previously.

What is more interesting is that many are shared with cerebral neoplastic processes as well. This suggests that there may be a future role for targeted medical therapies based on the understanding of the abnormal molecular pathways initiated and sustained by these active lesions. Around 900 genes have been shown to have altered expression in AVMs.[26,28] Detailing the molecular factors implicated in the embryological development of cerebral vessels is beyond the scope of this chapter. However, a few of those factors that have abnormally high expression in AVMs when compared to normal brain tissue have been noted here.[26]

VEGF (vascular endothelial growth factor) has multiple subtypes that have been seen in increased amounts not only in AVMs but in the surrounding tissue. Additionally, VEGF receptors are noted to have altered expression patterns in AVMs. Normally, VEGF variants are expressed in high levels during embryonic development. They play a key factor in angiogenesis, vascular proliferation, and capillary migration. VEGF expression is normally suppressed in adulthood but can be rapidly increased by HIF-1 (hypoxia-induced factor) in response to a low oxygen microenvironment.

ANGs (angiopoetins) regulate the recruitment of smooth muscle cells and pericytes to endothelial cells are thought to promote vascular stabilization during angiogenesis.

FGFs (fibroblast growth factors) are thought to help differentiate progenitor cells to angioblasts during vasculogenesis. The differentiation of fibroblasts to smooth muscle cells is thought to be regulated by bFGF (basic fibroblast growth factor); it may participate in the arterialization of AVM veins.

The congenital theory of development can imply that an AVM begins as a response to some environmental abnormality during development or that a genetic alteration was initially responsible. In the case of the latter, genetic alterations may be sporadic or familial. Several genetic disease syndromes have been associated with an increased predisposition to harbor AVMs such as Wyburn-Mason syndrome, Sturge-Weber disease, and ataxia-telangiectasia.[24,26]

Osler-Weber-Rendu disease, also known as *hereditary hemorrhagic telangiectasia*, is an autosomal dominant disorder with variable penetrance. Genetic analysis has isolated two sources for mutation: *HHT1* is found on chromosome 9q and *HHT2* is found on chromosome 12q. Incidence for AVM in *HHT1* mutations is approximately 10 times higher than that for *HHT2*, which shows that different genetic mutations alter the risk of developing AVMs based on the function each encoded protein has during development.[29] In addition to known hereditary disorders, there have been AVM cases among families, suggesting a multifactorial genetic patterning to formation.

PHYSIOLOGY

The physiology of AVMs can be generally categorized into those of the malformation itself and those of the surrounding brain structures. Understanding the hemodynamics of arteriovenous shunts is a key concept.

Intracranial hemorrhage from an AVM is thought to occur when a vessel within the circuit ruptures. Typically this vessel is thought to be within the nidus or a draining vein, though an arterial feeder bleed may be possible. It is difficult to localize the exact source of hemorrhage within an AVM using current imaging modalities. Hemorrhage will occur when the stress exhibited within a vessel wall exceeds the limit for structural integrity. This may occur from either a decrease in the structural integrity limit of the wall or an increase in the stress delivered. The structural integrity limit of the wall depends on the material of the wall itself. The stress delivered depends on the pressure within the vessel along with the radius and the thickness of the vessel. Changes to the vessel shape and material composition can occur chronically over time as a result of biological processes, and pressure changes can vary relatively quickly. Aneurysms, for example, are biological processes that are known to increase the risk of rupture within an AVM by changing the structure and material composition of the vessel wall itself.

The hemodynamics of AVMs is a subject of continuing study. It is difficult to model an AVM using fluid dynamic models given their individual variability. Some electrical network analogies have been described in the literature in order to help conceptualize individual elements within a complex system.[30,31] For the scope of this chapter, it may be simpler to reduce the concept into flow rates and pressures through three structures—the feeding artery, the nidus, and the draining vein—of an AVM with one of each. In this model, for conservation of mass, any flow increase to one structure will be the same to all. Flow increase may be achieved, however, through increased feeding arterial pressure, decreased draining pressure, or decrease in the vascular resistance of the AVM by enlargement of the nidus. A nidus can enlarge by increasing the diameter of existing vessels or generating new ones. Note that if a nidus increase can bring about decreased vascular resistance, the feeding artery's pressure can either drop or its flow rate can increase until a new equilibrium is reached. For pressure to increase in a nidus, flow can be increased by increasing pressure in the feeding artery or flow can be decreased by increasing pressure (indirectly by increasing distal resistance) in the draining vein. This model neglects the fact that many AVMs are not so simple. Also, there is the possibility of capacitance, that is, the ability of the nidus to increase flow without necessarily increasing vascular resistance or, therefore, pressure.

With these concepts in mind, some general hemodynamic considerations in AVM therapies are as follows: (1) Decreasing flow is best effected by obstructing feeding arteries, and (2) decreasing flow by obstructing veins will increase intranidal pressures and, therefore, bleeding risk (Fig. 14.5).

Another hemodynamic consideration is that of the surrounding brain tissue. Increased shunting by a lower vascular resistance within an arteriovenous shunt does not occur in isolation. The congenital nature of the AVM implies that the surrounding normal brain tissue has developed with relatively lower vascular resistance than what would have normally occurred. As a result, the vascular beds of normal brain parenchyma surrounding the AVM are perfused at lower local arterial pressures. From this concept, two ideas have developed.

First, as the vascular resistance from the arteriovenous shunt decreases (possibly as a result of nidus enlargement), arterial blood will preferentially flow toward the shunt unless the normal brain tissue can reduce its resistance as well. This situation can progress until the normal brain can no longer match the arteriovenous shunt and becomes underperfused,

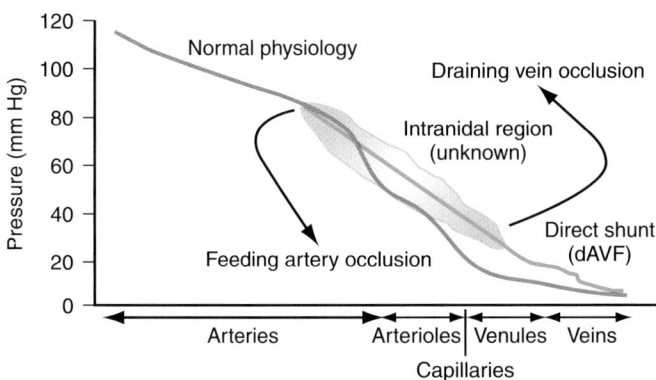

FIGURE 14.5 Conceptual comparison of intravascular pressure in a normal vascular bed versus an arteriovenous shunt. Normal vessels have high resistance in the arterial system causing significant pressure drops by the time blood reaches the capillary bed. Most arteriovenous shunts, by contrast, likely sustain higher pressures with associated higher vascular wall stresses. For a plexiform arteriovenous malformation (AVM), the pressures within the nidus cannot be measured but are likely variable depending on individual intranidal vessels. A direct shunt, by contrast, will experience a linear drop in pressure between the artery and vein. Occluding a feeding artery should bring down intranidal pressures but venous occlusion can do the opposite, thereby increasing risk of rupture.

causing neurological dysfunction. This phenonemenon, known as *vascular steal*, has been difficult to definitively demonstrate.[22] However, there are studies showing that patients with AVMs harbor neuropsychological dysfunction possibly as a result of this phenomenon.[32-34]

The second idea to develop from the arteriovenous shunting is that as adjacent tissues develop with lower perfusion pressures, they lose their ability to autoregulate their blood flow in response to normal pressure changes. Consequently, when the arteriovenous shunt is removed iatrogenically, overall systemic vascular resistance is increased, allowing for normal physiological perfusion pressures. As these capillary beds are not used to higher pressures, they tend to become hyperemic with increased risk for postresection hemorrhage. This phenomenon is known as *normal perfusion pressure breakthrough* (NPPB).[35]

Both of these phenomena have several common points. First, their existence is debated in the literature at the clinical and laboratory level. Second, their pathophysiology is related to the magnitude of arteriovenous shunting and they are therefore more likely to be encountered in larger AVMs. Finally, functional MRI (fMRI) has been used to assist in identifying eloquent brain structures for tumor surgery planning. One should be aware that fMRI utilizes cerebral blood flow changes at the microcirculatory level to determine functional brain activation. Because autoregulation is disrupted in normal brain tissue surrounding AVMs, however, this modality may produce false results (see Fig. 14.3).

EPIDEMIOLOGY AND NATURAL COURSE

The rarity of AVMs combined with their long period of clinical silence makes it difficult to estimate the overall prevalence of this disease. Two reviews, published in 2000[36] and 2001,[37]

highlighted the flaws with previous prevalence estimates along with difficulties in obtaining good estimates. Specifically, older prevalence estimates (500-600 per 100,000 population) were based on autopsy data, a source that is inherently biased. Another estimate (140 per 100,000 population) originated from an inappropriate analysis of data from the Cooperative Study of Intracranial Aneurysms and Subarachnoid Hemorrhage. Determining the true prevalence of AVMs would likely require MRI screening of more than 1 million asymptomatic persons to achieve reasonable confidence intervals. Estimates of incidence have been made by observing the specific geographic populations over time. These separate studies were reviewed[37] to find an incidence of approximately 1 per 100,000 person-years. The New York Islands AVM Study, published in 2003, found an average AVM detection rate of 1.34 per 100,000 person-years. The incidence of first ever hemorrhage was 0.51 per 100,000 person-years.[38]

For any patient presenting with an AVM, the risks of treatment should be weighed against the alternative of no intervention. Though extremely rare, AVMs have been known to spontaneously regress.[39,40] A small nidus and single draining vein were common factors. There has been an association between smaller AVMs and increased risk of rupture. This association may be attributable to higher feeding pressures in smaller AVMs.[41]

There have been numerous attempts to provide better assessments of the lifetime risk for hemorrhage. The oldest and most widely reported study from 1990 utilized prospective data on 160 Finnish patients followed for a mean period of 23.7 years.[42] Key characteristics of the patients in this study were that (1) they were the unoperated cohort of a total population of 262 AVM patients, and (2) they were all symptomatic (71% hemorrhage, 23% seizures, 6% other). The study reported an annual hemorrhage rate of 2% to 4% per year with a combined rate of morbidity and mortality to be 2.7% per year and mean time to hemorrhage of 7.7 years. Also, different initial presentation did not apparently change risk of hemorrhage.

In 2008 two studies were published on the Finnish AVM cohort.[43,44] The first was a comparison of long-term excess mortality against the general population. It showed that excess mortality rate was highest among patients with no treatment, but also that partially treated AVMs had a comparatively lower excess mortality rate. There was no excess mortality among the completely treated AVM group after 1 year. The second study was a natural history of 238 untreated patients for a mean period of 13.5 years. It showed the annual hemorrhage risk to be 2.4%. Importantly, however, the study showed that there is a higher hemorrhage risk of 4.7% in the first 5 years after diagnosis compared to 1.6% after 5 years. A multivariate analysis showed hemorrhage risk factors to include previous rupture, infratentorial and deep location, and large size.

The cumulative probability of an annualized risk for expected years of remaining life can be determined using the formula $p = [1 - (\text{risk of no hemorrhage})^n]$, where n is the number of years of expected life remaining.[45] The cumulative probability can also be simply approximated with the linear formula of $p = (105 - \text{age})/100$ (Fig. 14.6).[46]

In discussing possible treatment options with asymptomatic patients, there is always the difficulty of performing a

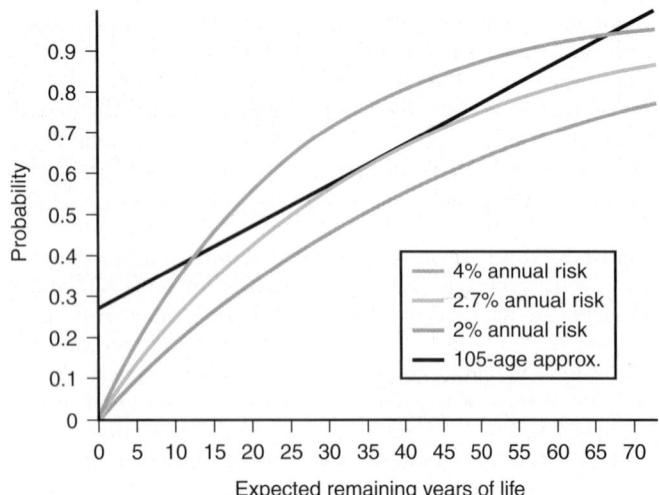

FIGURE 14.6 Applying the law of multiplicative probability, one can construct a risk curve for hemorrhage based on the expected years of life remaining using the various annual risks reported.[42] If one assumes a life expectancy of 78 years, the linear formula of "105 – Age" approximates the 2.7% per year risk profile between the ages of 25 to 55 when most arteriovenous malformations present themselves.[46]

potentially morbid procedure for a statistical probability. A study in 2005 showed that patients with AVMs that have hemorrhaged are less likely to worsen clinically after treatment because of the injury already caused by the hemorrhage, but elective AVM surgery is associated with a greater chance of clinical decline from baseline.[47] It would be ideal to have an accurate assessment of risk for an otherwise asymptomatic patient, whose AVM may have been detected by imaging modalities that were not in existence when the Finnish Database Study commenced. All studies to date have been biased toward symptomatic patients, the major symptom being hemorrhage. The ARUBA study, which began in 2008,[48] was designed to test the null hypothesis that any treatment offers no difference in the risk of death or symptomatic stroke, and no better functional outcome than does conservative management at 5 years from discovery of an unruptured AVM. Although the study is ongoing, the limitation of a 5-year follow-up has been called into question by the Finnish Database Study,[44] as evidence of benefits of partial treatment were seen after 5 to 7 years. The average interval between hemorrhages was noted to be 7 years.

Arteriovenous Malformations in the Pediatric Population

In the pediatric population, AVMs are the most likely pathology in spontaneous intracerebral hemorrhage.[49,50] As most AVMs are likely to present in the adult years, those that present in the pediatric age group usually have relatively more morbid sequelae that can have devastating consequences. Hemorrhage is the most likely presenting symptom, followed by seizures, congestive heart failure, and neurological deficit. Congestive heart failure is a symptom

seen mostly in the newborn population and is secondary to the large amount of left-to-right cardiovascular shunting that occurs from a clinically symptomatic AVM. This is most common in the distinct variety of AVM called the *vein of Galen malformation*. These newborns tend to have a poor prognosis, although recent advances in critical care support and neuroendovascular techniques have improved long-term outcomes.[51]

Surgically resected AVMs in the pediatric population have occasionally been observed to recur;[52] these patients, therefore, need long-term follow-up. A possible hypothesis involves the earlier mentioned concept of microshunting that is not apparent on angiography but that enlarges over time. This idea is also consistent with the observation that many pediatric AVMs grow in volume and degree of arteriovenous shunting.

Although hemorrhage is usually the presenting symptom in this group, patients overall tend to have a better recovery from initial deficits. Because of this and the higher lifetime risk of recurring hemorrhage from a pediatric AVM, it is necessary to consider aggressive treatment. Microsurgical resection with preoperative embolization, if necessary, is the preferred treatment unless the potential risk of neurological deficit is extremely high. The outcomes are excellent in children in our experience as well in that of others.

Arteriovenous Malformations and Pregnancy

As they are thought to be congenital lesions, AVMs are likely present during a woman's reproductive years. During pregnancy total blood volume can increase by up to 40% while cardiac output can increase by up to 60% to match the increasing vascular bed demanded by the fetus.[53] Arterial pressures can vary during pregnancy; however, hypertension can occur near delivery. Although these hemodynamic alterations during pregnancy have been thought to play a participating role in the occurrence of AVM hemorrhage, it is unclear as to whether there is an increased statistical risk. It is, however, believed that pregnancy does increase the risk of hemorrhage. It generally tends to occur in the second and the third trimesters and the early postpartum period.

If a pregnant patient presents with a hemorrhage from an AVM, the risk of rebleed during the same pregnancy can be up to 27%;[54] this risk can be mitigated only with total resection of the AVM. Treating an AVM during pregnancy, however, entails risks to both mother and fetus. Given its risks to the fetus and its slow rate of occlusion, radiosurgery is not a viable option during pregnancy. Endovascular therapies, even as an adjunct, pose the added risks of exposing the fetus to radiation, intravenous (IV) contrast agent, and embolic solvents. Therefore, microsurgical resection may be the only tool if the patient wishes to have treatment before delivery. In general, definitive treatment of the AVM should be deferred until after the pregnancy is over. The patient needs to be followed in a high-risk pregnancy setting and delivered by cesarean section.

If a patient presents with a life-threatening intracranial hemorrhage, immediate surgical evacuation is necessary for stabilization. Otherwise, a careful discussion with the patient and the family should be done regarding the risks of hemorrhage and disability with intervention. Pregnant

FIGURE 14.7 **A,** Posterior fossa arteriovenous malformation with flow-related, pedicular artery aneurysm arising from the left superior cerebellar artery. **B,** Endovascular occlusion of the aneurysm was safely achieved, leaving the nidus to be treated by a surgical modality later with less operative exposure.

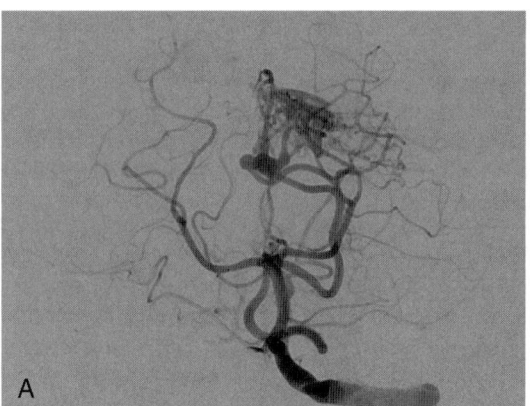
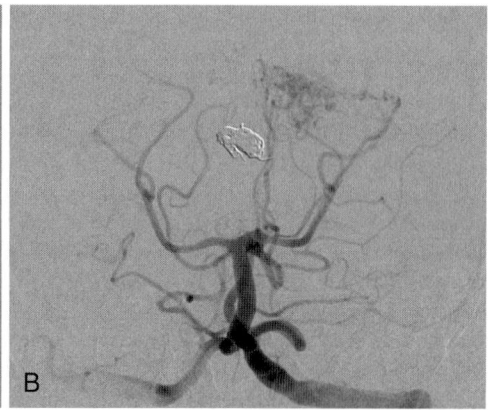

patients with unruptured AVMs should consider definitive treatment after parturition. These patients may present with seizures that are best controlled medically with anticonvulsants. The patient should be made aware that although these medications may pose a minimal teratogenic risk, especially in the first trimester, they provide the safest option for both mother and child as opposed to immediate surgical treatment.[54]

Arteriovenous Malformations and Aneurysms

AVMs presenting with aneurysms pose a special challenge because both are vascular pathological lesions with potentially devastating consequences. However, there is a definite relationship between the two.[55] The increased flow associated with AVM vessels is thought to predispose them to aneurysm formation because their walls will experience higher shear stress. Generally aneurysms with AVMs can be characterized into four types:[56] (1) unrelated to flow vessels (remote); (2) arising at the circle of Willis origin of a vessel supplying the AVM (proximal); (3) arising from the midcourse of a feeding pedicle (pedicular); and (4) arising from within the nidus itself (intranidal). The latter three types can be classified as "flow-related" aneurysms.

The variability in structures of AVMs has made their behavior with aneurysms difficult to predict. Nevertheless, aneurysm rupture is a possible clinical consequence that patients should be aware of. The risk of a ruptured aneurysm should always be kept in mind when evaluating a patient with intracranial hemorrhage. In this setting, a neurosurgeon may not have the luxury of a multidisciplinary team and should, therefore, be prepared. There are some general principles to note. First, a four-vessel cerebral angiogram, CTA, or MRA with adequate visualization of all major arteries should always be attempted to rule aneurysms out. Second, the risk of aneurysm rerupture is higher in the acute setting and the risk of morbidity and death from an aneurysmal subarachnoid hemorrhage is higher compared to an AVM. Third, most aneurysms can be secured using surgery or endovascular coiling, but the resectability of AVMs is not always assured. Fourth, flow-related aneurysms associated with AVMs have been known to regress spontaneously after AVM resection.[57] Finally, if an AVM bleeds, there may be morphological changes to the nidus and associated vessels that preclude an accurate characterization in the acute setting. With these

principles in mind the important questions to ask during an evaluation for hemorrhage are as follows:

1. Where is the aneurysm (as defined in the preceding paragraph)?
2. Which pathological entity was responsible for the hemorrhage? If there is subarachnoid blood, one may suspect the aneurysm; however, one cannot rule out a nidus on the cortical surface. If there is uncertainty, one should assume the aneurysm has ruptured.
3. Is the AVM sufficiently visualized?
4. If it is well visualized, can it be safely treated surgically?

If the AVM is surgically treatable and the aneurysm can be secured, then it is advisable to treat both in the same setting. If there is any question, however, to the resectability of the AVM, then it is advisable to treat the aneurysm by any means acutely and leave the nidus alone for later, multidisciplinary management (Fig. 14.7).

Intranidal aneurysms are a special case. First, as they can reside within a nidus, they can be difficult to visualize on any imaging modality. Second, it can be difficult to diagnose an intranidal aneurysm rupture as a cause for hemorrhage. Third, its location within the nidus means that any surgical or radiosurgical treatment will deal with it simultaneously. Therefore, an AVM with an intranidal aneurysm should be treated together surgically. If radiosurgery is being considered or if the nidus is considered unresectable, one should consider a limited endovascular embolic therapy with the goal of occluding the arterial pedicle that feeds the aneurysm. In unruptured patients it is unclear if intranidal aneurysms increase the risk of future hemorrhage.

TREATMENT

Patients presenting with hemorrhage need treatment based on the degree of hemorrhage and the neurological status. Unlike an aneurysm, the risk of immediate rebleeding is relatively low, but early treatment without advanced understanding of the specific AVM characteristics can be dangerous. Therefore, unless there is a life-threatening hematoma requiring immediate surgical evacuation, treatment of an AVM is delayed to allow time for the hemorrhage to resolve and the AVM to stabilize its architecture for treatment planning. This allows for the brain swelling to improve, so there is better tolerance for surgical manipulation. It also allows for better assessment of the nidus whether looking at microsurgery or radiosurgery as the definitive treatment. If the patient is neurologically deteriorating, urgent intervention is necessary. Immediate treatment of hydrocephalus with a ventriculostomy may be indicated. A CTA can give a good idea about the nidus if it is large enough. If the neurological condition allows, an angiogram is desirable. Preferably one would decompress the hematoma while avoiding the AVM. Attempting to more completely remove the hematoma can result in bleeding from the nidus or premature venous rupture. In case of significant brain swelling, adding a dural patch and leaving a large bone flap out is extremely helpful. It is preferable to wait 4 to 6 weeks before undertaking the definitive treatment. The likelihood of rebleeding, though possible, is extremely rare.

When considering definitive treatment, the following options are available:

1. Medical or symptomatic management
2. Embolization
3. Microsurgery
4. Radiosurgery
5. Multimodality therapy

The treatment decision requires that multiple factors be considered, and each patient requires individualized assessment. It is best to have a multidisciplinary team consisting of a vascular neurosurgeon, neuroendovascular specialist, and radiation oncologist. The main considerations are as follows:

1. Size of AVM
2. Location
3. Vascular anatomy
4. Age
5. Medical condition

Medical Management

Medical management or nonintervention is indicated when the patient may have suffered a devastating neurological deficit. The malformation may be very extensive, located deep in the brain, with blood supply primarily from deep perforating vessels, which are not amenable to endovascular or radiosurgical treatment. Very advanced age would also be a consideration for symptomatic therapy. Obviously poor medical condition, such as advanced heart disease, respiratory insufficiency, or cancer with metastasis, would be a contraindication to a definitive AVM treatment. Symptomatic treatment refers to management of nonhemorrhagic sequelae such as AEDs for seizure control.

Embolization

The advancement of applications in interventional neuroradiology has led to its application in the treatment of AVMs.[58,59] Although the treatment of certain AVMs may be possible with interventional techniques alone and the technologies are evolving, embolization is not yet considered an exclusive general treatment for most AVMs for two reasons. First, AVMs that are embolized have a rate of permanent morbidity between 4% and 14%.[60] Second, if the goal of AVM cure is considered to be complete obliteration of the nidus with

no remaining arteriovenous shunting, then current techniques are not yet at the point where *any* vessel of *any* size and location can be safely embolized without risk of perforation or cerebral infarcts. Additionally, attempting to arrest all arteriovenous shunting visualized on angiography can result in eventual reconstitution of shunting by recanalization or de novo vascular development, depending on the embolized vessel's reaction.

The general technique of AVM embolization is similar to that of aneurysm or tumor embolization. Using transfemoral access, the intracerebral vasculature is accessed with a microcatheter. Selected feeding arteries are isolated and various agents are delivered in an attempt to reduce the arteriovenous shunt. An overall danger to avoid throughout the procedure is the avoidance of premature venous outflow occlusion, which can cause AVM rupture. This is especially difficult in endovascular cases because a well-occluded shunt may not allow for adequate visualization of the draining veins and the lack of surgical access precludes quick control of a bleed.

Because embolization is usually done as part of a multimodality approach, it is important that the embolization plan be discussed with the neurosurgeon and radiosurgeon prior to commencing the procedure in order to understand the goals of embolization, which can vary depending on the subsequent treatment. For example, a radiosurgeon may want overall nidus volume reduction as a primary goal in order to bring it within the limits of safe radiation dosing. The tradeoff, however, may be to complicate the overall geometric shape of the nidus beyond the ability of a radiation delivery device, such as the gamma knife. For microsurgery, preoperative embolization can offer several options. In addition to nidus reduction, one may attempt to reduce the overall flow of the arteriovenous shunt by occluding the largest feeders in order to reduce the risk of blood loss during the surgery. Finally, one may attempt to embolize the feeding arteries that may be deemed too difficult to access during surgery.[61] Typically these arteries lie deep to the nidus during exposure and may hinder its manipulation. The vessels may vary, depending on which approach the surgeon is considering, so it is difficult to consider general "rules" for the best vessels to embolize. The tradeoff of embolization is that total occlusion may induce normal perfusion pressure breakthrough, especially in large AVMS. Staged embolization over multiple sessions may overcome this problem and can be considered an advantage compared to microneurosurgery because it is easier to perform these minimally invasive procedures multiple times. Another tradeoff to consider is that large amounts of embolic material in the nidus may hinder intraoperative mobilization by making it too stiff. One of the advantages of AVM resections over neoplasms is that they are generally more compressible and, if carefully manipulated, can be moved more easily than a meningioma, for example.

Embolic Agents

Several types of agents have been used in endovascular embolizations of AVMs.[62] It is important for neurosurgeons to have a basic idea of their capabilities and limitations in order to effectively communicate with their interventional colleagues in deciding the best possible treatment. Embolic agents generally can be classified into three categories: occlusive devices, microparticles, and liquids.

Occlusive Devices

Occlusive devices include balloons for large vessel occlusions, braided silk threads which are highly thrombogenic, and coils. Fibered coils, in particular, are usually platinum coils with polyester fibers attached to increase thrombogenicity. Coils can be used to permanently occlude larger arterial feeders. They can also be used via a transvenous route in the case of dAVFs to more safely occlude a fistula.[62]

Particles

Many earlier reports of embolizations used particles, specifically, polyvinyl alcohol (PVA) (Counter PVA particles, Boston Scientific, Fremont, CA). These particles are irregularly shaped and can have slight variations in size such that a selection of 50-µm particles can range from 50 to 100 µm. Selected sizes generally range from 45 to 1180 µm.[63] Appropriate particle size selection should be considered in AVMs because of the need to avoid having particles that are too small to lodge within the nidus. A fistulous connection, for example, is generally too large for any particles. In AVMs one can never know the exact sizes of the largest and smallest nidus vessels.

In general, the technique of particle embolization involves mixing with contrast material before injecting. During injection, it is of paramount importance that the particles do not reflux into *en passage* or transit vessels and occlude capillary beds of normal brain tissue; this is difficult to ascertain, however, as the particles themselves are radiolucent.

Particle embolization of AVMs has slowly fallen out of favor as early experiences showed a high recanalization rate after angiographically confirmed obliteration. Histological analysis of embolized vessels showed a heterogeneous mixture of particles with thrombus. Embospheres (Biosphere Medical, Rockland, MA) are trisacryl gelatin microspheres of uniform size and spherical shape and may better "pack" vessels than PVA particles. Another difficulty noted with particulate embolization was the lack of being able to tell whether the particles were lodged in the nidus or simply obstructed the feeding artery. If the latter, a patent nidus may simply recruit new vasculature by the mechanisms of angiogenesis and arteriogenesis mentioned earlier. It is possible that the early dismal results of AVM recanalization by exclusive embolic therapies were attributable to this. However, it is more important to realize this is a long-term deficiency. Hence, particle embolization may not be suitable as part of a combined treatment with radiosurgery. On the other hand, particle embolization may allow for a more pliable nidus intraoperatively and may, thus, be a benefit when performed shortly in advance of microsurgical resection.

Liquids

Two liquid agents are currently in use in the United States for embolization: NBCA and EVOH (Onyx). The primary difference is in their mechanical properties for delivery. It is advisable to observe the delivery of these agents in the interventional suite to get an idea of their capabilities and weaknesses (Fig. 14.8).

N-Butyl cyanoacrylate (NBCA) (Trufill NBCA Liquid Embolic, Cordis Endovascular) is a monomer stabilized in a

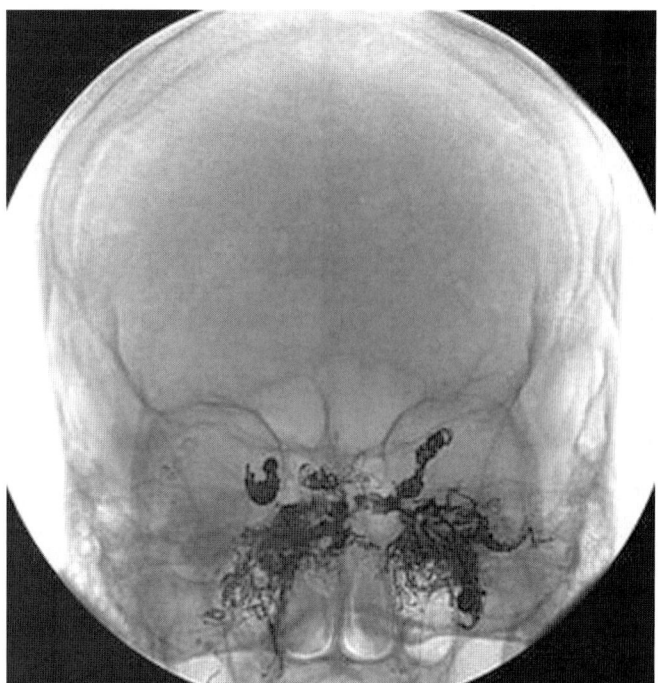

FIGURE 14.8 Digital fluoroscopic image of a skull after successive endovascular treatments using both coils and liquid embolic agents. The patient was being treated for a transosseus arteriovenous malformation.

hydrophobic ethiodol solution mixed with tantalum for radiopacity; it is also used as a fast-acting skin adhesive (Indermil) and is a chemical variant of superglue. On contact with an ionic solution such as blood, NBCA polymerizes to form a solid cast that strongly adheres to surrounding structures such as the endothelium of a nidus vessel. The rate of polymerization can be manipulated by varying the amount of ethiodol, and this property can be used to plan the amount of penetration. As an example, a fast-flowing fistulous connection may require instant polymerization on exiting the delivery catheter but a large, plexiform nidus may require more time for the liquid to cast the distal portions of the vascularized pedicle. Critical events during the procedure include prevention of polymer flowing past the shunt into the venous circulation, risking pulmonary embolism, as well as rapid removal of the catheter following delivery to avoid refluxing polymer adhesion. Although older than EVOH, NBCA enjoys widespread usage from continued experience along with a microcatheter delivery system that allows for easier manipulation than EVOH in tortuous AVM feeders.[63,64]

EVOH (ethylene and vinyl alcohol) is also known as Onyx (Micro Therapeutics, Irvine, CA). It is a copolymer that is mixed with tantalum powder and dissolved in DMSO (dimethyl sulfoxide). On injection, the copolymer precipitates as the DMSO diffuses, in a lava-like manner. The outer portion remains nonadhesive but solidifies as the central core continues to flow. This pliable effect can be used in a slower, more controlled manner to selectively embolize the vasculature over a longer period of time. The DMSO solvent can remain in the patient's system for several days with a distinctive odor. Patients should be reassured that it is safe in therapeutic quantities.[63,65]

Timing Between Embolization and Surgery

In the case of a combination of embolization followed by a surgical procedure, the timing between the procedures is a continuing question. Staging an embolization over multiple sessions may be necessary if there is a large arteriovenous shunt. However, if vascular pedicles are slowly taken out by embolization, more time may be required for the autoregulation in the brain surrounding the AVM to assume a new equilibrium. While surgery is delayed, embolization can alter the hemodynamics of an AVM nidus and the risk of hemorrhage is increased.

Microsurgery

Preoperative Management and Anesthesia

Prior to general anesthesia induction, it is important to communicate to the anesthesiologist the unique nature of AVM surgery and the risk for hemorrhage. For every procedure, an arterial line is a requirement. The use of central lines can be reserved for large AVMs, extended procedures, or patient positions in which an air embolism is a concern. The use of saline instead of lactated Ringer's solution is advised because the latter can cause edema if the blood-brain barrier is disrupted. Maintenance of the hematocrit above 30% is an advisable intraoperative goal and the patient should have compatible blood available for transfusion. When potential excessive bleeding is anticipated, a cell saver should be set up along with the availability of other blood products such as fresh frozen plasma and platelets. The use of volume expanders such as hetastarch can interfere with platelet function and prolong coagulation times and should, therefore, be avoided. For cerebral edema, the anesthesiologist should maintain a $PaCO_2$ of 30 to 35 mm Hg. Mannitol can be given in doses up to 1 g/kg for cerebral volume reduction if needed. As it takes approximately 15 minutes to take effect, the surgeon should plan its administration around the time the bone flap is turned. Lasix can be given simultaneously to enhance its effect.

Positioning

The general principles to keep in mind when positioning and designing a craniotomy are similar to those for any intracranial mass lesion. First, a lesion should ideally be perpendicular to the surgeon's line of sight with the caveat that no unresectable structure is interposed. Second, the working corridor should be as short as possible to allow for minimal retraction and a comfortable working length. Third, gravity should be kept in mind as an aide to retraction and drainage. A special consideration to be added in positioning for an AVM is the locations of the arterial feeders, which must be isolated and eliminated before the nidus can be resected. Therefore, a larger craniotomy can sometimes be necessary to assist in locating these feeders, as well as having a broader perspective of the malformation.

General Surgical Principles

The microsurgical resection of an AVM must take into consideration the complex nature of its feeding arteries and draining veins. Because this is a three-dimensional structure that is generally approachable by a limited number of angles, it is critical to have in mind which structures one should be seeing at each level of the procedure. Bear in mind that angiographic pictures only relay two-dimensional projections and a good neurosurgeon must use his or her mind's eye to visualize that structure from a different perspective.

The first objective in any AVM resection is the identification of the general location of the nidus. MRI is a useful tool for navigation, especially for those AVMs that are deeply situated. Although one can use preoperative imaging along with general anatomical knowledge, frameless stereotactic guidance is another useful tool.

Knowing where the nidus is, one next should attempt to localize all the major feeding arteries and draining veins with the goal of isolating the arteries only and disconnecting them from the nidus. Ideally, the surgeon should study the preoperative angiogram to know not only the location of these arteries but also the order in which he or she plans to encounter them during the approach. Occasionally, for large, diffuse AVMs, angiographic planning is limited by rapid nidus opacification. In this case, there are some general concepts one should keep in mind during the dissection. First, the ectatic, high blood flow and irregular pattering of AVM vessels generally give them a different appearance under direct visualization compared to normal cerebral vessels. Second, feeding arteries can usually be distinguished from draining veins not by sight, as the veins will usually have arterialized blood, but by noting if the distal vessel collapses with gentle occlusion. Third, unless there is definite evidence on an angiogram that an artery is a direct nidus feeder, the surgeon should always secure the feeding artery as close to the nidus as possible to ensure this is no *en passage* artery feeding normal brain.

Securing the individual vessels can be done with bipolar coagulation. However, the pathological nature of the AVM vessel wall may not allow it to be sufficiently coagulated to withstand arterial pressures. At the same time, many vessels may have walls that are too thin to close for coagulation. In many neurosurgical procedures, surgeons often place the bipolar tips in close approximation with the open vessel, usually a vein, in between the vessel wall while the electrical field generated by the tip delivers enough energy into the thin vessel walls to allow for coagulation. It is important to realize that this effect may be mitigated in AVM vessels by high blood flow transferring energy out of the vessel walls, thereby keeping them at a subcoagulation temperature. Therefore, arterial aneurysm clips should always be loaded and ready for use, especially for larger feeding arteries. For smaller vessels, Sundt vascular microclips were designed for this purpose and could be used. Another issue to consider during small vessel coagulation is that excessive bipolar usage or premature disconnection can cause a small vessel to retract into normal parenchymal tissue. Again, although in many other neurosurgical procedures, placing cotton with gentle pressure and patience may arrest this bleeding, the high flow associated with AVMs may not allow this technique to work. In the majority of instances it is feasible to occlude the vessels with bipolar coagulation by keeping the power low and occluding the vessel gradually. In our own experience it has been rarely necessary to use the clips. Occasionally, however, a larger feeder may be occluded with a temporary aneurysm clip while the actual smaller feeding vessels are isolated and occluded.

With the arteries identified and secured, dissection of the nidus can begin. Ideally, one should try to move around the nidus to separate it from the surrounding brain superficially and progress around the edges with minimal manipulation of either the brain or nidus. There may be difficulty in developing a surgical plane between the nidus and surrounding brain tissue. If the patient has had a previous hemorrhage, there is usually a residual margin, which can be a good starting point for dissection. The hemorrhage plane rarely envelops the entire nidus. Often during a surgical approach, one encounters the hemorrhage cavity with a portion of the nidus found on one side. While proceeding with the nidus dissection, one should maintain a uniform depth with circumferential separation to avoid encountering a poorly visualized vessel without the luxury of a mobilized nidus. It is possible that encountering excessive bleeding may mean that one's dissection plane has penetrated the nidus. In this case, the surgeon should attempt to dissect a wider margin or reassess anatomical landmarks to ensure he or she is not straying off course.

Unlike a tumor, it is impossible to attempt to internally debulk the nidus in hopes of mobilizing its boundaries during surgery. It is difficult to judge the flow patterns within the nidus intraoperatively based on the feeding arteries that have been secured and one cannot be assured of easy hemostasis once the nidus has been penetrated. One advantage of surgical manipulation of a nidus compared to a solid tumor, however, is that its dynamic nature makes it relatively more compressible than the surrounding normal brain tissue. As more feeders are isolated and secured, the intranidal pressure can decrease and allow for more manipulation. One unfortunate side effect of nidus embolization is that the liquid embolic agents, when solidified, reduce this compressibility. However, embolized sections of the nidus can be removed provided there is no collateral circulation, although one must exercise extreme caution in that the forces required to break apart the embolized nidus are large and can easily rip apart vessels attached to the remaining, vascularized, portion.

Deep arteries are generally encountered last. In general, a still well-vascularized nidus can be lying between the surgeon and these vessels. Embolization can help minimize the difficulties with securing larger vessels. Small deep perforators, such as lenticulostriate arteries, however, are difficult to embolize preoperatively and even coagulate intraoperatively for the reasons previously mentioned. Excessive bipolar coagulation usage can cause retraction into eloquent tissue and significant neurological morbidity.

As individual arteries are secured from the AVM, one can notice the gradual loss of arterialized blood in the nidus and draining veins. One of the principles of AVM resection is that the draining veins be preserved at all costs to avoid an intranidal pressure increase, which may facilitate rupture. Often, however, this is impractical, especially if the veins are superficial to the nidus, thereby tethering it in a way that prevents easy manipulation. In these situations, one must use judgment to determine what would be gained by prematurely disconnecting a vein. Ideally, the last structures to be secured before removing the nidus are the draining veins. When resecting the nidus and securing the draining veins, one should exercise caution to note if small feeding arteries are still attached.

During surgical resection, there is always the possibility of intraoperative hemorrhage. It is important to know the cause of hemorrhage in order to secure it as quickly as possible because these bleeds can precipitate large blood loss. Hemorrhage can, of course, come from the nidus itself as a result of trauma during manipulation or spontaneous rupture. If this is the case, the most appropriate initial action is to rapidly place a cotton ball over the location with the least pressure possible to arrest or even slow down the blood loss enough to visualize its source for focal hemostasis. If the hemorrhage source appears to be deep within the nidus, it is inadvisable to explore the nidus itself because of the risk of creating multiple hemorrhages that are difficult to control. Rather, rapid isolation of the suspected vascular pedicle should be attempted while anesthesia is notified of the blood loss. Surgical assistants should exercise caution with excessive suctioning because a nidus or arterialized vein can easily tear again.

If the bleeding cannot be localized to a focal point within the nidus, then the arterial feeders should be reexamined to ensure one did not reopen. As mentioned earlier, smaller arterial feeders may retract into the parenchyma, preventing easy visualization. Alternatively, hemorrhage may originate from normal perfusion pressure breakthrough in the surrounding parenchyma, which may manifest first by rapid edema. However, as mentioned earlier, in our own experience this is rare if at all present. This situation usually is the result of having a portion of the nidus outside the line of resection.

Blood pressure reduction and packing of the surgical cavity may assist in localizing the hemorrhage, followed by more aggressive surgical exploration, knowing that the tradeoff is increased morbidity.

Surgical Approaches

Even though many of the small, deeper malformations are currently being treated with radiosurgery, they are also treatable microsurgically and actually successfully. For deeper AVMs surgical approaches generally fall into three categories: transcortical, transcortical-transventricular, or interhemispheric (Table 14.4).[66,67] The presence of intraventricular hemorrhage from a deep AVM usually requires a transcortical-transventricular or an interhemispheric route. Each approach has advantages and complications. Cortical incisions risk injury to eloquent cortex and epileptogenesis. Interhemispheric routes offer limited, deep exposure of medial structures with risks to bridging veins and complications associated with callosotomy. Transventricular routes can cause bleeding into the CSF circulation, risking hydrocephalus and chronic shunt dependence.

Postoperative Management

Patients should be admitted to the intensive care unit (ICU) for at least 24 hours with continued arterial blood pressure control and neurological checks. Depending on the size of the AVM, its location, the surgical approach, and the patient's neurological status, continued ICU observation may be indicated. It is generally advisable to undergo an angiogram to confirm total resection of the AVM prior to discharge. If the resection was incomplete, a reopening of the craniotomy can be done during the same admission. Postoperative complications include hemorrhage, seizures, cerebral edema, and postsurgical infarcts especially related to venous occlusions.

TABLE 14.4 Surgical Approaches to Deep Arteriovenous Malformations (AVMs) with Intraventricular Hemorrhage

Approach	AVM Location
Transcortical-Transventricular Approaches	
1. Middle frontal	Caudate head; anterolateral thalamus
2. Parietal	Posterolateral thalamus; trigone
3. Middle temporal	Trigone
4. Anterior and inferior temporal	Trigone
5. Temporoparietal	Trigone
6. Occipital	Trigone
Interhemispheric Approaches	
1. Transcallosal (rostrum)	Caudate head; anteromedial thalamus; anterior third ventricle
2. Transcallosal (splenium)	Posteromedial thalamus; posterior third ventricle
3. Retrocallosal	Parasplenial-retrosplenial; medial occipital horn
Transcortical Approaches to Nonhemorrhagic Deep AVMs	
1. Middle frontal	Dorsal AVMs (caudate head)
2. Orbitofrontal	Anterior perforated substance; deep basal ganglia
3. Transinsular	Putamen; external capsule
4. Combined middle frontal transsylvian	Dorsal AVMs

Radiosurgery

Stereotactic radiosurgery has been recognized as a major treatment modality for AVMs. The goal of radiosurgery is delivery of sufficient ionizing radiation to the complete nidus volume to obliterate arteriovenous shunting. The major advantage of radiosurgery is the ability to treat the AVM without a craniotomy, and thus, radiosurgery has been proposed as an ideal alternative to microsurgery in patients with comorbid conditions as well as those harboring AVMs that may be difficult to resect. Obliteration rates can vary from 60% to 85% and are highly dependent on the nidus size.

There are drawbacks to radiosurgery for AVMs, however. First, as the radiation induces a biological effect that is dependent on cellular mitosis, there is a considerable delay of 2 to 5 years between treatment and nidus obliteration. During this time, there is no reduction in the risk of hemorrhage. Applying the 2.7% annual rate[42] leaves a 2- to 5-year actuarial risk of 5.3% to 12.7%; note that this risk would be even higher if the AVM has recently ruptured. In a similar manner, the potential morbidities from radiosurgery may develop over time. Complications not related to the AVM include the effects of radiation delivery to surrounding functional tissue. These effects have been studied more in relation to treatment for neoplastic diseases and include postradiation edema, cyst formation, and radionecrosis.

When discussing radiosurgery with a patient it is important that the patient realize that a risk that is spread out over 2 years should be weighed against the upfront risk of possible surgical resection that would, if successful, obliterate the risk of hemorrhage immediately. On the other hand, the risk of complications secondary to surgical or endovascular treatment, such as normal perfusion pressure breakthrough or premature venous occlusion, is minimal.

High-dose radiation is believed to induce an inflammatory response in the vascular walls of the nidus with loss of endothelium and proliferation of smooth muscle cells.[29] Because the AVM is a biologically dynamic structure, it has the ability to compensate if the radiation dose is insufficient. Radiosurgeons typically prescribe an isodose shell, defined as a set of all points within a plan that receive the same radiation dose. The objective is to match the minimum isodose shell to the periphery of a nidus. As an example, a nidus border that is set to 18 Gy to the 70% isodose line means that the periphery of the nidus will receive 18 Gy while points interior will receive up to $18/0.7 = 25.7$ Gy. The dose delivered to the periphery is highly correlated to the rate of obliteration. Typically, an AVM with a small, compact nidus will be easily covered by an isodose conformation. As the volume becomes higher the radiosurgeon must either decrease the radiation delivered to the periphery of the nidus by reducing the isodose shell (risking nonobliteration) or increase the overall amount of radiation (risking increased complications). A nidus volume that is less than 3 mL or a nidus that is smaller than 2 cm in its largest dimension, therefore, is a good predictor of successful AVM obliteration.[68-70] Other factors include sharp delineation of the nidus border on imaging, younger age, fewer draining veins, and hemispheric location.[71]

A potential complication of radiosurgery is the inaccurate localization of the nidus for targeting. Older treatments based on angiography for stereotactic localization of the nidus suffered from the modality's lack of allowing for adequate, three-dimensional dose planning of complex shapes. MRI can identify a nidus location with good spatial resolution and should be used along with an angiogram for stereotactic targeting. However, as most AVMs present with hemorrhage, it is important to realize that the mass effect from the hemorrhage may distort the nidus or even occlude a related blood vessel to the point that sufficient visualization for targeting is unobtainable in any modality. In this case, one should repeat the relevant studies after a period of about 4 to 6 weeks to let the nidus achieve a stable geometry before radiosurgery is performed.

A conservative definition of radiosurgery treatment failure would be persistent arteriovenous shunting demonstrated on angiography 5 years after treatment. Options for therapy include revisiting multimodality treatment.[72,73]

DURAL ARTERIOVENOUS FISTULAS

As mentioned earlier, dAVFs (also called dAVMs) are not thought to be congenital, but acquired. The dura is a vascularized structure that has a blood supply that is distinct from the rest of the brain. Most dAVFs occur adjacent to the venous sinuses.[74] The dural walls form several sinuses functioning as conduits for cerebral venous drainage. There is the opportunity for arteriovenous shunting between the arterial vessels supplying the dura and the sinuses themselves. A simple conceptualization of the formation of a dural arteriovenous shunt may be the rupture of a small artery due to a trauma that, in other compartmentalized tissues, may tamponade itself.

The relatively low pressure of the adjacent venous drainage, however, leads to a high-flow fistula that is unable to spontaneously thrombose. Infection may pose a similar effect. Most fistulas, however, are idiopathic. Adjacent venous sinus thrombosis has been known to be related to dAVFs and has been theorized to be the triggering factor.[75] Thrombosis may precipitate dissolution of microvessels within the sinus secondary to venous hypertension or the release of pro-angiogenesis factors. Like brain AVMs, these fistulas are biologically active and thus are able to recruit additional arterial supply (including intracranial arteries) over time. Despite their acquired nature, however, they are rarer than AVMs, usually composing 10% to 15% of all high-flow arteriovenous shunts. Most are seen in the region of the transverse and sigmoid sinuses.[76] Other locations include the cavernous, straight, petrosal, and superior sagittal sinuses. Carotid cavernous fistulas (CCFs) have been classified into four types based on the feeding arteries involved.[77] The type A variant, involving direct communication between the internal carotid artery and cavernous sinus, can usually be brought about by trauma or a cavernous carotid aneurym. However, types B, C, and D can be considered dAVFs based on the supply from meningeal internal carotid artery branches (B), meningeal external carotid artery branches (C), or both (D).

Like the AVM, the main morbidity risk of dAVF is intracranial hemorrhage from rupture. Unlike an AVM, however, dAVFs do not usually have a well-defined nidus. This difference may make their pathological behavior similar to that of a fistulous brain AVM. Another difference with brain AVMs is that the anatomical presentation influences the risk of rupture. The mechanical strength of the vessel wall of the dural sinuses is much larger than that of an intracranial vein, allowing the sinus to withstand arterial pressures with minimal risk of rupture. The risk of hemorrhage and neurological deficit is increased, however, with cortical vein involvement.[74] This has led to classification schemes based more on patterns of venous drainage than size, shape, or location. The Borden and Cognard classification systems (Table 14.5) are commonly used.[74,78] Although the Borden scheme is simpler, the advantage of the Cognard scheme is that it uses the dynamics of angiography to incorporate the direction of venous flow in the sinus which may cause venous congestion to cortical veins that are not exhibiting reflux.[74,78] Proper classification is important in order to assess the necessity of treatment.

Other clinical findings in patients with dAVF include bruit, pulsatile tinnitus, headache, papilledema, seizures, or neurological deficit. In CCFs, increased intraocular pressures can lead to visual deficits and may necessitate an emergent therapy. Because a significant proportion of these lesions have associated complete or partial thrombosis of the involved sinuses, the intracranial pressure can be significantly increased, leading to associated symptoms, especially papilledema. It also results in rather bizarre venous drainage patterns, as evident by Cognard classification.

The routine MRI may not show sufficient changes to suspect the diagnosis of a smaller fistula. One has to pay special attention to flow voids on the surface of the brain or in the soft tissues. Routine MRA may also miss the lesion unless it is of significant size. Visualization of a sinus on an MRA should raise the possibility. The source images of an MRA are actually very useful not only in suspecting the diagnosis, but also

TABLE 14.5 Classification Systems for Dural Arteriovenous Fistulas with Recommended Treatment Strategy

Type	Venous Drainage Pattern	Recommendation
Borden Classification		
I	Into venous sinus or meningeal vein	Observation
II	Into venous sinus with cortical venous reflux	Treatment
III	Into cortical veins only	Treatment
Cognard Classification		
I	Into venous sinus with antegrade flow	Observation
IIa	Into venous sinus with retrograde flow	Treatment if symptomatic
IIb	Into venous sinus with antegrade flow and cortical venous reflux	Treatment
IIa + IIb	Into venous sinus with retrograde flow and cortical venous reflux	Treatment
III	Into cortical veins only	Treatment
IV	Into cortical veins only with venous ectasia	Treatment
V	Into spinal perimedullary vein	Treatment

getting an estimation of feeders and drainage. The ones associated with ectasia and venous aneurysms are much more easily visualized on T2 MRI sequences.

It is critical to make the distinction between dAVFs with direct sinus drainage versus associated or direct cortical venous drainage (Fig. 14.9). Treatment decisions, being dependent on making this distinction, require absolutely detailed selective and superselective angiography including the external carotids as well as vertebral arteries. This also allows for the assessment in planning the treatment, if felt necessary.

As in the case of brain AVMs, the treatment of dAVFs requires a multimodality effort with goals of relieving symptoms and reducing the risk of intracranial hemorrhage. Characterization of the symptoms as benign or aggressive can also help with decision making. Options for treatment include observation in patients with type I dAVFs with benign symptoms. Occasionally pulsatile tinnitus can be so debilitating that treatment is sought. The fistula in these patients involves either the transverse sigmoid sinus or the bone itself. The treatment here requires resection of the sinus or removal of the involved bone. These patients should be monitored, however, to ensure that the dAVF does not progress into a more aggressive variant.

Treatment concepts center on whether the fistula can be successfully occluded or not. Here, both endovascular and microsurgical techniques can be used to occlude the arterial feeders and the venous drainage. It is tempting to initially plan transarterial obliterations using endovascular and surgical approaches. However, several caveats apply: First, arterial feeders may be too small and numerous to successfully catheterize. Second, not all arterial feeders may be seen on angiogram. In addition, the dAVF is a biologically dynamic pathological process that can recruit new arterial feeders to

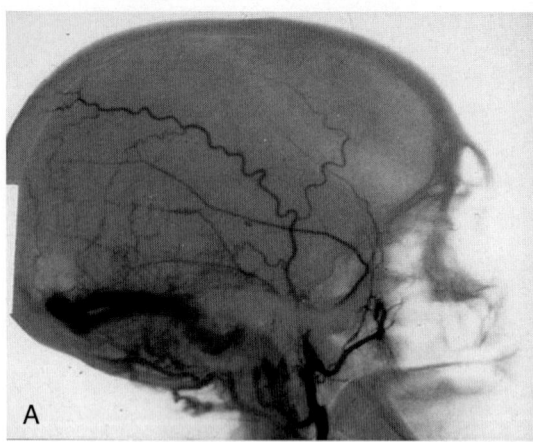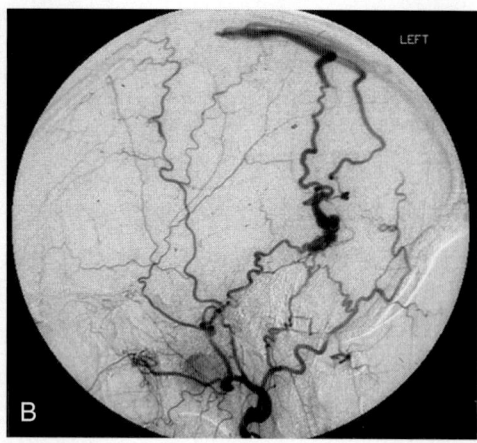

FIGURE 14.9 A, Dural arteriovenous fistula (dAVF) showing cortical venous reflux from the superior sagittal sinus. **B,** A different patient showing a dAVF without cortical venous reflux. The presence of cortical reflux in the first patient increases the risk of intracerebral hemorrhage, but the second patient can be managed conservatively.

the fistula and they may not be as accessible, especially if only partial occlusion or simply proximal occlusion of large feeders is accomplished. The liquid embolic agents are providing better means of transarterial embolization. The risk to the cranial nerves needs to be kept in mind because these nerves derive their blood supply from the external carotid branches such as the ascending pharyngeal arteries. Similarly, unusual anastomoses between the external and internal carotid branches (e.g., middle meningeal) require identification to avoid inadvertent passage of embolic material into the internal carotid circulation, risking neurological deficits.

Both microsurgical and endovascular techniques can take advantage of transvenous routes to occlude the outflow of a fistula, thereby facilitating its thrombosis. This approach differs from brain AVMs in that fistulas do not have a nidus that risks rupture from pressure increases brought on by obstruction of its drainage. Occlusion can be performed to the sinus, cortical veins, or both. When occluding cortical veins involved in the fistula, it is important that the point of occlusion be at the point where they enter the dural sinus to avoid subjecting the remnant veins to higher pressures from the fistula. This approach follows the same principle used in spinal dAVF to take away the venous hypertension. Transvenous approach is most applicable to the dAVFs involving the cavernous sinus. It is important to monitor intraocular pressure and avoid visual loss. A potential complication from transvenous occlusion is venous congestion and infarction of normal brain tissue. In case of excessive large sinus occlusion, venous infarction or hemorrhage can result in major morbidity or even death. Therefore, collaborative effort between a neurovascular surgeon and endovascular specialist is critical. A vessel or sinus that has retrograde drainage is not participating in normal functions and thus can be occluded. Balloon occlusion testing for venous drainage is not as predictable as its arterial counterpart, though one can use a catheter to measure the changes in upstream pressure during occlusion with the idea that a significant rise in pressure predicts increased risk of infarction. If a sinus cannot be occluded, a secondary option is to detach all cortical veins receiving reflux drainage to reduce the risk of intracranial hemorrhage by converting the fistula to a type I variety.

The dAVFs involving the skull base and the tentorium are often extremely complex, in the case of both arterial supply and venous drainage. The arterial supply to the tentorial lesions is typically dual (i.e., from external carotid branches as well as

internal carotid). There can also be feeders from branches of the vertebrobasilar circulation. The internal carotid branches usually come from the meningohypophyseal trunk or the meningeal branches of the ophthalmic artery. These branches are usually not amenable to transarterial occlusion and require microsurgical occlusion. The surgical approaches need to be individualized and one can take advantage of different skull base approaches.[79] The fistulas affecting the skull base itself have their own special features. The ones involving the bone lateral to the jugular and hypoglossal foramina can be easily eliminated by intra-arterial embolization followed by removal of the affected bone.[80-82] On the other hand, when the clivus is involved there is arterial supply from both sides and often very small branches, making complete obliteration literally impossible.

At times dAVFs are multiple and even bilateral with one side having cortical drainage while the other is a Borden type 1 fistula. Treatment needs to follow the same principles as outlined earlier. As is evident, dAVFs have wide variation of presentation, arterial supply, and venous draining, posing challenges in diagnosis and treatment decisions. A multidisciplinary approach in evaluation and treatment is critical, and patients are best treated at institutions having such teams.

SUMMARY

AVMs that were once considered incurable are now being treated using multidisciplinary modalities. Future research directed at the natural course of these lesions along with their biological development and responses to interventions should give both neurosurgeons and their patients a better idea of what to expect in dealing with this unique but potentially devastating disease.

SELECTED KEY REFERENCES

Cognard C, Gobin YP, Pierot L, et al. Cerebral dural arteriovenous fistulas: clinical and angiographic correlation with a revised classification of venous drainage. *Radiology.* 1995;194(3):671-680.

Joint Writing Group. Reporting terminology for brain arteriovenous malformation clinical and radiographic features for use in clinical trials. *Stroke.* 2001;32(6):1430-1442.

Ondra SL, Troupp H, George ED, Schwab K. The natural history of symptomatic arteriovenous malformations of the brain: a 24-year follow-up assessment. *J Neurosurg.* 1990;73(3):387-391.

Pollock BE, Flickinger JC, Lunsford LD, et al. Factors associated with successful arteriovenous malformation radiosurgery. *Neurosurgery.* 1998;42(6):1239-1244:discussion 1244-1247.

Spetzler RF, Martin NA. A proposed grading system for arteriovenous malformations. *J Neurosurg.* 1986;65(4):476-483.

Please go to expertconsult.com to view the complete list of references.

15 Cavernous Malformations Management Strategies

Aimee Two, Ali K. Ozturk, Murat Gunel

CLINICAL PEARLS

- Cerebral cavernous malformations (CCMs) are vascular lesions that contain a compact bundle of pathological capillary vessels without brain parenchyma between the vessels. CCMs are relatively common, affecting approximately 1 in every 200 individuals and accounting for 8% to 15% of all vascular malformations of the central nervous system (CNS). The majority of lesions occurs in the brain, with most being located in the supratentorial compartment and the minority infratentorially, to include the brainstem. Approximately 3% to 5% are discovered as intramedullary spinal CCM.

- Despite the high prevalence of CCM, most lesions are asymptomatic, being discovered incidentally, if ever. Only 20% to 30% of CCM patients will be symptomatic in their lifetimes, presenting to medical attention most commonly during their third to fifth decades of life with symptoms such as headaches, seizures, and focal neurological deficits due to lesion expansion following such events as thromboses and hemorrhages.

- Cavernous malformations can be either familial or sporadic. The familial form of the disease often manifests as multiple lesions in the setting of a family history of neurological disease. In the sporadic form, patients rarely have more than two lesions, and family history is typically absent. Mutations in three genes, *CCM1*, *CCM2*, and *CCM3*, have been discovered as being responsible for the familial disease, accounting for 96% of all mutations. De novo occurrence of lesions can occur and may impact long-term outcome.

- Complete surgical resection of CCM is the only management strategy that is curative. Medical management is limited to seizure control and symptomatic relief of headaches.

- The indication for radiosurgery treatment is controversial. In contrast, successful lesion resection immediately eliminates a patient's hemorrhage risk, but up to 80% of patients achieve seizure control postoperatively. The main goal in managing CCM is to balance the risks of surgery with those of the natural history of the disease. Because both of these factors vary significantly, each CCM patient must be considered on an individual basis.

- The most serious complications of CCM natural history is intracerebral hemorrhage. Patients with posterior fossa cavernomas are reported to be 6.75 times more likely to present with a bleed and the rehemorrhage rate is higher than that for lesions in other locations. Not only were these repeat hemorrhages common but brainstem cavernomas can result in debilitating deficits due to the high density of critical tracts and nuclei in this region.

- As a result of devastating outcomes with untreated cavernomas in high-risk regions, surgical treatment must always be considered for these select patients. Four major criteria assist in determining which patients with infratentorial lesions are appropriate surgical candidates: (1) lesions that rise to the pial surface based on T1-weighted MRI, (2) lesions with repeated hemorrhages causing progressive neurological deficits, (3) lesions with acute hemorrhage extending outside the lesion capsule, and (4) significant mass effect produced with a large intralesional hemorrhage. Surgery is considered only when total resection can be achieved, because lesion remnants can grow and hemorrhage as well.

DESCRIPTION

Cerebral cavernous malformations (CCMs), or cavernomas, are vascular lesions consisting of a compact bundle of dilated capillary-like channels lacking intervening neural parenchyma. They typically range in size from 1 mm to several centimeters and can be found anywhere in the central nervous system (CNS) as well as in other organs such as the skin and eye. Histologically, the lesions are composed of a single layer of endothelial cells and lack structural elements found in mature vessels, including smooth muscle and elastin. Other elements usually found in the blood-brain barrier, including astrocytic foot processes and pericytes, are also diminished or completely absent.[1-3] Macroscopically, the lesions appear reddish purple.

They are often multilobulated and can be encapsulated by a variable layer of fibrous adventitia, giving them their characteristic mulberry-like appearance.

Cavernous malformations can be either familial or sporadic. The familial form of the disease usually manifests as multiple lesions in the setting of a family history of neurological disease. In the sporadic form, patients rarely have more than two lesions, and family history is typically absent. Mutations in three genes, CCM1, CCM2, and CCM3, have been discovered as being responsible for the familial disease, accounting for 96% of all mutations.

Radiographically CCMs are best detected on magnetic resonance imaging (MRI), where they appear as a mixture of high and low T1 and T2 signal intensity surrounded by hemoglobin degradation products. These different components give lesions a characteristic popcorn appearance, with a surrounding hemosiderin ring due to chronic bleeds, that appears hypointense both on T1- and T2-weighted imaging. Because computed tomography (CT) findings for cavernomas are nonspecific, this imaging modality is less useful for detection. Angiography is similarly of little diagnostic help because lesions are usually angiographically occult. After a hemorrhage, however, developmental venous anomalies (DVAs) can be detected on angiography and should alert the clinician to a concomitant cavernoma, which frequently coexists with DVAs.

CCMs are relatively common, affecting approximately 1 in every 200 individuals and accounting for 8% to 15% of all vascular malformations of the CNS.[4,5] The majority of lesions occurs in the brain, with 63% to 90% of these being located in the supratentorial compartment and 7.8% to 35.8% infratentorially.[4,6] Between 9% and 35% of infratentorial lesions are located in the brainstem.[6]

Despite the high prevalence of CCM, most lesions are asymptomatic, being discovered incidentally, if ever. Only 20% to 30% of CCM patients will be symptomatic in their lifetimes, presenting to medical attention most commonly during their third to fifth decades of life with symptoms such as headaches, seizures, and focal neurological deficits due to lesion expansion following such events as thromboses and hemorrhages.[7] Asymptomatic patients will also occasionally present to health care providers after having one or multiple CCMs detected incidentally on imaging studies obtained for other purposes. Given this highly variable presentation and disease progression in patients with CCM, choosing the appropriate management strategy can be challenging. This chapter will explore the different treatment options available for CCM and provide suggestions as to the appropriate management in different circumstances. Before doing so, however, the natural history of these lesions will be discussed, as sound understanding of the natural history of the disease is paramount in any decision-making process with regard to treatment.

NATURAL HISTORY

The natural history of CCM can vary widely among patients. Although once believed to be congenital, it is now recognized that CCM can also occur de novo.[8] Once present, these lesions are dynamic, expanding as lesions thrombose and hemorrhage,

and regressing as they recanalize and as blood products from hemorrhages are resorbed.[8,9] The most common symptom reported in these patients is seizures, which are especially common with frontal or temporal lobe lesions.[10] Cavernoma lesions are typically surrounded by reactive gliosis which, at least in certain cases, is thought to serve as an epileptogenic focus. The estimated annual seizure risk is approximately 1% to 2%, and in patients with supratentorial lesions several seizure types including simple, complex partial, and generalized have been reported.[10,11]

Gross apoplectic hemorrhages are the most severe presentation of CCM. Because cavernomas are low-flow, low-pressure lesions, most bleeds are relatively small and result from blood extravasation from the leaky vascular channels of the lesion. Larger bleeds can and do occur, though, with an annual hemorrhage risk ranging between 0.25% and 6% depending on a variety of factors.[11] Larger and deeper lesions have been reported to have an increased bleeding risk, as do lesions in older patients, pregnant patients, and patients who have suffered a previous bleed.[7,12] Asymptomatic patients or those presenting with seizures typically have the lowest risk, which usually ranges from 0.4% to 2% annually.[12] Symptoms from a hemorrhage are typically maximal at the time of the bleed and gradually improve as the hemorrhage undergoes organization and resorption. With repeat hemorrhages, however, neurological deficits often worsen, and the risk that such deficits will become permanent increases.[13] Progressive neurological deficits are usually the most common presenting symptom of infratentorial CCM. Because this region has a higher density of eloquent neural structures compared to supratentorial regions, lesions here usually become symptomatic at smaller sizes.[14]

MANAGEMENT OPTIONS

Current medical literature recognizes four options for managing CCM: expectant management, medical management, surgical resection, and stereotactic radiosurgery. Understanding which technique or combination of techniques is appropriate for a particular patient depends on a variety of factors and will be discussed in a later section. The current section will focus on describing the four available options as well as highlighting some of their pros and cons.

Expectant Management

Expectant management consists of regular radiographic follow-up of lesions, usually every 1 to 2 years. Because MRI is the best modality for visualizing CCM, it is the imaging technique of choice when following lesions expectantly. Each new MRI is compared to prior ones in order to detect evidence of lesion changes over time. Of particular interest are signs of lesion expansion or hemorrhage. If present, there may be a need for intervention, especially for those lesions located in neurologically high-risk areas. For patients who are not operative candidates owing to their age or because of significant medical comorbid conditions, expectant management may be the only option. Asymptomatic patients, especially those with lesions in eloquent brain regions, are also best managed nonoperatively.

Medical Management

Options for medically managing cavernomas are unfortunately limited. There is no medical cure for cavernomas, so current medical therapy is limited to providing symptomatic relief through analgesics for headaches and antiepileptic medications for seizure control. Not all patients' seizures can be controlled by antiepileptics, though, and therefore, surgical intervention should be considered for patients with seizures refractory to pharmacological agents. Similar to patients being managed expectantly, these patients should also be followed with regular MRIs, and particular attention should be given to scans if patients have had changes in their symptoms despite taking their medication regularly as prescribed.

Recent in vitro and in vivo studies on animal models have shown activation of Rho GTPases in CCM lesions, suggesting that statin therapy, which is known to inhibit signaling through these molecules, might have a role in medical treatment.[15] However, clinical trials are needed to test the validity of statin treatment in CCM patients.

Surgical Resection

Complete surgical resection of CCM is the only management strategy that can be fully curative. Not only does a successful lesionectomy immediately eliminate a patient's hemorrhage risk, but up to 80% of patients achieve seizure control postoperatively.[16] As the most invasive treatment option, however, surgical resection is also the riskiest, with potential complications including permanent neurological deficits and even death. When offered to appropriate patients, however, surgical interventions usually have good outcomes. A brief explanation of the techniques employed in surgical resection of CCM is provided here.

Once the decision to treat surgically has been made, a preoperative MRI is essential for understanding the anatomy of the lesion. This anatomy is important in order to determine the operative approach that will best allow for removal of the lesion while minimizing contact with normal brain tissue and preserving potential branches of a DVA that does not appear to be draining the lesion. Because surgery is not usually considered for infratentorial lesions unless hemorrhage from the lesion reaches the pial surface based on T1-weighted thin-cut MRI, a clue to the location of most cavernomas arising in this area will be identifiable upon brain exposure. By following the track from the hemorrhage, it should be possible to visualize the lesion. For lesions that are not immediately visible upon exposure of the brain, intraoperative MRI with stereotactic images can also be useful in localizing lesions.

Having exposed the lesion, the next step in surgical resection is to enter and shrink the lesion using bipolar cauterization. The contracted cavernoma must then be dissected from the surrounding neural tissue, a process that is often made easier by the presence of a gliotic pseudocapsule around the lesion that can provide a circumferential surgical plane, before its removal. Following excision of the cavernoma, a decision must be made regarding the pseudocapsule. In supratentorial lesions, this area is generally removed provided it is not in or near a critical structure. In general, because the gliotic tissue of the pseudocapsule is thought to serve as an epileptogenic focus, the benefits of removing this tissue in symptomatic

patients could outweigh the risks associated with leaving these regions intact. For infratentorial lesions, however, the pseudocapsule is generally left intact.

Finally, before closing, the area should be examined for evidence of satellite lesions and cavernoma remnants, all of which should be resected to prevent lesion recurrence. Care should be taken, however, to preserve any associated branches of nearby DVAs, as their destruction may lead to venous infarcts with potential significant neurological deficits.

Stereotactic Radiosurgery

The use of stereotactic radiosurgery in the treatment of CCM remains controversial.[14] As the only intervention available for cavernoma treatment aside from open surgery, radiosurgery seems like an attractive alternative for patients who are either not surgical candidates or who have lesions in surgically inaccessible areas. Current imagining techniques are unable to detect complete lesion occlusion, though, making it impossible to determine whether or not this treatment modality is curative.[17] Efficacy therefore must be based on clinical data such as postprocedural hemorrhage rates or on histological results such as specimens that show complete occlusion following radiosurgical intervention. Several studies have looked at these parameters following radiosurgical intervention, but none of them has found evidence supporting the cure of CCM with this procedure. Although some studies report decreased hemorrhage rates following radiosurgery,[18,19] others, including some of the same studies, report an increased complication rate following this intervention, such as permanent neurological deficits.[20-22] Furthermore, patients in one study had to undergo open surgical resection of their lesions after radiosurgery failed to eliminate their cavernoma.[21]

In terms of histological studies, evaluation of resected cavernoma specimens from patients who had undergone radiosurgery anywhere from 1 to 10 years prior failed to show complete obliteration of their lesions. Instead, the main finding in these specimens was changes consistent with fibrinoid necrosis.[23]

Based on the preceding summarized data, radiosurgery does not appear to be an effective treatment strategy for CCM and should be used only in highly selected, if any, cases.

MANAGEMENT DECISIONS

The main goal in managing CCM is to balance the risks of therapy with those of the natural history of the disease. Because both of these factors can vary greatly among patients, each case must be considered on an individual basis. The following section will further explore the different factors that contribute to these risks and provide suggestions on appropriate management techniques.

One of the most serious complications of CCM is intracerebral hemorrhage. Patients with posterior fossa cavernomas are reported to be 6.75 times more likely to present with a bleed than those with lesions in other locations.[24] In addition to this increased initial bleeding risk, several studies have found an increased rehemorrhage rate among these patients. Not only were these repeat hemorrhages common, but 21% to 50% of rehemorrhages from brainstem cavernomas resulted

TABLE 15.1 Annual Hemorrhage Rates and Events Due to Cerebral Cavernous Malformations by Location*

Location	Hemorrhage Rate (%/yr)	Event Rate (%/yr)
Infratentorial	3.8	10.6
Supratentorial	0.4	0.4
Deep	4.1	10.6
Superficial	0	0

*An *event* refers to neurological deterioration, defined as subjective worsening (new or increased neurological symptoms) accompanied by objective worsening of neurological findings, with or without radiologically proven hemorrhage.
Modified from Porter PJ, Willinsky RA, Harper W, Wallace MC. Cerebral cavernous malformations: natural history and prognosis after clinical deterioration with or without hemorrhage. J Neurosurg. 1997;87:190-197.

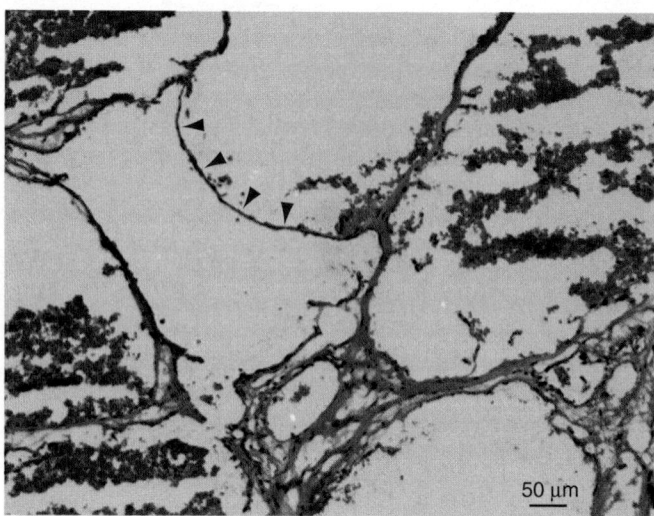

FIGURE 15.1 Histological picture of a human cavernous malformation shows a single layer of endothelial cells (*arrowheads*) surrounding sinusoidal spaces with thrombosed red blood cells within them. Note the lack of normal brain parenchyma within the lesions. Hematoxylin and eosin (H&E) stain. Scale bar represents 5 µm. *(Courtesy of Dr. Angeliki Louvi, Yale University School of Medicine.)*

in debilitating deficits[25,26] owing to the high density of critical tracts and nuclei in this region (Table 15.1).

Given this potential for devastating outcomes with untreated cavernomas in these high-risk regions, surgical treatment must always be considered for these patients. However, the locations of these lesions also make the surgery higher risk, and this risk needs to be weighed heavily against the natural course of the disease when deciding whether to operate. In the acute setting, if a patient's neurological status is rapidly deteriorating from mass effect related to a hemorrhage, immediate surgery might be warranted. In all other settings, four major criteria have been developed to assist in determining which patients with infratentorial lesions are appropriate surgical candidates: (1) lesions that abut the pial surface based on T1-weighted MRI, (2) lesions producing repeated hemorrhages causing progressive neurological deficits, (3) lesions with acute hemorrhage extending outside the lesion capsule, and (4) significant mass effect produced with a large intralesional hemorrhage. In addition, surgery is considered only when total resection can be achieved because lesion remnants can grow and hemorrhage as well. A study by Porter and associates looked at the results of 86 patients with brainstem cavernomas who satisfied these surgical criteria and underwent resection of their lesions. Thirty-five percent of these patients suffered temporary or permanent morbidity or death, with permanent or severe deficits occurring in 12%. The overall mortality rate was 8%, with 3.5% of deaths being surgically related. Nonetheless, patients undergoing surgery seemed to do better than those receiving conservative management. At late follow-up, 87% of surgically treated patients reported doing the same or better than before surgery, compared to 58% of patients in the nonsurgical group having this outcome. In addition, only 10% of surgical patients were worse at this late follow-up, as opposed to 42% of those not receiving surgery. Although risky, surgery is therefore justified in these cases.[6] Gross and colleagues performed a systematic review of 78 studies that looked at CCM of the brainstem. Of the 745 cases examined, 683 (92%) of the cavernomas were completely resected. Although early postoperative morbidity rates ranged from 29% to 67%, it was often temporary. Of the 683 patients who received surgery, 85% had clinical improvement, 14% had deterioration of their symptoms, and 1.9% died as a result of complications related to surgery.[27] These results suggest that, although risky, surgery benefits a

majority of patients and might therefore be justified in carefully selected symptomatic patients.

Supratentorial lesions are reported to have a lower hemorrhage rate[28] (Fig. 15.1, see Table 15.1). Although infrequent, however, overt hemorrhages might occur. In these situations, patients are usually taken to surgery based on their rate of neurological decline as well as the foreseeable consequences of mass effect from the bleed. Blood may interfere with the ability to visualize the cavernoma on imaging, in which case surgery may be deferred if the patient does not require immediate surgical decompression. In all other cases, two options can be considered. In the first, the patient can undergo elective exploratory surgery soon after the event, especially when the clot is subacute and thus soft. Otherwise, the patient can be managed expectantly until the diagnosis is confirmed.

More commonly, though, lesions in this location are associated with seizures. Antiepileptic drugs have traditionally been the initial management strategy for such patients, with surgery being considered for patients with seizures that are refractory to medication or that intensify during pharmacological treatment. Using this treatment approach, 65% of the 168 patients with supratentorial lesions in one study were free from their disabling seizures 3 years after surgery, with half of them remaining seizure free for this entire period.[29] A few other studies suggest that this outcome can be improved with earlier surgical intervention. In one study, 100% of patients who had developed epilepsy within 2 months of surgery were completely free of seizures postoperatively. Patients who waited between 2 and 12 months and greater than 12 months after the onset of epilepsy to undergo surgery had seizure control rates of 76% and 52%, respectively.[30] Regardless of when surgery is done, outcomes are usually good. For patients with solitary, superficial supratentorial CCM, the risks of surgical resection of cavernomas outside highly eloquent areas are only slightly higher than those of general anesthesia in trained hands. Furthermore, in the study of 168 patients discussed

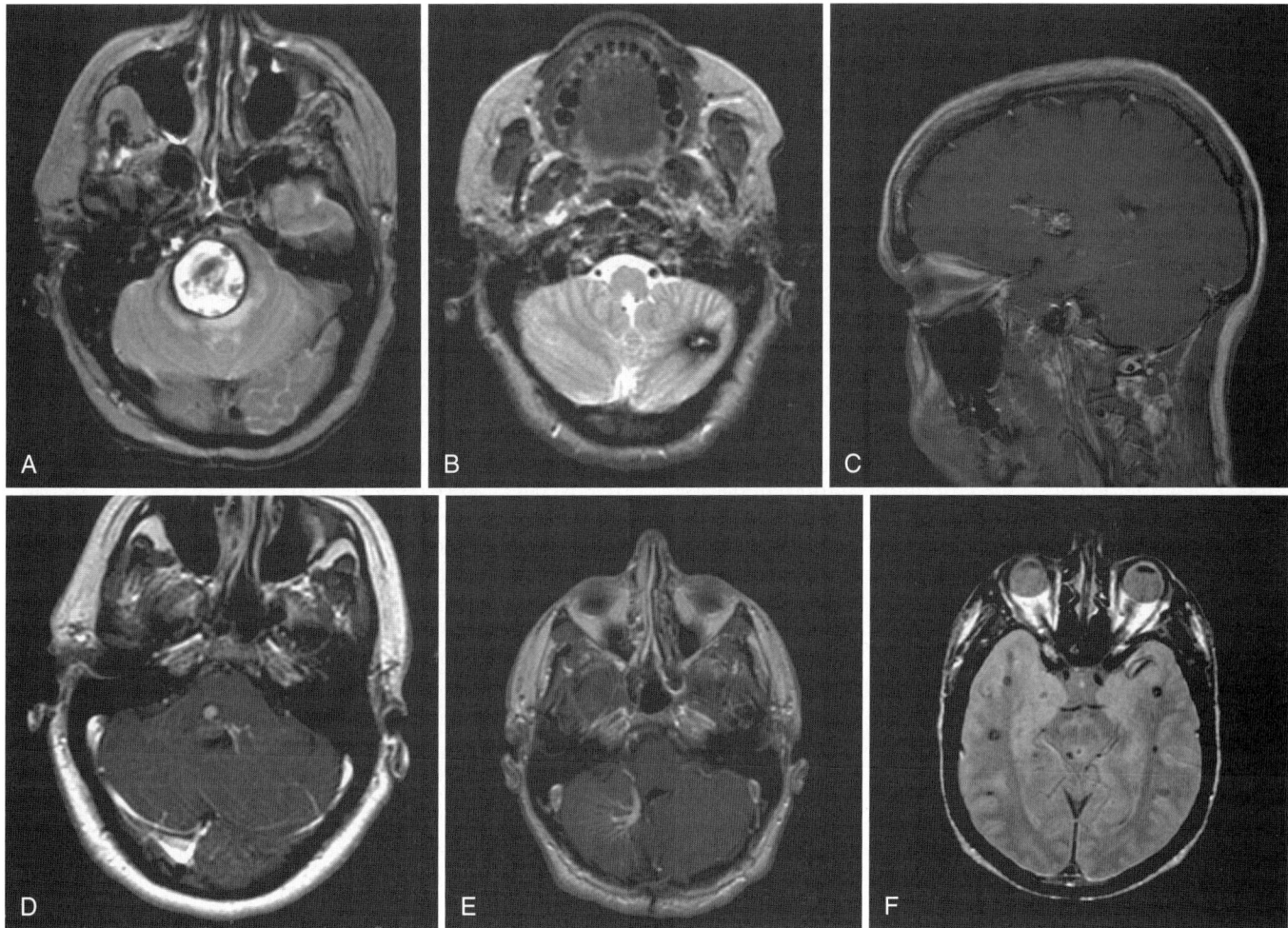

FIGURE 15.2 Axial T2-weighted images show a large pontine (**A**) and cerebellar (**B**) cavernous malformations with surrounding hemosiderin rings. Sagittal (**C**) and axial (**D**, **E**) T1-weighted images after gadolinium administration demonstrate supratentorial (**C**) and infratentorial (**D**, **E**) cavernomas with associated developmental venous anomalies (DVAs). Although the two frequently coexist, only the DVA will typically be apparent on traditional angiography, and this finding should alert the clinician to a potential concomitant cerebral cavernous malformation (CCM) (**F**). Gradient echo image demonstrates numerous small cavernous malformations in this Hispanic patient who was found to harbor a mutation of the *CCM1* gene. Multiple lesions are typical for familial cases of CCM.

previously, which is one of the largest studies of supratentorial cavernomas, no deaths occurred, and mild postoperative neurological deficits were seen in only 12 patients.[29]

Another factor to consider when operating on patients with seizures is whether or not to resect any gliotic or hemosiderin-stained tissue surrounding the lesion. Although some studies report complete resolution of seizure activity with pure lesionectomies, others report a higher rate of seizure control with removal of additional elements surrounding the lesion. In a study of 31 patients, 64% of the 14 who underwent excision of the hemosiderin ring in addition to a lesionectomy were categorized as Engel class I (free of disabling seizures) 1 year later. Only 53% of patients who had undergone either a lesionectomy or a lesionectomy plus partial removal of the hemosiderin ring fell into this category. Fifty-nine percent and 46%, respectively, were still in this group 3 years postoperatively[31] (Fig. 15.2). Another study had similar results, with 77.8% of patients being classified as Engel type Ia (free of all seizures) after a complete lesionectomy plus hemosiderin ring resection compared to 65.7% of those in the lesionectomy-only group,

but the additional benefit of the hemosiderin ring resection was only seen in a subset of patients who received surgery within 2 years of their seizure onset[32] (Table 15.2).

Although most CCMs are located in the brain, intramedullary spinal cavernomas account for 3% to 5% of lesions.[33-35] These cavernomas can occur alone or in combination with cerebral lesions. Lesions are typically located in the thoracic cord, with cervical cavernomas being second most common, and lumbar or conus rare. Spinal CCMs usually present with a slowly progressive myelopathy causing deficits in sensation, motor skills, or both.[36] Acute presentations of focal neurological deficits can also occur as a result of hematomyelia, intralesional hemorrhage, and cord compression.[37] Although symptoms resulting from acute presentations often resolve spontaneously, those resulting from chronic myelopathy frequently do not improve even after surgery. Surgery will stop the progression of myelopathy, though, and therefore is warranted in symptomatic patients. In a chart review of 26 patients receiving surgery for spinal CCM, 12 (46%) were improved at long-term follow-up, 12 (46%) were unchanged,

TABLE 15.2 Complete Seizure Control (Engel Class 1a—Free from All Seizures) in Relation to Cerebral Cavernous Malformation (CCM) Location and Hemosiderin Ring Resection*

Hemosiderin Resection	CCM Location	ENGEL CLASS 1A		
		After 1 Year	After 2 Years	After 3 Years
Complete resection	Temporal	7/12 (58%)	5/12 (42%)	5/12 (42%)
	Parietal	0	0	0
	Frontal	2/2 (100%)	1/1 (100%)	1/1 (100%)
	Occipital	0	0	0
Partial or no resection	Temporal	5/8 (63%)	4/8 (50%)	1/7 (14%)
	Parietal	3/7 (43%)	1/6 (17%)	1/5 (20%)
	Frontal	0/1 (0)	0/1 (0)	0/1 (0)
	Occipital	1/1 (100%)	1/1 (100%)	0/1 (0)

*Rates of complete seizure control at 1, 2, and 3 years after resection, grouped by resection of hemosiderin ring and location of CCM31.

and only 2 (8%) had worsened neurological conditions.[36] Surgery therefore might be the best option to prevent disease progression in select cases in order to potentially improve the patient's condition.

Although less common than symptomatic patients, asymptomatic patients are often referred for management after a lesion is found incidentally on imaging studies. Because it is unknown whether these patients will ever become symptomatic, choosing a management strategy can prove to be difficult. Provided that there is no evidence of bleeding, expectant management is usually the initial recommended management for these patients.

SPECIAL CONSIDERATIONS

While the preceding guidelines apply to the majority of patients with CCM, several patient groups require special consideration. These patients will be discussed in this section.

Older patients and those with significant comorbid conditions represent one group requiring special consideration. These patients usually have a high surgical risk and therefore may not be suitable candidates for surgery. Expectant or medical management may therefore be a better option for these patients unless the risks of intervention are justified, such as repetitive bleeds with progressive decline in neurological function or life-threatening hemorrhages.

Another group requiring special consideration is patients with multiple lesions. Almost all cases of familial CCM and a small percentage of patients with sporadic cavernomas might have more than one lesion. Treatment of these patients should be handled expectantly, with intervention being reserved for symptoms that can be attributed to a specific lesion that is clinically active. For patients experiencing progressive neurological deficits, imaging can be helpful in determining which lesions may be active based on size changes over time. Seizure types and auras, as well as monitoring devices, can be helpful in identifying particular lesions that are symptomatic in patients presenting with seizures. If the clinically active seizures can be determined using these tools, surgical intervention may be warranted. In a recent study of 63 patients with medically refractory CCM, 11 patients had multiple lesions, with a mean of 3.7 lesions per patient. All of these patients had only one epileptogenic zone, and removal of the cavernoma at this site resulted in nine patients being classified as Engel class Ia and two as Engel Ib (free of disabling seizures) or IVc (seizure worsening postoperatively) 2 years later.[38] Unfortunately de novo occurrence of lesions is common in these patients and can have a negative impact on the patient's long-term outcome.

Genetic screening of patients with a family history of CCM is not recommended.[39] The three genes currently recognized as being responsible for cavernous malformation account for 96% of familial mutations, making it possible that a fourth gene has yet to be discovered and consequently would not be detected during genetic screens.[40] A study of 20 families affected by cavernomas failed to detect mutations in any of the three cavernous malformation genes in 12 of the families.[41] Furthermore, the origin of sporadic CCM is unknown, and could be related to environmental factors either alone or in combination with genetic factors. Patients with a positive cavernoma family history should obtain an MRI if they experience any symptoms commonly associated with cavernomas, including headaches, seizures, and focal neurological deficits, or if they are diagnosed with a cerebral hemorrhage. In addition, genetic counseling should be offered to these patients.

CONCLUSION

The natural history of CCM can differ greatly among patients depending on various factors, including the location, biological state, and genetic background of the patient. Choosing an appropriate management strategy can therefore be difficult because different patients can be subject to vastly different clinical courses. In general the best treatment strategy is the one that minimizes the risks associated with the disease's natural history while also having a low procedural risk. Therefore, infratentorial lesions with high rates of devastating hemorrhage are often treated surgically, and supratentorial lesions commonly causing seizures can either be treated medically or surgically depending on the patient's surgical risks and seizure control. In experienced hands, outcomes from these procedures generally have low morbidity and mortality rates, and these statistics will only further improve as research provides new insight to the disease's natural history and the long-term outcomes of different treatment options.

SELECTED KEY REFERENCES

Baumann CR, Acciarri N, Bertalanffy H, et al. Seizure outcome after resection of supratentorial cavernous malformations: a study of 168 patients. *Epilepsia.* 2007;48:559-563.

Brown Jr RD, Flemming KD, Meyer FB, et al. Natural history, evaluation, and management of intracranial vascular malformations. *Mayo Clin Proc.* 2005;80:269-281.

Kondziolka D, Lunsford LD, Flickinger JC, Kestle JR. Reduction of hemorrhage risk after stereotactic radiosurgery for cavernous malformations. *J Neurosurg.* 1995;83:825-831.

Porter RW, Detwiler PW, Spetzler RF, et al. Cavernous malformations of the brainstem: experience with 100 patients. *J Neurosurg.* 1999;90:50-58.

Tu J, Stoodley MA, Morgan MK, Storer KP. Ultrastructural characteristics of hemorrhagic, nonhemorrhagic, and recurrent cavernous malformations. *J Neurosurg.* 2005;103:903-909.

Please go to expertconsult.com to view the complete list of references.

16 Spontaneous Intracerebral Hemorrhage

Alan Hoffer, Justin Singer, Nicholas C. Bambakidis, Warren Selman

CLINICAL PEARLS

- Hemorrhagic stroke accounts for 10% of all strokes. Strokes are the third leading cause of death and the main cause of long-term disability in the United States.

- Spontaneous intracerebral hemorrhage (ICH) is most commonly caused by chronic hypertension and occurs in penetrating arteries in the basal ganglia, thalamus, pons, and cerebellum. However, other causes, such as vascular malformations, tumors, and amyloid angiopathy, should always be considered.

- The presentation of ICH depends on its location, with neurological deficits being specific to the function of the brain involved. A decreased level of consciousness can occur with

- large lesions that cause herniation or lesions in the posterior fossa that result in brainstem dysfunction or hydrocephalus.

- The prognosis for ICH depends on the location and size of the hemorrhage, the age of the patient, and the degree of neurological impairment at the time of presentation.

- Medical therapy can try to prevent expansion of the hematoma, but emergent surgical evacuation should be considered for patients with rapid deterioration.

BACKGROUND AND EPIDEMIOLOGY

Spontaneous intracerebral hemorrhage is defined as a non-traumatic hemorrhage into brain parenchyma. The clinical significance of *intracerebral hemorrhage* (ICH), also known as *hemorrhagic stroke,* can be more clearly understood when it is viewed as a subtype of stroke. According to the National Vital Statistics Report, stroke is the third leading cause of death in the United States, behind only heart disease and cancer, and is responsible for nearly 6% of total deaths on an annual basis.[1] ICH accounts for approximately 10% of all strokes with an annual incidence between 15.9 and 32.9 per 100,000.[2] A sharp increase in incidence occurs in patients more than 75 years old and the incidence is even higher in patients older than 85, with reported incidence rates as high as 309.8 per 100,000, nearly seven times greater than the rate in the general population.[3] Though less frequent than ischemic stroke, the overall mortality rate of ICH is significantly greater, with 30-day mortality estimated at 44% to 52% and half of all deaths occurring within the first 2 days of hemorrhage.[4-6] The national cost of first-time strokes has been estimated at $40.6 billion, with more than $6 billion accounting for aggregate lifetime cost.[7] Of the $40.6 billion, only 45% of the cost was attributable to acute stroke care, with more than 47% of the total cost coming from long-term ambulatory and nursing care. Of all patients with ICH, only 20% have been noted

to be functionally independent 6 months after their stroke.[5] Although these statistics underscore the significant economic burden of ICH, they fail to emphasize the immeasurable emotional and social impact of ICH. It is essential to note, however, that since 1958, there has been a general annual decline in stroke deaths nationally. Between 2005 and 2006, there was a 6.4% decrease in stroke deaths.[1] This decline is attributable to significant improvements in treatment of modifiable risk factors related to cardiovascular and cerebrovascular health. Still, the rate of ICH is expected to increase in the future as a result of increasing population age.

PATHOPHYSIOLOGY

ICH may be classified as primary or secondary, depending on the etiology of the hemorrhage. Primary ICH most commonly results from chronic arterial hypertension. It occurs in small perforating arteries, typically at bifurcations from larger cerebral arteries where a pressure gradient is transmitted from the larger vessel to smaller, susceptible vessels. Small perforating vessels with diameters of 50 to 700 μm are often the offending vessels and may have multiple sites of rupture.[8] Hypertension is the most important risk factor for ICH, with nearly 60% of patients with ICH in a prospective study having elevated blood pressure.[9] Hypertensive bleeds are noted to occur more

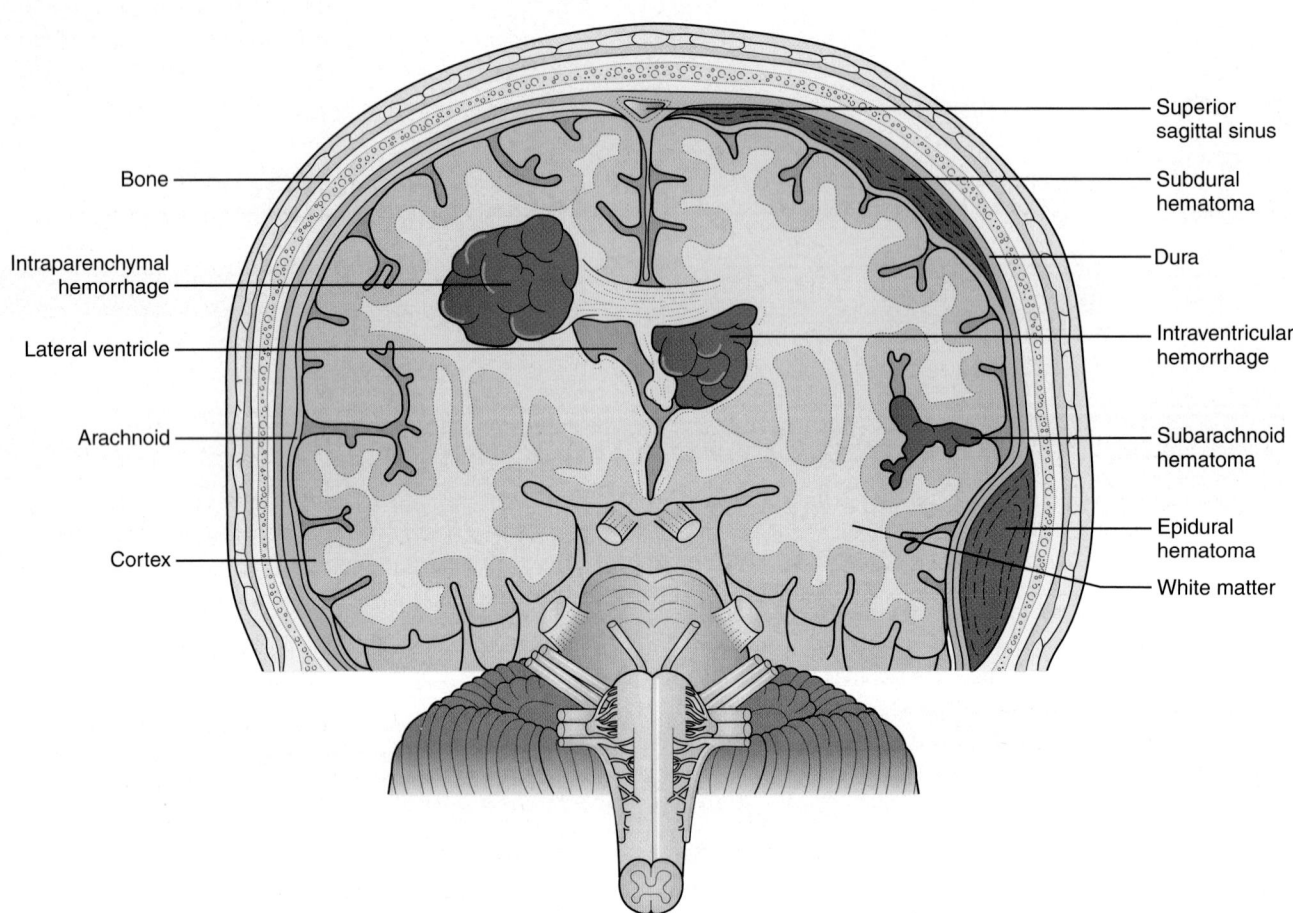

Bone

Intraparenchymal
hemorrhage

Lateral ventricle

Arachnoid

Cortex

Superior
sagittal sinus

Subdural
hematoma

Dura

Intraventricular
hemorrhage

Subarachnoid
hematoma

Epidural
hematoma

White matter

FIGURE 16.1 Common sites of hypertensive intraparenchymal hemorrhage.

frequently within deep gray matter structures, most commonly the basal ganglia, followed by the thalamus, pons, and the cerebellum (Fig. 16.1). Lobar hemorrhages, however, are not infrequent. Of all ICHs, one population study reviewed the locations of cerebral bleeds and noted 49% were deep in location, 35% were lobar, 10% were in the cerebellum, and 6% were in the brainstem.[10]

Classically, hypertensive bleeds have been attributed to the rupture of miliary aneurysms as described initially by Charcot and Bouchard in 1868 from their postmortem analysis of hemorrhage cavities in autopsy specimens. Further research has clarified that the miliary aneurysms described by Charcot and Bouchard are in fact pseudoaneurysms or weaknesses in the perforating arteriole walls where there has been extravasated blood and accumulated fibrin.[11] Pathological analysis of vessels in ICH specimens and in patients with chronic hypertension has more clearly demonstrated the process of lipohyalinosis in which chronic hypertensive damage gives rise to intimal hyperplasia, fibrin deposition, and focal accumulation of fat-filled macrophages, ultimately leading to necrosis in the vessel walls.[11] These vessel changes are more commonly seen at sites of hemorrhages than miliary aneurysms and thus are believed to be the source.

After the inciting hemorrhage, blood disperses along surrounding fiber tracts in the parenchyma. In an estimated 10% to 15% of cases, blood will decompress from the parenchyma into the ventricular system, creating an intraventricular

hemorrhage.[12] Ultimately, the hemorrhage is self-contained by tamponade from the parenchyma adjacent to the bleed site and by activation of hemostatic pathways. Regions of brain surrounding a hemorrhage are often characterized by extensive inflammation, edema, apoptosis, and necrosis that may contribute to the neurological deficit. Moreover, increased intracranial pressure and herniation secondary to mass effect occur with particularly large-volume hemorrhages. The rate of expansion of a hemorrhagic lesion is also an important variable to consider. Rapidly expanding lesions cause greater direct injury to axons and tissues and therefore result in greater damage to adjacent neural structures than slowly expanding lesions.

Secondary ICH results from underlying lesions such as aneurysms, vascular malformations, coagulopathies, tumors, hemorrhagic conversion of ischemic infarcts, cerebral amyloid angiopathy, and drug-related hemorrhages. Common metastatic tumors that are prone to hemorrhage include melanoma, choriocarcinoma, and renal carcinoma. Lung and breast cancer should also be considered because of their high incidence in the population. Primary brain neoplasms associated with ICH include glioblastoma multiforme, oligodendroglioma, and ependymoma.[13] Although secondary ICH is less common, it is important to consider these causes in the differential diagnosis and work them up appropriately because they place patients at risk for recurrent hemorrhage with the potential for extensive morbidity and even death.

ETIOLOGY

Hypertension

Normal blood pressure is currently defined as systolic blood pressure (SBP) less than 120 mm Hg and diastolic blood pressure (DBP) less than 80 mm Hg. Hypertension is currently classified as four stages: prehypertension (120-139/80-89 mm Hg), stage 1 hypertension (140-159/90-99 mm Hg), stage 2 hypertension (160-179/100-109 mm Hg), and stage 3 hypertension (≥190/≥110 mm Hg). Multiple studies have verified the dramatically increased risk of ICH as it corresponds to increases in hypertensive stage.[9,14-16] One meta-analysis of 11 case-control studies reported an overall odds ratio of 3.68 for ICH in hypertensive patients. Relative risk for patients with high normal hypertension (130-139 mm Hg systolic or 85-89 mm Hg diastolic) was 2.2, 5.3 for stage 1 hypertension, 10.4 for stage 2 hypertension, and 33.3 for stage 3 hypertension, as described by Suh and colleagues.[16] Individuals with stage 3 hypertension are five times more likely to experience ICH than individuals with normal blood pressure or prehypertension. The rate of ICH increases 22% for every 10 mm HG increment of SBP.[9] Naturally, improvements in hypertensive management and available antihypertensive medications have aided in decreasing the incidence of intracerebral hemorrhage.[17]

Cerebral Amyloid Angiopathy

In the elderly population, cerebral amyloid angiopathy (CAA) is an important etiological factor for ICH, accounting for an estimated 5% to 10% of all cases.[18] CAA results from the deposition of β-amyloid in the media and adventitia of cerebral vasculature, including capillaries, arterioles, and even small to medium-sized cerebral arteries in the cerebral cortex, leptomeninges, and cerebellum. CAA is commonly associated with the gene encoding apolipoprotein E, and a familial syndrome has been described accounting for CAA-related hemorrhages in younger patients.[19] For every decade increase in age, there is a 1.97 relative risk increase for ICH and a three times and seven times increased incidence rate for patients aged 65 to 74 and greater than age 85, respectively.[14,20] ICH due to CAA is most commonly in lobar locations, classically in the posterior parietal and occipital lobes. Special consideration of CAA should be given for bleeds in these locations, especially in elderly patients.[12] Recurrent lobar hemorrhages are relatively common in CAA and account for substantial increases in morbidity and mortality rates. The 2-year recurrence rate of lobar hemorrhages in patients with known CAA is 28%.[21]

Anticoagulation Therapy

ICH is a common yet serious complication of anticoagulation therapy. Patients on oral anticoagulation therapy suffering from ICH typically have significant vasculopathy related to chronic hypertension or CAA.[22] There is a 1% per year increase in risk for ICH while on anticoagulation therapy, seven to ten times the rate in the normal population.[23] This increased risk is quite significant given the high mortality rate of ICH associated with anticoagulation therapy, which is approximately 70%.[24] Moreover, patients on oral anticoagulation therapy have a significantly greater hematoma volume than patients not on anticoagulation. Prompt recognition of ICH is essential in this patient population, with particular attention paid to correcting the coagulopathy and stabilizing hematoma expansion.

Drugs and Alcohol

Certain drugs are capable of causing spontaneous ICH. Those most commonly associated with ICH are sympathomimetic agents, such amphetamines, cocaine, and pseudoephedrine. Hemorrhages associated with sympathomimetic agents are often related to transient elevations in blood pressure, leading to arterial rupture. Additionally, transient hypertensive episodes associated with substance abuse may cause hemorrhage from an otherwise asymptomatic vascular lesion such as an aneurysm or arteriovenous malformation. In younger age groups, cocaine abuse is commonly associated with ICH and subarachnoid hemorrhage.[25] As such, underlying vascular pathology should still be considered in young patients with ICH.

Intravenous drug abuse is associated with ICH. Injection of nonsterile substances by intravenous drug abusers places these patients at risk for systemic bacteremia, which may result in chronic damage to small vessels and necrotizing angiitis, weakening arteriole walls and increasing the susceptibility for rupture. Moreover, these patients are at risk for mycotic aneurysms that are susceptible to rupture (discussed later in this chapter).

ICH has also been associated with alcohol consumption. Juvela and colleagues demonstrated an increased risk of ICH in patients who were moderate or heavy drinkers in a dose-dependent manner. A positive CAGE questionnaire* was associated with increased risk of ICH.[26] The exact pathophysiological mechanism by which alcohol contributes to ICH is not clear; however, alcohol-associated hypertension, impaired hemostasis, and decreased levels of clotting factors have been implicated.

Aneurysms

An aneurysm is formed from a defect in an arterial wall that allows the intima to protrude through the muscular layer of an artery. The etiology of the defect leading to aneurysm formation may be embolic, traumatic, neoplastic, or atherosclerotic.

Saccular Aneurysms

The majority of aneurysms are saccular aneurysms whose etiology may be a combination of congenital, hereditary, and acquired factors, including smoking and hypertension. The mortality associated with subarachnoid hemorrhage from a saccular aneurysm rupture is estimated to be between 40% and 50%, making this a grave disease.[27]

Saccular aneurysms are typically located at branch points of major cerebral arteries, usually arising from the vessels that form the circle of Willis. Saccular aneurysms may be associated with inherited conditions, including Ehlers-Danlos syndrome, adult polycystic kidney disease, and other conditions that predispose individuals to aneurysm formation because of intrinsic weaknesses in their vessel walls. In fact, 20% of patients with saccular aneurysms harbor more than just one. Additionally, lesions that alter cerebral

---

*Cut down, annoyed by criticism, guilty about drinking, eye-opener drinks (a test for alcoholism).

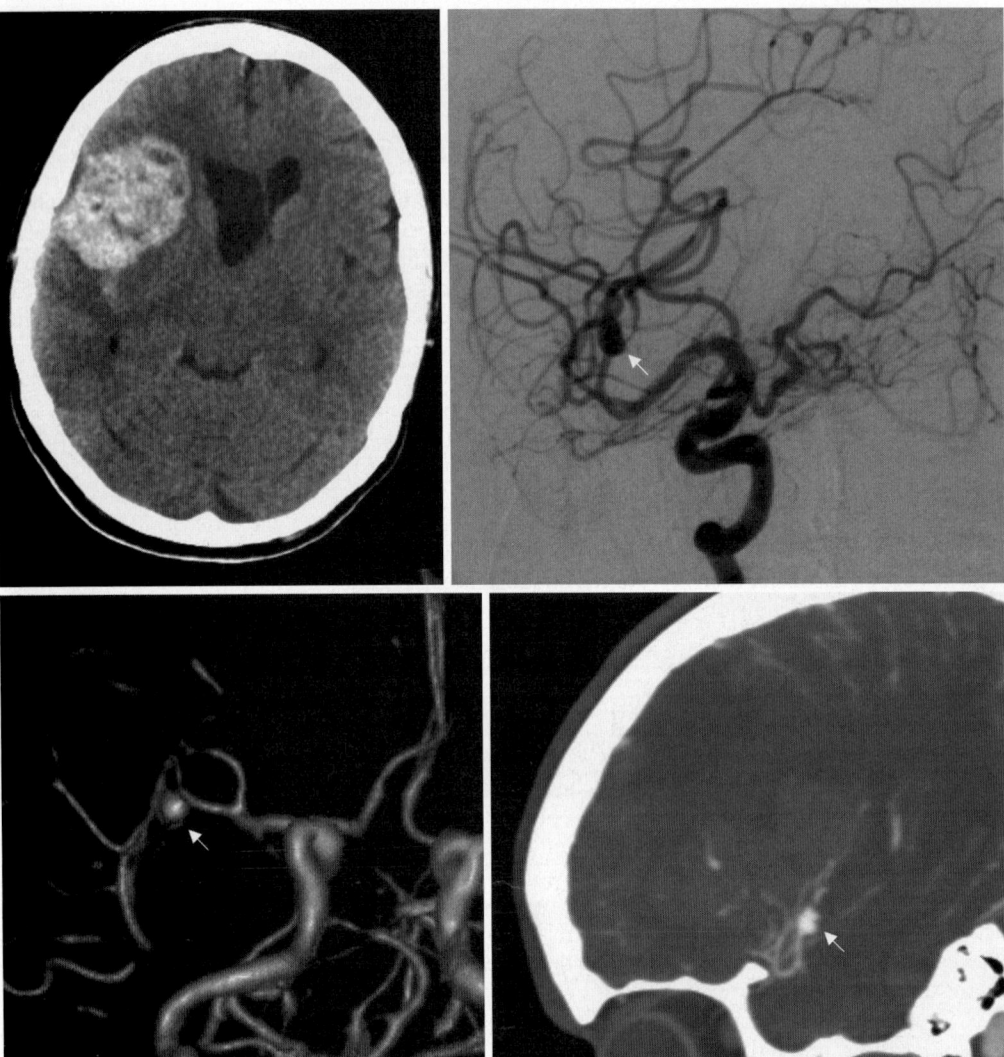

FIGURE 16.2 Ruptured aneurysm of the middle cerebral artery, causing intracerebral hemorrhage. The hyperdense signal on computed tomography (CT) demonstrates the acute hemorrhage. The aneurysm (*white arrows*) is visualized by catheter angiography (*top right*) and CT angiography (*bottom left and right*).

blood flow, such as tumors or vascular malformations, may lead to aneurysm formation. Bifurcations and trifurcations are particularly susceptible areas for aneurysm formation because these points experience a greater hydrostatic pressure owing to loss of laminar blood flow and greater turbulence. Although saccular aneurysm rupture usually leads to subarachnoid hemorrhage, intraparenchymal hematomas into adjacent brain are common (Fig. 16.2). The presence of an intraparenchymal hematoma after aneurysm rupture may play an important role in the need for and timing of surgical intervention.

The mean frequency of aneurysm occurrence is 5%, with a prevalence between 10 and 15 million people in the United States.[28] The annual rate of rupture of aneurysms has been quoted at between 0.3% and 1.3%, but estimates are highly variable.[27,28] There does appear to be a relationship between aneurysm size and annual rate of rupture, with a rate of rupture of aneurysms 10 mm or greater being slightly less than 1% per year and an astounding 6% rate of rupture in the first year for giant aneurysms measuring greater than 25 mm.[28] In an attempt to better elucidate this relationship, the International Study of Unruptured Intracranial Aneurysms Investigators (ISUIAI) performed a combined retrospective

and prospective multicenter study to examine the rupture rates. They found that risk of rupture was associated with aneurysm size and location, with small aneurysms (<7 mm) in the anterior circulation having an annual rupture rate of 0.05%. The risk increased with aneurysm size from 0.5% to 3% per year in 7- to 24-mm aneurysms and 8% per year for giant aneurysms. Aneurysms in the posterior circulation had an 8 to 14 times higher relative risk of rupture.[28,29] Although this study has been criticized for design, it reinforces the notion of size and location being major determinants in risk of rupture.

Mycotic Aneurysms

Mycotic aneurysms are a potentially life-threatening condition resulting from septic emboli. They commonly occur in smaller cortical arteries, where the emboli become lodged. Transmigration of infection through the arterial wall and extensive damage to the vessel media weaken the vessel wall, resulting in subsequent dilatation and rupture. Mycotic aneurysms are usually seen in the setting of bacterial endocarditis, with 30% of cases of bacterial endocarditis having neurological complications, including stroke and hemorrhage.[30]

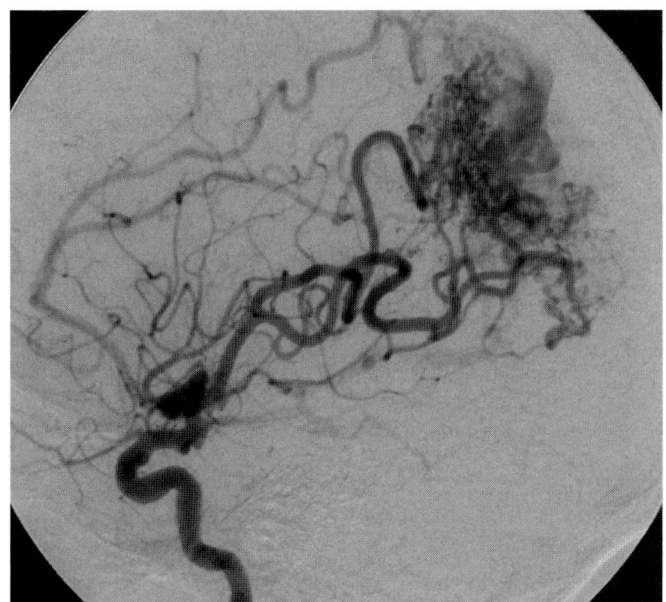

FIGURE 16.3 Catheter angiogram of an arteriovenous malformation, demonstrating the early filling of the lesion and the venous drainage system.

Atherosclerotic Aneurysms

Severe intracranial atherosclerotic disease, accompanied by chronic hypertensive vessel damage, leaves weakened vessels susceptible to aneurysm formation. The posterior circulation is usually involved, and rupture is uncommon.

Vascular Malformations

The most common and most clinically significant of the vascular malformations is the arteriovenous malformation (AVM). AVMs are congenital vascular anomalies consisting of a meshwork of vessels fed by one or more arteries that drain directly into the venous circulation (Fig. 16.3). As there is no flow through a capillary bed, the arterial pressure is transmitted directly into the venous system. AVMs carry a significant risk of bleeding. The annual risk of hemorrhage from an AVM is estimated to be 2% to 3% per year, with higher rates in patients with smaller AVMs, AVM-associated aneurysms, or deep venous drainage.[31] The most common presentation of AVMs is ICH, accounting for 69% of symptomatic cases.[32] Hemorrhages are most common during the second through fourth decades of life, as opposed to primary ICH, which is more likely to occur starting in the fifth decade of life. Traditionally, these lesions have been treated by open resection if the location and characteristics of the AVM are amenable. Recent advances in neurosurgery, including endovascular embolization techniques and stereotactic radiosurgery, have become useful tools in the treatment of this disease.

Other vascular malformations include cavernous malformations, venous angiomas, and capillary telangiectasias. Cavernous malformations and venous angiomas consist of large anomalous vessels in deep white matter. Cavernous angiomas differ from their venous counterparts in that they do not contain normal brain tissue between the abnormal vessels. Cavernous malformations rarely cause hemorrhages that result in clinical deficits; however, microhemorrhages are common and may increase the incidence of seizures in these patients. Capillary telangiectasias, which are mostly found in the brainstem and cerebellum, are characterized by small capillary-sized vessels and rarely bleed. Venous angiomas (now referred to as venous anomalies) in isolation are not associated with an increased risk of hemorrhage.

SIGNS AND SYMPTOMS

The presentation of patients with ICH is highly variable and depends on multiple factors, including the location and size of the hemorrhage. Neurological symptoms have a gradual onset over a period of minutes or hours, as opposed to the sudden onset of a subarachnoid hemorrhage or embolic event. Many of these patients may present with hemiplegia or other focal neurological deficits. Decreased level of consciousness and brainstem dysfunction are frequently seen with large hematomas, especially those located in the posterior fossa. Signs of increased intracranial pressure may include headache, nausea, and vomiting. One third of patients have seizure activity during presentation, often related to hemorrhages in lobar locations.[33] The symptoms of ICH may correspond to more than one vascular territory, allowing differentiation from patients with ischemic events who typically display symptoms confined to a single vascular territory. In addition, symptoms of ICH rarely regress in the acute phase of hemorrhage as is sometimes seen during the acute phase of an ischemic or embolic event.

There is substantial variability in the clinical presentation of ICH related to the exact location of the hemorrhage. Hemorrhages in deep locations involving the basal ganglia often present with hemiplegia, and thalamic involvement causes hemisensory deficits. Cortical bleeds often present with focal signs and symptoms, such as weakness, aphasia, and visual field defects, which correspond to the area of hemorrhage. Cerebellar hemorrhages frequently originate in the dentate nucleus and may efface or extend into the fourth ventricle. These hemorrhages typically exhibit classic cerebellar signs, including ataxia, nystagmus, and dysmetria. They may also produce nausea, vomiting, cranial nerve deficits, and decreased level of consciousness or coma if there is sufficient compression of brainstem structures or hydrocephalus.

Intraventricular hemorrhage (IVH), hydrocephalus, and herniation syndromes are of particular importance in ICH as they may be lethal to patients. Intraventricular extension of hemorrhage occurs in approximately 40% of patients with ICH and is associated with a mortality rate ranging from 45% to 80%.[12,10,34] Hydrocephalus can result either from the obstruction of the ventricular system by IVH (noncommunicating hydrocephalus) or blockage of cerebrospinal fluid (CSF) resorption at the arachnoid granulations by blood in the CSF (communicating hydrocephalus). Occasionally, mass effect in the cerebellum from a hemorrhage and associated edema may efface the fourth ventricle, causing an obstructive hydrocephalus without IVH. Patients with a decreased level of consciousness and severe neurological deficits out of proportion to the size of the bleed during and after their hospitalizations should be evaluated for IVH and hydrocephalus. Increased intracranial pressure due to hydrocephalus or from mass effect resulting from a rapid and large hematoma is a true neurosurgical emergency. In this clinical setting, immediate extraventricular drainage and surgical decompression may be indicated.

NATURAL HISTORY

It has been estimated by two population studies that between 20% and 40% of hemorrhages undergo volume expansion after the initial bleed.[35,36] Moreover, hematoma expansion has been shown to carry a fivefold increased risk of clinical deterioration and was associated with ICH-related death.[36] Brott and colleagues demonstrated that the majority of the hematoma growth occurred within 3 to 4 hours after hemorrhage onset and was similarly associated with neurological deterioration. Kazui and colleagues found that, in patients who had hematoma expansion, 36% had growth within 3 hours of onset, 16% had expansion between 3 and 6 hours after onset, 15% had growth between 6 and 12 hours, and only 6% had growth between 12 and 24 hours. Of note, no patients in the study had hematoma expansion between 24 and 48 hours after hemorrhage onset. The most rapid phase of hemorrhage, however, is still felt to occur within the first hour. It is important to note that 35% to 46% of patients with neurological deterioration did not have hematoma expansion and their deterioration was likely related to mass effect associated with edema, IVH, or hydrocephalus.[35,36] Nonetheless, clot stabilization is a priority of initial management of ICH, as hematoma expansion is associated with worse outcome.

As previously mentioned, the 30-day mortality rate of ICH is estimated at 44% to 52%.[4,5] Given the high mortality rate, many studies have investigated predictors of poor outcome in this patient population. Independent predictors of poor outcome include low Glasgow Coma Scale (GCS) scores at the time of presentation, age 80 or older, infratentorial origin, ICH volume, and the presence of IVH. Volume of intracerebral hemorrhage alone is a very strong predictor of the 30-day mortality rate.[37] Hemorrhages with volumes greater than 60 cm³ resulted in 30-day mortality rate of 93% for deep hemorrhages and 71% for lobar. Lethal volume of hemorrhage is variable and dependent on the location of the hemorrhage, with hemorrhages in the pons and cerebellum having significant mortality rates in hemorrhages greater than 5 cm³ and 30 cm³, respectively.[4]

In an effort to provide a more accurate determination of prognosis, mortality risk, and clinical course for patients with ICH, Hemphill and colleagues have devised the ICH score. The scale utilizes GCS scores, ICH volume, presence of IVH, infratentorial origin, and age older than 80 years at the time of presentation to stratify patient mortality risks. The scale was found to be an accurate tool for assessing 30-day mortality risk. In the study, no patient with an ICH score of 0 died, though the mortality rate was 100% for patients with a score of 5.[38]

DIAGNOSIS

While the importance of a thorough history and physical examination cannot be underestimated, imaging studies are the primary diagnostic tools for ICH. Computed tomography (CT) provides a rapid, sensitive means by which ICH can be diagnosed. Coagulated blood is hyperdense (bright) compared to the brain on CT imaging. As the hematoma ages and is broken down, the clot becomes less dense. In the subacute phase, it may appear isodense with the brain. In the chronic phase, it appears hypodense (dark), resembling CSF. In addition to elucidating the location, size, and shape of the hematoma, CT scanning is useful in demonstrating the presence of hydrocephalus and the extent of parenchymal shift associated with the hemorrhage. In some cases, it may assist in determining the cause.

Magnetic resonance imaging (MRI) is more sensitive than CT but takes significantly longer to obtain. Therefore, it is not a good tool for screening but should be reserved for situations in which a patient has been deemed clinically stable. The signal characteristics of ICH are complex. They are determined by the molecular constituents of the blood clot as they undergo catabolism from oxyhemoglobin to deoxyhemoglobin, intracellular methemoglobin, and extracellular methemoglobin (Fig. 16.4). The administration of intravenous contrast agents

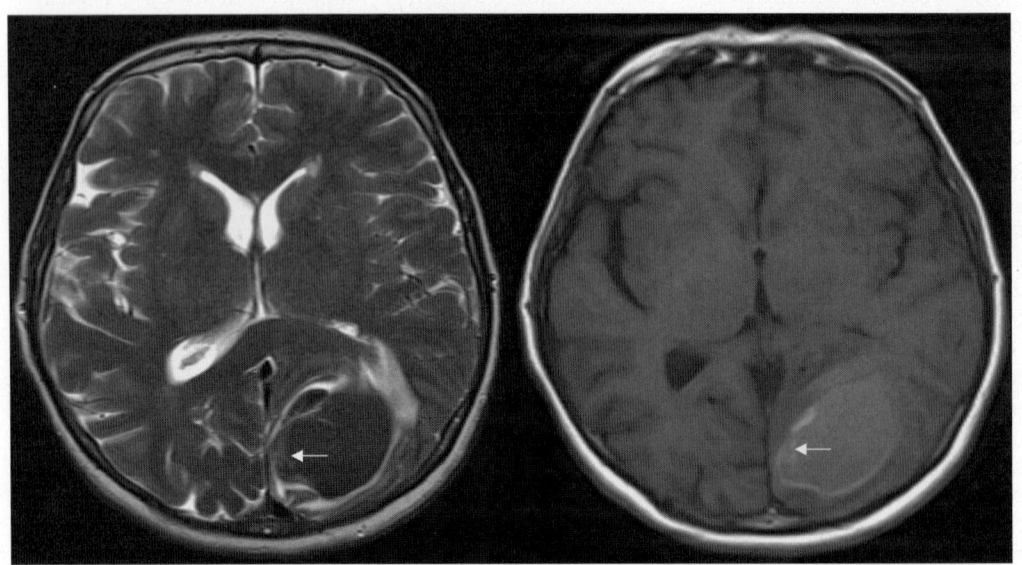

FIGURE 16.4 Magnetic resonance imaging of a hematoma as it matures from the acute to the subacute phase, demonstrated by the transition from intracellular deoxyhemoglobin to intracellular methemoglobin (*white arrows*).

may increase the sensitivity of MRI for underlying tumors or vascular malformations. It should be noted, however, that in many instances the hematoma can obscure the underlying anomaly. Waiting 3 to 4 weeks after the hemorrhage often allows enough resorption of the clot to visualize the lesion.

If a vascular malformation is suspected, cerebral angiography should be employed to evaluate for its presence and nature. It should be noted that 10% of vascular lesions are angiographically occult at the time of the first study. More recently, techniques for CT and magnetic resonance angiography have increased the detection of some vascular malformations, such as aneurysms and AVMs, without exposing patients to the risks of conventional angiography. These studies, particularly CT angiography, can be acquired rapidly in most patients with adequate kidney function and are of huge benefit for patients who require emergent evaluation prior to surgery. Catheter angiography should be reserved for cases in which noninvasive studies are negative but the clinical suspicion for a vascular lesion is high, or cases in which the nature of the lesion is not clearly demonstrated. Even if catheter angiography does not demonstrate a lesion, the study should be repeated after 7 days if a vascular malformation is suspected, as the consequences of not treating one may be fatal.

TREATMENT

Medical Management

The purpose of medical therapy in ICH patients is to stabilize the patient and eliminate any factors that may exacerbate the hemorrhage or its sequelae, including blood pressure control, reversal of coagulopathies, and treatment of intracranial hypertension. The medical care of patients with ICH is complex. Because of the potential for rapid neurological deterioration, these patients require admission to an intensive care unit (ICU). Being treated in an ICU and by physicians that specialize in neurological conditions has been shown to decrease the morbidity and mortality rates of ICH.[39]

Because hypertension increases the risk for hematoma growth, blood pressure monitoring and treatment play a central role in the care of these patients. The target for blood pressure after ICH is controversial. Although it has been shown that tighter control results in less hematoma growth, there is a concern for cerebral hypoperfusion, particularly in the region immediately surrounding the clot, resulting in ischemia. The current American Heart Association (AHA) guidelines for blood pressure control are as follows:

- If SBP is 200 mm Hg or mean arterial pressure (MAP) is 150 mm Hg, then consider aggressive reduction of blood pressure with continuous intravenous infusion, with frequent blood pressure monitoring every 5 minutes.
- If SBP is 180 mm Hg or MAP is 130 mm Hg and there is evidence of or suspicion of elevated intracranial pressure (ICP), then consider monitoring ICP and reducing blood pressure using intermittent or continuous intravenous medications to keep cerebral perfusion pressure 60 to 80 mm Hg.
- If SBP is 180 mm Hg or MAP is 130 mm Hg and there is no evidence or suspicion of elevated ICP, then consider a modest reduction of blood pressure (e.g., MAP of 110 mm Hg

or target blood pressure of 160/90 mm Hg) using intermittent or continuous intravenous medications to control blood pressure, and clinically reexamine the patient every 15 minutes.[37]

Several recent studies have examined whether or not stricter control is warranted. The Intensive Blood Pressure Reduction in Acute Cerebral Haemorrhage Trial (INTERACT) randomized 276 patients with spontaneous ICH, without an underlying tumor or vascular abnormality, to the parameters suggested by the 1999 AHA guidelines or a more intensively controlled group with SBP less than 140 mm Hg. The investigators found that the more intensively controlled group had less hematoma growth than the guideline group (11.9%, 8.3%, and 9.8% less at 24 hours, 72 hours, and over 72 hours, respectively).[40] Additionally, the Antihypertensive Treatment of Acute Cerebral Hemorrhage (ATACH) study sought to evaluate the safety and effectiveness of aggressive blood pressure reduction and identify an appropriate blood pressure target. Sixty patients were randomized into three groups (SBP targeted to 170-200 mm Hg, 140-170 mm Hg, and 110-140 mm Hg), and 3-month mortality rate was recorded. Although the study was not powered to compare the mortality rates between the three groups, all had lower than expected mortality rates.[41]

Although ICH itself can lead to devastating neurological injuries, it is worsened by the presence of coagulopathy. A number of etiologies exist for coagulopathy, but the most common is the use of anticoagulation and antiplatelet medications. Though they do not cause hemorrhages by themselves, they can significantly exacerbate the bleeding that occurs. Without the normal ability to clot, hematomas may continue to grow, worsening local tissue injury and ICP. The reversal of warfarin-induced anticoagulation may be achieved by administration of plasma, which contains the factors depleted by the medication. This is not without risk, however. Transfusion reactions and systemic volume overload are common. Although plasma is an effective means of restoring clotting factors, its usefulness may be limited by the time it takes to administer multiple units to a patient with severe coagulopathy who has evidence of significant mass effect from the hematoma. Studies are currently being undertaken to evaluate exogenous activated factor VII, a substrate whose endogenous counterpart allows the conversion of prothrombin to thrombin, almost immediately reversing the coagulopathy. Of note, activated factor VII has been studied in noncoagulopathic patients with ICH in a large randomized trial.[42] This study demonstrated that activated factor VII was able to decrease hematoma growth in a dose-dependent fashion but did not alter clinical outcome at 6 months.

One of the most serious complications of ICH is the development of intracranial hypertension, which can lead to global cerebral dysfunction and compression of critical structures. Treatment of intracranial hypertension includes simple measures, such as sedation and elevating the head of the bed, as well as more aggressive treatments, such as the use of osmotic diuretics, CSF drainage, paralysis, and decompressive craniectomy.

Surgical Management

Surgical management of ICH has traditionally been reserved for patients with ongoing neurological deterioration that require emergent relief of intracranial hypertension or decompression of vital structures. The extent to which clot evacuation ameliorates injury outside these conditions is not well understood. Numerous trials have looked at craniotomy as a treatment for ICH. The largest of these was the Surgical Trial in Intracerebral Hemorrhage (STICH) that randomized 1033 patients with supratentorial hemorrhages to early surgery (<72 hours) or medical management alone. No difference was found between the groups in the rate of mortality or good outcome at 6 months.[43] Trends were seen for improved outcome in younger patients, GCS scores at presentation, more superficial hemorrhages, and absence of intraventricular extension. These factors did not reach significance, though. Unlike supratentorial hemorrhages, patients with cerebellar hemorrhages clearly benefit from surgery. Because of the proximity of these hemorrhages to the brainstem and the fourth ventricle, any significant hematoma in the cerebellum should be evacuated emergently.

More recently, other surgical techniques have been developed to address ICH, including the stereotactic administration of the thrombolytic agents directly into the hematoma via indwelling catheters and stereotactic endoscopic clot evacuation. These promising procedures are currently being evaluated in multicenter randomized trials, including the Minimally-Invasive Surgery plus t-PA for Intracerebral Hemorrhage Evacuation (MISTIE) and Intraoperative CT-guided Endoscopic Surgery for ICH (ICES) trials, to determine their efficacy. In conclusion, we are still evolving both accepted and novel surgical and medical treatments for ICH to decrease the mortality, morbidity, and long-term disability associated with this common presentation of stroke.

SELECTED KEY REFERENCES

Anderson CS, Huang Y, Arima H, et al. Effects of early blood pressure-lowering treatment on growth of hematoma and perihematoma edema in acute intracerebral hemorrhage. *Stroke.* 2010;41:307-312.

Broderick JP, Brott TG, Duldner JE, et al. Volume of intracerebral hemorrhage. A powerful and easy-to-use predictor of 30-day mortality. *Stroke.* 1993;24(7):987-993.

Hemphill III JC, Bonovich DC, Besmertis L, et al. The ICH score: a simple, reliable grading scale for intracerebral hemorrhage. *Stroke.* 2001;32(4):891-897.

Kazui S, Naritomi H, Yamamoto H, et al. Enlargement of spontaneous intracerebral hemorrhage. Incidence and time course. *Stroke.* 1996;27(10):1783-1787.

Mendelow AD, Gregson BA, Fernandes HM, et al. Early surgery versus conservative medical management in patients with spontaneous supratentorial intracerebral hemorrhage in the International Surgical Trial in Intracerebral Hemorrhage (STICH): a randomized trial. *Lancet.* 2005;365 (9457):387-397.

Please go to expertconsult.com to view the complete list of references.

17 Endovascular Neurosurgery

Sabareesh K. Natarajan, Adnan H. Siddiqui, L. Nelson Hopkins, Elad I. Levy

CLINICAL PEARLS

- Endovascular neurosurgery has undergone tremendous expansion in the past two decades and is becoming a mainstay of treatment of cerebrovascular disease and other vascular disease of the head and neck as a primary or alternative treatment to open microvascular treatment.

- Endovascular techniques are used to treat a wide variety of cerebrovascular conditions that include severe symptomatic vasospasm after subarachnoid hemorrhage (SAH), arteriovenous malformation (AVM) and tumor embolization, cerebral aneurysm occlusion, and temporary or permanent balloon occlusion during parent vessel sacrifice.

- Endovascular therapy is expanding the time-window after stroke symptom onset for revascularization in patients with acute ischemic stroke. Clinical trials have established a benefit of intra-arterial thrombolysis (IAT) up to 6 hours after stroke symptom onset, with an increase in recanalization rates. The mechanical device trials show effectiveness of mechanical revascularization therapy up to 8 hours after stroke symptom onset.

- Endovascular treatment of intracranial aneurysms has undergone and continues to undergo improvements

- since the introduction of Guglielmi detachable coils for endosaccular occlusion of cerebral aneurysms in 1994. Current adjunctive techniques include balloon-assisted and stent-assisted coiling to improve the success rate of long-term occlusion of the aneurysm. Flow diversion for giant aneurysms may be a promising technology.

- Preoperative endovascular embolization of feeding arteries has rendered many previously difficult AVMs much easier to remove surgically. Only a minority of AVMs can be cured by endovascular embolization despite the significant advances in embolic material such as Onyx. Most intracranial tumor embolization procedures have been performed on neoplasms with robust vascular pedicles in order to decrease the blood loss during resection.

- Endovascular therapy is evolving and adds a plethora of tools and opens up multiple options with which to treat complex vascular lesions, in addition to microsurgical approaches. Currently, neurosurgeons who desire to be trained in treating the entire spectrum of cerebrovascular disease may pursue both microsurgery and endovascular neurosurgery training.

INTRODUCTION (Box 17.1)

The treatment of neurovascular diseases has been completely revolutionized with the introduction and growth of endovascular neurosurgery. Endovascular neurosurgery is becoming a primary treatment alternative to conventional open surgery for multiple neurovascular pathological conditions, including carotid and vertebral atherosclerotic stenosis, cervical vessel dissections, acute and chronic cerebral ischemia, intracranial aneurysms, arteriovenous malformations (AVMs), and dural arteriovenous fistulas (dAVFs). Endovascular revascularization has resulted in recanalization rates as high as 70% to 100% for acute large vessel occlusions responsible for ischemic stroke in patients in whom intravenous (IV)

tissue plasminogen activator (t-PA) therapy has failed or was contraindicated. Endovascular techniques are used to treat severe symptomatic vasospasm after subarachnoid hemorrhage (SAH), for tumor embolization, and for temporary or permanent balloon occlusion during parent vessel sacrifice. Neuroendovascular surgery is being increasingly integrated into the neurosurgical training curriculum. It is essential for future neurosurgeons to have a basic understanding of endovascular techniques and tools and have them as an option for treating cerebrovascular pathological conditions. In this chapter, we discuss the basics of arterial access, catheters for supra-aortic and intracranial access, access site management, and the rationale and techniques for the treatment of various cerebrovascular diseases.

BOX 17.1 Abbreviations Used

ACAS, Asymptomatic Carotid Atherosclerosis Study
ACST, Asymptomatic Carotid Surgery Trial
AVM, arteriovenous malformation
CAS, carotid angioplasty with stenting
CCA, common carotid artery
CE, Conformité Européenne
CEA, carotid endarterectomy
COCOA, Complete Occlusion of Coilable Intracranial Aneurysms Study
CT, computed tomography
DAC, distal access catheter(s)
dAVF, dural arteriovenous fistula
DMSO, dimethyl sulfoxide
DSMB, Data and Safety Monitoring Board
ECA, external carotid artery
ECST, European Carotid Surgery Trial
EVIDENCE, Endovascular Treatment of Intracranial Aneurysms with Pipeline versus Coils with or without Stents
FDA, Food and Drug Administration
F, French
GESICA Groupe d'Etude des Sténoses Intra-Crâniennes Athéromateuses symptomatiques
HR, hazard ratio
IA, intra-arterial
IAT, intra-arterial thrombolysis
ICA, internal carotid artery
ICH, intracranial hemorrhage
IDE, Investigational Device Exemption
ISR, in-stent restenosis
IV, intravenous
IVT, intravenous thrombolysis

MCA, middle cerebral artery
MERCI, Mechanical Embolus Removal in Cerebral Ischemia
MR, magnetic resonance
mRS, modified Rankin scale
NASCET, North American Symptomatic Carotid Endarterectomy Trial
NIH, National Institutes of Health
NIHSS, National Institutes of Health Stroke Scale
NINDS, National Institute of Neurological Disorders and Stroke
PED, Pipeline Embolization Device
PGLA, polyglycolic-polylactic acid
PITA, Pipeline Embolization Device in the Intracranial Treatment of Aneurysms
PROACT, Prolyse in Acute Cerebral Thromboembolism
PUFS, Pipeline for Uncoilable or Failed Aneurysms Study
PVA, polyvinyl alcohol
SAH, subarachnoid hemorrhage
SAMMPRIS, Stenting vs. Aggressive Medical Management for Preventing Recurrent Stroke in Intracranial Stenosis
SAPPHIRE, Stenting and Angioplasty with Protection in Patients at High Risk for Endarterectomy
SARIS, Stent-Assisted Recanalization in Acute Ischemic Stroke
SES, self-expanding stent
SWIFT, Solitaire FR with the Intention for Thrombectomy
TIA, transient ischemic attack
TIMI, Thrombolysis in Myocardial Infarction
TLR, target lesion revascularization
t-PA, tissue plasminogen activator
VA, vertebral artery
WASID, Warfarin vs. Aspirin for Symptomatic Intracranial Disease

GENERAL PRINCIPLES

Preprocedural Evaluation

Before the diagnostic angiogram or intervention is performed, a brief neurological examination is conducted. The patient is asked whether there is a history of reaction to iodinated contrast material. Femoral, dorsalis pedis, and posterior tibial pulses should be examined to identify iliofemoral disease and for comparison after the intervention. Laboratory test results, including renal function and coagulation parameters, should be reviewed. Oral foods and fluids, except medications, are withheld for 6 hours prior to the angiogram or intervention. One or two (for intervention) peripheral IV lines are started. A Foley catheter is placed if an intervention is planned. Conscious sedation is very commonly used for diagnostic angiograms and most interventions performed at our center. Midazolam and fentanyl are the common drugs used for conscious sedation. Intraprocedural monitoring is done with electrocardiograms, blood pressure readings, pulse oximetry, and frequent neurological examinations. Thigh-high sequential compression device sleeves are placed on the lower extremities for deep-vein thrombosis prophylaxis. If stent or flow-diversion device placement is planned, pretreatment with antiplatelet therapy may be indicated.

Antiplatelet Therapy

Patients scheduled to undergo elective stent or flow-diversion device placement receive aspirin (325 mg by mouth daily) and clopidogrel (75 mg by mouth daily) for a minimum of 4 days before the procedure. Those undergoing stenting on a more urgent basis receive aspirin (650 mg by mouth) and clopidogrel (600 mg by mouth) 4 hours before the procedure. If stenting is performed as an emergency bailout maneuver, we administer an intravenous bolus dose of glycoprotein IIb-IIIa inhibitor (180 mg/kg eptifibatide at our institution) and then clopidogrel (600 mg by mouth) and aspirin (650 mg by mouth) immediately after the procedure. Eptifibatide (2 mg/kg/minute) is continued as an intravenous drip for 4 hours after the procedure to allow the clopidogrel to reach therapeutic levels of platelet inhibition. In the rare case of a patient with an acutely ruptured aneurysm undergoing stent placement, the glycoprotein IIb-IIIa inhibitor can be given after the stent is in place and the first or second coil is in proper position. All patients with a stent or flow-diversion device are placed on clopidogrel (75 mg daily) for 3 months and aspirin (325 mg daily) for life.

Contrast Agents

Iohexol, a nonionic contrast agent, is the agent most commonly used for cerebral angiography. Patients with normal renal function can tolerate 400 to 800 mL of iohexol administered at a concentration of 300 mg/mL without adverse effects. Nonionic, low-osmolality contrast agents, such as iodixanol and iopromide, have been shown to be less renal-toxic when compared to iohexol.

Femoral Artery Puncture

The groin is prepared and draped in the usual sterile fashion. The femoral pulse is palpated at the inguinal crease, and local anesthesia is administered via infiltration of 2% lidocaine (5-10 mL) at the site of the planned groin incision. A 5-mm incision is made parallel to the inguinal crease. A Potts needle with the bevel facing upward is advanced at a 45-degree angle to the skin, pointing to the patient's opposite shoulder. On posteroanterior fluoroscopy, the femoral artery is located approximately 1 cm medial to the center of the femoral head. A single-wall puncture technique is performed by looking into the hollow of the needle for blood return; the needle is advanced 1 to 2 mm after blood is seen to maneuver the stylet into the vessel. A J-wire is gently advanced through the needle for 8 to 10 cm. For diagnostic angiography, the needle is exchanged for a regular 5-French (F) 10-cm sheath that is secured with a silk stitch. Sheaths are available in sizes of 4F and larger. The size refers to the inner diameter. The outer diameter is 1.5 to 2.0F larger than the stated inner diameter size. We are increasingly using a micropuncture technique for femoral puncture. In this technique, a 21-gauge needle is inserted in the same fashion as a Potts needle. A 0.018-inch microwire is inserted into the needle. The 21-gauge needle is exchanged for the dilator, and the dilator is exchanged for the sheath. The puncture hole is smaller with this technique and the technique gives a better "feel" of the vessel and needle entry.

For interventional procedures, a 6F sheath is used. Sheaths are also available in various lengths, most commonly 10 or 25 cm. The 25-cm version has the advantage that it bypasses any tortuosity in the iliac arteries. Having the distal end of the sheath in the aorta prevents any danger of injuring the iliac artery during catheter introduction through the sheath. Sheaths that are 90 cm in length, such as the Shuttle (Cook Inc., Bloomington, IN), can reach the carotid artery and can be used as a large-lumen guiding catheter or for added stabilization for a standard guiding catheter.

Radial or brachial artery access can be attempted if femoral artery access is not feasible.

Catheter Navigation

Guide catheters should be advanced over a hydrophilic wire to prevent trauma to the vessels. The tip of the wire is observed under direct fluoroscopic visualization. Slow twisting movements of the wire and observing the tip of the wire will help in identifying inadvertent pinning of the wire in the intima. The catheter-wire system should never be advanced with less than 8 to 10 cm of wire extending from the tip. The commonest catheter we use for supra-aortic cannulation is the Headhunter Multipurpose C catheter (Codman, Raynham, MA). A Simmons-2 or -3 guide catheter (Cordis, Warren, NJ) is used to access the left common carotid artery (CCA) in patients with a bovine arch configuration, with a tortuous arch, or who are older than 50 years.

Roadmapping

Roadmapping (superpositioning of previous contrast angiographic images with "live" or real-time fluoroscopic images) should be used when engaging the vertebral arteries (VAs) and the internal carotid artery (ICA) and external carotid artery (ECA). Roadmapping is essential during intracranial navigation. A "false roadmap" can be created using a regular digital subtraction angiogram; a frame from an angiographic run is selected and then inverted (i.e., vessels are turned white against a black background). This technique conserves contrast material and reduces the amount of radiation exposure.

Aortic Arch Imaging

The aortic arch is catheterized using hydrophilic wires and a soft-tipped guide catheter. The 0.035-inch angled Glidewire (Terumo Medical, Somerset, NJ) is soft, flexible, and steerable, and is the wire used most commonly for aortic arch catheterization. Aortic arch imaging is performed more often in older patients or patients with known variations of the supra-aortic vessel origins or ostial stenosis. A 4F or 5F pigtail-shaped catheter is guided over a hydrophilic wire into the ascending part of the aortic arch. The image intensifier is set to low magnification and rotated 30 degrees to the left. The patient's head is rotated to the left so that he or she is facing the image intensifier. A power injector is used to administer contrast material. A standard left anterior oblique view can be supplemented with a lateral view by rotating the image intensifier 30 degrees to the right to have a better three-dimensional (3D) orientation of the supra-aortic vessels to the arch.

Heparinization

A loading dose of heparin is administered intravenously (70 units/kg) after groin puncture, and 5 minutes later, the activated coagulation time is obtained. The guide catheter is placed in the ICA or VA only after a therapeutic level of heparinization has been achieved. The activated coagulation time should be kept between 250 and 300 seconds for the duration of the procedure. Continuous irrigation of the guide with heparinized saline (5000 units of heparin per 500 mL of saline) is important to avoid thrombus formation. A three-way stopcock connects the heparinized saline flush line to a rotating hemostatic valve to allow continuous infusion of saline through the guide and microcatheter while other devices are being inserted. More recently, we are using a COPILOT Bleedback Control Valve (Guidant Corporation, St. Paul, MN) in the place of a rotating hemostatic valve with the guide catheter because it has a one-way valve that prevents backbleeding from the rotating hemostatic valve during exchange of devices through the guide.

Carotid and Vertebral Artery Catheterization

For carotid artery catheterization, the innominate artery is engaged, and the wire is advanced superiorly into the right CCA, followed by the catheter. To engage the left CCA, the wire is brought inside the catheter, and the catheter is withdrawn and pointed to the left. If selective ICA catheterization is planned, angiography of the cervical carotid arterial system should be done to check for ICA stenosis. Once the CCA is catheterized, turning the head away from the side being catheterized facilitates catheterization of the ICA and turning toward the ipsilateral side facilitates ECA catheterization.

Intermittent "puffing" of contrast material once the catheter is in the subclavian artery will allow identification of the VA origin. A roadmap is made, and the wire is passed into the VA until the tip of the wire is in the upper third of the cervical portion of the vessel. Placing the wire relatively high in the VA provides adequate purchase for advancement of the catheter, helps straighten out any kinks in the artery near the origin, and facilitates smooth passage of the catheter past the entrance of the artery into the foramen tranversarium at the C6 vertebral level. Using roadmapping, the guide catheter is positioned in the distal extracranial VA, usually at the first curve (at C2).

Improved Distal Guide Access

The Neuron or Neuron-2 (Penumbra Inc., Alameda, CA) and Outreach (Concentric Medical, Mountain View, CA) distal access catheters (DACs) are special guide catheters that are relatively rigid proximally but very flexible distally (105 and 120 cm in length), allowing for very distal placement intracranially, with minimal trauma to the vessel. This type of catheter provides a very stable platform in tortuous vessels. We use a coaxial technique of advancing a microcatheter over a microwire through the Neuron/DAC into the target vessel distal to the desired final position of the guide catheter. The Neuron/DAC is then advanced over the microcatheter to its final position. A more substantial microcatheter, such as a Renegade (Boston Scientific, Inc., Natick, MA) or a Prowler Plus (Codman Neurovascular), can provide sufficient support to facilitate distal placement of the Neuron/DAC.

Intracranial Access

Intracranial access and intervention require a stable microwire-microcatheter system. Biplane or three-dimensional roadmapping is essential for safe and expeditious navigation. A wide variety of microwires are available, with differing properties such as size, softness, visibility on fluoroscopy, shapeability, steerability, trackability, and torque control. All microwires suitable for neuroendovascular procedures are hydrophilically coated to reduce friction. Wires can have a shapeable distal tip or may come preshaped. Microwires range from 0.008 inch for the Mirage (ev3, Irvine, CA), to a variety of 0.10-inch and 0.014-inch wires, up to the 0.016-inch Headliner (Terumo Medical Corporation, Somerset, NJ). The Transend EX 0.014-inch Platinum (Boston Scientific) and the Synchro-14 0.014 inch (Boston Scientific) are our main microwires for intracranial manipulations.

Microcatheters are of three types: over the wire (commonest), flow-directed, and steerable. With over-the wire microcatheters, a curved microwire is manipulated toward the target position and the microcatheter is passively advanced over the wire until it reaches the proper position. If Onyx (ev3) is contemplated as an embolic agent, a microcatheter that is compatible with dimethyl sulfoxide (DMSO) must be used. Flow-directed catheters (e.g., Magic microcatheter, A.I.T.-Balt, Miami, FL) are so flexible distally that the catheter tip is pulled

along by blood flow, making this a good choice for high-flow lesions, such as AVMs. Steerable catheters are over-the wire microcatheters (Enzo, Boston Scientific) with a steerable tip to allow access to difficult angulated branches. In our experience, these catheters are very rigid and we use them rarely. Two-marker, over-the-wire microcatheters, rather than single-marker catheters, are necessary for the use of detachable coils. The two markers in microcatheters used in detachable coils are 3 cm apart to determine that the coil is properly deployed.

Femoral Artery Access Site Management

Manual compression is typically used for management of the arteriotomy. The sheath is removed, and pressure is applied 1 to 2 cm above the skin incision. The pressure is usually applied for 15 minutes (40 minutes if the patient is taking aspirin or clopidogrel). The pressure is then slowly released, and a pressure dressing applied. A femoral artery clamp (e.g., Compressar, Instromedex, Hillsboro, OR) can be used instead of manual compression. Percutaneous femoral artery closure devices can allow the patient to ambulate sooner than is possible with compression techniques and can be helpful when the patient is receiving antiplatelet or anticoagulant medications. When a closure device is used, the patient should remain in a supine position for 2 hours.

ISCHEMIC STROKE INTERVENTION

Stroke remains the third most common cause of death in industrialized nations and the single most common reason for permanent adult disability.[1] Each year, approximately 795,000 Americans experience a new or recurrent stroke.[2] The estimated direct and indirect cost of stroke for 2010 is $73.7 billion.[2] The incidence of new or recurrent strokes per year is projected to rise to 1.2 million per year by 2025.[3]

The only medical therapy approved by the Food and Drug Administration (FDA) for acute ischemic stroke treatment until recently was IV recombinant t-PA (rt-PA) administered within 3 hours of symptom onset to patients eligible for thrombolysis.[4,5] The American Heart Association/American Stroke Association guidelines[6] recommend evaluating patients for consideration of IV t-PA therapy 3 to 4.5 hours after stroke symptom onset (on the basis of data from the European Cooperative Acute Stroke Study III).[7] Unfortunately, less than 1% of acute ischemic stroke patients in the United States receive t-PA, primarily because of a delay in presentation for treatment.[8] Early reocclusion following thrombolysis has been demonstrated by transcranial Doppler imaging to occur in 34% of patients receiving IV t-PA and may result in neurological worsening in many of these patients.[9-11] Recanalization rates after IV t-PA therapy for proximal, large vessel arterial occlusions are poor and range from only 10% for ICA occlusion to 30% for middle cerebral artery (MCA) occlusion.[12] IV thrombolysis (IVT) is not as effective in thromboembolic obstruction of these large, proximal vessels, as compared with more distal smaller vessels.[13] The outcome after large intracranial vessel thromboembolic occlusion currently remains dismal and is associated with high rates of morbidity and mortality.[14-17] Patients who do not meet the eligibility criteria for thrombolytic therapy, who fail to improve neurologically after thrombolytic therapy, or who improve and then worsen (patients with reocclusion) are currently candidates for endovascular revascularization therapies.

Endovascular Stroke Revascularization Techniques

Techniques for stroke revascularization can be classified as mechanical and pharmacological. Mechanical methods include microwire manipulation; snare; the current FDA-approved embolectomy devices, namely, the Penumbra (Penumbra Inc., Alameda, CA) and the Merci retriever (Concentric Medical Inc., Mountain View, CA); and stent-assisted or stent-platform-based stroke thrombectomy devices.

Time Window for Endovascular Stroke Therapy

Endovascular therapy is expanding the time window after stroke symptom onset for revascularization in patients with acute ischemic stroke The Prolyse in Acute Cerebral Thromboembolism (PROACT) trials[18,19] established a benefit of intra-arterial thrombolysis (IAT) up to 6 hours after stroke symptom onset, with an increase in recanalization rates. Flow is reestablished faster with mechanical revascularization strategies than with thrombolytics; thus, such strategies may increase the benefit of treatment, even when there is a delay in presentation for treatment. The Mechanical Embolus Removal in Cerebral Ischemia (MERCI),[20,21] Multi-MERCI,[22] and Penumbra[23] trials show effectiveness of mechanical revascularization therapy up to 8 hours after stroke symptom onset. There is increasing evidence that identification of potentially salvageable brain tissue with advanced magnetic resonance (MR) and computed tomography (CT) imaging may allow the selection of patients who can be effectively and safely treated more than 8 hours post ictus.[7,24-29]

Higher Recanalization Rate and Improved Outcome after Stroke Intervention

In MERCI,[20,21] Multi-MERCI,[22] and the combined analysis of data from the Interventional Management of Stroke I and II studies,[30] functional outcome (measured by modified Rankin Scale [mRS] score of ≤2 at 3 months) was significantly better and the 3-month mortality rate was significantly lower in patients who had thrombolysis in myocardial infarction (TIMI) scores 2 or 3 recanalization than in patients in whom vessels failed to recanalize after endovascular therapy. In a review of 53 studies that included 2066 patients, good functional outcome (mRS score ≤2) at 3 months was identified more frequently in patients with vessel recanalization than without vessel recanalization.[31] The 3-month mortality rate was reduced in patients in whom vessels were recanalized. Higher rates of recanalization were achieved with endovascular methods, particularly mechanical therapies, and consequently were associated with better outcomes.

Merci Device (Fig. 17.1 and Video 17.1)

The Merci retriever system has a flexible nitinol wire that assumes a helical shape once it emerges from the tip of the microcatheter. A microcatheter containing this wire is passed distal to the thrombus, the catheter is withdrawn, and the wire, in its helical configuration, ensnares the clot for removal from the vasculature. Vessels amenable to embolectomy with the Merci device include the ICA, M1 and M2 segments of the MCA, VA, basilar artery, and the posterior cerebral artery. The retriever is then retracted into the guide catheter under proximal flow arrest. FDA approval of the Merci device in 2004 was based on a review of data obtained in the multicenter MERCI trial that involved 141 patients (mean age, 60 years; mean National Institutes of Health Stroke Scale [NIHSS] score, 20) ineligible for standard thrombolytic therapy.[20,21] The Multi-MERCI trial[22] is a prospective, multicenter, single-arm registry that included 164 patients who were treated with different Merci retrieval systems (X5, X6, and L5).

Penumbra Device (Fig. 17.2 and Video 17.2)

The Penumbra System (Penumbra, Inc., San Leandro, CA) is the second FDA-approved mechanical treatment for acute stroke. The system primarily involves clot aspiration using a microcatheter attached to a powered aspiration pump that is capable of producing 25 mm Hg of suction. The separator is a soft wire with a 6-mm teardrop-shaped enlargement proximal to its tip and is inserted via the microcatheter to fragment the clot and keep the microcatheter tip from clogging. A major advantage over the Merci system is that the Penumbra System works at the proximal face of the clot, eliminating the need to blindly position the microcatheter distal to the occlusion. A prospective, single-arm, independently monitored trial was performed to assess the efficiency and safety of the Penumbra System.[23] In a prospective multicenter single-arm trial of 125 patients with acute stroke who underwent revascularization with the Penumbra device, TIMI 2 or 3 recanalization was achieved in 81.6% patients, with a symptomatic intracranial hemorrhage (ICH) rate of 11.2% and only 25% of patients achieving an mRS score of 2 or less.[32]

Stent-Assisted Thrombolysis

Self-expanding stents (SES) designed specifically for the cerebrovasculature are available. These stents can be delivered to intracranial target areas with a greater than 95% technical success rate with an increased safety profile because they are deployed at significantly lower pressures than balloon-mounted coronary stents.[33] With the stent-for-stroke technique (using Wingspan [Boston Scientific] and Enterprise [Codman Neurovascular] SES), vessel recanalization is instantaneous, and the chance of early reocclusion after treatment is decreased. Reocclusion after IVT (34%) and pharmacological IAT (17%) has been shown and is associated with poor outcome.[34]

For stent-assisted thrombolysis, standard femoral access is obtained, and a 6F (or larger) guide catheter is placed in the target vessel proximal to the occlusion. To minimize the release of distal emboli, the occlusion is crossed in a fashion similar to that used for the Merci clot retriever. First, a .014-inch steerable wire is softly advanced through the clot. A low-profile catheter is then advanced over the wire distal to the occlusion. Following microangiographic confirmation that the microcatheter is distal to the occlusion, an exchange wire is brought through the microcatheter and anchored distal to the occlusion. The microcatheter is removed, and the stent delivery catheter is delivered over the exchange wire. To minimize

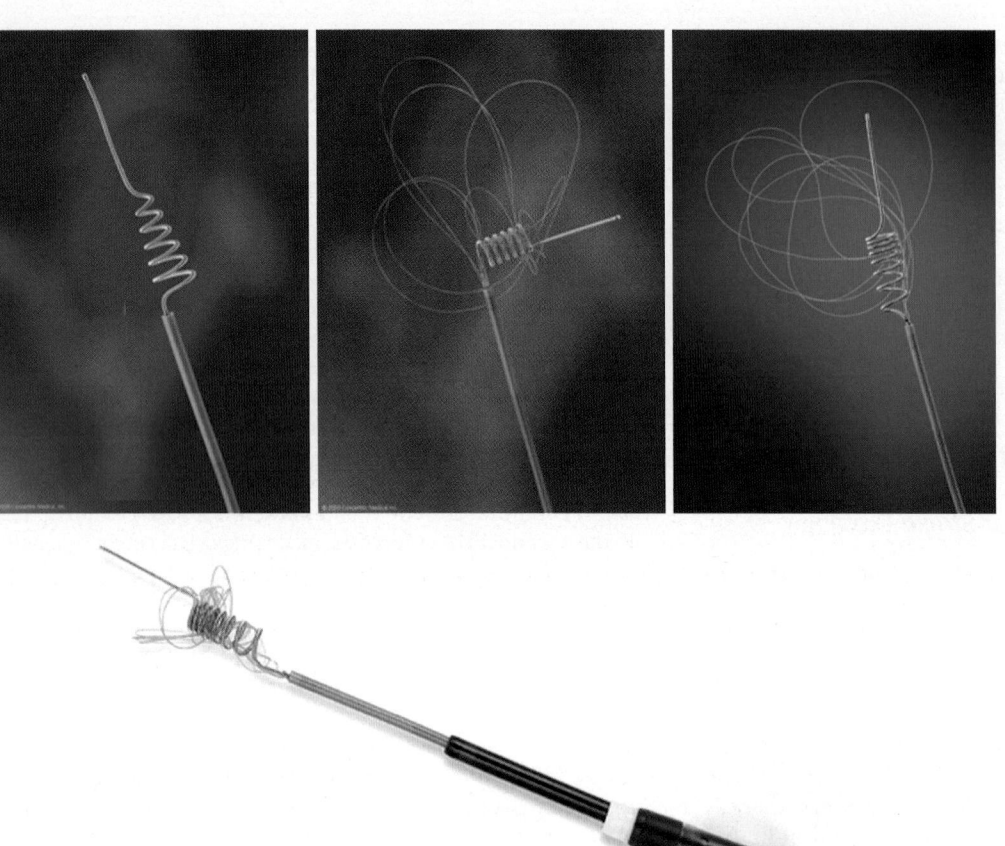

FIGURE 17.1 Types of Merci devices. Left, Type X. Middle, Type L. Right, Type V. Bottom, Catheter system. *(Courtesy of Concentric Medical, Mountain View, CA.)*

© 2009 Concentric Medical, Inc.

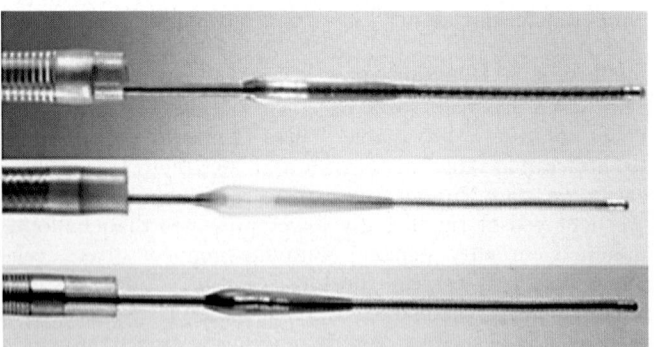

FIGURE 17.2 Penumbra device. Sizes are 026, 032, and 041, from bottom to top. *(Courtesy of Penumbra Inc., Alameda, CA.)*

the release of debris, the stent is deployed first distal to the occlusion (thus trapping any debris that may be later released between the stent and the vessel wall), then through the occlusion, and finally just proximal to the occlusion.

Several retrospective case series reported successful use of SES for acute stroke treatment, with higher rates of recanalization than other recanalization modalities.[35-37] Presently, SES are used only off-label under a humanitarian device exemption as a salvage therapy when current FDA-approved thrombectomy devices fail. On the basis of these preliminary data, we received FDA approval for a pilot study, Stent-Assisted Recanalization in Acute Ischemic Stroke (SARIS),[38] to evaluate the Wingspan stent for revascularization in patients who did not improve after IVT or had a contraindication to IVT. Average presenting NIHSS score was 14. Seventeen patients presented with a TIMI score of 0 and three patients with a TIMI score of 1. Intracranial SES were placed in 19 of 20 enrolled patients. One patient experienced recanalization of the occluded vessel during positioning of the Wingspan stent delivery system, prior to stent deployment. In two patients, the tortuous vessel did not allow tracking of the Wingspan stent. The more navigable Enterprise stent was used in both these cases. Twelve patients had other adjunctive therapies. TIMI 2 or 3 recanalization was achieved in 100% of patients; 65% of patients improved more than 4 points in NIHSS score after treatment. One patient (5%) had symptomatic ICH, and two had asymptomatic ICH. At the time of the 1-month follow-up evaluation, 12 of 20 (60%) patients had mRS scores of 2 or less and nine (45%) had mRS scores of 1 or less. Mortality rate at 1 month was 25%. None of these patients died because of stent-placement-related causes; all deaths were due to the severity of the initial stroke and associated comorbid conditions.

Stent-Platform-Based Thrombectomy Devices (Stentrievers)

The Solitaire FR Revascularization Device (ev3) (Figs. 17.3 and 17.4) and Trevo device (Concentric Medical Inc.) are recoverable self-expanding thrombectomy devices that

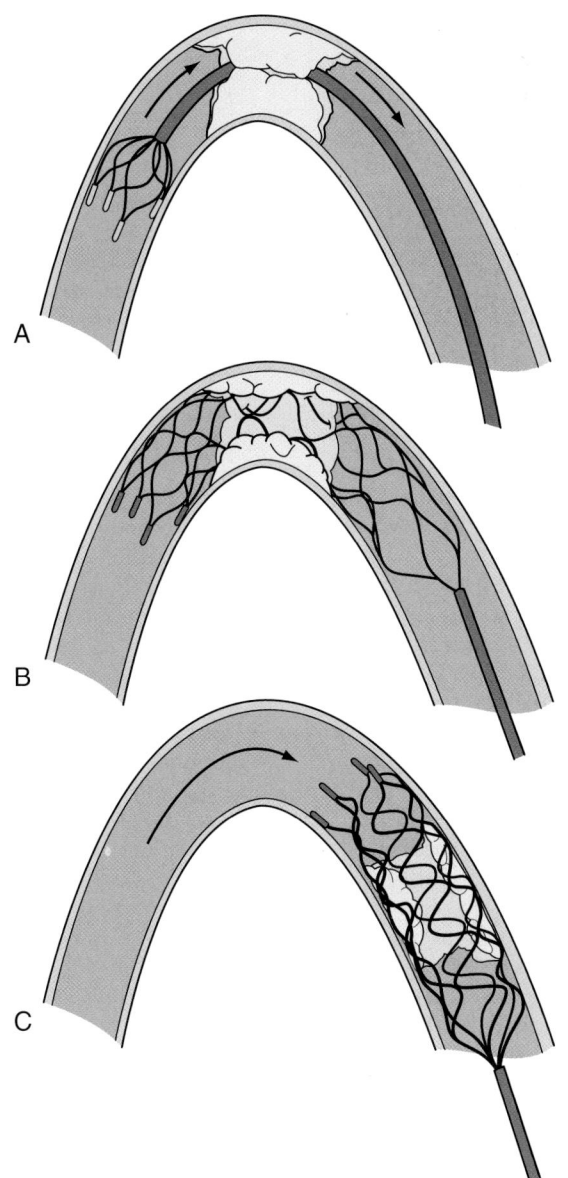

FIGURE 17.3 A, An occlusive clot in the vessel that has been crossed by the Rebar microcatheter (ev3, Irvine, CA). The microwire has been exchanged with the Solitaire device (ev3) that is being deployed in the direction shown by the arrows. **B,** The Solitaire device is completely deployed and pushes the clot to the side, restoring blood flow immediately in the occluded vessel. **C,** The Solitaire with the clot and the Rebar are pulled with the clot into the guide catheter with constant syringe aspiration from the guide catheter. *(From Natarajan SK, Siddiqui AH, Hopkins LN, Levy EI. Retrievable, detachable stent-platform-based clot-retrieval device (Solitaire FR) for acute stroke revascularization: first demonstration of feasibility in a canine stroke model. Vasc Dis Management 2010;7:E120-E125.)*

are being tested clinically in the United States and Europe, respectively, for acute ischemic stroke revascularization. The advantage of these devices is that they are fully recoverable, SES-platform-based devices that can be used for both temporary endovascular bypass and thrombectomy. The devices restore flow immediately and avoid the placement of a permanent stent, thus obviating the need for antithrombotic therapy

and the risk of in-stent stenosis. The Solitaire can be electrolytically detached like a coil in case a permanent stent is necessary, such as in the setting of an atherothrombotic lesion. The Solitaire FR With the Intention for Thrombectomy (SWIFT) trial is an ongoing multicenter randomized controlled trial that is testing the ability of the Solitaire FR device versus the Merci device to achieve TIMI 2 or 3 recanalization without symptomatic ICH. Two small preliminary studies with this device have shown promising results.[39,40]

Intra-arterial Pharmacological Thrombolysis

At our center, pharmacological thrombolysis is mainly used as an adjunct to primary mechanical therapy or in lesions that are inaccessible with currently available mechanical devices. To perform IAT, a microcatheter is placed proximal to or directly into the thrombus and rt-PA or eptifibatide is administered. Eptifibatide is used primarily when new thrombus formation is seen during the revascularization procedure, whereas rt-PA is used for distal unreachable clots and distal emboli after mechanical therapy.

Perfusion Imaging for Complication Avoidance and Patient Selection

Endovascular revascularization is an invasive procedure and is associated with acceptable complications in light of the morbidity and mortality risks associated with a major stroke if recanalization is not achieved. Despite aggressive revascularization with mechanical therapies, only up to 45% of patients recover to an mRS score of 0 to 2 at 3 months, and there is approximately an 8% to 10% procedure-related risk of symptomatic ICH, a potentially detrimental complication.[19-23,32,38] CT and MR perfusion imaging are utilized in attempts to differentiate the three zones of postischemia brain tissue that are critical for patient selection and complication avoidance, and thus the ability to discriminate among them with these modalities is envisioned to lead to an improvement in outcomes after endovascular stroke therapy in the future. The three zones are core (tissue that is dead), penumbra (tissue at risk of death if not revascularized/reperfused), and benign oligemia (tissue that will tolerate the reduced blood flow and will survive even without reperfusion, mainly dependent on collaterals). Currently, no imaging modality is capable of differentiating between penumbra and benign oligemia. MR-diffusion-weighted imaging and cerebral blood flow maps obtained with CT perfusion imaging are able to identify core tissue with acceptable false positive and false negative rates. At our center, we have found that core tissue in the basal ganglia region or a core occupying more than 30% of occluded territory presages a higher risk of symptomatic ICH after endovascular stroke intervention. Sophisticated and precise imaging is needed to identify these three territories after cerebral ischemia.

INTRACRANIAL ATHEROSCLEROSIS TREATMENT

Approximately 8% to 10% of ischemic strokes are attributable to intracranial atherosclerosis.[41,42] An estimated 40,000 to 60,000 new strokes per year in the United States are due to

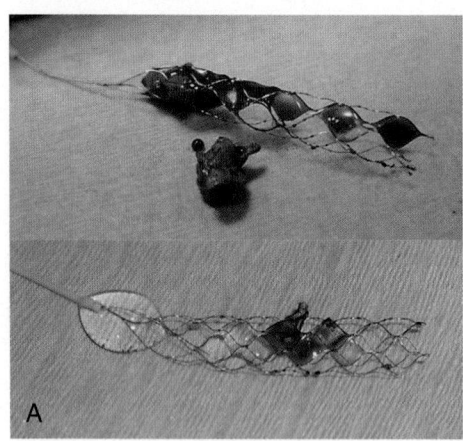
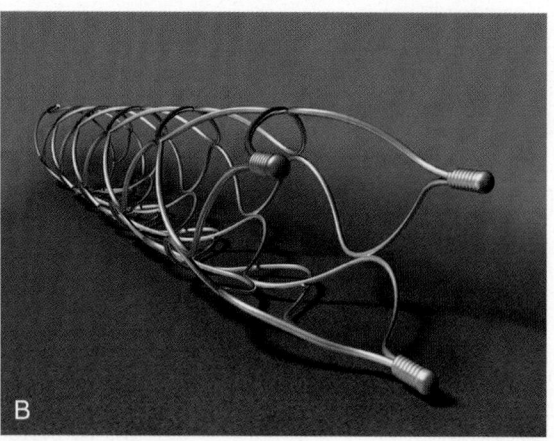

FIGURE 17.4 **A,** Solitaire FR device with retrieved clot (actual size). **B,** Solitaire FR. *(A from Natarajan SK, Siddiqui AH, Hopkins LN, Levy EI. Retrievable, detachable stent-platform-based clot-retrieval device (Solitaire FR) for acute stroke revascularization: first demonstration of feasibility in a canine stroke model. Vasc Dis Management 2010;7:E120-E125; B courtesy of ev3, Irvine, CA.)*

intracranial atherosclerosis.[43] In a study of patients with intracranial stenosis undergoing repeat angiography at an average interval of 26.7 months, 40% of lesions had stabilized, 20% had regressed, and 40% had progressed.[44] Stenosis progression, as detected by transcranial Doppler imaging, was an independent predictor of stroke recurrence.[45]

Need for Treatment

The most definitive study of symptomatic intracranial stenosis thus far is the prospective Warfarin versus Aspirin for Symptomatic Intracranial Disease (WASID) trial, which found an 11% to 12% first-year risk of ischemic stroke in territory attributable to the patient symptoms.[46] The majority of strokes (73%) in WASID patients were in the territory of the stenotic artery.[47] Patients in the Extracranial-Intracranial Bypass Study with MCA stenosis who were randomized to medical therapy had an annual ipsilateral ischemic stroke rate of 7.8%.[48,49] In the prospective, nonrandomized Groupe d'Etude des Sténoses Intra-Crâniennes Athéromateuses symptomatiques (GESICA), 102 patients with more than 50% symptomatic intracranial stenosis had "optimal" medical therapy, with a follow-up period of 23.4 months.[50] Among these patients, ipsilateral transient ischemic attack (TIA) occurred in 12.6% and ipsilateral stroke in 7.0%.

Endovascular Tools and Technique

The Wingspan Stent System with the Gateway percutaneous transluminal angioplasty balloon catheter was designed for the treatment of intracranial atherosclerotic stenosis and received FDA approval for this indication under the humanitarian exemption device provision in August 2005. Prestent dilation of the stenotic lesion is done with the angioplasty balloon and the stent, a self-expanding nitinol device, is then deployed (Fig. 17.5 and Video 17.3).

Essential devices for the angioplasty portion of the procedure include an exchange-length microwire, a microcatheter, and a balloon. Microwire properties that are most important for intracranial angioplasty are "beefiness," trackability, and torque control. A relatively soft distal tip is helpful as well to minimize the chances of vasospasm or perforation of distal vessels. We prefer to use the 0.014-inch, 300-cm Transend FloppyTip microwire (Boston Scientific) because it has superior torque control compared with other microwires. The 0.014-inch, 300-cm X-Celerator microwire (ev3) is another option; it has a soft tip, relatively supportive body, and is very lubricious. A low-profile, straight microcatheter, usually of any kind, is sufficient. The 1.7-F Echelon-10 microcatheter (ev3) can be pushed through tortuous and stenotic vessels better than other microcatheters.

The Gateway balloon is a modified version of the Maverick 2 Balloon Catheter (Boston Scientific) with silicone coating on the balloon and hydrophilic coating on the catheter to facilitate access. Radiopaque markers on the balloon permit visualization of the proximal and distal ends of the balloon during fluoroscopic imaging. With roadmap guidance, the balloon is advanced until the balloon markers are across the lesion. A guide catheter angiogram is performed with the balloon in position to confirm proper positioning. The balloon is slowly inflated to nominal pressure, at a rate of approximately 1 atm every 10 seconds, under fluoroscopy. When the balloon is fully inflated, it is left inflated for another 10 to 20 seconds and then deflated. A guide catheter angiogram is obtained prior to removal of the balloon.

The Wingspan is a 3.5F, nitinol, over-the-wire SES. The design of this stent is very similar to that of the Neuroform 2 stent (Boston Scientific), which will be described later. The Wingspan has four platinum markers at each end for visualization and is deployed from the delivery microcatheter (called the "outer body") with the "inner body"; the inner body is analogous to the "stabilizer" device that is used to deploy Neuroform stents. The rotating hemostatic valve is tightened on the inner body to prevent its migration, and the outer body of the Wingspan system is advanced over the exchange-length microwire. The inner body is advanced just proximal to the stent using the marker bands to identify the position of the stent. The outer body is pulled back to bring the outer body tip into position just past the region of stenosis. Holding the inner body in a stable position with the right hand, while slowly withdrawing the outer body with the left hand, results in deployment of the stent. The goal of therapy in these cases is to open the vessel to only 80% of its normal diameter.

Wingspan Studies

U.S. Wingspan Registry

In the U.S. Wingspan registry,[51-53] treatment with the stent system was attempted in 158 patients with 168 intracranial

FIGURE 17.5 **A,** A Gateway balloon (*top*) and a Wingspan stent (*bottom*). **B,** A critical atherosclerotic stenosis in an intracranial vessel. **C,** The Gateway balloon has been placed across the lesion, and the lesion has been predilated. **D,** Placement of a Wingspan stent system (undeployed) across the dilated segment. **E** and **F,** Deploying the Wingspan stent across the lesion. **G,** Arrows indicate the radial expansive force in the Wingspan stent. *(Courtesy of Boston Scientific, Natick, MA.)*

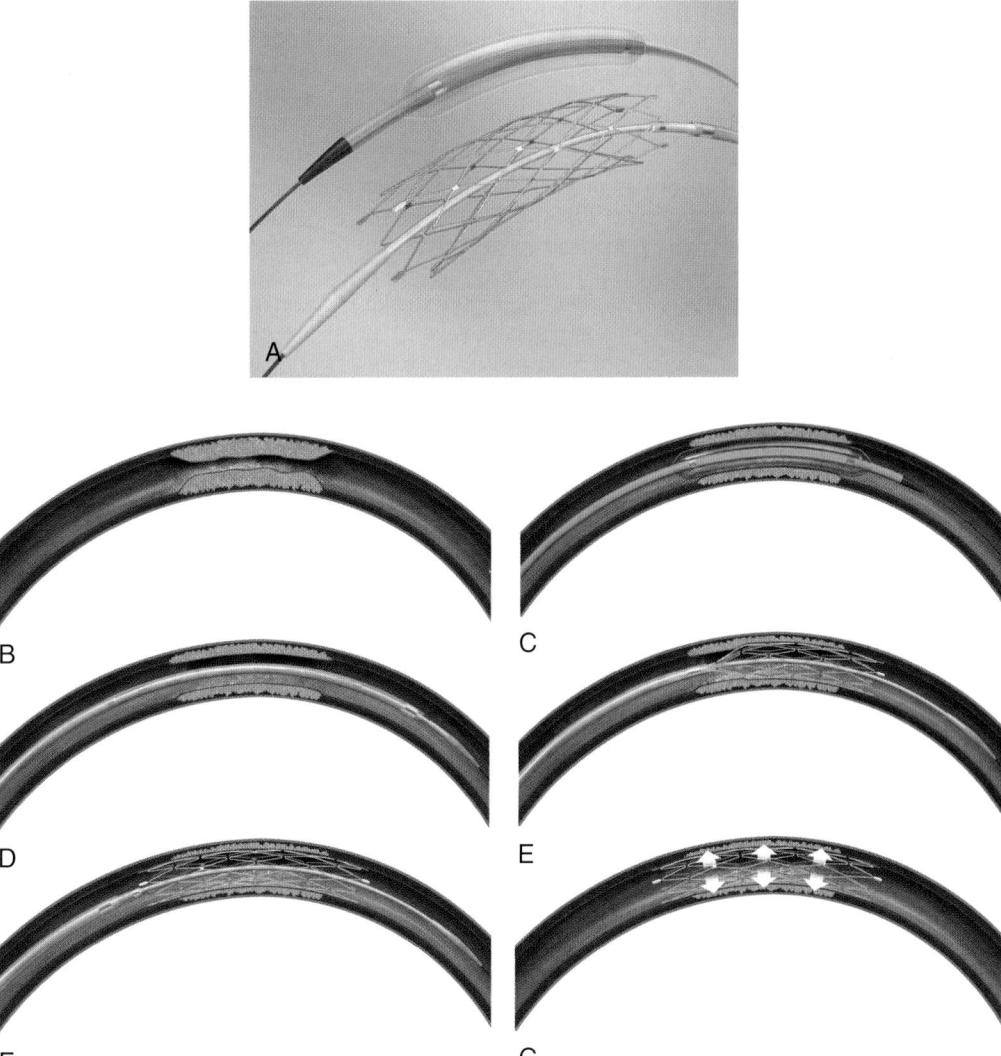

atheromatous lesions. Of these, 161 lesions were successfully treated (96.0%) during the first treatment session. Of the 168 lesions in which treatment was attempted, there were 9 (5.4%) major periprocedural neurological complications, 4 of which ultimately led to the death of the patient within 30 days of the procedure. The total periprocedural event rate was 12.5% (21 of 168 cases). Most postprocedure events (18 of 21) were related to definable (and potentially controllable) issues: early antiplatelet interruption (*n* = 6) and in-stent restenosis (ISR) (*n* = 13). Imaging follow-up was available for 129 treated lesions (75 anterior circulation, 54 posterior circulation). Thirty-six of 129 (27.9%) patients with imaging follow-up of treated lesions experienced ISR. Of these 36, 29 (80.6%) underwent target lesion revascularization (TLR) with angioplasty alone (*n* = 26) or angioplasty with restenting (*n* = 3). Post-Wingspan ISR was more common in patients younger than 55 years old (odds ratio = 2.6). This increased risk can be accounted for by a high prevalence of anterior circulation lesions in this population, specifically those affecting the supraclinoid segment. When patients of all ages were considered, much higher rates of both ISR (66.6% vs. 24.4%) and symptomatic ISR (40% vs. 3.9%) were associated with supraclinoid

segment lesions, by comparison with all other locations. Of the 29 patients undergoing primary TLR, 9 required one intervention for recurrent ISR, for a total of 42 TLR interventions. Only one major complication, a postprocedural reperfusion hemorrhage, was encountered during TLR (complication rates: 2.4% per procedure; 3.5% per patient). Angiographic follow-up was available for 22 of 29 patients after primary TLR. Eleven of 22 (50%) patients demonstrated recurrent ISR at follow-up angiography. Subsequently, 9 of these patients have undergone multiple re-treatments (6 patients had two re-treatments each, 2 had three re-treatments each, and 1 had four re-treatments) for recurrent ISR.

The 12-month follow-up results were recently published.[54] The average follow-up duration was 14.2 months with 110 patients having at least 12 months of follow-up. The cumulative rate of the primary endpoint (stroke or death within 30 days or ipsilateral stroke after 30 days) was 15.7% for all patients and 13.9% for patients with high-grade stenosis (70-99%). Thirteen ipsilateral strokes occurred after 30 days, and 3 of these patients died. Ten of 13 (76.9%) strokes occurred within the first 6 months of the stenting procedure, and no events occurred after 12 months. An additional 9 patients had ipsilateral TIA after 30 days. Most postprocedure events (86%) were related to in-stent restenosis ($n = 12$), interruption of antiplatelet therapy ($n = 6$), or both ($n = 1$).

Wingspan NIH Registry

In the Wingspan National Institutes of Health (NIH) registry,[37] 129 patients with symptomatic 70% to 99% intracranial stenosis were enrolled from 16 medical centers. The rate of technical success (stent placement across the target lesion with <50% residual stenosis) was 97%. The rate of any stroke, ICH, or death within 30 days or ipsilateral stroke beyond 30 days was 14% at 6 months. The rate of 50% or greater restenosis on follow-up angiography was 25% among 52 patients with follow-up. The NIH registry investigators published a posthoc analysis report of 158 of 160 patients who had successful placement for intracranial atherosclerotic lesions with 50% to 99% stenosis.[55] The primary endpoint (any stroke or death within 30 days or stroke in the territory of the stented artery beyond 30 days and up to 6 months) occurred in 13.9%. In multivariable analysis, the primary endpoint was associated with posterior circulation stenosis (vs. anterior circulation) (hazard ratio [HR] 3.4, $p = 0.018$), stenting at low enrollment sites (<10 patients each) (vs. high enrollment site) (HR 2.8, $p = 0.038$), 10 or fewer days from qualifying event to stenting (vs. ≥10 days) (HR 2.7, $p = 0.058$), and stroke as a qualifying event (vs. TIA or other cerebral ischemic event, such as vertebrobasilar insufficiency) (HR 3.2, $p = 0.064$).

SAMMPRIS Study

In 2007, the NIH approved funding for the multicenter, prospective, randomized Stenting vs. Aggressive Medical Management for Preventing Recurrent Stroke in Intracranial Stenosis (SAMMPRIS) study.[56] The hypothesis of the study is that "Compared with intensive medical therapy alone, intracranial angioplasty and stenting combined with intensive medical therapy will decrease the risk of the primary endpoint by 35% over a mean follow-up of 2 years in high-risk patients (patients with 70-99% intracranial stenosis who had a TIA or stroke within 30 days prior to enrollment) with symptomatic stenosis of a major intracranial artery." A total of 764 patients will be recruited within 30 days of TIA or stroke due to 70% to 99% stenosis of a major intracranial artery. The patients will be randomized to either stent treatment with the Wingspan intracranial stent and Gateway balloon system plus intensive medical therapy with management of blood pressure, lipids, and other risk factors for vascular events or to this intensive medical therapy alone. Each patient will be followed for a minimum of 1 year and a maximum of 4 years after randomization. On April 11, 2011, the National Institute of Neurological Disorders and Stroke (NINDS) issued an alert[57] to the SAMMPRIS investigators to stop enrollment in this trial because the last data and safety monitoring board (DSMB) review found that 14% of patients treated with angioplasty combined with stenting experienced a stroke or died within the first 30 days after enrollment compared with 5.8% of patients treated with medical therapy alone, a highly significant difference. The 30-day rate of stroke or death in the intensive medical treatment arm was substantially lower than the estimated rate of 10.7% based on historical control

subjects, most of whom received standard medical care. In addition, the 30-day rate in the stent group was substantially higher than the estimated rate of 5.2% to 9.6%, based on registry data. The SAMMPRIS Executive Committee was in agreement with NINDS and the DSMB that enrollment in the study should be stopped and that the trial data currently available indicate that aggressive medical management alone is superior to angioplasty combined with stenting in patients with recent symptoms and high-grade intracranial arterial stenosis. Follow-up of currently enrolled patients and a comprehensive analysis of the total trial dataset will be important in the final interpretation of this study.

CAROTID ANGIOPLASTY AND STENTING

Atherosclerotic disease in the carotid arteries is thought to be the cause in up to 30% of ischemic strokes.[41] The North American Symptomatic Carotid Endarterectomy Trial (NASCET),[58,59] Asymptomatic Carotid Atherosclerosis Study (ACAS),[60] Asymptomatic Carotid Surgery Trial (ACST),[61] and the European Carotid Surgery Trial (ECST)[62,63] established carotid endarterectomy (CEA) as an effective means of future stroke prevention in at-risk populations with significant carotid artery disease. Carotid angioplasty with stenting (CAS) was introduced as a less-invasive alternative to conventional CEA. With the subsequent development of distal embolic protection devices and stents for the carotid system, CAS became a promising and viable option for patients who were poor candidates for CEA.[64-66]

The major impetus for the advancement of CAS came with the publication of the results of the Stenting and Angioplasty with Protection in Patients at High Risk for Endarterectomy (SAPPHIRE) trial,[67] which demonstrated effectively that patients considered high risk for CEA were less likely to have complications if treated with CAS. This resulted in the approval of CAS by the FDA, Centers for Medicare & Medicaid Services, and Medicare as a viable option for such patients. More recently, an entirely new method of embolic protection achieved through flow reversal from the ICA into the arterial guide sheath, classified as proximal embolic protection, is being tested.[68]

Technique (Video 17.4) and Tools

An aortic arch angiogram is initially performed to define the atherosclerotic burden as well as the anatomical configuration of the great vessels, which allows the operator to predict the feasibility of carotid cannulation and select the devices needed for the procedure. Selective carotid angiography is then performed, and the severity of the stenosis is defined. The diameters of the CCA and ICA are measured with attention paid to determining a landing zone for the embolic protection device. Intracranial angiography is also essential before the intervention because the presence of tandem lesions should be considered in the management strategy as well as for comparison of pre- and post-intracranial angiograms to confirm the absence of any vessel dropout suggestive of embolism.

After completion of the diagnostic angiogram and positioning of the catheter in the CCA, roadmapping of the cervical carotid artery is performed. An exchange-length

0.035-inch wire is positioned in the ECA. The diagnostic catheter is exchanged over the wire for a 90-cm, 6F to 10F sheath that is then advanced into the CCA below the bifurcation. For patients who have undergone complete diagnostic cerebral angiography before the stenting procedure, a combination of a 6F, 90-cm shuttle over a 6.5F Headhunter 125-cm slip-catheter (Cook) or a 5F, 125-cm Vitek catheter (Cook) can be used. In these cases, the shuttle is introduced primarily in the femoral artery over a 0.35-inch wire and is parked in the descending aorta. The inner obturator and wire are removed. The 125-cm catheter is then advanced into the shuttle, and the target vessel is catheterized. The shuttle is brought over the wire and the catheter in the CCA. The size of the shuttle is usually dictated by the profile of the embolic protection device and compatibility with the stent system. An optimal angiographic view that maximizes the opening of the bifurcation and facilitates crossing of the stenosis should be sought. The lesion is crossed with the protection device. Predilation of the stenotic vessel segment is performed at the operator's discretion. We avoid predilation of the lesion whenever possible; however, if predilation is necessary, we prefer to undersize the balloon to simply facilitate crossing of the stent, usually using a 2- to 3-mm-diameter balloon. A 3- to 4-mm coaxial angioplasty balloon is advanced to the lesion over the 0.014-inch wire holding the protection device. On rare occasions, predilation needs to be performed before the introduction of an embolic protection device.

The diameter of the stent should be sized to the caliber of the largest segment of the carotid artery to be covered (usually 1-2 mm more than the normal caliber of the CCA). Oversizing of the stent in the ICA does not usually result in adverse events, but a tapered stent can better conform to the vessel wall. Particular attention should be paid to the selection of a stent that is long enough to cover the entire lesion.

After removing the stent system, poststent dilation is performed using a balloon with a diameter matching that of the ICA distal to the stent. A coaxial balloon is usually preferred for this purpose. The embolic protection device is then removed, using its retrieval catheter. (When a balloon occlusion catheter is used for cerebral protection, the embolic debris is aspirated before deflation and retrieval of the balloon.)

Embolic Protection Devices

All embolic protection systems currently on the market can be classified under three main groups, each with its own working principle: (1) distal occlusion balloons, (2) distal filters, and (3) proximal occlusion devices. With the distal occlusion devices, a balloon is inflated in the ICA between the lesion and the brain to block the blood flow toward the cerebrum. Consequently, debris cannot enter the cerebral vasculature during the procedure. The debris is aspirated and flushed, forcing it either into the ECA or out of the body, through a sheath in the CCA. Filtration systems function in the manner of an umbrella- or windsock-like filter hose, which are opened in between the carotid lesion and the brain to capture all debris during the CAS procedure. Together with the distal filter, the debris is removed at the end of the procedure. A distal filter can be mounted on a guidewire, on which it is directly brought in place and retrieved, or alternatively, can come with its own specific delivery and retrieval system. Proximal occlusion systems (Fig. 17.6) are characterized by two compliant

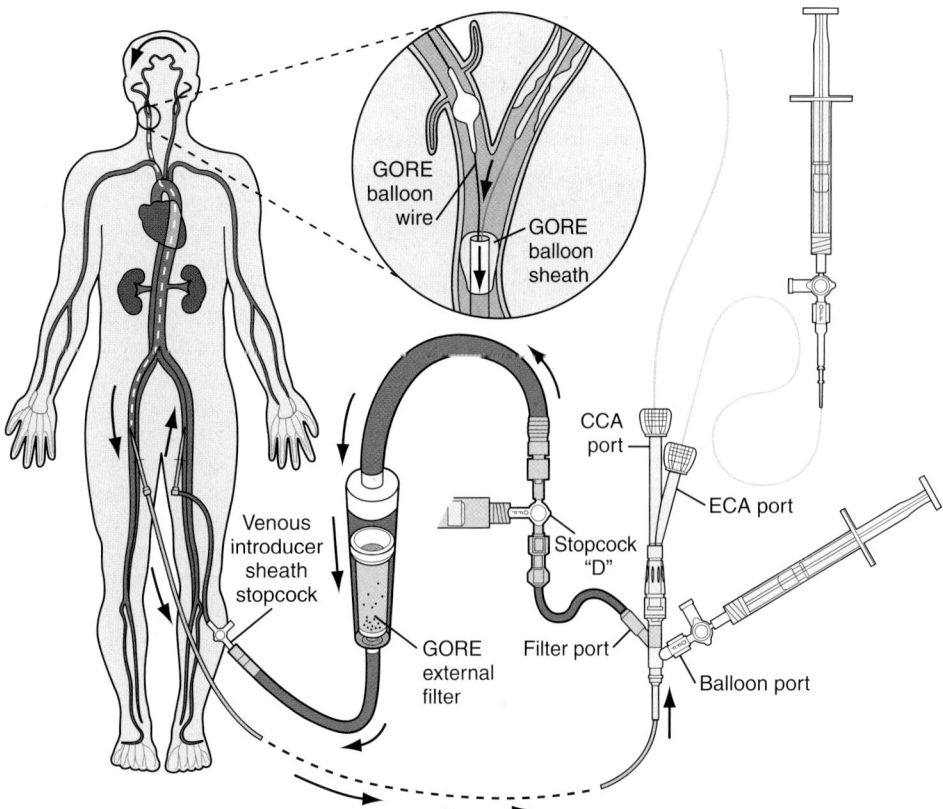

FIGURE 17.6 The Gore flow reversal device causes a no-flow or a reversed-flow pattern within the internal carotid artery (ICA) that prevents debris from entering the cerebral circulation. The advantage of the Gore device is that it provides embolic protection before crossing the lesion, although it requires favorable arch anatomy and a larger access sheath is needed for delivery. *(Courtesy of W.L. Gore & Associates, Flagstaff, AZ.)*

balloons to be inflated, one in the proximal CCA and one in the ECA. This double-balloon inflation creates either a no-flow or a reversed-flow pattern within the ICA, thereby preventing embolization of debris in the cerebral circulation. Proximal occlusion devices are especially attractive because complete cerebral protection is established before the device is passed across the lesion. The concerns associated with proximal protection devices are their large size (currently requiring 9F access to the femoral artery) and the concurrent delivery of a 9F system into tortuous CCAs.

INTRACRANIAL ANEURYSM TREATMENT

The overall prevalence of unruptured intracranial aneurysms in the general population is between 0.8% and 6%. The incidence of aneurysmal subarachnoid hemorrhage (SAH) is between 10 and 15 per 100,000 people per year. Endovascular treatment of intracranial aneurysms has undergone multiple changes since the introduction of Guglielmi detachable coils (Boston Scientific/Target, Fremont, CA) for endosaccular occlusion of these aneurysms in 1994. When there was a high recurrence rate for wide-necked aneurysms after simple coiling, adjunctive techniques including balloon-assisted and stent-assisted coiling were introduced. Onyx liquid embolic agent is being tested for aneurysm occlusion. The concept of flow diversion and parent vessel reconstruction without endosaccular occlusion of the aneurysm has gained momentum and has been useful in complex aneurysms that could not be adequately treated with previously available endovascular techniques. Flow-diversion devices are being widely tested for the safety and efficacy of aneurysm exclusion.

Aneurysm Coils

A coil consists of a fine platinum thread tightly looped around a thicker platinum wire. The coil is connected to a "pusher wire"; the attachment site is the location of the detachment mechanism, which may be electrolytic, thermal, or hydraulic in design. The coil and pusher wire come from the manufacturer in a slim plastic delivery sheath; the sheath is placed within the hub of the rotating hemostatic valve, and the coil and pusher wire are threaded together into the microcatheter.

The coil is designed to assume one of a number of shapes as it is pushed out of the microcatheter. Framing coils are three-dimensional coils designed to "frame" the aneurysm; that is, these coils are meant to "sphericize" the aneurysm with gentle outward radial force to permit packing with two-dimensional coils. Filling coils are intended to occupy space within the aneurysm after framing. These coils usually have a helical shape and are of intermediate stiffness. Finishing coils are the softest coils and are designed for final packing of the aneurysm and "finishing off" of the neck.

Observations of aneurysm recanalization after treatment with bare platinum coils led to the introduction of coils containing materials meant to enhance fibrosis within the aneurysm and decrease the chance of recanalization. Several "bioactive" coil systems are on the market currently; some contain polyglycolic-polylactic acid (PGLA) while others contain hydrogel. The PGLA polymer degrades by hydrolysis to glycolic acid and lactic acid, which promote fibrocellular proliferation. Matrix 2 (Boston Scientific) coils are platinum coils covered with PGLA. Cerecyte (Micrus Endovascular, Sunnyvale, CA) and Nexus (ev3) coils also incorporate PGLA. The HydroCoil® system (MicroVention, Inc., Aliso Viejo, CA) consists of platinum coils coated with an expandable hydrogel. The hydrogel provides a greater filling volume than bare platinum coils by filling the interstices of the coil mass. No firm scientific data yet exist to support one coil type over another.

Coiling Technique (Video 17.5)

Using roadmapping, the microwire and microcatheter are advanced to the target vessel. For an end-artery aneurysm (basilar-tip aneurysm, for example), the microwire is usually advanced directly into the aneurysm, followed by the microcatheter. For side-wall aneurysms, the aneurysm is usually accessed by guiding the microwire and microcatheter tip past the aneurysm neck. The microwire is pulled into the microcatheter, and the microcatheter is slowly pulled back, allowing the tip to flip into the aneurysm. When initially framing the aneurysm using a three-dimensional coil, it is often best to have the tip of the microcatheter at the neck of the aneurysm to allow the coil to assume its spherical shape, to keep the coil from protruding into the parent artery, and to maximize the number of loops of coil across the neck. During framing of the aneurysm, gentle movement of the microcatheter, either forward or backward, can help distribute the loops of the coil within the aneurysm in a more controlled fashion. Once the aneurysm is nicely framed, the microcatheter tip is placed centrally within the aneurysm and two thirds of the way to the top of the dome for added stability during the bulk of the filling phase of the procedure. During the finishing phase, the microcatheter may need to be repositioned several times to fill residual pockets within the aneurysm with coils.

Balloon-Assisted Coil Embolization (Fig. 17.7)

The use of balloons to occlude the aneurysm neck during coiling of wide-necked aneurysms was first described in 1994 by Moret and associates.[69] A 6F or larger guide catheter is required to accommodate both a balloon catheter and a microcatheter. A microcatheter is placed into the aneurysm fundus, and a balloon catheter is centered over the neck of the aneurysm. The balloon is subsequently inflated during placement of a coil and then deflated intermittently in between coils to allow antegrade flow. Sequential inflations and deflations are performed as additional coils are placed until the aneurysm is completely coiled, at which point the balloon is removed. The rationale behind this technique is that the presence of the balloon prevents distal embolization and conforms the coil mass to the shape of the balloon and that the coil mass shape becomes stable, thereby protecting the parent artery as the individual coils interlock. During the initial insertion of a coil, one should be careful to form a loop that directs the distal end of the coil away from the aneurysm fundus in order to limit the risk of aneurysm perforation during balloon inflation.

At our center, balloon assistance is used for cases of ruptured wide-necked giant aneurysms in which the use of antiplatelet agents is contraindicated and in which the deployment of a stent is not feasible. The number of patients in the second category is decreasing as more deliverable intracranial SES become available. We currently use the HyperGlide and HyperForm balloons (Micro Therapeutics, Irvine, CA) in such cases.

Balloon-Assisted Onyx Embolization (Fig. 17.8)

Onyx embolization for the treatment of intracranial aneurysms is an investigational procedure. Onyx is composed of an ethylene vinyl alcohol copolymer dissolved in DMSO and suspended in micronized tantalum powder (for visualization under fluoroscopy). The ethylene vinyl alcohol copolymer is infused through a microcatheter into an aqueous environment; the DMSO diffuses outward into the surrounding tissue, allowing the material to precipitate into a spongy, space-occupying cast. Onyx embolization of aneurysms requires a balloon-assisted technique to permit infusion of the material into the aneurysm without embolization into the distal circulation. DMSO-compatible devices must be used.

Patients are administered a loading dose of aspirin and clopidogrel prior to the procedure as described in stent-assisted coiling. A deflated compliant, DMSO-compatible balloon (Hyperglide, ev3) is placed in the parent vessel adjacent to the aneurysm. A DMSO-compatible microcatheter (Rebar, ev3) is navigated into the aneurysm. The balloon is inflated, and contrast material is gently injected through the microcatheter as a test to confirm that the balloon has made an adequate seal over the aneurysm neck. After the microcatheter is primed with DMSO, a Cadence Precision Injector syringe (ev3) is filled with Onyx and attached to the hub of the microcatheter. Onyx is injected under fluoroscopic observation at a rate of approximately 0.1 mL/minute or slower. The injection is continued and paused after each incremental volume of approximately 0.2 to 0.3 mL to allow the material to polymerize and to allow temporary balloon deflation. Several sequential reinflations and injections may be necessary.

At the completion of the embolization process, with the balloon deflated, the microcatheter syringe is decompressed by the aspiration of 0.2 mL of Onyx left in the microcatheter, which prevents dribbling of Onyx material during removal of the microcatheter. An interval of 10 minutes is allowed to elapse prior to microcatheter removal, in order to permit the

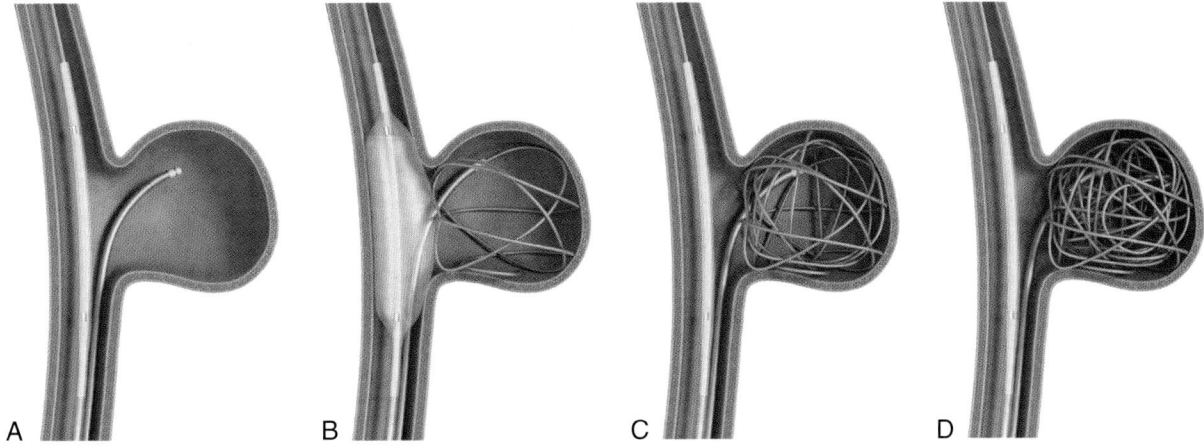

FIGURE 17.7 Balloon-assisted aneurysm coiling. **A,** Balloon catheter across the neck of the aneurysm; microcatheter in the aneurysm. **B,** The balloon has been inflated across the aneurysm neck, and the framing coil is being placed. **C,** The balloon is deflated after the framing coil is in place. **D,** Further coiling inside the frame with the balloon deflated. *(Courtesy of ev3, Irvine, CA.)*

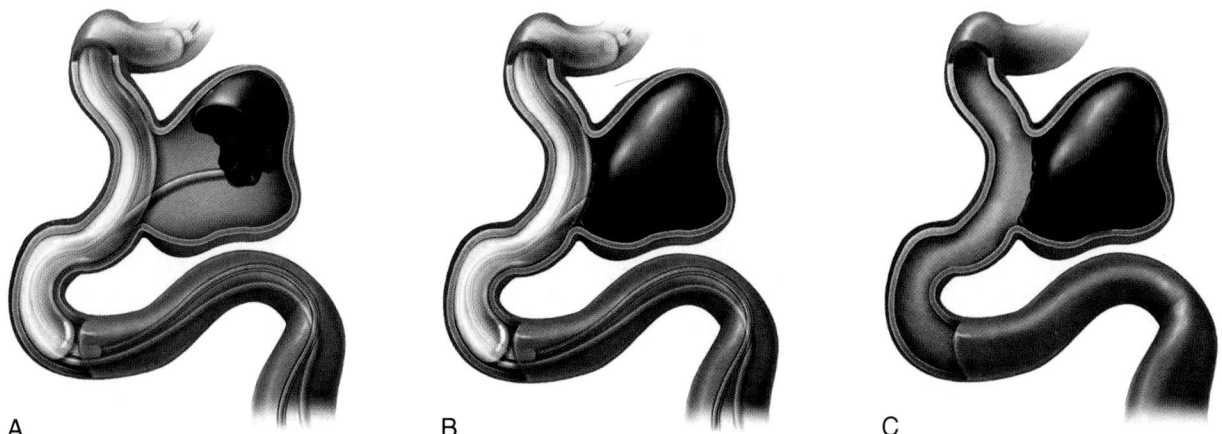

FIGURE 17.8 Balloon-assisted Onyx aneurysm embolization. **A,** A balloon has been inflated across the aneurysm neck, and Onyx is being injected through a DMSO-compatible microcatheter. **B,** Complete filling of the aneurysm with Onyx. **C,** The balloon has been removed, and the aneurysm is completely occluded with Onyx. *(Courtesy of ev3, Irvine, CA.)*

Onyx material to set within the aneurysm. As the microcatheter is withdrawn, the balloon is inflated a final time to stabilize the Onyx mass. The patient should be kept on an antiplatelet regimen for 1 month after the procedure.

In a multicenter investigation of cerebral aneurysm treatment with Onyx, the rate of permanent neurological morbidity was 8.3% (8/97 patients), and there were two procedural deaths.[70] The procedures for large and giant aneurysms were lengthy (up to 6 hours). Delayed occlusion of the carotid artery occurred in 9 (9%) of 100 patients. At the 12-month follow-up evaluation of 53 patients, 38 (72%) large and giant aneurysms were completely occluded. Re-treatment was performed in 9 (11%) of 79. Although some single-center studies show slightly better results,[71] in our opinion, the relatively high complication rate and high rate of delayed carotid artery occlusion do not justify this treatment in patients with unruptured aneurysms who cannot tolerate carotid artery occlusion. Currently, short-term results of Onyx occlusion for large aneurysms are not better than for selective coil occlusion, and the immediate and delayed complication rates are probably higher.

Self-Expanding Intracranial Microstents

Presently, there are two intracranial SES designed specifically for stent-assisted coiling of wide-necked intracranial aneurysms available in the United States: the Neuroform 3 stent (Boston Scientific) and the Enterprise Vascular Reconstruction Device and Delivery System (Codman Neurovascular). Both devices consist of a self-expanding nitinol stent that is deployed in the parent vessel adjacent to the aneurysm neck; the stent then acts as a scaffold to hold coils in place inside the aneurysm. Both devices are extremely navigable (compared to delivery of balloon-mounted coronary stents), and the Enterprise stent presents several benefits over the Neuroform stent,

including reconstrainability, a lower profile delivery system, and a technically less complicated deployment mechanism.

Recently, SES have begun to be viewed not only as adjunctive devices to support coiling but also as tools that could potentially support the long-term durability of coil embolization, particularly in difficult cases in which the aneurysm is prone to recurrence. This is because stents have several possible effects on the physiology and biology of the aneurysm–parent vessel complex: altering the parent vessel configuration and thus possibly altering intra-aneurysmal flow dynamics; disruption of the inflow jets; reduction in the vorticity and wall shear stress on the aneurysm wall and reduction of the water-hammer effect of the pulsatile blood flow that causes coil compaction by the tines of the stents; and providing a scaffolding and stimulus for the overgrowth of endothelial and neointimal tissue across the neck of the aneurysm, creating a matrix for "biological remodeling" in the region of the aneurysm neck.

Neuroform Stent (Fig. 17.9)

The Neuroform stent comes from the manufacturer preloaded in a 3F microdelivery catheter. A "stabilizer" catheter (also preloaded in the delivery microcatheter) is then used to stabilize and deploy the stent as the microdelivery catheter is withdrawn. The stent consists of a fine wire mesh that cannot be seen on standard fluoroscopy; however, the four platinum marker bands at each end can be seen. The devices come in sizes ranging between 2.5 and 4.5 mm in diameter and 10 and 30 mm in length. The recommended diameter for placement is 0.5 mm greater than the largest diameter of the parent artery to be stented. The length is chosen such that the stent extends for at least 5 mm proximal and distal to the aneurysm neck. The struts composing the stent measure approximately 60 μm in thickness. The interstices of the fully expanded stent are

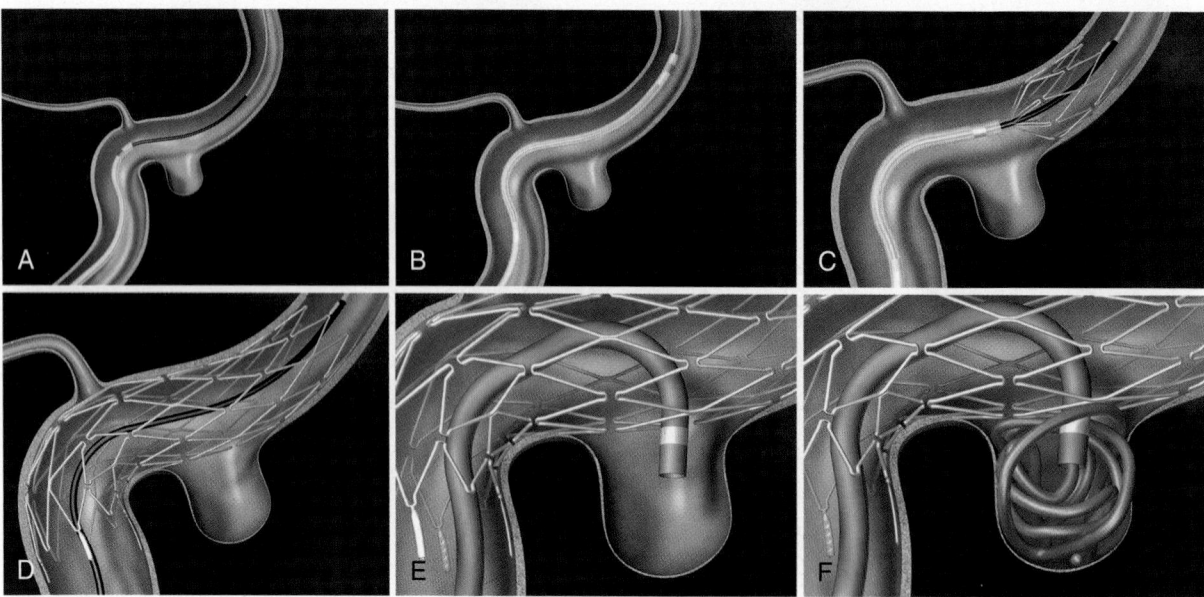

FIGURE 17.9 Neuroform stent-assisted coiling. **A,** The neck of the aneurysm is crossed by a microwire, and a Neuroform stent is advanced to the aneurysm. **B,** The stent has been placed, centered on the aneurysm neck. **C** and **D,** Deployment of the stent across the neck of the aneurysm. **E,** Placement of microcatheter through the stent tines into the aneurysm for coil embolization. **F,** Coil embolization through the microcatheter. *(Courtesy of Boston Scientific, Natick, MA.)*

large enough to accommodate a microcatheter tip size of 2.5F or less (realistically, <2.0F) for coiling.

A microcatheter and microwire (0.010 or 0.014 inch) are navigated past the aneurysm, using roadmap guidance. The microwire is removed and replaced with an exchange-length 0.014-inch microwire with a soft, J-shaped distal curve. The microdelivery catheter containing the Neuroform stent is threaded onto the exchange-length wire and advanced across the neck of the aneurysm. The stabilizer catheter is then held firmly in place as the microdelivery catheter is pulled back over the stabilizer and microwire, such that the stent is unsheathed. As the stent expands, the marker bands can be seen to spread. The microdelivery catheter and stabilizer are removed over the exchange-length wire. A standard-length microcatheter is advanced over the microwire until it is past the stent. The exchange-length microwire is removed and replaced with a standard-length microwire. The microwire and microcatheter are then guided through the stent and into the aneurysm for coiling.

Enterprise Stent (Fig. 17.10 and Video 17.6)

The Enterprise stent comes from the manufacturer within a plastic sheath (the "dispenser loop"). A delivery wire is preloaded within the stent, and both the stent and delivery wire come from the manufacturer in the dispenser loop. The delivery wire has three radiopaque zones: the proximal wire, the "stent positioning marker" (which indicates where the undeployed stent is loaded, and runs the length of the stent), and the distal tip. The Enterprise measures 4.5 mm in diameter when unconstrained and as such is indicated for use only in vessels measuring between 2.5 and 4 mm in diameter. The device comes in lengths of 14, 22, 28, and 37 mm. The struts of the Enterprise, like those of the Neuroform, are approximately 60 µm thick. The stent struts cannot be seen on standard fluoroscopy; each end of the four platinum marker bands can be seen, but these are considerably more difficult to visualize than the markers on the Neuroform stent. The interstices of the fully expanded Enterprise stent are large enough to accommodate a microcatheter tip with an outer diameter size less than or equal to 2.3F for coiling.

The Enterprise is a closed-cell stent; this design makes it reconstrainable. A Prowler Select Plus microcatheter (a 2.9F/2.3F proximal/distal outer diameter; 0.021-inch inner

diameter; Codman Neurovascular) and microwire (0.010 or 0.014 inch) are navigated past the aneurysm using a roadmap. The tip is positioned at least 12 mm distal to the neck of the aneurysm. The microwire is removed, and the Enterprise stent is inserted into the Prowler Select Plus microcatheter by placing the tip of the dispenser loop in the rotating hemostatic valve and advancing the delivery wire. The delivery wire can be advanced without fluoroscopy until the marker on the wire is at the rotating hemostatic valve. The marker on the delivery wire is 150 cm from the distal tip. The delivery wire and stent are then navigated into position across the aneurysm neck. The stent is deployed by holding the delivery wire firmly in place while carefully retracting the microcatheter. If the stent position is unsatisfactory, advancing the microcatheter may allow recapture of the stent. Stent recapture may be done provided that less than 80% of the stent has been deployed. If the proximal end of the stent-positioning marker is still within the microcatheter, the stent can be recaptured. The stent should be recaptured only once. If further repositioning is needed, the stent should be removed and a new one used. When the operator is satisfied with the position of the stent, the microwire and microcatheter are guided through the stent and into the aneurysm for coiling.

Indications for Self-Expanding Intracranial Microstents

The current indications for self-expanding intracranial microstents include stent-assisted coil embolization, rescue during embolization, and balloon-assisted coiling followed by stenting.

Stent-Assisted Coil Embolization

The most common technique at our center is trans-stent coiling in which the stent is placed across the neck of the aneurysm and coil embolization is performed after manipulation of a microcatheter. Trans-stent coiling may be performed at the time of the initial procedure or during a second procedure ("staged technique"), typically 4 to 8 weeks after stenting. Some operators prefer the staged technique to allow endothelialization of the stent prior to attempted coiling. The advantages of staging are that the stent is more stable after endothelialization, and the clopidogrel is most often discontinued before coiling.

The other technique used is a jailing technique in which a microcatheter is placed inside the aneurysm before stent deployment.[72] The jailing technique is not preferred because (a) there is a chance of displacement of the microcatheter during stent placement and (b) there is a higher chance of coil stretching or breakage because the coil can get caught between the stent and the vessel wall.

Rescue During Coil Embolization

If detached coils or entire coil mass prolapse into the parent vessel during the procedure, the stent is placed in the vessel either to replace the coils back in the aneurysm lumen or tack up the coils against the vessel wall and thus prevent further migration and distal emboli.[73,74]

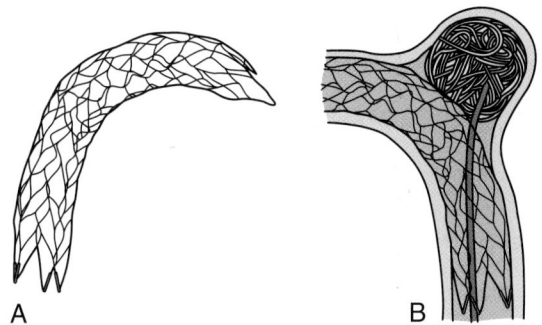

FIGURE 17.10 A, The Enterprise stent. **B,** Photograph taken after the stent has been deployed in an aneurysm phantom model; the aneurysm has been coiled. *(Courtesy of Codman Neurovascular, Raynham, MA.)*

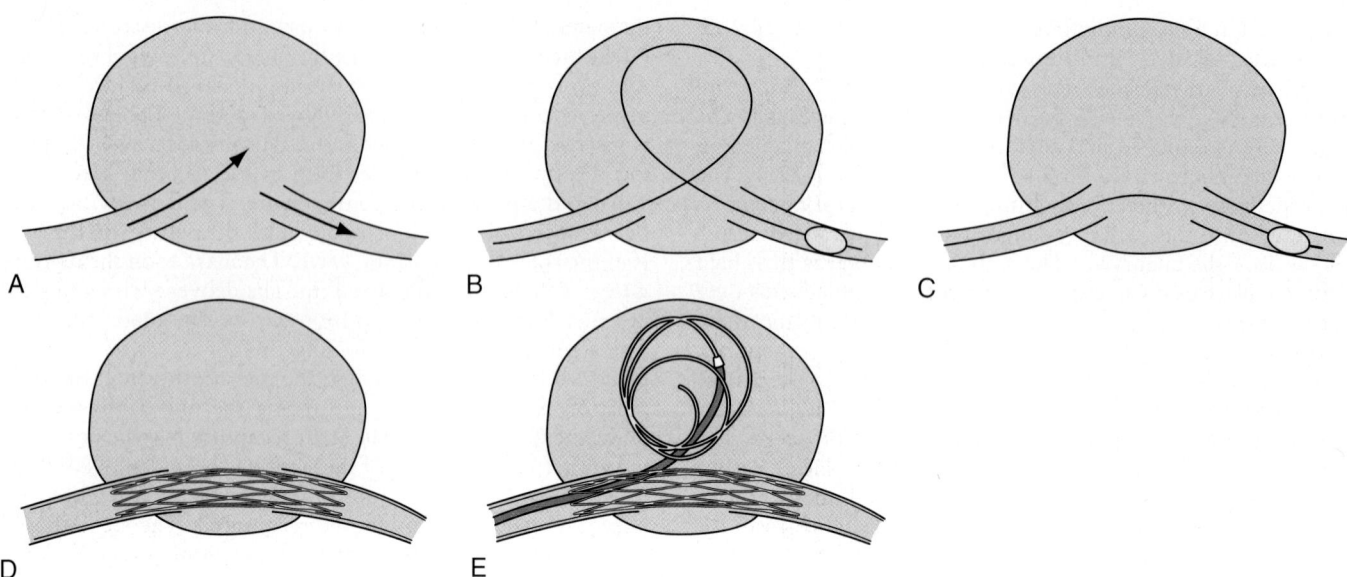

A

B

C

D

E

FIGURE 17.11 The balloon anchor technique. **A,** A fusiform aneurysm with different inlet and outlet flow directions. This makes directing the microwire into the distal parent vessel difficult. **B,** The microwire is allowed to follow the inlet flow and curve around in the aneurysm to exit at the outlet. **C,** A balloon is inflated in the distal parent vessel to serve as an anchor, and the wire is slowly pulled to bridge the neck of the aneurysm. **D,** A stent is placed across the aneurysm neck. **E,** Stent-assisted coiling of the aneurysm. *(From Snyder KV, Natarajan SK, Hauck EF, et al. The balloon anchor technique: a novel technique for distal access through a giant aneurysm. J NeuroInterventional Surg 2010;2:363-367, and Levi EI, Siddiqui AH, Crumlish A, et al. First Food and Drug Administration-approved prospective trial of primary intracranial stenting for acute stroke; SARIS [Stent-Assisted Recanalization in acute Ischemic Stroke). Stroke 2009;40:3552-3556.)*

Balloon-Assisted Coiling Followed by Stenting

Some operators prefer balloon-assisted coiling followed by self-expanding intracranial microstent placement because (a) the aneurysm neck-parent vessel interface is best seen during balloon-assisted coiling; (b) it allows adjustment of the coil mass to configure to the neck of the aneurysm and thus allows denser packing; (c) it pins the microcatheter and allows easier recatheterization if it is displaced; and (d) if there is intraprocedural perforation of the aneurysm, the balloon can be inflated to cause temporary flow arrest and allow time for reversal of heparin or further coiling to secure the bleeding.

Advanced Self-Expanding Intracranial Microstent Techniques Used in Complex Aneurysms

Balloon Anchor Technique for Difficult Distal Vessel Access (Fig. 17.11 and Video 17.7)

This technique is used in wide-necked aneurysms with a dominant flow jet that constantly directs any device used for distal vessel access into the aneurysm. This, coupled with the inability to achieve stable distal purchase of the access after it is obtained, often leads to abortion of the procedure. Distal parent vessel access was obtained by allowing the microwire to follow the local hemodynamics into a giant internal carotid artery aneurysm and around its dome into the distal vessel. An over-the-wire balloon inflated in the distal vessel followed by gentle retraction of the balloon catheter and microwire allowed only a wire bridge across the aneurysm neck, thereby allowing the stent catheter to be brought up in a standard fashion.

Y-Stent (Fig. 17.12)

This technique is most commonly used for bifurcation aneurysms arising from the basilar tip or carotid terminus. Two stents can be placed, the first extending out one limb of the bifurcation and the second introduced through the interstices of the first stent and extending into the other limb of the bifurcation. This configuration forms a Y-shaped construct at the bifurcation and provides very robust support for the coil embolization of terminal aneurysms.[75-77] This Y-stent technique has also been applied to treat middle cerebral artery aneurysms[76] and anterior communicating artery aneurysms.

Waffle-Cone Technique (Fig. 17.13)

In cases in which a Y-stent is not feasible, a stent may be deployed from the parent artery directly into the aneurysm (i.e., "intra-extra" aneurysmal stent placement or waffle-cone technique) to achieve parent artery protection. Using this technique, a single stent can be used to stabilize an intra-aneurysmal coil mass.[78] However, the final construct sets up a vector of flow redirection directly into the terminal aneurysm sac and actually disrupts flow into the bifurcation branches. One might expect that such a construct could lead to high rates of recanalization. In addition, if this technique fails or leads to recanalization, other available means of treatment (surgical clipping, endovascular therapy with balloon remodeling or Y-stent reconstruction) are made considerably more difficult, if not impossible.

Trans-Circle of Willis Stenting (Video 17.8A and B)

In some cases when Y-stenting is not feasible for terminal aneurysms, a stent can be placed across the circle of Willis

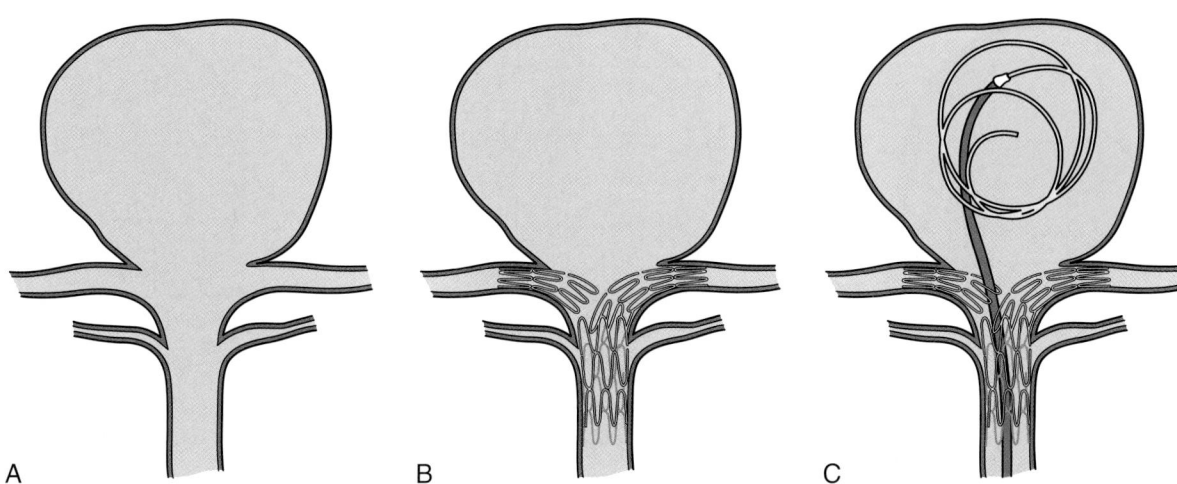

FIGURE 17.12 A Y-stent-assisted coiling procedure. **A,** Wide-necked basilar tip aneurysm. **B,** First, a stent is placed in one posterior cerebral artery (PCA) from the basilar artery (BA). Another stent is placed through the stent tines of the first stent into the other PCA from the BA. **C,** A microcatheter is brought in through the stent tines into the aneurysm, and a coil is deployed in the aneurysm sac.

from P1 to P1 via the posterior communicating artery, from A1 to M1 via the anterior communicating artery, or from the ipsilateral A1 to contralateral A1 via the anterior communicating artery.[79] This technique provides a means by which to achieve protection of both limbs of the bifurcation with a single self-expanding intracranial microstent.

Balloon In-Stent Technique

In a circumferential fusiform aneurysm with a large parent artery defect, a balloon-mounted coronary stent could be used to bridge the proximal and distal vessels, and a microcatheter placed outside the stent before balloon inflation can be used for coiling of the aneurysm around the balloon-mounted coronary stent. The main disadvantages are the difficulty in tracking the balloon-mounted coronary stents through the intracranial vasculature and the possibility of prolapse of the coil mass into the lumen of the stent. Self-expanding intracranial microstents cannot be used for the balloon in-stent technique as they tend to overexpand into the saccular component of the aneurysm, and it can become challenging to ascertain whether the embolization coils are being placed within the parent artery or within the saccular component of the aneurysm. In addition, self-expanding intracranial microstents are easily damaged and displaced; such migration can result in displacement of one end of the stent into the saccular component of the aneurysm. The recent development of flow-diverting devices has obviated the need to perform this technique.

Flow-Diverting Devices

The concept of parent vessel reconstruction is quickly advancing with the recent development of dedicated flow-diverting endovascular constructs designed for intracranial use. These devices primarily target parent vessel reconstruction, rather than endosaccular occlusion, as the means by which to achieve definitive aneurysm treatment. The current flow-diverting devices are high-metal surface area coverage, stent-like constructs that are designed to provide enough flow redirection, and endovascular remodeling to induce aneurysm thrombosis

without the use of additional endosaccular occlusive devices (i.e., coils). At the same time, the pore size of the constructs is large enough to allow for the continued perfusion of branch vessels and perforators arising from the reconstructed segment of the parent vessel.[80] Large or giant size or the presence of intra-aneurysmal thrombus, which are both factors typically associated with coil compaction and aneurysm recurrence, are not an issue with the flow-diverting devices, because no endosaccular coils are placed. In addition, as a purely "extrasaccular" treatment strategy, no direct catheterization or manipulation of the aneurysm sac is required with the flow-diverting devices, possibly reducing the likelihood of procedural rupture and potentially improving the safety of endovascular aneurysm treatment. The Pipeline Embolization Device (PED) (ev3) represents the first flow-diversion device used in humans. We have recently used the SILK flow-diverting device (BALT, Montmorency, France) in a patient (on a compassionate basis). Multiple other flow-diverting devices are currently in development and testing.

Pipeline Embolization Device (Fig. 17.14 and Video 17.9)

The PED is a cylindrical, stent-like construct composed of 48 braided strands of cobalt, chromium, and platinum. The device is packaged within an introducer sheath collapsed upon a delivery wire. The device is loaded into and delivered via the hub of a 0.027-inch internal diameter microcatheter that has been positioned across the neck of the aneurysm. Initially collapsed within the delivery sheath or microcatheter, the device is elongated approximately 2.5 times its deployed length when expanded to nominal diameter. As it is deployed, the device foreshortens toward its nominal length (which it achieves only if allowed to expand fully to its nominal diameter). Currently, the available devices range from 2.5 to 5 mm in diameter (in 0.25-mm increments) and 10 to 20 mm in length (in 2-mm increments). The deployed device is very flexible and conforms to the normal parent vessel anatomy, even in very tortuous vascular anatomy.

When fully expanded, the PED provides approximately 30% metal surface area coverage. When deployed in a parent

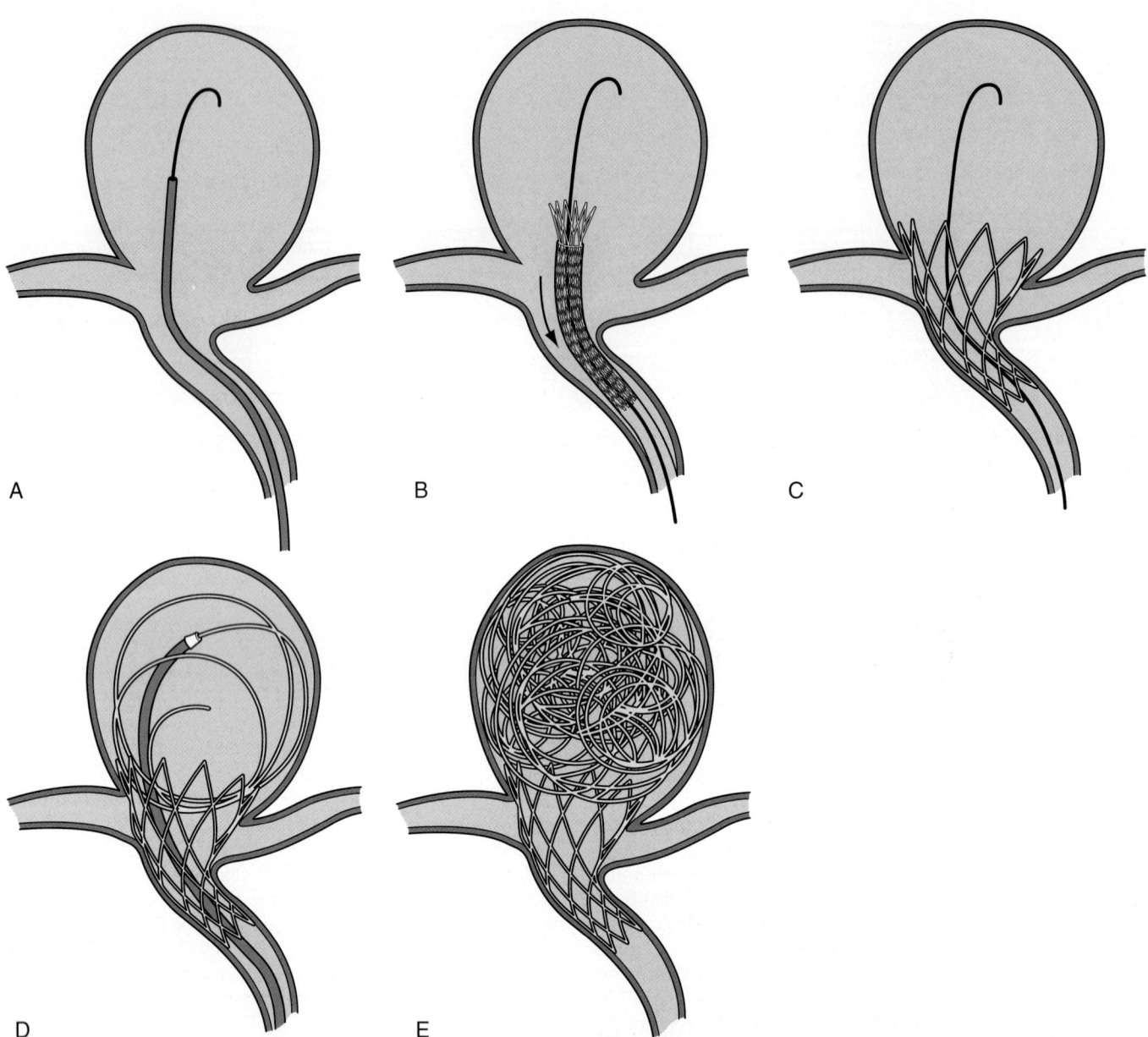

A

B

C

D

E

FIGURE 17.13 Waffle-cone technique. **A,** Catheter over wire. **B,** Neuroform stent (Boston Scientific, Natick, MA) being deployed in aneurysm. **C,** Stent deployed in aneurysm with microwire within the aneurysm. **D,** Microcatheter in aneurysm with coil being deployed. **E,** Coiled aneurysm with waffle-cone configuration. *(From Horowitz M, Levy E, Savageau E, et al. Intra/extra-aneurysmal stent placement for management of complex and wide-necked bifurcation aneurysms: eight cases using the waffle cone technique. Neurosurgery 2006;58(4 Suppl 2):ONS-26.)*

artery smaller than the nominal diameter of the device, the PED cannot fully expand, and as such, it deploys longer than its nominal length and yields a lesser metal surface area coverage. To augment surface area coverage, several devices can be overlapped, or an individual device can be deployed with forward pressure on the microcatheter. To achieve coverage of vessel defects measuring longer than 20 mm, multiple devices can be telescoped to reconstruct longer segments of the cerebrovascular anatomy. The tremendous versatility of the device essentially allows the operator to achieve reconstructions of most any segment of the cerebrovascular anatomy and allows some control of the metal surface coverage of different regions of the conglomerate construct. This control over the length, shape, and porosity of the final reconstructed vessel allows

the operator to build a "customized" implant for each patient treated.

By August 2010, 1178 aneurysms had been treated with the PED.[81] The Pipeline Embolization Device in the Intracranial Treatment of Aneurysms (PITA) trial was an industry-sponsored safety trial for the Conformité Européenne (CE) mark of approval. The trial comprised a prospective four-center, single-arm study with core laboratory image analysis. Thirty-one patients with unruptured wide-necked intracranial aneurysms in whom treatment with coil embolization had failed were enrolled. The mean aneurysm neck diameter was 5.8 mm, and the mean aneurysm diameter was 11.5 mm. The PED was used alone in 48% of patients and with coils in 52% of patients. Six-month imaging follow-up was conducted

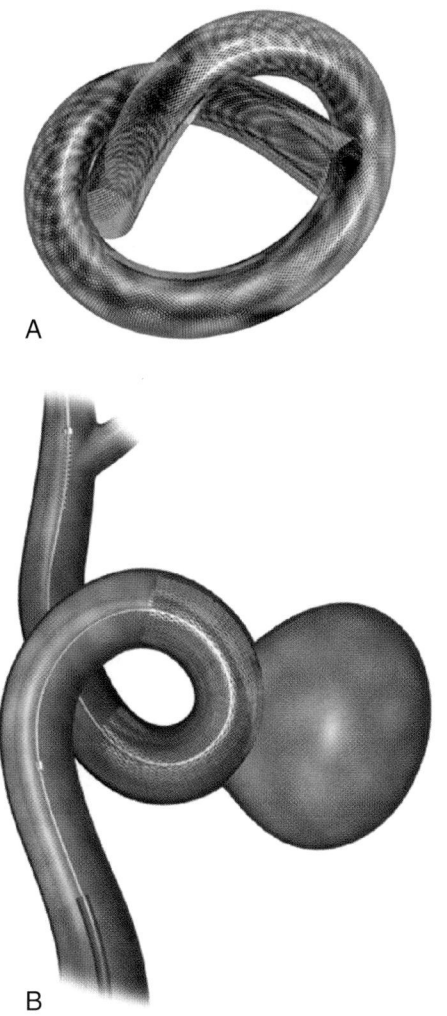

A

B

FIGURE 17.14 Pipeline Embolization Device (PED). **A,** The PED (ev3). **B,** The PED deployed across a wide-necked aneurysm. *(Courtesy of ev3, Irvine, CA.)*

in 96% of patients. Complete occlusion at 6 months was achieved in 93.3% of patients. At 6 months, the mortality and permanent morbidity rates were 0% and 6.5%, respectively.[82] This unprecedented rate of complete angiographic occlusion at follow-up surpasses any of the reported occlusion rates for aneurysms after endovascular therapy and far exceeds those rates reported for large or wide-necked lesions.

The Budapest single-center study, which was a continuation of the PITA study, confirmed the findings of that study.[83] A total of 19 large or giant wide-necked aneurysms were treated in 18 patients. Angiography at 6 months demonstrated complete occlusion in 17 aneurysms. Four neurological complications resulted in one patient (5.5%) with permanent morbidity and one (5.5%) death. Of the 17 ophthalmic arteries that were covered by a PED, one (5.9%) was occluded acutely, with visual deficit, and two (11.8%) were occluded in a delayed fashion, with no clinically detectable deficit. No other side branch occlusions were documented.

The Buenos Aires study,[84] a prospective single-center registry that comprised 53 patients with 63 intracranial aneurysms, also expanded on the PITA study and confirmed the findings

of the aforementioned two studies. Thirty-three (52.4%) aneurysms in the Buenos Aires study were small wide-necked aneurysms. Complete angiographic occlusion was achieved in 56%, 93%, and 95% of aneurysms at 3 months (n = 42), 6 months (n = 28), and 12 months (n = 18), respectively. There were no deaths; three patients (5%) with giant aneurysms experienced transient exacerbation of preexisting cranial neuropathies or headache. Five patients developed hematomas at the femoral puncture site.

The experience of the group at Hacettepe University (Ankara, Turkey) with the PED was presented recently.[85] The study comprised 129 patients with intracranial aneurysms treated with the PED. The 12-month occlusion rate was 95%. There was one (0.8%) symptomatic parent artery stenosis, four (3.2%) permanent morbidities, and one (0.8%) death. Again, the outcomes were similar to the other three reported studies.

The PED has also been used to successfully treat nonsaccular (fusiform or circumferential) aneurysms. Three such cases have been performed in North America under an FDA exemption.[86] All three lesions, which were judged to be untreatable with existing endovascular or open surgical technologies, were angiographically cured with PED treatment, without technical or neurological complications. In two cases, eloquent perforator or side-branch vessels were covered by the PED construct; and in both cases, vessels remained patent at angiographic follow-up. Two of these patients now have more than 1 year of clinical and angiographic follow-up and remain angiographically cured of their lesions and are without neurological symptoms.[85]

The Pipeline for Uncoilable or Failed Aneurysms Study (PUFS) was a U.S. investigational device exemption (IDE), nonrandomized, single-arm, multicenter premarket approval study using a historical control group.[87] PUFS enrolled 120 patients with large or giant (paraclinoid or cavernous) ICA aneurysms and 6-month data were available in 107 (89%) patients. After reviewing these data, the FDA on April 6, 2011, approved the PED "for the endovascular treatment of adults (22 years of age or older) with large or giant wide-necked intracranial aneurysms in the ICA from the petrous to the superior hypophyseal segments."[88,89]

The Complete Occlusion of Coilable intracranial Aneurysms (COCOA) study is an ongoing, randomized, multicenter U.S. IDE study comparing coiling to the PED for the treatment of small paraclinoid aneurysms (aneurysm diameter <10 mm and neck diameter <4 mm). The safety endpoint is death and ipsilateral stroke, and the effectiveness endpoint will be assessed on the basis of complete aneurysm occlusion at 6 months.

A multicenter randomized clinical trial has been planned to compare coiling and PED. This trial is the U.S. government-sponsored endovascular treatment of intracranial aneurysms with Pipeline versus coils with or without stents (EVIDENCE) trial. The aim is to recruit patients with intracranial aneurysms between 7 mm and 15 mm. The study protocol details have not yet been published.

SILK Flow-Diverting Device

The SILK device is similar to the PED and has 48 braided wires (44 nitinol and 4 platinum). It is available in 2.0- to 5.5-mm diameters (0.5-mm increments) and 15- to 40-mm lengths

(5-mm increments). The SILK device shortens by at least 50% when deployed. It comes prepackaged with a delivery system comprising a delivery wire and an introducer and a reinforced microcatheter for placement (Vasco + 21 2.4F for devices 2-4.5 mm in diameter and 3F for devices 5-5.5 mm in diameter; preshaped with a multipurpose distal curve). The SILK device is preloaded on the delivery wire inside the introducer. After microcatheter access to the aneurysm has been obtained, working projections and vessel measurements are taken for device sizing. The SILK device is transferred from the introducer into the hub of the microcatheter using a Y-connector and by gently advancing the delivery wire. The device is positioned past the aneurysm neck at least 1.5 times the diameter of the parent vessel. The delivery wire is gently pushed until the distal radiopaque end is out of the distal marker on the microcatheter. Withdrawing the microcatheter to deploy the SILK device to approximately 1 cm creates a fix-point on the delivery wire. This manipulation ensures that SILK does not move distally, which can result in the wire struts of the SILK damaging the vessel wall. Once the SILK is deployed by approximately 1 cm, the distal tip is positioned by simultaneously pulling on the catheter and delivery wire. The SILK device may be moved by pulling the delivery wire, as long as the distal ring of the catheter does not superimpose the marker on the delivery wire. If repositioning of the device is required, the catheter is gently advanced over the deployed SILK, the system is repositioned, and the device is re-deployed in the new location. The SILK is fully deployed when the marker of the delivery wire lines up with the distal ring of the catheter. It is then impossible to resheath the SILK. The delivery wire is pushed until its marker passes the catheter's marker by a minimum of 2 mm. The microcatheter is positioned distal to the stent to maintain access through the stent before removal of the delivery wire. The main advantages of the SILK device over the PED are the better translatability of the one-to-one movement of the microcatheter and the delivery system and the ability to recapture and reposition the system even up to 90% deployment. In our experience, the ability to recapture a flow-diverting device in our experience is very important. These devices frequently require repositioning because they foreshorten during deployment, and we often realize the final position of the stent only after it has been partially deployed.

The main limitations of flow-diverting devices when compared to intracranial SES are the efficacy and safety of their use in bifurcation aneurysms, as there is a potential for jailing of one limb of the bifurcation, and the lack of data regarding the safety of these devices in vessels rich with eloquent perforators. Available data in experimental animal models and in humans, especially with the PED, suggest that coverage with a single device is safe.

PARENT VESSEL SACRIFICE

Parent vessel sacrifice is still used as a last resort in giant aneurysms that are high risk for open surgical methods and cannot be safely excluded by currently available endovascular reconstructive techniques. Balloon test occlusion is performed concurrently if permanent vessel occlusion (endovascular or surgical) is considered as a treatment option or as a bailout maneuver. Currently, deconstructive strategies without a

bypass are used only as a bail-out when other treatment options are not available because all the temporary occlusion tests for the presence of collateral supply have false negative results; and there is a 16% to 20% chance of developing an ischemic event after carotid sacrifice even if balloon occlusion tests were negative.[90,91] If surgical bypass is planned, endovascular sacrifice should be performed promptly after the surgical procedure to minimize the risk of graft thrombosis due to low flow.

The key step in the sacrifice of a large vessel, such as the ICA or the VA, is temporary proximal flow arrest to prevent inadvertent embolization into the cerebral vasculature during the procedure. In general, the parent vessel should be occluded either at or immediately proximal to the lesion. Occlusion of the vessel can be accomplished with detachable coils or detachable balloons. Although detachable balloons are not commercially available in the United States at the present time, they are available in Europe and Japan.

Coil Occlusion

Guide catheter access to the parent vessel is established. A single 6F 90-cm sheath has an inner diameter large enough to accommodate two microcatheters, one for deployment of detachable coils and another for the balloon. Under roadmap guidance, the microcatheter to be used for coil deployment is positioned in the vessel where the occlusion is planned. A nondetachable balloon is positioned in the proximal segment of the vessel.

The balloon is inflated, and temporary flow arrest is confirmed with gentle injection of contrast material through the guide catheter under fluoroscopy. The first coil is deployed. The 0.018-inch system three-dimensional coils, with a diameter about twice the diameter of the target vessel, are usually effective. Prior to coil detachment, the balloon is briefly deflated to confirm that the first coil is stable. If there is no movement of the first coil with restoration of flow, the balloon is reinflated, and the first coil is detached. Additional coils are deployed as necessary to achieve tight packing of several centimeters of the vessel. The balloon is then deflated and final angiographic images are obtained.

Detachable Balloon Embolization

The Goldvalve detachable balloon (Acta Vascular/Nfocus Neuromedical Inc., Santa Clara, CA) is available in most of the world outside the United States, and the vendor is working on obtaining approval for the North American market. Complete stasis of flow can be achieved more rapidly with balloons than with coils, but balloons require more preparation prior to use. Occlusion of an artery with detachable balloons should always be undertaken with two balloons placed end to end, with the proximal balloon functioning as a "safety" balloon to minimize the chance of distal migration of the balloons.

A large guide catheter is required, often 7F or 8F (alternatively, a 6F or 7F, 90-cm sheath may be used). A balloon is chosen that is slightly larger than the diameter of the vessel to be occluded. The balloons are attached to their recommended delivery catheters. If the guide catheter is large enough, it is preferable to advance the two balloons simultaneously through the guide catheter and into the vessel in order to limit the risk of premature detachment. Ideally, the balloons should be positioned in a relatively straight segment of the vessel. When the balloons are in proper position, they are inflated with contrast material. If they are properly sized, they will flatten out and elongate as they are inflated. When the position and stability of the balloon appear to be satisfactory, the distal balloon is detached by slowly, gently pulling back on the balloon catheter. The proximal balloon is for flow arrest and is deflated and removed after the distal balloon is deployed.

INTRACRANIAL ARTERIOVENOUS MALFORMATION EMBOLIZATION

The prevalence of AVMs is estimated at approximately 0.01% of the general population, but reported rates range from 0.001% to 0.52%. Cerebral AVMs are detected at a rate of 1 per 1 million person-years and account for 2% of all hemorrhagic strokes. Given the relatively high rate of hemorrhage associated with AVMs without treatment and the prospect of cure with treatment, obliteration of these lesions is usually desirable. Surgical resection is favored for patients in good medical condition with a good life expectancy who harbor small to medium-sized AVMs in anatomically accessible locations within the brain. Both radiosurgery and endovascular embolization have important roles in AVM management. The former is a viable alternative to surgical resection when small lesions (<3 cm) are either deep or in eloquent areas. The latter is a useful adjunct in facilitating microsurgical or radiosurgical therapy and less often a primary cure.

Endovascular Embolization

Only a minority of AVMs can be cured by endovascular embolization. The ability to obliterate AVMs via the endovascular route has increased in conjunction with the use of Onyx for embolization. At our center, most AVMs are resected after endovascular embolization unless they are in deep, inaccessible, or eloquent locations, or unless we are convinced that the embolization is complete and that we will be able to evaluate the patient for follow-up on a regular basis. As a stand-alone therapy, endovascular embolization is not commonly a definitive treatment.

Preoperative endovascular embolization of feeding arteries has rendered many previously difficult AVMs much easier to remove surgically. In general, endovascular embolization is most useful for Spetzler-Martin grade III AVMs.[92] If endovascular access to the feeding vessels can be achieved without placing normal vessels at substantial risk, it can be used for lower grade AVMs as well.

The goal of preoperative embolization is to facilitate surgical resection. Preoperative embolization can facilitate surgery by (1) decreasing intraoperative bleeding and operating time; (2) embolizing surgically difficult areas, such as deep regions of AVM near the ventricles and areas of the AVM nidus bordering eloquent regions; and (3) delimiting very small AVMs that would be very difficult to identify in the parenchyma. The risks of embolization increase as the number of embolized pedicles increases and as the percentage of the AVM embolized increases. We traditionally embolize 30% to 50% of the AVM during a single sitting and bring the

patient back for additional sittings, if necessary, 4 to 6 weeks apart. It is important to tailor the endovascular procedure only to facilitate surgical resection and not to embolize the entire AVM nidus unless that is the original plan or there is evidence during the procedure that venous outflow has been compromised and therefore the patient will need emergent surgery immediately after embolization. During embolization, it is very important not to overshoot 50% of the AVM nidus at a sitting. Most important, it is critical to remain mindful of the venous outflow and its character and timing because any increase in delay or any changes in venous outflow can presage a hemorrhage. Because a decision to operate on an AVM on an emergency basis can be made during or after the intervention, we try to perform our embolization procedures during the initial half of the day so that surgical intervention, if necessary, may be done using routine daytime operating room personnel.

Technique of Embolization

At our center, most AVM embolizations are performed under conscious sedation to allow neurological examinations to be performed throughout the procedure. In addition, we routinely perform Wada testing in the arterial pedicle to be embolized to determine whether the AVM is located in an eloquent region or there is en passant supply from the selected pedicle. We most commonly use Onyx as the embolic agent during embolization procedures. After microcatheterization, often with a flow-directed microcatheter, we initially perform microruns to study the angioarchitecture in detail. The endovascular neurosurgeon must be aware of en passant feeders and critical feeders taking off proximal to the point of injection in order to judge the safest distance for allowable reflux of the embolic agent (Fig. 17.15A). We initially use Onyx-34 to create a plug around the microcatheter (Fig. 17.15B), and this facilitates the forward injection of Onyx-18. Oblique views are obtained to see the tip of the catheter clearly, so that the any reflux of the Onyx can be appreciated readily.

Once the microcatheter tip is in the desired position, the injection of the Onyx is carried out as follows: the microcatheter is flushed with 10 mL of normal saline; 0.23 mL DMSO is injected into a Marathon flow-directed microcatheter (ev3) to fill the dead space. DMSO is also used to wash the hub of the syringe to avoid the polymerization of Onyx (when it comes in contact with water). Onyx is aspirated into a 1-mL syringe. Meniscus-to-meniscus connection is made between the Onyx (in the syringe) and the DMSO (in the catheter hub). Onyx is then injected slowly at a flow rate of 0.1 mL/second to fill the microcatheter and replace the DMSO in the dead space. The embolic agent is released at the tip of the microcatheter under free-flow conditions and fills the nidus compartment directly in an antegrade fashion, with subsequent reflux into the feeding artery beyond the tip of the microcatheter (first penetration). The goal is to form a cast of Onyx around the tip of the microcatheter over a short distance, so that when the Onyx is injected, it flows forward into the AVM and not retrogradely into the feeding vessel. The injection procedure is then interrupted for up to 1 minute to allow the cast to form, and small volumes of the Onyx are injected per cycle until there is enough reflux to form an attenuated cast for

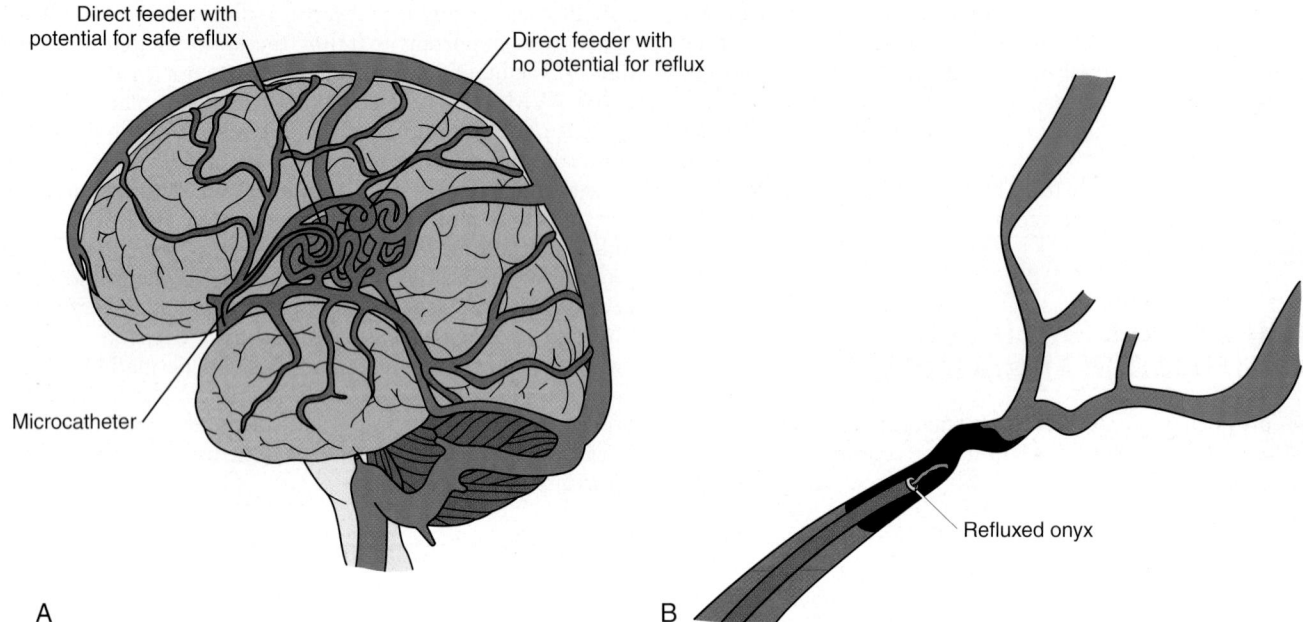

Direct feeder with
potential for safe reflux

Direct feeder with
no potential for reflux

Microcatheter

Refluxed onyx

A

B

FIGURE 17.15 **A,** Preferably, the direct feeder with the longest possible reflux distance should be chosen for Onyx (ev3, Irvine, CA) injection. **B,** Position of the microcatheter for Onyx embolization. Notice the reflux of Onyx around the tip of the microcatheter to form a plug. *(From Natarajan SK, Ghodke B, Britz GW, et al. Multimodality treatment of brain arteriovenous malformations with microsurgery after embolization with Onyx: single-center experience and technical nuances. Neurosurgery 2008;62:1213-1226.)*

a second penetration of the nidus. The maximum safe distance of reflux is usually approximately 2 cm or at least 1 cm distal to a cortical branch of the feeding artery. Careful repeated subtraction roadmaps allow better visualization of the regions of the AVM that are being embolized. We are currently using a triple coaxial guide system containing an Outreach DAC or a Neuron (Penumbra Inc.) catheter to allow more distal placement in order to perform better selective angiography and further selective MCA, posterior cerebral artery, or anterior cerebral artery catheterization to evaluate further details of the AVM with the remainder of the circulation subtracted. Further, in our experience, the use of a triple coaxial guide system greatly facilitates removal of the microcatheter from the Onyx plug after completion of the embolization procedure.

Intracranial Dural Arteriovenous Fistula Embolization

dAVFs account for 10% to 15% of all intracranial AVMs.[93] The venous drainage pattern is the most important predictor of the clinical behavior, and dAVFs with cortical venous reflux exhibit a much higher incidence of ICH or venous infarction. The annual mortality rate for dAVFs with cortical venous reflux may be as high as 10.4%, whereas the annual risk for hemorrhage or nonhemorrhagic neurological deficits during follow-up of nontreated lesions are 8.1% and 6.9%, respectively, resulting in an annual event rate of 15%.[94] Recent studies demonstrate evidence that the risk of bleeding for a dAVF with cortical venous reflux is less when the patient does not present with a hemorrhage or a nonhemorrhagic neurological deficit.[95,96] Strom and colleagues[96] report that asymptomatic versus symptomatic

dAVFs (in patients presenting with hemorrhage or neurological deficit) have annual hemorrhage rates of 1.4% versus 19%, respectively. Although small, these studies make the important point that the natural history may depend on the type of presentation.

With the advent of Onyx (ev3), most intracranial dAVFs can be successfully managed with endovascular techniques. Onyx is more often used for transarterial access when the ECA branches supplying a dAVF can be safely embolized. dAVF location close to dural venous sinuses also facilitates access and transvenous occlusion through the sinus, mainly with coils. The combination of transarterial and transvenous embolization results in higher obliteration rates than previously reported in series with only transvenous embolization.

Transarterial Embolization

A 6F guiding catheter (MPD; Codman Neurovascular) or a triple coaxial guiding system that allows more distal intracranial placement of the guide (Neuron-2, Penumbra, Inc.) is navigated into the target vessel. A DMSO-compatible catheter (Marathon or Echelon, ev3) with a microwire (Mirage or X-Pedion, ev3) is navigated into the feeding vessel of the dAVF as close to the nidus as possible and allowing for an adequate distance for reflux of the embolic agent. When there are multiple feeders, the feeder with maximum reflux distance from the skull base is chosen to decrease the chances of cranial nerve palsies. Embolization of the dAVF is then performed with Onyx-34 or Onyx-18 in the manner previously described for AVMs. The endpoint of the embolization is the angiographic obliteration of the fistula, with some filling of the draining veins. When the fistula is very complex, more than one session of Onyx embolization through multiple feeders is necessary. The average interval between such sittings is 2 to 4 weeks.

Transvenous Embolization

The transvenous route is mainly used for indirect ICA-cavernous sinus fistulas and some tentorial dAVFs. After diagnostic angiography, the femoral vein is punctured (usually on the contralateral side), and using roadmaps obtained from an IA injection, a 6F guiding catheter is placed in the internal jugular vein. Through this guiding catheter, the microcatheter is advanced through the inferior petrosal sinus or the superior petrosal sinus (or one of the clival veins) into the cavernous sinus, placing it as far anteriorly as possible. Occasionally, the superior ophthalmic vein or one of the facial veins (through the pterygoid plexus) and the contralateral inferior petrosal sinus are used to access the cavernous sinus. For tentorial dAVFs, the microcatheter is advanced through the draining vein, past the fistula, to the arterial side. Embolization is then performed with platinum coils or Onyx, using the appropriate microcatheter.

ENDOVASCULAR THERAPY FOR VASOSPASM

Symptomatic cerebral vasospasm (also known as *clinical vasospasm* or *delayed ischemic neurological deficit*) is the leading cause of death and disability in patients with SAH. Symptomatic vasospasm occurs in some 20% to 25% of patients.[97,98] Balloon angioplasty is an option for symptomatic vasospasm affecting intracranial arteries larger than 1.5 mm in diameter, such as the intracranial ICA, the M1, A1, and the VA and basilar arteries and P1 segments. The internal elastic lamina and smooth muscle cells are stretched and thinned during angioplasty. Dilation of the vessel segments is essentially "permanent" for the duration of the clinical vasospasm; vasospasm generally does not recur after angioplasty. Reversal of neurological deficits with angioplasty has been reported in 30% to 70% of patients who fail hypervolemic, hypertensive, and hemodilution (triple H) therapy.[99-101] Clinical improvement appears to be strongly dependent on the timing of the procedure, with significantly better results reported with angioplasty done within 24 hours[99] and within 2 hours[102] of the neurological change. An IA infusion of antispasmodic medications (verapamil, nimodipine, or nicardipine) can supplement angioplasty and can be used for the endovascular treatment of spasm of vessels distal to the circle of Willis that are too small for balloon angioplasty.

The balloons used for angioplasty are either compliant balloons, such as the HyperGlide (ev3) or HyperForm (ev3), or noncompliant balloons, such as the Maverick 2. Because noncompliant balloons are difficult to navigate into small distal vessels, angioplasty is usually limited to larger proximal vessels, where one is less likely to face problems. For most cases, the HyperGlide 4 × 10-mm balloon is most suitable. At our center, we use the Maverick 2 balloon as it has fixed size, and we undersize it to prevent complications. The microwire and balloon are advanced into the target vessel under roadmap fluoroscopy. The balloon is carefully and gently inflated under fluoroscopic visualization. In cases of severe spasm and constriction of the target vessel, pretreatment with an IA injection

of nitroglycerin (20 μg) may allow passage of the balloon. The drug is slowly infused through a microcatheter positioned in the proximal portion of the vessel.

TUMOR EMBOLIZATION

Most intracranial tumor embolization procedures have been done for neoplasms with robust vascular pedicles, such as meningiomas, hemangiopericytomas, and paragangliomas. Tumor embolization was primarily used for the reduction of blood loss during subsequent surgery. More recently, IA therapies for recurrent and malignant brain neoplasms have been reported. Although the results of these studies show promise, especially in that chemotherapeutic agents can be delivered to tumor beds while sparing patients from many of the systemic toxicities associated with the treatment, larger studies are needed. Controversy remains regarding preoperative embolization of meningiomas. Although there may be a role for preoperative embolization in cases in which large tumor vessels and significant vascular blushing are appreciated on angiography, many meningiomas may not be sufficiently vascular to warrant the risk and expense of preoperative embolization.

Embolic Agents

Several agents are currently used for tumor embolization and include polyvinyl alcohol (PVA), Gelfoam (Pfizer, New York, NY), coils, alcohol, and trisacryl gelatin microspheres. The goal of embolization is to saturate the tumor vascular bed with these agents and not simply to occlude large feeding arteries. Thus, the choice and order of embolic agents used are important when attempting to first saturate the fine network of vessels that supply the deepest regions of the tumor bed. Gelfoam powder, microspheres, and polyvinyl alcohol are available in particle sizes as small as 50 μm and as large as 1 mm. Smaller particles should be used during the initial stages of pedicle embolization as these can penetrate and occlude the fine, distal vasculature supplying the tumor bed. As these vessels become saturated with particles, larger particles can then be used to embolize more proximal, and therefore larger, vessels supplying the tumor. We caution that smaller particles have an increased risk of penetrating distal branches of normal parenchyma should reflux occur, as compared to larger particle that cannot penetrate the tumor bed beyond the more proximal vessels. Some interventionists advocate the use of microspheres during the later stages of tumor embolization as microspheres are less likely to occlude the catheter during slow injections because of their uniform nature. Although liquid embolic agents such as alcohol have been used for tumor embolization, this technique is typically reserved for embolization of distal vessels unreachable by microcatheters. Typically, a balloon is inflated proximal to the microcatheter tip to prevent reflux of the alcohol. Usually, less than 5 mL is needed to attain the desired effect of intimal disruption, inflammation, and tumor necrosis.

Potential Complications

With the variety of agents used for embolization of meningiomas, complication rates range from 0% to 9%. An uncommon but potentially devastating neurological complication is peritumoral or intraluminal hemorrhage from acute changes in the tumor blood supply. Often, a partially embolized tumor may hemorrhage into the tumor capsule or into portions of necrotic tumor. Other complications include the formation of iatrogenic fistulas, such as carotid-cavernous fistulas following vessel perforations. Infarctions to the retina or parenchyma tend to occur when anastomoses between the external carotid and internal carotid artery are poorly appreciated. Such anastomoses occur between the middle meningeal artery and the ophthalmic artery, between the ascending pharyngeal artery and the VA, between the occipital artery and the VA, between the accessory meningeal branches to the inferolateral trunk, and finally through persistent fetal anastomoses. It should be noted that parasagittal or convexity meningiomas may receive bilateral supply from the middle meningeal artery, and thus retinal infarctions may occur bilaterally via aberrant anastomoses.

Techniques for Complication Avoidance

Several techniques are employed by neurointerventionists to avoid some of the aforementioned complications. Following careful review of the patient's baseline angiograms, superselective microcatheterization is done to evaluate the blood supply of the tumor and anastomoses that would be potentially dangerous. Typically, a 6F guide catheter is advanced over a stiff 0.035-inch wire into the appropriate parent artery (ECA, ICA, or VA) in the cervical region. A microcatheter is then advanced over a steerable microwire into a tumor pedicle, and superselective angiography is performed to visualize any anastomoses with vessels supplying normal tissue. Lidocaine and methohexital are injected into the pedicle, and careful cranial nerve and other neurological testing is performed. Contrast material is mixed with the embolic agent of choice, and the pedicle is then embolized. Using negative roadmapping techniques, the operator may readily see subtle reflux of embolic agent proximal to the catheter tip. At this point, the catheter must be cleared of embolic material with saline. Care must be taken to avoid reflux of embolic material proximal to the catheter tip, which may lead to embolic agents entering vessels supplying brain parenchyma or the retina. Additionally, liberal angiography should be done to evaluate the angioarchitecture, as vessels previously absent on angiography may become apparent as blood is preferentially shunted through them.

Future Possibilities

The future of IA tumor therapy remains exciting, as clinicians try to bridge the utility of stereotactic radiosurgery, with the potential of endovascular surgery for local delivery of chemotherapeutic agents. The high incidence of metastatic brain neoplasms (approximately 150,000 to 200,000 are newly diagnosed annually), combined with the lack of effective treatments for glioblastoma multiforme, may allow such hybrid therapies to make a significant impact on this current health care dilemma. Radiation-sensitizing agents that have affinity for metastatic neoplasms to the brain, such as gadolinium texaphyrin, may be administered intra-arterially at higher doses than IV infusion affords, with avoidance of systemic effects. Following administration of these agents, patients would undergo stereotactic radiosurgery. With the aid of current advances in surface-coating techniques and materials, embolic agents may be potentially coated with antineoplastic agents and then directly injected into the tumor bed.

EPISTAXIS

Epistaxis is a common condition that can be managed conservatively in most cases. When these measures, including anterior and posterior packing of the nasal cavity, are unsuccessful at controlling the bleeding (in 5% of cases), interruption of the blood supply to the sinonasal area can be performed, either by surgical ligation or by transarterial embolization.

Embolization should be preceded by thorough diagnostic angiography. Aside from aiding with subsequent selective catheterization and embolization, such angiography may reveal significant anatomical anomalies, anastomoses, or an unsuspected cause of epistaxis. Taking these findings into account, the interventionist may decide to refrain from embolization or adjust the technique to minimize the risk of adverse events, which are mostly related to inadvertent embolization of the ICA or ophthalmic artery.

Endovascular treatment for nosebleeds usually consists of superselective catheterization with particle embolization of the nasal vessels, usually the sphenopalatine arteries. Complications can be minimized by careful attention to angiographic anatomy and awareness of dangerous anastomoses. Provocative testing with amobarbital and lidocaine prior to embolization is an added safety factor. The contralateral sphenopalatine artery is checked during the angiogram, even if the bleeding is obviously unilateral, because there can be side-to-side collaterals. Ethmoidal branches from the ophthalmic may be the cause of treatment failure after embolization of the internal maxillary artery. Embolization of the branches of the ophthalmic artery is not recommended because of the risk to vision and the availability of a fairly easy and safe surgical procedure to ligate these vessels. Accessory meningeal arteries may also rarely be a source of bleeding in epistaxis and can be embolized.

Materials frequently used for embolization include pledgets of gelatin sponge (Gelfoam); Gelfoam powder (Pfizer); PVA particles, ranging in size from 50 to 700 µm; platinum coils; or a combination of materials. Smaller particles (50-150 µm) are discouraged, because they are more likely to enter dangerous anastomoses. PVA particles, usually between 150 and 500 µm, with or without the subsequent addition of Gelfoam sponge pledgets or platinum coils, are the main embolic agents used.

CONCLUSION

Endovascular neurosurgery has undergone tremendous expansion in the past two decades and is becoming the mainstay of treatment of cerebrovascular diseases. The use of endovascular therapy for acute ischemic stroke revascularization has tremendously multiplied the endovascular neurosurgeons' patient base just by the sheer number of cases of acute and chronic ischemic stroke per year when compared with other cerebrovascular disease conditions that were traditionally treated by neurosurgeons. Endovascular therapy has also increased the disease entities that fall under the purview of neurosurgery including head and neck vascular lesions and disease of supra-aortic vessels. Endovascular neurosurgical therapy adds a plethora of tools and opens up multiple options with which to treat these complex lesions in addition to microsurgical approaches. It is important for a neurosurgeon to be "completely" trained (both in microsurgery and endovascular neurosurgery) if he or she wishes to specialize in treating cerebrovascular diseases. At present, multiple trials are attempting to establish the superiority of one of these treatment options over the other. However, we strongly believe that these are complementary therapeutic modalities that require evaluation by treating physicians with the intent to achieve the treatment goals with the least morbidity. We are excited and fortunate to be a part of and to contribute to this dynamic era of cerebrovascular neurosurgery.

SELECTED KEY REFERENCES

del Zoppo GJ, Higashida RT, Furlan AJ, et al. PROACT: a phase II randomized trial of recombinant pro-urokinase by direct arterial delivery in acute middle cerebral artery stroke. PROACT Investigators. Prolyse in acute cerebral thromboembolism. *Stroke.* 1998;29:4-11.

Levy EI, Siddiqui AH, Crumlish A, et al. First Food and Drug Administration-approved prospective trial of primary intracranial stenting for acute stroke: SARIS (Stent-Assisted Recanalization in acute Ischemic Stroke). *Stroke.* 2009;40:3552-3556.

Lloyd-Jones D, Adams RJ, Brown TM, et al. Heart disease and stroke statistics—2010 update: a report from the American Heart Association. *Circulation.* 2010;121:e46-e215.

National Institute of Neurological Disorders and Stroke rt-PA Stroke Study Group. Tissue plasminogen activator for acute ischemic stroke. *N Engl J Med.* 1995;333:1581-1587.

Yadav JS, Wholey MH, Kuntz RE, et al. Protected carotid-artery stenting versus endarterectomy in high-risk patients. *N Engl J Med.* 2004;351:1493-1501.

Please go to expertconsult.com to view the complete list of references.

CHAPTER 18

Cerebral Revascularization for Giant Aneurysms of the Transitional Segment of the Internal Carotid Artery

Jonathon J. Lebovitz, Jorge L. Eller, Justin M. Sweeney, Deanna Sasaki-Adams, Aneela Darbar, Sheri K. Palejwala, Anja-Maria Radon, Saleem I. Abdulrauf

CLINICAL PEARLS

- Giant transitional internal carotid artery (ICA) aneurysms incorporate the cavernous, clinoidal, and supraclinoidal segments of the ICA in their necks and are more than 2.5 cm in diameter.

- The natural history of intracavernous ICA giant aneurysms is relatively benign, compared to transitional segment giant ICA aneurysms. Unruptured giant aneurysms in this location had a rupture rate of 40% in 5 years, according to the International Study of Unruptured Intracranial Aneurysms.

- Elective occlusion of the ICA for treatment of aneurysms carries a significant stroke risk, even after a successful balloon test occlusion of the ICA.

- These aneurysms can be treated by the performance of a high-flow bypass graft (radial artery or saphenous vein) from the external carotid artery or the internal maxillary artery to the M2 divisions of the middle cerebral artery, with simultaneous proximal occlusion or trapping of the giant aneurysm. The procedure carries low mortality and morbidity rates, as shown in the authors' series of 55 patients with giant ICA transitional aneurysms.

- Flow diversion stents such as the Pipeline stent are being used for the endovascular treatment of unruptured giant ICA aneurysms. Longer follow-up is needed to evaluate the results and complications.

Transitional internal carotid artery (ICA) aneurysms incorporate the cavernous, clinoidal, and supraclinoidal segments of the ICA as portions of the neck of the aneurysm. In this chapter we will review the natural history of giant internal carotid aneurysms, present our treatment results, and discuss surgical procedures and related technical aspects in the treatment of these aneurysms.

Pure cavernous ICA aneurysms are a separate category of aneurysms that do not extend beyond the dural ring of the ICA. In the neurosurgical literature these aneurysms are considered benign, even when they are larger.[1] However, in our experience it is possible that when these aneurysms get significantly large, they can cause rupture through the middle fossa dura, causing hemorrhage and potentially death (Fig. 18.1).

NATURAL HISTORY

Unruptured giant intracranial aneurysms are being diagnosed more often as a result of the availability of better imaging techniques, and these lesions pose management problems for practitioners. The first series of giant aneurysms was presented in 1969 by Morley and Barr, who described giant aneurysms as greater than 25 mm.[2] Giant aneurysms are relatively rare, accounting for between 5% and 7% of aneurysms[3] in most series. Giant aneurysms have a female predominance with female:male ratios as high as 3:1 in some series[4] and most commonly present in the middle decades of life. Giant aneurysms are most frequently located on the ICA, specifically involving the paraclinoid segment 21% of the time.[5]

The natural history of giant aneurysms is one of a poor prognosis. Some have compared the fate of unruptured giant aneurysms to that of subarachnoid hemorrhage (SAH).[6] Patients often present with symptoms consistent with SAH or mass effect. The Italian cooperative study has shown a 28% mortality rate for untreated giant aneurysms compared to a 14% mortality rate for patients who received treatment.[7] In the same series, morbidity was seen in 48% of cases owing to aneurysm expansion. Giant aneurysms, not unlike other aneurysms, continue to enlarge over time. Expansion is thought to be from growth of the lumen or thrombus formation within the sac. This progressive enlargement often causes symptoms of mass effect.[8]

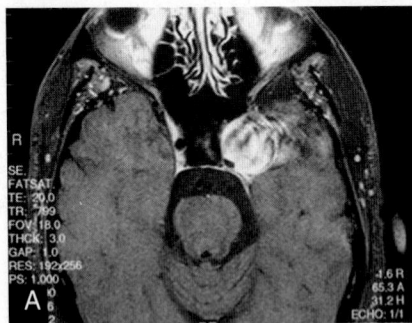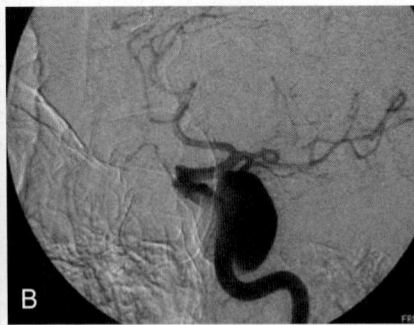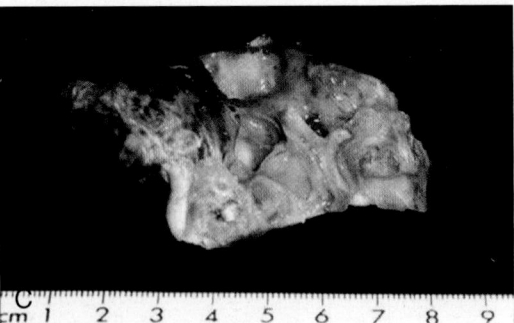

FIGURE 18.1 A, This 55-year-old patient presented with new-onset diplopia. T1 axial magnetic resonance image shows cavernous sinus aneurysm. **B,** Digital subtraction angiogram shows a giant cavernous internal carotid artery aneurysm (does not extend into the supraclinoidal segment). Following balloon test occlusion, that night the patient had an acute headache, and pupils became fixed and dilated. The patient subsequently died within 2 hours. **C,** Autopsy revealed rupture through the middle fossa dura into the temporal lobe.

Historically, it was thought that giant aneurysms were less prone to rupture; however, contemporary evidence suggests that this is inaccurate. Drake found that 62 of 174 cases did rupture.[9] Aneurysms that were 25 mm or more had a relative risk of rupture of 59.0 compared to aneurysms less than 10 mm.[10] Giant aneurysms had a 6% rupture rate in the first year compared to less than 1% for aneurysms less than 10 mm.[10] Patients with a giant aneurysm, but without previous SAH, were at a significantly increased risk for rupture based on size. The rupture rate was not dependent on the location of the aneurysm; all anterior circulation giant aneurysms were at increased risk of rupture.[3] Risk factors for aneurysm rupture include hypertension, current or former tobacco use, alcohol use greater than five drinks per day, and oral contraceptives.[10] It was thought that partially or completely thrombosed aneurysms would be less likely to rupture, thus not requiring treatment; however, in Drake's large series this was not the case.[9]

The International Study of Unruptured Intracranial Aneurysms (ISUIA) trial has shown that unruptured aneurysms overall do not pose as high a risk as once thought; and that treating aneurysms, specifically small ones, puts the patient at greater risk than watchful waiting. However, this advice should not be applied to the special case of giant aneurysms, in which "the natural history is ominous."[6] Morley and Barr's original series demonstrated similar findings, with an 80% mortality rate for untreated aneurysms. Other studies have also shown high 1-year mortality rates.[11] Peerless and associates found that 85% of patients with giant intracranial aneurysms were dead at 5 years.[12] Additionally, the ISUIA II trial found that the cumulative rupture rates for anterior circulation giant aneurysms with no previous history of SAH were 40%. Patients who do present with SAH are at increased risk of death compared to patients without SAH.[13] Figure 18.2 presents a case of a ruptured giant aneurysm without previous history of SAH 6 months after initial diagnosis.

Deliberate Internal Carotid Artery Occlusion

Traditional neurosurgical literature and practice have held a liberal view of ICA occlusion for the treatment of giant ICA aneurysms. Historically this has been accompanied by a relatively high risk of stroke following ICA occlusion (Table 18.1). With more recent improvements in the balloon test occlusion (BTO) paradigms, the risk is smaller but clearly not trivial.

Patients with giant ICA aneurysms are usually younger and have relatively fewer medical comorbid conditions when compared to patients with cervical carotid occlusive disease, and they face an insignificant risk after planned carotid sacrifice. Long-term effects of deliberate carotid occlusion are not well studied. The risks of forming additional aneurysms, developing hemodynamic ischemic disease, and potential cognitive disorders have to be taken into account when this decision is made. Therefore, it has been the practice of the senior author (SIA) to preserve ipsilateral hemispheric flow in the treatment of giant aneurysms, especially in younger patients, by performing a bypass procedure (Fig. 18.3).

TREATMENT OF GIANT INTERNAL CAROTID ARTERY ANEURYSMS

We performed a retrospective review of 55 consecutive patients treated at Saint Louis University Hospital from June 1999 to June 2007. The objectives of this study were to assess the use of high-flow extracranial-intracranial (EC-IC) bypass for the treatment of giant transitional ICA aneurysms, delineate the surgical mortality and morbidity rates, and determine the long-term efficacy of the treatment and the functional outcomes of these patients. All 55 patients had giant transitional ICA aneurysms. The mean aneurysm size was 34.7 mm (range 25 to 70 mm). The mean age was 46 years (range 30-64 years). The mean follow-up period was 34.7 months (range 1-76 months). The most common presenting symptoms were cranial neuropathy (42%), presence of headaches or incidental finding (40%), and subarachnoid hemorrhage (18%) (Fig. 18.4). The World Federation of Neurosurgical Societies (WFNS) grade was 0 in 81%, 1 in 15%, 2 in 2%, and 3 in 2% (Fig. 18.5). All 55 patients underwent a high-flow EC-IC bypass procedure prior to ICA ligation.

Surgical Techniques for Extracranial-Intracranial Bypass Procedure

Minimally Invasive Low-Flow Bypass

We rarely utilize low-flow bypass for giant aneurysms in which primary occlusion of the internal carotid artery is planned. In certain situations, such as elderly patients who pass balloon

FIGURE 18.2 A, A patient was diagnosed with ruptured giant aneurysm at an outside institution and conservative treatment was recommended. **B,** Patient was transferred to our institution 6 months after initial diagnosis with acute subarachnoid hemorrhage and intraventricular hemorrhage. Patient underwent angiography. **C,** During angiography, the aneurysm re-ruptured (see extravasation of blood). **D,** Postangiography computed tomography (CT) scan shows blood completely filling the lateral ventricles. The patient subsequently died.

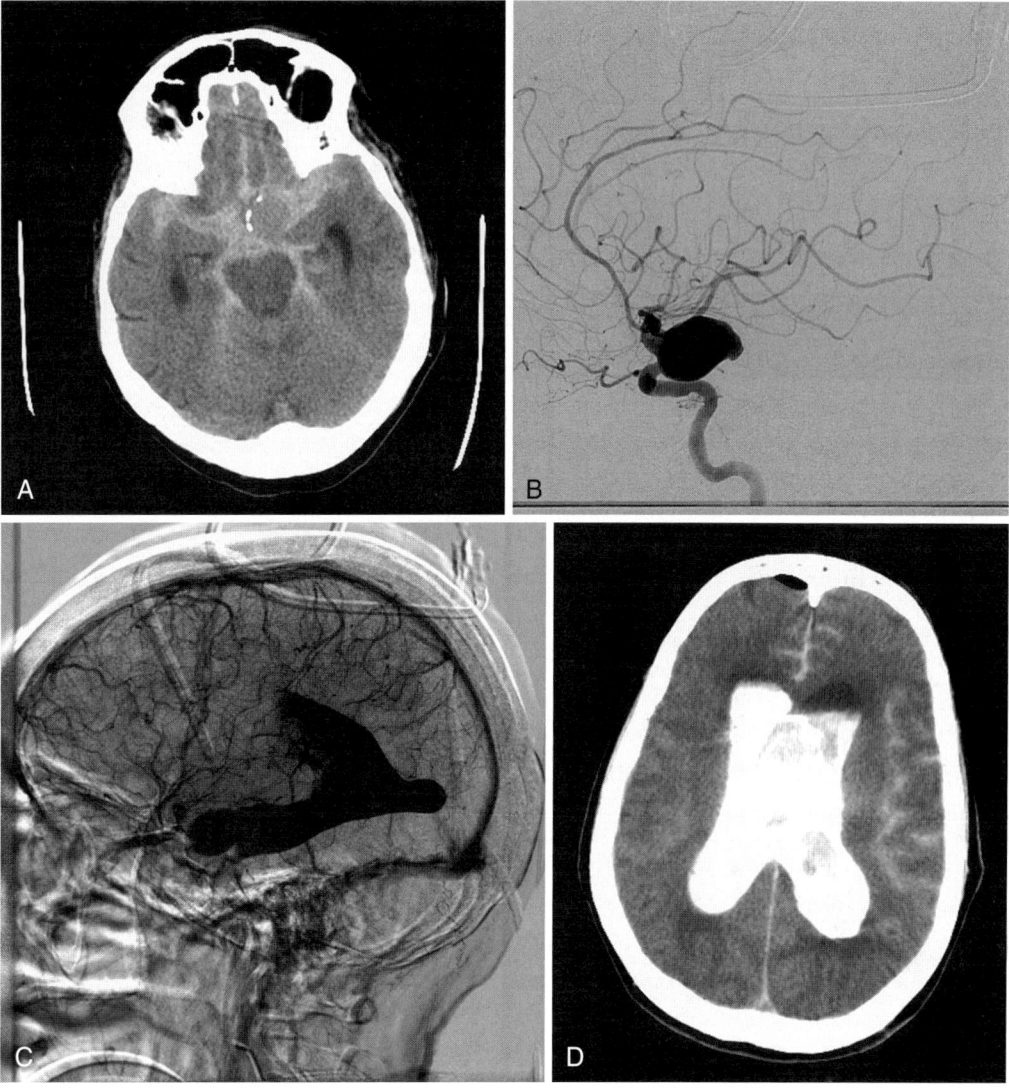

TABLE 18.1 Complications with Internal Carotid Artery (ICA) Sacrifice: Summary of Clinical Studies				
	COMPLICATION RATE (%)			
Study	**TIA**	**Stroke**	**SAH**	**Death**
ICA Ligation				
Sahs and Locksley, 1969		30%		20.7%
Roski et al. 1981	16.6%	16.6%	5.5%	5.5%
Intravascular ICA Occlusion				
Linskey et al. 1994		12.9%		3.2%
Larson et al. 1995	10.9%	3.6%	3.6%	5.4%

SAH, subarachnoid hemorrhage; TIA, transient ischemic attack.[14]
Data from Sahs AL, Perret GE, Locksley HB, et al, editors. Intracranial Aneurysms and Subarachnoid Hemorrhage: A Cooperative Study. Philadelphia: Lippincott, 1969.
Additional data from
  Roski et al. J Neurosurg 1981.[15]
  Linskey et al. Am J Neuroradiol 1994.[16]
  Larson et al. Neurosurgery 1995.[17]

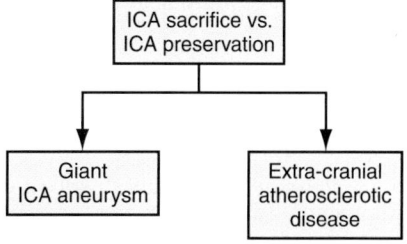

FIGURE 18.3 Internal carotid artery sacrifice versus internal carotid artery preservation.

test occlusion and SPECT (single-photon emission computed tomography) scanning, it may be reasonable to perform low-flow bypass to maximally minimize surgical morbidity.

Using a preoperative computed tomography (CT) angiogram that provides clear visualization of the superficial temporal artery (STA), including its frontal and parietal branches, we measure the diameters of these branches and identify the optimal vessel for use as a donor (Fig. 18.6). This enables us to plan a linear skin incision overlying the chosen donor vessel.

PRESENTING SYMPTOMS

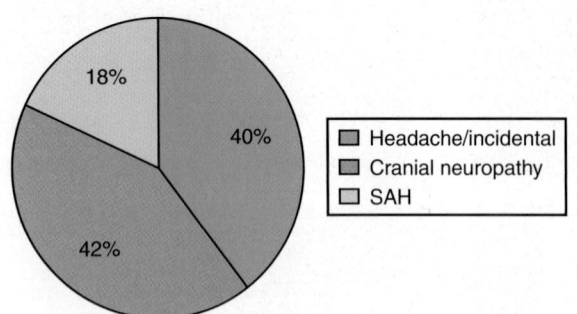

FIGURE 18.4 Percentage of patients initially presenting with headache, cranial neuropathy, and subarachnoid hemorrhage.

WFNS GRADE

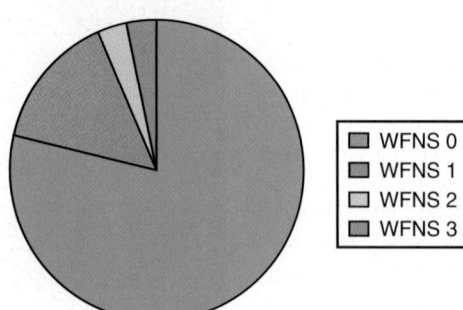

FIGURE 18.5 Initial WFNS (World Federation of Neurosurgical Societies) grade at presentation.

The bur hole/craniotomy can be planned preoperatively with the help of the stereotactically reconstructed model based on the CT angiogram. The recipient vessel is chosen based on its caliber and superficial location in the sylvian fissure (Fig. 18.7). The ideal recipient vessel is identified based on the review of the CT angiogram. Using CT angiography–based neuronavigation, the exact location of the bur hole/craniotomy is planned to overlie the selected recipient vessel and to be in the immediate proximity of the selected donor vessel (Fig. 18.8).

The incision is performed under the microscope, and the temporalis muscle is split vertically directly below the selected donor branch of the STA.

A bur hole is made and enlarged to the size of a very small craniotomy (~ 2-2.5 cm) under the microscope (Figs. 18.9 and 18.10), and the recipient vessel is exposed in the distal sylvian fissure over a length of 1 cm. A rubber dam is applied and the anastomosis is performed with a 9-0 nylon suture in a running fashion. The back wall is anastomosed first, followed by the front wall. Temporary clips are applied on the M4 recipient vessel during the anastomosis. Postoperatively, the patients are followed up with angiography (Fig. 18.11) or CT angiography (Fig. 18.12).[18]

Standard High-Flow Extracranial-Intracranial Bypass Technique

Craniotomy

Patients are started on acetylsalicylic acid (ASA) 81 mg daily for 3 days prior to the surgery. Intraoperative electroencephalogram (EEG), somatosensory evoked potentials (SSEPs), and motor evoked potentials (MEPs) are continuously monitored. A skull base approach, usually a cranio-orbital-zygomatic approach, is the senior author's preference to facilitate a wide access to the sylvian fissure and better exposure of the proximal supraclinoid ICA for possible proximal occlusion or trapping of the giant aneurysm. We prefer a single-piece craniotomy that entails an osteotomy of the superior and lateral orbital roofs. A high-speed drill is used to thin the zygomatic arch posteriorly which allows the radial artery to lie over the zygomatic arch without risk of kinking (Fig. 18.13A).

Cervical Carotid Exposure

The common, external, and internal carotid arteries (CCA, ECA, and ICA, respectively) are then exposed in the ipsilateral cervical region. A standard incision is performed anteriorly to the sternocleidomastoid muscle and the fascial planes of the neck are dissected until the vessels are properly exposed. Vessel loops are applied around the CCA, ECA, and the ICA. We recommend the use of the ECA as the site for the proximal anastomosis.

Radial Artery Graft Harvest and Tunneling

The radial artery is then harvested in the contralateral arm to serve as an interposition graft. It is the preference of the senior author to use radial artery as opposed to saphenous vein in order to minimize diameter mismatch between donor and recipient vessels and the graft. Prior to radial artery harvesting, an Allen's test is performed to assure proper palmar arch perfusion by the ulnar artery alone. The critical aspect of radial artery harvest is the length of the graft, which can be limiting. Obtaining maximal length is critical during this harvest. The superficial wall of the radial artery is marked with a marking pen prior to removal of the graft. This step is crucial to avoid graft rotation during the tunneling (Fig. 18.13B). Once the graft is harvested, it is placed in a heparinized saline solution. The graft is tunneled using a pediatric chest tube. The marked surface of the graft is kept most superficial.

Cervical Anastomosis

The proximal cervical anastomosis is performed first to minimize time of temporary occlusion of the ICA. The radial artery graft is placed opposite an area of the ECA where the proximal anastomosis is planned. Long temporary aneurysm clips are used for the ECA anastomosis. An end-to-side or end-to-end anastomosis can be performed between the radial artery and the ECA after temporary occlusion of this vessel. We prefer a running suture technique using 7-0 nylon or prolene stitches. We perform the "back" wall (i.e., the more difficult anastomosis) first followed by the front wall (Fig. 18.13E). When the anastomosis is completed, antegrade flow is confirmed in the graft followed by the placement of a temporary clip on the graft just distal to the anastomosis.

Intracranial Anastomosis

The site of the intracranial anastomosis is determined based on several factors: the intended revascularization territory, the size of donor and recipient vessels, the length of the graft, and the location of the aneurysm. Mild hypothermia is utilized. EEG burst suppression using pentobarbital is maintained during the temporary clipping period. A color background is placed underneath the recipient vessel. Temporary clips are

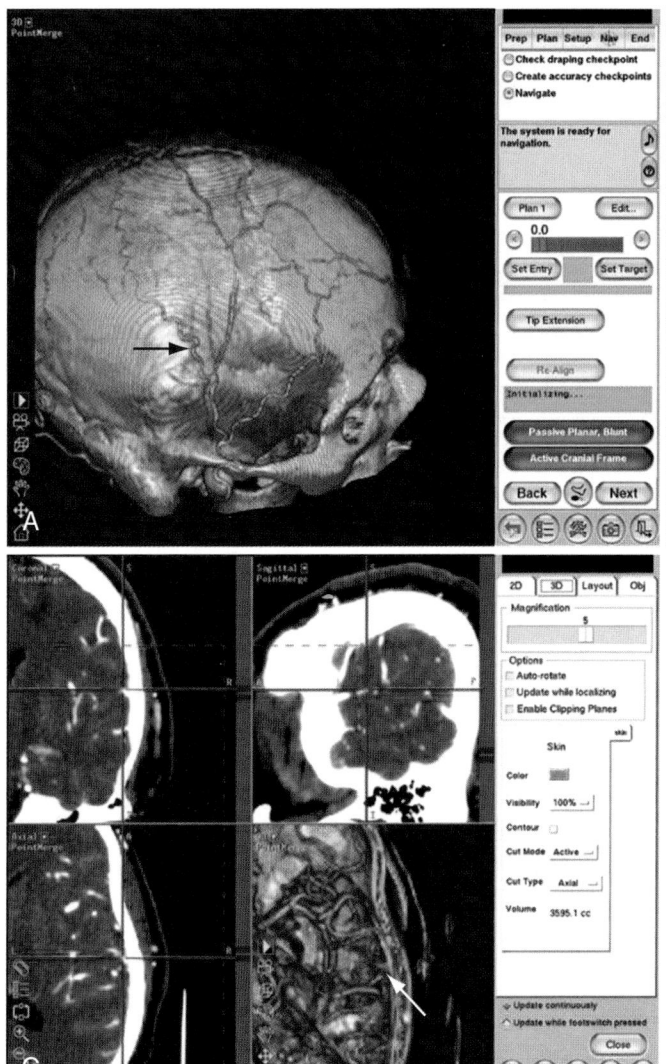

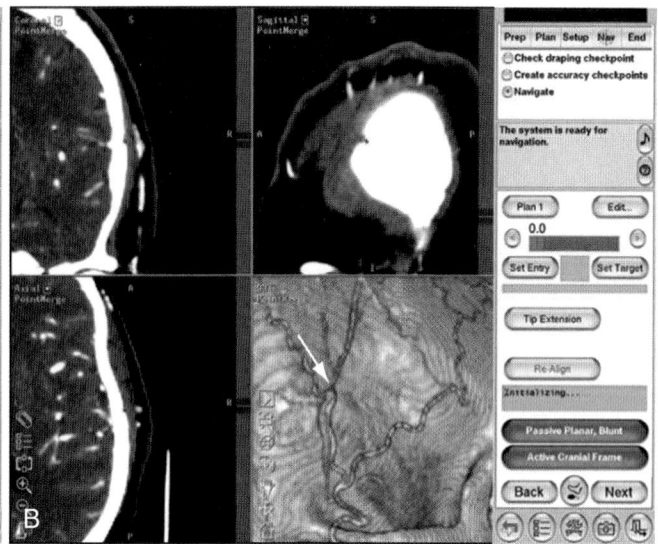

FIGURE 18.6 A, Image guidance workstation view of three-dimensional reconstruction of computed tomography (CT) angiogram showing the donor vessel, parietal branch of superficial temporal artery (STA) (*arrow*). **B,** Image guidance workstation axial, coronal, and sagittal and three-dimensional reconstruction CT angiogram views showing the preselected bur hole/craniotomy site (*red dots*). The overlying donor (*arrow*) and recipient vessels are seen on both sides of the bur hole location. **C,** Image guidance workstation axial, coronal, and sagittal and three-dimensional reconstruction CT angiogram views showing the middle cerebral artery (MCA) recipient vessel in the sylvian fissure (*arrow*). *(From Coppens JR, Cantando JD, Abdulrauf SI. Minimally invasive superficial temporal artery to middle cerebral artery bypass through an enlarged bur hole: the use of computed tomography angiography neuronavigation in surgical planning, J Neurosurg 2009;109(3):553-558, used with permission.)*

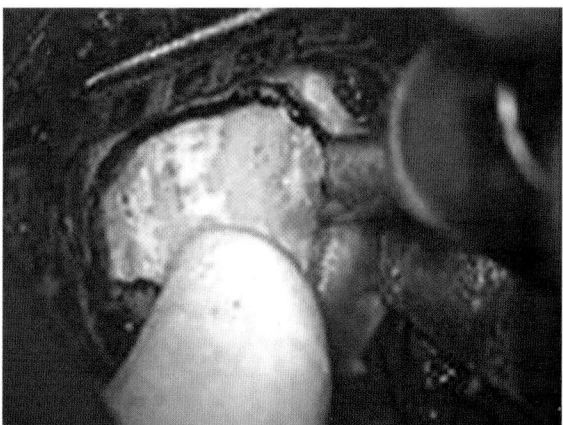

FIGURE 18.7 Intraoperative photograph obtained through the microscope while the bur hole/craniotomy was being performed. *(From Coppens JR, Cantando JD, Abdulrauf SI. Minimally invasive superficial temporal artery to middle cerebral artery bypass through an enlarged bur hole: the use of computed tomography angiography neuronavigation in surgical planning, J Neurosurg 2009;109(3):553-558, used with permission.)*

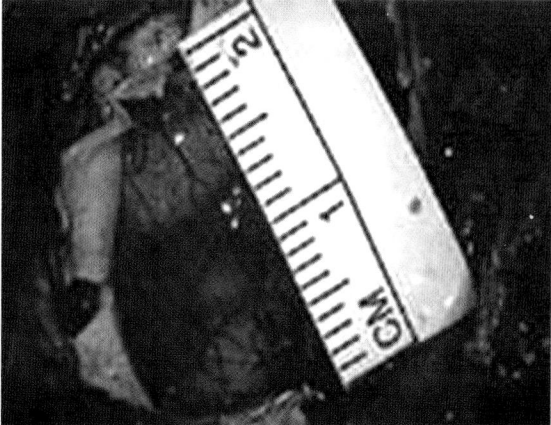

FIGURE 18.8 Intraoperative photograph obtained through the microscope demonstrating the maximum diameter of the bur hole/craniotomy to be approximately 2 cm. *(From Coppens JR, Cantando JD, Abdulrauf SI. Minimally invasive superficial temporal artery to middle cerebral artery bypass through an enlarged bur hole: the use of computed tomography angiography neuronavigation in surgical planning, J Neurosurg 2009;109(3):553-558, used with permission.)*

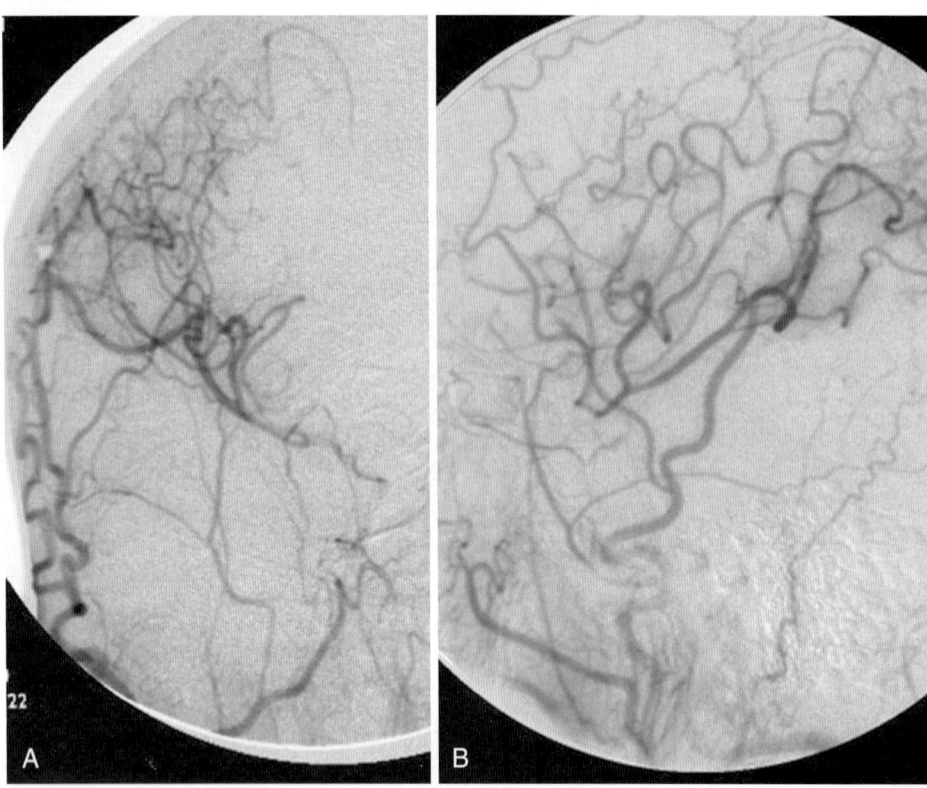

FIGURE 18.9 Anteroposterior (**A**) and lateral (**B**) views of the postoperative cerebral angiogram demonstrating the bypass in the form of an STA-MCA (M4 branch) anastomosis. MCA, middle cerebral artery; STA, superficial temporal artery. *(From Coppens JR, Cantando JD, Abdulrauf SI. Minimally invasive superficial temporal artery to middle cerebral artery bypass through an enlarged bur hole: the use of computed tomography angiography neuronavigation in surgical planning, J Neurosurg 2009;109(3):553-558, with permission.)*

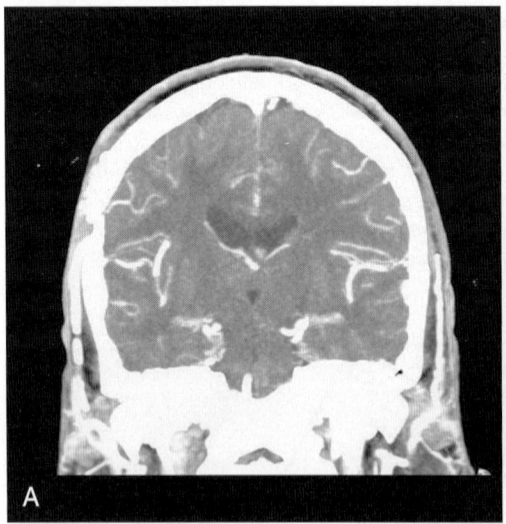
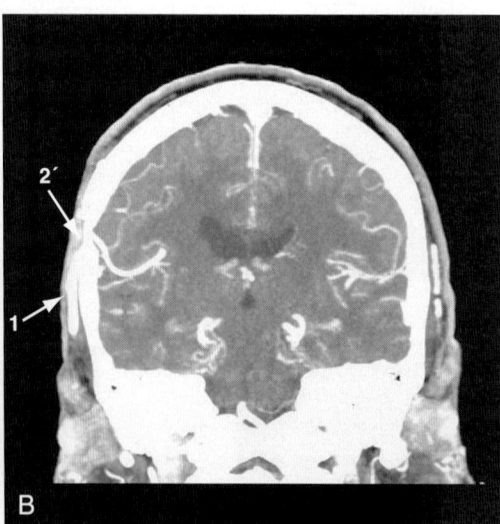

FIGURE 18.10 **A** and **B,** Sequential coronal computed tomography (CT) angiograms showing the STA-MCA bypass entering through a bur hole (<2.5 cm). Arrow 1 shows the SA, arrow 2 points toward the bur hole opening, and arrow 3 indicates the recipient MCA vessel. MCA, middle cerebral artery; STA, superficial temporal artery.

applied (Fig. 18.13C). An arteriotomy is made using an arachnoid knife. The arteriotomy is extended using microscissors to the width of the interposition graft lumen. The lumen of the interposition graft is expanded by "fish-mouthing" the opening. We used 9-0 nylon for M2 and M3 vessels and 8-0 nylon for the supraclinoidal ICA. A similar technique of "back" wall and "front" wall can be utilized as described previously for the cervical anastomosis (Fig. 18-13D).

Graft Inspection

Pulsatility of the graft is not enough to confirm graft patency. Micro-Doppler (Mizuho America, Inc., Beverly, MA) can be used. We now use indocyanine green (ICG) microscope-based

angiography routinely for these cases. If the latter technology is not available, intraoperative angiography, in our opinion, is critical before parent vessel occlusion is performed. Flow probe technology (Transonic Systems, Inc., Ithaca, NY) has allowed us to estimate the amount of flow (mL/minute) within the graft.

Parent Vessel Occlusion

Once the preceding steps, including intraoperative angiography, have documented flow in the graft, we then advocate parent vessel occlusion during the same surgical procedure, rather than delayed (staged) occlusion. In our opinion, the risk of graft occlusion would be high if competitive flow in

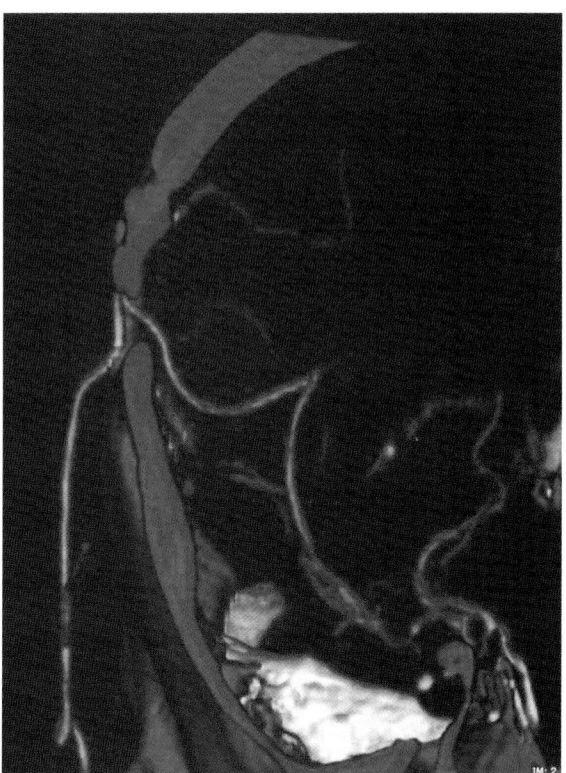

FIGURE 18.11 A three-dimensional reconstruction of the postoperative computed tomography (CT) angiogram demonstrating maturation of the extracranial-intracranial (EC-IC) bypass. *(From Coppens JR, Cantando JD, Abdulrauf SI. Minimally invasive superficial temporal artery to middle cerebral artery bypass through an enlarged bur hole: the use of computed tomography angiography neuronavigation in surgical planning, J Neurosurg 2009;109(3):553-558, with permission.)*

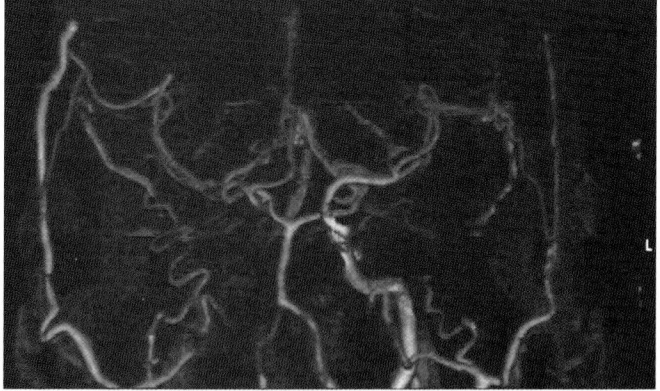

FIGURE 18.12 Computed tomography (CT) angiography three-dimensional reconstruction of the STA-MCA bypass using a minimally invasive technique. (Note the right carotid artery occlusion with which the patient presented.) MCA, middle cerebral artery; STA, superficial temporal artery.

the parent vessel were allowed to continue. We occlude the ICA at the level of the bifurcation in the cervical area and just distal to the giant aneurysm in the supraclinoidal portion of the ICA. The distal occlusion must be performed proximal to the anterior choroidal and dominant posterior communicating arteries.[19]

Minimally Invasive High-Flow Extracranial-Intracranial Bypass Technique

A new approach to performing high-flow EC-IC bypasses involves using the internal maxillary artery (IMAX) as the donor vessel. It has many potential advantages over the standard high-flow bypass technique, such as the closer proximity between donor and recipient vessels (which allows a much shorter graft with likely longer graft patency), the ability to perform an EC-IC bypass through a single craniotomy incision, with avoidance of both cervical incisions and need for tunneling the graft, and finally the possibility of making this procedure technically simpler and easier to perform.

The craniotomy is performed just as in a standard high-flow bypass and may require a skull base approach such as an cranio-orbito-zygomatic approach to allow easier access to the proximal supraclinoid carotid for aneurysm trapping or proximal internal carotid ligation. The radial artery is also harvested from the contralateral arm in the same fashion as with standard bypass procedures.

The IMAX exposure is performed through the same intracranial approach. The distal aspect of the IMAX, within the pterygopalatine fossa, is exposed to be used as the donor vessel. The head is rotated about 60 degrees to the contralateral side and the vertex is slightly tilted upward to allow a more lateral view toward the middle fossa floor. The dura is reflected away from the lateral wall of the middle fossa until both foramina ovale and rotundum are visualized. The greater wing of the sphenoid bone is drilled all the way down to the infratemporal crest to allow entry into the pterygopalatine fossa. The anteroposterior limits of this drilling are the sphenozygomatic suture anteriorly and a point where the greater sphenoid wing is crossed by an imaginary line drawn perpendicular to the foramen rotundum posteriorly.

Once within the pterygopalatine fossa, the fibers of the infratemporal head of the lateral pterygoid muscle are visualized and dissected until the IMAX is found surrounded by adipose tissue. The IMAX is usually located inferior to the maxillary nerve and lying on the posterior wall of the maxillary sinus. This technique provides very good exposure of the IMAX and its branches, which can then be mobilized successfully for an end-to-side anastomosis with the radial artery graft. The radial artery is then trimmed to reach the desired M3 recipient vessel within the sylvian fissure, where another end-to-side anastomosis is performed using the same technique already described for the standard bypass. (Figs. 18.14 and 18.15). Intraoperative indocyanine green angiography is used to demonstrate graft patency (Fig. 18.16).[20]

Results of Giant Aneurysm Series

The outcome of this series shows that 50 patients (91%) had a Modified Rankin Scale (MRS) score of 0 to 1, 2 patients (3.5%) had an MRS score of 2 to 3, and 3 patients (5.5%) had an MRS score of 4 to 5. Fifty-one patients (93%) had a Glasgow Outcome Scale (GOS) score of 5, 2 patients (3.5%) had a GOS score 3 to 4, and 2 patients (3.5%) had a GOS score of 1 to 2. At discharge from the hospital 49 (81%) patients went home, 4 patients (7%) went to rehabilitation facilities, and 2 patients (4%) went to nursing homes (Fig. 18.17).

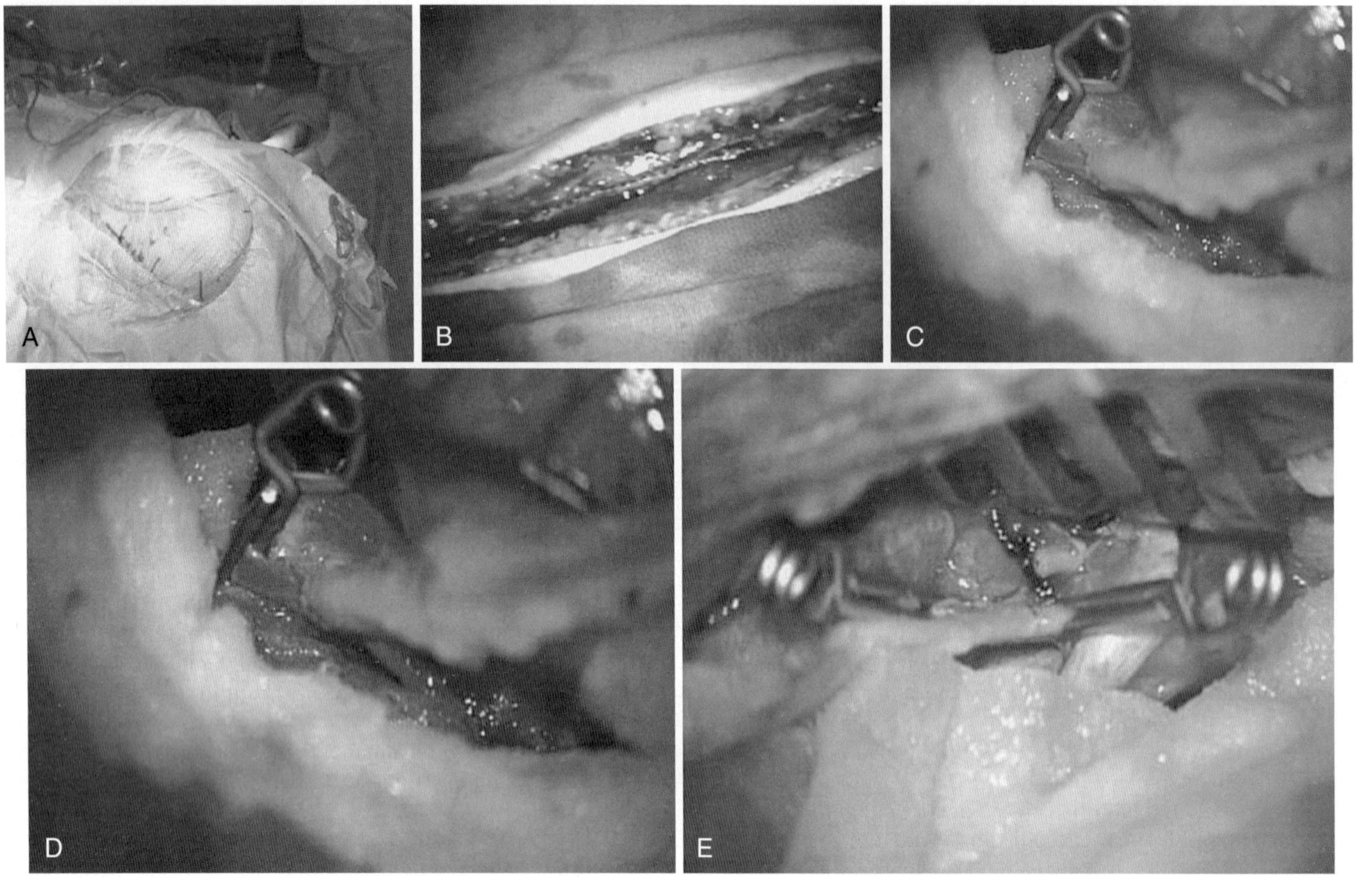

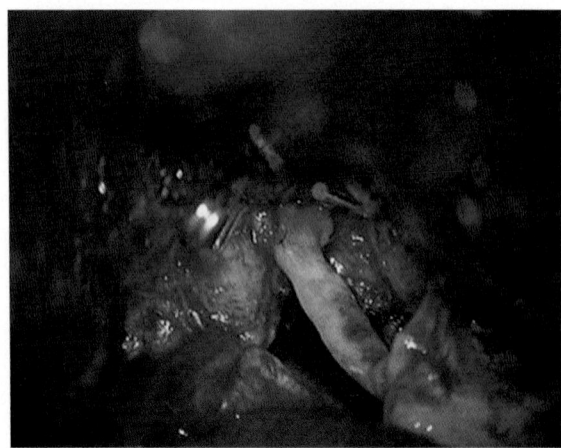 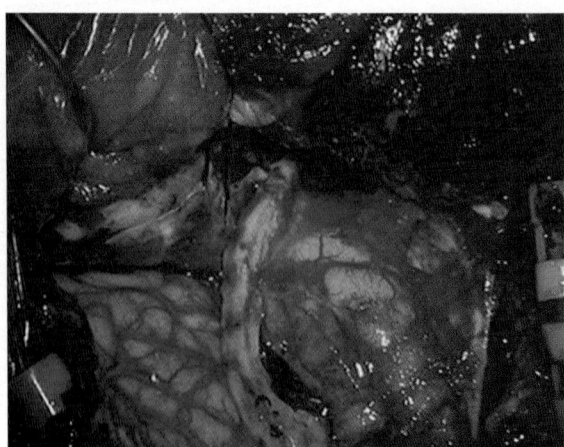

FIGURE 18.13 A, Operative photograph shows simultaneous planning for the craniotomy, cervical incision, and radial artery harvest. **B,** Operative photograph shows exposure of the radial artery with superficial marking. **C,** Trans-sylvian preparation for anastomosis. M3 recipient branch with temporary clips. Radial artery donor grafts are shown. **D,** Completed anastomosis is shown. **E,** Anastomosis of the radial graft to the external carotid artery (ECA) in the neck is shown. Temporary clips on ECA are shown. *(From Abdulrauf SI. Extracranial-to-intracranial bypass using radial artery grafting for complex skull base tumors: technical note, Skull Base 2005;15:207-213, used with permission.)*

FIGURE 18.14 Proximal radial artery graft to internal maxillary artery anastomosis. *(From Abdulrauf SI, Sweeney JM, Mohan YS, Palejwala SK. Short segment internal maxillary artery to middle cerebral artery bypass: a novel technique for extracranial-to-intracranial bypass. Neurosurgery 2011;68(3):804-809, used with permission.)*

FIGURE 18.15 Radial artery graft connecting the IMAX (*top*) to the M3 segment of the MCA (*bottom*). IMAX, internal maxillary artery; MCA, middle cerebral artery. *(From Abdulrauf SI, Sweeney JM, Mohan YS, Palejwala SK. Short segment internal maxillary artery to middle cerebral artery bypass: a novel technique for extracranial-to-intracranial bypass. Neurosurgery 2011;68(3):804-809, used with permission.)*

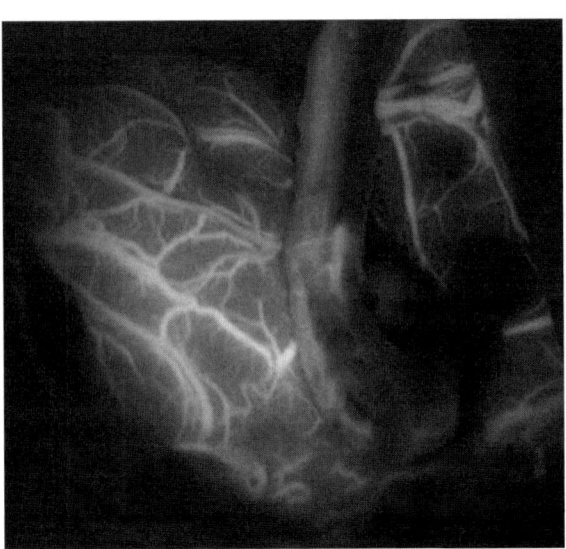

FIGURE 18.16 Intraoperative indocyanine green (ICG) angiogram showing patency of the radial artery graft. *(From Abdulrauf SI, Sweeney JM, Mohan YS, Palejwala SK. Short segment internal maxillary artery to middle cerebral artery bypass: a novel technique for extracranial-to-intracranial bypass. Neurosurgery 2011;68(3):804-809, used with permission.)*

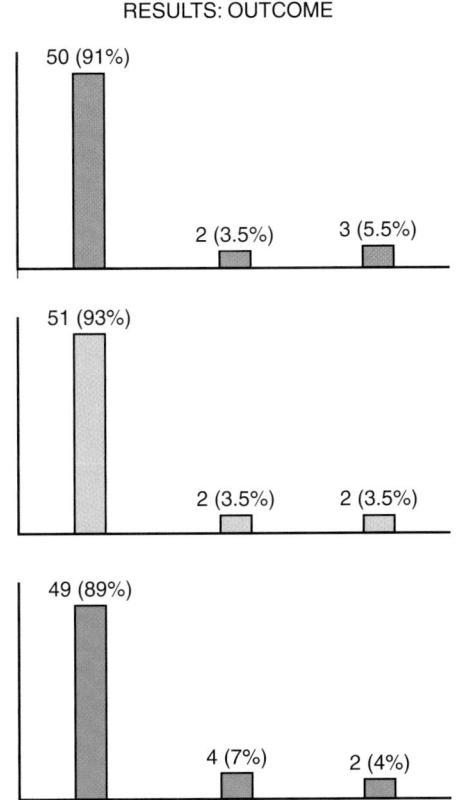

FIGURE 18.17 In this series 92.7% of patients had good Glasgow Outcome Scale (GOS) scores, 90.9% had none to no significant disability, and 89.1% went home. Only one patient died, which accounts for the 1.8% mortality rate.

Acute graft occlusion occurred in 4 patients (7.3%), and late graft occlusion in 4 patients (7.3%). The main complication/morbidity was cerebrovascular accident (CVA), which occurred in 4 patients (7.3%). Two patients had CVA secondary to acute graft occlusion, and 2 patients had CVA secondary to microsurgical manipulation of calcified aneurysms. Aneurysm recurrence was seen in only 1 patient (Fig. 18.18). One patient died from a pulmonary embolus at home 5 weeks after operation.

Treatment Options

Traditional treatment of giant aneurysms was direct microsurgical clipping, which continues to be a feasible option in certain cases. However, the risk of direct clipping of giant aneurysms is not low. Our review of major series of direct clipping of giant ICA aneurysms revealed a fair to poor outcome in approximately 18% of the patients. In these same series, the mortality rate was 11% (Table 18.2). Endovascular treatment of giant aneurysms also poses certain challenges. Our review of major series of coiling or stenting plus coiling of giant aneurysms reveals that approximately 42% of the aneurysms are completely occluded by the treatment. Thirty-seven percent of the aneurysms recanalize. Major morbidity rate was approximately 21% in these patients, and mortality rate was 15% (Table 18.3).

EC-IC bypass for giant aneurysms in the major published series shows relatively better outcomes than direct microsurgical clipping or endovascular treatment. Based on our review of these major series, excellent to good outcome was achieved on average in 84% of the patients. Significant morbidity was seen on average in 11% of the patients. On average, 5% of the patients died (Table 18.4).

Technical Aspects in High-Flow Extracranial-Intracranial Bypass Surgery

Atypical Appearance of Giant Aneurysms

Irregular appearance of the wall, or the pattern of more than one aneurysmal sac, ought to indicate partial calcification or thrombosis. The appearance of the aneurysm on cerebral angiography is a critical factor in decision making regarding treatment. In the experience of the senior author, complex aneurysms, including those with irregular appearance of the wall, outpouching within the dome, or the presence of calcification, may carry a higher risk with direct clipping. Partial thrombosis of the aneurysm may show a smaller aneurysm on angiography when compared to magnetic resonance imaging (MRI). Partially thrombosed aneurysms also carry a risk of embolic complications during microsurgical clipping or endovascular coiling (Fig. 18.19).

Aneurysm Size

The size of the aneurysm, although a critical factor when considering direct microsurgical clipping or endovascular coiling, is not an equally important factor when considering EC-IC bypass. In our opinion, for significantly large aneurysms, EC-IC bypass would be the least risky procedure (Fig. 18.20).

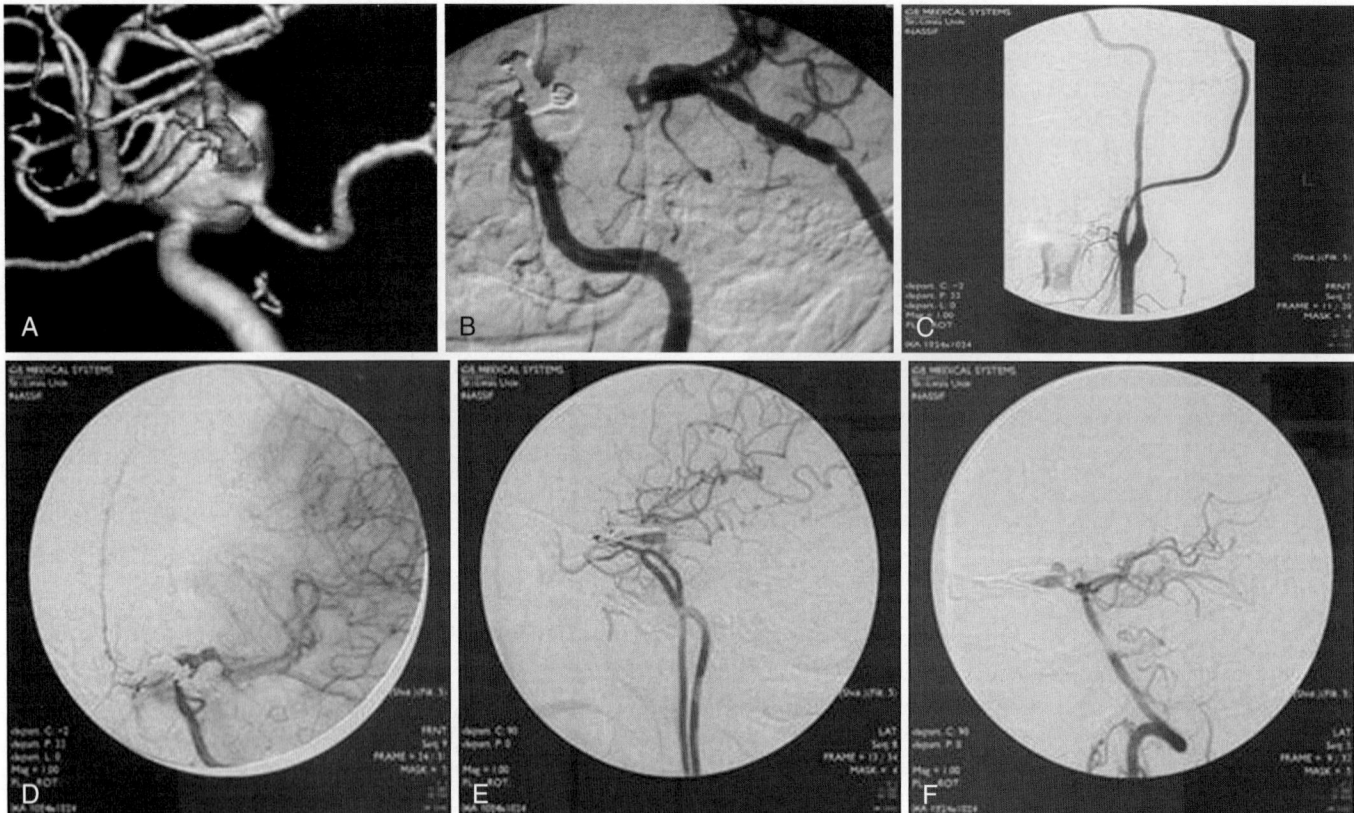

FIGURE 18.18 A, Fusiform aneurysm (involves the entire wall) of the left internal carotid artery (ICA) segment. Patient failed balloon text occlusion (BTO) within 60 seconds. **B,** Immediate postoperative angiogram showing graft with nonsymptomatic vasospasm. **C,** A 6-month follow-up angiogram showing end-to-end bypass (patient is asymptomatic.) **D,** A 1-year follow-up showing progression of disease into the distal ICA. **E,** Lateral view ICA injection showing the progression. **F,** Lateral view vertebral artery injection showing new formation of aneurysm in distal ICA.

Giant Cavernous Segment Internal Carotid Artery Aneurysm

The location of the aneurysm is an important factor when making decisions regarding treatment. Endovascular stenting plus coiling or EC-IC bypass are potential treatments of a giant cavernous segment aneurysm. Direct surgical clipping should not be considered in these cases, as it would almost certainly lead to ophthalmoplegia (Fig. 18.21).

End-to-Side versus End-to-End Proximal Anastomosis

For the proximal anastomosis, end-to-end or end-to-side are both reasonable options. The senior author prefers the use of the ECA as the donor vessel. This avoids temporary occlusion of the ICA during the procedure. The advantage of end-to-end anastomosis is, presumably, more vigorous flow into the graft. The disadvantage of end-to-end anastomosis is potential occlusion of ophthalmic vessel collaterals into the supraclinoidal carotid artery. End-to-side anastomosis, therefore, is a reasonable option and an easier procedure in comparison to end-to-end anastomosis (end-to-end may create a size mismatch, which may in certain situations be difficult to compensate for) (Fig. 18.22).

Competitive Flow

It is important to recognize that during intraoperative angiography the graft may only supply a single division of the recipient territory (i.e., a single M2 division). This should not be a concerning sign. In general, this is due to the fact that there is significant competitive flow coming through the anterior communicating artery from the contralateral side, which is protective, and the surgeon ought not to change the strategy during the case (Fig. 18.23).

Radial Artery Graft Enlargement

The diameter size of the graft as seen during intraoperative catheter or ICG angiography ought not be concerning as long as there is no occlusion or specific area of stenosis. In our experience, the graft will expand in diameter over time to accommodate for blood flow demand (Fig. 18.24).

Intraoperative Failure of Graft

In most situations in which the graft is not visible during intraoperative angiography, technical failure is assumed and the anastomosis, as well as the tunneling, ought to be

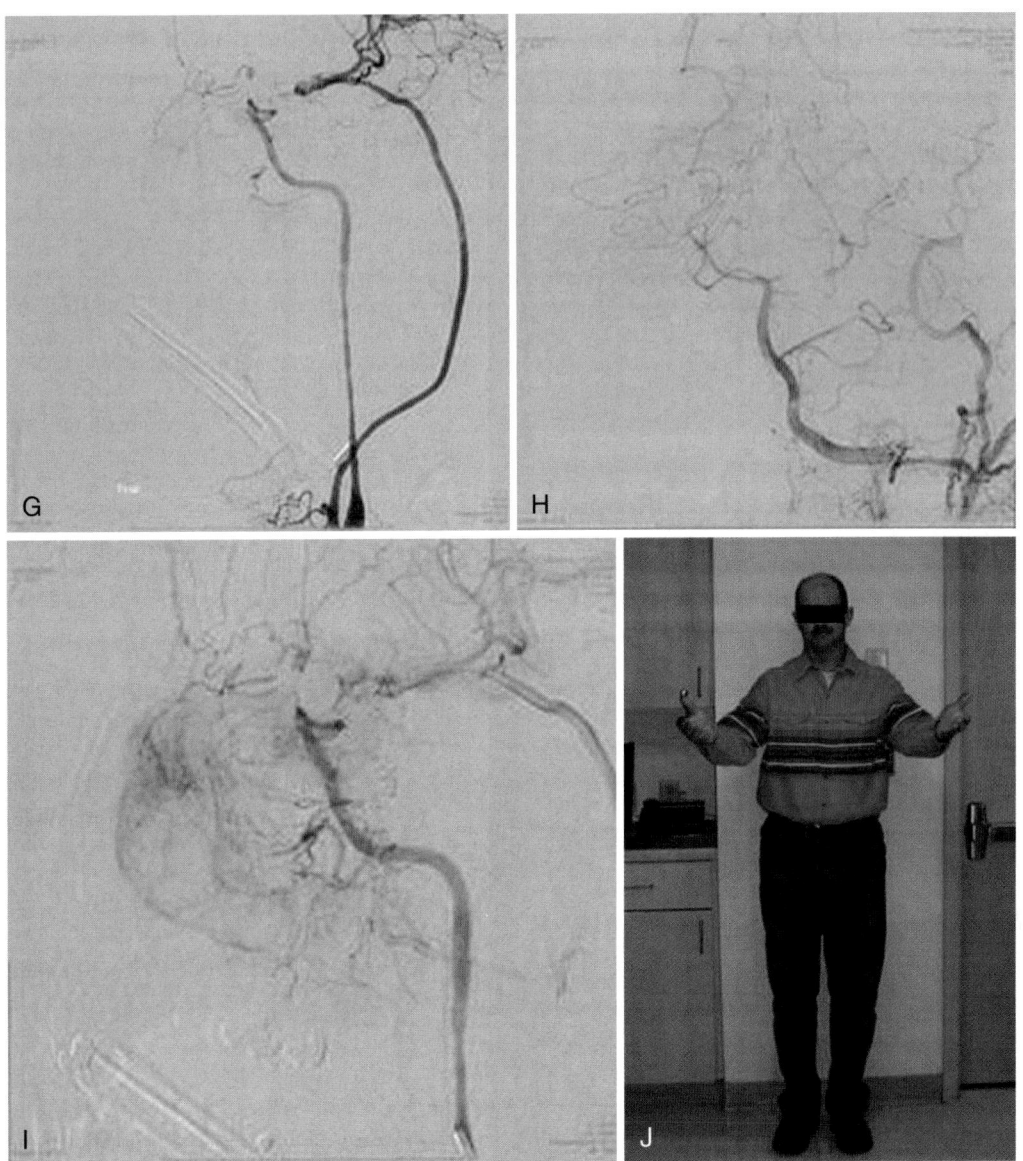

FIGURE 18.18, cont'd G, ICA injection following endovascular coiling of the aneurysm through the posterior communicating artery (PCA). **H,** Vertebral artery injection following endovascular coiling through the PCA. **I,** Common carotid artery (CCA) injection following coiling showing the bypass as well as complete resolution of the aneurysm. **J,** At 1-year follow-up patient is asymptomatic and aneurysm is completely treated.

TABLE 18.2 Outcomes with Direct Clipping of Giant Internal Carotid Artery (ICA) Aneurysms: Summary of Clinical Studies

		CLINICAL OUTCOME		
Study	No. of Patients	Excellent/Good	Fair/Poor	Death
Drake et al. 1979[9]	23	16 (70%)	4 (17%)	3 (13%)
Sundt and Piepgras. 1979[21]	47	40 (85%)	6 (13%)	1 (2%)
Heros et al. 1983[11]	25	20 (80%)	2 (8%)	3 (12%)
Symon et al. 1984[22]	9	5 (56%)	2 (22%)	2 (22%)
Yasargil et al. 1984[23]	10	8 (80%)	2 (20%)	0 (0%)
Batjer and Samson. 1994[24]	10	5 (50%)	4 (40%)	1 (10%)
Lawton and Spetzler. 1994[25]	34	25 (73%)	2 (6%)	7 (21%)
TOTAL	158	71%	18%	11%

TABLE 18.3 Outcomes with Endovascular Treatment of Giant Internal Carotid Artery (ICA) Aneurysms: Summary of Clinical Studies

Study	No. of Patients	Treatment	% Complete Occlusion of the Aneurysm	% Recanalized	% Morbidity	% Mortality	Follow-up Angio
Gruber et al. 1999[26]	12	Coil	42	37.5	33	33	24.3 mo
Hayakawa et al. 2000[27]	10	Coil	10	90	NS	NS	NS
Mawad et al. 2002[28]	11	Stent + Onyx	81	0	9	18	5 mo
Murayama et al. 2003[29]	19	Coil	25	58	NS	NS	NS
Sluzewski et al. 2003[30]	17	Coil	29	53	29	18	12.7 mo
Gonzalez et al. 2004[31]	29	Coil	24	NS	NS	NS	NS
Molyneux et al. 2004[32]	73	Balloon + Onyx	47	0	16	0	5 mo
Cekirge et al. 2006[33]	21	Stent + Onyx	76	20	19	5	12 mo
Jahromi et al. 2008[34]	16	Stent + coil	25	62.5	12.5	12.5	19.1 mo
TOTAL	208		40%	38%	20%	14%	13 mo

Angio, angiography; NS, not significant.

TABLE 18.4 Outcomes with Extracranial-Intracranial Bypass for Giant Internal Carotid Artery (ICA) Aneurysms

Study	No. of Patients	Graft Type	Excellent/ Good	Poor	Death	OUTCOME Acute Occlusion	Late Occlusion	Late Patency
Sundt and Piepgras, 1986[35]	NS (20)	SV	80%	15%	5%	13%	3%	84%
Lawton and Spetzler, 1996[36]	12	SV/ STA-MCA	93%	5%	2%	5%	3%	92%
Sekhar et al. 2001[37]	4	SV/RA	76%	12%	12%	25% SV 6% RA	NS	94% SV 100% RA
Jafar et al. 2002[38]	12	SV	90%	7%	3%	7%	0	93%
Tulleken et al. 2006[39]	34	SV	73.5%	20.5%	6%	NS	3%	97%
Abdulrauf, 2007[40]	55	RA	91%	7%	2%	7%	7%	86%
TOTAL	117		84%	11%	5%	8%	3%	90%

MCA, middle cerebral artery; NS, not significant; RA, radial artery; STA, superficial temporal artery; SV, saphenous vein.

reinvestigated. In patients who have passed the BTO, it is possible to have such significant competitive flow that the resistance in the graft cannot match the higher contralateral flow and the graft is not necessary. It is important to look at every step of the procedure to make sure that there is no technical failure before making any other decisions. If no technical failures are found and no changes in the patient's motor and sensory evoked potentials are detected, it is reasonable to leave the graft in place. In certain circumstances the graft may enlarge over time if demand is placed on it, while in other situations, the graft would be occluded without any neurological symptoms based on the fact that competitive flow was significantly strong and the graft was not needed to start with (Fig. 18.25).

Creation of a New Posterior Communicating Artery

EC-IC bypass surgery is an intellectual exercise given the complexity of the aneurysm. In certain situations an intraposition graft may be needed. In some cases an intracranial-to-intracranial bypass may be more appropriate than an EC-IC bypass. In other cases the creation of a new anterior

communicating or posterior communicating artery (using an interposition graft) may aid in the treatment of the specific of aneurysm, whether it is microsurgical or endovascular (Fig. 18.26).

The Length of the Graft and Risk of Occlusion

The length of the graft is also an important aspect. Additional unneeded length may lead to kinking in the cervical or cranial areas and could be a risk factor for graft occlusion. This aspect has to be inspected well during the operation, as this is an important variable in achieving success in EC-IC bypass surgery (Fig. 18.27).

Distal Anastomosis Size Mismatch

From a technical standpoint of the distal anastomosis, it is important to match the size of the donor and recipient arteries. In our opinion a significant size mismatch could have a higher risk of turbulent flow and subsequent thrombosis at the anastomosis site (Fig. 18.28).

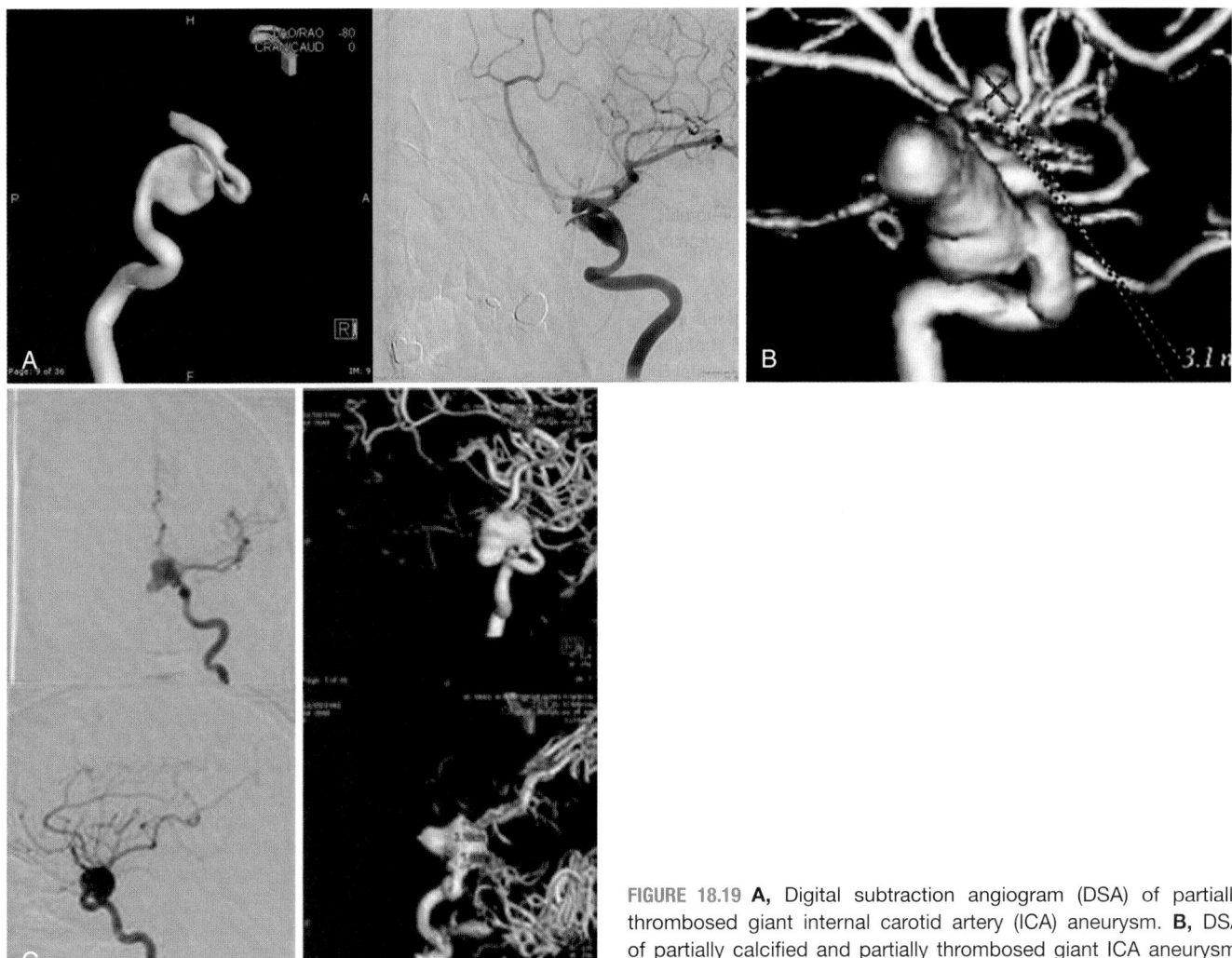

FIGURE 18.19 **A,** Digital subtraction angiogram (DSA) of partially thrombosed giant internal carotid artery (ICA) aneurysm. **B,** DSA of partially calcified and partially thrombosed giant ICA aneurysm. **C,** DSA of a partially thrombosed and partially calcified ICA aneurysm.

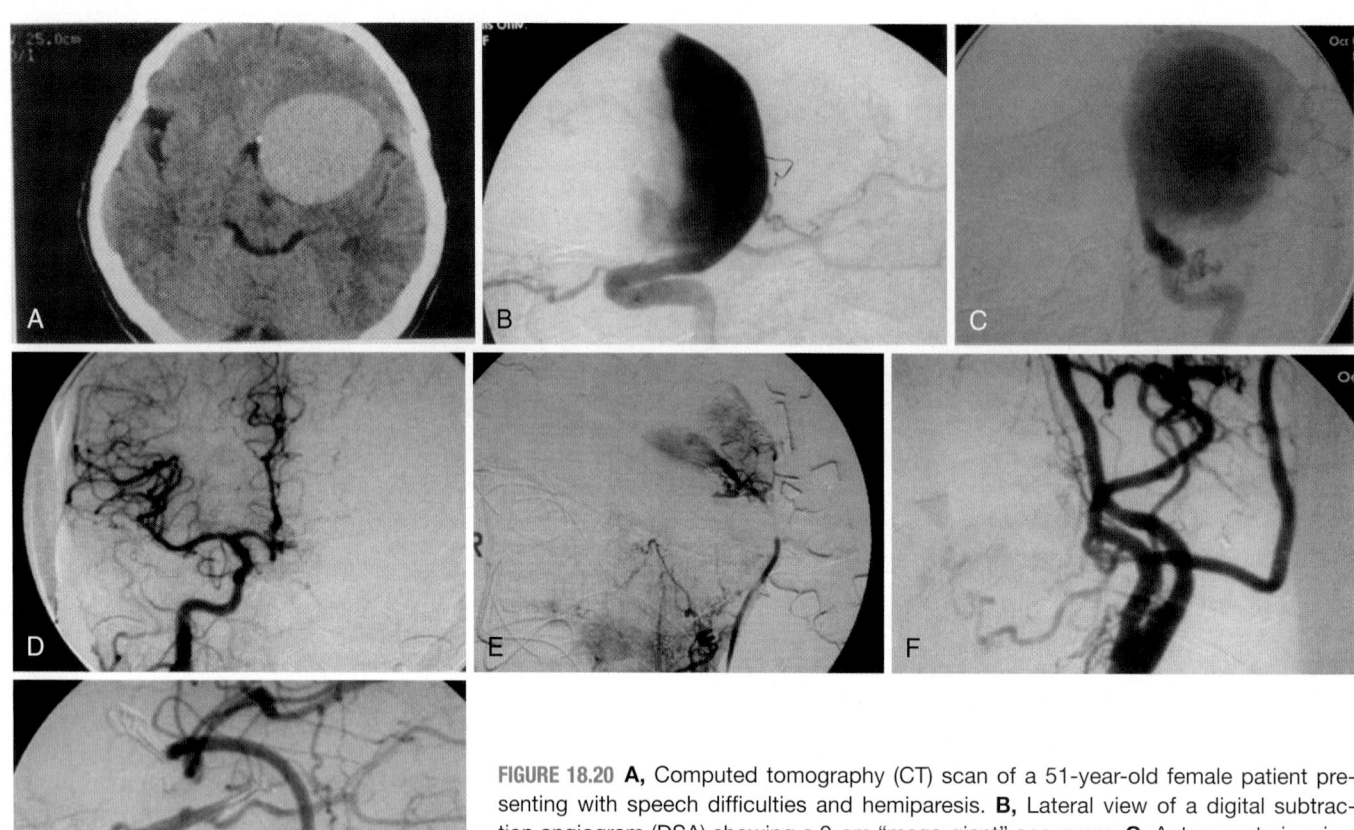

FIGURE 18.20 **A,** Computed tomography (CT) scan of a 51-year-old female patient presenting with speech difficulties and hemiparesis. **B,** Lateral view of a digital subtraction angiogram (DSA) showing a 9-cm "mega-giant" aneurysm. **C,** Anteroposterior view showing aneurysm. **D,** Contralateral DSA shows no flow through anterior communicating artery. **E,** Intraoperative angiogram showing radial artery to middle cerebral artery (MCA) bypass. **F,** Postoperative angiogram. **G,** Postoperative DSA showing bypass and clip reconstruction of the aneurysm and the preservation of the posterior communicating artery.

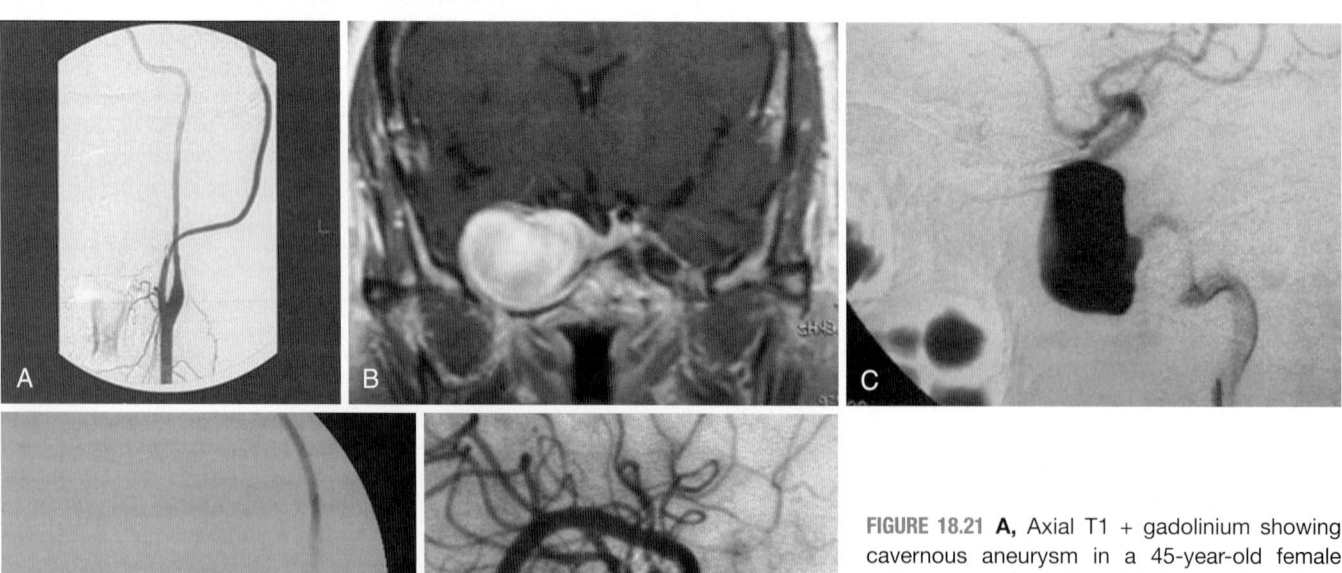

FIGURE 18.21 **A,** Axial T1 + gadolinium showing cavernous aneurysm in a 45-year-old female patient presenting with ophthalmoplegia. **B,** Sagittal T1 + gadolinium. **C,** Digital subtraction angiogram (DCA) of giant aneurysm. **D,** Intraoperative angiogram of internal carotid artery–radial artery graft. **E,** Postoperative angiogram showing radial graft and occlusion of the cavernous aneurysm.

FIGURE 18.22 **A,** End-to-side radial artery graft to the external carotid artery (ECA). **B,** End-to-end radial artery graft to the ECA.

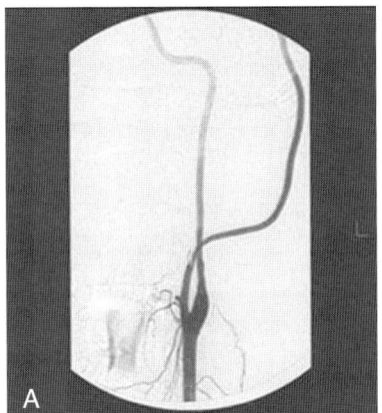
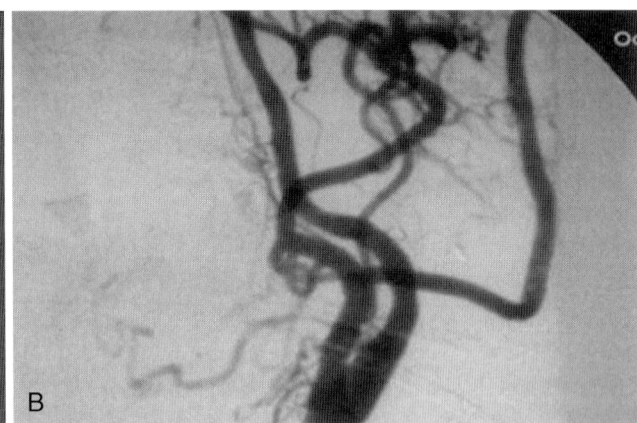

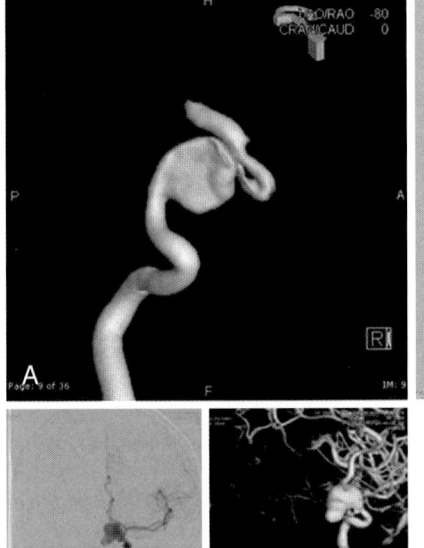
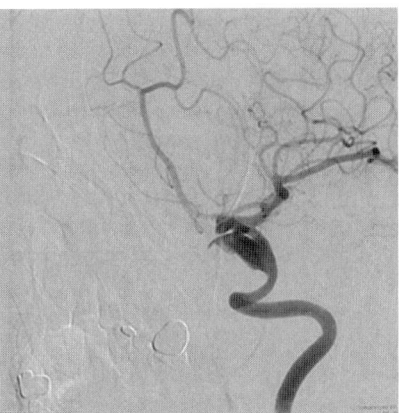
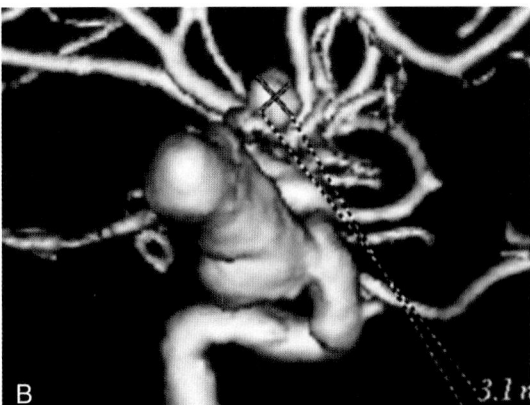

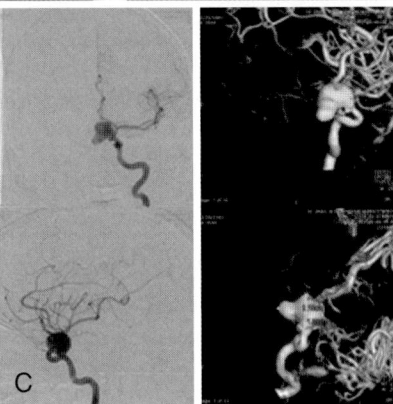

FIGURE 18.23 Intraoperative angiogram of an external carotid artery (ECA) to middle cerebral artery (MCA)–radial artery bypass showing flow into a single MCA division.

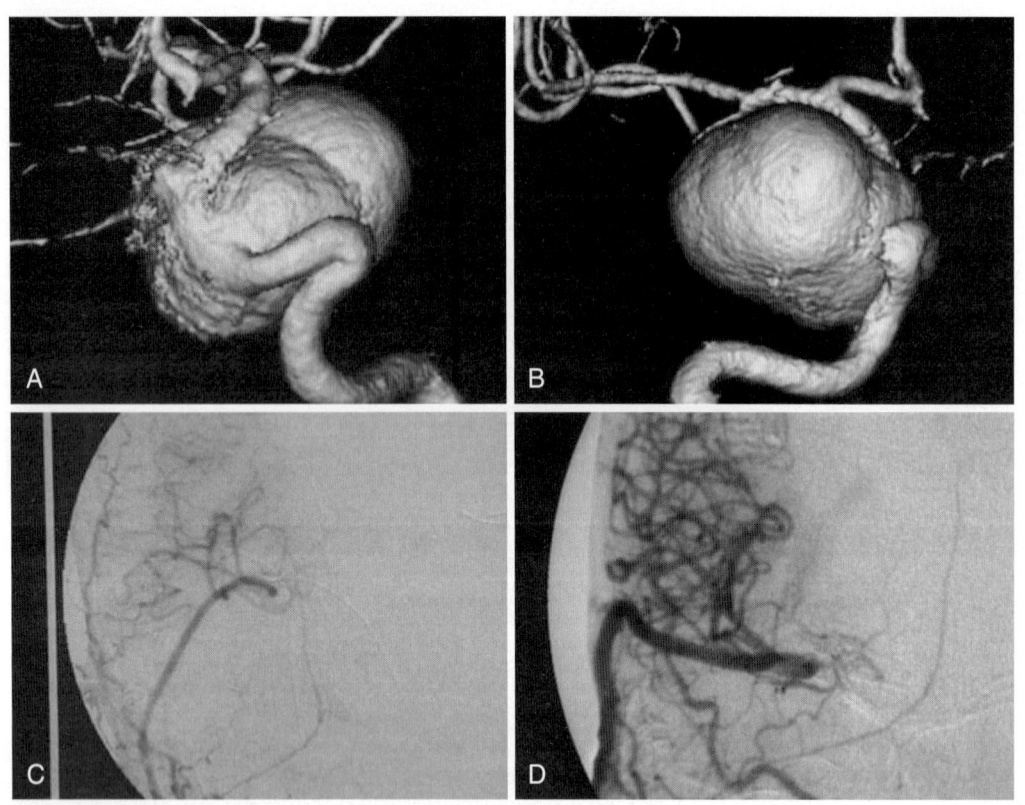

FIGURE 18.24 **A,** Lateral three-dimensional (3D) digital subtraction angiogram (DSA) reconstruction of a giant internal carotid artery (ICA) transitional segment aneurysm. **B,** Anteroposterior 3D DSA reconstruction of a giant ICA transitional segment aneurysm. **C,** Intraoperative angiogram showing the bypass and deliberate occlusion of the ICA. **D,** DSA at 1-year follow-up shows increased diameter of the graft.

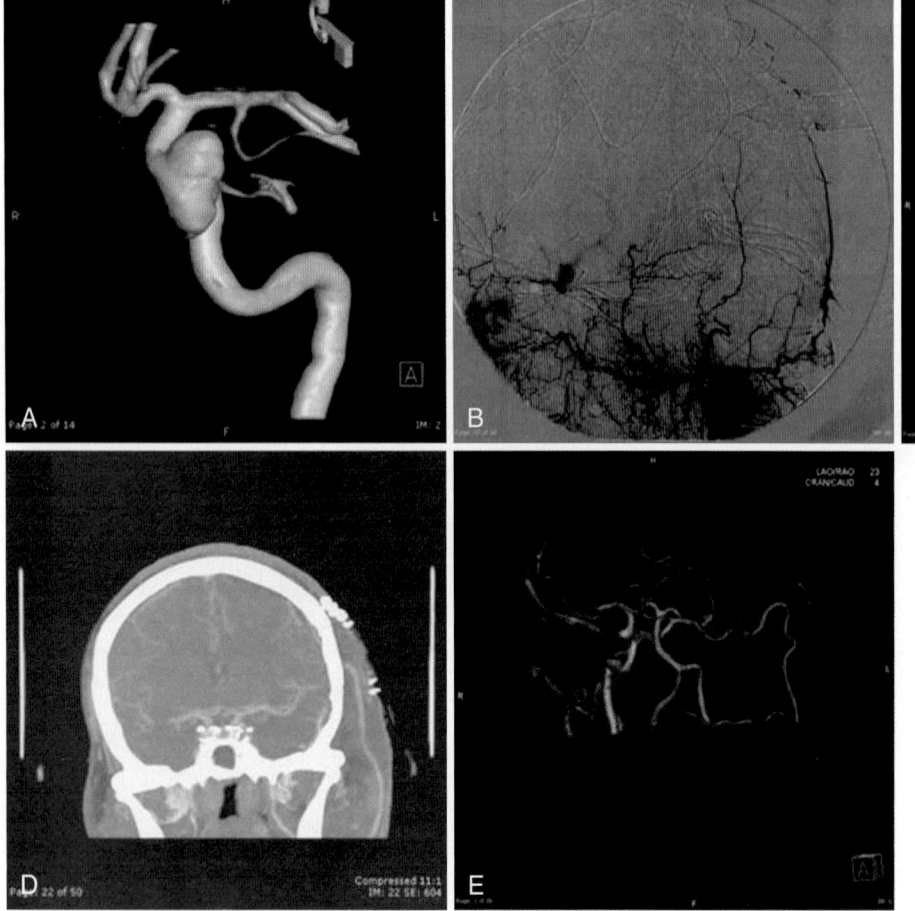

FIGURE 18.25 **A,** Three-dimensional (3D) digital subtraction angiogram (DSA) reconstruction of complex internal carotid artery (ICA) partial thrombosed aneurysm. **B,** Intraoperative failure to establish flow with no change in somatosensory evoked potentials (SSEPs) and motor evoked potentials. **C,** Immediate postoperative reconstruction showing graft is patent but small diameter. **D,** Immediate postoperative computed tomography angiogram (CTA) showing small diameter graft. **E,** A 3-month follow-up CTA reconstruction showing the expanded graft diameter.

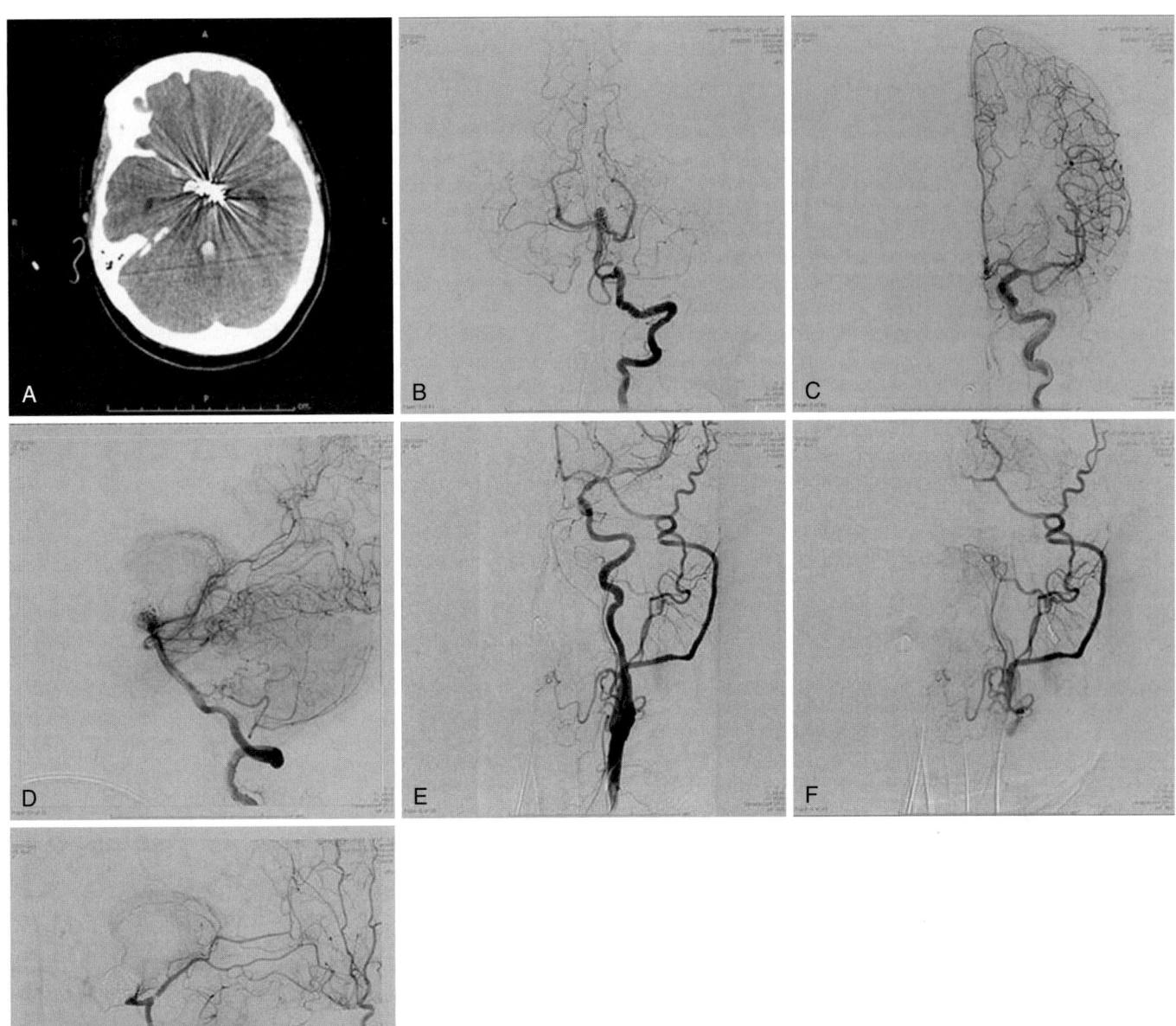

FIGURE 18.26 A, Patient with a third subarachnoid hemorrhage following previous endovascular coiling. **B,** Anteroposterior (AP) digital subtraction angiogram (DSA) showing the coil embedded in the left P1 segment. **C,** AP DSA of left ICA showing new posterior communicating artery (PCA). **D,** Vertebral artery DSA showing PCA flow completely dependent on the P1 segment. **E,** External carotid artery (ECA) to PCA bypass postoperative DSA showing graft. **F,** Postoperative DSA showing flow to the PCA. **G,** Postoperative lateral view of a PCA to radial artery graft showing PCA flow completely coming through the graft.

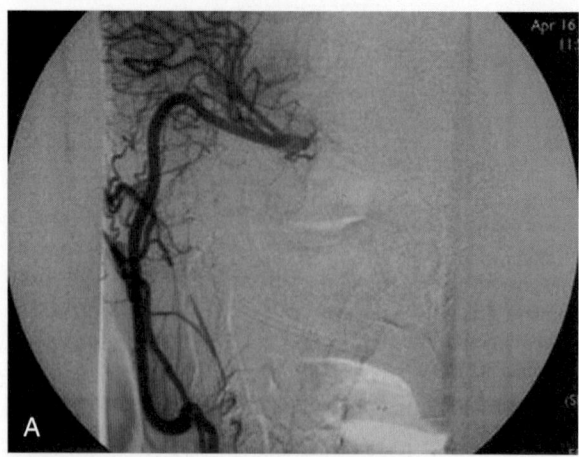
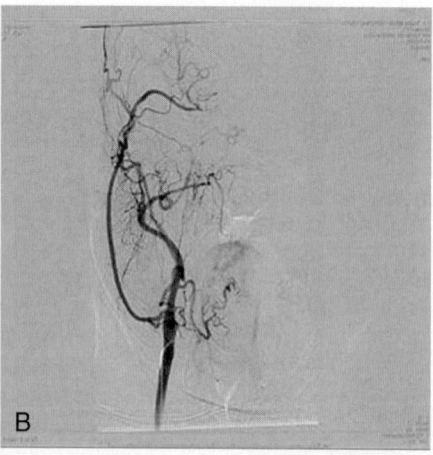

FIGURE 18.27 **A,** Digital subtraction angiogram (DSA) of the right common carotid artery (CCA) showing a radial artery bypass for a giant aneurysm. The graft redundancy in the cervical area may be risky from a kinking standpoint, as shown in this case. **B,** DSA of the right CCA showing a radial artery bypass for a giant aneurysm with ideal length of the graft that would minimize the risk of kinking.

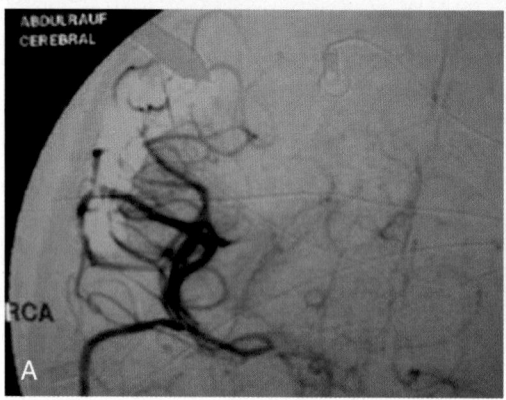
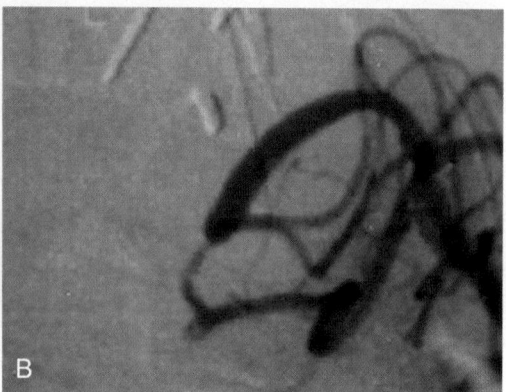

FIGURE 18.28 **A,** Digital subtraction angiogram (DSA) of a radial artery bypass to the middle cerebral artery (MCA) showing ideal size match. **B,** DSA of a radial artery bypass to the MCA showing significant size mismatch.

CONCLUSIONS

Giant intracranial aneurysms carry a high risk of morbidity and mortality. They are among the highest risk disease processes within the field of neurosurgery. These aneurysms are potentially curable. Advances in microsurgical clipping, endovascular treatments, and EC-IC bypass have all contributed to decreasing the morbidity rate of these treatment modalities.

Evolving techniques in EC-IC bypass have documented a measurable decrease in the morbidity of treating these complex lesions. Minimally invasive evolving EC-IC bypass techniques will add an additional armamentarium that will potentially lead to lower morbidity while still achieving a cure.

SELECTED KEY REFERENCES

Abdulrauf SI. Extracranial-to-intracranial bypass using radial artery grafting for complex skull base tumors: technical note. *Skull Base.* 2005;15(3):207-213.

Abdulrauf SI, Sweeney JM, Mohan YS, Palejwala SK. Short segment internal maxillary artery to middle cerebral artery bypass: a novel technique for extracranial-to-intracranial bypass. *Neurosurgery.* 2011;68(3):804-809.

Awad AI, Barrow DL, eds. *Giant Intracranial Aneurysms.* Park Ridge, IL: American Association of Neurological Surgeons; 1995.

International Study of Unruptured Intracranial Aneurysms Investigators. Unruptured intracranial aneurysms—risk of rupture and risks of surgical intervention. *N Engl J Med.* 1998;339(24):1725-1733.

Linskey ME, Sekhar LN, Hirsch Jr WL, et al. Aneurysms of the intracavernous carotid artery: natural history and indications for treatment. *Neurosurgery.* 1990;26(6):933-937:discussion 937-938.

Please go to expertconsult.com to view the complete list of references.

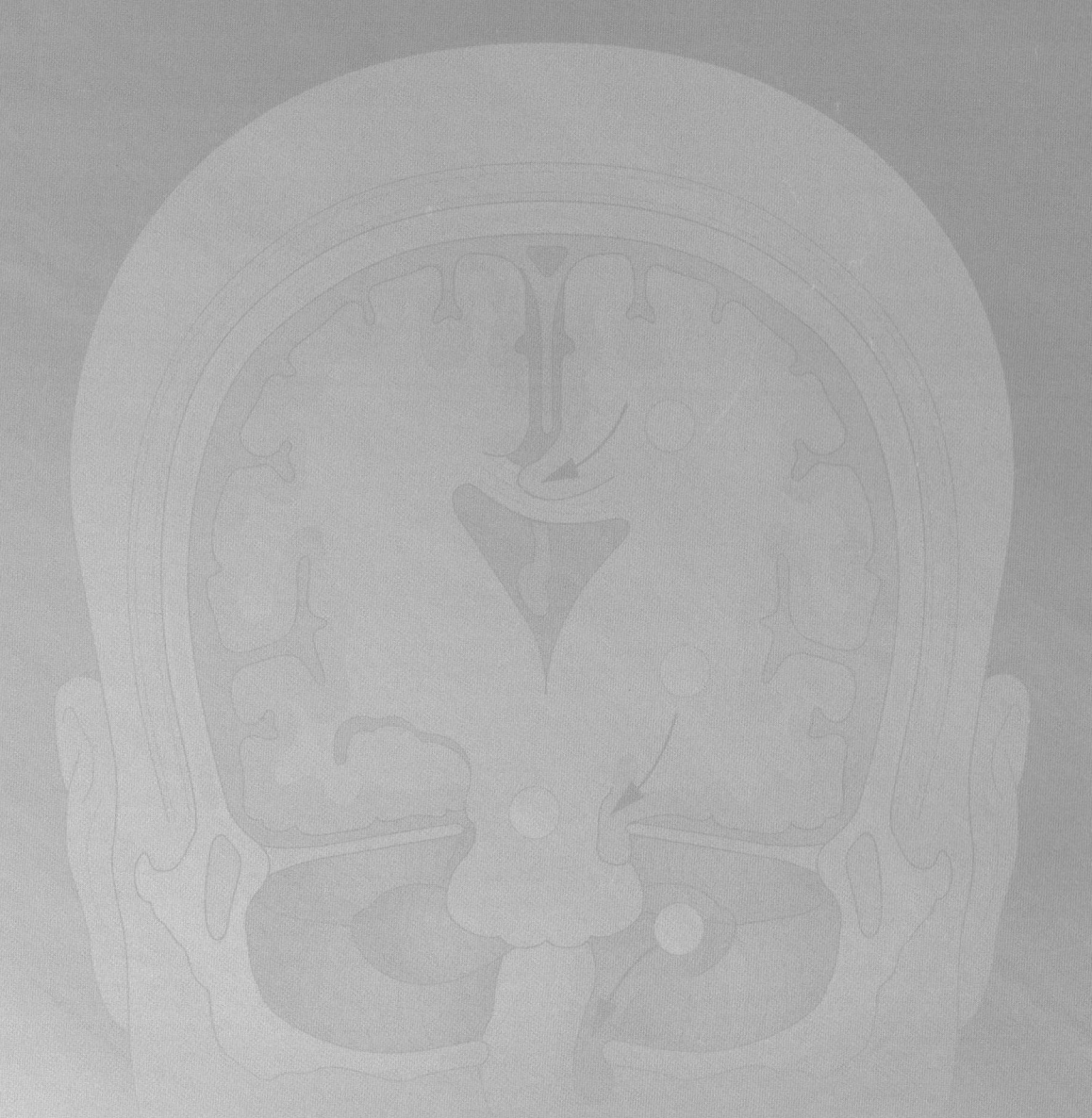

PART 4
Trauma

Intracranial Hypertension

Ryan Morton, Richard G. Ellenbogen

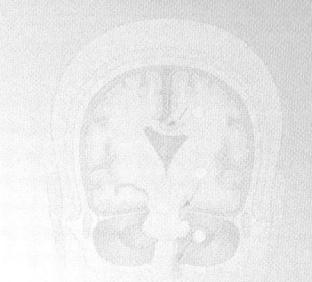

CLINICAL PEARLS

- States of impaired consciousness are expressed as numerical scores on the Glasgow Coma Scale (GCS), which is used worldwide and has prognostic and management implications.

- The key clinical signs that help in clinical assessment and determination of prognosis are the presence or absence of certain brainstem reflexes such as pupillary response, corneal reflex, oculocephalic and oculovestibular reflexes, and gag reflex.

- Computed tomography (CT) scan of the head remains a key imaging modality in the rapid assessment of a patient with impaired consciousness. Mass lesions that are directly responsible for intracranial hypertension should be surgically removed.

- Intracranial pressure (ICP) is generally monitored when the GCS score is less than 8 with an abnormal CT scan, although there is no class I evidence that mandates use of ICP monitors worldwide. A fiberoptic monitor is a good tool for measuring and managing increased ICP in an

unconscious patient. Fiberoptic ICP monitors have a low incidence of complication and infection in experienced hands. However, they do not give a therapeutic option for lowering ICP like a ventriculostomy catheter with external ventricular drainage does. Head of bed elevation, maintaining euthermia, sedation, analgesia, and mild hyperventilation can also have temporary therapeutic effects on elevated ICP.

- After conservative therapies have been exhausted, hypertonic saline may be as efficacious as mannitol and is associated with a lower overall incidence of comorbidity.

- Decompressive hemicraniectomy is a reasonable option in uncontrolled intracranial hypertension, especially if there is a mass lesion.

- Future studies are being undertaken to further elucidate the role of microdialysis and brain tissue oxygenation monitoring in the setting of intracranial hypertension.

The cranium is a rigid structure. The major intracranial contents are the brain (to include the neuroglial elements and interstitial fluid), blood (arterial and venous), and cerebrospinal fluid (Table 19.1). When a new intracranial mass is introduced, a compensatory change in volume must occur through a reciprocal decrease in venous blood or cerebrospinal fluid (CSF) to keep the total intracranial volume constant. This is the Monro-Kellie doctrine (Fig. 19.1), which has been confirmed by many experimental and clinical observations. Only in children, with open fontanelles and whose sutures have not yet fused, can the cranium itself expand to physically accommodate extra volume.

Compliance (dV/dP) is the change in volume observed for a given change in pressure. This represents the accommodative potential of the intracranial space. In clinical practice, however, what is actually measured is *elastance* (dP/dV). Elastance is the inverse of compliance and is the change in pressure observed for a given change in volume. It represents the resistance to outward expansion of an intracranial mass. The elastance curve (not compliance) is what is plotted in Figure 19.2. Although technically a misnomer, the term *compliance* is actually entrenched in the literature to describe the aforementioned phenomenon instead of using the proper term *elastance*. Because of this we, too, will conform to the traditional nomenclature for the rest of this chapter.

In accordance with the Monro-Kellie doctrine, several innate homeostatic mechanisms exist in an attempt to maintain intracranial pressure within the physiological range—generally considered less than 20 mm Hg in the acute inpatient setting. First, the venous system collapses easily and squeezes venous blood out through the jugular veins or through the emissary and scalp veins. Likewise, CSF can be displaced from the ventricular system through the foramina of Luschka and Magendie into the spinal subarachnoid space.[1] When these compensatory mechanisms have been exhausted, small changes in volume produce precipitous increases in pressure. This effect can be demonstrated experimentally by inserting a Foley catheter into the epidural space of a rat and gradually inflating a balloon with increasing volumes. The curve produced by plotting intracranial pressure against volume is the so-called compliance curve in Figure 19.2. The innate homeostatic pressure-buffering mechanism offered by displacement of CSF and venous blood keeps this curve flat until a "critical volume" is reached. After this critical volume, small volumetric changes result in precipitous increases in pressure, and intracranial hypertension naturally ensues. Brain parenchyma and arterial blood do not participate, to any significant extent, in the innate intracranial pressure-buffering mechanisms.

TABLE 19.1 Intracranial Contents and Their Respective Volumes		
Component	**Volume**	**Percentage of Total Volume**
Brain (70%) and interstitial fluid (10%)	1400 mL	80%
Blood	150 mL	10%
Cerebrospinal fluid	150 mL	10%
Total	1700 mL	100%

ACUTE INTRACRANIAL HYPERTENTION

Symptoms and Signs

The symptoms and "sine qua non" of acute increased intracranial pressure are altered levels of consciousness with progressive neurological decline and decreasing wakefulness, usually followed by obtundation. The obtundation is usually due to one of two causes: (1) compression of the suprameduallary reticular activating system or (2) bithalamic or bicortical damage. This is typically manifested by a Glasgow Coma Scale (GCS) score less than 8, irregular breathing patterns, posturing, and possibly pupillary inequality.

Cerebral Blood Flow

Normal cerebral blood flow averages 55 to 60 mL/100 g brain tissue per minute. In the gray matter the blood flow is 75 mL/100 g brain tissue per minute, whereas in the white matter it is around 45 mL/100 g brain tissue per minute. This flow is sufficient to meet the metabolic needs of the brain. The brain usually begins to show signs of ischemia at 20 mL/100 g/minute and permanent damage usually results when the blood flow drops below 10 mL/100 g/minute in most models. The most significant factor that determines cerebral blood flow at any given

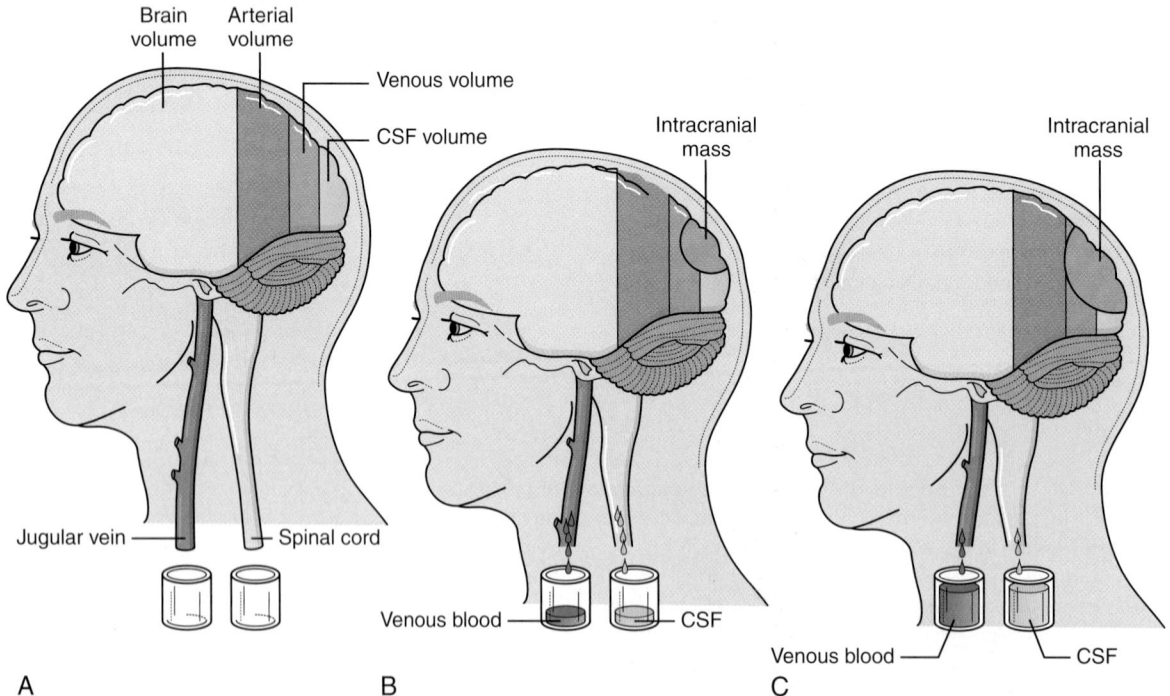

FIGURE 19.1 Monro-Kellie doctrine holds that total intracranial volume remains constant. **A,** Physiological state with normal intracranial pressure (ICP). The major intracranial components are brain (80%), arterial and venous blood (10%), and cerebrospinal fluid (CSF) (10%). The cranium is a rigid container, the intracranial volume is constant, and the normal intracranial contents are shown with ICP within physiological range (10 to 15 mm Hg). **B,** Intracranial mass with compensation (normal ICP). This patient has an intracranial mass (space-occupying lesion) of moderate size. Because intracranial volume is constant, the increasing volume caused by the mass is compensated by a decrease in the intracranial content. Venous volume decreases through egress of venous blood from the intracranial cavity into the jugular veins. CSF volume decreases because of egress of CSF through the foramen magnum into the spinal canal. The brain itself is nearly incompressible, and thus no significant change in its volume occurs; neither is there change in arterial volume. Intracranial volume is constant and there is no net rise in ICP (pressure buffering). **C,** Intracranial mass with decompensation and elevated ICP. The intracranial mass is much larger, beyond the pressure-buffering capacity of venous blood and CSF; there is a net rise in ICP.

time is the cerebral perfusion pressure (CPP). The CPP is the effective blood pressure gradient across the brain. CPP is the difference between the incoming mean arterial pressure (MAP) and the opposing intracranial pressure (ICP): CPP = MAP – ICP. The mean arterial pressure can be calculated in two ways: (1) the diastolic pressure plus one third of the pulse pressure (DP + ⅓PP) or (2) two thirds of the diastolic pressure plus one third of the systolic pressure (⅔DP + ⅓SP). The ICP has to be measured directly, which can be done with various devices and will be discussed later in this chapter. With increased ICP there is an obvious tendency for the cerebral perfusion pressure to decrease.

Three major factors regulate cerebral blood flow under physiological conditions: CPP, concentration of arterial CO_2, and arterial Po_2. The ability to maintain constant blood flow to the brain over a wide range of CPPs (50-150 mm Hg) is called *cerebral autoregulation*. When the CPP is low, the cerebral arterioles dilate to allow adequate flow at the decreased pressure. Conversely, an increase in CPP causes the arterioles to constrict and maintain the flow within physiological range (Fig. 19.3). Decreases in CO_2 tension in the blood (i.e., hyperventilation) causes diffuse vasoconstriction.[2] Vasoconstriction decreases both cerebral blood flow and cerebral blood volume in the brain. The risks and benefits of inducing hyperventilation are discussed under the treatment section at the end of this chapter. Lastly, severe hypoxia causes cerebrovascular dilatation. This effect only becomes apparent when the oxygen tension in the blood drops to 50 mm Hg and becomes maximal around 20 mm Hg.

Under certain pathological conditions cerebral blood flow cannot always be autoregulated.[3] When the CPP exceeds 150 mm Hg, such as in hypertensive crisis, the autoregulatory system fails. In this case there would be a passive increase in blood flow proportionate to the increase in systemic pressure,

causing an exudation of fluid from the vascular system with resultant vasogenic edema.[4] Additionally, certain toxins such as carbon dioxide can cause diffuse cerebrovascular dilatation and inhibit proper autoregulation.[5] Lastly, during the first 4 to 5 days of head trauma, many patients can experience a disruption in cerebral autoregulation; this is often observed in the pediatric population and may result in hyperemia.[6]

Disruption of cerebral blood flow autoregulation in the setting of trauma could potentially lead to severe alterations in CPP when a patient's brain is acutely injured.[7] When disrupted, cerebral blood flow would be directly proportional to CPP under a much larger range than normal. This is likely one of the contributing reasons why even one episode of hypotension in the patient with acute head injury may lead to significantly worse outcomes.[8] Thus, many institutions have adopted protocols to maintain a minimal CPP in the acute setting—usually around 50 to 60 mm Hg—and perhaps a maximum threshold of CPP if the intracranial hypertension can be linked directly to hyperemia.

Various ways to evaluate a patient's autoregulatory abilities have been developed to include computed tomography (CT) perfusion scans and transcranial Doppler (TCD) studies. Interpreting these studies, however, is a matter of current debate. Although still somewhat in its infancy, knowing the status of a patient's autoregulatory capacity in traumatic brain injury is beginning to shape individualized care in the intensive care unit (ICU).

Monitoring Intracranial Pressure

The most significant factor determining morbidity and mortality risk in patients with acute cranial neurosurgical disorders continues to be increased ICP. Continuous ICP monitoring is

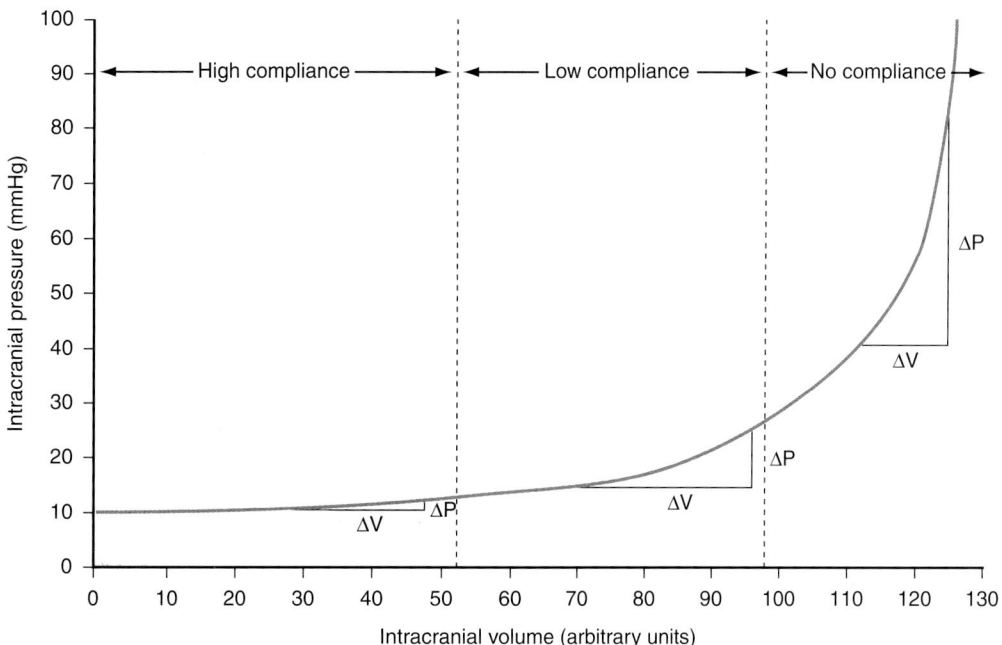

FIGURE 19.2 Pressure-volume curve. If an intracranial balloon is expanded slowly in a laboratory animal and the intracranial pressure (ICP) and the balloon's volume are plotted, an exponential curve results. In the initial phase there is virtually no increase in ICP because of the compensatory decrease in cerebrospinal fluid (CSF) and venous volumes; the compliance is high (elastance low). With further expansion of the balloon, the ICP begins to rise; compliance is low (elastance high). In the terminal stages, when the compensatory mechanisms are exhausted, there is a steep rise in pressure (no compliance, highest elastance).

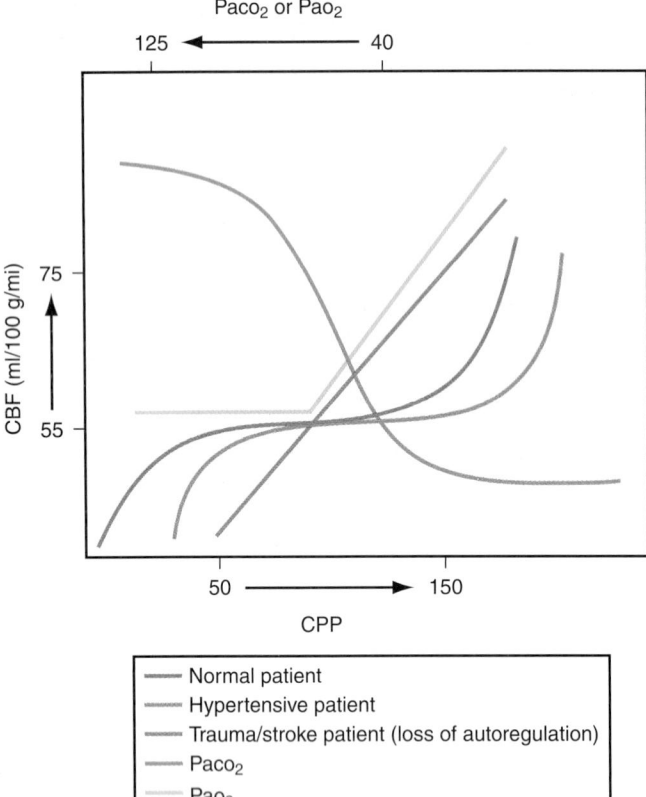

FIGURE 19.3 Three major factors regulate cerebral blood flow (CBF) under physiological conditions: cerebral perfusion pressure (CPP), concentration of arterial CO_2, and arterial Po_2. This graph can be read in regard to CPP to CBF, or Pao_2 and $Paco_2$ to CBF. The ability to maintain constant blood flow to the brain over a wide range of CPPs (50-150 mm Hg) is called *cerebral autoregulation*. Patients with hypertension have their autoregulatory curve shifted to the right. Trauma or stroke patients can have a loss of the normal sigmoidal shape to the autoregulatory curve. Additionally, decreases in CO_2 tension in the blood causes diffuse vasoconstriction. This decreases both cerebral blood flow and thus cerebral blood volume in the brain. Severe hypoxia causes cerebrovascular dilatation. This only becomes apparent when the oxygen tension in the blood drops to 50 mm Hg, and becomes maximal around 20 mm Hg.

very useful for assessing intracranial dynamics in patients with suspected intracranial hypertension. There are no clinical indicators that can be used in the early stage of rising ICP to forestall a further rise. Classical clinical indicators described in the literature (cranial nerve abnormalities, posturing, etc.) occur in the end stage and they are not sensitive enough to show subtle changes in pressure. The two most common indications for ICP monitoring are closed head injury and spontaneous subarachnoid hemorrhage.

Indications for Monitoring Intracranial Pressure

The advent of continuous ICP monitoring has improved outcomes in traumatic brain injury[9,10] by reducing the effects of secondary injury occurring after the initial brain insult. In the modern intensive care unit ICP monitoring in the adult patient with severe head injury is a recommended practice guideline

based on available clinical evidence. Indications of ICP monitoring following head injury include a GCS score between 3 and 8 and an abnormal CT scan. Unfortunately, no class I evidence is available regarding the use of ICP monitors in pediatric head injury patients. Nevertheless, strong evidence supports the association between elevated ICP and poor outcomes,[11] and aggressive treatment of elevated ICP is associated with the best clinical outcomes. ICP monitoring provides valuable data that can inform medical management.

Techniques of Monitoring Intracranial Pressure

Intracranial pressure is best measured directly and continuously from the cranial cavity. Although lumbar puncture can indirectly indicate ICP, it is neither safe nor accurate in the setting of intracranial hypertension as it might precipitate tonsillar/transtentorial herniation by increasing the pressure gradient between the cranial and spinal subarachnoid compartments.

There are two commonly used pressure-monitoring systems in contemporary neurosurgical practice. An intraventricular catheter connected to a manometer and a drainage system is the standard against which all other systems are compared.[12-14] The ventricular catheter ideally should be tunneled under the skin and brought out through a separate stab wound, well away from the ventricular entry site, to minimize the risk of infection. Infection is the most significant complication of intraventricular pressure monitoring. With the use of an electronic transducer, the waveform can also be monitored (Fig. 19.4). The major advantage of the method is that the ventricular catheter is used not only to measure the pressure, but also as a therapeutic modality allowing intermittent or continuous drainage of CSF when the pressure exceeds physiological limits.

A second method is the use of the fiberoptic transducer-tipped catheter system. The transducer-tipped catheter can be placed within the brain parenchyma or in the subdural space, depending on the surgeon's choice and the clinical situation.[15-17] The pressure monitor gives both digital readout and a waveform. The advantages of this system are that the zero point does not have to be reset with changes in head position because the pressure-sensing transducer is within the cranial cavity, and it is not susceptible to blockage by debris because it is not a fluid-coupled system. Also, insertion of a fiberoptic cable into the brain parenchyma is not affected by ventricular size or shift, which can make insertion of a ventricular catheter in the setting of intracranial hypertension quite trying. Lastly, the infection rates with fiberoptic probes are significantly lower than with ventriculostomy catheters, reported as less than 1% in one of the the largest reported series.[18] The disadvantages of this system, however, are (1) higher cost and (2) baseline drift, which means there is evidence that with prolonged fiberoptic monitoring the indicated pressures may become less accurate in an unpredictable fashion.[19,20]

Intracranial Pressure Waveforms

The waveform of normal ICP typically shows three components: the percussion wave (P1), the tidal wave (P2), and finally the dicrotic notch (P3) (Fig. 19.5A). Under physiological

FIGURE 19.4 Intracranial pressure (ICP) monitoring system using ventricular catheter, pressure transducer, manometer, and drainage bag.

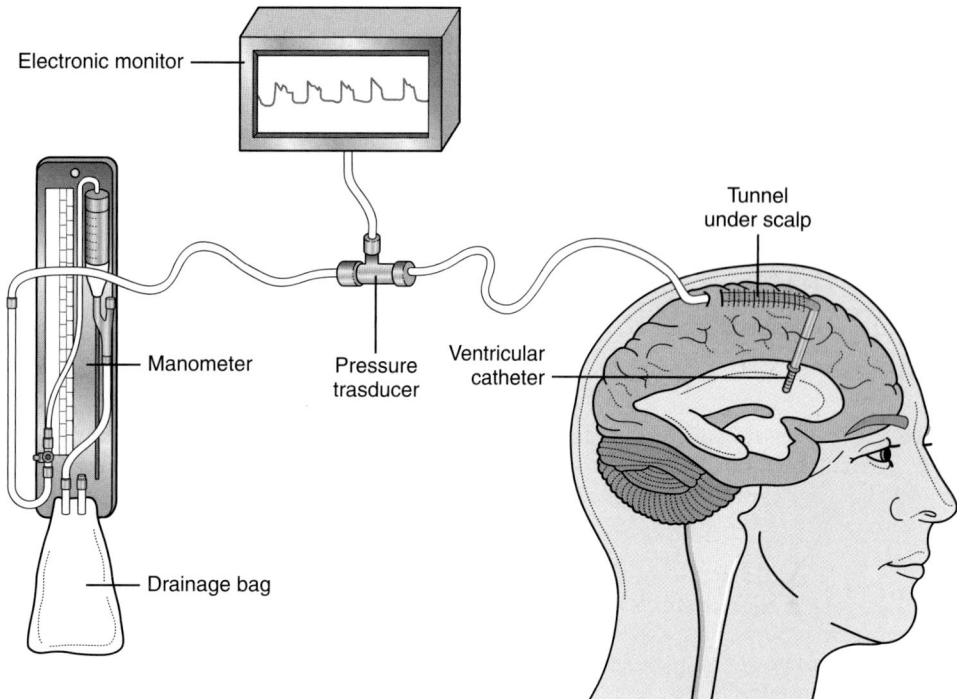

FIGURE 19.5 **A,** Intracranial pressure (ICP) waveform under physiological conditions. Three peaks are generally recognizable. The first, and usually tallest, is the percussion wave, followed by the tidal wave, the dicrotic notch, and the dicrotic wave. Note that the tidal and dicrotic waves have progressively lesser amplitudes than the percussion wave. **B,** Abnormal intracranial waveform with high ICP. The amplitude of the tidal wave exceeds the amplitude of the percussion wave.

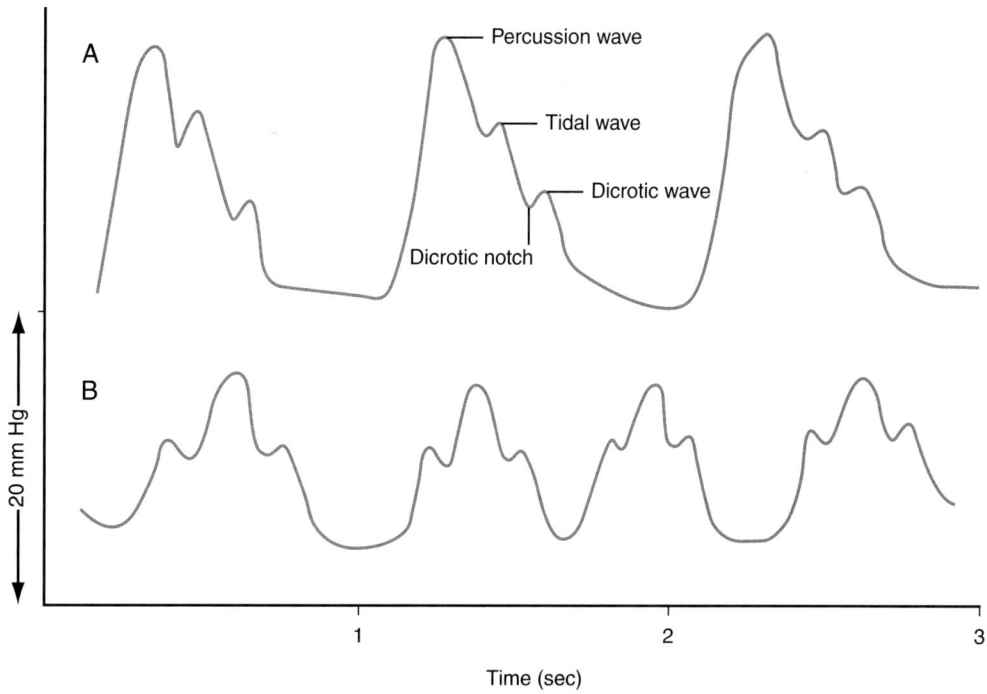

conditions P1 is the tallest and is thought to represent the pressure at peak cardiac systole transmitted throughout the choroid plexus. P2 follows P1 and its resultant smaller peak is thought to represent the filling of the intracranial arteries with systolic blood and results in a rebound increase in ICP from this increase in intracranial volume. Last is the dicrotic wave.

When the ICP rises and compliance decreases, one will observe P2 becoming taller than the P1. This is because a similar volume in intracranial arterial blood is now resulting in a

higher change in ICP (Fig. 19.5B). Such alterations in the morphology can give the treating physician further clues regarding not only the compliance but also the autoregulatory capacity of the brain.

When the ICP waveforms are registered over a period of time certain trends may become apparent[14] (Fig. 19.6). Plateau waves, or type A waves, are characterized by an abrupt elevation in ICP for 5 to 20 minutes followed by a rapid fall in the pressure to resting levels. The amplitude may reach as high as 50 to 100 mm Hg. Plateau waves may be clinically

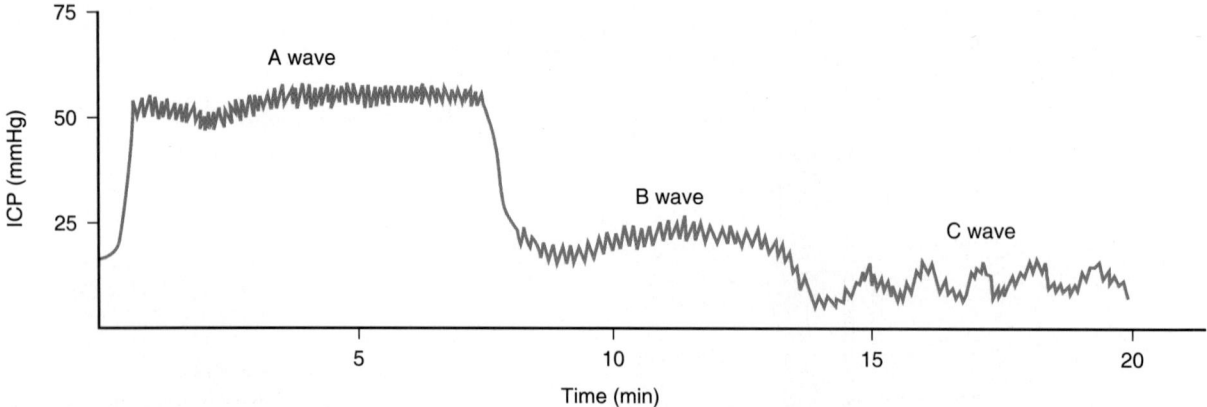

FIGURE 19.6 Examples of abnormal intracranial pressure (ICP) waveforms with trend recording. Plateau waves, or A waves, are character-ized by abrupt elevation in ICP for 5 to 20 minutes followed by a rapid fall in pressure to the resting level. Plateau waves herald neurological worsening. B and C waves have questionable clinical significance.

marked by a decreasing level of consciousness, restlessness, increased tone in the extremities, and tonic-clonic movements. Plateau waves may represent transient surges in ICP second-ary to increased cerebral blood volume likely related to CO_2 retention.

B waves, which have a frequency of 0.5 to 2 waves per minute, are related to rhythmic variations in breathing. The C waves are rhythmic variations related to the Traub-Meyer-Hering waves of systemic blood pressure and have smaller amplitude, with a frequency of about 6 per minute. B and C waves have questionable clinical significance, although there is some evidence that B waves may precede A wave formation.

Types of Brain Herniation

The brain is supported by dural folds that prevent undue movements of the brain within the cranial cavity (Fig. 19.7). There are two major dural folds—the *falx cerebri* and the *ten-torium cerebelli*. The falx cerebri is a sickle-shaped dural fold in the midline that separates the two cerebral hemispheres. The tentorium cerebelli is a tent-shaped dural fold that sepa-rates the occipital lobes from the posterior fossa structures. The tentorial incisura, or hiatus, is the dural opening that sur-rounds the rostral brainstem. Care must be taken during ICP management so as to not to exacerbate the pressure differ-ences between compartments and to inadvertently encourage herniation.

Cingulate Herniation

A focal mass lesion in the supratentorial compartment exerts progressive pressure locally on the ipsilateral hemisphere. The increase in ICP may not be uniform; it is greatest close to the mass, thus creating a pressure gradient. A supratentorial mass lesion may displace the cingulate gyrus, which is next to the free edge of the falx cerebri, and cause it to herniate under the falx to the opposite side. There is usually displacement of the ventricular system as well (Fig. 19.8). The anterior cere-bral artery may be compromised by the tight, sharp edge of the falx cerebri. There are no clinical signs and symptoms spe-cific to a cingulate herniation; however, an anterior cerebral

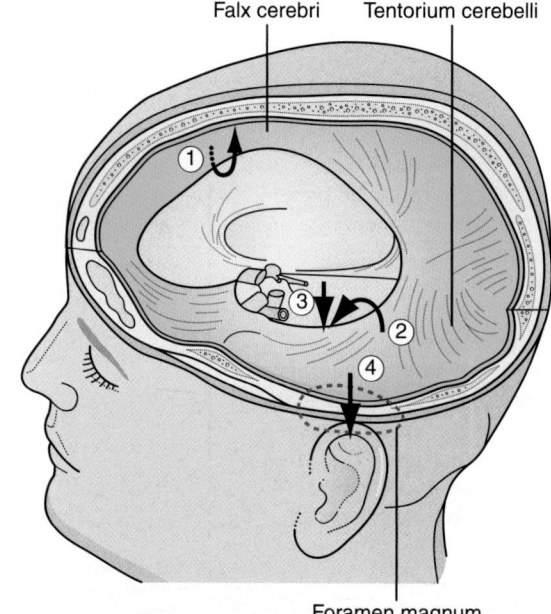

1 – Cingulate herniation

2 – Tentorial (uncal) herniation

3 – Central herniation

4 – Tonsillar herniation

FIGURE 19.7 Dural folds within the cranial cavity and associated her-niation sites.

artery stroke may result in a focal contralateral lower extrem-ity plegia.

Uncal Herniation

Uncal herniation is the most dramatic and most common herniation syndrome observed clinically. Uncal herniation is often seen with lesions of the middle cranial fossa such as acute epidural hematoma, subdural hematoma, temporal lobe contusions, or temporal lobe neoplasms. An expans-ile mass of the middle fossa causes the uncus, the most

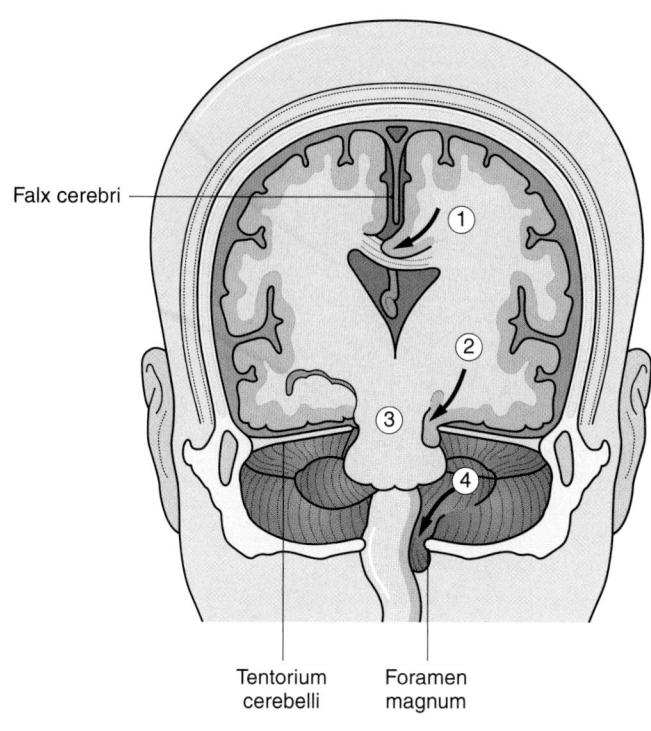

Falx cerebri

Tentorium   Foramen
cerebelli   magnum

1 – Cingulate herniation

2 – Tentorial (uncal) herniation

3 – Central herniation

4 – Tonsillar herniation

FIGURE 19.8 Types of brain herniation.

causing secondary infarction of the occipital lobe on one or both sides.

Central Transtentorial Herniation

In contrast to uncal herniation, which usually occurs from a mass lesion located near the tentorial hiatus, central transtentorial herniation occurs with mass lesions far removed from the tentorial hiatus, such as in frontal, parietal, or occipital areas. Bilateral mass lesions, such as subdural hematomas, can also cause central herniation. During central herniation, there is a downward displacement of the diencephalon and midbrain centrally through the tentorial incisura (see Fig. 19.8). The clinical syndrome in central herniation is not as easily recognizable as that of uncal herniation. The patients with central transtentorial herniation are obtunded, tend to have bilaterally small, reactive pupils, exhibit Cheyne-Stokes respiration, and may show loss of vertical gaze manifested as tonic downward gaze.

Tonsillar Herniation

Acute tonsillar herniation generally results from acute expansion of posterior fossa lesions. It may result from an ill-advised lumbar puncture in a patient with a mass lesion within the cranial cavity. The tonsils of the cerebellum herniate through the foramen magnum into the upper spinal canal, compressing the medulla (see Fig. 19.8). The manifestations of acute medullary compression are cardiorespiratory impairment, hypertension, high pulse pressure, Cheyne-Stokes respiration, neurogenic hyperventilation, and impaired consciousness. The patient may have a stiff neck or be in an opisthotonic position. Decorticate or decerebrate posturing may be present as well.

Upward Transtentorial Herniation

Acute upward cerebellar herniation occurs when the pressure in the infratentorial space exceeds the pressure in the supratentorial space. This can be iatrogenically caused from aggressive drainage of CSF from an external ventricular drain in the setting of a posterior fossa mass lesion. Upward transtentorial herniation does not have a clear-cut clinical syndrome, but results in obtundation, pupillary abnormalities, and posturing. Additionally, unilateral or bilateral superior cerebellar artery (SCA) infarctions could occur as the SCA becomes compressed against the bottom of the tentorium. As the SCA supplies the deep cerebellar nuclei, this would obviously portend a poor prognosis.

Treatment

With almost no exception, all patients with acute elevated ICP can be managed initially by the same conservative steps. First, the importance of elevating the head of the bed to 30 to 45 degrees cannot be overemphasized. This posture promotes venous drainage to enhance the innate compensatory mechanisms of the CNS. The neck should be kept straight and not allowed to kink over to any side. Second, normothermia should be achieved because an elevated brain temperature can increase metabolism, which can not only elevate ICPs but also promote ischemia. Lastly, sedation and analgesia are invaluable tools in the management of acute ICP. Propofol is the most commonly used sedating agent not only because of its

inferomedial structure of the temporal lobe, to herniate between the rostral brainstem and the tentorial edge into the posterior fossa (see Fig. 19.8). If the vector of pressure is more posterior, then the parahippocampal gyrus can herniate as well. In postmortem studies, a deep groove may be noticed at the lateral margin of the uncus as a manifestation of the herniation. In some instances, the displacement of the brainstem by the uncus may cause compression of the contralateral cerebral peduncle against the opposite tentorial edge, producing a paradoxical indentation called *Kernohan's notch*.

With uncal herniation, the clinical syndrome consists of the following triad: progressively impaired consciousness, dilated ipsilateral pupil, and contralateral hemiplegia. The impaired consciousness results from compression of the reticular activating system in the rostral brainstem. The dilated pupil is the result of compression of the ipsilateral third nerve, which carries the parasympathetic pupilloconstrictor fibers at the periphery. By injuring the pupilloconstrictor fibers there is unopposed dilation of the pupil. Contralateral hemiplegia results from direct compression of the ipsilateral cerebral peduncle, which carries corticospinal fibers innervating the contralateral side. When Kernohan's notch is present, the hemiplegia will be on the ipsilateral side from compression of the contralateral peduncle. In some patients with uncal herniation, the posterior cerebral artery may be compromised from compression in the ambient cistern,

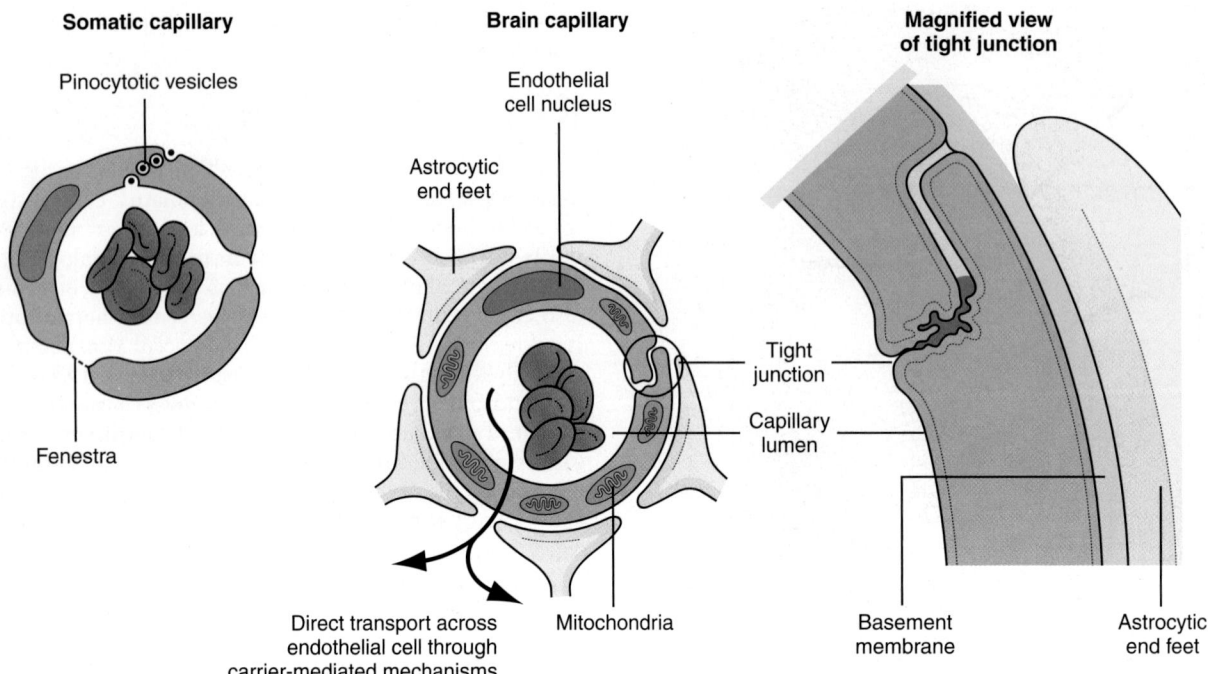

Somatic capillary

Pinocytotic vesicles

Fenestra

Brain capillary

Endothelial
cell nucleus

Astrocytic
end feet

Direct transport across
endothelial cell through
carrier-mediated mechanisms

Mitochondria

**Magnified view
of tight junction**

Tight
junction

Capillary
lumen

Basement
membrane

Astrocytic
end feet

FIGURE 19.9 Differences between somatic and brain capillaries. In the somatic capillary, fenestrations between endothelial cells allow free flow of plasma components into the tissues. In addition, there is bulky flow of plasma components across endothelial cells via pinocytotic vesicles. In the brain capillary, the endothelial cells are attached to each other by tight junctions. There are no intervening fenestrae. Certain selected plasma components cross the endothelial membrane if they are lipid soluble; others, such as amino acids and sugars, are transported across the endothelial cells through a carrier-mediated mechanism. The large number of mitochondria in the brain endothelial cells generate energy for active transport.

"quick on-quick off" effect but also because of its ability to lower cerebral metabolism. After these initial steps have been taken, further ICP therapy requires enhanced knowledge of physiology as described in the following section.

The Blood-Brain Barrier

In order to understand the optimal way to treat intracranial hypertension, knowledge of the components of the blood-brain barrier is paramount. Not all substances that are carried in the blood can reach the neural tissue—a barrier composed of astrocytic foot process wrapping around a capillary endothelium composed of tight junctions[4] (Fig. 19.9). These endothelial tight junctions are the barrier to the passive movement of many substances in order to protect the sensitive neural tissue from toxic materials. There are two mechanisms by which materials may be transported naturally across the endothelial cells. First, lipid-soluble substances can usually penetrate all capillary endothelial cell membranes in a passive manner.[21] Second, amino acids and sugars are transported across the capillary endothelium by specific carrier-mediated mechanisms.[22] The measurement of how easily something diffuses across the blood-brain barrier is called the *reflection coefficient*. A coefficient of 0 is complete passive diffusion; 1 indicates no passive diffusion.[23,24]

Decompressive Hemicraniotomy

The most direct way to normalize raised ICP to the physiological range is to eliminate its cause. If the increased pressure is the result of a mass effect, such as a blood clot, prompt evacuation

of the offending lesion will restore ICP to normal more effectively than any other measure. The goal of a decompressive craniotomy is to perform a robust craniotomy that extends from the frontal lobe to the occipital lobe and includes the temporal lobe so that uncal herniation can be alleviated. After the bone is removed, the dura is often flapped open and the mass lesion evacuated. The brain can then be covered with a dural substitute to permit expansion. The bone flap can be placed back or kept off depending on intraoperative findings and personal surgical preferences. If the bone flap is kept off, the dural substitute is then covered with the scalp and a subgaleal drain is usually placed (Fig. 19.10). The bone flap may be either placed in a subcutaneous abdominal pocket, or more commonly at the present, stored in a −80°C freezer in a sterile fashion. A cranioplasty or cranial bone replacement should be performed at a later date if the patient survives the acute injury.

The indications for performing this operation are most often (1) control of increased ICP that is recalcitrant to medical therapy and (2) progressively worsening neurological examination with evidence of massive hemispheric brain swelling, contusion, or intracranial blood or mass lesion. Despite the widespread use of decompressive hemicraniotomy worldwide,[25-27] no level I data are available that show its superiority over aggressive medical treatment. In fact, a recently published randomized control trial evaluated patients with *diffuse* brain swelling (i.e., *no mass effect*) with refractory ICP.[28] This study found that even though decompressive bifrontal craniectomy reduced ICP more than medical management, it did not translate in better outcomes and indeed appeared to actually worsen them in some circumstances. There are some critiques of this

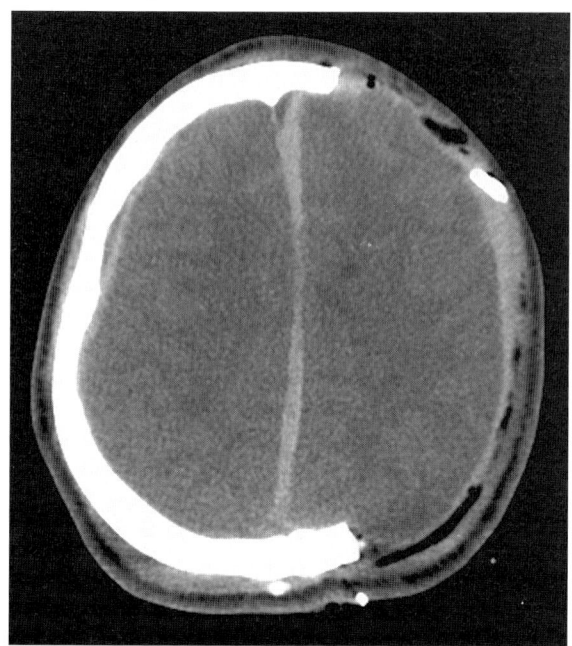

FIGURE 19.10 Decompressive hemicraniectomy. Note the extensive bony decompression from the frontal bone to the occiput and the remaining interhemispheric subdural hematoma. The brain parenchyma on the left can be seen protruding beyond the previous boney-boundary indicating how severe the intracranial hypertension was. The hyperdensity seen above the left frontal lobe is part of the Jackson-Pratt subgaleal drain.

trial, including the definition of "refractory ICP," but nonetheless, it reinforces that the use of decompressive hemicraniectomy in diffuse brain swelling is an area of controversy. In addition, surgery is obviously fraught with comorbidity, and thus, nonsurgical options is reasonable as a first-line therapy when there is no obvious mass lesion, contusion or intracranial blood. However, we still employ decompressive craniectomy in trauma patients who have failed medical therapy and have contusions and intracranial blood with elevated ICP. Indicated as a first-line therapy when there is no obvious mass lesion. These options are discussed in the following sections.

Hyperventilation

Hyperventilation causes a fall in ICP by reducing intracranial blood flow and blood volume through vasoconstriction. Hyperventilation is generally initiated for hyperacute management of increased ICP. Sustained hyperventilation in acute intracranial hypertension is a mode of therapy that has not been found to be beneficial and is actually contraindicated. In the setting of increased ICP, prolonged hyperventilation will promote ischemia through decreased cerebral blood flow supply. If undertaken, hyperventilation should be moderate, reducing the carbon dioxide between 30 and 35 mm Hg.

Mannitol

Mannitol is the osmotic agent universally used to treat cerebral edema.[29-31] Other osmotic agents such as urea and glycerol are no longer used in contemporary neurosurgical practice because of side effects such as hemolysis. Mannitol

decreases ICPs in two distinct mechanisms. First, when mannitol is initially delivered it creates an osmotic gradient from all body tissues into the intravascular space. This transiently increases intravascular volume and improves the rheology of cerebral blood. This transient increase in cerebral blood flow is thought to trigger the intrinsic autoregulatory mechanism of the intracranial vasculature (if it is intact) to vasoconstrict and decrease intracranial arterial blood volume. This decrease in blood volume translates into decreases in ICP, and is the mechanism that gives mannitol almost immediate efficacy in the setting of intracranial hypertension.

Once mannitol begins to circulate through the intracranial vasculature, the cumulative effects of the osmotic gradient can draw fluid from the brain interstitial space into the vascular space. Key to this process is intact tight junctions. If the tight junctions are not intact, mannitol will slowly permeate the neural tissue, preventing the formation of an osmotic gradient.

Mannitol is generally given in boluses rather than as a continuous drip. The usual dose is 0.25 g to 1 g/kg at 4- to 6-hour intervals. Mannitol boluses are generally effective for 48 to 72 hours. Its routine/scheduled use beyond 72 hour can become ineffective because mannitol's reflection coefficient is 0.9, meaning that even with an intact blood-brain barrier it will slowly leak into the interstitial fluid/brain parenchyma. Serum osmolality, kidney function, and electrolytes should be carefully monitored during mannitol therapy.

Hypertonic Saline

High-dose aliquots of hypertonic saline have recently emerged as a potential first-line therapy for elevated ICP. Thirty-milliliter boluses of 23.4% sodium chloride given through a central line over 15 minutes have been shown to be at least as efficacious as mannitol in multiple small prospective studies in lowering intracranial pressure.[32,33] The mechanism by which 23.4% saline works is similar to that of mannitol, in that it creates an osmotic gradient to draw fluid from the interstitial space of the brain across the blood-brain barrier and into the intravascular space.

The reflection coefficient of hypertonic saline is 1.0, meaning that if a patient's blood-brain barrier is intact it will not accumulate in the interstitial space/brain parenchyma. This makes hypertonic saline appealing for longer than 48- to 72-hour use. Also, unlike mannitol, hypertonic saline does not have a systemic diuretic effect and thus MAPs/CPPs are more stable during its use. Therefore, hypertonic saline is a potentially better alternative to treating a polytrauma patient's elevated ICP who may have concomitant systemic hypovolemia and hypotension. A single dose of 23.4% hypertonic saline does not seem to alter systemic sodium concentrations. However, with repeated use, bolus therapy of 23.4% saline can causes electrolyte abnormalities and thus potentially cardiac conduction abnormalities and should be monitored.

Loop Diuretics

Furosemide has been classically used as an adjunct to mannitol because it seems to have a synergistic effect. Furosemide alone, however, cannot be relied upon to reduce ICP. Because its primary action is on the kidney, it is not dependent on the intact blood-brain barrier for its effect. It is also possibly thought to reduce CSF production.

Ventricular Drainage

Drainage of CSF from the ventricular system is a simple, effective, and quick method of decreasing ICP. Ventriculostomy is supremely effective in two unique patient populations: acute subarachnoid hemorrhage and spontaneous/traumatic intraventricular hemorrhage. Providing an alternative pathway for CSF drainage in these patient populations can dramatically reduce ICP and result in a remarkably quick improvement in clinical examination.

Ventriculostomy drainage can also be used in the setting of trauma, not only to monitor pressure continuously but also to drain the ventricular to provide therapeutic effects.

Barbiturate Coma and Paralytics

Induction of coma with short-acting barbiturates or inducing chemical paralysis is a last and controversial resort in the medical management of raised ICP when all other conservative measures fail. Barbiturates decrease the ICP by several mechanisms. They inhibit the release of fatty acid perioxidation products by scavenging free radicals from the mitochondrial respiratory chain. They also inhibit cerebral metabolism and reduce cerebral blood flow. The most commonly used drug is thiopental, which is given in a loading dose of 3 to 10 mg/kg over a 10-minute period and a maintenance dose of 1 to 2 mg/kg/hour. The serum level should be maintained at 3 to 4 mg/L. Patients in barbiturate coma require intensive monitoring of hemodynamic function, ICP, and blood gases. Vasopressors may have to be administered if hypotension results. Barbiturate therapy is usually withdrawn when the ICP normalizes and there is a good intracranial compliance; no clinical indicators are available to dictate termination of therapy.

SUBACUTE TO CHRONIC INTRACRANIAL HYPERTENSION

Causes of subacute to chronic intracranial hypertension are mass lesions (tumors, chronic subdural hematomas, etc.) that not only increase intracranial volume but also can induce interstitial edema. The most common symptom of subacute/chronic elevations is headache that is generalized in nature and is worse in the morning—presumably because of the increase in CO_2 tension (from a physiological decrease in respiratory rate) and increased venous pressure from laying supine. The pain-sensitive structures within the cranial cavity are the dura and the blood vessels. Focal mass lesions that distort the dura and stretch the vessels tend to cause headache more frequently than diffuse generalized increases in ICP without focal mass effect, such as a pseudotumor cerebri or hydrocephalus. The headache, if present, may be associated with vomiting. The vomiting associated with increased ICP is usually not associated with nausea. Papilledema is another cardinal sign of increased ICP.[34]

A sixth cranial nerve/lateral rectus palsy is another classic sign of a subacute to chronic presentation of increased ICP. The long intracranial course of the abducens nerve makes it susceptible to injury from elevated ICP. The abducens nerve exits the ventral brainstem at the pontomedullary junction and travels in the subarachnoid space before ascending up the clivus to the petrous apex. Once at the petrous apex it travels beneath the petroclinoid ligament of Gruber before piercing the dura at Dorello's canal and entering the cavernous sinus. It travels through the cavernous sinus to the superior orbital fissure before entering the orbit. Elevated ICP is postulated to compress the abducens nerve at the petroclinoid ligament.

Cerebral Edema

Cerebral edema is a prominent cause of subacute to chronic intracranial hypertension. It may be defined as a state of increased brain volume as a result of an increase in water content. There are three types of cerebral edema (Table 19.2).

Vasogenic edema is the most common form of brain edema encountered in clinical practice (Fig. 19.11). It results from increased permeability of capillaries of the blood-brain barrier. The tight junctions between the endothelial cells become incompetent, allowing plasma filtrate to escape into the intercellular space[35-37] (Fig. 19.12). The phenomenon of contrast enhancement in CT and magnetic resonance imaging (MRI) scans is, in part, because of the breakdown of the blood-brain

TABLE 19.2 Types and Characteristics of Cerebral Edema

Characteristic	Vasogenic Edema (Extracellular Edema)	Cytotoxic Edema (Intracellular Edema)	Interstitial Edema
Pathogenesis	Increased capillary permeability	Cellular swelling (neuronal, glial, and endothelial cells)	Increased brain water due to impairment of absorption of CSF
Location of edema	Mainly white matter	Gray and white matter	Transependymal flow of CSF and interstitial edema in the periventricular white matter in hydrocephalus
Composition of edema fluid	Plasma filtrate containing plasma proteins	Increased intracellular water and sodium due to failure of membrane transport	CSF
Extracellular fluid	Increased	Decreased	Increased
Pathologic lesion causing edema	Primary or metastatic tumor, abscess, late stages of infarction, trauma	Early stages of infarction, water intoxication	Obstructive or communicating hydrocephalus
Effect of steroids	Effective	Not effective	Not effective
Effect of mannitol	Effective	Effective	Questionable

CSF, cerebrospinal fluid.

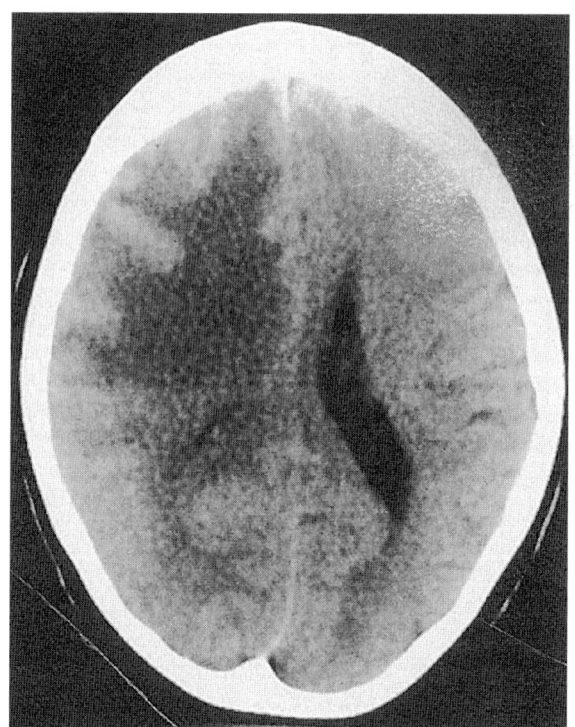

FIGURE 19.11 Computed tomography (CT) scan of a patient with vasogenic edema caused by metastatic tumor. Note that the edema involves predominantly the white matter.

barrier and resultant vasogenic edema. Vasogenic edema is most commonly seen with tumor, abscess, and chronic reaction to a blood clot. The edema is more marked in white matter than in gray matter.

Cytotoxic edema most commonly results from hypoxia of the neural tissue. The hypoxia affects the adenosine triphosphate (ATP)-dependent sodium/potassium pump mechanism in the cell membrane, promoting an accumulation of intracellular sodium and the subsequent flow of water into the cell to maintain osmotic equilibrium. Thus, the edema is primarily *intracellular* and affects virtually all cells, including the endothelial cells, astrocytes, and neurons. Because of the swelling of these cells, the interstitial space is considerably narrowed (see Fig. 19.12). The two most common causes of cytotoxic edema are tissue hypoxia and water intoxication. The CT scan commonly shows only subtle initial changes or no changes at all, indicative of cytotoxic edema in the early phases of ischemic stroke.

Interstitial edema results from transudation of CSF in obstructive hydrocephalus. It is best observed on CT or MRI scan as periventricular low-density areas because of the retrograde transependymal flow of CSF into the interstitial space of the white matter (Fig. 19.13). Interstitial edema is most commonly observed in the frontal region. This finding generally indicates active hydrocephalus requiring surgical therapy.

Treatment

Craniotomy

As previously mentioned, the most direct way to normalize raised ICP to the physiological range is to eliminate its cause.

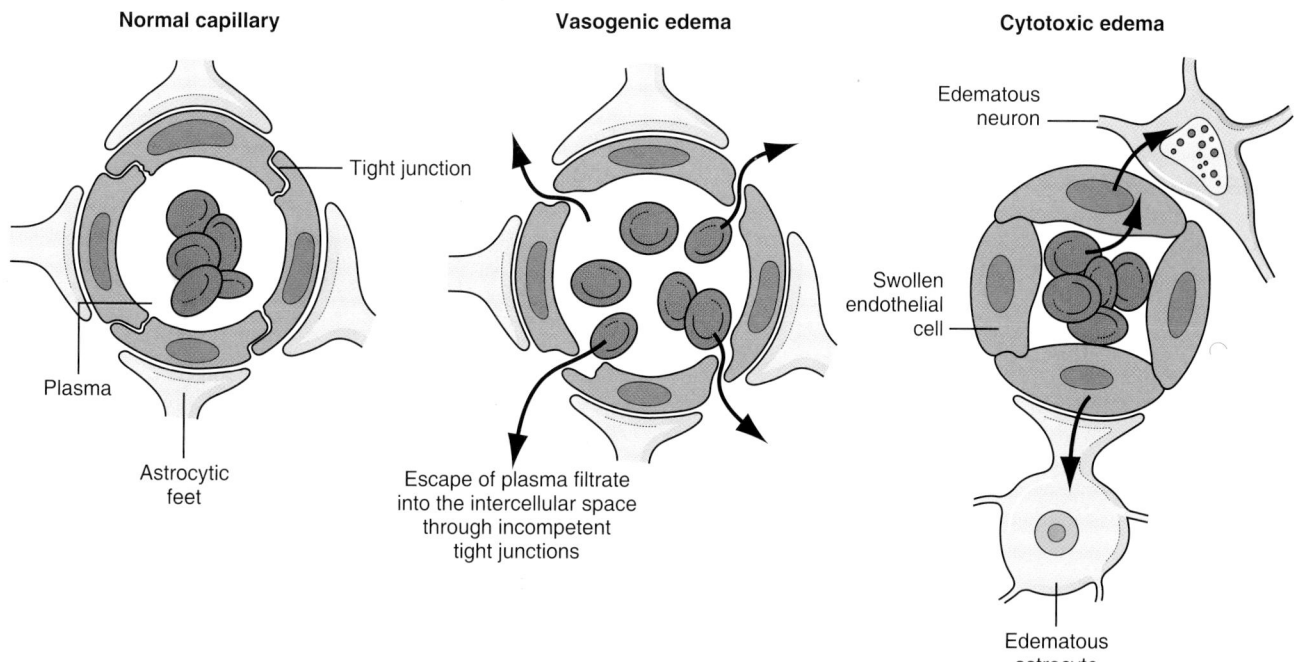

FIGURE 19.12 Normal appearance of a cerebral capillary contrasted with the changes that occur in vasogenic or cytotoxic edema. Under normal conditions, the intercellular tight junctions are intact. In vasogenic edema, the tight junctions are not competent, allowing leakage of plasma into the interstitial space. In cytotoxic edema, there is a primary failure of adenosine triphosphate (ATP)-dependent sodium pump mechanism resulting in intracellular accumulation of sodium and secondarily water.

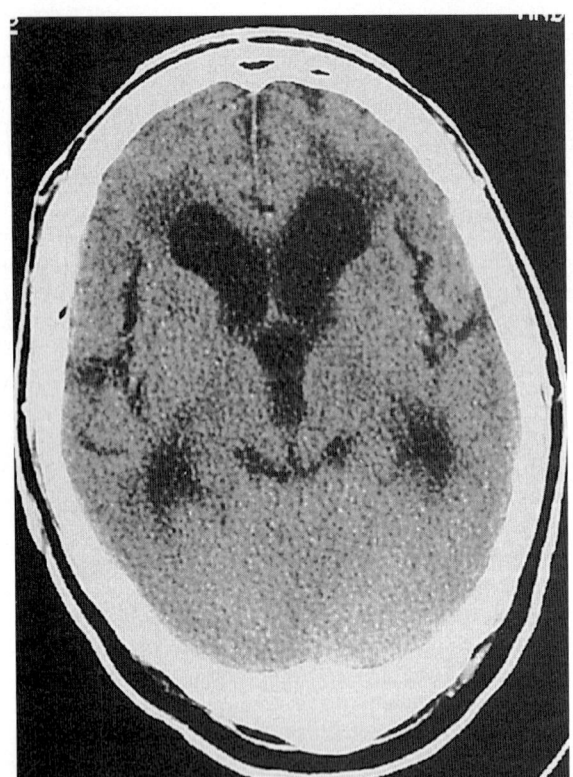

FIGURE 19.13 Computed tomography (CT) scan of a patient with active hydrocephalus showing periventricular low density representing transependymal flow of cerebrovascular fluid (CSF) (interstitial edema).

If the increased pressure is the result of a mass effect, such as a tumor or chronic subdural hematoma, prompt evacuation of the offending lesion will restore ICP to normal more effectively than any other measure. Ventriculostomy may also be used to stabilize ICP.

Steroids

Dexamethasone is used for treating chronic increases in ICP related to vasogenic edema caused by primary or metastatic neoplasms. It is ineffective in the management of cytotoxic edema related to head trauma or cerebral infarction. Steroids are thought to stabilize the cell membrane and restore the normal permeability of endothelial cells. This stability is brought about by inhibition of lysosomal activity, suppression of polyunsaturated fatty acid production that causes edema, and decrease of free radical production. The usual loading dose is 10 mg, given intravenously, followed by 4 mg every 6 hours. When the appropriate therapeutic goal has been achieved, the dose should be slowly tapered over a period of 3 to 4 days. Patients can make a remarkable neurological improvement on steroids if vasogenic cerebral edema is the main cause of the intracranial hypertension. Side effects include a relative leukocytosis, elevated systemic glucose, mildly increased blood pressures, stomach ulcers, immunosuppression, increased appetite, acute psychiatric disease such as mania or irritability, and osteoporosis with long-term use. If steroids are used for a protracted

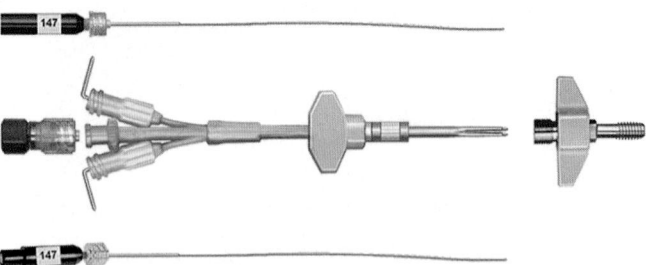

FIGURE 19.14 Licox probe insertion. *(Used with permission from Integra: www.integralife.com.)*

period, a long taper should be used rather than abrupt discontinuation to avoid complications with potential adrenal suppression.

NOVEL ADJUNCTIVE THERAPIES

In the setting of acute head trauma, much focus has now turned to prevention of secondary injury. This approach includes not only ICP control but also monitoring and attempted manipulation at cerebral oxygenation.

Brain Tissue Oxygenation Monitoring

A polarographic cerebral oxygen monitor (Licox system) can be placed to the brain parenchyma itself to monitor brain tissue oxygenation levels (Fig. 19.14). Several retrospective studies correlated poor outcome with low cerebral oxygenation (jugular saturation) and low values for partial pressure of oxygen in brain tissue ($Pbto_2$ (<10 mm Hg for >2 hours).[38-41,42] This finding opens up the possibility that therapeutric interventions to manipulate the $Pbto_2$ value could potentially alter the traditionally poor outcome in traumatic brain injury, notably the 36% mortality rate.[43,44] Indeed, several retrospective studies have suggested that active treatment of low $Pbto_2$ (defined as <20 mm Hg) does improve outcomes as measured on the Glasgow Outcomes Scale.[45,46] However, a few other papers suggest it does not and simply adds to the cost of care and stay in ICU.[47] The precise role of $Pbto_2$ measurement in management of ICP is evolving, and utility remains to be determined. However, its popularity in centers that manage a large population of head-injured patients has certainly expanded over the past decade.

There is no established or uniformly accepted algorithm to treat low $Pbto_2$. Strategies include increasing the CPP to 70 mm Hg to allow for increased cerebral blood flow (assuming ICP remains stable), transfusion to keep a hematocrit level above 30, optimization of cardiac output, and increasing the Fio_2 by intervals of 20% on the ventilator.

Microdialysis

Brain microdialysis is being used in some centers as a research tool to investigate brain metabolism in patients with increased ICP, stroke, vasospasm, and other brain insults.[48-52] The technique of cerebral microdialysis entails the implantation of specially designed catheters in the cerebral cortex to collect small-molecular-weight substances to help measure and identify neurotransmitters, peptides, and other substances. This research tool has clinical applications that are yet to be defined. The goal of this technique may be to identify the neurochemical milieu around the penumbra of trauma or stroke in order to devise better ways of protecting the undamaged cerebral cortex. Detailed discussion of this technique and its future uses is beyond the scope of this chapter.

Chemotherapy

Blood-brain barrier tight junctions can be transiently opened artificially by the intra-arterial injection of a bolus of an osmotic agent, such as mannitol, that dehydrates the endothelial cells or high-frequency ultrasound.[53] During this brief interval, which lasts for a few hours, certain chemotherapeutic or other agents can be administered that would not otherwise be able to cross the blood-brain barrier to reach the glia.

ACKNOWLEDGMENT

Setti Rengachary, MD, the late editor of this textbook, was an original author of this chapter. Many of the basic concepts and descriptions are his or adopted from his words, and he deserves credit for being the guiding force in the creation of this chapter, which has been significantly updated.

SELECTED KEY REFERENCES

Chesnut RM, Marshall LF, Klauber MR, et al. The role of secondary brain injury determining outcome from severe head injury. *J Trauma*. 1993;34:216-222.

Cooper JD, Rosenfeld JV, Murray L, et al. Decompressive craniectomy in diffuse traumatic brain injury. *N Engl J Med*. 2011;364(16):1493-1502.

Kerwin A, Schinco MA, Tepas 3rd JJ, et al. The use of 23.4% hypertonic saline for the management of elevated intracranial pressure in patients with severe traumatic brain injury: a pilot study. *J Trauma*. 2009;67:277-282.

Lundberg N. Continuous recording and control of ventricular fluid pressure in neurosurgical practice. *Acta Psychiatr Neurol Scand Suppl*. 1960;149:1.

Polin RS, Shaffey ME, Bugaev CA, et al. Decompressive bifrontal craniectomy in the treatment of severe refractory posttraumatic cerebral edema. *Neurosurgery*. 1997;41:84-100.

Please go to expertconsult.com to view the complete list of references.

CHAPTER
20 Closed Head Injury

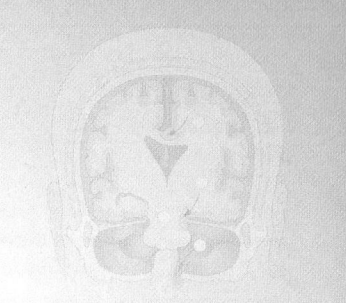

Clifford M. Houseman, Shawn A. Belverud, Raj K. Narayan

CLINICAL PEARLS

- The first priority in treating the head-injured patient is prompt physiological resuscitation—restoration of blood pressure, oxygenation, and ventilation and obtaining a postresuscitation Glasgow Coma Scale (GCS) score.

- Episodes of hypotension or hypoxia greatly increase risk of morbidity and death after severe head injury; therefore, even a single episode should be avoided if possible.

- Available literature indicates that glucocorticoids do not lower intracranial pressure (ICP) or improve outcome in patients with severe head injury; therefore, the routine use of steroids is not recommended.

- Mannitol is effective in reducing intracranial hypertension but is not to be used as a prophylactic treatment. Recent evidence suggests that hypertonic saline may be as effective, if not more effective, than mannitol for reduction of ICP and maintaining cerebral blood flow/cerebral perfusion pressure.

- Cerebral ischemia may be the single most important secondary event affecting outcome following severe traumatic brain injury (TBI); maintaining the cerebral perfusion pressure ideally greater than 60 mm Hg may help avoid both global and regional ischemia. However,

pushing the cerebral perfusion pressure much higher may have undesirable pulmonary effects. ICP monitoring as well as brain oxygen tension monitoring are associated with improved outcomes in TBI patients.

- Chronic prophylactic hyperventilation should be avoided during the first 5 days after a severe TBI, and particularly during the first 24 hours. Prophylactic hyperventilation therapy further reduces cerebral blood flow and thus has been associated with poorer outcomes. It should be used in an acutely deteriorating patient as a temporizing measure until a definitive treatment may be initiated.

- Antiepileptic medications show no reduction in late onset seizures (>7 days after injury). Dilantin or Keppra is recommended for the first 7 days after TBI to help reduce the risk of early onset seizure (<7 days after injury).

- The ventriculostomy remains the gold standard for ICP monitoring and is part of the treatment of elevated ICP. Brain oxygen tension monitors and temperature probes show promise with reductions in morbidity and mortality rates. More comprehensive monitors are under development.

Closed head injury or traumatic brain injury (TBI), with or without associated skull fractures and intracranial hemorrhages, remains a common clinical entity encountered by neurosurgeons. Although these injuries were most commonly seen in young patients, the aging of our population and the relatively common use of anticoagulation in the elderly have resulted in a second peak of TBI in the geriatric population. In either case, TBI remains a significant cause of death, disability, and cost to our society and affects up to 2% of the population each year.

Intracranial hemorrhages complicate 25% to 45% of severe TBI cases, 3% to 12% of moderate TBI cases, and 1 in 500 persons with mild TBI.[1] As the skull is impacted, the force is transmitted intracranially and brain movement can lead to disparate types of intracranial hemorrhages. These

hemorrhages include subdural hematomas, epidural hematomas, traumatic subarachnoid hemorrhages, intraparenchymal hemorrhages, intracerebral contusions, or combinations of the aforementioned.

Although controlled and strictly comparable data are hard to come by, it is evident that significant strides have been made in our understanding of this condition and in its management. The mortality rate from severe TBI has steadily decreased from 50% to 35% to 25% and even lower over the past three decades.[2] Difficult to prove conclusively, the likely causes of this decline include air bags, seat belts, and better-built cars; improved prehospital evaluation and resuscitation; rapid transport to trauma centers; prompt imaging and intervention; surgical decompression; and better neurological critical care. All of these efforts serve to limit secondary brain injury.

325

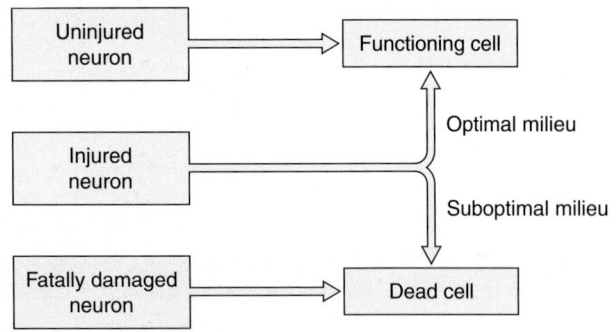

FIGURE 20.1 An optimal milieu must be maintained for healing in the injured brain.

The first evidence-based guidelines for the management of TBI patients were published in 1995,[3] with an updated version published in 2000.[4] Also in 2000, the Cochrane Library published a series of reviews that provided evidence-based standards and guidelines for the management of TBI patients.[5-7] The third edition of evidence-based guidelines for the management of severe traumatic brain injury were published in 2007, and are the most current and up-to-date recommendations on the management and treatment of TBI. Evidence-based guidelines for the management of penetrating head injury have also been published,[8] as well as guidelines for prehospital and pediatric TBI management.[9-11] The Brain Trauma Foundation (BTF) maintains and updates most of these guidelines every few years and they can be reviewed in full at the BTF website (www.braintrauma.org).

Better understanding of the pathophysiology of TBI has led to better neurological critical care aimed at the prevention of secondary injury to the at-risk brain (Fig. 20.1). Along with better monitoring techniques, this has translated into strict parameters for maintaining oxygen saturation and preventing hyponatremia and hyperglycemia. Unfortunately these parameters can often be difficult to control, as many trauma patients have other injuries as well that predispose them to hypoxia, hypotension, anemia, coagulopathies, intracranial mass lesions, and elevated intracranial pressure (ICP). The hallmark treatment of TBI is the monitoring and control of ICP.

While better critical care and physiological management have proved to be very valuable, pharmacological interventions have for the most part yet to be proved effective in the clinical setting. Despite promising results in animal models, clinical trials to date have not generated drug treatments with proven benefit.[12]

CLASSIFICATION

Although head injuries could be classified in several different ways, the most practical categorizations are based on mechanism, severity, and morphology (Fig. 20.2).

Mechanism

Head injury is classically categorized as "closed" or "penetrating" head injury. These categories are not necessarily mutually exclusive. For example, a depressed skull fracture with bone fragment extension into the brain may fit both descriptors.

For practical purposes closed head injury is typically used to describe head injury after falls, automobile accidents, and assaults, and penetrating head injury is used to describe gunshot wounds and stabbings. More recently two new categories have been developed: crush and blast. Crush injury can best be described as the cranium being held between compressive forces that subject the skull and intracranial contents to increasing pressures. This force, if significant enough, can lead to failure of the calvarium as a protective shell to the intracranial contents. Blast injury has recently been added as a separate category after the experience with improvised explosive devices (IEDs) in the recent Afghanistan and Iraq conflicts.

Severity

Prior to 1974, different authors used various terms to describe patients with head injury, making it virtually impossible to compare groups of patients from different centers. In 1974, Teasdale and Jennett,[13] by identifying the clinical signs that predicted outcome most reliably and that seemed to have the least interobserver variation, designed what has come to be known as the Glasgow Coma Scale (GCS). The introduction of the GCS (Table 20.1) brought some degree of uniformity into the head injury literature.[13] This scale has gained widespread use for the description of patients with head injuries and has also been adopted for the description of patients with altered levels of consciousness due to other causes.

Jennett and Teasdale defined coma as the inability to obey commands, to utter words, and to open the eyes.[14] A patient needs to meet all three aspects of this definition to be classified as comatose. In a series of 2000 patients with severe head injury, these authors observed 4% who did not speak but could obey commands and another 4% who uttered words but did not obey commands. Among patients who could neither obey nor speak, 16% opened their eyes and were therefore judged not to be in coma. Patients who open their eyes spontaneously, obey commands, and are oriented score a total of 15 points, whereas flaccid patients who do not open their eyes or talk score the minimum of 3 points. No single score within the range of 3 to 15 forms the cut-off point for coma. However, 90% of all patients with a score of 8 or less, and none of those with a score of 9 or more, are found to be in coma according to the preceding definition. Therefore, for all practical purposes, a GCS score of 8 or less has become the generally accepted definition of a comatose patient.

The distinction between patients with severe head injury and those with mild to moderate injury is thus fairly clear. However, distinguishing between mild and moderate head injury is more of a problem.[15] Somewhat arbitrarily, head-injured patients with a GCS score of 9 to 13 have been categorized as "moderate," and those with a GCS score of 14 or 15 have been designated "mild." Authors have variably classified the GCS 13 patients with the mild or moderate TBI groups, but studies suggest that patients with a GCS of 13 at admission fit better into the moderate rather than mild TBI group. Eighty percent of head injuries are categorized as mild, 10% as moderate, and 10% as severe. Williams and colleagues reported that the neurobehavioral deficits in patients with mild head injury (GCS 14 or 15) and an intracranial lesion on initial computed tomography (CT) scan were similar to those in patients with moderate head injury (GCS 9 to 13), but

FIGURE 20.2 Classification of head injury.

By mechanism			
	Closed		High velocity (auto accidents)
			Low velocity (falls, assault)
	Penetrating		Gunshot wounds
			Other open injuries

By severity
Mild: GCS 14–15
Moderate: GCS 9–13
Severe: GCS 8 or less, comatose

By morphology			
	Skull fractures	Vault	Linear or stellate
			Depressed or nondepressed
		Basilar	With/without CSF leak
			With/without nerve VII palsy
	Intracranial lesions	Focal	Epidural
			Subdural
			Intracerebral
		Diffuse	Mild concussion
			Classic concussion
			Diffuse axonal injury

patients with mild head injury uncomplicated by an intracranial lesion on CT scan did significantly better.[16]

Morphology

The advent and easy attainability of CT scans in most centers has revolutionized the evaluation and treatment of the head injury patient. It is rare in current practice for patients to receive exploratory bur holes/craniotomy as described historically. Frequent CT follow-up is essential as the morphology of the head injury patient evolves over hours, days, and even weeks. For a morphological description, head injury can be described into two broad categories as skull fractures and intracranial lesions.

Skull Fractures

In current practice in developed countries, CT scans are the imaging study of choice and plain skull films are rarely obtained. Skull fractures may be seen in the cranial vault or skull base, may be linear or stellate, and may be depressed or nondepressed (Fig. 20.3). Basal skull fractures are harder to document on plain x-ray films and usually require CT scanning with bone-window settings for identification. Another indication of covert skull fracture is the presence of pneumocephalus, which can be readily identified on CT scan.

The clinical signs of a basal skull fracture include cerebrospinal fluid (CSF) leakage from the nose (rhinorrhea) or ear (otorrhea), blood behind the eardrum (hemotympanum), bruising behind the ear (postauricular ecchymoses or Battle's sign), and bruising around the eyes (periorbital ecchymoses or raccoon eyes). The presence of these clinical signs should increase the index of suspicion and help in the identification of a basal skull fracture. Most require no treatment, but persistent CSF leakage may require operative repair.

A depressed skull fracture may cause pressure on the brain or a dural breach. As a general guideline, fragments depressed more than the thickness of the skull require elevation. Open or compound skull fractures have a direct communication between the scalp laceration and the cerebral surface because the dura is torn. They require early surgical repair and appropriate antibiotic coverage. Outcome after a depressed skull fracture is based on the degree and location of the underlying injury to the brain.

A linear vault fracture increases the risk of intracranial hematoma. For this reason, the detection of a skull fracture on plain skull radiograph always calls for a CT scan of the head and generally warrants admission to the hospital for observation.

Fractures can also involve the anterior or posterior tables of the frontal sinus. These fractures can lead to inadequate drainage and recurrent sinusitis if the communication between the sinus and nasal cavity (nasofrontal outflow tract) is obstructed. Furthermore, if the posterior table is violated with obstruction of the nasofrontal outflow tract, there is an increased risk of intracranial infections. Treatment of such fractures should be based on the fine cut CT bone window findings, patency of the nasofrontal outflow tract, and cosmetic deformity caused by the fracture.[17,18]

Intracranial Lesions

Intracranially lesions may be broadly classified into focal or diffuse injuries. It is not uncommon to for these types of injuries to coexist. Focal lesions include epidural hematomas, subdural hematomas, and contusions/intracerebral hematomas. Diffuse brain injury, also referred to as *diffuse axonal injury*, may have a relatively benign-appearing CT scan (Fig. 20.4A); however, small punctate hemorrhages may be noted particularly at midline structures. Patients with diffuse axonal injury typically have a poor neurological examination with altered sensorium or even deep coma out of proportion to the findings on their imaging workup.

Epidural Hematoma (Fig. 20.4B)

This type of bleeding is located between the inner table of the skull and the dura. Most commonly these hemorrhages are located in the temporal or temporoparietal region and are classically associated with tearing of the middle meningeal artery secondary to calvarial fracture. Most epidural hematomas are related to arterial bleeding; however, in up to one third of the cases an epidural may be associated with bleeding from the bone. Epidural hematomas may also occur from tearing of the middle meningeal vein, diploic veins, or venous sinuses, particularly in the parieto-occipital area or the posterior fossa.

TABLE 20.1 Glasgow Coma Scale (GCS)	
Scoring Component	**Points Assigned**
Eye opening (E)	
Spontaneous	4
To call	3
To pain	2
None	1
Motor response (M)	
Obeys commands	6
Localizes pain	5
Normal flexion (withdrawal)	4
Abnormal flexion (decorticate)	3
Extension (decerebrate)	2
None (flaccid)	1
Verbal response (V)	
Oriented	5
Confused conversation	4
Inappropriate words	3
Incomprehensible sounds	2
None	1

Scoring
GCS sum score = (E + M + V); best possible score = 15; worst possible score = 3.

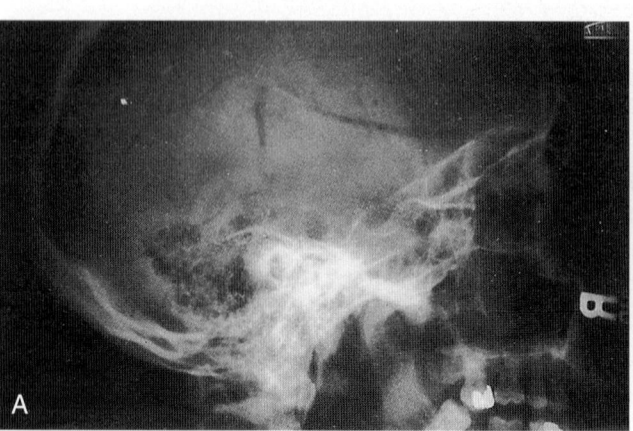

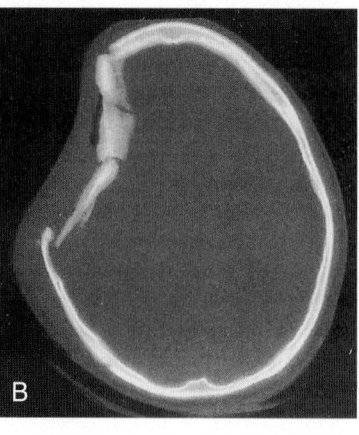

FIGURE 20.3 **A,** Linear skull fracture; **B,** depressed skull fracture.

Nonsurgical epidural hematomas are reported in 2.7% to 4% of TBI patients.[10,19-22] In patients presenting with coma up to 9% may harbor an epidural hematoma. Epidural hematomas tend to affect patients between 20 and 30 and are most commonly seen in traffic accidents (53%), falls (30%), and assaults (8%).[10] The mortality rate in all age groups and GCS scores undergoing surgery for epidural hematoma is approximately 10%.[10] More specifically in patients not in coma the mortality rate approximates 0%, for obtunded patients it is 9%, and for patients presenting in coma it approaches 20%.

Subdural Hematoma (Fig. 20.4C)

Subdural hematoma (SDH) is a much more common entity, with reports of 12% to 29% of patients with severe TBI having an associated SDH on initial imaging.[10] The BTF review of surgical subdural hematomas showed that in 2870 patients 21% presented with SDH. They occur most frequently from a tearing of bridging veins between the cerebral cortex and the draining sinuses. However, they can also be associated with lacerations of the brain surface or substance. A skull fracture may or may not be present and the mechanism is often age dependent. Younger patients (18-40 years) presented with SDH after motor vehicle accident (MVA) (56%), with only 12% presenting after

a fall.[23] In patients older than 65 the opposite is seen, with SDH seen in 22% of MVAs and 56% of falls, often seen in those on anticoagulants used in the management of other chronic disease processes.[23] The brain damage underlying acute SDHs results from direct pressure caused by the hematoma, brain swelling, increased intracranial pressure, or diffuse axonal injury as a result of mechanical distortion of the brain parenchyma. The injury in patients with SDH is usually much more severe, and the prognosis is much worse compared to epidural hematomas. MVA is described as the mechanism of injury in 53% to 75% of patients who are comatose with SDH. The mortality rate in a general series may be around 60% but can be lowered by very rapid surgical intervention and aggressive medical management.[24] Multiple studies show that the morbidity and mortality rates are increased if the surgery is performed after 3 to 4 hours, and the timing of acute SDH surgical intervention should be done within 2 to 4 hours of TBI if possible.[10]

Contusions/Intracerebral Hemorrhage (Fig. 20.4D)

Pure cerebral contusions are fairly common, found in 8% of all TBI[10,25] and 13% to 35% of severe injuries.[10] The incidence is much more apparent as the quality and number of CT scans increase. Furthermore, contusions of the brain are

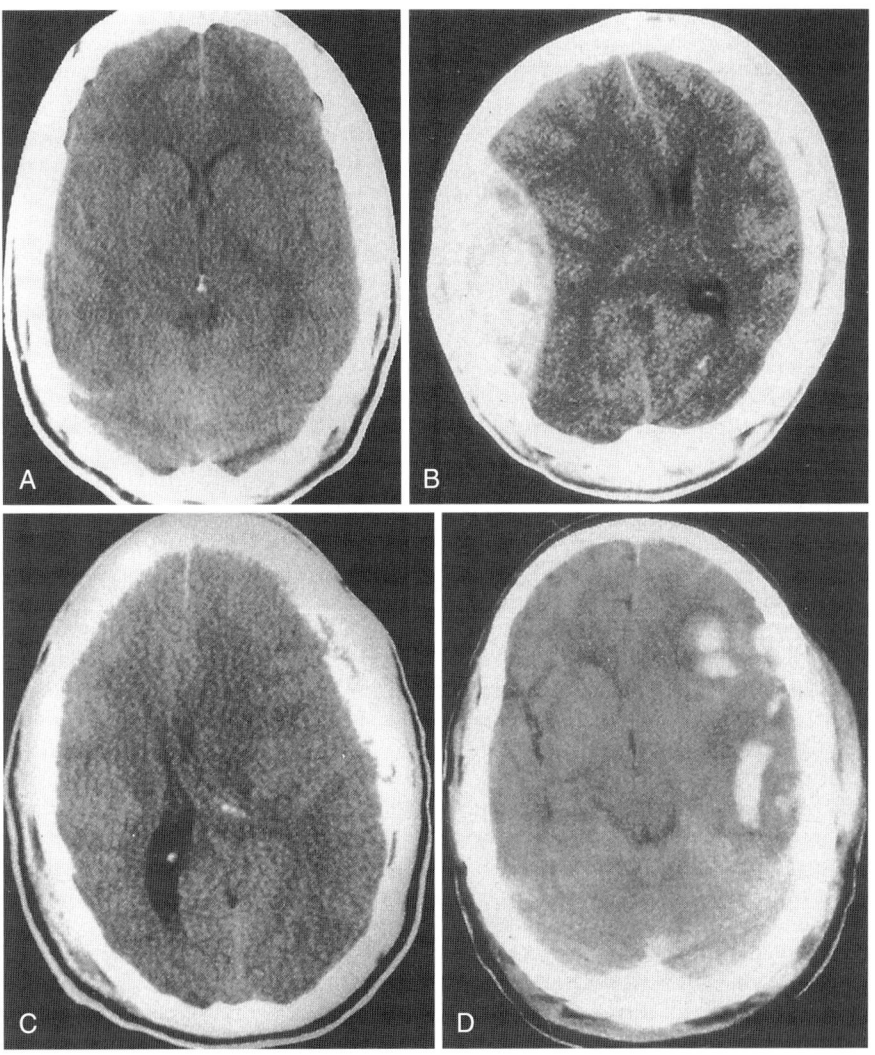

FIGURE 20.4 **A,** Diffuse brain injury; **B,** epidural hematoma; **C,** subdural hematoma; and **D,** intracerebral hematoma.

often concomitant with SDH. The vast majority of contusions occurs in the frontal and temporal lobes, although they can occur at almost any site, including the cerebellum and brainstem. The distinction between contusions and traumatic intracerebral hematomas remains somewhat ill-defined. The classic "salt and pepper" lesion is clearly a contusion, but a large hematoma clearly is not. However, there is a gray zone, and contusions can, over a period of hours or days, evolve into intracerebral hematomas.

Management of the intracerebral hematoma is dependent on the neurological status of the patient. Rapid surgical evacuation decompression is recommended if there is a significant mass effect (generally, a 5-mm or greater actual midline shift). The current BTF guidelines state that patients with parenchymal mass lesions and signs of progressive neurological deterioration related to the lesion, refractory intracranial hypertension, or signs of significant mass effect on CT should be treated operatively. Also in patients with GCS scores of 6 to 8 with frontal or temporal contusion greater than 20 cm³ with midline shift greater than 5 mm or cisternal compression on CT scan, and patients with any lesion greater than 50 cm³ in volume should be surgically treated.[10]

Conservative management may be utilized in patients with no neurological compromise, no signs of elevated intracranial pressure, and no CT scan evidence of significant mass effect. These patients should be managed with intensive monitoring, serial imaging, and a constant vigilant neurological examination.

Diffuse Injuries

Diffuse brain injuries form a continuum of progressively severe brain damage caused by increasing amounts of acceleration-deceleration injury to the brain. In its purest form, diffuse brain injury is the most common type of head injury.

A mild concussion is an injury in which consciousness is preserved, but there is a noticeable degree of temporary neurological dysfunction. These injuries are exceedingly common and, because of their mild degree, are often not brought to medical attention. The mildest form of concussion results in transient confusion and disorientation without amnesia. This syndrome is usually completely reversible and is associated with no major sequelae. Slightly greater injury causes confusion with both retrograde and post-traumatic amnesia.

A classic cerebral concussion is that post-traumatic state that results in loss of consciousness. This condition is always accompanied by some degree of retrograde and post-traumatic amnesia, and the length of post-traumatic amnesia is a good measure of the severity of the injury. The loss of consciousness is transient and reversible. The patient has returned to full consciousness by 6 hours, although it is usually much sooner. Although the great majority of patients with classic cerebral concussion have no sequelae other than amnesia for the events relating to the injury, some patients may have more long-lasting and sometimes significant neurological deficits.

Diffuse axonal injury is the term used to describe a prolonged post-traumatic state in which there is loss of consciousness from the time of injury that continues beyond 6 hours. This phenomenon may further be broken down into mild, moderate, and severe categories.[26] Severe diffuse axonal injury usually occurs in vehicular accidents, comprising about 36% of all patients with diffuse axonal injury. These patients are rendered deeply comatose and remain so for prolonged periods

of time. They often demonstrate evidence of decortication or decerebration (motor posturing) and often remain severely disabled, if they survive. These patients often exhibit autonomic dysfunctions such as hypertension, hyperhidrosis, and hyperpyrexia, and were previously thought to have primary brainstem injury. It is now believed that diffuse axonal injury throughout the brain is the more common pathological basis.

EVALUATION

Mild Traumatic Brain Injury

Approximately 80% of patients presenting to the emergency room with head injury fall under the category of mild TBI. These patients are awake but may be amnesic for events surrounding the injury with a GCS score of 14 or 15. There may be a history of brief loss of consciousness, which is usually difficult to confirm. The issue is often confounded by alcohol or other intoxicants.

Most patients with mild head injury make "uneventful recoveries" but often suffer mild neurological sequelae that can be identified when given in-depth neuropsychological testing. Furthermore, about 3% of patients deteriorate unexpectedly, and can become neurologically devastated if the decline in mental status is not noticed early.[27] How can a physician guard against such an occurrence? Early CT scanning of all patients with a history of a TBI is generally advisable, although the classic struggle between "cost-effective" and the "best possible" management is clearly evident here, and practice varies in different centers.

In 1999, a Task Force on Mild Traumatic Brain Injury was devised under the support of the European Federation of Neurological Societies. The efforts of the task force produced the recommendations for the initial management of mild traumatic brain injury (Fig. 20.5).[28] Since their recommendations, further work has been done in the evaluation and treatment of mild TBI.

In the head-injured patient, skull x-ray films may be examined for the following features: linear or depressed skull fractures, position of the pineal gland if calcified, air-fluid levels in the sinuses, pneumocephalus, facial fractures, and foreign bodies. However, the routine ordering of skull films has in most instances become obsolete with the availability of CT scanners. Studies comparing skull radiography with CT have shown a low sensitivity and specificity of the presence of a skull fracture on skull radiographs for intracranial hemorrhage.[29] A meta-analysis confirmed that skull radiography is of little value in the clinical assessment of mild TBI.[30]

Hence, CT is considered the gold standard for the detection of intracranial abnormalities after mild TBI. It is recommended for those with loss of consciousness or post-traumatic amnesia and is considered mandatory in all patients with GCS scores of 13 or 14, or in the presence of risk factors.

The cervical spine and other parts must undergo x-ray studies if there is any pain or tenderness. Non-narcotic analgesics are preferred, although codeine may be used if there is an associated painful injury. Tetanus toxoid must be administered if there are any associated open wounds. Routine blood tests are usually not necessary if there are no systemic injuries and the patient is not on anticoagulants. A blood alcohol level and urine toxic screen can be useful both for diagnostic and for medicolegal purposes.

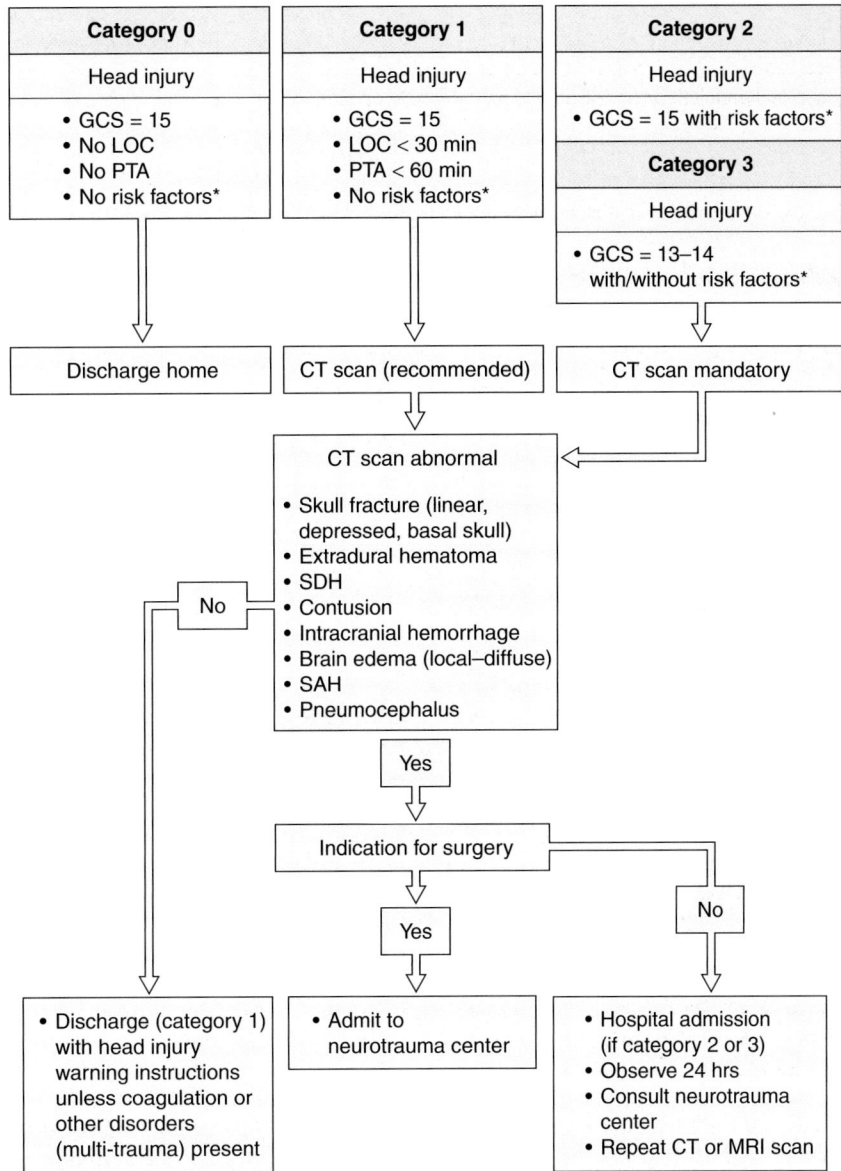

FIGURE 20.5 Algorithm for management of mild head injury. *Risk factors include ambiguous accident history, continued post-traumatic amnesia, retrograde amnesia more than 30 minutes, clinical signs of skull fracture, headache, vomiting, focal neurological deficit, seizure, age younger than 2 years and older than 60 years, coagulation disorder, or high-energy (speed) accident.

Moderate Traumatic Brain Injury

Patients with moderate head injury constitute approximately 10% of head injury patients seen in the emergency room. They are still able to follow simple commands but are usually confused or somnolent and may have focal neurological deficits such as a hemiparesis. In patients with mild or moderate head injury, extracranial injuries play a significant role in the overall outcome. Approximately 10% of these patients will deteriorate and lapse into coma. Therefore, they should be managed as patients with severe head injuries, although they are not routinely intubated (Fig. 20.6).

On admission to the emergency room, a brief history is obtained and cardiopulmonary stability is ensured prior to neurological assessment. A CT scan of the head is obtained in all moderately head-injured patients. In a review of 341 patients with a GCS score of 9 to 12, 40% of cases had an abnormal initial CT scan and 8% required surgery.[31] The patient is admitted for observation even if the CT scan is normal. If the patient improves neurologically and a follow-up CT scan of the head shows no surgical mass lesion, he or she may be discharged from the hospital over the next few days. On the other hand, if the patient lapses into coma, the management principles described for severe head injury are adopted.

Severe Traumatic Brain Injury

Severe TBI patients are those who are unable to follow simple commands even after cardiopulmonary stabilization. Although this definition includes a wide spectrum of brain injury, it identifies the patients who are at greatest risk of suffering significant morbidity and even death. We believe that in such

Definition	
The patient may be confused or somnolent but is still able to follow simple commands (GCS 9–13)	
Initial work up	
Same as for mild head injury, except that baseline blood work (CBC, Chem 7, PT/PTT) may be obtained	
CT scan of the head is advisable in all cases	
Admission for observation is the safest option, even if the CT scan is normal	
After admission	
Frequent neurologic checks	
Follow-up CT scan if condition deteriorates or preferably prior to discharge	
If patient improves (90%)	**If patient deteriorates (10%)**
Discharge when stable Follow-up clinic	If the patient stops following simple commands, repeat CT scan and manage per severe head injury protocol

FIGURE 20.6 Algorithm for management of moderate head injury.

patients a "wait and see" approach can be disastrous and that prompt diagnosis and treatment are of the utmost importance (Box 20.1).[24,32,33]

MANAGEMENT OF SEVERE TRAUMATIC BRAIN INJURY

Airway

A frequent concomitant of a severe TBI is transient respiratory arrest. Prolonged apnea may often be the cause of "immediate" death at the scene of an accident. If artificial respiration can be instituted immediately, a good outcome is possible.[34] Apnea, atelectasis, aspiration, and adult respiratory distress syndrome are frequently associated with severe head injury, and by far the most important aspect of the immediate management of these patients is the establishment of a reliable airway. *Patients with severe TBI should be intubated early.* One hundred percent oxygen is then used for ventilation until blood gases can be checked and appropriate adjustments of the FiO_2 made. There is little danger of oxygen toxicity even when 100% oxygen is used for less than 48 to 72 hours.

Blood Pressure

Hypotension and hypoxia are the principal enemies of the head-injured patient. It has been shown that the presence of hypotension (systolic blood pressure <90 mm Hg) in severe TBI patients increases the mortality rate from 27% to 50%.[35] Furthermore, it was found that 35% of patients arriving at major trauma centers are hypotensive. While the airway is being established, another group of emergency room personnel should be checking the patient's pulse and blood pressure and taking steps to obtain venous access.

If the patient is hypotensive, it is vital to restore normal blood pressure as soon as possible. Hypotension is usually not the result of the brain injury itself, except in the terminal stages when medullary failure supervenes. Far more commonly, hypotension is a marker of severe blood loss, which may be either "overt" or "occult," or possibly both. One must also consider associated spinal cord injury (with quadriplegia or paraplegia), cardiac contusion or tamponade, and tension pneumothorax as possible causes. While efforts are in progress to determine the cause of the hypotension, volume replacement should be initiated.

The importance of routine abdominal paracentesis in the hypotensive comatose patient has been demonstrated historically.[36] In most trauma centers today either high-resolution rapid CT scan or ultrasound (focused assessment with sonography for trauma, FAST) is an acceptable option to rule in or rule out intra-abdominal injury. It must be emphasized that *a patient's neurological examination is meaningless as long as he or she is hypotensive.* Time after time, we have seen hypotensive patients who are unresponsive to any form of stimulation revert to a near-normal neurological examination soon after normal blood pressure has been restored.

Cardiopulmonary Stabilization

Brain injury is often adversely affected by secondary insults. In a study of 100 consecutive patients with severe brain injury evaluated on arrival in the emergency room, 30% were hypoxemic (Po_2 <65 mm Hg), 13% were hypotensive (systolic blood pressure <95 mm Hg), and 12% were anemic (hematocrit <30%).[37] It has subsequently been demonstrated that hypotension at admission (systolic blood pressure <90 mm Hg) is one of three factors in severe head injury with a normal CT scan (the other two being age over 40 years and motor posturing) that, when noted at admission, are associated with subsequent ICP elevation.[38] High ICP is in turn associated with poorer outcome. Subsequent analyses have also confirmed a strong association between hypotension and worse outcomes in patients with severe head injury.[39]

Initial Management of Severe Head Injury

Definition
The patient is unable to follow even a simple command because of impaired consciousness.

Management
History
Age of patient and type and time of accident
Drug or alcohol intake
Neurological deficit progression
Progression of vital sign changes
Vomiting, aspiration, anoxia, or seizures
Past medical history, including medications and allergies

Cardiopulmonary Stabilization
Airway: intubate early
Blood pressure: normalize promptly using normal saline or blood
Catheters: Foley, nasogastric tube
Diagnostic films: cervical spine, chest, skull, abdomen, pelvis, extremities

General Examination
Vital signs
Trauma survey
Open wounds, lacerations, abrasions
Obvious deformities and abnormalities
General state of patient

Emergency Measures for Associated Injuries
Tracheostomy
Chest tubes
Neck stabilization: hard collar, Gardner-Wells tongs, traction
Abdominal paracentesis

Neurological Examination
Eye opening
Motor response
Verbal response
Pupillary light reaction
Oculocephalics (doll's eye)
Oculovestibulars (caloric)

Therapeutic Agents
Sodium bicarbonate, phenytoin, mannitol, hyperventilation

Diagnostic Tests
CT scan, MRI scan, CTA/MRA, air ventriculogram, or angiogram (in descending order of preference)

CT, computed tomography; CTA/MRA, computed tomographic angiography/magnetic resonance angiography; MRI, magnetic resonance imaging.

Therefore, it is imperative that cardiopulmonary stabilization be achieved rapidly.

Catheters

A Foley catheter (16 to 18F for average adults) should be carefully inserted and a urine sample should be sent for urinalysis and toxic screen when appropriate. Gross hematuria, in the absence of local trauma, suggests renal injury and is an indication for an abdominal CT scan and an emergency intravenous pyelogram. Mild hematuria may be secondary to traumatic catheterization, renal contusion, or, rarely, a dissecting aortic

aneurysm. Special attention must be paid to maintaining accurate records of fluid intake and output, especially in children and the elderly. In addition to ensuring fluid balance, such records help assess blood loss and monitor renal perfusion.

A nasogastric tube, preferably a Salem sump (double-lumen plastic catheter), should be inserted and connected to a wall suction unit. Potential, albeit rare, complications of this procedure, such as intracranial passage of the tube secondary to a basal skull fracture or those with a history of transnasal skull base surgery, must be kept in mind. In patients with anterior basal skull fractures it is probably wise to pass the tube under direct vision with a laryngoscope or to pass it through the mouth.

Diagnostic Radiographs

As soon as the preliminary steps toward cardiopulmonary stabilization have been taken, diagnostic radiographs should be obtained. Cervical spine films (cross-table lateral and anteroposterior) or a thin-cut cervical spine CT scan are the first to be taken in the severely traumatized patient and must be read by a knowledgeable reader before the patient's neck can be moved. Features to look for in this study are loss of alignment of the vertebral bodies, bony fractures or compressions, loss of alignment of the facet joints, and prevertebral soft tissue swelling (more than 5 mm opposite the C3 vertebral body is significant). Every effort must be made to visualize the lower cervical levels (C6-T1); these are often obscured by the shoulders, especially in heavy-set patients. On plain films, fracture-subluxations at these levels may be overlooked if the films are not repeated with caudal traction on both arms and greater x-ray penetration (Fig. 20.7).[40] If these maneuvers also fail, a "swimmer's view" lateral film can be obtained. If any of these films shows any of the abnormalities listed here, the neck must remain immobilized in a hard collar (Philadelphia, Aspen, or Miami J) pending further studies (high-resolution CT scan). In many centers, plain films of the cervical spine have been replaced by a thin-cut CT scan as the initial study.

Cervical spine CT is indicated for the unconscious patient with suspicious or inadequate cervical radiographs and with all cervical fractures or suspected fractures on initial plain films. Several studies have demonstrated the value of the full CT scan, with sagittal and coronal reconstructions, for the exclusion of significant spinal injury.[41] Widening, slippage, or rotational abnormalities of the cervical vertebrae suggest soft tissue injury. An absence of such signs appears to exclude significant instability. Additional modalities, such as magnetic resonance imaging (MRI), can also be employed, although these studies are not generally used as initial studies.

If a cervical spine fracture does exist, either computed tomography angiography (CTA) or magnetic resonance angiography (MRA) may be ordered in specific cases in order to evaluate the carotid and vertebral artery to exclude vascular injury. It is important to rule out these injuries as arterial dissection or occlusion may to lead to ischemic stroke or cerebral hypoperfusion.

The chest film is useful in ruling out endotracheal tube malposition, pneumothorax, hemothorax, lung contusion, hemopericardium, rib fractures, thoracic spine fractures, and other thoracic injury that may have a bearing on patient management.

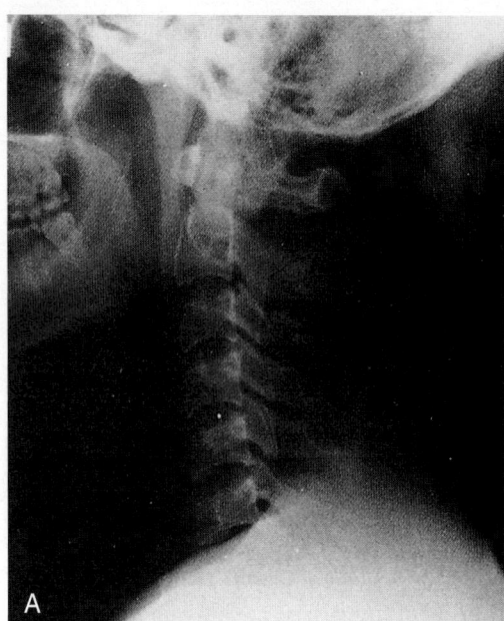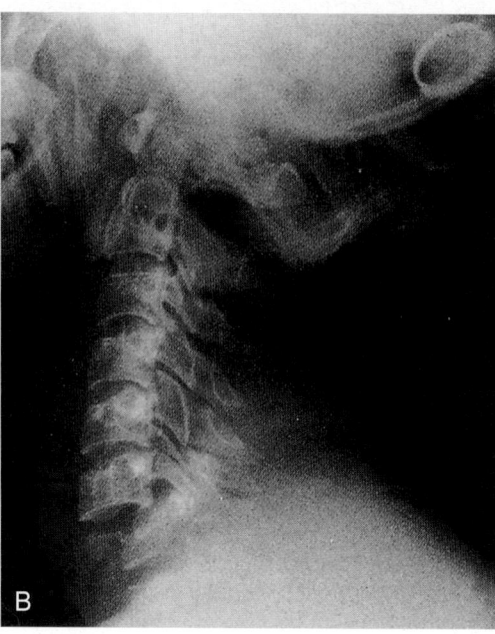

FIGURE 20.7 A, The lower cervical spine is obscured by the shoulders. **B,** Traction on the shoulders reveals a fracture-subluxation at C6-C7.

Although skull films (anteroposterior and lateral) have been overshadowed by CT scanning, they can be helpful in identifying maxillofacial injuries, depressed skull fractures, and penetrating injuries. The presence of pneumocephalus or an air-fluid level in one of the sinuses can alert the clinician to a basal skull fracture.

A single anteroposterior abdominal film (kidney, ureter, and bladder; KUB) may be taken in trauma patients. This film may help identify large retroperitoneal hematomas, lumbosacral spine fractures, distended viscera, and possibly subdiaphragmatic air.

Anteroposterior and lateral pelvic films may also be obtained, looking for pelvic injuries, which may be the site of significant blood loss. The extremities may be studied whenever indicated to rule out fractures or subluxations.

In most trauma centers today CT scanning is readily available and trauma patients meeting the indications for imaging workup will receive a CT scan of the head, neck, chest, abdomen, and pelvis as indicated, after being evaluated and stabilized by the trauma team.

General Examination

During the process of cardiopulmonary stabilization, the clinician conducts a rapid general examination looking for other injuries. In one series of severe TBI patients, more than 50% had additional major systemic injuries requiring care by other specialists (Table 20.2).[37] One must check for head and neck, thoracic, abdominal, pelvic, and spinal injuries, and injuries involving extremities.

Neurological Examination

As soon as the patient's cardiopulmonary status has been stabilized, a rapid and directed neurological examination is performed (Box 20.2). Although various factors may confound

TABLE 20.2 Frequency of Systemic Injuries in Patients with Severe Head Injury*

Type of Injury	Incidence (%)
Long-bone or pelvic fracture	32
Maxillary or mandibular fracture	22
Major chest injury	23
Abdominal visceral injury	7
Spinal injury	2

*$N = 100$.
Modified from Miller JD, Sweet RC, Narayan RK, Becker DP. Early insults to the injured brain. JAMA 1978;240:439-442.

an accurate evaluation of the patient's neurological state (e.g., hypotension, hypoxia, intoxication, sedation or paralytic agents), valuable data can nevertheless be obtained. If a patient demonstrates variable responses to stimulation, or if the response on each side is different, the best response appears to be a more accurate prognostic indicator than the worst response. To follow trends in an individual patient's progress, however, it is better to report both the best and the worst responses. In other words, the right-side and left-side motor responses should be recorded separately.

One should not limit the examination to the GCS. Other important data in the initial assessment of patients with impaired consciousness are the patient's age, vital signs, pupillary response, and eye movements.[42] The GCS score provides a simple grading of the arousal and functional capacity of the cerebral cortex, and the pupillary responses and eye movements serve as measures of brainstem function. Advanced age, hypotension, and hypoxia all adversely affect outcome. Indeed, there is considerable interplay between all these factors in determining the ultimate outcome in the severe TBI patient.

Glasgow Coma Scale score
Pupillary response to light
Eye movements
Oculocephalic (doll's eye)
Oculovestibular (caloric)
Motor power
Gross sensory examination

Pupils

Careful observation of pupil size and response to light is important during the initial examination (Table 20.3). A well-known early sign of temporal lobe herniation is mild dilatation of the pupil and a sluggish pupillary light response. Compression or distortion of the oculomotor nerve during tentorial-uncal herniation impairs the function of the parasympathetic axons that transmit efferent signals for pupillary constriction, resulting in mild pupillary dilatation. Sometimes, bilateral miotic pupils (1-3 mm) can occur in the early stages of herniation as a result of compromise of the pupillomotor sympathetic pathways originating in the hypothalamus, permitting a predominance of parasympathetic tone and pupillary constriction. In either instance, continued herniation causes increasing dilatation of the pupil and paralysis of its light response. With full mydriasis (8- to 9-mm pupil), ptosis and paresis of the medial rectus and other ocular muscles innervated by the oculomotor nerve appear. A bright light in a darkened room is always necessary to determine pupillary light responses. A magnifying lens such as the +20-diopter lens on a standard ophthalmoscope is helpful in distinguishing between a weak and an absent pupillary light reaction, especially if the pupil is small. A computerized pupillometer underwent clinical testing, but the results were reportedly unclear.[43]

Recognition of additional pupillary disorders that can occur in an unconscious patient is useful in the examination of the patient with head trauma. Disruption of the afferent arc of the pupillary light reflex within the optic nerve is detected by the swinging flashlight test. As the flashlight is swung from the normal eye to the injured eye, injury to the optic nerve is indicated by a paradoxic response of the pupil: dilatation rather than constriction. This paradoxic pupillary dilatation is termed an *afferent pupillary defect* or *Marcus Gunn pupil*, and in the absence of opacification of the ocular media it is unequivocal evidence of optic nerve injury.

Bilaterally small pupils suggest that the patient has used certain drugs, particularly opiates, or has one of several metabolic encephalopathies, or a destructive lesion of the pons. In these conditions pupillary light responses can usually be seen with a magnifying lens. Unilateral Horner's pupil is seen occasionally with brainstem lesions, but in the trauma patient attention should be given to the possibility of a disrupted efferent sympathetic pathway at the apex of the lung, base of the neck, or ipsilateral carotid sheath. Midposition pupils with variable light responses can be observed in all stages of coma. Traumatic oculomotor nerve injury is the diagnosis in patients with a history of a dilated pupil from the onset of injury, an improving level of consciousness, and appropriate ocular muscle weakness. A mydriatic pupil (6 mm or more) occurs occasionally with direct trauma to the globe of the eye. This traumatic mydriasis is usually unilateral and is not accompanied by ocular muscle paresis. Finally, bilaterally dilated and fixed pupils in patients with head injury may be the result of inadequate cerebral vascular perfusion caused by hypotension secondary to blood loss or elevation of intracranial pressure to a degree that impairs cerebral blood flow. Return of the pupillary response may occur promptly after the restoration of blood flow, if the period of inadequate perfusion has not been too long.

Eye Movements

Ocular movements are an important index of the functional activity that is present within the brainstem reticular formation. If the patient is sufficiently alert to follow simple commands, a full range of eye movements is easily obtained, and the integrity of the entire ocular motor system within the brainstem can be confirmed. In states of depressed consciousness, voluntary eye movements are lost and there may be dysfunction of the neural structures activating eye movements. In these instances, oculocephalic or oculovestibular responses are used to determine the presence or absence of an eye movement disorder. If a neck fracture has been excluded, function of the pontine gaze center is quickly ascertained by the oculocephalic maneuver.

The oculovestibular response can be tested with ice water and only a small expenditure of time. Obstructions within the external auditory canal due to blood or cerumen must be removed, and ocular movement may be limited in patients with orbital edema. In alert patients, cold caloric stimulation causes fast-phase nystagmus in the direction opposite to the tonic eye deviation. The mnemonic "COWS" (cold opposite, warm same) refers to this phenomenon. However, in comatose patients, functional suppression of the reticular activating system is reflected by the absence of nystagmus in response to caloric stimulation so that only the tonic eye deviation is seen (cold same). Thus, irrigation with cold water in a comatose patient causes ipsilateral deviation of the eyes toward the stimulated side.

TABLE 20.3 Interpretation of Pupillary Findings in Patients with Head Injury

Pupillary Size	Light Response	Interpretation
Unilaterally dilated	Sluggish or fixed	Cranial nerve III compression secondary to tentorial herniation
Bilaterally dilated	Sluggish or fixed	Inadequate brain perfusion Bilateral cranial nerve III palsy
Unilaterally dilated	Cross-reactive (Marcus Gunn)	Optic nerve injury
Bilaterally miotic	May be difficult to determine	Drugs (opiates) Metabolic encephalopathy Pontine lesion
Unilaterally miotic	Preserved	Injured sympathetic pathway (e.g., carotid sheath injury)

While oculocephalic and caloric testing is being performed, infranuclear, internuclear, and supranuclear ocular motility disorders are recognizable. A destructive lesion of a frontal or pontine gaze center results in tonic overaction of the opposite frontal-pontine axis for horizontal eye movement. This overaction results in ipsilateral deviation of the eyes with frontal lobe lesions, and contralateral gaze deviation with pontine lesions.

Third and sixth cranial nerve palsies are generally not difficult to recognize in patients with head injury. Fourth cranial nerve palsies cannot ordinarily be identified in coma because of the select action of the superior oblique muscle. In alert and recovering patients, however, superior oblique paresis causes troublesome double vision, especially with downward and inward gaze. Head tilt opposite the side of the paretic muscle lessens the diplopia, while ipsilateral tilt of the head increases it. Internuclear ophthalmoplegia is suggested by select adduction paresis without additional involvement of the pupil, lid, or vertical muscles innervated by the third nerve. This ophthalmoplegia results from disruption of the ipsilateral medial longitudinal fasciculus that connects the oculomotor subnucleus for medial rectus neurons to the contralateral horizontal gaze center. Either bilateral or unilateral internuclear ophthalmoplegia may be seen, depending on the extent of the brainstem trauma.

Motor Function

The basic examination is completed by a gross test of motor strength, although severely head-injured patients are not sufficiently responsive for such a determination to be reliably made. Each extremity is examined and graded on the internationally used scale shown in Table 20.4. Furthermore, stimuli to assess patients should be standardized. In assessing for localization the elbow should be bent at 90 degrees with the forearms resting on the patient's chest. If the patient is able to bring the hand at or above the chin, localization should be noted. To assess withdraw, deep nailbed pressure to the second digit is done to test for any movement away from the noxious stimulus. Assessing the lower extremities for withdraw is difficult to differentiate from reflexive triple flexion and thus has diminished validity.

Diagnostic Procedures

As soon as a patient's cardiorespiratory condition has been stabilized and a preliminary neurological examination completed, it behooves the physician to rule out the presence of an intracranial mass lesion. The patient is by this time intubated, often paralyzed with a paralytic agent, and on mechanical

TABLE 20.4 Motor Function Scale	
Component	**Points Assigned**
Normal power	5
Moderate weakness	4
Severe weakness (antigravity)	3
Severe weakness (not antigravity)	2
Trace movement	1
No movement	0

ventilation. This prevents the patient from straining and moving around, thus avoiding intracranial pressure surges and greatly enhancing the quality of the diagnostic studies. Needless to say, CT scanning has rendered all other diagnostic tests virtually obsolete. However, other tests have to be used in certain instances either to substitute for CT scanning or, as in the case of angiography, to obtain certain supplemental data.

Computed Tomography

CT scanning is clearly the procedure of choice in the evaluation of the head-injured patient and has probably significantly improved outcome after head injury.[44] It is strongly recommended that an emergency CT scan be obtained as soon as possible (preferably within half an hour) after admission with a severe head injury. Centers dealing with a large number of such patients must make arrangements to have CT technicians in the hospital on a 24-hour basis, or within easy accessibility in an emergency. CT scans should also be repeated whenever there is a change in the patient's clinical status or an unexplained rise in intracranial pressure.

In a prospective study of CT scan abnormalities in 207 patients with severe TBI, we found the initial CT scan to be normal in 30% of cases. The remaining 70% of patients had CT scan abnormalities: low-density lesions in 10%, high-density nonsurgical lesions in 19%, and high-density lesions requiring surgery in 41%.[32]

Edema is seen on CT as a zone of low density associated with mass effect on the adjacent ventricles reflected as compression, distortion, and displacement of the ventricular system. The edema may be focal, multifocal, or diffuse. With diffuse cerebral edema it may be hard to appreciate the lower density because no area of normal brain density is available for comparison. In such cases there is usually bilateral ventricular compression which may be so gross that the ventricular system is not seen, especially in children. The picture of diffuse brain swelling on CT can be secondary to edema or vascular engorgement (hyperemia).

Cerebral contusions are seen as nonhomogeneous areas of high density, often interspersed with areas of low density ("salt and pepper" appearance). The CT appearance results from multiple small areas of hemorrhage within the brain substance, associated with areas of edema (see Fig. 20.4D). The margin is usually poorly defined. A mass effect is often seen, although this appearance may be minimal. Depending on the extent of hemorrhage, the degree of edema, and the time course, a contusion may appear predominantly dense or lucent.

Although it is not always possible to differentiate between subdural and epidural hematomas on CT, the latter are typically biconvex or lenticular in shape, because the close attachment of the dura to the inner table of the skull prevents the hematoma from spreading (see Fig. 20.4B). Approximately 20% of patients with an extracerebral hematoma have blood in both the epidural and subdural spaces at operation or autopsy. Because there is little chance of epidural blood mixing with CSF, these lesions appear as uniformly dense collections and are rarely isodense. However, they may develop in a delayed fashion, especially after evacuation of a contralateral "balancing" lesion.

The typical subdural hematoma is more diffuse than an epidural hematoma and has a concave inner margin that follows the surface of the brain (see Fig. 20.4C). The distinction between acute, subacute, and chronic lesions is somewhat arbitrary. However, most acute subdural hematomas are hyperdense, most subacute lesions are isodense or of mixed density, and most chronic hematomas are hypodense as compared with brain tissue. Effacement of the cerebral sulci over the convexity and distortion of the ipsilateral lateral ventricle may suggest the presence of an isodense hematoma.

Traumatic intracerebral hematomas are usually located in the frontal and anterior temporal lobes, although they can occur in virtually any area. The majority of hematomas develops immediately after the injury, but delayed lesions are often noted, usually within the first week. They are high-density lesions and are usually surrounded by zones of low density caused by edema. Traumatic hematomas are more often multiple than hematomas from other causes.

Traumatic intraventricular hemorrhage was previously believed to have a uniformly poor prognosis but this is no longer considered true. It is frequently associated with parenchymal hemorrhage. The blood becomes isodense relatively rapidly and often disappears completely within a couple of weeks. If indicated, a ventriculostomy may be placed in the less bloody ventricle and CSF drainage can be used to monitor and reduce intracranial pressure and drain away the blood.

Acute obstructive hydrocephalus may develop secondary to a posterior fossa hematoma that obstructs the ventricular pathways. However, delayed hydrocephalus is far more common, occurring in about 6% of patients with severe head injury. This communicating hydrocephalus results from blood in the subarachnoid space and is often evident by the fourteenth day after injury, although it can certainly become evident later.

Acute ischemic infarction appears as a low-density area compared with the adjacent brain. The infarction may be detectable on CT scan within 24 hours of onset and over 60% are clearly seen by 7 days. Contrast enhancement improves the diagnostic yield by nearly 15%, and MRI is even more sensitive.

Overall, a noncontrast CT scan of the brain is a quick and accurate diagnostic tool for initial and serial assessment in TBI patients. Furthermore, studies have shown that CT can also be used as a prognostic tool in TBI.[10,45-47] Predictive value can be maximized by taking all protocols into account, using a combination of the group as a tool to help prognosticate patient outcome including at least the following parameters: status of basal cisterns, midline shift, traumatic subarachnoid or intraventricular hemorrhage, and presence of different types of mass lesions.[48]

Ventriculography

As an historical note, ventriculograhy was once used prior to the era of CT scanning to help identify mass lesions causing ventricle compression and shift. In current practice, there is essentially no indication for ventriculography.

Angiography

Again, prior to the advent of CT scanning, angiography was once used to diagnose mass lesions and shift of the brain by examining the pattern of the blood vessels and looking for

shift or displacement. In patients with neck injuries or skull base fractures near the carotid canal, angiography may be performed for diagnosis and possible treatment of carotid or vertebral injuries, such as dissection. Angiography may still be useful in the diagnosis of patients with Horner's syndrome, dysphagia, hemiparesis, obtundation, and monoparesis when CT scanning does not illicit an abnormality. With the advent of CTA and MRA true invasive cerebral angiography is not used as much, with the newer tests being less invasive and having less risk.

Computed Tomography Angiography

Patients who have skull base fractures through the petrous bone, cervical trauma, or cervical fractures through the transverse foramen are at risk for carotid and vertebral artery dissection. CTA offers a rapid means of cervical and intracranial vascular injury assessment while the patient is the emergency department.[49-52] Contraindications to CTA use include allergies to iodine-based contrast dye as well underlying renal disease. Most centers have protocols in place to guide specific criteria in regard to dealing TBI with such patients.

Magnetic Resonance Imaging

A wide range of CT findings in patients with closed head injury can represent a specific GCS score. Furthermore, repeat CT scans offer a cumulative risk or iatrogenic pathology because of the radiation used to obtain the images.[53] The use of MRI in TBI patients can help in diagnosis, especially in those with nonspecific CT findings. Particularly helpful imaging sequences include diffusion-weighted imaging (DWI), susceptibility-weighted imaging (SWI), diffusion tensor imaging (DTI), MRI spectroscopy, and functional MRI with established protocols.[54-56]

Intracranial Pressure

Since the early 1970s, there has been an increasing interest in ICP monitoring and control This has been associated with progressive evolution of related technology. However, the intraventricular catheter (or ventriculostomy) remains the most widely used and most useful device for measuring ICP and helping in its control and for maintaining cerebral perfusion pressure.[57,58]

Cerebral perfusion pressure (CPP) is the mean arterial blood pressure minus ICP. Because cerebral ischemia may be the single most important secondary effect affecting outcome following severe TBI, it is useful to follow CPP rather than ICP alone.[59] The guidelines have recommended maintaining CPP at a minimum of 60 mm Hg to possibly help in the avoidance of both global and regional ischemia. Conversely, too great a CPP may also have a deleterious effect, particularly with respiratory complications.

Head injury is the most common indication for ICP monitoring. As a general rule, patients who can follow simple commands need not be monitored and may satisfactorily be followed clinically. In patients who are unable to follow simple commands and have an abnormal CT scan, the incidence of intracranial hypertension is high (53-63%), and monitoring is warranted.[38] Severe TBI patients with normal CT scans generally have a lower incidence of elevated ICP (approximately 13%) unless they have two or more of the following adverse features at admission: systolic blood pressure less than 90 mm Hg, unilateral or bilateral motor posturing, or age over 40 years. In the presence of these adverse features, the incidence of intracranial hypertension (even in patients with normal CT scans) is as high as in those with abnormal CT scans on admission.[38] Compression or absence of basal cisterns has also been associated with elevated ICP.[60]

Normal ICP in a relaxed or paralyzed patient who is neither hypotensive nor hypercarbic is 10 mm Hg (136 mm H_2O) or less (1 mm Hg = 13.6 mm H_2O = 1.36 cm H_2O). Pressures in the range of 10 to 20 mm Hg (136-272 mm H_2O) may occur with moderate disturbances of intracranial volumes; pressures greater than these herald an intracranial hematoma, diffuse brain swelling, or both.

Most dangerous traumatic intracranial mass lesions shift the midline 5 mm or greater. This is invariably associated with an elevated ICP unless a CSF leak is present. Significant temporal lobe lesions may cause only a minimal shift of the midline, but the ICP may be elevated and the third ventricle, if seen, will often be shifted more than the lateral ventricles. If there is little or no midline shift, the ICP is elevated, and the patient is not hypercarbic, then either there are bilateral mass lesions or there is significant diffuse brain swelling.

When intracranial pressure demonstrates an upward trend, certain basic items should be checked. The neck should be in a neutral position to facilitate venous drainage. In most cases, having the head end of the bed elevated approximately 30 degrees is useful.[61] The calibration of the system must be checked, and one should confirm that the transducer is level with the foramen of Monro. If the patient is fighting the ventilator, he or she should be sedated or chemically paralyzed. If these measures are not adequate, various methods exist to reduce the ICP, including ventricular drainage, mannitol, and hyperventilation.

New technology now allows one to monitor cerebral oxygenation, via the LICOX CMP System. The purpose of this triple-lumen bolt system is to provide additional data including brain tissue oxygenation (P_{BTO_2}) and temperature as well as ICP in patients in whom cerebral hypoxia and ischemia are a concern. Mean normal brain tissue oxygen pressure is greater than 30 mm Hg (range 25-50 mm Hg) with ischemia reported at ranges less than 8 to 12 mm Hg and cell death at less than 5 mm Hg.[62]

Because the duration and severity of cerebral tissue hypoxia correlates with unfavorable outcomes in severe TBI, this could prove a valuable tool in management and possibly in predicting outcome. The monitor is able to indicate cerebral tissue perfusion status local to the sensor placement, although local brain oxygen levels may not reflect what is happening in the rest of the brain. In the recent literature brain tissue oxygenation monitoring and treatment have shown promise in decreasing morbidity and fatality associated with traumatic brain injury.[63-65]

GUIDELINES FOR TREATMENT

It is difficult to lay down hard and fast rules regarding the management of a disease as diverse as head injury. The primary aim to treatment is to prevent secondary damage to an already injured brain. Nevertheless, in 1995 a document was developed by the Brain Trauma Foundation that established treatment protocols for the management of TBI.[3,4] This document was the result of a joint effort between the Brain Trauma Foundation and the American Association of Neurological Surgeons. A panel of expert neurosurgeons with specific interests in the care of patients with severe head injury examined the available data on TBI. Recommendations of care were formulated relying on scientific evidence rather than expert opinion. The recommendations were classified as level I, II, or III, reflecting the degree of clinical certainty. Table 20.5 presents an outline of these recommendations.[3,4] The Brain Trauma Foundation updated these guidelines in 2007.[9] These updates will be applied to the following treatment recommendations and are included in Table 20.5.

MEDICAL THERAPY

Blood Pressure and Oxygenation

A significant portion of brain injury patients have hypotension and hypoxia in the prehospital and hospital setting. These confounding factors increase the resultant secondary brain injury. Presently the exact level of hypotension that is detrimental to outcome is unknown; however, systolic blood pressure (SBP) less than 90 mm Hg is the currently used definition of hypotension. The level of hypoxia is similarly unknown; however, the definition is apnea cyanosis in the field or a Pao_2 less than 60 mm Hg. Clinical studies have yet to show a decrease in morbidity and mortality rates in TBI patients when these factors are corrected. Currently there are insufficient data to support level I recommendations. There is level II evidence for monitoring blood pressure and avoiding hypotension defined as SBP less than 90 mm Hg.[9] Level III evidence exists for oxygenation monitoring and avoidance of hypoxia (Pao_2 <60 mm Hg or O_2 saturation <90%).[9]

Hyperosmolar Therapy

Classically the hyperosmolar therapy for elevated intracranial pressure consisted of mannitol. Recent literature has supported the use of hypertonic saline as a trauma resuscitation fluid, as well as a therapy for treating elevated ICP.

The indications for mannitol are as a one-time dose to lower ICP while obtaining further diagnostic studies or while waiting for definitive treatment. Mannitol has been used on an intermittent basis on a more prolonged timeline for the treatment of elevated ICP. There are few human trials that validate the currently used regimens of mannitol in most centers.

Mannitol's physiological effect relies on its ability to expand plasma, reduce hematocrit, and increase deformability of erythrocytes, reducing blood viscosity and increasing cerebral oxygenation delivery. Mannitol's effect takes place between 15 and 30 minutes while plasma gradients are established. Mannitol should be used with caution in patients with renal issues or on nephrotoxic drugs as serum osmolality rises and patients are at risk for acute tubular necrosis. Serum osmolality should not generally be allowed to go much above 320 mOsm/L, if possible, to avoid systemic acidosis and renal failure. There is clinical and laboratory evidence to suggest

TABLE 20.5 Level I (Standards), Level II (Guidelines), and Level III (Options) Recommendations in the Care of the Head-Injured Patient*

Application/ Indication	Level I	Level II	Level III
Trauma systems and the neurosurgeon	Insufficient data	All regions in the United States should have an organized trauma care system.	As delineated in the ACS Committee on Trauma Resources for Optimal Care of the Injured Patient, 1993: neurosurgeons should have an organized and responsive system of care.[40] Neurosurgeons should initiate neurotrauma care planning (prehospital management and triage), maintain call schedules, review trauma care records for quality improvement, and participate in trauma education.
Brain-specific treatments during initial resuscitation	Insufficient data	Insufficient data	The first priority is complete and physiological resuscitation. No specific treatments should be directed at intracranial hypertension in the absence of signs of transtentorial herniation or progressive neurological deterioration not attributable to extracranial explanation. If present, the physician should treat aggressively with rapid hyperventilation and mannitol under conditions of adequate volume resuscitation. If signs of expanding mass lesion or neurological deterioration. Recent literature indicates that hypertonic saline may be the resuscitation fluid of choice in trauma patients with head injury.
Resuscitation of blood pressure and oxygenation	Insufficient data	Blood pressure should be monitored and hypotension (SBP <90 mm Hg) avoided.	Oxygenation should be monitored and hypoxia (Pao_2 <60 mm Hg or O_2 <90%) avoided.
Hyperosmolar agents	Insufficient data	Dosage is .5 gm/kg to 1 gm/kg for mannitol use. Arterial hypotension (SBP <90 mm Hg) should be avoided.	Restrict mannitol use before ICP monitoring to patients with signs of transtentorial herniation or progressive neurological deterioration not attributable to extracranial causes. Further studies on hypertonic saline and mannitol are needed to determine ideal treatment of elevated ICP.
Hypothermia	Insufficient data	Insufficient data	Pooled data indicated that prophylactic hypothermia is not significantly associated with decreased mortality rate in comparison with normothermic control subjects. Preliminary findings point to a greater decrease in mortality risk with maintenance of target temperatures for more than 48 hours. Prophylactic hypothermia is associated with significantly higher GOS scores when compared with scores for normothermic control subjects.
Infection prophylaxis	Insufficient data	Periprocedural antibiotics for intubated patients should be administered to reduce incidence of pneumonia. This does not change length of stay or mortality risk. Early tracheostomy should be performed to reduce mechanical ventilation days. This does not alter mortality risk or the rate of nosocomial pneumonia.	Routine ventricular catheter exchange or prophylactic antibiotic use for ventricular catheter placement is not recommended to reduce infection. Early extubation in qualified patients can be done without increased risk in pneumonia.
DVT prophylaxis	Insufficient data	Insufficient data	Graduated compression stockings or intermittent pneumatic compression stockings (IPC) are recommended, unless contraindicated secondary to lower extremity injury; they should be continued until ambulation. Low-molecular-weight heparin or low-dose unfractionated heparin should be used in combination with mechanical prophylaxis; there is an increased risk for expansion of intracranial hemorrhage if present. Insufficient data are available to recommend preferred agent, dose, or timing of pharmacological initiation of DVT prophylaxis.

Continued

TABLE 20.5 Level I (Standards), Level II (Guidelines), and Level III (Options) Recommendations in the Care of the Head-Injured Patient*—cont'd

Application/ Indication	Level I	Level II	Level III
Indications for ICP monitoring	Insufficient data	ICP should be monitored in all salvageable patients with severe TBI (GCS 3-8) and an abnormal CT scan, defined as a scan showing contusions, edema, herniation, hematomas, or compressed basal cisterns.	ICP monitoring is indicated in patients with severe TBI and two or more of the following features: (1) age >40 years, (2) unilateral or bilateral motor posturing, or (3) SBP <90 mm Hg.
ICP monitoring technology	Insufficient data	Insufficient data	Currently the ventriculostomy catheter connected to an external strain gauge is the most accurate, low-cost, and reliable method of monitoring ICP. Parenchymal ICP monitors cannot be recalibrated during monitoring and have negligible drift. The drift is independent of the duration of monitoring. Subarachnoid, subdural, and epidural monitors are less accurate.
ICP treatment threshold	Insufficient data	ICP treatment should be initiated at an upper threshold of 20 mm Hg.	A combination of ICP values and clinical and brain CT findings should be used in the decision making for duration and type of ICP-lowering therapy.
CPP	Insufficient data	Aggressive attempts to maintain CPP >70 mm Hg with fluids and pressors should be avoided owing to associated risk of ARDS.	CPP <50 mm Hg should be avoided. CPP optimal target value lies between 50 and 70 mm Hg. Patients with intact cerebral autoregulation tolerate higher CPP values. Ancillary monitoring of cerebral parameters such as cerebral blood flow, cerebral oxygenation, or cerebral metabolism facilitates CPP management.
Brain oxygen monitoring and thresholds	Insufficient data	Insufficient data	Jugular venous saturation (<50%) or brain tissue oxygen tension (<15 mm Hg) are treatment thresholds. Jugular venous saturation or brain tissue oxygen monitoring measures cerebral oxygenation. Recent small reports show a decreased mortality risk with treating decreased cerebral oxygen values.
Anesthetics, analgesics, and sedatives	Insufficient data	Prophylactic administration of barbiturates to induce EEG suppression is not recommended. High-dose barbiturate administration is recommended to control elevated ICP refractory to maximum standard medical and surgical treatment. Hemodynamic stability is essential before and during barbiturate therapy. Propofol is recommended for the control of ICP but not for improvement in mortality risk or 6-month outcome. High-dose propofol can produce significant morbidity (propofol infusion syndrome).	None

TABLE 20.5 Level I (Standards), Level II (Guidelines), and Level III (Options) Recommendations in the Care of the Head-Injured Patient*—cont'd

Application/Indication	Level I	Level II	Level III
Nutrition	Insufficient data	Replace 140% of resting metabolism expenditure in nonparalyzed patients and 100% of resting metabolism expenditure in paralyzed patients using enteral or parenteral formulas containing at least 15% of calories as protein by day 7 after injury.	The preferable option is use of jejunal feeding by gastrojejunostomy, owing to ease of use and avoidance of gastric intolerance.
Antiseizure prophylaxis	Insufficient data	Prophylactic use of phenytoin or valproate is not recommended for preventing late PTSs. Anticonvulsants are indicated to decreased the incidence of early PTS (<7 days from injury). Early PTS is not associated with worse outcomes.	Phenytoin and carbamazepine have been demonstrated to be effective in preventing early PTSs. Levetiracetam has more recently been used in patients with TBI and shows promise to be as effective as phenytoin in preventing early PTSs, although further large-scale studies are needed.
Hyperventilation	Insufficient data	Prophylactic hyperventilation (Paco$_2$ < 25 mm Hg) is not recommended.	Hyperventilation therapy may be necessary for brief periods when there is acute neurological deterioration or for longer periods if there is intracranial hypertension refractory to sedation, chemical paralysis, CSF drainage, and osmotic diuretics. Jugular venous oxygen saturation, arteriojugular venous oxygen content differences, and cerebral blood flow monitoring may help to identify cerebral ischemia if hyperventilation, resulting in Paco$_2$ values <30 mm Hg is necessary. More recently, brain tissue oxygen tension monitoring has been suggested also to be of benefit in evaluating brain oxygen delivery. Hyperventilation should be avoided in the first 24 hours after brain injury, when cerebral blow flow often is critically reduced and autoregulation is disrupted.
Glucocorticoids	The use of glucocorticoids is not recommended for improving outcome or reducing ICP in patients with severe head injury. In patients with moderate to severe TBI, high-dose methylprednisolone is associated with increased mortality risk and is contraindicated.	None	None

ACS, American College of Surgeons; ARDS, acute respiratory distress syndrome; CPP, cerebral perfusion pressure; DVT, deep vein thrombosis; EEG, electroencephalogram; GCS, Glasgow Coma Scale; GOS, Glasgow Outcome Scale; ICP, intracranial pressure; PTSs, post-traumatic seizures; SBP, systolic blood pressure; TBI traumatic brain injury.
Updated by the Brain Trauma Foundation, 2007.

that long-term, repeated use of mannitol can worsen brain edema and hence reverse the initial beneficial effect.[27] Mannitol has been shown to have an effect on ICP lasting from 90 minutes to 6 hours or more.

Recently studies on small volume resuscitations have shown the therapeutic effectiveness of hypertonic saline (HS) administration. Hypertonic saline solutions were administered in poly-trauma patients with hemorrhagic shock, and the subset of patients in the group with TBI showed an increase in survival and stabilization of hemodynamic properties.[9] As a result of this finding, other studies have been conducted showing its utility in the treatment of elevated ICP in trauma, subarachnoid hemorrhage, stroke, and other pathological insults.

The effect of HS on ICP is theorized to come from mobilization of water across the blood-brain barrier, decreasing cerebral water content. HS also increases plasma volume and cerebral blood flow. HS must be used with caution in patients with underlying cardiac or pulmonary issues as they are at risk for pulmonary edema. It must also be used with caution in patients with hyponatremia because rapid correction may lead to central pontine myelinolysis.

The theoretic advantage of using HS therapy over mannitol lies in the fact the HS pulls water intravascularly, increasing blood pressure and maintaining cerebral perfusion. Mannitol has the unfortunate result of diuresis and potential decrease in blood pressure, decreasing cerebral perfusion pressure.

Current Brain Trauma Foundation guidelines show level II evidence for mannitol's effective control of raised ICP at doses between 0.25 mg/kg to 1 g/kg of body weight.[9] Level II evidence exists to avoid hypotension (SBP <90 mm Hg).[9] Recent studies of HS show its utility in a continuous infusion form or as bolus treatment form equivalent to or superior to mannitol for refractory elevated ICP.[66-69] More studies need to be performed to evaluate mannitol versus HS with respect to clinical outcome after TBI.

Furosemide

Furosemide (Lasix) has been used alone and in conjunction with mannitol in the treatment of raised ICP. It has been shown that diuresis can be enhanced by the combined use of these agents with more pronounced and consistent brain shrinkage. A dose of 0.3 to 0.5 mg/kg of furosemide given intravenously is reasonable. When using diuretics the blood pressure must be monitored closely to prevent hypotension. This drug is not commonly used in TBI management at present.

Prophylactic Hypothermia

The utility of hypothermia in TBI has inconsistent results in the medical literature. During the BTF review of the literature mortality rate was affected only by the duration of cooling, which meant a decrease in mortality rate if cooling was for more than 48 hours.[9] Target cooling temperatures or rate of rewarming had no effect on outcome. The pathophysiological theory behind this treatment is that ICP can be decreased by decreasing brain metabolic demand.

Interpretation of trials involving hypothermia is difficult secondary to confounding factors affecting outcome. It appears that patients who are treated with hypothermia have a trend to more favorable outcome, Glasgow Outcome Scale

scores of 4 to 5. Currently there are no level I or level II recommendations for this treatment. A Cochrane Database review in 2009 found no evidence that hypothermia is beneficial in the treatment of head injury. Hypothermia may be effective in reducing death and unfavorable outcomes for traumatic head-injured patients, but significant benefit was only found in low-quality trials.[9] High-quality trials found no decrease in the likelihood of death with hypothermia, but this finding was not statistically significant and could be due to the play of chance.[9] Hypothermia should not be used except in the context of a high-quality randomized controlled trial with good allocation concealment.[9]

Infection Prophylaxis

In polytrauma patients the risk of infection can be increased significantly secondary to intubation, invasive lines, and placement of intracranial monitors. Infections can be broken down into infection/colonization of ICP monitors and infection/colonization of peripheral lines/pneumonia. Most trials of prophylactic antibiotics have shown selection of more virulent gram-negative organisms. Currently BTF guidelines recommend at a level II the use of periprocedural antibiotics for intubation to reduce the incidence of pneumonia.[9] This does not change length of stay or mortality rates. Early tracheostomy reduces mechanical ventilation days, but it does not alter mortality rate or nosocomial pneumonia rate. There is level III evidence against the routine use of prophylactic antibiotics for ventricular catheter placement.[9] There is currently level III evidence against the routine use of ventricular catheter exchange to prevent infection.[9]

Deep Venous Thrombosis Prophylaxis

The risk of developing deep venous thrombosis (DVT) in the absence of prophylaxis was found to be 20% after severe TBI in a study by Kaufman and associates.[70] This risk is related to systemic trauma as well as the relative period of immobility these patients face. DVTs of the distal lower extremity veins tend to be clinically silent and tend to stay that. Proximal lower extremity DVTs are more likely to produce symptoms clinically and result in pulmonary embolism (PE). The treatment of DVT and PE in the TBI patient is complicated by the uncertainty of the safety of anticoagulation, specifically in postcraniotomy patients or those with intracerebral hemorrhage from their trauma.

Prophylaxis options can be considered in two categories: mechanical versus pharmacological. These can be thought of in a graduated fashion ranging from graduated compression stockings, intermittent pneumatic compression stockings, and finally anticoagulant medications (low-dose heparin and low-molecular-weight heparin).

In studies comparing pharmacological versus mechanical treatment for the prevention of DVT, pharmacological treatment is more efficacious in preventing DVT but there is a trend toward increased risk of intracranial bleeding.[9] There are no current recommendations as to the timing or optimal dosing of pharmacological prophylaxis in neurosurgical patients with the current evidence.

Current BTF guidelines show level III evidence for graduated compression stockings or intermittent pneumatic compression stockings unless lower extremity injury prevents their use.[9] Low-molecular-weight heparin or low-dose unfractionated heparin should be used in combination with mechanical prophylaxis, but there is an increased risk for expansion of intracranial hemorrhage. There are currently no timing recommendations for the initiation of pharmacological DVT prophylaxis.

Intracranial Pressure Monitoring

With the relatively recent understanding of the evolution of brain injury starting at impact and continuing through as secondary insults in the following hours and days the management has taken shape in attempts to prevent these secondary injuries. This understanding has led to protocols to prevent hypotension, hypoxia, and anemia as discussed earlier and maintaining CPP. As discussed earlier the mean arterial pressure minus the ICP equals the CPP. The main way to ensure adequate CPP is to monitor arterial pressure and ICP.

Monitoring ICP can be used to monitor patients for worsening intracranial injury, help predict outcome, calculate CPP, and if ventriculostomy is used, therapeutic CSF drainage. When comparing patients with ICP monitoring to prior reports of patients without monitoring, monitored patients have improved outcome.[9]

Monitoring options include intraparenchymal monitors (Camino monitor), ventriculostomy catheter, and brain oxygen tension monitor (Licox). Ventriculostomy remains the gold standard, as it can monitor ICP as well as drain fluid as a therapeutic treatment to lower elevated ICP. The Licox monitor has the ability to measure ICP as well as brain oxygenation. The utility of these measurements has shown decreased morbidity and mortality rates in the recent literature, as discussed earlier.

Currently BTF guidelines show level II evidence for placing an ICP monitor in all salvageable patients with severe TBI defined by a postresuscitation GCS score of 3 to 8 and an abnormal CT scan of the head.[9] An abnormal CT of the head is defined as one showing hematomas, contusions, swelling, herniation, or compressed basal cisterns.[9] Current level III evidence exists for ICP monitoring in patients with severe TBI with a normal CT and two or more of the following: (1) age over 40 years, (2) unilateral or bilateral motor posturing, or (3) systolic blood pressure less than 90 mm Hg.[38] These three factors were found to have higher incidence of elevated ICP in patients with normal admission CT scan.

Intracranial Pressure Monitor Technology

As stated in the previous section different types of intracranial monitors exist. The ideal monitor should have several useful qualities including ease of insertion, safety of insertion, accuracy, reliability, cost effectiveness, and the need for minimal troubleshooting. The Association for the Advancement of Medical Instrumentation (AAMI) was developed in association with a neurosurgery committee. This association led to the development of the American National Standard for Intracranial Pressure Monitoring Devices. The job of this standard is to provide labeling, safety, and performance requirements of intracranial monitors. According to the AAMI standard, ICP monitors should have (1) pressure ranges of 0 to 100 mm Hg, (2) accuracy ±2 mm Hg in the range of 0 to 20 mm Hg, and

(3) maximum error of 10% in the range of 20 to 100 mm Hg.[9] The current ICP monitors work via external strain, catheter tip strain, or catheter tip fiberoptics. Catheter tip fiberoptics are calibrated prior to intracranial insertion and are at risk for measurement drift and possible inaccurate readings.

Current available ICP monitors were ranked based on accuracy, reliability, and cost. The order of ranking is as follows: (1) intraventricular devices (fluid-coupled catheter), (2) intraventricular devices (microstrain gauge or fiberoptic), (3) parenchymal pressure transducers, (4) subdural devices, (5) subarachnoid fluid couple devices, and (6) epidural devices.[9]

The ventricular catheter connected to an external strain gauge remains the most cost effective and reliable method of ICP monitoring.[9] However, solid state monitors such as the Camino or Codman systems are generally reliable, although they cannot be recalibrated once they have been inserted.

Treatment Thresholds and Optimal Cerebral Perfusion Pressure

The threshold to treat elevated ICP should be based on the patient's CT scan, clinical picture, and ICP number. Multiple small studies show the optimal treatment window to be between 15 and 25 mm Hg. It is important to emphasize that patients with temporal hematomas or posterior fossa hemorrhages may have deceptively low ICP despite being under neurological duress. Current level II evidence recommends treating patients with ICP greater than 20 mm Hg with ICP lowering measures.[9]

The management paradigm of elevated CPP (>70 mm Hg) for treatment of TBI became popular in the late 1980s. It has since been found that the optimal CPP ranges between 50 and 70 mm Hg.[9] Currently level II evidence recommends keeping CPP less than 70 mm Hg because systemic complications are increased when the CPP is elevated above this level. Current level III evidence suggests a CPP less than 50 mm Hg should be avoided; the optimal range is somewhere between 50 and 70 mm Hg.[9] Ancillary monitoring of blood flow, oxygenation, or metabolism helps to facilitate on a patient-by-patient basis the optimal CPP.

Brain Oxygenation Monitoring and Threshold for Treatment

In recent years the monitoring of cerebral oxygenation has taken form in two different ways: (1) brain oxygenation monitoring probes, and (2) jugular venous oxygen monitoring. Other novel monitoring techniques have been developed but have yet to be substantiated in clinical studies. Abnormal venous jugular oxygen levels have been correlated with poor outcomes. High and low values have been associated with poor outcomes, which is believed to be related to brain metabolism. Venous jugular oxygenation is more helpful when arteriojugular difference in oxygenation is measured, most likely giving a more accurate picture of cerebral metabolism.

Multiple studies have shown that a diminished oxygenation of brain tissue (as measured by the partial pressure of oxygen in brain tissue, P_{BTO_2}) is correlated with poorer outcomes and death.[63-65] Treatments to keep P_{BTO_2} greater than

25 mm Hg along with CPP and ICP management have shown decreased mortality rates when compared to outcomes of treating CPP and ICP alone.[63-65]

Even though treatments to maintain cerebral oxygenation seem promising there is only level III evidence for jugular venous monitoring and brain tissue oxygen tension monitoring.[9] Treatment thresholds are less than 50% for jugular venous saturation and more than 15 mm Hg for brain tissue oxygenation.[9]

Anesthesia, Analgesics, and Sedatives

It has been long understood that pain and agitation may raise ICP in the TBI patient. Pain medications and sedatives have often been used to calm patients to prevent a dangerous rise in ICP that may be associated with severe agitation. Barbiturates have been used since the 1930s with the knowledge of their ability to lower ICP.[71] Barbiturates are also known to decrease cerebral metabolism having a cerebral protective effect.[72,73] The use of barbiturates couples blood flow to cerebral metabolism, decreasing blood flow where metabolism is low and shunting blood flow to areas where metabolism is high.

Prophylactic administration has not proved to be effective in preventing elevated ICP. The Cochrane group reviewed two randomized controlled trials of barbiturate use showing no evidence of improved outcomes in severe TBI. They also found that there was a 25% chance of hypotension when receiving barbiturates, offsetting any effect of ICP lowering. To monitor for appropriate sedation patients are placed on electroencephalograph (EEG) monitoring. Dosing to burst suppression reduces cerebral metabolism to maximal reduction.

Propofol has more recently been studied because of its quick onset of action, and its short duration of action allows quick neurological assessment. Studies have shown that propofol does have a minimal effect at lowering ICP, and one study reported high-dose propofol showing a favorable neurological outcome when compared to a low-dose propofol.[74] Propofol must be used with caution, especially in high doses, as some patients develop propofol infusion syndrome, which may lead to death.

BTF guidelines currently have level II evidence that *prophylactic* administration of barbiturates to burst suppression is not recommended. High-dose barbiturate treatment is recommended for refractory ICP control; however, hemodynamic stability must be maintained and improved outcomes have never been proved.[9] Propofol is recommended for the control of ICP, but not for improvement of 6-month outcomes.[9]

Nutrition

It is known that patients with TBI have dysfunction of metabolism. These patients require a higher nitrogen intake as their nitrogen balance becomes negative. Studies show that TBI patients' caloric intake had a mean increase of 140%. Studies have shown a decreased mortality rate when full caloric replacement is achieved by 7 days. Typically to reach this goal caloric replacement begins around 72 hours after injury.

There are three ways to initiate early feeding: gastric, jejunal, and parenteral. It is important to maintain normoglycemia in head injury patients as hyperglycemia has been associated with worse outcomes.

Current level II evidence recommends that patients should be fed full caloric replacement by 7 days after injury.[9]

Antiseizure Prophylaxis

The role of prophylactic anticonvulsants in patients with severe head injury has been more clearly defined with the advent of the published guidelines. Post-traumatic seizures are classified as "early," occurring within 7 days of injury, or "late," occurring more than 7 days after the injury.[75,76] It is desirable to prevent early and late seizure activity, although these medications have been associated with adverse and neurobehavioral ill effects. The classic study by Jennett[77] found post-traumatic epilepsy to occur in about 5% of all patients admitted to the hospital with closed head injuries and in 15% of those with severe head injuries. Three main factors were found to be linked to a high incidence of late epilepsy: early seizures occurring within the first week, an intracranial hematoma, or a depressed skull fracture. Recent updates show that post-traumatic seizures are also associated with GCS scores less than 10, penetrating head wound, or a seizure within the first 24 hours. Although certain earlier studies were unable to show significant benefit of prophylactically administered anticonvulsants, a double-blind study of 404 patients with severe head injury, who were randomized to receive phenytoin or placebo beginning within 24 hours of injury and continuing for 1 year, found that phenytoin reduced the incidence of seizures in the first week after injury but not thereafter.[78] This study appears to justify stopping prophylactic convulsants after the first week in most cases. In patients who have had a seizure, anticonvulsants are continued for at least a year.

With the recent use of Keppra (levetiracetam) as an antiepileptic, with its relatively low side effect profile, studies have been done to evaluate its efficacy compared to the gold standard Dilantin (phenytoin). It does appear to be as effective as Dilantin at preventing early seizures with a lower side effect profile.[79,80] Larger scale studies will need to be done to confirm this finding. It should also be noted the Keppra had a tendency to show more seizure activity on EEG analysis in one study.[79]

Current BTF recommendations show level II evidence that Dilantin and valproate are not indicated to prevent *late* onset seizure activity.[9] Level II evidence shows that antiepileptic medication is indicated to prevent early onset seizure (within 7 days); however, early onset post-traumatic seizure have not been proved to be associated with worse outcomes.[9]

Hyperventilation

Hyperventilation has been used in the treatment of severe TBI for the past 20 years. Recent pathophysiological understanding of TBI and the mechanism of ICP lowering of hyperventilation have put it under recent scrutiny. Hyperventilation decreases ICP by decreasing CO_2 leading to cerebral vasoconstriction. This in turn leads to decreased cerebral blood flow (CBF). Aggressive sustained hyperventilation may lead to cerebral ischemia and stroke, especially in the severe TBI patient who may already have alterations in CBF and autoregulation.

Hyperventilation does have utility in the deteriorating TBI patient as a temporizing measure until more definitive treatment of elevated ICP may be implemented.

Current BTF recommendations show level II evidence against the routine use of prophylactic hyperventilation to $Paco_2$ less than 25 mm Hg.[9] Level III evidence exists that hyperventilation may be used as a temporizing measure in the acutely deteriorating patient.[9] Hyperventilation should be avoided in the first 24 hours after TBI when CBF may be critically reduced. If hyperventilation is used, there is level III evidence for jugular venous oxygen monitoring or brain tissue oxygen tension monitoring.[9]

Steroids

While steroids are clearly useful in reducing the edema associated with brain tumors, their value in head injury is not clear. In fact, most studies to date have not demonstrated any beneficial effect associated with steroids in terms of either ICP control or improved outcome from severe head injury. Furthermore, there is some evidence that steroids may have a deleterious effect on metabolism in these patients. It is possible that very high doses of particular steroids may have a beneficial effect in certain subsets of head-injured patients. However, currently available steroids in standard dose regimens have not proved to be valuable in severe head injury.

Level I evidence currently recommends against the routine use of steroids for improving outcome or reducing ICP.[9] It has been shown in patients with moderate to severe TBI on high-dose methylprednisolone that mortality rate is increased.[9]

SURGICAL THERAPY

Indications for Surgery

An important reason for operating on a mass lesion is a midline shift of 5 mm or more. Such a shift may be demonstrated by CT scan, occasionally by angiography or ventriculography. Most epidural, subdural, or intracerebral hematomas associated with a midline shift of 5 mm or more are surgically evacuated. In a patient who has a small hematoma causing less than 5 mm shift and is alert and neurologically intact, a conservative approach is justified. However, the patient may deteriorate, and very close observation is vital. Should there be any change in mental status, a repeat CT scan should be obtained immediately.

Our policy is to operate on all comatose patients with an intracranial mass lesion and 5 mm or more of midline shift unless they are brain-dead. This policy is based on evidence that some patients with bilaterally nonreactive pupils, impaired oculocephalic responses, and decerebrate posturing can nevertheless make a good recovery. In one series, 3 of 19 such patients who were treated maximally ended up in the "good" or "moderately disabled" category, despite the foreboding constellation of signs.[81]

The management of brain contusions is somewhat less clear-cut. Galbraith and Teasdale,[82] in their series of 26 patients with acute traumatic intracranial hematomas who were managed without surgery, found that all patients with ICP greater than 30 mm Hg eventually deteriorated and

required surgery. In contrast, only one patient with ICP less than 20 mm Hg deteriorated. Patients in the 20 to 30 mm Hg range were about evenly divided between the surgical and nonsurgical groups.

We have recently analyzed our experience with 130 head-injured patients with pure contusions who were managed with CT scanning and ICP monitoring as needed.[83] This study showed that patients with brain contusions who could follow commands at admission did not require ICP monitoring and, as a rule, did well with simple observation. However, those who could not follow commands (in the absence of a focal lesion in the speech area) often had intracranial hypertension and needed to have their ICP monitored. The majority of these patients who had a midline shift of 5 mm or more required surgery.

It has been demonstrated conclusively that patients with a large (over 30 mL) temporal lobe hematoma have a much greater risk of developing tentorial herniation than those with a frontal or parieto-occipital lesion.[84] The bias should therefore tilt toward early surgery in such cases.

Once a decision has been made as to whether the patient is a surgical candidate or not, he or she is promptly moved to the operating room or to the neurosurgical intensive care unit (NICU), respectively. If the patient is harboring a mass lesion, mannitol (1-2 g/kg) should be administered en route to the operating room. In addition, the patient can be hyperventilated briefly to achieve an arterial PCO_2 of 25 to 30 mm Hg. As in all the maneuvers undertaken thus far, time is of the essence. The sooner the mass lesion is evacuated, the better the possibility of a good recovery.[24] If, on the other hand, no surgical lesion is found, the patient is carefully monitored in the NICU, both clinically and with various physiological parameters, notably ICP recordings and serial CT scans. Any rise in ICP above 20 mm Hg that cannot be readily explained and reversed or any deterioration in neurological status warrants prompt repetition of the CT scan followed by appropriate corrective measures.

Because there is great concern about increased ICP as a result of a mass lesion, the anesthetic agents that are used in head-injured patients preferably should not increase the ICP. Nitrous oxide has only a slight vasodilatory effect and generally does not cause a significant ICP increase. It is therefore considered a good agent for use in the head-injured patient. A commonly used combination is nitrous oxide with oxygen, intravenous muscle relaxant, and propofol. Hyperventilation and mannitol prior to and during induction can blunt the vasodilatory effect and limit intracranial hypertension to some degree while the cranium is being opened. If, during surgery, malignant brain swelling occurs that is refractory to hyperventilation and mannitol, pentobarbital in large doses (5-10 mg/kg) should be used. This agent can cause hypotension, especially in hypovolemic patients, and should therefore be used with caution.

Subdural Hematomas

Acute subdural hematomas may result from bleeding from lacerated brain, ruptured cortical vessels, or an avulsed bridging vein. The most common sites for brain injury are the inferior frontal lobes and the anterior temporal lobes. In the surgical management of subdural hematomas, a large fronto-temporoparietal question mark–shaped incision is recommended. This allows the surgeon to deal with bleeding near the midline as well as to débride effectively parts of the frontal, temporal, and parietal lobes as needed. If the patient is deteriorating rapidly, a quick temporal decompression can be performed via a small craniectomy before opening up the rest of the flap. This maneuver could reduce the probability of tentorial herniation. A generous subtemporal craniectomy may be useful in postoperative ICP control. The role of decompressive craniotomy with removal of the bone flap and creation of a dural pouch to allow brain swelling is currently being examined.

Epidural Hematomas

Epidural hematomas are most often located in the temporal region and often result from tearing of the middle meningeal vessels due to a temporal bone fracture. Venous epidural hematomas may occur as a result of a skull fracture or an associated venous sinus injury. These tend to be smaller and usually have a more benign course. Such hematomas often present several hours or days after the initial injury and can be managed nonsurgically. However, usually an epidural hematoma represents a surgical emergency and should be evacuated as rapidly as possible. Every effort should be made to relieve the pressure as soon as possible. A more localized craniotomy flap is warranted for epidural hematomas.

Contusions/Intracerebral Hematomas

Contusions are most often located in the anterior and inferior frontal lobes as well as the anterior temporal lobes. Quite commonly, the CT appearance of a contusion evolves over several days so that what are initially small "salt and pepper" lesions coalesce to form hematomas. This phenomenon is also termed *delayed traumatic intracerebral hematoma*. Patients who are awake and alert but demonstrate cerebral contusions can be managed without surgery in the vast majority of cases.[83] However, patients who are comatose and have a significant midline shift usually need surgery. Between these two extremes, there are patients who demonstrate alterations in levels of consciousness or focal neurological deficits; in these, the decision to undertake surgical débridement is not always easy. As a general rule, débridement of the left frontal and temporal lobes is undertaken more reluctantly because the speech area is on this side.

Depressed Skull Fractures

A skull fracture is considered significantly depressed if the outer table of the skull lies below the level of the inner table of the surrounding bone. Sometimes such depression may not be evident on plain radiographs, but it is usually seen clearly on the CT scan. Most closed depressed fractures occur in young children and may be of the ping-pong ball variety. Surgery may be undertaken in such cases for cosmetic reasons or because of brain compression. In compound depressed fractures, the wounds are often dirty and contaminated. Hair, skin, or other foreign debris may be insinuated between the depressed bone fragments. Therefore, except in the simplest of injuries, the use of the operating room for the closure of such wounds is recommended.

Venous Sinus Injuries

Injuries of the major venous sinuses are among the most difficult problems a neurosurgeon has to face. As a general rule, ligation of the anterior third of the superior sagittal sinus is tolerated well; ligation of the posterior third is most likely to produce massive venous infarction of the brain. Ligation of the middle third of the superior sagittal sinus has somewhat unpredictable effects. A dominant transverse sinus usually cannot be safely ligated. Although the use of shunts in the repair of these major sinuses has been often described, in our experience simple pressure with the use of hemostatic agents is much more practical in the majority of cases.

Posterior Fossa Hematomas

Posterior fossa hematomas, fortunately, are less common than supratentorial hematomas. In general, an aggressive surgical approach is recommended for most of these lesions because the patient can deteriorate very rapidly. Because it generally takes longer to expose the posterior fossa and because the brainstem structures are likely to suffer irreversible damage from a shorter period of compression, the surgeon does not have much leeway in terms of time.

PROGNOSIS

The Glasgow Outcome Scale (GOS) has been widely accepted as a standard means of describing outcome in head injury patients. This is a simple five-point scale (Table 20.6).[85] These categories are sometimes lumped together as either favorable outcomes (G, MD) or unfavorable outcomes (SD, V, or D). Post-traumatic amnesia is a fairly good prognostic indicator of outcome. First described by Russel in 1932, post-traumatic amnesia is defined as the duration of time from the point of injury until the patient has continuous memory of ongoing events. In most cases, the retrospective measurement of post-traumatic amnesia is unreliable. Therefore, Harvey Levin developed the Galveston Orientation and Amnesia Test (GOAT) to provide an objective reliable measurement of post-traumatic amnesia. The duration of post-traumatic amnesia has proved to be highly correlated with ultimate functional outcomes.[86]

Several statistical studies have reported the use of various prognostic indicators for predicting outcome in severe head injury. Because of unexpected medical and surgical complications and the inherent unpredictability of disease, there is no

TABLE 20.6 Glasgow Outcome Scale (GOS)	
Good recovery (G)	Patient returns to preinjury level of function
Moderately disabled (MD)	Patient has neurological deficits but is able to look after self
Severely disabled (SD)	Patient is unable to look after self
Vegetative (V)	No evidence of higher mental function
Dead (D)	

absolutely unfailing prediction system. Based on experience with a large group of patients, an algorithm has been developed for approximate expected outcomes associated with certain prognostic features.[87] An attempt to predict mortality with 100% certainty appeared to work in one center.[88] However, when this system was applied to other patient populations, some patients who were predicted to die based on this scale instead survived.[89]

This highlights the difficulty in making foolproof predictions of outcome in patients with head injury. Nevertheless, certain broad predictions can be made based on the patient's initial examination and this can be valuable in counseling the family.

SELECTED KEY REFERENCES

Bullock MR, Chestnut R, Ghajar J, et al. Surgical management of TBI author group. *Neurosurgery.* 2006;58(suppl 3): S1-S62.

Bullock R, Chestnut RM, Clifton G, et al. Guidelines for the management of severe head injury. *J Neurotrauma.* 2000;17:449-627.

Chestnut RM, Ghajar J, Maas AIL, et al. Early indicators of prognosis in severe traumatic brain injury. *J Neurotrauma.* 2000;17:557-590.

Feldman Z, Narayan RK. Intracranial pressure monitoring: techniques and pitfalls. In: Cooper PR, ed. *Head Injury.* 3rd ed. Philadelphia: Williams & Wilkins; 1993:247-274.

Oddo M, Levine JM, Frangos S, et al. Effect of mannitol and hypertonic saline on cerebral oxygenation in patients with severe traumatic brain injury and refractory intracranial hypertension. *J Neurol Neurosurg Psychiatry.* 2009;80(8):916-920.

Temkin NR, Dikmen SS, Winn HR. Posttraumatic seizures. *Neurosurg Clin North Am.* 1991;2:425-435.

Please go to expertconsult.com to view the complete list of references.

CHAPTER
21   Penetrating Brain Injury

Michael Cirivello, Randy S. Bell, Rocco A. Armonda

CLINICAL PEARLS

- In the presence of penetrating brain injury, the first step is to initiate advanced trauma life support resuscitation with early transportation to definitive care.

- The major principles of management of penetrating brain injuries include early decompression with conservative débridement of the brain. Surgeons should avoid disrupting functional eloquent cortex when chasing deep-seated fragments. In addition, it is important to identify and remove superficial expanding hematoma and foreign material, reconstruct the anterior skull base, and attempt a watertight dural closure.

- One should attempt to avoid secondary injury (i.e., meningitis, seizures, delayed vasospasm, and thrombo-embolic stroke) through protocol-driven neurocritical care, which includes monitoring intracranial pressure and drainage of cerebrospinal fluid.

- It is essential to maintain a high suspicion for acute and delayed neurovascular injuries (i.e., traumatic aneurysms) with subsequent endovascular evaluation and treatment when indicated.

- Delayed or immediate restoration of normal anatomy can be accomplished through craniofacial reconstruction techniques.

Penetrating brain injury (PBI) is a neurosurgical problem that presents a host of management challenges depending on its mechanism, location, and ensuing complications. Good outcomes for those who survive the initial injury can depend not only on accurate and early surgical intervention but also on the ability to provide high-level neurocritical care in a timely fashion. Epidemiologically, penetrating head injury (PHI) and trauma, in general, affect a younger demographic worldwide, and as a result such injury carries a high socioeconomic burden.

The modern treatment of PBI has developed predominantly from military experience, beginning with Dr. Harvey Cushing's classification of head injuries from World War I, and continues today with lessons learned from penetrating trauma in Operation Enduring Freedom (OEF) and Operation Iraqi Freedom (OIF). Although it may be argued that the mechanism of both civilian and military PHI constitutes the same traumatic forces, we must be careful to generalize recommendations for treatment and draw distinctions where appropriate. The goal of this chapter is to provide a historical overview of penetrating injury, look at prognosis of PBI in civilian and military populations, review patterns of injury, and provide recommendations for management based on the current literature.

HISTORICAL BACKGROUND

No discussion of the neurosurgical management of penetrating brain injury is complete without first acknowledging Dr. Harvey Cushing's contributions during World War I. His landmark 1918 *British Journal of Surgery* article consisted of a retrospective review and classification of 219 cranial injuries and associated rates of mortality.[1] In this paper he advocated aggressive débridement of necrotic tissue, removal of all in-driven debris, and meticulous scalp and dural closure. With this strategy he was able to decrease the incidence of brain abscesses and thereby lower the operative mortality rate from 55% to 29% within a 3-month period (Table 21.1).

This approach continued throughout World War II and was refined by Dr. Donald Matson in his classic monograph published in 1958.[2] Matson described the principal tenets of performing initial lifesaving interventions, preventing infection, preserving neurological function, and restoring normal anatomy. These strategies hold as true today as then and have developed into modern advanced trauma life support (ATLS) guidelines,[3] aseptic surgical techniques, prevention of secondary injury through neurocritical care, and craniofacial reconstruction.

Cushing's strategy of débridement continued to be applied in both the Korean War and the Vietnam conflict where early experiences with less aggressive approaches were met with higher infection rates and increased mortality rates.[4-6] It was not until the Israel/Lebanon conflict of 1982, when computed tomography (CT) first became routine in the assessment of head injury, that a more conservative approach was advocated in favor of brain preservation. This approach was validated by 6 years of follow-up in the studies by Brandvolt and associates and Levi and colleagues and by 8 years of follow-up in a similar group of patients from the Iran-Iraq war of 1986 by Amirjamshidi and co-workers revealing no statistically significant increase in delayed infection or seizure disorders.[7-9] A report of early experience with conservative débridement in Operation Desert Storm continued to find similar results[10] (Fig. 21.1).

In 1995, the Brain Trauma Foundation developed the first traumatic brain injury (TBI) guidelines with the assistance of international experts in the field to address the need for protocol-driven health care based upon the most current scientific literature. In 2001, guidelines for the care of PBI were created toward the same end with the support of the Brain Injury Association, the International Brain Injury Association, the American Association of Neurological Surgeons (AANS), and members of the Congress of Neurological Surgeons (CNS). These guidelines stand as the most comprehensive evidence-based evaluation of interventions specific to the care of PBI and are summarized in Table 21.2.[11] It is worth mentioning, however, that despite the exhaustive literature search used to develop the guidelines, no recommendation achieves a level beyond that of *option* and this underscores the need for further research. No level I or II data exist on the subject.

Craniofacial injuries sustained during OEF and OIF have resulted in further modifications to the management of patients with severe PBI.[12-18] Although aggressive débridement of the brain is no longer used, early and aggressive cranial decompression with subsequent watertight dural closure is the current accepted practice (see Fig. 21.1).[18] This strategy affords the patient protection from significant elevations in intracranial pressure (ICP) during the long flights, unaccompanied by neurosurgeons, from operative theaters back to the United States. This initial stabilization is then followed by protocol-driven neurocritical care aimed at preventing secondary neurological decline and maximizing neurological recovery. Though the data are still under review, preliminary analysis appears favorable[15,19] (Fig. 21.2).

PROGNOSIS

Civilian PBI has high mortality rates that remain refractory to medical and neurosurgical advances based on the most recent case series.[20,21] The mortality rate in most retrospective cohorts is greater than 70% owing in large part to the higher percentage of gunshot wounds (see Fig. 21.2), suicides, and the ubiquitous absence of cranial protection (helmets) compared to military injuries.[22-26] Other variables that differentiate these two groups are presented in Table 21.3. The reported civilian mortality rates from gunshot wounds to the head (GSWH) in the literature range from 23% to 92% with those series on the lower end including a number of cases without dural violation.[27-29] Death from PBI occurs shortly after injury with 70% of patients succumbing after the first 24 hours[23,25] (Table 21.4).

Prognostic indicators were classified as a separate section in the 2001 PBI guidelines and are summarized in Table 21.4.[11] Of these factors and consistent with data in other forms of TBI, a postresuscitation Glasgow Coma Scale (GCS) score stands as the most reliable predictor of death and other unfavorable outcomes.[30] This measure is a consistent predictor for both civilian and military populations but appears to have the greatest correlation with civilian mortality. In series segregating out patients with poor presenting neurological function or upon subgroup analysis of those with GCS scores of 3 to 5, mortality rate rises to 87% to 100%.[25-31] A recommended triage for both military and civilian patients is located in Figure 21.3.

Because of the many dissimilar characteristics between civilian and military populations it has been difficult to correlate the weight of certain prognostic factors and to compare treatment measures across groups; however, a recent study by Dubose and associates compared the epidemiology and outcomes of military and civilian severe TBI.[19] The Joint Trauma Theater Registry (JTTR) database and the American College of Surgeons' National Trauma Data Bank (NTDB), both the largest patient databases of their kind, were queried for severe TBI and PBI. Subgroup analysis then selected for isolated PBI from gunshot wounds and statistically matched counterparts across the same period of 2003 to 2006. The results showed a threefold increase toward neurosurgical

Grade	Description	No. of Patients	Mortality Rate (%)
I	Scalp lacerations with intact skull	22	4.5
II	Wounds with skull fractures/intact dura/with or without depression	54	9.2
III	Wounds with depressed skull fracture/dural laceration	18	11.8
IV	Wounds (guttering type) with in-driven fragments, usually protruding brain	25	24
V	Penetrating wound, lodged projectile, brain usually protruding	41	36.6
VI	Wounds penetrating ventricles with either (a) bone fragments or (b) projectiles	14 (a) 16 (b)	42.8 100
VII	Wounds involving orbitonasal or auropetrosal region with extruding brain	15	73.3
VIII	Perforating wounds, cerebral injury severe	5	80
IX	Craniocerebral injury with massive skull fracture	10	50

TABLE 21.1 Cushing's Classification of World War I Injuries

Modified from Cushing H. A series of wounds involving the brain and its enveloping structures. Br J Surg 1918;5:558-684.

intervention in the JTTR group compared with civilian, particularly in the way of ICP monitoring (13.8% vs. 1.7%). Outcomes showed a tenfold decrease in mortality rate in the JTTR over their NTDB counterparts (5.6% vs. 47.9%). Although a dramatic difference in mortality rates between these populations is not new, this study excludes the confounding differences in explosive fragment PBI and GSWH injuries and allows for a more direct comparison of pertinent factors.

To make these populations truly comparable, however, the high rate of suicides and point-blank injuries in the civilian population needs to be accounted for in the analysis. In the most recent case series of civilian GSWH, Hofbauer and colleagues analyzed the impact of shooting distance on mortality rate in contact, near-contact, intermediate range, and at distance.[21] Those at intermediate and long distances had a 0% mortality rate of 19 patients treated. In contrast, the contact group showed mortality rates of 91% with self-inflicted

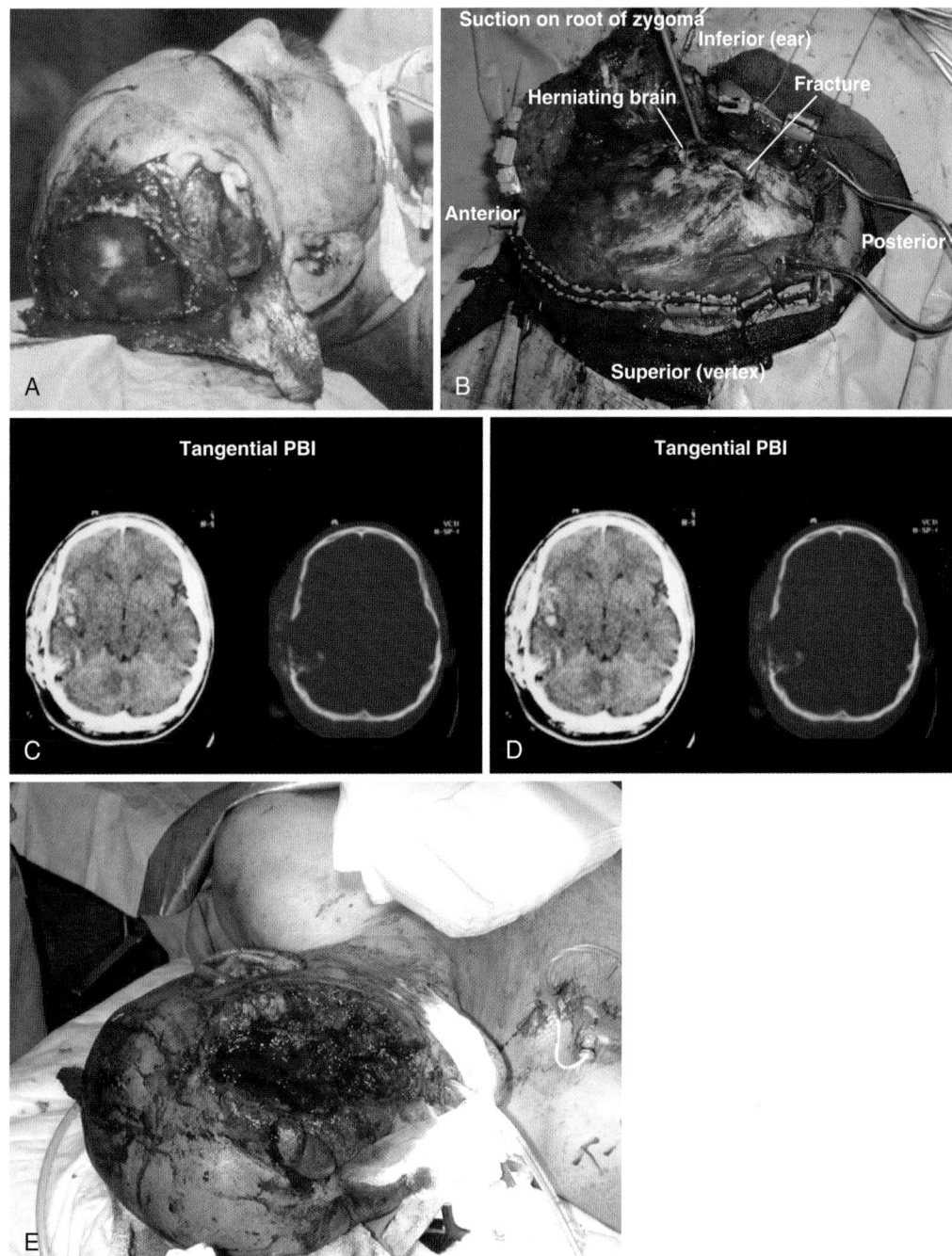

FIGURE 21.1 **A,** Tangential penetrating injury with posterior entry. **B,** Patient was immediately taken for decompressive hemicraniectomy for elevated intracranial pressures. **C** and **D,** Axial noncontrast computed tomography (CT) scan demonstrating superficial scalp hematoma, with comminuted bony fracture and underlying hemorrhagic contusion. No midline shift, preservation of the basal cistern, without a focal mass lesion.

Continued

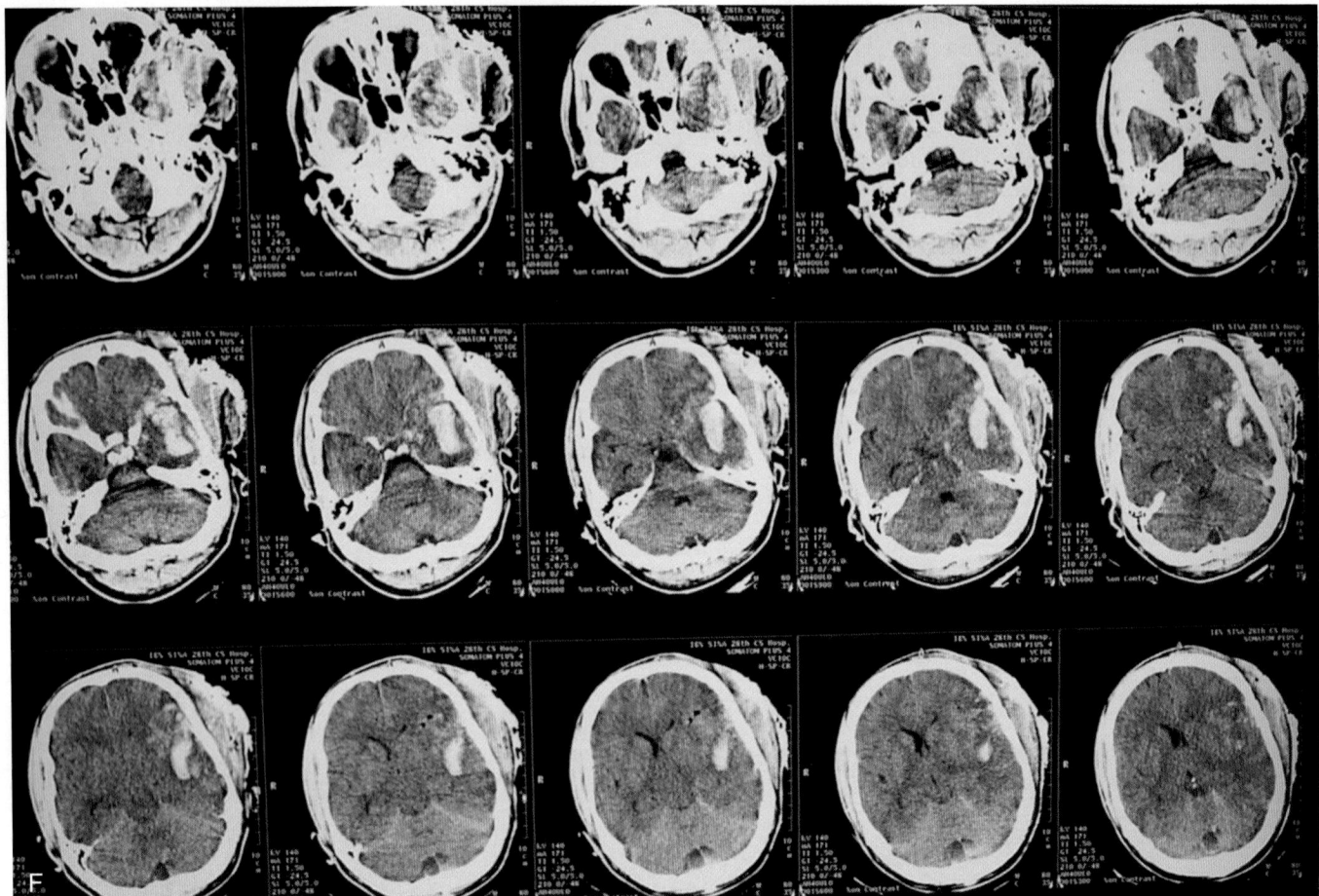

FIGURE 21.1, cont'd **E** and **F,** Severe lateral temporofacial explosive blast injury with significant disruption of anatomical continuity, tissue loss, associated traumatic orbital injury, with left hemispheric edema, midline shift, obliteration of ambient cisterns, and focal temporal lobe hematoma. Patient responded well to left hemicraniectomy, evacuation of temporal lobe hematoma, left orbital enucleation, and staged skull base repair. Incision was placed in midline with large left posterior auricular curve toward the mastoid tip away from the zone of injury. After hemicraniectomy, duraplasty, skull base repair with split-thickness bone graft from the cranial plate of the hemicraniectomy, with tissue closed up to the zygoma separating the lateral facial component, followed by initial wound packing in the infratemporal portion, wound was later definitively closed after subsequent débridements.

wounds (n = 46) and 100% with non-self-inflicted wounds (n = 4). Until variables of mechanism and modes of injury can be more appropriately matched, treatment effects across civilian and military PBI will be difficult to discern (Figs. 21.4 and 21.5).

PATHOPHYSIOLOGY

The pathophysiology of penetrating head injury is in many ways similar to all forms of severe brain injury. Injury can be classified as either primary (directly resulting from the penetrating force) or secondary (injury sustained from complications of the initial penetrating injury). Initial neurological cell death occurs immediately adjacent to the trajectory of the penetrating object (see Fig. 21.4). Subsequent cell death can occur as a result of increased ICP, mass effect from space-occupying lesions, stroke from initial vessel injury (see Fig. 21.5) or delayed ischemic neurological deficits resulting from traumatic vasospasm (Fig. 21.6), complications from infection,

uncontrolled seizure activity, and delayed hydrocephalus.[32-38] Surgical and critical care management strategies must therefore be directed at mitigating complications from the secondary neurological injury described here[37,38] (Fig. 21.7).

MECHANISMS OF PENETRATING BRAIN INJURY

Open head injury mechanisms have been described in various systems of classification from high and low velocity to blunt, explosive, penetrating, and perforating. For the purpose of this discussion, anything related to gunshot wounds to the head will be explicitly defined, and penetrating fragment injuries will be referred to as explosive or blast fragmentation injuries. Blunt injuries will include open, comminuted, and depressed skull fractures with indriven bone fragments as the result of a nonpenetrating external force (i.e., "under the body armor," Fig. 21.8). Discussion concerning nonprojectile penetrating injuries

TABLE 21.2 2001 Guidelines for the Management of Penetrating Brain Injury

Topic	Conclusion	Recommendation Level
I. Antibiotic prophylaxis	The use of prophylactic broad-spectrum antibiotics is recommended for patients with PBI.	Option
II. Seizure prophylaxis	The use of prophylactic antiseizure medications in the first week after PBI is recommended to prevent early post-traumatic seizures.	Option
III. ICP monitoring	Early ICP monitoring is recommended when the clinician is unable to assess the neurological examination accurately or if CT scans suggest elevated intracranial pressure. The need to evacuate a mass lesion is unclear.	Option
IV. Management of CSF leaks	Surgical correction is recommended for CSF leaks that do not close spontaneously, or are refractory to temporary CSF diversion. During the primary surgery, every effort should be made to close the dura and prevent CSF leaks.	Option
V. Neuroimaging	CT scanning of the head is strongly recommended. Angiography is recommended in PBI when a vascular injury is suspected. Routine MRI is not recommended for use in the acute management of missile-induced PBI.	Option
VII. Surgical management	Evacuation of hematomas with mass effect, conservative débridement of missile tract without retrieval of remote fragments, débridement of nonviable scalp, bone, or dura before primary closure, and watertight repair of open-air sinus injuries is recommended.	Option
VIII. Vascular complications	CT angiography and/or conventional angiography should be considered when vascular injury is suspected. If traumatic intracranial aneurysm (TICA) or arteriovenous fistula (AVF) is identified, surgical or endovascular management is recommended.	Option

CSF, cerebrospinal fluid; CT, computed tomography; ICP, intracranial pressure; MRI, magnetic resonance imaging; PBI, penetrating brain injury.
Modified from Aarabi B, Alden TD, Chestnut RM, et al. Management and prognosis of penetrating brain injury. J Trauma 2001;51:3-43.

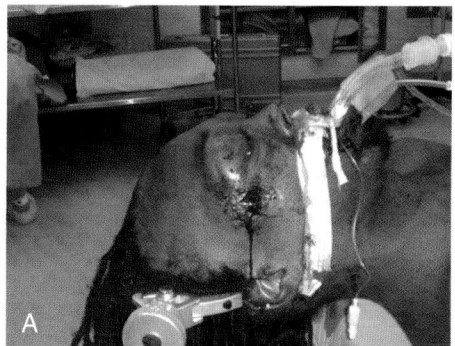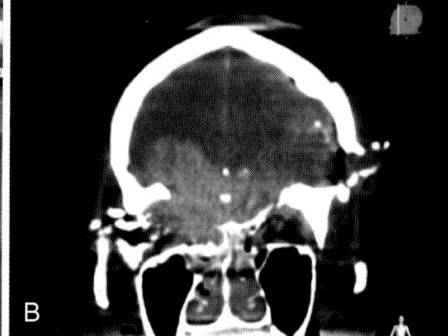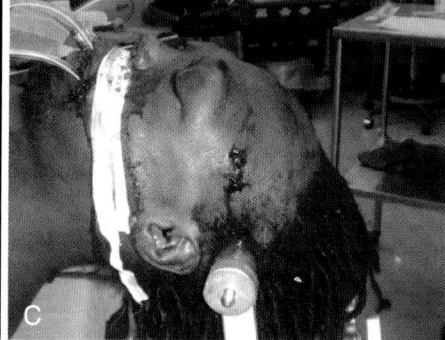

FIGURE 21.2 **A,** Victim of a point blank attempted homicide evidenced by powder burns at the entry site. At the initial physical examination, this bihemispheric gunshot wound to the head (**A** and **B**) appears to cross the zona fatalis, but the computed tomography (CT) scan (**C**) instead reveals a more anterior trajectory. This information led to the appropriate course of decompression and aggressive management, subsequently resulting in a favorable outcome.

TABLE 21.3 Comparison of Civilian and Military Penetrating Brain Injury

Factor	Civilian	Military
Population	Heterogeneous	Homogeneous (younger overall age)
Mechanism	Gunshot/suicide	Blast/shrapnel
Environment	Modern sanitation	Possibly contaminated
Prehospital care	Variable	Immediate
Tertiary care	Hours	Variable
Injury severity score (ISS)*	Low	High

(i.e., stab wound from knives or sticks) will be excluded given the relative infrequency in the referenced studies. As previously mentioned, the most common mechanism shared between civilian and military populations are GSWH. The lethality of GSWH is greater than the vast majority of penetrating blast fragment injuries and has been assumed to be partially responsible for the disparity of favorable outcomes in the civilian population. The ratio of fragment to GSWH, approximately 7:2, remains relatively consistent among wartime conflicts.[1,2,4,5,7,8,15,31]

Ballistics, or the study of the dynamic properties of a projectile, is useful to understand when reconstructing what occurred at time zero of the impact.[39] Terminal or wounding ballistics is perhaps even more relevant to the neurosurgeon as it describes how the projectile behaves after impacting tissue. Kinetic energy (KE), also known as wounding energy, is the quantity of energy that a projectile transfers to the brain

TABLE 21.4 Prognostic Variables

Topic	Conclusion	Data Class
I. Age	Age > 50 years is associated with higher rate of mortality, but significance is unclear.	III
II. Cause of injury (suicide)	Self-inflicted GSWH carry a higher rate of mortality than those for other causes.	II
III. Mode of injury	Perforating wounds have a higher mortality rate than tangential or penetrating PBIs.	III
IV. Caliber of weapon	No demonstrated effect.	
V. Hypotension	Hypotension is associated with increased mortality rate.	III
VII. Coagulopathy	Coagulopathy is associated with increased mortality rate.	III
VIII. Respiratory distress	Respiratory distress is associated with increased mortality rate.	III
IX. GCS	In civilian injuries, low GCS score correlates with higher mortality rate and unfavorable outcome. In military injuries, low GCS score correlates with unfavorable outcome.	I (civilian) III (military)
X. Pupil size and response	The presence of bilateral fixed and dilated pupils is highly predictive of fatal outcome.	III
XI. ICP	High ICP is predictive of higher mortality rate.	II

GCS, Glasgow Coma Scale; GSWH, gunshot wounds to the head; ICP, intracranial pressure; PBI, penetrating brain injury.
Modified from Aarabi B, Alden TD, Chestnut RM, et al. Management and prognosis of penetrating brain injury. J Trauma 2001;51:44-86.

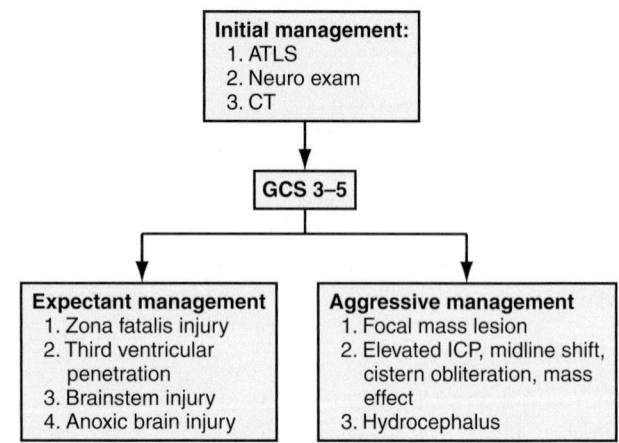

FIGURE 21.3 Triage flow chart for prognosis and management of penetrating brain injury.

and creates damage. Kinetic energy is calculated by the equation $KE = (Mass)(Velocity)^2$, revealing the relative weight that velocity conveys to a missile's wounding potential.

In low-velocity wounds, the injury is made primarily by the projectile itself, crushing tissue within its immediate trajectory in creating the permanent cavity. High-velocity wounds, in contrast, create a more complex pattern of injury based on the whether the projectile penetrates or perforates the cranial vault and the degree of the KE imparted to the tissue. The KE of a perforating wound can be calculated as equal to $(Mass)(Impact velocity - Exit velocity)^2$. The release of KE into tissue causes a phenomenon of cavitation: a brief, compressive force that expands tangentially from the tract of primary injury, generating a destructive wake. After the KE is depleted, and the cavity has expanded to its maximal size, the area begins to collapse under negative pressure and may suck in surrounding debris. The cavity may then subsequently undergo further expansions and contractions in decreasing amplitudes depending on the viscoelastic properties of the tissue. In inelastic tissue, such as brain, the permanent cavity can become tenfold larger than the diameter or profile of the offending projectile.

Other characteristics of a projectile include caliber, shape, yaw, precession and nutation, and ballistic coefficient. A round's caliber is defined by the internal diameter of the weapon's barrel, therefore representing the widest diameter of the bullet. This is can be measured in both inches (.45) and millimeters (9-mm) and essentially approximates the bullet's mass. The shape of a projectile may be sharp or round nosed, or may be completely spherical as is the case in some explosive munitions. The shape will be the main determinant of the other following characteristics. Yaw is the rotation of a bullet around its long axis. As the yaw of a projectile increases to 90 degrees, the size of the permanent cavity, and therefore tissue destruction, is maximized. The potentially large discrepancy between in-flight yaw and tissue-travel yaw explains why an exit wound may be many times larger than the entry wound. The precession and nutation are the circular motions of a projectile in flight and contribute more to in-flight stability than impact damage. The ballistic coefficient, or drag, is the force that resists a bullet's forward velocity. This, along with initial velocity, will determine the effective range of the weapon. Other factors not discussed are fragmentation and explosive potential, ricochet (Fig. 21.9), jacketed versus unjacketed rounds, and hollow-nosed or soft-pointed cartridges.

MANAGEMENT RECOMMENDATIONS IN THE SETTING OF PENETRATING BRAIN INJURIES

Evaluation, Diagnostics, and Medical Management

A penetrating brain injury can be an overwhelming "shock to the senses," blinding the examiner from identifying other additional life-threatening issues. As a general management pearl, focusing solely on the head injury to the exclusion of a more meticulous systematic evaluation is to be avoided. A thorough review of the entire patient as recommended by the primary and secondary survey of ATLS will prevent this trap. Thinking of the examination and injury analysis as a complete "crime scene investigation" will allow the examiner to consider the details of the mechanism involved and record them for later consideration in the management of the patient.

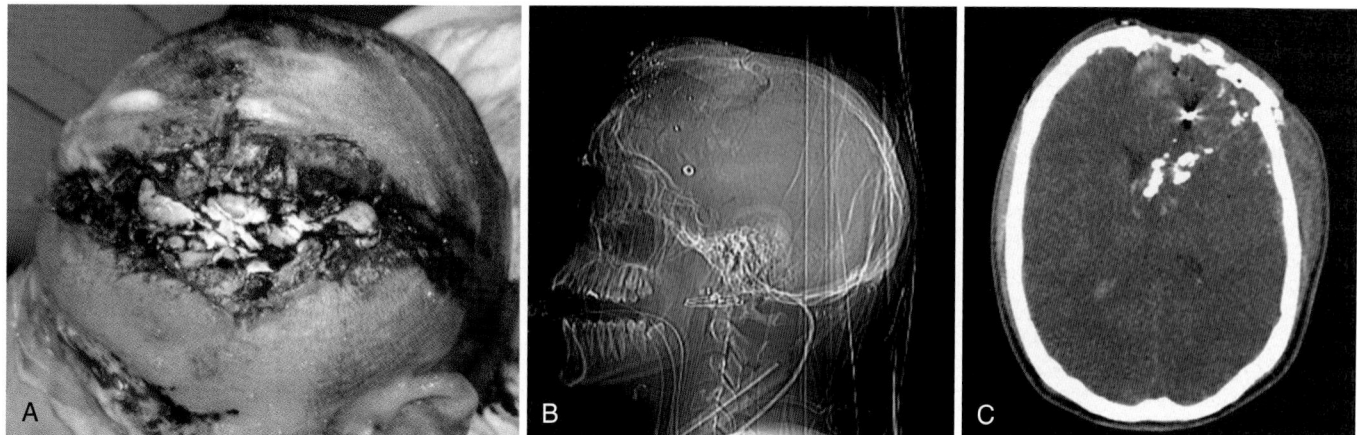

FIGURE 21.4 **A** to **C**, Severe penetrating brain injury caused by pistoning of the patient's Kevlar helmet upon impact of a nonpenetrating high-velocity round. These "under the body armor" wounds share a similar mechanism and pattern as Cushing's "guttering" injuries, but they may be from a variety of orientation angles at impact.

FIGURE 21.5 **A** and **B,** Computed tomography (CT) scan of the pilot in Figure 21.10 reveals the degree of bone fragmentation resulting in a secondary projectile phenomenon. Bony fragments drove into the depths of the sylvian fissure, resulting in stenosis and occlusion of the middle cerebral artery major divisions and a large hemispheric infarct.

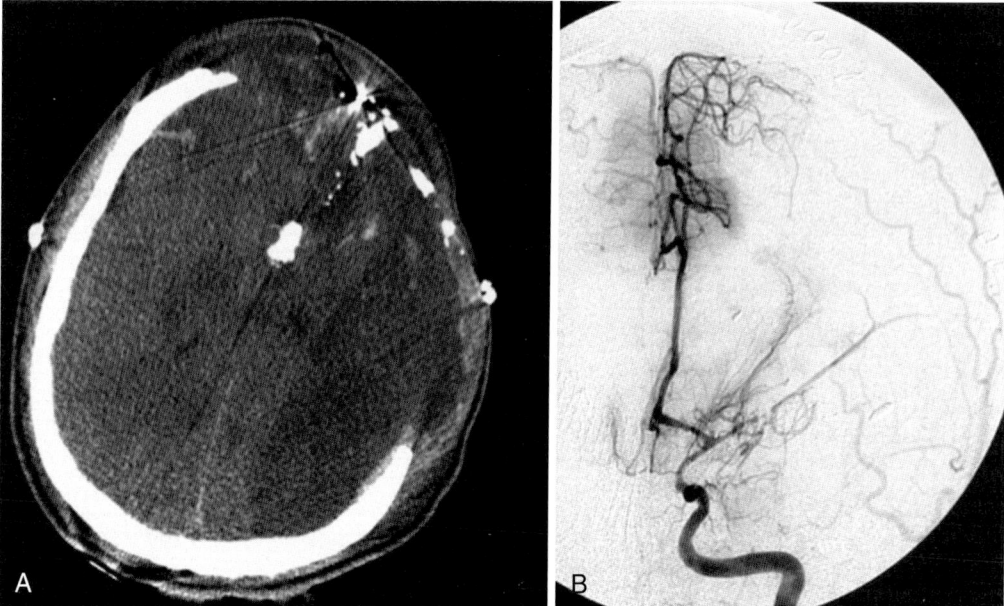

In the setting of multitrauma, concomitant thoracic, abdominal, and cranial trauma may require simultaneous intervention. The recent combination of abdominal ultrasonic FAST (focused assessment with sonography for trauma) examinations in conjunction with head CT scans in the trauma bay can avoid significant treatment delays in the radiology suite. Alternatively, imaging done in the operating room with the use of a mobile CT scanner can facilitate diagnoses in patients too hemodynamically unstable to be transported to radiology. Individuals with multiple missile injuries should be triaged with a low threshold for immediate surgery if major visceral injury is suspected. If a neurological examination is not obtainable, the placement of a ventriculostomy or ICP monitor is advised to better manage the effects of intracranial hemorrhage or cerebral edema.[40]

Imaging modalities such as three-dimensional CT volumetric reconstruction is a luxury in some environments but is helpful for fragment path delineation and re-creation of the zone of injury. Standard CT stands as the most common and useful

tool when evaluated penetrating brain injury. It allows for the analysis, with rapid precision, of the trajectory path, resultant intracranial hemorrhages, concomitant orbital and skull base fractures, and associated disrupted structures.[41] The addition of CT angiography, when available, helps provide a reasonable initial assessment of vascular injuries. It may direct the clinician to proceed to angiography if further concern exists (Figs. 21.9 and 21.10). The role for immediate angiography is presented in Box 21.1. When evaluating the CT, questions specifically to be answered include the following:

1. Does the injury include the vascular structures, skull base, ventricles, orbits, or cranial nerves?
2. Does it cross the zona fatalis or brainstem?
3. Is there evidence of anoxic brain injury or diffuse axonal injury?

Remember that fragments can also be dynamic particles and positional movements may be missed between static CT images. When trying to determine if a projectile is still mobile,

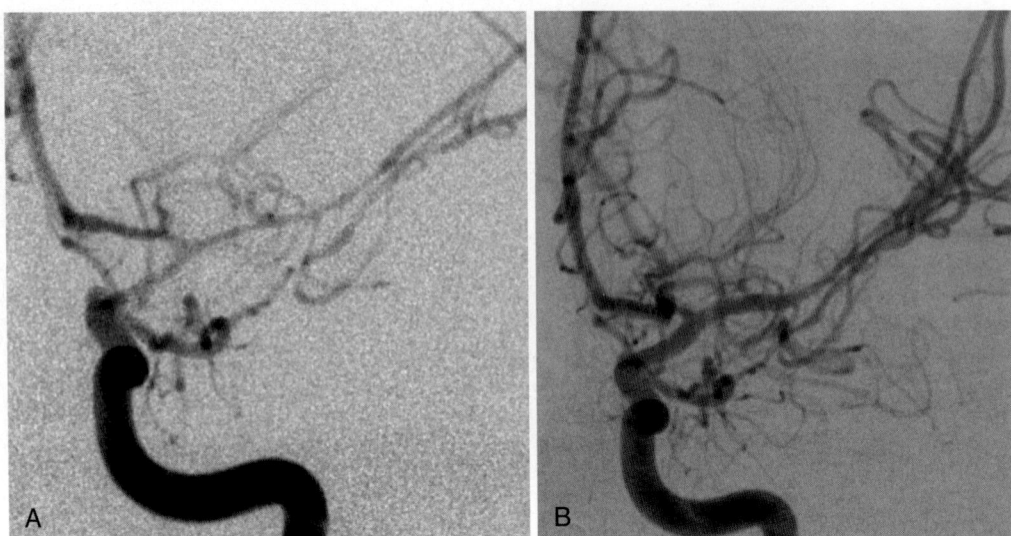

FIGURE 21.6 Post-traumatic vasospasm in penetrating brain injury before (**A**) and after (**B**) being treated successfully with intra-arterial nicardipine and angioplasty. Vasospasm was picked up on serial transcranial Doppler (TCD) examination when velocities in the M1 and M2 branches exceeded 250 and Lindegaard ratios became greater than 5. The patient had a poor neurological examination and already had scattered areas of ischemic infarct on computed tomography (CT) scan; therefore, intervention was felt to be warranted. Post-treatment velocities fell to just over 100 and the Lindegaard ratio dropped to less than 3.

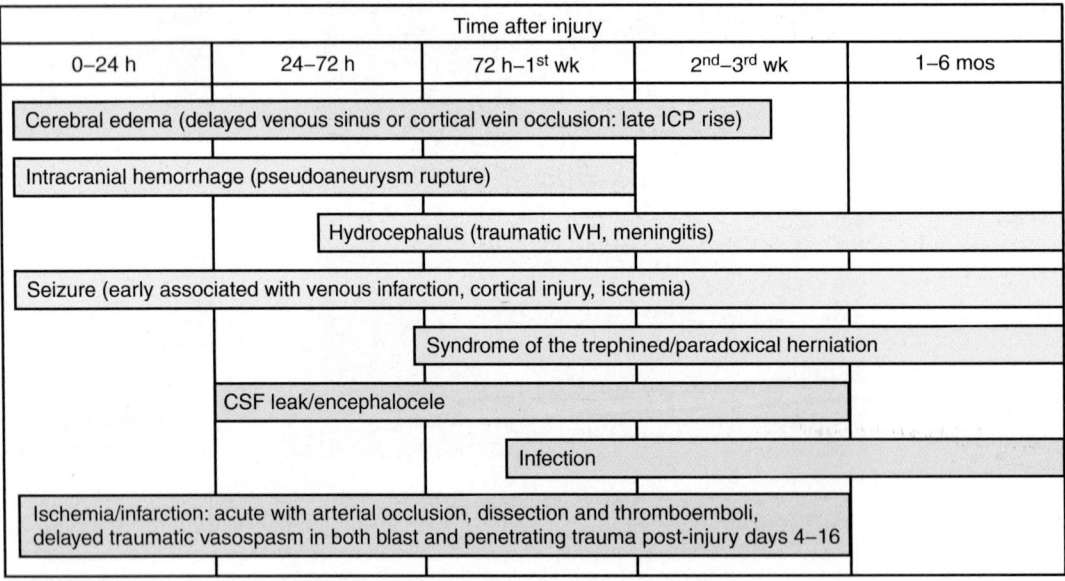

FIGURE 21.7 Complications of penetrating brain injury.

flexion and extension plain skull radiographs may be useful. Because of the mechanism of injury and the high likelihood of retained fragments with ferromagnetic properties, magnetic resonance imaging (MRI) is not recommended as an initial imaging modality in PBI (see Box 21.3).

Outside the need for immediate operative intervention, patients with penetrating brain injury should initially be managed by applying fundamental critical care principles.[37,38,40] After establishing basic life support and applying initial resuscitation via ATLS guidelines, obtaining an accurate initial neurological examination is most essential next step. In the ensuing time course, avoidance of hypoxia and hypotension is critical, as is fluid resuscitation with efforts taken to avoid hypotonic fluid administration. Efforts to monitor and mitigate the effects of elevated ICP should proceed rapidly following admission depending on the patient's physical examination.

Surgical Management

The tenets of surgical treatment should be directed at preventing secondary insults due to raised ICP, delayed infection, and ischemia. Common neurosurgical management principles include brainstem decompression, reducing ICP, restoring anatomical continuity, and obtaining hemostasis. For injuries in which a focal insult has occurred, such as an open depressed skull fracture, débridement of the entry wound with fracture elevation may be all that is necessary. In patients with hemispheric or global injury, evacuation of mass lesions

FIGURE 21.8 Artist's rendition of an "under the body armor" injury. **A,** Point of contact with subsequent pistoning of the inner helmet table. **B,** In-driven bone fragments with vessel laceration. **C,** Pseudoaneurysm formation.

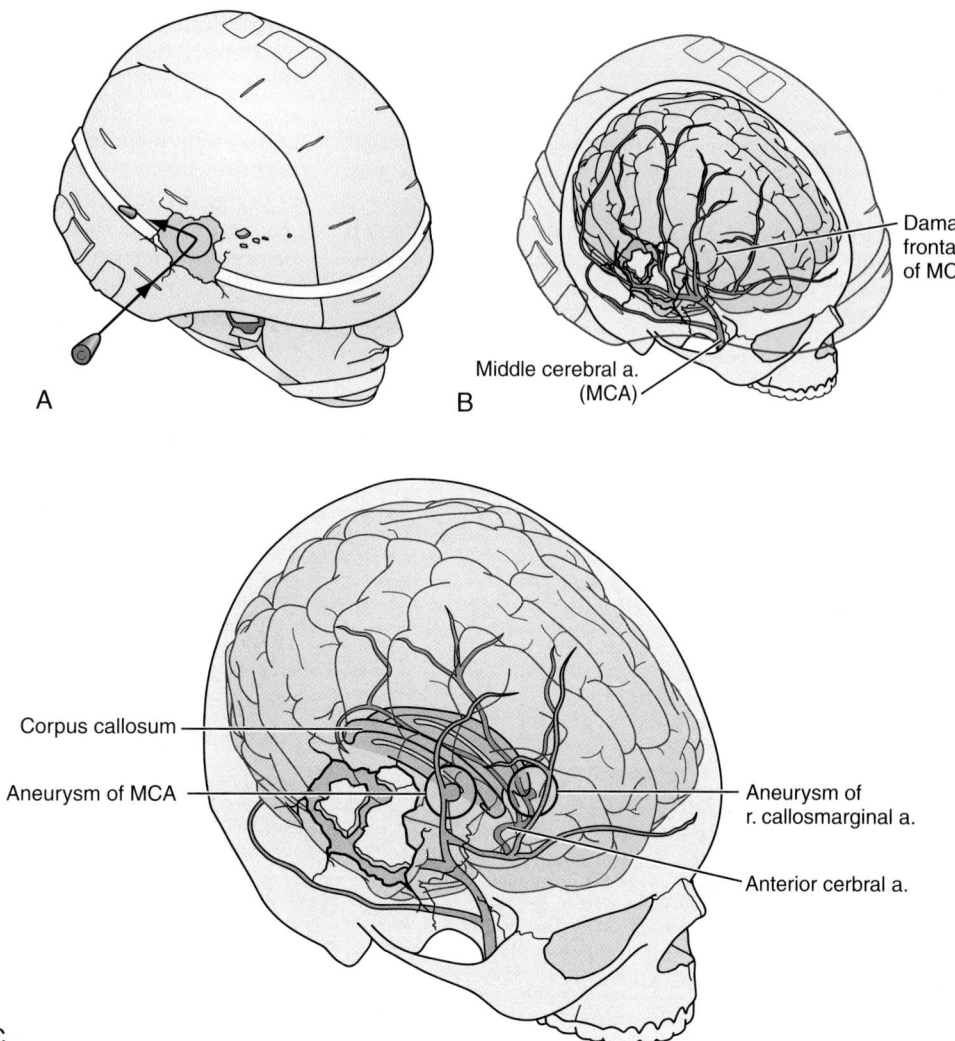

Damaged frontal br. of MCA

Middle cerebral a. (MCA)

A

B

Corpus callosum

Aneurysm of MCA

Aneurysm of r. callosmarginal a.

Anterior cerbral a.

C

(hematoma) should be performed in conjunction with a large decompressive craniectomy to ameliorate secondary cerebral edema and ICP elevations. Early obliteration of basal cisterns, loss of sulcal and gyral pattern, midline shift not explained by associated mass lesion, or hemispheric edema are indicative of a diffuse insult with a less clear role for intervention. Surgical recommendations specific to PBI are summarized in Box 21.1.

The role for removal of deep embedded fragments has been discussed at length and attempts should be tempered by the potential for associated injury caused by deep tract dissection.[7-10] Only superficial fragments that readily present themselves at the cortical surface or that can be dislodged with gentle irrigation should undergo primary débridement. Delayed fragment removal (metal, bone, or environmental elements) is indicated in certain situations and categorized in Box 21.2.

Preoperative Planning

Avoidance of iatrogenic injury is always of paramount importance to the neurological surgeon. Violation of major venous sinuses and cortical veins are complications that can arise when performing large decompressions. Awareness of alterations in normal anatomy and an evaluation of the fragment or missile pathway should always precede intervention. A plan should provide for a rim of bone around the major venous sinuses to allow for dural tuck-up sutures if a tear of the transverse or sigmoid sinus is suspected. If a depressed bone fragment compromises the venous sinus, this bone should be carefully elevated with a bone flap that encompasses the surrounding bone and allows direct repair if necessary. The use of muscle, fascia, dura, vein, and synthetic allograft has been described for sinus repairs and all are effective in many circumstances.[42] Preserving normal venous outflow is essential in these cases and should be confirmed by CT angiography or cerebral angiography. Delayed venous occlusions may result in a poor outcome with subsequent venous infarction, swelling, bleeding, neurological deterioration, and death. The role for anticoagulation in PBI-related sinus occlusion has not been well studied.

Those penetrating wounds without exit may have resulted from significant ricochet on the inner aspect of the calvarium. This has been reported in up to 30% in autopsy series.[43] These rounds may then travel in an opposite direction and penetrate another intracranial compartment or stop at a dural margin. Special consideration should be given to injuries that cross two dural compartments, in particular those that penetrate from the posterior fossa to the supratentorial space. These rounds may require staged decompressive procedures to access separate mass lesions or mitigate ICP elevations in different compartments. In rare situations, a delayed venous infarction may result in supratentorial ICP elevations in a trajectory that crosses the tentorium from a posterior fossa entry (see Fig. 21.8). Typically the posterior fossa should be decompressed first, given the proximity to the brainstem and the potential for immediate death, followed by supratentorial decompression if necessary (see Fig. 21.8).

Operative Techniques

The hazards of poor surgical management in these injuries include improperly fashioning an incision using the traumatic scalp laceration, poor hemostasis, inadequate initial repair of skull base defect, and generally inadequate cranial decompression (Fig. 21.11). Basing an incision behind the zone of injury allows placement of a large craniotomy or craniectomy incision in normal tissue whose healing properties are not compromised. This avoids delayed wound breakdown, CSF leakage, and related infections.

In the operating room, the patient should be positioned in such a manner that allows for proximal carotid exposure if

a skull base arterial injury is suspected. This should be done pre emptively if a fracture or fragment penetration includes the petrous pyramid, sphenoid bone, anterior clinoid, or optic strut (Fig. 21.12). Preparation for a potential donor bypass graft would include having the contralateral leg prepped with saphenous vein marked or arm preparation for possible radial artery graft. Additional foresights include having a Doppler readily available to delineate the superficial temporal artery before skin incision.

Injuries that include the frontal sinus or an anterior skull base defect may require autologous fascia or fat to close the defect. This may involve prepping the lower leg for harvesting of the fascia lata, an excellent autologous dural substitute, and the abdomen for a fat graft. Other considerations for incorporating the abdomen into the surgical field are for possible implantation of a postcraniectomy bone flap. It is important that the right anterior abdominal wall be used in lieu of the left to avoid the potential compromise of a percutaneous gastrostomy site. Implanting the bone flap prevents the autologous bone from being separated from the patient, allowing it to remain sterile, viable, and available. Alternatively, the autologous bone can be split and used for immediate reconstruction of the cranial base or orbital bandeau. If possible, this measure allows a more solid foundation for future cranial

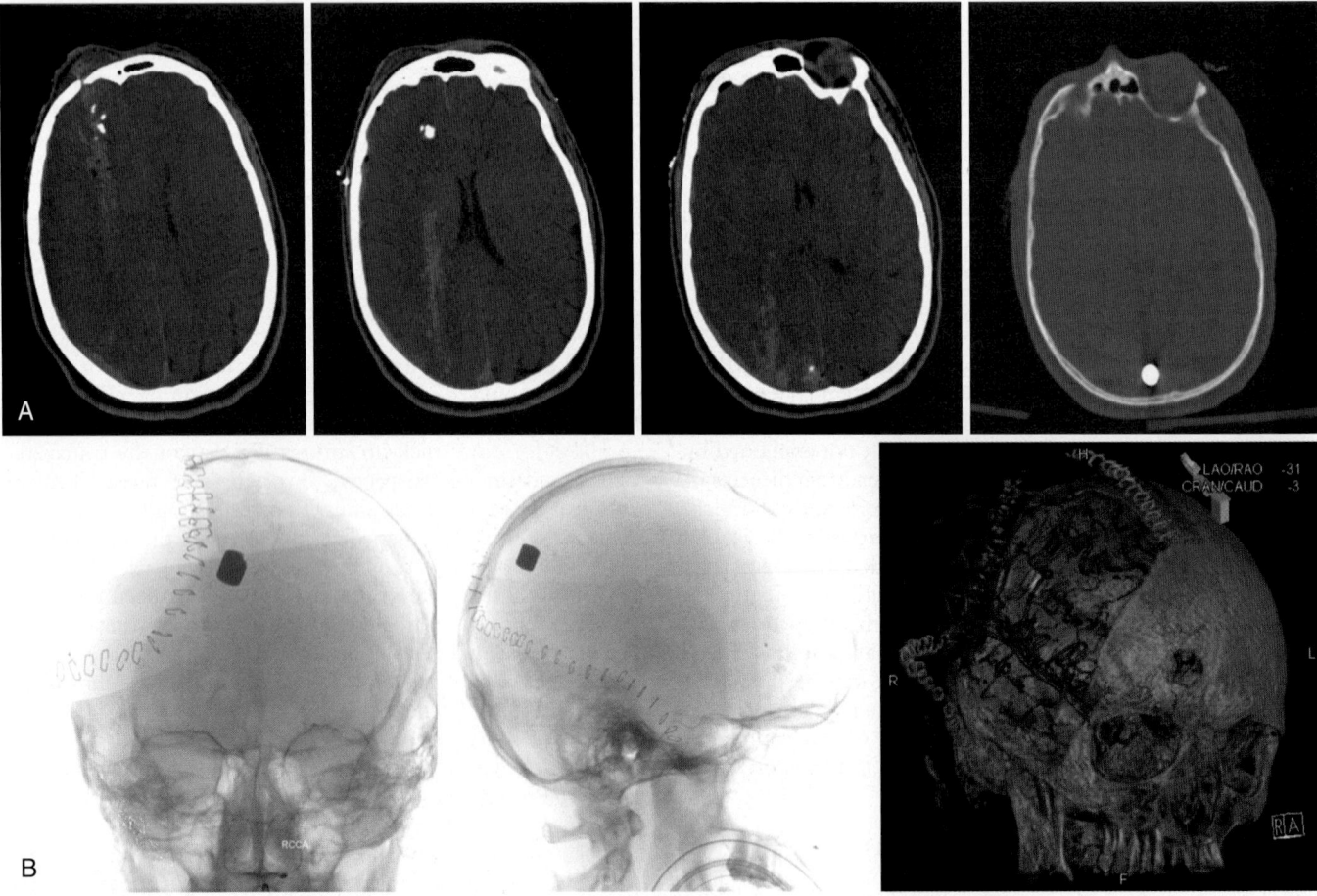

FIGURE 21.9 A, Soldier with right frontal entry wound and complete anteroposterior penetration through the right hemisphere. Subsequent ricochet placed the projectile just lateral to the posterior sagittal sinus. Immediate decompression resulted in a postresuscitation Glasgow Coma Scale (GCS) score of 11 with improvement to 15 after extubation. Angiogram revealed no vascular injury; plain skull radiographs and postangiography volumetric reconstruction are shown in **B.**

vault reconstruction and helps to prevent a possible CSF leak or encephalocele.

Endovascular Considerations

In addition to decompression and reconstruction of the cranial vault, adjunctive endovascular procedures may be required to prevent delayed ischemic or hemorrhagic deterioration. In some cases CT angiography may not demonstrate peripherally located small aneurysms or those hidden in venous contamination, bone, or metal scatter artifact. Modern digital subtraction cerebral angiography will demonstrate these smaller aneurysms more effectively and may allow for immediate treatment if necessary. The indications for immediate angiography are discussed in Box 21.3[12-14,16,17,44,45] (Figs. 21.13 and 21.14).

In some circumstances, an intraoperative cerebral angiogram can be coordinated to facilitate a simultaneous cranial decompression and cerebrovascular intervention. This proves essential in scenarios that include associated penetrating head and neck injuries, allowing for identification of the cervical vasculature injury in parallel with a timely cerebral decompression. The details to be considered in a well-orchestrated operation include (1) employing radiology technicians facile with the use of fluoroscopy, (2) use of a radiolucent headholder before pinning, (3) appropriate prep and draping for femoral arterial sheath placement, and (4) positioning the patient in a 180-degree turn from anesthesia. In this manner the surgical/endovascular team has access to the groin, neck, and cranial vault. The C-arm is then brought in at the head, directly in line with the patient, to allow the simulation of biplane positions (Fig. 21.15).

Delayed cerebral angiograms should also be considered in those patients who demonstrate a neurological deterioration that may be related to development of cerebral vasospasm, venous sinus occlusion, or de novo pseudoaneurysm formation in previously occluded branches. In the intensive care unit (ICU), morning sedation holidays with diligent neurological examinations and daily monitoring of transcranial Doppler (TCD) prove to be our least invasive and most

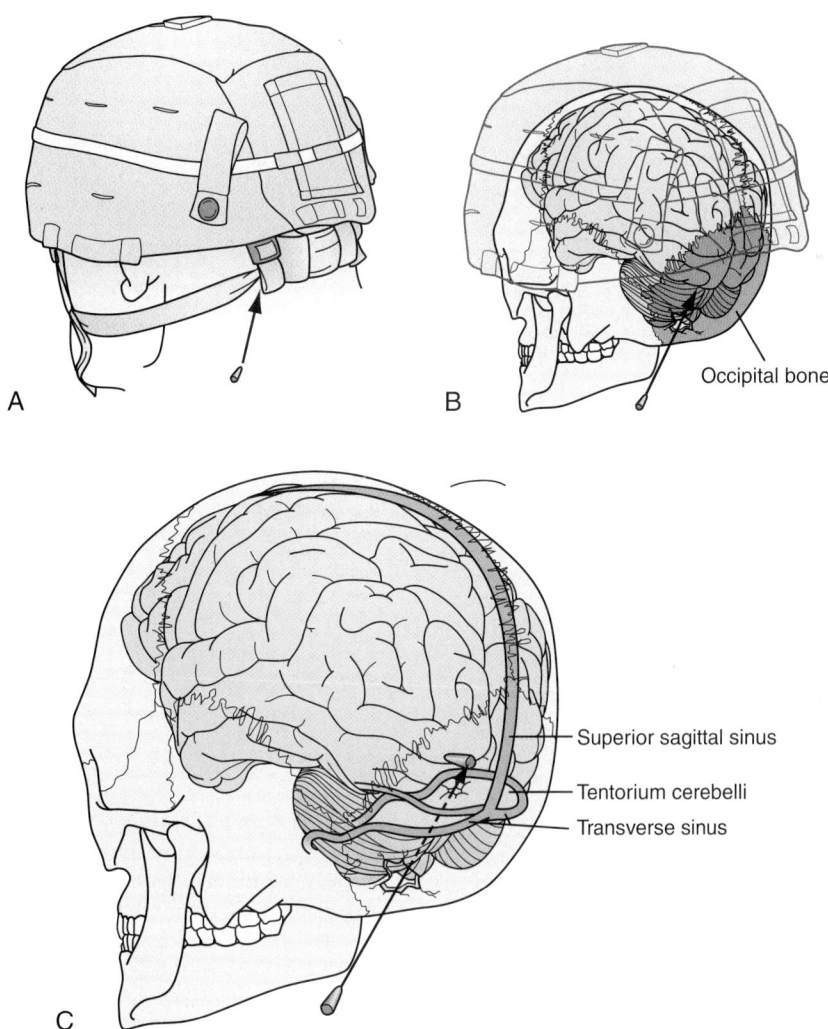

FIGURE 21.10 **A** to **D,** Helicopter pilot shot by sniper round while attempting to leave a hostile LZ. The bullet entered at left occiput, penetrated the left posterior fossa with a climbing trajectory, crossed the tentorium cerebelli, and came to rest in the right occipital lobe after ricocheting off the inner table. The patient was reportedly able to safely land the helicopter before losing consciousness. Immediate decompression of the posterior fossa was performed.

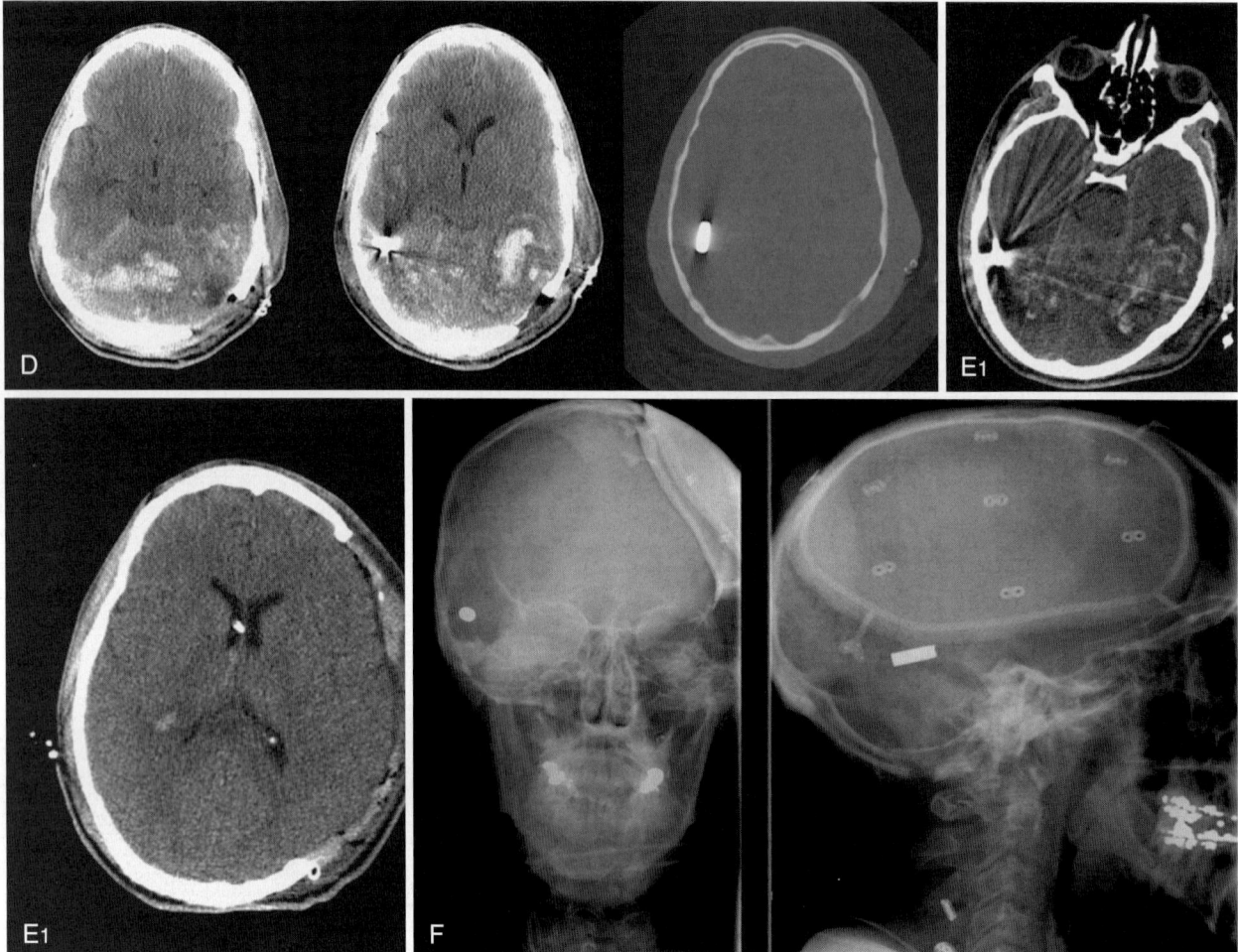

FIGURE 21.10, cont'd Secondary to increased intracranial pressure refractory to medical management, a decompressive hemicraniectomy was completed (**E**). The patient subsequently made a remarkable recovery, attaining a Glasgow Outcome Scale (GOS) score of 4 and returned months later for his cranioplasty (**F**).

BOX 21.1   Surgical Recommendations for Penetrating Brain Injury

1. Avoid use of the entry/exit wound when planning scalp incision.
2. Identify global/hemispheric injuries and role for large decompressive craniectomy.
3. Separate cranial-facial-orbital compartments with autologous bone or titanium mesh for support and watertight repair with dural substitutes.
4. Initiate early repair and fixation of the orbital bandeau to support future cranial vault reconstruction.
5. Perform conservative débridement of the trajectory path and imbedded fragments.
6. Consider intraoperative cerebral angiography in patients with combined penetrating neck and brain injury.

BOX 21.2   Criteria for Intracranial Fragment Removal

1. Fragment movement
2. Abscess formation
3. Vascular compression
4. Ventricular obstruction (hydrocephalus)
5. Heavy metals identified in cerebrospinal fluid

CONCLUSION

Penetrating brain injury is a high-mortality emergency for the neurological surgeon. Advances that have improved the outcomes in the military population include better prehospital care in the field, a more standardized approach to the treatment of PBI, and early neurosurgical intervention to include ICP monitoring, early decompression, reconstruction of the anterior skull base, and watertight dural closure. The use of endovascular techniques has increased our ability to manage vascular complications as a result of PBI. In time, measures learned from the treatment of PBI in the military population may be conferred to civilian patients provided they survive their initial injury and ensuing field and emergency room resuscitations.

reliable measures toward detection of such events. In the future, noninvasive near-infrared cerebral oximetry, cerebral blood flow probes, xenon CT, CT perfusion, continuous electroencephalography (EEG), and brain tissue oxygen probes may allow earlier and more sensitive identification of these problems.

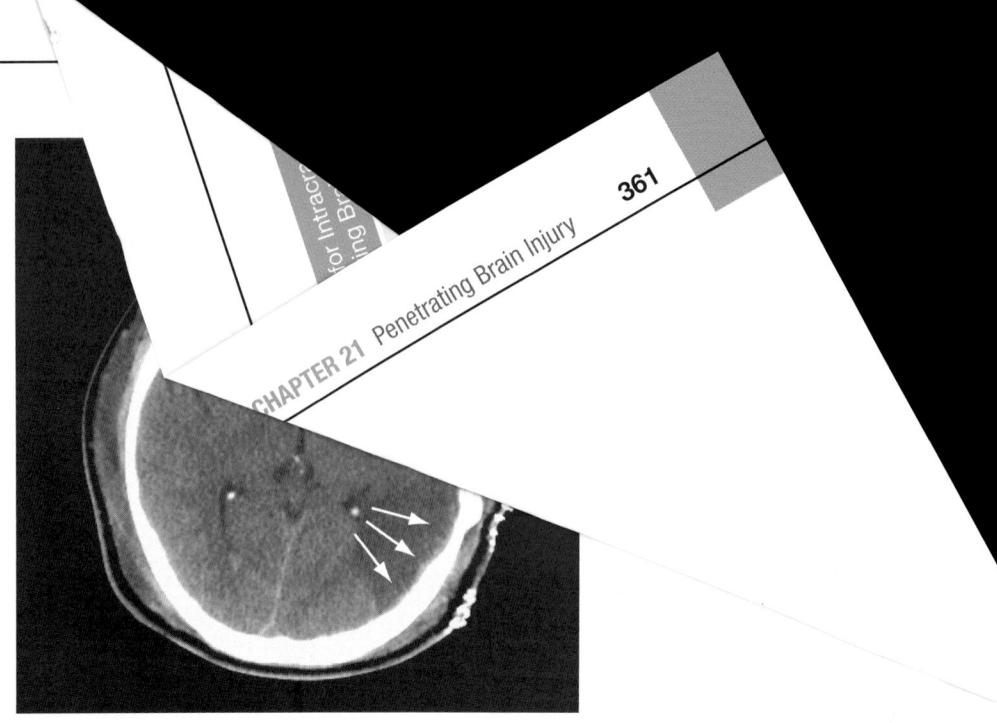

FIGURE 21.11 A soldier decompressed secondary to a fragmentary penetrating brain injury from a roadside IED (improvised explosive device) blast. Recommended hemicraniectomy size measures 15 cm in the anteroposterior dimension by 12 cm in the superoinferior dimension; inadequate bone removal at the inferior and posterior aspects of this frontotemporoparietal hemicraniectomy likely resulted in the observed area of infarct.

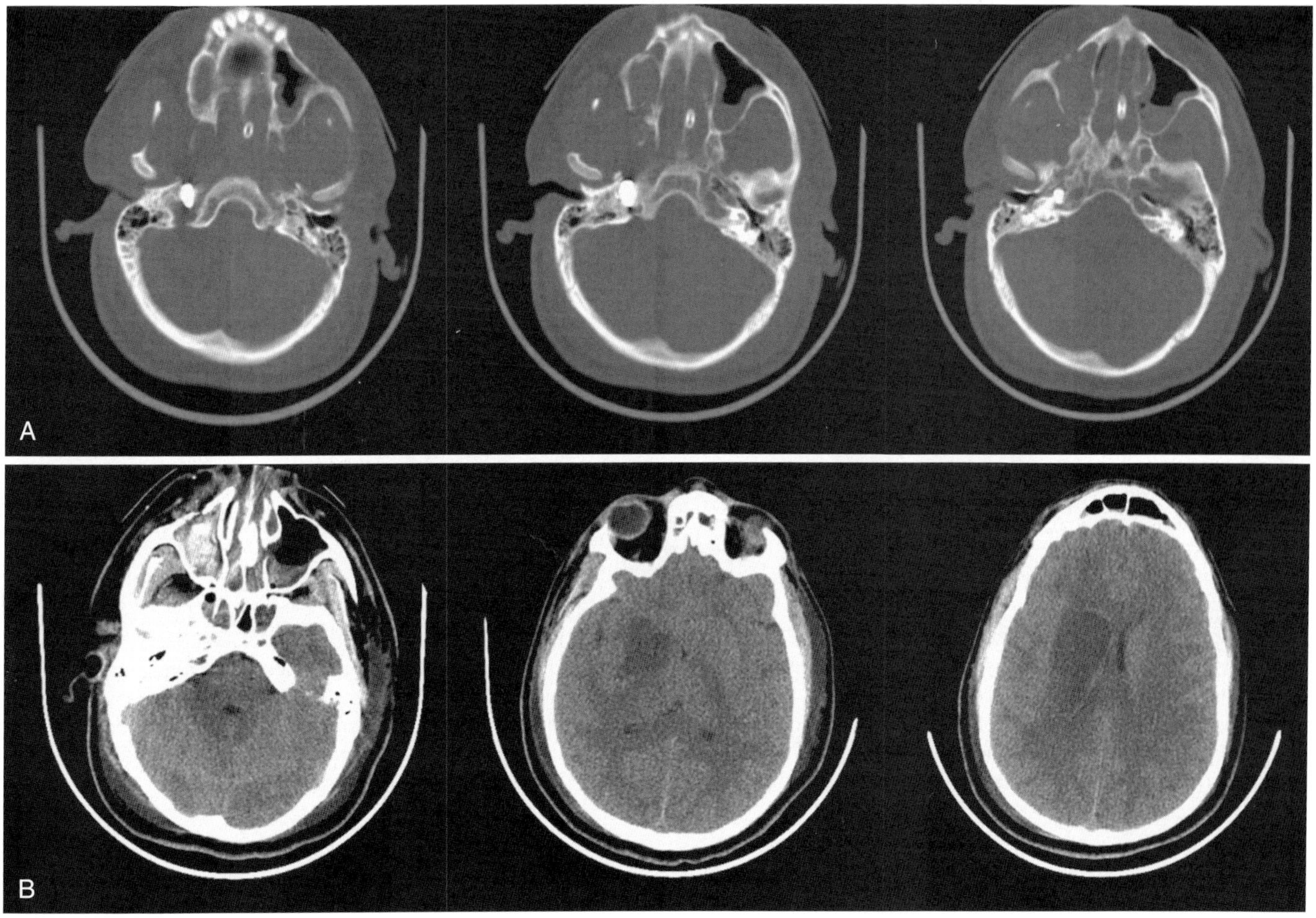

FIGURE 21.12 Patient with a bullet lodged in the petrous carotid demonstrated on bone windows (**A**) subsequently causing stump emboli and infarct (**B**).

...ial Angiography Following
...un Injury

...y through pterion, orbit, or posterior fossa
...agment with intracranial hematoma
...erebral artery sacrifice or pseudoaneurysm at the
...of initial exploration
...blast-induced penetrating injury with Glasgow Coma Scale
score <8
5. Transcranial Doppler or computed tomography angiographic
evidence of severe vasospasm

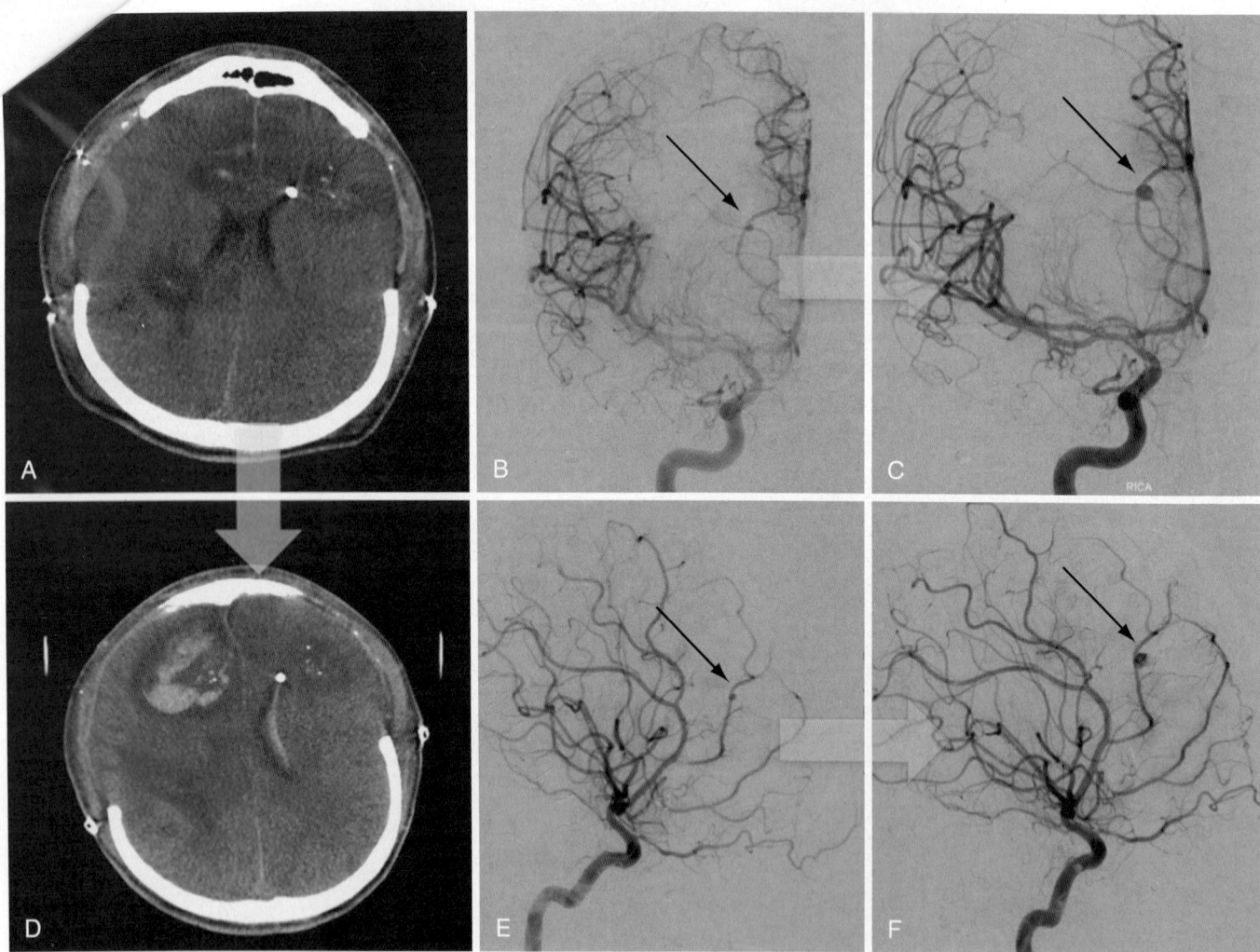

FIGURE 21.13 A, A patient sustained multiple penetrating fragments from an IED (improvised explosive device) blast requiring a bifrontal craniectomy and ventriculostomy placement. **B** and **C,** Six days later on initial angiographic evaluation a small 2-mm right pericallosal pseudoaneurysm was identified and initially managed without intervention; 72 hours later the patient became bradycardic with blood draining from his ventriculostomy. **D,** A repeat noncontrast head computed tomography (CT) scan shows a new right frontal hemorrhage. **E** and **F,** Repeat angiogram reveals pseudoaneurysm enlargement to 8 mm.

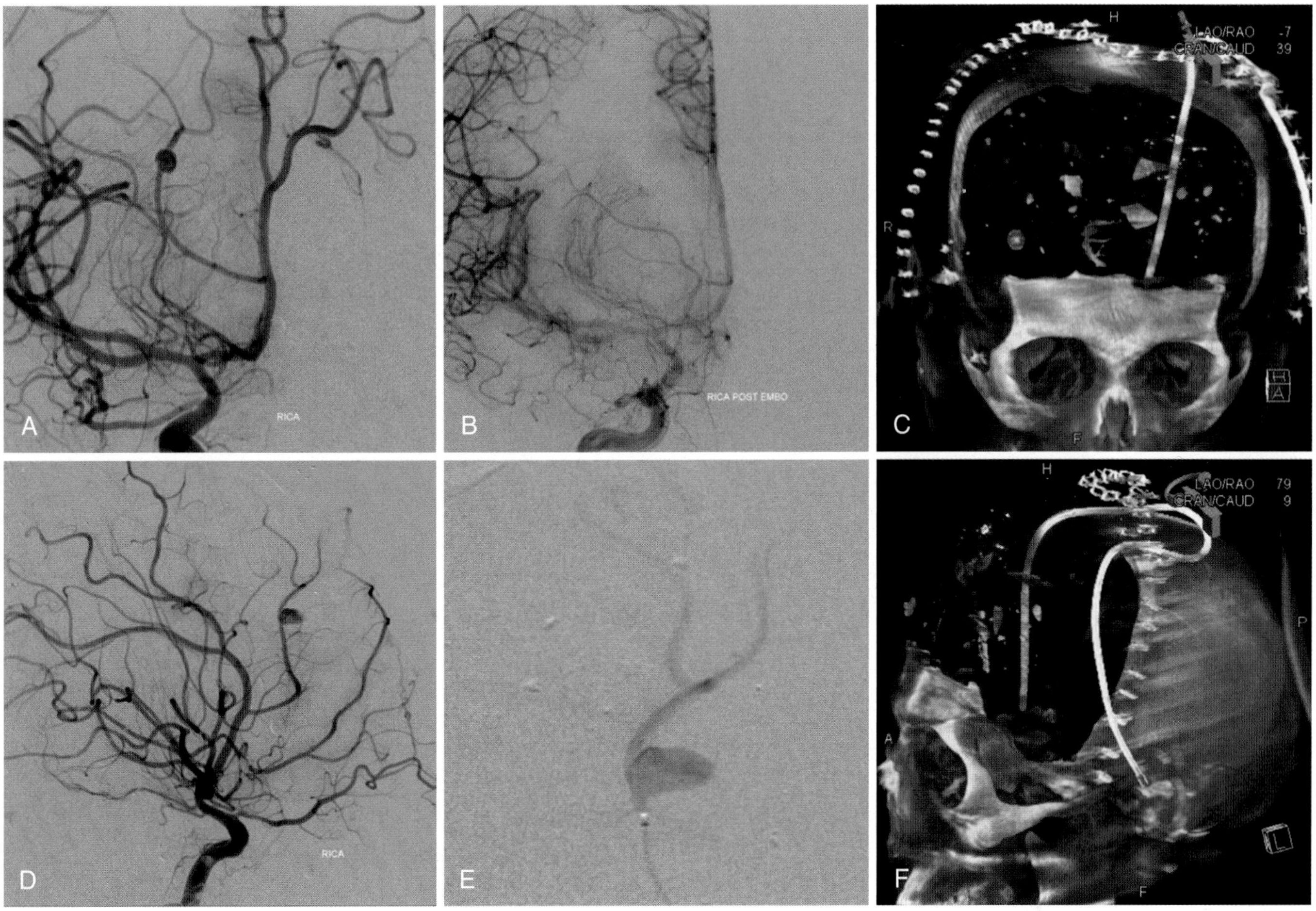

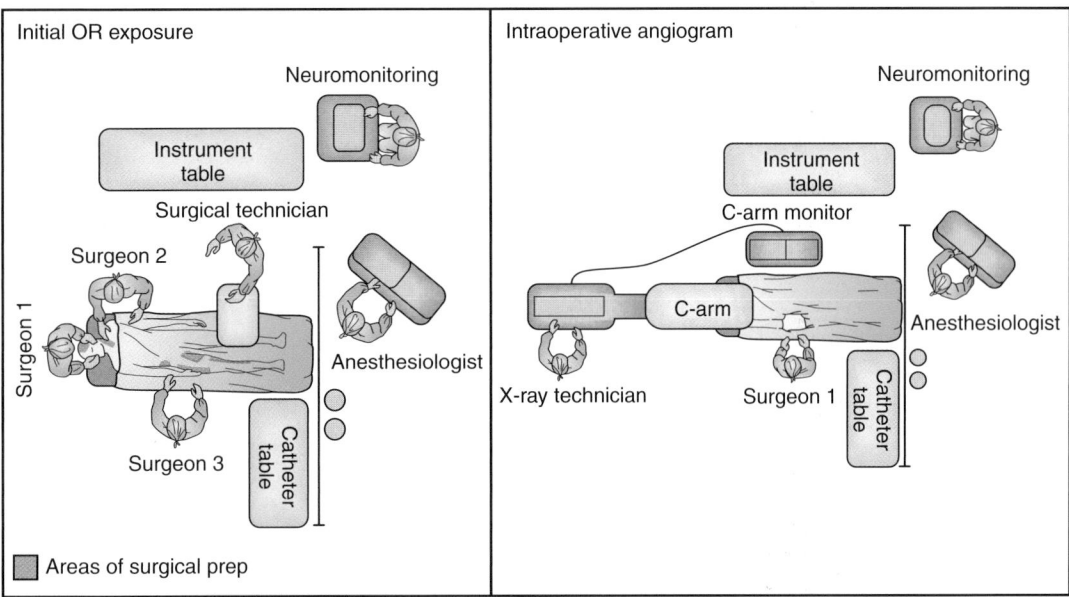

FIGURE 21.14 Same patient from Figure 21.8, preembolization (**A** and **B**) and after PAO and embolization with Onyx (**C** and **D**). The black arrows indicate the enlarged pseudoaneurysm, the empty arrows the subtracted Onyx cast, and the white arrows differentiate the cast from in-driven bone fragments on the dyna computed tomography (CT) scan (**E** and **F**).

FIGURE 21.15 Operating room layout showing Surgeon 1, proximal cervical carotid exposure, and Surgeon 2, cranial exposure. Intraoperative brachiocephalic angiogram position facilitates C-arm positioning, anesthesia, and neuromonitoring. Insure radiolucent table, headholder with reversal of the table positioning of the table pedestal to allow movement of the C-arm. Angiography table has basin, closed manifold system with contrast, saline flush, and femoral sheath in-place, with two continuous pressurized heparin flushes for both guide catheter and femoral sheath. Anesthesia should be oriented to the set are maintained, palpable pulses present in the lower extremity, a set of clear plastic drapes extend from the edge of the catheter table to the opposite side referred to as a "shower curtain."

SELECTED KEY REFERENCES

Aarabi B, Alden TD, Chestnut RM, et al. Management and prognosis of penetrating brain injury. J Trauma. 2001;51:3-86.

Bell RS, Vo AH, Neal CJ, et al. Military traumatic brain and spinal column injury: a 5-year study of the impact of blast and other military grade weaponry on the central nervous system. *J Trauma.* 2009;66(Suppl 4):S104-S111.

Bullock MR, Povlishock JT. Guidelines for the management of severe traumatic brain injury. *J Neurotrauma.* 2007;24(1):11-106.

Cushing H. A series of wounds involving the brain and its enveloping structures. Br J Surg. 1918;5:558-684.

Matson D. The Management of Acute Craniocerebral Injuries Due to Missiles. Washington, DC: Office of the Surgeon General, Department of the Army; 1958.

Please go to expertconsult.com to view the complete list of references.

22 Traumatic Skull and Facial Fractures

Fred H. Geisler, Eduardo Rodriguez, Paul N. Manson

CLINICAL PEARLS

- Linear skull fractures do not require stabilization or treatment when the scalp is closed. Depressed skull fractures may need exploration depending on the extent of the injury to the underlying brain, frontal sinus, or facial bones. Closed depressed fractures are usually repaired for cosmetic reasons. Compound depressed skull fractures with brain involvement are often neurosurgical emergencies. It becomes an emergency to treat the underlying brain injury, perform a watertight closure of the dura, and débride the devitalized scalp.

- Growing skull fractures, although rare, occur in children under 2 to 3 years of age and require surgical repair. If there is a tear in the dura accompanying a skull fracture after trauma, the pressure of the brain pulsations in a growing brain may enlarge the fracture and dural opening. The brain can herniate through this skull defect, causing a pulsatile mass under the scalp.

- Basilar skull fractures may present with periorbital ecchymoses, hemotympanum, or ecchymosis over the mastoid. The management of these fractures is usually

conservative unless a cerebrospinal fluid (CSF) leak is present. Many traumatic CSF leaks will spontaneously resolve in a week. Those that do not may be managed by CSF drainage, or in some cases surgical repair to avoid infection, once the location of the leak is identified.

- Frontal sinus fractures can be diagnosed on computed tomography (CT) and are managed differently depending on whether the frontal or posterior wall is disrupted. Orbital fractures are managed based on the extent of the injury to the globe, optic nerve, and orbital contents. Patients with a fluctuating or worsening visual acuity will require decompression of their optic nerve and relief of globe pressure. There are two indications for surgery of orbital "blow-out" fractures: (1) muscle or ligament entrapment with diplopia or (2) enophthalmus (backward dislocation of the globe) caused by prolapse of the orbital contents through the fracture. Le Fort fractures are often injuries to the entire midface region. Their surgical management depends on the extent and stability of the maxillary fracture.

SKULL FRACTURES

Skull fractures are classified in three ways: by pattern (linear, comminuted, depressed), by anatomical location (vault convexity, base), and by skin integrity (open, closed). The pattern of a skull fracture is affected by two factors. The first factor is the force of impact. A linear fracture results first at a point of weakness when the skull structure fails to undergo further elastic deformation as a response to impact; the fracture typically starts at the point of weakness in response to the maximal stress (the point of weakness is often remote from the actual impact point) and then extends to the point of impact. A comminuted fracture results when the impact force is sufficient to break the bone into multiple pieces under the point of impact and further through areas of weakness. Comminution absorbs the force of the injury. With even larger impact energies, the comminuted pieces can be driven inward to create a

depressed fracture and may penetrate the dura and cortical surface of the brain.

The second factor is the ratio of the impact force to the impact area. If the impact, even one of high energy, is dispersed over a large area, as in a blunt head injury to an individual wearing a motorcycle helmet, it often produces no skull fracture, even though the brain may be severely injured. Parenthetically, it should be noted that some helmets, by the efficiency of their very force-transferring protection, have created basal skull fractures by transferred energy absorbed from protection of the vault and face and then transmitted through the mandible via the chin strap to the skull base. However, if the impact, even one of low energy, is concentrated in a small area, such as from a hammer blow, it often produces a small depressed fracture with multiple linear skull fractures radiating from the site of impact.

The location of a skull fracture is classified by its geography in two distinct areas: the skull convexity (generally termed *skull vault fracture*) or the base of the skull (generally termed *basilar fracture*). Any of the two areas can occur singly or in combination. The pattern may also become more comminuted with increasing energy forces. A skull fracture can be further classified as "open" or "closed" by the presence or absence, respectively, of an overlying scalp laceration. In addition, a fracture extending into the skull base with violation of the paranasal sinuses, the nose, middle ear, or mastoid structures is also considered an "open" fracture.

Linear Skull Fractures

A linear skull fracture is a single fracture line that goes through the entire thickness of the skull.

Diagnosis

Although it is generally accepted that clinical indications for radiological examination include loss of consciousness, retrograde amnesia, discharge from nose or ear, drainage from eardrum, dislocation of the middle ear structure or hemotympanum, positive Babinski reflex, or cranial nerve abnormalities, controversy exists (based on a cost-benefit analysis) regarding the use of plain x-rays to diagnose linear skull fractures. The patient's eventual neurological outcome depends largely on the brain injury, rather than on the presence of a skull fracture per se. However, for a few patients radiological examination may make a crucial difference. For example, a linear fracture crossing the path of the middle meningeal artery in even a mild head injury indicates risk for late neurological deterioration from an epidural hematoma. Furthermore, computed tomography (CT) scans of the skull may detect depressed fractures, puncture wounds, and intracranial foreign objects that might otherwise elude physical examination. In practice a CT scan should be obtained in most cases; however, plain skull radiographs usually add little information. Medicolegally, it is usually best to obtain a CT scan, especially if the patient has an equivocal history or if there is evidence of a cognitive issue or indication of a significant force of injury.

Management

Linear skull fractures require no stabilization or exploration when the scalp is closed, and when there is no evidence of epidural hematoma or underlying dural or cortical injury. Even when a scalp laceration is present, very seldom is surgical exploration with bone removal necessary. Exceptions would include a machete injury to the skull producing a linear skull fracture with underlying dural laceration and brain damage. The skull fracture does, however, show that significant head trauma has occurred, and a careful assessment of the brain, facial structures, and cervical spine is required. Open linear fractures are débride of foreign material, devitalized soft tissue, and bone fragments; preferably, the damaged soft tissue at the edges of the laceration is excised to healthy, noncontused bleeding tissue (if the tissue excision can be tolerated and will permit primary closure) and the laceration is closed after thorough cleansing. If there is insufficient vascularized soft tissue present to permit excision of the contused devitalized tissue, a rotation flap and skin graft to the donor area may have to be considered (Fig. 22.1).

Growing Skull Fractures in Children

A rare complication after linear skull fracture in young children (usually younger than 2 or 3 years) is a "growing" skull defect at the fracture site. In these cases, the dura is torn under the linear skull fracture. The pathogenesis is thought to be an expanding pouch of arachnoid passing through the torn dura and skull fracture, acting as a one-way valve that traps

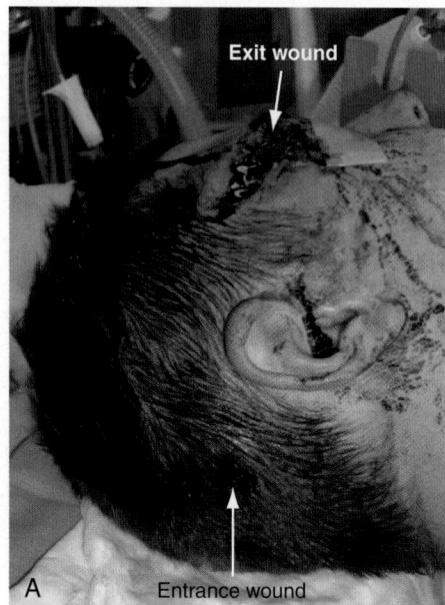
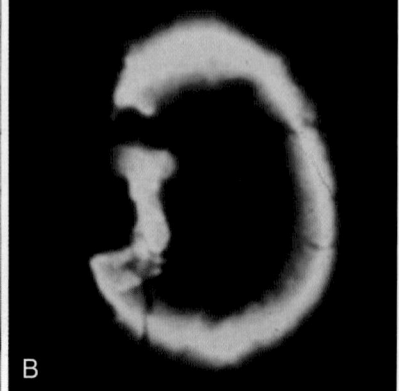
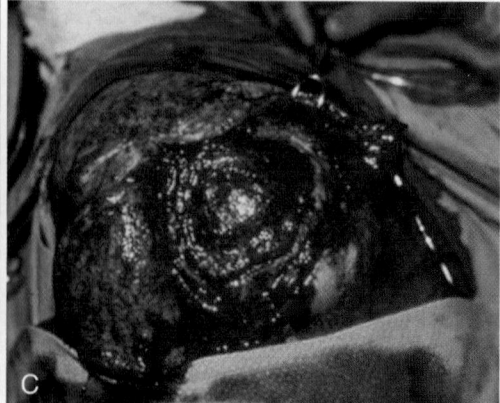

FIGURE 22.1 Open skull fracture (**A**) with tissue loss (**B**) sufficient that an immediate (**C**) scalp rotation flap had to be performed to achieve scalp closure.

cerebrospinal fluid (CSF) and causes progressive pressure erosion of the fractured edges to enlarge the fracture. Alternatively, the growth of the brain, which produces pulsating, spreading tensile pressure forces on the edges of an unrepaired dural laceration, may also cause a skull defect to enlarge. These vectors of force by the brain may sometimes cause herniation through the skull defect, causing a new neurological deficit (Fig. 22.2). These lesions are surgically repaired with closure of the dura or with a dural patch and replacement or repair of the bone defect. Some surgeons routinely take a skull film at 1 year after linear skull fracture treated nonoperatively to detect such growing skull fractures. For this reason it is worthwhile for the primary care doctor to examine the scalp and skull of any child with a known skull fracture under the age of 2 or 3.

Comminuted Fractures

A comminuted fracture occurs when multiple linear fractures radiate from the point of impact. Some of the fracture lines may involve the suture lines (diastatic fracture) or may stop at them. Around the point of impact there may be free fragments of bone.

Diagnosis

Diagnosis is made on skull radiographs and CT of the head with bone windows.

Management

If the skin is closed, and no depression of bone fragments greater than the thickness of the skull is demonstrated on CT, management is as that for linear skull fractures. However, in many of these cases, surgery is performed for the underlying intracranial injury, such as an epidural hematoma (Fig. 22.3). After the intracranial injury has been corrected, the bone

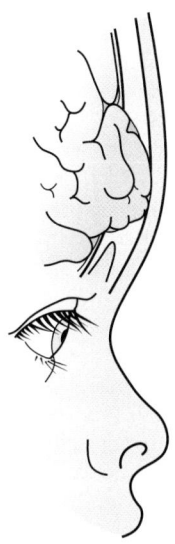

FIGURE 22.2 "Growing"" skull fracture in a child. The mechanism is a closed skull fracture that tears the dura. The pressure of the pulsating brain creates slow erosion of the bone, creating a bone and dural defect. Repair of the dura and cranioplasty is required.

fragments are primarily replaced as a bone cranioplasty after cleaning.

Missing bone can be replaced with a titanium mesh screen. If the skin is open, and free bone fragments are present, cleansing or débridement of the contaminated fragments is performed, before dural and scalp closure (Fig. 22.4). Bone too contaminated may be discarded, and a titanium screen is then used to span the bone defect (Fig. 22.5).

Depressed Skull Fractures

In a depressed skull fracture, the greatest bone depression can occur at the interface of fracture and intact skull or near the center of the fracture if several fragments are displaced inward. Impacted fractures may be "wedged" into position by blocked bone edges.

Diagnosis

Some patients with depressed skull fractures experience initial loss of consciousness and neurological damage owing to the force transferred from the impact through the skull and into the brain. However, 25% of patients experience neither loss of consciousness nor neurological deficit. Another 25% of patients experience only brief loss of consciousness. Although the diagnosis of a depressed skull fracture is often indicated on routine skull radiographs by an area of double density (overlying bone fragments) or by multiple or circular fractures, the full extent and depth of injury are rarely appreciated with a CT scan. Physical examination is more difficult in the presence of scalp mobility and swelling. Scalp mobility can result in nonalignment of the sheared layers of the scalp or a scalp laceration and can therefore simulate, under palpation, the sense of a skull fracture; normal skull under a scalp laceration also does not exclude a depressed fracture 1 or 2 cm from one edge of the laceration. Furthermore, post-traumatic swelling of the scalp minimizes the palpable and visual appearance of the step-off at the bony edges, preventing accurate clinical assessment of the extent of a skull deformity or displacement for the first few days.

CT is the diagnostic method of choice. When image display windows are adjusted to optimize bony detail, they display the position, extent, and number of fractures as well as the presence and depth of depression. With the imaging windows set to optimize intracranial contents, the same CT scan also allows assessment of the underlying brain for contusion or hematoma, small bone fragments, or foreign bodies as well as other intracranial trauma. Occasionally, coronal CT images through fractures near the vertex of the head or extending into the skull base are used to supplement the standard CT images, because the depth of a depression is more accurately measured on CT images perpendicular to the depression.

Management

Combined therapy of depressed fractures of the cranial vault extending to involve the frontal sinus or facial bones is covered in the sections on facial fractures. When a depressed skull fracture on the convexity also includes facial fractures, the intracranial injury is typically repaired first with removal of intracerebral hematoma and repair of dural laceration if present (Figs. 22.6 and 22.7).

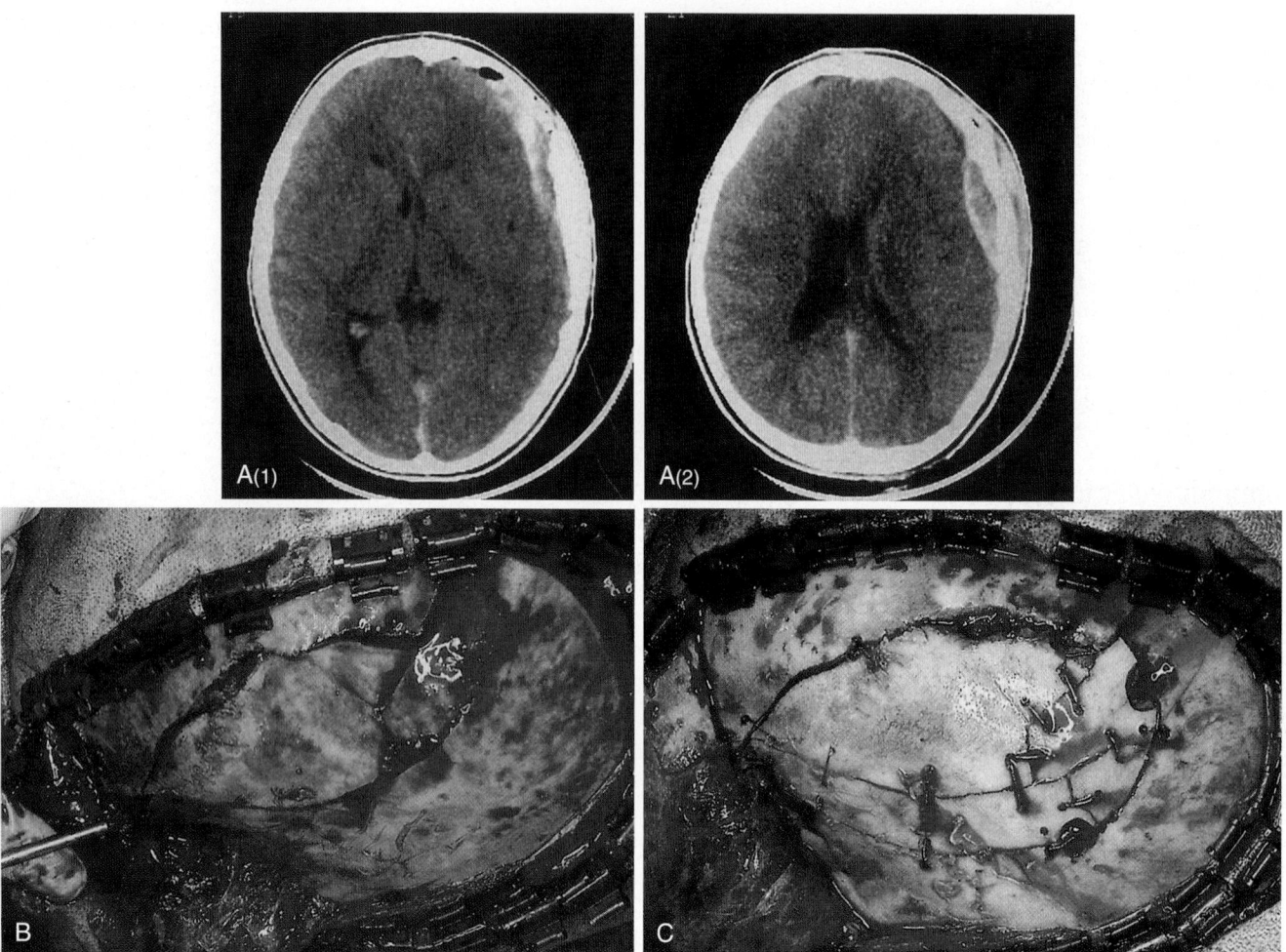

FIGURE 22.3 Comminuted minimally depressed open skull fracture with underlying epidural hematoma. **A,** Computed tomography (CT) scan through the center of the depressed region. Note the small amount of air at the anterior edge of the epidural hematoma. **B,** Intraoperative view of the depressed bone before evaluation. **C,** The bone was removed, sutured together, and replaced as a cranioplasty. The epidural hematoma was removed after the bone fragments had been removed.

Although a focal neurological deficit from the cortex directly under a depressed skull fracture is occasionally improved by elevation of the bone fragments (presumably by increasing local cortical blood flow), elevation usually produces no neurological change, implying that the initial impact produces the major cortical damage responsible for the brain deficit. The brain dysfunction usually undergoes a neurological recovery phase of several weeks to months, similar to that after a stroke or head injury without a depressed fracture. Likewise, the incidence of epilepsy after a depressed skull fracture is determined by the cortical damage at the time of impact. Therefore, the treatment of depressed skull fractures is based on relieving pressure on the brain (initiating neurological recovery), minimizing epilepsy, correcting cosmetic deformity, and preventing infection.

In closed, depressed fractures, the major indication for surgery is usually cosmetic, with the procedure performed on an elective basis in the first few days after the trauma, once the patient is cleared for elective anesthesia. The greatest cosmetic deformity occurs in the forehead. Exploration is more urgent for a large, closed depressed fracture when the radiological appearance suggests dural laceration, brain penetration,

simultaneous frontal sinus fracture, mass effect, or underlying hematoma. The hematoma is evacuated, the dura is repaired, and the bone fragments are replaced and held in position with small plates and screws.

A compound depressed fracture is a neurosurgical emergency because of the risk of bacterial infection of the cranial cavity. The initial surgery is performed within 24 hours and usually within the first 12 hours. The major objectives are removal of contaminated bone fragment and foreign material; débridement of devitalized scalp, dura, and brain; and provision of a watertight closure of the dura. Often, foreign material or hair wedged between bone fragments cannot be seen through the overlying scalp incision, so simple irrigation and closure may be inadequate for débridement of foreign material. Dural closure is essential to prevent CSF leaks from the wound and brain herniation into the fracture area. Dural closure is essential to prevent CSF leaks from the wound and brain herniation into the fracture area. Dural closure also presents intracranial spread of infection from a scalp wound. Reconstruction of the calvarium is performed during the initial surgery if considered safe: otherwise a cranial defect is left and the cosmetic repair is performed later. The major reasons to consider deferred

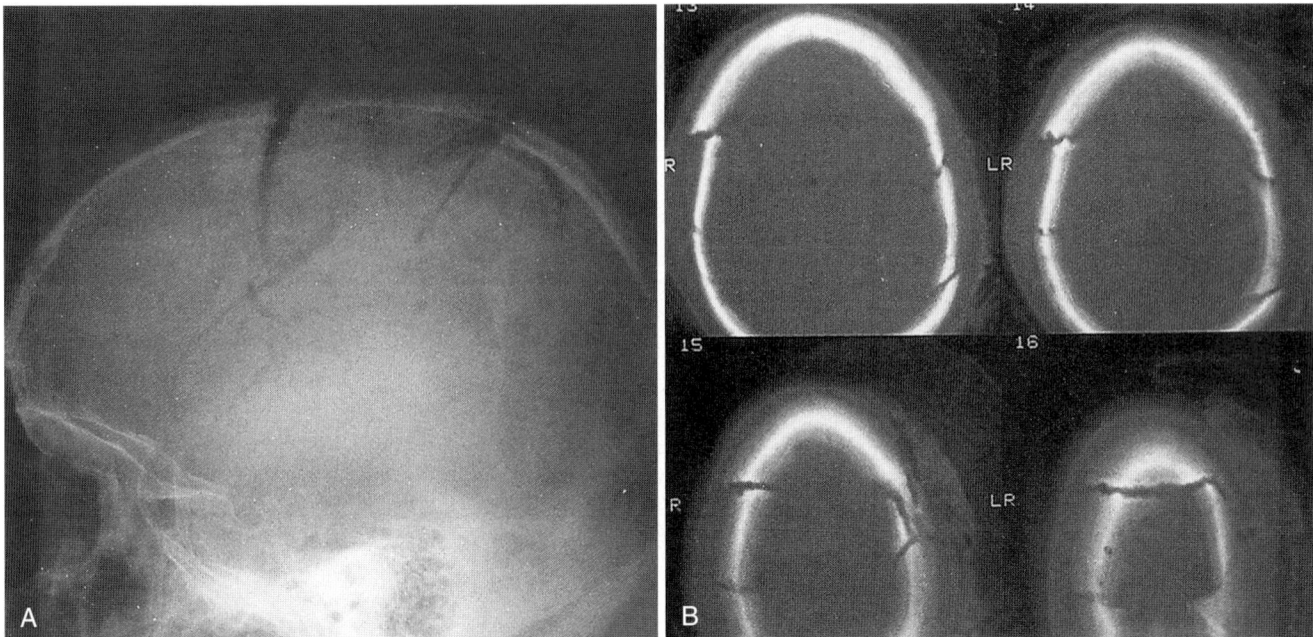

FIGURE 22.4 Comminuted skull fracture involving a diastatic fracture of both coronal sutures and additional fractures of the frontal and parietal bone bilaterally. In this case, the skin was open and cerebrospinal fluid was coming from the wound. **A,** Lateral radiograph demonstrating the comminuted fracture. **B,** Computed tomography scan with bone windows near the top of the head showing the comminuted fracture.

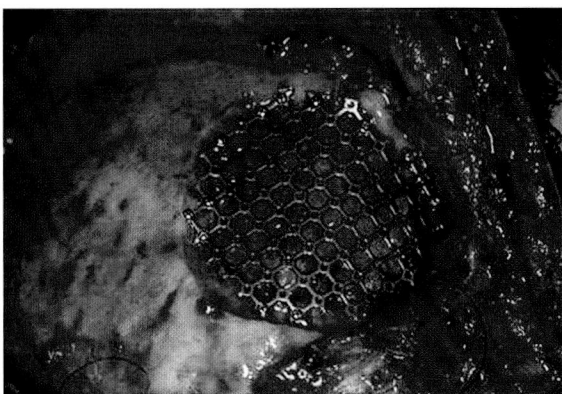

FIGURE 22.5 A titanium screen can be used to span a bone defect when autologous bone cannot be used because it is contaminated and must be discarded.

calvarial reconstruction are to shorten additional anesthesia and blood loss by major head injury or multitrauma, especially with hemorrhage; gross contamination of wounds where the bone fragments cannot be adequately cleaned; and a delay of more than 24 hours for the initial surgery.

The scalp laceration associated with a compound depressed skull fracture is usually stellate and may contain areas of contused/devitalized tissue. These areas require débridement to normal vascularized scalp to allow prompt healing and prevent breakdown of the partially viable scalp covering the fracture site (see Fig. 22.1). Scalp breakdown can many times be treated locally but occasionally will require early flap coverage. If early flap coverage is not successful, the replaced cranial bone may require débridement of any dead or nonviable necrotic bone or portion of the skin flap; a subsequent flap rotation and delayed cranioplasty will be required in stages.

Depressed Fractures over Dural Sinuses

Depressed skull fractures over a venous sinus require special handling. Surgical elevation of these fractures may involve massive blood loss if a depressed fragment has been plugging a sinus tear. There are two strategies for management. The fracture can be carefully elevated, attempting to gain control of the venous sinus as soon as possible, preparing for significant transfusion requirements. If the fracture site is not grossly contaminated with foreign material, or will not cause a major cosmetic or functional deformity, or not cause intracranial hypertension secondary to sinus occlusion, such fractures are managed with scalp débridement alone and irrigation, followed by serial CT scans for signs of brain abscess for at least a year. A delayed cranioplasty may then be required for contour. The management of these fractures requires both judgment and experience as no definite rules apply to the variation of presentations.

Basilar Skull Fractures

Fractures of the base of the skull occur in 3.5% to 24% of head-injured patients. This wide variation results from differences in study populations and the difficulty in obtaining radiographic verification of the fractures. Linear fractures in the skull base carry a risk of meningitis, whereas this risk is extremely low in fractures of the convexity unless the scalp, bone, and dura are all violated. The dura is easily torn in a basal skull fracture; this places the subarachnoid space in direct contact with the paranasal sinuses or middle ear structures, providing a pathway for infection. For example, a persistent fistula allows a continuous CSF leak, and bacterial colonization of the meninges will eventually develop.

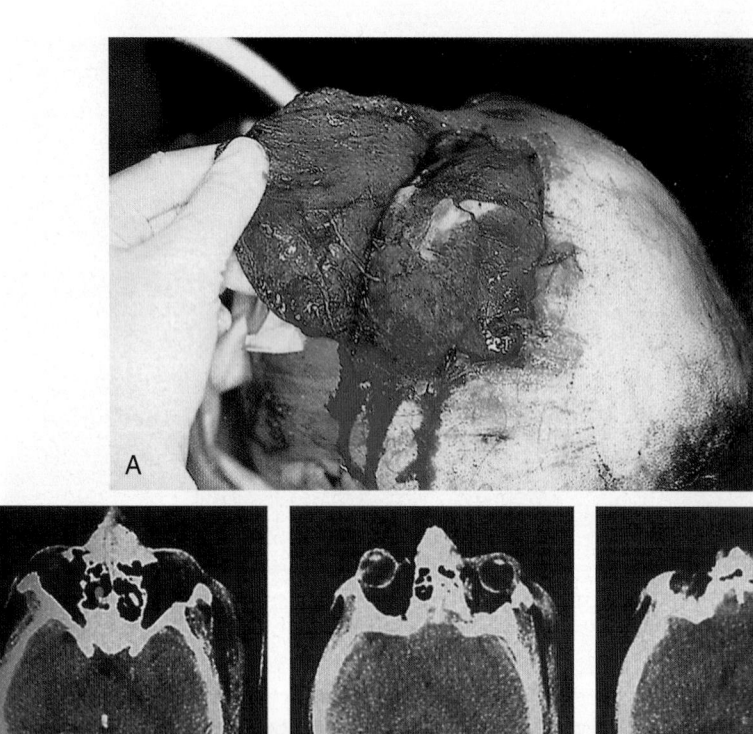

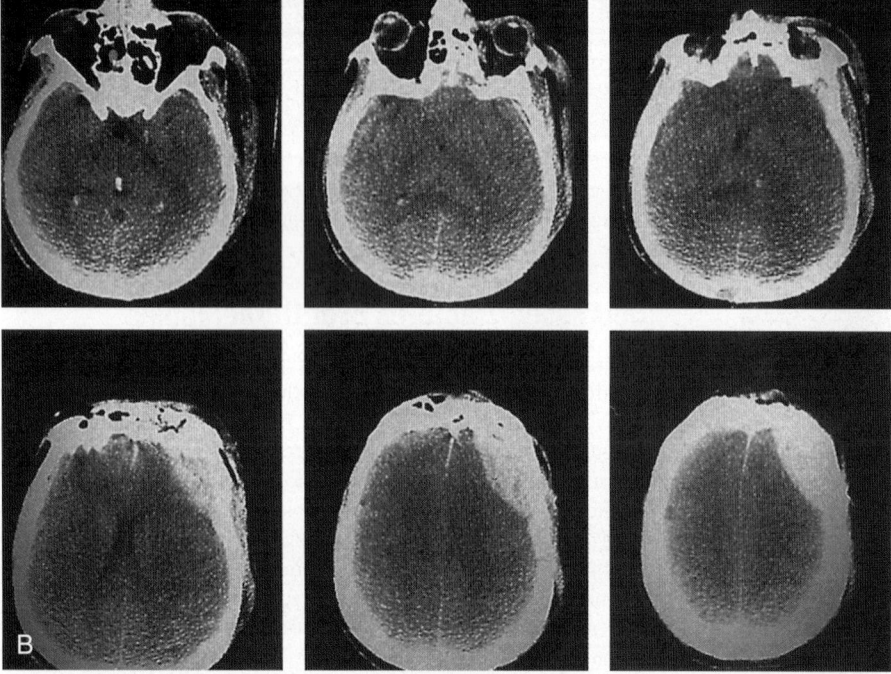

FIGURE 22.6 Open frontal and facial fracture. **A,** View of frontal skull fracture under the wound. **B,** Computed tomography scan showing the epidural hematoma under this open skull fracture.

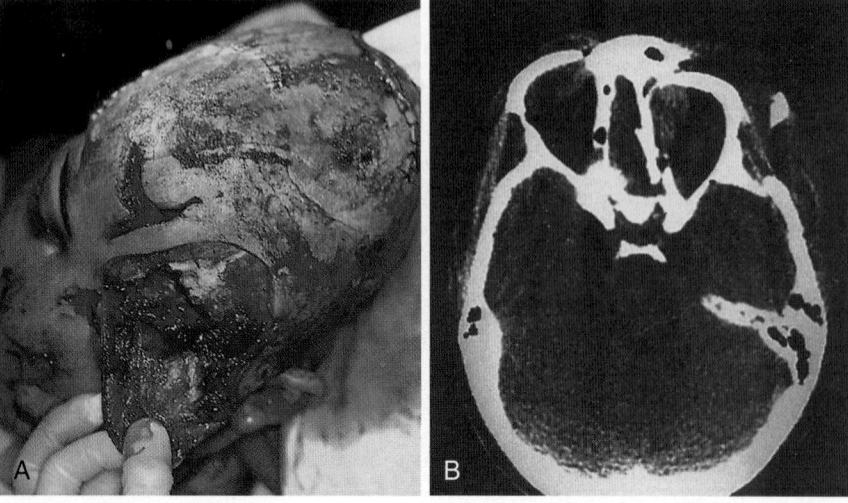

FIGURE 22.7 Open dressed skull fracture involving the frontal bone with extensive fractures and displacement of bones of the orbit and ethmoid region. **A,** Presenting scalp laceration. **B,** Computed tomography scan at the level of the orbit demonstrating extensive orbital and ethmoid fractures with displacement of the bony facial structures.

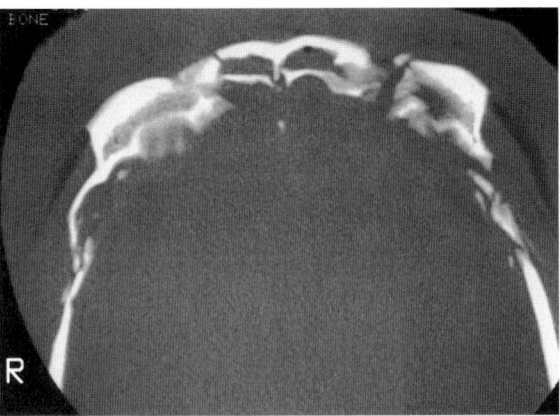

FIGURE 22.8 Type III frontobasilar fracture involves both the lateral and the central segments of the anterior skull.

Petrous bone fractures can either be either longitudinal or transverse, relative to the long axis of the petrous pyramid. Longitudinal fractures are more common and usually involve the tympanic membrane or external ear canal, thereby producing otorrhea. Transverse fractures result from higher-energy impacts and can damage middle ear ossicles or the facial nerve. These fractures occur with or in continuity with linear, comminuted, or depressed skull fractures and not infrequently are large linear extensions of vault fractures, crossing the base of the anterior and middle cranial fossae (Fig. 22.8).

Diagnosis

Clinical signs of basal skull fractures include bilateral periorbital ecchymoses (spectacle hematoma) (Fig. 22.9), anosmia, or CSF rhinorrhea for anterior skull base fractures, as well as hemotympanum, blood in the external auditory canal, seventh or eighth cranial nerve palsies, ecchymoses over the mastoids (Battle's sign), or CSF otorrhea for temporal bone fractures (Fig. 22.10). Frequently, the CSF leak is first detected several days or weeks after the trauma. This delay often occurs because the CSF leak was hidden in bloody nasal discharge from facial fractures, or less frequently, it is the result of delayed development of hydrocephalus with rupture of the arachnoid at the fracture site. A larger clear ring surrounding a central blood-tinged clot when a few drops of bloody discharge are placed on a paper towel indicates that CSF is probably mixed with the blood. This sign (the "double ring") can also be noted on the patient's pillow during rounds.

Basal skull fracture with CSF rhinorrhea is common after head injury and has an estimated incidence in the United States of 150,000 cases per year. A clear, watery nasal discharge containing glucose indicates CSF rhinorrhea. An intermittent CSF leak from the paranasal sinuses can often be demonstrated by having the patient sit on the edge of the bed with the head close to the knees for 2 minutes and watching for clear fluid to drip from the nose. CSF mixed with blood may form a halo on a piece of gauze it touches. Testing for beta-2 transferrin presence in the fluid confirms the protein found almost uniquely in CSF.

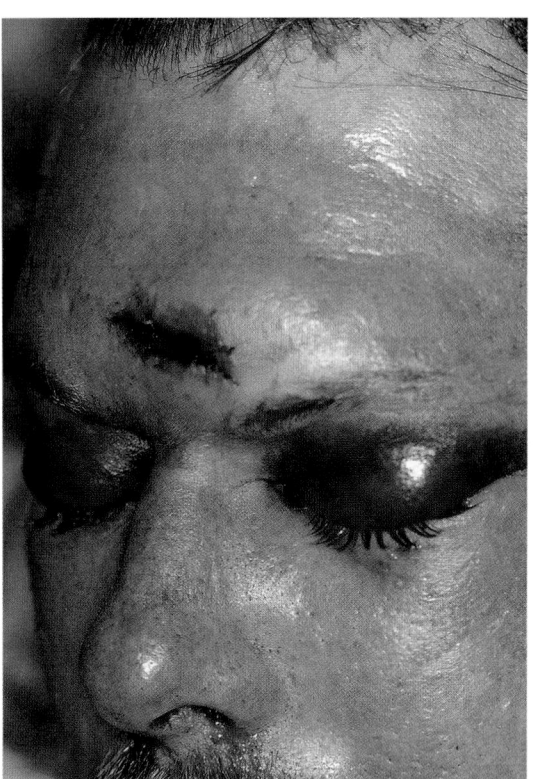

FIGURE 22.9 Bilateral spectacle hematoma from an open frontal sinus anterior skull base fracture.

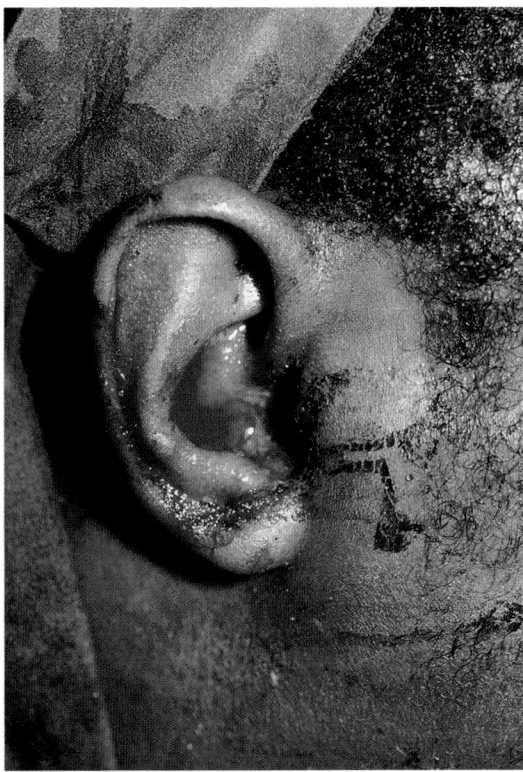

FIGURE 22.10 Cerebrospinal fluid leaks from the ear canal and a hematoma is visible in the postauricular area. These are signs of a fracture at the junction of the middle and posterior cranial fossa.

Management

Basal skull fractures are managed depending on whether a CSF leak is present. A patient with a basal skull fracture but no leak is observed for 2 to 3 days. During this time, repeated checks for rhinorrhea and otorrhea are made to verify the absence of a CSF leak. Otorrhea is more likely than rhinorrhea to resolve spontaneously. Because antibiotics are not effective in preventing meningitis over a prolonged interval and select for resistant organisms if an infection occurs, "prophylactic" antibiotics are not used on a prolonged basis in patients with basal skull fractures. When definitive closure of a leak is performed, perioperative antibiotics are utilized.

A CSF leak is managed initially by observing the amount of leakage and monitoring for signs of infection: change in temperature, altered mental status, or increased white blood cell count. Radiographic or imaging studies may indicate the area and size of the defect, which may suggest the likelihood of spontaneous closure. Most traumatic CSF leaks resolve spontaneously within the first week. If the leak persists beyond 5 to 7 days, lumbar punctures are performed daily for 3 days, removing 30 to 50 mL of spinal fluid each time, attempting to decrease the CSF pressure.

If spinal taps fail to stop the leak, spinal drainage can be used for 72 hours with the patient in a 30-degree head-up position. Should pneumocephalus develop during the course of the CSF drainage, the drainage procedure is terminated and the dural leak is surgically closed. CSF leaks refractory to spinal fluid drainage require surgical closure; the exact site of the leak is determined preoperatively from a CT scan with water-soluble intrathecal contrast or from a nuclear cisternogram with nasal pledgets for small or questionable leaks. A CT scan of the base of the skull can provide additional details of the pattern and size of the bone spicules in the fracture.

CSF otorrhea usually occurs through a fracture in the petrous bone with perforation of the tympanic membrane, although it can occasionally take place through a laceration of the external canal via fractured mastoid air cells. If the tympanic membrane remains intact, CSF that has gained access to the middle ear can flow through the eustachian tube and present as rhinorrhea. In these cases, the CT scan typically images a fracture in the temporal bone and fluid in the mastoid air cells and middle ear. Blood from the ear canal or a tympanic canal laceration may also be caused by a temporomandibular joint injury or dislocation, either of which may produce some of the same symptoms (bloody fluid from the ear canal).

A patient with CSF otorrhea often presents with hearing loss from blood in the external ear canal. Irrigation and probing of the ear in cases of suspected otorrhea are not indicated initially because they increase the risk of infection. Such a patient is managed by placing a loose-fitting sterile gauze pad over the ear; the pad is changed every nursing shift and saved as an indicator of the amount of drainage from the ear. Most cases of otorrhea stop spontaneously within the first few days. A detailed auditory, vestibular, and facial nerve function examination is performed initially and 6 to 8 weeks after trauma to diagnose abnormalities and determine treatment or sequence progress.

Patients with basilar skull fracture who have immediate complete facial nerve paralysis and temporal bone fracture are considered for high-dose steroid treatment or surgical exploration to decompress or graft the nerve. Patients with delayed onset of the facial paralysis or those who initially have only facial paresis are treated with steroids, and observed, because some spontaneous recovery frequently occurs.

MAXILLOFACIAL INJURIES

Skull and maxillofacial fractures often coexist after head trauma. For instance, fractures of the frontal bone or basilar skull commonly extend into the orbit, and midfacial fractures frequently accompany frontal skull, frontal sinus, or orbital fractures. In addition, fractures through the skull into the nasal sinuses can cause dural lacerations with CSF leak or pneumocephalus. When maxillofacial injury is suspected on physical examination, a CT scan of the face is the most useful diagnostic test and should be obtained at the time of the initial radiographic survey. Facial CT scans should consist of bone and soft tissue windows and axial and coronal sections.

Assessment

The events of the injury should be ascertained and a complete history of the accident or injury should be reached as described by the emergency medical technician, patient, or family members. A thorough facial physical examination is performed in sequence, concentrating on functional deficits in areas of injury. Consultations from specific specialists, such as an ophthalmologist, are also obtained. Cranial nerve abnormalities may also accompany facial fractures; oculomotor deficit, facial sensory deficit, and visual deficit are some common symptoms.

Soft tissue injury implies the possibility of damage to deeper structures, which should be presumed until appropriate examination excludes them. Hematomas are usually diffuse, and not amenable to aspiration, but localized hematomas can be aspirated or removed to facilitate healing. Lacerations should be carefully debrided and repaired after damage to bones and deep soft tissue structures has been determined.

The facial bones should be examined in a methodical sequence from top to bottom. Symptoms that imply bone injury include soft tissue injury (contusion, laceration, hematoma), bone movement, crepitation, localized tenderness, discomfort, numbness in the distribution of a cranial sensory nerve, paralysis in the distribution of a cranial motor nerve, malocclusion, visual acuity disturbance, diplopia, facial deformity or asymmetry, intraoral lacerations, fractured or avulsed teeth, air in soft tissues, and bleeding from the nose or mouth. The examiner should palpate the symmetry of the facial bones, comparing both sides. In all cases reference to old photographs (such as a driver's license) are valuable aids in documenting a preexisting facial deformity or in establishing a change from previous appearance. Dental malalignment (malocclusion) is an index of bone or tooth fracture, edema, or temporomandibular joint injury.

Facial sensation is noted in the supraorbital, supratrochlear, infratrochlear, infraorbital, and mental nerve regions of the trigeminal nerve distribution for both pinprick and light touch sensation. Diminished sensation in the distribution of a specific sensory nerve indicates injury from transaction, impact, or continued compression of the nerve as the result

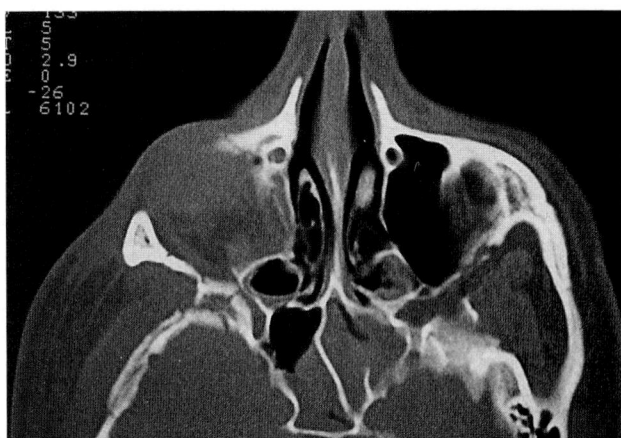

FIGURE 22.12 Axial window of an orbital fracture. The globe is prolapsing into the floor defect.

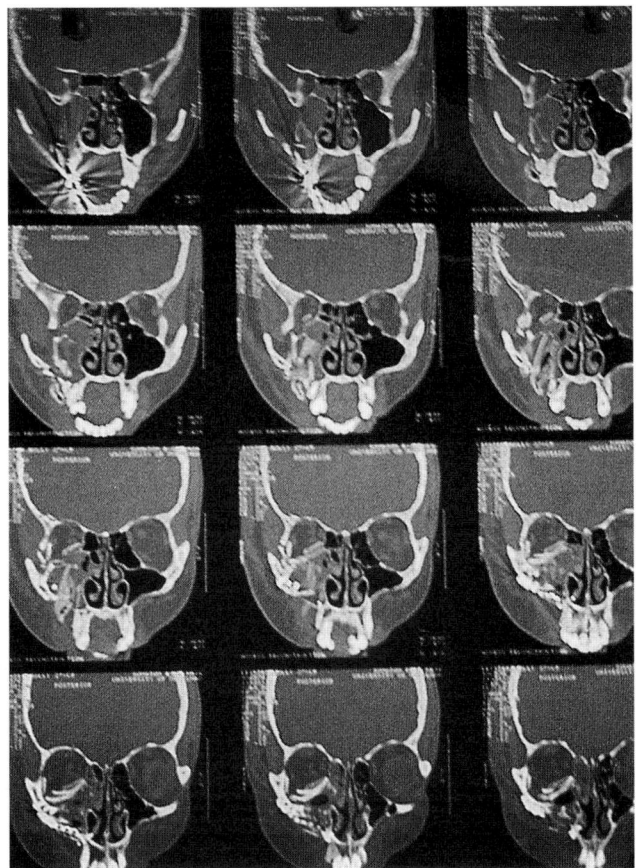

FIGURE 22.11 Two-dimensional facial computed tomography (CT) scans are essential in facial fracture evaluation. They can be rapidly obtained after the CT evaluation of the brain. Axial and coronal windows should be obtained through the entire area of the injury. Here, coronal CT scans demonstrate reduction of a zygomatic fracture by plate and screw fixation and orbital floor bone grafting.

of a fracture. The facial nerve is tested by comparing facial expression bilaterally. Extraocular movements and pupil response are compared, evaluating symmetry, pupil size, and the speed of pupil reaction bilaterally to both direct and consensual responses to light.

Emergency treatment is immediately directed toward life-threatening events such as (1) airway obstruction, (2) bleeding (major hemorrhage from the scalp or face), and (3) aspiration (prevented when the airway is maintained by orotracheal intubation, although occasionally an emergency cricothyroidotomy is required). The stability of the cervical spine is assessed in every patient with head trauma during this phase.

The early management of maxillofacial injuries is based entirely on a good clinical examination and facial CT scans (Fig. 22.11). Soft tissue windows are necessary on the CT scan to evaluate the brain and orbital soft tissue fully. Axial (Fig. 22.12) and coronal CT bone windows (direct or reformatted) are crucial to reveal details of fractures of the upper face and orbit. Coronal sections (Fig. 22.13) begin with the nasal pyramid and continue posteriorly through the orbital apex. Axial scans begin at the superior aspect of the skull and progress through the brain with standard axial brain imaging. The size and spacing of the cuts at the level of the frontal sinus are reduced to 5 mm or less to obtain the required detail.

When a mandible fracture is suspected, the axial CT scanning is continued through the entire mandible and temporomandibular joints, visualizing both the horizontal and vertical portions of the mandible and the temporomandibular joints. Although three-dimensional reconstruction with shading (Fig. 22.14) adds spatial information, it does not provide the detail of two-dimensional axial and coronal images. In some cases, special reconstructions, as one performed in the longitudinal axis of the optic nerve in orbital injury, provide additional information.

Associated Conditions

Respiratory Obstruction

Facial injuries can impair breathing in several ways. Fractures or avulsed teeth, broken dentures or bridgework, and foreign objects displaced into the airway must be removed. Facial fracture segments may be sufficiently displaced to compromise the airway. In addition, facial bleeding can contribute to aspiration and respiratory obstruction. Patients with combinations of burns and fractures of the upper and lower jaws; fractures of the nose, maxilla, and mandible; or fractures of the mandible that result in significant bleeding into the floor of the mouth and neck all may have respiratory obstruction. Noisy respiration, stridor, hoarseness, drooling, inability to swallow or handle oral secretions, sternal retraction, and cyanosis all herald impending death from respiratory obstruction, and immediate intubation or tracheostomy is therefore required. The use of plate and screw fixation for facial fracture reduction has allowed intermaxillary fixation to be discontinued postoperatively for many patients. Tracheostomy therefore may often be avoided with the use of rigid fixation.

Profuse Hemorrhage

Cutaneous bleeding that accompanies facial lacerations is usually controlled with digital pressure, which allows precise identification of the bleeding vessel for control or ligature. Blind probing in facial tissue or unselective cautery or ligature placement can damage branches of the facial nerve and should be avoided.

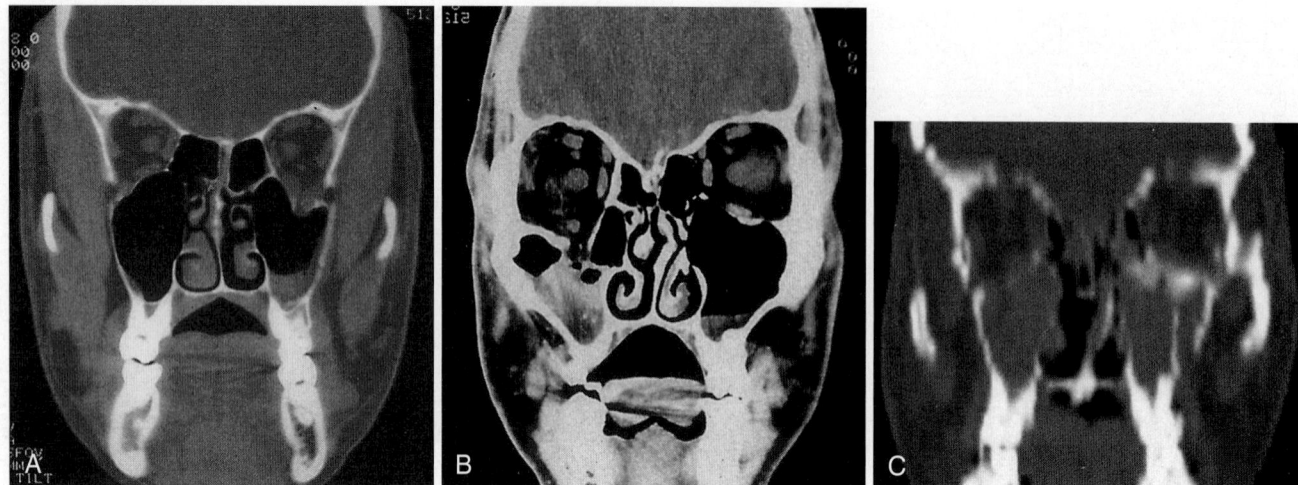

FIGURE 22.13 Direct coronal windows are preferable for evaluation of the orbit, sinuses, and palate. Both soft tissue (**A**) and bone (**B**) windows should be obtained for the orbit. Two blow-out fractures are seen. In **A** the inferior rectus muscle is adjacent to the fracture. In **B** soft tissue windows clearly show the inferior meatus muscle adjacent to the fracture. **C,** Reformatted images may be obtained where the direct coronal image is not possible. Their clarity depends on the axial cuts.

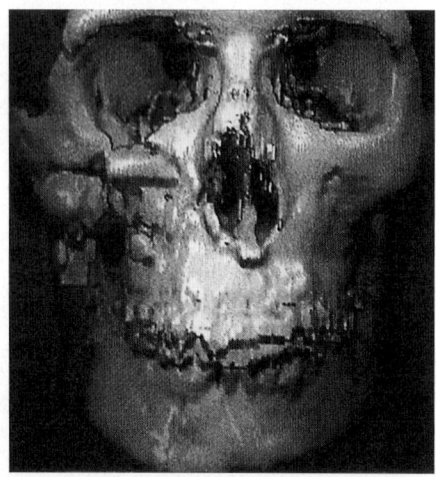

FIGURE 22.14 Three-dimensional computed tomography (CT) scans add spatial perspective, but they do not replace two-dimensional CT scans and are not essential for fracture repair. A depressed zygomatic and orbital fracture is seen.

Bleeding from closed maxillofacial injuries usually results from fractures involving the sinuses. Bleeding from the nose (epistaxis) occurs with nasal, zygomatic, orbital, frontal sinus, nasoethmoidal, maxillary, and cranial base fractures. Although profuse nasopharyngeal hemorrhage usually accompanies Le Fort maxillary fractures, epistaxis is a nonspecific indication of many types of midfacial fractures. Usually the hemorrhage is self-limiting. Several maneuvers control the hemorrhage when required, including anteroposterior nasal packing, manual repositioning of the maxilla, the application of intermaxillary fixation (rest position of the maxilla), or an external facial compression (Barton) dressing.

If profuse nasopharyngeal hemorrhage from closed fractures does not respond to the preceding measures, arterial embolization or arterial ligation can be performed. An angiogram is obtained to determine the major source of bleeding.

In Le Fort fractures bleeding usually involves the branches of the internal maxillary artery. This artery can be embolized or selectively ligated directly through the back wall of the maxillary sinus, or arterial ligation of the external carotid and superficial temporal arteries (both) on the ipsilateral side usually reduces such bleeding substantially. Arterial ligation is rarely necessary.

Because bleeding abnormalities are noted early in patients with cerebral injuries and facial fractures, replacement of depleted coagulation factors is based on assessment of coagulation factors in hemorrhaging patients.

Aspiration

Aspiration of blood, saliva, and gastric contents frequently accompanies maxillofacial injuries and can obstruct respiration and cause pulmonary parenchymal damage. Endotracheal intubation or tracheostomy is the definitive treatment.

Coma and Brain Injury

Coma or unconsciousness should not prevent or delay the treatment of facial fractures; many patients with facial fractures are in a coma for several weeks before waking up. In patients with maxillofacial fractures, neurological deficits from frontal lobe symptoms may be subtle or absent despite contusions imaged on brain CT scans. Confusion, somnolence, personality change, irritability, and difficulty in thinking are some of the milder symptoms of frontal brain contusion. In patients with Glasgow Coma Scale scores of 14 or less, and especially when traumatic brain abnormality is visualized on CT scan, an intracranial pressure monitoring device may be employed in those patients who require anesthesia. A fiberoptic intracranial pressure (ICP) monitor or intracranial ventricular pressure monitor is used in the operating room during the facial repair, thus allowing optimal modification of the anesthesia and if necessary CSF drainage in patients in whom multiple injuries require early surgical intervention.

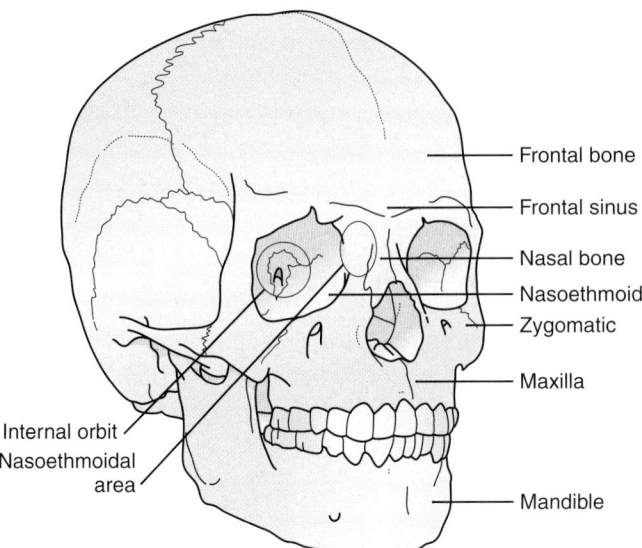

FIGURE 22.15 The anatomical regions of the face are shown. They include the frontal bone, the frontal sinus, the nose, the nasoethmoidal area, the zygoma, the internal orbit, the maxilla, and the mandible.

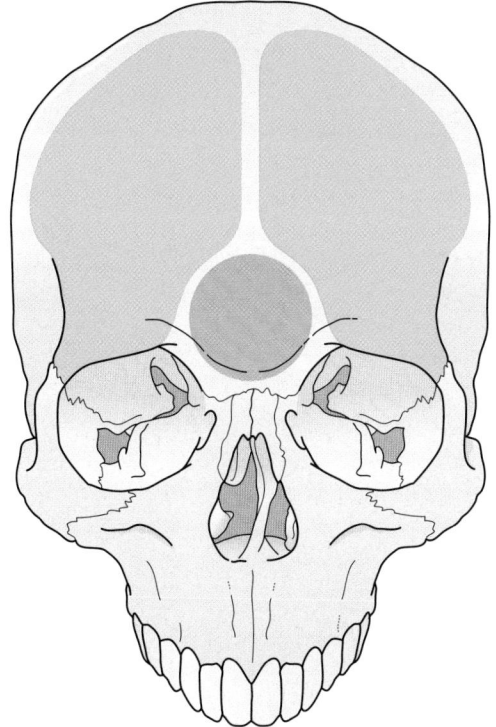

FIGURE 22.16 The divisions of the frontal bone area are shaded. They include the central (frontal sinus) area (*blue*) and, laterally, the frontal-temporal-orbital region (*green*), which extends to the coronal suture. Fractures often involve two of three areas of the frontal skull.

Facial Fracture Classification by Anatomical Region

The treatment of maxillofacial fractures is organized by anatomical region (Fig. 22.15). The frontal bone region includes the frontal bone, the supraorbital rims bilaterally, and the frontal sinus (Fig. 22.16). The upper midface region includes

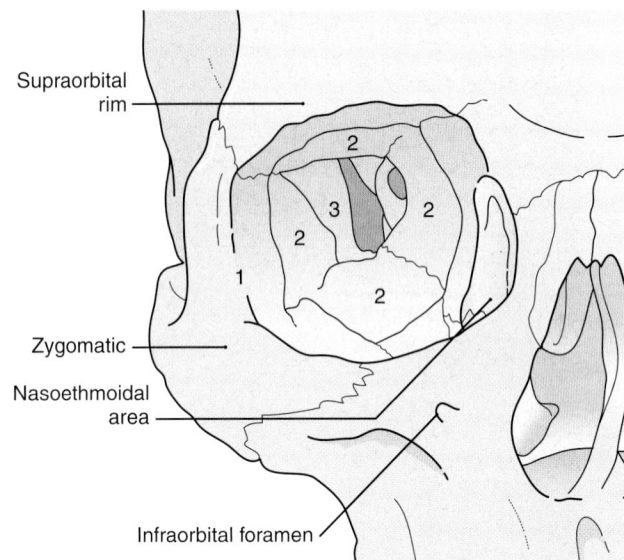

FIGURE 22.17 The orbit consists of three sections from anterior to posterior: (1) the thick rim anteriorly; (2) the thin middle section; and (3) the thick posterior third of the orbit. The posterior portion of the orbit represents the cranial base. The orbital rim can be conceptualized in three regions: superiorly, the supraorbital rim; inferiorly and laterally, the zygomatic region; medially, the nasoethmoidal area.

the zygoma laterally, the internal orbital area, and the nasoethmoidal area centrally. The lower midface consists of the maxillary alveolus. The mandible consists of the horizontal portion containing the teeth and the vertical portion that includes the angle, ramus, coronoid, and condylar process. The pattern and displacement of the fractures in each anatomical region determine treatment. Orbital fractures are classified by their position on the orbital rim and by their involvement of the internal section of the orbit. Orbital rim fractures are divided into supraorbital, the nasoethmoid medically, and the zygomatic region inferolaterally (Fig. 22.17). The section of the internal orbit consists of the orbital floor, the lateral orbit, and the medial (ethmoidal) orbit. Maxillary fractures are classified according to the patterns of Le Fort, based on the fracture's location in the maxilla where it is separated from intact upper facial units.

Fractures of the Frontal Bone and Supraorbital Area

Fractures of the frontal bone area frequently extend to the orbital roof, frontal sinus, and nose. A fracture in this area implies the possibility of injury to the dura and to the frontal lobes. CSF rhinorrhea and pneumocephalus may be present. Because of its strength, the frontal bone is involved in only 5% to 10% of all fractures. Fractures that simultaneously involve the cranium and the orbit are high-energy injuries, and soft tissue damage is more severe. Major injuries to the brain and the cervical spine frequently accompany these fractures, and contusions of the forebrain and orbital contents are routine.

The frontal and ethmoid sinuses render the frontal bone more vulnerable to injury and infection. Each major segment of the frontal sinus (generally two) has a "duct" (usually a broad ostium) that communicates with the middle meatus of the nose.

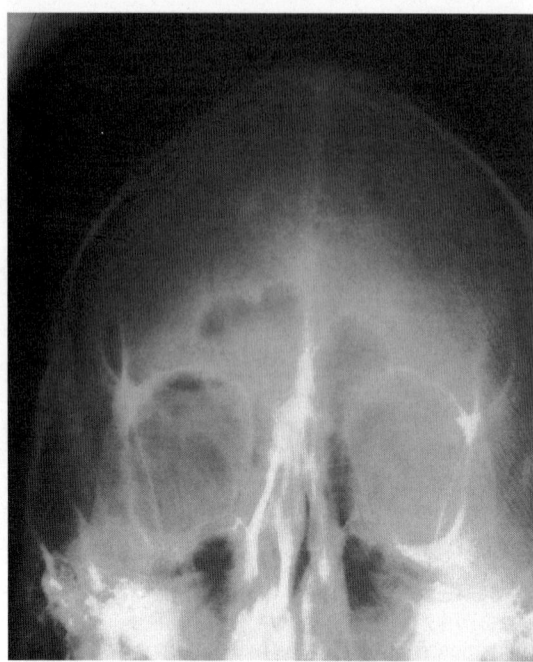

FIGURE 22.18 A fracture and frontal sinus duct obstruction are visible on this plain film. A mucocele might have a similar appearance.

Sinus injury may therefore result in duct obstruction after fracture, mucosal edema, or damage (Fig. 22.18). A cyst-like structure called a *mucocele* (obstructed mucous cyst) sometimes follows mucosal injury; depending on size, it may create eroding bone pressure and penetrate into the orbit or intracranial cavity. Surgery at a later time is necessary to remedy either of these conditions, as symptoms of pain and sinusitis will persist. Because the posterior wall of the frontal sinus is in contact with the dura, any infection in that area represents an extradural abscess. Posterior wall fractures of the frontal sinus are often accompanied by dural tears. Many of these tears extend along the anterior frontobasilar region of the skull to cause CSF leak or pneumocephalus. A small CSF leak is often masked by epistaxis in the early days after facial injury. When fractures in the posterior wall of the frontal sinus or the anterior base of the skull are noted, a CSF leak should be suspected.

Fractures of the frontal bone commonly extend within the cranial sutures and then involve other regions. When the fracture extends into the supraorbital region, the bone is usually depressed downward and posteriorly, compressing the orbital contents and producing a downward and forward dislocation of the globe (Fig. 22.19). With more limited injuries, linear frontal skull fractures may extend into the orbit and along the cranial base. These fractures can create a CSF leak or obstruct sinus drainage by edema or bone displacement. As fracture patterns become more complex and severe, bone displacement occurs. The anterior base of the skull and the roofs of the orbit are comminuted, and linear fractures extend from the anterior through the middle cranial fossa. The anterior and middle sections of the orbit displace, absorbing energy, and linear fractures extend from the displaced bone through the posterior portion of the orbit and into the middle cranial fossa. These fractures can account for basilar CSF leaks, pituitary

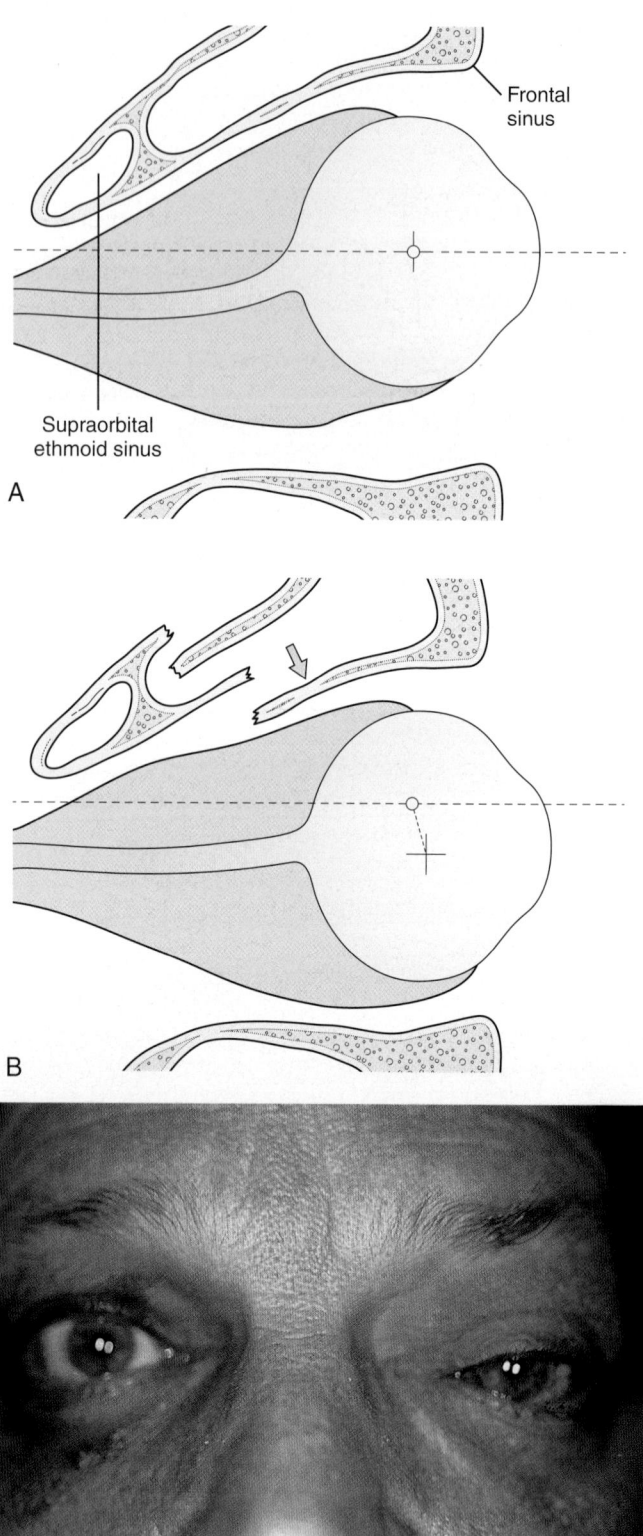

FIGURE 22.19 In the supraorbital fracture, posterior and inferior displacement of the superior orbital rim produces downward and forward dislocation of the globe. **A,** The normal configuration of the superior orbit. **B,** Dislocation of the superior orbital rim and globe displacement. **C,** A patient with a displaced supraorbital fracture producing inferior globe displacement.

disturbances, and dizziness from involvement of the temporal bone and vestibular structures.

Diagnosis

The most common clinical signs of fractures of the frontal bone are a bruise or hematoma over an area of blunt injury and, less often, a laceration of the brow or the central forehead. CT scans occasionally show a posterior wall fracture of the frontal sinus without accompanying anterior wall fracture. Fractures of the orbit usually result in palpebral and subconjunctival hematomas. A step deformity or irregularity in the orbital rim may be appreciated on palpation, but swelling may obscure the irregularity. If periorbital swelling is severe, complete ptosis exists. If the lid cannot be opened voluntarily, it should be opened manually to inspect the globe for integrity. Visual acuity should be assessed and extraocular muscle motion should be evaluated where possible.

Evaluation of the visual system is critical. Supraorbital fractures, for example, represent 10% of all periorbital fractures but account for 30% of serious eye injuries. The most common serious injuries to the globe are rupture, retinal detachment, and vitreous or anterior chamber hemorrhage. The presence of globe injury modifies fracture treatment by severely limiting manipulation; avoidance of any pressure on the globe may take precedence over bone reconstruction. Visual acuity and pupil response are documented before and after any surgical treatment using a Rosenbaum pocket visual screening card. If this is not possible, the pupillary response to light is evaluated both directly and consensually. Inability to move the globe into a particular field of gaze indicates either a cranial nerve palsy or interference with an extraocular muscle secondary to contusion, local nerve injury, or incarceration of an extraocular muscle or its adjacent soft tissues.

Fractures of the roof of the orbit usually produce a temporary paresis of the levator muscle that results in post-traumatic ptosis. This palsy may persist for months; no treatment to elevate the lid further is indicated until all chance of spontaneous recovery has been permitted (at least 6 months). Partial or complete spontaneous recovery usually occurs. The superior rectus muscle is usually undamaged in fractures of the superior orbit, but occasionally paresis occurs and mimics incarceration of the inferior rectus muscle (failure to elevate the globe). These conditions are differentiated by the combination of radiographic evaluation, forced-duction testing, and formal eye muscle evaluation. Entrapment of the levator or superior rectus muscles rarely occurs in orbital roof fractures.

Supraorbital fractures involving the orbital rim are usually displaced inward and downward (see Fig. 22.19), producing a forward and downward displacement of the globe. The globe occasionally bulges forward so that the eyelids cannot close completely. In such cases urgent facial fracture reduction is required to protect the cornea. Fractures of the orbital roof may have a linear extension that enters the superior orbital fissure or optic foramen. Visual acuity is affected if the optic nerve is compressed by a displaced fracture fragment or by edema or nerve shearing, in which case direct pupillary response to light on the injured side is slower than the direct pupil response on the other side. A superior orbital fissure syndrome may also be present, consisting of variable palsy of extraocular muscle motion (cranial nerves III, IV, VI), ptosis, global proptosis,

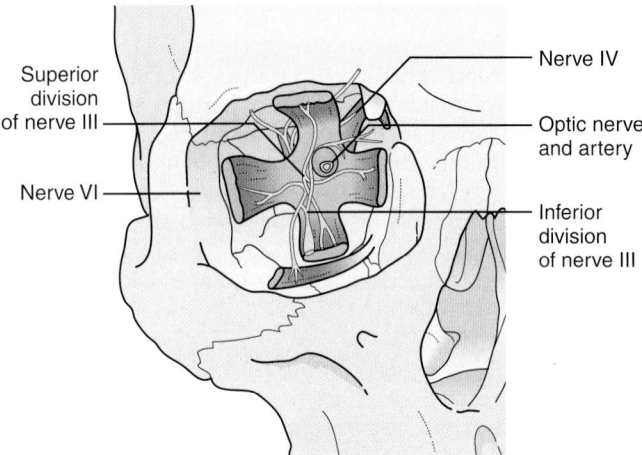

FIGURE 22.20 The contents of the superior orbital fissure include cranial nerves III, IV, and VI, the ophthalmic division of (trigeminal) cranial nerve V, and vascular structures. The optic foramen is contained within the lesser wings of the sphenoid and admits the optic nerve and ophthalmic artery.

and anesthesia in the first division of the trigeminal nerve (the ipsilateral forehead) (Fig. 22.20 and see section on Orbital Fractures). Patients may experience numbness in the distribution of the supraorbital and supratrochlear nerves, which is usually transient, although lacerations in the area frequently divide the nerve, producing permanent numbness.

Management

Displacement of the roof and rim of more than 4 or 5 mm produces a depression and a forward movement in globe position; release of the pressure on the globe or the nerves may improve function. Open skull fractures require débridement, repair of dural lacerations, evacuation of epidural hematomas, and appropriate surgical procedures for frontal lobe injury. Bone fragments are cleaned of mucosa and debris, and antiseptic irrigation is used. The frontal skull can be reconstructed primarily by linking the bone fragments with wires or plate and screw fixation, stabilizing the pieces securely.

Frontal Sinus Fractures

Fractures of the frontal sinus may involve the anterior wall, the posterior wall, or both. Fractures that obstruct the nasofrontal duct must be treated by eliminating the function of the sinus. Fractures that depress only the anterior wall of the frontal sinus are repaired for esthetic reasons. The symptoms of a frontal sinus fracture include localized bruising, hematoma, or lacerations; the fracture often extends into the orbit, producing both palpebral and subconjunctival hematomas (spectacle hematoma).

Diagnosis

Frontal sinus fractures are diagnosed on CT scan noting fractures of the front wall, back wall, duct, or both walls. Displacement of bone of the posterior wall more than the thickness of the bone wall usually indicates an underlying dural laceration.

Management

Localized fractures of the anterior wall are managed by returning the bone fragments to the proper position and debriding any devitalized mucosa. If the nasofrontal duct is intact, fluid will flow freely into the nose; replaced bone fragments are

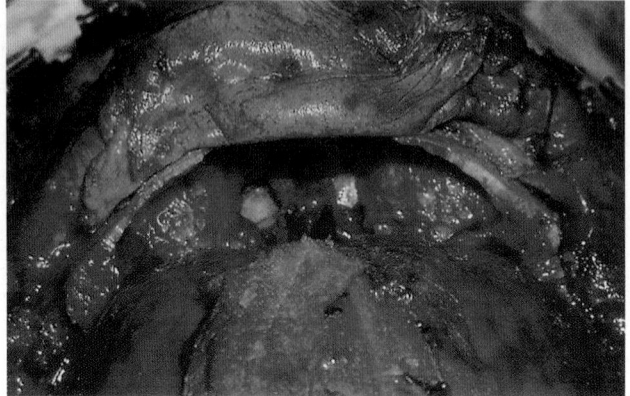

FIGURE 22.21 The nasofrontal duct should be plugged with several layers of bone graft. Bone provides strong structural material to close the opening between the intracranial cavity and the nose. Muscle and fascia deteriorate rapidly and do not provide stability.

stabilized with plate and screw fixation. If the posterior wall is involved, the integrity of the dura is usually assessed by direct inspection at operation. Significant fractures of the anterior and posterior walls are best managed by intracranial exposure and débridement of small bone fragments, and defunction of the sinus. If the posterior wall of the sinus is removed, the sinus is "cranialized" by completely removing the mucosa and plugging the nasofrontal duct with several layers of bone grafts. A sheet bone graft is placed over the bone plugs and over the involved ethmoid sinuses (Fig. 22.21). Involved sinus must be debrided to minimize infection and delayed mucocele formation because obstruction of an ethmoid sinus produces an orbital or epidural abscess. The anterior wall of the frontal sinus is then reconstructed. Complete removal of sinus mucosa requires mucosal stripping and light burring of its bone fragments as the mucosa has minute invaginations (foramina of Breschet) into the bone.

Less complicated frontal sinus fractures may be managed by another more limited procedure which defunctionalizes the sinus "obliteration." When fractures compromise nasofrontal duct function, the sinus mucosa should be removed and the walls of the sinus should be burred to bleeding bone. The nasofrontal duct is then plugged with several layers of bone plugs taken from the calvaria, and the remainder of the sinus is filled with bone shavings (Fig. 22.22). Unfortunately,

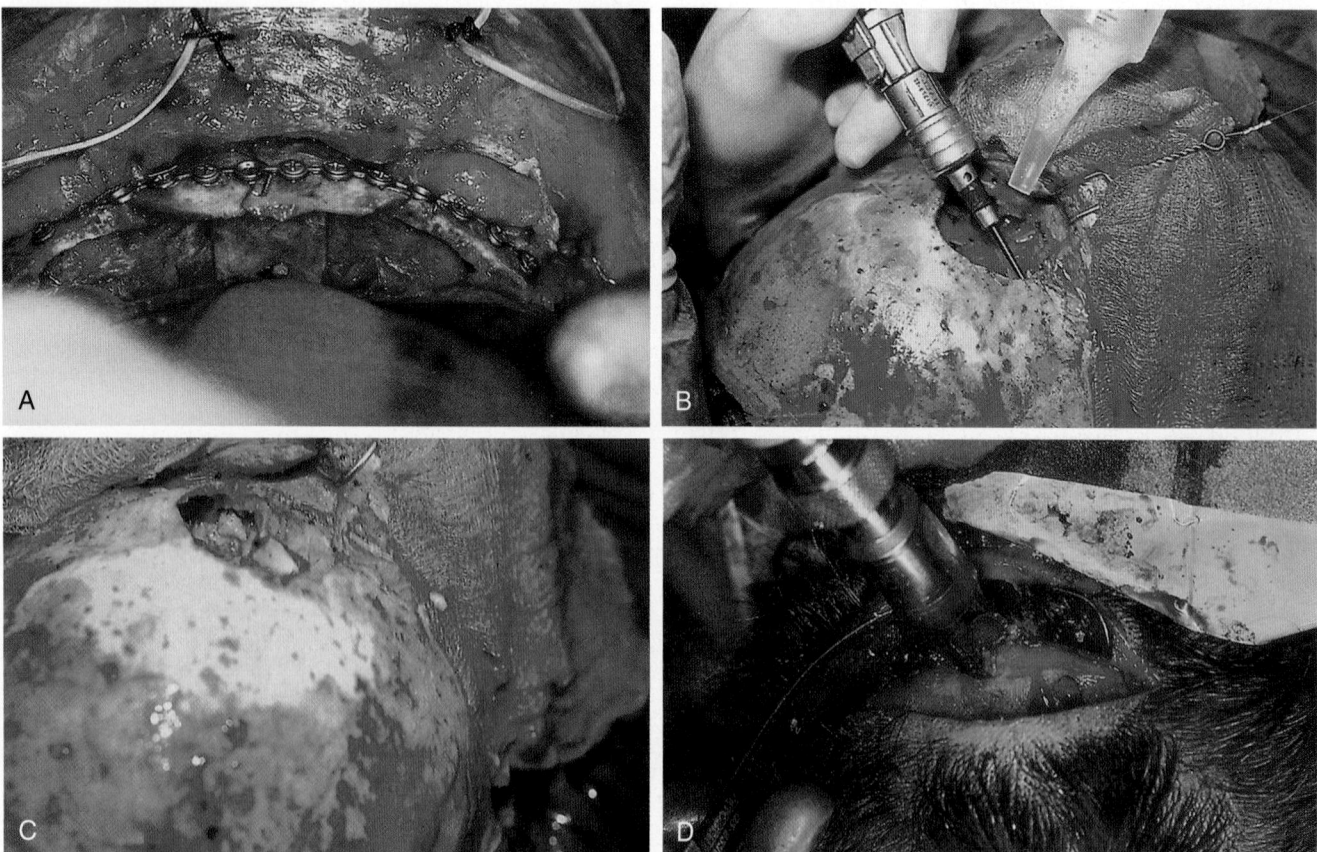

FIGURE 22.22 **A,** A sheet bone graft should be laid across the plugged frontal sinus ducts to cover previously cleansed and débrided fractures involving the cranial base and ethmoidal sinuses. This layer is not watertight but begins to develop its own partition between the intracranial cavity and the nose. **B,** In cases in which the sinus cavity is to be obliterated, the mucosa is thoroughly removed. The walls of the sinus should be burred lightly to eliminate areas where mucosa extends along the veins into the bony walls of the sinus cavity. After nasofrontal duct obliteration with bone plugs, the sinus cavity can be obliterated with particulate bone graft (**C**) taken from the parietal area with a craniotome (**D**).

regrowth of frontal sinus mucosa may occasionally occur, or the development of a cyst in a lacerated area of mucosa may produce a mucocele. Surgical intervention may be required for infection or erosion of the cyst into adjacent structures.

Orbital Fractures

The supraorbital rims are weakened centrally by the presence of the frontal sinus. The supraorbital rim extends to join the temporal bone and the zygoma (see Fig. 22.17). The orbit cavity itself has three sections (see Fig. 22.17): the anterior or rim, the middle, and the posterior orbit. The midsection of the orbit can be divided into four regions (see Fig. 22.17) and the rim into three sections. Fractures occur first in the thin bone of the middle third of the orbit, then the rim. This sequence protects the posterior orbit fractures from much displacement.

A blow to the lateral aspect of the upper face can fracture both the supraorbital rim and the zygoma. Cranio-orbital injuries call for both neurosurgery and orbital reconstruction. Zygomatic fractures usually extend from the junction medially with the maxilla at the infraorbital rim through the inferior and lateral orbit. Medially, the fracture often involves the canal for the infraorbital nerve, which is located 8 to 10 mm inferior to the lower orbital rim, parallel to the medial aspect of the cornea. A fracture here produces numbness in the infraorbital nerve distribution.

The nasoethmoidal orbital region represents the medial rim and medial wall of the orbit (Fig. 22.23). Posteriorly, the ethmoid air cells weaken the nasoethmoidal region, one of the thinnest portions of the orbital wall. Fractures involving the medial orbital rim displace the bone bearing the attachment of the medial canthal tendon posteriorly and laterally, which may also block the lacrimal system, resulting in tearing. Displacement of the medial orbital rim or the infraorbital rim and floor of the orbit alters the medial attachment of the eyelids and the suspensory ligaments of the globe, permitting globe and canthal ligament dystopia and telecanthus, which can be detected on physical examination.

The orbital roof is composed of the greater and lesser wings of the sphenoid. It separates the anterior cranial fossa from the orbital contents. Medially, at the frontal sinus, the orbital roof thins, becoming almost transparent. The attachment of the superior oblique tendon immediately behind the rim is often a separate small fragment in fractures. Diplopia produced by interference with superior oblique function is difficult to remedy. The surgeon must be aware of this attachment and carefully avoid injury by making dissection exactly subperiosteal beyond the confines of the muscle. The frontal sinus is extremely variable in size and shape, and asymmetry is the rule. It does not develop until the teenage years and thus is absent in the pediatric trauma victim.

The medial wall of the orbit is formed by the thin orbital plate of the ethmoid bone. This bone is reinforced by septa within the ethmoid sinus, which gives it some additional strength (see Fig. 22.23). The lateral wall of the orbit consists of the orbital process of the malar bone anteriorly and the greater wing of the sphenoid posteriorly (Fig. 22.24). The zygomaticosphenoid suture is involved in all zygoma fractures with the exception of those confined to the zygomatic arch. Its broad surface forms an excellent area for confirmation of proper zygomatic alignment at the time of reduction. With

more comminuted orbital fractures, displacement of multiple walls of the orbit contributes to dramatic orbital deformity. Because soft tissue orbital deformity is not entirely reversible with secondary corrections, the emphasis is on immediate anatomical reconstruction.

The lateral canthal ligament is attached with the lateral aspect of the eyelids to the zygoma at Whitnall's tubercle, which is a shallow bulge behind the internal aspect of the lateral orbital rim about 10 mm inferior to the zygomaticofrontal suture. The anterior limb of the lateral canthal tendon is continuous with the galea, and the posterior limb joins the lateral extension of the levator tendon and Lockwood's suspensory ligament in its attachment to Whitnall's tubercle (Fig. 22.25). The extraocular muscles travel close to the orbital walls in the posterior half of the orbit, In the anterior half of the orbit, they are protected from orbital wall fractures only by a thin cushion of extramuscular cone fat. Thin "muscular cheek ligaments" extend from the extraocular muscles diffusely to the

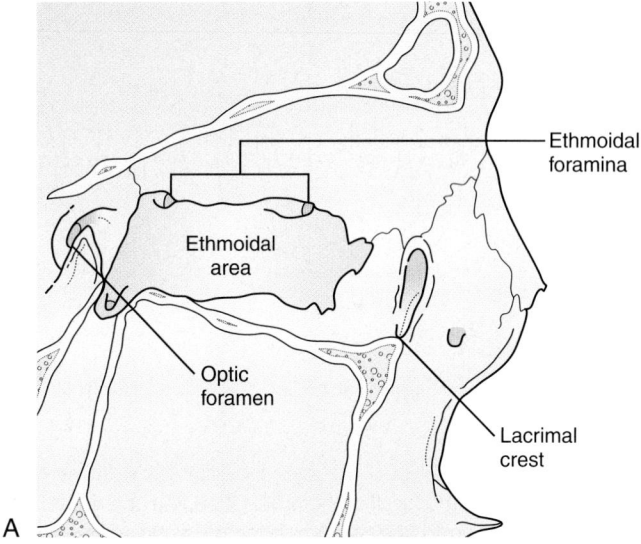

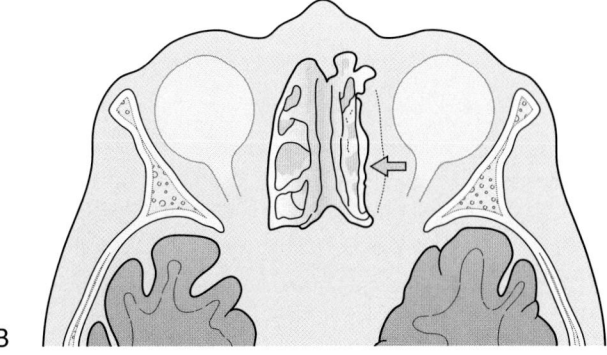

FIGURE 22.23 **A,** The medial wall is the thinnest bone of the orbit but, reinforced by septa within the ethmoid sinus, it is stronger than its thickness implies. The anterior and posterior ethmoidal foramina, located toward the upper portion of the medial orbital wall, are on the same level as the optic canal. These neurovascular foramina can be used as landmarks to direct the surgeon, warning to protect the optic nerve canal, which is 5 mm from the posterior ethmoid foramen. **B,** Fractures of the ethmoid frequently show symmetrical compression. Reconstruction involves bone grafting to the normal contour.

orbital walls (Fig. 22.26). The fine ligament system, described by Leo Koorneef (see Fig. 22.26), diffusely interconnects the soft tissue of the orbit to provide structural continuity among all the orbital tissues, such as fat, muscle, periosteum, and globe. This interconnection of all orbital soft tissue is why diplopia (extraocular muscle restriction) occurs if a particular section of orbital fat is trapped in a fracture by virtue of these connections. The entrapped fat and ligament system, in the absence of actual extraocular muscle incarceration, may cause diplopia.

The orbital floor is one of the weakest portions of the orbit. There is an initial concave section of the floor immediately behind the inferior orbital rim, and then a convex constriction of the orbit posteriorly. This complex orbital shape must be re-created when reconstructing the orbit. Because the

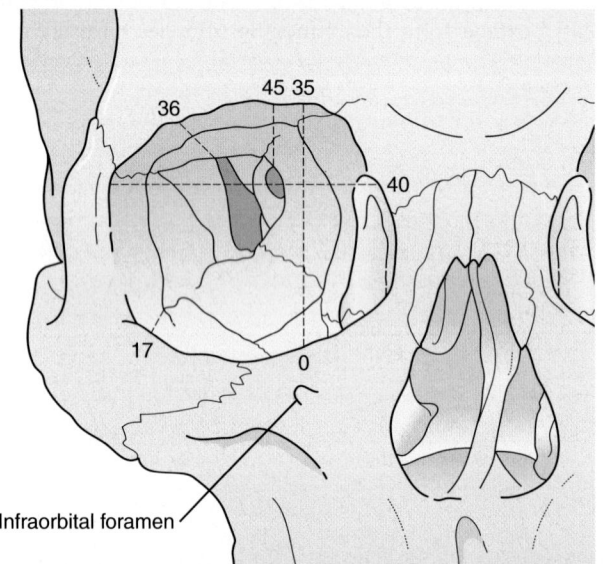

FIGURE 22.24 The lateral wall of the orbit. Often, the anterior portion of the greater wing of the sphenoid fractures and is involved in expansion of the orbital cavity. The distances of the various structures from the rim are shown.

complex curves of bone in relation to the soft tissue determine globe position (Fig. 22.27), it is extremely important to mimic the exact curvature of the middle portion of the orbit and the position of the orbital rim in reconstruction. The concave orbital roof must be reconstructed in its exact arching anatomical position, or the globe will be displaced inferolaterally. The orbital roof is convex from anterior to posterior, and from medial to lateral.

The posterior third of the orbit contains the optic foramen, the superior orbital fissure, and the posterior aspect of the inferior orbital fissure. The superior orbital fissure is bounded by the greater and lesser wings of the sphenoid (see Fig. 22.20). Linear fractures are commonly seen in the posterior portion of the orbit; however, displacement of bone is less common. Usually, the anterior and middle sections of the orbital bones displace, acting as a "shock absorber" protecting posterior orbital bone from severe displacement.

The inferior orbital fissure separates the orbital floor from the lateral orbital wall. It contains veins, the infraorbital artery and nerve, and the zygomaticofacial nerve.

Diagnosis

A mobile or absent orbital roof may allow pulsating exophthalmos, in which cerebral pulsations are transmitted to the globe and its adnexal structures. This is corrected by reconstruction of the roof, separating the orbit from the intracranial contents with a bone graft.

Fractures involving the orbital roof and middle cranial fossa may sometimes create a communication (carotid-cavernous sinus fistula) between the carotid artery and the cavernous sinus. A traumatic carotid-cavernous fistula is usually accompanied by severe visual and cranial nerve disturbances. Marked chemosis, globe prominence, extraocular muscle palsy, and blindness are usually present. The fistula is confirmed by arteriography; attempts to obliterate it involve intravascular radiographic embolization techniques.

The most common reason for visual acuity deficit after trauma is optic nerve injury. Shearing, contusion, or compression may be involved. These injuries may occur with or

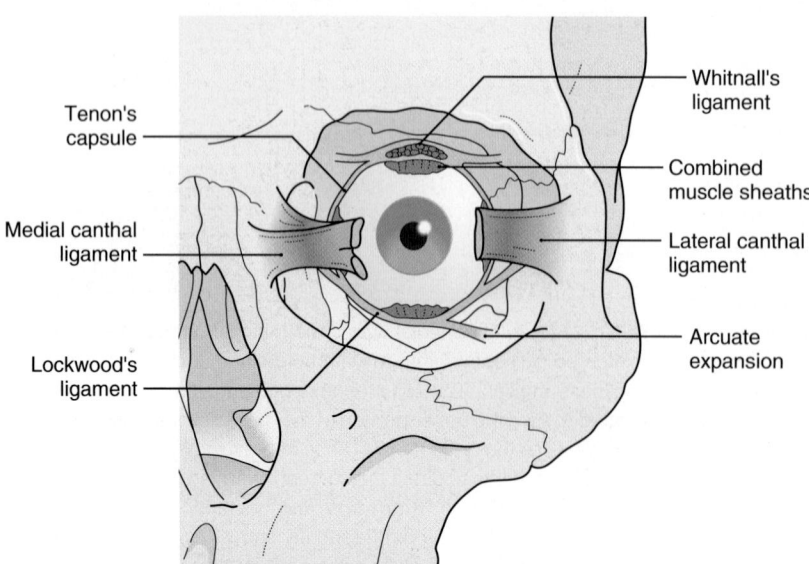

FIGURE 22.25 The fascial sling for globe support. The globe has been removed. Medially and laterally, the medial and lateral canthal ligaments provide attachments for structures that provide anterior globe support. Indicated are Lockwood's ligament, supporting the globe inferiorly, the medial and lateral canthal ligaments, and behind them, medial and lateral cheek ligaments. Superiorly, Whitnall's ligament is present. The combined muscle sheaths also attach to the globe and provide a relative sling for fat and globe support. These ligaments and their sheaths join to Tenon's capsule.

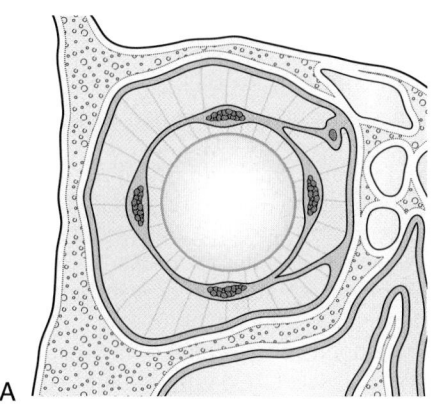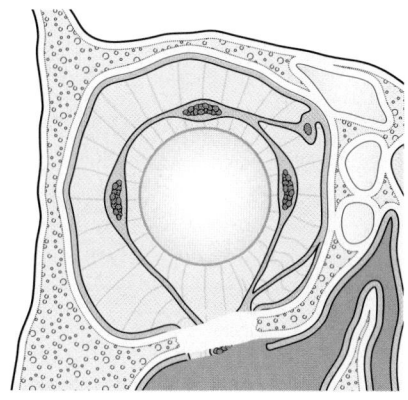

FIGURE 22.26 Entrapment of the fine ligament system described by Leo Koorneef may produce limitation of extraocular motion. **A,** The normal system of ligaments that diffusely connect the bony walls of the orbit to the extraocular muscles and the globe. **B,** An orbital floor fracture has trapped fat and its interconnecting ligaments in the fracture site. Ocular motility may be impaired by impingement of the fine ligament system. *(After Koorneef L. Current concepts in the management of blow-out fractures. Ann Plast Surg 1982:9:185-199.)*

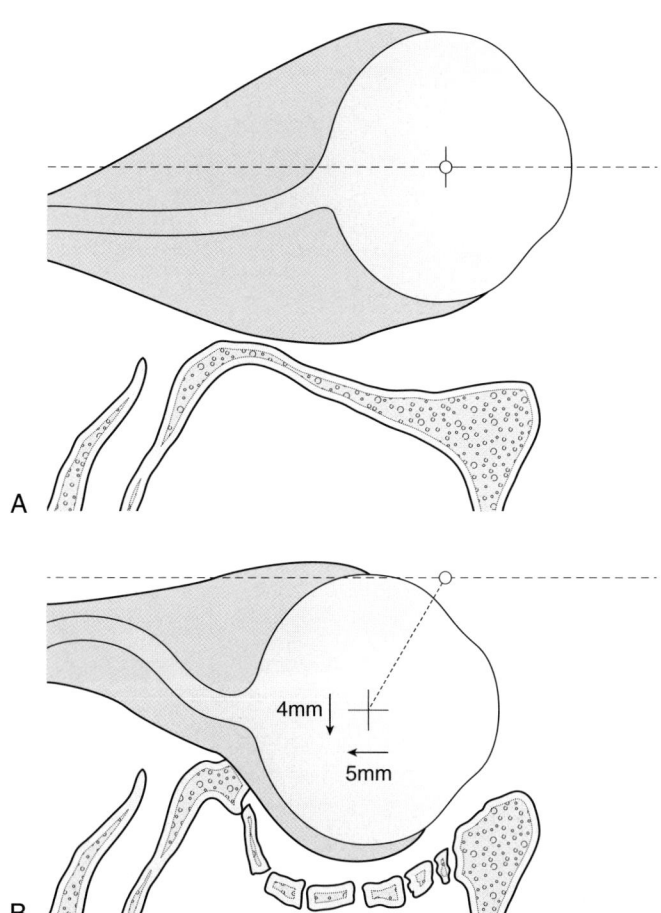

FIGURE 22.27 The curves of the orbit in the longitudinal axis of the optic nerve. The normal configuration (*top*) and the usual configuration in enophthalmos (*bottom*) of the orbital floor are indicated. An intact ledge of bone is present in the posterior orbit and provides a guide for the floor reconstruction. First, the orbital rim should be properly positioned. The intact posterior ledge of bone provides a scaffold for bone support between the rim and the posterior orbit. The soft tissue prolapsing into the maxillary sinus must be elevated, restoring globe position.

without demonstrated fractures of the optic canal. If vision is lost at the moment of impact, decompression of an optic canal fracture usually does not increase the chance of visual recovery. Frequently, steroids are employed but recently their efficacy has been questioned. When bone displacement that compromises the optic canal is demonstrated, or if fluctuating or deteriorating visual deficit is seen, then optic canal decompression should be considered. Immediately after an optic nerve injury, the optic disk usually looks normal. A patient with visual loss may present with a Marcus Gunn pupil, in which the reaction to consensual constriction is present but the reaction to direct stimulus is reduced. Swinging a light from one eye to the other demonstrates paradoxical pupillary dilatation in the affected eye (Fig. 22.28).

Atrophy of the optic disk does not appear until 1 month after an optic nerve is injured, so it cannot be used as an acute indication of optic nerve damage. If vision is initially present after an injury and then deteriorates, swelling from hemorrhage and edema may be compromising the optic canal, compressing the optic nerve. Surgical decompression or medical (high-dose steroids) decompression are indicated on an emergency basis for such delayed nerve function loss. Some feel that optic nerve injury with no light perception should be treated routinely with canal decompression, but the prognosis for this injury remains poor no matter what is done.

Nasoethmoid Orbital Fractures

The nasoethmoid orbital fracture consists (in its simplest form) of injury to one or both frontal processes of the maxilla (medial orbital rims) with their attached canthal ligaments and the nose. The frontal process of the maxilla is the lower two thirds of the medial orbital rim. When this is fractured, the medial canthal ligament is displaced because of its attachment to the fractured bone segment. Nasoethmoid fractures often extend to adjacent areas, including the supraorbital region, the frontal sinus, the zygoma and inferior orbital rim, the medial internal orbit, and the orbital floor.

These injuries, which may cause significant long-term deformity of telecanthus and enophthalmos, are often initially obscured by swelling. Patients usually present with bleeding

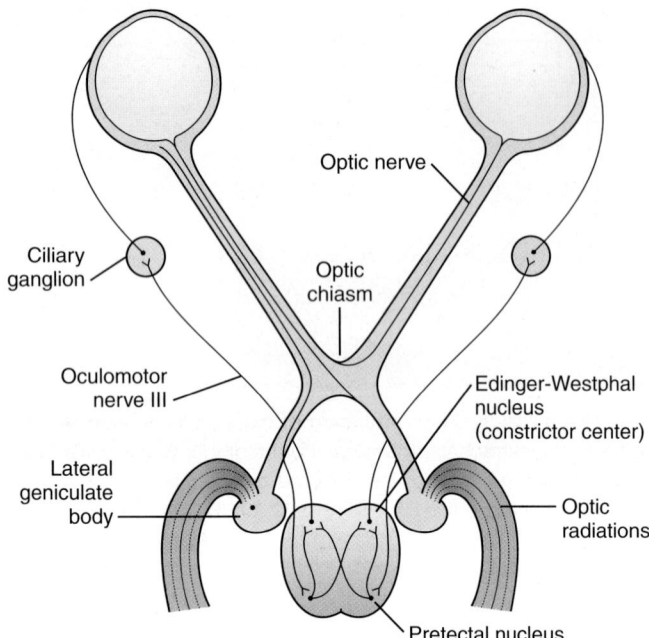

FIGURE 22.28 The normal pupil reflex pathway and the relation for the Marcus Gunn pupil. In the normal eye, light striking the retina produces an impulse in the optic nerve that travels to the pretectal nucleus, both Edinger-Westphal nuclei, via nerve III to the ciliary ganglion and papillary constrictor muscles. In lesions involving the retina or optic nerve back to the chiasm, a light in the unaffected eye produces consensual constriction of the pupil of the affected eye, but a light in the affected eye produces a paradoxic dilatation of the affected pupil. *(After Jabaley ME, Lerman M, Saunders HJ. Ocular injuries and orbital fractures: a review of 199 cases. Plast Reconstr Surg 1975:56:410.)*

from the nose, a nasal dislocation, and bilateral periorbital and subconjunctival hematomas (Fig. 22.29). The nasal deformity consists of depression of the nasal dorsum and foreshortening of the nose, with an increased angle between the columella and the lip. Severe dislocation of the septum and nasal septal perforation are often present. Forty percent of nasoethmoid fractures are unilateral, and because of their proximity to the frontal sinus and the dura, a CSF leak may be present. Nasoethmoid fractures produce tearing by compromising the drainage of the lacrimal system as it passes through the maxilla. On palpation, pain and tenderness are found over the frontal process of the maxilla, and the palpating finger, inserted deeply over the medial canthal ligament, discloses bony crepitus, movement, and tenderness. Telecanthus may be present if the medial orbital rim fracture fragment has been dislocated laterally, in which case the palpebral fissure shortens.

Diagnosis

The presence of a nasoethmoid fracture can be determined by a bimanual examination (Fig. 22.30). A palpating finger is placed deeply over the canthal ligament opposite a clamp placed intranasally, and the "central" (canthal ligament containing) bone fragment is moved between the finger and clamp. Movement confirms a mobile base fracture.

On CT scan, fractures surround the lower two thirds of the medial orbital rim, medial and inferior internal orbital fractures are present, and the inferior orbital rim, piriform aperture, nose, and internal angular process of the frontal bone at the glabella are fractured.

Lacrimal system injury should be suspected in lacerations of the medial portion of the eyelids. The lacrimal system may

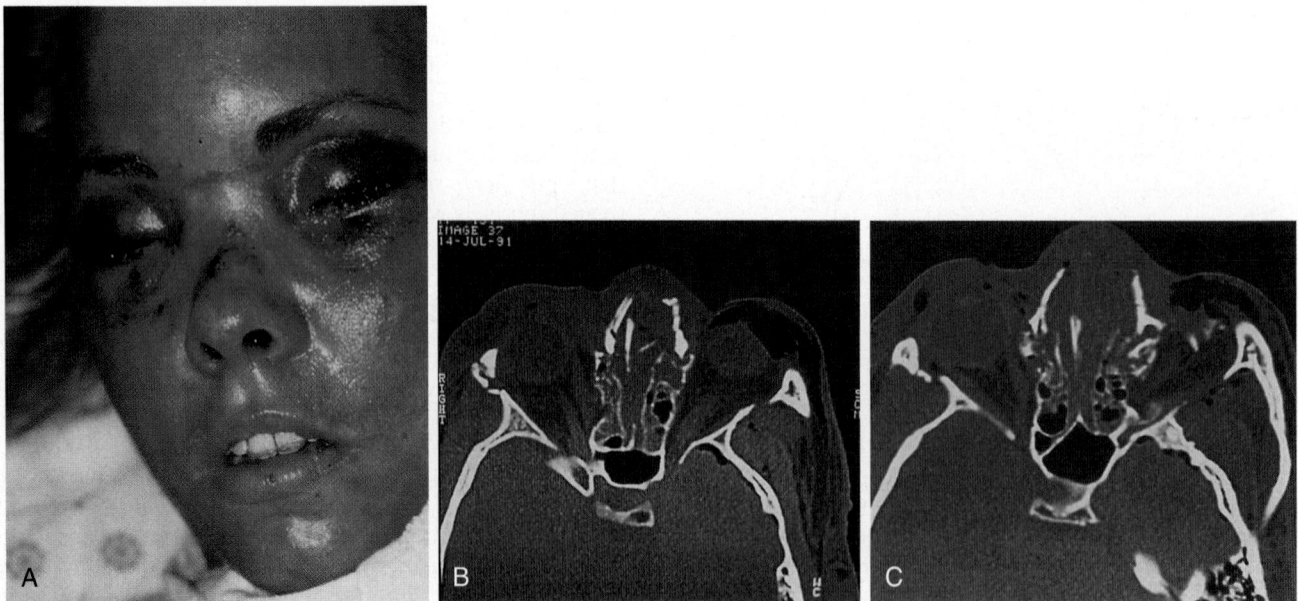

FIGURE 22.29 **A,** In most patients with nasoethmoidal fractures, severe midfacial injury is obvious. Bilateral periorbital hematomas are routine. Here, the nose has literally been driven into the midface and is depressed along its dorsum with foreshortening of the length (increased angle between the lip and columella). **B** and **C,** Computed tomography scans of the nasoethmoidal orbital fracture demonstrate comminution of the entire medical orbit and nose.

also be compromised by fractures involving the bone surrounding the nasolacrimal duct. If the lacrimal system is transected, fluid emerges from a laceration on irrigation of the system with saline by a catheter placed through the lacrimal punctum in the lower lid.

Management

Nasoethmoid orbital fractures require a definitive open reduction consisting of interfragment wiring and plate and screw fixation of the assembled fragments. In some situations, this can be accomplished through a laceration or local incision; otherwise, a broad exposure must be provided by a coronal incision (Fig. 22.31), bilateral lower eyelid incision, and gingival buccal sulcus incision. Usually, the surgeon is careful to avoid detaching the canthal ligament from the bone during fracture reduction. If the canthal ligament is detached by the injury, it must be reattached after assembly of the bone fragments to the proper area of the medial orbital rim. A separate set of transnasal wires, again passed posterior and superior to the lacrimal fossa through the nose, connect the canthal ligament to the bone in its proper position (Fig. 22.32) after the bone reduction. Contoured bone grafts are used to reconstruct the medial and inferior internal orbit (Fig. 22.33). Long straight bone grafts are used to provide contour and to add dorsal height to the nose. These bone grafts are taken from the calvarium, the iliac crest, or a split rib.

If a fracture compromises the lacrimal system, replacement of bone into its normal position is the initial treatment. If the

lacrimal system is transected, a direct repair of lacrimal canalicular transaction is performed with fine sutures under magnification over fine tubes (0.025 in; 0.6 mm). Both the upper and lower puncta should be intubated and the tubes should be brought into the nose through the nasolacrimal canal. They should remain in place for several months to splint the lacrimal system repair.

Fractures of the Orbital Floor

The bony orbital space is a modified cone or pyramid. Fractures of the inferior portion of the orbital floor often extend 30 to 35 mm behind the rim. The presence of the intraorbital nerve canal weakens the orbital floor. Fractures of the rim and floor usually impair the function of the nerve, producing hyperesthesia of the upper lip, ipsilateral nose, and anterior maxillary teeth.

The most frequent fracture of the internal orbit is the blow-out fracture, which is usually confined to the floor and the lower portion of the medial wall (Fig. 22.34). A depressed fracture of this section of the orbit allows the orbital tissue to be displaced downward into the maxillary and ethmoid sinuses. Medial, inferior, and posterior dislocation of the globe occurs. If fat is trapped in the fracture, it may interfere with the motion of the globe because of the fine internal ligament system of the orbit linking all soft tissue (see Figs. 22.34 and 22.26). Less commonly, the inferior rectus muscle may be directly trapped in a small fracture, leading to restriction of globe movement. Patients with orbital fractures usually present with a history of a blunt injury to the orbit. They may have double vision when looking either upward or downward. Extraocular range of motion may be limited. Periorbital and subconjunctival hematomas are present and there may be numbness in the infraorbital nerve distribution. It is imperative that the globe be examined; the possibility of hyphema, retinal detachment, or globe rupture exists with any fracture involving the orbit.

The possible presence of an intraorbital foreign body should also be considered. Orbital fractures are accompanied in 10% to 15% of cases by a globe injury. The visual system and globe are evaluated by visual acuity, visual fields,

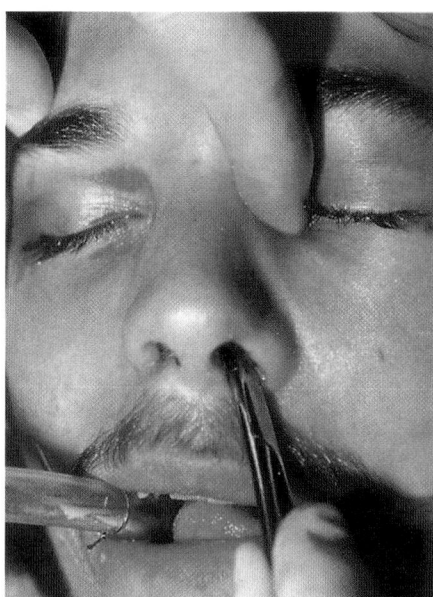

FIGURE 22.30 The bimanual examination is performed by placing a clamp inside the nose with its tip immediately adjacent to the attachment of the canthal ligament on the frontal process of the maxilla. It is important that the clamp *not* be placed beneath nasal bones or a false positive diagnosis of a nasoethmoidal fracture will be obtained. A palpating finger is placed externally deeply over the canthal ligament. If the frontal process of the maxilla can be moved between the clamp and the palpating finger, a nasoethmoidal fracture is present. Mobility requires surgical reduction.

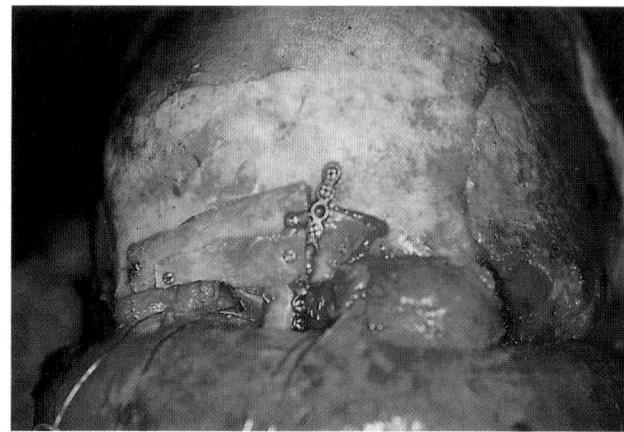

FIGURE 22.31 Exposure of the entire medial (nasoethmoidal orbital) section is provided by a coronal incision with dissection of the supraorbital area, orbital roofs, and lateral orbit.

funduscopic examination, extraocular motion, and intraocular pressure.

Diagnosis

When an orbital floor fracture is accompanied by diplopia, the "forced-duction" test is used to confirm incarceration of orbital soft tissues in the fracture site. Absence of rotation on attempted globe rotation documents muscle or extraocular system tissue restriction. A "force-generation" test provides additional information by demonstrating "pull" generated by extraocular muscles when the globe is held by forceps and globe rotation is attempted by the patient. Globe entrapment by tethering soft tissue occurs most frequently with small orbital fractures. Enlargement of the orbital volume is generally produced by large fractures; globe dystopia and enophthalmos are the result of significant orbital cavity enlargement.

Enophthalmos denotes the backward dislocation of the globe into the orbit (Fig. 22.35). Large fractures of the orbital floor allow the orbital soft tissue to prolapse backward, downward, and medially, resulting in a loss of globe support and a change in globe position. The position of the globe on physical examination is best compared by assessing symmetry in the patient with an inferior view (Fig. 22.36) or with Hertel exophthalmometry. The trauma of the injury may produce periorbital fat atrophy, which may cause globe malposition. Acutely, periorbital injuries produce hemorrhage and edema. Initially, proptosis or exophthalmos appears. Acute enophthalmos is unusual and indicates a dramatic enlargement in the orbit. If the globe prolapses away from the lids, lubrication of the cornea cannot be accomplished; this is an urgent indication for orbital wall repair. Enophthalmos is usually accompanied by inferior displacement (globe dystopia). Posterior displacement of the globe produces a supratarsal hollow and ptosis of the upper eyelid.

Management

In many cases, the symptoms of a small internal orbital fracture resolve substantially within a short period. Frequently, double vision is the result of muscular contusion and resolves with observation. Surgery is usually indicated for double vision only when it occurs in a functional field of gaze and is the result of incarceration of the muscle or the ligament system. There are thus two indications for surgery for blow-out

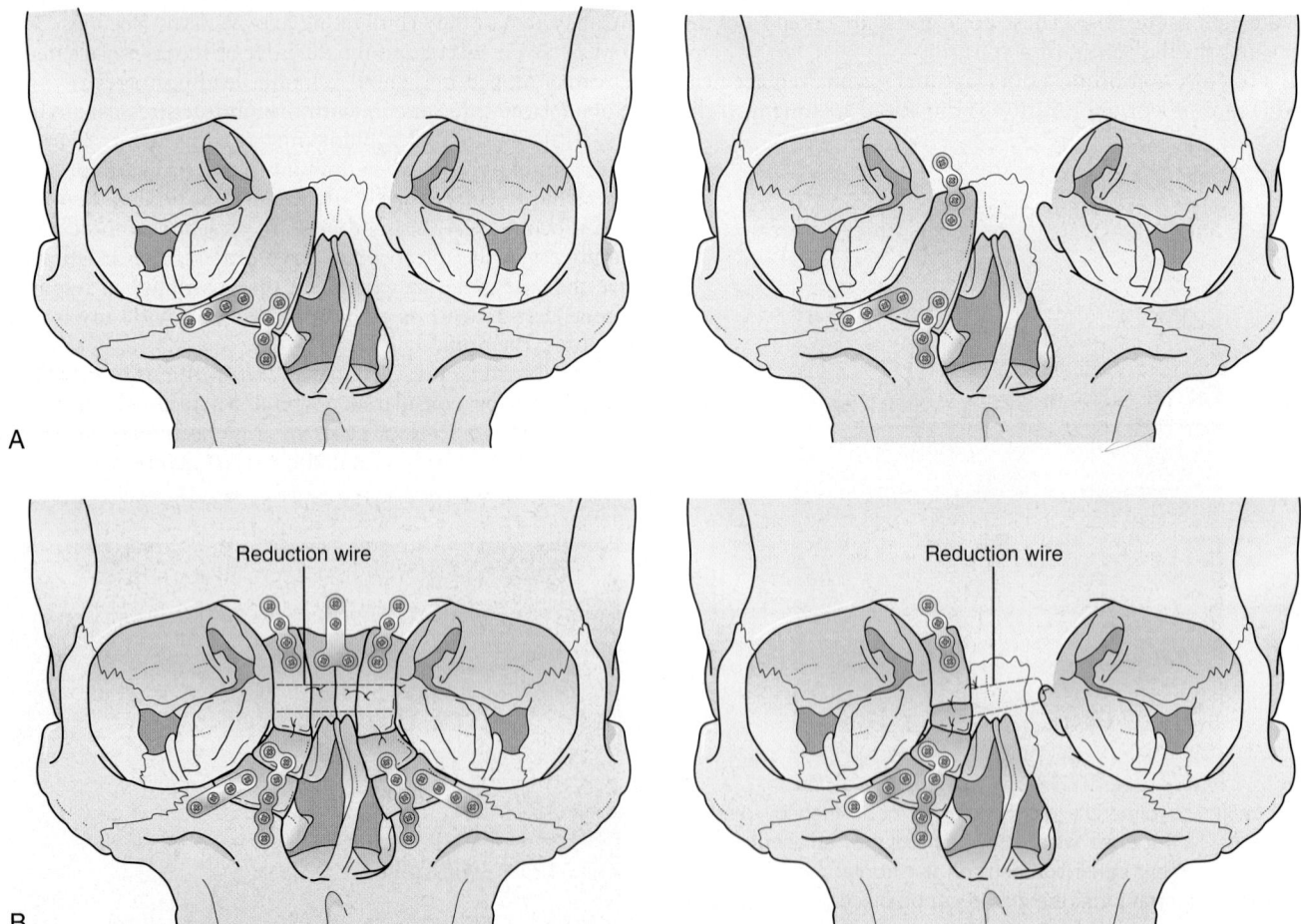

FIGURE 22.32 **A,** Treatment of a simple nasoethmoidal orbital fracture by plate and screw fixation. Noncomminuted fractures can be treated in this fashion. **B,** Comminuted fractures require a thorough connection of all fragments with interfragment wires. The essential step in the treatment of a nasoethmoidal orbital fracture is to pass a wire between both medial orbital rim segments. This wire is passed transnasally posterior and superior to the lacrimal fossa.

fractures: muscle or ligament entrapment confirmed by CT scan and forced-duction examination, and enlargement of the orbit sufficient to produce enophthalmos. This generally requires more than 2 cm² of orbital floor involvement, with displacement of that section more than 3 to 4 mm. The size of the fracture can be accurately estimated on CT scans. The orbit should be reconstructed by bone grafts or alloplastic material placed over the edges of the orbital defect so as to support the orbital contents (see Fig. 22.33).

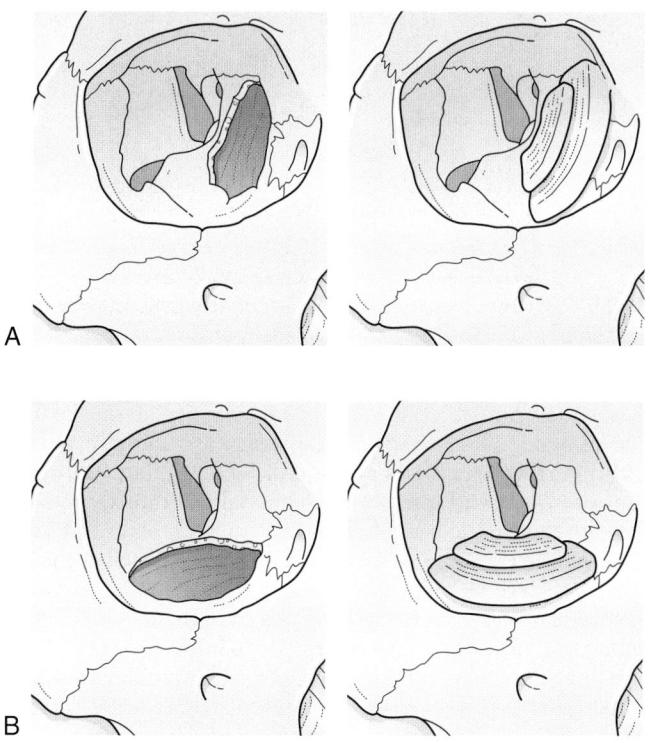

FIGURE 22.33 The usual internal orbital fractures involving the orbital floor (**A**) and the medial orbital wall (**B**). Bone grafts can be used to restore internal orbital integrity.

Le Fort Maxillary Fractures

Fractures of the maxilla involve not only the lower maxilla but often the entire midfacial region. These fractures are termed *Le Fort maxillary fractures* after the classification used by René Le Fort (Fig. 22.37), who described the three "great lines of weakness" of the maxilla through which fractures commonly occur.

Diagnosis

In 10% of the Le Fort fractures the maxillary alveolus itself is split, usually in a sagittal (longitudinal) direction (Fig. 22.38), increasing instability and making preservation of normal occlusion a challenge. Lower maxillary fractures are diagnosed by malocclusion and maxillary mobility. Upper maxillary fractures are diagnosed by maxillary mobility, malocclusion, periorbital hematomas, nasopharyngeal bleeding, pain, and the symptoms of zygomatic, orbital, and nasoethmoidal fractures. Examination for maxillary mobility is essential to confirm the presence of a Le Fort fracture. The level at which the mobility occurs indicates the level of the Le Fort fracture. The maxilla should be grasped with one hand while the head is stabilized with the other. The level at which the mobility occurs indicates the level of the Le Fort fracture. Multiple Le Fort fracture levels may be seen in the same patient. Occasionally, Le Fort fractures are not mobile; they may be either impacted or incomplete.

Management

The principal treatment of Le Fort fractures is intermaxillary fixation with the maxilla in occlusion with the mandible. Initial stabilization is generally accomplished by ligating the arch bars to the upper and lower teeth and connecting the maxillary and mandibular arch bars with intermaxillary wires. Fracture sites at the various levels of the midface (as defined by CT scans) are aligned, and then the nasofrontal and zygomaticomaxillary buttresses (Fig. 22.39) are reconstructed with direct plate and screw fixation.

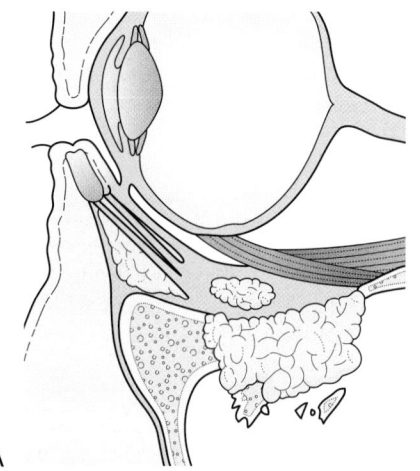
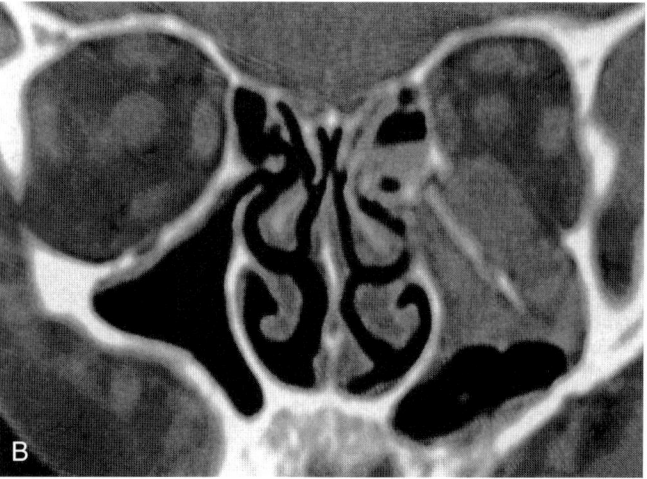

FIGURE 22.34 **A** and **B**, An orbital blow-out fracture involving the thin portion of the orbital floor. Fat and its interconnecting fascia are trapped among the blow-out fragments and limit the excursion of the inferior oblique and inferior rectus muscles. Diplopia may be present from muscle restriction in either up- or downgaze.

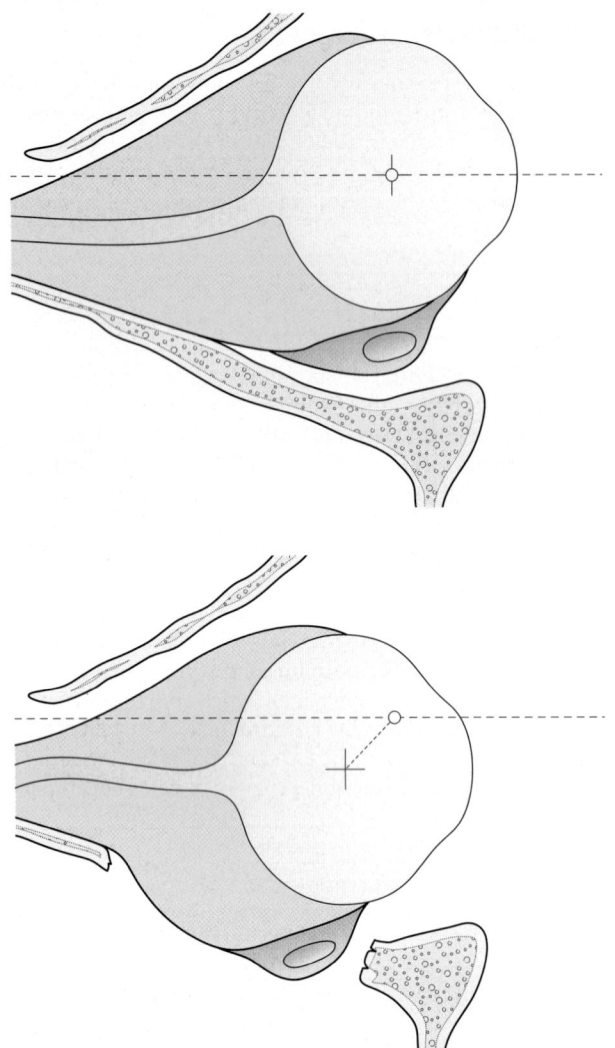

FIGURE 22.35 The orbit's enlargement allows displacement of the globe backward and downward to produce enophthalmos.

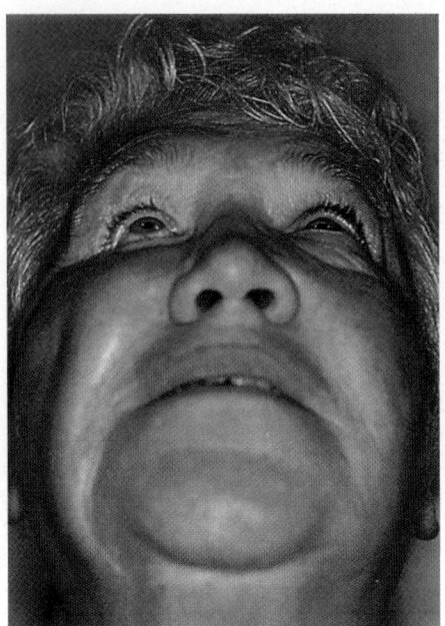

FIGURE 22.36 Enophthalmos is most accurately assessed by comparison of globe position from an inferior perspective.

This eliminates or decreases the need for intermaxillary fixation postoperatively.

A Le Fort I fracture is treated by placing the patient in intermaxillary fixation, exposing the four Le Fort I level buttresses, reducing the fracture, and using direct plate and screw fixation over the buttress fractures (Fig. 22.40). Bone grafts should span bone gaps of more than 3 to 5 mm.

Le Fort II fractures are treated by placing the patient in intermaxillary fixation. The fracture fragments are aligned and stabilized with direct plate and screw fixation (Fig. 22.41). Orbital floor defects are spanned with bone grafts, or perhaps with alloplastic implants for smaller defects. If rigid fixation is used, intermaxillary fixation may frequently be discontinued early postoperatively. Normal occlusion must be confirmed carefully for a 4- to 12-week period postoperatively. Patients with intermaxillary fixation require a liquid diet and should be placed on a soft diet when it is discontinued. The upper nose may need direct fixation through a coronal incision, and the lower orbital rims are reduced and stabilized through bilateral lower eyelid incisions.

Le Fort III fractures are treated with surgical approaches to zygomatic, nasoethmoidal, and orbital floor fractures and these fractures are connected to the maxilla at the Le Fort I level (Fig. 22.42). Again, fragments are initially aligned with interfragment wires and stabilized with plate and screw fixation. A sagittal fracture of the maxilla is directly reduced through the palatal laceration or incision with plate and screw fixation (see Fig. 22.38). A small plate is also placed at the piriform aperture to unite the two maxillary alveolar segments. In some cases, an acrylic splint is placed in the palatal vault to reduce the occlusal relationships. A "panfacial fracture" (Le Fort fractures, plus fractures of the nasoethmoidal and mandibular areas) is shown repaired with plate and screw fixation (Fig. 22.42B). The mandibular subcondylar and symphysis fractures were stabilized prior to the fixation of the Le Fort fracture.

Fractures of the Nose

A fracture of the nose may involve the cartilaginous nasal septum, the bony septum, the bony nasal pyramid, or the upper or lower lateral cartilages.

Diagnosis

Two types of dislocations occur in the nasal fractures (see Fig. 22.33): (1) posterior dislocation (shortening or flattening of the nose, resulting in a wider nasal bridge); and (2) lateral dislocation (deviated nose). Any patient with a nasal fracture should have the nasal airway inspected. If a significant hematoma exists along the septum, it should be drained to prevent cartilage necrosis. Patients with nasal fractures usually have swelling over the external surface of the nose. A small laceration is often the clue to the presence of a fracture. Pain, crepitation, and periorbital ecchymoses are present but not confirmed sharply to the insertion of the orbital septum as in periorbital fracture. The most reliable sign of a nasal fracture is epistaxis. Radiographic evaluation of the nose is best

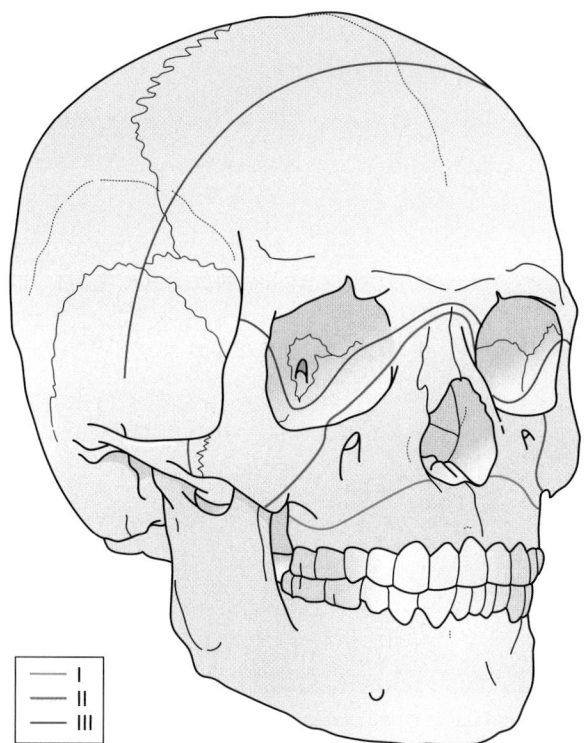

FIGURE 22.37 Le Fort fractures. Le Fort, on the basis of cadaver experiments, identified thinner areas of the midfacial skeleton that fracture more commonly. Often, combinations of fractures are seen. The Le Fort I fracture travels horizontally across the base of the piriform aperture, separating the lower portion of the maxillary sinuses from the upper midfacial skeleton. On the Le Fort II injury, a pyramidal lower facial segment is separated from the upper cranial facial skeleton. The fracture travels laterally at the Le Fort I level, then travels upward through the inferior orbital rims medially, and through either the cartilaginous portion of the nose or the nasofrontal junction centrally. In the Le Fort III injury, the cranium is separated from the midfacial skeleton through the internal orbital margins of the zygoma. The fracture begins at the zygomaticofrontal suture, extends down the junction of the greater wing of the sphenoid with the orbital process of the zygoma, crosses the orbital floor to travel up the medial orbital wall, comminutes the nasoethmoid region and the nasofrontal junction, and similarly transects the contralateral orbit. In practice, it is usual to see the Le Fort fracture level higher on one side than the other. Commonly, Le Fort III superior level injuries occur on one side with a Le Fort II superior level injury on the other side.

performed with a CT scan, which can confirm the nasal fracture and also rule out the possibility of adjacent fractures.

Management

The treatment of nasal fractures generally involves a closed reduction under local or general anesthesia. The septum is replaced into its proper position with Asch forceps. The nasal bones are first outfractured by levering the nasal bone outward to complete the fracture (releasing incomplete components of the fracture) and then digitally remolding the nasal bones into their proper positions. A Doyle nasal splint (containing an airway) supports the reduction of the nasal septum and minimizes bleeding. An external metal or plaster splint is placed over the

nasal pyramid for 1 week to protect the nose during the healing period. Nasal fractures frequently display residual mild deformity after this initial "closed" management. If the airway remains compromised by a deviated septum, a formal septal resection to improve respiratory symptoms may be performed after 3 to 6 months. Residual deformity of the nasal pyramid requires late osteotomy of the nose (formal rhinoplasty).

Fractures of the Zygoma

The zygoma forms the lateral and inferior portion of the orbit and supports the lateral areas of the upper midface (Fig. 22.43). The prominent position of the zygoma makes it a frequent recipient of traumatic dislocation. A fracture usually involves the entire zygoma, but may less commonly involve the zygomatic arch alone, which produces a minimal depression in the lateral cheek. Depression of the zygomatic arch may interfere with movement of the coronoid process of the mandible, a symptom requiring reduction. Because complete zygomatic fractures involve the lateral and inferior internal walls of the orbit, they may produce ocular symptoms that require treatment.

Diagnosis

The symptoms of zygomatic fractures are shown in Figure 22.44. The lateral canthus, which attaches to the frontal process of the zygoma, may be dislocated inferiorly, producing an antimongoloid slant to the palpebral fissure. Either swelling or dislocation of the zygoma may interfere with motion of the coronoid process by producing a mild temporary interference with occlusion. Hematomas are observed in the cheek, periorbital area, and upper gingival buccal sulcus. Orbit symptoms produced by the fractures include diplopia, ocular dystopia, and lower eyelid dislocation. Palpation of the orbital rim may demonstrate a "step" deformity or depression. Palpation of the malar eminence, when compared with the normal side, demonstrates retrusion. With a medially dislocated zygomatic fracture, the orbital volume may be constricted, resulting in exophthalmos. With laterally or inferiorly dislocated zygomatic fractures, the orbital volume increases, and enophthalmos occurs.

Zygomatic fractures should be evaluated with axial and coronal CT scans (including both soft tissue and bone windows) for evaluation of the orbital soft tissue and its relation to the fracture.

Management

Treatment of fractures of the zygoma involves reduction, accomplished through lower eyelid and gingival buccal sulcus incisions, and immobilization with interfragment wires stabilized with plate and screw fixation. Thin bone grafts may be required to replace damaged sections of the zygomaticomaxillary buttress, inferior rim, or walls of the orbit. If the zygomatic arch is laterally dislocated, a coronal incision aids reduction. The coronal incision or an upper lid incision exposes the frontal process of the zygoma.

Initially, dislocated fragments of the zygoma are repositioned and aligned by drilling holes adjacent to the fractures and linking the fragments with small interfragment wires. The fracture fragments are held in position while rigid internal fixation is performed using small plates and screws (Fig. 22.45).

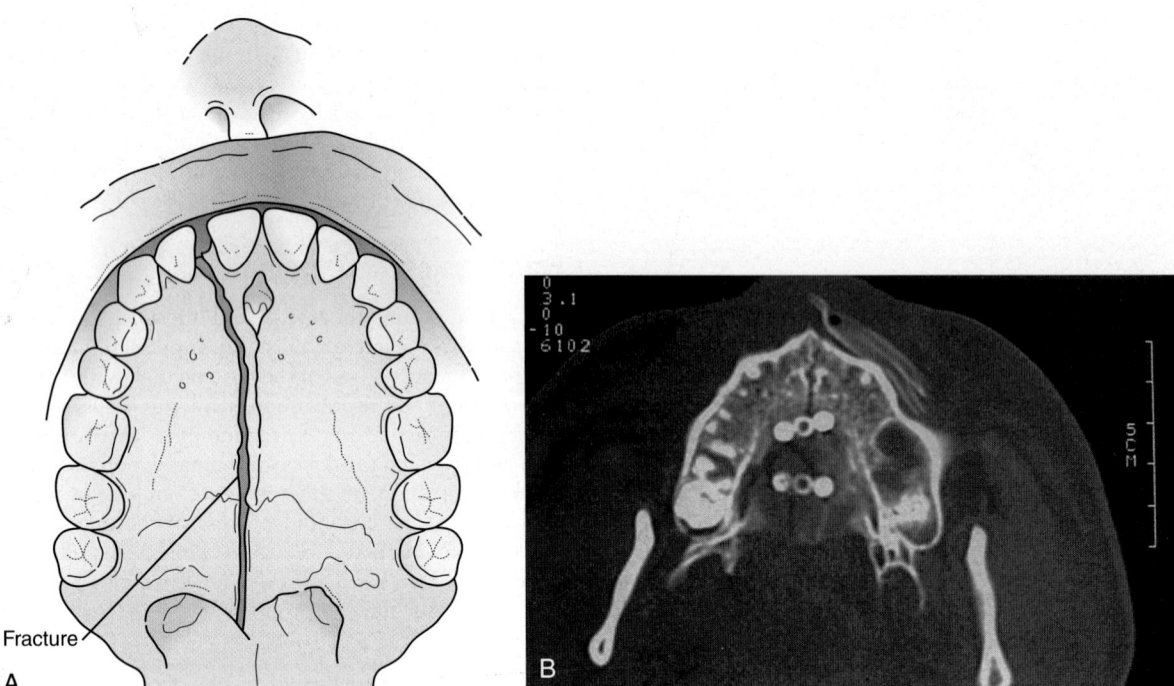

FIGURE 22.38 A, Sagittal fracture of the maxilla. **B,** Open reduction and internal fixation using small plates and screws is being performed in the roof of the mouth for this sagittal fracture of the palate.

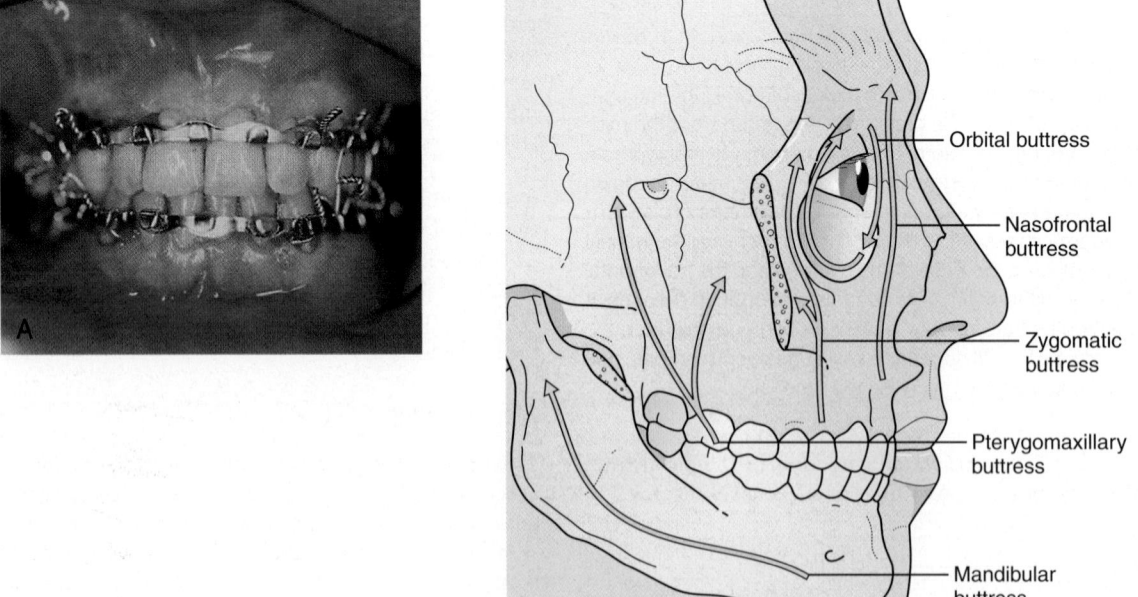

FIGURE 22.39 A, Treatment of a Le Fort fracture begins with intermaxillary fixation. **B,** The internal buttress system of the maxilla must be restored by assembling the fragments and stabilizing them with interfragment plate and screw fixation. Here anterior, middle, and posterior maxillary buttresses are seen. The anterior and posterior buttresses are stabilized with rigid fixation, and the posterior buttress by intermaxillary fixation to an intact mandible.

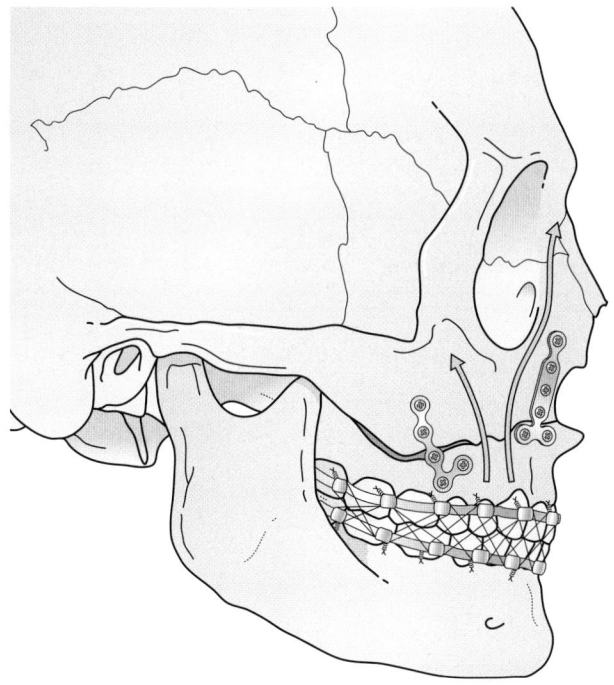

FIGURE 22.40 Diagram of Le Fort I fracture treatment.

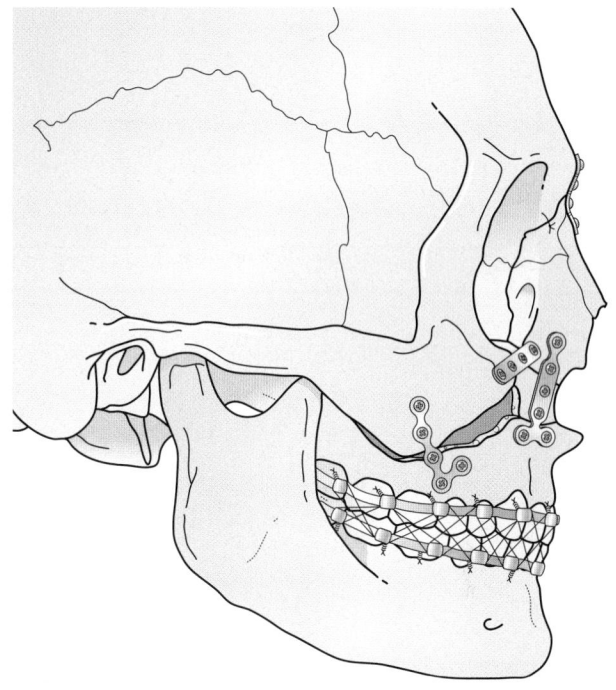

FIGURE 22.41 Diagram of Le Fort II fracture treatment.

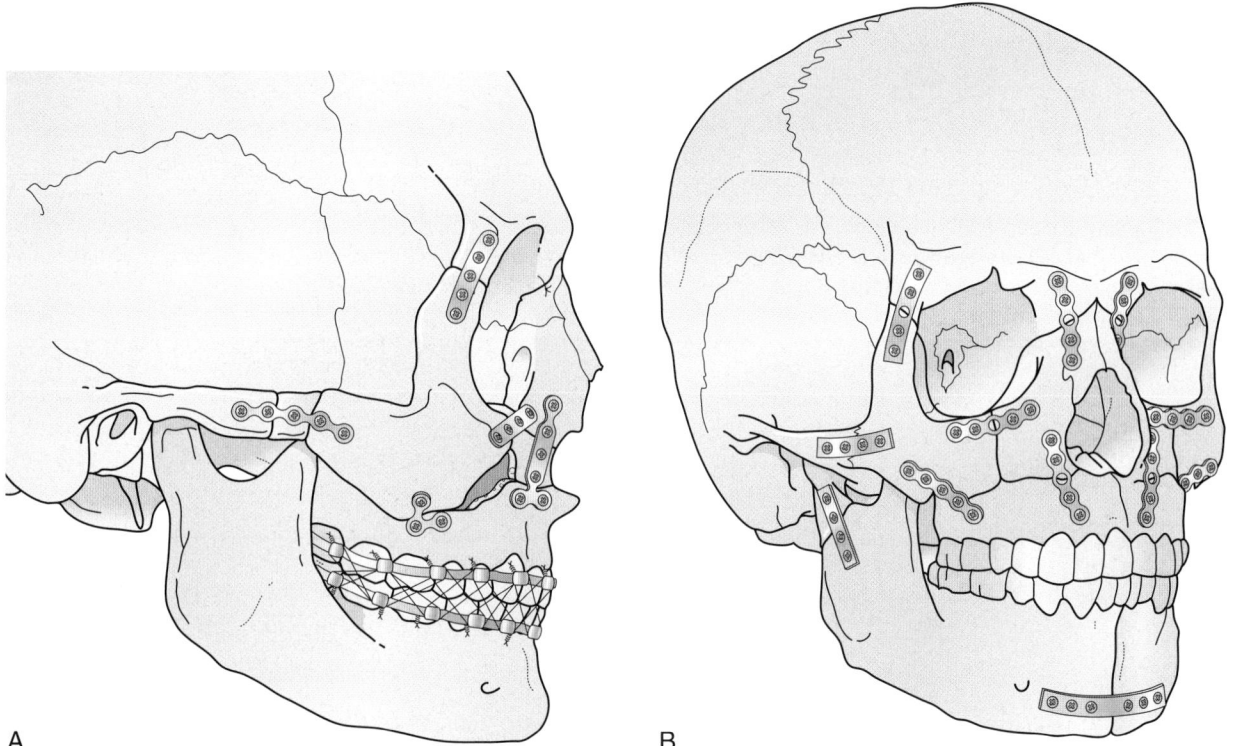

A

B

FIGURE 22.42 **A,** Diagram of Le Fort III fracture treatment using plate and screw fixation. **B,** Diagram of treatment of panfacial (Le Fort plus mandible) fractures.

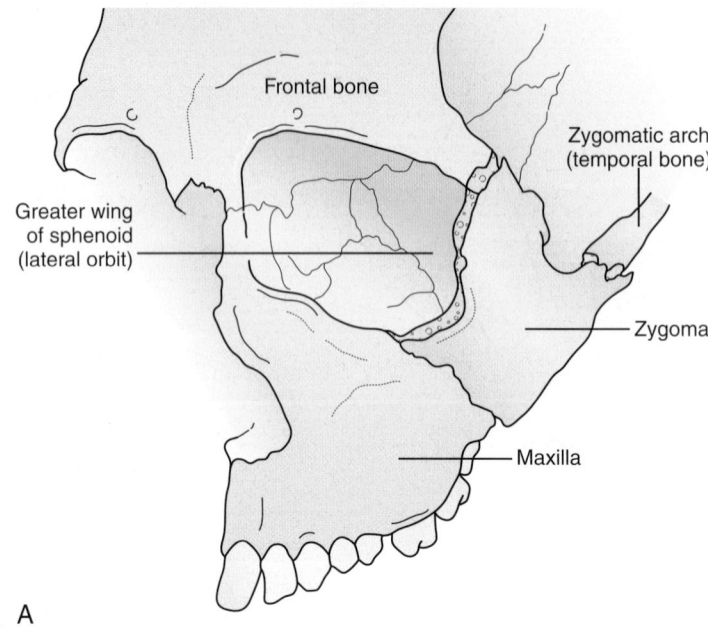

A

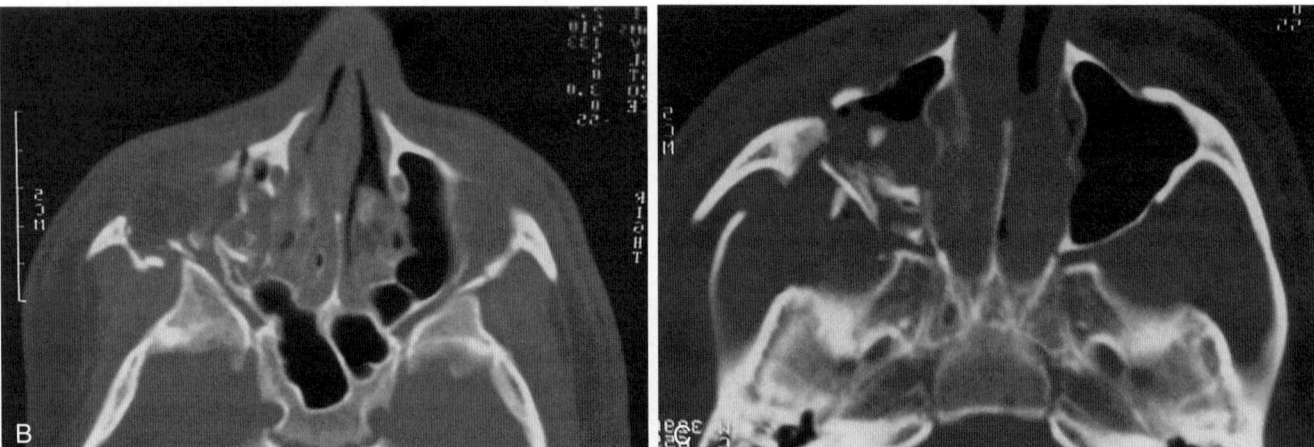

B

C

FIGURE 22.43 Fracture-dislocation of the zygoma. **A,** The zygoma attaches to the frontal bone superiorly to the temporal bone through the zygomatic arch, to the maxilla medially and inferiorly, and to the greater wing of the sphenoid through the lateral orbit. All of these surfaces must be aligned in fracture reduction. **B** and **C,** A typical fracture dislocation of the zygoma is seen in these computed tomography scans.

In figure A the following labels appear: Frontal bone, Zygomatic arch (temporal bone), Greater wing of sphenoid (lateral orbit), Zygoma, Maxilla.

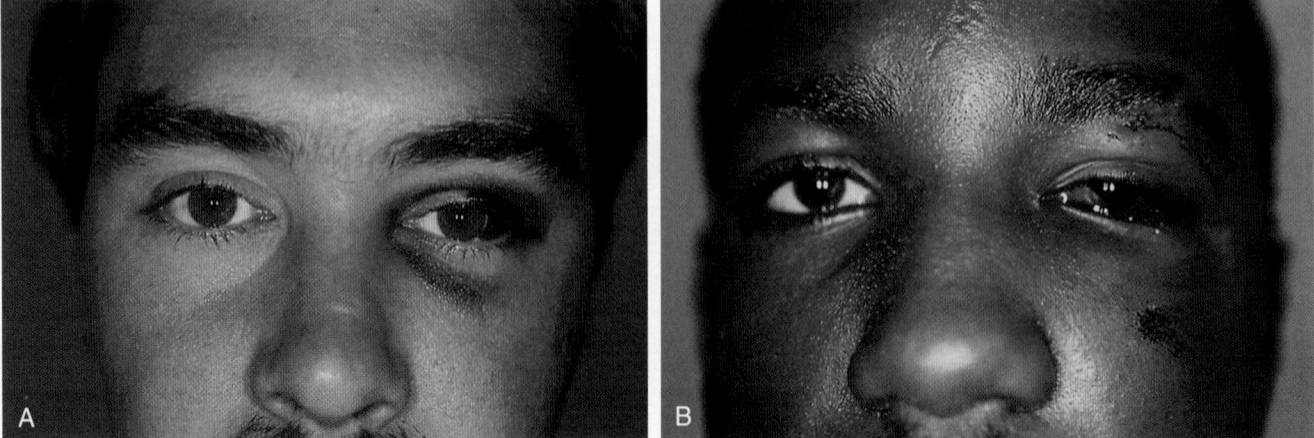

A

B

FIGURE 22.44 **A** and **B,** The symptoms of zygomatic fractures almost always include the combination of periorbital and subconjunctival hematomas. Posterior displacement of the malar eminence, a palpable step deformity in the orbital rim, and numbness in the distribution of the infraorbital nerve are frequently present. Bleeding from the ipsilateral nose occurs if the fracture extends into the ipsilateral maxillary sinus. The congested swollen conjunctiva in **B** is a warning of retrobulbar hematoma and possible globe injury.

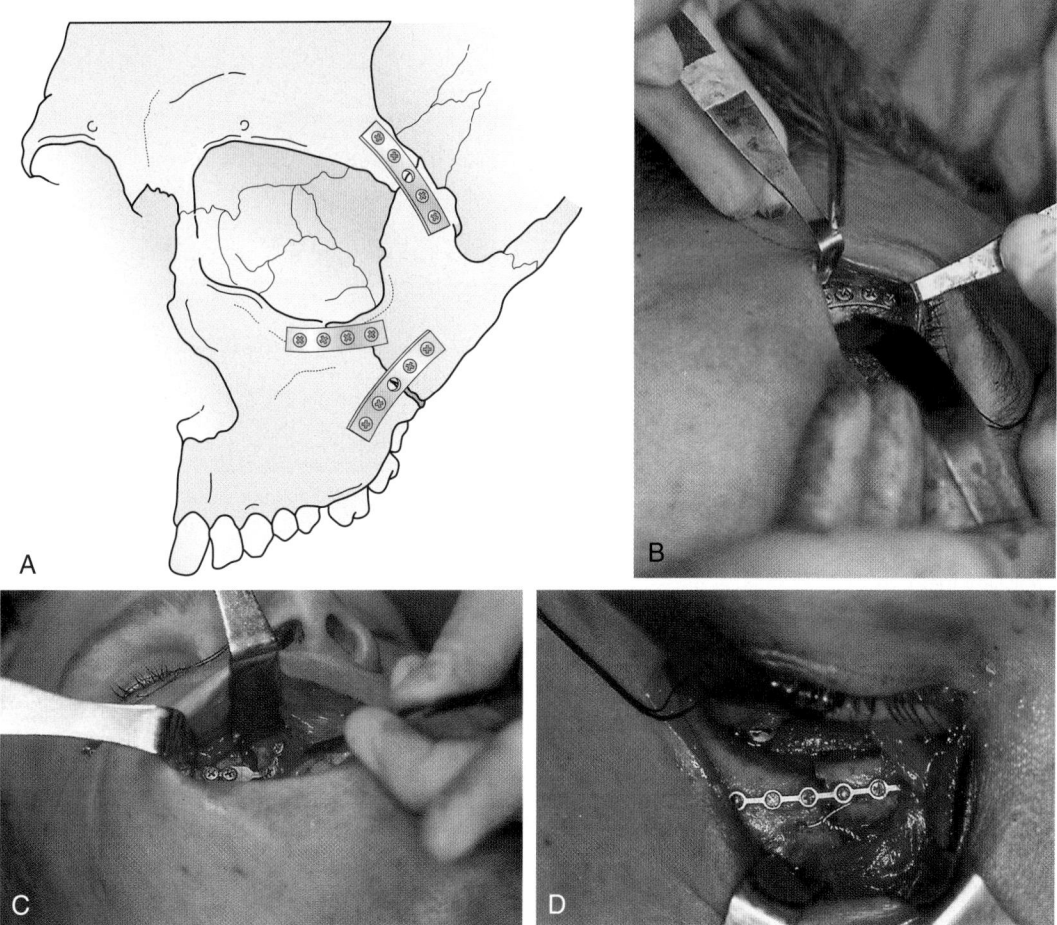

FIGURE 22.45 **A,** Diagram of an open reduction and internal fixation of the zygoma. **B,** A strong midface plate is placed at the zygomatico-frontal suture and a thinner microsystem plate at the inferior orbital rim (**C**). Depending on the comminution of the fracture, the surgeon may need to plate the zygomaticomaxillary buttress or the zygomatic arch (**D**).

If the lateral canthus is detached in the reduction, it should be replaced after bone assembly.

For a medially dislocated fracture of the zygomatic arch, whether isolated or occurring simultaneously with other fractures of the zygoma, a small incision can be made in the temporal hair and the "Gilles" approach used to elevate the zygomatic arch into its proper position. An elevator is placed beneath the temporalis muscle fascia directly on the temporalis muscle, which easily slides under the arch, and the zygomatic arch is levered into its proper position.

Fractures of the Mandible

Mandibular fractures are common facial injuries because the mandible's prominent position renders it susceptible to trauma. Frequently, multiple fractures are present in the same mandible. Mandibular fractures may be classified as "closed" or "open" and by anatomical location. Mandibular areas such as the subcondylar region, the region of the angle, or the cuspid region (the latter two being weakened structurally by the molar and cuspid teeth, respectively) are well-known anatomical areas. The edentulous mandible most commonly fractures in the body and angle region followed by the subcondylar area.

Diagnosis

The diagnosis of the mandibular fracture is suggested by malocclusion, pain, swelling, tenderness, crepitus, fractured teeth, gaps or discrepancies in the level of the dentition, asymmetry of the dental arch, presence of intraoral lacerations, broken or loose teeth, or numbness in the distribution of the mental nerve. An odor is frequently present. Fractured, missing, or dislocated teeth are frequently seen. An "open bite" occurs if the fracture sufficiently dislocates a segment of jaw so that the teeth cannot be brought into occlusion (Fig. 22.46). The open bite may occur anteriorly, laterally, or bilaterally. On opening, the jaw may deviate toward one side because of the fractures in the subcondylar area, which prevent the balancing effect of the lateral pterygoid muscle. Fractures in the condylar and subcondylar area may result in a laceration of the ear canal that produces bleeding, confusing the injury with that of a middle cranial fossa fracture. Instability of the alveolar section of the mandible relative to the mandibular body implies the presence of an alveolar fracture. Separation of the alveolus from the basilar bone of the mandible creates dramatic dental instability.

The mandible has strong muscular attachments that contribute to displacement after injury. The direction of the

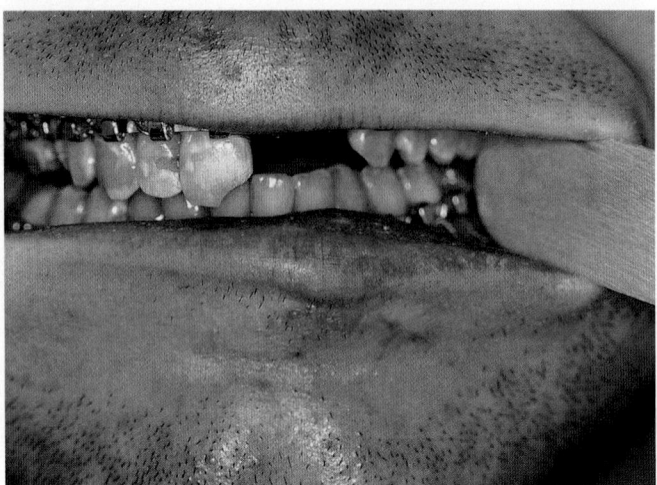

FIGURE 22.46 "Open bite" after mandibular fracture treatment. The front teeth cannot be brought into full occlusion because displaced posterior aspects of the mandible block its full motion and alignment with the maxillary teeth.

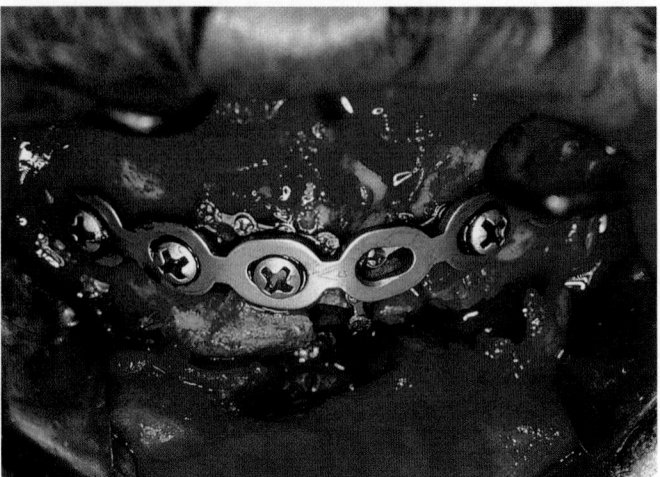

FIGURE 22.47 Rigid fixation in a mandibular fracture utilizes small and large plates for stabilization of all the segments.

fracture line may oppose fracture displacement produced by the muscles. The Panorex radiograph uses a rotating x-ray tube to obtain a circumferential view for an excellent evaluation of the entire mandible in a single plane. Lateral oblique, posteroanterior, and Towne's skull views are used to demonstrate the mandible on plain films. A CT scan provides one of the most accurate evaluations of a mandibular fracture but can occasionally miss nondisplaced fractures. CT scans also demonstrate the course of the fracture through the bone, which is essential for treatment planning.

Management

The treatment of mandibular fractures depends on the state of the dentition and the location of the fracture. It begins with closure of intraoral and extraoral lacerations and the application of arch bars and intermaxillary fixation to bring the teeth into occlusion (Fig. 22.47). In some cases, an acrylic splint can be applied to the teeth temporarily to align them. Some fractures are treated with intermaxillary fixation alone for 4 to 6 weeks after "closed reduction." For displaced fractures in both the horizontal and vertical portions of the mandible, direct open reduction of the fracture with plate and screw fixation is the preferred treatment. A plate is placed along the inferior border of the mandible, avoiding the mental nerve and tooth roots (Fig. 22.48). At least two screws are placed to each side of the fracture in stable bone.

The angle region may be treated intraorally, with an intraoral incision, or for more comminuted fractures, extraorally, such as an incision in the upper neck in the hyoid crease or retromandibular area. Fractures of the condyle that require open reduction are treated with a preauricular approach, protecting the facial nerve. Mandibular fractures may be prone to complications such as nonunion, delayed union, and infection. Antibiotics are generally indicated at the time of the fracture reduction in fractures that include the dentition.

Facial Fractures in Children

Less than 5% of all facial fractures occur in children: of that 5%, most occur in those over 5 years of age. The bones of children are less brittle than those of adults, and they displace without fracture in many cases. Fracture healing progresses more rapidly in children than in adults. Sinuses are small and therefore do not weaken the bony structure of the midface. The treatment of fractures in the upper face of a child follows the same principles described for adults. The emphasis is on early or immediate treatment because healing occurs rapidly. It may be difficult to reduce a Le Fort fracture after even 1 week. Intermaxillary fixation is often difficult to apply in children because of mixed dentition and inadequate root structure of the teeth and the shape of the crowns, which produces difficulty in ligating teeth. Arch bars may have to be supported by piriform aperture wires, circummandibular wires, or suspension wires for stabilization. The application of acrylic splints to the dentition can facilitate reduction of the fracture. The use of miniature plate and screw fixation systems in children is preferred. The long-term efficacy of resorbable plates in pediatric facial fractures has yet to be defined. Healing times are shorter in children. Because of the prominence of the frontal skull in children, frontal skull and supraorbital fractures are frequent in the young (0-5 years) age group. Orbital floor fractures are not frequent because of the small size of the maxillary sinus. The frontal sinus is absent in young children. Healing times are generally significantly reduced in children. One would like to minimize the use of fixation materials that will remain because of a possible role in localized growth restriction (perhaps 5%).

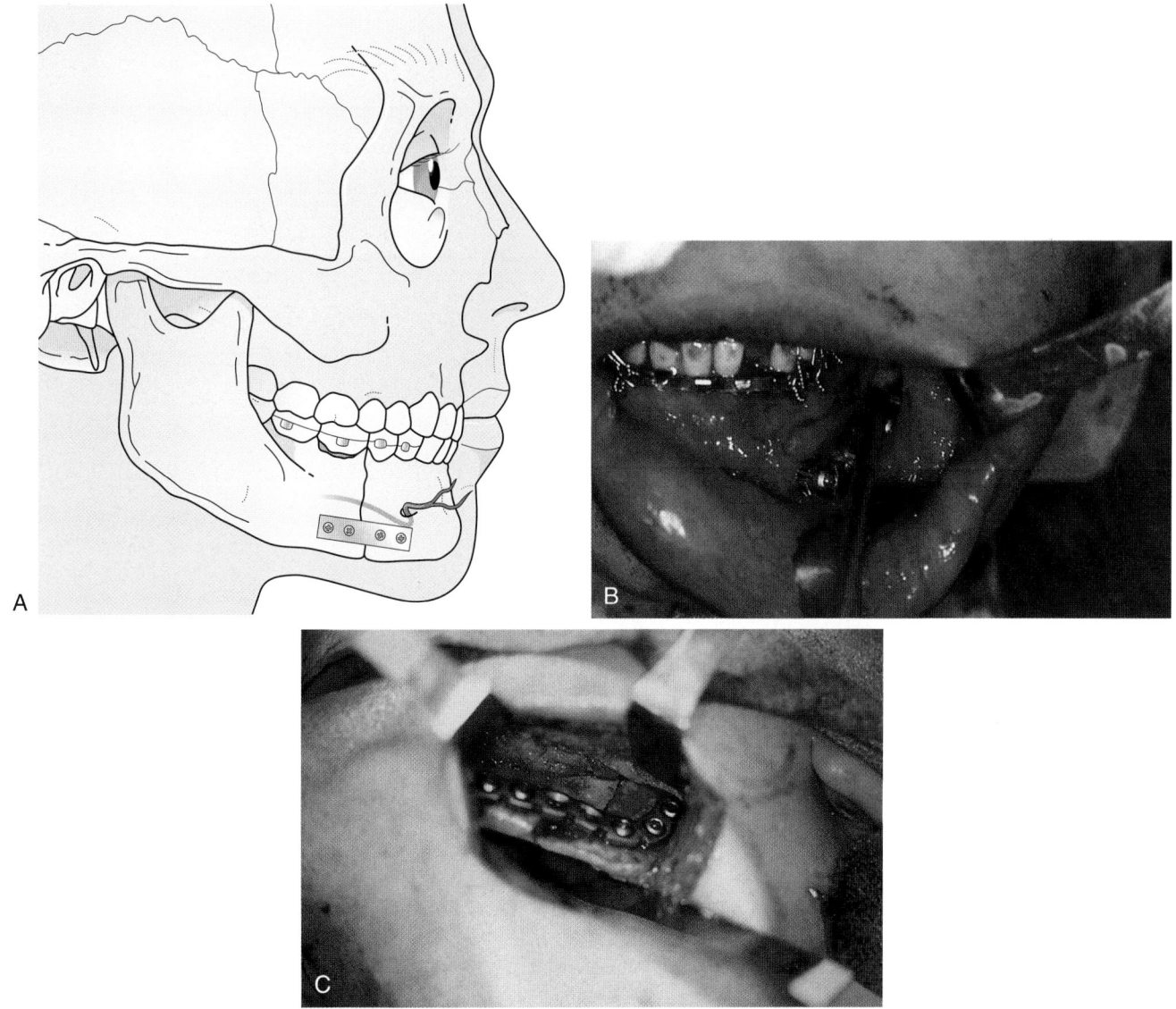

FIGURE 22.48 **A,** A fracture of the mandibular body is treated with a compression plate along the inferior border of the mandible. **B,** An intra-oral exposure is used for plate and screw fixation of a fracture of the mandibular symphysis. **C,** Plate and screw fixation of a mandibular angle fracture through an external incision in the upper neck.

SELECTED KEY REFERENCES

Clark N, Birely B, Manson PN, et al. High-energy ballistic and avulsive facial injuries: classification, patterns, and an algorithm for primary reconstruction. *Plast Reconstr Surg.* 1996;98:583-601.

Gruss J. Advances in craniofacial fracture repair. *Scand J Plast Reconstr Hand Surg.* 1995;27(Suppl):67-81.

Manson PN, Stanwix M, Yaremchuk M, et al. Frontobasilar fractures: anatomy, classification and clinical significance. *Plast Reconstr Surg.* 2010;124:2096–2016.

Rodriguez ED, Stanwix MG, Nam AJ, et al. Twenty-six-year experience treating frontal sinus fractures: a novel algorithm based on anatomical fracture pattern and failure of conventional techniques. *Plast Reconstr Surg.* 2008;122(6):1850-1866.

Please go to expertconsult.com to view the complete list of references.

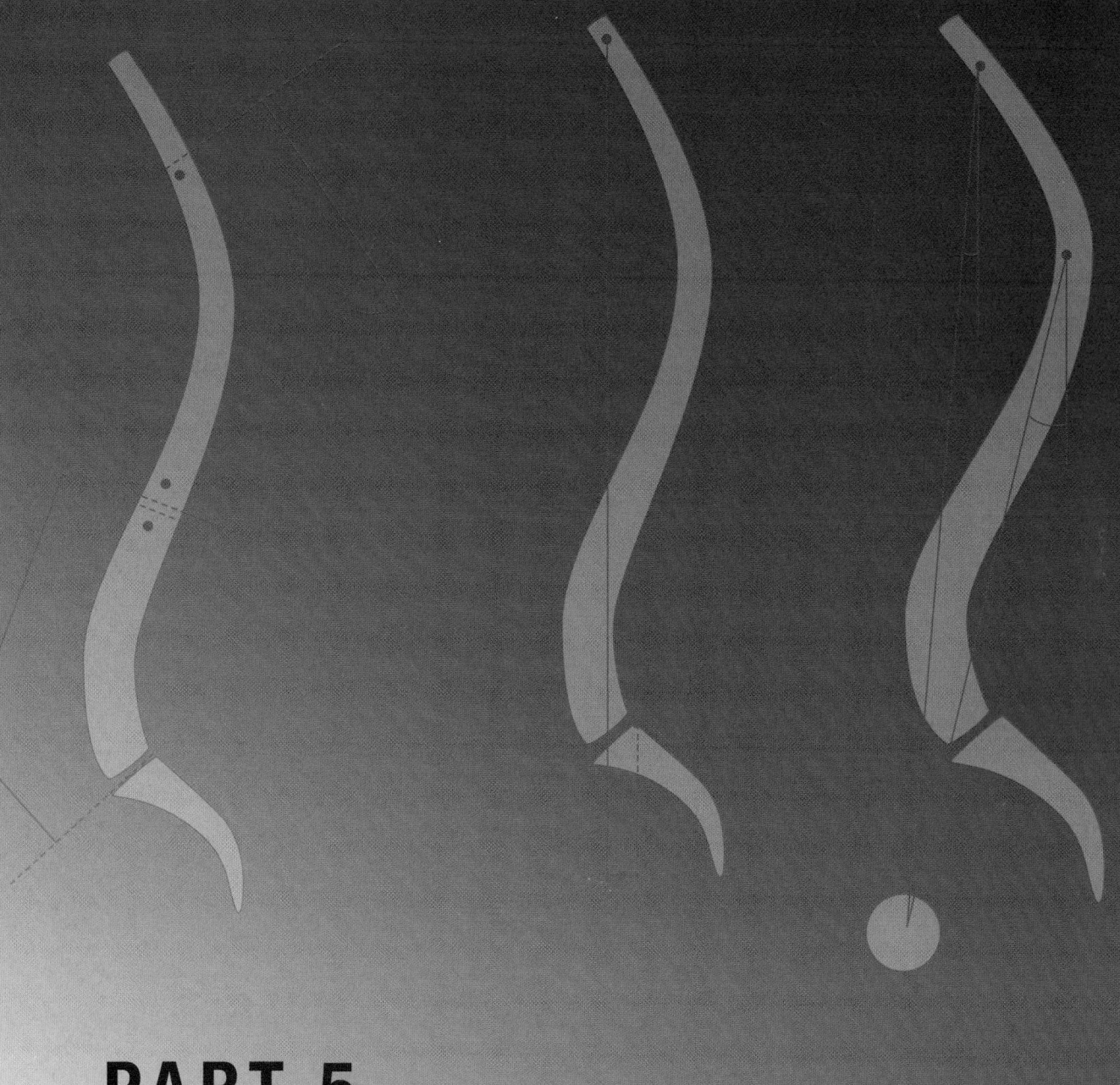

PART 5
Spine

23 Injuries to the Cervical Spine

M. Yashar S. Kalani, Aristotelis S. Filippidis, Nicholas Theodore

CLINICAL PEARLS

- The cervical spine is mobile and highly prone to traumatic injury.

- Early immobilization of the cervical spine and its thorough evaluation with imaging allow identification of a cervical injury and minimize further injuries related to the clinical evaluation of patients.

- The clinician should always search for clinical and imaging signs of ligamentous injury.

- Injuries can be classified as bony, ligamentous, or both according to various classification schemes described in

the text. The type of injury and its degree of stability dictate the intervention, which may include conservative management with external immobilization or aggressive management, including open or closed reduction, or internal stabilization and fusion.

- Spinal cord injury may present in a delayed fashion. In all cases of incomplete spinal cord injury, early reduction, when appropriate, should be considered.

The cervical spine is the most mobile portion of the spine and the most common site of spinal injuries. The relative traumatic involvement of different spinal levels is shown in Table 23.1. Nearly 12,000 to 14,000 spinal cord injuries occur each year in the United States.[1-6] Cervical spine trauma accounts for almost 1.5% of all pediatric trauma admissions.[7] Nearly 10,000 patients die each year as a result of an injury to the spinal cord.[5,8-11]

The most common mechanisms of injury to the cervical column are motor vehicle accidents, falls, and sports. Teens and young adults ranging in age between 15 and 30 are the most frequently injured population.[2,5,12-14] Falls account for 18% to 30% of cervical spine injuries in the younger age group (<8 years) and for 11% in the older age group (>8 years). Sports injuries are more prevalent in the older group (20-28%) and uncommon in the younger group (3%).[15,16] Nonaccidental trauma and penetrating injuries are also found in small numbers of very young children and adolescents, respectively.

The cause of spinal injury varies with age, and particularly with gender. Males are three to four times as likely to sustain an injury as females. Fractures are the most common injury pattern in all age groups, although ligamentous disruptions and dislocations are more prevalent in the young. Upper cervical spine injuries (C1-C4) are almost twice as common as lower cervical injuries (C5-C7).[1,17-19] Subluxation injuries without fracture and spinal cord injuries without radiographic abnormality (SCIWORA) are less common in adults and are more likely to occur in younger patients.[17,18,20]

NEUROLOGICAL INJURY

As many as 15% of patients who sustain a traumatic spinal injury will sustain a neurological injury as a result.[5,14] Injuries to the cervical spine, in particular, result in a much higher incidence of injury to the spinal cord than injuries at any other spinal level. The incidence of spinal cord injury ranges from 2% to *nearly* 100% of cervical spine injuries, depending on the cervical level involved, with an incidence of 40% to 60% overall (Table 23.2).[1,2,5,8-12,21,22] The incidence of spinal cord injury associated with cervical fractures is likely to be underestimated because some patients may die before reaching medical attention. This situation is particularly true of atlanto-occipital dislocations, in which 25% of patients may die as a result of respiratory arrest before evaluation.[4,5,14]

The level and mechanism of the spinal injury, the force involved, and the patient's age and medical status have important influences on the extent of neurological injury following trauma. In particular, conditions such as ankylosing spondylitis or Down syndrome, which have a significant effect on the relative rigidity (or laxity) of the spinal column, may predispose affected individuals to neurological injury.[5,14] Furthermore, the status of the patient after spinal injury can influence neurological injury, mainly through the deleterious effect of hypotension or hypoxia.[3,5,13,14] The American Spinal Cord Injury Association (ASIA) scale[23] is a clinical assessment tool that offers a detailed overview of the extent and type of spinal cord injury in an efficient and easy to apply format (Fig. 23.1).

TABLE 23.1 Incidence of Adult Spine Injuries

Spinal Segment Level of Injury	Incidence
Cervical	60%
Thoracic	8%
Thoracolumbar	20%
Lumbar	10%
Sacral	2%

TABLE 23.2 Cervical Spine Injury and Neurological Deficit

Injury Level	Incidence of Neurological Deficit
Atlanto-occipital dislocation	Up to 100%
Atlas	1-2%
Axis	10%
C3-T1	6%
Unilateral cervical facet dislocation	60%
Bilateral cervical facet dislocation	Up to 100%

General Principles

Given the significant incidence of spinal injury, clinicians must maintain a high index of suspicion for potential spinal injury in all trauma patients. All trauma patients should be immobilized until an appropriate and thorough evaluation of the spine for fractures or instability is completed. Ideally, immobilization should be initiated at the trauma scene and maintained during triage, resuscitation, and primary and secondary surveys. The primary trauma survey places special emphasis on the airway, breathing, and circulation (ABCs of resuscitation). In patients improperly immobilized, the primary survey can exacerbate existing cervical spine injuries in nearly 10% of the cases.[4,5]

In 2002 the Joint Section on Disorders of the Spine and Peripheral Nerves of the American Association of Neurological Surgeons (AANS) and the Congress of Neurological Surgeons (CNS) published specific evidence-based guidelines for the management of acute cervical spine and spinal cord injuries.[24] We have adopted these guidelines and discuss them here.

Imaging

In a trauma situation, the evaluation for cervical injury usually begins with a cross-table lateral radiograph (Fig. 23.2A). A swimmer's view may be added to visualize the cervicothoracic junction and the top of the T1 vertebral body (Fig. 23.2B).[5,14,25] The combination of a cross-table lateral and swimmer's view has an 85% sensitivity and a negative predictive value of 97% for fracture.[25,26] An open-mouth odontoid view should be obtained to assess the C1-C2 vertebrae and articulations and is particularly valuable for assessment of the odontoid process (Fig. 23.2C). If an open-mouth view cannot be obtained for whatever reason, the pillar (oblique) view can be utilized to demonstrate the odontoid process. The anteroposterior view is often ignored by inexperienced clinicians, but it can identify injuries with a rotatory component,

such as unilateral facet dislocations, that may not be readily apparent on lateral films. With the use of the anteroposterior, lateral, and open-mouth odontoid views, the sensitivity and negative predictive values of the series are 92% and 99%, respectively.[25-27] Adding oblique views to the standard series does not increase the sensitivity.[28]

The use of computed tomography (CT) has become commonplace in the evaluation of the trauma patient and is particularly useful for evaluating the occipitocervical and the cervicothoracic junctions. However, the routine use of CT in the trauma setting is difficult to recommend as there have been no direct comparisons with plain radiographs.[29,30] Areas identified as possible injury on plain radiographs should be further investigated with CT with fine sections through the suspicious area (Fig. 23.3A).[14,25] Reconstructions in the sagittal and coronal planes may further help define the nature of the injury (Fig. 23.3B and C).[25] Determining the level of trauma may be difficult in SCIWORA patients. In these cases, the neurological examination is critical in evaluating the appropriate level to be studied.[17] The evaluation can also be conducted by the use of magnetic resonance imaging (MRI).[31] Approximately 10% of patients with a cervical spine fracture have a second associated, noncontiguous vertebral column fracture; therefore, a complete radiographic assessment of the entire spinal column is warranted.[5,14] The exceptions to early CT after the initial lateral radiographs have been obtained are patients with an obvious facet fracture-dislocation injury.[21] These patients may benefit from early reduction of the fracture and realignment of the cervical spine as long as rostral injuries, especially injuries to the craniocervical junction, are ruled out. Three-dimensional CT can be useful in the evaluation of complex cervical spine fractures and particularly in operative planning (Fig. 23.3D).[32]

The debate over the most appropriate workup for cervical spine injury in an asymptomatic trauma patient has resulted in several guidelines to minimize the cost and radiation exposure to patients.[33] According to the Guidelines from the AANS/CNS Joint Section, trauma patients who meet the following criteria do not require x-ray evaluation of the cervical spine: (1) normal neurological examination and a Glasgow Coma Scale (GCS) score of 15, with no delayed or inappropriate responses, (2) not intoxicated, (3) no neck pain or midline tenderness, and (4) no significant distracting injury such as long-bone fracture or visceral injury.[34] Symptomatic patients who do not meet these criteria should undergo a full radiographic assessment of the cervical spine.

Alternatively, the Canadian C-spine rules can be applied as a guideline to minimize the use of radiographs in the evaluation of alert and stable trauma patients when cervical spine injury is a concern.[31,35]

MRI is an extremely useful tool in the assessment of patients with a cervical spine injury and may identify injuries, such as disk herniations and ligamentous injuries, not seen on plain radiograph or CT. MRI provides a longitudinal assessment of the spine and spinal cord with views in the axial, sagittal, and coronal planes (Fig. 23.4).[5,10,14,25,36-38] MRI may be the only imaging modality on which an abnormality is found in patients with SCIWORA, because ligaments, soft tissues, and neural elements can be imaged with superior detail. Hematomas within the spinal canal will not be identified on plain radiograph and may even be missed on CT but are readily

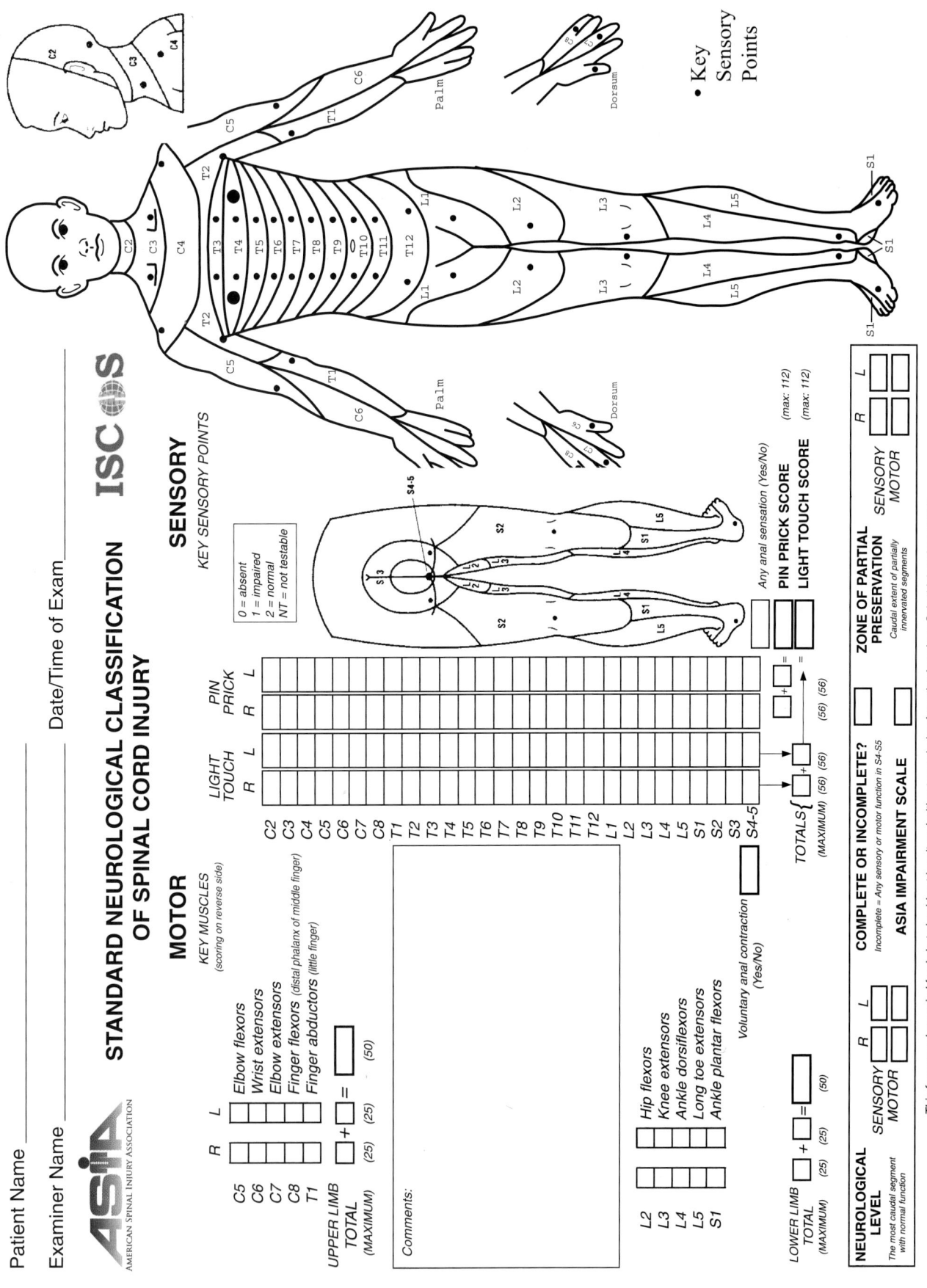

FIGURE 23.1 The American Spine Injury Association (ASIA) scale for spinal cord injury. (Used with permission from the American Spinal Injury Association.)

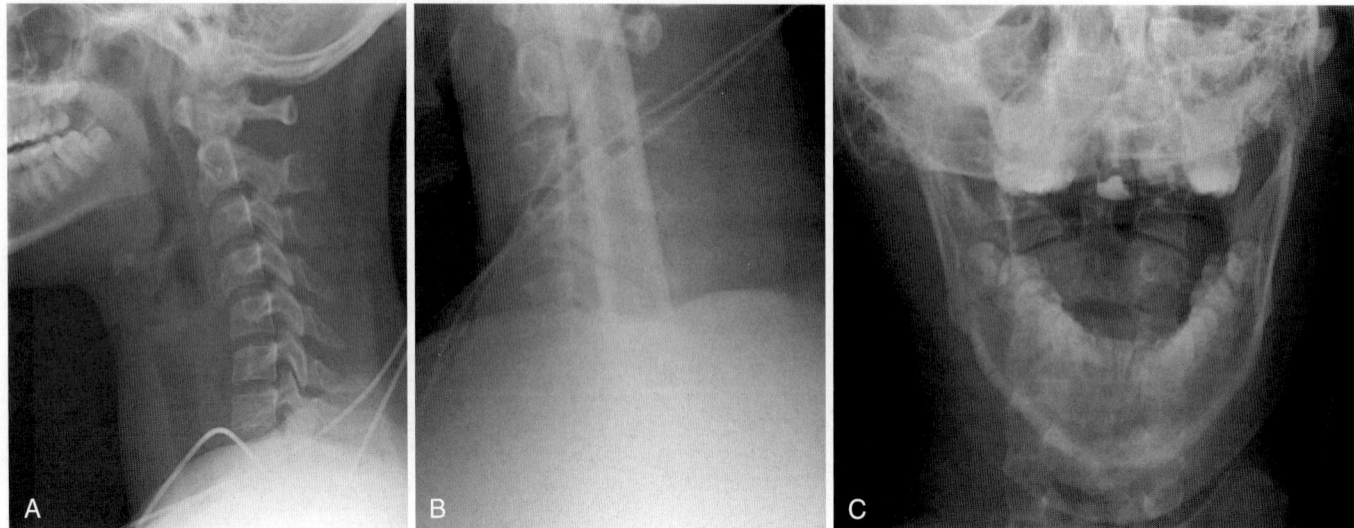

FIGURE 23.2 Cross-table lateral (**A**) and swimmer's view (**B**) radiographs are important tools for the initial workup of the trauma patient with a suspected cervical spine injury. **C,** The addition of an open-mouth odontoid view can reveal possible odontoid fractures that could be missed on the other two views. *(Used with permission from Barrow Neurological Institute.)*

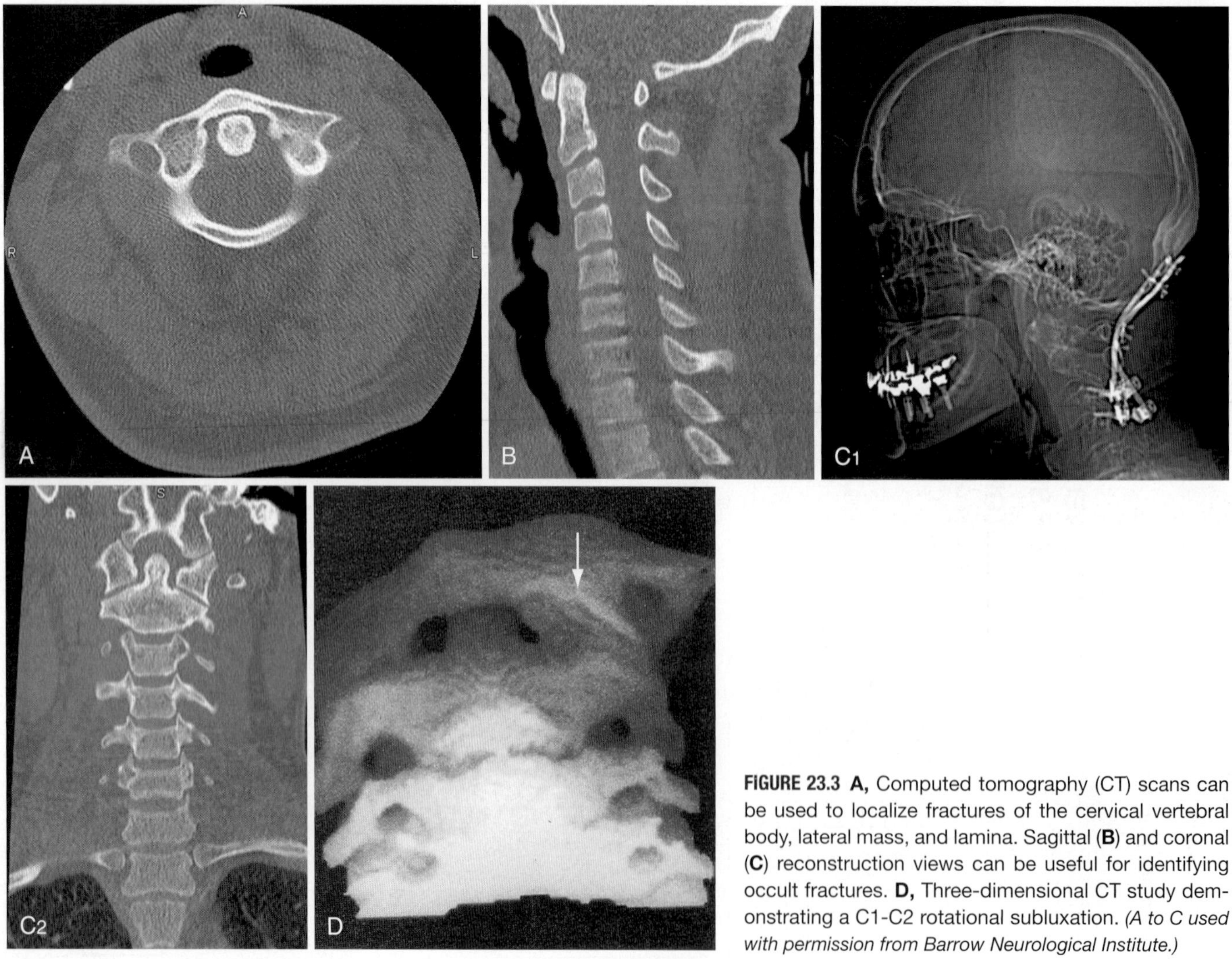

FIGURE 23.3 A, Computed tomography (CT) scans can be used to localize fractures of the cervical vertebral body, lateral mass, and lamina. Sagittal (**B**) and coronal (**C**) reconstruction views can be useful for identifying occult fractures. **D,** Three-dimensional CT study demonstrating a C1-C2 rotational subluxation. *(A to C used with permission from Barrow Neurological Institute.)*

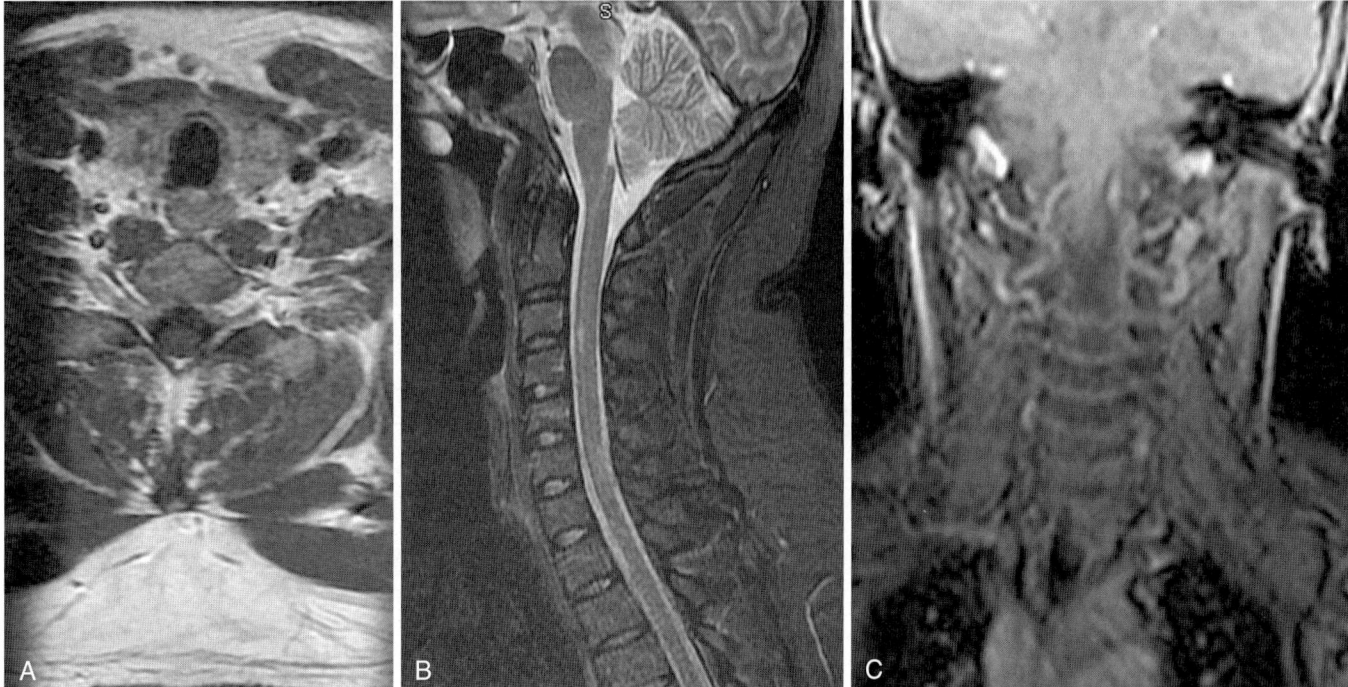

FIGURE 23.4 A, Magnetic resonance imaging (MRI) is a powerful tool for assessing cervical spine integrity. Sagittal (**B**) and coronal (**C**) reconstructions can be used to assess ligamental stability and to assess for disk protrusion and compromise of the cervical canal. *(Used with permission from Journal of Neurosurgery.)*

identified on MRI.[10,37,39] Although MRI is extremely sensitive for ligamentous injury, it cannot be used alone to diagnose an "unstable" injury.[35]

In the case of cervical trauma but no demonstrable fracture or dislocation injury on the initial standard cervical spine x-ray and CT studies, flexion and extension lateral cervical spine views are important additions to the radiographic assessment. Dynamic flexion-extension views may determine the presence of subluxation injuries or abnormal ligamentous laxity in patients who have persistent post-traumatic neck pain.[5,14] In the obtunded or unconscious patient, flexion and extension may be performed under fluoroscopy and may detect a previously unrecognized injury, although its clinical significance is uncertain.[40,41] Fluoroscopy is probably indicated only in patients with high-risk injuries such as high-speed motor vehicle accidents, falls over 3 m, major associated injuries, or vehicle crashes involving a death at the scene, because low-risk injuries have only a 0.2% incidence of cervical spine injury.[42] MRI can be performed in flexion and extension, a technique that may be useful in identifying positional subluxation or compression of the cervical spinal cord in select cases.[25,37,38]

MANAGEMENT

Atlanto-Occipital Dislocation

Traumatic atlanto-occipital dislocation (AOD) is associated with a high incidence of neurological morbidity and mortality.[39,43-48] The mechanism and amount of force required to disrupt the atlanto-occipital junction are often fatal to victims of this type of injury. Historically, AOD injuries were deemed uncommon. More recent autopsy reports indicate that AOD accounts for 6% to 8% of all traffic fatalities. Of cervical spine injury-related deaths, 20% to 30% are the result of AOD.[49-51] Given recent advances in the diagnosis and management of AOD, as many as 20% of survivors with this type of injury have a favorable functional outcome if therapy and immobilization are instituted promptly (Fig. 23.5).[35,39,43-47]

A classification scheme for the types of AODs describes anterior (type I), longitudinal (type II), and posterior (type III) dislocations based on the movement of the occiput with respect to the cervical spine (Fig. 23.6).

Once the examination or mechanism of injury suggests a case of AOD, strict cervical spine precautions are mandatory to prevent further complications. The use of rigid collars, which further distract the occipitoatlantal joint, should be discontinued. We prefer to use sandbags on either side of the patient's head with taping to immobilize the patient and have had excellent success using this method. Another method of immobilization is the use of early halo fixation once the diagnosis of AOD is confirmed. A halo vest provides immediate immobilization and can be quite effective during positioning and intubation of the patient for surgical fixation.

On the basis of class III evidence, *The Guidelines for the Management of Acute Cervical Spine and Spinal Cord Injuries* recommend applying the Harris method to a plain lateral cervical radiograph to recognize AOD. Since the publication of these guidelines, several groups have documented the use of CT as the diagnostic imaging of choice in patients suspected of having AOD.[31,52-54] Based on these studies a basion-dens interval (BDI) (with 10 mm as the cutoff) and the occipital condyle-C1 interval (CCI) (>4 mm is abnormal) are the diagnostic

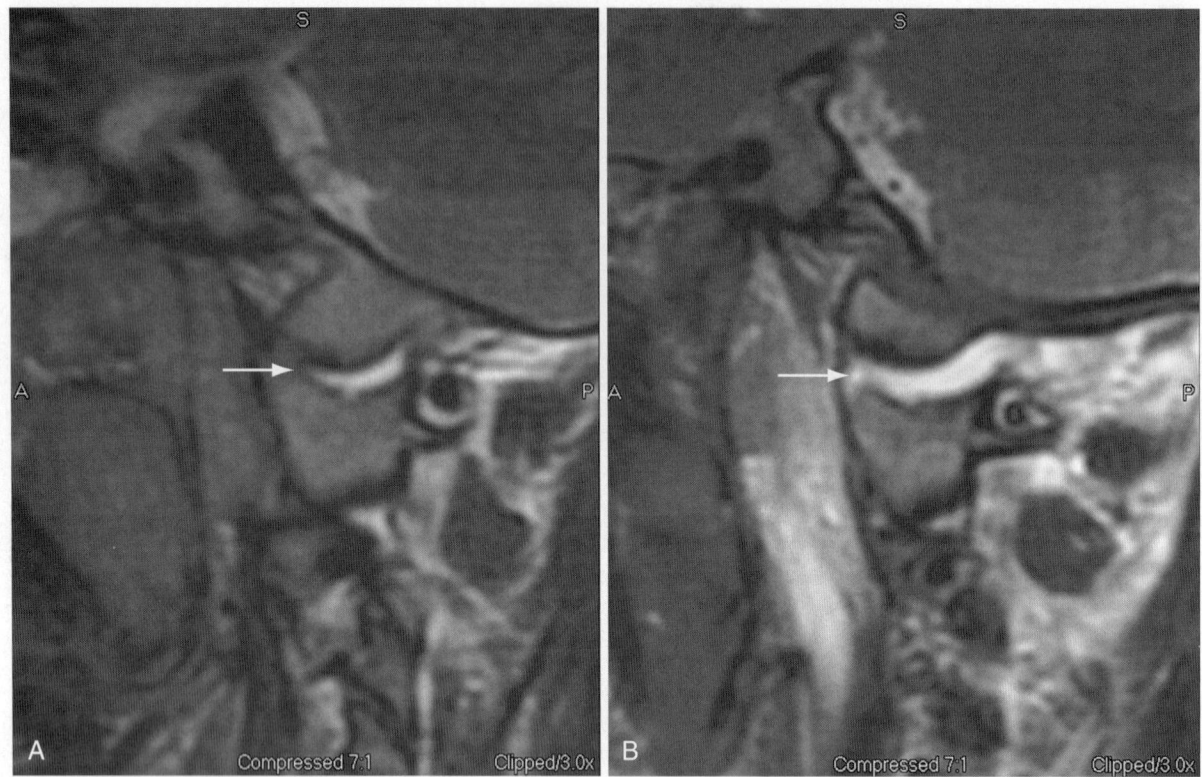

FIGURE 23.5 Sagittal T2-weighted magnetic resonance images demonstrating abnormal high signal intensity (*arrows*) in the atlanto-occipital joints on the right (**A**) and left (**B**) sides consistent with atlanto-occipital dislocation. *(Used with permission from Journal of Neurosurgery.)*

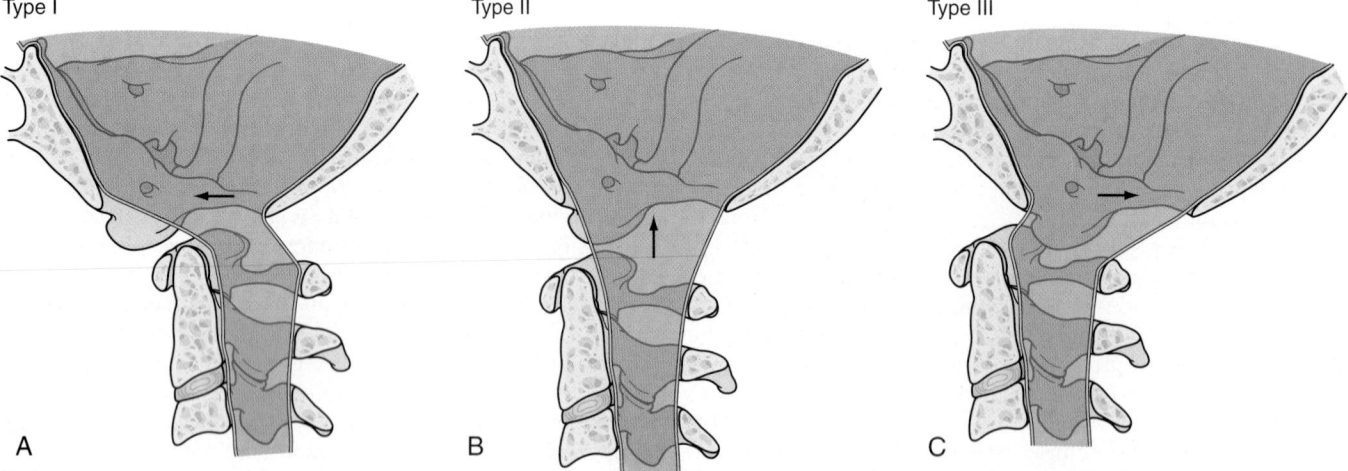

FIGURE 23.6 Classification system for atlanto-occipital dislocation (AOD). **A,** Type I or anterior dislocation of the occiput with respect to the atlas. **B,** Type II or vertical displacement. **C,** Type III or posterior displacement. *(Redrawn with permission from Barrow Neurological Institute.)*

tests of choice.[53] It should be emphasized that AOD is a highly unstable injury and can be missed on any imaging modality if normal alignment is temporarily restored. MRI can be an important adjunct in the diagnosis of this condition.[35]

Our treatment paradigm for AOD is based on the recommendations from the largest published series of AOD patients (Table 23.3). Grade I injuries are those with "normal" BDI and CCI (Fig. 23.7) and equivocal MRI findings such as high posterior ligamentous or occipitoatlantal signal and mild to no signal change at the occipitoatlantal joint. In this population,

nonoperative management with a halo or collar is adequate. Grade II injuries are defined by a minimum of one abnormal finding on CT-based criteria or grossly abnormal MRI findings in the occipitoatlantal joints, tectorial membrane, or alar or cruciate ligaments. Effective surgical stabilization of these patients requires open reduction and internal fixation (ORIF) from the occiput to the upper cervical spine.[39,43-45] Fixation can be achieved with one of several types of instrumentation (Fig. 23.8) and must be supplemented by allograft or autogenic bone to provide long-term stability.

TABLE 23.3 Treatment Algorithm for Atlanto-Occipital Dislocations

Study	Grade	CT/Radiographic Findings	MRI Findings	Provocative Traction Results	Treatment
Horn et al., 2007	I	Normal based on established criteria (Powers' ratio, BDI, BAI, X-line, CCI)	Moderately abnormal (high signal in posterior ligaments or occipitoatlantal joints)	NA	External orthosis
	II	≥1 abnormal finding based on established criteria	Grossly abnormal findings in occipitoatlantal joints, tectorial membrane, alar ligaments, or cruciate ligaments	NA	Internal fixation

BAI, basion-axial interval; BDI, basion-dens interval,; CCI, condyle-C1 interval; CT, computed tomography; MRI, magnetic resonance imaging; NA, not applicable; X-line method, craniometric parameter based on plain radiograph findings and used to diagnose atlantoccipital dislocation.

Modified from Horn EM, Feiz-Erfan I, Lekovic GP, et al. Survivors of occipitoatlantal dislocation injuries: imaging and clinical correlates. J Neurosurg Spine 2007;6(2):113-120. Used with permission from *Journal of Neurosurgery.*

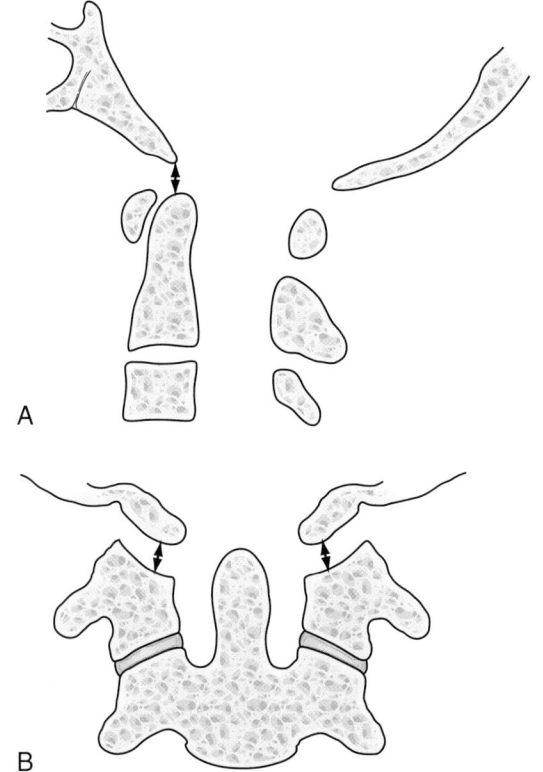

FIGURE 23.7 Drawings illustrating cervical radiographic techniques for the diagnosis of atlanto-occipital dislocation (AOD). **A,** Basion-dens interval (BDI) is abnormal in the presence of a displacement between the basion and the dens exceeding 10 mm in adults or more than 12 mm in the pediatric population. **B,** A distance of more than 2 mm in adults or 5 mm in pediatric patients between the occipital condyle and the superior articular facet of the atlas is considered an abnormal condylar gap. *(Redrawn with permission from Barrow Neurological Institute.)*

Occipital Condyle Fractures

Occipital condyle fractures (OCFs) are frequently missed on plain radiographs. With almost universal use of CT scans of the occipitocervical junction in the evaluation of trauma patients, these injuries are now being recognized with increased frequency.[55] The true prevalence of OCF is unknown, but most authors have concluded that it is probably more common than typically realized.[4,5] The reported incidence of OCF ranges from 4% to 19%, with a mean age of presentation of 32.4 years (range, 7 months to 88 years) and a male predilection of 2:1.[56]

OCFs commonly occur as isolated injuries.[28,29,57] The presence of a retropharyngeal hematoma on a lateral cervical radiograph may be the only clue that serious craniovertebral insult has occurred.[58-60] Based on CT-based anatomical studies, Anderson and Montesano have classified these fractures (Fig. 23.9).[61] Type I fractures (axial load and comminuted fractures) and type II fractures (extension of a skull-base fracture) are usually considered stable if isolated. Thus, symptomatic treatment is indicated and may include external immobilization in a collar.[62] Type III injuries (avulsion of a condylar fragment by the alar ligament) may be unstable and require rigid external immobilization in a collar or halo or even ORIF, if other injuries such as atlantoaxial instability are present.[62] Patients not treated may develop lower cranial nerve palsies, which still have a significant chance of resolving with immobilization.[63]

The need for surgical intervention to treat OCF is rare, and conservative management of all isolated OCFs is generally supported, even in cases of brainstem compression with neurological injury. Bilateral OCF can represent a unique presentation of AOD and needs to be evaluated carefully.[35]

Atlas Fractures

The atlas is the first cervical vertebra (C1) and bridges the occiput with the axis, the second cervical vertebra (C2), and the rest of the cervical spine.[64] The position of the atlas and its ring shape make it vulnerable to a number of different fracture patterns. Fractures of the atlas account for 3% to 13% of all cervical spinal injuries.[65,66] Injuries to C1 are mostly isolated, but 40% to 44% are associated with fractures of C2.[65] Owing to the wide spinal canal at the level of C1, a neurological injury in the region is rare. Atlas fractures can be observed in various patterns and multiple classification schemes exist. The one used most commonly is the classification first presented by Jefferson[67] and later modified by Gehweiler and associates[68] (Fig. 23.10). In this modified classification scheme, type I fractures involve only the posterior arch. Only the anterior arch is involved in type II fractures. In type III fractures the

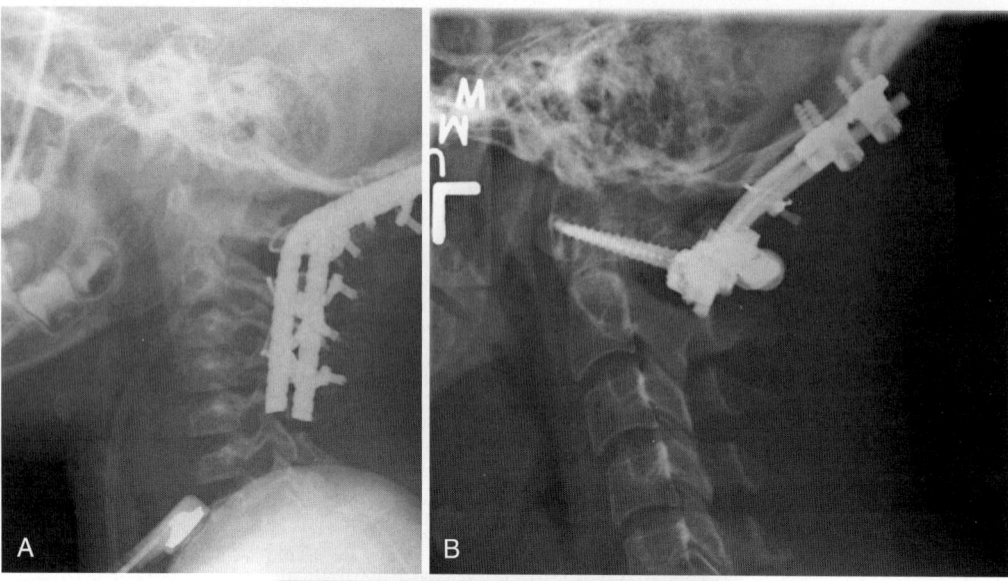

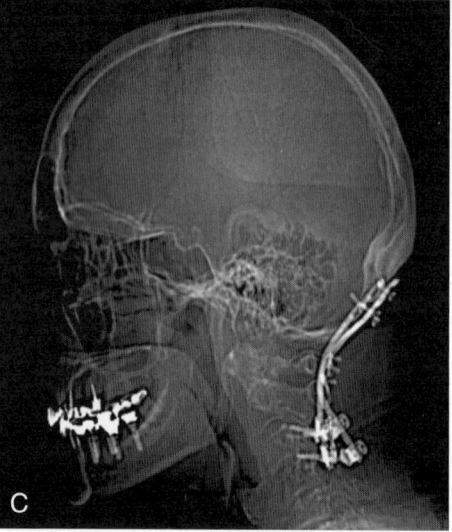

FIGURE 23.8 Surgical stabilization was achieved with occiput-to-C4 titanium rod fixation and autograft fusion. **A,** Lateral radiograph after occiput-to-C4 fusion in a patient whose vertebral artery anatomy was unfavorable for C2 screw placement and sublaminar wiring of C1 and C2 to the rod for extra stability. **B,** Lateral radiograph showing occipitocervical fusion with occipital keel screws and C1 lateral mass screws, sparing the atlantoaxial joint. **C,** Lateral radiograph after occiput-to-C4 fusion with keel screws and C3-C4 screws sparing the C1-C2 levels. *(Used with permission from Barrow Neurological Institute.)*

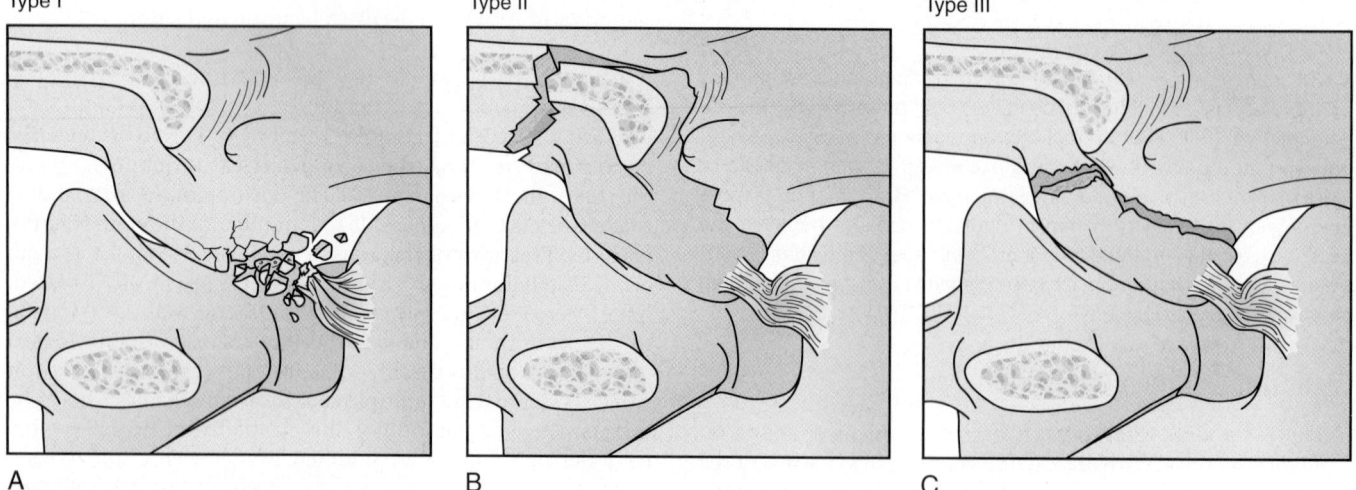

FIGURE 23.9 **A** to **C,** The various types of occipital condyle fractures based on the Anderson and Montesano classification system. *(Redrawn with permission from Barrow Neurological Institute.)*

FIGURE 23.10 A to **G,** Types of C1 fractures based on the Jefferson classification. A class I Jefferson fracture involves the posterior ring (**A**), and a class II Jefferson fracture involves the anterior ring (**B**). Type III Jefferson fractures involve both anterior and posterior rings (**C** to **E**), and type IV Jefferson fractures are crush injuries involving the lateral mass (**F** and **G**). *(Redrawn with permission from Barrow Neurological Institute.)*

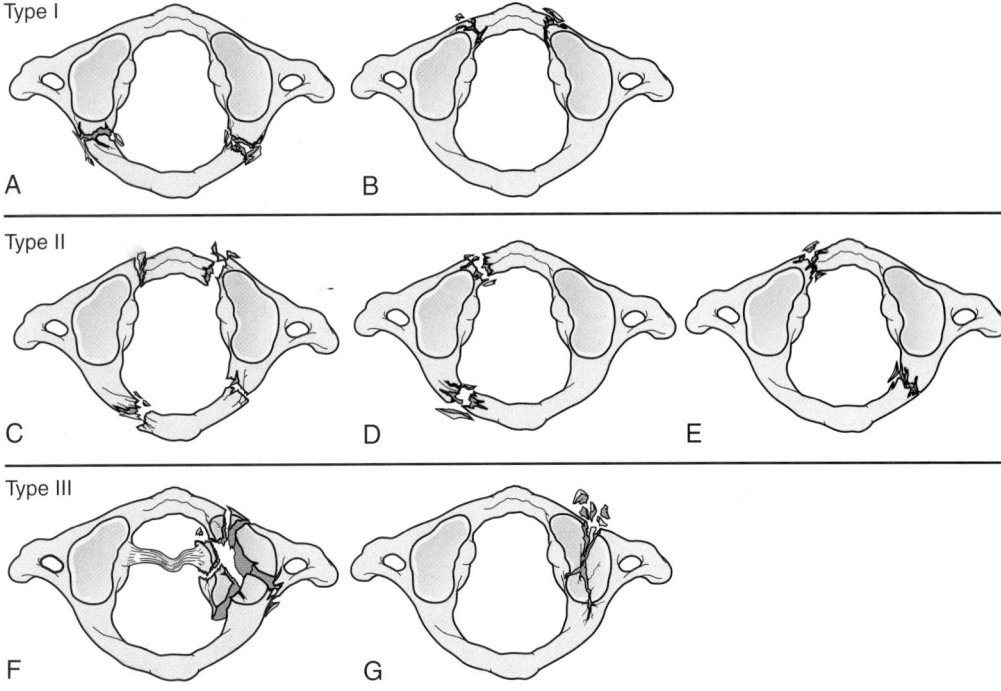

posterior arch is fractured bilaterally, and there is an associated unilateral or bilateral anterior arch fracture. The classic Jefferson fracture is a type III atlas burst fracture. In this case the lateral masses are displaced laterally. The classic Jefferson fracture is the most frequent fracture pattern of C1, and it is caused by axial loading of the atlas. Type IV fractures involve the lateral mass, and type V fractures are transverse anterior arch fractures. Congenital abnormalities of the C1 ring can be mistaken for a fracture in some cases and MRI can be used in these cases to assess the affected area for edema within the bone.

Apart from the bony fractures of C1, the integrity of the transverse atlantal ligament (TAL), which is a key factor in determining the stability of atlas fractures, should always be assessed.[69] The classic *rule of Spence* assesses the extent of lateral mass displacement (of C1 with respect to C2) on spine radiographs to provide evidence for the appropriate treatment modality.[70] The combined sum of the displacement of both lateral masses of C1 on C2 is measured on open-mouth odontoid or coronal CT. If the combined sum of the displacement is 6.9 mm or greater, it is presumed that the TAL is incompetent and the fracture is considered unstable. In the era of CT and MRI, Dickman and co-workers demonstrated that 61% of TAL ruptures could be missed by using the rule of Spence; therefore, they proposed a new classification system for TAL ruptures (Fig. 23.11).[69] Disruption at the midportion of the TAL or at the insertion of the medial tubercle is considered a Dickman type I disruption, which cannot be healed by external immobilization alone. Dickman type II TAL disruption involves purely bony avulsions and can potentially be treated by external immobilization alone.

The treatment of atlas fractures relies only on level III evidence data from published series (Fig. 23.12). In general, isolated fractures can be treated with cervical immobilization alone if the transverse ligament is intact. If the transverse ligament is disrupted, both cervical immobilization alone or surgical fixation and fusion are reasonable options.[64] Fractures of the anterior or posterior arch are treated with a rigid cervical orthosis. Fractures of the anterior and posterior arches (burst) with an intact TAL can be treated with a rigid cervical orthosis or halo brace. Both anterior and posterior arch fractures (burst) that are unstable (TAL disrupted) can be treated with a halo brace but usually require C1-C2 stabilization and fusion. Depending upon the extent of injury to C1, occipitocervical fixation may be indicated. Comminuted lateral mass fractures require a rigid cervical orthosis or a halo brace. In all cases, 8 to 12 weeks of immobilization are recommended. When a surgical solution is indicated, the approach is determined by the extent of C1 injury. An unstable unilateral ring or anterior C1 ring fracture requires C1-C2 fusion, while multiple ring or posterior ring fractures may require occipitocervical fusion.

Axis Fractures

Fractures of C2 account for 18% of all cervical spine traumatic injuries.[4,12,14,19,21,71,72] Odontoid process fractures are the most common C2 fracture, representing approximately 60% of fractures at this level. The rates of neurological deficit and acute injury mortality associated with axis fractures are 8.5% and 2.4%, respectively.[73] Autopsy studies have revealed that a significant proportion of deaths at the scene of traffic accidents are associated with fractures of the upper cervical spine; of these, axis fractures are estimated to range from 25% to 71%.[50,74-76]

The Anderson-D'Alonzo classification of odontoid fractures is presented in Table 23.4 and Figure 23.13.[77] Type I odontoid fracture is the rarest and involves an isolated odontoid tip fracture. Type II is the most common and involves the base of the odontoid tip. The type IIA fracture is the only widely accepted modification to the Anderson-D'Alonzo nomenclature and includes comminution associated with a

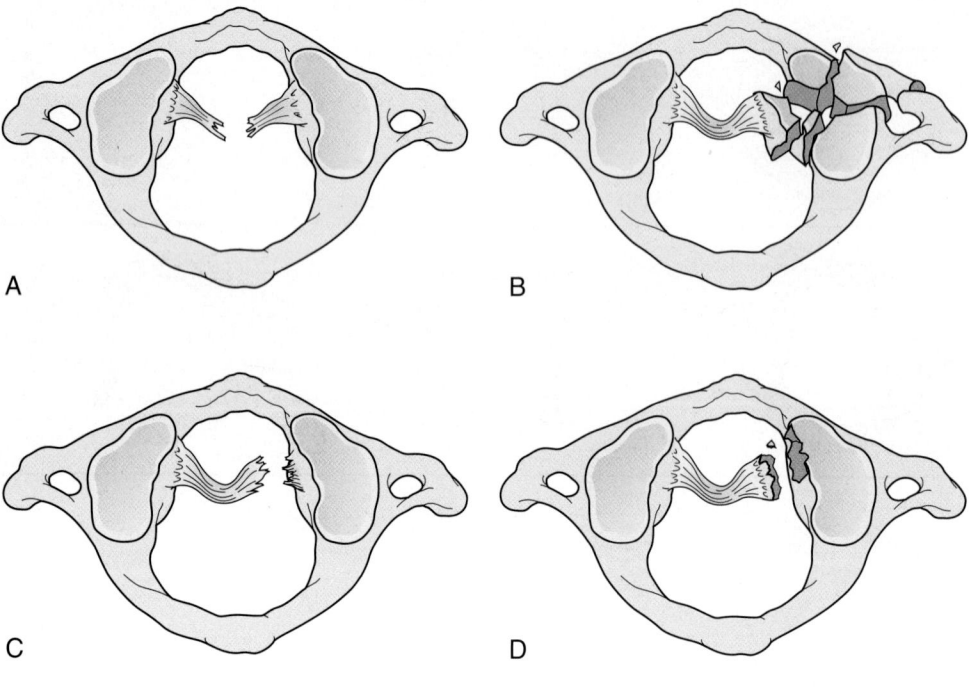

A

B

C

D

FIGURE 23.11 **A** to **D**, Dickman modification to the Jefferson classification system, taking into account the integrity of the transverse ligament. Both disruption of the midportion of the transverse ligament (**A**) and at the insertion of the medial tubercle (**B**) represent Dickman type I fractures and cannot heal without surgical intervention. Bony avulsions (**C** and **D**) represent Dickman type II fractures and have a good chance of healing when treated with external immobilization. *(Redrawn with permission from Barrow Neurological Institute.)*

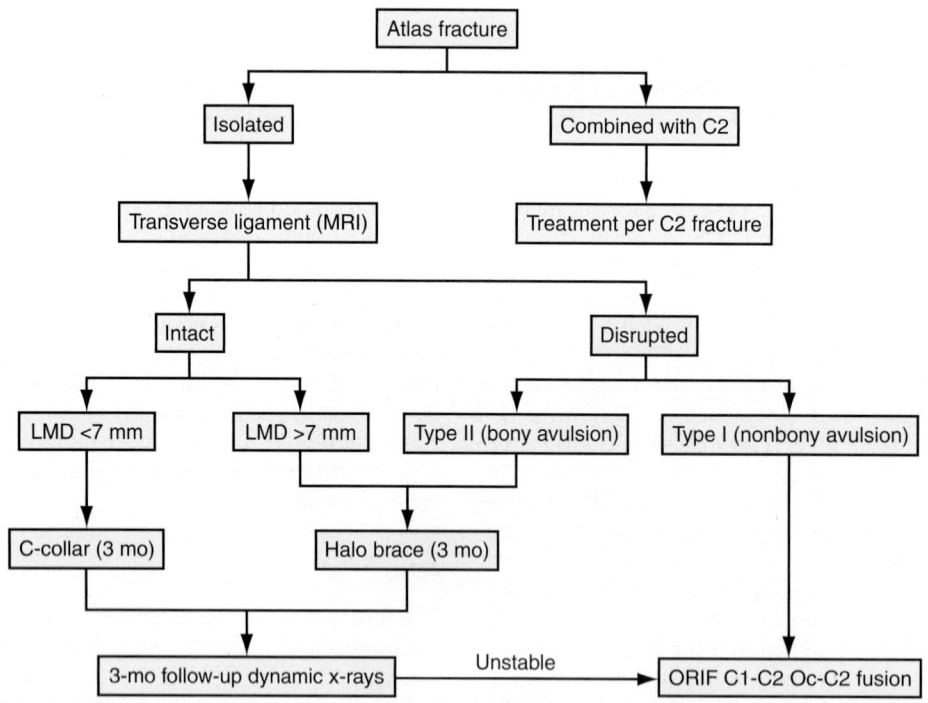

FIGURE 23.12 Treatment algorithm for atlas fractures. C, cervical; LMD, lateral mass displacement; mo, month; MRI, magnetic resonance imaging; Oc, occiput; ORIF, open reduction internal fixation. *(Redrawn with permission from Barrow Neurological Institute.)*

TABLE 23.4	Anderson and D'Alonzo Classification of Odontoid Fractures
Type	**Fracture Location**
I	Tip of odontoid
II	Base of odontoid
IIA*	Type II with bony chips
III	Base of odontoid into body of C2

*Hadley and associates added type IIA in 1988: Hadley MN, Browner CM, Liu SS, Sonntag VK. New subtype of acute odontoid fractures (type IIA). Neurosurgery 1988;22(1 Pt 1):67-71.

type II fracture; this type accounts for about 5% of odontoid fractures. Type III odontoid fractures represent one third of all odontoid injuries and involve a fracture that extends through the vertebral body of C2.[4,12,14] Odontoid type I and type III fractures are usually treated with rigid external immobilization. Type III fractures have a 97% fusion rate in a halo vest.[4,12,14,71,72] In contrast, odontoid type II fractures, which are more difficult to treat, are associated with a nonunion rate as high as 40% when treated with external immobilization alone.[4,12,14,19,72] Type II fractures with less than 5 mm of dens displacement are good

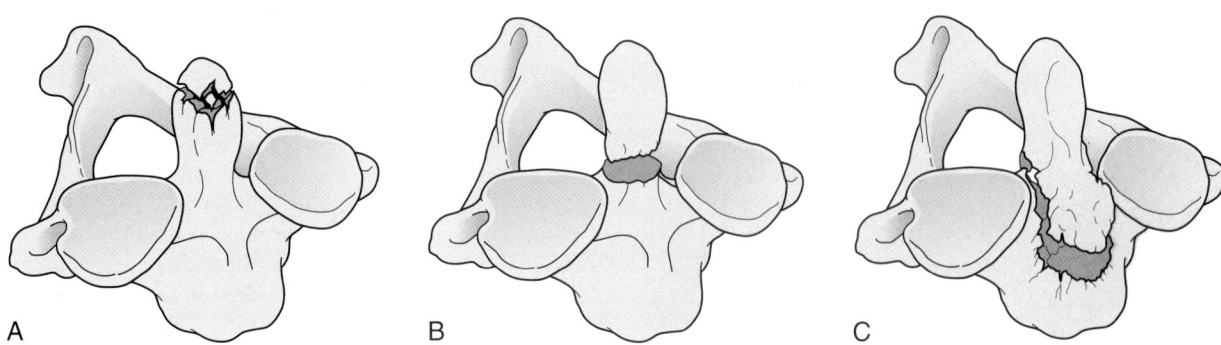

FIGURE 23.13 Anderson and D'Alonzo classification of odontoid fractures. **A,** A type I odontoid fracture involves only the tip of the odontoid. **B,** A type II fracture extends to the base of the odontoid. **C,** A type III fracture extends to the body of the C2 vertebra. *(Redrawn with permission from Barrow Neurological Institute.)*

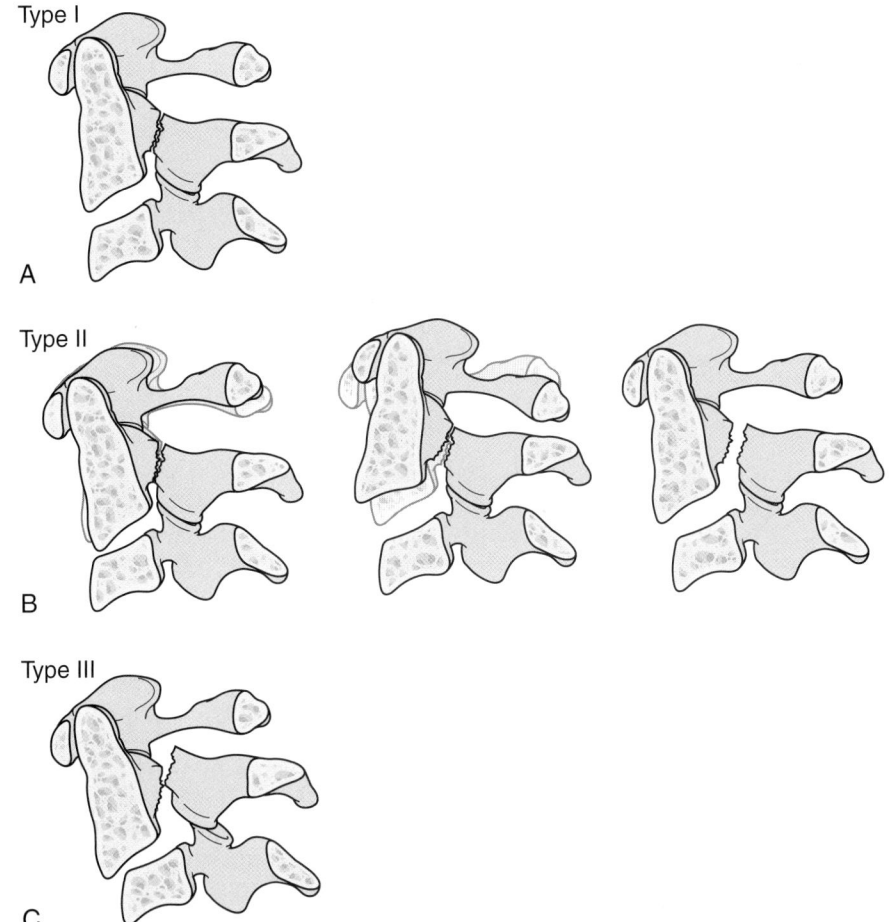

Type I

A

Type II

B

Type III

C

FIGURE 23.14 Effendi classification of hangman's fractures. A type I hangman's fracture (**A**) is a nondisplaced fracture, a type II (**B**) shows anterior displacement, and a type III (**C**) shows facet dislocation at C2-C3 with an anterior fragment in a flexed position. *(Redrawn with permission from Barrow Neurological Institute.)*

candidates for halo stabilization. However, the rate of failure associated with external immobilization alone of those with more than 5 mm of dens displacement is greater than 86%; therefore, these fractures should be addressed surgically.[4,12,14,72,78] Compared with younger patients, patients older than 50 years of age have a 21-fold greater incidence of nonunion with type II odontoid fractures; thus, primary treatment with surgery should be considered.[79] Type IIA odontoid fractures should also be treated with early surgery.

Surgical operations include anterior odontoid screw fixation or posterior atlantoaxial fusion.[14,80]

Hangman's fractures, or bilateral fractures of the pars interarticularis (also referred to as *traumatic spondylolisthesis of the axis*), represent 4% of all cervical spine fractures and 20% of all axis fracture injuries.[4,12,14,19,81] Hangman's fractures are associated with a low rate of neurological injury.[82] Effendi and colleagues classified hangman's fractures into nondisplaced fractures (type I), fractures in which the anterior

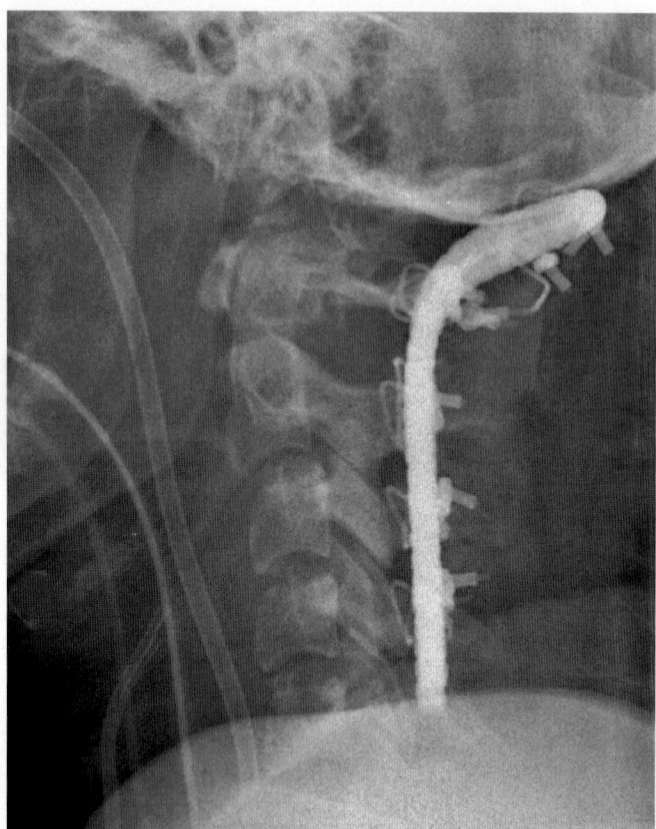

FIGURE 23.15 Lateral postoperative radiograph demonstrating the construct for an occipitocervical fusion. *(Used with permission from Journal of Neurosurgery.)*

fragment is displaced (type II), and fractures in which the anterior fragment is in a flexed position and a C2-C3 facet dislocation (type III) is present (Fig. 23.14).[83] Types I and II hangman's fractures are well treated with external immobilization with a halo vest or rigid collar.[4,12,14,84] Type III hangman's fractures should be preferentially treated with open surgery.[85-87] Levine and Edwards further modified the Effendi classification to include the degree of angulation into the grading system.[88] The combination of the Effendi and Levine systems is the most popular system for grading hangman's injuries. If there is evidence of C2-C3 subluxation and instability with any subtype of axis fracture, surgical repair should be performed because these fractures have a high rate of nonunion with nonoperative therapy.[4,12]

Fractures involving the body, pedicle, lateral mass, laminae, and spinous process of C2 account for nearly 20% of fractures at this level.[14,71,84] Fractures of the C2 vertebral body are usually treated conservatively.[89,90]

Combination fractures of the atlas and axis comprise 4% of all cervical spine fractures. In general, the type of C2 fracture dictates the type of intervention in combined fracture situations. Surgical options include posterior C1-C2 fusion,[91] transarticular screws,[92] anterior odontoid screw fixation,[93] C1-C3 posterior fusion, or occipitocervical fusion (Fig. 23.15).[94,95] Anterior approaches to C1 and C2 include odontoid screw fixation (Fig. 23.16) for odontoid fractures and C2-C3 interbody fusion with anterior plating for hangman's fractures.[4,96,97]

C3-T1 Injuries

The third cervical vertebra is an uncommon site for isolated injury, accounting for less than 1% of all cervical spine injuries.[4] Fractures of C3 associated with C2 fractures (usually of the hangman's variety) are slightly more common and may involve the lamina and spinous process of C3. C3 may be relatively protected from injury because it is situated between the more vulnerable C1-C2 complex and C5-C6, which is the area of greatest flexion and extension in the cervical spine.[4,71]

Almost 75% of all cervical spine fractures occur between C4 and T1.[1,4] The most common level of cervical vertebral fracture is C5, and the most common level of subluxation injury is the C5-C6 interspace.[1,4,5] Fractures of the vertebral bodies are the most common type of injury to occur in the subaxial cervical spine. In decreasing order of frequency, subluxations, facet dislocations, and laminar, pedicular, or spinous process fractures can also occur. It is possible to have a purely ligamentous injury without fracture or dislocation. Subluxation associated with vertebral body fracture results in a high incidence of spinal cord injury.[5,9,11,21] Patients suffering bilateral facet dislocations have a nearly 100% incidence of neurological injury, and the incidence in those with unilateral facet dislocations is 80%.[21] Of particular importance, most injuries with unilateral dislocations are root injuries, while the most common neurological injury associated with bilateral facet dislocations is a complete spinal cord injury.

In designing the optimal regimen for the management of patients with C4-T1 spinal injuries, it is important to consider the following factors: the mechanism of injury, the type of injury, the extent of the neurological deficit, and the type of material (e.g., hematoma, bone fragments, or disk material) that may be compressing the spinal cord.[4,5,14,57,71,98,99] These injuries can be classified according to the system proposed by Allen and co-workers that includes distraction/flexion (including facet dislocation), compression/flexion/vertical compression, extension, and subluxation injuries.[100]

General management principles of spinal cord injury also apply for subaxial cervical spinal injuries. Specifically, C3-T1 fracture or subluxations should undergo early reduction and realignment as well as operative decompression of injuries with nonreducible compression of the spinal cord, especially for patients with incomplete spinal cord injuries. Patients with undisplaced vertebral body fractures or isolated posterior element fractures will usually heal with external immobilization alone. Facet dislocations that have been successfully reduced can heal with nonoperative immobilization if there is an associated facet fracture rather than a pure ligamentous injury. Patients treated with nonoperative immobilization need to be followed with serial and dynamic imaging to ensure delayed instability has not developed. If the fracture or subluxation cannot be reduced by closed manipulation, open reduction and repair are required, again more urgently if the patient has an incomplete neurological injury. Operative fixation is also indicated for patients who have failed to heal with external immobilization alone. Patients with pure ligamentous injuries should be considered for primary operative repair as the likelihood of healing without surgery is small.

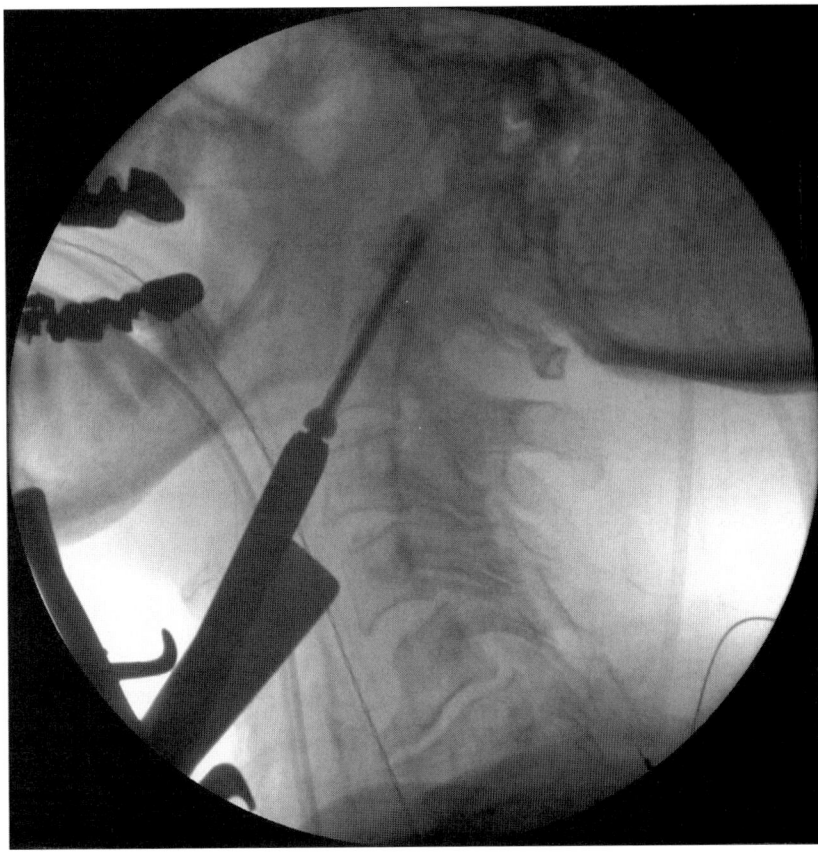

FIGURE 23.16 Lateral postoperative radiograph demonstrating odontoid screw fixation of C1-C2. *(Used with permission from Barrow Neurological Institute.)*

The surgical approach chosen for patients with subaxial spinal injuries must account for the potential need for decompression of the spinal cord or spinal roots as well as the need for stabilization and fusion.[4,5,14,57,98,99] In general, anterior pathology is approached anteriorly and posterior pathology is approached posteriorly, although there are exceptions. Posterior reconstructions may include decompression of the spinal cord and nerve roots if needed, with stabilization using a variety of wiring and screw fixation techniques that must be augmented by a bony fusion.[4,57,101,102] Ventral stabilization can be performed following corpectomy or diskectomy with an interbody graft and anterior plate (Fig. 23.17).[4,99]

Almost one third of patients with facet-dislocation injuries fail initial closed reduction.[21] One third of patients will fail to maintain alignment with external immobilization alone, with pure ligamentous disruption being a predictor of failure.[21,103] Anterior and posterior stabilization procedures have a high chance of successful fusion; only 2% to 5% of cases are associated with postoperative instability.[104-108] Indications for surgical therapy include nonreducible spinal cord compression with deficit, ligamentous injury with facet instability, kyphosis 15 degrees or greater, vertebral body compression of 40% or more, and subluxation of 20% or more.[109]

Overall, cervical vertebral compression injuries have a 5% incidence of instability when treated with external immobilization alone.[104,110] The incidence of fractures of the extension type associated with instability may be as high as 24%, and that of subluxation-type fractures may be even higher.

Whiplash Injury

The cervical spine is the most mobile segment of the human spine. This property makes it quite vulnerable to injury caused by high- or low-energy forces. Any traumatic injury to the soft tissues of the cervical spine resulting from hyperextension, hyperflexion or rotation of the neck without associated fracture, dislocation, or intervertebral disk herniation is defined as "a whiplash injury."[111] The structures vulnerable to this type of injury are the cervical musculature, ligaments, intervertebral disks, facet joints, and branches of the cervical spinal nerves such as the occipital nerve. Of all traffic accidents 90% occur at speeds less than 14 mph with whiplash injury to the cervical spine being especially common in injuries involving a rear-end collision.[112] Interestingly, the clinical picture can be acute with symptoms clearly related to cervical spine injury or can show an insidious, delayed course presenting with cognitive defects, chronic headaches (4.6% of whiplash patients), and even lower back pain.[112,113]

The severity of whiplash injuries can be approached though the simple clinical grading system proposed by the Quebec Task Force.[114] Type I whiplash injuries involve neck pain, stiffness, or tenderness with no clinical signs of cervical spine injury. To the previous group, type II injuries add signs of decreased range of motion (ROM) of the cervical spine with point tenderness. Type III injuries manifest with neck complaints (as in type I injuries), decreased ROM, point tenderness, and neurological signs such as decreased

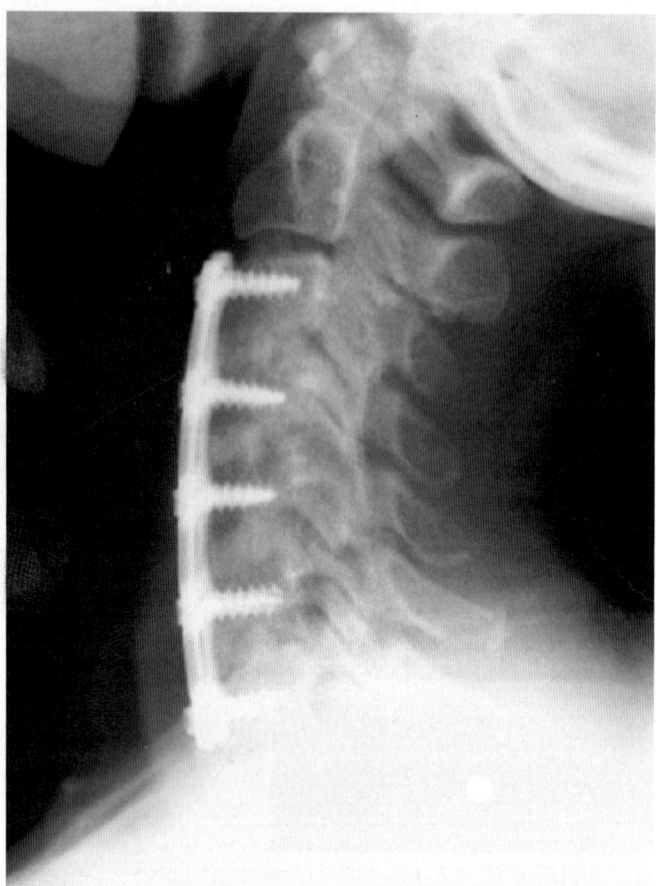

FIGURE 23.17 Lateral postoperative radiograph demonstrating cor-pectomy and fusion of the cervical spine. *(Used with permission from Barrow Neurological Institute.)*

or absent deep tendon reflexes, muscle weakness, and sensory deficits.

The treatment of whiplash injury and associated disorders involves a multimodal approach because many of these patients demonstrate signs of depression or deficits in their ability to work in conjunction with physical signs and symptoms.[112,114,115]

Cervical Spinal Cord Injuries

The goals in cervical spinal cord injuries are mainly the reduction of neurological deficits and pain, the prevention of disabilities and deformities, and finally the restoration of the previous functional level. Complete spinal cord injuries have limited potential to reach those imposed targets because of extended disruption of the neural circuits and fixed neurological deficits. Incomplete spinal cord injuries have greater ability to achieve some of their previous functional level owing to neural plasticity, but these patients must be protected from the devastating results of a secondary insult to the spinal cord.

The time frame for intervention is critical and the level of care needed is demanding. All acute spinal cord injury patients should be admitted to the intensive care unit. Spinal cord perfusion is precious and must be maintained in the acute setting to preserve function in areas at risk for secondary injuries. Consequently, the mean arterial blood pressure

should be maintained at 85 to 90 mm Hg or higher for the first week after injury. Any drop of pressure below that limit should be corrected rapidly with pressors (such as dopamine) or fluids to avoid compromising spinal cord blood flow. Signs of a complete spinal cord injury associated with neurogenic shock indicate a poor prognosis as far as recovery of neurological function is concerned.[21] Maintaining oxygenation and meticulous monitoring with clinical evaluations and neuroimaging studies are also critical. The use of high-dose steroids in the setting of spinal cord injury previously was considered to be the standard; however, the utility of the protocol has recently been subjected to serious criticism.[116-118] Currently, high-dose steroids are an option (level III evidence) in the management of spinal cord injury and should be given within 8 hours of injury if at all. Many centers have abandoned the use of corticosteroids as a thoughtful review of the literature has seriously questioned their efficacy. Level I evidence supports deep venous thrombosis preventive strategies in patients with a spinal cord injury and should be followed meticulously. This approach includes stockings, compression devices, and anticoagulation.

Other factors that may be associated with the extent of neurological deficits include the force of the initial injury; the presence of continued spinal cord compression by bone, disk, or hematoma; and the presence of an irreducible spinal deformity.

Some authors have stated that the neurological outcome of a cervical spinal cord injury may be optimized by initial attempts at closed reduction followed by the institution of rigid external immobilization.[14,21] Early closed reduction of these injuries with cranial-cervical or manual traction offers the possibility of recovery of neurological function in select patients, particularly those with incomplete neurological injuries.[21] There is an 80% success rate with these maneuvers, a 1% chance of permanent neurological injury, and a 2% to 4% chance of transient neurological change.[119] Only two well-documented cases have ascribed neurological injury to a herniated disk during reduction maneuvers.[120,121] The presence of a herniated disk, which may be found in 46% of cases on prereduction MRIs, may reflect a pseudodisk and does not predict neurological outcome.[121,122] The overwhelming majority of compression in the case of bilateral locked facets is due to bone. Thus, obtaining a prereduction MRI does not increase the safety of the procedure and may delay therapy.[119]

The timing of cervical spinal cord decompression appears to be important with respect to subsequent recovery of neurological function in certain patients, because of focal compressive injury. These patients may benefit from early surgery and stabilization, although no randomized controlled trials have confirmed this possibility.[123-125] A recent meta-analysis of the timing of decompressive surgery after traumatic spinal cord injury indicated that early surgical intervention should be considered for every patient with compressive injury within 8 to 24 hours of an acute spinal cord injury.[126] Evidence is also available on the safety of early surgery (<72 hours) in patients with spinal cord injury after hemodynamic optimization. Urgent reduction of bilateral locked facets in a patient with incomplete tetraplegia is also indicated.[126,127]

A small subset of adult patients will have signs of a spinal cord injury but no fracture or subluxation demonstrable on radiograph or CT. This scenario, which is much more common in children than in adults, is referred to as SCI-WORA (spinal cord injuries without radiographic abnormality).[128] Presentation may be delayed and caution is needed in managing children who initially present with mild neurological dysfunction, even if they may be neurologically normal when examined. Children initially cleared of spinal column injury who have subsequently returned with signs of spinal cord injury have been reported.[18,20,128,129] These patients, as in all patients with spinal cord injury, must be properly immobilized and evaluated with CT, MRI, and dynamic x-rays. Some evidence suggests that somatosensory evoked potentials are useful in identifying the extent of injury and in predicting the expected neurological recovery.[17,18,20] Poor prognostic indicators include a complete neurological injury and age less than 4 years.[17,20]

Evidence also suggests that MRI may be able to predict outcome, with a normal scan being predictive of an excellent neurological outcome.[130] Based on MRI data five subgroups of patients with SCIWORA can be identified: complete transection, major hemorrhage, minor hemorrhage, edema only, and normal. Appropriate therapy includes rigid immobilization in a collar, restriction from activities that may result in further injury, and follow-up examination that should include flexion and extension views. Current recommendations are for 12 weeks of rigid immobilization followed by another 12 weeks of restricted activity, although achieving these goals in children can be challenging.[131] Several investigators have described delayed SCIWORA injuries and recurrent spinal cord injuries among patients who presented with SCIWORA injuries but recovered and were cleared of vertebral column injury on their initial hospital evaluation.

CONCLUSIONS

The cervical spine, owing in large part to its inherent mobility, is the most common site of traumatic spinal column injuries. It is critical to follow established guidelines for early immobilization, thorough evaluation for injuries, and early intervention in cases of identified damage. Treatment of patients with cervical spine injuries should be individualized based on the type of injury and the need for conservative versus aggressive therapy and early surgical intervention.

ACKNOWLEDGMENT

This chapter contains material from the second edition, and we are grateful to the original authors for their contribution.

SELECTED KEY REFERENCES

Anderson LD, D'Alonzo RT. Fractures of the odontoid process of the axis. *J Bone Joint Surg Am.* 1974;56(8):1663-1674.

Dickman CA, Mamourian A, Sonntag VK, Drayer BP. Magnetic resonance imaging of the transverse atlantal ligament for the evaluation of atlantoaxial instability. *J Neurosurg.* 1991;75(2):221-227.

Effendi B, Roy D, Cornish B, et al. Fractures of the ring of the axis. A classification based on the analysis of 131 cases. *J Bone Joint Surg Br.* 1981;63-B(3):319-327.

Gehweiler Jr JA, Clark WM, Schaaf RE, et al. Cervical spine trauma: the common combined conditions. *Radiology.* 1979;130(1):77-86.

Sonntag V, Hadley M. Management of upper cervical spinal instability. In: Wilkins R, ed. *Neurosurgery Update.* New York: McGraw Hill; 1991:222-223.

Please go to expertconsult.com to view the complete list of references.

24 Thoracolumbar Spine Fractures

Edward M. Marchan, George M. Ghobrial, James S. Harrop

CLINICAL PEARLS

- The thoracolumbar junction is a flexible transition region in the spine, susceptible to injury due to transfer of kinetic energy.

- Clinicians should maintain a high suspicion of injury with thoracolumbar trauma because the incidence of a second vertebral fracture is 10% to 15%, and soft tissue injury may be as high as 50%.

- The most common mechanism of abdominal injuries is distraction or seat-belt injuries. Blunt abdominal aortic dissections are associated with distraction-rotational injuries of the thoracolumbar region.

- The three-column model of spine injury suggests that when all three columns are injured surgery may be necessary.

- Goals of surgery should be restoration of stability, balancing of opposing biomechanical forces, and decompression of the spinal canal with the aim to improve neurological outcome.

- Dorsal decompression via multilevel laminectomy alone after thoracic and thoracolumbar injuries has been shown to be ineffective and should not be performed as an isolated treatment strategy. Pedicle screw fixation provides for instrumentation of vertebrae with fractured or absent laminae, with purchase through all three columns. Increased rigidity by pedicle screw fixation permits fewer segments of fixation, leading to the preservation of more motion segments.[1]

Approximately 160,000 patients a year in the United States suffer traumatic spinal column injuries, with 10% to 30% of them having a concurrent spinal cord injury.[1-4] Although the majority of these injuries involves cervical (C1-C2) and lumbar (L3-L5) spine fractures, 15% to 20% of traumatic fractures occur at the thoracolumbar junction (T11-L2), whereas 9% to 16% occur in the thoracic spine (T1-T10).[5,6] Paraplegia secondary to thoracic fractures have a first-year mortality rate of 7%,[3,7] illustrating the devastating effects of thoracolumbar trauma.

The thoracic spine and thoracolumbar junction presents a unique regional anatomy, with resulting biomechanical characteristics that predispose this area to traumatic injury. Primary goals in thoracolumbar trauma patients are prompt recognition and treatment of associated injuries and expeditious stabilization of the spine and protection of the neural elements.

BIOMECHANICS

Forces along the long, rigid kyphotic thoracic spine catalyze an abrupt switch into the shorter, mobile lordotic lumbar spine at the thoracolumbar junction (Fig. 24.1). Biomechanically, this transition zone is susceptible to injury and is the most commonly injured portion of the spine. High-energy trauma (motor vehicle accidents) is the leading cause of injury over this region, followed by falls and sports-related injuries.[8] Owing to the higher energy mechanisms of injury, additional organ systems are often injured in up to 50% of thoracolumbar trauma patients.[8]

The vertebral body is the primary load-bearing structure of the spine, with the intervertebral disk transferring all forces applied to the adjacent vertebral bodies.[9,10] The annulus fibrosus of the intervertebral disk supports a significant portion of all applied axial and lateral loads and resists tension and shearing.[11] The spinal ligamentous structures are essential in maintaining overall sagittal balance. The posterior longitudinal ligament (PLL) is a relatively weak ligament that provides some restriction to hyperflexion, along with the ligamentum flavum. The thick anterior longitudinal ligament (ALL) functions in resisting spinal hyperextension and distraction.[12]

The thoracic spine differs from the remainder of the spinal column because it is supported by and maintains articulations with the ribs. The intact rib cage increases the axial load-resisting capacity of the thoracic spine by a magnitude of four. The rib cage and facet articulations limit rotation, and therefore most thoracic spine fractures occur from a flexion or axial compression force vector.[13] The majority of stability in flexion is provided by the costovertebral articulations.[14,15] A significant factor in the degree and extent of fracture character is the rate of force impact loading.[16]

The thoracolumbar vertebrae are at an increased risk for developing compression fractures after trauma as a consequence of axial loads resulting from the natural kyphotic curvature of the thoracic spine.[17] The kyphotic posture results in the placement of axial forces on the ventral portion of the vertebral body. If the strength of the ventral vertebral body is exceeded, a fracture of the vertebral body occurs, resulting in a vertebral compression fracture (VCF). The traumatic forces may also exceed the strength of the dorsal vertebral body and ligamentous elements, resulting in disruption of the dorsal tension band.

The osseous structures, ligaments, rib cage, and inherent anatomy impart great integrity on the thoracic and lumbar spine. The great kinetic energy needed for a fracture to the spine here is dissipated on impact through the soft tissue and viscous elements contained within and around the thoracic cavity, resulting in a high incidence of concurrent injuries. The incidence of concurrent injuries is reported to be greater than 80%, and these injuries involve the thorax, appendicular skeleton, and abdominal region.[18-20] These high-energy impacts also affect remote areas from the trauma, such as the cranial vault.

Petitjean and associates[18] reported a 65% incidence of head injuries after high-velocity impacts, which resulted in incomplete thoracic spinal cord injury with 12% of these injuries classified as severe (Glasgow Coma Scale [GCS] score less than 8).[18]

Tearing or rupture of the aorta, with associated hemodynamic compromise, has been associated with thoracic vertebral fractures.[18,21-23] Hemothorax in up to one third is another comorbidity.[24,25] Pulmonary injuries have been reported in 85% of patients and typically consist of pulmonary contusions.[26] Infrequently, perforation of the esophagus and tracheal injuries have also been associated with thoracic fractures.[27-29]

The thoracolumbar region is more vulnerable to concurrent injuries than the thoracic region because it is not provided the protection of the thoracic rib cage. Typically these injuries consist of hollow viscous injuries, such as intestinal perforations, mesenteric avulsions, or solid organ injuries.[18,26,30]

The most common mechanism of abdominal injuries is distraction or seat-belt injuries.[18,26,31] Blunt abdominal aortic dissections are associated with distraction-rotational injuries of the thoracolumbar region.[2,31] Multiple-level thoracic and lumbar fractures are also associated with a high incidence of abdominal injuries.[2]

Axial load injuries, particularly in patients who have jumped or fallen and landed on their feet, may manifest as both thoracolumbar fractures and calcaneal fractures. Miller and colleagues reported a 48% incidence of concurrent abdominal injuries associated with transverse process fractures.[32] Therefore, a physician treating vertebral column injuries must be aware of not only the presence of spinal fractures but also the possibility of concurrent, nonspinal, soft tissue and bony injuries.

RADIOGRAPHIC EVALUATION

In trauma patients, fractures are commonly missed in the early resuscitative period. Reportedly, between 5% and 15% of multisystem trauma patients have occult fractures missed on initial evaluation.[33-35] Composing a minor proportion of traumatic fractures, thoracic spine fractures are extremely difficult to visualize compared to other vertebral or appendicular fractures. Approximately 20% to 50% of superior thoracic spinal fractures are not diagnosed by admission plain radiographs.[5,20,36] Therefore, all suspected spinal trauma admissions should be immobilized until a thorough and detailed spinal evaluation can be performed. If appropriate stabilization precautions are not taken in this patient population, unforeseen neurological compromise may result.[6]

Initial radiographic assessment includes anteroposterior (AP) and lateral spine films assessing for loss of vertical body height, fracture of the pedicles, increased interpedicular distance, transverse process or rib fractures, and malalignment of vertebral bodies. One should examine the lateral radiograph for loss of body height, disruption of rostral or caudal end plate, dorsal cortical wall fracture with retropulsed bone, fracture of spinous processes, widening of interspinous distance, and subluxation or angulation of vertebral bodies.[37] Malalignment in the AP plane is suggestive of fracture dislocation.[38-40] The Cobb angle may also be calculated, for assessment of deformity.[41]

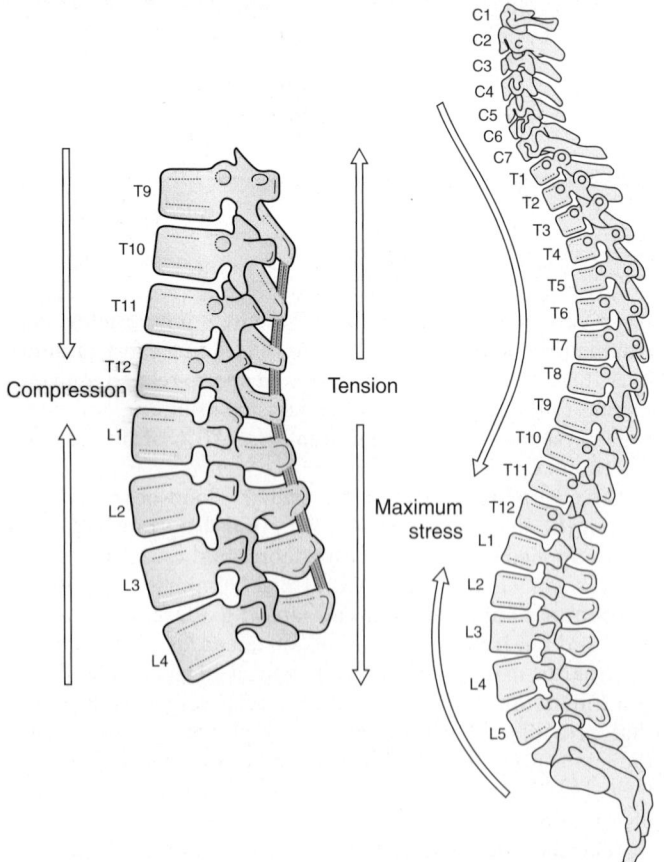

FIGURE 24.1 Transfer of stress forces to the thoracolumbar junction. Biomechanical transfer of energy places the thoracolumbar junction under increased stress, resulting in a high incidence of fractures compared to other areas of the thoracic and lumbar spine.

The Cobb angle is a measurement commonly used for evaluation of coronal spinal curves in scoliosis on an AP radiographic projection. When measuring the Cobb angle, first one must identify the apical vertebra of the curve in question. This is the vertebra that is the most displaced and rotated from the midline alignment. The end or transitional vertebrae are also identified from the curve above and below the apical vertebra. The end vertebrae are defined as the most superior and inferior vertebrae that are least displaced and least rotated but still present in the deformity's curve. Two lines are drawn, one along the superior end plate of the superior end vertebra and a second line drawn along the inferior end plate of the inferior end vertebra. Because these lines typically will not meet in the space provided, unless they are severe curves, perpendicular lines are drawn. The angle between the intersecting perpendicular lines is the same as the original lines and is referred to as the *Cobb angle* (Fig. 24.2).

In the presence of a vertebral body injury, the entire spine should be imaged in an orthogonal manner because of the high incidence (5% to 20%) of noncontiguous spinal fractures.[19,42-44] Radiographically, a typical superior end plate thoracic fracture has loss of vertebral height, with or without malalignment, a widened paraspinal line, and possibly a widened mediastinum.[20] Difficulties in imaging the upper thoracic region (T1-T4) have led to decreased reliance on diagnosis with plain films. Computed tomography (CT) is more sensitive in detecting fractures than plain radiographs.[45] CT is particularly adept at showing the integrity of the middle column, the degree of canal compromise, as well as subluxations or fractures of facets and lamina.

Sagittal reconstructions are helpful in visualizing flexion-distraction injuries and fracture dislocations. CT image reconstruction is also invaluable at the cervicothoracic junction because of the overlay of the scapula, shoulders, and surrounding tissues. In the obtunded patient this technique has been reported to identify more than 10% of fractures not visualized on plain radiographs.[46] CT, however, has a limited capacity to visualize disk herniations, epidural or subdural hematomas, ligamentous disruption, or spinal cord parenchymal changes.[47]

Magnetic resonance imaging (MRI) has further improved the ability to visualize and comprehend the pathological anatomy of the soft tissue, ligamentous, intervertebral disk, and neural element disruption that occurs after spinal injury. MRI has supplanted CT myelography as the imaging tool of choice of the neuraxis, because it is faster, is noninvasive, and allows improved visualization of the spinal cord parenchyma.[48,49]

MRI evaluation is especially useful at the thoracolumbar junction because of the variable location of the cauda equina and conus medullaris in the adult population at this level.[50] A neurological examination can be difficult to interpret at the conus/cauda equina transition level, as a result of the presence of lumbar spinal nerve sparing, the presence of concurrent injuries, sedation, in-dwelling catheters, and delayed reflex recovery. Accurate neural visualization may help in clarifying the pathological anatomy in this clinical situation.

CLASSIFICATION OF THORACOLUMBAR FRACTURES

Injuries to the thoracic and lumbar spine account for more than 50% of all spinal fractures and a large portion of acute spinal cord injuries.[51] Given this frequency and the significant impact of these injuries, significant advancements have been made in the surgical treatment of thoracolumbar trauma. Nonetheless, although there has been progress in the invention and continued evolution of spinal instrumentation and surgical techniques, medical decision making in spine trauma remains controversial.

A number of classification systems have been developed in an attempt to better define thoracolumbar trauma and aid treatment decision making. These systems are typically based on either anatomical structures (the Denis three-column system) or on proposed mechanisms of injury (Ferguson and Allen).[52,53]

One of the earliest classifications of spinal fractures was by Watson-Jones in 1931, which was based primarily on diagnosis and treatment of flexion injuries.[54] This was followed by Nicholl[55] who developed the first detailed thoracic and thoracolumbar spinal fracture classification scheme and attempted to define unstable versus stable fractures after trauma in a series of flexion and flexion-rotation injuries.[55] Later, Holdsworth[56] (Fig. 24.3) further studied the

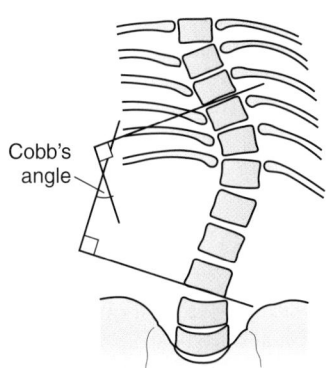

FIGURE 24.2 The Cobb angle.

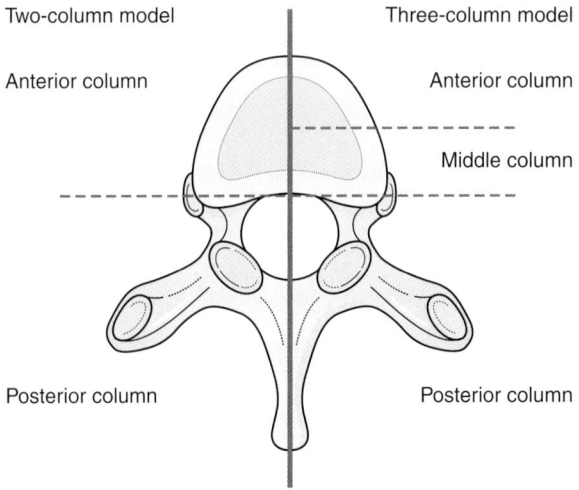

FIGURE 24.3 Two-column model (Holdsworth) compared with three-column model (Denis).

importance of the spinal ligamentous complexes after thoracolumbar junction injuries and classified fractures according to their mechanism of injury into four main types: flexion, flexion and rotation, extension, and compression. Holdsworth[56] further classified these fractures as unstable if the posterior ligamentous complex, consisting of the intervertebral disk, spinous ligaments, facet capsules, and the ligamentum flavum, was disrupted.[57]

Kelly and Whiteside[58] reported that without dislocation of the dorsal elements of the spinal column neurological injuries rarely occur. They classified fractures based on structural criteria and considered the spine to consist of not one, but rather two separate supportive columns. The primary ventral column is composed of the vertebral bodies, and a second structural column consists of the posterior neural arches and ligaments. Later, Louis[59] further modified this structural classification scheme by proposing a third column. Louis' three-column concept consisted of one ventral column and two dorsal columns involving each facet articulation.

Denis used the enhanced CT imaging techniques, along with in vitro biomechanical data, to further modify the spinal column theories into a different three-column classification scheme (see Fig. 24.3). In this classification the ventral column consists of the ALL, the anterior annulus fibrosis, and the anterior half of the vertebral bodies. The middle column consists of the PLL, the dorsal annulus fibrosis, and the dorsal half of the vertebral bodies. Lastly, the posterior column, analogous to what Holdsworth defined as the dorsal ligamentous complex, consists of the bony neural arch, posterior spinous ligaments, and ligamentum flavum, as well as the facet joints. According to the Denis classification scheme, rupture of the dorsal ligamentous complex creates instability only if and when there is concurrent disruption of at least the PLL and dorsal annulus.[53]

Denis defined failure of the anterior column alone under compression (compression fracture) with an intact posterior column as a stable fracture. Burst fractures were defined as being generated through an axial compressive load, and involved failure of the anterior and middle columns. Severe tensile injuries resulted in seat-belt fracture or flexion-distraction injuries, which involve a disruption of the posterior and middle columns with an intact anterior column that serves as a fulcrum or hinge. The last category in Denis' scheme is fracture dislocations, which are defined as a mechanical failure of all three columns, which makes them extremely unstable injuries (see Fig. 24.3).

Denis organized instability into three categories: mechanical, neurological, or both mechanical and neurological. Mechanical instability may result in a late kyphotic deformity. For instance, a seat-belt or severe compression fracture with compromise to the dorsal ligamentous complex may result in the spinal column falling into kyphosis, rotating around the intact middle column because of the deficient dorsal tension band.

External immobilization, and when appropriate, operative reduction and stabilization, may prevent this deformity progression. Neurological instability may occur after a severe burst fracture in which the middle column has ruptured under axial loads. This disruption and retropulsion of bone fragments into the spinal canal predisposes these patients to an increased risk for neurological injury, especially with increased spinal motion. Denis reported that 20% of patients with severe burst fractures and dorsal ligamentous injuries who were treated nonoperatively with external immobilization developed a subsequent neurological deficit. Neurological and mechanical instability may develop after a burst fracture or fracture/dislocation, with or without an initial neurological deficit. These injuries are very unstable and, according to Denis' analysis, require decompression and internal stabilization.

McCormack and co-workers[60] created a classification system based on a load-sharing principle that uses a graded point system based on the integrity of the vertebral bodies or anterior and middle column. Points are based on the amount of vertebral body comminution, spread of fragments at the fracture site, and the amount of corrected traumatic kyphosis.[61,62] This classification scheme assists the surgeon in deciding if ventral spinal support is necessary after dorsal instrumentation, based on the premise that inadequate anterior column support will result in excessive loads being transferred to the dorsal elements (and instrumentation), thus increasing the risk for failure.

Vaccaro and associates[63] proposed the thoracolumbar injury severity score (TLISS) in 2005, designed to simplify the classification of thoracolumbar injury and increase consistency of treatment among surgeons. This system helped address many of its predecessor's limitations.[64-67] The TLISS system defines injuries according to injury morphology, and now for the first time combined with both the PLL status and the neurological status of the patient.

The TLISS was designed to aid in medical decision making by providing both diagnostic and prognostic information with a weighted injury severity score. Stable injury patterns (TLISS < 4) may be treated nonoperatively with brace immobilization and active patient mobilization. Unstable injury patterns (TLISS > 4) may be treated operatively with the guiding principles of deformity correction, neurological decompression if necessary, and spinal stabilization followed by active patient mobilization.[64,67]

So far, the TLISS system has shown good to excellent intra- and interobserver reliability in a number of countries, among spine surgeons, and throughout a spectrum of spine treatment providers with varying levels of experience.[64] A study of 71 cases of thoracolumbar traumatic fracture was given to five spine surgeons, along with details of the TLISS and instructions for scoring, finding a 96.4% agreement among surgeons.[63] Furthermore, use of the TLISS has yielded more than a 90% agreement in the management of thoracolumbar trauma across a number of providers.[68]

Although the TLISS system has demonstrated success, there are inherent limitations. To date, many of the investigations into the TLISS system have been performed by individuals involved with its development.[69] Additionally, a prospective application of the TLISS system and severity score to the treatment of spinal injuries is needed to define any improvements in care and patient outcomes compared with conventional systems.

FRACTURE MANAGEMENT

No definitive treatment algorithm has been universally accepted for this spinal disorder, despite the numerous classification systems that exist. Stability of the vertebral column over the thoracic and thoracolumbar region, like the remainder of the spine, is dependent on the integrity of the osseous and ligamentous components. One difficulty in treating these fractures is that the definition of instability of the spine is difficult to assess, based on clinical and radiographic findings.

Nonoperative treatment is indicated for stable injuries without the potential for progressive deformity or neurological injury. One-column injuries such as compression fractures and posterior element fractures are stable by definition and can be treated nonoperatively unless excessive kyphosis is noted, which raises concern for increased pain and deformity in the future.

Treatment of two-column injuries, such as burst fractures, depends to a significant extent on the neurological status. In neurologically intact patients, nonoperative treatment is generally recommended consisting of bedrest, early mobilization in a thoracolumbosacral orthotic (TLSO) brace, and continued close monitoring for increased kyphosis and neurological changes.[70] Defino and Canto demonstrated an excellent reduction of sagittal deformity on 2-year follow-up of 20 patients.[71]

The most devastating complication of nonoperative treatment is the development of neurological deterioration. It appears that the rate of neurological worsening lies between 0% and 20%. A low potential for chronic or glacial instability still remains. Glacial instability usually presents as mechanical pain but could also present as a neurological deficit.

Burst fractures, as defined by Denis, are vertebral body fractures involving the anterior and middle columns, such that the ALL and vertebral body, including the dorsal vertebral body cortex, are disrupted. As stated before, a burst fracture in a neurologically intact patient without posterior ligamentous or dorsal element fractures is usually considered a stable injury. Burst fractures are inherently more stable because of the presence of the costovertebral ligamentous complex, along with the support of the rib cage.[72]

Brown and colleagues[73] advocated nonoperative treatment of burst fractures with less than 50% of vertebral body collapse, less than 30 degrees of kyphotic deformity, and no more than 3 cm of offset from the standard sagittal vertical angle on lateral scoliosis films. These recommendations are supported by the findings of Cantor and associates.[42] Brown's management protocol recommended immediate casting of the hemodynamically stable patient in a hyperextension body cast, followed by serial radiographs. Early mobilization was associated with reduced hospital stays and costs.

Nonoperative management therefore may be used in the neurologically intact patient, even with a large degree of spinal canal stenosis from retropulsed bone fragments, as long as there is no significant kyphosis representing significant disruption of the dorsal osteoligamentous complex.[74] However, if there is a decline in the patient's neurological status during nonoperative treatment, operative intervention is indicated in the presence of documented instability or neural compression.[75]

Siebenga and co-workers[76] demonstrated the benefits of surgery in 34 patients with AO type A fractures without neurological deficits (compression fractures) who were randomized to short-segment posterior stabilization (Fig. 24.4) versus orthosis predominantly at the thoracolumbar junction. Superior correction of the kyphotic deformity in the surgical arm and functional outcome scores (Visual Analog pain score) were found. A higher percentage of patients in the surgical

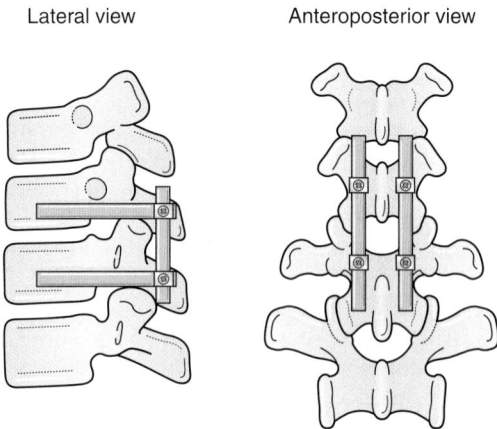

Lateral view   Anteroposterior view

FIGURE 24.4 Short-segment posterior instrumentation with pedicle screws.

arm had returned to work at follow-up, in accordance with the findings of several nonrandomized trials.[76] This differed from the earlier works of Wood and associates[77] finding no difference in outcome when comparing operative and nonoperative treatment of neurologically intact burst fractures.

In general there are only a handful of strict surgical indications for thoracolumbar burst fractures. Those burst fractures which are severe and have a neurological deficit with canal compromise should be operated on. Moreover, in those patients neurologically intact, but who have evidence of loss of disruption of the PLL, inferred from greater than 25 degrees of kyphosis on radiographs or direct visualization of rupture of the PLL on fat-suppressed sagittal T2-weighted MRI, surgery is warranted.

Distraction injuries, seat-belt injuries, and Chance fractures require surgical stabilization because of loss of integrity of the posterior column in order to restore the posterior tension band. Translation injuries, rotational injuries, and those that shatter through the disk space and ligamentous complexes from ventral to dorsal always require surgical stabilization.

Harrington rods were the first spinal implants widely used for the treatment of vertebral fractures.[77] Unfortunately, this artificially applied distraction force can result in the loss of the normal spinal curvature, now working at a biomechanical disadvantage.[78,79] Newer segmental instrumentation systems were initially developed for scoliosis. Maximization of fixation was achieved by instrumenting across all three vertebral columns, which resulted in a relatively low incidence of fixation failure. Compression, distraction, and translation are all possible within the same construct.

Pedicle screw fixation allowed for instrumentation of vertebrae with fractured or absent laminae, with purchase through all three columns, an improvement on previous segmental fixation devices. Increased rigidity necessitates fewer segments of fixation, leading to the preservation of more motion segments. Preservation of motion is most important in the cervical and lumbar segments.[72] Surgeon preference often plays a role, as does fracture morphology. Timing of surgery becomes an important issue in the treatment of thoracic spine fractures. Progressive neurological deficit in the presence of canal compromise is an accepted indication for immediate decompression and stabilization. Some studies suggest that patients with thoracic spine fractures treated within

72 hours, irrespective of concomitant injuries, do much better physiologically postoperatively than those in whom stabilization is delayed. Boerger and colleagues[80] showed in a meta-analysis that patients with an incomplete neurological deficit who underwent an operative decompression and stabilization procedure in less than 72 hours had enhanced neurological recovery compared to nonoperatively treated patients.[80,81]

Flexion-distraction injuries result in disruption of the posterior and middle columns in tension.[82] Very often, the anterior column remains intact, acting as a hinge. Surgical intervention for these fractures typically involves a posterior approach. Anterior approaches (Fig. 24.5) are not routinely used in these injuries, to preserve the intact anterior column.[83]

Fracture-dislocation injuries have a significant distraction component and differ from seat-belt-type injuries in that there is a large rotatory or torque component that causes a disruption of all three spinal columns.[52] As a result, they carry a high incidence of complete spinal cord injury. Therefore, the main objective of surgical intervention is solely to provide posterior stabilization, facilitating early mobilization and rehabilitation. Anterior decompression and stabilization (see Fig. 24.5) are performed following posterior surgical realignment of the fracture in rare instances in which partial neurological deficit exists in the presence of significant anterior neural compression.[84,85] Chapman and co-workers reported in their series that a "lapbelt-sign" had a positive predictive value of 0.69 and a negative predictive value of 0.91 for intra-abdominal injury, illustrating the high morbidity rate in flexion-distraction injuries.[86]

When partial neurological deficit is present, seen often with burst fractures, improving residual canal compromise is also the goal of surgery. Laminectomy with transpedicular decompression also can improve the canal clearance achieved through a posterior approach. The ventral approach is particularly useful for decompressing midline ventral lesions and correcting severe kyphotic deformities.[80,87-89]

Dorsal decompression via multilevel laminectomy alone after thoracic and thoracolumbar injuries has been shown to be ineffective and should not be performed as an isolated treatment strategy.[89,90] Loss of the dorsal tension band and instability, along with the potential progression of a kyphotic deformity, may ensue. The immediate result of removing the

dorsal osseous components is dorsal migration of the spinal cord if the spine has a lordotic alignment.

The osseous structures are fused concomitantly with posterior instrumentation. Some surgeons fuse only the injured vertebral segments with subsequent staged removal of hardware. Other surgeons fuse the entire length of the instrumentation. This results in loss of motion at additional segments. As mentioned, this is of less importance in the thoracic spine. With modern segmental fixation, fewer segments need to be instrumented to provide stability, and generally, the entire instrumented region is fused.[91]

Minimally invasive surgery (MIS) is seeing increased use in North America in tandem with the development of easier to implement systems. In a review of over 138 papers in the literature it has been cited that the average blood loss is 1 L and the anterior and posterior approach infection rate is 0.7% and 3.1%, respectively.[92]

Less commonly, anterior MIS procedures are implemented endoscopically. Posterior percutaneous pedicle screw instrumentation accounts for the majority of MIS procedures, along with balloon-assisted techniques. In higher energy burst fractures, the risk of epidural extrusion of cement and dorsal displacement of posterior bony fragments is relevant.[92,93] Lastly, there is a paucity of level 1 or 2 evidence comparing MIS with open techniques.

SUMMARY

The care of patients with thoracolumbar spine trauma with or without neurological deficits has evolved dramatically over the past 30 years. The development of more effective instrumentation techniques coupled with the establishment of spinal injury care centers where immediate treatment and rehabilitation can be administered successively has definitely improved the care of these patients. Despite these advances, the majority of patients with thoracolumbar injuries are still treated nonoperatively with cast or brace immobilization and early ambulation. More aggressive treatment is guided by the use of classification systems that detail the mechanism of injury, the degree of compromise of spinal structures, and the potential for late mechanical instability or neural injury. Guidelines

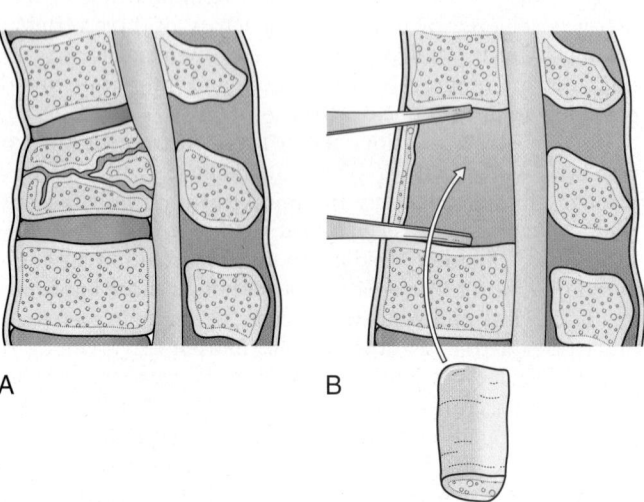
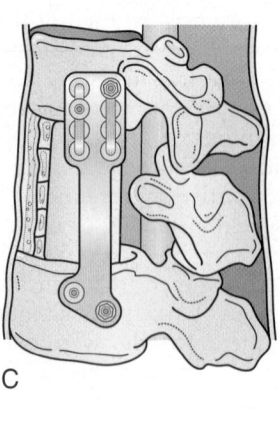

A   B   C

FIGURE 24.5 Anterior corpectomy with fusion and hardware.

such as the TLISS system are now in place to help the clinician make better educated decisions as to which patients to treat operatively and which to manage nonoperatively. As we have seen here, there is no clear consensus as to the absolute indications for surgical intervention in patients with many types of thoracolumbar fractures.

SELECTED KEY REFERENCES

Denis F. The three column spine and its significance in the classification of acute thoracolumbar spinal injuries. *Spine*. 1983;8(8):817-831.

Haber TR, Filmy WT, O'Brien M. Thoracic and lumbar fractures: diagnosis and management. In: Bridwell KH, DeWald PR, eds. *The Textbook of Spinal Surgery*. Philadelphia: Lippincott; 1991:857-910.

Patel AA, Dailey A, Brodke DS, et al. Spine trauma study group. Thoracolumbar spine trauma classification: the thoracolumbar injury classification and severity score system and case examples. *J Neurosurg Spine*. 2009;10(3):201-206.

White AA, Panjabi MM. *Clinical Biomechanics of the Spine*. Philadelphia: JB Lippincott; 1978.

Wood K, Buttermann G, Mehbod A, et al. Operative compared with nonoperative treatment of a thoracolumbar burst fracture without neurological deficit. A prospective, randomized study. *J Bone Joint Surg Am*. 2003;85A(5):773-781.

Please go to expertconsult.com to view the complete list of references.

25 Intradural Extramedullary and Intramedullary Spinal Cord Tumors

Michaël Bruneau, Florence Lefranc, Danielle Balériaux, Jacques Brotchi

CLINICAL PEARLS

- Surgery is the initial and primary treatment of choice in most spinal tumors.

- Intradural extramedullary spinal tumors, mostly benign peripheral nerve sheath tumors and meningiomas, carry an excellent prognosis. Surgery allows most of the time complete resection and neurological improvement or recovery.

- The main objective should be preserving the patient's functional condition and making an accurate diagnosis. Postoperative results depend on the preoperative neurological status, the tumor grade, tumor location, and the surgical team's experience.

- Many intramedullary spinal tumors, such as ependymomas, astrocytomas, and some of nonglial origin, have a favorable prognosis because they may be completely resected based on the favorable surgical plane between the tumor and spinal cord.
  - As soon as patients are symptomatic surgery should be considered. Functional recovery depends significantly on

the preoperative neurological condition. The better the preoperative function, the better the chance of a good long-term outcome.
- A wide differential diagnosis should be considered on all intramedullary lesions prior to surgery. Some lesions may not be neoplasms based on clinical presentation or imaging. Inflammatory diseases, infections, and demyelinating disease should be considered and ruled out after a careful preoperative evaluation.
- If a cleavage plane between tumor and spinal cord is not clear, especially in infiltrating tumors such as some astrocytomas, it may be wise to discontinue the resection because it can be detrimental for the patient's neurological function. In addition, motor evoked potentials are of great value in determining when the resection should be redirected or terminated.
- Radiation therapy should be limited to malignant tumors. Incompletely resected benign tumors can be followed with surveillance scans and reoperated upon if there is progression.

INTRADURAL EXTRAMEDULLARY TUMORS

Incidence and Types

Spinal intradural extramedullary tumors (SIEMTs) are primarily peripheral nerve sheath tumors (PNSTs) and meningiomas in similar numbers.[1] In the largest reported study on SIEMTs, nerve sheath tumors and meningiomas accounted for almost 70% of all lesions.[1] Other SIEMTs and lesions include arachnoid cysts, hamartomas, and ependymomas, with an incidence between 5.5-7.5% each.[1] The differential diagnosis for SIEMTs and lesions is broad and includes angioblastoma, cavernoma, chordomas, dermoid, epidermoid, exophytic astrocytoma, germinoma, hemangiopericytoma, lipoma, lymphoma, malignant teratoma, medulloblastoma, melanocytoma, melanoma, metastasis, myxoma, neuroblastoma, and sarcoma.[1,2]

In about 50% of cases, SIEMTs are located at the thoracic level.[1] Lesions with an extradural extension are seen at the

cervical level in more than half of patients.[1] Benign nerve sheath tumors are the most common SIEMT and are associated with extradural extension with an approximate incidence of 77%.[1] Meningiomas, hamartomas, and sarcomas are other SIEMTs with extradural extension.[1]

Peripheral Nerve Sheath Tumors

Most schwannomas are purely intradural but 15% have an extradural component, being either solely extradural or both intra- and extradural. These tumors originate from the dorsal sensory nerve root.[3] Typically, these lesions are well encapsulated and rarely include a cystic portion. In contrast, neurofibromas are not well encapsulated and rarely occur alone. Multiple plexiform neurofibromas are usually seen with neurofibromatosis type 1 (NF1), a genetic disorder associated with mutations of chromosome 17.[4-6] Diffuse plexiform neurofibromas are detected clinically and radiologically, respectively, in 26.3% and 50% of the patients with NF1.[6] They appear in early childhood and have a variable growth pattern. Lesions may grow rapidly until adolescence and then become quiescent.[6] The presence of a tumor is not an indication for surgery. Resection is indicated in NF1 patients if the tumor is growing or is causing progressive neurological deficits. In 2% to 5% of the cases, malignant changes may be observed with rapid expansion of the tumor mass.[6] Surgery can be challenging in malignant tumors when the tumor is attached and infiltrates surrounding soft tissue. Neurofibromatosis type 2 (NF2) is another genetic condition associated with chromosome 22 anomalies.[6] The clinical picture of NF2 may include SIEMTs such as schwannomas, neurofibromas, and meningiomas in 30% of patients.[6] Pathologically, nerve sheath tumors are subdivided according to the WHO (World Health Organization) classification into schwannomas (WHO grade I), neurofibromas (WHO grade I), and malignant peripheral nerve sheath tumors (WHO grade III/IV).

Meningiomas

Spinal meningiomas commonly occur in middle-aged patients with a predilection for women.[7] Most of the sporadic meningiomas are solely intradural. Of those remaining, one third are intra- and extradural and two thirds are primarily extradural.[8] These lesions have a strong tendency to develop at the thoracic level with a frequency reported in the literature between 55% and 83%.[7,9-11]

Clinical Picture

Most patients present with a long history of progressive symptoms and neurological deterioration because SIEMTs are slow-growing tumors. It is uncommon for a patient to abruptly deteriorate due to spontaneous tumor hemorrhage with spinal compression. SIEMTs appear with signs and symptoms indicative of upper and lower motor neuron involvement, related to the severity of the nerve root insult and spinal cord compression. In half of the cases, the first symptom reported by patients with SIEMTs is pain.[1] The tenderness and pain are characteristically increased at night or in the supine position and are relieved after returning to an upright position. Pain is often described along a radicular dermatome but can also reach varying distribution. It is usually described as a dull, aching sensation, and less frequently as burning. Radicular involvement results in lower motor neuron dysfunction, with weakness, sensory disturbances, hyporeflexia, atrophy, and fasciculation at the affected level. Myelopathic symptoms are correlated with the severity, level, and site of spinal cord compression. Nerve sheath tumors typically compress the lateral aspect of the spinal cord and are therefore more likely to be associated with the development of a Brown-Sequard syndrome. Upper motor neuron deficits manifest by gait ataxia and spasticity of the affected extremities. Hyperreflexia as well as other pyramidal signs such as the Hoffman and Babinski signs may be detected upon clinical examination. Patients present with pain, gait ataxia, motor weakness, and sensory deficits in 70% to 77% of the cases, and dysesthesias and sphincter disturbances are found in about 40%.[1]

Preoperative Imaging

Magnetic resonance imaging (MRI) is currently the gold standard method for imaging. MRI provides accurate diagnoses and delineates the soft tissue components.[12,13] Gadolinium administration highlights enhancing portions of the tumor. MR myelography is a special study that is particularly useful for showing small schwannomas.[13]

On MRI, schwannomas and meningiomas often appear as isointense to the spinal cord on T1-weighted images (WI). On T2-WI, schwannomas are most often hyperintense, as opposed to meningiomas that appear isointense.[13] After gadolinium administration both lesions enhance intensely and homogeneously.[13] A cystic component and hemorrhagic foci may be noted in schwannomas or neurofibromas, respectively, in 40% and 10% of the cases.[13] Less frequently than with cranial lesions, there is often a characteristic dural tail associated with spinal meningiomas.[3]

The computed tomography (CT) scan enables detection of calcifications as well as of spinal canal and neural foramen enlargement in cases of extradural extension.[13] CT angiography (CTA) and MRI angiography (MRA) provide relevant information for cervical dumbbell-shaped neurofibromas that develop in close proximity to the vertebral artery (VA).[14] Conventional angiography has a few indications for some of these tumors. It is helpful for providing relevant information about the anterior spinal artery at the cervical level[14] and the Adamkiewicz artery at the thoracolumbar junction. CT myelography is invasive and thus not as useful as MRI. It is no longer recommended as the primary imaging modality.[13]

Surgery

The surgical approach should be adjusted according to the presumed diagnosis and tumor location. The surgical strategy of a PNST is different from that with a meningioma. First, PNSTs most often develop on the anterolateral aspect of the spinal cord, mainly at the cervical level, inducing a posteromedial displacement of the neuraxis. Second, few of them are solely intradural/extramedullary lesions; numerous are dumbbell-shaped lesions extending into the vertebral foramen. Third, at the cervical spine level, their vascular supply from the vertebral artery (VA) requires special considerations.[14]

Peripheral Nerve Sheath Tumors

Several surgical techniques have been described for PNST resection. These lesions are accessed using a posterolateral approach, as described for meningiomas. The posterolateral approach through a laminectomy is adequate for the resection of the intradural component. In the case of cervical PNST extending through the vertebral foramen and in close proximity to the VA, the posterior approach has several drawbacks.[14] First, a significant portion of the facet must be resected to reach the foraminal component of the tumor. This may potentially cause postoperative instability requiring fusion.[15] Second, the VA providing the tumor blood supply is reached at the end of the surgical procedure, precluding any devascularization of the tumor supply before the final surgical step.[14] Moreover, without proximal control of the VA, the risk of VA damage is higher.[14] Finally, it often results in leaving tumor remnant that remains vascularized, and thus has a potential to grow in the future. For some anterior lesions, the anterolateral approach may be useful in select patients. It allows for complete devascularization of the tumor at the beginning of the procedure, cutting down on blood loss. Then, tumor resection can most often be completed in a single surgical step.[14] The intradural component of the lesion may be accessed through the enlarged vertebral foramen that may be drilled out slightly. This tailored opening rarely destabilizes the spine and subsequent fusion is not uniformly required. The primary reason for a fusion is a history of previous laminectomy, which completely removes the facets. The anterolateral approach requires VA control, which requires experience. However, this approach is safe and associated with low morbidity rate in experienced hands;[15,16] the incidence of permanent deficits drops to less than 3%.[15,16] The main risk is a postoperative Horner syndrome.

The Anterolateral Approach with Vertebral Artery Control for Cervical Dumbbell-Shaped Tumors (Fig. 25.1)

Preoperatively, the VA position has to be anticipated by an MRA or CTA: anatomical variations must be ruled out, as well as VA displacement induced by the tumor.[17,18] The tumor

often grows at the posterior VA aspect therefore pressing on the artery anteriorly or anteromedially. The patient is placed in the supine position, with head lying on a small cushion, slightly extended with a tape passing under the chin and turned to the contralateral side at 30 degrees.[15,16] Fluoroscopy is used to check the correct level. Electrophysiological monitoring (consisting of motor and somatosensory evoked potentials [MEP, SSEP] and electromyography [EMG]) is maintained throughout the surgical procedure. The skin incision follows the medial border of the sternomastoid muscle. After division of the platysma, the dissection is pursued medially to the medial border of the sternomastoid muscle and laterally to the internal jugular vein. The carotid-jugular sheath is left undissected and is retracted medially. Dissection of the sympathetic chain is an important step in avoiding the main complication of this approach, which is Horner syndrome. The sympathetic chain must be differentiated from the longus colli muscle (LCM) and retracted laterally using stitches applied on the LCM aponeurosis that has been divided medially to the chain. At the C6-C7 level, the thoracic duct on the left side or the accessory thoracic duct on the right side must be preserved to avoid a leak.[19,20] After its exposure, the LCM must be resected. In order to prevent VA injury, the LCM must be resected down

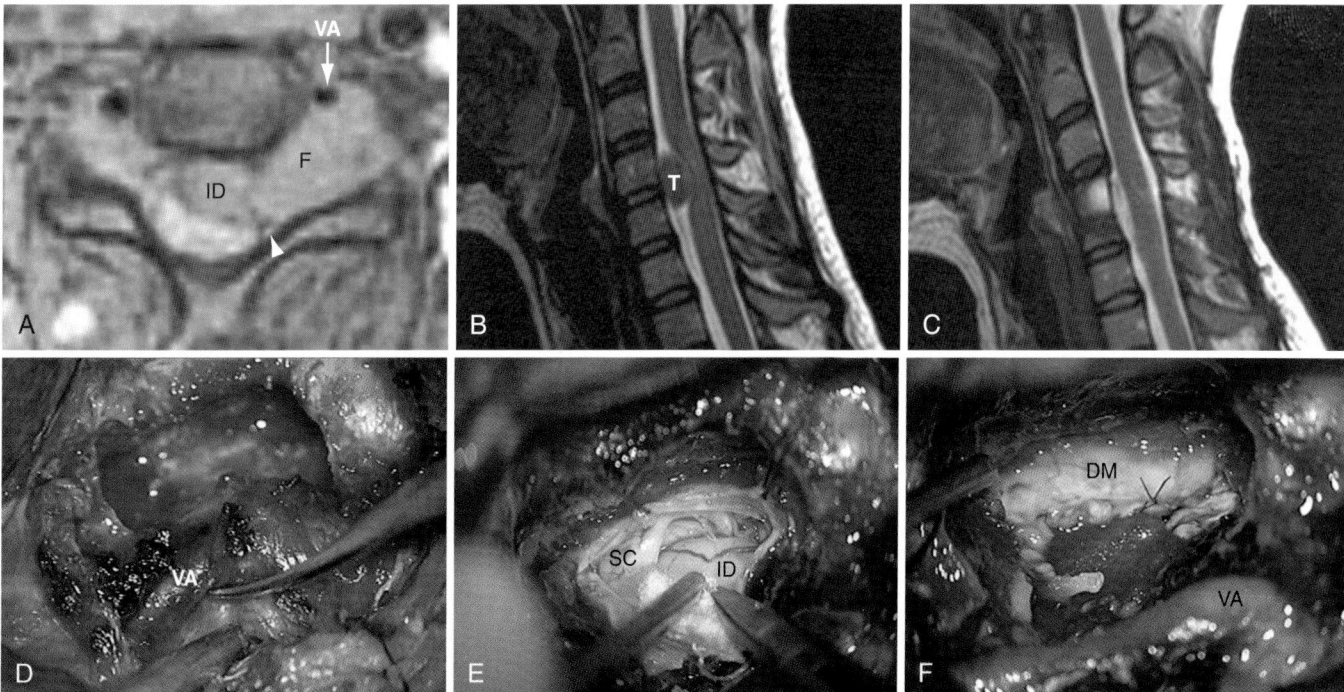

FIGURE 25.1 A C4-C5 dumbbell-shaped neurofibroma resected using a lateral approach with control of the vertebral artery. **A** and **B**, Preoperative magnetic resonance (MR) axial and sagittal T2-weighted images (WI). The tumor (*T*) extends from the intervertebral foramen (*F*) to the intradural compartment (*ID*) through the dura mater (*arrowhead*), severely compressing the spinal cord. The tumor has developed close to the posterior aspect of the vertebral artery (VA). **C**, Postoperative MR T2-WI as diagram B after complete resection of the tumor. The spinal cord has recovered an almost normal shape but there is a small ill-defined high signal intensity area in the cord, without any clinical consequences, corresponding to a sequellar lesion due to chronic cord compression by the tumor. **D** to **F**, Perioperative views. **D**, A partial oblique corpectomy has been carried out to expose the anterior aspect of the dura mater. The vertebral artery is lifted up from the tumor. Working laterally to the vertebral artery allows for resecting the foraminal portion of the lesion. **E**, The intradural component is exposed after opening the dura mater. The lesion may be carefully separated from the spinal cord (SC). **F**, View at the completion of the procedure. Dura mater closure requires a patch. *Parts E and F reproduced with permission from Bruneau M, George B. Surgical technique for the resection of tumors in relation with the V1 and V2 segments of the vertebral artery. In: George B, Bruneau M, Spetzler RF, eds. Pathology and Surgery around the Vertebral Artery. Paris: Springer; 2011, Chap. 14.*

to the transverse processes above and below the level of tumor. It is safe because, in the absence of anatomical variations, the VA is protected inside the bone of the transverse foramen.[15-18] Afterward, the muscle is resected along the lateral border of the cervical vertebrae. From an anatomical point of view, it must be pointed out that, between C6 and the foramen magnum, a venous plexus enclosed inside a periosteal sheath surrounds the VA. The periosteal sheath is continuous with the periosteum of each transverse process. It means the periosteal sheath should be left intact inside the transverse foramen. It can be achieved only by performing a subperiosteal dissection of the anterior branch of the transverse process with a smooth spatula before resecting the bone with a Kerrison rongeur.[15,16] In case of tearing of the periosteal sheath, troublesome venous bleeds may arise but can easily be controlled by direct bipolar cauterization of the sheath itself or packing with resorbable cellulose.[15,16] At this point, the VA is controlled from above and below the tumor. The vertebral foramen, already enlarged by the tumor, may be made slightly larger by drilling. The tumor feeders will be cauterized during the separation between the anterior aspect of the nerve root and the VA posterior border, facilitating further tumor resection.[15,16] In the case of a schwannoma, the tumoral nerve root fascicle may be separated from the normal nerve roots. The nerve root may be sacrificed if there is already a neurological deficit by nerve root involvement.[14] Intraoperative stimulation may provide additional relevant information for this decision.[14] Pursuing a lateromedial tumor resection will allow entrance into the intradural compartment. The dura mater opening through which the tumor has passed may be enlarged as much as necessary to provide the appropriate intradural exposure. The use of an ultrasonic aspirator (the Cavitron ultrasonic aspirator, CUSA) is helpful for debulking the lesion.[14] The tumor should then be cautiously separated from the spinal cord using a microsurgical technique.

At the completion of the surgery, the dura should be closed with a 4-0 to 6-0 nonresorbable running suture, with a dural patch to close a defect, if necessary. Sealing with fibrin glue and packing with fat and muscle are recommended. A lumbar drainage may also be required for 72 hours to prevent cerebrospinal fluid (CSF) leak or a pseudomeningocele.

Meningiomas (Fig. 25.2)

In the case of meningiomas, the tumor origin can be found anywhere along the surface of the dura. A general rule is that the neuraxis is displaced to the side opposite to the tumor origin. Therefore, posterior meningiomas put pressure on the spinal cord anteriorly and for this reason are better approached directly with a laminectomy. Posterolateral and lateral meningiomas displace the neuraxis anteromedially and medially, respectively. A posterolateral approach is advocated, by laminectomy possibly extended on the tumor side to the medial aspect of the facets. With anterolateral meningiomas, the posterior displacement of the neuraxis requires a more location-specific approach because surgical access is limited. In this situation, we still advocate a posterior approach, extended laterally on the side of the tumor, but the lateral surgical corridor must be enlarged by dividing dentate ligaments. With that maneuver, most lesions can be adequately resected. Rare reports have advocated the use of an anterior approach for anterior meningiomas.[21] This anterior approach is considered safe and has several theoretical advantages: a large bony window of access, extradural cauterization of the anterior blood supply, direct visualization of the entire tumor ventral to the spinal cord, and tumor resection without spinal cord manipulation; but it is nevertheless associated with drawbacks, such as the need for fusion and a more challenging access route.[21] It is nevertheless associated with drawbacks such as the need for fusion and a more challenging access route. The depth and narrowness of the working channel present a significant technical challenge. In addition, dural closure is also very difficult, resulting in a higher probability of CSF leakage.[21]

The Posterior Approach

The patient is placed in the prone position under continuous electrophysiological monitoring, especially for cervical lesions. At this level, we use a Mayfield head holder and are careful to position the head in a neutral position to avoid tumor-induced spinal cord compression. Fluoroscopy is used to accurately target the pathological levels. Usually, only two vertebrae must be exposed. The laminectomy may be extended laterally to facets on the side of the tumor. The dura mater is usually incised longitudinally over the tumor. The dural edges are retracted laterally with several 4-0 silk sutures. Lateral lesions may require section of the dentate ligaments to provide exposure. Sutures from dentate ligament to opposite dura keeps the surgical space open and offers good control of anterior dura as a result of gentle rotation of the spinal cord. Great care must be taken to avoid any traction or compression on the spinal cord itself. Cottonoids are placed at each end of the tumor to avoid intradural soiling. Most of the time, the arachnoid can be separated and the resection completed in the extra-arachnoidal plane. The tumor surface is cauterized and incised with a knife or microscissors. Samples are sent to the pathologist for immediate analysis. In lateral meningiomas, the tumor debulking is performed with either microinstruments

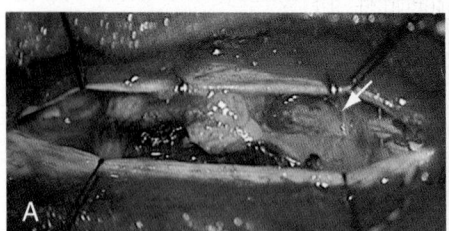 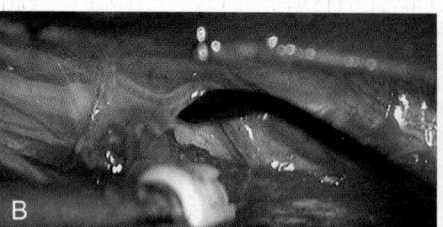 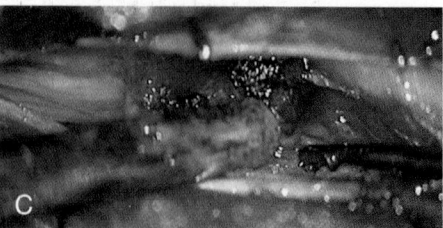

FIGURE 25.2 Lateral thoracic meningioma. **A,** The tumor has been devascularized by coagulation and divided along its base of insertion. The arachnoid layer *(arrow)* has been attached to the dura mater with a clip to resect the lesion in the extra-arachnoidal plane. **B,** Spinal vessels must absolutely be respected to avoid spinal vascular injury. A major vessel is separated from the tumor. This vessel remains protected by the arachnoid. **C,** At the completion of the tumor resection, the dura mater is cleansed from any tumor residue and coagulated. *(Used with permission from Hôpital Erasme, Université Libre de Bruxelles.)*

or an ultrasonic aspirator, starting along the dural base if possible. Bleeding of feeding vessels is gently controlled with bipolar cauterization. In this way, the tumor is progressively devascularized and becomes mobile. The pressure at the tumor–spinal cord interface and at the dural insertion base is then released. Shrinkage of the tumor by electrocautery may also help to keep the plane open. Only vessels supplying the tumor should be sacrificed. Progressively, the dural base may be divided, resulting in tumor devascularization. Nevertheless, we advise keeping a small dural attachment until the tumor is completely released from the spinal cord. Otherwise, the lesion may become too mobile, thereby increasing difficulties and risks in completing the dissection of the spinal cord–tumor interface. At the completion of surgery, the dural base should be either cauterized or resected. The choice is guided by the location of the pathological dura and the possibilities of performing a watertight reconstruction. Resection and reconstruction with a patch graft is advised for posterior and posterolateral lesions. Contrarily, we advise only coagulating anterior or anterolateral dura mater portions. Cauterization instead of resection of the dura mater is not associated with a higher risk of recurrence.[9,11,22] Finally, the intradural compartment is copiously washed with a normothermic saline solution. The dura mater is closed with a 5-0 nonabsorbable running watertight suture to prevent CSF leakage. The aponeurosis is also closed with a watertight running suture to avoid a CSF leak. Drains may be inserted at the level of the muscular layer.

Postoperative Outcome

Short-term outcome after the resection of SIEMTs is usually excellent, with the neurological condition generally improving significantly.[2] Resolution of preoperative deficits has been noted in about 80% of the cases.[7,8] The patient's neurological condition remains stable in 14% of patients and few deteriorate.[7] Several factors influence the outcome such as the preoperative neurological status, the duration of preoperative symptoms, and the type of surgical resection.[7] The histological characteristics of the tumor may influence the long-term outcome: the psammomatous type is associated with a less favorable neurological outcome than the nonpsammomatous type. Psammomatous tumors consist essentially of acellular concretions, rendering blood vessels and spinal roots extremely adherent.[8] Location of the tumor below C4 and posteriorly or laterally in the intradural compartment is, however, a favorable factor.[8] Complete tumor resection is possible in 96% to 97% of the cases[7,22] and is associated with a recurrence rate of 6% after 15 years of follow-up. Subtotal resection of a tumor resulted in recurrence in 17% of the cases.[22] Serious complications may develop in case of perioperative vascular or medullar injuries but are unusual. Physical therapy hastens neurological recovery. Most patients can resume a normal or nearly normal neurological condition. A gratifying quick recovery may be observed within the first 6 weeks after surgery, but progressive recovery may be expected by 1 year after surgery. We see patients at 6 months, 1 year, and 2 years with performance of an MRI and then every 5 years in the absence of recurrence.

Radiation Therapy

When dealing with a malignant PNST, current consensus advocates postoperative radiation therapy (RT), started as soon as possible after surgery even if resection margins are tumor free.[23,24] The role of radiotherapy in the management of spinal meningiomas is controversial. The slow indolent growth of these lesions and the risk associated with irradiating the vicinity of the spinal cord are confounding issues.[7] Several indications for adjuvant radiation therapy have been proposed: early recurrence after total or subtotal resection, partial resection, and high-risk surgical treatment.[7] If possible, we prefer repeat surgery over radiation for recurrence.

INTRAMEDULLARY SPINAL CORD TUMORS

Surgery on spinal cord intramedullary tumors (SCIMTs) has been refined over the past few decades. The pioneering work of Elsberg[25] and subsequently of many others such as Cooper,[26] Epstein and Epstein,[27] Guidetti and associates,[28] McCormick and colleagues,[29] Malis,[30] Stein and McCormick,[31,32] and many others[33,34] have greatly contributed to advancing the microsurgical technique and success in removing spinal cord lesions. Several tools have added safety features to the microsurgical resection of these lesions. The advent of MRI has definitively improved diagnosis accuracy. The introduction of ultrasonic aspiration (CUSA) and intraoperative electrophysiological monitoring has modified the surgical approach and improved safety and outcome significantly.

Incidence and Types

With an incidence in adulthood of 2% to 4% of all central nervous system tumors, SCIMTs are considered rare.[30,32,35-37] Three main groups of SCIMTs can be distinguished: tumors of glial origin, tumors of nonglial origin, and other mass lesions.

Tumors of Glial Origin

These tumors primarily consist of ependymomas and astrocytomas.[13,38] Other glial tumors such as oligodendrogliomas are rare.[39]

Ependymomas

Spinal cord ependymomas are the most frequent SCIMTs in adult patients. They may reach considerable size prior to diagnosis. The majority of spinal cord ependymomas in adults have a good prognosis because usually they can be completely removed and are primarily grade II by the WHO classification. In the literature, the rate of complete removal varies from 69% to 97%.[40-42] The vast majority of patients, 48% to 75%, are stabilized after the radical surgical resection, thereby highlighting the need for timely surgery in case of neurological deterioration.[41-45] The overall rate of neurological improvement for this patient population varies between 10% and 40%.[41-45] A rate of postoperative deterioration has been reported in the literature between 9% and 15%.[41-45] Subtotal resection has been reportedly associated with a lack of clinical improvement,[43] and incomplete resection is the most important factor correlating with tumor recurrence.[41,46,47] The 5- and 10-year survival rates are respectively quoted between 83% to 96% and 80% to 91%.[40,42,43,45,48,49]

Astrocytomas

Spinal cord astrocytomas represent more than 80% of the SCIMTs in children,[43] and in adults astrocytomas are the second most common type of tumor.[43] Only 10% to 17% of astrocytomas in childhood are anaplastic lesions or glioblastomas, whereas in adults, the percentage is higher, 25% to 30%.[28,34,43,50-53] In large studies, the proportion of pilocytic astrocytomas varies greatly from more than 30% to 60%.[42,43] By their nature, grade II to IV tumors are infiltrating. Therefore, in contrast to ependymomas, radical resection of astrocytomas is not always possible. Surgery consists of removing as much tumor as possible. In some instances, one can only perform biopsy or decompression with duraplasty. In the literature, the rate of complete and subtotal removal varies between 11% to 31% and 21% to 62%, respectively.[42,43,54] The pathological diagnosis of pilocytic astrocytoma and surgical experience are factors associated with higher rates of complete resection.[42,43] Low spinal level (conus), malignancy, and adult onset are considered important factors associated with a higher tumor recurrence rate.[43] The degree of resection, and spinal canal decompression via tumor debulking, have not been found to be directly related to progression-free survival or overall survival in many studies.[26,32,43,50,52,55,56] In low-grade astrocytomas, the 5- and 10-year survival rates range from about 77% to 82%.[43,56] These rates drop, respectively, to 27% and 14% for malignant astrocytomas.[43,56]

Gangliogliomas

Gangliogliomas are very uncommon lesions mainly reported as case reports and a few studies.[57,58] These lesions are mainly encountered in children and young adults.[57] In a large series of 56 patients, complete or subtotal resection has been achieved in 82%, and 18% of the patients had a 5-year survival rate of 88% and a progression-free survival rate of 67%.[57]

Factors Determining Outcome

The major determinant of long-term patient survival is based on the histological characteristics of the tumor. The 5-year progression-free survival (PFS) rate drops from 78% for low-grade gliomas to 30% for high-grade gliomas.[50] A longitudinal database (Surveillance, Epidemiology, and End Results [SEER] database) encompassing 26% of the U.S. population was published in 2010 and included 1814 patients with spinal cord gliomas.[59] In this study, age, histology, and grade were defined as significant predictors of outcome.[59]

Tumors of Nonglial Origin

From this group of nonglial spinal cord lesions, hemangioblastomas and cavernomas are the most frequently encountered. These vascular benign tumors are characteristically well delineated and sometimes multifocal.

Other lesions such as metastases, epidermoids, dermoid cysts, lipomas, intramedullary schwannomas, PNETs, and teratomas may also be encountered.[13,43,55] In addition to these rare lesions, we have also encountered lymphomas and neuroglial cysts.

Hemangioblastomas

Hemangioblastomas are highly vascular lesions that represent almost 2% to 15% of SCIMTs in some studies.[42,43,60-63] These lesions consist of two main components: (1) large vacuolated stromal cells that have been identified as the neoplastic cell of origin and (2) a rich capillary network.[64] Hemangioblastomas are often observed as encapsulated lesions abutting the

pia, especially at the posterior or posterolateral aspect of the spinal cord close to the dorsal root entry zone. They may also be encountered anteriorly or in intramedullary sites.[43,60,63] Radicular arteries or anterior branches feed these lesions.[65] Despite being histologically benign, spinal hemangioblastomas may be associated with significant neurological morbidity, often secondary to associated cyst and syrinx (present in 80-90% of the cases) and edema.[60] En bloc surgical resection is the treatment of choice, associated with excellent neurological outcome. Patients with incidental asymptomatic solitary lesions may be followed.[60] Surgery is indicated as soon as symptoms develop or sequential MRI demonstrates tumor or cyst growth.[43] For patients with von Hippel-Lindau (VHL) disease and multiple lesions, the timing of surgery remains open to debate.[63] Some authors operate on asymptomatic patients if they exhibit radiological progression before significant neurological deficits occur.[63] Follow-up of patients with VHL disease, and associated neoplasms such as pheochromocytoma and renal and pancreatic cancer, should be performed at regular intervals with spinal and brain MRI studies.[43,66]

Cavernomas

Intramedullary cavernomas accounted for 3% to 16% of intramedullary lesions in large studies.[42,43,61,67] Cavernous malformations are well-circumscribed lesions consisting of closely packed, capillary-like vessels, without intervening brain or spinal tissue.[67] The clinical presentation may vary. Some patients may present with gradual neurological deterioration explained by repeated hemorrhages. Others exhibit slow progressive deterioration induced by small hemorrhages and increasing gliosis, or with acute onset and significant neurological deterioration due to spontaneous hemorrhage.[67-72] When an intraspinal cavernoma is discovered, a survey of the entire central nervous system is advised.[67] Approximately, 40% of patients with a spinal cavernoma may also have a synchronous intracranial lesion.[73] In our practice, removal of intramedullary cavernomas is indicated in two circumstances: (1) symptomatic lesions or (2) asymptomatic lesions, if the cavernoma is easily accessible, specifically posteriorly and/or abutting the pial surface. This surgical attitude is controversial for asymptomatic patients[68,69] but it is supported by some in the literature.[43,74] The annual rate of hemorrhage in symptomatic intramedullary cavernous malformations ranges from 1.4% to 4.5% but rises to 66% in the case of previous bleeding.[72,75] Most lesions can be completely removed with concomitant clinical improvement. An improved postoperative outcome is obtained if symptoms have existed for less than 3 years.[72]

Associated Diseases

Most SCIMTs develop sporadically; only a minority is associated with genetic diseases. Hemangioblastomas are a component of von Hippel-Lindau disease. Ependymomas and astrocytomas are associated with neurofibromatosis type 1 and 2.[43,60,63,76,77] Overall, SCIMTs are noted in these genetic disorders in approximately 20% of the patients.[60,78] Intraspinal mass lesions such as hamartomas, dermoid cysts, and dermal sinus tracts are associated with spinal dysraphism.[43,79-82] Demyelinating disease may present as a mass lesion with histological features identical to those seen in the brain. Sarcoidosis has also been described as a primary spinal cord lesion.

Spinal cord involvement in sarcoidosis is rare, occurring in less than 1% of patients with sarcoidosis.[83] Any isolated spinal cord intramedullary lesion that is diffusely enhanced and not associated with a mass effect should be investigated for inflammatory disease.

Clinical Expression

There is no typical presentation for spinal cord tumors (SCIMTs). An important characteristic in distinguishing them from demyelinating diseases should be addressed. Intermittent symptom regression and progression is never noted in SCIMTs.[43] The clinical course is often insidious and progressive over years. In fact, in 80% of the patients, tumors grow slowly and most of them are benign lesions.[13,43] Episodic deteriorations or abrupt onset may also be encountered especially as a result of hemorrhage. Spinal subarachnoid hemorrhage originates predominantly from arteriovenous malformations that mimic a tumor[84] but also rarely from hemangioblastomas.[85] Hydrocephalus induced by SCIMTs has been reported in the literature.[86,87] We have also encountered a malignant intramedullary tumor with associated leptomeningeal dissemination.[88] For this reason, a child presenting with hydrocephalus of unknown origin should have a spinal MRI to rule out an SCIMT.[87]

Adults more often complain of pain as a first symptom (35%), while children are more likely to present with motor weakness (42%).[43] In descending order of frequency, patients may present with sensory disorders, gait ataxia, motor deficits, and sphincter disorders. In children under 3 years of age, in descending order, the clinical presentation may include progressive motor regression/weakness, torticollis, gait abnormalities, and kyphoscoliosis.[89] The presentation is most often directly related to the level of the lesion. In large studies, the cervical cord is involved in 30% to 56% of the cases, the cervicothoracic cord in 17% to 25%, the thoracic cord in 17% to 49%, and the remaining ones occur in the conus area.[42,61,90,91] However, it is possible for cervical intramedullary tumors to present without sensory or motor deficit in the upper extremities, and the patients with a conus tumor may not suffer from sphincter dysfunction. An aspecific presentation is inevitably associated with a diagnostic delay after the first symptom, with a mean time of 1 to 3 years depending on the tumor's growth rate.[13,43] The most useful clinical classification system is that reported by McCormick.[29] In this clinical/functional classification system, grade I corresponds to a patient neurologically intact, with mild focal deficit not significantly affecting function of involved limb, with mild spasticity or reflex abnormality, or normal gait.[29] In grade II, the patient presents with sensorimotor deficit affecting function of involved limbs, mild to moderate gait impairment, severe pain or dysesthetic syndrome impacting patient's quality of life; he or she still functions and ambulates independently. In grade III, he or she suffers from more severe neurological deficit, requires cane/brace for ambulation or significant bilateral upper extremity impairment; he may or may not function independently.[29] In grade IV, the patient has severe deficit and requires wheelchair or cane/brace with bilateral upper extremity impairment; he or she is usually not independent.[29] This classification takes into account both sensory and motor functions to rate the patient's clinical status at the time of the surgery and during follow-up.

Diagnosis

Preoperative Imaging

MRI is currently the gold standard for accurately diagnosing any SCIMT and determining the extent, location, and characteristics of the tumor in preparation for surgery. In our department, the role of standard x-ray studies and CT scan has been reduced to a few indications such as assessing spine stability or bone structure, especially for patients who need a re-exploration.

A complete MRI workup requires T2- and T1-WI with and without gadolinium sequences in at least two planes (sagittal and axial).[13] The slice thickness should be of less than 3 mm and a large visual field should be used to encompass the entire spinal cord.[13] Full spinal axis imaging allows ruling out transitional bone anomalies especially in thoracic tumors to accurately locate pathological levels under fluoroscopy at the beginning of the surgery. Several aspects of the tumor and its characteristics should be evaluated in order to determine the preliminary diagnosis and surgical plan. On axial images, it can be determined whether the lesion is centrally located or eccentric, with a possible exophytic component. The demarcation from the normal spinal cord tissue can also sometimes be determined. Enhancement after gadolinium administration directs the surgical trajectory and gives information on tumor vascularity as well as the spinal cord–tumor interface.

Cysts are commonly observed in association with the solid portion of the tumor. Two large categories of cysts should be distinguished: tumor cysts and polar cysts. Each type of cyst requires a different operative strategy and each is associated with a different prognosis. The wall of a tumor cyst typically enhances after contrast administration. Their contours are usually well defined and their signal is usually different from that of CSF, because their content is rich in protein or contains blood products. However, the wall of polar cysts, also called *satellite cysts*, does not enhance after contrast injection. These cysts may develop at both poles, on either side of the solid portion, appearing round and under tension. Their signal intensity is comparable to that of CSF. During surgery, they are discovered outside the tumor and will progressively shrink and disappear within a few months after surgery.

On MRI, intramedullary ependymomas appear as well-circumscribed lesions, typically located at the center of the spinal cord because they originate from ependymal cells lining the central canal.[12,92,93] Their signal can be variable on T1-WI and hyperintense on T2-WI. Typically, ependymomas enhance homogeneously after gadolinium injection.[13] Four patterns of contrast enhancement have been determined by Miyazawa and co-workers[94]: homogeneous pattern, heterogeneous pattern, heterogeneous with cyst wall enhancement, and enhanced nodule on the cyst wall. Associated satellite cysts are present in 60% of the cases.[13,43] On T2 sequences, it is interesting to look for hypointense signal at both poles of the solid portion of the tumor, called the "cap-like" appearance. In our experience, although this finding is not pathognomonic, it is observed in only 30% of ependymomas and 12% of hemangioblastomas. It has been correlated histologically and intraoperatively with areas of chronic hemorrhage with hemosiderin deposits or high protein substances and sometimes is referred to as *Froin's syndrome*.[13]

Astrocytomas often appear hypointense on T1-WI and hyperintense on T2-WI.[13] FLAIR (fluid-attenuated inversion recovery) images and T2 sequences can be helpful in delineating the precise extension of an astrocytoma whose borders are not well demarcated due to its infiltrative nature. A cystic component is depicted in 27% to 42%[13,43] of the tumors and is associated with hydromyelia in about half of the cases.[13] Grade II astrocytomas generally do not enhance after gadolinium administration.[13] Conversely, pilocytic astrocytomas and high-grade lesions that appear more heterogeneous with necrotic and cystic regions enhance intensely.[13] Gradient echo T2-WI is a useful sequence for determining hemorrhagic zones within the lesion.[13] Regardless of typical radiological appearances, the distinction between astrocytomas and ependymomas remains difficult and demands histological analysis. MRI can predict but not definitively ascertain the precise diagnosis. For this reason, the potential degree of resection cannot be predicted preoperatively.

On the contrary, MRI has a high degree of accuracy with nonglial tumors. The nodule of an hemangioblastoma appears classically iso- to hypointense on T1-WI and iso- to hyperintense on T2-WI.[13] Homogeneous uptake is evident after gadolinium injection. Proton density imaging and T2-WI are appropriate for delineating enlarged feeding arteries, rich tumor vascular networks, and dilated draining veins.[13] An associated cyst has been found in 88% of the cases in large studies.[43] MRA with a contrast-enhanced bolus for three-dimensional T1-weighted sequences may currently identify some feeding arteries and large draining veins. Angiography is considered only when preoperative embolization is required to reduce the risk of bleeding during surgery.

Cavernous malformations have a characteristic appearance on MRI. A cavernoma is composed of mixed signal intensities, surrounded by a hemosiderin hypointense ring. Completing the preoperative workup with a brain MRI is advocated because synchronous lesions are often noted and confirm the diagnosis.[13]

Magnetic Resonance Tractography

This method, which is based on diffusion tensor imaging techniques, is still in evolution. It holds potential for analyzing spinal cord fiber displacement or disruption from tumors or non-neoplastic lesions.[95,96] Secondary alterations to white matter tracts can be reliably displayed and could therefore become of great value for planning treatment and follow-up.[96]

Preoperative Diagnostic Pitfalls

A wide differential diagnosis should be entertained in order to adopt the appropriate treatment strategy for lesions in the spinal cord. In some circumstances, associated conditions provide crucial information to focus the diagnosis and rule out an intramedullary tumor. Intramedullary bacterial, fungal, or parasitic abscesses should be in the differential diagnosis in the presence of systemic disease or immunocompromised patients. In contrast to SCIMTs, a rapid clinical deterioration is observed in infections.[97] If symptoms develop abruptly, a medullary infarction is suspected.[98] Multiple sclerosis can mimic an intramedullary tumor, especially active lesions that enhance on MRI.[55] If there is any doubt, complete central

nervous system screening for concomitant lesions should be performed by MRI. If other lesions are not discovered, but the clinical presentation is one of intermittent neurological deficits, demyelinating disease is not ruled out. Further testing is required.[43] A cerebrospinal fluid examination to look for oligoclonal bands and serum markers may be helpful.[55] If there is continuing doubt about a demyelinating diagnosis, and the neurological presentation is not progressive or atypical for neoplasm, a repeat MRI in a few weeks is a reasonable plan. Indeed, the signal characteristics of the lesion on MRI may change in the case of demyelinating or inflammatory disease. Neoplastic disease is unlikely to change in a short interval, unless there is a highly malignant tumor.[43] Spinal cord edema and rim-like contrast enhancement may also be seen in the case of subacute necrotizing myelopathy. In this disorder, spinal cord atrophy develops over time.[97]

In a study of nine patients undergoing surgery for neoplastic-like lesions reported by Lee and associates,[99] the histological examination of the surgical specimens showed demyelinating lesions, sarcoidosis, amyloid angiopathy, and a group of non-neoplastic inflammatory cells of unknown etiology. The most consistent finding that the author reported for differentiating non-neoplastic lesions from neoplastic ones was the absence of or minimal spinal cord expansion on preoperative MRI in non-neoplastic lesions.[99]

Biopsy

In some lesions, when the diagnosis cannot be defined based on clinical data, blood work or CSF samples, and MRI, a biopsy may be helpful for diagnosing granulomatous disease such as sarcoidosis, tuberculosis, brucellosis, and histoplasmosis, which can affect the spinal cord.[99-103] These lesions often have systemic manifestations[97] but even without them, the diagnosis cannot be made with an MRI alone, and thus, a biopsy is necessary.[104] In these disorders, surgery should be limited to a biopsy; nodule resection may indeed be linked with neurological worsening.[103] Then, a steroid-based treatment offers a good prognosis,[105] although a relapse may occur when steroids are discontinued.[106]

Two conditions often lead to diagnostic errors after biopsy: small sample size and location of the biopsy. Indeed, the small size of a biopsy specimen may limit the accuracy of the diagnosis. We strive to provide a sample that is sufficient to assist the pathologist in making the correct diagnosis without injuring the patient. Second, the biopsy diagnosis depends on the sample location. For example, intense reactive gliosis around a lesion (e.g., arterio-venous malformations or hemoblastomas) can be mistaken for a glioma.

Surgical Considerations

The most important factor in determining the long-term neurological and functional outcome following surgery is the patient's preoperative neurological status.[43,61,107] Therefore, we advise surgery in the presence of neurological deficits or decline. Serial monitoring for asymptomatic individuals is also critical. Patients with either no deficits or only mild deficits prior to surgery are unlikely to experience permanent deficits in a meticulously planned and executed surgery, reinforcing the importance of early diagnosis and treatment.[50] Complete resection is attempted with ependymomas, hemangioblastomas, and cavernomas, as opposed to astrocytomas. Currently, the vast majority of well-demarcated tumors are potentially curable with a good quality of life. A carefully planned strategy should be adopted for the first surgical procedure. The patient's prognosis is directly related to the results of the first surgery; a second surgery after an unsuccessful attempt usually results in neurological worsening due to damage caused by dissection of scar tissue or trying to discern unrecognizable surgical planes.

Intraoperative Monitoring

Intraoperative monitoring of the functional integrity of the spinal cord during intramedullary procedures has been recognized as a promising adjunct that may help in intraoperative decision making and in prediction of neurological outcome.[108,109] Historically, somatosensory evoked potentials (SSEPs) were the first to be used, but motor evoked potentials (MEPs) have become more popular, useful, and technically accessible to surgeons. The continuation of the SSEPs should encourage pursuing an aggressive resection, but the loss of SSEPs is often of little value in anticipating postoperative motor deficits. In contrast, MEPs correlate more closely with the postoperative motor function. Loss of MEP waveform and a 50% reduction of the D wave seems to represent a critical points.[61,109] In this situation, we wait for a few minutes to see if the waveform recovers, which is often the case, and then continue resection in another part of the tumor where there may be a good plane of cleavage. If the lesion is infiltrative or the MEP waveform does not improve or deteriorate, surgical judgment and experience becomes paramount in the decision on whether to curtail the operation or not.

Patient Positioning

The patient is always positioned prone on cushions in such a way that the abdomen and thorax remain free from any pressure. We are not in favor of the sitting position when dealing with SCIMTs, even for lesions located at the cervicomedullary junction.

General anesthesia is induced using intravenous opioids and continuous propofol. Blood pressure is monitored with an arterial line and kept close to preoperative baseline levels during the procedure. Halogenated volatile anesthetics should be avoided because they interfere with SSEPs. Intubation is facilitated with short-acting muscle relaxants administered at induction and discontinued quickly afterward to allow for MEP monitoring.

A three-point head fixation device is always used for cervical or upper thoracic lesions, taking care to avoid inadvertent cervical flexion and pressure on the face. Head positioning is crucial in SCIMT surgery. Usually the head is placed in a neutral position as long as SSEPs remain stable. The head should be elevated above the level of the heart to decrease venous pressure and not be overflexed because it could increase spinal cord compression. Prior to surgery, baseline SSEPs and MEPs are recorded. In our practice, a bolus of methylprednisolone (30 mg/kg) is injected, according to the spinal cord trauma protocol (30-mg/kg bolus followed after 1 hour by 5.4 mg/kg/hour during 23 hours).

Surgical Approach

A midline skin incision is performed, extending one level above and below pathological levels. The aponeurosis is divided and paravertebral muscles are retracted symmetrically. A laminectomy is most often performed in adults and a laminotomy is preferred in children, especially at the cervical level. In infants, when possible, we perform a unilateral soft tissue dissection and a unilateral laminotomy. Bone opening is limited to one level above and one level below the solid portion of the tumor but for very extensive tumors, requiring extensive laminectomy or laminotomy, for children as well as adults, we recommend leaving in place one posterior arch every five to six levels. Bone should always be gently and patiently removed with high-speed drill or Kerrison thin-clamp in order to avoid any stress to the already compressed spinal cord. The articular facets should be kept intact to diminish the probability of postoperative kyphosis. Before opening the dura mater, meticulous hemostasis should be obtained to avoid any intradural soiling, especially because the tumor is at the deepest part of the surgical field. For this reason, the soft tissue dissection is preferably performed with monopolar cautery. Bone wax is applied on the edges of the bone opening. Careful epidural hemostasis is necessary, with insertion of small pieces of resorbable cellulose under cottonoids, because any epidural bleeding will increase after the dural incision and CSF drainage.

Dural and Arachnoid Incisions

We always open the dura under microscopic magnification, keeping the arachnoid intact if possible. The dural edges may be sutured either to adjacent muscles or retracted with simple sutures. Even if this latter technique is often used, the former one has the advantage of significantly enlarging the narrow and deep surgical space. The arachnoid is subsequently opened separately with microscissors, and delicately freed from the posterior and lateral aspects of the spinal cord. Keeping the arachnoid layer intact will allow reapproximation at closure. Careful inspection of the spinal cord under magnification may show some subpial discoloration induced by the underlying tumor. Most of the time it is not required but with any doubt about the tumor location, we use ultrasonography to localize solid and cystic tumor sections.

Ependymomas and Astrocytomas (Figs. 25.3 and 25.4)

Intramedullary Dissection

At this point, it should be decided whether the approach will be midline between the posterior columns or directly on the lateral aspect of the spinal cord, such as the dorsal root entry zone. Most often, a standard midline dissection is preferred, but the strategy should be adapted to the tumor. Indeed, in gliomas, we almost always perform a midline approach with gentle separation of posterior columns in the posterior median sulcus,[34,38,44] except on rare occasions when a lesion is located eccentrically and comes up to the pial surface of the cord, making entry much more direct.

Identifying the midline can be challenging in some patients. It can be especially troublesome when working on astrocytomas that develop asymmetrically. If the problem

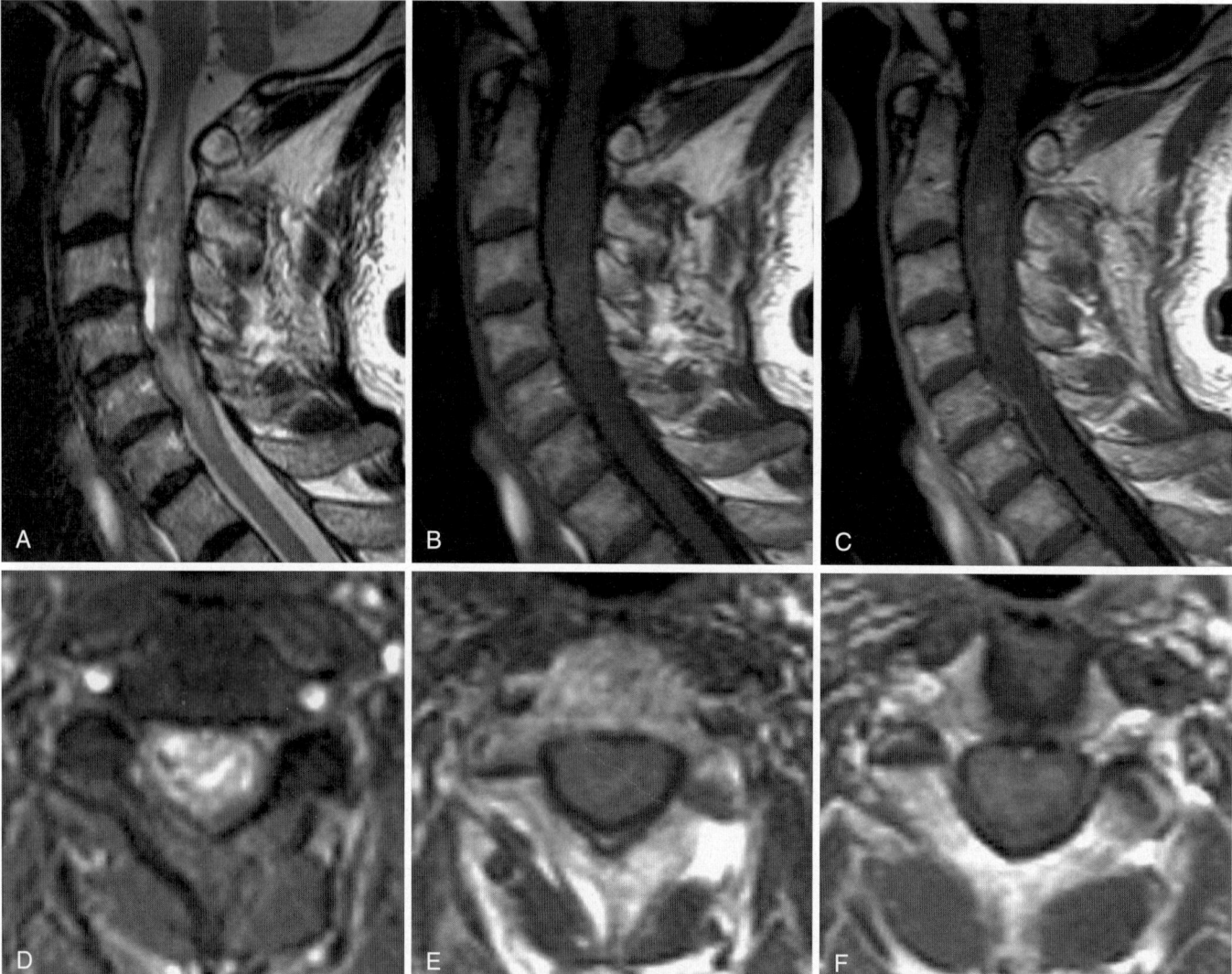

FIGURE 25.3 Cervical ependymoma. **A** to **F,** Preoperative magnetic resonance (MR) sagittal and axial T2-weighted images (WI) (A and D); T1-WI before (B and E), and after (C and F) gadolinium injection. The tumor is centrally located within the cord. It has an inhomogeneous signal behavior being mainly hypersignal on T2-WI and T1-WI and enhancing strongly after contrast injection.

cannot be solved, two pearls may be very helpful. First, the midline can be delineated after looking for it above or below the tumor where the spinal cord is normal. Second, the median sulcus can be recognized by the convergence of vessels toward the midline. Under high magnification with the microscope, the very tortuous posterior spinal vein running over the posterior median sulcus can be localized. Sometimes, vessels of varying size run longitudinally over the dorsal columns and have to be dissected and mobilized laterally to expose the sulcus. All of the narrowest arterial or venous structures in the sulcocommissural region should be dissected carefully and spared. Opening the midline implies careful retraction of the dorsal columns and progressive opening with microinstruments along the length of the solid portion of the tumor. These maneuvers open the spinal cord like the pages of a book. The process is pursued until the entire extent of the tumor is visualized as well as rostral and caudal cysts, if present.

Pial Retraction

Pial retraction is obtained with tensionless 6-0 sutures holding the median pia mater attached to the dural edges. This maneuver greatly improves intramedullary exposure and decreases repetitive trauma that may be caused by the tumor dissection. This handling is secured by SEP monitoring that must remain stable during this step. No pial traction is needed in the rare case in which the pressure of the tumor itself keeps the posterior columns separated.

Tumor Biopsy

As soon as the tumor is reached, a sufficient portion must be sampled with forceps and scissors, without applying cauterization. The pathologist immediately examines this biopsy. Then, we take some time before proceeding with surgery until we find out the results. Indeed, tumor removal should sometimes be discontinued early if there is an infiltrating or a malignant tumor, or a nontumoral process such as sarcoidosis.

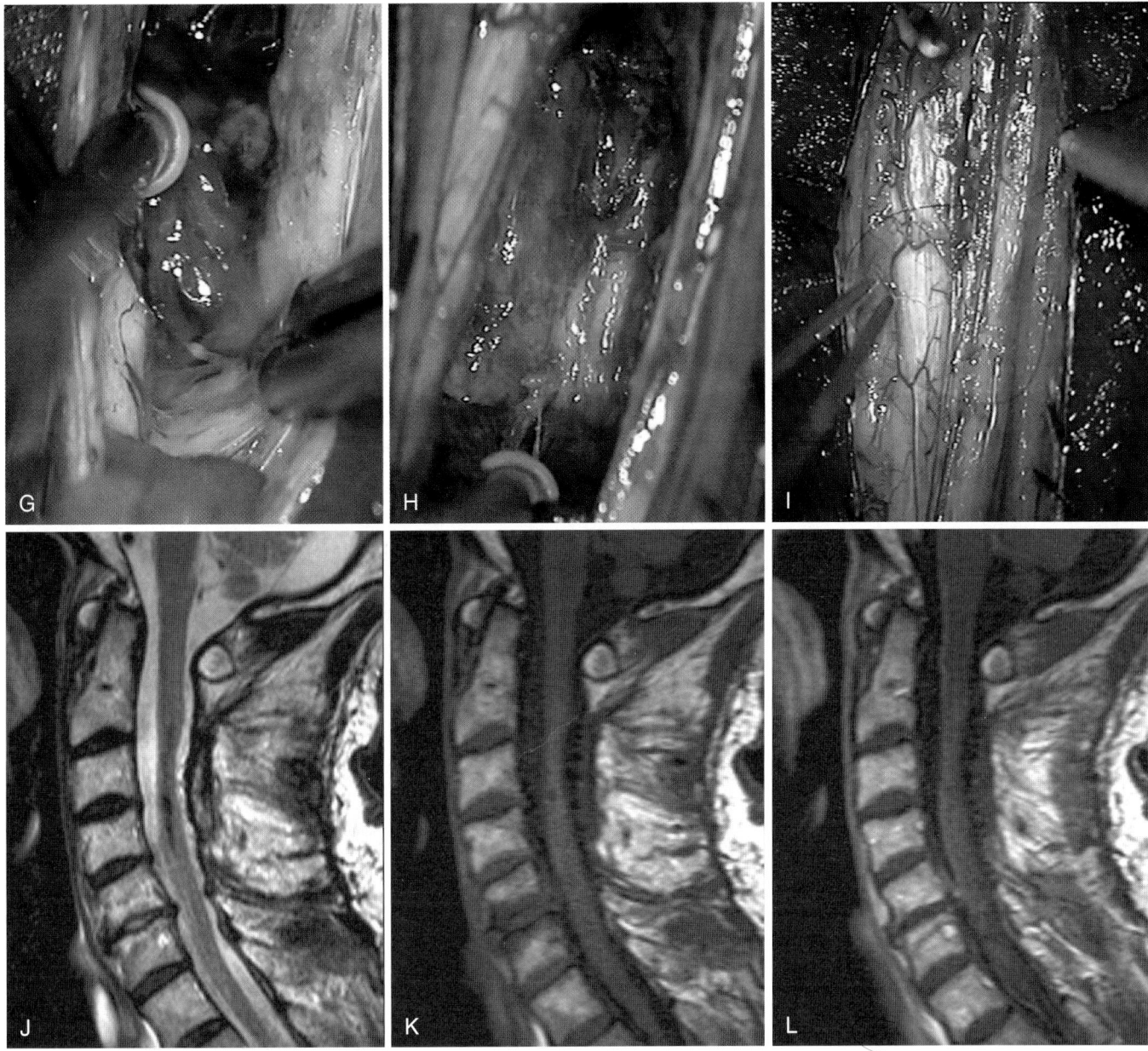

FIGURE 25.3, cont'd G to **I,** Perioperative views. **G,** A plane of cleavage exists allowing separation of the tumor from the spinal cord tissue. **H,** Great care must be taken while resecting the anterior aspect of the lesion, close to anterior spinal artery branches. **I,** The spinal cord is closed at the completion of the procedure. **J** to **L,** Postoperative views (of A to C) after complete tumor resection. *(Used with permission from Hôpital Erasme, Université Libre de Bruxelles.)*

Tumor Debulking

At this point, the same technique is adopted with ependymomas and astrocytomas. The tumor should be debulked before looking for a cleavage plane. This point is crucial in avoiding any traction or pressure on the spinal cord itself. Reducing the tumor volume is carried out using a CUSA. Intratumoral resection is completed from inside out. Drainage of a cyst or an intratumoral hematoma, whenever present, may facilitate the spinal cord relaxation.

The CUSA is used in a very controlled fashion to "paint" the tumor out of spinal cord. The surgeon should be being compulsive about respecting the tumor versus spinal cord plane and stay within the tumor until the tumor needs to be gently peeled or suctioned off the surrounding walls.

Cleavage Plane Dissection

When the tumor has been debulked, it is essential to look for a tumor spinal cord cleavage plane. This plane exists in most ependymomas[29,38,44,77,110] and in about 30% to 40% of astrocytomas.[38,52,110,111] Finding the cleavage plane makes tumor removal more successful. The cleavage plane is observed as a color change between the tumor and the spinal cord. In our practice, the best dissection is preferably made with two microforceps. Very commonly, we dissect the spinal cord from

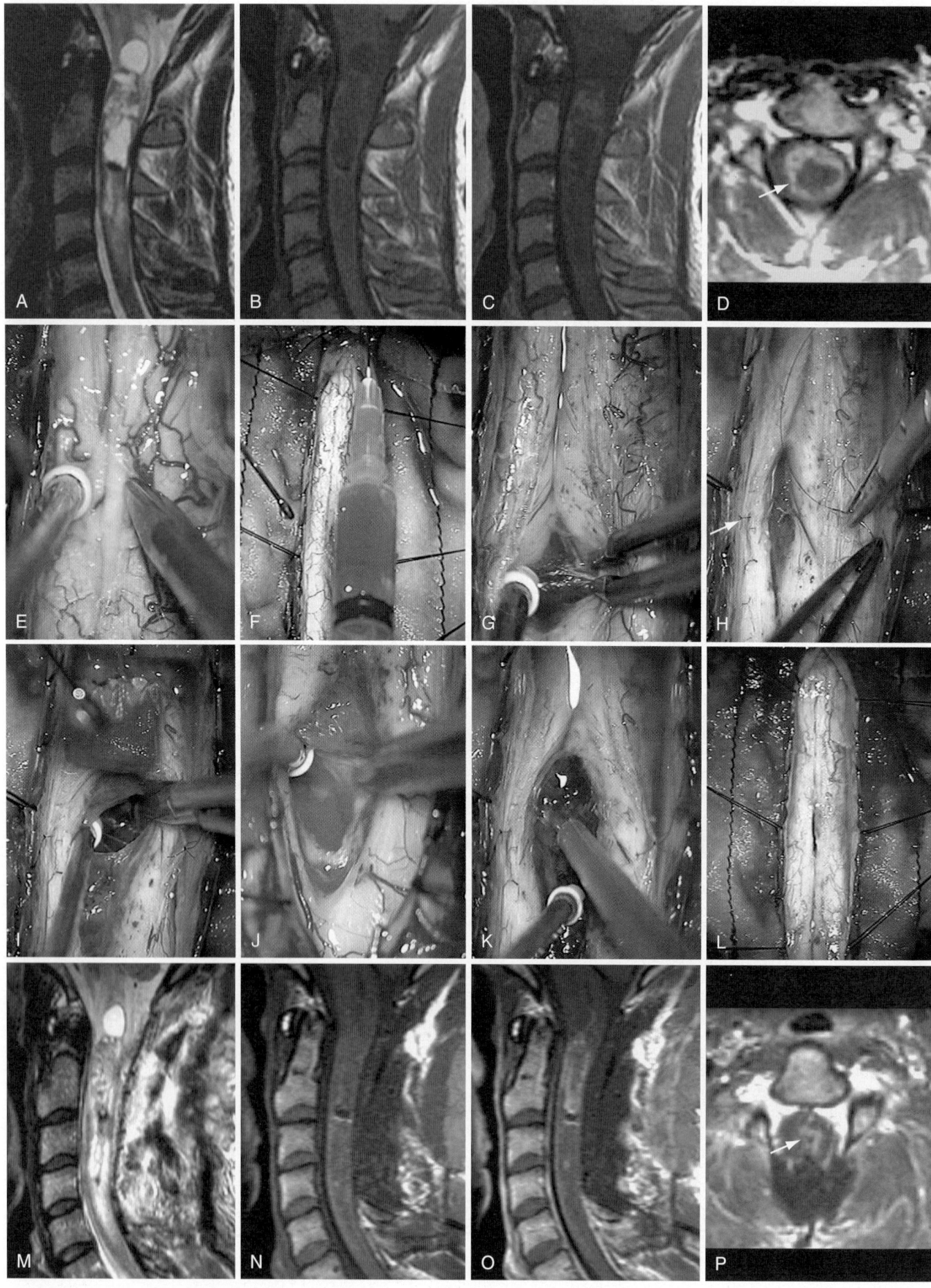

FIGURE 25.4 Cervical astrocytoma. **A** to **D,** Preoperative magnetic resonance (MR) T2-weighted images (WI) (**A**); T1-WI before (**B**) and after (**C** and **D**) gadolinium administration. Arrow indicates the lateral margin of the tumor. The tumor has multiple cystic and enhancing solid components. Signs of chronic hemorrhage are seen on the T2-WI. **E** to **L,** Perioperative views. **E,** The posterior columns are gently separated. **F,** Puncture of intratumoral cysts facilitates the spinal cord opening. **G,** The tumor appears. **H,** The arachnoid is sutured on the dural edges to maintain the spinal cord open like a book. **I** and **J,** Intratumoral cysts are opened. **K,** The tumor is debulked with an ultrasonic aspirator. **L,** View at the completion of the procedure. The tumor can only be partially removed. **M** to **P,** Postoperative views. The tumor volume has been significantly reduced (*arrow* on P is located at the periphery, as on D). *(Used with permission from Hôpital Erasme, Université Libre de Bruxelles.)*

---

the tumor, holding in the left hand an atraumatic sucker. We also regularly use cotton strips moistened with normothermic saline. If the tumor is encapsulated or not too friable, its margins can be grasped. Frequently, some parts of the tumor are more difficult to dissect than others. Instead of continuing, we recommend switching work areas. We recommend the same procedure when there is change or decrement in the SSEPs or MEPs waveforms. We will only come back to a tenacious area after further cytoreduction.

If the cleavage plane is not clear, especially in infiltrating tumors, we will discontinue the resection since it may be detrimental for the patient's neurological function. At this moment, MEPs are of great value in determining when the resection should be terminated, always keeping in mind that the patient's quality of life is the main surgical priority. If no plane of separation is found between the cord and tumor, as is often the case with astrocytomas, an aggressive surgery should be avoided to preserve the patient's neurological condition. In case of associated nonenhancing cyst on MRI, removal is considered complete when the cyst is fenestrated and the normal spinal cord is observed through the transparent cyst wall, as the cyst wall is similar to that seen in syringomyelia cavities.

Vascular Pedicle Section

The management of vascular pedicles supplying a tumor represents the final challenge because these pedicles are connected to the anterior spinal artery, which one should always avoid injuring. Careful cauterization and division of all small arterial feeders makes hemostasis trouble-free. In fact, no bleeding remains at the end of the procedure when a complete macroscopic resection has been achieved. Small spinal cord vessels coagulate spontaneously, so it is unusual to need to cauterize outside the tumor margin.

Hemangioblastomas (Fig. 25.5)

Approach

Hemangioblastomas are essentially located near the pial surface, lying over or inside the spinal cord. If the lesion is entirely inside the spinal cord, the lesion is accessed through the midline, as described previously. If the lesion is observed directly on the pia dorsally it is approached straight on.[112] If present, we always take advantage of a huge and tense syrinx cyst associated with hemangioblastomas by gently puncturing the fluid with a 22-gauge needle; it collapses the spinal cord and gives ideal access to the solid tumor nodule through the transparent puncture site.[113] In case of huge hemangioblastomas, the surgeon must be particularly cautious to avoid any

cauterization of the draining vein at the beginning of the procedure. Interrupting venous outflow will induce hyperpressure inside the malformation and uncontrollable tumor bleeding. When the tumor is located ventrally, we use the same approach as described earlier for anterior/ventral meningiomas.

Resection

Biopsy or tumor debulking is to be avoided in hemangioblastoma to avoid massive bleeding, which could compromise the surgical procedure. Under microscopic magnification, tumor limits are defined. In fact, we look for a region on the surface with scarce vessels to be our starting dissection point. The cleavage plane remains distinct as long as bleeding does not interfere with the dissection. Slight tumor retraction obtained by gentle coagulation on its surface can be helpful for detaching the lesion from the cord. This maneuver is best completed with nonstick bipolar forceps or irrigating bipolars. After a step-by-step technique consisting of repeated cauterization and division of vascular connections, the lesion becomes devascularized prior to sacrifice of the draining vein. This vein should be interrupted only at the end of the procedure. We then finish the resection by carefully rolling out the tumor from its last spinal cord attachment. In this condition, we also advocate closing the arachnoid layer over the surgical field once the tumor is resected to prevent tethering the spinal cord against the dura.[38]

Cavernomas (Fig. 25.6)

Like hemangioblastomas, cavernomas are usually encountered close to the pial surface. If the lesion is located on the anterolateral aspect of the spinal cord, access becomes possible by dividing one or two dentate ligament attachments and gently rotating the spinal cord with 6-0 silk sutures applied to the ligaments. In this fashion, most anterolateral lesions are discovered through the transparent pia mater.[38,114] We approach these lesions directly, through a limited opening of the pia, maintained if necessary with 8-0 silk sutures.

Like hemangioblastomas, cavernomas are best removed most of the time "en bloc." Nevertheless, in rare circumstances, reducing the volume of large cavernomas with the ultrasonic aspirator may be necessary. Then, with gentle cauterization on its surface, the lesion is shrunk in order to release the pressure on the lesion–spinal cord interface and assist in its dissection. In some huge cavernomas, it may even be indispensable to use strategies combining different approaches (posterior and anterolateral) in the same surgical procedure.

In hemangioblastomas and cavernomas, we do not close the spinal cord opening, but we do close the arachnoid layer.

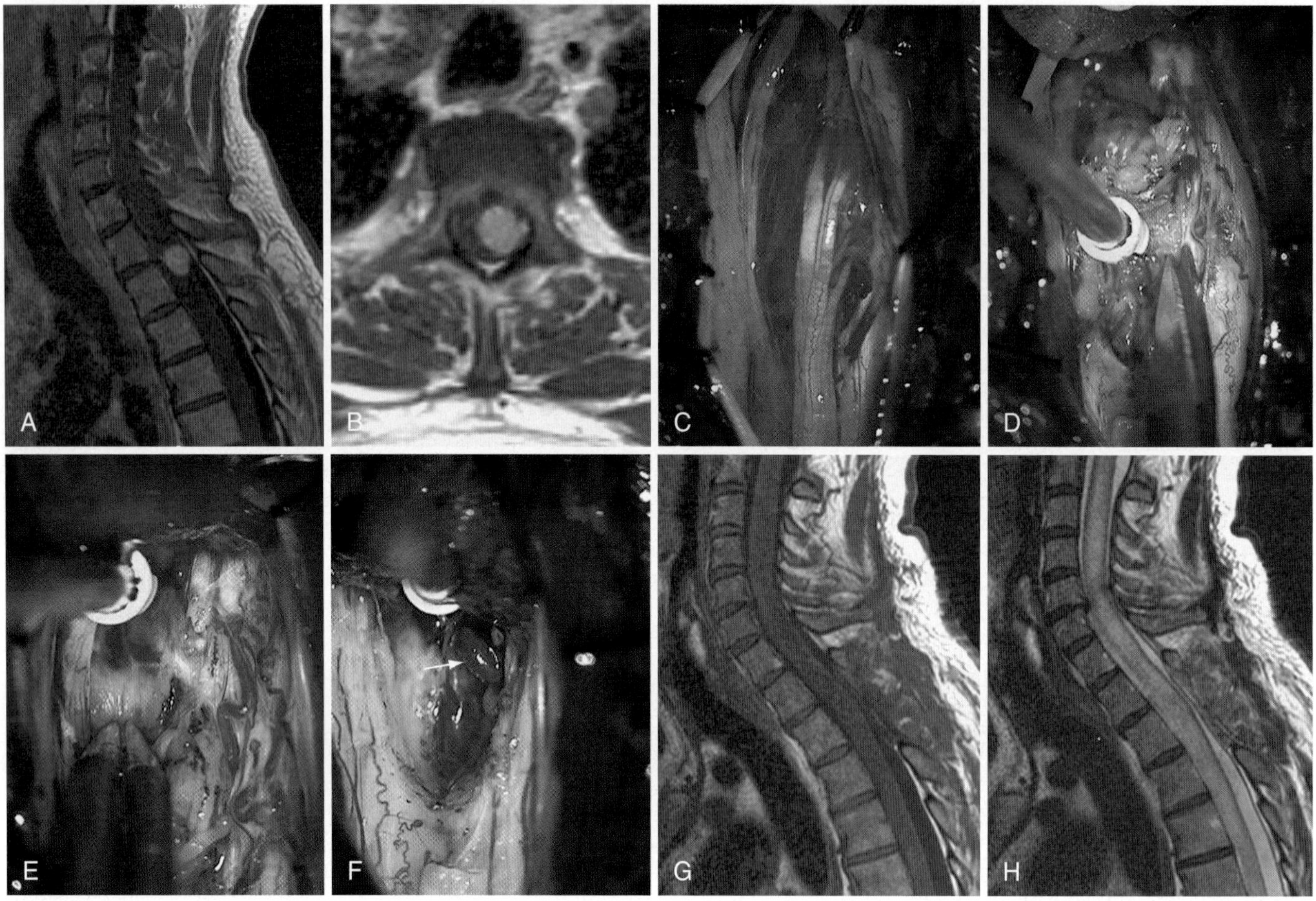

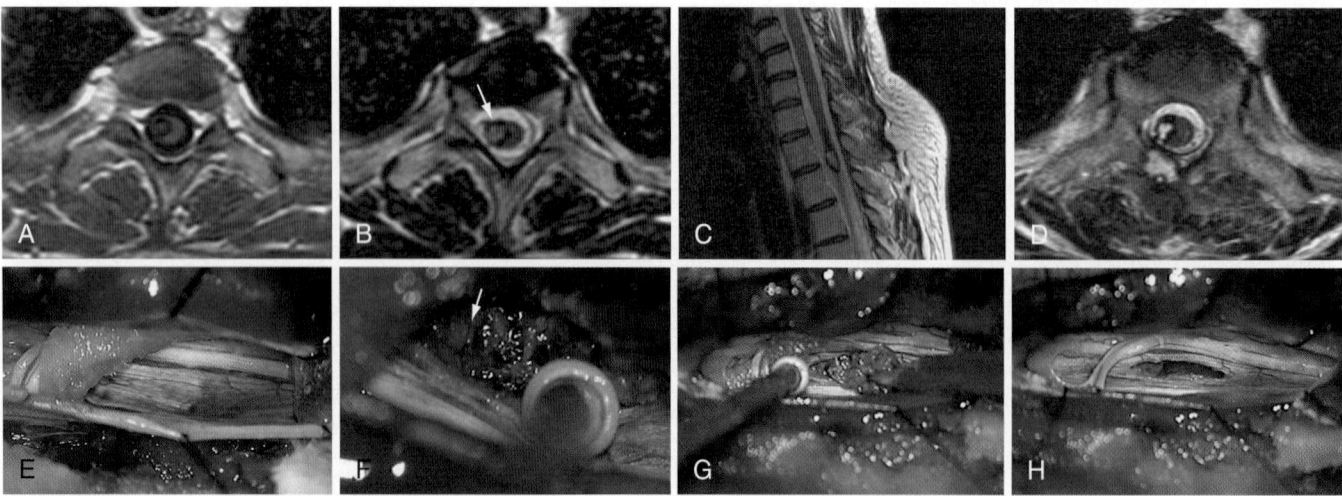

FIGURE 25.5 T1-T2 hemangioblastoma. **A** and **B,** Preoperative gadolinium-enhanced magnetic resonance (MR) T1-weighted images (WI). **C** to **F,** Perioperative views during "en bloc" removal. The draining vein *(arrow)* can be divided only at the final step. **G** and **H,** Early postoperative MR T1- and T2-WI confirm the complete resection. The extensive hypersignal areas seen on T2-WI sequences corresponding to the classically observed huge peritumoral edema will disappear within a couple of months. *(Used with permission from Hôpital Erasme, Université Libre de Bruxelles.)*

FIGURE 25.6 Thoracic lateral spinal cord cavernoma. **A** to **C,** Preoperative magnetic resonance (MR) image. Arrow shows the hemosiderin ring. **D,** Postoperative axial MR T2-weighted images (WI) of B. The tumor has been completely resected but the hyposignal of the hemosiderin ring remains. **E** to **H,** Perioperative views. **E,** The lesion appears as a discoloration visible through the arachnoid layer. The nerve root is protected by a cottonoid. **F,** The lesion is gently separated from the spinal cord. The lesion-spinal cord interface is underlined with the arrow. **G,** En bloc removal is carried out. **H,** Final view. *(Used with permission from Hôpital Erasme, Université Libre de Bruxelles.)*

Closure

At the completion of a tumor resection, pial traction sutures are divided to release the dorsal columns. After complete tumor resection, we reapproximate the cord with nonabsorbable 6-0 pial sutures, gently approximating both posterior columns together. The arachnoid may also be partially reconstituted with the same suture, if the layer has been preserved at the opening. This arachnoid closure is most often possible because the cord volume is smaller than at the beginning. However, in cases of partial or subtotal removal, we only close the dura mater.

In all cases, the dura is closed in a watertight fashion with a 5-0 nonabsorbable running suture. A duraplasty should be carried out if only a biopsy was possible. In the case of laminotomy, the bone is replaced, taking care to prevent any spinal cord compression. Spacers can sometimes be useful for increasing the spinal canal volume. Wound drain without suction is placed in the muscular layer for 2 days. Paraspinal muscles are reapproximated with sutures. The fascia is, on the other hand, tightly closed with a running resorbable suture. Subcutaneous tissue and skin are closed in two layers. When surgery is performed at the cervical level, the patient is progressively awakened and extubated in the intensive care unit where he or she stays for monitoring for one night. If the lesion is at the thoracic level, the patient is awakened and extubated in the operating room and placed in the recovery room for a few hours before going back to the hospital floor.

Postoperative Course

Patients are often aware of the temporary decrement in sensory and motor deficits below the level of the lesion and must be reassured that recovery is possible and likely. They also receive analgesics and anti-inflammatory drugs to alleviate often distressing but temporary pain in the limbs and spine. Early postoperative mobilization is advocated to achieve better functional results.

Results

Mortality Rate and Complications

In our personal study of 440 patients with spinal cord tumors, the early surgical mortality rate was 1.6%, and it was 0% from the last 225 cases. Surgical complications have no effect on the mortality rate. These complications include the following: hematoma at the operative site or epidural hematoma, arachnoiditis, sepsis, meningocele, CSF fistulas, pulmonary embolism, perforated gastric ulcer, and cervical kyphosis after laminectomy.

The risk of *postlaminectomy spinal deformity* is well known, especially in children. Risk factors often responsible for postoperative deformities are young age, the presence of preoperative spinal deformity, cervical laminectomy including C2, laminectomy involving at least six vertebrae, anterior and posterior column involvement, and malignant neoplasm. In order to reduce this risk, injury to the facet joints should be avoided. In children, osteoplastic laminotomy is an option that should be considered; however, it does not assure spinal stability in all patients. Close clinical and radiological monitoring until the end of the child's growth period is suggested.

Functional Results

Upon awakening from surgery, many patients are very anxious and complain of discomfort, more so than for any other surgical procedures. Indeed, patients may feel pain everywhere, and suffer diffuse hyperesthesias and paresthesias. They may avoid movement because their position sense is affected. Muscle and spinal pain complete this clinical picture, which lasts for several days and is unfortunately not uniformly responsive to the usual analgesic drugs. The severity of the postoperative picture is closely tied to the extent of surgery.

Prior to discharge, a basic functional evaluation is performed according to the four-tier system proposed by McCormick and colleagues[29] to document and follow motor and sensory function over time. Immediately after surgery, it is not unusual for nearly all patients to worsen in comparison to their preoperative status. They should be aware that these deficits may be transitory and are not related to their long-term outcome. However, at 3 months, the neurological situation becomes more or less definitive.

The postoperative outcome based on 3 months after surgery is correlated with the preoperative one. We have seen, according to the McCormick's preoperative levels, the following outcomes:

- In preoperative grade I patients, 95% were unchanged and 5% worsened.
- In preoperative grade II patients, 7% improved, 86% were unchanged, and 7% worsened.
- In preoperative grade III patients, 28% improved, 53% were unchanged, and 19% worsened.
- In preoperative grade IV patients, none except one child improved. Most remained unchanged.

Our results confirm that SCIMTs, if possible, be operated on at clinical grade I or II to attain the best results.

Follow-up

Within 48 hours of surgery, all patients undergo an early MRI examination. This is of particular importance to show any residual tumor and as a basis of assessment for subsequent lesion progression or recurrence during the patient's follow-up. Diagnosis of residual tumor is easily made when the lesion was enhanced after contrast injection prior to surgery. However, the diagnosis becomes more difficult if there was no enhancement preoperatively. In those patients the determination is often based primarily on the persistence of areas of hyperintense signal on T2-WI. We recommend seeing the patient for an MRI examination on a yearly basis. Even when the tumor has been completely removed, subsequent examinations are still necessary to exclude any tumor recurrence for several years.

Relevance of Radiotherapy

It is our opinion there is no indication for radiotherapy (RT) in benign SCIMTs even after incomplete removal, recurrence, or progression. Our personal opinion is based on a follow-up for over 5 years in 193 patients who had surgery either on a low-grade ependymoma (122 patients) or on a low-grade astrocytoma (71 patients), without adjunctive RT. We observed 5 recurrences (3 astrocytomas after respectively

5, 6, and 7 years and 2 ependymomas after 18 and 19 years) in those whose tumors were completely removed (110 ependymomas and 29 astrocytomas).

In fact, in our series, even low-grade astrocytomas that were partially removed have a very indolent evolution. Seventeen tumors remained stable in spite of partial removal; a few showed a slow MRI evolution without any clinical consequences. Furthermore, we have faced very difficult technical challenges when reoperating on several patients sent from other institutions who had previously received RT after biopsy or partial removal. All have worsened after our surgery in contrast to those who did not receive RT. When we are facing a recurrence or tumor progression in an astrocytoma, without any option for reoperation, we prefer to start with chemotherapy first (temozolamide). Unfortunately, in malignant gliomas the treatment is still only palliative such as with brain tumors. Contrary to low-grade spinal astrocytomas, in which we do not recommend postoperative adjunct RT, we recommend it, as do others,[115] for malignant spinal gliomas. Regardless of which treatments are used—repeated surgery, radiation, or chemotherapy—the prognosis is poor and the disease is usually fatal in 9 months to 4 years.

CONCLUSIONS

Microsurgical excision of most SIEMTs and SCIMTs yields a good prognosis by an experienced team, especially because many of these tumors are benign and are amenable to resection.

Surgery is the initial and primary treatment of choice in most spinal cord tumors. The main objective should be preserving the patient's functional condition. Postoperative results depend on the preoperative neurological status, the tumor grade, tumor location, and the surgical team's experience.

SELECTED KEY REFERENCES

Bruneau M, George B. Surgical technique for the resection of tumors in relation with the V1 and V2 segments of the vertebral artery. In: George B, Bruneau M, Spetzler RF, eds. *Pathology and Surgery Around the Vertebral Artery.* Paris: Springer; 2010, Chap. 14.

Fisher G, Brotchi J. *Intramedullary Spinal Cord Tumors.* New York: Thieme; 1996.

Klekamp J, Samii M. Extramedullary tumors. In: Klekamp J, Samii M, eds. *Surgery of Spinal Tumors.* Berlin: Springer; 2007:143-320.

Klekamp J, Samii M. Intramedullary tumors. In: Klekamp J, Samii M, eds. *Surgery of Spinal Tumors.* Berlin: Springer Verlag; 2007:120-131.

McCormick PC, Torres R, Post KD, et al. Intramedullary ependymoma of the spinal cord. *J Neurosurg.* 1990;72(4):523-532.

Please go to expertconsult.com to view a complete list of references.

26 Treatment of Spinal Metastatic Tumors

Ilya Laufer, Marcella A. Madera, Daniel Sciubba, Ziya L. Gokaslan

CLINICAL PEARLS

- Histology plays paramount role in determination of tumor treatment. After a thorough radiological evaluation of the extent of systemic and spinal disease, a percutaneous computed tomography–guided biopsy is frequently the next step in the diagnostic algorithm, because 10% to 20% of the spine metastases have no known primary source. Determination of tumor histological type is of critical importance in determining the appropriate subsequent treatment.

- Treatment of metastatic spine tumors optimally requires a multidisciplinary approach that involves surgeons, radiation and medical oncologists, radiologists, and rehabilitation medicine physicians. However, the general treatment goal of patients with spinal metastases is palliation, because spinal metastases usually signal advanced metastatic disease with little hope of cure. Mechanical instability and high-grade cord compression secondary to solid tumors may require surgical decompression and stabilization as part of the palliative plan as long as survival time anticipated from the systemic neoplastic disease is greater than 3 months.

- The choice of surgical strategy and approach for spinal metastases remains predicated on the surgeon's comfort, training, and experience. The definition of mechanical instability in patients with metastatic spinal tumors

has recently been elucidated by an expert panel. The same stability classification used in trauma should not be applied to metastatic cases. Movement-related pain or pain relieved with recumbence may be considered to be a symptom of instability. Lytic lesions, subluxation and progressive deformity, extension into the posterior elements, and lesions that occupy more than 50% of the vertebral body and are accompanied by loss of height are also judged to be associated with instability. These symptoms and signs of instability and progressive neurological compromise may lead the treatment team to recommend surgical stabilization.

- When a ventral surgical approach for decompression and stabilization is employed, an anterior plate spanning one level above and one level below the vertebrectomy defect is generally used in order to buttress the cage or cement reconstruction. In posterior decompression, lateral mass or pedicle instrumentation is usually employed, spanning at least two levels above and below the tumor.

- Stereotactic spinal radiosurgery may provide excellent tumor control rates in radioresistant tumors. Radiosensitive tumors, such as lymphoma, multiple myeloma, plasmacytoma, and small cell lung carcinoma may be treated with radiation therapy even in the presence of cord compression.

Physicians will make over 1.5 million new diagnoses of cancer in 2010 in the United States, and over 500,000 people are expected to die from cancer in 2010 [fact sheet 2010]. Five-year survival rates in patients with cancer have improved to 68% (1999-2005) from 50% (1975-1977) as treatment techniques have advanced [fact sheet 2010]. Spine metastases, the most common site of bone metastasis, occur in 30% to 90% of terminal cancer patients.[1-3] As patients continue to live longer with cancer, it is likely that spine metastatic disease rates will continue to climb.

The most common primary tumors that give rise to spine metastases are breast, lung, and prostate cancers, reflecting the high prevalence of these tumors.[3] These primary tumors

may spread to the spine through the arterial or venous systems, by direct extension, or via cerebrospinal fluid (CSF). Hematogenous spread (arterial or venous) is thought to be the most common route by which primary tumors metastasize to the spine. Because the vertebral bodies have an extensive arterial blood supply, tumor cells from distant primary lesions can travel to the spine and initiate metastatic disease.[4] Venous spread occurs by flow through Batson's plexus, the longitudinal network of valveless veins that connects vertebral veins with many venous beds (caval, portal, azygous, intercostal, pulmonary, and renal). Primary tumors may also spread by direct extension; lung cancer can extend posteriorly to the thoracic spine or superiorly to the cervical spine. Pelvic or abdominal cancers (prostate, bladder, and colorectal) can locally invade the lumbar or sacral spine. Metastasis through the CSF can occur spontaneously or after surgery for brain lesions. Multicentric disease (i.e., tumor in multiple vertebrae) can result from any of these mechanisms of spread.

The location of spine metastases may be extradural, intradural-extramedullary, and intramedullary, with most occurring in the extradural space. This spread is usually in the vertebral body and may include extension to the posterior elements. The extradural compartment also includes the epidural space and paravertebral space, both of which can contain tumor as it extends from bone. The most common levels for spine metastases, in descending order of frequency, are the thoracic, lumbar, cervical, and sacral regions of the spine. Intradural metastases, whether intra- or extramedullary, are very rare but result from spread through the CSF.

PRESENTATION

Metastatic tumors can cause any neurological or structural symptom associated with spine pathology in general. The spine not only protects the neural elements but also provides mechanical support to the body. Pathology in the spine can affect either or both of these basic functions of the spine. Loss of integrity of the spine due to metastasis may cause the patient back pain, radicular pain, paresis, paralysis, numbness, bowel or bladder dysfunction, myelopathy, fractures, or spinal deformity. In addition to spine-related symptoms, patients with metastatic disease may have global symptoms such as weight loss, fatigue, and other organ system abnormalities.

Pain

Pain, the most common first presenting symptom of spine metastasis, can have different mechanisms depending on the tumor's interaction with the bony spine or the neural elements, and 83% to 95% of patients with spinal metastases complain of pain. Because pain often precedes other neurological symptoms, it should be carefully evaluated by clinicians.[5,6] If tumor compresses a nerve root, pain that is burning and radiates down the leg in a dermatomal distribution (radicular pain) is a common symptom. If tumor causes a pathological fracture or collapse of a vertebral body, that collapse can narrow the foramina and cause radicular pain, or it may cause mechanical pain. Mechanical pain typically is worse with loading of the spine during sitting or standing, and it often does not improve with anti-inflammatory medications. Local or biological pain may also be experienced by patients with spine metastases; it is usually described as a deep ache that is worse at night. This type of pain can improve with anti-inflammatory medications or corticosteroids, and it is likely due to inflammation in the spine due to the presence of tumor. Tenderness to palpation over the spine may be evident on physical examination due to local pain from periosteal stretching and inflammation. Treatment of spine metastases often includes a goal of treatment of the patient's pain, and the type of pain a patient experiences may guide that treatment. Local pain is often palliated with radiation treatment; mechanical pain may be best addressed with bracing or surgical stabilization.

Neurological Dysfunction

The second most common group of symptoms that patients with spinal metastases complain of is neurological deficit.[7] Weakness in upper or lower extremities may result from epidural compression of the spinal cord, individual nerve roots, or the cauda equina by tumor. Tumor or fractured bone fragments may impinge on neural structures, and patients may also complain of autonomic problems including bowel, bladder (usually urinary retention), or sexual dysfunction. Asking patients directly about these problems should be routine, as the symptoms might not be revealed on initial history gathering. Without treatment, motor dysfunction usually progresses to paralysis. Dermatomal changes in sensation, including anesthesia, hyperesthesia, and parasthesia, usually occur with motor dysfunction and pain. Patients with spinal cord compression may complain of sensory abnormalities in a band-like distribution across the chest or abdomen. Myelopathy also results in hyperreflexia from chronic spinal cord compression. Diagnosis before these neurological deficits occur is important because neurological prognosis is related to the amount of neurological function at the time of diagnosis.[4] Pain is usually experienced before a neurological deficit, but because of the extremely common prevalence of back pain in the general population, metastatic spine disease can be missed until deficit occurs. Any patient with a known history of cancer and a new complaint of back or neck pain should be thoroughly evaluated for spinal metastatic disease. As the thoracic spine is the most common location for metastasis to the spine, and degenerative problems there are less common, pain in the thoracic spine should cue clinicians to consider a neoplastic process in patients with new-onset thoracic pain.

DIAGNOSIS

Patients with a newly diagnosed spinal lesion require a thorough diagnostic workup, which begins with a history and physical examination. Patients without cancer diagnosis require a standard evaluation and management of back pain, which would likely include initial observation and conservative treatment without extensive imaging or invasive diagnostic procedures. However, certain signs and symptoms may increase the probability of a neoplastic process and merit a more aggressive initial evaluation. Fatigue and unintended weight loss may result from a systemic process such as cancer. Furthermore, history of human immunodeficiency virus (HIV), chronic inflammatory conditions, smoking, hazardous occupational exposures, and familial cancer history increases the likelihood of a neoplasm. Nocturnal or morning back pain elevates the suspicion for neoplasm, and progressive pain during the course of the day is generally more indicative of degenerative lesions. In patients with a previous diagnosis of cancer, any back pain or neurological deficit should prompt a diagnostic evaluation in order to determine if the patient harbors any metastatic lesions. Prior to any decision regarding treatment, a thorough oncological staging evaluation must be performed according to the histology-specific protocols. Hematological, electrolyte, endocrinological, and cancer marker aberrations may aid in the diagnosis of tumor histological type and stage.

Imaging Studies

Plain radiographs often serve as an initial imaging evaluation of a patient with back pain, owing to their low cost and widespread availability. These studies may help in identifying significant abnormalities such as compression fractures, scoliosis, large lytic or sclerotic osseous lesions, and radiopaque extraossous lesions. However, in order to be apparent on plain radiographs, the lesions must reach a significant size, thereby making these studies a fairly insensitive modality in tumor diagnosis.[8] Although radiographs may be an appropriate initial study in patients without history of cancer, they should not be used as a screening or diagnostic modality in patients with an elevated suspicion of spine tumors.

Multidetector computed tomography (CT) scanners provide a rapid high-resolution image of the spine and surrounding structures. The availability of two- and three-dimensional reconstructions allows easy localization and visualization of lesions that are hyper- or hypodense in relation to the surrounding structures. The lesions appear lytic, sclerotic, or mixed and this information may aid in the determination of the potential stability of the spine. The great definition of the osseous anatomy also aids in operative planning, allowing precise measurements of the screw length and diameter suitable for each vertebral body, as well as the trajectory of the screw insertion. CT imaging is also invaluable in imaging instrumentation position and the degree of osseous fusion. Finally, injection of dye into the subarachnoid space during CT myelography allows precise definition of the CSF surrounding the cord and nerve roots. This technique is invaluable in diagnosing neural element compression in the setting of instrumentation that creates ferromagnetic artifact on magnetic resonance imaging (MRI) or in patients who cannot undergo MRI. It has become a standard component of treatment planning for spine stereotactic radiosurgery in patients with spinal hardware.

Universal nuclear body scans have become a standard component of histological staging for certain cancers. Nuclear scintigraphy (bone scan) permits detection of osseous remodeling throughout the skeletal system and has been reported to have 62% to 89% sensitivity in detection of spinal metastases.[9] However, it is not specific for neoplasms and cannot differentiate tumors from regions of infection and inflammation. Furthermore, in order for a neoplasm to be detected on a bone scan, active osseous remodeling must be taking place, which is not always the case in sclerotic neoplasms. Single-photon emission computed tomography (SPECT) permits improved differentiation of neoplastic from inflammatory processes, because it detects the metabolic components of the lesion.[10,11] It allows three-dimensional imaging of the lesion with sensitivity and specificity superior to standard bone scans. Finally, positron emission tomography (PET) using fluoride-18 (^{18}F-PET) and ^{18}F-fluorodeoxyglucose (^{18}FDG-PET) provides a sensitive screening modality for neoplastic lesions through the body. ^{18}F-PET detects regions of fluoride uptake and thereby skeletal remodeling. ^{18}FDG-PET detects regions of high glucose uptake in the skeletal system and the soft tissues, thereby detecting hypermetabolic lesions that may signify a neoplastic, degenerative, inflammatory, or infectious process. However, correlation with concomitant MRI and CT scans generally allows high diagnostic specificity. Furthermore, ^{18}FDG-PET has been shown to be a highly sensitive and specific screening modality in patients with solid tumors harboring spinal lytic and mixed lesions.[12] The decreased sensitivity of ^{18}FDG-PET in detection of sclerotic lesions may be associated with the acellular and therefore low metabolic nature of these lesions. PET imaging may also aid in the selection of biopsy targets in the setting of multiple lesions, because lesions with higher metabolic activity will likely produce higher diagnostic yield due to their high cellularity.

MRI remains the gold standard in spine imaging and in detection of spinal metastases. MRI has superior sensitivity and specificity in screening for vertebral metastases, allowing precise delineation of their size, quantity, and location. It furthermore provides thorough information about the surrounding soft tissues that include the spinal cord and nerve roots, ligaments, meninges, interverterbal disks, and paraspinal musculature. In addition to the standard T1- and T2-weighted sequences with gadolinium injection, fat suppression and diffusion-weighted sequences may provide additional information about the acuity and etiology of visualized fractures. MRI allows excellent visualization of the spinal cord and nerve roots and any compression that may result from epidural tumor extension. T2 hyperintensity of the cord signifies cord edema and may indicate increased severity of compression.

Percutaneous CT-guided biopsy is a frequent step in the diagnostic algorithm, because 10% to 20% of the spine metastases have no known source and determination of tumor histological type is of paramount importance in determining the appropriate treatment.[13] Furthermore, in patients with distant cancer history a biopsy may be required in order to rule out a second malignancy. Modern large-bore needle biopsy techniques have excellent diagnostic yield and are generally performed as an outpatient procedure. Caution must be exercised when interpreting negative biospsies of blastic lesions, because they may be falsely negative owing to their acellular nature. Such patients may merit additional follow-up in order to monitor these lesions clinically and radiographically.

Metastases that originate from hypervascular primary tumors generally require preoperative digital subtraction angiography and embolization. Angiography allows evaluation of the vascularity and the blood supply of the tumor and delineation of the location of the artery of Adamkiewitz. Renal, thyroid, hepatocellular, neuroendocrine tumors and tumors that contain "angio" or "hemangio" in their name should generally undergo angiography and embolization when possible. Complete and even partial preoperative embolization of vascular tumors has been shown to significantly decrease intraoperative blood loss.[14-16]

MANAGEMENT

Advances in modern surgical technique, radiation delivery technology, and pharmacotherapy have extended the life expectancy and improved the life quality of cancer patients. Today, treatment of metastatic spine tumors requires a multidisciplinary approach that involves surgeons, radiation and medical oncologists, radiologists, and rehabilitation medicine physicians. However, the general treatment goal of patients with spinal metastases is palliation, because spinal metastases usually signal advanced metastatic disease with little hope of cure. Thus, patients succumb to systemic complications of visceral metastases and successful treatment of metastatic spinal tumors has not been convincingly shown to extend survival. The explicit goals of treatment of spinal metastatic tumors include preservation or restoration of neurological function, spinal stability and pain control, with minimal hospital stay and morbidity.

Modern treatment paradigms must incorporate surgical, radiation, and chemotherapeutic treatment options. One of the suggested treatment frameworks incorporates four considerations: neurological, oncological, mechanical, and systemic (NOMS).[17] Spinal metastases frequently present with epidural extension resulting in cord and nerve root compression. The degree of epidural extension may dictate the possible treatment options, with patients with high-grade cord compression and myelopathy usually requiring surgical decompression. Several grading schemes have been used in the metastatic literature in order to describe the degree of epidural tumor extension. The Weinstein-Boriani-Biagini staging system divides the vertebral body into 12 radiating zones and five concentric layers in the axial plane.[18] However, this system was initially designed to describe primary spinal tumors, and its application in the treatment of spinal metastases relies on the assumption that similar surgical principles may be applied to primary and metastatic tumors. A 6-point scale devised specifically for the purpose of describing the degree of epidural spinal cord compression secondary to spinal metastases was recently validated by the Spinal Oncology Study Group (SOSG).[19] In this scale, the grade of 0 is assigned to bone only lesions, grade 1 is assigned to lesions with epidural extension but without cord compression, grade 2 is assigned to lesions causing cord compression but with CSF still visible around the cord, and grade 3 is assigned to lesions causing cord compression without CSF visible around the cord. Grade 1 lesions are further subdivided into three categories depending on the degree of epidural extension. Grades 2 and 3 tumors may result in neurological deficits and myelopathy and, with the exception of very radiosensitive tumors, generally require surgical decompression.

Tumor histological type plays a crucial role in appropriate selection of therapy. Small cell lung carcinoma and hematological malignancies such as lymphoma and plasmacytoma are exquisitely sensitive to radiation therapy and chemotherapy, and therefore usually do not require surgical decompression.[20] Solid metastatic tumors display a range of radiosensitivity, with breast cancer being moderately sensitive, colon and non-small cell lung carcinomas being moderately resistant, and thyroid, renal, melanoma, and sarcoma metastases being highly radioresistant. The degree of radiosensitivity and the aggressive nature of the tumors should play an important role in determining the type of radiation treatment and the degree of surgical intervention that the patient will receive. Thus, a radiosensitive tumor without high-grade cord compression may respond well to conventional external beam radiation therapy (cEBRT) and not require surgical intervention, but a radioresistant tumor will likely require an operation in order to decompress the spinal cord and to provide adequate space between the tumor and the cord in order to deliver stereotactic radiosurgery (SRS). Of course, each patient and each case of metastatic tumor must be analyzed on its individual clinical characteristics and the collective evaluation and experience of the treating team of physicians and surgeons.

Metastatic tumors frequently invade and weaken the vertebral bodies and pedicles, thereby undermining the mechanical stability of the spine. Radiation therapy and chemotherapy cannot restore spinal stability, and patients who manifest evidence of instability require instrumented stabilization, regardless of tumor histological type or their neurological status. The definition of mechanical instability in patients with metastatic spinal tumors remains controversial. Previous definitions of spinal instability in the setting of metastatic disease relied on the three-column spinal model developed by Denis and attempted to modify this model in order to apply it to cancer patients.[21] However, the Denis model was developed to define instability in the setting of spinal trauma and the mechanics and the extent of injury to the osseous and ligamentous structures, as well as the healing potential, are drastically different in the settings of trauma and spinal metastases. Activity-related neck or back pain is generally accepted as one of the defining symptoms of mechanical instability. The SOSG expert panel has recently defined *spine instability* as "loss of spinal integrity as a result of a neoplastic process that is associated with movement-related pain, symptomatic or progressive deformity, or neural compromise under physiological loads."[22] The panel developed a 6-point Spine Instability Neoplastic Score (SINS), which incorporates multiple radiographic parameters in addition to the presence of mechanical pain (Table 26.1). Junctional tumor location was considered to be the most unstable, followed by the mobile (C3-C6, L2-L4), semirigid (T3-T10), and rigid spine (S2-S5). Movement-related pain or pain relieved with recumbence was considered to be a symptom of instability. Lytic lesions, subluxation and progressive deformity, extension into the posterior elements, and lesions that occupy more than 50% of the vertebral body and are accompanied by loss of height were also judged to be associated with instability.

Finally, the systemic considerations must be taken into account when determining the optimal treatment plan for the patient. The extent of medical comorbid conditions and systemic tumor burden must not preclude the patient from undergoing general anesthesia and surgery that will likely last for several hours and may include significant blood loss and hemodynamic shifts. Furthermore, it is generally accepted that the life expectancy of the patient should exceed 3 months in order to justify surgical intervention.

Surgery

The most convincing data supporting surgical decompression resulted from a prospective randomized trial conducted by Patchell and associates.[23] The trial included patients with solid metastatic spinal tumors causing spinal cord compression, which was defined as any degree of cord displacement. The patients had to have at least one neurological sign or symptom, which may have been pain, and could not be paraplegic longer than 48 hours. The trial excluded patients with radiosensitive tumors such as hematological and germ cell malignancies and patients with previous radiation that precluded the study radiation dose. Patients were randomized to two trial groups: the first group received 30 Gy fractionated radiation therapy and the second group first underwent surgical decompression followed by radiation. The study was stopped at the midpoint of the enrollment owing to the clear superiority of the surgery group

TABLE 26.1 Spine Instability Neoplastic Score (SINS)

Location	
Junctional (occiput-C2, C7-T2, T11-L1, L5-S1)	3
Mobile spine (C3-C6, L2-L4)	2
Semirigid (T3-T10)	1
Rigid (S2-S5)	0
Pain	
Yes	3
Occasional pain but not mechanical	1
Pain-free lesion	0
Bone lesion	
Lytic	2
Mixed (lytic/blastic)	1
Blastic	0
Radiographic spinal alignment	
Subluxation/translation present	4
De novo deformity (kyphosis/scoliosis)	2
Normal alignment	0
Vertebral body collapse	
>50% collapse	3
<50% collapse	2
No collapse with >50% body involved	1
None of the above	0
Posterolateral involvement of spinal elements	
Bilateral	3
Unilateral	1
None of the above	0
Status	**Total Score**
Stable	0-6
Indeterminate	7-12
Unstable	13-18

Adapted from Fisher CG, DiPaola CP, Ryken TC, et al. A novel classification system for spinal instability in neoplastic disease: an evidence-based approach and expert consensus from the Spine Oncology Study Group. *Spine.* 2010;35(22):E1221-1229.

in the ability to ambulate, duration of ambulation, maintenance of continence, decreased use of opioids and corticosteroids, and extended survival. The limitations of the study include randomization of patients with instability to the radiation arm as well as the surgery arm, outdated spinal stability criteria, low benchmark for ambulation (only four steps), and lack of requirement for instrumented stabilization in the surgery arm.

Several grading systems have been devised in order to tailor the extent of surgical intervention to the expected survival of the patient. Tomita and colleagues proposed a 10-point scale that considered three prognostic factors: tumor histological type, the extent of visceral metastases, and the number of skeletal metastases.[24] They recommended that patients with slowly growing tumors (breast, thyroid) and moderately growing tumors (renal, uterus) and solitary spine metastases undergo en bloc tumor excision. Patients with rapidly growing tumors (lung, stomach) and patients with more extensive visceral and skeletal burden were recommended a spectrum of intralesional excision, palliative decompression, or supportive care. Tokuhashi and co-workers proposed a similar scale which in addition to the above-mentioned factors included the general performance status of the patient and the extent of neurological deficits.[25] They used these factors in order to estimate the expected survival and recommended that

patients with longer than 1-year survival should undergo excisional surgery (goal of en bloc spondylectomy), and patients with expected survival between 6 months and 1 year should undergo palliative surgery (piecemeal cord decompression and stabilization).

The choice of surgical strategy and approach for spinal metastases remains predicated on the surgeon's comfort and training. The vertebral body represents the most common site of spinal metastases. Thus, anterior approaches often provide the most direct access to these tumors. The transcervical approach provides direct access to the subaxial cervical spine and most spine surgeons are facile with this approach. The transoral and transmandibular approaches have been traditionally used in order to access the craniocervical junction and the atlantoaxial spine; however, recently transnasal and transcervical approaches have also been employed in order to access these regions. Manubriotomy, sternotomy, or the trapdoor approach may be required in order to provide ventral access to the upper thoracic spine (T1-T4). However, the great vessels and mediastinal contents generally complicate ventral access to the upper thoracic spine. The above-mentioned complex anterior approaches to the craniocervical junction and the upper thoracic areas are generally used in order to treat primary tumors, since the palliative nature of metastatic tumor treatment rarely justifies the potential morbidity of these approaches. A thoracotomy provides direct vertebral body access at the T5-L1 levels.[26,27] Access to T5-T7 usually requires sacrifice of the rib one level above the target vertebral level, and access to T8-L1 requires sacrifice of the rib two levels above. In order to visualize T11-L1 vertebral bodies, the diaphragm usually has to be reflected. The retroperitoneal approach provides ventral access to L2-L5 and sacral regions. Head and neck, thoracic, general, and vascular surgeons may be required to provide these ventral approaches, and are recommended if the patient had previous radiation, anterior surgery, or extensive tumor burden ventral to the spine.

Patients with limited lung capacity and previous neck, thoracic, or abdominal surgery or radiation may not be optimal candidates for anterior approach surgery. Posterior approaches provide direct access to the spinal cord and thereby allow direct decompression without extensive osseous work.[28,29] While the posterior approach is rarely employed in order to access cervical vertebral bodies, costotransversectomy and transpedicular approaches provide access to the thoracic and lumbar vertebral bodies. In the thoracic spine, nerve roots below T2 may be sacrificed in order to obtain posterolateral access to the anterior column. In the lumbar spine, the nerve roots must be preserved and may be retracted medially in order to provide ventral access.

Combined anterior and posterior approaches may be implemented in order to achieve circumferential cord decompression and spinal reconstruction. Although en bloc tumor resection may be achieved via a posterior approach in the lumbar spine, a combined anterior-posterior approach is generally required in the thoracic spine. Combined approaches are generally associated with higher surgical morbidity.[30]

Vertebral body reconstruction may be accomplished with the help of Steinman pins with polymethylmethacrylate (PMMA), PMMA in a chest tube, mesh or expandable titanium cages, or polyetheretherketone (PEEK) cages.[31]

When a ventral approach is employed, an anterior plate spanning one level above and one level below the vertebrectomy defect is generally used in order to buttress the cage or cement reconstruction. In posterior decompression, posterolateral lateral mass or pedicle instrumentation is usually employed, spanning at least two levels above and below the tumor.

Vertebroplasty/Kyphoplasty

Vertebroplasty involves injection of PMMA into the vertebral body through a percutaneously placed transpedicular needle. During kyphoplasty, prior to PMMA injection, a balloon is inflated inside the vertebral body in order to attempt to restore vertebral body height. Both procedures have been shown to successfully control back pain in patients with spinal metastases. The suggested mechanisms of action include thermoablation of pain receptors secondary to the heat dissipated by the injected cement and to partial restoration of stability in a fractured vertebral body. Patients with back pain but without cord compression or gross instability that requires surgical stabilization may undergo vertebroplasty or kyphoplasty in order to provide pain relief in conjunction with radiation or medical therapy. Although successful tumor treatment with radiation may provide eventual pain control after several weeks, vertebroplasty generally has an instantaneous or rapid onset of effect. Extravasation of the cement into the vasculature or into the spinal canal represents the largest proportion of procedure-related complications. Furthermore, cement may embolize into the lungs and other distal organs. However, these are generally radiographic findings without clinical consequences. In a series of 56 patients, 84% reported significant or complete pain relief without significant complications related to the procedure.[32] Furthermore, prophylactic vertebroplasty may be performed in patients undergoing stereotactic radiosurgery.[33] This may be an appropriate treatment in patients with lytic lesions that occupy a large portion of the vertebral body who are at high risk for fracture after radiation treatment.

ADJUVANT THERAPIES

Radiation Therapy

Modern radiation therapy allows precise and safe delivery of radiation to spinal tumors, and available treatments range from conventional fractionated schemes to high-dose stereotactic radiosurgery. Maranzano and Latini prospectively evaluated 209 patients with a wide range of primary histological types that received cEBRT with a dose of 30 Gy in two fractionation schemes. Seventy-six percent of patients were ambulatory after treatment, with 51% of nonambulatory patients regaining ambulation.[34] Importantly, the results varied dramatically, depending on the histological type, with breast, lymphoma, and plasmacytoma responding to radiation much better than liver, bladder, or renal cancers. Thus, cEBRT remains an important treatment component for radiosensitive tumors, whether used as primary treatment or as a postoperative adjunct. Because cEBRT delivers radiation to a wide field surrounding the tumor, it is important to wait at least 2 to 4 weeks prior to initiating postoperative radiation in order to avoid wound-healing complications. Furthermore, preoperative cEBRT has been shown to be associated with significant elevation in the wound complication rate.

Tumors that display poor response to conventional fractionated schemes generally respond well to single-fraction high-dose therapy delivered during spinal stereotactic radiosurgery treatments. Gerszten and associates used CyberKnife technology to treat 60 renal cell carcinoma spinal metastases, most of which failed cEBRT.[35] Pain control was achieved in 89% of the treated cases. Subsequently, a larger series that included 93 renal metastases, treated by the same group, displayed an 87% radiographic tumor control rate.[36] The same series also included 38 melanoma lesions, which showed 96% pain control and 75% radiographic control rates. Furthermore, Yamada and colleagues prospectively followed 103 radioresistant metastatic tumors treated with image-guided radiation therapy (IGRT).[37] The overall actuarial tumor control rate was 90% after a median follow-up of 15 months, with tumors receiving 24-Gy single-fraction treatments showing better control rates than tumors that received lower doses. Spinal stereotactic radiotherapy allows delivery of high doses of tumoricidal radiation with outstanding spatial precision, generally requiring as little as 2 mm between the cord and the tumor. Furthermore, patients may undergo spinal stereotactic radiosurgery shortly before or after surgery without the wound complications associated with cEBRT.[38]

Chemotherapy

Advancements in chemotherapeutic agents have played a large role in prolongation of survival and occasional cure of many cancers. However, spine metastases generally appear to be resistant to chemotherapy and represent a manifestation of advanced cancer with multiple systemic metastases. However, certain tumor histological types such as superior sulcus tumors, germ cell tumors, high-risk neuroblastomas, Ewing's sarcomas, and osteogenic sarcomas have been shown to benefit from neoadjuvant chemotherapy followed by resection.[39-41] Neoadjuvant therapy with etoposide and cisplatin has dramatically improved the potential for negative-margin resection of superior sulcus non-small cell lung tumors and has improved survival.[39]

In patients with breast or prostate cancer antihormone therapy has been shown to successfully treat patients with appropriate hormone receptors expressed by their tumors. Letrozole, anastrozole, and exemestane, which are aromatase inhibitors, and tamoxifen, which is a selective estrogen receptor modulator (SERM), have been effective against breast tumors.[42] Androgen suppression with gonadotropin-releasing hormone (GnRH) and flutamide has been successful in treating men with prostate cancer.[43] Unfortunately, spine metastases generally occur during or after treatment with these agents and are therefore tumor clones that are resistant to hormone therapy.

Bisphosphonates

Cancer patients frequently have poor bone quality secondary to radiation, chemotherapy, long-term glucocorticoid therapy, decreased activity, and advanced age. Furthermore, many spine metastases manifest as lytic vertebral lesions, thereby predisposing patients to pathological fractures. Bisphosphones, which inhibit osteoclastic activity and suppress bone resorption, have been shown to reduce the fracture risk, relieve local pain, and decrease hypercalcemia in patients with breast cancer, multiple myeloma, and other lytic histological types.[44]

Corticosteroids

Corticosteroids remain an integral part of pharmacotherapy in patients with spinal metastases. Their anti-inflammatory effects provide pain relief in patients with biological tumor-related back pain. Furthermore, they may reduce cord edema secondary to cord compression and have been shown to improve neurological function in animal models of metastatic cord compression.[45,46] Initial animal studies used very high doses (96 mg/day), but further studies failed to show a difference in functional outcome after treatment with high (100 mg) and low (10 mg) doses.[47] Furthermore, in lymphoma and multiple myeloma patients, corticosteroids play a role in oncolytic treatment of the tumors.

Analgesia

Patients with spinal metastases exhibit a broad range of pain syndromes that may be associated with tumor-related inflammation, instability, or compression of the spinal cord or nerve roots. Inflammation may be effectively treated with steroids, which may be weaned after treatment with radiation or chemotherapy. Mechanical pain or symptomatic cord compression generally requires surgery. However, in patients who are not surgical candidates analgesia plays an important role in their management and may be the primary goal of palliative treatment of hospice patients. Analgesics are generally administered in a stepwise fashion, with a spectrum from nonsteroidal anti-inflammatory drugs (NSAIDs) to potent opioids and from oral to intravenous delivery. In the treatment of neuropathic pain, anticonvulsants, neuroleptics, and topical lidocaine may be more successful than opioids. In more severe pain syndromes, rhizotomy, cryoablation, or intrathecal delivery of opioids may be required. Many of the above-mentioned medications may result in alteration of mental status, sedation, gastrointestinal complications such as nausea and constipation, and physical dependency.

CONCLUSIONS

Current treatment of spinal metastases requires a multidisciplinary approach in order to optimize therapy for individual tumor histological types. Although many tumors require surgical intervention to restore spinal stability or to provide cord decompression, radiation and chemotherapy may successfully treat other tumors, thereby avoiding surgery. Surgeons must be facile with anterior, posterior, and lateral approaches and a wide range of surgical techniques that include spinal instrumentation and microsurgical, minimally invasive, open and percutaneous techniques in order to tailor the operation to each patient. Furthermore, fractionated, hypofractionated, and single-fraction radiation schemes and various radiation delivery methods provide a broad range of radiation therapies available for the treatment of spinal metastases. Future research directions include standardization of indications for surgery and radiation, prospectively collected evidence evaluating the quality of life after treatment of spinal metastases, and further refinement of surgical and radiation technology and of chemotherapy in order to provide curative treatment of cancer.

SELECTED KEY REFERENCES

Fisher CG, DiPaola CP, Ryken TC, et al. A novel classification system for spinal instability in neoplastic disease: an evidence-based approach and expert consensus from the Spine Oncology Study Group. *Spine*. 2010;35(22):E1221-E1229.

Fourney DR, Gokaslan ZL. Anterior approaches for thoracolumbar metastatic spine tumors. *Neurosurg Clin North Am*. 2004;15(4):443-451.

Gerszten PC, Burton SA, Ozhasoglu C, Welch WC. Radiosurgery for spinal metastases: clinical experience in 500 cases from a single institution. *Spine*. 2007;32(2):193-199.

Gokaslan ZL, York JE, Walsh GL, et al. Transthoracic vertebrectomy for metastatic spinal tumors. *J Neurosurg*. 1998;89(4):599-609.

Patchell RA, Tibbs PA, Regine WF, et al. Direct decompressive surgical resection in the treatment of spinal cord compression caused by metastatic cancer: a randomised trial. *Lancet*. 2005;366(9486):643-648.

Tomita K, Kawahara N, Kobayashi T, et al. Surgical strategy for spinal metastases. *Spine*. 2001;26(3):298-306.

Please go to expertconsult.com to view the complete list of references.

27 Spinal Cord Injury

David W. Cadotte, Michael G. Fehlings

CLINICAL PEARLS

- Spinal cord injury (SCI) is a problem in both the developed and developing countries and is associated with significant morbidity and long-term human and financial costs.

- Spinal cord injury is a medical emergency. Patients suffering from this injury should be treated in specialized centers with strict adherence to proper clinical examination, imaging, and medical and surgical therapies.

- SCI is a result of primary damage to neural structures and vasculature, followed by secondary damage from physiological insults such as hypotension and hypoxia and resultant cytotoxic swelling and death of neurons and glial cells.

- There have been a multitude of strategies of neuroprotection and repair in SCI and can be found in Box 27.2.

- Spinal shock is represented by depressed or absent spinal reflexes below the injury site. Neurogenic shock after trauma results from disruption of the sympathetic nervous system usually at T6 or higher, which may lead to hypotension and may be difficult to distinguish from hypovolemic shock. The optimal treatment of neurogenic shock is restoring intravascular volume; if symptoms of neurogenic shock persist, vasopressors such as dopamine may be useful.

- Central cord syndrome is often the result of a traumatic spinal cord contusion and affects the central part of the spinal cord. This can cause loss of bilateral pain and temperature sensation and loss of motor function at the level of the lesion and below.

- Early closed reduction of bilateral locked facets in an awake patient, who can participate in a neurological examination, may relieve spinal cord compression and restore normal alignment.

- The use of methylprednisolone as a neuroprotective agent in acute SCI shows moderate benefit in terms of neurological outcome but the benefits of its administration should be considered against the risks associated with medical comorbid conditions in individual patients.

- There are several indications for surgical decompression in SCI. The first is to treat spinal instability caused by fractures and ligamentous injury that may cause further neurological damage. There is some evidence, albeit controversial or evolving, that surgical decompression within 24 hours may improve neurological outcome in some patients with isolated SCI, especially those with cervical SCI who are deteriorating neurologically.

Spinal cord injury (SCI) can result from a traumatic event, such as a motor vehicle accident or penetrating assault, or a chronic progressive disorder such as cervical spondylitic myelopathy. In either case the neural elements of the spinal cord, including both the gray and white matter of the spinal cord and the exiting nerve roots, become damaged to the point of causing neurological deficit in the patient. In this chapter we will focus on traumatic SCI. We will highlight the pathophysiological events that occur as a direct consequence of trauma and the biological mechanisms that follow this event. We will then provide an overview of some of the research that is being done to understand the reasons why neurological deficit occurs following trauma, beyond the obvious destructive forces, and discuss attempts at resolving these mechanisms in order to restore neurological function. Lastly, we will discuss the clinical management of the SCI patient with an emphasis on how specialized treatment is geared at minimizing neurological deficit. These specialized treatment options are the result of extensive studies into the pathophysiological mechanisms presented in the first portion of this chapter and represent important advances in translational research—the notion that understanding a disease process at its most fundamental level can result in treatment strategies that will ultimately improve the quality of life for patients and their families.

To frame the concepts of SCI—from pathophysiology to translational research to clinical practice—it is important to understand the reasons for undertaking such an endeavor. Spinal cord injury has been studied at a population level in order to understand the incidence, prevalence, and economic costs of this devastating event. These studies tend to come from developed countries that have the financial resources to conduct such research, but this problem certainly does not respect borders. In fact, the frequency of neurotrauma in the developing world is estimated to be higher than in the developed world for reasons such as poor quality of roads, unsafe driving practices, old vehicles without seatbelts or airbags, and a greater proportion of relatively inexpensive transportation such as small motorcycles. Nonetheless, the estimated incidence in the developed world is in the range of 11.5 to 53.4 people per 1 million population.[1] This number must be interpreted with caution as some authors point out that the actual incidence may be on the higher side because an unknown number of patients suffering SCI die at the scene of the accident without ever being examined or treated in a hospital.[2] Another study estimated that approximately 48% to 79% of individuals die either at the scene of the accident or on arrival to hospital.[3] This study was performed in the mid-1970s and most surgeons treating this disease would agree that the number of patients who die is likely less today, mainly as a result of an improved understanding of the cardiorespiratory complications that can arise following injury and advanced intensive care units that are well versed in managing these complications.

One way to comprehend the costs involved in treating a person with SCI is to imagine that a 25-year-old sustains an injury and becomes completely dependent on family and the health care system from this point forward in life. One study estimated that the total cost would be in the range of $3 million (U.S. dollars),[4] not to mention the impact of this event on the person's family and peers. The average age of SCI patients is the late 20s and early 30s and tends to occur more commonly in males. Going back to our example, this event therefore affects people as they are starting their careers and families. A lack of income combined with insurmountable medical costs translates into financial and emotional hardship. Depression and forms of psychological distress are common in this patient group. In well-developed health care systems support networks exist to aid patients and families through the life that they could not have imagined. In third world countries, patients and families are left to their own devices. From either case comes a drive to understand the pathobiology of this devastating condition and hopefully offer treatment strategies. In the pages that follow, we will systematically discuss the events that occur following a traumatic accident—from the shear forces that destroy white matter tracts to the cellular mechanisms that result. With this as a foundation we will discuss different translational research programs that are under way to minimize neurological deficit and hopefully offer neuroregenerative strategies in the near future. Lastly we discuss how a detailed understanding of the pathophysiology of this condition has led to clinical treatment strategies. These strategies are an essential knowledge base for any medical student or resident interested in the treatment of this devastating condition.

PATHOPHYSIOLOGY

Acute traumatic injury to the spinal cord can come in the form of a blunt mechanism, such as an acrobat falling onto a hard surface or a person thrown from a car during an automobile collision, or a penetrating injury such as a stab or gunshot wound. The forces involved in each of these events are transmitted to the spinal column and if great enough result in disruption of the bony and ligamentous structures and in damage to the neural elements. Damage to the spinal cord or the

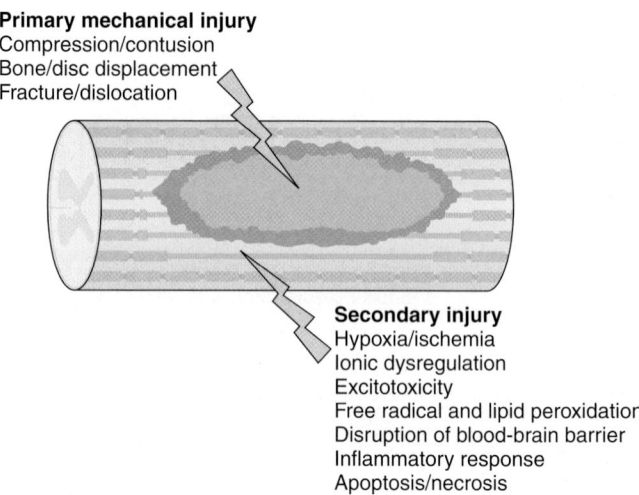

Primary mechanical injury
Compression/contusion
Bone/disc displacement
Fracture/dislocation

Secondary injury
Hypoxia/ischemia
Ionic dysregulation
Excitotoxicity
Free radical and lipid peroxidation
Disruption of blood-brain barrier
Inflammatory response
Apoptosis/necrosis

FIGURE 27.1 Following a primary mechanical injury, numerous secondary mechanisms result in ongoing damage to the spinal cord and minimize the chance for recovery.

exiting nerve roots can result in motor, sensory, or autonomic dysfunction. In an attempt to delineate the precise cause of neurological dysfunction researchers have divided the temporal sequence of destructive events into primary and secondary injury. *Primary injury* refers to the destructive forces that directly damage the neural structures such as the shear force tearing an axon or direct compressive force occluding a blood vessel, resulting in ischemia. These destructive primary mechanisms not only result in instantaneous damage to neurons and blood vessels but also initiate a cascade of cellular mechanisms that result in ongoing damage to the neural structures, termed *secondary injury*. In fact, in cases of ongoing primary injury, for example, in the setting of a fracture dislocation where the bony spinal column is displaced and physically pushed up against the spinal cord, these cellular mechanisms are thought to be locked into the "on" position until such physical forces are removed either by closed reduction or surgically. Secondary injury may persist from hours to weeks to years following primary injury. A great deal of work has gone into the detailed understanding of these cellular cascades and along with this work has come an appreciation for the destructive effects of the mechanisms and the role of potential therapeutics to halt these cascades. In the remainder of this section we will highlight the most important secondary mechanisms of injury (Fig. 27.1) and in the section titled "Translational Research" we will discuss some of the therapeutic targets that resulted from these basic science discoveries.

Secondary injury stems from any aberrant physiological or physical force and results in further tissue damage and potential exacerbation of primary injury. Two of the easiest physiological parameters to recognize are hypotension and hypoxia. Both of these conditions are relatively common in trauma patients, who often sustain concomitant injuries and blood loss. Both are also amenable to medical management shortly after the patient arrives at the hospital. Specific treatment options will be discussed later; here we highlight the importance of these two causes of secondary injury and the fact that they further exacerbate secondary cellular cascades. Both global hypotension and hypoxia add to the overall effect of hypoperfusion to the damaged area of the spinal cord. Several other mechanisms add to hypoperfusion including disruption of the microvasculature, loss of normal autoregulatory mechanisms, and increased interstitial pressure.[5-7] The effects of this ischemic insult are cytotoxic cell swelling of both neurons and glial cells; as a downstream effect of this, blockade of action potentials has been demonstrated as a result of axonal swelling.[8]

Ionic dysregulation and excitotoxicity are closely linked events that contribute to tissue damage. Calcium dysregulation in particular has been widely linked to cell death through a number of different processes including calpain activation, mitochondrial dysfunction, and free radical production.[9] Whether calcium dysregulation or disruption of other ionic gradients occurs, loss of ionic homeostasis is central to both necrotic and apoptotic cellular death. Excitotoxicity results from activation of glutamate receptors via the influx of both sodium and calcium ions. As cell death occurs, either through the process of necrosis or apoptosis, extracellular glutamate levels rise presumably due to the failure of energy-dependent transporters such as the Na^+/K^+-ATPase membrane transporter.[10] In the next section we will discuss how antagonists of NMDA (N-methyl-D-aspartic acid) receptors are potential targets of translational research in order to minimize cellular death.

Free radical–mediated secondary injury occurs through the process of lipid peroxidation that ultimately results in disruption of axons and death of both neurons and glial cells. Considering the mechanism of free radical damage, peroxynitrite and other reactive oxygen species act through a chain reaction that ultimately destroys cellular membranes and leads to cell lysis, organelle dysfunction. and calcium dysregulation.[11] This, in turn, adds to the ionic dysregulation described in the preceding paragraph. Free radicals have been measured in the damaged tissue of experimental models and are found to be elevated for approximately 1 week following injury, returning to preinjury baseline only after 4 to 5 weeks.[12] Examples of these free radicals include hydrogen peroxide, hydroxyl radical, nitric oxide, and the superoxide radical. Specific radicals, such as peroxynitrite, have been directly liked to the activation of apoptotic cascades in rat SCI models.[13] As with NMDA receptors, free radical oxygen species become a potential target of translational research. If one is theoretically able to mediate the level of these dangerous compounds, could one not prevent the degree of secondary damage that occurs following SCI? This idea will be expanded on in the translational research section below.

Tight junctions between endothelial cells act as an interface between the systemic circulation and the central nervous system. Known as the blood-brain barrier (BBB), it also functions in the spinal cord and acts as a selective barrier that allows passage of solutes such as glucose while maintaining impermeability to macromolecules and infectious agents such as bacteria. Endothelial cells and astrocytes are normally bridged by tight junctions and are interspersed with very selective transmembrane proteins to allow the passage of vital molecules and ions. With the destructive forces that accompany SCI comes the destruction of the BBB. This can result either from direct mechanical destruction, such as damaged blood vessels and spinal cord parenchyma, or from destruction at a cellular level. The latter is best understood as a result of the effects of numerous inflammatory mediators on the endothelial cells that disrupt the normally impermeable barrier. One way researchers have studied this effect is through the use of a compound called *horseradish peroxidase*. When injected into the peripheral circulation of a normal animal, this compound does not cross the fortress of the BBB and remains in the systemic tissues. When injected into animal models of SCI, the compound was found to permeate into the CNS at a peak time of 24 hours following injury. Such permeability was persistent for up to 2 weeks following injury.[14] A number of compounds have been identified that are thought to contribute to this ongoing permeability following injury, each of which is related to the secondary mechanisms of SCI. Inflammatory mediators affecting vascular permeability include tumor necrosis factor-α (TNF-α) and interleukin 1β (IL-1β) and both have been shown to be unregulated following SCI.[15,16] Other compounds that play a role include matrix metalloproteinases, histamine, and reactive oxygen species including nitric oxide.[12]

The inflammatory reaction following SCI has received a renewed interest in recent years largely because of what is thought of as the dual nature of the immune response. On the one hand inflammatory mediators seem to be responsible for the ongoing destruction of tissue, and on the other hand they seem to be clearing cellular debris and optimizing the environment for regenerative growth. Several noncellular mediators are involved in the cascade, the most prominent of which are TNF-α, interferons, and interleukins.[17] Cellular mediators following SCI include both resident microglia and peripheral inflammatory cells. A few of the well-characterized examples, mainly from studies in the rodent population, include astrocytes, T cells, neutrophils, and invading monocytes.[18] A great example of this dual nature of protection and destruction comes from studies involving TNF-α, which has been demonstrated to be significantly unregulated following SCI.[19] Subsequent studies involved the application of neutralizing antibodies to TNF-α following experimental injury, resulting in improved neurological function.[20] However, TNF-α-deficient mice have been shown to have higher numbers of apoptotic cells, increased lesion size, and worse function following SCI when compared to wild-type mice.[21] This demonstrates the complexity of the inflammatory cascade in SCI and should point the novice reader in the direction of thinking beyond the notion of one type of molecule causing destruction; rather, one must view the many players as acting in a complex pattern, some of which may aid in optimizing function and others that may result in ongoing destruction. The role of research in this field is to tease out these details and provide specific targets for translational research that aim to optimize the potential for recovery.

Cellular death via the apoptotic pathway is thought to play little role in the fate of neurons[22] but a considerable role in the fate of oligodendrocytes[23] following SCI. Although it may be difficult to demonstrate the apoptotic mechanism of neuronal death in human SCI, there is some evidence for its role in animal models.[24] In contrast, the apoptotic mechanism of oligodendrocyte death has been convincingly demonstrated and its mechanism at least partially elucidated. Following SCI, microglia are activated within the first 2 to 48 hours and express the Fas ligand.[25] This ligand has a receptor largely expressed on the oligodendrocyte, and communication occurs via the p75 neurotrophin receptor.[26] The interaction of the Fas ligand and its receptor initiate apoptosis by way of the caspase cascade that ultimately results in proteolysis, DNA cleavage, and cellular death. This pathway has been the target of translational research strategies and will be expanded on in the next section.

In contrast, cellular death via the necrotic pathway has been demonstrated in both the neuronal and non-neuronal cell populations. Several of the secondary mechanisms of injury previously discussed, such as hypoperfusion and excitotoxicity, culminate in the necrotic death of neurons. Oligodendrocytes are also susceptible to this death pathway and the loss of this cell type has the consequence of axonal demyelination. This demyelination, in combination with other insults on the neuronal processes such as lipid peroxidation and ischemic swelling, results in death of the associated neuronal cell bodies.[27] Animal studies have provided evidence that preserved axons represent a critical therapeutic target in order to regain neurological function.[28] In stark contrast to this, postmortem human studies have failed to identify demyelinated axons[29] and may represent an important disconnect between animal and human pathology following SCI.

Primary and secondary injuries are conceptual frameworks that divide the temporal sequence of events following SCI. This framework provides a basis for research into the complex pathways that are activated in response to trauma, some of which may result in optimizing the local environment for neurological recovery and others that have deleterious side effects. The pathological processes that occur at the cellular level include ischemia, vasospasm, ion-mediated cellular damage, excitotoxicity, oxidative cellular damage, neuroinflammation, and cellular death. Each of these processes involves complex cascades of events. As research continues into each of these cascades different targets for intervention are discovered. In the paragraphs to follow we will highlight some of these targets and explain how they may eventually prove to be beneficial in treating persons that suffer an SCI.

TRANSLATIONAL RESEARCH

As previously stated, an in-depth understanding of secondary mechanisms of SCI has led to identification of numerous possible targets for prevention of this secondary damage and possible regeneration of partially damaged neural circuits. Here we will review a number of agents that are currently under investigation. Broad categories include neuroprotective agents (minocycline and riluzole), myelin-associated inhibitors of neural regeneration (ATI355 and Cethrin), and cellular transplantation strategies (activated autologous macrophages, bone marrow stromal cells, and human embryonic stem cells). This list is by no means exhaustive. Numerous other strategies have been attempted in the past and many lessons have been learned—both positive and negative. Readers interested in a recent history of translational research in the field of SCI are referred to a recently published open source review.[30] Alongside developments in neurobiology have come advances in clinical management and operative strategies. In a similar fashion to the scrutiny of drug delivery trials, these clinical and surgical options have also been the focus of clinical trials and extensive review to determine if their effects provide

---

BOX 27.1	Selected Neuroprotective Approaches, in Early Phase Clinical Trials, with a Potential Role for Improving Outcomes in Spinal Cord Injury

Riluzole
Minocycline
Polyethylene glycol/magnesium
Hypothermia

---

better outcomes for patients. Research that has gone into blood pressure management, methylprednisolone therapy, closed reduction of bilateral locked facets, and early surgical decompression will be discussed in the following section on clinical management.

Neuroprotective Agents

Several promising neuroprotective strategies are under investigation (Box 27.1); two of these are reviewed in greater detail here. Minocycline is a tetracycline derivative that has been of interest to neuroscience for quite some time. It has been shown to have neuroprotective properties in a diversity of animal models, including those that aim to study stroke, Parkinson's disease, Huntington disease, amyotrophic lateral sclerosis (ALS), and multiple sclerosis.[31] As a result of its promise in these conditions, its potential application was carried over to the realm of SCI. Initially studied in animal models, its benefit became apparent in improved neurological outcomes[32] and its mechanism of action was thought to be a result of decreased microglia activation and antiapoptotic pathways mediated by the inhibition of cytochrome *c* release. Because of its extensive use in other neurological conditions, and promise in animal models of SCI, at least two clinical trials are under way to test the efficacy of minocycline in human SCI.

Riluzole is a benzothiazole anticonvulsant that has been in clinical use for greater than a decade. Used primarily in patients with ALS, it has been shown to prolong the lives of persons by 2 to 3 months.[33] Relevant to our earlier discussion of ionic dysregulation as a secondary means of injury, riluzole is thought to act by blocking voltage-sensitive sodium channels, whose overactivity after trauma has been associated with neural tissue destruction. In addition, riluzole has been shown to block presynaptic calcium-dependent glutamate release, whose deleterious effects have been discussed. Multicenter clinical trials are under way to study this agent. Its dosing will be similar to that for ALS patients and the duration will be 10 days. This duration was decided as a direct effect of studies into secondary injury cascades, where results indicate that sodium- and glutamate-mediated damage persists for that time period—an excellent example of how translational research is the direct result of thorough and comprehensive basic science research.

A nonpharmacological means of neuroprotection currently under study in the SCI population is hypothermia. Cooling the human body to slow metabolism and enzymatic processes is certainly not new in clinical medicine. However, its application for SCI has received recent attention likely due to new methods that allow for easy and faster cooling via a femoral sheath catheter. A recent retrospectively designed study[34] demonstrated the safety of this method and gathered

> **BOX 27.2** Selected Molecular/Pharmaceutical Strategies with a Potential Role for Improving Outcomes in Spinal Cord Injury by Influencing Regeneration or Plasticity
>
> Nogo-A monoclonal antibody (ATI335)
> Cethrin
> Rolipram
> Lithium carbonate
> Chondroitinase ABC

> **BOX 27.3** Selected Cellular and Bioengineered Strategies with a Potential Role for Improving Outcomes in Spinal Cord Injury
>
> Cellular strategies either in phase I clinical trials or destined for phase I clinical trials
> Neural stem cells
> Oligodendroglial precursor cells
> Schwann cells
> Olfactory ensheathing cells
> Bioengineered strategies in late stage preclinical trials or early phase I studies
> Cethrin
> Transcriptional factors to up regulate vascular endothelial growth factor (ZFP-VEGF)

preliminary data with regard to cooling temperature, time to target temperature, duration of cooling, and any adverse events. The long-term follow-up of these patients compared to control subjects will be necessary to demonstrate any functional benefit.

Myelin-Associated Inhibitors of Neural Regeneration

Many regenerative strategies for the treatment of SCI are under investigation; the most prominent molecular and pharmaceutical strategies are listed in Box 27.2 and selected cellular and bioengineered strategies are listed in Box 27.3. Here, we further discuss the evolution of this field along with two therapeutic agents. The notion that the central nervous system cannot regenerate axons after injury was convincingly disproved in the 1980s[35] and with numerous other studies after this. Axons, however, do not typically regrow after injury for the many reasons discussed in the secondary injury cascade. Of the innate mechanisms that stunt this growth are the myelin-associated proteins whose activity has been directly linked to a lack of regenerative capacity. Many inhibitors of myelin-associated proteins have been researched in cell culture and animal models and two have been the focus of investigation in clinical trials: ATI335 and Cethrin.

ATI335 has a rich history ranging from basic laboratory science through animal models and into the realm of translational research. CNS myelin, at this time known to be an inhibitor of axonal growth, was biochemically separated into component proteins.[36] Antibodies to these proteins were then developed and applied to in vitro models that demonstrated their ability to diminish the inhibitory effects of myelin.

Subsequent animal models demonstrated improved neurological outcomes with administration of these antibodies.[37] After a flurry of excitement in the animal world, Nogo was characterized as the target antigen and human antibodies were subsequently developed. These antibodies were demonstrated to promote axonal growth and functional recovery in primate models of SCI. Clinical trials began shortly thereafter and are currently under way in both Europe and Canada.

Myelin inhibitors of axonal growth are known to signal through the *Rho* cascade. Briefly, Rho is a guanosine triphosphatase that, when activated, binds to Rho kinase (ROCK). ROCK, in turn, is a key regulator of axonal growth cone dynamics and cellular apoptosis. Disruption of this cascade has been shown to facilitate axon growth and functional recovery in mice.[38] Initial studies made use of a toxin produced by *Clostridium botulinum* termed *C3 transferase*, a specific inhibitor of Rho. Eventually, a recombinant protein was created, commercialized, and brought to clinical trial. Cethrin is a combination of this recombinant protein and fibrin glue—the mixture is applied directly to the dura at the time of surgical decompression of SCI. Initial results of a multicenter phase I/IIa trial are becoming available and appear promising in terms of neurological recovery. A phase II study is being planned.

CELLULAR TRANSPLANTATION STRATEGIES

Up to this point we have discussed how secondary mechanisms following SCI result in a hostile environment that prevents recovery of neural function and may lead to damage beyond the original injury. We then discussed how a detailed understanding of these secondary mechanisms has led to various research strategies aimed at combating these cascades in hopes of optimizing spinal cord recovery. In the next few paragraphs we will discuss the idea behind cellular transplantation, a concept that transcends the notions of optimizing the spinal cord for natural recovery and introduces cell types with the goal of integrating these cells within spinal circuits and allowing for neurological recovery. Many different cell types have been studied. Here we will focus on three: activated autologous macrophages, bone marrow stromal cells, and human embryonic stem cells. Although the theory surrounding transplantation strategies sounds promising, the experimental results have been humble. Nonetheless, it is hoped that careful attention to the barriers will lead to a successful treatment strategy in the near future.

Activated Autologous Macrophages

It has been realized for about 2 decades that macrophages play a vital role in the regeneration of peripheral nervous function and that this role does not exist in the central nervous system. Following injury to a nerve in the peripheral nervous system, macrophages are recruited to the site of injury and are responsible for clearing myelin debris and optimizing the local environment for regeneration. In order to capitalize on this finding in the central nervous system, researchers attempted to take autologous macrophages from SCI patients, activate them with peripheral myelin, and inject them into the damaged area of the spinal cord shortly after injury. The initial results were promising, although only a small number of individuals received treatment. Owing to financial circumstances, the trial was never expanded beyond the initial study. This strategy once again highlights a bridge between understanding the secondary mechanisms of damage, in this case how central myelin acts to inhibit neural regeneration and repair, and the development of potential therapy. Hopefully this promising strategy will be revitalized and studied in a larger population.

Bone Marrow Stromal Cells

The use of bone marrow stromal cells aims to take advantage of a relatively accessible multipotent stem cell that has the potential to differentiate and integrate into existing spinal circuits and result in neural recovery. A number of groups around the world are reporting the use of these cells including scientists from Korea, China, Russia, the Czech Republic, and Brazil. To date, the trials have been small and are often not blinded, prompting cautious interpretation of the results. Nonetheless, researchers report significant neurological recovery after direct injection of this cell type in the damaged area of the spinal cord. Researchers in Prague, Czech Republic, did have blind assessors evaluate patients at follow-up in terms of both the ASIA (American Spinal Injury Association) scale and electrophysiologically. Significant improvement was noted in patients who received therapy within 3 to 4 weeks of injury but not in those who were in the chronic stages of injury.[39]

Human Embryonic Stem Cells

Although human embryonic stem cells are theorized as one of the more promising strategies in cell replacement in the spinal cord, there are a number of hurdles that must be overcome. This cell type is first cultured in vitro and the purity of these cultures is paramount and somewhat challenging. In addition, viral contamination via delivery vectors and the acquisition of membrane polysaccharides that may react with the host immune system are all concerns that are being addressed. Significant advances have been made in this field, mainly out of the University of California at Irvine,[40,41] and are currently being evaluated by the Food and Drug Administration (FDA) in the United States. The goal of this therapy is to achieve differentiation of these stem cells into oligodendrocytes that would aid in remyelination of spared but demyelinated axons. This represents a promising avenue of research in the decades to come.

Each of these translational research concepts is extremely important in the overall undertaking to prevent neurological decline and optimize a hostile environment for recovery, and several translational ideas have already made their way into mainstream clinical practice. These practices include maintenance of blood pressure, methylprednisolone therapy, early closed reduction of bilateral locked facets, and early surgical decompression. Each of these topics will be briefly reviewed in the next section on clinical management.

CLINICAL MANAGEMENT

A patient who sustains an SCI has often sustained concomitant injuries and may be medically unstable; in fact, the treating physician may not recognize the presence of SCI immediately.

Adherence to Advanced Trauma Life Support (ATLS) protocol is essential. Airway, breathing, and circulation (ABCs) are of paramount importance, followed by the treatment of any immediate life-threatening condition. If there is concern that any one of these domains is unstable, it should be revisited before moving on. Hypotension, in particular, must be observed for an ongoing secondary SCI can result. Following stabilization of the patient, the treating physician should then proceed with the neurological examination. This comes in the form of testing for motor power, sensory impairment, and reflexes including rectal tone. This examination should be documented on the standard ASIA forms.[42] Following a detailed examination, and assuming the finding of a deficit, imaging of the spinal column with computed tomography (CT) scan and imaging of the spinal cord with magnetic resonance imaging (MRI) should follow in short order. To frame the concepts of SCI, refer to Figure 27.2, which displays the MRI of an 18-year-old male subject who sustained an SCI. Also shown in this figure is the method for calculating the maximal spinal canal compromise and the maximal cord compression—two measurements that are useful for quantifying the degree of injury.[43] In the remainder of this chapter we will review the following important concepts that are essential to understand in order to properly care for the SCI patient: spinal shock, neurogenic shock, spinal cord syndromes, evidence for early closed reduction of bilateral locked facets, evidence for methylprednisolone therapy, and evidence for early surgical decompression.

Spinal Shock

Spinal shock is a term used to describe depressed spinal reflexes caudal to the injury site following SCI. This is an important concept to understand because the initial neurological examination may not be an accurate reflection of disrupted neuronal circuits, including those that control motor and sensory pathways. Normally, these reflex pathways receive continuous input from the brain. When this tonic input is disrupted, the normal reflex pattern is disrupted and can vary from areflexic through to hyperreflexic depending on the time since the original injury. Clinically, this translates into the potential for a misleading representation of deficits if spinal reflexes are absent following injury. It is therefore recommended that patients be examined not only on presentation to the treating physician but also at the 72-hour mark following injury.

Neurogenic Shock

Neurogenic shock is a potentially life-threatening condition and must be managed as such. Without a clear understanding of this condition inappropriate management of a trauma patient, who often suffers concomitant hemodynamic instability, could be fatal. Neurogenic shock is defined as disruption of the sympathetic nervous system with preserved parasympathetic activity. This typically occurs with patients suffering a severe SCI at the level of T6 or higher. Disruption of the sympathetic division of the autonomic nervous system affects three areas of the cardiovascular system: coronary blood flow, cardiac contractility, and heart rate. With preserved parasympathetic activity this translates clinically into bradycardia

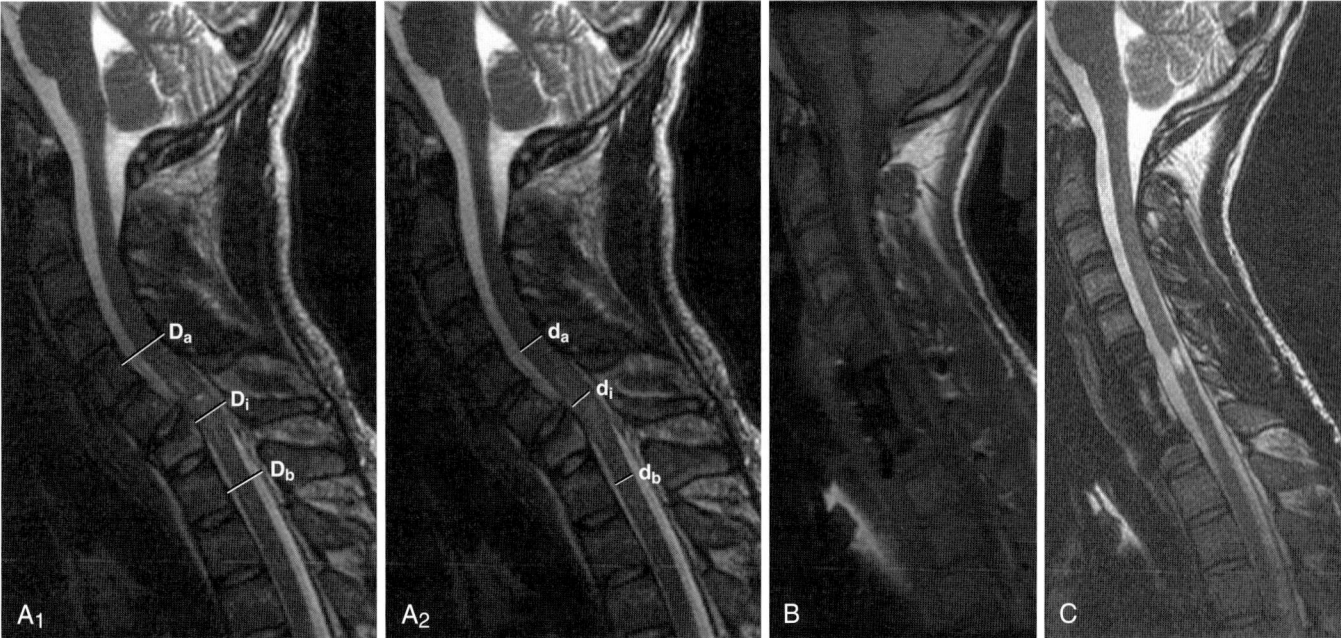

Maximum canal compromise

$$\left(1 - \frac{D_i}{(D_a + D_b)/2}\right) \times 100\%$$

Maximum cord compression

$$\left(1 - \frac{d_i}{(d_a + d_b)/2}\right) \times 100\%$$

FIGURE 27.2 Preoperative T2-weighted (**A₁** and **A₂**) and postoperative T1-weighted (**B**) and T2-weighted (**C**) MRI studies of an 18-year-old man who sustained a spinal cord injury after being involved in a motor vehicle accident. A_1 illustrates how to calculate maximal canal compromise (MCC): D_i is the anteroposterior canal diameter at the level of maximum injury, D_a is the anteroposterior canal diameter at the nearest normal level above the level of injury, and D_b is the anteroposterior canal diameter at the nearest normal level below the level of injury. A_2 illustrates how to calculate the maximum spinal cord compression (MSCC): d_i is the anteroposterior cord diameter at the level of maximum injury, d_a is the anteroposterior cord diameter at the nearest normal level above the level of injury, and d_b is the anteroposterior cord diameter at the nearest normal level below the level of injury. **B** and **C** illustrate the effect of decompressive surgery on relieving spinal cord compression and restoring normal alignment.

(and possibly other cardiac arrhythmias) in the setting of profound hypotension. A prudent clinician must look for these characteristics in combination, as many trauma patients are hypotensive as a result of blood loss or intravascular hypovolemia but will mount an appropriate tachycardic response.

The treatment of neurogenic shock is therefore quite difficult. Although it is theoretically possible to distinguish between hypovolemic and neurogenic shock, clinically this distinction is not so clear. In fact, acute trauma patients sustaining a high cervical SCI may suffer from both conditions. It has therefore been recommended by the Consortium for Spinal Cord Medicine to rule out other causes of shock before assuming a diagnosis of neurogenic shock. The practical treatment of these patients rests on initially restoring intravascular volume and if symptoms of neurogenic shock persist, vasopressors (such as dopamine) should be used. The goal of treatment in the first week after sustaining an SCI is to maintain a mean arterial blood pressure of 85 mm Hg.

Spinal Cord Syndromes

One should be aware of the terminology used to describe deficits and identify different spinal cord syndromes in order to localize the lesion to a particular area of the spinal cord and a particular level.

Paresis is a term used to describe weakness or partial paralysis. For example, *hemiparesis* describes weakness on one side of the body. In contrast, both *paralysis* and the suffix *-plegia* refer to no movement. For example, *hemiplegia* refers to no movement on one side of the body. Keeping these terms in mind, we turn our attention to spinal cord syndromes that occur when a select region of the spinal cord is damaged, resulting in a predictable pattern of neurological deficit. These syndromes are expanded on in the paragraphs that follow and are depicted in Figure 27.3, along with a description of the ASIA impairment scale.

Transverse spinal cord lesions disrupt all motor and sensory pathways at and below the level of the lesion. There is a sensory level that corresponds to the level of the lesion.

Hemisection of the spinal cord, commonly referred to as *Brown-Sequard syndrome*, is characterized by damage to one half of the spinal cord and all motor and sensory pathways at that level and neurological deficits at and below that level. This results in ipsilateral upper motor neuron weakness and ipsilateral loss of vibration and position sense at and below the level of lesion. There is contralateral loss of pain and temperature sensation below the level of the lesion. There may also be ipsilateral loss of pain and temperature sensation at the level of the lesion for one or two spinal segments if the lesion has damaged posterior horn cells before fibers have crossed to the other side.

ASIA IMPAIRMENT SCALE		
ASIA Grade	Complete or incomplete	Description
A	Complete	No motor or sensory function is preserved in the sacral segments S4-S5
B	Incomplete	Sensory but not motor function is preserved below the neurological level and includes the sacral segments S4-S5
C	Incomplete	Motor function is preserved below the neurological level, and more than half of the key muscles below the neurological level have a muscle grade less than 3
D	Incomplete	Motor function is preserved below the neurological level, and at least half of key muscles below the neurological level have a muscle grade of 3 or more
E	Incomplete	Motor and sensory function are normal

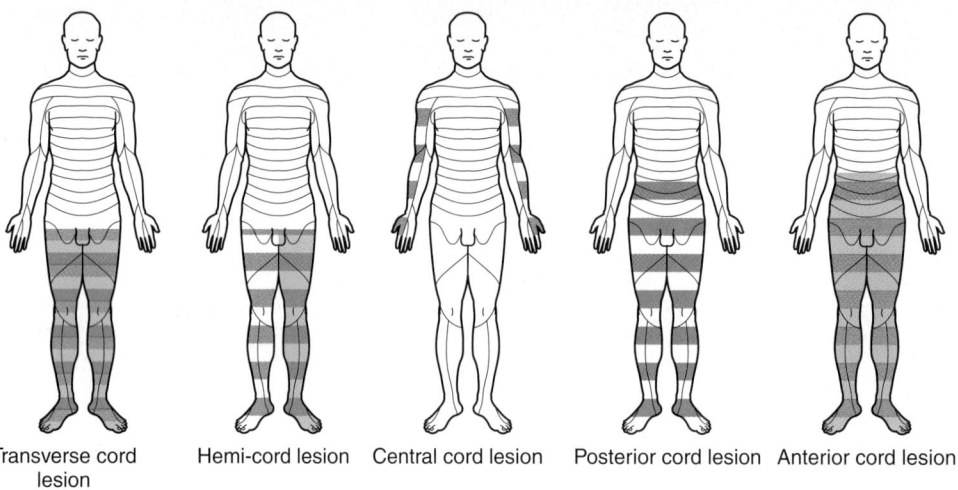

Transverse cord lesion   Hemi-cord lesion   Central cord lesion   Posterior cord lesion   Anterior cord lesion

■ Loss of vibration and position sense   ■ Loss of pain and temperature sense   ■ Loss of motor power

FIGURE 27.3 The ASIA impairment scale is outlined (*top*) along with spinal cord syndromes (*bottom*). Central cord syndrome is representative of a small lesion. If the central cord lesion were large, one would expect involvement of the motor and vibration/position sense systems (see text for further explanation). Motor power is graded according to the following scale: 0 = total paralysis, 1 = palpable or visible contraction, 2 = active movement, full range of motion, gravity eliminated, 3 = active movement, full range of motion, against gravity, 4 = active movement, full range of motion, against gravity, and provides some resistance, 5 = active movement, full range of motion, against gravity, and provides normal resistance, NT = not testable because the patient is unable to reliably exert effort or the muscle is unavailable for testing due to factors such as immobilization, pain on effort, or contracture. Sensory testing is graded according to the following scale: 0 = absent, 1 = impaired, 2 = normal, and NT = not testable.

Central cord syndrome is commonly caused by a traumatic spinal cord contusion, posttraumatic syringomyelia, or a medullary spinal tumor. This lesion tends to affect pathways that are in the immediate vicinity of the central portion of the spinal cord, and the symptoms differ depending on the size of the lesion. Small lesions affect spinothalamic fibers that cross in the ventral commissure and cause bilateral regions of suspended sensory loss to pain and temperature. If the lesion is larger, anterior horn cells, corticospinal tracts, and posterior columns may be affected. Loss of these pathways respectively results in lower motor neuron deficits at the level of the lesion, upper motor neuron signs below the level of the lesion, and loss of vibration and position sense below the level of the lesion. In addition to suspended pain and temperature loss with small lesions, larger lesions can result in complete loss of pain and temperature sensation below the level of the lesion if the anterolateral pathways are compressed from a medial

aspect. Given the spinal cord laminations, sacral sparing is observed.

Posterior cord syndrome involves bilateral loss of vibration and position sense below the level of the lesion as a result of disruption of the posterior columns. If the lesion is large enough, one may observe upper motor neuron signs below the level of the lesion, indicating involvement of the lateral corticospinal tracts. In addition to traumatic injury, vitamin B_{12} deficiency or tertiary syphilis can cause isolated involvement of the posterior columns.

Anterior cord syndrome results in loss of pain and temperature sensation below the level of the lesion (spinothalamic pathways), lower motor neuron signs at the level of the lesion (anterior horn cell damage), and upper motor neuron signs below the level of the lesion (lateral corticospinal tracts). In addition, urinary incontinence is common because of the ventral location of the descending pathways controlling sphincter function. Common causes of this syndrome include trauma and anterior spinal artery infarct.

Evidence for Early Closed Reduction of Bilateral Locked Facets

As mentioned earlier, imaging of the spinal column with CT scan and the spinal cord and soft tissues with MRI should follow clinical examination. These imaging modalities provide essential information that determines subsequent steps in management. In the setting of severe flexion injuries, disruption of the anterior, middle, and posterior columns along with the ligamentous joint capsules can occur. This is an extreme example on the spectrum of flexion injuries and usually results in quadriplegia. CT imaging reveals the inferior articular facets from one vertebral body to be dislocated anteriorly with respect to the superior facets of the adjacent vertebra. MRI is necessary to investigate the degree of neural element involvement and the degree of ligamentous compromise.

Treatment of this injury usually begins with closed reduction of the facet dislocation; whether or not one investigates the cervical spine with MRI prior to this maneuver is a controversial issue. An important qualifying factor in this situation is that the patient must be awake, alert, and able to participate in repeated neurological examinations. This notion rests in the dictum of "do no harm to your patients." Early closed reduction of bilateral locked facets aims to relieve severe spinal cord compression in the setting of significant ligamentous damage by restoring normal bony alignment. The technique should be performed in a monitored setting and involves applying either Gardner-Wells tongs or a halo crown as a rigid fixation device to the skull and applying a traction force. Increasing weight is added over time while neurological status is monitored for stability and lateral radiographs are used to follow the bony anatomy. The goal is to obtain reduction of the cervical facets. A postreduction MRI should be obtained to rule out disk herniation. This maneuver should only be performed in specialty centers with surgeons experienced in its application. Under no circumstances should this maneuver delay operative management. The evidence for this technique was recently reviewed and consisted of a number of class II and III studies, with retrospective and prospective designs.[44] The results of these studies varied from neurological deterioration to no neurological change to neurological improvement. In order to further distill the controversy, several authors reported that the method is safe and that neurological decline is often transient and improves with removal of added weight. Furthermore, a number of studies report neurological improvement that led to the recommendation of early closed reduction as a clinical guideline in patients with bilateral locked facets and an incomplete tetraplegia or in those with deteriorating neurological status.

Evidence for Methylprednisolone Therapy

The use of methylprednisolone as a neuroprotective agent to mitigate the deleterious effects of secondary injury is still controversial. It has been shown to offer modest benefit in terms of neurological outcome following SCI.[45] The National Acute Spinal Cord Injury Study (NASCIS) aimed to investigate the question of whether or not patients would benefit from its administration. In the paragraphs that follow we will review the results of this study along with the method and dose by which physicians administered the drug in each trial.

NASCIS was designed as a multicenter trial and was completed as three separate trials: NASCIS I, NASCIS II, and NASCIS III. The first study compared low- and high-dose methylprednisolone (no placebo), the second trial was randomized and controlled with a placebo, and the third trial compared the effects of 24- versus 48-hour treatment. NASCIS I randomized SCI patients into two cohorts: the first group received a 100-mg loading dose of methylprednisolone followed by 25 mg every 6 hours for 10 days, and the second group received a 1000-mg loading dose of methylprednisolone followed by 250 mg every 6 hours for 10 days.[46] There were no differences in neurological outcome between the two groups at 1 year after injury. NASCIS II investigated a 30-mg/kg bolus of methylprednisolone over 1 hour followed by 5.4 mg/kg/hour over the following 23 hours and included a placebo group and naloxone administration group. The reason for the higher doses (in comparison to NASCIS I) involved the analysis of animal research that suggested a therapeutic benefit only above a certain threshold. Results from the overall group showed no significant differences in neurological outcome at 6 months; a subgroup analysis demonstrated improved motor and sensory outcomes in patients receiving methylprednisolone within 8 hours of injury.[47] NASCIS III examined outcomes in acute SCI patients receiving a 30-mg/kg bolus of methypredniosolone followed by 5.4 mg/kg/hour for either 23 hours or 47 hours. Patients treated with methylprednisolone for 48 hours had better neurological outcomes in comparison to the other treatment groups if therapy was initiated within 3 to 8 hours of injury; however, the 48-hour regimen was associated with increased risk of sepsis and pneumonia.[48] Following the completion of each of these studies, Bracken conducted a reviewed along with two other independent trials and concluded that high-dose therapy was safe and afforded a modest benefit in terms of neurological outcome.[49]

Clearly the results were not overwhelmingly in favor of methylprednisolone administration and there is still considerable debate as to whether or not it should be used. Furthermore, if a practicing physician decides to use this therapy, there is debate as to which administration protocol should be used. The senior author of this chapter has published his protocol for administering methylprednisolone following acute SCI based on the timing of administration.[45] Patients with acute nonpenetrating SCI should receive methylprednisolone as per the NASCIS II protocol if started less than 3 hours after injury. If started between 3 and 8 hours after injury, then the NASCIS III 48-hour protocol should be applied. If therapy cannot be administered within 8 hours of injury, or there is a penetrating SCI, then methylprednisolone should not be administered for neuroprotection. The decision to administer methylprednisolone must account for patient medical comorbid conditions. For example, the risks of administration may outweigh the benefits in a patient with diabetes mellitus and a complete thoracic SCI injury. Blood glucose levels must be carefully monitored during the course of methylprednisolone therapy, and hyperglycemia aggressively managed with an insulin infusion.

Evidence for Early Surgical Decompression

The concept of surgical decompression for SCI has received a great deal of attention in the past 2 decades largely because of the research questions posed around the concepts of secondary injury. It is important to consider the fact that there may be several indications for surgery following traumatic SCI—first and foremost is spinal instability caused by torn ligaments and bony fracture. There is little controversy over the need for surgical stabilization in this setting. The other, and the focus of this section, is surgical decompression that aims to improve neurological outcome without a strong indication for the treatment of spinal column instability. As mentioned earlier, physical compression of the spinal cord is responsible for triggering an ongoing series of deleterious cascades, and surgical decompression aims to relieve this compression. Evidence is mounting for improved outcomes in this setting and we will review these concepts here.

One of the parameters to consider when studying the effect of surgical decompression after SCI is the timing of this decompression. There is no definition of this timing although most authors and spinal surgeons would agree that early surgery is that which is performed within 24 hours of initial injury. A great deal of the preclinical animal literature focuses on timing of surgical decompression at much earlier times following injury, in the range of 8 to 24 hours. These animal studies consistently report improved neurological outcomes with early decompression. There have been a number of recent systematic literature reviews that address previous preclinical and clinical research.[44,50,51] Perhaps the main force behind these reviews is not only to get a firm grasp on what has been accomplished to date but to form a clear rationale for proceeding with clinical trials in the future. Preliminary results from the Surgical Treatment of Acute Spinal Cord Injuries Trial (STASCIS) indicate that decompression within 24 hours of injury may actually improve outcome in patients with isolated SCI.[52] Based on both animal studies and recent clinical investigations guidelines have been formed that recommend surgical decompression within 24 hours for cervical SCI. Very early decompression, within 12 hours of injury, should be strongly considered for patients suffering incomplete cervical SCI or those who are deteriorating neurologically.

CONCLUSIONS

Throughout the course of this chapter we have discussed how rigorous study of SCI has led to a detailed understanding of the pathophysiological mechanisms that follow a traumatic event. The paradigm of secondary injury has opened the door for many research projects ranging from apoptosis to neuroprotection. Each of these research avenues has, in turn, resulted in translational research initiatives aimed at preserving and restoring neurological function. Lastly, many of these translational ideas have resulted in clinical practices that result in better outcomes for patients that suffer an SCI. We have therefore presented a spectrum of thought, ranging from the molecular level to cellular interactions to the neurological movement and sensation that is transmitted through the spinal cord. It is through these research programs and their clinical application that we are able to advance science and our understanding of how to repair the spinal cord or prevent further neurological damage after SCI.

SELECTED KEY REFERENCES

Fehlings MG, Baptiste DC. Current status of clinical trials for acute spinal cord injury. *Injury.* 2005;36(Suppl 2): B113-122.

Fehlings MG, Perrin RG. The timing of surgical intervention in the treatment of spinal cord injury: a systematic review of recent clinical evidence. *Spine.* 2006;31:S28-35:discussion S36.

Hawryluk GW, Rowland J, Kwon BK, Fehlings MG. Protection and repair of the injured spinal cord: a review of completed, ongoing, and planned clinical trials for acute spinal cord injury. *Neurosurg Focus.* 2008;25:E14.

Miyanji F, Furlan JC, Aarabi B, et al. Acute cervical traumatic spinal cord injury: MR imaging findings correlated with neurologic outcome—prospective study with 100 consecutive patients. *Radiology.* 2007;243:820-827.

Tator CH, Koyanagi I. Vascular mechanisms in the pathophysiology of human spinal cord injury. *J Neurosurg.* 1997; 86:483-492.

Please go to expertconsult.com to view the complete list of references.

28 Syringomyelia

Spyros Sgouros

CLINICAL PEARLS

- The presence of syringomyelia requires lifelong neurological follow-up with repeat magnetic resonance imaging scans.

- When a patient with Chiari I or Chiari II malformation, with hydrocephalus and syringomyelia, has deteriorated radiologically, the shunt should be investigated first before any treatment for syringomyelia is considered.

- Chiari I patients with syringomyelia require decompression of the cerebrospinal fluid (CSF) obstruction at the craniovertebral junction.

- Treatment of syringomyelia caused by trauma requires decompression of the CSF at the level of the deformity or block followed by spinal stabilization, when clinically indicated. Treatment with a syringosubarachnoid or syringopleural shunt may stop the progression of the syrinx and neurological deterioration but the long-term prognosis remains guarded.

- Chiari II malformation is very different from that of Chiari I with respect to syringomyelia management.

Syringomyelia is the cystic cavitation of the spinal cord extending over a distance of more than two spinal segments. The syringomyelia cavity contains fluid with a consistency similar or equivalent to that of cerebrospinal fluid (CSF). The term is derived from the word *syrinx,* an ancient Greek word meaning wooden reed or tube (also describing a wooden ancient Greek musical organ, pan pipes, similar to a flute), and the word *myelos,* meaning the spinal cord. The word *syrinx* has its origins in Greek mythology in the tale of a beautiful and chaste nymph, Syrinx, being pursued to the river-bank by Pan, an amorous creature, half man and half goat. Syrinx, the nymph, in order to escape the approaching Pan, turned to the river nymphs for assistance. They turned her into a bundle of hollow reeds, which Pan cut down to make pan pipes. This new musical instrument of hollow tubes played plaintive music as the frustrated god's breath blew over them. These pan pipes are known as syrinx. The word *syringe* is derived from this term, denoting a hollow tube.

The condition, syringomyelia, was described in 1876 by Leyden[1] and in 1891 by Abbe and Coley.[2] Although several theories had been proposed in the 1960s and 1970s on the pathophysiology surrounding the formation and propagation of syringomyelia, the real progress came after the advent of magnetic resonance imaging (MRI) in the past decade, which facilitated noninvasive high-definition imaging of the condition, and later with the development of dynamic in vivo imaging of CSF movement.

Syringomyelia is most frequently associated with hindbrain herniation. Hindbrain herniation, or Chiari I malformation, is the herniation of the cerebellar tonsils for 5 mm or more beyond the foramen magnum below a line connecting the basion and opisthion (Figs. 28.1 to 28.3). In large clinical series 50% to 80% of patients with symptomatic Chiari I malformation (CMI) have syringomyelia. However, because these series contained only symptomatic patients it is difficult to know the precise incidence of syringomyelia among all patients with Chiari I malformation. It is unclear also if syringomyelia represents an evolutionary stage in the natural history of the Chiari I malformation or it starts ab initio, from the beginning of the creation of the malformation. In most patients, Chiari I malformation is regarded as congenital. It is unclear if the malformation changes with time, if the cerebellar herniation increases. Certainly, from studies in asymptomatic patients and from the author's unpublished experience of following over 20 asymptomatic children for many years with yearly MRI scans, in most patients the cerebellar herniation does not increase with time.[3,4] Very few occasions of spontaneous resolution of Chiari I malformation have been reported.[5] On the other hand, syringomyelia frequently changes with time. Acquired Chiari I malformation can develop following lumbar shunt placement or failure of a ventricular shunt, if the hindbrain is pulled down through the foramen magnum.[6,7] Syringomyelia may be associated also with various other conditions such as spinal arachnoid cysts; traumatic paraplegia (Fig. 28.4); postinfectious, postinflammatory, or tuberculous meningitis; chemical insults following use of intrathecal agents, antibiotics, or myelographic contrast agent Myodil-Pantopaque; epidural abscess; Pott's disease; and idiopathic meningeal fibrosis. In addition, various forms of spinal dysraphism such as spinal lipoma (Fig. 28.5), diastematomyelia (Fig. 28.6), recurrent tethering after myelomeningocele repair (Fig. 28.7), thickened filum terminale, rare malformations

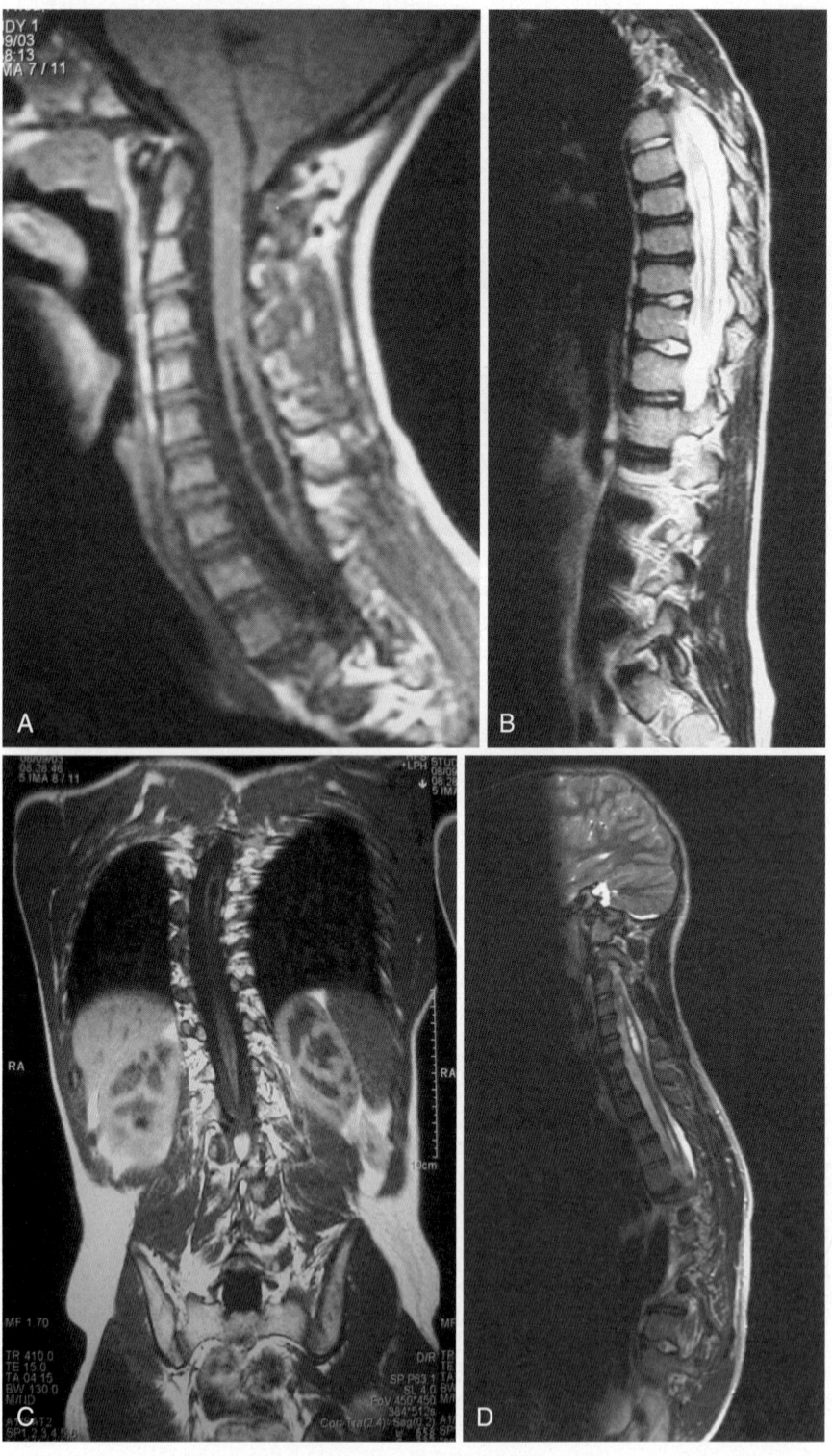

FIGURE 28.1 Chiari I malformation, syringomyelia, and scoliosis. Magnetic resonance images of a 12-year-old boy who presented with progressive scoliosis and a limp. **A,** Head T1-weighted sagittal sequence. There is cerebellar tonsillar herniation below the foramen magnum down to the lower border of the arch of C1, and an extensive syringomyelia with septations in its cavity, that commences at the level of C4. **B,** Spine T2-weighted sagittal sequence. The syringomyelia cavity extends down to the lower thoracic spine. It is difficult to calculate the lower level, as the spine is not seen in one image due to the scoliosis. **C,** Spine T1-weighted coronal sequence. There is significant scoliosis and the syringomyelia cavity is seen in the midthoracic region. **D,** Postoperative spine T2-weighted sequence, 1 year after craniovertebral decompression. The syringomyelia cavity has decreased in size in comparison to the image in B.

affecting the foramen magnum region such as achondroplasia, posterior fossa arachnoid cysts, Chiari II malformation, syndromic craniosynostosis, osteogenesis imperfecta, mucopolysaccharidosis, and spinal cord tumors can also be associated with syringomyelia (Fig. 28.8).

Syringomyelia affects commonly the cervical and upper thoracic spinal cord, although it can extend throughout the entire spinal cord, creating a holocord syringomyelia (see Figs. 28.3B and 28.5). If untreated, it follows a progressive and often relentless course over a number of years. Usually the neurological deterioration is gradual, but sudden deterioration has been described. The neurological function of arms and legs is at risk and patients in whom, despite treatment, the syringomyelia cavity continues to extend end up quadriplegic.

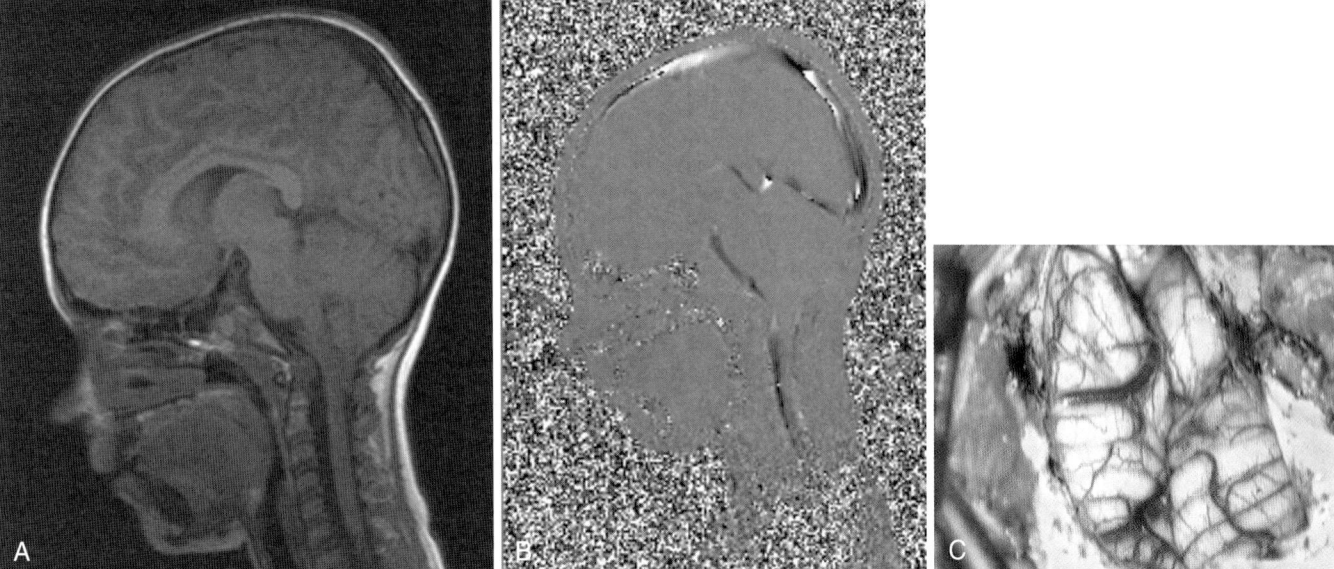

FIGURE 28.2 Chiari I malformation without syringomyelia. Magnetic resonance images of a 12-year-old boy who presented with occipital headaches, severe enough to miss significant time from school. **A,** Head T1-weighted sagittal sequence. There is significant cerebellar tonsillar herniation below the foramen magnum down to the upper border of the lamina of C2. **B,** Head cardiac gated phase contrast cine sequence. There is reduced cerebrospinal fluid flow in the posterior aspect of the foramen magnum. **C,** Operative photograph taken through the microscope during craniovertebral decompression. The patient is in prone position, so the top of the head is toward the bottom of the photograph. The view is that of the region of the foramen magnum after opening the dura and the arachnoid. Toward the top of the image the two cerebellar tonsils are seen, protruding well below the foramen magnum. For orientation, the "burned" edges of the dura either side toward the top of the photograph are the site of the dural venous sinus, commonly seen in children and young adults, which have been coagulated for hemostasis, marking the level of the foramen magnum. The tips of the tonsils are well into the upper cervical subarachnoid space.

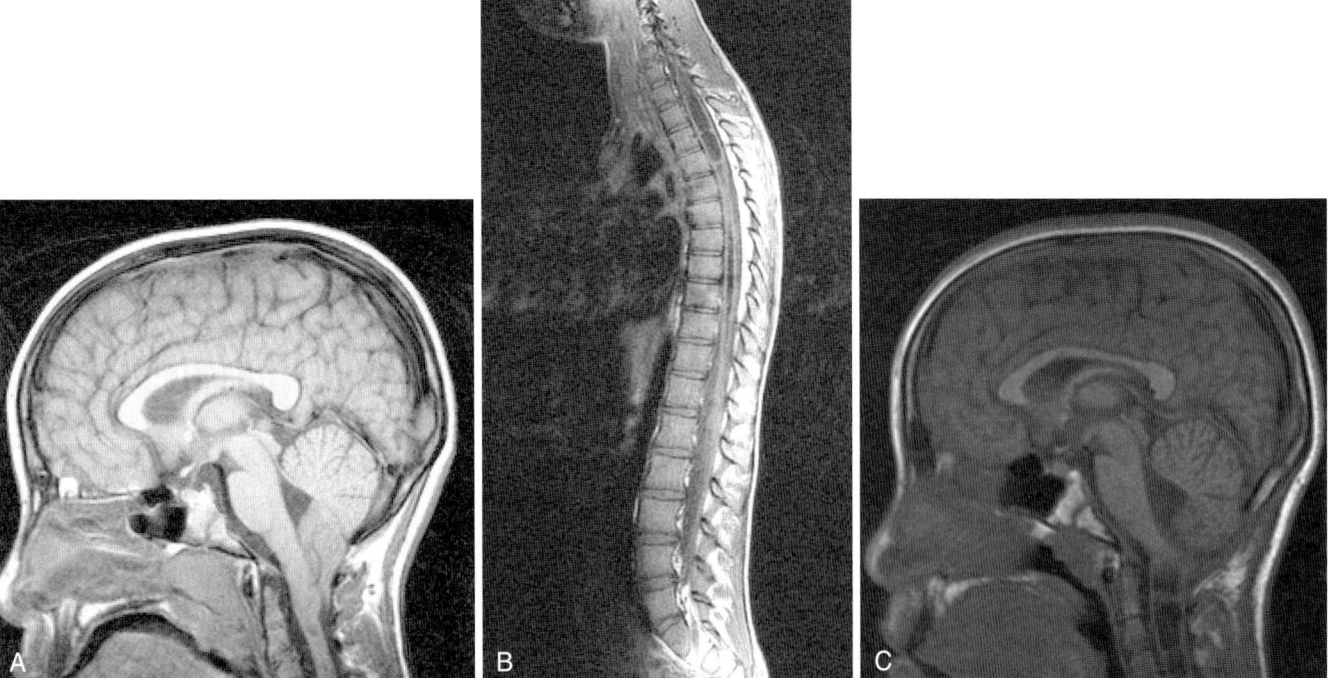

FIGURE 28.3 Syringomyelia that progressed to syringobulbia. Magnetic resonance images of an 11-year-old boy who presented with weakness of the right upper limb. **A,** Head T1-weighted sagittal sequence. There is significant cerebellar tonsillar herniation below the foramen magnum down to the lamina of C2. **B,** Spine T1-weighted sagittal sequence. There is extensive syringomyelia cavity down to T10 at least. The patient had craniovertebral decompression. He developed postoperative cerebrospinal fluid (CSF) leak and meningitis that was treated with antibiotics and lumbar punctures to relieve the CSF pseudomeningocele. **C,** Head T1-weighted sagittal sequence 6 months after operation. There are adhesions—arachnoid fibrosis at the craniovertebral junction—which cause tethering of the dorsal aspect of the lower medulla and upper cervical cord to the operation site. The syringomyelia cavity has extended cranially (compare with image in A) and is invading the lower medulla.

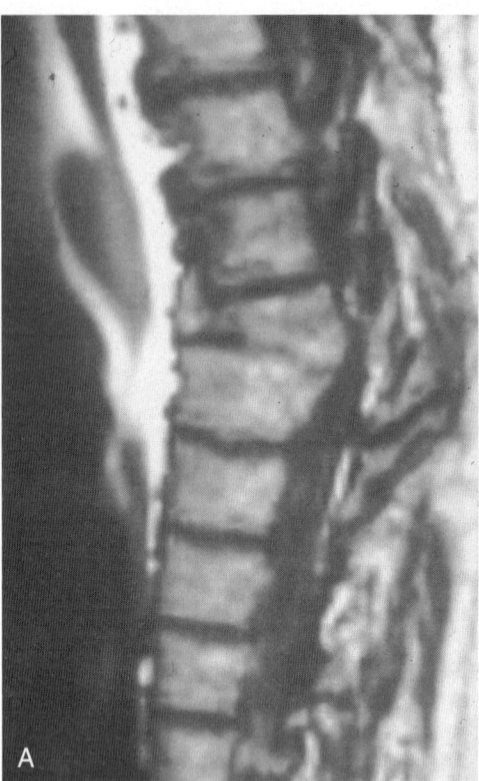
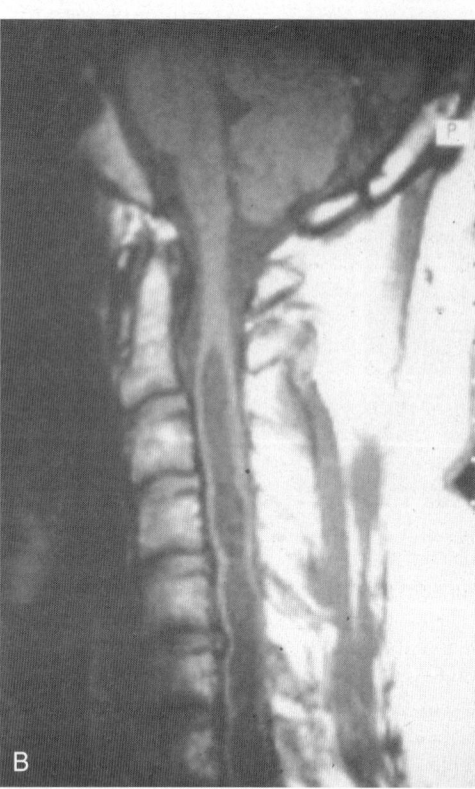

FIGURE 28.4 Post-traumatic syringomyelia. Magnetic resonance images of a 36-year-old man who suffered a motor vehicle accident that led to spinal injury and paraplegia. **A,** Spine T1-weighted sagittal sequence. There is wedge fracture of the body of T7 and corresponding fracture of the upper-posterior aspect of the body of T8. There is corresponding narrowing of the spinal canal and compression of the spinal subarachnoid space. **B,** Cervical spine T1-weighted sagittal sequence. There is a significant syringomyelia cavity extending cranially up the level of C2.

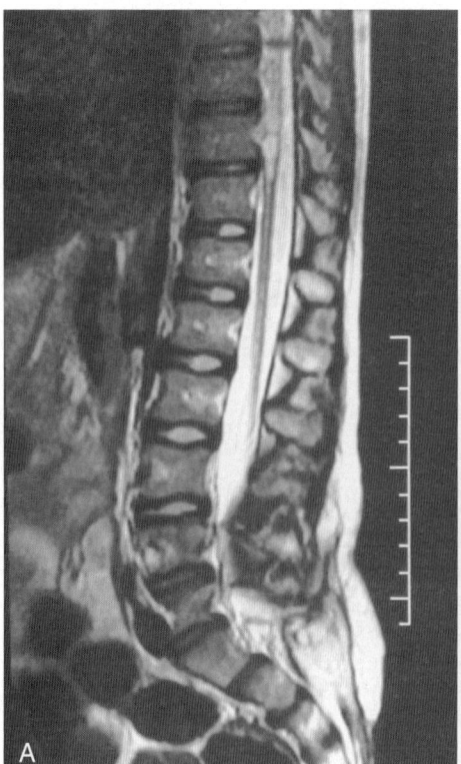
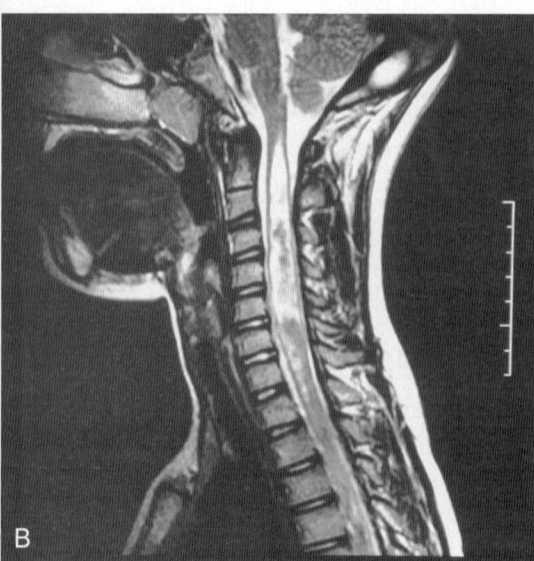

FIGURE 28.5 Syringomyelia with spinal lipoma. Magnetic resonance images of a 9-year-old boy who had surgical untethering for spinal lipoma at the age of 1 year, and now his walking has been deteriorating for several months. **A,** Lumbar spine T2-weighted sagittal sequence. There is tethering of the lower spinal cord at the region of the lower lumbar-sacral spine, at the site of the previously operated spinal lipoma. At the level of T10 there is the lower end of a syringomyelia cavity. **B,** Cervical spine T2-weighted sagittal sequence. The syringomyelia cavity extends cranially up to the level of C2; essentially, it is a holocord syringomyelia.

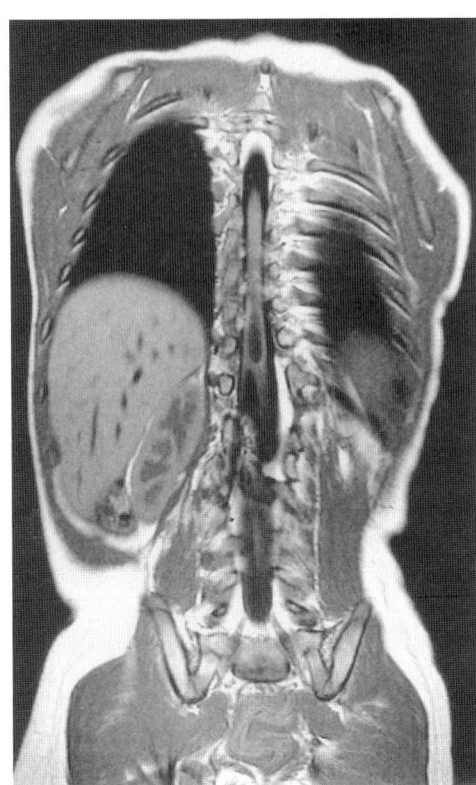

FIGURE 28.6 Syringomyelia with diastematomyelia. Spine T1-weighted coronal magnetic resonance image of a 6-year-old girl who had a hairy patch in the midline of the back at the level of the upper lumbar spine and developed a limp in her walking. There is a bony spur in the region of L1, which splits the spinal cord in two hemicords. Just cranially to the cord split there is a syringomyelia cavity, extending for two spinal levels.

The cavity may extend both proximally and distally and the tension of the fluid inside it continues to increase. Longstanding syringomyelia provokes gliosis formation in the cavity walls and the surrounding cord. Gliosis formation has been seen in postmortem examinations, in which the cavity walls are seen to be clearly lined by gliotic tissue.[8] A drain inserted in the syringomyelia cavity may be encased by gliotic tissue.[8] Even though surgical treatment may lead to radiological collapse of the syringomyelia cavity, sometimes this is not associated with clinical improvement. Gliosis inside the cord may lead to progressive neurological loss even after successful surgery and collapse of the cavity.[9] The syringomyelia cavity can reach the upper cervical cord and medulla, becoming syringobulbia (Fig. 28.3C); it may cause deterioration of neurological function in the arms and eventually affect the function of the lower brainstem, producing bulbar palsy, respiratory failure, and death.

EPIDEMIOLOGY

The incidence of Chiari I malformation in the general population is estimated at 7%, but not all subjects are symptomatic. The increasing use of MRI scanning in the investigation of headaches has led to an increase in the incidence of this diagnosis. It is unclear, though, what percentage of patients with radiological evidence of Chiari I malformation have symptoms attributable to it. Syringomyelia has a prevalence of 8.4 cases per 100,000 population. It is estimated that in the United States, 21,000 Americans suffer from syringomyelia. More accurately, the figure is likely to be considerably higher, as even today, despite the wide availability of MRI scanning, the condition is underdiagnosed. The incidence of post-traumatic syringomyelia is around 1% to 3% of cases of paraplegia with a male predominance and relatively young age, and parallel to the incidence or trauma for age and gender.[10-12] Why so few patients develop syringomyelia following spinal cord injury is not known. The average time between spinal injury and symptomatic presentation is 7 years (range: 3 months to 30 years). Post-traumatic syringomyelia is rare in children.

PATHOPHYSIOLOGY OF SYRINGOMYELIA

In the majority of patients syringomyelia is associated with an obstruction of CSF flow in the subarachnoid space. Surgical treatments are designed to remove such a subarachnoid obstruction. In most patients the block in CSF flow is in the region of the foramen magnum and is due to hindbrain hernia (Chiari I and Chiari II) or in other sites in any of the other conditions mentioned before.

The mechanism of formation of syringomyelia has not been adequately explained yet. Most of the studies that attempt to explain the development of syringomyelia focus on the model of hindbrain hernia in Chiari I malformation. In experimental studies, dye injected in the spinal subarachnoid space has been found in the central canal, believed to have traveled there along the Virchow-Robin spaces beside the vessels of the cord. It is unclear when and how the creation of the cavity commences.[13] There are reports of a presyringomyelia state seen in MRI scans of patients with Chiari I malformation, with upper cervical spinal cord swelling, which subsequently developed into syringomyelia.[14-16] These reports are very few, in contrast to the very high numbers of patients with established syringomyelia that have been reported and are seen in clinical practice. This by implication may signify that the presence of a presyringomyelia state may be the exception rather than the rule. Several theories have been proposed on the formation and propagation of syringomyelia. The most notable ones, in chronological order, are Gardner's hydrodynamic theory, Williams' theory of "pressure dissociation," and Oldfield's theory of increased subarachnoid CSF pressure wave:

- In the 1960s Gardner observed that in patients with hindbrain hernia the foramen of Magendie was partially obstructed by a membrane. He believed that fluid entered the central canal in the obex at the floor of the fourth ventricle due to the "water hammer" effect of the arterial pulsations on CSF flow. Fluid accumulated inside the central canal creating the syringomyelia cavity—communicating syringomyelia or hydromyelia.[17,18] This led to the surgical concept of obex plugging, where a piece of muscle or cotton wool was used to plug the obex. Syringomyelia not communicating with the central canal was called *noncommunicating*. MRI studies have shown that in the majority of the patients there is no direct communication between

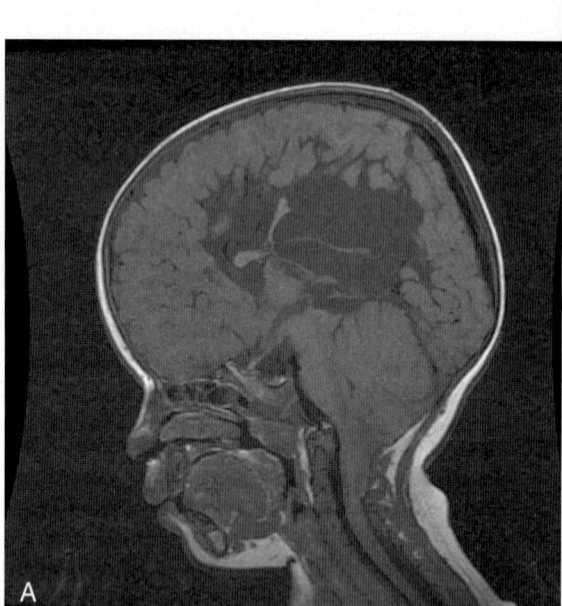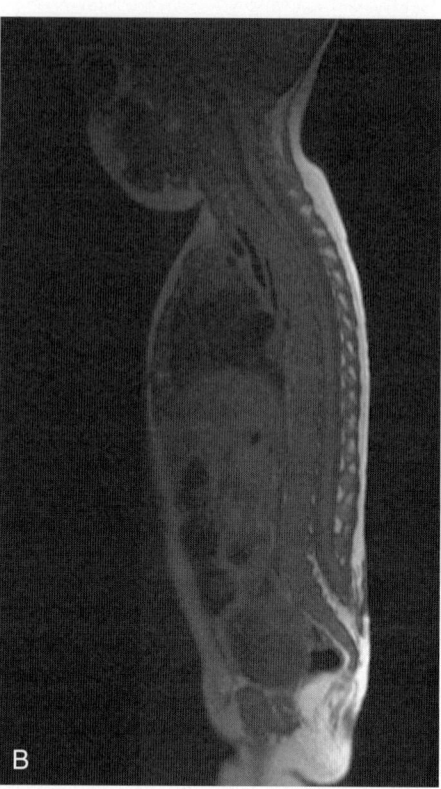

FIGURE 28.7 Syringomyelia with Chiari II malformation. Magnetic resonance imaging (MRI) studies of a 7-year-old boy who was born with myelomeningocele and Chiari II malformation. He had closure of the myelomeningocele at birth and placement of a ventriculoperitoneal shunt for hydrocephalus. Owing to the low level (lumbosacral) of the myelomeningocele, he developed to become fully ambulant, walking with no support. For the last 4 months prior to this MRI examination, he has been complaining of pain in his legs and deteriorating walking. **A,** Head T1-weighted sagittal sequence. There is a Chiari II malformation, with cerebellar herniation down to the level of C3. Other features of the Chiari II malformation are seen such as hypoplastic corpus callosum, small posterior fossa, caudal migration of the medulla, and hypertrophic interthalamic adhesion. **B,** Spine T1-weighted sequence. There is a syringomyelia cavity extending from T2 to T7.

the obex and the syringomyelia cavity. Cardiac gated cine phase contrast MRI (cine PC-MRI) studies have shown that during systole the syrinx cavity contracts, whereas if Gardner's theory was correct it should expand under the force of inflowing CSF. Gardner's theory is regarded as imperfect and the term *communicating syringomyelia* has been used with less frequency. The technique of obex plugging has fallen out of favor, if for no other reason than the material used to plug the obex caused significant arachnoid fibrosis and adhesions, with subsequent recurrence of the syringomyelia.

- In the early 1980s Williams described the concept of "pressure dissociation" between the subarachnoid CSF spaces of the head and the spine secondary to the block of hindbrain hernia, based on in vivo CSF pressure measurements and in vitro biomechanical studies, which he performed.[19] Every time a Valsalva maneuver takes place (e.g., coughing) the pressure from the chest and abdomen is transmitted to the spinal canal through the valveless venous plexus around the vertebral bodies. Normally, pressures are equalized within the spine rapidly. In the presence of a partial subarachnoid block, fluid is forced upward past the block more efficiently than it can run down again. This leads to a collapsed theca below the block, which exerts a suction effect on the spinal cord (the "suck" mechanism).

Fluid that has entered the cord cavity can extend the cavity (the "slosh" mechanism).[9,20,21] Williams' theories were partly verified by MRI scan observations, and Williams' demonstrations of his "suck and slosh" theory with models were impressive. Using cine PC-MRI it has been shown that in the presence of hindbrain hernia CSF movement in the region of the foramen magnum differs between systole and diastole. However, Williams' observations of pressure differential were not confirmed by other studies of intraoperative CSF pressure measurements.[22] It is possible that the sitting position he used to obtain his readings contributed to exaggerated cranial-spinal pressure difference readings, owing to CSF leakage from the site of the spinal measuring needle.

- Using preoperative PC-MRI scanning and intraoperative CSF pressure measurements in patients with syringomyelia and Chiari I malformation, Oldfield's group observed that CSF velocity was increased at the foramen magnum but CSF flow was decreased. Cervical subarachnoid CSF pressure was increased, spinal CSF compliance was decreased, and syrinx CSF flowed caudally during systole and cranially during diastole.[22,23] They surmised that the prolapsed cerebellar tonsils act like a piston, partially occluding the subarachnoid space, and create a state of increased subarachnoid pressure waves, which compress the spinal cord

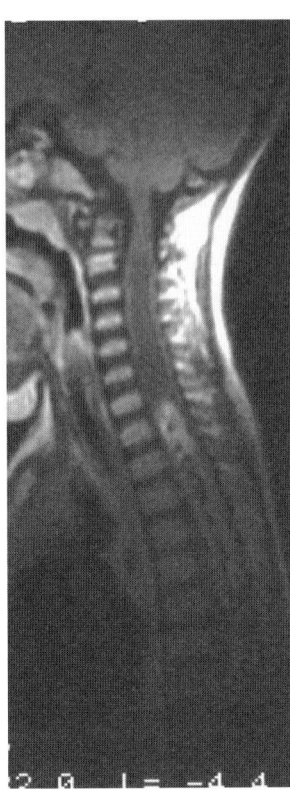

FIGURE 28.8 Syringomyelia with spinal cord astrocytoma. Spine T1-weighted sagittal sequence with intravenous contrast agent in a 5-year-old girl who presented with back pain and a limp. There is a contrast-enhancing intramedullary spinal cord tumor at the levels T8-L1. Cranially to the tumor there is a large syringomyelia cavity extending up to C2. The tumor was excised and proved to be grade II astrocytoma.

from without and force CSF into the syrinx cavity and propagate it with each heartbeat.

All these theories do not explain precisely how and where CSF enters the cord and the mechanism of formation of septations inside the syringomyelia cavity. In the past decade, research with in vitro computer simulations using parameters gained from MRI has focused on the hydrodynamic properties of CSF, how they are altered in the presence of a subarachnoid block, and how the spinal cord viscoelastic properties relate to these changes.[24-31] It is hoped that as our noninvasive imaging of CSF flow evolves, more insights will be gained on the formation and propagation of syringomyelia.

In patients who suffer spinal cord trauma, cord contusion leads to edema, blood effusion, and subsequent cord liquefaction during the first few months after injury in up to 50% of patients. Subsequently, cavity formation results and may be referred to as the *primary cyst*.[32-34] Commonly, the cyst at the site of the injury is separated from the syringomyelia cavity by an intact septum. The syringomyelia cavity may decompress above and below the injury site following treatment, but the primary cysts may remain unchanged.[35,36] As the acute injury settles, inflammation is followed by adhesions in the subarachnoid space and gliosis in the cord. Obstruction of the CSF pathways may be compounded by narrowing of the bony

spinal canal from the spinal fracture. Fluid may enter the cord at the fracture site, which is often thin-walled.

Syringomyelia is associated with other pathological conditions such as dysraphic states, spinal cord tumors, and spinal arachnoid cysts. There is no unifying, satisfactory explanation of how CSF enters the spinal cord, and it may be analogous to the situation in hindbrain-related syringomyelia, but that remains unproved. The presence of arachnoid adhesions appears to be an important event in the formation of syringomyelia. The presence of syringomyelia associated with tethered cord or low-lying cord from a thickened filum terminale is difficult to explain applying the concept of subarachnoid CSF block. Thus, the exact pathophysiology of a terminal syrinx or dilatation of the central canal associated with a low-lying spinal cord remains unknown.

Posterior Fossa Volume

The pathophysiology of syringomyelia and Chiari I malformation is often studied together, as the latter is the most common coexisting pathological condition with the former. The theory that a small posterior fossa is implicated in the cause of hindbrain hernia has been pursued for many years. It is a very obvious suggestion, as it is unlikely that Chiari I patients have "excess" cerebellar tissue compared to normal control subjects. It follows logically that some patients may have a smaller posterior fossa, which is unable to accommodate the normal volume of cerebellum. Early two-dimensional studies on lateral skull radiographs demonstrated that the height or the area of the posterior fossa is small in patients with Chiari I malformation.[37,38] Recent studies used advanced image analysis techniques to calculate posterior fossa volume in computed tomography (CT) or MRI scans.[39-41] The researchers conclude that the posterior fossa is smaller than normal in patients with Chiari I malformation due to presumed maldevelopment of the occipital enchondrium. This finding supports to a large extent the widespread philosophy of surgical treatment of hindbrain hernia with craniovertebral decompression to provide the cerebellum with more room, that has evolved in the past two decades.

Careful appraisal of all these studies demonstrates that none has separated patients with Chiari I according to the presence of syringomyelia. In fact, in most studies the patients with syringomyelia form the majority of the sample. A study that focused on the pediatric age group demonstrated that patients with Chiari I alone have posterior fossa of normal volume, whereas patients with Chiari I and syringomyelia have posterior fossa volume significantly smaller than normal.[42] The difference in posterior fossa volume ratio according to the presence of syringomyelia was more pronounced in children who presented before the age of 10 years and smaller in those presenting after the age of 10 years. After the age of 10 years there is no significant change in the growth of the cranium overall, and little change in the growth of the skull base.[43] These findings challenge the view that the development of syringomyelia represents an evolutionary stage of the Chiari I malformation. From personal observations, although new development of syringomyelia can be seen after craniovertebral decompression as a result of arachnoiditis, in patients who did not have syringomyelia at presentation, such development has not been seen in nonoperated patients with

Chiari I malformation alone. Currently, there are no sizeable reports in the literature of patients with nonoperated Chiari I malformation, who have been followed for a very long time, to clearly define the risk of developing new syringomyelia. On the other hand, the phenomenon of acquired Chiari I malformation in different circumstances (e.g., following lumbar or ventricular shunting) is well recognized.[6,7]

It has been proposed that in most cases from the beginning of the creation of their malformation patients either have normal posterior fossa and Chiari I malformation only with no syringomyelia, or small posterior fossa and syringomyelia, resulting in "loss" of CSF in the spine, in a situation similar to patients with Chiari II malformation in which the open myelomeningocele is associated with true loss of CSF and small posterior fossa. This view is strengthened by the observation that children with syringomyelia and brainstem descent had even smaller posterior fossas. At present it would be difficult to establish whether the two subtypes of Chiari I malformation represent differences in phenotypic expression, with the syringomyelia subgroup being the more severely affected by the underlying process, or whether they are two different malformations within the Chiari malformation spectrum.

There is increasing evidence that the mechanism of symptoms creation in Chiari I malformation is probably not volume related. Even in patients with syringomyelia, it has been noticed that in a small proportion of patients symptoms and radiological signs have not responded following suboccipital craniectomy, leading certain authors to conclude that the underlying mechanism causing the syringomyelia is not volume related. The presence of normal posterior fossa in Chiari I alone does not explain the development of tonsillar herniation. It could be postulated that localized venous hypertension and possible altered geometry of the posterior fossa[43,44] could initiate the downward migration, which subsequently is perpetuated by CSF movement and impaction. Personal observations during foramen magnum decompression operations for Chiari only in the absence of syringomyelia indicate that soon after dural opening and division of arachnoidal adhesions that link the impacted tonsils to the surrounding structures, the cerebellar tonsils usually ascend to their natural position, without the need for further coagulation or resection. Thus, it appears that foramen magnum decompression probably works by allowing disimpaction of the tonsils from the craniovertebral junction, rather than "enlarging" the posterior fossa, as the tonsils never move to occupy the newly enlarged cisterna magna, but ascend to a normal location. In that line, there is a universal tendency for reduction of the size of the craniectomy in the foramen magnum.

CLINICAL FEATURES

Presenting Symptoms

Patients can have symptoms and signs from the cerebellum and the lower cranial nerves in the presence of Chiari I malformation or syringobulbia and from long tracts originating from the syringomyelia. The symptoms can be grouped into those of pain, sensory and motor deficits, and disordered autonomic functions. Severity of symptoms can vary and there

are patients who remain completely symptom free for long time periods.

Patients with hindbrain hernia–related syringomyelia often present with symptoms from the Chiari I malformation and the syringomyelia is discovered when an MRI scan is performed on suspicion of hindbrain hernia. Symptoms associated with Chiari I malformation include headaches that are usually occipital but not uncommonly poorly localized, and worse on physical exertion and straining; occasionally clumsiness and poor coordination with hands; and ocular symptoms such as blurred vision, diplopia, or oscillopsia. Other rare symptoms relevant to the Chiari I malformation are dizziness, unsteadiness (disequilibrium), tinnitus, vertigo, hyperacusis, nystagmus, dysphagia, sleep apnea, dysarthria, tremor, facial pain or numbness, shortness of breath, and syncopal (drop) attacks.

Symptoms relevant to the presence of syringomyelia include weakness or clumsiness from arms and legs, which may not be following a myotomal distribution; paresthesias, dysesthesias, and pain, which may not be following a dermatomal distribution; unsteady gait; muscle atrophy; and spasticity. Pain is commonly a prominent feature. In a small percentage of patients there may be urinary and fecal incontinence and impotence in male patients. The location of symptoms may not be correlated with radiological findings. They can be strikingly unilateral even though the syrinx may appear to occupy the central part of the cord on imaging. Syringobulbia can be life threatening. The commonest symptom of syringobulbia is spreading facial numbness. Swallowing and voice may also be affected, then vision, hearing, and finally respiratory function. Nocturnal hypoventilation has been described in the presence of syringomyelia not extending to the medulla.[45]

It should be emphasized that a significant proportion of patients with radiologically identified Chiari I malformation do not experience any symptoms and their malformation was identified incidentally during investigations for other reasons.[3,4] A large study of 22,591 MRI scans identified 175 patients with Chiari I malformation and 14% of them were completely asymptomatic.

Clinical Examination Findings

In patients with Chiari I malformation or syringobulbia clinical examination findings include lower cranial nerves and cerebellar signs. In patients with syringomyelia long tract signs are common. Neuro-ophthalmological findings include impaired visual acuity, extraocular muscle palsy, nystagmus, and papilledema in a small minority.[46] Ophthalmological assessment is of paramount importance in patients with Chiari I malformation. Other signs from lower cranial nerves include facial sensory loss, sensorineural or conductive hearing loss, impaired vestibular function, vocal cord palsy, and impaired gag reflex. Cerebellar signs such as dysmetria or truncal ataxia are not uncommon.

Clinical examination findings associated with syringomyelia include weakness of arms and legs, not always following a myotomal distribution, and sensory deficits over arms and legs, not always following dermatomal distribution. Unilateral weakness of one upper limb, not infrequently associated with a sudden strain and associated pain, is commonly seen. The small muscles of the hand are often affected first and wasting of the first dorsal interosseous muscle between the fingers and the thumb may be an early finding. The triceps or the shoulder musculature could be affected before the hand. In advanced cases it is not uncommon to find claw deformity in the hand with wasting of all the forearm and arm musculature. Sensory loss can be of spinothalamic or dorsal column type, occasionally in patchy distribution. It is usually unilateral and tends to involve the upper limb early, progressing by an increase of the density of the deficit more often than by anatomical extension. It can even be variable throughout the course of the day, and is presumably related to a variable state of filling of the syrinx. The traditionally described pain/temperature dissociation that is loss of pain and temperature sensation with preserved light touch and joint position sense is rare. Muscular atrophy and fasciculation can be seen as well as dystrophic (Charcot) joints. Hyper- or hyporeflexia can be present depending on the level of syringomyelia.[47,48] Asymmetry is not uncommon and certain reflexes may be unexpectedly spared. Spasticity can affect upper and lower limbs. Scoliosis is a common finding with syringomyelia in young children, and is seen often in previously undiagnosed young adults as well.[49-53] Short neck and low hairline are seen in patients with basilar invagination. Horner syndrome is seen infrequently. Gross disturbance of sweating can occur.[54] Dry skin or hyperhidrosis can be observed, usually symmetrically in the lower half of the body, although the upper limbs may be affected in an asymmetrical distribution with facial involvement at times, and unequal pupils may be the only feature.

In patients with spinal cord injury incomplete paraplegia that deteriorates or the development of new autonomic features may be associated with syringomyelia. The most important features are those that ascend. Descending syringomyelia is rarely diagnosed. In complete paraplegia, improvement of leg spasms could imply downward extension of the syringomyelia. So also could alteration of sweating patterns and impairment of other autonomic functions such as bladder and bowel control and sexual function. Pain is common in post-traumatic syringomyelia, and a paraplegic complaining of severe pain has syringomyelia until proved otherwise.[9-12,35,36,55-59] It is frequently associated with straining and progression of neurological deficit. Although it is commonly experienced at the level of the deficit, it can affect sites above or below that level and can be misleading. It can be confused with chest or abdominal disease. Not infrequently it is soon replaced by dysesthetic sensory loss.

In general, in the presence of syringomyelia new contralateral symptoms in a patient, who had drainage treatment for a deteriorating syrinx and has been stable for a while, could imply the excavation of a new cavity alongside the previous one.

DIAGNOSIS

Once a patient is suspected of having the diagnosis of syringomyelia, MRI scan is the investigation of choice and confirms the diagnosis in most cases. In the pre-MRI era, CT scan with intrathecal metrizamide was employed, acquiring late views to view contrast material in the syringomyelia cavity. Postmyelography CT scan remains useful in patients with severe claustrophobia or magnetic implants. Plain radiographs of the spine are useful in patients with scoliosis and when a bony malformation of the craniocervical junction is suspected. Whenever the issue of possible instability arises, flexion-extension views can provide more information on spinal stability. In patients with post-traumatic syringomyelia, plain films often show post-traumatic kyphosis and associated narrowing of the spinal canal.

Radiology

MRI scanning shows the Chiari malformation and the extent of the syringomyelia cavity and haustrations, especially in T2-weighted sequences.[34,60,61] Around 15% of patients have hydrocephalus. Other pathological conditions are clearly demonstrated. The syrinx in children with profound scoliosis can be difficult to visualize in MRI scanning (see Fig. 28.1). Because the curvature of the spine can be extensive it may not be possible to have the entire spinal cord in a single sagittal view, and it may be difficult to correctly count the vertebral levels and identify the full extent of the syrinx (see Fig. 28.1B and C). Children with significant scoliosis can have syringomyelia in the absence of Chiari I malformation. Post-traumatic syringomyelia and its relation with primary cysts shows well in MRI scans (see Fig. 28.4), although in some patients with extensive spinal fractures it may be difficult to identify the complexity of the bony injury. Spinal lipomas (see Fig. 28.5) and diastematomyelia (see Fig. 28.6) are clearly seen. In patients with spinal lipoma there may be the need to obtain fat suppression sequences to visualize the relation between lipoma and spinal cord better, in preparation for a cord untethering. In patients with diastematomyelia, commonly the syringomyelia cavity is not extensive. Spinal cord tumors are clearly identified in contrast-enhanced MRI sequences (see Fig. 28.8). Whenever a patient is found to have syringomyelia in the absence of a clearly identifiable associated lesion, contrast-enhanced sequences should be obtained to exclude the presence of spinal cord tumor. In a small minority of patients no associated lesion is identified. Information relating to the CSF circulation can be obtained with cardiac gated cine PC-MRI (see Fig. 28.2B). In current clinical practice the value of cine-MRI is limited in the influence it may have in clinical decisions. The utility of this tool is evolving in the study of CSF movement and its correlation with clinical symptoms and outcome.[62-68] Sequential MRI is useful in assessing the results of treatment or in observing the evolution of the symptoms and deciding when radiological progression may indicate a need for surgical intervention.[69,70]

Neurophysiological Tests

Nerve conduction studies, brainstem evoked potentials, spontaneous electromyography (EMG), motor evoked potentials (MEPs), and somatosensory evoked potentials (SSEPs) have been used in the study of patients with syringomyelia.[71,72] It has not been easy to use such tests to tailor the indication for surgery, as normal neurophysiological tests do not imply absence of threat of neurological deterioration. Usually these tests are abnormal when clinical symptoms or signs have been established. Nevertheless, they may prove useful in the follow-up of patients treated surgically. SSEPs, EMG, and MEPs can be useful intraoperatively in selected cases with tumors, syringomyelia, and other spinal cord anomalies.

CONTROVERSIES IN MANAGEMENT

While the diagnosis is easily done today with the relatively common availability of MRI scanning, it is less easy at times to decide what the optimal treatment strategy is for the individual patient. Considerable controversy still surrounds the management of hindbrain hernia and syringomyelia, and this debate is largely due to the uncharted natural history of the condition. Inevitably, any discussion of the management of syringomyelia involves intimately the management of Chiari I malformation. The Chiari II malformation has special issues for consideration and will be discussed separately.

Controversy surrounds the following issues:

1. When does hindbrain hernia/Chiari I malformation need surgical treatment?
2. When does syringomyelia need surgical treatment?
3. What is the best surgical treatment for the management of hindbrain hernia?
4. What is the best surgical treatment for the management of syringomyelia?
5. What is the best management of recurrent syringomyelia?
6. What is the best management of the associated hydrocephalus?

NATURAL HISTORY

Hindbrain Hernia

There are no prospective, nonoperative studies outlining the natural history of hindbrain hernia and syringomyelia. In surgical series of patients with symptomatic hindbrain hernia the incidence of syringomyelia varies from 55% to 85%,[9,61,73-79] but inevitably all such series have a highly selected population. There are very few studies following "asymptomatic" patients.[4] The absence of such data is largely due to historical reasons: before the advent of MRI it was very difficult to diagnose hindbrain hernia and syringomyelia. Since the introduction of MRI, the condition is diagnosed more frequently, and the clinicians have adopted a wide variety of successful surgical and conservative approaches. Neurosurgeons who see larger numbers of patients with these conditions tend to appreciate more common signs and symptoms such as motor and sensory deficits or tussive headaches.

The general attitude is that a completely asymptomatic Chiari I malformation can be managed conservatively and followed closely.[80] The difference of opinion among clinicians rests on what constitutes asymptomatic hindbrain hernia. In most patients who provide a history, there is clear evidence of tussive, cough-, or exercise-induced headache or occipital pain. Some even admit to arm pain on exertion. In small children, motor developmental delay of mild degree is frequently seen in both arm dexterity and fluency of walking. Such cases should be seen as symptomatic patients and considered for potential treatment. Other more subtle symptoms and signs can go unnoticed unless a longitudinal approach is adopted. It should be remembered that intracranial hypertension can be otherwise "silent" and only manifest with papilledema on funduscopic examination. It is the author's belief that the incidence of truly asymptomatic hindbrain hernia is smaller than stated. Instead, there is a spectrum of symptom intensity and symptoms may change or develop in time, and the neurosurgeon's decision to operate or not is relevant to his or her expertise in the field and willingness to follow these patients over the long term.

Syringomyelia

Similar to hindbrain hernia, the natural history of untreated syringomyelia is not charted conclusively. It is considered that syringomyelia deteriorates with time, but the speed with which this deterioration takes place is unknown.[81] When faced for the first time with a patient with syringomyelia, it is difficult to postulate on the risk of sudden neurological deterioration, although such a complication is well documented albeit rare. Similarly, in the presence of a large syringomyelia cavity, it is not known what percentage of patients develop symptoms over what time frame. Whereas the typical symptoms and signs of syringomyelia are readily appreciated, the subtler ones are easier to miss. Mild scoliosis and very subtle motor developmental delay in very young children are important. Long-standing syringomyelia leads to gliosis in the spinal cord and irreversible neurological damage. Thus, it would be reasonable to have a low threshold for considering treatment when syringomyelia is discovered.

SURGERY

Indications for Surgical Treatment

- In patients with Chiari I malformation only, and no syringomyelia, the presence of occipital headaches, cough induced or deteriorating, and possibly other cerebellar symptoms is an indication for surgical treatment with craniovertebral decompression. Other subtle symptoms should be considered individually.
- In patients with Chiari I malformation and syringomyelia, the presence of relevant symptoms and clinical findings, as discussed previously, constitutes an indication for surgical treatment with craniovertebral decompression. A distended syringomyelia occupying the cervical cord, even if asymptomatic, merits surgical treatment, as it potentially threatens vital neurological functions. In contrast, the patient with a small, two-level cavity and no relevant symptoms can be watched with repeat MRI scans annually.
- The presence of scoliosis in children, even in the absence of other neurological symptoms, requires surgical treatment to stabilize the progression of scoliosis. Most orthopedic surgeons would not contemplate surgical correction of scoliosis in the presence of untreated syringomyelia, as the risk of postoperative paraplegia or quadriplegia is significant.
- Patients with post-traumatic syringomyelia merit early surgery because syringomyelia can expand silently and insidiously, compromising residual neurological function. Surgical decompression at the site of the subarachnoid block is recommended, which is commonly the fracture site.
- In patients with spinal dysraphism, syringomyelia rarely constitutes an urgent indication for surgery. An expanded syrinx may be the result of a shunt failure, which needs to be addressed first. Patients with symptoms from

spinal cord tethering and a new syrinx may need surgical treatment.

- Patients with spinal cord tumors require surgical excision for their tumor, which leads to reduction of the syringomyelia cavity.[82] Recurrence of syringomyelia commonly implies tumor recurrence or CSF block, or arachnoiditis at the level of the previous surgery.
- Patients with spinal arachnoid cysts commonly have neurological symptoms from cord compression and require surgical excision or drainage of the cyst.[83,84]
- Patients with postinflammatory syringomyelia present particular difficulties because commonly they have significant neurological deficits from their condition even before syringomyelia develops. This is not always easy to appreciate if the development of radiological syringomyelia is associated with the development of new symptoms. When a clear link is established between radiological and clinical deterioration, surgery should be pursued. If such a clear link is not apparent, a period of observation and regular repeat scanning may be preferable.
- Patients with recurrent syringomyelia and unclear neurological signs require careful assessment. Repeat surgery for such patients often has guarded results and caution should be exercised. Often an initial period of observation and repeat MRI scans is a good strategy, reserving surgery for when there is a clear clinical or radiological deterioration.

The challenging patients are those with unremarkable symptoms and whose syringomyelia is not progressing or has only moderate distention. In patients with post-traumatic syringomyelia, and incomplete paraplegia, indications for surgery can be difficult to discern. There is a risk of allowing further deterioration to occur by not intervening surgically. It is not uncommon for a patient who has what appears to be a stable syringomyelia, not increasing in size over a number of years, to develop rapid clinical deterioration. On the other hand, there is a complication rate associated with any operative procedure, and it is often difficult to justify surgery in stable patients. As the natural history of syringomyelia can be variable, it is recommended to err toward early surgical treatment, as it is likely that untreated patients will deteriorate. In general, it is believed that early surgery offers better long-term results.[9,21,36] Patients with recurrent syringomyelia, years after an initial successful surgical treatment and unclear neurological signs, require careful assessment and pose a significant dilemma. Repeat surgery for such patients often has guarded results and caution should be exercised. Often an initial period of clinical observation and repeat MRI scans is a good initial management strategy, reserving surgery for when there is a clear clinical or radiological deterioration.

Surgical Strategy

- Patients with Chiari I malformation (with or without syringomyelia) require craniovertebral decompression as the first procedure.
- Patients with post-traumatic syringomyelia require surgical decompression at the site of the subarachnoid block.
- Patients with dysraphic states require cord untethering or craniovertebral decompression relevant to their pathological condition as the first procedure.

- Patients with post-inflammatory syringomyelia need careful radiological evaluation to appreciate the site of the subarachnoid block, and surgical strategy is then tailored accordingly.

Surgical Management of Chiari I Malformation

Craniovertebral decompression for Chiari I malformation includes occipital craniectomy and removal of the arch of C1 at least, depending on the extent of the hindbrain hernia.[20,80,85-101] This aims to remove the block of CSF flow in the craniovertebral junction due to the prolapsed tonsils. The size of the craniectomy has been decreasing over the years, and now a craniectomy flap of 3 × 3 cm is regarded as satisfactory; larger defects are associated with cerebellar slumping.[69] This operation leads to clinical improvement of symptoms in 80% of patients and to radiological improvement of syringomyelia in up to 70% of the patients.[102] Syringopleural or syringosubarachnoid shunts used as primary treatment have a very poor long-term success rate in the presence of an active subarachnoid block, which acts as a filling mechanism for the syringomyelia.[8,103-107]

Controversy exists on whether the arachnoid mater should be opened. Most neurosurgeons prefer to open the arachnoid. The proponents of opening the arachnoid maintain that dissection of the arachnoid adhesions on the foramen magnum safeguards against recurrence. The proponents of leaving the arachnoid intact believe that breaching the arachnoid can promote creation of further adhesions owing to the intraoperative spillage of blood. Essentially, the decision focuses on opening the dura or not, as commonly during dural opening the arachnoid is breached and has to be opened widely. Recently, intraoperative ultrasound scanning (US) has indicated that absence of CSF flow at the foramen magnum after craniectomy may be an indication for opening the arachnoid membrane and is used by several neurosurgeons routinely.[108] Utilization of intraoperative ultrasound is not regarded as mandatory, though. Recently, the technique of extradural decompression has been revisited with claimed satisfactory results, especially in young children.

Another controversial issue is the use of a duraplasty graft to enlarge the cisterna magna after lysis of the arachnoid adhesions versus closure of the craniectomy without duraplasty, by closing the overlying muscles and leaving the dura open, thus creating a pseudomeningocele.[9,21,80,85,93,109-112] When performing duraplasty, some surgeons prefer to use pericranial graft, harvested from the occipital area just above the craniectomy site, and others prefer to use artificial graft. The use of a duraplasty decreases the incidence of CSF leak but often adequately treats the associated syringomyelia. In patients who do not receive a duroplasty, the risk of a CSF leak is higher, but the possibility of recurrence or failure to adequately treat an associated syrinx decreases.

Patients who have craniocervical instability in the context of syndromes affecting the craniocervical junction (e.g., Morquio syndrome, achondroplasia) may need simultaneous atlanto-occipital fixation in the same operation after the craniovertebral decompression.[74,113,114] A small group of patients have anterior compression from basilar invagination and should be considered for anterior decompression transorally.[115]

Surgical Management of Post-Traumatic Syringomyelia

In the 1970s and 1980s syringosubarachnoid and syringopleural shunts were used widely but in the 2000s long-term effectiveness has been questioned.[11,55,87,105,106,116-122] A variety of complications and infection have been observed. The drain functions for some time, the cord collapses around it, and the draining holes become occluded by gliotic tissue. Subsequently the syringomyelia recurs if the filling mechanism has not been corrected.[8] The current treatment of post-traumatic syringomyelia is decompressive laminectomy and subarachnoid space reconstruction by lysis of arachnoid adhesions at the fracture site.[9,35,36,57,83,94,123,124] This operation should not be performed before issues of spinal stability have been addressed. This technique results in radiological improvement of the syringomyelia in up to 80% of the patients.

In the late 1980s and early 1990s attempts were made to treat post-traumatic syringomyelia with omental grafting.[125] This operation involved laparotomy first in order to harvest a vascularized pedicle of omentum, which was subsequently tunneled under the skin to the spine and was laid over the injured spinal cord at the injury site, which was exposed by laminectomy. These operations were associated with high morbidity and low success rates in controlling the syringomyelia and have been abandoned.

Surgical Management of Residual or Recurrent Syringomyelia

When an initial decrease of syringomyelia size has been observed, followed by recurrence, reexploration of the craniovertebral junction, opening of the arachnoid, and extensive dissection of the adhesions in the regions of all the foramina of the fourth ventricle are required.[126,127] This surgical strategy is associated with an average success rate (60%). Surgical variations include the use of stents in the foramen magnum to avoid recurrent adhesions. Although the author does not favor stents in this region, they have been reported to offer good long-term control of the syringomyelia. A significant problem with stents in the foramen magnum is the high risk of migration into the brainstem, which causes significant neurological deterioration. If that fails, then as a last measure a syringopleural or subarachnoid shunt could be attempted. These shunts enjoy an average chance of radiological improvement (around 50-60%) but lower than average chance of clinical improvement (around 10-20%).[128] However, often, they are the last resort to avoid clinical deterioration in a patient with an expanding syrinx. Insertion of a syringopleural or syringosubarachnoid shunt requires laminotomy in the site of the widest diameter of the syrinx and intradural exposure of the spinal cord. A midline myelotomy is performed. It is recommended to use a fine ultrasound probe prior to performing the myelotomy, to confirm the most dilated location of the syrinx. However, often ultrasound is not needed as the syrinx can dilate the cord so much that the pial surface becomes translucent, making placement of the myelotomy easier. After a small myelotomy is performed, a T-shaped catheter is inserted in the syrinx cavity and secured with pial fine sutures. The other end is placed in the subarachnoid space or threaded toward the chest wall in the midaxillary line and in the pleural cavity. As all shunts, syringomyelia shunts have similar mechanical and infectious risks.

The use of endoscopic techniques to break down septations inside the syringomyelia cavity was in vogue in the 1990s with resurgence of neuroendoscopy but has no rationale based on any pathophysiological observations. It has only modest impact on the size of the syringomyelia and has been abandoned in the 2000s, even in the phase of dramatic expansion of neuroendoscopy.

The presence of persistent syringomyelia despite adequate craniovertebral decompression may indicate underlying intracranial hypertension.[124,127,129] Invasive intracranial pressure (ICP) measurement may be required to investigate and resolve this issue. In the presence of ventriculomegaly and raised intracranial pressure, ventriculoperitoneal shunt may eventually help resolve the persistent syringomyelia if all other measures have failed.[79]

Overall, patients with recurrent syringomyelia or recurrent arachnoiditis in the region of the foramen magnum pose significant challenge on their long-term management, and in general they do not have good long-term outcome, as they continue to deteriorate over a number of years.[130]

Recurrent post-traumatic syringomyelia after initially successful surgical treatment requires repeat exploration of the fracture site and lysis of adhesions. This procedure tends not to have good long-term success, but the surgeon has to pursue surgical treatment in order to arrest continuing clinical deterioration. Similarly, recurrent postinflammatory syringomyelia poses a formidable surgical challenge as the results of repeat surgery are not rewarding.

Management of the Associated Hydrocephalus

The connection between hydrocephalus and syringomyelia has not been elucidated fully yet. Traditionally hydrocephalus is treated first, before a craniovertebral decompression. From cine PC-MRI there is evidence that hydrocephalus is due to fourth ventricle obstruction. When ventricular shunting is performed first, the syringomyelia cavity reduces in size but the need for craniovertebral decompression is not avoided. Recently, endoscopic third ventriculostomy has been used to treat hydrocephalus, with good results in terms of syringomyelia resolution.[131,132]

In patients with a ventriculoperitoneal shunt and syringomyelia that has been controlled, recurrence of the syringomyelia implies shunt obstruction until proved otherwise. Shunt revision should be performed first before any other surgery is contemplated.

Complications

The complication rate for craniovertebral or spinal decompression is low. Perioperative fatality is rare. Wound infection, CSF leak, meningitis, subdural hematoma, urinary tract infection, and thromboembolic complications have been observed at a low rate. Self-limiting aseptic meningitis affects many patients after craniovertebral decompression, more often when the arachnoid has been opened. A very small percentage of patients suffer catastrophic complications such as posterior fossa hematoma, transverse sinus thrombosis, or brainstem infarction due to posterior inferior cerebellar artery damage. Cerebellar sag or slump has been reported as a delayed side effect of cranioveretebral decompression. It was more common in the 1980s to 1990s and presented with intractable headaches and lower cranial nerve signs. In recent years there has been a tendency for smaller occipital craniectomy, which has reduced the incidence of this complication.

Treatment Outcome

Up to 80% of patients with hindbrain-related syringomyelia experience clinical improvement after craniovertebral decompression. Most symptoms improve, but an unfortunate minority experience long-standing incapacitating chronic headaches, often associated with radiological presence of arachnoid adhesions at the region of the foramen magnum. Established neurological deficits associated with syringomyelia such as sensory loss and weakness improve little. Muscle wasting and severe lower cranial nerve palsies do not improve. Early myelopathy improves variably. Established spasticity improves little and often other surgical options have to be employed (e.g., intrathecal baclofen).[133]

In paraplegics several problems may persist despite resolution of syringomyelia. Loss of pain sensitivity leads to trophic changes in skin or joints. Damage to joints without pain sensation may be severe, leading to neuropathic or Charcot joints. In the shoulder the head of the humerus may rapidly absorb. The elbow joint can develop osteophytes and limitation of movement. Paraplegic patients have increased risk of developing cervical spondylosis, possibly related to increased use of their arms as a result of the paraplegia.

Syringomyelia improves after craniovertebral decompression in 70% of the patients, although in the majority of them a residual cavity remains, albeit considerably smaller than preoperatively. Around 15% of patients have no change in the size of the syringomyelia cavity, but it does not deteriorate with time either. Up to 15% of the patients do not experience any postoperative radiological decrease of the syringomyelia. Most of them end up having reexploration of the craniovertebral junction or the spinal decompression site and division of residual arachnoid adhesions with variable result. Patients with recurrent syringomyelia or recurrent arachnoiditis in the foramen magnum or the spinal decompression site tend to deteriorate with time.

Despite radiological control of the syringomyelia, a significant number of patients continue to deteriorate clinically, possibly due to progressive gliosis around the syringomyelia cavity walls.

INTRACRANIAL HYPERTENSION AND SYRINGOMYELIA

Intracranial hypertension may be more common among children with isolated Chiari I malformation than previously realized.[134,135] Routine systematic detailed ophthalmoscopy can detect papilledema, which if left untreated can cause blindness. There have been reports of an incidence of up to 13% of papilledema in patients with hindbrain hernia with or without syringomyelia, and some patients may have raised intracranial hypertension without papilledema.[135] The incidence of intracranial hypertension in the absence of papilledema remains unknown and may well be more frequent than initially thought. The realization that intracranial hypertension may be present in patients with syringomyelia is fairly recent, and it is possible that those who do not demonstrate resolution of syringomyelia despite apparently successful surgery may well harbor raised ICP. More research is expected to illuminate this aspect of syringomyelia in the future.

SYRINGOMYELIA WITH CHIARI II MALFORMATION

In similarity to Chiari I malformation, the majority of patients born with myelomeningocele have hindbrain herniation of varying extent as part of the Chiari II malformation, which is a complex anatomical malformation involving all the brain, not only the hindbrain. Nevertheless, there are many anatomical and physiological differences between the two types of Chiari malformations, and the theoretical models that explain syringomyelia creation and propagation in Chiari I malformation do not easily apply to patients with Chiari II malformation. To date, there is no detailed investigative work in the literature that attempts to explain the formation of syringomyelia in Chiari II patients. All evidence is based on clinical retrospective observations. Some of the main differences between the two malformations are noted in the following list:

1. In Chiari II malformation most of the prolapsed cerebellar tissue is part of the vermis and not the tonsils, as the malformation is created in utero before formation of the cerebellar tonsils. Often, the lower medulla and part of the fourth ventricle are also below the foramen magnum. Whereas in Chiari I the mobile tonsillar tissue can move as a "piston" with every cardiac cycle and "plug" the foramen magnum, in Chiari II the hindbrain hernia contains less "mobile" structures, such as the vermis and the lower medulla, so the analogy may not be appropriate.
2. In support of the previous point, during craniovertebral exploration, in patients with Chiari II malformation there are always significant and dense arachnoid adhesions in the region of the foramen magnum and foramina of Magendie and Luschka, much more than in patients with Chiari I malformation. This is evident even in children who are only a few weeks old at operation.
3. The majority of patients with Chiari I malformation are symptomatic from it, whereas the majority of patients with Chiari II malformation do not experience symptoms directly caused by the malformation unless they present with stridor at birth.[80,136]
4. Most patients with Chiari I malformation and syringomyelia will require surgical treatment at some stage of their disease. In the context of Chiari II malformation the coexistence of syringomyelia can vary between 40% and 90% in different reports,[101,137-142] but only a third of them require treatment for syringomyelia.[138]
5. In the context of Chiari I malformation, although the phenomenon of progressive development of syringomyelia has been well described, in most patients syringomyelia is present ab initio, at the first clinical presentation,[76] and very often is responsible for the symptoms. In the context

of Chiari II malformation, syringomyelia may be present at birth, and commonly expands many years later, probably as a manifestation of recurrent spinal cord tethering or insufficient shunt function. The average age of children with Chiari II who have symptomatic syringomyelia is between 4 and 7 years.[101,138-142]

6. In patients with Chiari I malformation and syringomyelia, hydrocephalus is rare. In contrast, in most patients (80-90%) with Chiari II and syringomyelia there is long-standing hydrocephalus, which has been treated in the first few weeks of life with a ventriculoperitoneal shunt.[136,143]

There has been no study demonstrating a correlation between the extent of herniation of the hindbrain and the incidence of syringomyelia. In recent years, prenatal repair of myelomeningocele has been performed, and this has been shown to lead to improved motor outcomes and reduced need for ventriculoperitoneal shunting.[144] A recent randomized controlled trial showed improved motor outcome and reduced need for shunting in children who had prenatal repair of myelomeningocele, but there was an increased maternal and fetal risk of serious complications such as preterm delivery and uterine dehiscence.[145] Nevertheless, as this treatment has been performed for less than two decades and in only three centers worldwide, it is unclear if it leads also to reduced syringomyelia incidence in these patients.

Commonly, patients who had closure of myelomeningocele at birth and have Chiari II malformation, hydrocephalus, and syringomyelia have been stable for many years and at some stage, they present with gradual progressively deteriorating neurological symptoms and signs related to bulbar, long tract, or bladder function.[101,129,138-142] Bulbar symptoms include respiratory distress, stridor or sleep apnea, vocal cord paresis, difficulty in swallowing, episodes of aspiration, impaired gag reflex, and oculomotor paresis with squint or diplopia and nystagmus. Motor symptoms and signs include deterioration of leg function in ambulatory patients with progressive difficulty in walking and clumsiness or even spasticity, and if the cervical spinal cord is affected there may be new problems in the upper limbs with clumsiness in fine hand movements and dexterity (e.g., deterioration of writing pattern). Sensory symptoms include new pain or deterioration of previously existing pain in trunk and lower limbs, altered sweating pattern especially below the level of the paraplegia, and patchy altered sensation in a nondermatomal distribution. Patients who have intact bladder function can develop deterioration of the micturition pattern. Many paraplegic patients with spina bifida have scoliosis, and the development of syringomyelia can coincide with deterioration of the scoliotic curve.[146]

In patients with Chiari II malformation the causative link of such symptoms with syringomyelia is not always obvious or firm. Patients with Chiari II, hydrocephalus, and a shunt often develop many of the symptoms outlined previously even in the absence of syringomyelia when their shunt is malfunctioning, and they improve after successful shunt revision. Even scoliosis deterioration has been reported in association with shunt malfunction.[147] Moreover, most patients who had repair of myelomeningocele at birth have the radiological appearance of a tethered cord at the repair site in MRI scans. Regardless of how successful and anatomically correct the repair has been, the spinal cord never ascends to its correct level and

always appears attached to the area of the repaired defect. This situation becomes established in the first few weeks after the repair and remains unchanged even when the patient is clinically very well and stable.

The presence of syringomyelia is easily diagnosed in the sagittal spinal T1- and T2-weighted MRI scans in patients with Chiari II (see Fig. 28.7). In contrast to Chiari I–related syringomyelia which is most often cervical in location, in Chiari II the center of gravity of the cavity is located usually in the thoracic cord. It can be either "segmental," occupying a few segments of the spinal cord, or "holocord," occupying the entire spinal cord. Although in Chiari II the syringomyelia cavity is commonly longer than in Chiari I, its transverse diameter is usually less than that seen in cavities associated with Chiari I malformation. Rarely, the syringomyelia cavity is in the cervical cord and threatens to become syringobulbia.

Occasionally, the presence of syringomyelia is discovered incidentally, in the course of such a routine MRI scan.[138] These patients tend to have mild to moderate syringomyelia. In the absence of symptoms, and if the cavity's transverse diameter is less than half the width of the spinal cord, most often we would elect to avoid surgery and instead observe at first and repeat the scan in a few months, before we decide to consider surgical treatment. Clinically "silent" syringomyelia cavities often remain radiologically stable and do not require treatment for years. In most units, though, routine MRI scans of patients with Chiari II malformation are not performed, reserving that examination for when new clinical problems arise.

In most cases, the presence of new neurological symptoms prompts an MRI scan, which can demonstrate syringomyelia. It is difficult to determine whether the clinical symptoms are due to the syringomyelia, the hydrocephalus, or the tethered cord. This dilemma has created inconsistencies in the management of patients with Chiari II and syringomyelia. There are no agreed protocols or robust evidence originating from randomized studies on how these patients should be managed,[148] and different schemes and algorithms have been suggested based on clinical series, often reflecting prevailing tendencies at the time and the difference in experience, training, and attitude. Although there have been many attempts to classify and group different neurological symptoms, the situation is even more confusing with scoliosis, as there is no clear evidence if its deterioration is directly related to syringomyelia.[146]

If the syringomyelia is extensive, with transverse diameter more than half of the width of the spinal cord, and appears threatening, in association with the onset of new symptoms, then surgical action is required.

It is universally accepted that in a patient who has had treatment for hydrocephalus with a ventriculoperitoneal shunt and now presents with clear neurological deterioration and significant syringomyelia, the shunt must be investigated first, and even in the absence of ventriculomegaly or symptoms of raised ICP, shunt revision should be performed to exclude shunt malfunction and establish a functioning shunt.[101,137-142] In most patients, shunt revision leads to improvement of the clinical symptoms and radiological improvement of the syringomyelia or at worst stabilization, thus not requiring any further surgical measures. Recently, endoscopic third ventriculostomy (ETV) has been tried when a patient presents with blocked shunt, in order to remove the shunt completely, with some success.

In a small proportion of patients the ventricles have been either normal or borderline enlarged at birth and these patients have not had surgical ventricular drainage procedures.[144] An even smaller proportion has moderate ventriculomegaly without symptoms of raised pressure, which represents a state of arrested hydrocephalus and is not treated surgically in most cases. Patients who have syringomyelia and have not had shunts before, in the presence of moderate ventriculomegaly, should be considered for surgical drainage of the ventricles. Most surgeons would insert a ventricular shunt, although in the past few years there have been reports of successful treatment and resolution of the syringomyelia cavity with ETV.[131]

After surgical treatment of hydrocephalus, in the presence of clinical improvement, even if the syringomyelia cavity has not reduced in size it is best to avoid immediate surgical action; observe for a while instead and repeat the MRI scan to verify that the syringomyelia cavity remains stable. The remaining treatment options have increasing difficulty and complexity and a significant complication risk, and thus, careful consideration should be given before further surgical action is taken.

If hydrocephalus treatment (shunt revision/insertion or ETV) has not resulted in clinical or radiological improvement, craniovertebral decompression should be performed to establish CSF circulation in the craniocervical junction if the predominant symptoms are those of craniovertebral junction compression, and tethered cord release should be undertaken if the predominant symptoms are those of bladder dysfunction.[101,141] Both surgical options have significant challenges.

Craniovertebral decompression in Chiari II malformation is considerably more difficult than in Chiari I, as part of the contents of the hindbrain hernia is not only the cerebellum but also the lower medulla. It is not uncommon for the fourth ventricle to be at the level of the foramen magnum or even lower. The hindbrain hernia can extend down as low as C4-C5. When C1-C2 laminectomy has been performed and if the dura is opened, care should be taken as dissection may result in early access and exposure of the floor of the fourth ventricle. If the surgeon is opening the dura, care must be taken to ensure that durotomy is below the low-lying torcular. In some patients, a surgeon may elect not to open the dura and just perform a bony decompression as the results can be catastrophic if care is not taken to avoid the low-lying sinuses. Inadvertent damage to the brainstem can have severe neurological side effects and bulbar palsy. At the end of the procedure, if the dura is opened, closure is performed either with duraplasty from pericranium or artificial material, or by leaving the dura open in the pseudomeningocele technique as for Chiari I. Craniovertebral decompression in patients with Chiari II has mixed results.[129,138] Severe bulbar symptoms tend not to improve and long-tract signs show moderate improvement. Bilateral vocal cord paresis and very young age are poor prognostic factors.[129] When craniovertebral decompression is performed for syringomyelia, especially in the absence of bulbar symptoms, results are better with good chance of success, over 60%.

If despite all these measures, the clinical symptoms and the radiological appearances of syringomyelia persist, insertion of a syringopleural or syringosubarachnoid shunt could be considered.[107,138-140] The use of syringomyelia shunts is controversial. Many authors have suggested them as an early surgical option, before craniovertebral decompression.[137,141] There is no conclusive evidence on the best time to use them. There have been reports of good result in spina bifida patients.[107] Nevertheless, in the analogy of Chiari I malformation, if a syringomyelia shunt is inserted before addressing the block at the foramen magnum, the beneficial effect tends to be short lived.[8]

For paraplegic wheelchair-bound patients with severe bladder and bowel disorder and with relentlessly deteriorating syringomyelia, the option of cordotomy and terminal ventriculostomy exists. This was practiced infrequently in the 1970s to 1980s but has fallen out of favor because of its amputating nature and is not performed today.

SELECTED KEY REFERENCES

Armonda RA, Citrin CM, Foley KT, Ellenbogen RG. Quantitative cine-mode magnetic resonance imaging of Chiari I malformations: an analysis of cerebrospinal fluid dynamics. *Neurosurgery.* 1994;35:214-224.

Gardner WJ, Angel J. The mechanism of syringomyelia and its surgical correction. Clin Neurosurg. 1959;6:131-140.

Milhorat TH, Chou MW, Trinidad EM, et al. Chiari I malformation redefined: clinical and radiographic findings for 364 symptomatic patients. Neurosurgery. 1999;44:1005-1017.

Oldfield EH, Muraszko K, Shawker TH, Patronas NJ. Pathophysiology of syringomyelia associated with Chiari I malformation of the cerebellar tonsils. Implications for diagnosis and treatment. J Neurosurg. 1994;80:3-15.

Sgouros S, Williams B. A critical appraisal of drainage in syringomyelia. J Neurosurg. 1995;82:1-10.

Williams B. Simultaneous cerebral and spinal fluid pressure recordings. Cerebrospinal dissociation with lesions at the foramen magnum. Acta Neurochir. 1981;59:123-142.

Please go to expertconsult.com to view the complete list of references.

Craniovertebral Junction: A Reappraisal

Atul Goel

CLINICAL PEARLS

- Atlantoaxial joint opening, manipulation, and direction fixation form important components of treatment of craniovertebral instability.

- Lateral masses of C1 and C2 are firm and largely cortical in nature and provide a solid ground for screw fixation.

- For atlantoaxial dislocation, atlantoaxial fixation should be done.

- Reduction of basilar invagination can be performed by distraction of the facets of the atlas and axis in a specific group of patients.

- Syringomyelia is always a secondary phenomenon. The primary cause should be identified and appropriately treated. Direct manipulation of the syrinx can be harmful.

The craniovertebral junction is elegantly designed and structured to provide strength and free movements to the most mobile and stable region of the body. A direct inspection of the joints in a cadaver will reveal that the ligaments in the region of the occipitoatlantal joint are so strong that it will take considerable effort and heavy and sharp instruments to dislodge the joint, the effort being significantly greater than for any other joint of the body. The human spine mimics a pillar that bifurcates in its upper part to support the roof. The facets of atlas and axis and the occipital condyles form the superior bifurcation of the vertical pillar formed by the vertebral bodies of the spine, giving the "human spinal pillar" a Y-shaped design. Craniovertebral instability is more often a result of involvement of the pillar, and manifests by abnormalities in the atlantoaxial facet articulation. The majority of craniovertebral instability is related to the atlantoaxial joint, and a small minority of cases have instability related to the occipitoatlantal joint.

The surgical management of craniovertebral anomalies is complex due to the relative difficulty in accessing the region, critical relationships of neurovascular structures, and the intricate biomechanical issues involved.

CRANIOVERTEBRAL ANOMALIES

The subject of craniovertebral junction anomalies has been under discussion and evaluation for over a century. A number of classical reviews have attempted to clarify a variety of complex associated issues. Despite the volumes of publications on the subject, it appears that the last word has not yet been said. A large array of complex bony and neural anomalies has been described in this region. The issues in the management include consideration for decompression of the region and provision

of firm and stable fixation that is able to bear the stresses and strains of movements, distraction, and compression. If correct and timely treatment is provided to these patients a satisfying long-term outcome can be obtained.

ATLANTOAXIAL DISLOCATION

Atlantoaxial dislocation (AAD) can be due to a number of etiological factors. The dislocation can be of a *mobile and reducible* type or of a *fixed or irreducible* type. In the more common form of AAD, the atlas dislocates over the axis. In cases with occipitalization of the atlas, the head and atlas form one unit and the axis and the rest of the spine form the other unit. The odontoid process of the axis is normally in close approximation with the anterior arch of the atlas. In AAD, the head and atlas dislocate ventrally on the axis on flexion of the head, widening the atlantodental interval and reducing the diameter of the spinal canal, with consequent pressure on the cervicomedullary junction cord. The dislocation increases on flexion of the head and reduces in extension in the mobile variety of AAD. In the fixed or irreducible variety, the dislocation persists entirely or at least partially on full extension of the head.

Mobile and Reducible Atlantoaxial Dislocation

In the year 2001, we analyzed 160 cases with mobile and reducible AAD treated in our department during the years 1988 to 2001.[1,2] In the series, the etiological factor for the dislocation included Morquio's disease (9 cases), Down syndrome (8 cases), and craniosynostosis (5 cases). Although trauma leads to mechanical disruption of ligaments of the region, in "congenital" dislocation and dislocation related to known syndromes, laxity or incompetence of the ligaments is more often the cause. In several cases, the exact differentiation between a congenital and an acquired cause is difficult to decipher. The range of mobility of the dislocation is in general significantly higher in cases with congenital dislocation than in cases with trauma-related dislocation.

Clinical Features

Pain in the upper part of the neck and restriction of neck movements are common symptoms. The patient may give a history of an injury that flexed the head and neck (as when he is hit on the back of the head) as the precipitating factor. Weakness and spasticity of all limbs can follow the event of trauma. A range of motor and sensory deficits can occur. The sensory deficits are relatively less severe. Severe injuries to the cervicomedullary cord may produce respiratory paralysis, coma, and even death.

Investigations

Radiographs showing the lateral views of the atlantoaxial region with the head and neck flexed and extended confirm the diagnosis. Dynamic computed tomography (CT) scans with appropriate reconstruction images show the dislocation clearly. Magnetic resonance (MR) and CT angiography can show the relationship of the vertebral artery to the facets of C2 and C1. Such information can be crucial when lateral mass fixation techniques are employed. Magnetic resonance imaging (MRI) can provide useful information regarding the nature of soft tissue alterations.

Surgical Treatment

The treatment of patients with atlantoaxial instability is a surgical challenge, and achieving a successful outcome for these patients is gratifying. The complications of surgery, however, are potentially lethal. Various methods of fixation have been described and used successfully in the treatment of patients with atlantoaxial instability. The techniques of craniovertebral fixation evolved during the twentieth century as the anatomy and biomechanics of the craniovertebral region became clearer.

The aim of surgery in general is to restore normal or the best possible alignment and to achieve stability of the atlantoaxial joint. The techniques of fixation for atlantoaxial dislocation can be divided into *midline procedures* that involve fixation of the arch of the atlas with the lamina of the axis and *lateral mass fixation procedures*. *Midline* methods of fixation include use of interlaminar clamps, Gallie's posterior C1-C2 sublaminar wiring,[3] Brooks-Jenkins fusion,[4] and the Sonntag technique of sublaminar wiring.[5] *Lateral mass fixation* procedures include Goel's C1 lateral mass and C2 pedicle/pars screw fixation (interarticular)[1,2] and the Magerl's C1-C2 transarticular technique.[6]

Metal implants and fixation methods provide an initial period of fixation of the region, facilitating bony fusion. Bony fusion takes about 3 months and the metal implants should be strong enough to hold the region for that period. It ultimately depends on bony fusion to provide stability to the region. Bone harvested from the patient's own iliac crest has been identified

by several authors to be superior to any other form of bone graft or artificial material. Compromise on using the type of bone graft can lead to inadequate fusion, a phenomenon that can mar the entire operative procedure. Multiple pieces of corticocancellous bone graft should be placed in the craniovertebral region after elaborately preparing the host bone. The movements in the atlantoaxial region occur in the atlantoaxial joint. Any method of stabilization that directly fixes the joint and is segmental in nature has superiority over methods that employ fixation remote to the site of maximum movements and those that attempt to fix multiple bone segments. The lateral mass fixation techniques[7] have been identified to be philosophically superior and biomechanically stronger to the techniques that involve fixation of the midline structures such as lamina and arch of atlas.

Craniovertebral Junction and Related Anatomy

The C1 and C2 vertebrae are called "atypical vertebrae" and have a unique shape and architecture and a characteristic vertebral artery relationship. Injury to the artery during surgery can lead to catastrophic intraoperative bleeding, and compromise to the blood flow can lead to unpredictable neurological deficits, which will depend on the adequacy of blood flow from the other arteries of the brain.

The vertebral artery adopts a serpentine course in relation to the craniovertebral region. The artery has multiple loops and an intimate relationship with the atlas and axis bones. We observed a wide variability of the course of the artery in our specimens. The shape, size, and location of the vertebral artery groove on the inferior aspect of the superior articular facet of the C2 and over the posterior arch of the atlas have wide variations. The vertebral artery during its entire course is covered with a large plexus of veins. The venous plexuses are the largest in the region lateral to the C1-C2 joint. After a relatively linear ascent of the vertebral artery in the foramen transversarium of C6 to C3, the artery makes a loop medially toward an anteriorly placed superior articular facet of the C2 vertebra, making a deep groove on its inferior surface. The extent of medial extension of the loop varies. The distance of the artery from the midline of the vertebral body of C2 as would be observed during a transoral surgical procedure is an average of 12 mm.[8] The vertebral artery loops away from the midline underneath the superior articular facet of the C2.

The dens or the odontoid process is flanked by two large, superior facets, extending laterally onto the adjoining pars interarticularis and articulating with the inferior atlantal facets. The superior facet of the C2 vertebra differs from the facets of all other vertebrae in two important characteristics. First, the superior facet of C2 is present in proximity to the body when compared to other facets, which are located in proximity to the lamina. Second, the vertebral artery foramen is present partially or completely in the inferior aspect of the superior facet of C2, but in other cervical vertebrae, the vertebral artery foramen is located entirely in relation to the transverse process. Unlike superior facets of all other vertebrae, they do not form a pillar with the inferior facets, being considerably anterior to them. The pedicle of the C2 vertebra is relatively small. The course of the vertebral artery in relation to the inferior aspect of the superior articular facet of the C2 makes it susceptible to injury during transarticular and interarticular

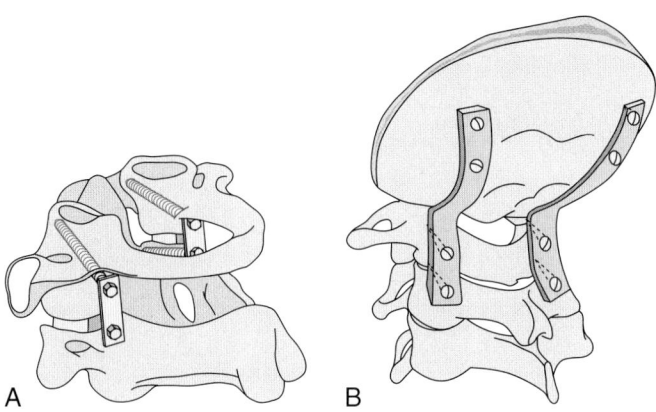

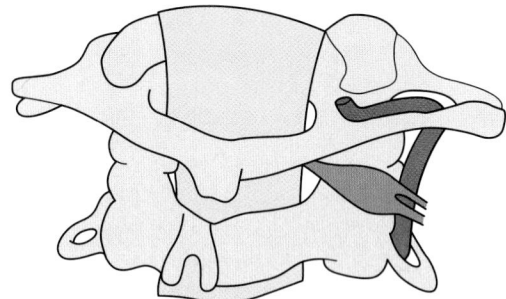

FIGURE 29.3 Drawing showing the relationship of the C2 ganglion, vertebral artery, and atlantoaxial joint.

FIGURE 29.1 A, This drawing shows the Goel technique of atlantoxial fixation using plates and screws. The atlantoaxial joint is opened, articular cartilage is widely denuded, and the joint space is filled with bone graft. **B,** In the occipitocervical fixation, the occipital end of the plate is fixed with the help of screws. The cervical end of the plate is fixed with lateral mass of C2 alone or of both C1 and C2.

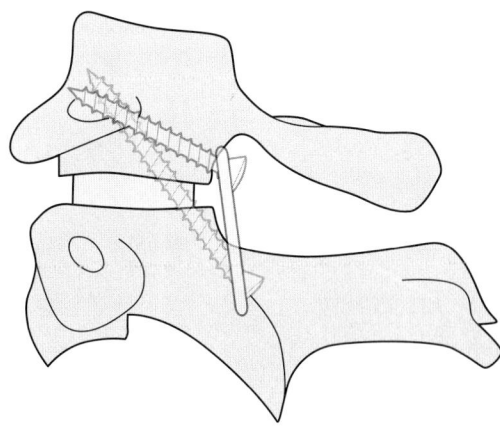

FIGURE 29.4 In the "double insurance" method of fixation the screw in C2 is placed in a transarticular method of fixation.

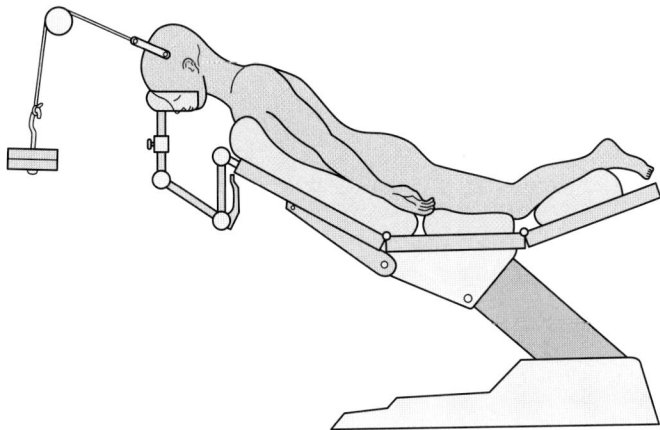

FIGURE 29.2 Position of the patient under cervical traction. The head end of the table is elevated by approximately 35 degrees.

screw implantation techniques. The average distance of the artery from the ganglion is 7.5 mm. This finding suggests that the dissection around the lateral end of the ganglion should be carefully done.

The inferior facet of the atlas is almost circular in most of the vertebrae without any significant difference in the mean anteroposterior and transverse (15 mm) dimensions. The thickness of the inferior facet under the posterior arch of the atlas is on average 3.5 mm. The thickness of the posterior arch of the atlas separating the vertebral artery groove from the inferior facet is about 3.5 mm.

Lateral Mass Plate (or Rod) and Screw (Monoaxial or Polyaxial) Fixation (Figs. 29.1 to 29.6)[1,2]

Cervical traction is set up prior to induction of anesthesia and the weights are progressively increased to approximately 5 to 8 kg or one sixth of the total body weight. The patient is placed prone with the head end of the table elevated to about 35 degrees (see Fig. 29.2). Cervical traction stabilizes the head in an optimally reduced extension position and prevents

any rotation. The traction also ensures that the weight of the head is directed superiorly toward the direction of the traction and pressure over the face or eyeball by the headrest is avoided. The head is in a "hanging" position, the headrest being placed only for additional or minimal support. Elevation of the head end of the table, which acts as a countertraction, helps in reducing venous engorgement in the operative field. The suboccipital region and the upper cervical spine are exposed through an approximately 8-cm longitudinal midline skin incision centered on the spinous process of the axis. The spinous process of the axis is identified, and the attachment of paraspinal muscles to it is sharply sectioned. The large second cervical ganglion is closely related to the vertebral artery on its lateral aspect (see Fig. 29.3). It is first exposed widely and then sectioned sharply. This procedure provides a wide exposure of the lateral masses of the atlas and axis. Bleeding from the large venous sinuses in the region and in the extradural space can be troublesome. Packing of the region with Surgicel and Gelfoam can assist in the control of venous bleeding. The joint capsule is cut sharply, and the articular surfaces of the joint are exposed. The adjacent synovial articular surfaces of the atlantoaxial joint are decorticated widely with a microdrill, and pieces of bone harvested from the iliac crest are stuffed into the joint space. The lateral aspect of the lamina and a part of the pars of the axis are drilled to make the posterior surface of the lateral mass of the axis relatively flat so that the metal plate can be placed snugly and parallel to the bone. Drilling also helps in reducing the length of the plate and in placing

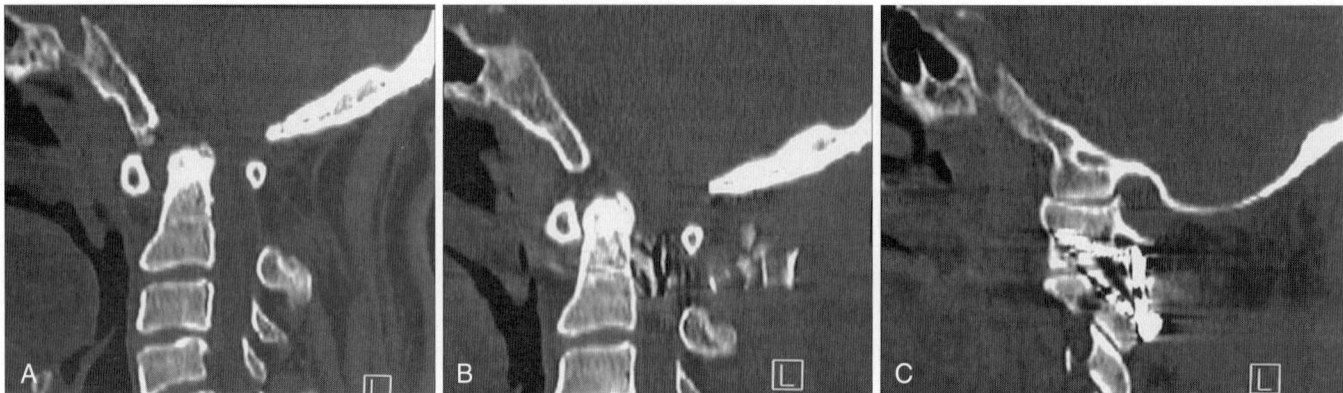

FIGURE 29.5 A, Lateral radiograph shows mild basilar invagination and atlantoaxial dislocation. The pathological change is related to degenerative arthritis of the atlantoaxial joint. **B,** Postoperative computed tomography (CT) scan shows reduction of the atlantoaxial dislocation. **C,** CT scan reconstruction image through the atlantoaxial joint shows the "double insurance" plate and screw fixation.

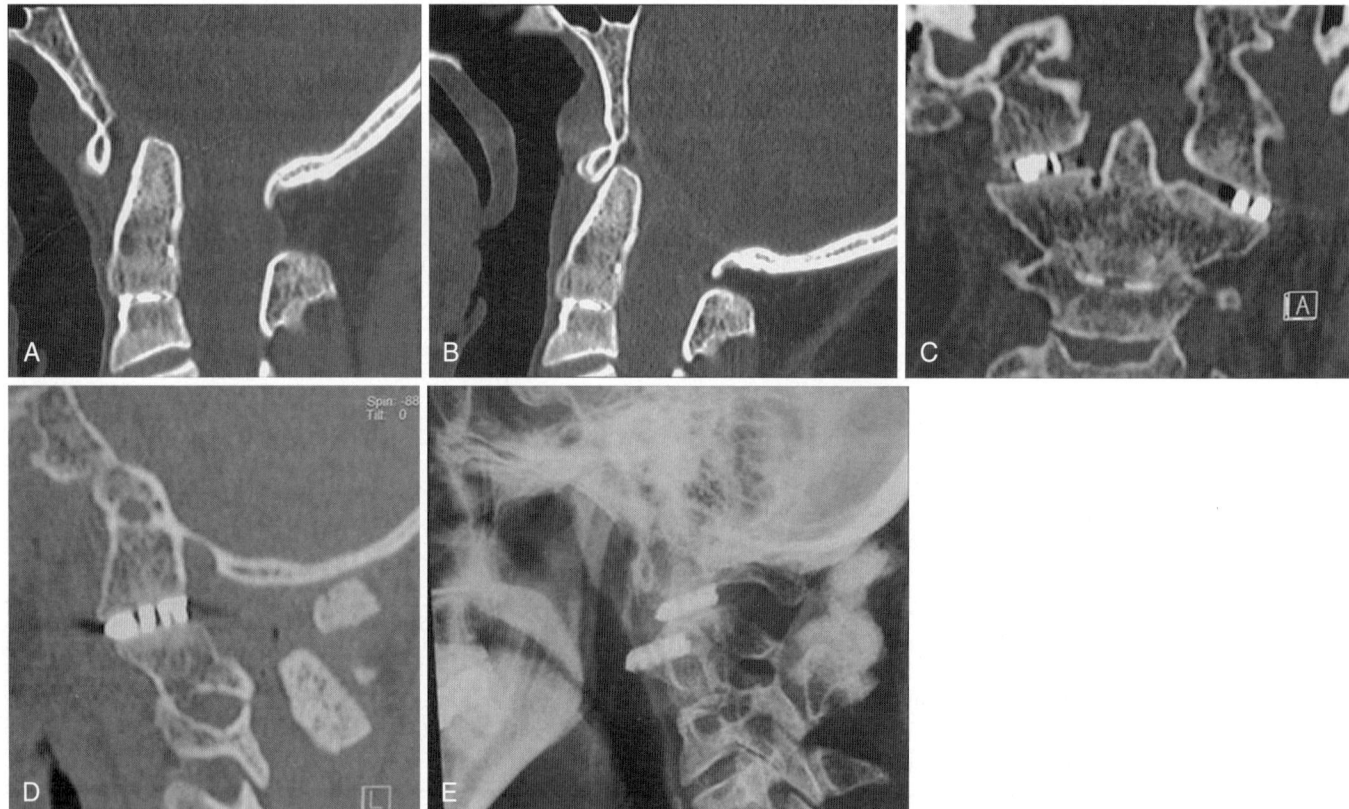

FIGURE 29.6 A, Computed tomography (CT) scan with the head in flexed position shows atlantoaxial dislocation. **B,** CT scan with the head extended shows reduction of the dislocation. **C,** Coronal image of CT scan shows spiked spacers within the atlantoaxial joint. **D,** Sagittal image shows the spacer within the joint. **E,** Lateral radiograph shows the atlantoaxial fixation using spacers.

the screw more superiorly and almost directly into the lateral mass of the axis. Actual vertebral artery exposure is unnecessary either lateral to the pars of the axis or superior to the arch of the atlas.

Screws are implanted into the previously created guide holes in the lateral mass of the atlas and axis through a two-holed (approximately 2 cm in length) metal (stainless steel or titanium) plate. First, a screw is placed into the atlas. It is directed at an angle of approximately 15 degrees medial to the sagittal plane and 15 degrees superior to the axial plane. The preferred site of screw insertion is at the center of the posterior surface of the lateral mass, 1 to 2 mm above the articular surface. Whenever necessary, careful drilling of the inferior surface of the lateral aspect of the posterior arch of the atlas in relation to its lateral mass can provide additional space for the placement of the plate and screw implantation. The screw may even be implanted by choosing an insertion point on the articular surface of the lateral mass of the atlas. Such a site is useful more frequently in children than in adult patients. Screws can also be implanted into the facet of the atlas through the lateral aspect of the posterior arch of the atlas. Owing to the intimacy of vertebral artery relationships, screw implantation in the axis is relatively unsafe and needs to be precise. It was observed that the screw implantation in the superior facet of the C2 vertebra has to be sharply medial and directed toward the anterior tubercle of the C1 for transarticular fixation and toward the vertebral body of C2 for interarticular fixation. The pars interarticularis can be divided into nine quadrants;[9] the superior and medial compartments can be used for the interarticular technique of screw implantation. Neuronavigation can be of assistance in identifying the best and the safest trajectory of the screw. The direction of screw implantation must be sharply medial and superior and should be toward the superior aspect of the body of the axis vertebra toward the midline. The medial surface of the pedicle of the axis is identified before the implantation of the screw. The screw is directed at an angle approximately 25 degrees medial to the sagittal plane and 15 degrees superior to the axial plane. The angle of screw insertion varies, depending on the local anatomy and the size of the bones. The quality of cancellous bone in the lateral masses of the atlas and axis in the proposed trajectory of screw implantation is generally good, providing an excellent purchase of the screw, and avoids the vertebral artery. The screws used are 2.9 mm in diameter in adult patients and 2.7 mm in diameter in pediatric patients. The length of the required screw is calculated on the basis of the size of the lateral masses observed on the preoperative radiological studies. The approximate lengths of the atlas screws are 26 to 28 mm in adults and 22 to 26 mm in children. The screws in the atlas and axis are almost similar in their length. The lateral masses of the atlas and axis are firm and cortical in nature, and, although preferable, it is not mandatory that the screws engage both the posterior and anterior cortices. If the screw traverses beyond the anterior cortex, it will lie harmlessly in the anteriorly displaced soft tissue. Injury to the critical neurovascular and pharyngeal wall is possible in such a situation but is extremely rare. Intraoperative fluoroscopic control and navigation were found to be helpful but not essential in determining the state of the screws. Large pieces of corticocancellous bone graft from the iliac bone are then placed over the adequately prepared posterior elements of atlas and axis. After the wound is closed, cervical traction is discontinued. The patients are mobilized as soon as possible and advised to wear a hard cervical collar for 3 months.

Complications

The most dreaded complication of the procedure is injury to the vertebral artery. The vertebral artery can be injured during the process of lateral dissection of the C2 ganglion. The other potential site of injury is at the insertion of the screw in the axis. In the latter situation, to control the bleeding, one has to pack the bleeding bone hole with bone wax. One can then prepare for an alternative site of screw insertion or use an alternative method of atlantoaxial fixation. Screw implantation can be completed through the same site on some occasions.

The lateral mass plate and screw fixation technique can provide an opportunity to manipulate the atlas and axis

independently by obtaining fixation points in their strongest elements and hence has very versatile applications.

Magerl's Technique[6]

Magerl's technique of fixation involves use of transarticular lateral mass screws. This technique also involves stabilization of the joints and is a popular and satisfactory method of stabilization.

Double Insurance Fixation[10]

An alternative method of atlantoaxial fixation that combines the transarticular method of fixation and the interarticular fixation technique can be used. The technique combines the biomechanical strengths of both of the more commonly used techniques of fixation and provides maximal stability to the implants (see Figs. 29.4 and 29.5).

Joint Jamming Technique[11]

Jamming of spiked spacers within the atlantoaxial joints can provide a satisfactory method of atlantoaxial fixation. The joint jamming technique can be suitable in cases in which the atlantoaxial dislocation is not remarkably mobile as is usually encountered in cases with congenital atlantoaxial dislocations. Such a method of fixation can usually be employed as a supplement to other techniques of fixation.

Use of Spinous Process and Lamina for Insertion of Axial Screws[12]

Placement of screws in the large and stubby spinous process of the axis can be a useful method. Insertion of the screw in the spinolaminar junction or in the lamina has been described to provide a stable fixation point.

Treatment of Irreducible or Fixed Atlantoaxial Dislocation

Direct distraction of facets of atlas and axis and placement of bone graft within it, with or without additional support of metallic spacers, can result in significant or complete reduction of dislocation. Subsequent atlantoaxial fixation that can sustain the reduction is then carried out. Transoral decompression of the odontoid process followed by posterior fixation is also a useful method of treatment, particularly when the surgeon is not familiar with lateral mass fixation and distraction procedures.

BASILAR INVAGINATION

Basilar invagination forms a prominent component of the craniovertebral anomalies. Chiari malformation and syringomyelia are commonly associated with basilar invagination and are the soft tissue components of the dysgenesis. Plain radiological and tomographic parameters have been principally used to diagnose basilar invagination for many years. There has been a renewed interest in the normal anatomy and pathological lesions of the craniovertebral junction with the development of imaging by high-resolution CT scan and MRI. Dynamic MRI and CT scans have helped in the evaluation of the pathology of basilar invagination, in the assessment of biomechanics of the joints, and in the formulation of a rationale for the surgical strategy. Despite the clarity of imaging, controversy regarding the management of basilar invagination continues. Even the natural history has not been clearly elucidated in the literature. The surgical indications for a given approach together with the timing of the surgical stages are still under discussion.

Pathogenesis

Several theories have been suggested to elucidate the probable cause and origin of basilar invagination. Most of these theories point toward embryological dysgenesis, genetic abnormalities, and viral infections.[13-16] Several authors, for over a century, have thought that deformation had a mechanical cause and therefore applied the name: "impressio baseos cranii" (Berg and Retzius, 1855, cited by Virchow, 1876),[17] or basilar impression.[18] Grawitz (1880)[19] believed that basilar invagination was often a result of under- or maldevelopment of the craniovertebral transition region. A range of malformations is frequently associated with anomalies of the atlas and axis, some of which may be quite atypical, and with fissures or defects and bone projections from the spinal column in the craniovertebral transition zone. The latter anomalies were grouped together by von Torklus and Gehle (1970) as suboccipital dysplasias.[18] Basilar invagination can be secondary to abnormally inclined alignment of the facets of the atlas and axis.[20] The progressive slippage of the atlas over the axis secondary to this malalignment, a process similar to spondylolisthesis in the lumbosacral spine, results in invagination of the odontoid process into the craniocervical cord.[20,21] Short neck, low hairline, web-shaped neck muscles, torticollis, reduction in the range of neck movements, and several such physical variations have been described as hallmarks of basilar invagination for over a century. A number of bone fusion deformities and platybasia have also been recorded. Neck pain, muscle spasms, and restriction of neck movements are frequently noted and suggest instability of the region. Degeneration of the atlantoaxial joint and primary or secondary destruction of the facets of atlas or axis can lead to superior and posterior migration of the odontoid process and result in basilar invagination and fixed or irreducible atlantoaxial dislocation. Such involvement of the lateral masses can result in laxity of the posterior atlantoaxial or retro-odontoid ligaments that result in retro-odontoid pannus or "tumor-like" or "osteophyte-like" formation.

Classification into Groups I and II

In 1997, we presented a classification system for basilar invagination that divided it into two discrete categories. This classification helped in clarifying the understanding of the pathology and pathogenesis of the anomaly, in the selection of the surgical treatment, and in prediction of the outcome.[22] Based on a single criterion of the absence or presence of Chiari malformation, the anomaly was classified into groups I and II, respectively.

Essentially, group I included cases in which there was invagination of the odontoid process into the foramen magnum and indented into the brainstem. The tip of the odontoid process distanced itself from the anterior arch of the atlas or the inferior aspect of the clivus. The distancing of the

odontoid process from the anterior arch suggested the presence of instability in the region and atlantoaxial dislocation. The angle of the clivus and the posterior cranial fossa volume were essentially unaffected in these cases. In group II, on the other hand, the assembly of the odontoid process, anterior arch of the atlas, and the clivus migrated superiorly in unison, resulting in reduction of the posterior cranial fossa volume, which was the primary pathology in these cases. The Chiari malformation or herniation of the cerebellar tonsil was considered to be a result of reduction in the posterior cranial fossa volume. In 1997, Goel first defined the clinical implication of association of small posterior cranial fossa volume and Chiari malformation.[22]

Classification into Groups A and B

In our 2004 study, we identified a subgroup of patients in whom there was clear radiological evidence of instability of the region that was manifested by distancing of the odontoid process away from the anterior arch of the atlas, and the radiological features matching those of group I cases. Considering this current evaluation we have proposed a *new classification for basilar invagination* into two groups based on parameters that determined an alternative treatment strategy.[23,24] In group A basilar invagination there was a "fixed" atlantoaxial dislocation and the tip of the odontoid process "invaginated" into the foramen magnum and was above the Chamberlain line,[25] McRae line of the foramen magnum,[26] and Wackenheim's clival line.[27] The definition of basilar invagination of prolapse of the cervical spine into the base of the skull, as suggested by von Torklus,[18] was suitable for this group of patients (Fig. 29.7A). In group B basilar invagination the odontoid process and clivus remained anatomically aligned despite the presence of basilar invagination and other associated anomalies. In this group, the tip of the odontoid process was above the Chamberlain line but below the McRae and Wackenheim's lines (Fig. 29.7B). The radiological findings suggested that the odontoid process in group A patients resulted in direct compression of the brainstem. Essentially, in group A basilar invagination, the pathogenesis appeared to be mechanical instability of the region that was manifested by the tip of the odontoid process distancing itself from the anterior arch of the atlas or the lower end of the clivus. In some group A patients there was Chiari malformation, and this feature differentiates the present classification from the earlier classification. In this group, the atlantoaxial joints were "active" and their orientation was oblique, as shown in Figure 29.8A, instead of the normally found horizontal orientation. Similarities of such a position of the C1-C2 facets with spondylolisthesis in the subaxial spine can be seen. It appears that the atlantoaxial joint in such cases is in an abnormal position and progressive worsening of the dislocation is probably secondary to increasing "slippage" of the facets of the atlas over the facets of the axis. In group B, the pathogenesis appeared to be congenital dysgenesis, and atlantoaxial joints were normally aligned or were entirely fused. The pathogenesis of basilar invagination appears to be different in the two groups. Understanding of these two types of basilar invaginations is crucial in understanding the various management issues involved.

FIGURE 29.7 A, Computed tomography (CT) scan shows group A basilar invagination. **B,** CT scan shows group B basilar invagination.

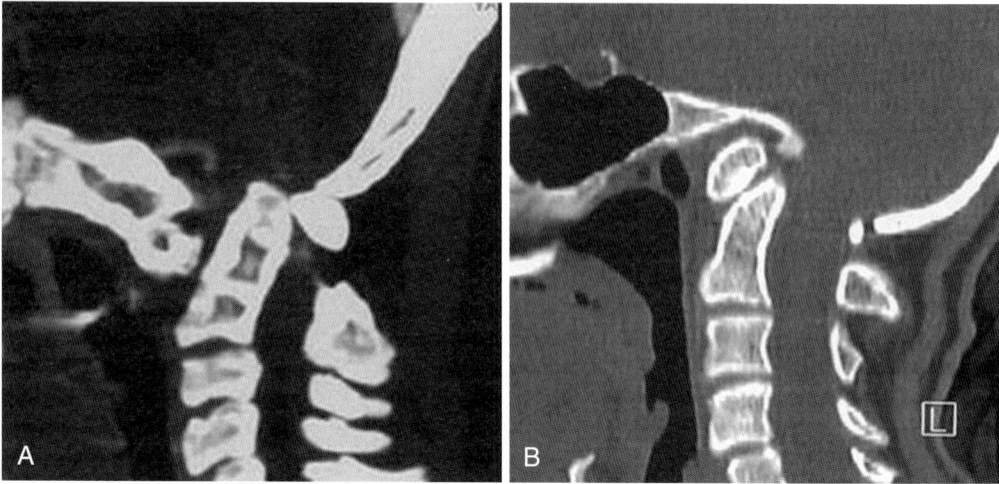

FIGURE 29.8 A, Drawing of the Goel modified omega angle. A line (A) is drawn along the hard palate. Another line is drawn that is parallel to line A that travels through the midpoint of the base of the C3 vertebral body. The angle of the odontoid process to this line is the omega angle. **B,** Drawing of the parameters used to measure the occipitocervical length (B) and the neck length (C). Line A is the tuberculum sella–torcula line.

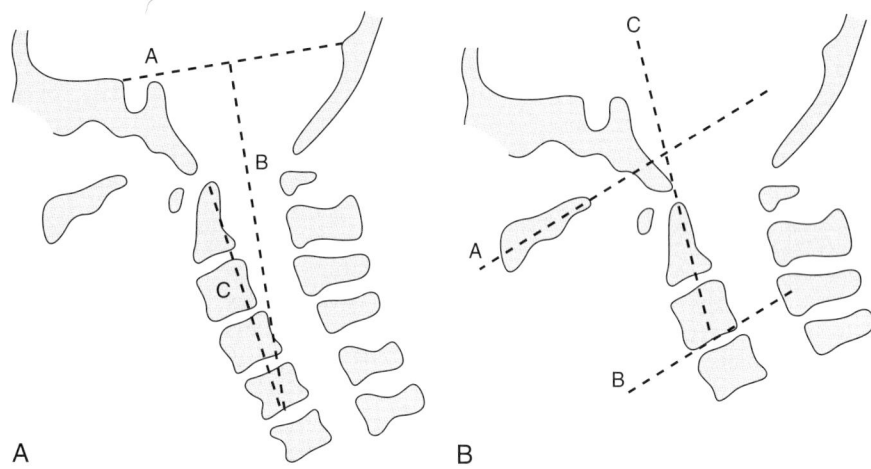

Vertical mobile and reducible atlantoaxial dislocation occurs when there was basilar invagination when the neck was flexed, but the alignment was normal when the head was in an extended position.[28] Although such mobility is only rarely identified, it does indicate the need for dynamic flexion-extension studies to preoperatively assess the craniovertebral instability. Vertical dislocation is due to incompetence of the atlantoaxial joint and lateral masses.

Diagnosis and Clinical Features

The majority of patients with group A basilar invagination (58%) had a history of minor to major head injury prior to the onset of the symptoms. The pyramidal symptoms formed a dominant component. Kinesthetic sensations were affected in 55% of these patients. Spinothalamic dysfunction was less frequent (36%). Neck pain was a major presenting symptom in 77% of cases. Torticollis was present in 41% of cases.[23] The analysis of radiological and clinical features suggests that the symptoms and signs were a result of brainstem compression by the odontoid process. The presentation was relatively acute in group A cases but it was long-standing and slowly progressive in group B cases. In group B cases, the onset of symptoms and their evolution were insidious.

Precipitating Factors

Trauma of varying severity was a noteworthy precipitating factor in group A cases.[29,30] Trauma seldom plays any major role in precipitating the symptoms in group B cases. The fact that trauma influenced the acute development of symptoms pointed toward an element of instability of the craniovertebral region in group A patients.

Associated Clinical Features

Mere inspection of the patients with basilar invagination was of diagnostic value in the majority of cases in both the groups. However, short neck and torticollis were more frequently encountered in cases with group A basilar invagination. The symptoms and signs in group B basilar invagination appeared to be directly related to the "crowding" of neural structures at the foramen magnum. Although the dimensions of the foramen magnum were large and sometimes larger than even in a normal state, the volume of its contents and probably the "pulsatile" compression of the structures at the foramen magnum resulted in neurological symptoms.[31] The markedly reduced girth of the brainstem in group A cases clearly showed that direct compression of the brainstem by the odontoid process caused the neurological symptoms. Central cord symptoms and related signs were noted in cases associated with syringomyelia.

Radiological Criteria

The Chamberlain Line

Basilar invagination was diagnosed when the tip of the odontoid process was at least 2 mm above the Chamberlain line.[25] Measurement of the Chamberlain line on lateral sagittal reconstruction pictures of CT scan and sagittal MRI were seen to be reliable and accurate. The analysis of basilar invagination in the two groups on the basis of the Chamberlain line suggested that the basilar invagination is much more severe in group B than in group A.

Distance Between the Odontoid Tip to the Pontomedullary Junction

The distance of the tip of the odontoid from the pontomedullary junction, as observed on MRI, is a useful index to define the reduction of the posterior cranial fossa bone size.[25] The distance was markedly reduced in group B cases but it was relatively large in group A cases.

Atlantodental or Clivodental Interval

In group A cases, it was seen that the odontoid process migrated superiorly and posteriorly into the foramen magnum and distanced itself from the anterior arch of the atlas and the inferior end of the clivus. As judged from the atlantodental or clivodental interval, there was an element of "fixed" atlantoaxial dislocation in these cases. Actual mobility of the atlantoaxial joint on flexion and extension of the neck can be demonstrated only rarely. In group B the alignment of the odontoid process with the anterior arch of the atlas and with the inferior aspect of the clivus remains normal and there is no instability.

Wackenheim's Clival Line

Wackenheim's clival line is a line drawn along the clivus. The tip of the odontoid process was significantly superior to Wackenheim's clival line in group A cases. In group B cases, the relationship of the tip of the odontoid process and the lower end of the clivus and the atlantodental and clivodental interval remained relatively normal. In a majority of these cases, the tip of the odontoid process remained below Wackenheim's clival line[4,27] and McRae's line of the foramen magnum.[26] The basilar invagination thus resulted from the rostral positioning of the plane of the foramen magnum in relation to the brainstem.

Platybasia

A line is drawn along the anterior skull base. The angle of this line to the clivus is referred to as the "basal angle." Reduction of the basal angle is referred to as "platybasia." Platybasia does not directly result in any neurological symptoms, but it participates with basilar invagination in critically reducing the posterior cranial fossa volume.

Posterior Cranial Fossa Volume

The Klaus' height index,[32] measured on MRI, was seen to be much more accurate than the conventional measurements based on plain radiographs. The tentorium could be clearly identified on MRI and the distance of the tip of the odontoid from the line of the tentorium indicated the height of the posterior cranial fossa. On the basis of Klaus' index, the posterior fossa height was found to be markedly reduced in group B cases but it was only moderately affected in group A cases.

Omega Angle

Although not frequently used, the omega angle, or the angulation of the odontoid process from the vertical as described by Klaus, was found to be a useful guide.[32] Goel described a modified omega angle as the measurement of the angle from the vertical and noted it was affected by the flexion and extension of the neck.[22] A line was drawn traversing through the center of the base of the axis parallel to the line of the hard palate. The line of the hard palate was unaffected by the relative movement of the head and the cervical spine during the movement of the neck in these "fixed" craniovertebral anomalies. Facial hypoplasia or hard palate abnormality was not seen in any case in this series and did not affect the measurements. The omega angle depicted the direction of displacement of the odontoid process. The omega angle was severely reduced in group A cases but it was much larger in group B cases. The reduction in the omega angle in group A cases depicted that the odontoid process had tilted toward the horizontal and was posteriorly angulated in group A cases, but it was near vertical and superiorly migrated in group B cases (Fig. 29.9).

Brainstem Girth

The effective brainstem girth measured on MRI is a useful additional parameter.[22] Although the brainstem girth is markedly reduced in group A cases, the girth is only marginally affected or unaffected in group B cases, indicating thereby that there is no direct brainstem compression as a result of the odontoid process in the latter group.

Occipitalization of the Atlas

Occipitalization of the atlas associated with basilar invagination was noted first by Rakitansky (cited by Grawitz 1880)[19] and has since been referred to frequently.[19,25,26,33,34] Many authors have regarded assimilation as a characteristic feature of basilar invagination. The assimilation of the atlas can be partial or incomplete.

Neck Size

Measurement of craniovertebral height can be done using a modification of Klaus' posterior fossa height index.[13,22,32] The cervical height was measured from the tip of the odontoid process to the midpoint of the base of the C7 vertebral body (see Fig. 29.9). *Direct physical measurement* of the neck length can be a useful parameter. The parameter of direct physical measurement of the neck length from the inion to the tip of the C7 spinous process can be useful.[13,35] *Cervical lordosis* is

FIGURE 29.9 A, Computed tomography (CT) showing group A basilar invagination. **B,** Sagittal cut through the atlantoaxial facet joints. The angulation of the joint and the listhesis of C1 over C2 can be appreciated. **C,** Postoperative CT scan showing reduction of basilar invagination. **D,** Sagittal cut through the atlantoaxial joint, showing the spacer and fixation by plate and screws.

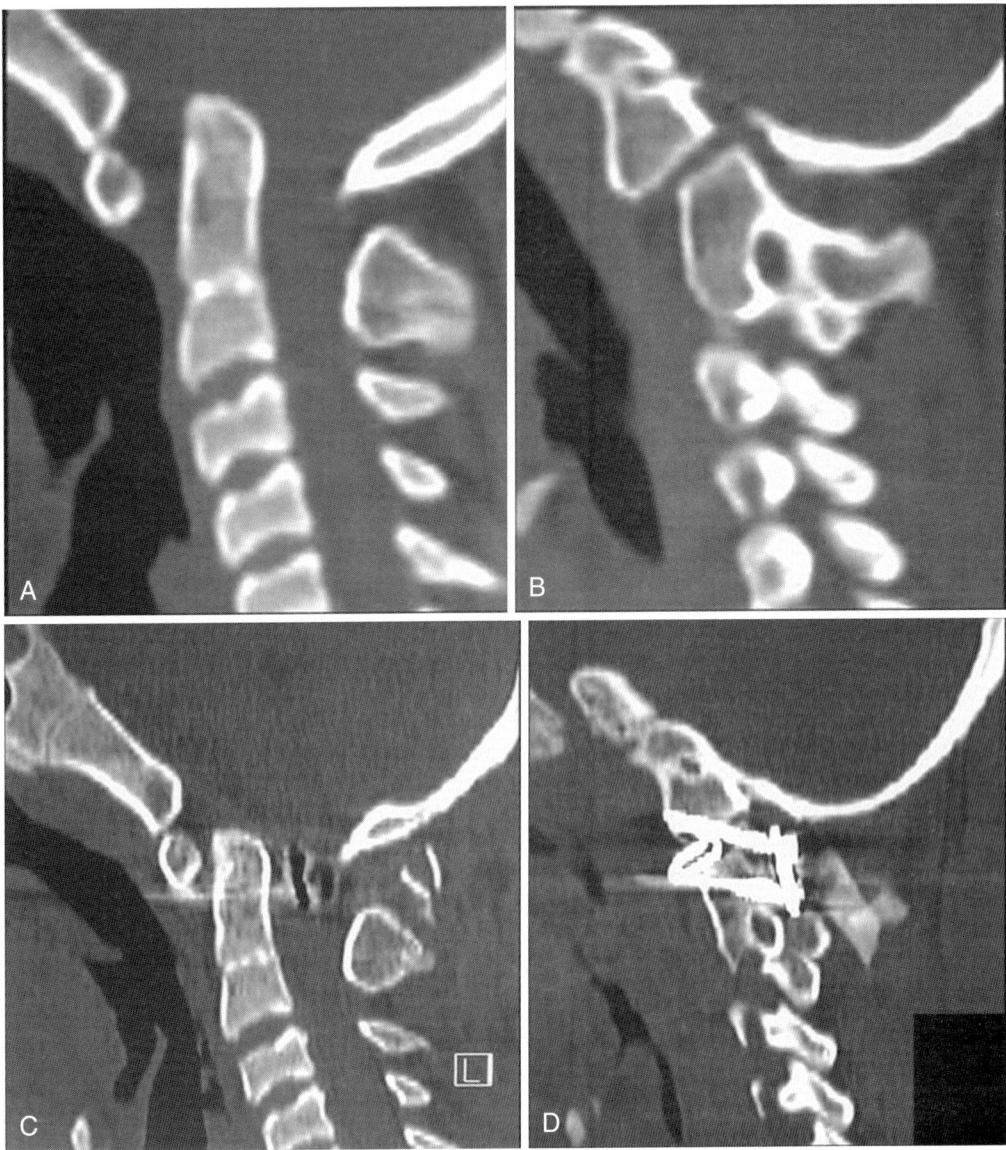

evaluated with a modification of the Klaus omega angle[13,32] and a modified omega angle.[22]

Surgical Management

Craniovertebral Realignment for Group A Basilar Invagination

The conventional form of treatment of group A basilar invagination is a transoral decompression[22,23,36] that is followed by posterior occipitocervical fixation. However, the long-term clinical outcome following the twin operation of transoral decompression followed by posterior stabilization was seen to be inferior to the clinical outcome following surgery that involves craniovertebral realignment without any bone, dural, or neural decompression. An attempt can be made to reduce basilar invagination by performing occipitocervical fixation following institution of cervical traction.[22,36] However, all our cases treated in this manner subsequently needed transoral decompression as the reduction of the basilar invagination

and of atlantoaxial dislocation could not be sustained by the implant. The technique of craniovertebral realignment by wide removal of the atlantoaxial joint capsule and articular cartilage by drilling and subsequent distraction of the joint by manual manipulation provides a unique opportunity to obtain reduction of the basilar invagination and of atlantoaxial dislocation.

Technique of Craniovertebral Realignment

This operation is suitable for patients with group A basilar invagination. The exposure of the atlantoaxial joint in cases with basilar invagination is significantly more difficult and technically challenging when compared to a normally aligned atlantoaxial joint encountered during the treatment of post-traumatic instability. The joint is rostral in location and the microscope needs to be appropriately angled. The atlantoaxial facet joints are widely exposed on both sides after sectioning of the large C2 ganglion. The joint capsule is excised and the articular cartilage is widely removed using a microdrill. The joints on both sides are distracted using an osteotome. The flat

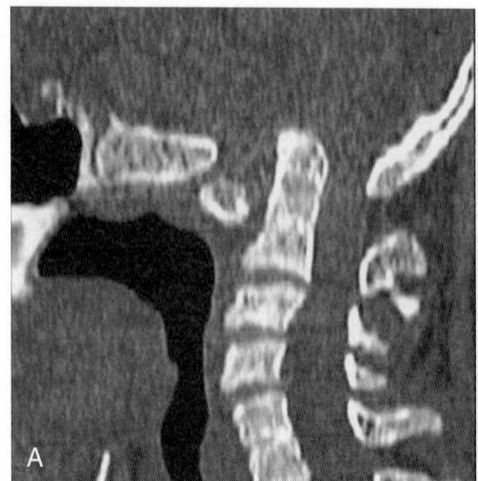 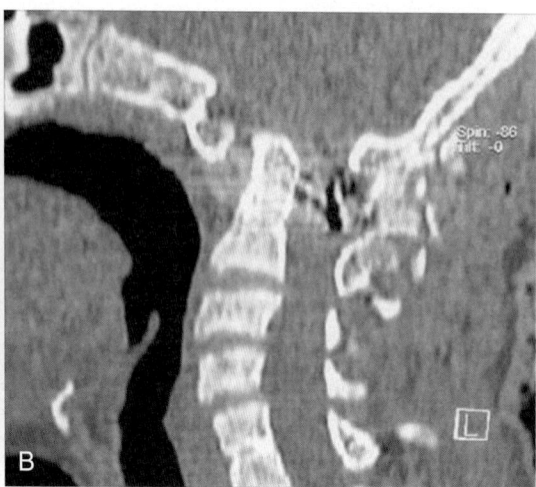

FIGURE 29.10 A, Computed tomography (CT) scan showing group A basilar invagination. **B,** Postoperative scan showing reduction of basilar invagination.

edge of the osteotome is introduced into the joint and it is then turned vertical to effect distraction. The status of the dislocation and of basilar invagination is evaluated by intraoperative radiographic control. Corticocancellous bone graft harvested from the iliac crest is stuffed into the joint in small pieces. Specially designed titanium spacers are used in selected cases as strut graft and impacted into the joints to provide additional distraction and stability. Subsequent fixation of the joint with the help of interarticular screws and a metal plate provides a biomechanically firm fixation and sustained distraction. Holes in the titanium metal spacer provide space for bone fusion. The fixation is seen to be strong enough to sustain the vertical, transverse, and rotatory strains of the most mobile region of the spine. Postoperatively the traction is discontinued and the patient is placed in a four-post hard cervical collar for 3 months during which all physical activities involving the neck are restrained (Figs. 29.8 to 29.10).

Reversibility of Musculoskeletal Changes Following Surgery[13]

A number of bone and soft tissue anomalies are associated with basilar invagination. These include short neck, torticollis, platybasia, cervical vertebral body fusion (Klippel-Feil abnormality) including assimilation of atlas, spondylotic spinal changes, and restriction of neck movements. A number of these abnormalities were seen to be reversible following decompression and stabilization of the region. Considering that several physical features associated with this group of basilar invagination are reversible, it appears that the pathogenesis in such cases may be more due to mechanical factors rather than to congenital causes or embryological dysgenesis. The common teaching on the subject is that the short neck and torticollis are a result of embryological dysgenesis and effectively result in indentation of the odontoid process into the cervicomedullary cord. However, it appears that it is the cord compression due to indentation by the odontoid process that is the primary event and all the physical alterations and bony abnormalities, including the short neck and torticollis, are secondary natural protective responses that aim to reduce the stretch of the cord over the indenting odontoid process. Pain, restriction of neck movements, and hyperlordosis of the neck indicate the presence of instability of the

craniovertebral junction. All of these natural responses probably allow the cord a relatively stretch-free traversal over the indenting odontoid process. Reduction of the disk spaces, osteophyte formation, incomplete and complete cervical fusions, and alterations in the craniospinal and cervical angulations appear to be directly related to the reduction in neck length. The reduction in the disk-space height and fusions are more prominently seen in the upper cervical vertebrae. It appears that cervical fusions and assimilation of the atlas may be related to long-standing and progressive reduction in the disk-space height.

Foramen Magnum Decompression for Group B Patients

Foramen magnum bony decompression appears to be ideal for group B basilar invagination. The procedure resulted in amelioration of symptoms and at least an arrest in the progression of the disability. Driesen (1960) reported that during operations for craniovertebral anomalies, he often had to remove noticeably thickened pieces of bone from the posterior edge of the foramen magnum.[30] In our cases, the suboccipital bone and posterior rim of the foramen magnum and the dura overlying the herniated cerebellar tissue were thin in a significant number of cases. This probably was related to the chronic pressure changes secondary to the reduced posterior cranial fossa volume. The bulbous lipping of the posterior rim of the foramen magnum represents the rudiments of the posterior arch of the atlas assimilated into the occipital bone.[16] Various authors have recommended that to achieve maximal decompression, it is necessary to open the dura mater and to cut all constrictive dural and arachnoidal bands. Some authors have recommended leaving the dura open while others have recommended the placement of a graft. Current papers do not recommend resection of the herniating tonsils[37] or even sectioning of adhesions around them. The fact that dural opening was not necessary while performing posterior fossa or foramen magnum decompression was first described by Goel and co-workers in 1997.[22] This finding was based on the understanding that the dura is an expansile structure and cannot be a compressive factor.[22,38] Opening of the dura is not only unnecessary but also subjects the patient to an increased risk of cerebrospinal fluid fistula. It makes an otherwise simple surgery into a relatively complex and dangerous surgical maneuver.

Syringomyelia

Syringomyelia is a frequently encountered clinical and radiological entity. It is associated with a range of pathological conditions that include congenital craniovertebral anomalies, tumors, infections, trauma, and spinal deformities. Syringomyelia is rarely or never an acute phenomenon and is generally encountered in long-standing and persistent space-occupying or space-reducing lesions and in situations with subtle but persistent instability. Obstruction to the normal flow of spinal or cranial CSF by post-traumatic or infective arachnoiditis is also a less frequently encountered cause of syringomyelia. Acute injuries, acute infections, rapidly growing malignant tumors, mobile dislocations, and acute post-traumatic deformities are generally not associated with syringomyelia. The clinical presenting features are long-standing and relentlessly progressive. Syringomyelia or "hydrocephalus of the cord" is never a primary phenomenon. It is always secondary to an obvious or an unidentified pathological cause.[38,39] The understanding of the pathophysiology of syringomyelia is crucially important to design a suitable treatment strategy and prognosticate the ultimate outcome. All attempts must be made to identify and treat the primary pathological cause. Syrinx drainage as a primary procedure may not be considered a therapeutic option. Syrinx drainage or shunting without dealing with the primary pathological cause can result in disastrous clinical consequences.

Basilar Invagination and Syringomyelia

Basilar invagination and the associated basal maldevelopment and the resultant reduction in the posterior cranial fossa volume are the primary pathological events in syringomyelia. There is usually no demonstrable structural abnormality of the brainstem, cerebellar hemisphere, or fourth ventricle, suggesting that the neural development in these patients remains unaffected in the embryonic dysgenesis. The presence of the normal bulk of the cerebellum in the reduced volume posterior cranial fossa results in the herniation of a part of the cerebellum into the foramen magnum, an entity labeled as Chiari I malformation. Essentially it appears that syringomyelia is a tertiary event to the primary basilar invagination and secondary to Chiari malformation. Long-standing pulsatile pressure of the herniated tonsil into the foramen magnum can result in compression of the cervicomedullary cord. Apart from physical attempts to increase the volume of the foramen magnum by bone erosion and membranous thinning and expansion, formation of syringomyelia probably provides a cushioning counterbalance of fluid from the spinal end so that the pressure of the tonsils on the cervicomedullary cord is minimized. The signs and symptoms related to the syrinx are more predominant than those related to brainstem compression by the tonsillar herniation. It could be that the primary aim of the entire process of syrinx formation is to reduce the compression of the brainstem at the level of the foramen magnum by the herniating cerebellum.

Rationale of Treatment

Treatment strategy in such cases should be directed toward increasing the posterior cranial fossa volume by posterior fossa volume expansion or foramen magnum decompression. Logue reported 75 patients treated with craniovertebral decompressions for Chiari malformations and syringomyelia.[40] The patients were divided into two groups: one was treated with bone decompression alone, leaving the arachnoid intact, and one group was treated with Gardner's procedure of opening the fourth ventricle and plugging the upper cervical canal. They concluded that muscle plugging did not seem to change the results. Levy and associates also concluded along the same lines.[41] Logue and Edwards noticed that there was no significant need for performing a syringosubarachnoid shunt following craniovertebral decompression.[40] Various subsequent studies have questioned the need for a syrinx drainage surgery following foramen magnum decompression. Di Lorenzo and colleagues concluded from their study that "conservative" craniocervical decompression should be considered the first option in the treatment of syringomyelia-Chiari I complex.[42] The routine of opening of the posterior cranial fossa dura, resection of the cerebellar tonsils, arachnoidal sectioning, and syringostomy is unnecessary. It appears that if the primary problem of basilar invagination is dealt with early in the course of the disease, the secondary and the tertiary events will spontaneously regress.[43] Craniovertebral realignment by atlantoaxial facet distraction can be a philosophical approach to treatment in cases having group A basilar invagination, Chiari malformation, and syringomyelia (Fig. 29.11). When there is syringomyelia and Chiari malformation but no definite basilar invagination, efforts can be made to identify the cause of the Chiari malformation.[44,45] In such cases, it might be possible that the cerebellar mass is larger than normal. Even in such cases, volume expansion of the posterior cranial fossa is required. The theory that dura or dural bands can act as a compressive factor appears unacceptable and does not correlate well with the pathogenic events. The dura is an expansile structure and may never be a compressive factor.[46,47]

Primary syringomyelia, in which the cause is not identifiable, is a relatively complex clinical situation. The syringomyelia in such cases simulates "normal pressure hydrocephalus." The intrasyrinx pressure is relatively low in such cases and the results of any kind of treatment are far from gratifying.

Syringomyelia secondary to primary cord pathology such as a tumor or kyphosis also appears to be a secondary and a "protective" phenomenon. Treatment in such cases should be directed toward treatment of the disease and not toward the treatment of syringomyelia.[44] Our observation is that if the syringomyelia is treated without dealing with the primary pathological cause, more often than not the outcome is poor and the patient can be harmed.

DEGENERATIVE ARTHRITIS

Like all other joints of the body, atlantoaxial joints are also subject to arthritis. With the general aging of the population, the issue of arthritis is becoming more relevant. Osteoarthritis of the atlantoaxial joint is a well-defined phenomenon that eventually results in atlantoaxial instability. The process of joint degeneration and instability is a progressive phenomenon and extends over several months to years. This instability is probably the result of degeneration of the articular cartilage, reduction of the joint space, and secondary incompetence of the ligaments controlling the movements.[48-51]

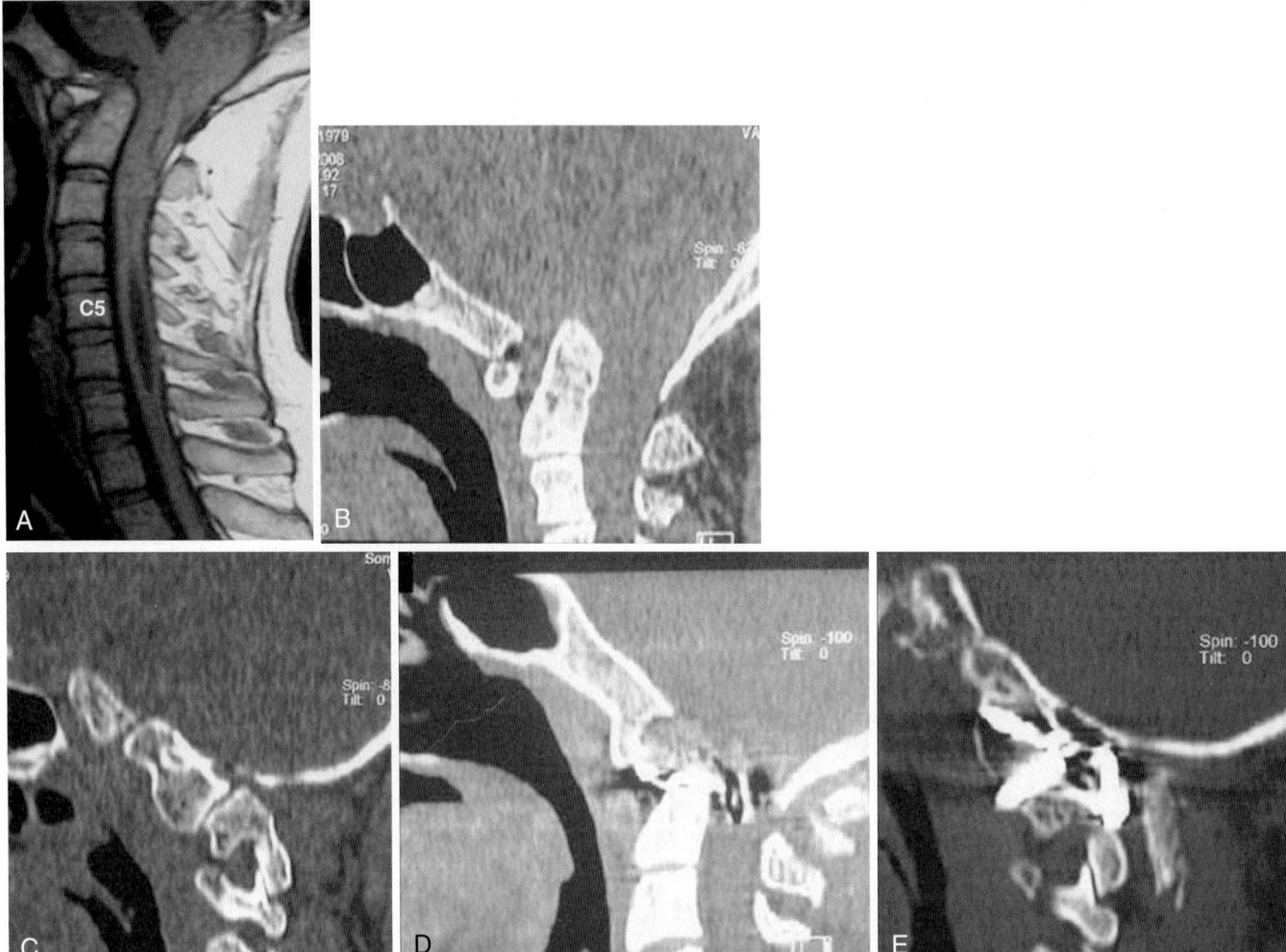

FIGURE 29.11 A, T1-weighted MRI showing group A basilar invagination, Chiari 1 malformation, and associated syringomyelia. **B,** CT scan showing group A basilar invagination, occipitalization/assimilation of the atlas. **C,** CT scan with the sagittal section passing through the facets showing "listhesis" of facet of atlas over facet of axis. **D,** Postoperative CT scan showing craniovertebral realignment. The odontoid process has significantly migrated away from the cord. **E,** Postoperative CT scan showing spacer within the atlantoaxial facet joint and plate and screw fixation of the atlantoaxial region.

Clinical Features

Pain in the neck on movement often forms the earliest and most prominent symptom. The more classical pattern of presentation is of an elderly patient presenting with symptoms of pain in the neck on movements and restriction of neck movements and gradually progressive quadriparesis over a few days to several months. The incidence and severity of quadriparesis vary in different reports and this variation reflects the duration of the disease before the diagnosis is clinched. Sensory symptoms are relatively mild and typically include bilateral upper and lower extremity paresthesias and kinesthetic sensation deficits. History of mild to moderately severe trauma a few days to several years prior to diagnosis may be present in a substantial number of patients and in most of these cases, the symptoms in general progress from the time of trauma. Palpable crepitus with motion has also been identified as a presenting symptom.[52] Carrying of heavy weights over the head has also been incriminated to cause increased incidence of cervical spondylotic changes and also basilar invagination.[53]

Radiological Features

Among the more constant radiological features is reduction of the height of lateral mass complex due to reduction of joint space. Erosion of bones of the lateral masses of atlas and axis and of the body is usually observed in more chronic situations.[54] Degenerative erosion of the facets of the atlas and axis, of the odontoid process and body of the axis, and periodontoid ligamentous degenerative changes are also frequent.

The term *basilar invagination* in cases with a variety of forms of craniovertebral arthritis has been used synonymously with the terms *cranial settling* or *vertical odontoid migration*.[23,24,53] The basilar invagination is only mild to moderate in cases with degenerative arthritis. This is in variance with the basilar invagination observed in cases of rheumatoid arthritis wherein the superior migration of the odontoid process is significantly more due to the more severe lateral mass bone collapse.

Atlantoaxial joint arthritis is expected to eventually result in atlantoaxial instability. The dislocation may only be partially reducible due to the presence of nonyielding tissues around the odontoid process. The subtlety of instability may make the diagnosis difficult in some cases.

Degenerative pannus, also termed as *articular, ganglion, synovial,* or *juxta-facet cyst,* may arise from the degenerating synovial lining of any joint in the body.[55-58] Pannus related to atlantoaxial joint arthritis probably represents degenerative ligaments and secondary "osteophyte-like" tissue formation in the periodontoid region.[50,59] Degenerating tissues are typically isointense on T1-weighted images and iso- to hypointense on T2-weighted images and do not enhance on contrast administration. In some cases, the retro-odontoid mass may give a "tumor-like" (pseudotumor) appearance resulting in posterior "buckling" of the posterior longitudinal ligament or the tectorial membrane and indentation of the cord substance.[51] The retro-odontoid ligamentous hypertrophy appears to be related to laxity of ligaments due to reduced atlantoaxial height and secondary to progressive degenerative changes in the region. The pathogenesis of the degenerative changes simulates to an extent the formation of posterior osteophytes in cases with spinal degeneration. It appears that the presence of retro-odontoid ligamentous degenerative hypertrophy in an elderly patient can be diagnostic evidence that suggests atlantoaxial instability, even when such instability is not clearly visualized on radiological imaging. In general, it is observed that retro-odontoid ligamentous degenerative changes are identified and are thicker in cases in which the atlantoaxial instability is less marked and the entire degenerative process was more chronic in nature. As opposed to cases having rheumatoid arthritis where the process is more chronic or long-standing, the bone destruction of the facets of the atlas and axis and osteomalacia are not as pronounced in cases of degeneration-related arthritis. Degeneration of the atlantodental joint may be observed in a minority of patients. Cervical spondylotic degenerative disease is likely to be present in varying degrees in the rest of the spine in most cases.

Surgery (see Fig. 29.5)

For basilar invagination and retro-odontoid ligamentous hypertrophy, transoral decompression or subsequent posterior fixation has been the treatment protocol.[52,60] Although some surgeons still prefer to resect the retro-odontoid degenerative mass,[52] the current consensus appears to be that in such cases stabilization of the atlantoaxial joint is sufficient and results in regression of the retro-odontoid mass. Some surgeons advise incorporation of the occipital bone and cervical vertebrae up to C3 and C4 in the occipitocervical fixation and feel that such a fixation is necessary to avoid "cranial settling."[50,60] However, such an extended fixation does not seem to be necessary. The lateral mass plate and screw method of fixation can be useful. An attempt may additionally be made to distract the facets and restore the height of the lateral mass by impaction of bone chips harvested from the iliac crest alone or by additional impaction of spiked metal spacers.[51] Distraction of the facets not only assists in the reduction and fixation of the atlantoaxial dislocation and basilar invagination but also stretches the buckled posterior spinal ligaments that appear to have a role in the pathogenesis of retro-odontoid ligamentous degenerative hypertrophic mass. Upon opening the joint,

the presence of a relatively rough and pale yellow articular surface devoid of end plate, reduction of the joint space, and evidence of instability of the region are the more prominent observations. On reviewing the postoperative images, it was apparent that in all cases there was reduction of atlantoaxial dislocation and of basilar invagination. The postoperative reduction of the dislocation was significant but incomplete in about half the cases in which the reduction of the dislocation was incomplete during preoperative evaluation. This was probably due to the presence of nonyielding periodontoid ligamentous degenerative mass. Despite the incomplete reduction, the treatment resulted in an immediate postoperative and sustained neurological recovery. This improvement appeared to be related to elimination of abnormal mobility, realignment of bones, and probably by reduction of the indentation by the retro-odontoid mass. Postoperative CT scan showed evidence of reduced soft tissue shadow in the periodontoid space.

Anterior Transoral Release Followed by Posterior Atlantoaxial Fixation

As the reduction of the dislocation was incomplete in a proportion of cases, the craniovertebral region can be approached transorally in the first stage of operation. The operation involves decompression and radical resection of compressive degenerative tissue in the periodontoid region, without resection of any part of the bone. Reduction of the dislocation is confirmed on radiological imaging. The patient is then turned prone and a posterior fixation is completed. This strategy of treatment appears to be a viable option in the treatment of arthritis-related "fixed" atlantoaxial dislocation.

RHEUMATOID ARTHRITIS AFFECTING CRANIOVERTEBRAL JUNCTION

Seropositive rheumatoid arthritis has been identified in approximately 0.9% of the white adult population of the United States and 1.1% of the adult population in Europe.[59,61] Of these, as many as 10% of patients may need an operation for craniovertebral region instability. Rheumatoid arthritis is a disease of the articular capsule and bones forming the atlantoaxial joint. The articular capsule and the subcapsular bone may be affected leading to varying degrees of subluxation and basilar invagination. Such a joint can lead to "lateral mass collapse," as has been identified by some authors in similar cases.[53,59,61] The term *basilar invagination* in cases with rheumatoid arthritis has been used synonymously with the terms *cranial settling* or *vertical odontoid migration*.[53,62,63] Basilar invagination is commonly associated with atlantoaxial dislocation and the complex results in a significant degree of neck pain and myelopathy, adding considerably to the disability secondary to involvement of other joints.

Surgery

A variety of instrumentation and methods have been adopted to secure the occipitocervical fixation. Recently, a number of authors have reported success after transarticular atlantoaxial fixation.[64,65] For basilar invagination, transoral decompression and subsequent posterior fixation have been accepted treatment protocols. Menezes and co-workers observed that traction in cases with basilar invagination and atlantoaxial subluxation results in a significant improvement in the craniovertebral alignment.[53]

Craniovertebral realignment and stabilization without any bone decompression can be successful. Wide removal of atlanto-axial joint capsule and articular cartilage by drilling and subsequent distraction of the joint by manual manipulation provided a unique opportunity to obtain reduction of the basilar invagination and of atlantoaxial dislocation. The use of spiked spacers provided distraction and stability to the region. In selected cases, the stability to the region was such that no additional fixation procedure was felt necessary. Maintenance of the joint in a distracted and reduced position with the help of bone graft and metal spacers and subsequent fixation of the joint with the help of interarticular screws and a metal plate provided a biomechanically firm fixation and sustained distraction.

Retro-Odontoid Pannus

Pannus has uniformly been recognized to be secondary to an inflammatory response in cases of rheumatoid arthritis. However, it appears that reduction of the height of the lateral mass pillar secondary to bone destruction and reduced joint space can result in buckling of the retro-odontoid ligaments, giving a "pannus-like" formation. Surgery that involves restoration of the height of the lateral mass can lead to immediate reduction of the size of the pannus.[66,67]

TUBERCULOSIS OF CRANIOVERTEBRAL JUNCTION

Tuberculosis of the craniovertebral junction usually occurs secondary to a primary focus elsewhere in the body. Osteoligamentous destruction and deformities leading to a range of clinical presenting symptoms have been recorded in cases with tuberculosis involving the craniovertebral junction. The understanding of the site of involvement of the tuberculosis in the craniovertebral junction, the pattern of its spread, and nature of its pathogenetic effects on the osteoligamentous assembly is crucial for defining the strategy of the management. It has to be understood that tuberculosis involves the bone primarily and that ligaments are affected only secondarily. Bones are involved by destruction, and the ligaments are involved by displacement and disruption.

Natural Course of Disease

The general pattern of progression of craniovertebral tuberculosis can be divided into three stages.

Stage 1

In this stage there is unilateral involvement of the cancellous part of the facet of the atlas. There is no destructive deformation in this stage. Less frequently, there may be isolated and unilateral involvement of the cancellous part of the facets of the axis or of the odontoid process. Inflammatory granulomatous reaction is present, and caseous necrosis may be seen.

Granulation tissue is usually located around the involved facet. The other parts of the atlas (or axis) bone and the contralateral facet are not involved.

In this stage, the patient has pain in the neck and restriction of neck movements. Systemic symptoms such as loss of weight, loss of appetite, and fever are usually present.

Stage 2

In this stage the disease progresses to involve the atlantoaxial joint by destructive necrosis and inflammation. The joint involvement is a result of extension of the inflammatory reaction. The destruction involves the atlantoaxial joint complex, and in addition it extends to other parts of the atlas or axis bones. Tuberculous inflammation may extend widely. The contralateral joint is still unaffected in this stage. The incompetence of the joint and osseous destruction and the adjoining ligamentous disruption in such a situation has been known to result in atlantoaxial dislocation. The atlantoaxial dislocation is probably a result of ineffectiveness of the alar and transverse ligaments as their bone attachment site is destroyed. As the contralateral atlantoaxial joint is normal, the atlantoaxial dislocation is of "fixed" and rotatory variety, and grossly mobile and reducible dislocation is never or seldom encountered. The facet of the atlas may be collapsed. Prevertebral or extradural spinal caseous necrosis or pus formation is usually encountered. On imaging, the joint space on the involved side is seen to be reduced or absent, but on the contralateral side it is normal.

In this stage, the patient has pain in the neck, neck muscle spasm, and severe restriction of neck movements. Torticollis is characteristic and is the most prominent symptom. Torticollis appears to be a natural defense process, wherein the neck turns to the contralateral side in an attempt to reduce all weight bearing by the affected lateral mass and the joint and protect the cord from compression by the infective granulation.

In this stage, the patient may or may not have neurological symptoms or deficits.

Stage 3

The disease involves the contralateral atlantoaxial joint and other bones and joints in the region. Evidence of instability of the craniovertebral junction is usually seen. In this stage, the patient usually has a neurological deficit.

Indications for Surgery

Neurological deficits are notably delayed and less pronounced despite the aggressive destruction and deformation by the disease. The disease is initially unilateral and the contralateral atlantoaxial joint is spared till late in the disease process. Owing to the relative stability of the craniovertebral region despite the unilateral facetal destruction and the effectiveness of modern antituberculosis drugs, surgery can be delayed or avoided. The extent and nature of involvement of the joints are determining factors for the need for any kind of surgery for stabilization of the region. Surgery for evacuation of pus or granulation tissue is seldom required. Despite the extensiveness of the bone destruction and inflammation, the patient is usually neurologically quite stable, and the systemic symptoms are not pronounced till late in the disease process. In the absence of progressive neurological symptoms and in the presence of an intact contralateral atlantoaxial joint, surgery can be avoided. The patient needs to be placed on antituberculosis drugs. In addition, the patient will need a firm four-poster cervical collar and all activities related to neck movements and weight bearing should be avoided for at least 3 months or till there is evidence of bone healing and regression of symptoms.

Surgery is indicated less frequently and may be required in stages 2 and 3 of the disease. The most positive indication for surgery includes the presence and progression of neurological deficits. Radiological deformity in the presence of intact neurological condition may only be a marginal indication of surgery. A more crucial issue is to identify and relate the problem to tuberculosis and differentiate the lesion from several tumor-like pathological situations.

If the disease is localized to the atlantoaxial region, surgery can involve fixation of the contralateral atlantoaxial joint by the lateral mass plate and screw fixation. Our experience suggests that even if the fixation is done by this method unilaterally, it is strong and provides a stable craniovertebral junction. Incorporation of the occipital bone in the fixation is seldom necessary. However, in the presence of gross and bilateral destructive disease, occipitocervical fixation can be a useful alternative.

Lateral Dislocation of the Facet of the Atlas Over the Facet of the Axis

In the presence of destruction of the facets of the atlas and axis on one side, it appears that the alar and transverse ligaments can become unilaterally incompetent. The shift of balance on the contralateral side and the obliquity of the inclination of the facet of the atlas in the atlantoaxial joint can result in its lateral dislocation over the facet of the axis. Distraction of the facets of the atlas and axis, reduction of lateral dislocation,

and unilateral fixation of lateral masses can result in effective stabilization of the region.

Long-Term Outcome After Conservative Treatment

The effectiveness of drugs usually begins at about 3 weeks of treatment. Pain reduces and the systemic symptoms begin to abate. Over the period, the patient recovers and the neurological symptoms and deficits abate to varying degrees. Fibrous reunion of the region and of the joint usually occurs over the period and normality of the joint movements is at least partially restored. Patients nonresponsive to drug treatment will usually continue to have progressive destructive necrosis, deformity, and instability.

SELECTED KEY REFERENCES

Goel A, Bhatjiwale M, Desai K. Basilar invagination: a study based on 190 surgically treated cases. *J Neurosurg.* 1998;88: 962-968.

Goel A, Laheri VK. Plate and screw fixation for atlanto-axial dislocation. Technical report. *Acta Neurochir (Wien).* 1994;129:47-53.

Goel A, Sharma P. Craniovertebral realignment for basilar invagination and atlantoaxial dislocation secondary to rheumatoid arthritis. *Neurol India.* 2004;52(3):338-341.

Goel A, Shah A. Reversal of longstanding musculoskeletal changes in basilar invagination after surgical decompression and stabilization. *J Neurosurg Spine.* 2009;10(3):220-227.

Goel A. Treatment of basilar invagination by atlantoaxial joint distraction and direct lateral mass fixation. *J Neurosurg Spine.* 2004;1(3):281-286.

Please go to expertconsult.com to view the complete list of references.

30 Degenerative Spine Disease

James K.C. Liu, Edward C. Benzel

CLINICAL PEARLS

- Degeneration in the spine is a naturally occurring process that can be understood through the "three-joint complex," which is composed of the intervertebral disk and the two dorsal articulating joints. Degeneration of any one joint leads to degeneration of the other two, initiating a cascade that leads to spinal degenerative disease.

- A detailed history and neurological examination can be used to isolate the level at which the underlying disease originate. Understanding the presenting symptoms can help to understand the degree of degeneration present and then start to formulate the most efficient treatment plan.

- Conservative treatment is a feasible first course of action to treat the clinical manifestations of first-onset degenerative spine disease. The most commonly accepted modalities range from anti-inflammatory therapy to exercises designed to increase muscle strength and relieve joint loading.

- Surgical intervention to treat symptoms that result from degenerative spine disease include diskectomy, laminectomy, and fusion procedures. Despite continuing controversy surrounding which procedure is most effective in providing long-term relief, the authors believe that the best course is to understand the underlying disease and select the least invasive procedure to target that pathological area.

- Fusion remains a heavily debated topic. Multiple studies have been performed to evaluate the benefits of fusion in the spine, none of which have provided definitive class I evidence to indicate a clear benefit. However, in addition to the class II and III evidence showing some benefit in selected patients, spine fusions may be indicated based on the need to create stability in an unstable region of the spine.

Back pain is the one of the most common reasons for primary care physician outpatient visits in the United States. A survey performed in 2002 reported that approximately 26% of Americans had low back pain and 14% had neck pain.[1] In 2002, 890 million office visits were due to back pain. As may be expected from these statistics, the cost associated with the diagnosis and treatment of spine-related problems is astronomical. The *Journal of the American Medical Association* reported $86 billion in health expenditures in 2005 devoted to spine-related problems. This amount was an increase of 65% from 1997.[2]

The process that leads to the development of neck and back pain can be segmented and categorized into acquired and congenital/developmental processes. This chapter focuses on the naturally occurring events that lead to degeneration of the spine.

ANATOMY AND PHYSIOLOGY OF SPINE DEGENERATION

Three-Joint Complex

An understanding of the process of spinal aging involves an understanding of the relevant anatomy of the affected spine. In order to understand the sequence of events that leads to degeneration of the spine, efforts have been made to deconstruct the spine in order to demonstrate the nature of the degenerative process, for such a process begins in one segment of the spine and then spreads to adjacent segments.

The Kirkaldy-Willis three-joint complex theory deconstructs the spine into three joints that are affected in the degenerative process. At each level of the spine there exists the "three-joint complex," composed of the intervertebral disk

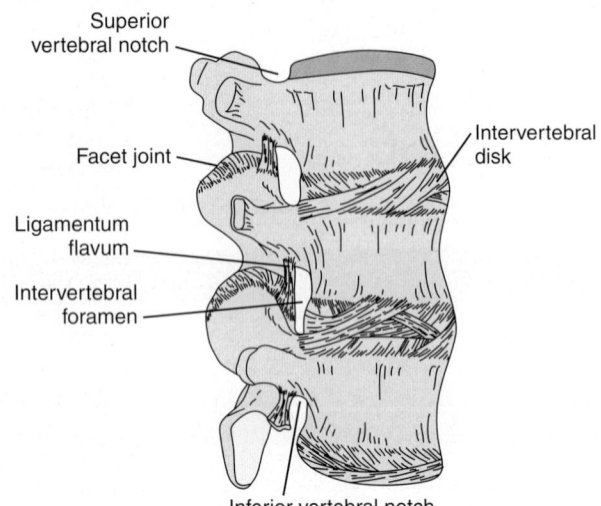

Superior
vertebral notch

Facet joint

Ligamentum
flavum

Intervertebral
foramen

Intervertebral
disk

Inferior vertebral notch

FIGURE 30-1 Three-joint complex. Each motion segment is composed of a three-joint complex, which consists of one intervertebral disk space and two dorsal zygapophyseal joints. Degeneration in one of these joints often leads to accelerated degeneration in the adjacent joints. This results in a relatively predictable progression of degeneration.

and two dorsal zygapophyseal joints.[3] Kirkaldy-Willis proposed that the three joints are linked, in that degeneration of one joint leads to degeneration of the other two joints, and ultimately results in the global manifestations of degenerative spine disease (Fig. 30.1).

Degeneration, as stated, typically begins in one joint. This, in and of itself, may lead to clinical manifestations. It, however, is the interplay of the three-joint complex as a whole that leads to degenerative disease, as it typically presents in the clinical setting. The three-joint complex is first examined individually here, and then a discussion of the interaction of pathological changes that lead to spinal stenosis follows.

Disk Degeneration

The intervertebral disk has three components: the nucleus pulposus, which is surrounded by the annulus fibrosis, and the cartilaginous end plates.[4] The nucleus pulposus is a semi-gelatinous structure situated near the center of the disk complex. It is a remnant of the notochord and is composed mainly of mucopolysaccharides with salt and water. The surrounding annulus fibrosis is a multilayered circular structure that surrounds the nucleus pulposus. It is composed of fibrocartilaginous lamellae and is stiffer than the nucleus. It is usually thicker ventrally than dorsally.[4]

The process of disk degeneration is a part of the natural aging process. Repetitive loading results in forces that foster degeneration. As part of the normal aging process, the intervertebral disk becomes desiccated as collagen and proteoglycans are replaced with fibrous tissue. As axial pressure continues to be repetitively applied to the disk, the less compliant annulus fibrosis develops circumferential tears that are most frequently observed in the dorsolateral aspect of the annulus.[5] These tears can enlarge and eventually develop into radial tears. These tears are areas through which the nucleus

pulposus may herniate. Since the nucleus pulposus is situated relatively dorsal in the disk space, herniation typically occurs dorsally into the spinal canal. The presence of the posterior longitudinal ligament forces disk herniations laterally. The aforementioned anatomical and biomechanical factors often lead to the common classical dorsolateral disk herniation.

Annular tears also lead to a weakening of the annulus fibrosus and to circumferential bulging of the annulus, which in turn results in a loss of disk height. Disk bulging can lead to osteophyte formation at the attachment of the annulus to the vertebral body. This contributes to narrowing of the central canal, as well as the neural foramen.

Dorsal Joint Degeneration

The dorsal aspect of the intervertebral joint is composed of articulating facets from the superior and inferior vertebral segments. The joints are diarthrodial joints with articular cartilage, a synovial membrane, and a capsule.[6] Studies have shown that natural aging of the dorsal joints passes through a progression that includes synovial reaction, fibrillation of the articular cartilage, osteophyte formation, and ultimately, laxity of the joint capsule. This inevitably results in instability of the joint complex and can lead to subluxation of the joint. Osteophytic formation from the joint protruding into the spinal canal can also contribute to stenosis, particularly in the lateral recesses of the spinal canal.

Combined Three-Joint Complex Degeneration

The three-joint complex degeneration concept implies that the individual aging process of the intervertebral disk and dorsal facet joints are interlaced to contribute to the clinical manifestation of spondylosis. As disk degeneration occurs, loss of disk height contributes to subluxation of the dorsal joints. The instability caused by the loss of disk height compounds the natural process of facet joint degeneration, which includes capsular laxity. Eventually, subluxation of the dorsal joints can occur. This results in subluxation of the rostral vertebral body ventrally with respect to the caudal vertebral body (spondylolisthesis). Such translation of the vertebral segments can result in further narrowing of the neural foramina, manifesting as lateral nerve root entrapment. Lateral nerve root entrapment can also result from loss of disk height. Disk resorption reduces the rostral-caudal dimension of the neural foramina, thus further contributing to this presentation.

Three Stages of Degenerative Spine Disease

Using the three-joint complex as a basis for degenerative spine disease, Kirkaldy-Willis categorized the degeneration of the spine into three stages to rationalize the natural history of spine degeneration, as well as to provide an algorithm to tailor treatment for each stage (Fig. 30.2).

The Dysfunction Stage

The first stage is that of dysfunction. The clinical manifestations both clinically and physiologically are minor at this stage. This stage is characterized by synovial reaction in the dorsal joints and small tears in the intervertebral disks.

THREE JOINT COMPLEX DEGENERATION

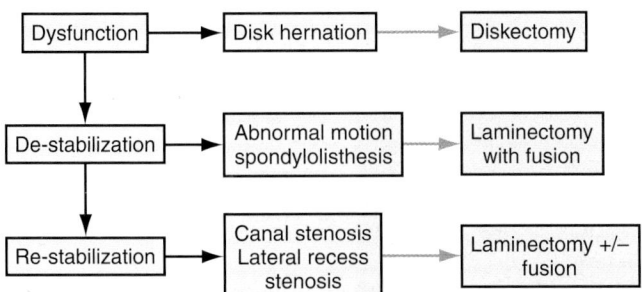

FIGURE 30.2 The three stages of degenerative spine disease. The first stage is dysfunction, which results primarily in simple disk herniations, often necessitating a surgical diskectomy. Progression of the degenerative process results in destabilization and abnormal spinal motion. This may necessitate the performance of a fusion procedure to stabilize the spine. The most advanced stage of degeneration is that of restabilization. The spine become more stable due to osteophyte formation, but in doing so creates a central and lateral recess stenosis, which often necessitates decompression, with or without a supplemental fusion. Red arrows designate the most likely surgical strategy for each phase of the degenerative process.

Clinical symptoms present at this stage are typically minor or absent and are best treated conservatively.

The Destabilization Stage

The second stage is the destabilization stage or rather the stage of instability. Kirkaldy-Willis defines this stage as being associated with greater degeneration in the three-joint complex, manifesting as laxity and subluxation in the dorsal joints and progressive disk degeneration. As its name implies, this stage is characterized by abnormal spinal motion. As segmental degeneration continues, the natural mobility of the spine is gradually lost. This is further compounded by advanced disk degeneration and loss of disk height, which can lead to spondylolisthesis. This creates a dysfunctional mechanical environment in the region of the motion segment, hence the term *dysfunctional motion segment*. Treatment options for spondylolisthesis include core strengthening and flexibility programs that are designed to stabilize or normalize the dysfunctional motion segment and strategies that are designed to immobilize the spine (dysfunctional motion segment), with or without restoration of the intervertebral height, and fusion of abnormal motion segments.

The Restabilization Stage

The third stage is restabilization. In this, the most advanced stage of degeneration as defined by Kirkaldy-Willis, spine instability is actually reduced via osteophyte formation secondary to a prior increased joint laxity and loss of disk interspace height. Clinically, resolution of symptoms can occur due to a gradually decreased spinal motion. The instability observed during the destabilization stage can be replaced by radiculopathy from spinal nerve entrapment or claudication symptoms from central canal and lateral recess stenosis.

CLINICAL PRESENTATION

The manifestation of clinical symptoms depends upon the type and degree of ongoing degeneration. A careful history and clinical examination enables the examiner to determine the stage of degeneration and the underlying disease. Determining the fundamental disease process facilitates the formulation of a focused plan of treatment, without the performance of unnecessary surgical intervention, to prevent advanced symptomatic segmental degeneration.

The first stage of degeneration as described by Kirkaldy-Willis, dysfunction, is characterized in the disk joint by annular tears and herniation of the nucleus pulposus. This leads to intervertebral disk herniation, one of the most common reasons for back pain, leg pain, and spine surgery. Disk herniation typically occurs in the dorsolateral aspect of the disk interspace. The strength of the posterior longitudinal ligament causes a paramedian migration and herniation of the nuclear material, which may result in impingement of a single nerve root, causing pain known as *radiculopathy*. Compression of the nerve root typically manifests as pain, but can also result in numbness or weakness in the distribution of the affected nerve root.

With cervical spine involvement, the patient often complains of a shooting pain that travels from the shoulder to the fingers. The exact location of the shooting pain can help to isolate the level of the disk herniation. Cervical disk herniations most often occur at the C5-C6 and C6-C7 levels.[7] In the lumbar spine disk herniations most commonly occur at the L4-L5 interspace[8] and manifest as shooting pain that often begins in the buttock region and passes down the legs, with or without extension into the feet. Once again, the distribution can help to localize the level of herniation. Thoracic disk herniations are much less common than cervical or lumbar disk herniations. In a study of 82 patients with thoracic disk herniations, 76% of the presenting complaints consisted of pain. Of the patient who presented with pain, 41% presented with localized back pain, thus relegating surgical management to the "precarious" category in most clinical cases.[9]

Further degeneration, resulting in further diffuse disk bulging into the spinal canal, combined with osteophyte formation from dorsal joint laxity and inflammation of the ligamentum flavum, can lead to circumferential spinal canal narrowing manifesting as neurogenic claudication. Neurogenic claudication manifests as pain that is exacerbated by walking or standing, and relieved with postural changes that allow increasing the diameter of the spinal canal or neural foramina. The affected patient often reports that pain is relieved when in the sitting position. Also, patients report that walking while leaning forward, often supporting their weight while pushing a shopping cart, allows for relief of back pain ("shopping cart sign"). An important distinction must be made between neurogenic claudication and vascular claudication. Vascular claudication is a result of vascular insufficiency and manifests as leg pain with motion that is relieved by rest. It is important to properly assess the vascular supply by inspecting distal pedal pulses in order to differentiate between the two entities. In addition, other clinical observations may be used to differentiate the two diagnoses. For example, pushing a shopping cart (i.e., "shopping cart sign") does not relieve vascular claudication symptoms. Other manifestations of vascular disease

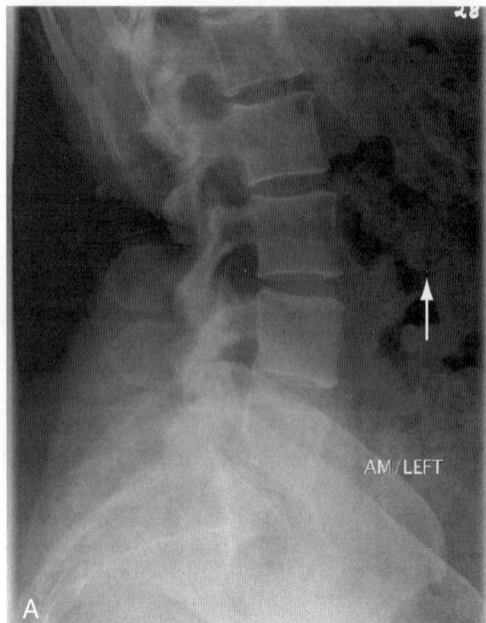
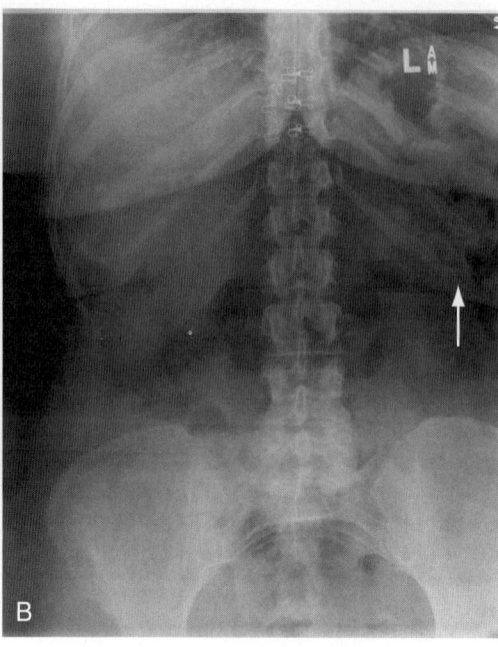

FIGURE 30.3 Lateral (**A**) and antero-posterior (**B**) plain radiograph views of the lumbar spine. Plain radiographs are effective in evaluating for alignment of the spine in both the sagittal and coronal orientation. The intervertebral height (**A**) is an indication of degenerative disk disease.

should be sought as well, including loss of foot/toe hair, skin discoloration, and a clinical history of other disorders and risk factors associated with ischemic vascular disease.

The degenerative process advances in the destabilization stage and involves laxity of the dorsal joints, which, in turn, leads to joint subluxation. This subluxation, combined with advanced disk degeneration resulting in disk desiccation and narrowing of the intervertebral space, can lead to slippage of one vertebral body relative to another, or spondylolisthesis. Spondylolisthesis manifests as instability of the joints, which, in turn, leads to abnormal or dysfunctional motion. The result of this process can eventually lead to mechanical back pain. Mechanical back pain is defined as pain that results from activity and is relieved with rest. This pain is attributed to joint instability and abnormal motion of one vertebral body upon another, which can be the result of the degenerative changes described previously but can also result from traumatic or congenital causes. The treatment for mechanical back pain includes restoration of stability to the segment through fusion and fixation.

DIAGNOSTIC FINDINGS

The initial evaluation of back and leg pain begins with static plain radiographs (Fig. 30.3). Static radiographs provide an evaluation of spinal alignment and the intervertebral disk spaces. An assessment of an affected intervertebral space serves to provide a rough estimation of the extent of disk degeneration, and therefore desiccation, that is present at a given level. Static radiographs consisting of flexion and extension views of the cervical or lumbar spine can reveal loss of normal alignment during motion. Such may be indicative of dorsal, or even ventral, joint instability.

Computed tomography (CT) provides a very useful evaluation of the bony anatomy (Fig. 30.4). CT is effective in evaluating for bony osteophytes, presence of calcification,

and dimensions of bony architecture that may be required for surgical planning. CT myelography is an effective alternative to assess the neural elements when magnetic resonance imaging (MRI) is either contraindicated (due to medical implants) or would be less efficacious owing to artifact from previous instrumentation. CT myelography can detect central as well as foraminal stenosis.

MRI is widely considered the gold standard for the imaging evaluation of spinal canal stenosis (Fig. 30.5). MRI can most effectively visualize the soft tissues surrounding the spinal canal, as well as the intervertebral disks, ligamentum flavum, and facet joints. In degenerative spine disease, the location of disk herniation can be evaluated. The origin of the spinal canal stenosis, whether from the intervertebral disks, hypertrophy of the posterior longitudinal ligament or of the ligamentum flavum, or facet hypertrophy, can be specifically localized by MRI.

Diskography is a more invasive diagnostic strategy. At times, when the clinical presentation does not match the findings on the aforementioned routine imaging techniques, or indeterminate findings on standard imaging modalities are present, some feel that diskography may be used to identify and characterize the disease. Diskography involves injecting contrast material into the intervertebral disks in question. The amount of contrast agent tolerated by a disk is an indication of degeneration. A normal cervical disk may tolerate 0.2 to 0.5 mL of fluid, whereas a degenerated disk can accept 0.5 to 1.5 mL of fluid.[10] If the pain produced following contrast injection is concordant with the typical pain experienced by the patient, the injected level is considered by some to be the pathological segment. Disk pressure at which pain is elicited is also used to predict the pathological level, because damaged disks allegedly produce pain at lower pressures than normal disks.[11] The effectiveness of diskography to predict positive surgical outcomes is controversial at best, with varying predictive reliability. One of the greatest criticisms of diskography is that the grading system employs a subjective criterion for

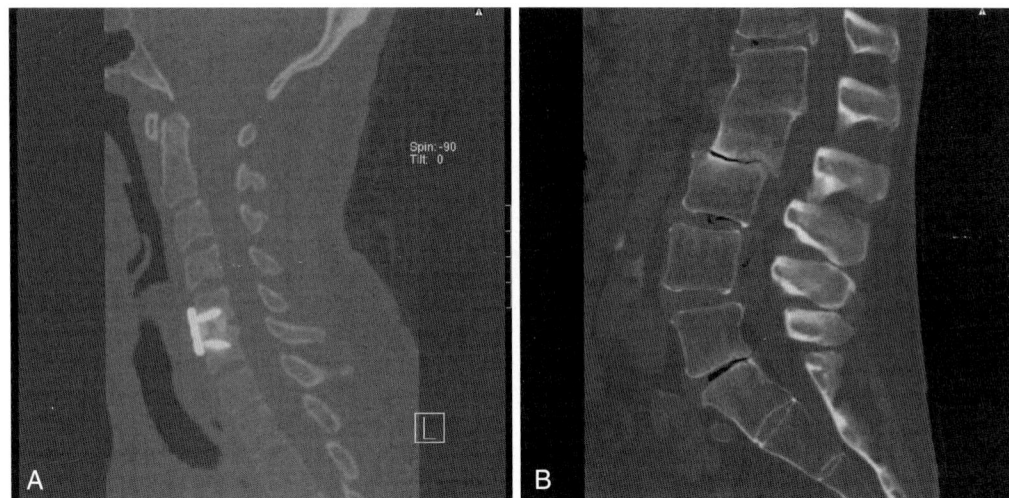

FIGURE 30.4 Computed tomography (CT) of the cervical and lumbar spine. CT scans are effective for evaluating bony structure in the spine. In the CT scan of the cervical spine (**A**), a single-level ventral fusion with plating has been performed. CT is more effective compared to magnetic resonance imaging (MRI) for evaluating instrumentation due to the lack of artifact on CT imaging. Successful fusion can also be effectively evaluated by CT imaging by observing whether the interbody graft is consistent with the vertebral bodies above and below. Careful assessment of the bony anatomy is required when instrumentation is planned. Autofusion of the spine as seen in the lumbar spine (**B**) at the L1-L2 level can be detected on CT and provides useful information prior to surgical intervention.

FIGURE 30.5 Severe lumbar spine degenerative changes. The sagittal view (**A**) magnetic resonance imaging (MRI) displays multilevel stenosis from anterior and posterior disease as well as loss of intervertebral disk height. Axial view (**B**) shows facet hypertrophy with edema in the facet joints indicated by the hyperintensity.

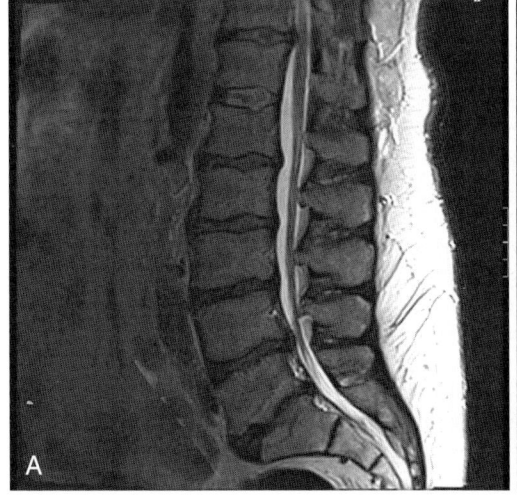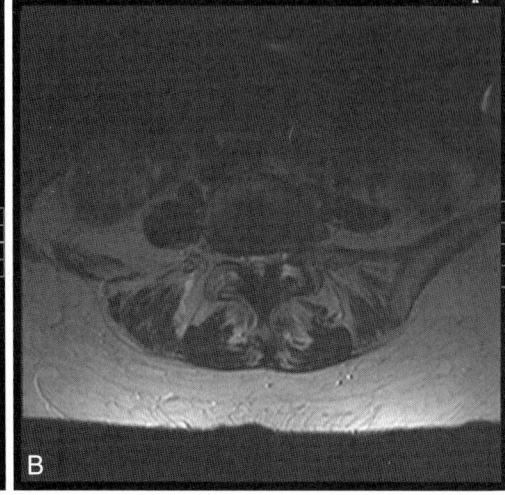

pain, and therefore can be skewed, depending on the patient and the examiner. It is emphasized that diskography should be used with the understanding that it does not provide clinically proven diagnostic utility.

TREATMENT OPTIONS

Nonoperative Management

Conservative management plays a significant role in the management of degenerative spine disease. Studies of the natural course of spinal stenosis have shown that up to 47% of patients with symptoms of lumbar spinal stenosis, including neurogenic claudication and radiculopathy, had improvement of symptoms without any intervention.[12] Although the physiology of spontaneous improvement of symptoms of spinal stenosis is unclear, it has been postulated that progressive disk dehydration may lead to shrinking of the disk and a decrease in nerve root compression.[13]

Medical treatment of degenerative spine disease ranges from symptomatic relief to reduction of inflammation. Narcotics can be effective for controlling back or extremity pain, but these drugs represent short-term resolutions, because they only postpone the inevitable course of the degenerative disease, whether it is toward improvement or further worsening of symptoms.

Nonsteroidal anti-inflammatory medications have been shown to be effective in providing relief for acute back pain.[14] Narcotic medication can be used to supplement those drugs when there is more severe pain, but the effectiveness of narcotics only serves to mask the degenerative process until it progresses or improves spontaneously. Furthermore, narcotic medications often contribute to the perpetuation of the cyclical process leading to the development of a chronic pain syndrome in patients who do not improve. Their use, therefore, should be very carefully considered.

Other medical treatments include muscle relaxants. Muscle relaxants have shown benefit for the treatment of acute neck and back pain.[15] Systemic oral steroids have also been utilized for the treatment of radicular pain. Some think that the anti-inflammatory effects may reduce nerve root irritation, although several studies have not demonstrated a proven clinical effect.[16-18]

A critical tool for nonoperative management of degenerative spine disease is physical reconditioning, often via the employment of a physical therapist. The goal associated with the application of self-induced physical focuses in order to strengthen core muscle groups is to help alleviate pathological loading of the affected dysfunctional joints. Flexibility exercises play an integral role as well. Improving segmental flexibility at adjacent segments can diminish pain and help preserve normal motion.

Epidural steroid injections (ESIs) have been shown to be effective, particularly for radicular pain. The anti-inflammatory effects of the steroids are likely to be effective against the chemoinflammatory responses emanating from a herniated disk. As expected from its mechanism of action, the effects of ESIs are usually acute and, hence, short term in nature. Because they do not alter the overall progression of the spine degeneration, their temporary clinical benefits are limited, and therefore, they serve best when used to supplement the use of an alternative conservative treatment, such as physical therapy.

Facet joint injections remain a controversial mode of treatment for back pain. Injections are composed of a long-acting local anesthetic, combined with steroids. Studies have reported no evidence of clinical improvement of back pain,[19] with only 33% of patients reporting greater than a 50% relief of pain.[20] This approximates results that are consistent with the placebo effect. The key to the efficacy of facet injections may reside in the proper selection of patients with the so-called facet syndrome. Lippitt defined the manifestations of the facet syndrome as "pain in the hips and buttocks area, cramping thigh pain, and back stiffness that is worse in the morning, without lower extremity paresthesias." One of the alleged key signs associated with the facet syndrome is the observation that the pain is exacerbated with lumbar spine extension.[21] A factor that may confound the efficacy of facet joint injections is the likelihood that injected material may leak out of the facet joint. This leaking may result in direct nerve root block or diffusion of anesthetic material into the paraspinous soft tissues. Such "leakage" would obviously skew outcomes. Nevertheless, facet joint injection persists as a popular therapeutic and diagnostic modality.

One of the less understood therapies patients have often attempted prior to their presentation to a spine specialist is spinal manipulative therapy (SMT). SMT is primarily provided by chiropractors, but can also be administered by physical therapists and osteopathic physicians. Manipulation can be categorized into three main types of therapies: therapeutic massage, mobilization, and manipulative procedures. These manipulation techniques range from the application of pressure isolated to the paraspinal musculature to maneuvers that stress the spinal joints and ligaments. The therapeutic benefit

of SMT stems from the hypothesis that neck or back pain is caused by either a limited range of motion or abnormal dorsal intervertebral joint motion. A natural joint motion consists of an active range of motion, followed by a passive range of motion that can be reached with external mobilization. A dysfunctional joint leads to pain because it is unable to reach the entire range of motion. SMT "resets" the joint by extending the joint beyond the passive range of motion, into the "paraphysiological range of motion." This stresses the joint to its limit, just short of joint disruption. At this point, joint cavitation occurs, and the often encountered sounds of joint mobilization, which are likely the result of gas released into the joint space,[22] occur. The effectiveness of spinal manipulation has been questioned, and definitive clinical studies that show significant long-term improvement are lacking. Clinical evidence indicates that there may be short-term relief for the management of low back pain, but there is no evidence of significance that demonstrates efficacy.[23] One of the difficulties associated with assessing the effectiveness of SMT is related to the fact that there exists no universal treatment strategy—the types and numbers of treatments administered vary most dramatically across the board.

Operative Treatment

Surgical treatment options for degenerative spine disease range widely in complexity and may correlate with the extent of disease progression. Via the matching of the clinical evaluation with imaging findings, the disease can be isolated and the most appropriate nonsurgical or surgical approach chosen and employed.

In the initial stage of spinal degeneration, disk desiccation leads to predominantly dorsolateral disk herniations causing radicular symptoms (Fig. 30.6). Single-level disk herniations can be treated nonoperatively or with cervical or lumbar diskectomy. The latter are relatively "simple" operations that are associated with a relatively high degree of short-term success. Long-term success is more variable.

More complex pathological processes may require surgical decompression via laminectomy or surgical stabilization. The options are myriad. The decision to fuse should not be taken lightly, however. A failed instrumented lumbar fusion often results in further surgery and chronic pain. Such patients are very difficult to manage moving forward.

Diskectomy

Diskectomy procedures can be typically categorized into ventral and dorsal approaches. In the cervical spine, the ventral approach is often utilized because of its ability to decompress broad-based disk herniations. The ventral approach is performed through a paramedian incision that requires little muscle splitting, which leads to a relatively low amount of postoperative pain and morbidity. The most commonly encountered postoperative complication is dysphagia secondary to retraction of the esophagus, which has been shown to occur in anywhere from 1% to 79% of cases following anterior cervical procedures, but dramatically improves in the majority of cases.[24] The other main consideration of the ventral cervical approach, and possibly a contraindication to the approach, is damage to the recurrent laryngeal nerve resulting

FIGURE 30.6 Single-level disk herniation in the cervical (**A**) and lumbar spine (**B**).

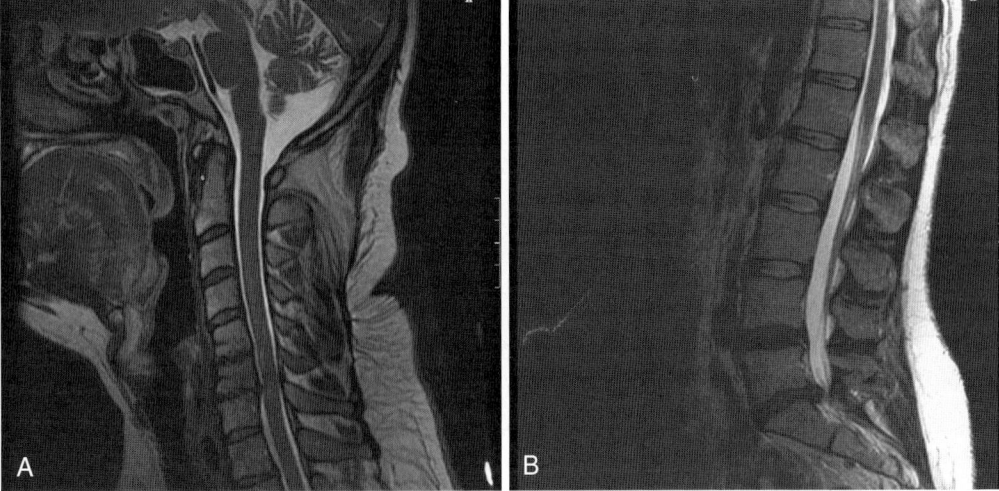

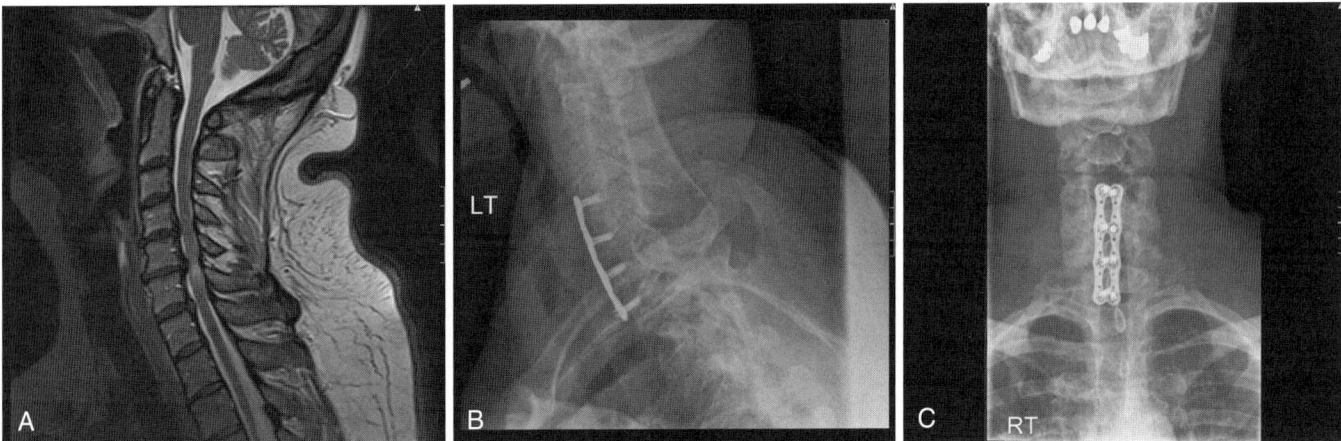

FIGURE 30.7 Sagittal magnetic resonance imaging (MRI) of the cervical spine (**A**) indicating multilevel stenosis primarily from disk herniations. A three-level anterior diskectomy and fusion procedure was performed. Postoperative radiographs (**B** and **C**) show a three-level fusion with ventral plating.

in vocal cord paralysis. This paralysis has also been shown to improve with time in the majority of cases[25] (Fig. 30.7).

The dorsal approach to the cervical spine has also been shown to be effective in eliminating unilateral nerve root compression. The technique is effective for eliminating posterolateral disk herniations either through foraminotomies with or without a diskectomy procedure. The dorsal approach eliminates the morbidity associated with the ventral approach, mainly dysphagia, and risk to the ventral neurovascular structures, but requires muscle splitting, which can add a variable amount of postoperative pain. Simple foraminotomies and diskectomies also do not require fusion, theoretically decreasing risk of adjacent segment degeneration. Minimally invasive techniques have been developed to reduce the amount of muscle dissection carried out and have shown to have up to a 97% success rate alleviating radiculopathy symptoms.[26]

Diskectomy procedures in the lumbar spine can also be categorized into anterior and posterior approaches, although unlike the cervical spine, the posterior approach is the more often utilized. Lumbar diskectomies involve a unilateral muscle dissection exposing the lamina of the given level to allow a hemilaminectomy, through which the herniated disk

is removed. The Spine Patient Outcomes Research Trial (SPORT) was a prospective, randomized trial that evaluated lumbar diskectomies against nonoperative treatment.[27] This trial concluded that patients undergoing lumbar diskectomies enjoyed reduction of pain, improvements in physical functioning, and a greater improvement in their disability index than patients undergoing conservative treatment. Given the presence of the cauda equina in the lumbar region as opposed to the spinal cord present in the cervical region, the posterior approach is more versatile in the sense that even more centralized disk herniations can be decompressed owing to the amount of manipulation that can be tolerated by the thecal sac.

Laminectomy

Laminectomies decompress the spine via the removal of the lamina and spinous process. Laminectomy can be applied equally in the cervical, thoracic, and lumbar spine, typically for multilevel reduction of spinal canal stenosis. In the cervical spine, multilevel laminectomy has been shown to be effective particularly for canal decompression resulting in cervical

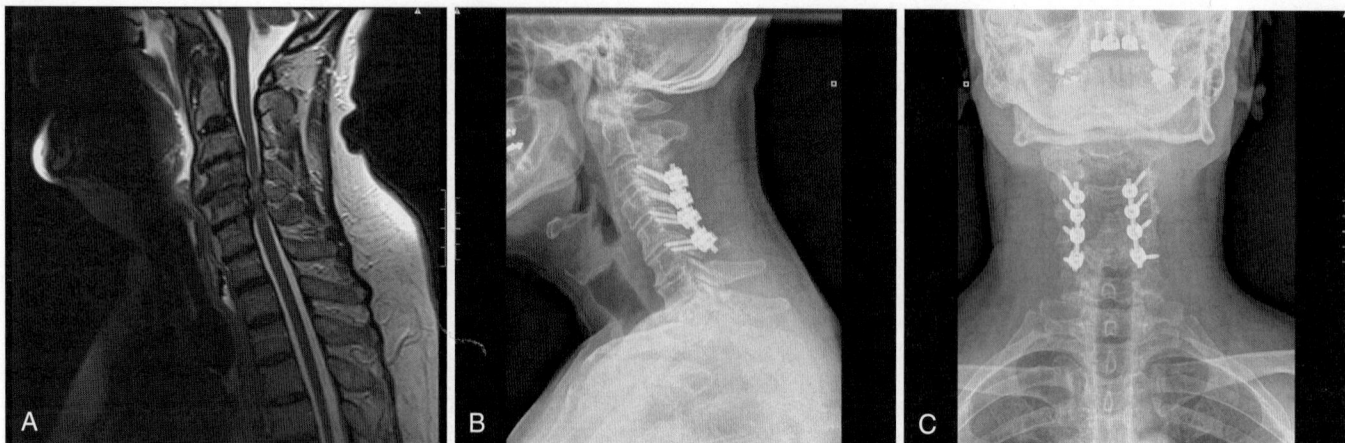

FIGURE 30.8 Multilevel cervical stenosis viewed on sagittal magnetic resonance imaging (MRI) (**A**). Laminectomies were performed from the C3 to C6 levels and fused with lateral mass screws. Postoperative lateral and anteroposterior (AP) radiographs are shown (**B** and **C**).

spondolytic myelopathy, as well as for other pathological disorders such as ossification of the posterior longitudinal ligament. Although shown to be effective in improving signs of myelopathy, the development of postoperative kyphosis has been reported to be between 14% and 47%.[28] This has led to the use of cervical laminectomy combined with fusion and laminoplasty. Although all three techniques have been shown to be effective in decompressing the spinal canal, laminectomy with fusion and laminoplasty have become more commonplace owing to their reduced incidence of postoperative kyphosis.

Laminoplasty involves detachment of the lamina on only one side by creating a trough, and thinning the lamina on the contralateral side to allow for "hinging" at the attached lamina site. This allows the detached lamina to be elevated and secured using small bone grafts to maintain the decompressed state. The preservation of the posterior elements has been shown to effectively decompress the spinal canal without the consequences of fusion such as loss of range of motion and adjacent segment degeneration. In one study, laminoplasty was shown to be associated with a 27% improvement in preventing the incidence of postoperative kyphosis.[29]

Laminectomy in the lumbar spine is most common procedure performed by spine and neurological surgeons. Laminectomy alone in the lumbar spine is most effective for neurogenic claudication resulting from spinal stenosis. Lumbar laminectomy involves removal of the lamina as well as performing a medial facetectomy to eliminate lateral recess stenosis.

Fusion

Fusion remains a heavily debated topic. Multiple studies have been performed to evaluate the benefits of fusion in the spine, none of which has provided definitive class I evidence to indicate a clear benefit. The consideration to perform a fusion is typically based on the need to create stability in an unstable region of the spine. In the cervical spine, fusion can be considered for ventral and dorsal approaches. A review of 13 class II and III studies comparing the outcome of anterior cervical diskectomies with and without fusion performed by Matz and associates, demonstrated that there was no clinically significant advantage of including fusion. Only two class III studies demonstrated that anterior cervical diskectomy alone had a short length of hospital stay and operative time.[30] Fusion has become a commonplace procedure with cervical laminectomies owing to the incidence of postoperative kyphosis (Fig. 30.8). Although no class I or II evidence exists to support the use of cervical laminectomy with fusion, there is class III evidence to indicate that fusion reduces postoperative kyphosis.[28,31,32]

A great deal of controversy surrounds the indications for fusion in the lumbar spine. The indication for fusion is typically during the end of the second stage of the Kirkaldy-Willis process, which is the phase of maximal destabilization. Degeneration of the joint complexes and disk space leads to excessive movement of one vertebral body upon another, creating mechanical back pain. The pain created is partially axial pain caused by disk degeneration and abnormal joint motion but can also have a radicular component due to foraminal stenosis and nerve root entrapment during mobility. Lumbar fusion can be used to augment the transition to the second stage of spinal degeneration into the third stage, restabilization. Fusion typically involves a laminectomy to decompress the spinal canal and the lateral recess (Fig. 30.9). Autograft bone is used either in the dorsolateral spaces or the interspaces to facilitate bony fusion while the construct immobilizes the spinal segment. There are no clear data to support the presumption that fusion results in better outcomes compared to simple laminectomy alone. A multicenter trial is currently underway to compare fusion with laminectomy alone for grade I spondylolisthesis.[33]

FIGURE 30.9 Sagittal magnetic resonance imaging (MRI) of the lumbar spine (**A**) showing a grade I spondylolisthesis at the L4-L5 level. This patient was treated with decompression fusion at those levels (**B**).

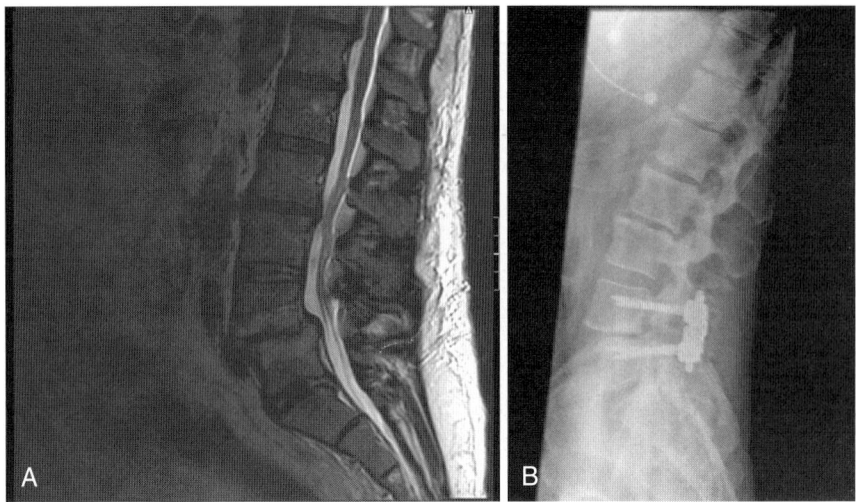

SELECTED KEY REFERENCES

Ghogawala Z. Spinal laminectomy vs. instrumented pedicle screw fusion. Available at http://www.spine-slip-study.org/2.

Johnsson KE, Rosen I, Uden A. The natural course of lumbar spinal stenosis. *Clin Orthop Relat Res.* 1992;279:82-86.

Ritchie JH, Fahrni WH. Age changes in lumbar intervertebral discs. *Can J Surg.* 1970;13(1):65-71.

Weinstein JN, Lurie JD, Tosteson TD, et al. Surgical versus non-operative treatment for lumbar spinal stenosis: four-year results of the spine patient outcomes research trial. *Spine.* 2010;35(14):1329-1338.

Yong-Hing K, Kirkaldy-Willis WH. The pathophysiology of degenerative disease of the lumbar spine. *Orthop Clin North Am.* 1983;14(3):491-504.

Please go to expertconsult.com to view the complete list of references.

Pediatric and Adult Scoliosis

David W. Polly Jr., A. Noelle Larson (Part I)
Frank Schwab, Benjamin Blondel, Virginie Lafage (Part II)

CLINICAL PEARLS

- The clinician must be alert for any evidence of underlying neurological disease, including asymmetrical abdominal reflexes, abnormalities on neurological examination, or a cavovarus foot deformity. On radiographs, hyperkyphosis over the apex of the curvature, an unusual curve pattern, marked trunk shift, a left thoracic curve, or lack of curve rotation may indicate an underlying neurological condition. These patients should undergo magnetic resonance imaging (MRI).

- Patients presenting with significant pain, those who have rapid progression, and children younger than 10 years of age should also have an MRI screening of the entire spine prior to initiation of treatment.

- Shoulder asymmetry, unilateral Sprengel's deformity, spasm from acute pain, or a leg-length discrepancy can give the false clinical appearance of scoliosis. Standing full-length scoliosis films are the gold standard for diagnosis.

- Bracing and surgery are the mainstays of treatment for scoliosis. Treatment must be tailored to the patient and family. Bracing is typically indicated in growing children with

- progressive curves measuring 20 to 45 degrees. In attempts to prevent curve progression, bracing is most effective in skeletally immature patients (Risser 0, 1, or 2) and in females who are less than 12 months past menarche. Casting is well tolerated in the young child and may be a preferable technique over bracing because of compliance. It has been shown to be curative in some cases of infantile scoliosis.

- When the curve magnitude exceeds 50 degrees in adolescent idiopathic scoliosis, surgical treatment is offered, typically with posterior spinal fusion.

- Adult scoliosis has a wide range of causes; most cases appear to relate to the degenerative process of aging or adolescent scoliosis in an adult. Other causes of deformity include osteoporosis, trauma, infection, and iatrogenic factors.

- Treatment for adult scoliosis is driven by the patient who wishes to regain function without pain. Correction of sagittal plane balance is essential to obtaining satisfactory results in this treatment.

PART I. SCOLIOSIS IN THE PEDIATRIC PATIENT

Scoliosis represents a complex three-dimensional deformity of the spine and thorax.[1,2] Scoliosis is defined as a coronal deformity of the spine with a Cobb angle measuring greater than 10 degrees (Fig. 31.1).[3] Small-magnitude curves may progress during periods of skeletal growth.[4] Larger curves may continue to increase, even in adulthood.[5,6] Thus, a pediatric patient with scoliosis should be followed until skeletal maturity, and young adults with large untreated curves should be monitored periodically for curve progression.

Congenital, neuromuscular, and idiopathic curves are commonly diagnosed in childhood. Congenital scoliosis results from malformation of the vertebral elements, either due to failure of formation or failure of segmentation. A hemivertebra with a contralateral bar results in the greatest risk of

curve progression.[7] Particularly in small children, it is difficult to predict which congenital curves will be progressive and will subsequently require surgical intervention. Because of a high associated risk, all children with congenital scoliosis require evaluation for concomitant renal, cardiac, and intrathecal abnormalities. Owing to the structural abnormalities, bracing in congenital scoliosis is typically not indicated. Neuromuscular curves are those associated with an underlying neurological difference, either structural (Chiari malformation, syrinx, tethered cord, diastematomyelia) or systemic (e.g., cerebral palsy, Charcot-Marie-Tooth disease, muscular dystrophy, neurofibromatosis). As idiopathic scoliosis is a diagnosis of exclusion, neurological causes for the deformity must be ruled out by medical history, clinical examination, radiographs, and in selected cases, axial imaging.

Idiopathic scoliosis is the most common type of scoliosis in children. Based on age at diagnosis, idiopathic scoliosis is traditionally classified into infantile (age less than 3 years),

ADOLESCENT IDIOPATHIC SCOLIOSIS

Coronal Cobb measurement technique
Proximal thoracic (PT), main thoracic (MT), and
thoracolumbar/lumbar (TL/L) curves

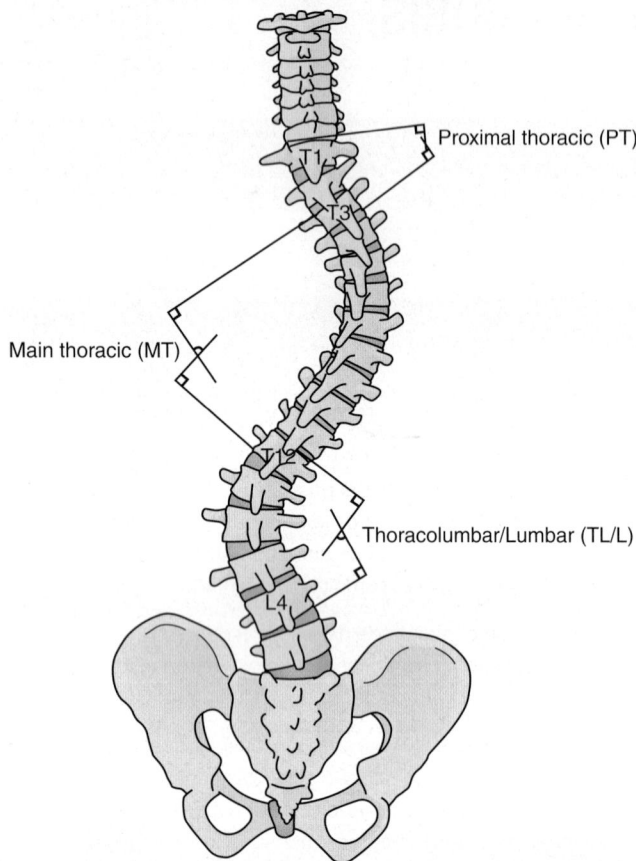

Proximal thoracic (PT)

Main thoracic (MT)

Thoracolumbar/Lumbar (TL/L)

FIGURE 31.1 Measurement of the Cobb angle to determine the coronal magnitude of the curve. The two most tilted vertebrae are identified, and a line is drawn marking the angle of the end plate. The angle between the end plates is then measured. To facilitate measurement of the angle, it is also possible to drop a perpendicular line from the end plate and measure the angle subtended by the perpendiculars.

juvenile (age 3 to 10 years), and adolescent (age greater than 10 years). More recently, the term *early-onset scoliosis* has been used for spinal deformities in children under the age of 5 years, including both idiopathic, congenital, and neuromuscular curves, in order to acknowledge the special challenges of treating very young children with scoliosis.[8] Infantile neuromuscular scoliosis is frequently progressive, but if the curve is flexible it may be effectively managed with bracing and casting (Fig. 31.2).[9] Idiopathic infantile scoliosis is more common in males than females, and patients may present with a left-sided curve. Factors associated with progressive infantile idiopathic scoliosis include age at treatment, rib vertebral angle greater than 20 degrees, a phase II rib, or a curve greater than 60 degrees.[9-11]

Although the cause of idiopathic scoliosis is unknown, family members of affected patients have an increased risk of developing scoliosis, reflecting a genetic component to the disease.[12-14] Several genes have been associated with familial scoliosis.[15,16] The incidence of adolescent idiopathic scoliosis

(AIS) with a curvature greater than 30 degrees ranges from 1 to 3 in 1000 children.[17-23] Small curves are common in both males and females, although progression is more common in female children.

Natural history studies of scoliosis reveal the greatest morbidity from early-onset scoliosis, with higher mortality rates and decreased pulmonary function for thoracic curves.[24] One series of patients with untreated juvenile and adolescent scoliosis revealed only one death from cor pulmonale, and overall mortality rates similar to those for the average population.[6] Back pain could not be correlated with the severity of the deformity, although patients with lumbar curves had more back pain.[6] Patients with thoracic curves have been noted to have poor pulmonary function because of decreased lung volumes from the coronal plane deformity.[6,25] Thoracic curves measuring 70 degrees may result in noticeable changes on pulmonary function testing, and curves greater than 100 degrees may result in clinical symptoms.[24]

Curves are at risk for progression during periods of rapid skeletal growth, specifically the first 2 years of life and the adolescent growth spurt.[4] There is increased risk of curve progression for large curves and for skeletally immature patients (Table 31.1).[4] Bone age, peak height velocity, Risser sign, and elbow and hand maturity indices may aid in determining risk of curve progression.[26-30] Active investigation is under way to identify genetic markers that would assist in predicting curve progression.[31] For adolescent idiopathic scoliosis, thoracic and double curve patterns are at higher risk of progression than thoracolumbar curves.[4] Curves less than 30 degrees at skeletal maturity are thought to be mostly stable and unlikely to progress over time.[5,32] Curves greater than 50 degrees at skeletal maturity commonly progress at a rate of up to 1 degree per year for thoracic curves.[5,32] Curves between 35 and 50 degrees at skeletal maturity present a diagnostic dilemma due to insufficient clinical data and should be followed radiographically into adulthood.

Indications

Bracing and surgery are the mainstays of treatment for scoliosis. Treatment must be tailored to the patient and family. Bracing is typically indicated in growing children with progressive curves measuring 20 to 45 degrees.[33] In attempts to prevent curve progression, bracing is most effective in skeletally immature patients (Risser 0 or 1, 2) and in females who are less than 12 months past menarche.[33] Numerous types of braces have been described,[34-38] but a TLSO (thoracic lumbar spine orthosis) is commonly used.[33] Brace wear has been shown to be efficacious if the brace is worn.[39,40] The brace is discontinued at the completion of growth. Casting is well tolerated in the young child and may be a preferable technique over bracing owing to derotational molding of the deformity and improved compliance.[9,10] It has been shown to be curative in some cases of infantile scoliosis, although in some instances these curves are self-resolving.[9]

When the curve magnitude exceeds 50 degrees in AIS, surgical treatment is offered, typically with posterior spinal fusion. Fusion of smaller curves can be considered in skeletally immature patients who have been documented to have significant progression or in patients who find the appearance and trunk shift unacceptable. Pain is not typically an indication for

FIGURE 31.2 A, A 14-month-old child presenting with 70 degrees right thoracic curvature. **B,** Significant improvement in standing film in Mehta cast. Long-term results of this technique in large magnitude curves are unpredictable, although this serves as an effective delay tactic.

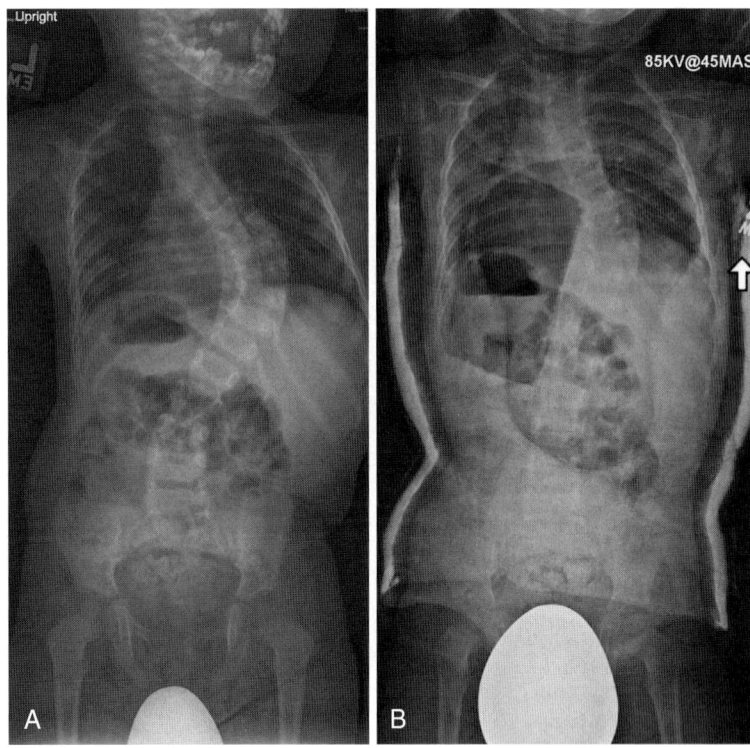

TABLE 31.1 Adolescent Idiopathic Scoliosis Treatment Algorithm

Growing Child

Open triradiate cartilage, Risser 0, 1, peak height velocity of 8-10 cm/year growth[42]
- Curves 5-19 degrees have a 22% chance of progression.[4]
- Curves 20-29 degrees have a 68% chance of progression.[4]

Curve Size*	Treatment	Follow-up Interval
≤25 degrees	Observation	4-6 months
25-45 degrees	Bracing (may consider in Risser 0 at 20-25 degrees with documented progression)	4 months
>45 degrees	Surgery—consider anterior release with open triradiate cartilage	

Adolescent Nearing Maturity

Closed triradiate, Risser 3-4, postmenarchal females
- Curves 5-19 degrees have a 2% chance of progression.
- Curves 20-29 degrees have a 23% chance of progression.

Curve Size*	Treatment	Follow-up Interval
≤30 degrees	Observation	12 months to document no progression
35-45 degrees	Consider bracing, efficacy not determined	4 months if braced 6-12 months otherwise
>50 degrees	Surgery	

Skeletally Mature Child

Risser 5, menarche + 2 years in females, cessation of growth[5,6]
- Large thoracic curves >50 degrees may progress up to 0.5-1 degree/year.[5,6]
- Lumbar curves >40 degrees may progress.[5]
- Curves <30 degrees are unlikely to progress.[5]

Curve Size*	Treatment	Follow-up Interval
≤50 degrees	Observation	1-2 years
>50 degrees	Surgery	

*Measurement variability for Cobb angle is reported at ±5-6 degrees.[75,76]

Note: Superscript numbers refer to references for this chapter, listed online.

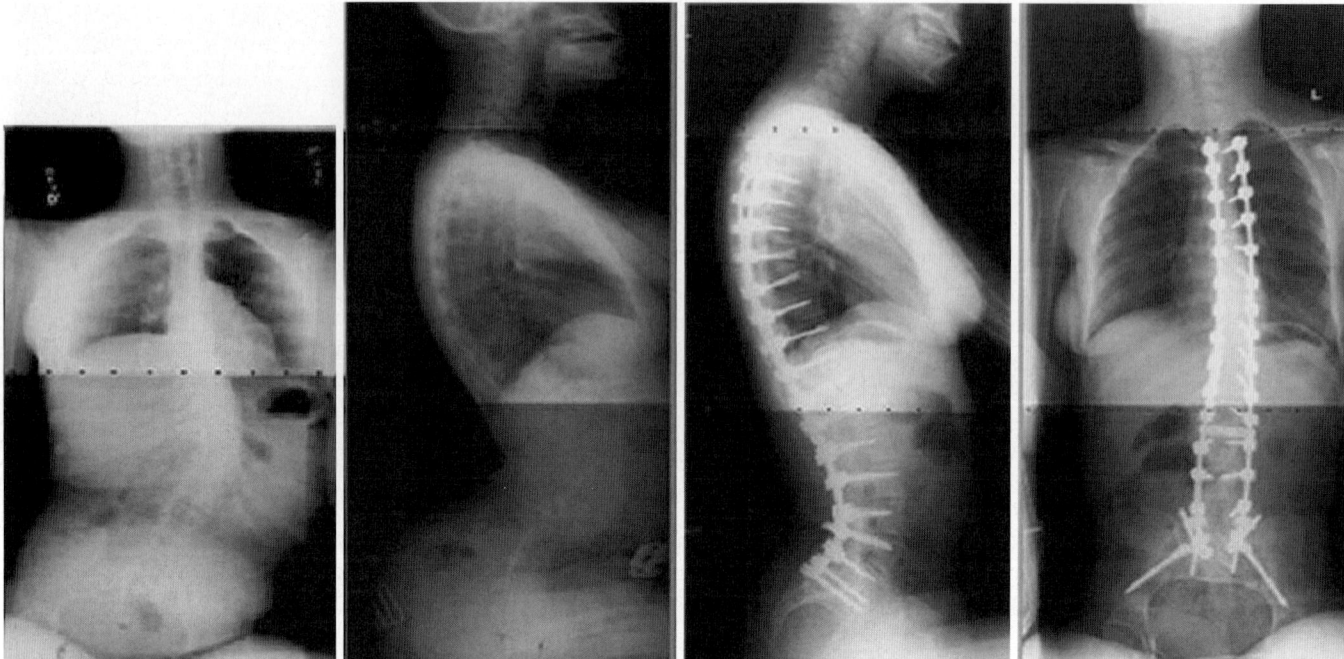

FIGURE 31.3 Patient with neuromuscular scoliosis preoperatively and following posterior spinal fusion from T3 to the sacrum with pedicle screw instrumentation.

surgery. Patients with severe deformity or who are skeletally immature (open triradiate cartilages) may also be treated with anterior release or posterior fusion to improve correction and prevent subsequent rotational and coronal or "crankshaft" deformity.[41-44] In the era of pedicle screw fixation, the necessity of anterior procedures is debated in the literature and may be a matter of surgeon preference.[45] Anterior release, fusion, and instrumentation in the thoracic spine may be performed through a thoracotomy or through a thoracoscopic approach.[46,47] Anterior procedures, particularly open surgery, may result in decreased pulmonary function.[46-48] Large curves and complex deformities can also be addressed by osteotomies through a posterior approach to achieve satisfactory correction. These procedures may include, in order of increased correction and neurological risk, Ponte/Smith-Peterson osteotomies, pedicle subtraction osteotomies, and vertebral column resections.[49-51]

Neuromuscular scoliosis is guided by similar treatment principles. Progressive imbalance from muscle weakness or spasticity may result in a sweeping thoracolumbar or C-type curvature and subsequent pelvic obliquity, truncal shift, and difficulty with wheelchair seating and caregiving.[52,53] The role of bracing in the neuromuscular population is not well defined, but may be a helpful delay tactic. Custom wheelchair seating systems can also serve as an external brace in many instances. Surgical management is indicated when bracing or wheelchair positioning can no longer accommodate the patient's deformity and the curve progresses to greater than 50 degrees (Fig. 31.3).[52] Smaller curves may continue to progress in adult patients with neuromuscular scoliosis, although curves greater than 50 degrees increase at a faster rate.[54] Patients with underlying cardiac or pulmonary deficits as classically seen in Duchenne muscular dystrophy may benefit from early surgery performed for smaller magnitude curves rather than waiting for the curve to progress while the patient's medical

status deteriorates.[55] New corticosteroid treatment protocols for Duchenne muscular dystrophy may redefine these indications.[56] Surgical treatment of nonambulatory patients typically involves fusion from the upper thoracic spine to the pelvis, although recent literature has shown improved mobility in paraplegic children fused to L5. Long-term results from this technique are not established. In ambulatory patients with an underlying neuromuscular condition, longer fusions are typically indicated to avoid subsequent decompensation.

Early-onset scoliosis has unique considerations. Thoracic fusion in a small child is unacceptable and may later lead to thoracic insufficiency syndrome and significant shortening of the trunk. Delay tactics include casting, bracing, and halo gravity traction.[9] When curves do not respond to these measures, surgical intervention may be undertaken to prevent curve progression and allow for spinal growth.[57,58] Several growing spine systems are in use, including growing spine-based and rib-based devices.[57,59-62] There is limited consensus as to the indications and applications of these devices. These are seen as a last resort because the child is then committed to twice yearly lengthening procedures and a high rate of complications, including infection, wound problems, early unintended fusion, implant failure, and rarely neurological complications.[57] A planned definitive fusion is performed at the completion of the lengthening procedures. For growing rods, a dual-rod construct has been shown to have fewer complications and improved correction, although a single rod can be used in conjunction with a brace.[60,63] The implants are frequently quite prominent. Prior to initiating surgical treatment, nutritional and medical status must be optimized. Large curves result in increased work of breathing and energy expenditure. Thus, children with significant deformity are often malnourished and require dietary supplementation and in many instances gastrostomy tube placement to improve soft tissue coverage and reduce wound complications.

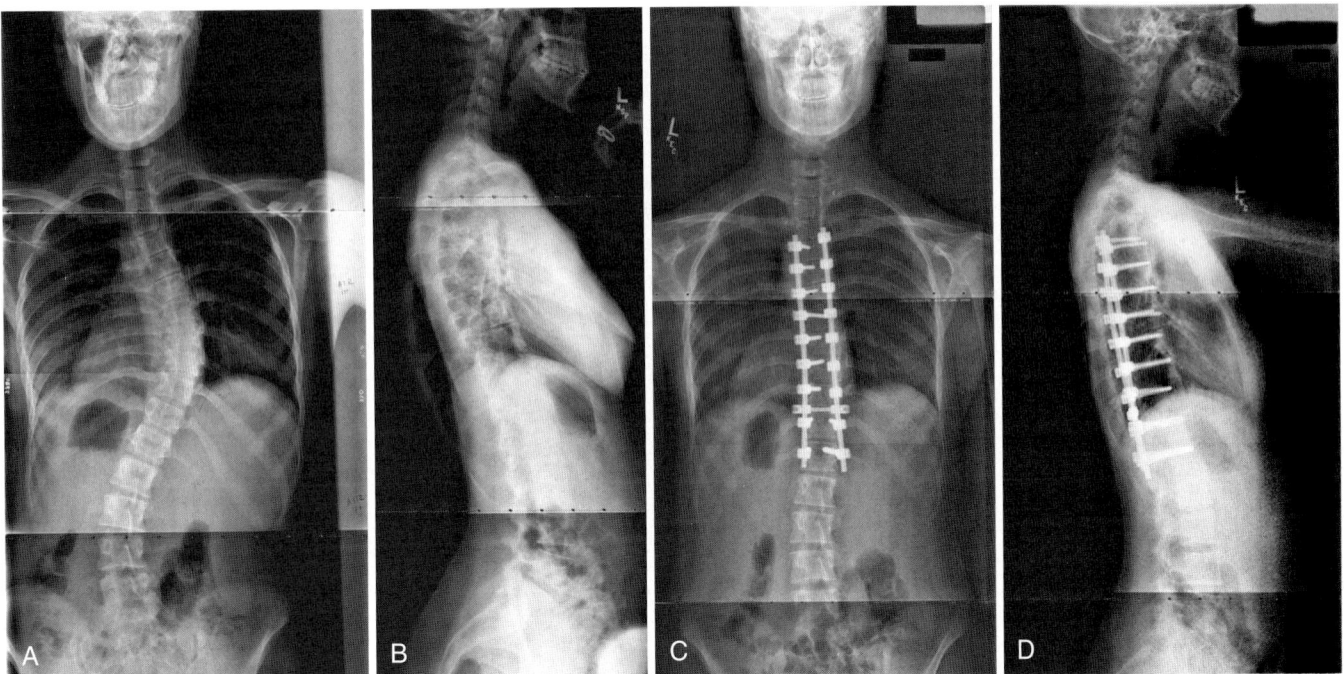

FIGURE 31.4 A, Posteroanterior (PA) standing scoliosis film in a patient with adolescent idiopathic scoliosis. **B,** Lateral spine film reveals hypokyphosis over the region of the curvature. **C,** Postoperative PA and, **D,** lateral views following pedicle screw fixation.

Diagnosis

Scoliosis is typically painless in the pediatric population, and children for the most part are asymptomatic. Mild back pain, however, is not uncommon. Screening examinations by pediatricians or school nurses frequently result in referrals. Parents may notice shoulder, scapula, or waist asymmetry, particularly if they are attuned to the diagnosis by a family history of scoliosis.

All patients with presumed idiopathic scoliosis should be evaluated with a medical history, complete neurological examination, and radiographs. A family history should be taken for scoliosis or a history of underlying neurological abnormalities. Females should be asked about age at menarche, because this landmark is an excellent predictor of skeletal maturity. On physical examination, the patient's back should be carefully examined for asymmetry, trunk shift, and sagittal plane alignment. AIS is balanced in the coronal plane and typically hypokyphotic, so the presence of kyphosis or excessive truncal shift is an indication for axial imaging[64] (Fig. 31.4). Asymmetrical abdominal reflexes may be associated with a neural axis abnormality.[65] The Adams' forward bend test may reveal a thoracic or lumbar rib prominence resulting from rotational deformity. The pelvis should be assessed for an occult leg-length discrepancy, which may give the appearance of scoliosis. The skin should be examined for masses, café au lait patches, and axillary or inguinal freckling indicative of neurofibromatosis. A hairy patch, dimple, or pigmentation over the lumbosacral region suggests spinal dysraphism. The patient should be examined for excess ligamentous laxity or pectus deformity, raising the possibility of an underlying syndrome.

Neural axis abnormalities are found in 13% to 26% of patients with juvenile scoliosis and 2.6% to 14% of patients with adolescent-onset scoliosis.[65-67] Up to 50% of patients with a left thoracic rather than right thoracic curve may have an underlying neural axis abnormality.[67-69] As many as 20% to 50% of children with infantile scoliosis may have an underlying neural axis abnormality.[67,70] No difference in treatment outcome has been reported based on the presence of a neurological abnormality, although a large syrinx, tethered cord, or Chiari malformation may require surgical intervention (Fig. 31.5).[69] In some instances, scoliosis may improve after treatment of the neural axis abnormality, but this is not predictable.

Standing posteroanterior (PA) and lateral spine images should include the neck, clavicles, and pelvis. A lateral image should be taken at presentation in order to document the sagittal plane alignment and rule out congenital deformity. Subsequently, the curve can be followed by standing PA imaging unless there is a concern for kyphoscoliosis.

The idiopathic scoliosis curve types have been classified by King and associates[71] and more recently by Lenke and colleagues (Fig. 31.6).[72] These classifications assist in choosing fusion levels and help identify idiopathic curve types for research purposes. With the Lenke classification, premeasured radiographs have high inter- and intrarater reliability,[72,73] although there is only poor to good interobserver reliability on unmeasured radiographs.[73,74] Cobb angle measurement error among different observers is 5 to 6 degrees; thus, more than 5 degrees increase in curve size is necessary in order to document curve progression.[75,76] Digital imaging systems may improve measurement accuracy.[75,76] Children who may be candidates for treatment should be followed with radiographs several times annually during periods of rapid growth.

Evidence-Based Medicine

Treatment for scoliosis includes observation, bracing or casting, and surgery. There are no studies that support the use of activity modification, manipulation, exercises, physical

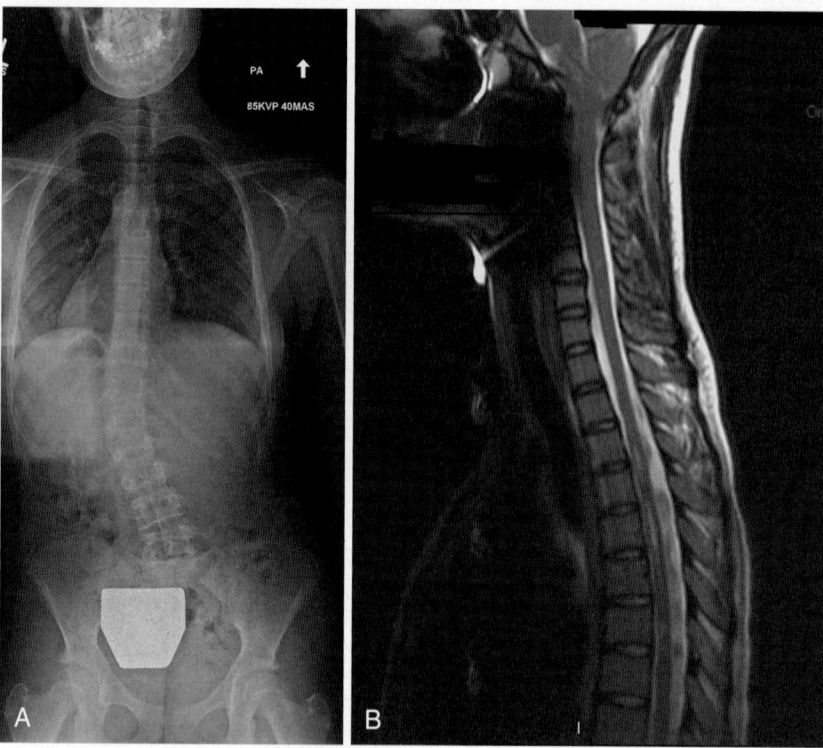

FIGURE 31.5 Scoliosis with a syrinx. **A,** Postero-anterior (PA) scoliosis film of a female patient presenting with deformity, back pain, and headaches. **B,** Magnetic resonance (MR) image of the spine reveals a syrinx and Chiari malformation.

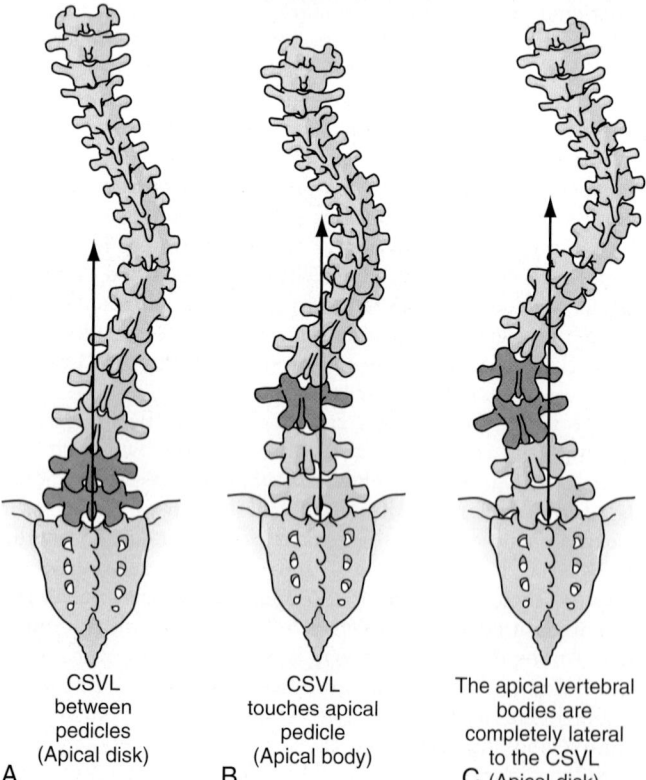

| CSVL between pedicles (Apical disk) | CSVL touches apical pedicle (Apical body) | The apical vertebral bodies are completely lateral to the CSVL |
| A | B | C (Apical disk) |

FIGURE 31.6 Lumbar modifier for the Lenke classification. The lumbar modifier is determined by the relationship of the pedicles in the lumbar curve to the central sacral vertebral line (CSVL).

therapy, or electrical stimulation for the correction of scoliosis.[77-80] Casting has been shown to be efficacious for infantile curves at high risk of progression. Braces, if worn consistently, may prevent curve progression.[39,40]

Surgical treatment is undertaken to prevent further curve progression, but has the added benefit of deformity correction. The importance of specific correction objectives are debated among surgeons and include coronal plane correction, restoration of thoracic kyphosis and lumbar lordosis, sagittal balance, and vertebral derotation.[81] Beginning with Harrington rods, a variety of implants have been used including hooks, wires, and screws.[82] Pedicle screws are now the gold standard due to no violation of the canal, superior rotational and curve correction, resulting improvements in pulmonary function tests (PFTs).[82-85] Pedicle screws can be placed using anatomical, fluoroscopic, or computed tomography (CT)-guided navigation.[86] The role of intraoperative CT is under development, but may be of great assistance in complex deformity and congenital cases when the anatomical landmarks are unreliable. Posterior spinal fusion for scoliosis results in improved patient perception of appearance and improved functional outcome scores. Long fusions limit spine motion and have the theoretical risk of increased stress and degenerative changes at adjacent motion segments.[87]

Selection of fusion level and density of implants is subject to significant variability in practice and is beyond the scope of this text.[71,88,89] Definitions of the end, neutral, and stable vertebrae may aid in selection of fusion levels (Fig. 31.7). Occasionally, levels can be preserved in thoracolumbar curves by using an anterior versus posterior approach. Bracing or casting is not routinely recommended postoperatively because new fixation techniques are quite sturdy and reliable.

Complications can be limited by diligent preoperative planning and clear communication with the medical and anesthesiology teams. The complication rates for posterior

ADOLESCENT IDIOPATHIC SCOLIOSIS
End, neutral, and stable vertebrae

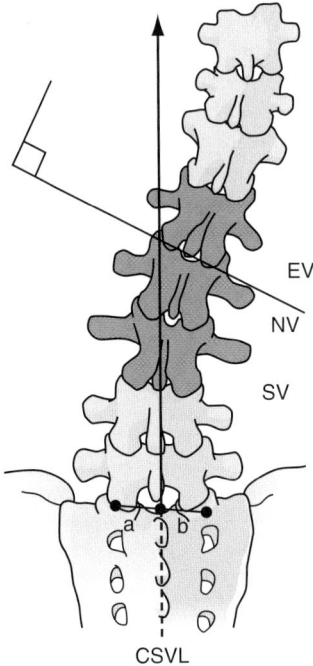

FIGURE 31.7 End, neutral, and stable vertebrae. The end vertebrae (EV) are the most tilted vertebrae, which are selected for measurement of the Cobb angle. The neutral vertebra is the most cephalad vertebral body below the end vertebra with no rotation (pedicles appear symmetrical). The stable vertebra (SV) is the most cephalad vertebral body below the end vertebra which is bisected by the central sacral vertebral line (CSVL).

spinal fusion is reported at 5% to 15% for idiopathic scoliosis patients[90-92] and 28% to 33% for neuromuscular scoliosis patients.[93,94] Higher complication rates are associated with prolonged surgical and anesthetic time, increased blood loss, hybrid constructs, and renal disease.[90,92] Growing spine patients face a 48% complication rate.[60] All patients should have blood products available. Tranexamic acid may help reduce blood loss.[95] Thoracic surgery should be performed with intraoperative somatosensory evoked potentials (SSEPs) and motor evoked potentials (MEPs) in collaboration with a neuromonitoring team and neurologist.[96] These tests require special anesthetic techniques such as total intravenous anesthesia. The Stagnara wakeup test can be used in instances when signals cannot be obtained in the patient and serves as a secondary method to assess neurological function intraoperatively. From an anesthesia standpoint, significant lead time may be required. The airway should be carefully protected, and the wound should be filled with saline to prevent pulmonary air embolus from deep inspiration at the time of the wakeup test. Forceful injection of thrombin products into the pedicle tract has been reported to cause neurological injury and should be avoided.[97] Neurological deficit can present in a delayed fashion postoperatively, likely due to vascular effects on the spinal cord.[98] Cases with osteotomies, high blood loss, and preoperative kyphosis or myelopathy are at greater risk of neurological complication. Thus, for high-risk procedures, careful postoperative monitoring, maintenance of blood pressure with fluid or in some instances with pressors, and adequate maintenance of hemoglobin should be ensured.

Conclusion

Scoliosis is the most common spinal deformity in the pediatric population. Advances in instrumentation and monitoring have rendered posterior spinal fusion a safe, reliable treatment to provide deformity correction and prevent curve progression in adulthood. Further work is ongoing about the role of intraoperative imaging. Early-onset scoliosis is a field with a wide variety of treatment techniques and limited consensus on the optimal surgical indications or implants. Although significant progress has been made in the treatment of scoliosis, much work remains to be done, both to better understand the cause of scoliosis and to improve the surgical treatment of the disorder.

PART II. ADULT SPINAL DEFORMITY: CONSIDERATIONS IN EVALUATION AND TREATMENT

Spinal deformity in the adult is increasingly recognized as a significant health care issue. With an aging population there are also increasing functional expectations of an older population in Western societies. The costs of caring for the elderly who lose autonomy due to spine deformity are substantial. Pain and disability are closely associated with spinal deformity in the adult population. One prevalence study[99] reports a 60% rate of spine deformity in a population over 60 years of age.

The treatment of adult spinal deformity (ASD) has received rather sparse attention compared to deformity in the pediatric population. Despite the large number of adults affected by spine deformities and the high potential for marked loss of function,[100] adult deformity remains poorly understood. Progress in research is hampered by the diversity of disorders associated with spinal deformity in the adult, the lack of a coherent system for classifying patients, and until recently, poorly understood correlations between deformity parameters and patient-reported disability.

This section of the chapter will summarize the efforts to date that have determined important correlations between health-related quality of life (HRQOL) measures and radiographic parameters as well as outline classification approaches and alignment guidelines related to ASD. The current state of the art will be presented as well as ongoing work that is certain to impact our management of the often complex situation in adult patients affected by a spinal deformity.

Key Radiographic Parameters and Health-Related Quality of Life

Although ASD has a wide range of causes, most cases appear to relate to the degenerative process of aging (de novo degenerative spinal deformity, or DDS) or adolescent scoliosis in an adult (ASA).[101] Other causes of deformity include osteoporosis, trauma, infection, and iatrogenic factors. For DDS and ASA, the two largest categories, a common pathway appears to lead to pain and loss of function.

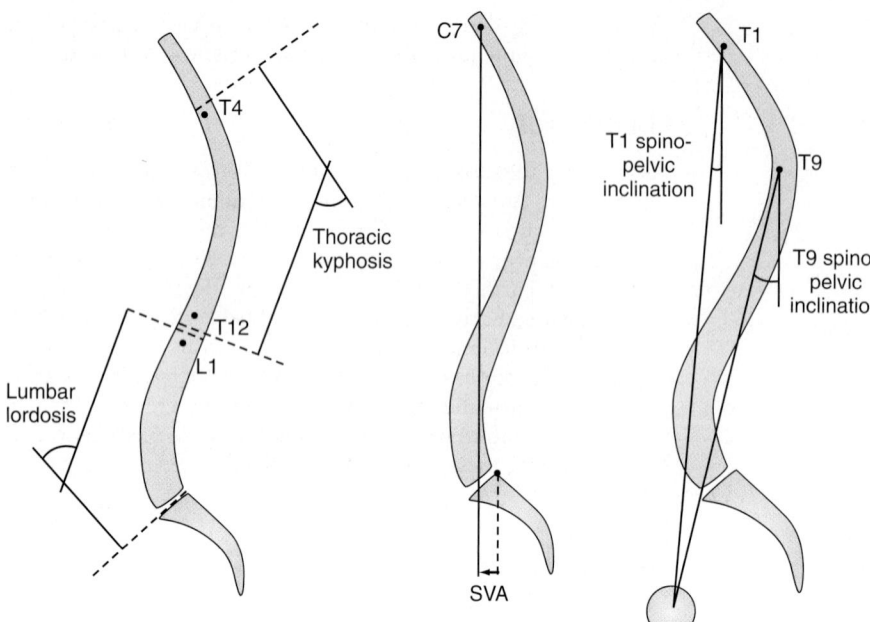

FIGURE 31.8 Sagittal spinal radiological parameters. *Thoracic kyphosis* is measured from the superior end plate of T4 to the inferior end plate of T12. *Lumbar lordosis* is measured from the superior end plate of L1 to the superior end plate of S1. *Sagittal vertical axis* (SVA) is defined as the horizontal offset from the posterosuperior corner of S1 to the vertebral body of C7. *T1 spinal-pelvic inclination and T9 spinal-pelvic inclination* are defined as the angle between the vertical plumbline and the line drawn from the vertebral body center of T1 or T9 and the center of the bicoxofemoral axis.

Many clinicians have investigated the regional and global alignment in the normal (asymptomatic) adult population[102-108] (Fig. 31.8). These data are helpful in understanding normative ranges but offer limited value in understanding disability related to ASD. However, a study by the Spinal Deformity Study Group (SDSG),[109] including 947 adults with spinal deformity, set out to answer this key question. Data from their multicenter prospective database were analyzed for HRQOL/radiographic correlation. All patients had radiographic analysis: frontal Cobb angle, deformity apex, lumbar lordosis, intervertebral subluxation. Health assessment included the Oswestry Disability Index (ODI) and Scoliosis Research Society instrument (SRS). Patients were classified by deformity apex, lordosis (T12-S1), and intervertebral subluxation. The correlation analysis revealed that HRQOL was driven by several key parameters (in the following order): global sagittal alignment (sagittal vertical axis, SVA), loss of lumbar lordosis (LL), intervertebral subluxation. This data set did not include pelvic parameters, which subsequently emerged as being critical to understanding ASD. In a recent investigation by Lafage and co-workers[110] radiographic pelvic parameters were established as an integral component in patient-reported function in the setting of spinal deformity.

Several authors have described the pelvis as a regulator of the sagittal plane alignment, and extensive studies have been conducted to understand the relationship between pelvic parameters and spinal alignment. Radiographic parameters of pelvic alignment (Fig. 31.9) have now emerged as essential components of the global standing alignment,[108,111-114] and their clinical relevance is briefly summarized here:

- *Pelvic tilt* (PT) is defined by the angle between the vertical and the line through the midpoint of the sacral plate to the femoral head axis; it is commonly reported as a compensatory mechanism: when the spine tilts forward (age-related change, sagittal imbalance, loss of lordosis, increase of kyphosis) the subject will try his or her best to maintain an economic posture and to keep the spine as vertical as possible (i.e., bring the spine over the pelvis).

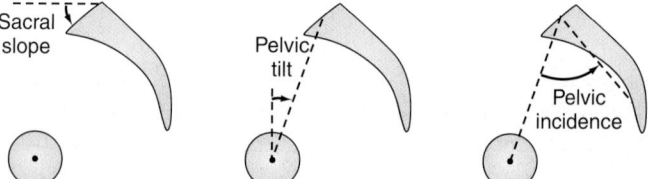

FIGURE 31.9 Pelvic parameters. *Pelvic tilt* is defined by the angle between the vertical and the line through the midpoint of the sacral plate to the femoral head axis (retroversion is then measured as a pelvic tilt increase, anteversion as a pelvic tilt decrease). *Sacral slope* is defined as the angle between the horizontal and the sacral plate. *Pelvic incidence* is defined as the angle between the perpendicular to the sacral plate at its midpoint and the line connecting this point to the femoral head axis. Pelvic incidence = Pelvic tilt + Sacral slope.

One way to maintain this spinal-pelvic alignment is to retrovert the pelvis (increase of pelvic tilt), which may be seen as a backward rotation of the pelvis around the hips.
- *Pelvic incidence* (PI) is defined as the angle between the perpendicular line to the sacral plate at its midpoint and the line connecting this point to the femoral head axis. This is a morphological parameter of primary importance because of its correlation with ideal lumbar lordosis. In a simplified formula lumbar lordosis should be within 9 degrees of PI (LL = PI ± 9) degrees.
- *Sacral slope* (SS) is defined as the angle between the horizontal and the sacral plate; this last parameter completes the geometric relationship where PI = PT + SS. Normative values and age-related changes of the pelvic parameters are provided (Table 31.2).

Classification

To date, plain x-ray films remain the basis for diagnostic approaches to many orthopedic disorders. Although newer imaging modalities have emerged, substantial variation in interpretation of information related to spinal diseases exist.

TABLE 31.2 Normative Values for Radiographic Sagittal Key Parameters

Parameter	NORMATIVE VALUES REPORTED IN DIFFERENT SERIES					
	Schwab et al., 2006[108]	Berthonnaud et al., 2005[103]	Vialle et al., 2005[114]	Legaye et al., 1998[112]	Boulay et al., 2006[118]	Roussouly et al., 2006[113]
No. of subjects	75	160	300	49	149	153
Age	49.3 yr (18-80)	25.7 ± 5.5 yr (20-70)	35 yr (20-70)	24.0 ± 5.8 yr (19-50)	30.8 ± 6.0 yr (19-50)	27 yr (18-48)
M:F ratio	0.56	0.95	0.63	0.56	0.52	0.52
SVA	-20 ± 30	—	—	—	—	35.2 ± 19.4 (-18.1-80.8)
T1 SPI	—	—	-1.4 ± 2.7 (-9.2-7.1)	—	—	—
TK (T4-12)	41 ± 12	47.5 ± 4.8 (22.5-70.3)	40.6 ± 10.0 (0-69)	~43.0 ± 13.0	53.8 ± 10.1 (33.2-83.5)	46.3 ± 9.5 (23.0-65.9)
LL (L1-S1)	60 ± 12	42.7 ± 5.4 (16-71.9)	60.2 ± 10.3 (30-89)	~60.0 ± 10.0	66.4 ± 9.5 (44.8-87.2)	61.2 ± 9.4 (39.9-83.7)
PI	52 ± 10	51 ± 5.3 (33.7-83.7)	54.7 ± 10.6 (33-82)	~52.0 ± 10.0	53.1 ± 9.0 (33.7-77.5)	50.6 ± 10.2 (27.9-82.8)
PT	15 ± 7	12.1 ± 3.2 (-5.1-30.5)	13.2 ± 6.1 (-4.5-27)	~11.0 ± 5.5	12.0 ± 6.4 (-2-30)	11.1 ± 5.9 (-2.8-23.7)
SS	30 ± 9	39.7 ± 4.1 (21.2-65.9)	41.2 ± 8.4 (17-63)	~40.0 ± 8.5	41.2 ± 7.0 (0.6-19.7)	39.6 ± 7.6 (17.5-63.4)

LL, lumbar lordosis; M:F, male-to-female; PI, pelvic incidence; PT, pelvic tilt; SS, sacral slope; SVA, sagittal vertical axis; T1 SPI, T1 spinal-pelvic inclination; TK, thoracic kyphosis.

Note: Studies cited in column heads are listed in the online references for this chapter.

In terms of establishing a classification of adult deformity it may be ideal to base this principally on x-ray image information to remain simple in form and reliable in application.

Given that treatment for adults with deformity is driven by the patient who wishes to regain function without pain, a classification of adults must take this as a basis upon which to build categories. It is not reasonable to transpose classification efforts applied to AIS because the treatment concerns are of a very different nature. Pain and disability are rarely noted in AIS.

A significant advance in the classification of scoliotic deformity is attributed to Lenke and colleagues.[72] In a 2001 publication, this classification offered an updated approach to AIS which was more comprehensive than the King classification[71] and offered sagittal plane consideration. Furthermore, the new AIS classification offered guidelines on surgical fusion levels using segmental fixation.

The classification of adult scoliosis[115] is clearly more complex than approaches to AIS. Adult deformity covers a broad range of segmental, regional, and global expression (Fig. 31.10). The treatment is driven by disability and pain and not simply by radiographic appearance. The latter has thus made it difficult to arrive at a clinically relevant x-ray classification. One of the first studies aimed at isolating the pain generator in adult scoliosis was published in 2002.[116] This work by Schwab and associates launched an ongoing effort at reconciling HRQOL measures and radiographic presentation of adult deformity. The approach has led to the Schwab-SDSG classification of which the basic structure hinges on the following:

- Basic coronal curve locations and basic patterns (single vs. multiple)
- A principally sagittal plane deformity category
- Regional and global modifiers with three grades tied to HRQOL

All aspects of the classification found a basis in HRQOL analysis. The cutoffs between groups within each modifier were determined by the HRQOL measures, splitting the population into discrete groups by clinical impact of each modifier parameter. Description of the classification is summarized in Table 31.3.

Alignment Goals When Treating Adult Spinal Deformity

Spinal-pelvic realignment is a complex undertaking. Other than decompression and stabilization of spinal segments (which is beyond the scope of this chapter) realignment of the sagittal spinal-pelvic axis is of primary importance during surgical treatment of symptomatic ASD. As outlined previously, normative data from an asymptomatic population may provide insight into ranges for regional and global alignment during standing posture. However, for optimal clinical outcomes, treatment should be adapted to a given individual based upon specific realignment needs.

Tailoring patient-specific treatment involves the crucial PI-LL relationship, wherein ideal lumbar lordosis is proportional to pelvic morphology quantified as pelvic incidence (PI). Additionally, alignment parameters driving pain and disability, namely, sagittal vertical axis (SVA) and PT, need to be addressed. The surgical method of realignment (i.e., pedicle subtraction osteotomy versus a Smith Peterson osteotomy, intervertebral spacer, rod contouring) remains of secondary importance to the primary goal: obtaining surgical realignment objectives. As a general concept and pragmatic tool for clinical application, spinal-pelvic realignment objectives involve attention to the following three key parameters[117] (Fig. 31.11):

- SVA: Global spinal realignment should attempt to obtain a postoperative SVA less than 50 mm. Restoration of SVA

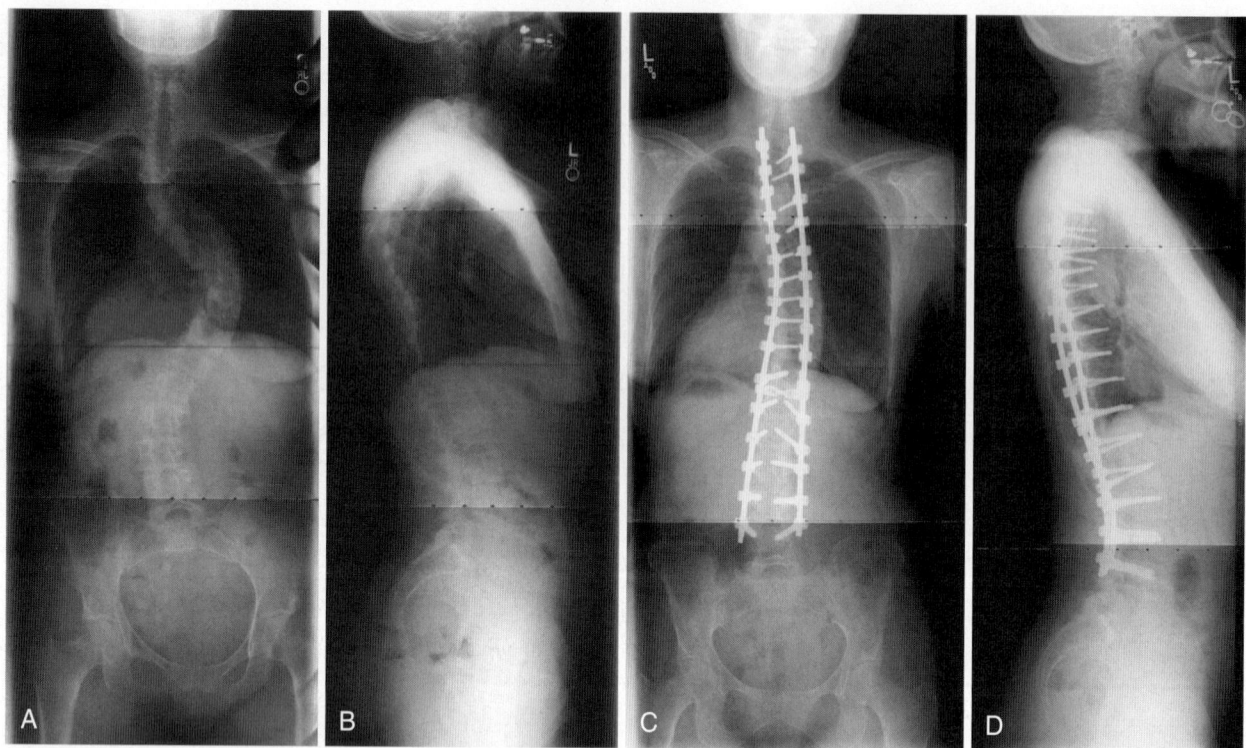

FIGURE 31.10 Adult scoliosis. Preoperative PA (**A, B**) and lateral views (**C, D**) show both coronal and sagittal plane deformity.

TABLE 31.3	Schwab-SDSG Adult Spinal Deformity Classification
Type	**Location of Deformity***
Type I	Thoracic-only scoliosis (no thoracolumbar or lumbar component)
Type II	Upper thoracic major, apex T4-8 (with thoracolumbar or lumbar curve)
Type III	Lower thoracic major, apex T9-T10 (with thoracolumbar/lumbar curve)
Type IV	Thoracolumbar major curve, apex T11-L1 (with any other minor curve)
Type V	Lumbar major curve, apex L2-L4 (with any other minor curve)
Type K	Deformity in the sagittal plane only
Lordosis Modifier	**Sagittal Cobb Angle: T12 to S1**
A	Marked lordosis >40 degrees
B	Moderate lordosis 0-40 degrees
C	No lordosis present <0 degrees
Subluxation Modifier	**Maximum Value: Frontal or Sagittal Plane (Anterior or Posterior)**
0	No subluxation
+	Subluxation 1-6 mm
++	Subluxation >7 mm
Global Balance Modifier†	**C7 Offset From Posterior Superior Corner of S1: Sagittal Plane**
N	0-4 cm
P	4-9.5 cm
VP	>9.5 cm

*Apical level of the major curve *or* sagittal plane only.
†N, normal; P, positive; VP, very positive.
SDSG, Spinal Deformity Study Group.

facilitates level gaze and achievement of a physiological standing posture. An SVA less than 50 mm brings the plumbline behind the femoral heads to relieve the complaint of "falling forward." Clinically, this threshold has been met with better HRQOL scores. Similarly, the reference T1 – SPI < 0 degrees may be used. Both parameters outline the same principle.

- **PT:** Pelvic realignment should attempt to obtain a postoperative PT less than 25 degrees. Attention to PT, as outlined by clinical data, is necessary to obtain optimal outcomes. Additionally, PT realignment restores appropriate femoral-pelvic-spinal alignment required during efficient ambulation (need an extension reserve to clear the step). Realignment of the SVA less than 50 mm in the setting of an elevated PT means the ASD patient is still compensating for residual structural spinal deformity. This parameter independently has been shown to correlate to impairment in walking tolerance and therefore should be realigned appropriately.
- **LL = PI ± 9 degrees:** Finally, to achieve patient-specific alignment treatment LL = PI ± 9 degrees may pragmatically be used. Increasing the angulation of the hypolordotic spine to match the patient's spinal-pelvic morphological type (i.e., PI) assures appropriate lordotic alignment. This chain of correlation has been extensively studied by many authors.[108,111,118,119] as it relates to the subject's morphological type.[113]

Predicting Outcome Related to Surgery for Adult Spinal Deformity

In building predictive models of outcome from surgery it is key to identify what combination of patient characteristics (including Schwab classification modifiers) and treatment options can be used to predict which patients will meet an outcome threshold for success.[120] Previous work by the SDSG on

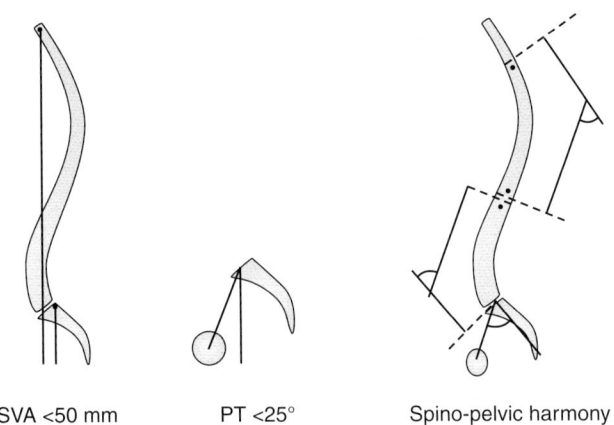

SVA <50 mm   PT <25°   Spino-pelvic harmony
                                      LL = PI ± 9°

FIGURE 31.11 Realignment objectives in the sagittal plane. SVA <50 mm, PT <25 degrees, and LL = PI ± 9 degrees sets the stage for achievement of a successful harmonious spinal-pelvic realignment. LL, lumbar lordosis; PI, pelvic incidence; PT, pelvic tilt; SVA, sagittal vertical axis.

TABLE 31.4 Strength of Predictive Models[1] Meeting MCID Threshold[2]*

Outcome Score[1]	% Correct Classification by Model	Area Under ROC Curve
SRS pain	81.10%	0.864
SRS appearance	75.40%	0.838
SRS pain and appearance	78.10%	0.845
SF-12v2 PCS	77.90%	0.862

*0.80 and above is considered good discrimination.

MCID, minimal clinically important difference; SF-12v2 PCS, Medical Outcomes Study, short-form, version 2, physical component summary; ROC, receiver operating characteristic; SRS, Scoliosis Research Society.[1,2]

TABLE 31.5 Summary of Post–Scoliosis Surgery Treatment Groups Likely to Reach MCID (Success) or Unlikely to Do So (Poor Outcome)

	Groups Less Likely to Reach Threshold Improvement	Groups With Higher Chance of Reaching Threshold Improvement
SF-12v2 PCS MCID summary	Apical level III Marked lordosis No subluxation Negative sagittal balance Baseline PCS ≥35	Apical level IV Subluxation + or ++ Positive sagittal balance Surgery involved osteotomy Surgery involved fixation to sacrum Baseline PCS <35
SRS combined pain/appearance MCID summary	Apical level III Marked lordosis No subluxation Negative sagittal balance	No lordosis Subluxation ++ Circumferential surgery Surgery involved osteotomy
SRS pain MCID summary	Apical level III Marked lordosis No subluxation Negative sagittal balance Posterior-only surgical approach No fixation to the sacrum	Apical level IV Subluxation ++ Circumferential surgery Surgery involved osteotomy Baseline PCS <35
SRS appearance MCID summary	Apical level V Surgery involved fixation to sacrum	No previous surgery Apical level IV Baseline PCS ≥35

MCID, minimal clinically important difference; SF-12v2 PCS, Medical Outcomes Study, short-form, version 2, physical component summary; SRS, Scoliosis Research Society.

minimal clinically important difference (MCID) has identified improvement thresholds for discriminating between patients who report being satisfied with surgical results and those who report being less than satisfied. Based upon those identified thresholds, binary logistic regression was used to examine how adult classification types and surgical strategy combine and interact to predict successful surgical outcomes. A second approach was to employ multiple linear regressions. For both binary and logistic regression, predictor variables included all classification types, all treatment options within surgery, patient age, gender, BMI (body mass index), previous surgery, and baseline health status. Backward and stepwise techniques were used to eliminate redundant predictor variables.

An analysis of patients most and least likely to reach an MCID can be drawn from the predictive models. It was found that in addition to the classification modifiers, baseline HRQOL was associated with higher chance of a poor outcome (Tables 31.4 and 31.5).

Conclusion

Adult spinal deformity is emerging as an important health care issue of the twenty-first century. This is due in part to increased awareness of its clinical impact, as well as the aging population in Western societies combined with functional expectations. Correction of sagittal plane balance is essential to obtaining satisfactory results in treatment.

SELECTED KEY REFERENCES

Danielsson AJ, Nachemson AL. Back pain and function 23 years after fusion for adolescent idiopathic scoliosis: a case-control study-part II. *Spine.* 2003;28(18):E373-383.

Lenke LG, Betz RR, Harms J, et al. Adolescent idiopathic scoliosis: a new classification to determine extent of spinal arthrodesis. *J Bone Joint Surg Am.* 2001;83-A(8):1169-1181.

Lenke LG, Kuklo TR, Ondra S, Polly Jr DW. Rationale behind the current state-of-the-art treatment of scoliosis (in the pedicle screw era). *Spine.* 2008;33(10):1051-1054.

Lonstein JE, Carlson JM. The prediction of curve progression in untreated idiopathic scoliosis during growth. *J Bone Joint Surg Am.* 1984;66(7):1061-1071.

Schwab F, Farcy JP, Bridwell K, et al. A clinical impact classification of scoliosis in the adult. *Spine.* 2006;31(18):2109-2114.

Weinstein SL, Ponseti IV. Curve progression in idiopathic scoliosis. *J Bone Joint Surg Am.* 1983;65(4):447-455.

Please go to expertconsult.com to view the complete list of references.

CHAPTER 32

Acute Nerve Injuries

Lynda J-S Yang

CLINICAL PEARLS

- Efficient identification of the injured nerve(s) and characterization of the nature and severity of injury facilitate the optimal evaluation and treatment of acute peripheral nerve injuries: obtaining a pertinent history and performing a directed physical examination are paramount. Each peripheral nerve is composed of fibers from more than one spinal nerve root; correspondingly, each spinal nerve contributes fibers to more than one peripheral nerve. Consequently, whereas spinal nerve lesions manifest in the clinical picture of radiculopathies with dermatomal sensory disturbances and mild to moderate weakness of muscles supplied by the spinal nerve, peripheral nerve lesions manifest in more precise borders of sensory disturbances acutely and more severe atrophy and paresis of muscles supplied solely by the peripheral nerve as time elapses.

- Use of electrodiagnostic and radiographic studies can augment the clinical evaluation when performed at the appropriate time and for specific indications. For example, the presence of intraoperative nerve action potentials (NAPs) across an involved segment implies that neurolysis alone is adequate for neural recovery.

- A preganglionic injury implies injury proximal to the dorsal root ganglion with permanent paralysis of the muscles innervated by the avulsed roots, complete sensory loss of the corresponding dermatomes, and most importantly, the preclusion of spontaneous recovery. A postganglionic injury potentially retains function of the cell body within the ventral horn of the spinal cord, and these neurons may regenerate axons in the appropriate conditions.

- Surgical options for nerve repair/reconstruction include neurolysis, nerve repair with and without graft, and nerve transfers. Direct (end-to-end) repair is possible only if a short nerve gap exists after resection of the nonfunctioning neural segment. Direct repair is preferred over indirect (graft) repair because of better functional results. Tension across the repair must be avoided to reduce the risk of failure of functional regeneration.

- Management of patient expectations is critical because recovery after nerve injury can take months to years. Nerve repair/reconstruction can be augmented with muscle/tendon transfers to maximize functional outcome.

Acute peripheral nerve injury may result from penetrating trauma, blunt trauma, compression, electrical and iatrogenic causes. The peripheral nerve is severed sharply in 30% of soft tissue lacerations,[1] or it can remain grossly in continuity but with varying degrees of intraneural trauma from contusion and stretch. In 15% of nerve injuries associated with a potentially transecting mechanism, the peripheral nerve is only partially severed.[2] Despite appearances, the injured peripheral nerve ultimately manifests in sensory and motor disturbances. The subsequent evaluation and treatment of acute peripheral nerve injuries rely upon the efficient identification of the nerve and the site affected and the characterization of the nature and severity of the injury. The challenge to the nerve surgeon remains in the optimal management of nerve injuries that will maximize functional outcomes.

EVALUATING THE PATIENT WITH AN ACUTE PERIPHERAL NERVE INJURY

A thorough understanding of the relevant anatomy and physiology aids the surgeon's abilities to optimally manage the acute nerve injury via a pertinent history and directed physical examination. The history and physical examination can then be supplemented with electrodiagnostic and radiographic studies.

Anatomy and Physiology

A few basic principles underlie the anatomy of the peripheral nervous system. Each peripheral nerve is composed of fibers from more than one spinal nerve root; correspondingly, each

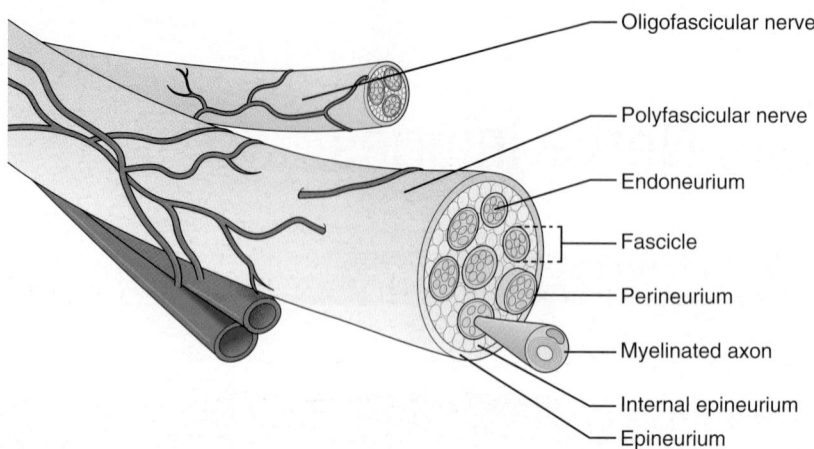

- Oligofascicular nerve
- Polyfascicular nerve
- Endoneurium
- Fascicle
- Perineurium
- Myelinated axon
- Internal epineurium
- Epineurium

FIGURE 32.1 Microscopic anatomy of the peripheral nerve.

spinal nerve contributes fibers to more than one peripheral nerve. Consequently, whereas spinal nerve lesions manifest in the clinical picture of radiculopathies with dermatomal sensory disturbances and mild to moderate weakness of muscles supplied by the spinal nerve, peripheral nerve lesions manifest in more precise borders of sensory disturbances acutely and more severe atrophy and paresis of muscles supplied solely by the peripheral nerve as time elapses.

The microscopic anatomy of the peripheral nerve comprises nerve fibers, fascicles, connective tissue (epi-, peri-, and endoneurium), blood vessels, lymphatics, and nervi nervorum (Fig. 32.1). Although the fascicular pattern may change as the nerve courses more distally, the general structure of the nerve remains constant. After a peripheral nerve is injured, a coordinated sequence of events occurs to remove the damaged tissue and ultimately initiates the regenerative process. When the nerve is disrupted, the severed ends retract owing to the elasticity of the endoneurium. Trauma to the vasa nervorum leads to robust inflammation triggering fibroblasts to proliferate to form the basis for a dense scar at the injury site: in the most severe cases, the nerve ends become markedly disorganized, with fibroblasts, macrophages, capillaries, Schwann cells, and collagen fibers within which the regenerating axons form disorganized masses known as *neuromas*. The degree of damage sustained by the proximal segment and neuronal cell body depends on the distance of the zone of injury from the cell body. The nucleus migrates to the periphery of the cell and select cytoplasmic elements (e.g., Nissl granules, endoplasmic reticulum) undergo chromatolysis. Cell survival relies upon the Schwann cells and trophic molecules present in the immediate environment.

Conversely, the distal portion of the axon undergoes Wallerian degeneration within hours after injury; this granular disintegration of the cytoskeleton and axoplasm occurs over several days to weeks, yielding empty endoneurial tubes. Early after injury, until the distal axons are totally degenerated, motor conductivity and sensory nerve potentials still can be observed in the distal segment; therefore, electrodiagnostic studies, used to predict severity of the lesion and to guide treatment recommendations, should not be performed within the first several weeks after injury.

When a peripheral nerve is injured, the accompanying muscle is denervated. Denervation leads to a series of structural changes and atrophy of the muscle if neural regeneration does not occur. Atrophy is seen as a mean 70% reduction in the cross-sectional area after 2 months.[3] Sodium channels regress toward embryonic forms with altered biochemical properties, and acetylcholine receptors redistribute to cover the entire muscle surface. This supersensitivity to acetylcholine manifests clinically as spontaneous uncoordinated muscle activity, otherwise known as *fibrillation*. Death of muscle fibers generally does not occur, but when it does, dropout occurs between 6 and 12 months after denervation.

Pertinent History of Injury

Pertinent history regarding the timing and location of the motor and sensory disturbances is critical for an accurate assessment of the acute nerve injury. For instance, an immediate neurological deficit coincident with the injury implies direct involvement of the peripheral nerve at the site of injury. In contrast, a delayed neurological deficit implies consequent involvement of the peripheral nerve, as with reduction of fractures, injections, or tourniquet application. If the motor and sensory disturbance progressively worsens, an enlarging adjacent lesion compromising the nerve (such as a hematoma, pseudoaneurysm, or pressure from a cast or splint) must be considered and urgently addressed. Additionally, with time, a bony callus can form causing a progressive neurological deficit such as in tardy ulnar palsy.

The description of the mechanism of injury can also yield information about the severity of injury to the nerve and guide treatment. For instance, if the injury involved low/no impact such as a fall from a standing position, neurapraxia will be the likely result. In contrast, if there is high impact as in extreme sports or high-speed motor vehicle accidents, then the likely injury is axonotmesis or neuronotmesis. This classification of nerve injury described by Seddon and associates in 1943[4] and expanded by Sunderland and colleagues in 1951[5] (Fig. 32.2) remains useful today, although most injuries occur along the continuum of pure grades.

Nerve injuries can also be classified as preganglionic or postganglionic, with profound surgical implications (Fig. 32.3). A preganglionic injury implies injury proximal to the dorsal root ganglion with permanent paralysis of the muscles innervated by the avulsed roots, complete sensory loss of the corresponding dermatomes, and most importantly, the preclusion

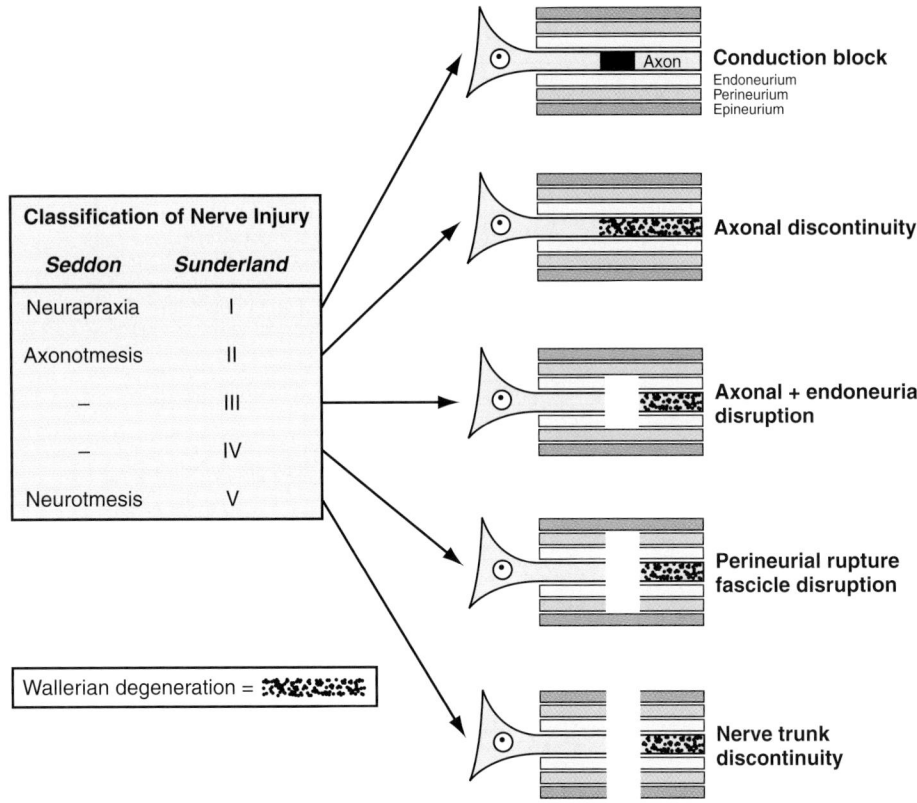

FIGURE 32.2 Seddon and Sunderland classifications of nerve injuries.

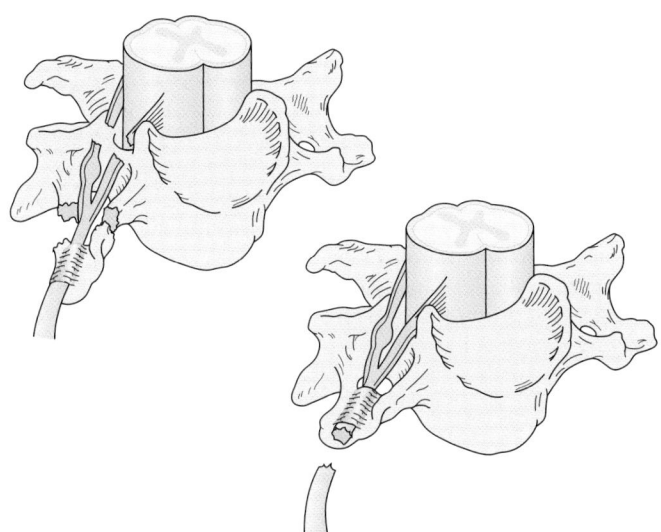

FIGURE 32.3 Pre- and postganglionic nerve injury.

of spontaneous recovery. A postganglionic injury potentially retains function of the cell body within the ventral horn of the spinal cord and these neurons may regenerate axons in the appropriate conditions. Acute nerve injuries can be classified as open or closed. Open injuries include sharp lacerations and missile wounds whereas closed injuries include traction or compressive injuries. Current guidelines recommend early repair (days) of clean, sharp nerve lacerations, and the delayed (weeks) repair of ragged or dirty nerve lacerations. Missile wounds with vascular injury should be explored acutely. Early

intervention is generally not recommended in closed injuries because of the potential for neurapraxic injury. Spontaneous regeneration, when it occurs, generally yields superior functional outcomes when compared to iatrogenic repair or reconstruction. Consideration of the clinical implications of these issues led to an algorithm for the surgical management of peripheral nerve and brachial plexus injuries[6] (Fig. 32.4).

Directed Physical Examination

The directed physical examination can be divided arbitrarily into several parts (Box 32.1). Inspection and observation initiate the examination. The presence of bruises, abrasions, and obvious lacerations can lead the examiner to the site of nerve injury: for example, road rash over the shoulder implies an upper brachial plexus injury, whereas road rash in the axilla extending along the chest wall implies a lower brachial plexus injury. Likewise, Horner's sign (ptosis, meiosis, anhydrosis) is indicative of a potential proximal T1/lower trunk brachial plexus lesion. Significant swelling can imply musculoskeletal injury such as a ruptured muscle/tendon in addition to the nerve injury in the absence of motor function. As described earlier, the observation of fasciculations and atrophy with time are also consistent with peripheral nerve injury.

An assessment of the relevant vasculature is a critical part of the directed physical examination because of the adjacent course of nerves and vessels. For example, the cords of the brachial plexus surround the axillary artery, and the median nerve courses adjacent to the brachial artery. Injury to the vessel can indicate simultaneous injury to the nerve, and the integrity of both should be assessed in the acute situation.

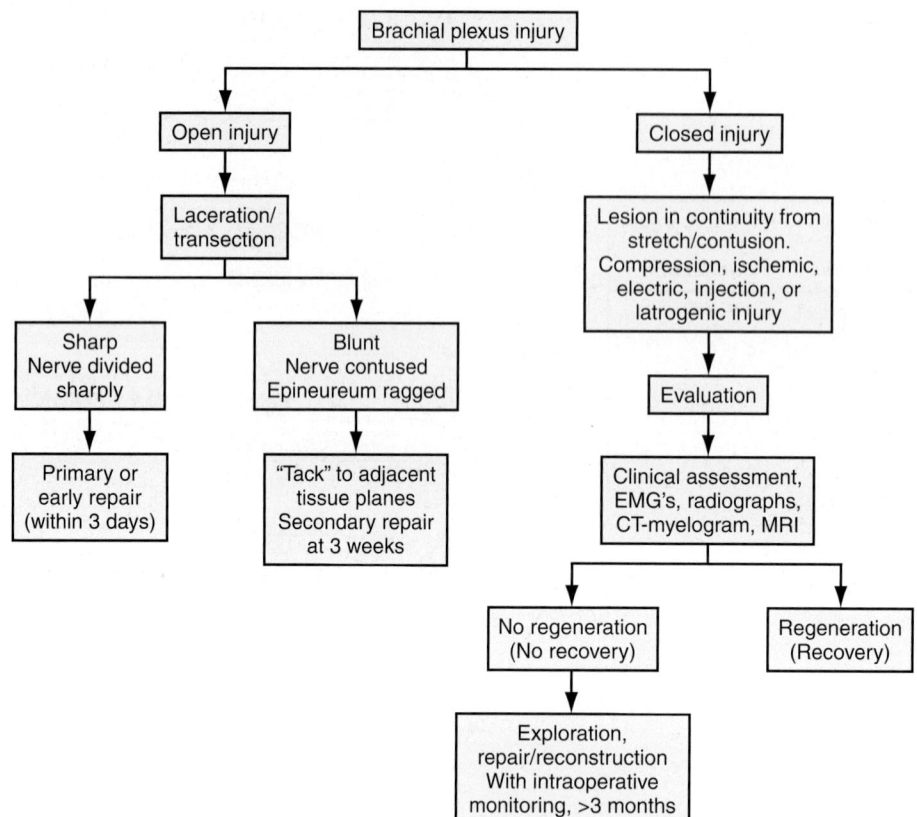

FIGURE 32.4 Algorithm for surgical management of peripheral nerve and brachial plexus injuries. *(Modified from Dubuisson A, Kline DG. Indications for peripheral nerve and brachial plexus surgery. Neurol Clin 1992;10(4):935-951.)*

BOX 32.1	Parts of the Directed Physical Examination for Nerve Injury

Inspection, observation
Vascular assessment
Motor examination including range of motion
Sensation and autonomic function
Tinel's sign
Assessment of diaphragm (phrenic nerve injury)

The motor examination should be conducted in the context of range of motion. If the range of motion is acutely compromised, musculoskeletal injury should be considered and motor power can be difficult to assess. To assess nerve function, there is no substitute for a thorough motor examination; the complete description of the motor examination lies outside the scope of this chapter but can be found in *Aids to the Examination of the Peripheral Nervous System*,[7] among other texts.[8] The importance of a thorough assessment of relevant muscles cannot be overemphasized because the standard cursory trauma examination can be misleading. Muscles in the distribution of noninjured nerves can simulate the motor function of the injured nerve to the inexperienced examiner: abduction of the fingers (ulnar nerve) can be mistaken for extension of the fingers (radial nerve), leading to the incorrect conclusion that the radial nerve is intact. A systematic examination of all muscles supplied by the relevant nerve(s) can preclude such errors.

The testing of sensory function is important but is often difficult and can be misleading. Observations should be made in the autonomous zones where the overlap in the innervation from adjacent nerves is minimal.

The presence of Tinel's sign can be indicative of a regenerating nerve, but whether the regeneration will be adequate to confer functional movement cannot be ascertained. Tinel's sign indicates an ectopic mechanosensitivity and can be used to assess the growth of a nerve; the expected progression is 1 mm per day distally in accordance with the extending axon. Failure of Tinel's sign to progress at the expected rate would suggest the need for surgical exploration.

Ancillary Studies

Electrodiagnostic studies (EDS) can aid in defining the site of injury and the potential for reinnervation of affected musculature. Baseline EDS are best performed 3 or more weeks after injury for reasons described earlier. Serial EDS can document clinically significant regeneration. Lack of innervation of paraspinal muscles implies a proximal injury. Sensory nerve action potentials (SNAPs) and somatosensory evoked potentials (SSEPs) are also useful in determining the site of injury; presence of a normal SNAP in the absence of SSEPs implies a preganglionic injury.

Radiographic studies may include long bone, cervical spine, and chest radiographs, which can reveal associated fractures, and in the case of brachial plexus injury, can demonstrate an elevated hemidiaphragm (phrenic nerve injury).

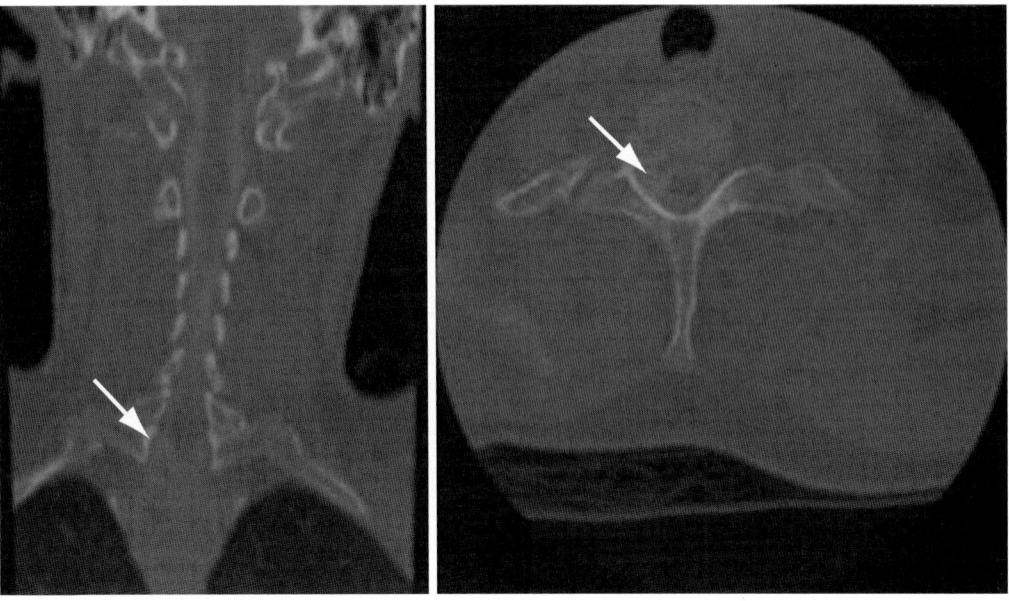

FIGURE 32.5 Postmyelogram computed tomography scan demonstrating pseudomeningocele *(arrows)*.

Postmyelogram computed tomography (CT) and magnetic resonance imaging (MRI) can be used to detect pseudomeningoceles (Fig. 32.5), which are often associated with preganglionic injuries. The present resolution provided by standard imaging techniques is yet unable to demonstrate direct evidence of the site and severity of nerve injury.

SURGICAL NERVE REPAIR/ RECONSTRUCTION

When operative treatment is contemplated, the surgeon should understand the patient's expected goals and address them if they are unreasonable. The patient and surgeon should agree on the reconstructive priorities when spontaneous recovery of function is unlikely. Patience from both the patient's and practitioner's perspective is needed during the recovery period.

The goal of surgical repair is to restore continuity between the proximal and distal nerve segments to restore innervation of target end organs in the absence of spontaneous recovery. Ideally, direct coaptation is preferred. However, if a significant gap exists between the proximal and distal nerve segments, nerve repair using an interposition graft or nerve transfer must be employed.

Surgical Options

Neurolysis is the removal of scar tissue from around the nerve (external neurolysis) or between fascicles (internal neurolysis) if the nerve is injured asymmetrically. Dissection is started with proximal and distal uninjured nerve ends toward the involved injured segment. Intraoperative EDS can determine if the injured segment can conduct electric signal. The presence of nerve action potentials (NAPs) across an involved segment implies that neurolysis alone is adequate for neural recovery (Fig. 32.6).[9]

Direct (end-to-end) repair is possible only if a short nerve gap exists after resection of the nonfunctioning neural

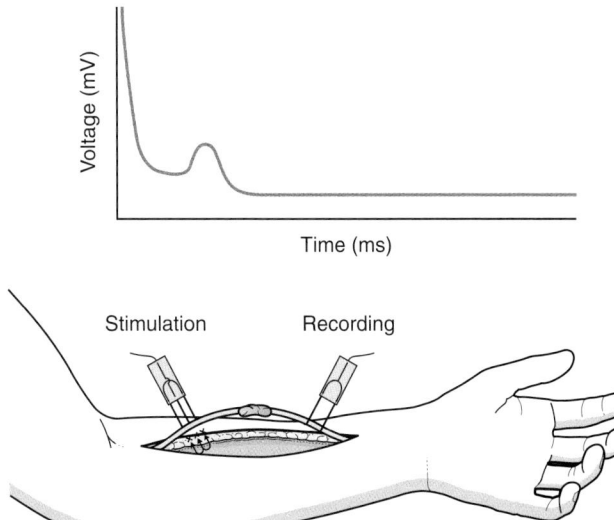

FIGURE 32.6 Nerve action potential electrodiagnostic tracing. *(From Spinner RJ, Kline DG. Surgery for peripheral nerve and brachial plexus injuries or other nerve lesions. Muscle Nerve 2000;23(5):680-695.)*

segment. Direct repair is preferred over indirect (graft) repair because of better functional results. Tension across the repair must be avoided to reduce the risk of failure of regeneration. Reducing tension across the repair can be achieved with proximal and distal mobilization of the nerve and optimal position of the surrounding soft tissues/bony elements to shorten the nerve gap distance. Direct repair is performed by coapting the ends with sutures if the repair crosses tissue planes, or by approximating the ends with tissue-fibrin glue if the repair lies within a tissue plane.

Graft (indirect repair) is needed when the gap that exists after resection of the nonfunctioning neural segment is too large for direct approximation without tension (Fig. 32.7). The length of the graft should be the length of the gap plus 10%. Autograft is usually used and derived from sural nerve,

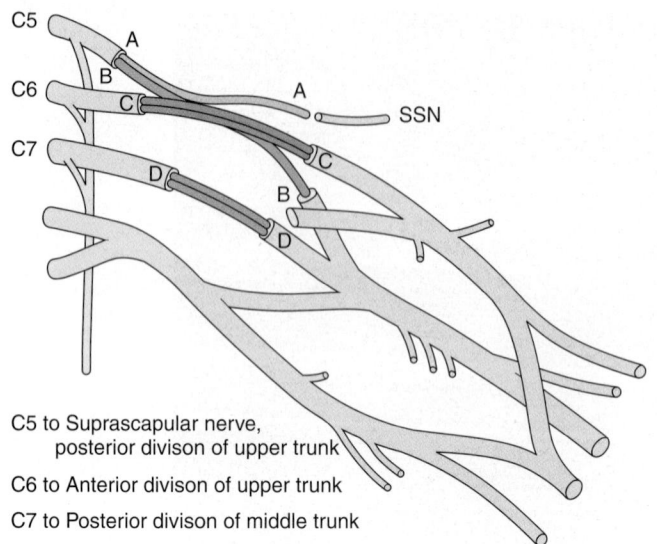

C5 to Suprascapular nerve,
   posterior divison of upper trunk

C6 to Anterior divison of upper trunk

C7 to Posterior divison of middle trunk

FIGURE 32.7 Graft repair of an injured brachial plexus.

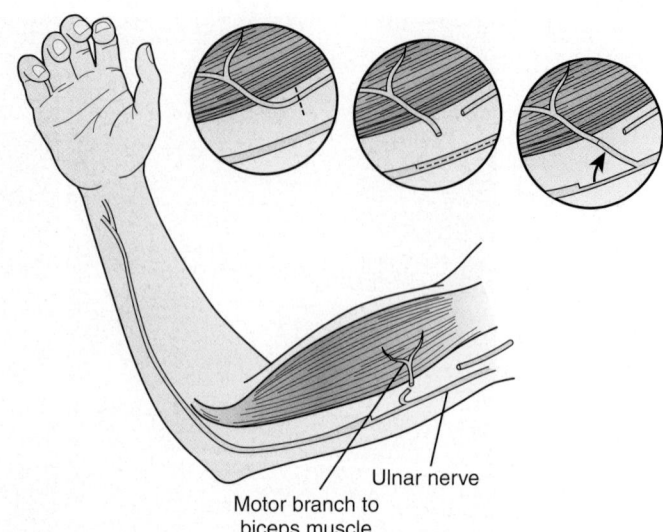

FIGURE 32.8 Transfer of ulnar nerve fascicle to musculocutaneous nerve.

medial antebrachial cutaneous nerve, or superficial radial nerve because these small-caliber grafts achieve better results (faster revascularization) than larger-caliber grafts.[10] Coaptation of the ends of the graft to the proximal and distal stumps is similar to that used for the direct repair. Artificial grafts are under active investigation but are not yet routinely used for repair of major nerves.

Nerve transfers/neurotization have augmented the surgical arena for the treatment of peripheral nerve injuries, particularly of brachial plexus injuries, especially in the context of avulsion (preganglionic) injury.[11,12] Nerve transfers have changed the outlook for the "unrepairable" injuries to "reconstructable" injuries by coapting a proximal functional nerve donor with a distal denervated nerve to reinnervate the latter with healthy donor axons. Popularized nerve transfer techniques include neurotization of the spinal accessory to the suprascapular nerve[13-16] or radial branch to axillary nerve[17,18] to achieve shoulder abduction and intercostal,[19-21] medial pectoral,[22,23] phrenic,[24,25] or ulnar fascicular nerve transfer to the musculocutaneous nerve (Fig. 32.8)[26,27] for elbow flexion. Recovery of the translated function appears to rely upon cortical plasticity.[28]

Postoperative Care

After nerve repair/reconstruction, appropriate joints can be immobilized for 3 to 6 weeks to allow the nerve suture lines to heal. Afterward, physical/occupational therapy is recommended for range of motion (prevent contractures) as well as for maintaining strength in the unaffected muscles and the affected muscles when reinnervation occurs. Patients should be informed that recovery is a long process, which may last several years. The treatment of pain with Neurontin/Lyrica, certain tricyclic antidepressants, and other agents, or later by neurosurgeons employing dorsal root entry zone (DREZ) procedures can aid in recovery. Documenting recovery following

peripheral nerve repair/reconstruction relies upon clinical and electrophysiological examinations. Additional augmentation of function via muscle/tendon transfers may be considered for those who are motivated to request other treatment options to maximize the functional outcome.

Outcomes After Nerve Surgery

Outcomes for functional repair of sharp lacerations of the median and radial nerves have been reported to be as high as 91% in contrast to 73% for ulnar nerves; similarly, for graft repair, functional outcomes were better for the median (68%) and radial nerves (67%) than for ulnar nerves (56%).[29] Outcomes for ulnar fascicular transfer to the musculocutaneous branch to biceps has been reported at 75% for antigravity elbow flexion with an average time for reinnervation at 5 months.[27]

CONCLUSION

Peripheral nerve injuries can be devastating to the patient's normal functional status, and the long-term implications of these injuries are often not understood by the patients or their families. Maximal functional outcomes rely on communication between the patient and the surgeon to manage expectant goals and to adapt to unrecoverable functional deficits. These injuries present challenging entities for the managing health care practitioner: the treating practitioner must rely upon an understanding of the anatomy, clinical acumen, appropriate use of ancillary radiographic and electrodiagnostic studies to determine the proper course, and timing for offering surgical options. With improved microsurgical techniques, potential development of pharmacological agents, and the increasingly creative reconstructive options offered by multidisciplinary collaborative teams, the outlook for patients suffering acute nerve injures will continue to improve.

CHAPTER 33

Entrapment Neuropathies

Mikhail Gelfenbeyn, Henry Marsh

CLINICAL PEARLS

- Entrapment neuropathy occurs when a peripheral nerve is subjected to repetitive movement in a constricted space. Conservative treatment involves reducing the movement; surgical treatment enlarges the space.

- Carpal tunnel syndrome is by far the most common entrapment neuropathy and the commonest cause of neurological symptoms in the hand. The symptoms are not always confined to the hand and can spread proximally.

- In cubital tunnel surgery, when comparing simple ulnar nerve decompression versus anterior subcutaneous

- transposition techniques, one can expect similar outcomes but fewer complications with simple ulnar decompression.

- Diagnosis of entrapment neuropathy can usually be made from the clinical history, and can then be confirmed by physical signs, electromyography, nerve conduction studies, and magnetic resonance imaging (MRI).

- Surgery for entrapment neuropathy is indicated if conservative measures fail or if the clinical picture is one of severe compression with significant pain and muscular weakness and wasting.

Some peripheral nerves, irrespective of whether they are motor, sensory, or of mixed type, pass through narrow, constricted areas in the arms or legs. Under certain circumstances, these nerves are susceptible to compression at these sites,[1-3] and this compression can eventually clinically manifest as *entrapment neuropathy*.[4-6] Entrapment of nerves usually occurs as they pass beside a joint, such as the elbow, wrist, or hip and only very occasionally elsewhere in the limbs. This, along with the fact that entrapment neuropathy seldom occurs in the head or trunk, suggests that repetitive motion is a major factor that precipitates entrapment in an anatomically constricted segment.

Two types of physical constrictions predispose to entrapment neuropathy. The first type (Fig. 33.1A) is a fibroosseous tunnel. The space available for the nerve within the tunnel becomes constricted either because the contents of the tunnel become larger or hypertrophic, as when a patient with tenosynovitis has carpal tunnel syndrome, or because the walls of the tunnel encroach upon the tunnel's lumen, as when fractured fragments of a carpal bone displace into the carpal canal. Compression of a nerve in a tunnel is an example of *static* compression. The second type (Fig. 33.1B) involves *dynamic* compression of the nerve as it passes through a fibrotendinous arcade. The nerve is flanked by two bellies of a muscle that under static conditions do not compress the nerve. When they contract, however, they cause a shutter-like closure of the arcade, compressing the nerve. For example, this can occur at the arcade of Frohse in the

supinator muscle, the two heads of the flexor carpi ulnaris at the entrance to the cubital tunnel, or the two heads of the flexor digitorum sublimis forming the "sublimis bridge."

PATHOLOGY OF NERVE COMPRESSION[7]

The pathophysiological changes following nerve compression[8-21] are dependent on the degree, rate, and duration of compression. Loss of function of the nerve as a result of compression is manifested clinically by motor paralysis, paresthesia, or numbness. In physiological terms, mild and brief compression produces a transient and reversible conduction block within the nerve. Sustained compression over a long period causes structural changes. Not all components of the nerve are equally susceptible to a given degree of compression. Nerve fibers that have a greater amount of epineurium compared to the nerve fascicles are less susceptible to compression than those with larger fascicles and scanty epineurium (Fig. 33.2). Also, within a given nerve, not all fibers undergo degenerative changes to the same extent. The superficially located fibers tend to bear the brunt of the compression, while the central fibers are relatively spared. Large, heavily myelinated fibers subserving light touch and motor function are more sensitive to compressive changes than unmyelinated fibers subserving pain sensation.

Impediment to microvascular flow appears to be a major factor in the pathophysiology of nerve impingement.[7] Capillary blanching and venular obstruction herald progressive

515

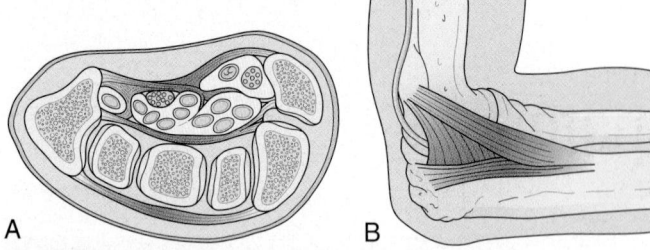

FIGURE 33.1 A, Example of a fibro-osseous tunnel—the carpal tunnel at the wrist. The median nerve and the tendons of the long flexor muscles are the main contents of the tunnel. **B,** Example of fibrotendinous arcade—the cubital canal at the elbow. The ulnar nerve enters the fibroaponeurotic arcade formed by the two heads of the flexor carpi ulnaris (Osborne's ligament).

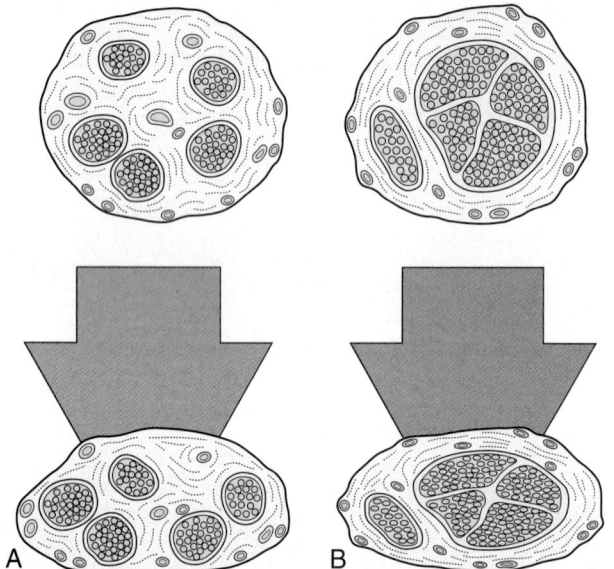

FIGURE 33.2 Nerves having a greater amount of epineurium (**A**) are less susceptible to compression than those having scanty epineurium (**B**).

compression. This leads to nerve ischemia, which in turn leads to endothelial impairment and progressive edema; the edema compounds the ischemia and swelling of the nerve (Fig. 33.3). Critical swelling of a nerve within the constraints of its surroundings may lead to further nerve compression, a phenomenon that can be called a *mini-compartmental syndrome.*

Nerve compression blocks axonal transport. The antegrade transport from the nerve cell to the axon toward the synapse can be divided into fast and slow components; the fast component carries the membrane-associated materials and the slow components carry the cytoskeletal proteins. Nerve compression impedes both the fast and slow components of the antegrade flow, resulting in a swelling of the nerve proximal to the compression as a result of the damming up of the moving axoplasm within the fibers. Thus, the distribution of cytoskeletal elements, axolemma constituents, and the transmitter substances required for synaptic conduction are all impaired by a block of antegrade flow. Retrograde axonal flow from the synaptic level to the cell body of the nerve is similarly blocked by compression of the nerve. This results in a loss of transfer of neuronotropic factors to the nerve cell body. The impairment of retrograde axonal transport results in certain changes in the nerve cell body comparable to those that occur after peripheral nerve section (wallerian degeneration). Thus, changes noted in the cell body are an eccentric nucleus, dispersion of Nissl substance (chromatolysis), and a decrease in nuclear and whole cell volumes. The overall result of the impediment to axoplasmic flow is impaired membrane permeability and conduction block.

With acute and severe compression one observes a characteristic sequential invagination or telescoping of the myelin sheath (Fig. 33.4). The polarity of invagination is reversed at the edges of the compression. With chronic compression, segmental demyelination occurs within the compressed segments, accounting for the slowing of conduction velocity of the nerve. In the early phases, the nerve fibers distal to the compression show normal morphology. With sustained compression, axolysis occurs within the compressed segment, leading to distal wallerian degeneration.

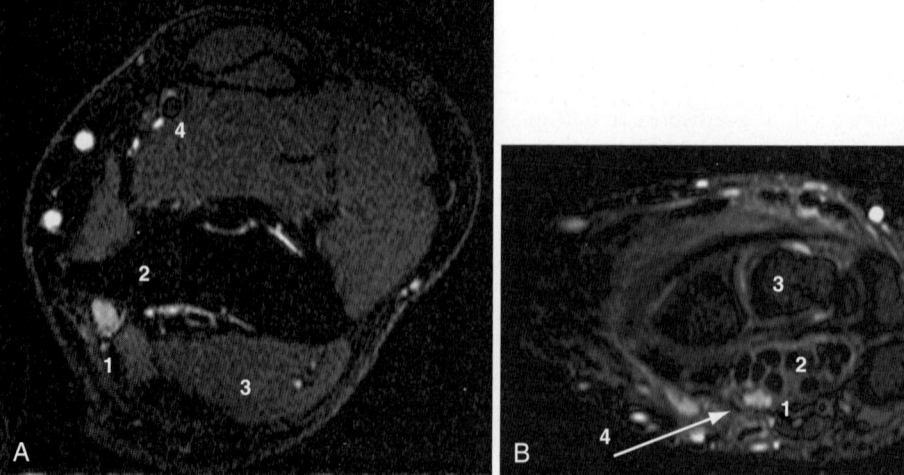

FIGURE 33.3 A, Magnetic resonance imaging (MRI) of right elbow showing ulnar neuropathy at the cubital canal (enlarged ulnar nerve with high short tau inversion recovery (STIR) signal). *1,* Ulnar nerve; *2,* medial epicondyle of humerus; *3,* triceps; *4,* brachial artery. **B,** MRI of the wrist showing median nerve changes (increased STIR signal) characteristic for carpal tunnel syndrome. *1,* Median nerve; *2,* tendons of flexor digitorum superficialis and profundus; *3,* carpal bones; *4,* flexor retinaculum.

DOUBLE CRUSH SYNDROME

If a nerve is compressed proximally, its distal part is more susceptible to compression than a normal nerve would be, because the antegrade axonal flow is blocked by the first compression. In a similar manner, if there is distal compression, the nerve cell body undergoes degeneration more quickly if a second compression is present proximally, because of impediment of retrograde flow. This latter syndrome is called a *reverse double crush syndrome.*[22]

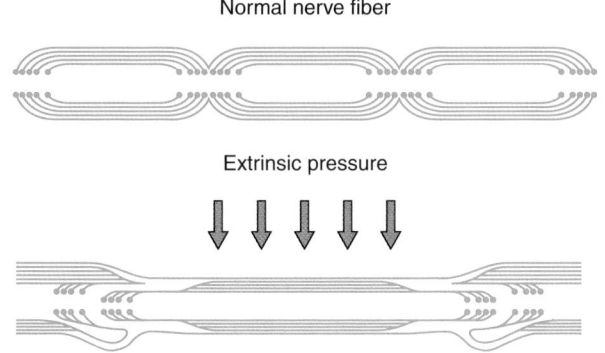

Normal nerve fiber

Extrinsic pressure

Compressed nerve fiber

FIGURE 33.4 Telescoping of myelin sheath with acute and severe nerve compression.

NERVE COMPRESSION SYNDROME IN DIABETICS

Patients with diabetic neuropathy are more susceptible to compression, presumably because of accumulation of sorbitol, a metabolite of glucose, and the formation of endoneurial edema.

THE ENTRAPMENT SYNDROMES

The entrapment sites, the nerves involved at each site, and the corresponding syndromes are listed in Table 33.1. This chapter will cover the most common entrapment syndromes: carpal tunnel syndrome, cubital tunnel syndrome, meralgia paresthetica, suprascapular nerve entrapment, and tarsal tunnel syndrome. Some patients can develop multiple entrapment neuropathies.[23]

TABLE 33.1 Entrapment Syndromes

Affected Location/ Structure	Nerve Entrapped	Compressing Element	Clinical Syndrome
Supracondylar region	Median nerve	Ligament of Struthers or supracondylar spur	High median entrapment neuropathy
Elbow	Median nerve	Bicipital aponeurosis (lacertus fibrosus), hypertrophic pronator teres muscle, or tendinous arch of flexor digitorum sublimis (the "sublimis bridge")	Pronator syndrome
Forearm	Anterior interosseous nerve	Variable anatomical abnormalities such as fibrous bands arising from pronator teres or flexor digitorum sublimis muscles; often no anatomical abnormalities may be demonstrated	Anterior interosseous nerve syndrome
Wrist	Median nerve	Carpal canal or element of its contents	Carpal tunnel syndrome
Elbow	Ulnar nerve	Variable: most commonly, the fascial band binding the two heads of the flexor carpi ulnaris	Cubital tunnel syndrome, tardy ulnar palsy
Wrist	Ulnar nerve	Guyon's canal syndrome	Guyon's canal syndrome
Forearm	Posterior interosseous nerve	Arcade of Frohse	Posterior interosseous nerve entrapment syndrome
Forearm	Posterior interosseous nerve	Variable	Resistant "tennis elbow," radial tunnel syndrome
Forearm	Superficial radial nerve	Variable; commonly, extrinsic compression or trauma; sometimes the deep fascia of the forearm between the extensor carpi radialis longus and brevis muscles	Superficial radial nerve syndrome
Neck	Brachial plexus	Cervical rib or fibrous band or scalenus anterior muscle	Thoracic outlet syndrome
Hip	Lateral femoral cutaneous nerve	Inguinal ligament and associated fasciae	Meralgia paresthetica
Knee	Peroneal nerve	Variable	Peroneal neuropathy
Ankle	Posterior tibial nerve	Tarsal tunnel	Tarsal tunnel syndrome
Shoulder	Suprascapular nerve	Suprascapular notch/foramen	Suprascapular nerve entrapment
Thigh	Saphenous nerve	Deep fascia roofing Hunter's canal	Saphenous nerve entrapment

Carpal Tunnel Syndrome[24]

The carpal tunnel syndrome[25-27] is the most common entrapment neuropathy encountered in clinical practice. It results from compression of the distal median nerve within the carpal tunnel, located in the proximal part of the palm of the hand.[28] The carpal tunnel is bounded dorsally by the carpal bones and ventrally by the transverse carpal ligament. The carpal bones form a shallow trough that is converted into a tunnel by the carpal ligament. The contents of the tunnel are the median nerve and tendons of the long flexor muscles (see Fig. 33.1A). Any lesion affecting the synovial sheath tends to compromise the cross-sectional diameter of the carpal canal and may induce compressive neuropathy.[29] Recent studies that include magnetic resonance imaging (MRI) and computed tomography (CT) scans show that patients with carpal tunnel syndrome tend to have small carpal canals. The small size of the carpal canal, measured by the decrease in its cross-sectional diameter, is a congenital or developmental phenomenon.[30] Its small size in women may account for their higher incidence of carpal tunnel syndrome.

Clinical Features[31]

Women are more commonly affected than men, by a ratio of 7:3. Most patients are middle-aged at the onset of symptoms. The predominant symptom is an aching, burning, tingling, numb sensation in the hand, ordinarily in the lateral half of the hand and the outer three or four digits.[32] Frequently there may be an aching pain in the proximal forearm or even in the arm up to the shoulder and it can lead to confusion with cervical radiculopathy. Patients typically wake up at night with increased pain, and they may shake their hand to obtain relief. The symptoms are often bilateral. With severe or advanced compression patients complain of weakness of grip and a tendency to drop things.

In the early stages of the syndrome, at which time most patients are seen in contemporary practice, there are few objective findings. Two mechanical tests can be performed. Tinel's sign may be elicited by lightly tapping over the median nerve at the wrist crease, which results in a tingling in the distribution of the median nerve if positive. Phalen's test consists of asking the patient to flex the wrist to 90 degrees for about 60 seconds, which will precipitate paresthesia in the distribution of the median nerve if positive.[33-35] Neither test is conclusive and both results are often absent. Perception of light touch, pinprick, and two-point discrimination in the tips of the fingers in the median nerve distribution may be impaired. In advanced cases there may be atrophy of the thenar muscles, especially in the abductor pollicis brevis. A recently proposed scratch collapse test for evaluation of carpal and cubital canal syndrome may be a significant addition for clinicians but it needs to be evaluated by independent reviewers.[36]

The clinical history, especially of nocturnal pain, is usually the most reliable diagnostic clue. There are several local and systemic risk factors that precipitate the symptoms of carpal tunnel syndrome (Table 33.2).[37-44]

Diagnosis

The most important diagnostic tests are electromyography and study of nerve conduction velocity.[45] The earliest and most significant finding is the prolongation of sensory latency due to demyelination. The sensory evoked response will show diminution of amplitude and may even be absent. Motor latency abnormalities occur late in the course of the disease. Needle electromyography may show loss of motor unit potentials and the presence of denervation potentials in the median-innervated muscles in the thenar eminence due to axonal loss. Clinically it corresponds to the impairment of two-point discrimination.

Treatment

Current management strategies based on the evidence-based medicine approach were summarized in the American Academy of Orthopaedic Surgeons practice guidelines published in 2009[46] and are summarized in Table 33.3.[47-51]

In early cases with minimal symptoms or in individuals in whom the syndrome is expected to be transient, conservative treatment should be instituted. This consists of a wrist splint in neutral position at night (initial relief in approximately 50%), a course of vitamin B_6, and anti-inflammatory drugs. Injection of local anesthesia and steroids around the median nerve may be beneficial,[52,53] but accidental injection directly into the nerve may result in annoying paresthesias in the distribution of the median nerve.

Surgical therapy is indicated when conservative measures fail.[51] The surgical procedure can be performed by either the open method[54] or an endoscopic technique.[55] The steps in the surgical sectioning of the transverse carpal ligament are shown in Figure 33.5. Usually local or regional anesthesia (Bier block) is used. General anesthesia may be used if the patient is extremely nervous.

Endoscopic section of the carpal ligament has recently been introduced.[55] The advantages are that the postoperative recovery period is shorter, a sensitive scar in the palm of the hand is avoided, and the structural integrity of the carpal tunnel mechanism is minimally disturbed. However, there is a greater risk of injury to the ulnar artery and to the sensory branch of the median nerve serving the middle and ring fingers. With any technique the patient should be instructed to move the fingers postoperatively to minimize scar formation.

Good outcome is to be expected in at least 85% to 90% of the cases but if there is significant weakness and wasting at the time of presentation the results are less satisfactory. Relief of typical nocturnal pain is usually immediate.[56]

Cubital Tunnel Syndrome

The cubital tunnel syndrome[57-80] results from entrapment of the ulnar nerve at the elbow. The cubital tunnel is located on the medial side of the elbow joint. It is a fibro-osseous tunnel that is roofed by the aponeurotic attachment of the two heads of the flexor carpi ulnaris and a tough fascial band that bridges these two heads, also known as the *Osborne's ligament*[74,75] (see Fig. 33.1B). The floor is formed by the medial ligament of the elbow joint. During flexion of the elbow, the volume of the cubital tunnel decreases; the reverse happens in extension. This is because the points of attachment of the flexor carpi ulnaris, that is, the medial epicondyle and the olecranon process, are farthest apart during flexion. Thus, there is more tension on the

TABLE 33.2 Risk Factors in the Pathogenesis of Carpal Tunnel Syndrome

Local Factors	Systemic Factors
Increased volume of the contents of the carpal canal	Increased susceptibility of nerves to pressure
Hypertrophic tenosynovitis	Alcoholic or diabetic polyneuropathy
Masses: neurofibroma, hemangioma, lipoma, ganglion cyst, gouty tophus, xanthoma	Hereditary neuropathy with liability to pressure palsies
Anomalous muscles and tendons[40]	Amyloidosis
Persistent median artery with or without thrombosis, aneurysm, arteriovenous malformation	Proximal lesions of the median nerve ("double crush" syndrome)
Acute palmar space infections	Other polyneuropathies
Hemorrhage[43]	Factors unique to women
Reduction in the capacity of the carpal canal	Pregnancy and lactation[41,43]
Congenitally small carpal canal[30]	Menstrual cycles
Idiopathic or familial thickening of the transverse carpal ligament[39]	Contraceptive pills
Malunion or callus following Colles' fracture or fracture of the carpal bones	Menopause
Unreduced dislocations of the wrist or intercarpal joints	Toxic shock syndrome
Improper immobilization of the wrist ("cotton loader position")	Eclampsia
Compression by cast	Other hormonal factors
Exostoses	Myxedema
Other local factors	Acromegaly
Burns at the wrist	Other systemic factors
	Obesity
	Raynaud's disease
	Athetoid-dystonic cerebral palsy
	Long-term hemodialysis[41,44]
	Inflammatory and autoimmune disorders
	Rheumatoid arthritis[37]
	Dermatomyositis
	Scleroderma
	Polymyalgia rheumatica
	Metabolic disorders
	Mucopolysaccharidoses
	Mucolipidoses
	Amyloidosis
	Chondrocalcinosis
	Gout

TABLE 33.3 Management of Entrapment Syndromes: Evidence-Based Medicine Results

Study/Review	Conclusions
Carpal Tunnel Syndrome	
Ono S, et al. Optimal management of carpal tunnel syndrome.[47] (A review of RCTs and systematic reviews.)	A trend toward recommending early surgery for cases with and without median nerve denervation.
Jarvik JG, et al. Surgery versus non-surgical therapy for carpal tunnel syndrome: a randomized parallel-group trial.[51]	Symptoms in both groups improved, but surgical treatment led to better outcome than that with nonsurgical treatment. However, the clinical relevance of this difference was moderate.
Cubital Canal Syndrome	
Bartels RHMA, et al. Prospective randomized controlled study comparing simple decompression versus anterior subcutaneous transposition for idiopathic neuropathy of the ulnar nerve at the elbow.[48]	The outcomes were equivalent, but simple decompression was associated with fewer complications. Use of this approach is advised even in the presence of (sub)luxation.
Chung K. Treatment of ulnar nerve compression at the elbow.[49] (A review of RCTs and systematic reviews.)	Different transposition techniques (subcutaneous and submuscular) yielded results similar to those with simple decompression. All mentioned randomized controlled trials had relatively small samples.
Tarsal Tunnel Syndrome	
Patel AT, et al. Usefulness of electrodiagnostic techniques in the evaluation of suspected tarsal tunnel syndrome: an evidence-based review.[50]	Nerve conduction studies may be useful for confirming the diagnosis of tibial neuropathy at the ankle (recommendation level C).

fascial band between these two heads, which increases the pressure on the cubital tunnel.

Clinical Features

The major presenting symptoms are weakness and atrophy of the intrinsic muscles of the hand and tingling and numbness in the medial two fingers. The onset of symptoms is generally insidious. Men are affected three times more commonly than women. An obvious etiological factor, such as an old, healed, supracondylar fracture, a ganglion cyst of the elbow, or synovitis, is sometimes evident. In the majority of instances, however, there is no apparent cause. The presence of a rare anomalous muscle, anconeus epitrochlearis, is an uncommon cause.

On objective testing there is weakness of the ulnar-innervated muscles in the hand, including the palmaris brevis, abductor digiti quinti, opponens digiti quinti, flexor digiti quinti, adductor pollicis, the medial two lumbricals, and all of the interossei. The flexor carpi ulnar is generally not affected because the fibers that subserve the motor innervation are thought to be very deep within the nerve and thus less susceptible to compression than the more superficial fibers to the intrinsic muscles. Provocative maneuvers, such as flexion of the elbow (stretching the ulnar nerve) or gentle direct compression on the ulnar nerve above the medial epicondyle, can reproduce typical symptoms and support the diagnosis.

Froment's sign is elicited by asking the patient to grasp a piece of cardboard between the index finger and thumb against resistance. In patients with weakness of the adductor pollicis there will be flexion of the first interphalangeal joint and the thumb.

Diagnosis

The characteristic electrodiagnostic finding is a delay in the conduction velocity in the ulnar nerve across the elbow. The sensory latency is prolonged, and the amplitude of the motor response in the abductor digiti minimi is decreased. A needle examination of the ulnar-innervated muscles may show denervation potentials. A special inching technique as well as MRI help to detect ulnar nerve entrapment across the elbow. A three-grade scale of the severity of ulnar entrapment at the elbow was proposed by McGowan.[71]

Tardy ulnar paralysis should be differentiated from lesions in the spinal cord affecting the C8, T1 segments, such as syringomyelia, spinal cord tumor, or amyotrophic lateral sclerosis, and extradural spinal lesions, such as cervical disk disease or

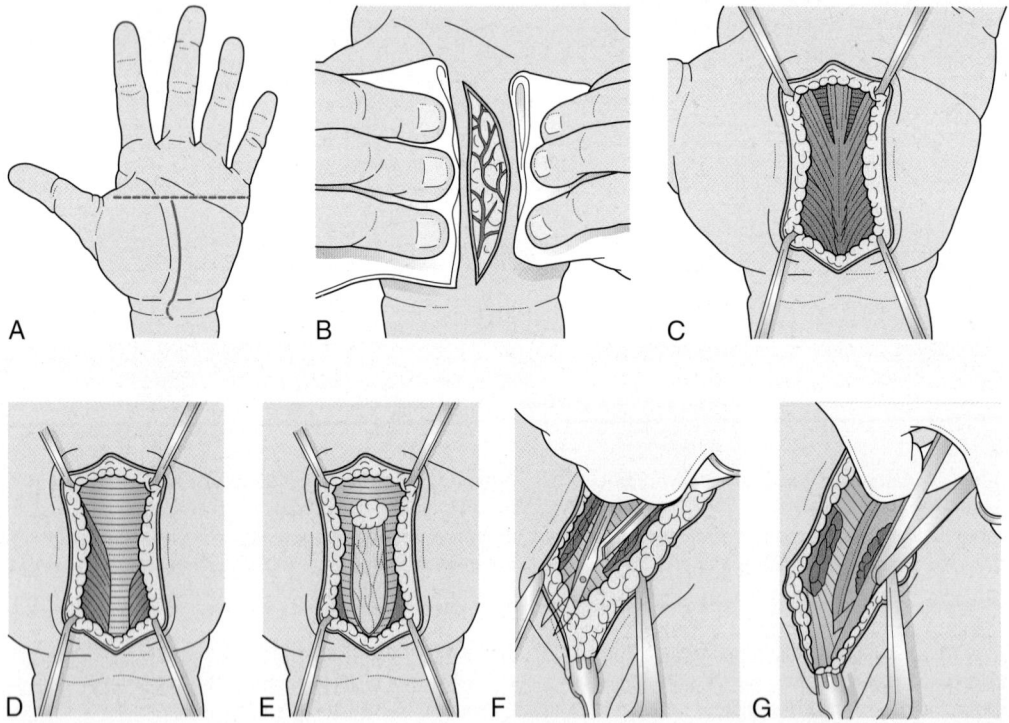

FIGURE 33.5 A, The skin incision extends from the wrist crease to a point in the midpalm in line with the fully extended thumb (*horizontal interrupted line*). An optional extension may be carried out in the distal forearm (*curvilinear interrupted line*) to facilitate exposure of the proximal part of the transverse carpal ligament and the distal part of the deep fascia of the forearm. Note that the main skin incision is not in the palmar skin crease but just medial to it. **B,** Protrusion of exuberant palmar subcutaneous fat after the skin incision is made. **C,** Exposure of the palmar aponeurosis. **D,** Exposure of the transverse carpal ligament after midline section and retraction of the palmar aponeurosis. The distal margin of the transverse carpal ligament can faintly be seen blending with the deep fascia of the palm. The proximal part of the transverse carpal ligament is covered by the hypothenar and thenar muscles. In many instances (not shown in this illustration) they may meet and interdigitate in the midline, blocking the transverse carpal ligament from view. **E,** About 80% of the transverse carpal ligament has been divided, exposing the median nerve. Note the constant fat globule superficial to the median nerve at the distal end of the exposure. **F,** Proximal skin is undermined with retraction to facilitate exposure of the proximal part of the transverse carpal ligament. **G,** Section of the most proximal part of the transverse carpal ligament and the distal deep fascia of the forearm.

spondylosis, neurofibroma, or meningioma. Lesions of the brachial plexus involving the lower trunk or the medial cord (Pancoast tumor), entrapment of the ulnar nerve distally at the wrist (Guyon's canal), and polyneuropathy should also be ruled out.

Treatment

In early, minimally symptomatic cases, a conservative approach is recommended. The patient should wear an elbow pad for protection against direct pressure to the nerve and avoid excessive flexion of the elbow and strenuous exercise for some time, especially sports with maneuvers that involve vigorous throwing, such as baseball. In persistent or highly symptomatic cases, surgical options should be considered. There is no other entrapment neuropathy for which the surgical options are more controversial than cubital tunnel syndrome. The available surgical methods are listed in Box 33.1. The simplest and most satisfactory procedure for uncomplicated cases is cubital tunnel release.[81] Excellent to good pain relief has been demonstrated in 75% to 90% of patients. Recovery of muscle weakness usually takes many months and does not always

BOX 33.1	Surgical Options for Treating Cubital Tunnel Syndrome

Simple in situ decompression
Medial epicondylectomy
Subcutaneous anterior transposition
Intramuscular anterior transposition
Submuscular anterior transposition

occur in severe cases. (The steps of the procedure are shown in Fig. 33.6.) In more involved cases complicated by elbow-joint abnormality, malunited fractures, or other abnormalities, the nerve may be transposed anterior to the elbow joint into the subcutaneous, intramuscular, or submuscular planes. Results of the recent prospective randomized controlled study comparing simple decompression with anterior subcutaneous transposition showed similar outcomes but fewer complications with decompression. It also was associated with lower cost.[48]

Meralgia Paresthetica

Meralgia paresthetica[82-84] is a syndrome caused by the entrapment of the lateral femoral cutaneous nerve of the thigh in the inguinal region. The name refers to the burning sensation that affected individuals complain of in the anterolateral thigh (*meros*, thigh; *algos*, pain).

The lateral femoral cutaneous nerve of the thigh arises from the lumbar plexus, emerges at the lateral margin of the psoas major muscle, descends obliquely downward and forward under the iliac fascia, pierces the inguinal ligament near the anterior superior iliac spine, courses under the fascia lata for about 5 cm, and then becomes subcutaneous by piercing the fascia lata (Fig. 33.7A). It innervates the skin of the anterolateral aspect of the thigh and the gluteal region (Fig. 33.7B and C).

Entrapment of the nerve occurs in the inguinal region at the point where it pierces the inguinal ligament. Obese individuals with a pendulous, flabby anterior abdominal wall are more prone to this disorder. Persons who spend much of the day walking or standing, such as patrolmen, postal workers, and traveling salesmen, are also more susceptible. Patients complain of a tingling, crawling, pricking, "pins and needles" sensation in the anterolateral thigh. Varying degrees of sensory

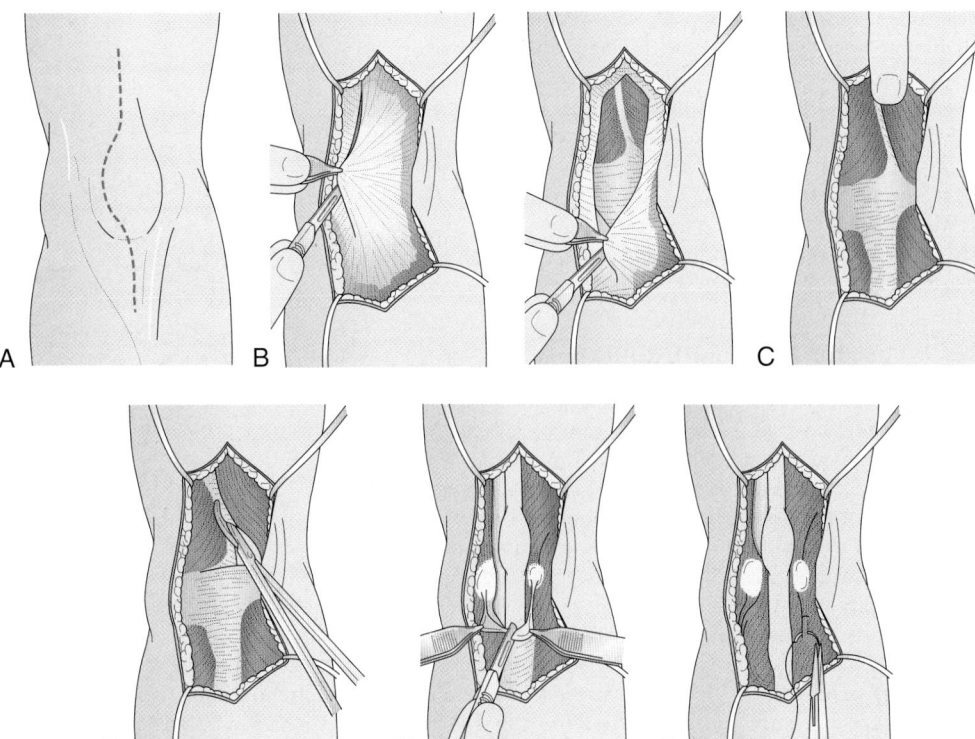

FIGURE 33.6 **A,** Skin incision for decompression of the ulnar nerve. Note that the incision stops short of the basilic vein. **B,** Incision of the deep fascia of the arm and forearm. **C,** Digital palpation of the medial intermuscular septum and the ulnar nerve in the arm. **D,** Section of the fascia over the ulnar nerve. **E,** Section of the dense fascia spanning the two heads of the flexor carpi ulnaris; a bulbous enlargement of the ulnar nerve is noticeable. **F,** The cut edges of the fascia are sewn over the flexor muscle on either side to prevent re-formation of the cubital tunnel.

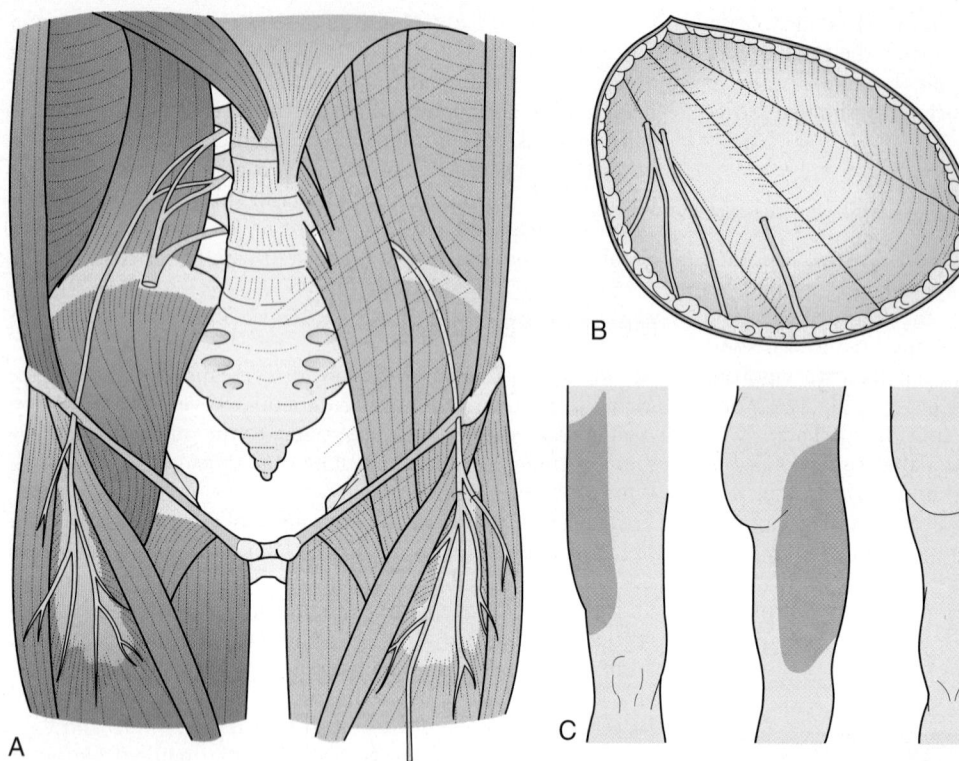

A

B

C

FIGURE 33.7 A, Origin, course, and distribution of the lateral femoral cutaneous nerve of the thigh. On the right side of the specimen, the psoas major muscle and the fasciae have been removed. Not all branches of the lumbar plexus are shown. **B,** Anatomy of the lateral femoral cutaneous nerve in the thigh. **C,** Distribution of the lateral femoral cutaneous nerve in the thigh.

loss may be present in the anterolateral thigh. Because the affected nerve is a purely cutaneous nerve, there are no motor abnormalities or reflex changes. Indeed, if they are present an alternative diagnosis should be entertained.

Electrodiagnostic tests are not helpful in establishing the diagnosis of meralgia paresthetica—they are used instead to exclude other disorders that involve the lumbosacral plexus or the cauda equina. The best test for confirmation of the clinical impression is a diagnostic nerve block, performed by injecting 5 mL of 0.5% lidocaine with epinephrine just medial to the anterior superior iliac spine. Complete relief of symptoms is generally predictive of a good operative result. The recently proposed pelvic compression test is supposed to release the nerve and provide relief of pain (Fig. 33.8).[85] It will also predict the result of surgery. The technique of sectioning of the inguinal ligament and decompression is shown in Figure 33.9.

Suprascapular Nerve Entrapment

Suprascapular neuropathy[86-88] results from injury to the suprascapular nerve and is typically due to direct compression or stretching that occurs with retraction of a large rotator cuff tear. The typical presentation includes deep and throbbing pain, located along the superior border of the scapula, and weakness of shoulder abduction despite a strong deltoid muscle (supraspinatus) and external rotation (infraspinatus). Muscle atrophy may be noticeable.

Of the two potential sites of constriction, the suprascapular notch is more common than the spinoglenoid notch (Fig. 33.10). The injury to the nerve at the suprascapular notch affects both supraspinatus and infraspinatus muscles but at the spinoglenoid notch only the infraspinatus.

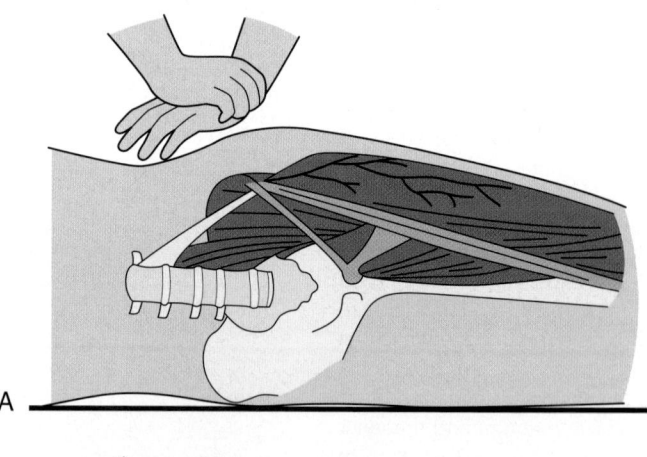

A

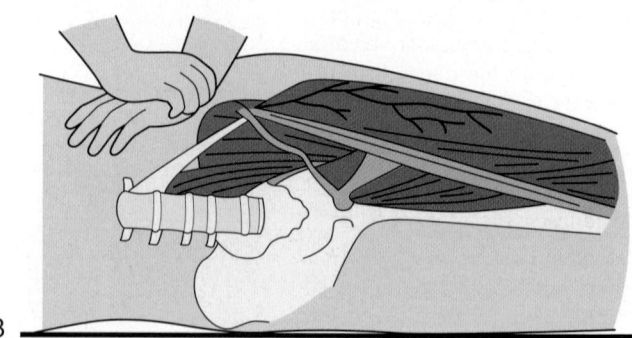

B

FIGURE 33.8 Pelvic compression test for meralgia paresthetica. **A,** The patient is positioned on his or her side on an examination couch. **B,** Downward pressure is applied and maintained for approximately 45 seconds. After 30 seconds, the patient is asked whether or not the symptoms have eased. A positive response constitutes a positive test result.

FIGURE 33.9 A, Skin incision conventionally used to expose the lateral femoral cutaneous nerve. **B,** Skin incision preferred by the author. **C,** Section of the fascia lata at the anterior border of the sartorius. **D,** Section of the superficial portion of the inguinal ligament. **E,** Section of the fascial bands posterior to the nerve.

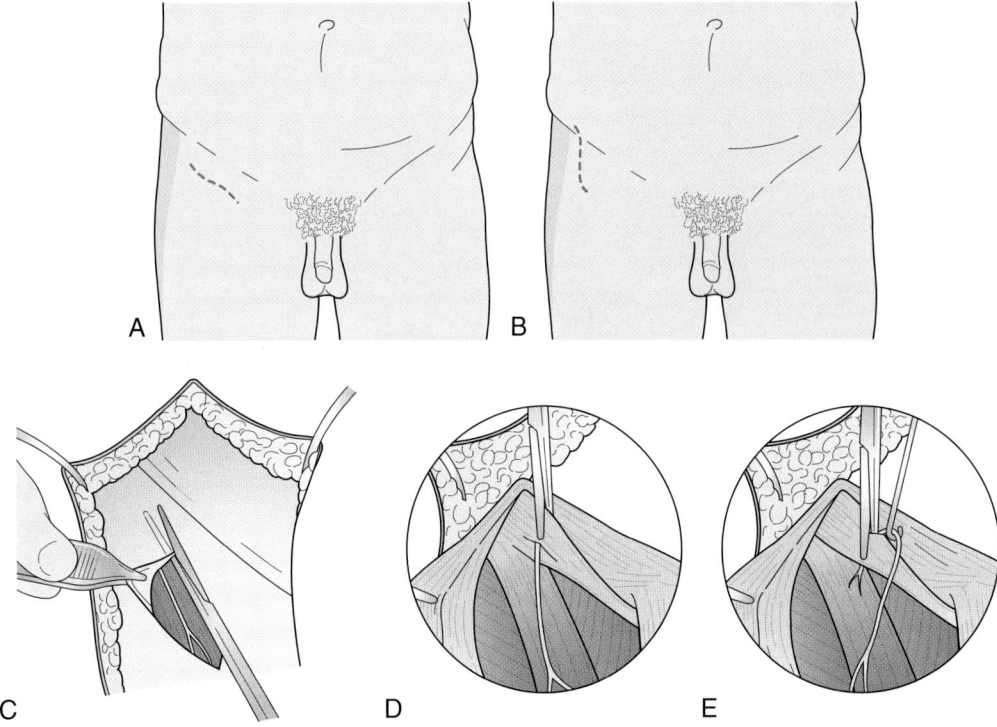

A   B   C   D   E

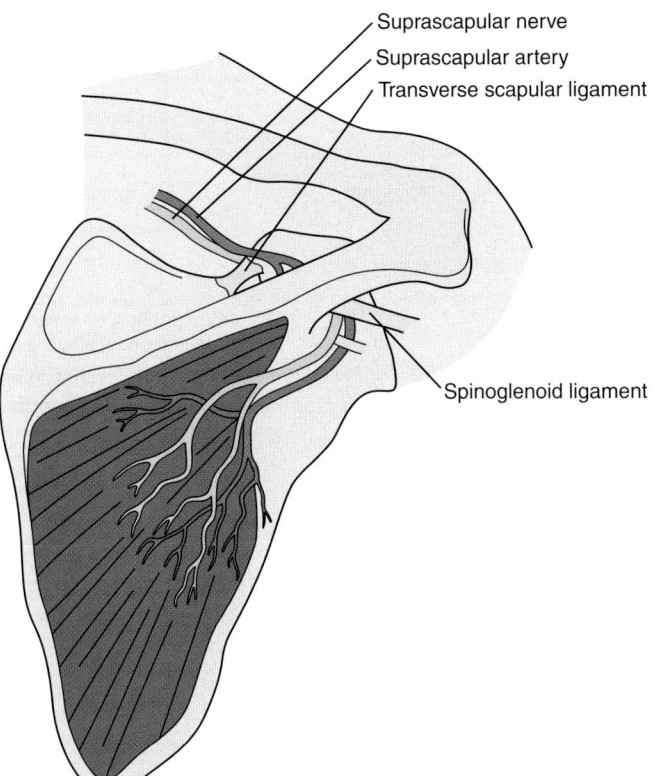

Suprascapular nerve
Suprascapular artery
Transverse scapular ligament
Spinoglenoid ligament

FIGURE 33.10 Suprascapular nerve anatomy.

Differential diagnosis includes various musculoskeletal conditions involving the shoulder as well as cervical radiculopathy affecting the C5 and the C6 roots, axillary neuropathy and neuralgic amyotrophy. Suprascapular entrapment neuropathy has often been overlooked as a source of shoulder pain.[88]

Additional diagnostic studies may include plain radiographs (to visualize the suprascapular notch), CT (looking for possible fractures, exuberant callus formation, osseous dysplasia, bone tumor, osseous variants of the suprascapular notch, ossification of the transverse scapular ligament), and MRI to evaluate the labrum, associated cysts, rotator cuff tendons, muscle fatty infiltration, or atrophy. Electromyography and nerve conduction studies may demonstrate denervation of the supraspinatus and infraspinatus muscle with resultant fibrillations and sharp waves. With nerve conduction velocity studies, the motor conduction velocities of the suprascapular nerve provide a latency value from the Erb point to the supraspinatus and infraspinatus muscles as well as a latency value between the muscles. Bilateral studies may be useful to enable a comparison of values.

The initial treatment for most isolated suprascapular nerve lesions not associated with a space-occupying lesion or a rotator cuff tear is advice to the patient about changing activities, taking nonsteroidal anti-inflammatory drugs, and using physical therapy.

Operative treatment may include decompression of the suprascapular nerve with or without repair of associated shoulder abnormalities. Decompression of the suprascapular notch can be done in an open fashion (Fig. 33.11)[87] or arthroscopically. At the time of this writing there are no prospective studies comparing operative and nonoperative treatment.[88]

Tarsal Tunnel Syndrome

Entrapment neuropathy of the tibial nerve is relatively rare. Consequently, it is often misdiagnosed. The most common site of tibial mononeuropathy is at the level of the tarsal tunnel where the tibial nerve can be compressed posterior and

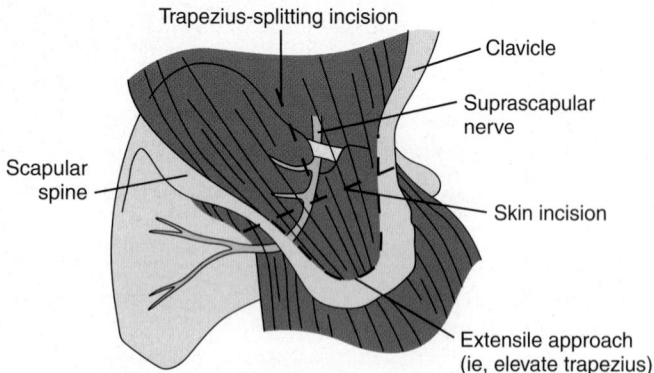

FIGURE 33.11 Open decompression of the suprascapular nerve at the suprascapular notch. With a posterior approach, a patient is placed prone with head supported by a horseshoe brace. Skin incision may be perpendicular or parallel to the scapular spine. After splitting the trapezius muscle, the supraspinatus muscle is then identified and divided in a similar fashion. Next, the suprascapular vessels are identified in their course above the transverse scapular ligament. At this point, a surgeon should be able to identify the nerve running under the ligament and dissect it. Then the ligament should be transected safely with a scalpel. *(From Laxton AW, Midha R. Suprascapular nerve palsy. In Midha R, Zager E, editors. Surgery of Peripheral Nerves. New York: Thieme; 2008.)*

inferior to the medial malleolus (Fig. 33.12). The typical constellation of symptoms includes pain and numbness in the sole of the foot and a sensation of tightness, cramping pain, and worsening of symptoms with prolonged standing or walking.[50]

The diagnosis is usually based on positive Tinel's sign and objective sensory loss in the territory of any of the terminal branches of the tibial nerve. The value of electrodiagnostic studies was recently evaluated but it was concluded that it was only of level C (poor evidence).[50]

As with other entrapment neuropathies, surgery should be considered when conservative treatment has failed or when there is a mass lesion. The technique involves exploration of the tarsal tunnel and release of the flexor retinaculum. As well as decompressing the tarsal tunnel roof, any space-occupying lesion should be removed. It is extremely important to follow the medial and the lateral plantar nerves well into the plantar aspect of the foot to check for any compression of these nerves by the abductor hallucis muscle or other fibrous bands. If these compressed nerves are encountered, they should be also released. An endoscopic technique has also been described.[89]

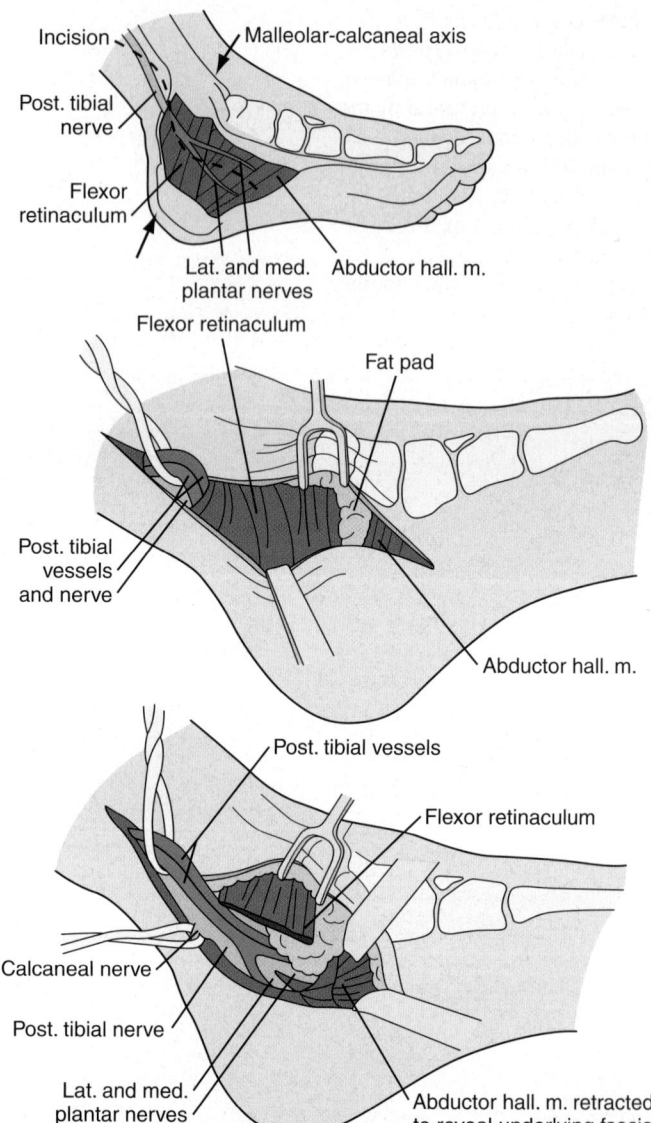

FIGURE 33.12 Relationship of the tibial nerve and its branches to the flexor retinaculum and abductor hallucis muscle and operative technique for treatment of tarsal tunnel syndrome.

ACKNOWLEDGMENT

The authors would like to acknowledge the late editor Setti Rengachary, MD, as one of the original authors of this chapter.

SELECTED KEY REFERENCES

American Academy of Orthopaedic Surgeons Work Group Panel. Clinical practice guidelines on the treatment of carpal tunnel syndrome. Available at www.aaos.org/research/guidelines/CTStreatmentguide.asp. Accessed Dec. 6, 2010.

Chung K. Treatment of ulnar nerve compression at the elbow. *J Hand Surg Am.* 2008;33:1625-1627.

Huang JH, Zager EL. Mini-open carpal tunnel decompression. *Neurosurgery.* 2004;54:397-400.

Jimenez DF, Loftus T. Endoscopic carpal tunnel release. In: Midha R, Zager E, eds. *Surgery of Peripheral Nerves.* New York: Thieme; 2008:100-104.

Ono S, Clapham PJ, Chung KC. Optimal management of carpal tunnel syndrome. *Intern J Gen Med.* 2010;3:255-261.

Please go to expertconsult.com to view the complete list of references.

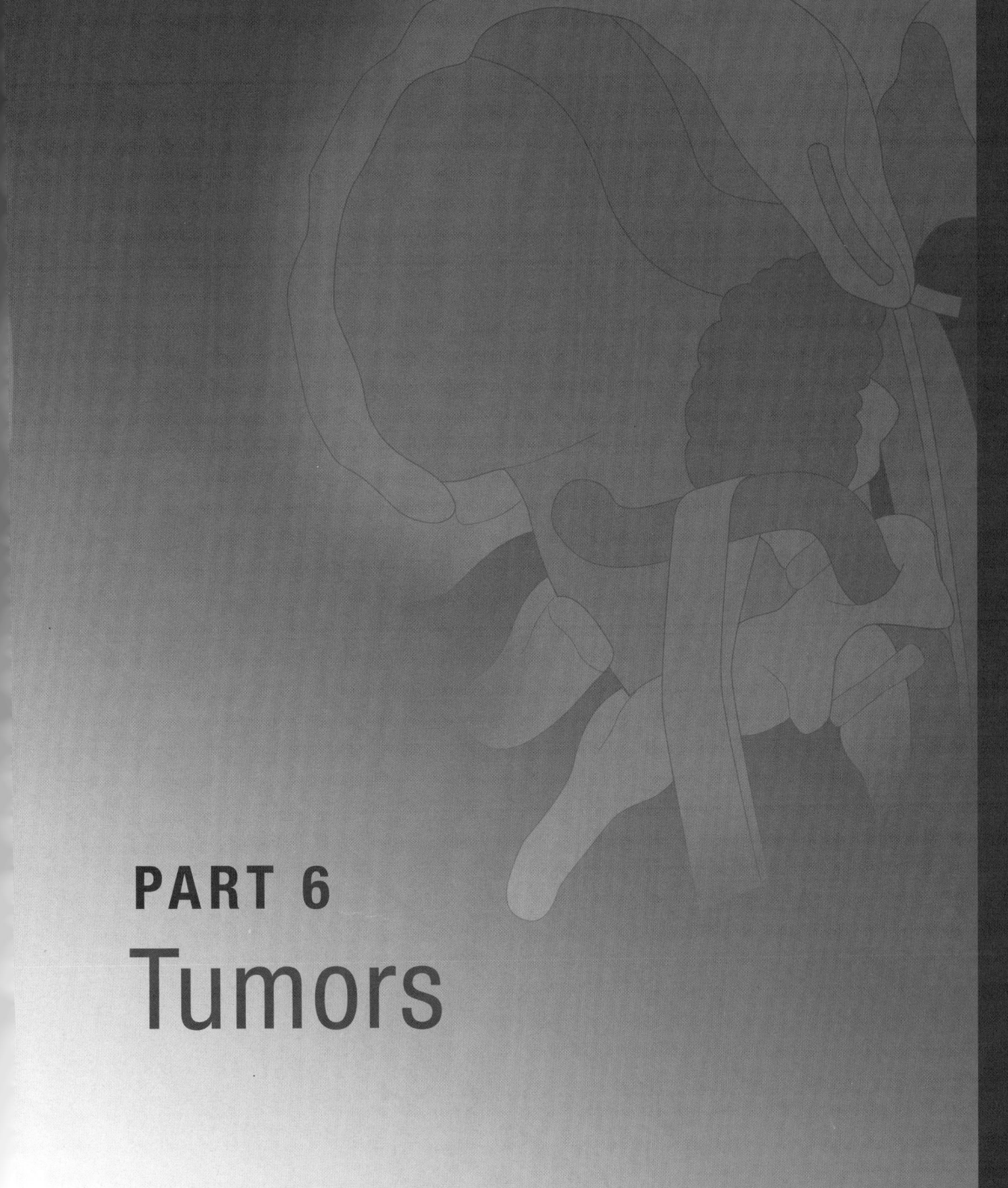

PART 6
Tumors

Low-Grade and High-Grade Gliomas

Nader Sanai, Mitchel S. Berger

CLINICAL PEARLS

- Low-grade gliomas (LGGs) account for 15% of primary adult tumors diagnosed, and in adults they mainly occur in supratentorial areas, particularly in the insular and supplementary motor areas.

- LGGs comprise astrocytomas, oligodendrogliomas, and oligoastrocytomas.

- Factors such as age less than 40 years, Karnofsky performance scale (KPS) score of 70 or greater, absence of contrast enhancement, and oligodendrogliomas are associated with a better prognosis for LGGs.

- The extent of surgical resection probably correlates with a better survival for LGGs, but resection must be tempered by their location close to the eloquent area. Motor-sensory mapping, language mapping, and diffusion tensor imaging should be used to assess tumors adjacent to critical regions.

- Postoperative radiotherapy is often used for LGGs and provides improved progression-free survival but does not extend overall survival.

- A better response to chemotherapy is seen in patients with oligodendrogliomas, which exhibit combined 1p/19q loss of heterozygosity.

- High-grade gliomas (malignant gliomas and glioblastoma multiforme [GBM]) may arise in progression from low-grade astrocytic tumors (secondary GBMs) or as de novo lesions (primary GBMs). There are distinct genetic differences between these two groups of tumors.

- Factors such as a younger age group, lower tumor histological grade, and higher KPS score are associated with a better prognosis for high-grade gliomas.

- The extent of resection (absence of class 1 evidence) has a probable influence on survival. Both radiotherapy and temozolomide chemotherapy significantly increase survival time of these patients.

- Advances in molecular markers may open avenues for new therapies.

LOW-GRADE GLIOMAS

A Perspective on Management

There are currently a number of considerations involved in the management of patients with low-grade gliomas (LGGs), which, for the purposes of this discussion, will be defined as World Health Organization (WHO) grade II gliomas. Advances in tumor biology, neuroimaging, and treatment paradigms have enabled the neurosurgeon to approach these patients with a better understanding of the disease entity and its natural history. However, many controversial issues remain unanswered. Diagnostic strategies previously considered reliable for LGG patients, including structural magnetic resonance imaging (MRI) and stereotactic biopsy, have more recently been shown to vary substantially with regard to specificity, sensitivity, and sampling error. Surgical management paradigms are also shifting, as mounting

evidence now highlights the predictive value of volumetric tumor burden for patient survival, the role of greater extent of resection in reducing malignant transformation rates, and the influence of tumor eloquence in determining resectability. Additionally, LGG-associated seizures are increasingly considered as a key determinant of quality of life, with electrocorticography being used as an effective surgical adjunct in this regard when seizures are medically refractory. Adjuvant therapies are also under renewed scrutiny. Although the utility of radiation therapy is clear, the timing and type of chemotherapy remain somewhat uncertain, as does the role of new molecular therapeutics. Taken together, these new innovations and controversies define the modern era of LGG management. Here we review the current literature in an effort to highlight high-impact developments that are changing our view of LGGs, as well as the pivotal studies that should guide neurosurgeons as they consider these many issues.

Epidemiology

LGGs are not uncommon, representing 15% of all primary adult brain tumors diagnosed each year. They are most frequent among white men and typically affect patients at a younger age than high-grade gliomas (fourth vs. sixth decade of life). Even though LGGs are diffusely distributed along a variety of supratentorial regions, they have a particular predilection for the insula and supplementary motor area. In contrast, LGGs rarely involve the cerebellum, brainstem, or spinal cord, as is commonly found in children. Most patients initially present with relatively good neurological function, and seizures are the most common symptom at presentation (80%). The only definite risk factor for LGG is previous exposure to ionizing radiation.[1] Hereditary factors do not play a substantial role in the development of LGGs, although these tumors are more common in patients with neurofibromatosis type 1 and Li-Fraumeni syndrome. From 15% to 20% of individuals with neurofibromatosis type 1 develop LGGs affecting the optic nerves, optic chiasm, and hypothalamus (optic pathway gliomas). Most of these gliomas are classified as WHO grade I tumors, although grade II LGGs can also occur in these locations.[2]

The etiology of adult LGGs is largely unknown and is thought to be multifactorial; various genetic, infectious, and immunological factors have been implicated. Glioma epidemiology studies have revealed few consistent findings, possibly because of small sample sizes in individual studies and differences between studies in patients, tumor types, and methods of classification. Individual studies generally have lacked samples of sufficient size to examine interactions, but larger consortium efforts have outlined several potential risk factors for gliomagenesis and outcome.[1] Data from the Surveillance, Epidemiology, and End Results (SEER) Program indicated that African Americans had similar or poorer survival than whites,[3] but those results were adjusted incompletely for important prognostic factors (e.g., age at diagnosis, treatment patterns, and tumor histological types). After adjustment, African Americans had a 40% higher risk of death from low-grade tumors compared with non-Hispanic whites.[4] Likewise, risks from specific neurocarcinogens have yet to be identified; however, the continued occurrence of brain tumor clusters leaves open the question of the effect and extent of their exposures. Observations of an association between drinking water and brain tumors suggest that ingestion of an environmental contaminant has an impact,[5-7] perhaps from chlorinated sources like chloroethane, a by-product of sewage treatment, or nitrate/nitrite contamination of drinking water supplies.

Recent epidemiological studies have also reported that adults with low- as well as high-grade gliomas are 1.5- to 4-fold less likely than control subjects to have allergies, which ranks the lack of allergies among the most consistent risk factors for glioma reported to date. In addition, an inverse relationship exists between immunoglobulin E (IgE), a biomarker for atopic allergy, and glioma risk. Interestingly, the strongest IgE-glioma association has been observed among the least prevalent allergen—food IgE. Low- and high-grade glioma patients with elevated levels of IgE are associated with an approximately 8 months' longer survival than individuals with lower or undetectable levels, demonstrating the potential clinical significance of such correlates.[8]

Classification

Tumor histological type remains the WHO's current standard for diagnosing glioma grade and subtype. As with all primary brain tumors, gliomas are classified according to their predominant cell type and graded based upon the presence or absence of necrosis, mitotic figures, nuclear atypia, and endothelial cell proliferation. Although grade I and II lesions are both categorized as LGGs, they follow radically different clinical courses and, for the purposes of this review, we will focus only on WHO grade II oligodendrogliomas, astrocytomas, and oligoastrocytomas that occur in adults. Among WHO grade II astrocytomas, cellularity is moderately increased and nuclear atypia is occasional, but mitoses, endothelial proliferation, and necrosis are not present. The prognostic value of defining subcategories of gliomas based upon these features remains unclear; nevertheless three histological subtypes are described: fibrillary, gemistocytic, and protoplasmic neoplastic astrocytes define these subtypes, each embedded in a loosely structured and microcystic tumor matrix. Fibrillary astrocytomas, the most frequent variant, demonstrate low cellularity with minimal nuclear atypia. Neoplastic fibrillary astrocytes are typically seen on a background of loosely structured tumor matrix that is extensively microcystic and expresses the intermediate filament marker, glial fibrillary acidic protein (GFAP), diffusely. Gemistocytic astrocytomas are histologically characterized by plump, glassy, eosinophilic cell bodies of angular shape. These gemistocytes consistently express GFAP, and the presence of abundant, compact glial filaments in the cytoplasm is also evident on electron microscopy. Interestingly, gemistocytic astrocytomas are reportedly more prone to malignant transformation than other histological counterparts, raising the possibility that they are not biologically low-grade gliomas and may belong in the high-grade glioma category. Protoplasmic astrocytomas, the rarest histological subtype, contain small-bodied astrocytes with few processes and scant GFAP expression. Mucoid degeneration and microcystic formation are common characteristics as well.

Oligodendrogliomas occur in the white matter and cortex of the cerebral hemispheres and show a monotonous pattern on low power with occasional nodules of higher cellularity. Unlike WHO grade II astrocytomas, the presence of low mitotic activity, vascular proliferation, and necrosis, including pseudopallisading necrosis, are insufficient by themselves to elevate the grade of WHO grade II oligodendrogliomas. Their nuclei are round and regular, and clear perinuclear halos are present in most paraffin-embedded specimens. This typical "fried egg" appearance is a formalin fixation artifact and is therefore not seen in frozen sections, smears, or rapidly fixed specimens. Oligoastrocytomas are a recognized category of LGGs, but are ill-defined, prone to subjectivity, and based on an unproven concept of dual differentiation of astrocytoma and oligodendroglioma as neoplastic processes.[9] Histologically, they are defined by a mixture of cells, some with oligodendroglioma features, and others resembling diffuse astrocytomas. Currently, there are no standardized immunohistochemistry or molecular panels to distinguish oligoastrocytomas from other LGGs.

Clinical Presentation

Patients with LGGs present with signs and symptoms of disease related to direct parenchyma infiltration; local tumor effects due to edema, hemorrhage, or tumor mass; or intracranial hypertension mediated by mass effects or ventricular obstruction. Although the onset of symptoms can be subtle and insidious, when patients become symptomatic, seizure is the most common presenting sign, occurring in up to 80% of cases;[10] this is probably due to the superficial localization and low growth rate of the tumor in many cases. Other, less common clinical presentations include headache, lethargy, and personality changes, although these symptoms, caused by raised intracranial pressure, are rare.

Prognostic Factors

Although substantial heterogeneity exists when profiling LGG patient outcome, several clinical factors are known to be predictive. Chief among those is age over 40 years, a predictive factor identified in multivariate analyses from two large, prospective trials.[11,12] Age at the time of LGG diagnosis is not only inversely correlated with time to progression, but tumor proliferative index may be higher among those older than 40 years as well.[13] Although the biology behind this association is unclear, one possibility is that age-related impairment of DNA repair mechanisms and the resulting acquisition of mutations may promote rapid progression after transformation occurs. Clinical presentation is another strong prognostic factor, as neurologically intact patients presenting with isolated seizures typically have a better performance status and overall prognosis. LGG patients who present with seizures also tend to be younger and have smaller tumors than those without seizure.[14]

An LGG preoperative prognostic scoring system developed at the University of California at San Francisco (UCSF) assigns a prognostic score based upon the sum of points assigned to the presence of each of the four following factors (1 point per factor): (1) location of tumor in presumed eloquent cortex, (2) Karnofsky performance scale (KPS) score 80 or less, (3) age more than 50 years, and (4) maximum diameter more than 4 cm. Cox proportional hazard modeling was used to confirm that the individual factors were associated with shorter overall survival (OS) and progression-free survival (PFS); and Kaplan-Meier curves estimated OS and PFS for the score groups.[15] Low-risk tumors are considered grades 0 or 1, and high-risk tumors are grade 4. This scoring system accurately predicted OS and PFS in a multi-institutional population of LGG patients.[16]

The median survival for oligodendrogliomas is approximately 15 years, a better prognosis than for astrocytomas, which have a median survival of 10 years.[17] Gemistocytic astrocytomas, a subtype of grade II astrocytomas, are more aggressive than predicted by grade.[18] Large tumors, nonlobar gliomas, and tumors that cross the midline are associated with a short survival and a high rate of malignant transformation.[11] Preoperative tumor burden is also associated with less extensive resection, which in turn portends poorer outcome.[19] Proliferative index has also been inversely related with LGG outcome, as has contrast enhancement.[20]

Recent work in glioma outcomes research also suggests that more unconventional factors may play a role in LGG patient outcome. For example, among patients with non-anaplastic oligodendroglial tumors, younger age and surgical resection versus biopsy were significantly associated with better survival, as expected. Interestingly, however, those patients who were college graduates also showed significantly better survival in age-adjusted comparisons.[21] Further consideration of impact of marital status, education, and other social factors in glioma survival may be warranted, as these factors also appear to be significant in predicting high-grade glioma outcome.

Efforts to synthesize LGG risk factors into distinct prognostic classes have led to four categories of patients: (1) younger patients (18-40 years of age) with a good performance status (KPS score $\geq$ 70) have a median survival of more than 10 years; (2) younger patients with a poor performance status (KPS score < 70) and older patients (>40 years of age) with a good performance status and no contrast enhancement had a median survival of more than 7 years; (3) older patients with a good performance status and with contrast enhancement had a median survival of less than 4 years; and (4) older patients with a poor performance status had a median survival of only 12 months.[22] It remains unclear, however, how tumor extent of resection impacts the predictive value of each category following resection because it was not evaluated in that study.

Similarly, the EORTC (European Organization for Research and Treatment of Cancer) developed a prognostic scoring system based on two large, randomized, multicenter trials with more than 600 patients.[11,12] In their multivariate analysis, age older than 40 years, astrocytic tumor type, tumor size greater than 6 cm, tumor crossing the midline, and neurological deficit at diagnosis were retained in the model. A favorable prognostic score was defined as no more than two of these adverse factors and was associated with a median survival of 7.7 years. The presence of three to five prognostic factors was associated with a median survival of 3.2 years (95% confidence interval [CI] = 3.0, 4.0).

Diagnostic Imaging

The 1.5-tesla MRI remains the imaging gold standard for noninvasive identification and diagnosis of LGGs, although the emergence of 3-tesla magnets has improved image resolution considerably.[23] LGGs are characteristically homogeneously isointense to hypointense on T1-weighted images and hyperintense on T2-weighted images. The epicenters of low-grade astrocytomas are typically within the white matter, whereas oligodendrogliomas can be more superficial and will occasionally expand the adjacent gyrus. Contrast enhancement is uncommon, but more often is seen in oligodendrogliomas (25-50%). Calcifications are apparent in 20% of lesions and are characterized by foci of high T1 and low T2 signals. Vasogenic edema and mass effect are uncommon because of the slow-growing nature of these tumors. Rarely, large LGGs will involve three or more cerebral lobes (gliomatosis cerebri). Diffusion tensor imaging has proved to be an essential adjunct to structural imaging for both preoperative planning and intraoperative neuronavigation. Specification of functional tract deflection around a lesion can not only alter the operative approach, but can dictate the limits of resection. Modalities such as functional magnetic resonance imaging (fMRI) and magnetoencephalography (MEG) can aid in preoperative planning by identifying these functional pathways, although these techniques remain too imprecise for complex functions such as language mapping, as their sensitivity (positron emission tomography [PET], 75%; fMRI, 81%) and specificity (PET, 81%; fMRI, 53%) remain suboptimal.[24-27] For the identification of peritumoral language pathways, direct intraoperative stimulation mapping remains the gold standard. Intraoperative MRI is another operating room technology that may impact LGG outcome. Through real-time guidance, it allows for localization of tumors and their margins, and facilitates continuous assessment of surgical progress. Studies of LGG patients who underwent resection in an intraoperative MRI suite report encouraging results in terms of achieving greater extent of resection.[28,29]

However, using standard structural imaging paradigms, the decision to presume low-grade histological type on the basis of a nonenhancing lesion is a common mistake. For patients with supratentorial mass lesions that exhibit the typical imaging features of LGG, structural MRI has a false positive rate as high as 50% when attempting to predict the histological diagnosis of astrocytoma.[30] This risk of anaplasia in MRI nonenhancing lesions increases significantly with patient age.[31] Thus, observation of LGGs is not a prudent option, and early tissue diagnosis is essential. These misleading imaging features are likely due to the intrinsic heterogeneity of LGGs, a characteristic evident on physiological MRI such as magnetic resonance spectroscopy (MRS), which can demonstrate pockets of high-grade populations nested within the tumor stroma.[32] Thus, stereotactic biopsies should be planned using MRS guidance to target putative high-grade components in nonenhancing tumors.

Next-generation structural MRI technologies have recently focused on preoperatively defining LGGs. Microscopic molecular movement of water in tumor tissue reflects tissue properties that include varying levels of structural alterations, tumor cellularity, and vasogenic edema. Diffusion-weighted MRI (DWI) uses strong gradients to probe the structure of biological tissues at a microscopic level by measuring the brownian motion of water molecules. Acquiring data with gradients in three directions allows the calculation of the apparent diffusion coefficient (ADC), while acquiring data with gradients in six or more directions allows the calculation of the ADC and the fractional anisotropy (FA). Recent work using these emerging imaging paradigms attempted radiographic prediction of specific LGG subtypes. Interestingly, initial attempts demonstrated a significant difference in the ADC and FA values between newly diagnosed patients with grade II oligodendrogliomas and astrocytomas, and patients with the heterogeneous grade II oligoastrocytomas had values that fell in between.[33] However, although ADC has been suggested to correlate to cell density in a mixed population of glioma patients, it remains unclear whether this parameter is what drives its correlation with specific LGG subtypes.

The emergence of physiological imaging techniques has indeed added a new dimension to LGG diagnosis and targeting.[34] Proton MRS imaging (¹H-MRSI) is another emerging modality that identifies the distribution of cellular metabolite levels. Five classes of molecules are generally observed in brain spectra: N-acetylaspartate (NAA); free choline and choline-containing compounds, including phosphocholine and glycerophosphocholine (Cho); creatine and phosphocreatine (Cr); lactate (Lac); and lipid (Lip). Using MRS, typical spectra of LGG include a dominant choline peak (reflecting increased membrane synthesis) with low-intensity N-acetylaspartate (reflecting decreased neuronal elements) and no quantifiable lipid or lactate (suggesting an absence of necrosis or hypoxia, respectively; both features of high-grade gliomas). The choline peak may be associated with cellular density and cellular proliferation, thereby improving selection of targets for biopsy. Normalized creatine/phosphocreatine levels (tCr) of LGGs are a significant prognostic factor for progression-free survival, as well as malignant progression-free survival.[35] Newly introduced three-dimensional (3D) techniques allow whole anatomical regions to be quantified metabolically, correlating well with the region of T2 hyperintensity, as well as with tumor extension along white matter tracts.[36] Three-dimensional MRS may also have the potential to evaluate the proliferation activity of LGGs and identify potentially more aggressive clinical behavior.[37] There is less convincing evidence, however, that MRS is sufficient for monitoring and follow-up of patients with suspected LGG.[38] In some instances, MRS can also be used to discriminate radiation necrosis from tumor progression, as well as to monitor treatment progress.[39]

Among low-grade astrocytomas, measurement of relative cerebral blood volume (rCBV) derived from dynamic susceptibility-weighted perfusion contrast-enhanced MRI (DSC-MRI) correlates well with tumor behavior and patient survival.[40] For these tumors, rCBV specifies regional tumor vascularity and expression of vascular endothelial growth factor (VEGF), two critical factors driving tumor growth.[41] Most low-grade astrocytomas demonstrate slightly higher rCBV than normal tissue (1.5), with an increase in rCBV (1.75-2.0) indicating the evolution of a more aggressive tumor and often preceding the emergence of enhancement.[42] Low-grade astrocytoma rCBV measurements also correlate well with time to progression, raising the possibility that DSC-MRI can predict the risk of transformation.[43] In contrast, however, low-grade oligodendrogliomas have a paradoxically high rCBV, confounding the strict reliability of this modality for preoperative assessment. Similar MRI techniques such as quantitative analysis of whole-tumor gadolinium enhancement are also predictive of malignant transformation for likely the same reasons.[44]

Radiographic quantification of tumor metabolism cannot only identify malignant transformation in LGG,[45] but it can also be employed to guide stereotactic biopsies. On positron emission tomography (PET) using fluorodeoxyglucose (¹⁸F-FDG), LGGs are hypometabolic, a feature that commonly distinguishes them from high-grade gliomas. In contrast, uptake of radiolabeled amino acids is increased in approximately two thirds of LGGs, and a prognostic role for amino acid PET in LGG has been proposed. O-(2-¹⁸F-fluoroethyl)-L-tyrosine (¹⁸F-FET) is a new PET tracer that, in contrast to other amino acid tracers, fulfills all requirements for routine clinical application, similar to the widely used ¹⁸F-FDG. Accordingly, recent work indicates that baseline amino acid uptake on ¹⁸F-FET PET and a diffuse versus circumscribed tumor pattern on MRI are strong predictors for the outcome of patients with LGG.[45] A comparable technique using 3′-deoxy-3′-¹⁸F-fluorothymidine (FLT), FLT PET, is a useful marker of cellular proliferation that correlates with regional variation in cellular proliferation; however, it is unable to identify the margin of LGGs.[46]

Surgery and the Value of Extent of Resection

In the past 2 decades, mounting evidence in the literature suggests that a more extensive surgical resection of LGG is associated with a more favorable life expectancy. In addition to providing longer overall survival, more aggressive resections for LGG can also influence the risk of malignant transformation, raising the possibility that a surgical intervention can alter the natural history of the disease.[47] These associations are evident not only within the general hemispheric LGG population,[19,48] but also for specific LGGs limited to certain subregions, such as insular LGGs.[49,50] An overall review of the modern neurosurgical literature reveals 24 studies[12,19,20,28,49,51-69] since 1990 that have applied statistical analysis to examine the efficacy of extent of resection in improving survival and delaying tumor progression among LGG patients. Six of these studies included volumetric analysis of extent of resection.[12,28,49,57,60,70] Of the nonvolumetric studies, 15 demonstrated evidence supporting extent of resection as a statistically significant predictor of either 5-year survival or 5-year progression-free survival. These studies were published from 1990 to 2009 and most commonly employed a combination of multivariate and univariate analyses to determine statistical significance. Interestingly, of the three nonvolumetric studies that did not support extent of resection as a predictor of patient outcome, none of these reports evaluated progression-free survival, but instead focused solely on 5-year survival.

Special Considerations: Malignant Transformation

Malignant degeneration of LGGs is a special consideration for these patients, as it carries with it a dramatically worse prognosis. Interestingly, the documented incidence of LGG transformation ranges from 17% to 73% in clinical studies published over the previous 15 years,[19,20,48,64,67,71-75] suggesting a high level of variability. Defining the timing of this phenomenon is equally elusive, as reported median intervals range from 2.1 to 10.1 years based upon studies published in the past 15 years.[19,20,48,67,76,77] Several recent studies have examined malignant transformation in the context of extent of resection, reasoning that the risk of progression increases with tumor burden. In a study of hemispheric LGGs, greater preoperative tumor volume was significantly associated with shorter malignant progression-free survival,[19] suggesting that larger tumors at presentation may have an inherently faster growth rate, and thus recur faster in the setting of a gross total resection or continue to grow faster in the setting of a subtotal resection. Tumor growth rates were also studied among 143 consecutive adult LGGs, in which a median survival of 5.16 years was associated with a growth rate of 8 mm per year or more and a median survival of more than 15.0 years was seen with a growth rate less than 8 mm per year.[78] Others have also evaluated LGG growth rate, demonstrating that sequential measurement of LGG volume allows accurate determination of growth rates and identification of patients whose tumors are at high risk for early transformation.[79] Six-month

tumor growth also may help to predict outcome in patients with LGG better than parameters derived from perfusion- or diffusion-weighted MRI.[80] Similarly, within the insula, the interval to malignant progression among grade II gliomas is longer in patients who have undergone greater resections.[49] As with hemispheric LGGs, the volume of residual tumor in the insula serves as a predictor of malignant transformation. Thus, these studies represent a potential shift in our concept of aggressive glioma resection, as the ability to manipulate the natural history of these tumors makes a case for earlier intervention and argues against the validity of a simple biopsy procedure or a wait-and-watch approach.

Mapping Functional Pathways

The principle that patient outcome improves with greater extent of resection must be tempered by the potential for functional loss following a radical resection. To this end, MRI neuronavigational techniques not only facilitate greater resection, but embedding of DTI-based tractography can prevent inadvertent resection of adjacent subcortical pathways.[81,82] In a recent study of 238 glioma patients randomized to DTI-based imaging versus traditional MRI neuronavigation without DTI, postoperative motor deterioration occurred in 32.8% of control cases, whereas it occurred in only 15.3% of the study cases. Among LGGs in this study, the findings did not impact patient survival, but demonstrated the utility of this technology in maximizing tumor resection while minimizing morbidity. Similarly, for patients with gliomas that are located within or adjacent to the rolandic cortex and, thus, the descending motor tracts, stimulation mapping of cortical and subcortical pathways enables the surgeon to identify these descending motor pathways during tumor removal and achieve an acceptable rate of permanent morbidity in these high-risk functional areas.[83-85] In a recent study where 46.1% of LGGs had a complete resection, new immediate postoperative motor deficits were documented in 59.3% of patients in whom a subcortical motor tract was identified intraoperatively and in 10.9% of those in whom subcortical tracts were not observed. However, permanent deficits were observed in 6.5% and 3.5%, respectively.[84] In another study of subcortical motor pathways in 294 patients who underwent surgery for hemispheric gliomas, 14 patients (4.8%) had a persistent motor deficit after 3 months. Interestingly, patients whose subcortical pathways were identified intraoperatively were more prone to develop an additional transient or permanent motor deficit (27.5% vs. 13.1%).[85] In another study with an 87% gross or subtotal resection rate, the overall neurological morbidity rate was 5% after using cortical motor mapping.[86] Thus, collectively the recent literature suggests that intraoperative motor mapping can safely identify corridors for resection, as well as define the limits of tumor resection.

Importantly, prediction of cortical language sites through classic anatomical criteria is inadequate in light of the significant individual variability of cortical organization, the distortion of cerebral topography from tumor mass effect, and the possibility of functional reorganization through plasticity mechanisms. A consistent finding among all cortical language stimulation studies has been significant individual variability.[87] Specifically, speech arrest is variably located and can go well beyond the classic anatomical boundaries of Broca's area for motor speech.[87] This variability has also been further confirmed by studies designed to preoperatively predict the location of speech arrest based upon the type of frontal opercular anatomy.[88] Similarly, for temporal lobe language sites, the distance from the temporal pole to the area of language function can vary from 3 to 9 cm.[89] Neural plasticity mechanisms also introduce an element of unpredictability to functional pathway localization. The capacity for the brain to reorganize itself is critical for the process of functional recovery in patients following central nervous system injury. Interestingly, more progressive lesions such as LGGs also induce large-scale functional reshaping. This reorganization is thought to explain why slow infiltrative LGGs within the eloquent areas often do not induce detectable neurological deficits[90] and must be anticipated when reoperating on patients with LGGs within or near functional pathways.[91]

Furthermore, because functional tissue can be located within the tumor nidus, the standard surgical principle of debulking tumor from within is not always safe.[92] In the largest reported series of intraoperative language mapping for gliomas, 4 of 243 surviving patients (1.6%) had a persistent new language deficit at 6 months. Among LGGs, the gross total resection rate was 51.6%, suggesting that intraoperative language mapping remains the most effective technique in maximizing resection while minimizing language morbidity.[87] In a recent LGG study designed to identify prognosticators of survival and tumor progression, four variables (areas of eloquence, patient age >50 years, KPS score ≤80, and lesion diameter >4 cm) were predictive of survival on multivariate analysis and were incorporated into a scoring system (UCSF Low-Grade Glioma Scoring System)[15] that was externally validated.[16] Importantly, the predictive value of tumor eloquence made evident in this study demonstrates the need for mapping functional pathways whenever an LGG is presumed eloquent. Consequently, preliminary evidence suggests that the utilization of intraoperative stimulation mapping in the resection of eloquent LGGs is associated with an improvement in overall survival.

Adjuvant Treatment

The determination of adjuvant treatment of LGG is still challenging and is based mainly on the best definition of prognostic factors. While watchful waiting remains an option for low-risk LGG patients, the optimal treatment has yet to be defined for those at risk of rapid progression and malignant transformation. In a recent prospective trial of 111 RTOG LGG patients, preoperative tumor diameter 4 cm or greater, astrocytoma/oligoastrocytoma histological type, and residual tumor 1 cm or greater according to MRI each was predictive of significantly higher recurrence rates.[69] Many clinical trials are evaluating adjuvant treatments stratified by these risk groups.

Chemotherapy

The role of chemotherapy for LGG remains to be defined. Several recent studies have explored upfront treatment (i.e., immediately following resection) of newly diagnosed LGGs with chemotherapy using either procarbazine/CCNU/vincristine (PCV) or temozolomide.[93-96] Collectively, these phase II trials provide little conclusive evidence for clinical efficacy in terms of overall survival, although measuring response in the absence of contrast enhancement is a challenge. In select instances, preliminary evidence suggests that temozolomide is associated with improved quality of life, better seizure control, and longer progression-free survival.[93,97,98] Furthermore, in a limited trial of 16 low-grade oligodendroglioma patients, data suggesting improved tumor control rates were also reported using PCV chemotherapy.[94] However, whether there is a true advantage in treating patients with upfront chemotherapy compared to initial radiotherapy is currently under investigation. Consequently, it remains controversial whether upfront chemotherapy should be offered to LGG patients, although for patients with bulky disease or neurological deficit, this is a reasonable strategy prior to implementation of radiotherapy.

For temozolomide, early data suggest that the best responders, if any, appear to be patients with oligodendrogliomas and mixed oligoastrocytomas. Combined 1p/19q loss of heterozygosity is significantly associated with a higher rate of and longer response to the methylating agent temozolomide.[99] The EORTC study 26971 on first-line temozolomide chemotherapy demonstrated this with a reported 50% response rate for recurrent oligodendroglioma patients.[100] Dose-intense continuous dosing schedules have also been investigated and were proved to be feasible.[101,102] Using a prolonged temozolomide schedule, patients with progressive or recurrent LGGs also have an overall response rate of 30% and a progression-free rate of 56.7%.[103]

Among PCV chemotherapy trials, the RTOG study 9802 randomized high-risk patients (age >40 or subtotal resection) to postoperative radiotherapy with or without subsequent adjuvant PCV. After stratification by age, histological type, KPS score, and presence/absence of contrast enhancement, patients were randomized to either radiotherapy alone (54 Gy) or radiotherapy followed by six cycles of standard dose PCV. With a median follow-up of more than 4 years, no advantage for the administration of PCV was evident, even in the group of high-risk LGG patients.[104] Ongoing clinical trials are evaluating the role of concurrent and adjuvant temozolomide for high-risk patients with LGG.

Radiation Therapy

Radiation therapy is often used postoperatively for many LGG patients. The EORTC study 22845 revealed an advantage for immediate postoperative radiotherapy in terms of progression-free survival (5.3 years compared with 3.4 years), but not for overall survival, among LGG patients.[105] The factors that influence the timing of radiation therapy relate to speed of progression and the possibility of late toxicity to normal brain. Higher doses of radiation (>45-50 Gy) have also failed to demonstrate an improved outcome and are associated with increased late toxicity.[11] In an ongoing international study (EORTC 22033–26033), LGG patients with high-risk disease or with progressive tumors are randomized between primary radiotherapy or primary chemotherapy with low-dose temozolomide for up to 1 year (12 cycles). In addition to clinical factors, these patients are stratified according to 1p/19q status and their tissue will also be surveyed for other molecular markers of interest in the hopes of generating a predictable profile for radiation response. Beyond fractionated radiotherapy, stereotactic radiosurgery has also been raised as a possibility for treating LGGs, although no data exist to support this strategy beyond small, retrospective case series.[106-110]

HIGH-GRADE GLIOMAS

Pathogenesis

Glioblastoma multiforme (GBM) may arise through two distinct pathways of neoplastic progression. Tumors that progress from lower grade (II or III) astrocytic tumors, termed *secondary* or *type 1 GBMs*, typically display both well-differentiated and poorly differentiated foci. Secondary GBMs develop in younger patients (fifth to sixth decade), with time to progression from lower-grade lesions ranging from months to decades. In contrast, primary type 2 GBMs develop in older individuals (sixth to seventh decade), have short clinical histories (less than 3 months), and arise de novo without any evidence of a lower-grade precursor. Primary and secondary GBMs also harbor distinct molecular genetic abnormalities: Primary GBMs are characterized by relatively high frequencies of EGFR amplification, PTEN deletion, and CDKN2A (p16) loss, whereas secondary GBMs often contain TP53 mutations, especially those involving codons 248 and 273 or G:C → A:T mutations at CpG sites.[111]

Pathology

Even within the conventional GBM category, the cellular composition is heterogeneous and may include fibrillary, gemistocytic, and occasional giant cells. Neoplastic fibrillary astrocytes contain enlarged, elongated to irregularly shaped, hyperchromatic nuclei, scant cytoplasm, and variable glial fibrillary acidic protein (GFAP)—immunoreactive processes that form a loose, fibrillary matrix. Such tumors may also harbor mucin-rich microcystic spaces. Because of cross-sectioning of spindled or cylindrical nuclei, neoplastic fibrillary astrocytes may also appear to have occasional rounded nuclear profiles, raising the differential diagnosis of high-grade oligodendroglial neoplasms (WHO grade III anaplastic oligodendroglioma and WHO grade III anaplastic mixed oligoastrocytoma). Nevertheless, a significant fraction of cells should have classic cytological appearance (e.g., round uniform cells with sharp nuclear membranes and bland chromatin) before one invokes an oligodendroglial component in the diagnosis.[112]

Multimodal Management

In general, high-grade gliomas (HGGs) have a poor prognosis, are rapidly progressive, and are resistant to therapy. Their infiltrating nature means they cannot be completely excised and the majority will recur within 2 cm of their original location. Median survival is around 1 year for GBM, 2 years for anaplastic astrocytoma (AA), and 5 years for anaplastic oligodendroglioma (AO). Management is based around symptomatic relief and increasing survival. The first option is surgery, which is usually required in some form for histological diagnosis. This may entail a biopsy or more likely aggressive resection. Radiotherapy is the treatment

with the greatest evidence base for effect and this is now part of standard management, resulting in an increase in median survival from 3 to 4 months to 9 to 10 months.[113] The other principal therapy is glucocorticosteroids, which have an important role in the reduction of peritumoral edema and can produce a marked improvement in neurological symptoms and survival by themselves.

Chemotherapy has been used as part of initial therapy as either single-agent or multiagent regimens to try to maximize penetration through the blood-brain barrier and tumor responsiveness. A meta-analysis of chemotherapy in HGG has demonstrated an improvement in survival with PCV chemotherapy (HR [hazard ratio] 0.85 CI [confidence interval] 0.78 to 0.92, $P < 0.0001$) with an overall improvement of 2 months in median survival to 12 months. It is not clear whether the gain in survival reflects a useful period of good quality of life. In grade III gliomas two recent randomized controlled trials did not demonstrate an increase in survival with PCV.[114,115] Temozolomide is effective as primary therapy for GBM. It prolongs survival and time to progression without a significant risk of early adverse events. It appears to be most effective in young and fit patients with GBM who have had debulking surgery. These results are based on two randomized controlled trials of 703 patients in total.[116,117] Temozolomide is also effective as therapy for recurrent disease, where it increases time to progression without an increase in adverse events. There are still some reservations with these data as the trials were not blinded or placebo controlled, while quality of life data could be further expanded upon.

The Value of Extent of Resection

Microsurgical resection remains a critical therapeutic modality for HGGs. However, there remains no general consensus in the literature regarding the efficacy of extent of resection in improving patient outcome. With the exception of WHO grade I tumors, gliomas are difficult to cure with surgery alone, and the majority of patients will experience some form of tumor recurrence.

For all HGGs, the identification of universally applicable prognostic factors and treatment options remains a great challenge. Among the many tumor- and treatment-related parameters, only patient age and tumor histological type have been identified as reliable predictors of patient prognosis, although functional status can also be statistically significant. While the importance of glioma resection in obtaining tissue diagnosis and to alleviate symptoms is clear, a lack of class I evidence prevents similar certainty in assessing the influence of extent of resection. In fact, despite significant advances in brain tumor imaging and intraoperative technology during the past 15 years, the effect of glioma resection in extending tumor-free progression and patient survival remains unknown.

Thus, beyond establishing the histological diagnosis and decompressing tumor mass effect, microsurgical resection of glioblastomas remains controversial in value. However, in the past decade, mounting evidence suggests that surgical extent of resection is associated with better glioblastoma patient survival. Although these data have helped establish a fragile, and frequently debated, consensus that glioblastoma resection improves patient outcome, the impracticality of conducting a randomized clinical trial limits our ability to quantify the value of greater tumor resection.

Among the 16 HGG studies demonstrating a statistically significant survival benefit with greater extent of resection, this prognostic factor was determined through univariate analysis in 11 studies. Additionally, multivariate analysis confirmed that extent of resection was a significant patient survival prognostic factor in 12 studies. Of note, three studies demonstrated conflicting statistical results between univariate and multivariate analyses of patient survival, although it was the authors' interpretation in all three series that their findings supported extent of resection as a predictor of survival. Time to tumor progression was another commonly used endpoint in extent of resection studies. However, only five studies demonstrated statistical significance through either univariate or multivariate analysis. Overall, however, our analysis of these 28 HGG studies strongly suggested an implicit benefit in terms of patient survival with greater extent of resection. Accordingly, the mean survival following gross-total versus subtotal resection in the HGG studies differed by nearly 3 months.

It is clear that a lack of class I evidence prevents the establishment of convincing criteria guiding either low- or high-grade glioma extent of resection. While careful analysis reveals a growing correlation between greater extent of resection and patient survival, it remains each practitioner's responsibility to determine if the magnitude and quality of evidence are sufficient to influence practice standards. In our practice, extent of resection is based on the functional nature of the tissue, not on its perceived biological aggressiveness.

Many critical questions remain unanswered in the literature regarding the value of extent of resection for HGGs. It is unclear whether the emerging correlation between aggressive glioma resection and survival holds true for both first-time and recurrent operations. The effect of extent of resection for different ages and histological subtypes must also be studied, although at least one study has addressed the former. Additionally, the question of the impact of surgical resection on patient survival must be asked in the context of current prognostic factors (e.g., 1p/19q and MGMT-methylation status) as well as in the context of specific adjuvant therapy regimens. Future studies linking extent of resection and outcome should use these markers as stratification factors in the analysis. Similarly, the efficacy of adjuvant therapies must also be studied in the context of extent of resection.

CONCLUSIONS

For the neurosurgeon, treatment of gliomas represents an opportunity to intervene early and impact outcome. Advances in molecular markers, diagnostic imaging, operative techniques and technologies, and adjuvant therapies have collectively pushed the envelope toward improved quality of life and survival. Stereotactic biopsy remains a source of sampling error, but can be enhanced through metabolic imaging. Extent of resection has been increasingly shown to correlate with improved outcome, as well as with better seizure control and reduced malignant transformation rates. Recent advances in our molecular understanding of the disease may open new avenues for novel therapy, including mTOR inhibitors currently in trial. Nevertheless, significant challenges remain; chief among them are the substantial clinical and biological heterogeneity that still exists within gliomas. Such limitations not only emphasize the need for further investigation into the tumor subsets, but also the value of clinical studies examining the forces shaping tumor recurrence and transformation.

SELECTED KEY REFERENCES

Abrey LE, Childs BH, Paleologos N, et al. High-dose chemotherapy with stem cell rescue as initial therapy for anaplastic oligodendroglioma: long-term follow-up. *Neuro-Oncology.* 2006;8:183-188.

Athanassiou H, Synodinou M, Maragoudakis E, et al. Randomized phase II study of temozolomide and radiotherapy compared with radiotherapy alone in newly diagnosed glioblastoma multiforme. *J Clin Oncol.* 2005;23:2372-2377.

Chaichana KL, McGirt MJ, Laterra J, et al. Recurrence and malignant degeneration after resection of adult hemispheric low-grade gliomas. *J Neurosurg.* 2009;111(2):203-210.

Claus EB, Black PM. Survival rates and patterns of care for patients diagnosed with supratentorial low-grade gliomas: data from the SEER program, 1973-2001. *Cancer.* 2006;106:1358-1363.

Karim AB, Afra D, Cornu P, et al. Randomized trial on the efficacy of radiotherapy for cerebral low-grade glioma in the adult: European Organization for Research and Treatment of Cancer Study 22845 with the Medical Research Council study BRO4: an interim analysis. *Int J Radiat Oncol Biol Phys.* 2002;52:316-324.

Please go to expertconsult.com to view the complete list of references.

35 Metastatic Brain Tumors

Juanita M. Celix, Daniel L. Silbergeld

CLINICAL PEARLS

- A metastatic brain tumor means that the patient has stage IV cancer, with median survival of under 1 year.

- When a patient presents with a new brain metastasis, without a known primary site, the chance of finding the primary tumor during the patient's lifetime is approximately 50%.

- As long as brain metastases undergo some form of treatment, the vast majority of patients will succumb to progression of systemic disease as opposed to brain metastases.

- Therapies for brain metastases are roughly equivalent, with local recurrence rate of 40% to 50% at 1 year. Therefore, the choice of therapy must be tailored to the individual patient, taking into account Karnofsky performance scale (KPS) score, medical comorbid conditions, systemic disease status, number of metastases, size and location of metastases, and symptoms.

- It is essential that treatment decisions for this lethal disease be made as a multidisciplinary team of oncologists, radiation oncologists, and neurosurgeons, as well as the patient and the patient's family.

Greater than half of all clinically diagnosed brain tumors in adults are cerebral metastases. Past estimates of the incidence of cerebral metastases were based on large population studies. Recent clinical series and autopsy studies demonstrate an increasing incidence of cerebral metastases, but the true incidence of cerebral metastases is difficult to ascertain. Estimates of the annual incidence of cerebral metastases in the United States range from 100,000 to 200,000 new cases, compared to fewer than 20,000 new cases of primary brain tumors. The apparent increase in the incidence of cerebral metastases may be due to a variety of factors. Improvements in systemic cancer treatments have increased the length of survival of many cancer patients, and advancements in cerebral imaging technology have augmented the ability to diagnose cerebral metastases. During the course of their lifetime 20% to 40% of patients with systemic cancer are diagnosed with cerebral metastases. Cerebral metastases are the presenting symptom of an undiagnosed primary cancer in at least 30% of patients and despite complete medical evaluation in 15% of patients a primary cancer will not be diagnosed. The use of magnetic resonance imaging (MRI) in the diagnosis of cerebral metastases has shown that greater than 60% of cancer patients with cerebral metastases have more than one metastatic brain lesion.

The histology and epidemiology of the primary cancer are the principal determinants of the frequency of cerebral metastases. Although the most common cancers diagnosed in adults in the United States are colorectal, prostate, breast, and lung, the two of these with the greatest proclivity to spread to the

brain are lung and breast. In decreasing order of relative frequency, the majority of cerebral metastases are due to lung, breast, melanoma, renal, and colon cancers. Primary lung cancer accounts for 30% to 60% of all cerebral metastases. Lung cancer is more frequently diagnosed in males, and as a result, primary lung cancer is the most common cause of cerebral metastases in males. Brain metastases from lung cancer are often synchronous at diagnosis. Breast cancer accounts for 10% to 30% of all cerebral metastases and is the most common cause of cerebral metastases in females. Unlike brain metastases from lung cancer, breast metastases to the brain are more often metachronous. Melanoma accounts for 5% to 20% of all cerebral metastases, while renal and colon cancer each account for 5% to 10% of cerebral metastatic disease. The tendency of a primary cancer to metastasize to the brain has a distinct order of relative frequency. The frequency of cerebral metastases for melanoma is greater than 50%, but the low incidence of melanoma relative to other cancers accounts for its lower overall relative frequency of all cerebral metastases. Lung cancer has the second highest overall tendency to metastasize to the brain. The frequency of cerebral metastases for lung cancer is 20% to 60%, but there is variability in the frequency of cerebral metastases based on lung tumor type. Small cell lung cancer and lung adenocarcinoma tend to metastasize to the brain more frequently than other types of lung cancer. Breast cancer has the third highest overall tendency to metastasize to the brain, with a frequency of 20% to 30%.

Metastatic brain tumors in children with a primary cancer are rare. The most common sources of cerebral metastases in the pediatric population are neuroblastoma, rhabdomyosarcoma, and Wilms' tumor.

CLINICAL PRESENTATION AND DIAGNOSTIC STUDIES

Brain metastases are most commonly parenchymal, but can also involve the ventricles, dura (most often with breast cancer), or leptomeninges. The major route of spread of metastatic brain tumors is hematogenous, and brain metastases often arise at the gray-white matter junction within the cerebral hemispheres, though brain metastases can occur in any part of the brain. The highest incidence of parenchymal brain metastases occurs in the distribution of the middle cerebral artery at the temporo-parieto-occipital junction, often near the eloquent cortex. Supratentorial metastases (80%) are more common than infratentorial metastases (15%). Within the posterior fossa in adults, metastatic brain tumors are the most common tumors. Therefore, a single cerebellar lesion in an adult is a metastasis until proved otherwise. Within the cerebellum, metastases can be located deep or hemispheric. Hematogenous spread of metastatic disease to the cerebellum can occur via the spinal epidural venous plexus or the vertebral arteries.

Similar to most primary brain tumors, metastatic brain tumors frequently present with slowly progressive signs and symptoms. Even with a history of treated cancer, there are no clinical findings that are specific for metastatic disease. Headache is the most common presenting symptom, occurring in 50% of patients. Nausea and vomiting may occur due to elevated intracranial pressure (ICP) from mass effect of the tumor or blockage of normal cerebrospinal fluid (CSF) drainage pathways. Focal neurological deficits, such as weakness, language difficulties, or cognitive impairment, will occur in up to two thirds of patients. This can be due to compression of brain parenchyma by the tumor mass or peritumoral edema, or compression of cranial nerves. Seizures occur in 15% to 20% of patients. Patients may present with symptoms of a transient ischemia attack (TIA) or stroke due to vascular compression or occlusion by the tumor or hemorrhage into the tumor. Intratumoral hemorrhage occurs in 5% to 15% of patients and is seen most frequently with metastatic choriocarcinoma (60-100%), melanoma (40%), and renal cell carcinoma. Mental status changes such as confusion, lethargy, apathy, and depression are not uncommon.

A complete history and physical examination is essential in the workup of a patient with a suspected metastatic brain tumor, because up to 30% of patients with no history of cancer will present with a cerebral metastasis. It is important to ask about constitutional symptoms, such as unintended weight loss, night sweats, loss of appetite, and so on. A family history of breast cancer and colorectal cancer may prove important. Any past history of cancer should be detailed, including stage at diagnosis and treatment, regardless of how remote the diagnosis, as approximately 90% of patients with newly diagnosed brain lesions and a known systemic cancer will prove to have metastases from the known cancer. Exposure to tobacco smoke and other toxins should be ascertained. Any abnormalities on routine screening evaluations, such as a Papanicolaou test, mammogram, or colonoscopy, should be investigated.

Screening of the most common primary sites—lung, breast, skin, kidneys, and colon—should include a chest radiograph, mammogram, skin survey, urinalysis, stool guaic test, complete blood count, and extended metabolic panel. An oral and intravenous contrast-enhanced computed tomography (CT) scan of the chest, abdomen, and pelvis is a routine diagnostic tool in many institutions. Radionuclide bone scan and positron emission tomography/CT (PET/CT) scan can be useful in detecting small malignancies or alternative biopsy sites. However, many cancers lack PET avidity, so the PET scan alone (rather than PET/CT) should be interpreted with caution.

CT is the most common initial imaging study to assess for an intracranial lesion. On a nonenhanced CT, cerebral metastases typically appear as isodense or hypodense mass(es) at the gray-white matter junction. Significant white matter edema is characteristic, but peritumoral edema can be variable. Intratumoral hemorrhage or hemorrhage into the surrounding parenchyma may be present and appears hyperdense. On a contrast-enhanced CT, cerebral metastases characteristically appear as round, well-circumscribed masses with peripheral enhancement. From 50% to 65% of cerebral metastases are solitary on CT. Gadolinium-enhanced MRI of the brain is much more sensitive than contrast-enhanced CT imaging in detecting cerebral metastases, particularly in the posterior fossa and brainstem. In 20% of patients with a single metastasis detected on CT, MRI, with the ability to detect lesions as small as 1 to 2 mm, will detect multiple metastases.

The best imaging tool for cerebral metastases is contrast-enhanced MRI (Figs. 35.1 and 35.2). On nonenhanced T1-weighted sequences, cerebral metastases generally appear isointense or hypointense. Certain metastases with intrinsically short T1, such as melanoma (due to the ferromagnetic melanin within the tumor), can appear hyperintense. Hemorrhage within the tumor will appear disorganized, with atypical evolution, and is best evaluated on T2-weighted gradient echo (GRE) sequences. On nonenhanced T2-weighted sequences, cerebral metastases generally appear hyperintense, but can be variable. Similarly, on FLAIR (fluid-attenuated inversion recovery) sequences the appearance of cerebral metastases can be variable, but is generally hyperintense. Both FLAIR and T2-weighted images usually demonstrate marked vasogenic edema. Tumor cysts and surrounding edema appear markedly hyperintense. The vast majority of cerebral metastases will enhance. On contrast-enhanced T1-weighted sequences cerebral metastases show strong enhancement in variable patterns. Cerebral metastases usually do not show restriction on diffusion-weighted imaging (DWI) sequences and exhibit elevated apparent diffusion coefficient (ADC) values. The differential diagnosis of cerebral lesions with imaging characteristics similar to cerebral metastases includes abscess, encephalitis, malignant glioma, radiation necrosis, thromboembolic stroke, demyelinating disease, and resolving hematoma. Multiplicity of lesions or location in the posterior fossa may increase the likelihood that the lesions are metastatic, rather than primary.

TREATMENT OPTIONS AND OUTCOMES

In general, cerebral metastases from systemic cancer are a harbinger of active systemic disease. With treatment, approximately 90% of patients with known brain metastases will

FIGURE 35.1 A, Axial contrast-enhanced T1-weighted magnetic resonance imaging (MRI) scan showing multiple non–small cell lung cancer metastases (right occipital and left temporal). Lesions are typically ring-enhancing and often multiple. **B,** Sagittal view of the left temporal lesion seen in A.

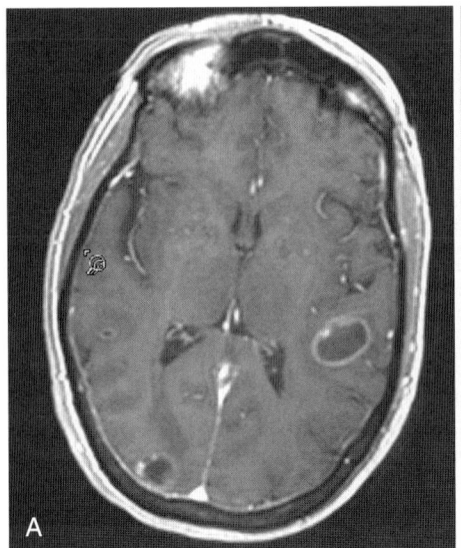
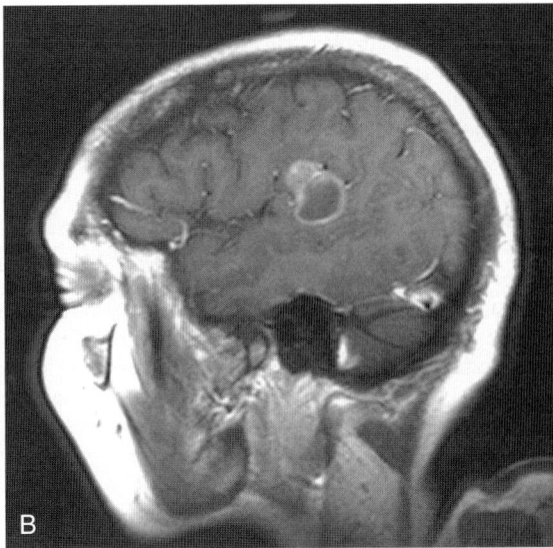

FIGURE 35.2 A, Axial contrast-enhanced T1-weighted magnetic resonance imaging (MRI) scan showing a solitary left frontal renal carcinoma metastasis. **B,** Fluid-attenuated inversion recovery (FLAIR) axial image showing the extensive vasogenic edema surrounding the lesion.

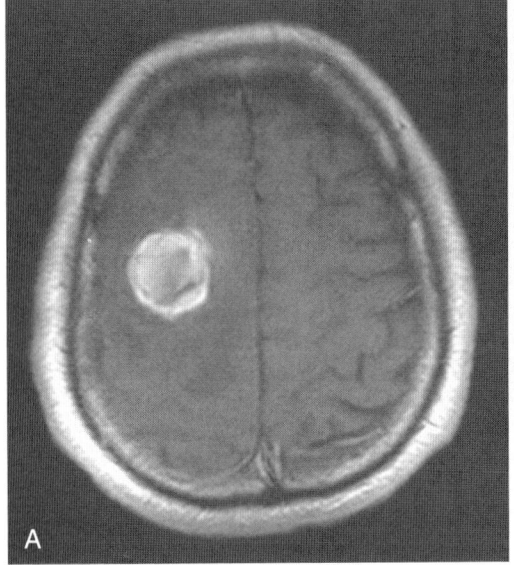
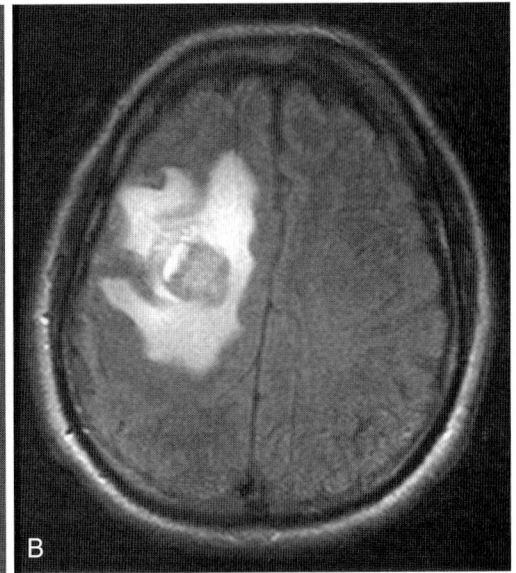

succumb to systemic disease progression, rather than cerebral progression. Cerebral metastatic disease is complex and there is no one optimal treatment algorithm. If neurological deficits are present at the time of diagnosis of cerebral metastases, the median survival in untreated patients is 4 to 6 weeks. There are several patient factors associated with improved survival regardless of treatment. Karnofsky performance scale (KPS) score greater than 70, age less than 60 years, isolated cerebral metastases, a single cerebral metastasis, absent or controlled primary disease, and longer than 1 year since diagnosis of primary disease predict a better prognosis. Even with comprehensive treatment, median survival is only approximately 6 to 8 months. Initial treatment of symptomatic cerebral metastases includes high-dose corticosteroid therapy to decrease the edema that commonly occurs. Because most cerebral metastases are accompanied by a considerable amount of reactive, vasogenic edema, steroid therapy can often improve neurological function. The use of corticosteroids alone doubles median survival to 8 to 12 weeks. In patients who present with seizure, an antiepileptic should be initiated. There is controversy, though, regarding routine seizure prophylaxis. Medical therapy can manage the symptoms of cerebral metastases, but the primary treatment options for definitive management include whole-brain radiation therapy, surgical resection, and stereotactic radiosurgery.

Whole-Brain Radiation Therapy

Since the 1950s, whole-brain radiation therapy (WBRT) has been used to treat cerebral metastases. Several studies have examined the role of WBRT in treating cerebral metastases. Studies by the Radiation Therapy Oncology Group (RTOG) established a median survival time of 4 to 6 months in cerebral metastases treated with WBRT. Additional studies demonstrated symptom improvement after WBRT. Cranial nerve deficits, symptoms of elevated intracranial pressure, headaches, and seizures have been shown to improve in 50% of patients after WBRT. Two separate studies from the RTOG identified favorable prognostic factors in patients with cerebral metastases treated with WBRT. Diener-West and colleagues used multivariate analysis and found a KPS score greater than 70, patient age less than 60 years, isolated cerebral metastases, and absent or controlled primary disease predictive of better survival.[1] Gaspar and colleagues used recursive partitioning analysis and identified the same patient-related factors to predict improved survival following WBRT.[2] The optimal WBRT dose-fractionation schedule was also assessed by the RTOG. Patients receiving higher-dose schedules of 20 to 40 Gy over a period of 1 to 4 weeks demonstrated greater duration of symptom improvement, shorter time of progression to improved neurological status, and greater rate of resolution of neurological symptoms compared to patients receiving ultrarapid schedules of 10 or 12 Gy in one or two fractions, respectively.[3] The common treatment schedule for WBRT is 30 Gy in 10 fractions.

WBRT to control micrometastases is typically recommended following surgical resection of cerebral metastases. In a study by Patchell and colleagues, WBRT following surgical resection of a single cerebral metastasis was shown to decrease the frequency of and time to recurrence of cerebral metastases, but did not influence the length of survival.[4] The common treatment schedule following surgery is 45 to 50 Gy plus a boost of 5 to 10 Gy for a total treatment dose of 55 Gy divided in low fractions of 1.8 to 2.0 Gy. The smaller daily fractions are recommended to reduce neurotoxicity. In patients who are not expected to live long enough to experience long-term radiation effects, higher daily fractions can be given. In the treatment of multiple cerebral metastases, a recent study by Kocher and colleagues assessed outcomes in patients with one to three cerebral metastases treated with surgical resection or stereotactic radiosurgery alone with or without adjuvant WBRT.[5] The addition of adjuvant WBRT in the treatment of multiple cerebral metastases reduced intracranial relapse and death due to a neurological cause, but did not improve functional independence or overall survival. Prophylactic WBRT is not commonly used in the treatment of most systemic cancers. It is reserved for patients with small cell lung cancer who are in complete remission after treatment. Studies of prophylactic WBRT for small cell lung cancer have demonstrated a 5% improvement in survival at 3 years and a 25% reduction in the incidence of cerebral metastases.

Short-term side effects of WBRT include headaches, nausea, vomiting, hair loss, scalp erythema, fatigue, and hyperpigmentation. Persistent fatigue coupled with irritability and anorexia can occasionally occur within weeks following WBRT. Long-term side effects, which include progressive dementia, ataxia, and urinary incontinence, can occur 6 to 36 months after WBRT.

Surgical Resection

Surgical resection is often considered the optimal treatment for symptomatic cerebral metastases. However, with surgery alone, there is approximately a 50% local recurrence rate at 1 year following a gross total resection. Patient selection is based on several factors, including the number, size, location, and histological type of cerebral metastases, as well as the patient's clinical condition. The number of cerebral metastases present is a principal factor in the decision

to treat with surgical resection. Conventionally, surgery has been reserved for patients with a single symptomatic cerebral metastasis in a surgically accessible location and an unknown primary diagnosis or primary disease known to be relatively radioresistant. Studies conducted in the 1990s demonstrated a benefit of surgical resection followed by WBRT for single cerebral metastasis compared with WBRT alone in patients with good neurological function. One of the decisive works in demonstrating improved survival after surgical resection was published by Patchell and colleagues. In this prospective randomized trial comparing surgical resection followed by radiation with WBRT alone in patients with a single cerebral metastasis, a KPS score greater than 70, and limited systemic disease, patients in the surgery and radiation group had longer survival, improved progression-free survival, and improved quality of life.[6] The benefit of surgery has not been shown in patients with poor functioning or extensive systemic disease. The role of surgical resection in patients with multiple metastases is unclear. For patients with multiple cerebral metastases, the classic surgical treatment strategy is for resection of only large lesions with symptomatic mass effect. There have been no prospective randomized studies, but there is evidence showing that patients with multiple or recurrent cerebral metastases may also benefit from surgical resection. A retrospective review was performed to assess survival, comparing patients with resection of all cerebral metastases to patients with resection of only one of multiple cerebral metastases, with a control group of patients with resection of a single cerebral metastasis. The result showed that resection of all of multiple cerebral metastases is as effective as resection of single cerebral metastases in prolonging survival, provided that all cerebral metastases are resected.

Cerebral metastasis size influences the decision to proceed with surgical resection, but it has not been shown to influence survival following surgery. Large cerebral metastases greater than 3 cm are generally considered too large to be treated with radiosurgery and are best treated with surgical resection. Small cerebral metastases less than 5 mm are typically treated with radiosurgery. These small lesions are usually asymptomatic and do not require surgical resection, or are difficult to locate during surgery. Cerebral metastases between 1 cm and 3 cm present a challenge. There is no good evidence to support either conventional surgery or radiosurgery, and the treatment decision is usually based on the patient's neurological function, extent of systemic disease, and surgical risk. The location of cerebral metastases also influences the decision to proceed with surgical resection. Lesions located deep within the brain, such as the thalamus, basal ganglia, and brainstem, or in eloquent cortex are generally not considered amenable to surgical resection.

The histological appearance of the primary disease is a significant factor in considering surgical resection for cerebral metastases. Lymphoma, small cell lung cancer, and germ cell tumors are sensitive to radiation and chemotherapy, and optimal treatment usually consists of fractionated radiation and chemotherapy. Melanoma, renal cell carcinoma, and sarcomas are generally resistant to radiation, and surgical resection is the preferred treatment for cerebral metastases. Breast and non–small cell lung cancer are moderately sensitive to radiation, and surgery is often a component of multimodality treatment.

The patient's overall clinical condition is an important factor in surgical decision making. The extent of systemic, or extracranial, disease and functional status as measured by the KPS score are the most important variables in determining the benefit of surgery. In patients with no systemic disease or systemic disease that is controlled, no leptomeningeal disease, and KPS score of 70 or greater, surgical resection of symptomatic cerebral metastases can provide a survival benefit and improved quality of life. Local recurrence rates following surgical resection and WBRT for a single cerebral metastasis are 10% to 20%.

Stereotactic Radiosurgery

Stereotactic radiosurgery is an alternative treatment option for cerebral metastatic disease and has been shown to be effective in the treatment of some cerebral metastases. Local control rates of 80% to 95% have been reported, though local recurrence/progression rates at 1 year, with radiosurgery alone, are more likely 40% to 50%. Radiosurgery is considered the preferred treatment choice for small cerebral metastases less than 5 mm, for cerebral metastases 1 to 3 cm in patients who are not good surgical candidates due to medical comorbid conditions, and for cerebral metastases in deep or eloquent brain locations. Cerebral metastases larger than 3 cm are generally not effectively treated with radiosurgery because the radiation dose must be decreased with increasing tumor size to prevent injury to adjacent brain. The consequence of decreased radiation dose to the tumor is decreased tumor control rates. There is considerable debate over the optimal treatment for cerebral metastases 1 to 3 cm in medically stable patients with good functional status. A few retrospective studies, comparing surgical resection to stereotactic radiosurgery in patients who were candidates for surgery, have produced mixed results. There is no good evidence to support stereotactic radiosurgery over surgical resection in this group of patients and the treatment decision is guided by the patient's clinical status and the risks and benefits of treatment. The risks of stereotactic radiosurgery include transient tumor enlargement early after radiosurgery, persistent peritumoral edema requiring long-term steroid treatment, and radiation necrosis with mass effect. These effects can be accompanied by hemorrhage, seizures, and worsening neurological function. Treatment with stereotactic radiosurgery can improve the symptoms associated with cerebral metastases, requires a shorter hospital stay, and avoids the morbidity associated with a craniotomy. The local recurrence rate after stereotactic radiosurgery is similar to the local recurrence rate for surgically treated cerebral metastases, and the median survival following radiosurgery ranges from 6 to 12 months.

Radiosurgery in combination with WBRT for treatment of single cerebral metastases may provide a survival benefit and result in treatment outcomes that are similar to surgical resection followed by WBRT. Andrews and colleagues demonstrated improved survival in patients with a single unresectable cerebral metastasis treated with WBRT and radiosurgery boost compared to WBRT alone.[7] In patients with multiple cerebral metastases, a randomized trial (Aoyama and colleagues) showed improved neurological function and local control in patients treated with radiosurgery and WBRT compared to WBRT alone, but there was no evidence for improved survival.[8] Stereotactic radiosurgery can also be utilized to treat recurrent cerebral metastases or persistent cerebral metastases following WBRT.

Clearly, treatment of brain metastases must be individualized. The neurosurgeon must take into account the type of cancer, recent systemic staging studies, patient KPS score, medical comorbid conditions, the number and location of metastases, the size of the lesions, and whether or not the tumors are symptomatic. Hence, a 4-cm solitary metastasis in the posterior fossa, with secondary hydrocephalus, would be considered a surgical lesion (assuming the patient could tolerate surgery). In contradistinction, a patient with 20 small brain metastases would be better served by radiotherapy. However, the patients whose situations fall between these two examples are the ones who require more complicated decision-making efforts on the part of the neurosurgeon, in concert with the patient and the treating oncology team. It is essential to bear in mind that median survival time is shorter than with glioblastoma, but the 5-year survival rate can be much higher (10-15%). Furthermore, it is important to remember that choice of treatment(s) of the brain metastases may have little impact on overall survival.

CONCLUSION

Cerebral metastatic disease represents a serious progression of systemic cancer. Advances in systemic cancer therapy that limit or stabilize systemic disease have allowed for more aggressive treatment of cerebral metastases. Currently, the most effective options for treatment of cerebral metastatic disease include whole-brain radiation therapy, surgical resection, and stereotactic radiosurgery. Despite maximal treatment, median survival in cerebral metastatic disease is still only 9 to 12 months, and even patients with the best prognostic indicators have limited long-term survival. One-year survival rate for a single cerebral metastasis is 40%, and the 2-year survival rate is 20%. Progressive systemic disease is the usual cause of death in the majority of patients with cerebral metastases. The most important prognostic indicators in patients with cerebral metastatic disease, regardless of treatment modality, are age, extent of systemic disease, and functional status. Both patient and disease characteristics will guide treatment decisions in regard to surgical resection and stereotactic radiosurgery in combination with WBRT. In patients with extensive systemic disease or poor functional status, treatment of cerebral metastases is palliative and should focus on optimizing quality of life. Future directions in the treatment of cerebral metastases will require continued investigation of the optimal combination of current therapeutic options as well as the development of new therapies.

SELECTED KEY REFERENCES

Gaspar LE, Mehta MP, Patchell RA, et al. The role of whole brain radiation therapy in the management of newly diagnosed brain metastases: a systematic review and evidence-based clinical practice guideline. *J Neurooncol.* 2010;96:17-32.

Kalkanis SN, Kondziolka D, Gaspar LE, et al. The role of surgical resection in the management of newly diagnosed brain metastases: a systematic review and evidence-based clinical practice guideline. *J Neurooncol.* 2010;96:33-43.

Linskey ME, Andrews DW, Asher AL, et al. The role of stereotactic radiosurgery in the management of patients with newly diagnosed brain metastases: a systematic review and evidence-based clinical practice guideline. *J Neurooncol.* 2010;96:45-68.

Sperduto PW, Chao ST, Sneed PK, et al. Diagnosis-specific prognostic factors, indexes, and treatment outcomes for patients with newly diagnosed brain metastases: a multi-institutional analysis of 4,259 patients. *Int J Radiat Oncol Biol Phys.* 2010;77:655-661.

Videtic GMM, Gaspar LE, Aref AM, et al. American College of Radiology appropriateness criteria on multiple brain metastases. *Int J Radiat Oncol Biol Phys.* 2009;77:961-965.

Please go to expertconsult.com to view the complete list of references.

36 Meningiomas

Federico Landriel, Peter Black

CLINICAL PEARLS

- Meningiomas are believed to derive from the arachnoid cap cells around arachnoid granulations near venous sinuses, cisterns, ventricles, and brain. They can be found anywhere there is known pia, arachnoid, or dura. These tumors exhibit a wide variety of behaviors from benign to extremely aggressive. The etiology of meningiomas is unclear but some are associated with genetic aberrations such as partial loss of chromosome 22, prior trauma, and radiation therapy.

- The latest World Health Organization (WHO) grading system of meningiomas evaluates these neoplasms from grades I to III. Grade I meningiomas have nine subtypes ranging from fibroblastic to psammomatous. Despite the different histological patterns there is no prognostic significance among the subtypes of grade I meningioma. Grade II represents an atypical meningioma and implies the presence of mitosis, or three or more of such features as increased cellularity, brain invasion, or necrosis. Grade III anaplastic malignant meningiomas are characterized by highly active mitosis, and their tumor cells resemble carcinoma or sarcoma. Metastases are rare in meningioma but can occur in the lungs, liver, bone, and heart.

- The treatment of meningiomas depends on a variety of factors such as their growth rate, radiological

characteristics, location, and patient clinical status and age. The advent of magnetic resonance imaging (MRI) has brought the age of more incidentally diagnosed lesions. The natural history of meningiomas varies, as do the growth rates. Some incidentally discovered meningiomas remain stable and can be observed, especially in elderly patients with few symptoms or signs. Meningiomas are symptomatic in a wide range of patient ages and locations and thus warrant excision. Total surgical excision of meningiomas is the treatment of choice.

- A wide spectrum of surgical approaches can be employed to radically excise a meningioma. Preoperative embolization can decrease intraoperative blood loss in selected patients. Postoperative radiation therapy, radiosurgery, and hormonal therapy is required for incompletely resected lesions or those with malignant characteristics.

- Simpson classification of meningioma provides a general estimate of recurrence after resection. The resection ranges from grade I resection, which is complete removal, to grade IV subtotal resection, and grade V, which is decompression of the tumor. The recurrence rates are as low as 9% for grade I resections and as high as 40% for grade IV resections.

In 1922, Harvey Cushing presented a series of 85 meningeal tumors in his Cavendish lecture and coined the term *meningioma* to describe these lesions.[1] Years later with Louise Eisenhardt, he created a definitive monograph on these tumors.[2] He believed that all meningeal tumors arose from the arachnoidal cap cells that are particularly abundant in the arachnoid granulations.

Meningiomas are the most common brain tumor and have a wide variety of clinical behaviors. Although most of them behave rather nicely, there are some that are extremely aggressive. Little is known about the reasons for this difference in natural history. The etiology of meningiomas remains unknown, but previous radiation therapy and monosomy or partial loss of chromosome 22 are important factors. Radiation therapy,

at a high or low dosage, can cause meningiomas even after several years of treatment.[3]

EPIDEMIOLOGY

Meningiomas constitute 15% to 20% of all primary intracranial tumors in surgical series, but their incidence in routine screening is 1 in 100 population. Their incidence increases with advancing age.[4] They predominantly affect women with an overall male-female ratio of 1:2.5. This difference is increased for intraspinal meningiomas with a ratio of 1:10 in comparison with an intracranial ratio of 2:3. Meningeal tumors are rare in children but tend to be more aggressive when they occur in children. They represent 0.4% to 4.1% of all childhood brain tumors and constitute 1.5% to 1.8% of all meningiomas.[5,6] Pediatric meningiomas tend to be more frequent in males with a male-female ratio of 1.2 to 1.9:1 and have a higher incidence of ventricular location.[7,8]

In one study, symptomatic meningiomas were encountered in 2.0 per 100,000 of the population and asymptomatic ones in 5.7 per 100,000, with an overall incidence of 7.7 per 100,000.[9]

GENERAL CLINICAL PRESENTATION

Meningiomas present with a wide variety of symptoms but many are asymptomatic. Signs and symptoms are related to the compression of adjacent structures. Depending on the area involved they may cause motor seizures and contralateral limb weakness (prerolandic cortex), sensory deficits and jacksonian seizures (postrolandic cortex), speech disturbance (Broca's or Wernicke's area), visual field impairment or behavioral disorders (large frontobasal tumors), anosmia (olfactory groove), obstructive hydrocephalus (intraventricular), limb weakness, numbness, or local pain (spinal).

IMAGING

Contrast-enhanced magnetic resonance imaging (MRI) scans with the addition of arterial and venous sequences are the most important studies to evaluate these tumors. Computed tomography (CT) may provide valuable information about bony anatomy. Three-dimensional (3D) MRI or CT scans provide useful information about tumor features and surrounding anatomy and are particularly useful for surgical planning.

Plain radiographs may demonstrate hyperostosis, irregular cortex, erosion, tumor calcifications, and enlargement of vascular grooves (middle meningeal artery).

Computed Tomography

Meningiomas on nonenhanced CT usually appear as well-circumscribed extra-axial lesions, hyperdense (70-75%), isodense (25%), or hypointense (1-5%) to adjacent parenchyma.[8] Calcifications ranging from microscopic psammoma bodies to dense sclerosis are found in 25% of patients. Necrosis, cysts, and hemorrhage are seen occasionally (8-23%).[8,10] With contrast agent, they usually enhance brightly.

Magnetic Resonance Imaging

T1-weighted imaging shows meningiomas as isointense or moderately hypointense to gray matter lesions. Calcifications and highly fibrous areas are hypointense. FLAIR (fluid-attenuated inversion recovery) is helpful to demonstrate edema, seen as a hyperintense signal in the adjacent parenchyma. T2-weighted imaging may present a wide range of possible signal intensities. Usually isointense or mildly hyperintense, it can show hypointensity if the meningioma is calcified or highly fibrous. Massive surrounding edema is seen as a hyperintense signal. Arterial feeders to tumor are seen as arborizing flow voids (hypointense). Pial blood vessels present as surface flow voids between tumor and parenchyma.[11] T2-weighted gradient echo (GRE) may "bloom" as parenchymal low signal, suggesting calcifications or intratumoral microhemorrhages.

T1 contrast enhancement shows meningiomas as heterogeneous clearly defined hyperintensive images. The "dural tail" may enhance in 35% to 80%, but is not specific.[11,12] Magnetic resonance (MR) angiography and venography are noninvasive options to demonstrate tumor blood supply, vascularization, drainage veins, and sinus compromise.

Functional MRI is based on increased brain hemodynamics in response to cortical neuronal activity due to certain stimulus performed during imaging. It can be helpful in surgical planning for localization of motor, sensory, and language regions. Diffusion may differentiate benign from atypical or malignant meningiomas.[13,14] Perfusion reveals differentials in relative cerebral blood volume, allows us to distinguish meningiomas from dural metastases,[15] and according to some authors also discerns typical from atypical histological grades.[8,16] Spectroscopy shows high choline peak, low or absent N-acetylaspartate (NAA) and creatinine levels, and variable amounts of lactate. Some of them also present high alanine and glutamate/glutamine levels on MR spectroscopy.[17]

Angiography

This invasive study is useful to demonstrate the meningioma primary blood supply, which is usually derived from dural arteries as branches of the external carotid artery. Feeding vessels could be bilateral, especially in falcine or parasagittal meningiomas. The degree of vascularization and major draining veins are also seen. The venous phase is important to evaluate sinus involvement and the presence of arteriovenous shunting. Angiography also allows the possibility to perform preoperative selective embolization, usually several days before surgery.

Positron Emission Tomography

The role of positron emission tomography (PET) in patients with meningiomas is still not clear. The benign variants of these tumors usually show isometabolism with [18F]-fluorodeoxyglucose (FDG) markers while atypical or anaplastic meningeal tumors may exhibit hypermetabolism.[18,19] FDG uptake in meningioma could be a predictive factor in tumor recurrence.[20] In one study FDG PET had 80% sensitivity but only 57% specificity for detecting meningiomas.[21]

Single-Photon Emission Computed Tomography/Scintigraphy

Meningiomas have many somatostatin receptors (SSr) and this is the base of the scintigraphy in which SSr-positive tumors can be imaged in vivo through single-photon emission computed tomography (SPECT). Octreotide is a somatostatin analog with high binding affinity for SSr subtype 2 and a longer plasma half-life than native somatostatin. Therefore, octreotide is a better SSr imaging agent than somatostatin.[22] Octreotide SPECT had 83% sensitivity and 27% specificity for identifying meningiomas.[21]

PATHOLOGY

Hormone Receptors

Meningioma growth may be related to hormonal status due to the presence of estrogen and progesterone receptors. The tumor may become clinically evident during pregnancy or in the luteal phase of the menstrual cycle.[23] The expression of progesterone receptors alone in a meningioma could be related to a favorable behavior. Absence of both progesterone and estrogen receptors or the presence of estrogen receptors alone correlates with aggressive clinical behavior, progression, and recurrence after complete surgical resection.[24] Despite the presence of these receptors, drug therapies targeting hormonal status have not been particularly successful.

Immunohistochemistry

In most cases, immunohistochemical staining is not needed for the diagnosis of meningiomas but may be useful in distinguishing certain tumor types from them. Meningiomas present focal positive staining with epithelial membrane antigen (EMA). This feature could be absent in World Health Organization (WHO) grade II and III variants. Nearly all subtypes exhibit vimentin diffuse positivity, but this is not pathognomonic of this tumor. They show variable positivity staining with S-100 protein and cytokeratin markers. The secretory variant of meningioma could have positive staining for carcinoembryonic antigen (CEA). This method could be helpful distinguishing meningiomas from schwannomas in small biopsies from difficult locations; immunoreactivity for S-100 protein is focal and generally low for meningiomas and strong and diffuse for schwannomas. EMA is commonly absent in schwannomas.

CLASSIFICATION

Histological subtypes are classified according to the most recent WHO grading system published in 2007[25] (Box 36.1). In the 2000 WHO classification of meningiomas, brain invasion was associated with aggressive behavior and increased probability of recurrence, but was not included as a diagnostic criterion for grade II or grade III tumor.[3] Perry and associates demonstrated that brain invasion indicated a greater likelihood of recurrence and felt that it should be considered one of the diagnostic features of grade II meningioma.[26] Following these findings, brain invasion by a meningioma is now an independent criterion for WHO grade II. Subtype classification does not appear to influence prognosis unless atypia or malignancy is evident.

Grade I

Grade I (benign meningiomas) is defined as the absence of criteria for grades II and III. The subtypes include meningothelial, fibroblastic, transitional, angiomatous, microcystic, secretory, lymphoplasmocyte-rich, metaplastic, and psammomatous variables. This subclassification into nine different subtypes has no prognostic significance but is useful in recognizing unusual histological patterns as meningiomas.

Grade II

Grade II (atypical meningiomas) implies the presence of 4 or more mitotic cells per 10 high-power fields or three or more of the following features: increased cellularity, high nuclear/cytoplasm ratio, geographic necrosis, prominent nucleoli, sheet-like growth, or brain invasion. There are also two morphological subtypes that are by their nature atypical:

Clear cell type is distinguished by lobulated or sheet-like proliferations of polygonal cells with clear, abundant glycogen cytoplasm (periodic acid–Schiff positive [PAS+]). This type is associated with a higher incidence of recurrence, frequently affects young patients, and commonly arises in spinal or cerebellopontine locations.[27]

Chordoid type is marked by the presence of cords of eosinophilic, epithelial-like, and vacuolated cells in a prominent myxoid background, similar to the appearance of chordomas. It is associated with chronic inflammation cell pattern, dysgammaglobulinemia, and microcytic anemia (features observed in Castelman's disease).[28] This variant also presents a high rate of recurrence after subtotal resection.[29]

Grade III

Grade III (anaplastic malignant meningiomas) is characterized by the presence of 20 or more mitoses per 10 high-power fields or obviously malignant cytological characteristics such as tumor cells resembling carcinoma, sarcoma, or melanoma. Again, certain types are typical:

Rhabdoid variant is characterized by rhabdoid-like cells with prominent eosinophilic cytoplasm, prominent nucleolus, and eccentric nuclei. This histological presentation has been associated with increased risk of recurrence and distant metastases.

Papillary type is composed of relatively uniform meningoendothelial cells disposed in a perivascular pseudopapillary pattern, resembling the perivascular pseudorosettes of ependymomas. It has aggressive behavior and a propensity to recur and metastasize. This histological pattern has a higher incidence of presentation in children and young adults.

Metastases

It is extremely uncommon for meningiomas to metastasize outside the nervous system. If metastasis occurs, it is generally associated with anaplastic or malignant patterns. The most common sites of metastasis include lungs, lymph nodes, liver, bones, and heart. Histologically benign meningiomas may also metastasize.

DECISION MAKING

The treatment of meningiomas depends on their natural growth rate, radiological characteristics, and location; the patient's clinical status; and an assessment balancing the potential morbidity of conservative versus invasive treatment. With the advent of better imaging techniques, more meningiomas are being incidentally discovered. Issues in decision making concerning proper management become particularly important.

In order to integrate these variables some treatment algorithms have been developed. Dr. Takeshi Kawase and his group (Adachi and associates[30]) in 2006 presented a set of rules for treating cranial base meningiomas. They give a score to each tumor based on predetermined risk characteristics:

- Attachment/size (0-2)
- Arterial involvement (0-2)
- Relation to brainstem (0-2)
- Cranial nerve involvement (0-2)

A higher score number (risk factor) implies a lower chance of complete resection.

Dr. Joung Lee[31] and his group at the Cleveland Clinic designed the "CLASS" algorithm for the treatment of all meningiomas. This algorithm compares negative features (comorbidity, location, and age) against benefits (size and symptoms) and assigns a score:

- Comorbidity (–2 to 0)
- Location (–2 to 0)
- Age (–2 to 0)
- Size (0 to 2)
- Symptoms and signs (0 to 2)

Patients with a score of +1 or higher had a 1.9% rate of poor outcome; those with a score of 0 to 1 had a 4% rate of poor outcome; and of those with a score of –2 or less, 15% had a poor outcome. Therefore, more negative features are related to an increased chance of having an undesirable postoperative outcome.

Even with these grading systems, the final management strategy for meningiomas should be based on the patient's age, general medical condition, and wishes for treatment.

CONSERVATIVE TREATMENT

Around two thirds of asymptomatic meningiomas do not continue to grow and may be observed at appropriate time intervals. Absolute growth rates of meningiomas vary between 0.03 and 2.62 cm^3 per year. Several studies following the behavior of asymptomatic meningiomas showed minimal growth during the follow-up period. In a retrospective study of tumor growth rate in 37 patients, 9 of the 37 (24.3%) showed tumor growth during a mean follow-up period of 4.2 years. Annual growth rates were calculated as the difference in tumor volume between the initial and latest imaging, divided by the time interval (years) between these determinations, with tumor growth defined as an annual increase in tumor volume more 1 cm^3 per year. In this study they associate the age of patients and the volume of the tumor at its initial diagnosis with growth rate increased. They concluded that young patients and those with large tumors should be carefully observed.[32] Nakamura and colleagues[33] studied 41 patients with asymptomatic meningiomas, reporting a majority (66%) of growth rates less than 1 cm^3 per year. They also correlated growth rate with patient age but did not consider initial tumor size as a predictive factor for tumor growth. Yano and Kuratsu in their study of surgical indications for asymptomatic meningiomas reported 37% of tumor growth during a period of observation of 3.9 years and only 6.4% becoming symptomatic.[34] Some authors recommend the surgical resection of meningiomas when the tumor growth rate is greater than 1 cm^3 per year.[32,33] Radiological features such as partial or complete calcification is related to slow growth rate or absence of it, so these tumors may be kept only under observation. Meningiomas that remain asymptomatic but show displacement and compression of delicate structures as spinal cord, optic nerve, chiasm, and brainstem, or with considerable surrounding edema, should be considered for early treatment. Observation alone, with periodic neurological and MRI evaluation follow-up, first at 3 months, second at 6 months, and then every year, is reasonable for asymptomatic or minimal symptomatic elderly patients with fewer than 10 to 15 years of remaining life expectancy.

SURGICAL TREATMENT

General Surgical Planning

Preoperative Embolization

The main goal of this procedure is to decrease intraoperative blood loss in meningiomas with high vascular supply. The superselective catheterization makes this procedure safer and allows for controlling the aggressiveness of embolization. The proximal occlusion of the tumor-feeding arteries only reduces the blood supply temporarily and collateral flow quickly develops. The time between embolization and surgery is controversial. The possibility of necrosis induced by vascular occlusion and therefore the softening of tumoral tissue should be compared to the increase of collateral supply development on time. The optimal interval could be between 3 and 9 days. Complications such as painful trismus, facial pain, scalp necrosis, ischemic stroke, and intratumoral hemorrhage could occur but are infrequent.

Neuronavigation

The principle of image guidance in neurosurgery is based on three-dimensional (3D) volumetric information obtained from preoperative CT, angiographic CT, and MRI images. The data are processed by graphic station software that provides high-resolution images in axial, coronal, and sagittal planes. This triplanar reconstruction can be rotated, segmented, and colored in real time. It is also possible to see through surfaces by turning them transparent, allowing the visualization in different depths. The image modality can be changed and adapted to each surgical step. CT is best for bone landmarks in the approach, angiographic CT is useful for vascular-bone relationships, and MRI is better to demonstrate soft tissue components and tumor removal.

The possibility of brain shift during tumor debulking may make the preoperative MRI no longer accurate. This can be solved with an intraoperative MRI. However, brain shift has a minimal impact in meningioma surgery because meningiomas are commonly attached to rigid structures such as dura or skull bone.

General Microsurgical Technique

Whenever possible, the dural origin of the tumor is primarily coagulated using the bipolar forceps to reduce tumor vascularization. After tumor capsule coagulation, internal debulking is performed by use of suction or ultrasonic aspirator. The cleavage plane between the tumor capsule and the underlying arachnoidal sheet must be identified, preserved, and followed as far as possible. The thinned tumor capsule is pulled toward the center of decompression and cottonoid pads are placed in the brain-tumor interface in order to protect the brain parenchyma from possible surgical trauma. Only confirmed feeding arteries are coagulated and divided. In large tumors portions of completely dissected and devascularized capsule can be removed to provide better visualization of deeper structures. These sequential steps of internal debulking, extracapsular dissection, and removal of dissected-devascularized capsule are repeated until the meningioma is totally removed. Whenever feasible all affected dura and bone surrounding the tumor are removed, preserving adjacent neurovascular structures. When total resection implies a significant risk of morbidity, subtotal removal must be considered, with further observation followed by reoperation or radiotherapy (RT) when the tumor is noted to be growing or causing new symptoms.

General Recurrence Rate

In 1957 Simpson[35] classified meningioma resection as follows: grade I, complete removal, including resection of dura and bone; grade II, complete tumor removal with coagulation of dural attachment; grade III, complete tumor removal without resection or coagulation of dural attachments; grade IV, subtotal removal; and grade V, decompression. This classification remains useful for evaluating recurrences. In Simpson's series, grade I through grade IV tumors had recurrence rates of 9%,

19%, 29%, and 40%, respectively, at a follow-up period of 10 years.

Considerations by Location

Convexity Meningiomas

Convexity meningiomas arise from any part of the cranial convexity without involving dural sinuses. They are frequently located around the coronal suture and frontotemporal junction. They can be totally removed including involved dura and bone with great chances of cure. They represent between 15% and 19% of all meningiomas.

Clinical Presentation

Over the prerolandic cortex they can cause contralateral palsy and motor seizures; if they are located posterior to the central sulcus they may present sensory deficits and jacksonian seizures. Speech disturbance is associated with compression of Broca's or Wernike's eloquent areas. Large frontobasal lesions are manifest by visual field impairment or behavioral disorders.

Evaluation

Classical radiological presentation often shows an extensive dural tail. Preoperative embolization is rarely used but could be helpful with meningiomas larger than 5 cm with hypervascular appearance in MR venogram. Neuronavigation could be used to localize small lesions and perform linear incisions for small centered craniotomies, especially in eloquent locations.

Options

Observation is acceptable in asymptomatic elderly patients with a tumor less than 3 cm in diameter and little edema. Stereotactic radiosurgery (SRS) as single treatment could be offered to symptomatic 3 cm or smaller tumors but surgical total resection is the gold standard. Postoperative radiation therapy may be offered to WHO grade II and III meningiomas.

Surgical Technique

Positioning. The patient is positioned in a way that the center of the tumor will be the highest point in the surgical field. The supine position is used for meningiomas located anterior to the coronal suture. Lateral or prone positions are reserved for tumors located behind the coronal suture or in the occipital convexity. The head is fixed with a three-point head rest. The patient's trunk and head are elevated 20 degrees.

Approach. Depending on the location and size of the lesion a linear or horseshoe incision is done with preservation of scalp vascularity. The scalp incision should extend at least 2 cm away from the craniotomy; this should allow extending the dura resection around 2 cm beyond the meningioma border. The pericranium is dissected from the skull and prepared for later grafting. Bur holes are placed around the tumor, and the dura is separated from the overlying bone with a blunt dissector. The bone flap is cut with a high-speed craniotome. Bleeding from bone edges is controlled with bone wax. The infiltrated dura or identified tumor-feeding vessels are coagulated.

Tumor Resection. The microscope may help for part of this resection but is usually not necessary. The dura is open at the tumor margin with minimal exposure of brain. Dural feeder vessels are coagulated and cut under direct visualization. The tumor is debulked and the capsule generally dissected from surrounding brain with care taken to avoid damage to vessels. The resected dura is replaced with pericranium or an artificial substitute.

Postoperative Care. Generally the patient is extubated before arriving to the intensive care unit (ICU). The patient spends the first 24 hours in the ICU and the next day is encouraged to ambulate.

Operative Results. In a series of convexity meningiomas Black and co-workers[36] reported no surgical fatality and no significant difference in morbidity between age groups younger and older than 65 years. The overall morbidity rate was 5.5%. The 5- and 10-year survival rate was 90% with overall recurrence rate of 4.3%. The 5-year recurrence rate for WHO grade I tumors was zero, for grade II 27.2%, and for grade III was 50%. In their series 15 patients (9%) underwent radiation therapy.

Complications. Neurological deficits arise from vascular injury or brain edema from manipulation or retraction.

Parasagittal Meningiomas

These meningiomas represent about 16.8% of meningiomas and are classified in relation to their location along the superior sagittal sinus (SSS) and its invasion. The anterior third extends from the crista galli to the coronal suture, the middle third from the coronal to the lambdoid sutures, and the posterior third from the lambdoid suture to the torcular. Sindou and associates have classified sinus involvement as follows:

Type I: Attachment to outer surface of the sinus wall
Type II: Fragment inside the lateral recess
Type III: Invasion of the ipsilateral wall
Type IV: Invasion of the lateral wall and roof
Types V and VI: Complete sinus occlusion, with or without one wall free, respectively[37]

To achieve a Simpson grade I or II radical resection, the infiltrated SSS should be removed with the tumor. They represent about 16.8% to 25.6% of all intracranial meningiomas.[38]

Clinical Presentation

Anterior third meningiomas usually cause headache, progressive mental deterioration, seizures, and possibly papilledema secondary to increased intracranial pressure. Motor or sensory focal seizures in the contralateral extremity are often seen in patients with meningiomas of the middle third. Tumors in the posterior third can produce homonymous hemianopia. Meningiomas arising from the anterior or posterior third have a more silent growth.

Evaluation

MR venography is not adequate to judge sinus patency, and angiography is the best study for surgical planning. However, the best test of patency may only be at surgery with tentative entry of the sinus. On angiography the arterial phase can predict the difficulty of dissection between the capsule and cortex when a pial vascular supply is identified. The late venous phase is important for evaluating sinus infiltration and the presence of collateral veins. Angiography may also allow embolization in vascular meningiomas. Navigation is very helpful in locating the tumor.

Pathology

The histological pattern in a reported series of 106 was 79.6% for WHO grade I tumors, 14.8% for grade II, and 3.7% for grade III meningiomas.[39]

Treatment

Observation is acceptable in asymptomatic elderly patients or with tumor less than 3 cm in diameter. The SSS total or partial invasion can be treated by radical resection of the sinus with or without venous reconstruction. Resecting the SSS is associated with an increased risk of intraoperative and postoperative hemorrhage, sinus occlusion, corticovenous thrombosis, and venous infarction leading to brain edema. A less aggressive surgical approach, with satisfactory long-term effect and fewer complications, is to resect the tumor up to the sinus wall and leave the sinus intact.[36] Residual tumor can be followed up and treated with radiosurgery at recurrence. Radiosurgery as first-line treatment can offer good results for tumors smaller than 3 cm.

Surgical Technique

Positioning. The supine position is used for meningiomas located in the anterior or middle third of the SSS. For middle third tumors, a useful position is to "hang" the head so the tumor side is down. The prone position is reserved for tumors located in the posterior third of the SSS.

Approach. At our center the skin and bone flaps are marked out with the assistance of neuronavigation. The craniotomy is done in two steps; elevating a bone flap on the tumor side 1 cm away from the SSS, then separating the dura from the overlying SSS and elevating the second bone flap on the contralateral side across the midline. Hemostasis of the SSS superior wall or major dural vessels is done with an oxycellulose packing or bipolar coagulation. Epidural bleeding is controlled with hitching sutures between dura and adjacent bone.

Microsurgical Resection. The dura is opened around the tumor under magnification, taking care not to compromise the afferent veins to the SSS. The tumor is dissected from the brain parenchyma using microsurgical techniques with careful preservation of the arachnoidal plane. Any tumor on the SSS wall is removed and the sinus wall is cauterized. The SSS is not opened or reconstructed.

Operative Results. In Black and co-workers'[36] series the anterior third of the SSS was involved in 12.8% of tumors, the middle third in 69.2%, and the posterior third in 17.9%. In 63.2% of patients there was total tumor resection, Simpson grades I and II. In 14 patients (36.8%) residual tumor was found on postoperative imaging, and 13.2% of those had tumor progression. Recurrence-free survival rate was 94.7% at 5 years.

Complications. Intraoperative bleeding can be reduced with the elevation of the patient head and compressive packing with absorbable hemostats. Brain swelling can be prevented with the preservation of the cortical vessels and avoiding brain retraction.

Falx Meningiomas

These meningiomas arise from the falx cerebri and tend to grow and compress the medial surface of the cerebral hemispheres. They can be classified according to involvement of the falx in longitudeal dimension. Like parasagittal meningiomas, they can be divided into anterior, middle, or posterior types. The classification proposed by Yasargil[40] separated them into outer falx meningiomas, which arise from the body of the falx, and inner falx meningiomas that arise adjacent to the inferior sagittal sinus (ISS). Falcine meningiomas represent 8.5% of all intracranial meningiomas.[41]

Evaluation

About 60% of falx meningiomas present the dural tail sign.[41] MRVA or angiographies are useful to determine the displacement or involvement of the anterior cerebral artery (ACA). The venous phase shows the SSS of ISS invasion and the localization of venous drainage.

Pathology

A transitional histological pattern is the most common subtype.[41]

Treatment

Observation with radiological following is preferable for asymptomatic and small lesions. If the meningioma involves the ACA a subtotal resection should be considered. Residual tumor can be treated with RT or SRS.

Surgical Technique

Positioning. Positioning is as used for parasagittal meningiomas; however, if the tumor is directly against the motor cortex a transcortical approach from behind the motor cortex might be useful.

Approach. A bicoronal craniotomy with navigation assistance is preferred. The bone flap should extend approximately 2.5 cm from the midline on each side.

Microsurgical Resection. Under magnification the dura is opened on the side of the larger component of the tumor or the side of the nondominant hemisphere. The dura is reflected and attached to the soft tissue. The medial aspect of the hemisphere is retracted to identify the SSS and the limits of the lesion. Afferent veins to the SSS should be respected. If it is possible, the falx is divided 1 cm away from the tumor limits to disrupt the blood supply. The internal debulking is performed to facilitate the capsule mobilization. Following the extra-arachnoidal plane the tumor is dissected from the brain parenchyma, taking care to preserve the ACA and its branches.

Operative Results. In the series of 68 patients presented by Chung and colleagues,[41] 85.2% had total resection with no evident recurrence and 92.6% achieved a good outcome (no neurological deficit or complications). SRS was performed as a postoperative adjunctive treatment in six patients.

Complications. Unilateral dural opening is preferred if it is possible to avoid bilateral infraction of bridging veins. If major arteries are encased in the tumoral tissue a subtotal resection followed by radiation therapy must be considered. In case of extreme bilateral edema the bone flap should not be repositioned after tumor resection.

Olfactory Groove Meningiomas

Olfactory groove meningiomas (OGM) arise in the midline of the anterior fossa, from the apophysis crista galli to the planum sphenoidal. Usually bilateral, they grow over the cribriform plate and frontosphenoidal suture. The invasion of the ethmoid bone and the paranasal sinuses makes a complete resection difficult and increases the chance for recurrence. Small meningiomas displace laterally the olfactory nerves and large tumors push them together with the optic chiasm into a posteroinferior direction. Blood supply of this tumor usually comes from ethmoidal branches of the ophthalmic artery, the anterior branch of the middle meningeal artery (MMA), and meningeal branches of the internal carotid artery (ICA). They represent 10% of all intracranial meningiomas.

Clinical Presentation

Common symptoms usually appear when the tumor is considerably large. Anosmia, headaches, seizures, and changes in personality are frequent. Visual deficits are almost always present, even with small tumors, generally as diminution of the acuity and restriction of the inferior field.

Evaluation

CT informs about erosion and hyperostosis of the anterior fossa bone. MRVA may show A2 segment of the ACA encased by the tumor.

Pathology

A psammomatous histological variant is commonly found in this location.

Treatment

Surgery is indicated in almost every case due to the size of the tumor at the time of diagnosis. Preoperative embolization is rarely indicated for the potential risk of occluding the ophthalmic artery and the consequent blindness. If major arteries are involved in the tumor mass, subtotal resection is recommended follow by RT or SRS in selected cases. Small, asymptomatic and commonly incidentally diagnosed meningiomas can be observed or treated with RT/SRS.

Surgical Technique

The frontotemporal (pterional) approach is preferred for small and medium-sized tumors and bifrontal craniotomy is recommended for large lesions.

Positioning. An external lumbar cerebrospinal fluid (CSF) drainage is placed to prevent or reduce brain retraction. For a frontotemporal approach the patient is placed in the supine position. The patient's trunk and head are elevated 20 degrees.

The head is turned to the contralateral shoulder, 30 degrees for more anterior lesions and 20 degrees for posterior tumors. The head is flexed, taking the chin to the ipsilateral clavicle and then slightly hyperextended so that the maxillary eminence reaches the highest point in the surgical field. For the bifrontal approach the patient is also placed in a supine position but with the head in a neutral position and minimally extended inferiorly.

Approach. In the frontotemporal (pterional) approach, the skin incision is begun 1 cm anterior to the tragus at the level of the zygomatic arch and is extended superiorly, then curving anteriorly from the superior temporal line to the midline, just behind the hairline, and extended behind. The scalp flap is reflected anteriorly with sharp dissection against the galea. The superficial and deep fascia of the temporalis muscle are incised 1 cm posterior and parallel to the course of the frontal branches of the facial nerve and retracted anteriorly with the skin flap. The temporalis muscle is incised posterior to the superficial temporal artery and lifted anteriorly and inferiorly using fish hooks to expose the roof and the lateral rim of the orbit. At the supraorbital ridge the supraorbital nerve and vessel run through the supraorbital foramen, and care must be taken to preserve them. The pericranium is dissected behind and incised as posteriorly as possible and then is reflected anteriorly over the scalp flap. A keyhole is placed behind the suture between the frontal bone and the frontal process of the zygomatic bone. Bur holes are made in the floor of the middle fossa and if it is necessary posterior to the superior orbital rim. The bone flap is done with a craniotome. The superior arch of the orbit may be removed for a wide exposure in large tumors. In the bifrontal approach the skin is cut posteriorly to the frontal hairline from zygoma to zygoma. The craniotomy is performed through bur holes placed on each side of the SSS with a high-speed drill. Approximately 1 cm of bone is left posteriorly to the orbital rim.

Microsurgical Resection. For the frontotemporal approach the dura is opened in a C-shape fashion with an anterior base along the sphenoid ridge. It is folded and anchored with sutures. Under magnification the sylvian fissure is dissected allowing the visualization and opening of the optic carotid and carotid oculomotor cisterns. The arachnoid membrane between the optic nerve and frontal lobe is incised and opened to allow the retraction of the frontal lobe and dissection from the tumor capsule. The internal debulking is performed with an ultrasonic aspirator or laser. Following this step the tumor capsule can be easily disected from the underlying brain. The blood supply is occluded along the base and the tumor capsule. With microdissection the tumor is removed. The dura attachment in the anterior fossa base is coagulated, the crista galli cuted and drilled. After hemostasis control the dural defect is closed in a watertight fashion with the vascularized pericranial flap, avoiding tension on the brain and allowing tenting to the bone flap to occlude dead space. If the frontal sinus is exposed it must be cranialized by removing its posterior wall. The frontonasal ostia are occluded with muscle and bone.

For the bifrontal approach the dura is opened in both sides of the SSS. The sinus is ligated or sutured and divided on its anterior third. The falx cerebri is cuted and with gentle retraction the tumor is exposed. Microsurgical tumor removal steps are followed as usual. The posterior surface of the tumor can be closely related to the ACA; care must be taken to avoid its injury. The frontotemporal artery is frequently attached to or encased in the tumor and should be released but can be sacrificed without consequence. After the tumor removal, the involved dura must be resected and coagulated. Hyperostotic bone should be drilled until normal bone is identified assessing the ethmoidal sinus in order to remove all invaded cavities. The dura defect must be closed in a watertight fashion to avoid CSF leakage.

Postoperative Care. External lumbar drainage may be left for 5 postoperative days. For patients with preoperative visual deficits a neuro-ophthalmological evaluation should be performed.

Operative Results. In Obeid and Al-Mefty's[42] series of 13 benign OGMs gross total resection was achieved in 93.3% of patients. Vision remained stable in six patients and improved in eight with no recurrence in a median follow-up period of 3.7 years. They reviewed the recurrence rate for OGMs reported in the literature and found that it ranged from 5% to 41%, and concluded that radical tumor resection, including the dural attachment and any involved bone during the initial surgery, is the best way to reduce the chances of recurrence.[42]

Complications. A vascularized pericranial flap is crucial for a proper reconstruction of the anterior cranial fossa; it must cover the frontal and ethmoid sinuses and be closed in a watertight fashion. The placement of an external lumbar drainage tube is mandatory to avoid brain retraction during surgery and help to prevent CSF rhinorrhea in the postoperative period. To prevent thrombophlebitis and pulmonary embolism, pneumatic compression thigh-high air boots should be used intra- and postoperatively. Bilateral subfrontal craniotomy with sectioning of the falx may improve the surgical field, allowing preservation of olfaction.

Tuberculum Sellae Meningiomas

Tuberculum sellae meningiomas (TSMs) arise from the dura of the tuberculum sellae, diaphragma sellae, chiasmatic sulcus, and limbus sphenoidale. Usually bilateral, they grow from the midline over one side. They can invade the suprasellar region as other meningiomas with different dural origins. TSM can be distinguished from OGM by the displacement of the optic nerves and chiasm. TSMs elevate the chiasm and optic nerves superolaterally, but OGMs displace the chiasm downward and posteriorly as they grow. TSMs represent 5% to 10% of all intracranial meningiomas.[43]

Clinical Presentation

The most frequent presentation of a TSM is optic atrophy with bitemporal hemianopia. The asymmetrical visual loss usually begins in an insidious way and progresses slowly. Other occasional symptoms include headache, mental status deterioration, seizures, anosmia, hyperprolactinemia due to pituitary stalk posterior displacement and compression, and hydrocephalus in cases of third ventricle compression.

Evaluation

Classical radiology presentation, CT images in coronal plane can show hyperostosis of the tuberculum sellae and chiasmatic sulcus. MRVA images provide information about ACA or ICA encasement or displacement often seen in these tumors. Ophthalmological evaluation must be considered.

Treatment

Surgery with total tumor resection must be considered as the first-line treatment before causing optic nerve and ICA involvement. TSMs are usually fed from the posterior ethmoidal artery, a branch of the ophthalmic artery. Preoperative embolization is not indicated for the potential risk of occluding the ophthalmic artery. In TSM encasing major arteries or the cavernous sinus subtotal resection followed by RT or stereotactic radiotherapy (SRT) should be considered. RT or SRT as the initial single therapeutic option is not usually indicated.

Surgical Technique

Bifrontal, frontotemporal, frontolateral, and the expanded endonasal approaches should be considered for these meningiomas.

Positioning. Bifrontal and frontotemporal pterional positioning and approach were described under surgical technique for OGM treatment. The frontolateral approach provides a more medial view of the clinoid and suprasellar region. The patient is placed in a supine position with the trunk and head elevated 20 degrees. The head is turned 10 to 20 degrees to the contralateral shoulder and slightly extended. The frontal lobes spontaneously fall downward because of gravity and allow less retraction to expose the anterior fossa.

Approach. The skin incision is made as in a pterional approach. The craniotomy is performed through a single bur hole at the orbital rim of the frontal bone behind the anterior temporal line. The inner table of the supraorbital ridge is drilled to make the frontal base flat and allow a better visualization of the anterior fossa. If the frontal sinus is opened during the craniotomy the mucosa must be removed completely and coagulated. Before removing the posterior wall, the frontonasal ostia are occluded with muscle and bone.

Microsurgical Resection. The dura is opened in a C-shape fashion with an anterior base along the supraorbital ridge. Under the microscope, the sylvian fissure is opened with a microsurgical technique. For frontolateral and frontotemporal (pterional) approaches the optic carotid and carotid oculomotor cisterns are identified and opened to release CSF and to achieve a better retraction of the frontal lobe. The tumor is identified medial to the ipsilateral optic nerve. Devascularization of the tumor is accomplished by coagulating the dural feeders and detachment from the dura base. The capsule is open to allow internal debulking. With delicate maneuvers the TSM is dissected from the frontal parenchyma until the optic chiasm and the contralateral optic nerve are visible. Small arteries arising from the medial wall of the ICA provide blood supply to the chiasm and optic nerves; their injury must be avoided—in fact, no vessels coming directly off the ICA should be coagulated. The posterior surface of the tumor can displace the pituitary stalk; care should be taken when this area is dissected.

If the tumor grows into the optic canal below the optic nerve, the optic canal is unroofed with a high-speed drill. After the tumor is removed the dura attachment is resected and coagulated. Bone invasion is drilled away.

Postoperative Care. Diabetes insipidus and hypopituitarism should be considered as possible postoperative complications. For patients with preoperative visual deficits a neuro-ophthalmological evaluation should be considered.

Expanded Endonasal Approach

Provide access to the anterior skull base extending from the crista galli to the foramen magnum;[44] all 12 cranial nerves and the carotid and vertebrobasilar arteries can be seen through the nose. This approach should be considered only for small TSMs measuring less than 4 cm owing to the limited lateral explosion. Tumors arising lateral to the optic nerve or beyond the midline of the superior orbit are best approached via craniotomy if the objective of surgery is total removal.[44] Neuronavigation is commonly used.

Positioning. The patient's head is tilted to the left shoulder and the face is turned approximately 20 degrees to the right side. Chlorhexidine 5% is applied in the face and nasal cavity for asepsis. Intranasal pledgets soaked with 0.02% oxymetazoline are used to decongest the mucosa. The abdomen is prepped with antiseptics for the potential use of a fat graft in the cranial base reconstruction.

Approach. In the binasal approach the endoscope is introduced into the right nostril at the 12 o'clock position to recognize the anatomical landmarks. Dissecting instruments are inserted through the left nostril. The middle nasal turbinate is the closest to the nasal septum. The right middle turbinate is removed while the left midde and inferior turbinates are outfractured. A posterior septectomy creates wide bilateral access to the sphenoid sinus rostrum, allowing access to the sinus cavity through the sphenoidal ostiums. The approach should be wide, involving a sphenoidal sinus and half of the other. The half is for allowing the endoscope to maneuver without competing for space, and the remaining sinus provides for unobtrusive movement of the bimanual instrumentation. The sellar floor is identified and opened with drill or rongeurs. In case of intradural extension, the exposed dura is coagulated and open.

Microsurgical Resection. The tumor microsurgical resection is followed as usual. Care should be taken in the dissection of critical vascular structures because of the limited control in the event of massive bleeding. The reconstruction of the cranial base is done with the use of a vascularized nasoseptal flap based on the sphenopalatine artery.

Postoperative Care. ATB therapy is used until the endonasal tamponades are removed 48 hours after the surgery.

Operative Results. In Nakamura and Samii's[43] series of 72 TSMs, total tumor removal could be achieved in 91.7% of patients (Simpson grades I and II). They found a visual improvement rate of 71% in small tumors (maximum diameter <3 cm) and 64% in larger tumors (diameter ≥3 cm) but the difference was not statistically significant. Recovery is thought to be related to tumor size, duration of visual symptoms, and patient edge. Gardner and associates'[45] series of anterior cranial base meningiomas resected endoscopically and endonasally reported that 85% of 13 patients underwent complete resection (Simpson grade I), and one patient underwent 95% resection. The remaining tumor had a 78% resection, based on volumetric analysis. The postoperative CSF leak rate of their entire series was 40%, mostly in TSMs.

Complications. To minimize brain retraction the sphenoid ridge must be drilled and flattened as far as possible. When the dural base and hyperostotic bone are drilled care should be taken to avoid opening the sphenoid sinus. In case of eventual opening a pericranial flap or fascia of the temporal muscle with addition of fibrin glue is used for covering the defect. The surgeon who performs endoscopic surgery for TSM removal must have significant technical experience to deal with critical encased vessels or tumor inside the optic canal. The dural opening cannot be closed by primary means; a vascularized nasoseptal flap should be used in every case to avoid CSF leakage. In the event a leak does occur immediate and early reexploration is recommended rather than diversion with a lumbar drain.[45]

Optic Nerve Sheath Meningiomas

Optic nerve sheath meningiomas (ONSMs) involve the optic nerve and the anterior visual pathways. They usually arise from the arachnoidal membrane of the intraorbital nerve and extend through the optic canal to the anterior fossa. Without treatment, slowly but progressive growth often results in unremitting visual loss. Schick and colleagues[46] classify the ONSM as three types:

Type I: Intraorbital lesions (Ia, flat extension around the optic nerve; Ib, bulbiform mass around the optic nerve; Ic, exophytic tumor around the optic nerve)

Type II: Intraorbital tumors with intracranial extension through the optic canal or superior orbital fissure (IIa, intraorbital growth through the optic canal; IIb, growth through the superior orbital fissure or cavernous sinus)

Type III: Intraorbital tumors with widespread intracranial tumor extension (IIIa, extension to chiasm; IIIb, extension to chiasm, contralateral optic nerve, and planum sphenoidale)

ONSMs represent approximately the 35% of all optic nerve tumors, 1% to 2% of all meningiomas, and 2% to 3% of all orbital tumors. ONSMs are unilateral; only 5% manifested bilaterally.

Clinical Presentation

Visual deterioration is the main symptom at presentation, consisting of progressive visual acuity decline, dyschromatopia, and finally complete loss of vision. Other common signs and symptoms are unilateral proptosis, afferent pupillary defect, scotomas, chemosis, pain, lower eyelid edema, and motility disturbance.

Evaluation

T1-weighted imaging CT with fat suppression is the gold standard for diagnosis of these tumors, especially for those with an intracanalicular or intracranial component. CT can show calcification of the nerve sheath or enlargement of the optic canal. Axial CT contrast-enhanced scans demonstrate hyperdense enhancement of the nerve sheath surrounding a hypodense optic nerve ("tram track sign"). Ultrasound imaging shows optic nerve sheath diameters up to 15 mm behind the globe.

Pathology

The most common histological presentations are meningothelial and transitional.[47] Aggressive tumors tend to infiltrate rather than compress of the globe or optic nerve.

Treatment

Observation must be considered in adults with good vision because of the slow growth behavior of these lesions. Observation without treatment should be followed with caution in pediatric and young patients in whom the tumor behaves aggressively. Complete surgical resection results in blindness in almost all cases, mostly caused by central retinal artery occlusion. Surgical treatment can be indicated for tumor intracranial extension, compressing the optic chiasm or the contralateral optic nerve. Complete neurectomy and tumor resection can be performed in patients with unilateral blindness accompanied by disfiguring proptosis. RT and SRT demonstrate stabilization and even improvement in vision and should be offered as primary therapy to patients with mild to moderate vision loss.

Schick and colleagues[46] recommended radiotherapy without biopsy for type Ia meningiomas; type Ib should be treated with surgery only if it is causing painful eye discomfort without useful vision. Otherwise, these tumors can be observed and treated with radiation once visual decline begins. Type Ic tumors with large exophytic portions should be treated surgically. Type IIa and IIb tumors causing visual impairment should be explored intradurally achieving decompression of the optic canal and superior orbital fissure (SOF). Subtotal resection must be followed by RT. Cavernous sinus involvement should be treated with RT. Type III tumors are operated on to prevent affecting the optic chiasm and contralateral optic nerve. The intraorbital portion should be treated with radiation once visual symptoms or signs occur.

Surgical Technique

The frontotemporal approach is used in almost all cases. The sphenoid ridge anterior clinoid process and optic canal are drilled without opening the dura. The drilling should begin laterally to avoid nerve injury. Finally, the optic canal is unroofed. Exophytic intraorbital tumor masses can be removed through a lateral orbitotomy.

Microsurgical Resection. The sylvian fissure aperture and the ipsilateral optic nerve and carotid cisterns are identified. The tumor capsule is coagulated and dissected around the dura of the optic canal. The falciform ligament of the ipsilateral optic canal is identified and opened to release the nerve. The optic nerve sheath is opened until the annulus of Zinn is reached; this maneuver expands the operative field mainly in the opticocarotid triangle, facilitating access to meningiomas in the suprasellar and subchiasmatic regions. The tumor among the infiltrated dura and the optic nerve is removed. Complete neurectomy and tumor resection are performed in blind patients with disfiguring painful proptosis. The intracranial tumor removal follows the classical steps of microsurgical resection.

Operative Results. Visual improvement after surgical treatment is unusual. In a large reported series of 79 patient with OSNM treated with surgery approximately 7.5% had visual improvement after surgery, 78.5% maintained their vision, and 14% suffered visual deterioration postoperatively.[46] Delfini and co-workers[48] reported that 11 (84%) of 13 patients treated with surgery for ONSM developed postoperative amaurosis. In a large review of meningiomas involving the orbit, Dutton[49] reported a mortality rate of 0%, the rate of operative complication was 30%, and the recurrence rate was 25%. Postoperative visual improvement was shown in only 5% of cases, in contrast with approximately 78% of patients experiencing no light perception. Recurrence rates for ONSMs have been reported to be 6.9% for WHO grade I, 34.6% for WHO grade II, and 72.7% for WHO grade III.

Complications. The most common complication of the surgical treatment of ONSM is visual loss; to avoid this complication care should be taken to preserve small feeding vessels to the optic nerve, chiasma, and the ophthalmic artery. Gentle maneuvers in the manipulation of the optic nerve should avoid the vasa vasorum vasospasm. If the ONSM infiltrates the optic nerve, resection should be limited to the exophytic part. Tumor rests involving the orbital apex, superior orbital fissure, and cavernous sinus should be treated with adjuvant RT.

Radiotherapy

RT demonstrates stabilization and even improvement in vision. In early studies Dutton reported outcomes for ONSM treated with RT: in 75% of cases visual acuity improved, in 8% vision remained stable, and in 17% vision declined. Turbin and Pokorny[47] reported 64 patients with ONSM managed with observation, surgery, surgery and adjuvant RT, or RT alone and concluded that treatment with RT alone resulted in the best long-term visual outcomes. They recommended fractionated external beam radiation between 50 and 55 Gy. However, 33% of these patients developed complications related to radiation. Complication rates improved with the introduction of precisely targeted radiation in the form of SRS or SCRT (stereotactic conformal radiotherapy). Andrews and associates,[50] in a series of 24 eyes treated with SCRT, used doses of 54 Gy and demonstrated visual improvement in 41.6%, stabilization in 50%, and complications in only 4%. Finally, Baumert and colleagues[51] reported on the fractionated SCRT treatment of 23 eyes with a mean follow-up period of 20 months and found 70% showed visual improvement and 22% had stable vision, and they reported the same complication rate of 4%. Fractionated SCRT has proved to be an important noninvasive treatment alternative for ONSM with preservation and improvement of visual function in approximately 80% of the patients.

Anterior Clinoidal Meningiomas

Anterior clinoidal meningiomas (ACMs) arise from the meningeal covering of the anterior clinoid process (ACP). Also called *medial sphenoid wing meningiomas*, they are considered one of the most challenging to treat because of failure of total removal,

high surgical mortality and morbidity rates, and a high rate of recurrence. Al-Mefty[52] classified clinoidal meningiomas based on their origin in three groups. In group I, the tumor origin is proximal to the end of the carotid cistern, and in its growth enwraps the carotid artery without intervening arachnoid. In group II tumors originate from the superior or lateral aspect of the anterior clinoid above the segment of the carotid invested in the carotid cistern and enwrap the carotid with intervening arachnoid. Finally in group III, tumors originate at the optic foramen, extending into the optic canal and the tip of the anterior clinoid process. Pamir and co-workers[53] combined the coronal diameter of the clinoidal meningiomas (suprasellar extension) with the classical Al-Mefty classification. They graded each tumor numerically to correspond to the classification of Al-Mefty and added a capital letter to represent the tumor size on coronal section. The letter A corresponds to a tumor measuring less than 2 cm, B applies to tumors between 2 and 4 cm, and C designates a tumor larger than 4 cm. Factors such as arachnoidal membrane covering of the tumor, size, and neurovascular relationship are important in determining the surgical resectability. ACMs represent 6.5% of all meningiomas and 24.5% of all meningiomas in the anterior fossa.

Clinical Presentation

Visual disturbances were present in 84% of patients. Visual loss preceded diagnosis by an average of 25 months.[52] Other common findings are optic atrophy, papilledema, seizures, headache, and oculomotor or trigeminal nerve impairment.

Evaluation

CT coronal scans may show hyperostosis of the ACP. MRVA or angiography demonstrates arterial displacement, encasement of major vessels, and tumor blood supply.

Pathology

Grade I histological type is found in more than 90% of the cases. Meningothelial variant is the most frequent appearance followed by the transitional pattern.

Treatment

Observation with radiological follow-up is preferable for asymptomatic and small tumors in gender patients. For young patients, surgery at the time of tumor diagnosis, regardless of the size, even in incidental tumors, should be considered. Subtotal resection followed by adjuvant RT must be considered in ACMs with significant adherence or invasion of the ICA, MCA, ACA, optic nerve, or cavernous sinus.

Surgical Technique

The frontotemporal approach is used.

Extradural Considerations. The sphenoid ridge is drilled out and a limited posterior orbitotomy is performed with the removal of the posterolateral orbital wall to completely decompress the superior orbital fissure. The optic canal is unroofed to avoid entering into the ethmoid or sphenoid sinus. The optic nerve is exposed and the dura is dissected from the ACP. The ACP and optic strut are drilled and gently fractured. The dura is opened in a C-shape fashion with an anterior base. Under microscopic guidance the dural incision is continued from the falciform ligament along the length of the optic nerve sheath extending to the annulus of Zinn. The intradural ICA is identified and with gentle maneuvers the tumor around the optic nerve is removed.

Microsurgical Resection. The tumor is dissected from the optic nerve and ICA following the arachnoidal plane. The anterior tumor capsule is coagulated and opened. Internal debulking allows an easier dissection of the tumor from the optic nerve and ICA. The sylvian fissure is opened and the frontal lobe is retracted. Meticulous care is taken to dissect the tumor from cerebral vessels. Large tumors may displace the pituitary stalk posteriorly, and this structure should be recognized and preserved. If the tumor invaded the cavernous sinus, the dural fold of the the oculomotor nerve is opened completely to allow decompression.

Operative Results. Al-Mefty[52] in his analysis of 24 patients achieved total resection in the 75%, with a low recurrence rate of 4% in a median follow-up at 57 months. Lee and associates[54] reported total resection rates of 72% in 42 patients with cavernous meningioma; 22 of them presented with visual deficits and 11 had visual improvement after surgery. No patient in their series showed loss of vision postoperatively.

According to the classification proposed by Pamir and coworkers[53] for a series of 43 cavernous meningiomas, 2 tumors were type IB (4.7%), 8 were type IIA (18.6%), 14 were type IIB (32.5%), 16 were type IIC (37.2%), and 3 (6.9%) were type IIIA. They achieved total surgical removal in 39 cases (90.7%). Vision improvement was found in 22 of the 26 patients who had visual problems, and none of the 43 patients presented with vision deterioration after operation. However, they reported a postoperative complication rate of 18% and a recurrence rate of 11% over a median follow-up period of 32 months.

Complications. Some authors believe that the intradural drilling of the ACP avoids the optic nerve stretch and possible injury. If a disruption into the ethmoid or sphenoid sinus occurs during the drilling stage, a small graft of temporalis muscle is used to cover the opening at the time of closure.

Spheno-Orbital Meningiomas

These tumors are essentially hyperostosing meningiomas en plaque arising from the dura of the lesser sphenoid wing with extension to the orbit. Aggressive bone infiltration usually leads to hyperostosis of the sphenoidal wing, orbital roof, lateral wall, and apex to the ACP and medial cranial fossa. The intracranial component can involve critical areas such as the optic nerve, ICA, or cavernous sinus. Spheno-orbital meningiomas (SOMs) represent up to 9% of all intracranial meningiomas

Clinical Presentation

The most common presentation of SOM is progressive exophthalmos (55-88%), visual impairment (32-78%), and ocular paresis (15-20%).[55-57]

Evaluation

MRI is the best study to evaluate tumor extension and its relationship with surrounding neurovascular structures. CT images can show typical hyperostosis in the sphenoidal wing, orbital roof, lateral wall and apex, ACP, optic canal, superior orbital fissure, and sphenoid or ethmoidal sinuses. Dural enhancement may be absent in contrast CT or MRI.

Pathology

Bone infiltration shows a histological periosteal pattern of hyperostosis. These tumors can have extensive intraosseous involvement without dural infiltration. In Shivastava and colleagues'[56] series all treated SOMs were low grade (WHO I), and the most frequently found variety was meningothelial.

Treatment

Observation with radiological follow-up is advisable for asymptomatic and small tumors in gender patients. Gross total resection is not possible due to frequent superior orbital fissure invasion. For Simpson grade II tumors, subtotal resection should be the main treatment. Owing to the slow growing nature of the SOM observation may be the best option for residual disease. Adjuvant RT should be offered to obtain radiological evidence of tumor progression.

Surgical Technique

The modified one-piece orbitozygomatic approach is preferred. The craniofacial approach is used only in cases of paranasal sinus involvement.

Positioning. The patient is placed in the supine position with the trunk and head elevated 20 degrees. The head is rotated 10 to 20 degrees to the contralateral shoulder and slightly extended.

Approach. A bicoronal incision is planned from the ipsilateral zygoma extending to the contralateral superior temporal line just behind the hairline. The skin flap is elevated and retracted anteriorly. An interfascial dissection is performed to protect the frontal branch of the facial nerve. The temporalis muscle is divided and reflected inferiorly. The anterior edge of the orbit, the foramen, and the supraorbital nerve are identified. The periorbita is dissected from the orbit ridge superiorly and laterally, and the supraorbital nerve is gently released from its notch or foramen. A keyhole is drilled behind the suture between the frontal bone and the frontal process of the zygomatic bone. Additional bur holes are made in the temporal bone and above the superior temporal line. The first cut is performed with a craniotome from the temporal squama bur hole and extended superiorly to the bur hole above the superior temporal line and anteriorly to the orbital edge, just lateral to the supraorbital notch. The next cut extends from the temporal squama bur hole anteriorly and parallel to the zygomatic arch and then turns superiorly toward the sphenoid ridge until stopped by the bony ridge. A cut then is made from the keyhole to the sphenoid ridge. The final cuts are made using the craniotome without the footplate. A cut is made through the orbital ridge and roof connecting with the first cut performed. Then a cut is made from the lateral orbital and frontal process of the zygoma to the keyhole, and finally, a superficial cut is made in the sphenoid spine allowing its fracture when the bone flap is elevated. Osteotomes are used to fracture the orbital roof and lateral wall. An anterior clinoidectomy with unroofing of the optic canal is performed in patients with visual deficits or intracanalicular tumor.

The bone infiltration is drilled away, and during this procedure the dura is left intact as long as possible.

Microsurgical Resection. The dura is opened in a C-shape fashion beyond the area of infiltration. The dura involvement is resected en bloc as far as possible, including the dura covering the sphenoid wing, temporal and frontal bone, and the outer layer of the cavernous sinus. The dura over the superior orbital fissure, tentorial notch, and trigeminal nerve branches remains intact after intensive coagulation. If the tumor infiltrated the periorbita, it is opened and partially resected. The intraorbital tumor component is removed, avoiding the injury of the lateral and superior rectus, the levator palpebrae superioris, and Zinn's annulus, which are sometimes infiltrated by the tumor. A pericranial graft is sutured to the dura margins at the frontal and temporal regions. If the pericraneal patch cannot be sutured in a watertight fashion it can be supplemented with dural graft and is placed under the frontal and temporal lobe. The epidural space is filled with fibrin glue to help seal the dural suture line. The bone flap is then replaced and if it is necessary the orbital roof or the lateral wall of the orbit are reconstructed with methylmethacrylate, titanium mesh, or hydroxyapatite.

Operative Results. In an early report, Carrizo and Basso[58] in a series of 25 patients presented postoperative improvement of exophthalmos without sequelae in 80% of the patients. Ringel and associates[57] presented a large series of 63 patients, with a median follow-up of 4.5 years, achieving proptosis improvement in 77%. Tumor residuals were found in 66%, of which 61% were stable and 39% were progressive. Scarone and colleagues[59] achieved a subtotal resection (Simpson grade II) in 90% of their patients. Radiological evaluation at a median follow-up of 61 months showed no contrast enhancement in 14 patients (47%), residual contrast enhancement without evolution in 13 (43%), and recurrence (new contrast enhancement) in 3 (10%). The exophthalmos improved at a median follow-up period of 61 months in 28 patients (93%).

Complications. Meticulous planning of the surgical approach will achieve better outcomes; lesions with paranasal sinus involvement may require a craniofacial approach and opening of the maxillary, sphenoid, and ethmoidal sinuses. Total gross resection is impossible without significant risk of serious neurological complications, so the dura over the superior orbital fissure, tentorial notch, and trigeminal nerve branches may remain intact in the dural resection stage. A lumbar drain can be used to decrease brain retraction and avoid postoperative CSF leakage.

Cavernous Sinus Meningiomas

Meningiomas involving the cavernous sinus (CS) are one of the most challenging tumors in regard to achieving radical surgical resection. They can arise and remain within the sinus, extend outside the sinus and infiltrate its lateral wall, or growth inside and outside the sinus. The true cavernous sinus meningiomas (CSMs) are seen infrequently; almost all the meningiomas that involve the CS arise in surrounding parasellar dura. Advances in skull base techniques allow surgical tumor resection in this area, previously considered inaccessible, although with significant morbidity, including hemorrhage, cranial nerve deficits, and ICA injury. RT in combination with microsurgical resection or alone has led to new treatment strategies for these tumors. In a large series of meningiomas involving the CS only 8% truly arise from the dural covering of the sinus.[60]

Clinical Presentation

The most common symptoms and signs are diplopia, exophthalmos, trigeminal nerve dysfunction, dizziness, seizures, and headache.

Evaluation

MRI shows a common sign of CSM, which is uneven narrowing of the siphon of the ICA, which is often encased by the tumor. This sign is rare in other tumors, such as, for example, pituitary adenomas with parasellar growth.

Pathology

Pathological classification of these tumors shows that 92.6% are WHO grade I (transitional 41%, meningothelial 23%, and angiomatous 22%), 5.4% are WHO grade II, and 2% are WHO grade III.[60]

Treatment

Primary management options range from observation to conservative surgical resection (without opening the sinus), aggressive surgical resection, RT, SRS, SCRT, and a combination of these therapies. Observation can be offered to asymptomatic elderly patients or those with minimal symptoms such as mild facial tingling or numbness. In young and asymptomatic patients with an extracavernous component, the natural growth rate of the disease and the pros and cons of the treatment options should be explained. Yano and Kuratsu[34] found a growth rate of 0.19 cm per year in 37.3% of patients, with a median follow-up greater than 5 years in their study of asymptomatic CSMs. Close observation followed by conservative surgical treatment if the patient becomes symptomatic should be considered in these patients. Conservative surgical resection as first-line treatment may be offered for CSM with visual or brainstem compression symptoms or with radiological evidence of progressive tumor growth. Adjuvant therapy with RT or SRS is used in selected cases.[60] For intracavernous meningiomas infiltrating the ICA or cranial nerves, SRS can be considered as the first-line treatment because of its long-lasting progression-free survival.[54,61]

Surgical Technique

A standard frontopterional approach is preferred.

Microsurgical Resection. The sylvian fissure is opened initially in order to avoid injuring the ICA. The tumor is debulked in order to expose the MCA branches surrounding the tumor capsule posteriorly. This maneuver will allow identification of the main trunk of the ICA. After identifying the ICA and the optic nerve, the tumor capsule is dissected from extracavernous structures. If it is applicable, decompression of the oculomotor and cranial nerves at their entry into the CS is performed, leaving the cavernous sinus unopened.

Operative Results. Pichierri and co-workers[60] in a series of 147 patients compared a group treated with open sinus surgery with a second group treated with closed sinus surgery. The mean follow-up time was 9.7 years. They found a statistical difference in postoperative morbidity rate between the two groups. Early postoperative morbidity rate was 62.5% for the first group and 31.7% for the second; permanent postoperative morbidity rates were 45.8% and 20.3%, respectively. They didn't find statistical differences in recurrence rates and progression between groups. Lee and associates[54] presented 159 patients, 52% of whom had SRS as their primary treatment. For this group, in 83 patients the control growth rate was 96.9% at 5 years. They concluded that SRS should be considered as the first-line treatment for tumors with a diameter less than 3 cm or volume less than 15 cm^3. Similar findings were reported by Nicolato and colleagues[61] showing an overall progression-free survival rate at 5 years of 96.5% in CSMs treated with SRS as the primary therapeutic option.

Sphenoid Wing Meningiomas

An early classification of sphenoid wing meningiomas (SWMs) designated them as (1) inner or clinoidal; (2) middle or alar; and (3) outer or pterional. The classification proposed by Pirotte and Brotchi[62] in 2008 distinguished them as (A) deep or clinoidal or sphenocavernous; (B) invading en plaque of the sphenoid wings; (C) invading en masse of the sphenoid wings, which combines the features of groups A and B; (D) middle ridge meningiomas; and (E) pterional or sylvian point meningiomas. Clinoidal meningiomas, also named *anterior clinoidal meningiomas* or *medial sphenoid wing meningiomas,* were already described. Middle and lateral SWMs are more surgically accessible and resectable than clinoidal meningiomas. They represent up to 20% of intracranial meningiomas.[63]

Clinical Presentation

Signs and symptoms of SWMs include diplopia, visual loss, dizziness, exophthalmos, retro-orbital pain, seizures, headache, and brain edema due to compression of the sylvian fissure veins.

Evaluation

CT and MRI may reveal an extensive dural invasion, "meningioma en plaque," characteristic hyperostosis, and invasion of the skull base, cavernous sinus, and craniofacial cavities, better seen in coronal slides. MRVA can show tumor vascularization, vascular supply branches, and compression of sylvian veins, allowing a safer surgical dissection.

Pathology

The vast majority (94%) of SWMs are histologically benign, WHO grade I.[63]

Treatment

Observation is preferred for asymptomatic elder patients. Surgical gross total resection is the gold standard treatment, even in asymptomatic young patients if the tumor progression may affect unresectable areas. RT must be considered as adjuvant therapy in selected cases with subtotal resection.

Surgical Technique

Most of these meningiomas are operated through a frontotemporal approach; if the tumor infiltrates the orbit, a modified orbitozygomatic approach may be considered.

Microsurgical Resection. For middle SWMs the dura attached is usually in the lesser wing. The sylvian fissure is opened with additional care in preserving the sylvian veins at their entry point into the sphenoparietal sinus. The following microsurgical steps are performed as usual. For lateral SWMs the modified orbitozygomatic approach is preferred. The bone infiltration is drilled away extradurally. The dura involvement is resected and if the tumor infiltrated the periorbita, that area is opened and partially resected, avoiding injury of the lateral and superior rectus, the levator palpebrae superioris, and Zinn's annulus, which are sometimes infiltrated by the tumor.

Operative Results. Pirotte and Brotchi[62] in their series reported no mortality or morbidity for the middle and lateral SWMs and total gross resection in all cases (Simpson grade I). The recurrence rate was less than 10%.

Complications. CSF leakage is avoided with a watertight closure of the dural defect with or without a pericranial patch. Fibrin glue may be used to seal the dura suture line. Postoperative edema can result in infarction of the sylvian veins. Meticulous study of the preoperative MRVA will reveal venous disposition; the lack of collateral veins enhances the preservation of the sylvian vein.

Petroclival and Upper Clival Meningiomas

Petroclival meningiomas (PCMs) arise from the upper two thirds of the clivus at the petroclival junction, medial to cranial nerves V, VII, VIII, IX, X, and XI. They can be located exclusively in the posterior fossa or extend to the middle fossa, prepontine cisterns, posterior CS, sphenoid sinus, and the foramen magnum inferiorly. PCMs may encase the basilar artery with its principal branches, the superior, anterior inferior, and posterior inferior cerebellar arteries; larger lesions can displace these vessels and brainstem to the contralateral side. Contrary upper clival meningiomas (UCMs) displace these neurovascular structures posteriorly. Approximately 3% to 10% of posterior fossa meningiomas are petroclival.

Clinical Presentation

The most frequent cranial nerves involved are the fifth, causing facial paresthesia, and the eighth nerve, leading to hearing loss. Facial nerve disturbance can occur in 30% to 50% of patients, and low cranial nerves are affected in approximately 30% of the cases.[64,65] Compression of the brainstem and cerebellum may present as gait disturbances and somatomotor and sensitive deficits.

Evaluation

CT scan may reveal bone erosion, hyperostosis, or both. Displacement and compression of normal structures are best demonstrated by MRI. Edema in the brainstem may be shown on T2-weighted imaging scans and implies disruption of the arachnoidal plane between the tumor and brainstem; thus, aggressive resection of the brainstem must be avoided.

MRVA and conventional angiography shows tumor vascularization degree, feeder branches, and displacement or encasement of the basilar artery and the principal branches. Angiography allows embolization of the tumor vascular supply, usually from the external carotid artery. As a distinctive sign the meningohypophyseal trunk (Bernasconi-Cassinari artery) may be enlarged.

Treatment

Observation is indicated in asymptomatic elderly patients or those with poor clinical status. Surgical treatment is considered in symptomatic lesions, even if they are small, because growth, albeit slow, can involve cranial nerves and vessels, making tumor dissection from these structures impossible. Subtotal resection should be achieved in cases of encasement or infiltration of critical neurovascular structures. Adjuvant RT is indicated in selective cases. SRS or fractionated SRT as primary therapy can be offered to patients with poor clinical status haven SWM that require treatment.

Surgical Technique: Fronto-Orbito-Zygomatic Approach

This approach with or without an anterior petrosectomy is preferred for PCMs with extension in the middle cranial fossa involving the posterior CS. This access provides a wide exposure of the middle fossa and early control of the ICA and should be considered for tumors across the middle line. Nevertheless, it does not allow an optimal visualization of the tumor in the infratentorial midline and the posterior fossa below cranial nerves VII and VIII or internal auditory meatus (IAM). This approach also implies a major manipulation of the trigeminal nerve and the possible lesion.

Positioning. The patient is positioned supine with the trunk and head elevated 20 degrees. The head is rotated 30 degrees to the contralateral shoulder, slightly extended, and fixed with a three-pin holder.

Approach. A classical pterional incision and skin flap are performed. The superficial and deep layers of the temporalis fascia are elevated with the skin flap to protect the frontal branch of the facial nerve. The zygomatic arch is incised obliquely at the most anterior and posterior ends and the temporalis muscle is elevated and retracted inferiorly. A fronto-orbito-temporal craniotomy is made. The great sphenoid wing, lateral orbit wall, and base of the middle fossa are drilled.

The dura along the floor of the middle fossa is elevated. By following the middle meningeal artery (MMA), the foramen spinosum is identified and the MMA is cut as it exits the foramen. Medial to the foramen spinosum, the greater and lesser superficial petrosal nerves are identified (GSPN, LSPN). Excessive retraction of the GSPN can cause facial nerve injury and anhidrosis. Dissection anterior to the foramen spinosum exposes the foramen ovale, foramen rotundum, and superior orbital fissure. The superior orbital fissure is opened. The horizontal portion of the petrous ICA lies deep and parallel to the GSPN and posteromedial to the foramen ovale and mandibular branch of the fifth nerve, and if it is necessary, it can be unroofed by using a diamond drill; however, it is not uncommon for the bony covering of the petrous carotid to be absent.

Microsurgical Resection. The dura is incised and the sylvian fissure is opened, exposing the ICA and olfactory, optic, and oculomotor nerves. The ICA, MCA, and ACA are carefully dissected from the tumor capsule, beginning from the noninvolved portion. The optic canal is drilled with diamond burs. The tumor in the middle fossa is removed, exposing the lateral wall of the CS. If the cavernous sinus is infiltrated, the extracavernous portion is removed and its lateral wall is coagulated. PCMs that extend anteriorly and infiltrate the superior orbital fissure, ICA, and second or third cranial nerves should be partially resected. For tumors extending posteriorly, the petrous apex is drilled medial to the ICA, extending from the trigeminal impression to the IAM, exposing the posterior fossa dura. The dura is then opened along the base of the temporal lobe. The superior petrosal sinus is coagulated and cut to allow opening of the tentorium and exposing the posterior fossa. The tentorium incision is made behind the entrance of the third cranial nerve in the CS. The exposed petrous dura and tentorium can be aggressively coagulated to devascularize the tumor. A wide exposure is achieved if the posterior clinoid process is drilled. Finally, the seventh and eighth cranial nerves with the basilar artery and its principal branches are dissected from the tumor capsule. No vessels coming directly off the basilar artery should be coagulated.

Posterior Petrosal Approach

This surgical corridor, also known as the *presigmoid retrolabyrinthine approach,* is used to expose tumors in the posterior fossa, lateral and inferior to the IAM. This approach offers a wide tumor exposure with minimal temporal lobe retraction and reduces the operating distance to the petroclival junction. The petrous resection is retrolabyrinthine, allowing for preservation of hearing and a more lateral view of the brainstem and petroclival groove. This approach requires the exposure and mobilization of the sigmoid sinus and may present a risk in patients with a dominant or single sigmoid sinus ipsilateral to the tumor, in patients with a transverse sinus that do not connect to the torcula, and in patients with the venous drainage through the tentorium. This approach does not provide a satisfactory exposure in patients with a high jugular bulb or a tumor located across the middle line of the clivus.

Positioning. The patient is placed in a supine position with the head rotated to the opposite side.

Approach. A curvilinear incision is made starting in the preauricular area, 4 cm above the zygomatic arch, passing 3 cm behind the ear, extending retroauricularly 2 cm behind the mastoid tip. The temporal fascia is incised and reflected inferiorly in continuity with the craniocervical fascia and sternocleidomastoid muscle. The temporalis muscle is cut along the superior edge of the skin incision and reflected inferiorly and anteriorly. Two bur holes above and two below the sigmoid sinus are placed, and a single bone flap is cut, exposing the middle and the posterior fossa.

The transverse-sigmoid sinus junction is exposed with the craniotomy. The cortical bone of the mastoid is drilled out and a mastoidectomy is performed, keeping the bony labyrinth intact. The presigmoid dura is exposed and the sigmoid sinus is skeletonized down to the jugular bulb. The dura is opened anterior to the sigmoid sinus, along the floor of the temporal fossa. The vein of Labbé must be identified at its insertion into the transverse sinus and preserved. The superior petrosal sinus is coagulated and ligated between two stitches, and is incised, allowing the connection with the anterior dura to be open. The tentorium is sectioned parallel to the transverse sinus and perpendicular to the superior petrosal sinus after the identification and preservation of the fourth cranial nerve insertion. The posterior temporal lobe is elevated and the sigmoid sinus is retracted posteriorly, allowing a wide exposure of the cerebellum.

Microsurgical Resection. The temporal lobe and the cerebellum are gently retracted, exposing the petroclival region from the third to eighth cranial nerves. The PCM is detached at its dural insertion; the capsule is coagulated and opened, allowing internal debulking. The tumor capsule is dissected from the cranial nerves and the basilar artery (BA) and its main branches. If the meningioma infiltrates the posterior portion of the CS, the extracavernous portion is resected, followed by coagulation of the CS external wall. All infiltrated petrous and clivus bone is drilled away. After tumor removal the dura is closed in watertight fashion. The mastoid air cells are closed with bone wax and the mastoid antrum with a muscle plug. The temporalis muscle flap is rotated to cover the exposed dura. The temporocraniocervical fascia and the sternocleidomastoid muscle are closed.

Combined Petrosal Approach

This approach is best for patients with large petroclival tumors and functional hearing. It provides the exposure of both anterior and posterior petrosal approaches with the preservation of hearing and facial nerve function. This option should be considered for tumors extending across the midline of the clivus with a significant amount of tumor in the posterior fossa below the IAM.

Positioning. The patient is placed in the park-bench position with the neck in slight flexion to open the occipitocervical angle. The thorax and head are elevated 15 to 20 degrees. The zygoma should be the highest point in the surgical field.

Approach. The skin incision consists of two limbs. The posterior limb incision is similar to that described for the posterior petrosal approach. The anterior limb begins 1 cm anterior to the tragus at the level of the zygomatic arch, continues anteriorly in a curvilinear fashion behind the hairline, and ends near the midline. The frontal skin flap is reflected anteriorly along with the temporal fascia to preserve the frontal branch of the facial nerve. The zygomatic arch is cut and the temporal skin flap is reflected inferiorly. The temporalis muscle is divided along the superior temporal line, leaving a fascial cuff for later repair, and reflected anteriorly and inferiorly. The craniotomy is similar to the posterior petrosal bone flap, although it is extended more anteriorly along the floor of the middle cranial fossa and the sphenoid wing. The cortical bone of the mastoid is drilled out and a mastoidectomy is performed keeping the bony labyrinth intact. The temporal lobe is carefully elevated and the anterior petrosectomy is performed as described earlier. The dura between the sigmoid sinus and petrous apex is exposed. A dural incision is made in the posterior fossa dura, anterior to the sigmoid sinus, and in the middle fossa dura,

superior to the petrosal sinus. This incision is prolonged posteriorly to the transverse sigmoid junction. Care is taken to avoid injuring the vein of Labbé. The superior petrosal sinus and tentorium are incised anteriorly to the incisura in a course directed posterior to the entry of the trochlear nerve into the tentorial edge. This approach allow the exposure of the medial temporal lobe, lateral pons, basilar artery, and cranial nerves III through VIII through the petrous bone anterior and posterior to the bony labyrinth.

Total Petrosectomy

This approach is indicated in patients with giant tumors crossing the middle line in the prepontine region and loss of hearing. The removal of semicircular canals and cochlea allows the widest exposure of the petroclival region; however, the risk of injuring the facial nerve during the drilling should not be despised. The initial surgical stages are similar to the combined petrosal approach. The external auditory canal is sectioned and closed in a blind sac. The mastoidectomy is followed by a labyrinthectomy and transposition of the facial nerve. The petrous apex and cochlea are drilled to complete the petrosectomy. After the tumor microsurgical resection the closure step is performed as usual, blocking the eustachian tube with a muscle plug and fibrin glue to avoid CSF leakage.

Complications. The increased risk of thromboembolic complications is avoidable by compression stocking and postoperative prophylaxis with low-molecular-weight heparin.

Operative Results. In a series of 97 patients with PCM presented by Al-Mefty and co-workers,[64] 28 patients were treated using the anterior petrosal approach, 27 with the posterior petrosal approach, 34 with the combined petrosal approach, and 8 underwent to a total petrosectomy. Eight patients presented with complications related to the approach. There were no cases of trigeminal neuralgia after the zygomatic anterior petrosal approach. Only 8% of the patients who underwent the posterior petrosal or combined petrosal approaches experienced hearing loss.

Petrosal Meningiomas

The cerebellopontine angle (CPA) meningiomas describe a group of tumors that compromise a common anatomical region, the CPA. These lesions may have their true origins in different locations, even outside the CPA. Because of their different clinical presentations and outcomes in relation to their site of origin,[66] they have been classified in reference to the internal auditory meatus (IAC) as anterior petrous meningiomas (group 1), tumors involving the IAC (group 2), superior petrous meningiomas (group 3), inferior petrous meningiomas (group 4), and posterior petrous meningiomas (group 5).[67] They are the second most frequent tumor in the CPA after vestibular schwannomas (10-15%), representing approximately 8% to 23% of all intracranial meningiomas.

Clinical Presentation

The main form of presentation is the hearing loss (73%), followed by vertigo, tinnitus, trigeminal dysfunction, and facial nerve dysfunction. The brainstem compression can cause gait disturbance and obstructive hydrocephalus in 10% to 20% of these patients.

Evaluation

CT is useful for demonstrating petrous bone, hyperostosis, pneumatization, and the surrounding venous sinus. MRI is best for visualizing tumor relationship with neurovascular structures. T2-weighted imaging helps to determine brainstem displacement and invasion of the IAC by the tumor. T2-weighted gradient echo (GRE) sequences may have potential value in differentiating vestibular schwannomas (VSs) from CPA meningiomas owing to the demonstration of microhemorrhages characteristics of VS. The dural tail sign also can help because it is often seen in meningiomas. In patients with neurofibromatosis type 2, a spine MRI should be performed because of possible associations with another central nervous system tumor.

Pathology

The most frequent histological presentation is WHO I type meningioma. The pattern may differ in relation to its localization, presenting 68% of meningothelial subtype in anterior petrosal meningioma, whereas 69% of posterior petrosal meningiomas and 62% of superior petrosal meningiomas had fibrous histological appearance.[68]

Treatment

Observation is preferred in asymptomatic elderly patients or those with poor clinical status. Surgery is considered the gold standard treatment in symptomatic lesions, even if they are small, because growth can encase the basilar artery and compress the brainstem and cranial nerves, making tumor dissection more difficult. If the adaptive limit of the brainstem structures is reached, then pial invasion and edema can lead to an acute clinical deterioration. Subtotal resection should be achieved in case of encasement or infiltration of cranial nerves or brainstem. Adjuvant RT is indicated in selected cases.

Surgical Technique

Positioning. The patient is placed in a supine, park-bench, or semisitting position. Intraoperative neurophysiological monitoring of the lower cranial nerves, somatosensory evoked potentials (SSEPs), and brainstem auditory evoked potentials are measured. Neuronavigation may be helpful to confirm the anatomical sinuses and bone landmarks.

Approach. A slightly curved skin incision is done, extending superiorly 2 cm behind the pinna, passing through the asterion and terminating 1 to 2 cm medial to the mastoid tip. The skin flap is elevated with the periosteum and held with a self-retaining retractor. The muscles are divided using monopolar cautery in line with the skin incision until the root of the digastric groove is visible. The asterion constitutes the superolateral limit of the craniotomy. A bur hole is made below the asterion to expose the transverse-sigmoid sinus junction and a suboccipital craniotomy 3 to 4 cm in diameter is performed with rongeurs or a high-speed drill. If the mastoid air cells are opened during the exposure they must be closed with bone wax. The dura is opened in a semicircular or L-shaped fashion along the transverse and sigmoid sinuses; in large lesions it

should extend caudally far enough to allow opening of the cisterna magna and release of CSF.

Microsurgical Resection. The arachnoid membrane is opened over the inferolateral cisterns and drains CSF to allow the cerebellum to relax. With gently oblique retraction on the cerebellum, the tumor capsule is exposed. The microsurgical principles of meningioma resection are applied. The anterior petrosal meningiomas are removed between the cranial nerve, mostly between the trigeminal and facial-vestibulocochlear nerves. The tumors from groups 2 to 5 should be debulked and reduced in size to identify these nerves. The IAC can be opened or invaded by the tumor, and frequently the posterior bony portion of the foramen should be drilled to access the tumor removal. The closure steps are followed as usual.

Operative Results. Nakamura and associates[67] present a series of 347 CPA meningiomas. Total tumor removal (Simpson grades 1 and 2) was achieved in 85.9% and subtotal removal in 14.1% of the patients, with best initial postoperative seventh and eighth nerve function in tumors located posterior and superior to the IAC. A good postoperative facial nerve function (House-Brackmann grade 1 or 2) was observed in 88.9% of patients with a mean follow-up time of 62.3 months. Hearing preservation among patients with preoperative functional hearing was documented in 90.8%. Similar findings were reported by Sade and Lee[68] in a group or 58 patients, with an informed gross total resection in 84% of the patients. New-onset hearing loss was present in 11% of patients. The best surgical results were also obtained with superior and posterior petrosal meningiomas.

Complications. Cranial nerve injury can be reduced with the routine utilization of neurophysiological nerve monitoring. Subtotal resection should be considered if the tumor infiltrates or encases neurovascular critical structures. In order to avoid CSF fistula, mastoid air cells must be waxed thoroughly and internal air cells exposed by drilling the posterior wall of the IAM, which must be sealed with small amounts of muscle plug and fibrin glue. Facial nerve paralysis can be managed with eyedrops and night-ocular occlusion. During the seventh nerve recovery, corneal ulcerations and conjunctivitis can be avoided with the subcutaneous insertion of a platinum plate into the superior eyelid. In the case of lower cranial nerve dysfunction, the preventive use of a nasogastric tube before extubation must be considered in order to avoid aspiration and consequently pneumonia.

Foramen Magnum Meningiomas

These tumors arise anteriorly from the inferior third of the clivus to the superior edge of the C2 body, laterally from the jugular tubercle to the C2 laminae, and posteriorly from the anterior border of the occipital squama to the spinal process of C2. The dentate ligament divided the foramen into anterior and posterior compartments. According to the insertion on the dura, foramen magnum meningiomas (FMMs) can be defined in the anteroposterior plane as anterior, if insertion is on both sides of the anterior midline; lateral, if insertion is between the midline and the dentate ligament; and posterior, if insertion is posterior to the dentate ligament.[69] The FMMs are located in the anterior face of the foramen in 70%, anterolateral in 21%, and posterolateral in 9% of the patients.[70] They represent 1.5% to 3.2% of all intracranial meningiomas.

Clinical Presentation
Frequent symptoms are cervical and occipital radicular pain, dizziness, dysphagia, dyspnea, hoarseness, long-tract deficits, muscular atrophy of limbs, and cerebellar ataxia.

Evaluation
CT axial scans may provide information about the size of occipital condyle and lateral mass of C1, and the angulations between these structures, important factors to be considered in the surgical planning. T2-weighted imaging is better to determine brainstem displacement and invasion; the encasement and narrowing of the vertebral artery (VA) is assessed with MRVA or angiography.

Treatment
Surgery is considered the gold standard treatment for FMM.

Surgical Technique
Positioning. Patients are placed in a ventral, park-bench, or sitting position. Intraoperative neurophysiological monitoring of the lower cranial nerves, SSEP, and brainstem auditory evoked potentials are measured. Neuronavigation may be useful to confirm the anatomical landmarks.

Approach. The posterior midline approach is preferred for posterolateral FMM. For anterior and anterolateral meningiomas a far-lateral retrocondylar approach is selected. In this surgical access the skin incision extends on the middle line, from C3-C4 superiorly to the occipital protuberance and curves laterally toward the mastoid process on the pathological side. The posterior muscles are detached along the occipital crest and retracted laterally to expose the occipital bone, the posterior arch of the atlas, and the C2 lamina, if required. The V3 segment of the VA running above C1 is identified and exposed in a subperiosteal plane from the midline of the posterior arch of the atlas laterally toward the atlas groove. The C1 posterior arch is removed up to its lateral mass. A retrosigmoid craniectomy is performed, including inferiorly the foramen magnum. The lateral extension of the occipital condyle is removed, and mobilization of the VA is established according to the position of the meningioma. In case of anterior FMM, the spinal cord is pushed posteriorly, so the surgical opening has to be enlarged laterally by drilling the medial side of the C1 lateral mass until the foramen transversarium is open. This maneuver allows displacing the VA to remove the posterior third of the occipital condyle. In the case of anterolateral meningiomas there is no need to move the VA or drill the occipital condyle because the spinal cord is displaced to the contralateral side. For FMMs involving the middle clivus, an extended far-lateral approach can be used; in that case the sigmoid sinus is unroofed and followed to the posterior aspect of the jugular foramen.

Microsurgical Resection. The dura is opened with a curvilinear incision starting at the inferolateral corner, then running vertically at a paramedian level and curving toward the superolateral corner. The arachnoid connections between the dura and the medulla are preserved to avoid an anterior fall of the

neuraxis during tumor resection. Lateral FMMs are directly devascularized and carefully removed in a piecemeal fashion. To access to anterior tumors, the two first dentate ligaments and sometimes first cervical nerve root have to be sacrificed to enlarge the surgical corridor. Care must be taken to preserve vessels coming directly from the VA. After tumor removal the dura is closed in a watertight fashion.

Postoperative Care. The patient is sent to the intensive care unit intubated, and if the cough and gag reflex is present on the next day the patient is extubated. If new lower cranial deficits are present, tracheotomy and nasogastric feeding must be considered.[70] Postoperative cranial nerve deficits require aggressive and early rehabilitation.

Operative Results. Wu and colleagues[70] presented a series of 114 patients with FMM. Gross total resection was achieved in 86.0% of patients and subtotal resection in 14.0%. Surgical mortality rate was 1.8%. Ninety-three patients were followed for a median period of 90.3 months: 59 (63.4%) had a normal life (Karnofsky performance scale [KPS] score 80-100), 28 (30.1%) had moderate disabilities (KPS score 50-80), and 6 (6.5%) presented with severe disabilities.

Jugular Foramen Meningiomas
Jugular foramen meningiomas (JFMs) arise on the jugular foramen (JF) dura and extend in the infralabyrinthine temporal bone and the middle ear; intracranially they may invade the skull base bone involving the jugular tubercle, hypoglossal canal, occipital condyle, and clivus. Extracranially they can compromise the parapharyngeal space encasing the carotid artery and jugular vein. The JF can be secondarily infiltrated by meningiomas arising from intracranial locations such as foramen magnum, petroclival region, CPA, and temporal bone. JFMs represent the third most common tumor of the JF after glomus jugulare tumors (GJTs) and lower cranial nerve schwannomas. They account for 0.7% to 4% of posterior fossa meningiomas and less than 1% of all intracranial meningiomas.

Clinical Presentation
The most common symptoms are hearing loss (52.3%), dysphagia (23.2%), and tinnitus (17.4%), followed by dysphonia, dizziness, ataxia, and cervical pain.[71]

Evaluation
On CT scans JFMs may show an irregular enlargement of the JF margins with a mixed permeative-sclerotic appearance, whereas GJTs present a permeative-destructive pattern. Schwannomas gradually enlarge the JF by pressure erosion conferring an expanded and scalloped but well-defined corticated margin.[72] The presence of dural tails, even when they are not pathognomonic of meningiomas, can be useful in the differential diagnosis. Another important differentiating characteristic seen in MRI scans is the absence of flow voids in the meningioma mass—this feature is often present in GJTs owing to their rich vascularization.[72]

Pathology
The frequency of histological subtypes is as follows: 88.5% WHO grade I, 6.5% WHO grade II, and 5% WHO grade III.[71]

Treatment
Even though observation can be considered for elderly asymptomatic patients, surgical total resection is the treatment of choice. Owing to the infiltrative behavior of these tumors, however, total resection is very difficult to achieve, and subtotal resection followed by adjuvant RT may be necessary.

Surgical Technique
There are several surgical approaches to JFMs. The petrooccipital transsigmoid (POTS) approach is preferred for preservation of middle and inner ear function without the need for facial nerve transposition.

Positioning. The patient is placed in the supine position with the head turned to the contralateral side.

Approach. A C-shaped incision is performed starting 3 cm over the auricle, extending 4 to 5 cm posteriorly, then curving inferiorly to the level of C1, and finally turning anteriorly to reach the posterior angle of the mandible. A musculoaponeurotic inferiorly based flap is made. After retracting the sternocleidomastoid muscle, the internal jugular vein is identified just anterior to the transverse process of the atlas. A retrosigmoid craniotomy is performed, followed by an extended mastoidectomy with skeletonization of the sigmoid sinus down to the jugular bulb. The posterior third of the condyle and the jugular tubercle are removed. A good landmark to use to limit the bony removal is the condylar vein. The hypoglossal canal is located at the junction of the posterior and middle thirds of the occipital condyle. The sigmoid sinus and the jugular bulb are completely unroofed up to the posterior semicircular canal. A retrolabyrinthine petrosectomy and dissection of the retrofacial and infralabyrinthine air cells is performed, taking care to preserve the cochlea intact. The internal jugular vein in the neck is ligated, and then the sigmoid sinus is occluded proximally and distally with two clips and opened.

Microsurgical Resection. The dura is opened with a horizontal incision, starting 3 cm posterior to the sigmoid sinus, traversing the sinus medial wall, and ending anteriorly at the level of the posterior semicircular canal. The jugular bulb is opened, allowing control of the foramen magnum. The tumor is carefully dissected from the surrounding lower cranial nerves. After tumor removal the superior and retrofacial air cells are closed with bone wax. The dura is closed in a watertight fashion and the dead space is filled with fat tissue.

Postoperative Care. Postoperative care is the same as that for foramen magnum meningiomas.

Operative Results. In a recent series of 13 patients presented by Sanna and co-workers[73] their findings showed gross total tumor removal (Simpson grades I and II) in 11 (84.6%) cases without evidence of tumor recurrence at a mean follow-up of 47 months. Good facial nerve function (grades I and II) was achieved in 46.1% of cases. A new deficit of one or more of the lower cranial nerves was recorded in eight (61.5%) patients. Ramina and associates[74] achieved gross total resection in 50% of their cases. Two patients died in the immediate postoperative period and four patients died because of disease progression, with a mean survival time of 35 months. They concluded that the incidence of postoperative deficit of cranial nerves is higher than in other benign tumors of the JF.

Tentorial Meningiomas
Yasargil's classification of tentorial meningiomas (TMs) defines eight types of tumors according to their location on the cerebellar tentorium. They were subsequently regrouped as follows:

Group I: Anteromedial, arising from the apex of the tentorial margin
Group II: Anterolateral, arising from the lateral aspect of the tentorial incisural margin
Group III: Intermediate, arising from the intermediate aspect of the tentorium remote from the incisura and the dural sinuses
Group IV: Posteromedial, arising from posteromedial aspect of the tentorium close to straight sinus or venous confluence at the torcula; this group also includes the falcotentorial and torcular meningiomas
Group V: Posterolateral, arising from the posterolateral aspect of the tentorium close to the sigmoid sinus[75-77]

TM represents 3% to 6% of all intracranial meningiomas.

Clinical Presentation
The most frequent symptoms are headache (75%), dizziness (49%), gait disturbance (45%), mental changes (12%), visual disturbance (11%), and hearing loss (9%).[75]

Evaluation
MRVA sequences are mandatory to achieve visualization of sinuses with partial or complete occlusion by tumor infiltration or compression.

Pathology
Grade I tumors represent approximately 95% of the histological pattern, grade II tumors account for 3.75%, and grade III accounts for 1.2%. The most frequent benign meningomas in these locations are fibroblastic and meningothelial.[75]

Treatment
Surgical excision is considered the best treatment.

Surgical Technique: Occipital Interhemispheric Approach
The occipital interhemispheric approach is preferred for group I, II, and III supratentorial meningiomas. The transtentorial access is indicated for group I, II, and IV tumors with supra- and infratentorial extension.

Positioning. The patient is placed in the semisitting position.

Approach. The head is slightly turned to the side of the lesion and fixed with a three-point headrest. A supraoccipital craniotomy is made exposing at its inferior margin the edge of the superior sagittal and transverse sinuses. For supra- and infratentorial tumors the exposure is completed by transection of the tentorium as far as the incisura, at least 1 cm parallel to the straight sinus.[76]

Microsurgical Resection. The occipital lobe is gently retracted laterally, allowing a wide exposure followed by coagulation of the surrounding falx and tentorium in order to reduce tumor vascularity. The meningioma is detached from its tentorial origin and resected. If the meningioma extends to the contralateral side it can be reached through a fenestration in the falx cerebri. In selected cases the tentorium opening will provide access to the pineal region and infratentorial portion of the tumor. Excessive occipital lobe retraction or venous injuries may result in postoperative hemiparesis or visual field deficits.[76]

Subtemporal Approach

The subtemporal approach can be used for group II supratentotrial meningiomas.

Positioning. The patient is placed in the supine position.

Approach. A standard subtemporal craniotomy is performed.

Microsurgical Resection. The temporal lobe is gently elevated to expose the tumor in the inner middle cranial fossa, and care must be taken to avoid injuring the vein of Labbé. Microsurgical steps of tumor removal are performed. The middle or inferior temporal gyrus resection may be considered in cases of difficult temporal lobe retraction due to tumoral compression or brain swelling.

Bioccipital-Suboccipital Approach

This access provides the exposure of the four quadrants of the torcula herofili. It is useful for treatment of group IV meningiomas.

Positioning. The patient is placed in the semisitting position.

Approach. A bioccipital and suboccipital craniotomy is performed on both sides of the midline, exposing the confluence of the venous sinuses.

Microsurgical Resection. After dura opening the occipital lobe ipsilateral to the largest portion of the meningioma is gently retracted to allow tumor exposure. After tumor internal debulking the falx is fenestrated to reach the contralateral tumor extension. The lesion is carefully detached from the torcula and straight and occipital sinus to achieve the removal of the infratentorial part of the tumor. The sinus walls are coagulated and left unopened if the tumor has partially occluded them. In the case of total occlusion the sinuses are removed.

Midline Supracerebellar Infratentorial Approach

This approach provides access to the tentorial incisura margin and the quadrigeminal cisterns. It is useful for infratentorial group I and IV meningiomas, and may allow removal of selected infra- and supratentorial tumors.

Positioning. The patient is placed in the sitting or park-bench position. Patients with a small posterior fossa usually have an almost vertical tentorial angle, making the supracerebellar infratentorial approach with the patient seated extremely difficult. In this situation the park-bench position should be considered or other approaches, such as occipital transtentorial trajectory, can be considered.

Approach. The head is placed in a neutral position and flexed about 15 degrees to position the tentorium in a horizontal plane. A U-shaped inferiorly based skin incision is made; after reflecting the musculocutaneous flap, a bilateral suboccipital craniotomy is performed from the confluence of the transverse sinuses and the torcula superiorly to approximately 2 cm above the foramen magnum. For larger lesions the foramen magnum can be included. The dura is opened and the occipital sinus is occluded with clips and cut. The dural flap is reflected superiorly.

Microsurgical Resection. The division of the bridging cerebellar veins may provide a wide surgical corridor to the tumor, allowing the cerebellum to fall down by gravity, although this step carries a major risk of cerebellar ischemia, so the veins should be preserved as far as possible. A wide exposure can also be obtained by placing the retractor blade over the tentorial surface. Care must be taken to preserve the vein of Galen, the basal vein of Rosenthal, the internal cerebral vein, and the straight sinus, usually displaced by anterior meningiomas. One disadvantage of this approach is the significant depth of the surgical field.

Paramedian Supracerebellar Infratentorial Retrosigmoid Approach

This approach provides access to the inferolateral part of the tentorium and to the CPA. It is preferred for infratentorial group II, III, and V meningiomas, and may allow the removal of selected infra- and supratentorial tumors.

Positioning. The patient is placed in the park-bench or semisitting position.

Approach. A slightly curved skin incision is done from the pinna to the mastoid tip. The asterion constitutes the superolateral limit of the craniotomy. A suboccipital craniotomy is performed, exposing the transverse-sigmoid sinus junction. The inferior and medial extension of the craniotomy depends of the tumor size. If the mastoid air cells are opened during the exposure they must be closed with bone wax. The dura is opened in a semicircular or L-shaped fashion along the transverse and sigmoid sinus; in large tumors the incision should extend caudally far enough to allow opening of the cisterna magna and release of CSF.

Microsurgical Resection. The inferolateral cerebellar cisterns are opened to drain CSF, allowing the cerebellum to relax. With gently oblique retraction on the cerebellum, the tumor is exposed. The draining veins from the superior cerebellar surface to the straight and transverse sinuses should be preserved. The microsurgical principles of meningioma resection are applied. The frequent presence of cerebellar parenchyma between the tumor and CPA cranial nerves provides a good cleavage plane and prevents their injury.

Operative Results. Bassiouni and colleagues[75] in a series of 81 TMs treated with surgery reported Simpson grades I and II resection in 91% of patients with permanent surgical morbidity and mortality rates of 19.8% and 2.5%, respectively. The recurrence rate was 8.6% in a mean follow-up of 5.9 years. Recently Shukla and co-workers[77] reported similar morbidity results with only 46% of a gross total resection of Simpson grades I and II tumors.

Intraventicular Meningiomas

Primary intraventricular meningiomas (IVMs) are uncommon lesions that are usually diagnosed when they have reached considerable size after several years of silent growth. They may arise either from the stroma of the choroid plexus or from rests of arachnoid tissue inside it. They represent about 2% of all intracranial meningiomas. Approximately 15% of the meningiomas in children and adolescents tend to occur in this location. Around 80% of these tumors are located in the lateral ventricles, 15% in the third ventricle, and the remaining 5% in the fourth ventricle.

Clinical Presentation

Common symptoms include headache occasionally related to head position changes, vomiting, visual impairment, vertigo, mental disturbance, and seizures. Frequent signs are papilledema, hemianopia, hydrocephalus, and motor deficits. Intraventricular and subarachnoid hemorrhage can be related to this tumor location.

Evaluation

In children the principal differential diagnosis of IVM is choroid plexus papilloma. CT may show IVM calcifications, which are helpful features to distinguish between these tumors. MRVA or angiography is mandatory to access IVM blood supply, grade of vascularization, and venous drainage.

Pathology

In a recent series all IVMs were WHO grade I; in the lateral ventricle five were angiomatous, three were meningothelial, and one was psammomatous. The sole third ventricle tumor was angiomatous. In the fourth ventricle one was fibroblastic and one was meningothelial.[78]

Surgical Technique

The approach is selected based on tumor locations; lateral ventricle tumors may be better accessed through an anterior transcallosal or parieto-occipital approach. Access to the anterior third ventricle can be achieved by expanding the anterior transcallosal approach. Posterior third ventricle meningiomas can be approached through a posterior transcallosal or supracerebellar infratentorial trajectory. Fourth ventricle meningiomas are usually resected via a medial suboccipital approach.

Anterior Transcallosal Approach

Positioning. The supine position is used.

Approach. A bicoronal incision behind the hairline and a parasagittal craniotomy are made, avoiding the bridging veins to the superior sagittal sinus if possible. Such locations are previously determined with MRI.

Microsurgical Resection. After opening the interhemispheric fissure, the pericallosal arteries on the surface of the corpus callosum are identified. A longitudinal midline incision of 10 to 15 mm is made into the corpus callosum. The lateral ventricle is opened with the consequent release of CSF, allowing for further relaxation of the brain. After tumor capsule coagulation internal enucleation followed by peripheral dissection is performed. The internal debulking is performed to allow better mobilization to expose its feeding vessels originating usually from the anterior choroidal artery. Feeding vessels and drainage veins are coagulated and divided. For anterior third IVMs, the tumor is reached via the transforaminal route. The foramina of Monro are usually already dilated because of pressure of the tumor, and thus the surgical dilation may be avoided.

Posterior Transcallosal Approach

Positioning. The patient is placed in the three-quarter prone position.

Approach. After parieto-occipital craniotomy, the dura is reflected toward the superior sagittal sinus.

Microsurgical Resection. Bridging veins are infrequent posteriorly but must be preserved. Under magnification the arachnoid below the falx is opened, allowing the identification of the distal branches of the ACA and occasionally the splenial branches of the PCA on the corpus callosum. Below the splenium and above the pineal gland the junction of the internal cerebral veins with the vein of Galen is seen. The posterior part of the corpus callosum is incised in the midline. This callosal incision opens the lateral ventricle and exposes the pulvinar, choroid plexus, and tumor.

Parieto-Occipital Transcortical Approach

Positioning. The patient is placed in the park-bench or prone position. The head is elevated 20 degrees.

Approach. A paramedian craniotomy is performed with neuronavigation assistance or centered in the parieto-occipital lobes. The dura is opened in a C-shape fashion and reflected toward the midline.

Microsurgical Resection. Under magnification a transcortical incision is made 4 cm from the interhemispheric fissure that begins 1 cm behind the postcentral fissure. The white matter is transverse before entering the ventricular surface. Once the tumor is identified the microsurgical steps are the same as for the transcallosal approach.

Midline Suboccipital Infratentorial Approach

The position and approach have already been described.

Microsurgical Resection. The fourth ventricle is exposed through a vertical incision of the cerebellar vermis. The tumor is debulked and coagulation of the vascular plexus coming from the choroid supply is achieved. The IVM is detached from the lower choroid tela or the choroid plexus, avoiding traction on the floor of the fourth ventricle.

Postoperative Care. An intraventricular drain may be considered for draining out the blood in the ventricular system and thus avoiding postoperative arachnoiditis and hydrocephalus.

Operative Results. Liu and associates[79] reported a series of 24 IVMs with total tumor removal in 87.5% of patients. No deaths or postoperative hydrocephalus occurred in their group although the morbidity rate was approximately 25%. Tumor recurrence rate was 8.3% in a follow-up period from 6 months to 15 years.

Cerebellar Convexity Meningiomas

True cerebellar convexity meningiomas (CCMs) are extremely rare lesions; usually their origin is related to sinuses and dural walls. These tumors have recently been classified as follows:

Group A: Pure convexity meningiomas arising from the dura over the posterior convexity of the cerebellum
Group B: Inferior peritorcular meningiomas arising from or invading the inferior wall of the torcular herophili or the medial transverse sinus
Group C: Parasinus meningiomas arising in the angle between petrous and convexity dura, including the wall of the sigmoid and transverse sinuses
Group D: Meningiomas with secondary invasion of cerebellar convexity/fossa

CCMs represent approximately 1.5% of all intracranial meningiomas.[80]

Clinical Presentation

Nonspecific symptoms are headache, cerebellar dysfunction, nausea, and vomiting. Large tumors may compress the brainstem and cranial nerves, causing classical symptoms and signs.

Evaluation

CT and MRI show the usual meningioma features. MRVA or conventional angiography should be considered to evaluate the blood supply, sinus occlusion, and venous relationship.

Treatment

Observation may be offered to elderly patients with asymptomatic lesions. Surgical excision is considered the best treatment.

Surgical Technique

Pure convexity meningiomas can be approached with a midline or paramedial suboccipital infratentorial trajectory. Microsurgical tumor removal is performed as usual.

Operative Results. In Delfini[80] and colleagues' series of 37 CCMs, total surgical resection was achieved in approximately 84% of patients. No postoperative morbidity or death was reported in the entire group. Tumor recurrence was 5.4% for the resection group and in one case treated with radiosurgery.

Spinal Meningiomas

Spinal meningiomas (SMs) are among the most frequently encountered primary spinal tumors. SMs arise at the junction of the spinal arachnoids and the dura of the nerve root sheath. They usually present as an intradural extramedullary tumor that grows from intradural attachments and tends to spread laterally in the subarachnoid space. SMs generally respect the pial layer of the spinal cord. SMs are mostly located dorsally to the spinal cord with a component that extends laterally. SMs account for 7.5% to 12.7% of all meningiomas. They represent 20% to 46% of all intradural extramedullary primary intraspinal tumors. Approximately 83% to 94% have an intradural component, 5% to 14% are extradural, and 10% may grow in both compartments. About 73% of spinal meningiomas occur in the thoracic spine, 16% are in the cervical location, and 5% arise in the lumbar region.[81]

Clinical Presentation

Local pain is frequently the initial symptom (radicular pain may occur but is less frequent compared to nerve sheath tumors) followed by sensitive motor deficits. Compression of the spinal cord can lead to myelopathy and Brown-Sequard syndrome. The involvement of the autonomic pathways can result in bladder or bowel dysfunction.

Evaluation

Plain radiographs should be obtained in all patients to evaluate bony anatomy and document the postoperative extent of bone resection or reconstruction. The best study is MRI: sagittal slices can show tumor location, myelomalacia, and syringomyelia; axial slices may demonstrate spinal cord displacement and nerve root involvement. Cranial MRI evaluation must be considered to search for intracranial meningiomas or hydrocephalus. The principal differential diagnoses of SMs are schwannomas, neurofibromas, and malignant nerve sheath tumors. The lack of dura tail enhancement and hyperintense appearance on T2-weighted imaging are typical features of schwannomas. In patients with contraindications for an MRI a CT myelography is useful.

Pathology

In a recent series of SMs presented by Sandalcioglu and coworkers,[81] 98.5% of the encountered tumors correspond to WHO grade I and 1.5% to WHO grade II. Of the benign meningiomas the psammomatous subtype appears to be most frequent.[82]

Treatment

Even though observation may be considered in asymptomatic patients, the gold standard of treatment is surgery.

Surgical Technique

Positioning. The patient is placed in the prone position, keeping the abdomen free of any pressure to reduce the epidural bleed. Somatosensory and motor evoked potentials are generally used. Dexamethasone is given preoperatively to decrease intramedullary edema. The skin incision is marked with fluoroscopy assistance.

Approach. Through a posterior approach a hemilaminectomy, laminectomy, or laminoplasty is performed. For lateral tumors, a hemilaminectomy is preferred. If the tumor has an intraforaminal extension a laminectomy with partial or complete facetectomy may be considered. Laminectomy provides a wide exposure for safer resection, but a multilevel laminectomy may cause instability, and in this case laminoplasty should be considered to avoid postoperative kyphosis and subluxation. For ventrally located tumor a more lateral approach is preferred, and the patient can be rotated away from the surgeon and additional bony resection by drilling the pedicles may aid anterior visualization.

Microsurgical Resection. Under magnification the dura is opened in a free border of the tumor and extended to the opposite margin. After tumor identification, the arachnoid plane is followed and resected to dissect the meningioma of surrounded structures. Large tumors must be debulked prior to complete total resection. In ventrally located SMs dividing the dentate ligaments or noncritical dorsal nerve roots may improve ventral exposure. The dural attachment is resected and margins are coagulated, allowing total tumor resection. Before closing, the intradural debris and blood are removed to decrease postoperative arachnoiditis, tethering, syringomyelia, and hydrocephalus.

Operative Results. Sandalcioglu and co-workers,[81] in their series of 137 SMs, reported complete surgical resection in 97% of patients and improved or unchanged neurological state in 96.2% of patients in a mean follow-up time of 61 months. Permanent operative morbidity and mortality rates were 3% and 0.8%, respectively. Recurrence rate was observed in 3% of patients after a mean follow-up period of 76.5 months. Schaller[82] demonstrated that the resection of psammomatous meningiomas of the spine is associated with a less favorable neurological outcome postoperatively than resection of spinal meningiomas of other pathological subtypes.

Conclusion

The decision to treat a meningioma is dependent on patient characteristics, tumor size, location, and associated symptoms. The main goal is to improve or preserve optimal quality of life, understanding the risks and benefits of conservative, surgical, and adjuvant treatment. The proper management of meningiomas must involve a multidisciplinary team approach to improve the effectiveness of therapies.

RADIATION THERAPY

Fractionated Radiotherapy

External beam radiotherapy has proved to be effective in the treatment of primary, unresectable, aggressive, residual, and recurrent meningiomas. Conventional fractionated radiation may be offered instead of surgery to patients with poor clinical status or unresectable meningiomas that involve critical central nervous system and vascular structures. Conventional fraction radiation doses between 50 and 55 Gy provide improvement of symptoms and tumor control up to 80% to 86% at 5 years.[83,84] In patients with aggressive meningiomas (grade II or III), even with a gross total resection, radiotherapy must be considered to reduce the high risk of recurrence.[84]

Radiation therapy may be offered as a standard adjuvant treatment following subtotal resection of selected meningiomas. External beam RT allows an 89% progression-free survival rate at 5 years for benign meningiomas with subtotal resection as compared with the 43% for those followed by observation only.[85,86] Several studies support the use of salvage RT in patients with (not previously irradiated) recurrent meningiomas and the treatment outcomes appear to be superior to those achieved with repeat resection alone.[84,86,87] Complications such as worsening of neurological symptoms,

radionecrosis, memory and cognitive deficit, and chronic otitis apparently decreased since the use of novel high-precision RT techniques such as stereotactic radiosurgery (SRS), fractionated stereotactic conformal radiotherapy (SCRT), proton beam radiotherapy (PBT), and intensity-modulated radiotherapy (IMRT).

Stereotactic Radiosurgery

This procedure delivers a single high dose of precisely targeted radiation; modalities include gamma knife, linear accelerator, proton beam, and the CyberKnife, a robotic radiosurgery system. Doses of approximately 15 Gy are equally efficacious to conventionally fractionated treatment and reduce the complication rate. The use of SRS in meningiomas smaller than 3 to 4 cm was associated with better local control.[88]

Fractionated Stereotactic Conformal Radiotherapy

This treatment modality advantage is the possibility of delivering higher doses but maintaining stereotactic accuracy. Numerous reports show optimal tumor control rate in short-term follow-up with doses ranging from 50 to 54 Gy.[89,90]

Intensity-Modulated Photon

IMRT is an advanced form of radiotherapy that delivers a conformal isodose of photon beams to a selected area.

Proton Beam Therapy

PBT delivers protons instead of radiotherapy photons. Protons are more conformal and homogeneous than photons and their use decreases the dose in surrounding tissue compared to photon beam therapy.[91] However, the treatment results of PBT appear to be similar to those for IMRT. A group from Harvard University reported the outcome of 46 patients treated with combined photon and proton beam radiation therapy for biopsied, resected, or recurrent meningiomas. The 5- and 10-year overall survival rates were 93% and 77%, respectively.[92]

CHEMOTHERAPY

Adjuvant chemotherapy treatment is generally ineffective against meningiomas. Many modalities have been tested including cytotoxic drugs, immunomodulation, molecular agents, and hormonal therapy. None of them has shown significant success. Conventional combined chemotherapy—cyclophosphamide, adriamycin, and vincristine—showed a modest activity against malignant meningiomas and may improve the median survival time.[93] Treatment with interferon alpha-2b has presented some success in preventing meningioma growth.[94] Hydroxyurea has also been suggested for treatment of unresectable and recurrent meningiomas.[95] This agent arrests meningioma cell growth in the S phase of the cell cycle as a result of DNA synthesis inhibition, therefore inducing apoptosis. Its early promise appears not to have held out over time, however.

SELECTED KEY REFERENCES

Igaki H, Maruyama K, Koga T, et al. Stereotactic radiosurgery for skull base meningioma. *Neurol Med Chir (Tokyo)*. 2009;49(10):456-461.

Nakamura M, Roser F, Michel J, et al. The natural history of incidental meningiomas. *Neurosurgery*. 2003;53:62-71.

Pamir N, Black P, Fahlbusch R. *Meningiomas: A Comprehensive Text*. New York: Elsevier; 2010.

Perry A, et al. Meningiomas. In: Louis DN, Ohgaki H, Wiestler OD, et al. eds. *World Health Organization Classification of Tumours of the Central Nervous System*. 4th ed. Lyon: IARC Press; 2007:164-172.

Yano S, Kuratsu J. Indications for surgery in patients with asymptomatic meningiomas based on an extensive experience. *J Neurosurg*. 200;105:538-543.

Please go to expertconsult.com to view the complete list of references.

CHAPTER 37

Tumors of the Pineal Region

Christian Matula

CLINICAL PEARLS

- Pineal region tumors account for about 1% of adult and 3% to 8% of all pediatric intracranial tumors. They are rare but surgically treatable tumors that require surgical expertise, experience, and multimodality therapy.

- The histological variety of pineal region tumors consists of several major categories: (a) germ cell tumors (germinomas), (b) nongerminomatous tumors (embryonal carcinoma, choriocarcinoma, and teratoma), (c) pineal parenchymal tumors (pineoblastoma, pineocytoma, and papillary tumor), (d) tumors of the supporting structures (meningioma, ependymoma, astrocytoma, mixed glioma, choroid plexus neoplasm), and (e) other tumor types (metastases, cysts, lymphoma, variable).

- Diagnostic workup includes a thorough clinical and neurological examination, magnetic resonance imaging (MRI), and serum markers. Serum markers when positive are best used to follow the tumor response to therapy. Diagnostic approaches to pineal region tumors include stereotactic biopsy, endoscopic biopsy, and open surgery. In many cases, symptoms are caused by compression of the neural

- structures or obstructive hydrocephalus. Concomitant hydrocephalus can be treated by an endoscopic third ventriculostomy with biopsy, ventricular diversion/shunting, or surgical removal of the tumor.

- Pineal region tumors can be removed with relatively low morbidity using a variety or combination of approaches. The most popular ones are a posterior fossa approach (infratentorial-supracerebellar), supratentorial approaches (occipital transtentorial), and posterior and anterior transcallosal approaches. Surgeons should be familiar with the anatomical structures in the pineal region and with the indications, limitations, risks, and benefits of each approach. Each tumor requires an individualized surgical and treatment approach.

- Multimodal treatments such as radiotherapy, chemotherapy, and radiosurgery in combination with open microsurgery or stereotactic or endoscopic surgery should be incorporated into any treatment paradigm based on the extent of resection and histological type of tumor.

Treatment of tumors in the pineal region remains one of the great intellectual and technical challenges to neurological surgeons. The mystique of the even nowadays poorly understood function of the pineal gland, the everlasting beauty of its anatomy, and the unbeatable elegance of the surgical approaches to this region have fascinated generations of neurosurgeons. When coupled with the currently satisfactory clinical outcomes in the hands of experienced neurosurgeons, the allure of microsurgery or endoscopy of pineal region tumors is understandable.

Advances in microsurgical techniques, imaging, anesthesia, and critical care medicine have led to a paradigm shift in the goals and approaches to treating pineal region tumors. Neuroendoscopic techniques (classical neuroendoscopic operations and endoscope-assisted or endoscope-guided procedures) continue to evolve and have helped further revolutionize this subject. They belong in the standard portfolio of the operative treatment of a pineal region tumor and have further improved outcome.

HISTORY

The mystique of the pineal gland's function and the challenge of operating in this region make it worthwhile to provide a brief overview of the relevant historical facts. The anatomists of ancient times knew about the pineal body and named it konareion because of its cone-shaped appearance. It was first described by Herophilus of Alexandria (325-280 BC). Like all his contemporaries, he believed the ventricles to be the "seat of spirits" and thought that the pineal body acted like a sphincter, regulating the flow of thoughts between the third and the fourth ventricles. Galen (129-201 AD) was most likely the first to hypothesize that the pineal body served as a gland. During Galen's time, the structures of the pineal region were compared with the external genital organs of men. They named the pineal body the "penis," the superior colliculi of the quadrigeminal plate "testes," and the inferior colliculli of the quadrigeminal plate "nates," simply based on their comparable appearance to these structures. Gibson, in 1763, would later recapitulate these ideas in his *Epitome of Anatomy*.

Vesalius (1514-1564) described the pineal gland as being "similar to a cone from a pine tree." His description in 1543 was the basis for the current name "pineal gland." Descartes (1596-1650) during the seventeenth century suggested that the pineal gland be named *epiphysis cerebri* as he thought it was the "seat of the soul." He suggested that the pineal body acted like a valve, regulating the passage of spirits between the ventricles. He conceived the human body as a machine controlled by the pineal gland, which activated all the organs. His descriptions in 1677 suggested that consciousness and the power of imagination were located in the pineal gland. The spiritual function played a decisive role in the neuroanatomy in the sixteenth and eighteenth centuries. The medical scientists at that time were seeking the "seat of the soul" and thought the pineal gland was a central component in combination with Lancisi's nerves (Giovanni Maria Lancisi, 1654-1720). "Brain science" was based on proving and confuting the theories of Galen. Many of his theories were based on the theory of animal spirits originally proposed by Herophilus of Chalcedon (335-280 BC), who is considered one of the pioneers in neuroscience and anatomy.

Medical history therefore has three hypotheses about the function of the pineal gland:

1. A mechanical function, serving as a sphincter between the third and fourth ventricles
2. A spiritual function, serving as a seat for the spirit and the soul
3. An organ with glandular function

In general, tumors of the brainstem, as well as in the pineal region, were considered to be inoperable until the later part of the twentieth century. There are only scattered reports on attempted or successful operations. In most cases, the patient died during the operation or shortly afterward. One of the first clinical reports of a pineal region tumor in the twentieth century was made by Cushing in 1904. He reported a bitemporal compression in a 28-year-old man with clinical evidence of a pineal region tumor. A few weeks later, the autopsy revealed the presence of a glioma of the quadrigeminal plate. The first direct surgical intervention was described by Horsley in 1905, and the first successful pineal region extirpation was described by Oppenheim and Krause in 1913. Since that time, a great number of neurosurgeons and investigators have written extensively on this topic, including McLean (1935), Dandy (1945), Pia (1954), Bailey (1964), Schmidek (1977), Pendl (1985), Schindler (1985), Slavin and Ausman (1991), and Tomita (2000), among others. More recent publications by Blakeley (2006), Kobayashi and Lunsford (2009), and some others are dealing with multimodal treatment options, including fractionated radiotherapy and multidisciplinary cooperation.

ANATOMY

The pineal region is defined as the area of the brain bordered superiorly by the splenium of the corpus callosum and the tela choroidea, inferiorly by the quadrigeminal plate and

midbrain tectum, anteriorly by the posterior parts of the third ventricle, and posteriorly by the cerebellar vermis as can be nicely shown in a midline sagittal section through the pineal gland and surrounding anatomical structures in an injected fixed human cadaver (Fig. 37.1). The pineal gland itself, as an invagination of the diencephalic ependymal roof between the habenular commissure and the posterior commissure, lies between the superior colliculi and basal to the splenium of the corpus callosum. It has a thin stalk to the epithalamus and developmentally is considered to be a paired structure. The neural connections with adjacent centers are the topic of discussion but have to be clarified. The pineal body itself has an average length of 7.97 mm (range 5.0-12.0 mm) and is 4.25 mm (2.5-7.0 mm) in height and width. It is oval in shape. The suprapineal recess projects posteriorly between the upper surface of the pineal gland and the lower layer of the tela choroidea in the roof. The stalk of the pineal body, from which the gland extends into the quadrigeminal cistern, has a cranial lamina and a caudal lamina. The habenular commissure, which connects the habenulae, crosses the midline over the cranial lamina, and the posterior commissure crosses the caudal lamina. The pineal recess projects posteriorly from the third ventricle into the pineal body between the two laminae. The posterior commissure forms the base of the triangular orifice of the aqueduct of Sylvius; the other two limbs are formed by the central gray matter of the midbrain. The quadrigeminal cistern is the subarachnoid space of the pineal region, and provides protection for the midbrain from the sharp edge of the tentorial notch. The arteries and veins inside the cistern are embedded in the firm arachnoidal septa. The quadrigeminal cistern communicates anteriorly with the cistern of the tela choroidea of the third ventricle, dorsally along the great vein of Galen with the dorsal cistern of the corpus callosum, laterally into the alae, caudally into the superior cistern of the cerebellum, which is formed by the medullary velum and the vermis, and anterodorsally into the ambient cistern. Through the latter cistern, the large arteries, the posterior cerebral artery and its branches, and the superior cerebellar artery approach the dorsal surface of the brainstem along the edge of the tentorium. The posterior border of the quadrigeminal cistern is formed by thickened opalescent arachnoid. Care must

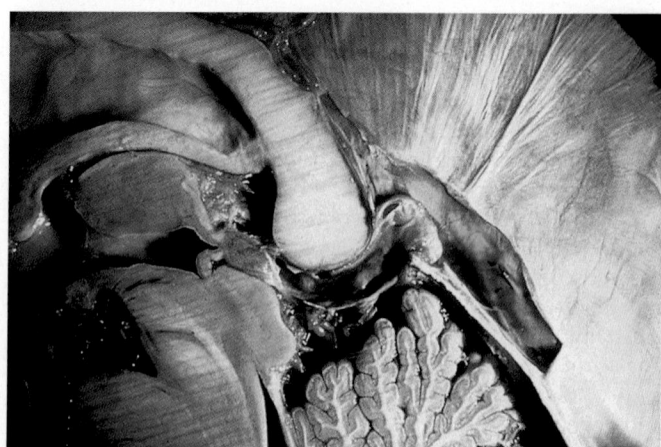

FIGURE 37.1 Midline sagittal section through the pineal region and related structures in a fixed human cadaver, vessels injected in red (arteries) and blue (veins).

be taken when dissecting this area because the vein of Galen and its tributaries lie immediately rostral. The mesencephalon with the pineal body has its arterial blood supply from various sources. Small vessels supplying the parenchyma of the cerebral peduncles and the rest of the midbrain arise from the posterior communicating artery as perforating branches forming an internal or direct system. The vascularization in situ can be shown using neuroendoscopic techniques in injected human cadavers (arteries red, veins blue) and gives an impression of the enormous variety of the vascular structure (Fig. 37.2). All these arteries widely anastomose with each other, which explains the rarity of infarcts in the mesencephalon and the relative tolerance of the midbrain to direct surgical intervention. The pineal body is supplied by the pineal artery, which originates from the medial posterior choroidal artery, arising from the posterior cerebral artery (PCA), and enters the gland through its lateral portion from both sides. The

great vein of Galen and its tributaries form a roof-like, dense venous network above the pineal body and the quadrigeminal plate, formed from the internal cerebral veins after they pass posteriorly through the tela choroidea and unite with the basal veins of Rosenthal. Other tributaries of the vein of Galen include the precentral cerebellar vein, internal occipital vein, posterior mesencephalic vein, and posterior ventricular vein. The straight sinus is formed by the joining of the great vein of Galen with the inferior sagittal sinus.

HISTOLOGY

The normal pineal gland contains pinealocytes derived from amino precursor uptake and decarboxylation (APUD) cells and glial cells (astrocytes). The pineal gland is usually calcified by the age of 16 and appears so on routine computed tomography (CT) scans. Pineal cysts can be found incidentally in magnetic resonance imaging (MRI) studies in about 1.1% to 4.3% and this incidence seems to be higher in females (~2.4%) than in males (~1.5%) (Fig. 37.3). They can be identified in patients of all ages, with an increased prevalence found in older patients and in approximately 25% to 40% of autopsies, albeit many of the pineal cysts are microcystic. Their etiology remains obscure and may be the result of ischemic glial degeneration or of sequestration of the pineal diverticulum. Usually they are benign, nonneoplastic and may contain clear, xanthochromic, sometimes hemorrhagic, fluid. In the majority of cases, they are asymptomatic and may be followed on serial MRIs. Only in very rare cases do they show an enlargement, and may become symptomatic by causing hydrocephalus through aqueductal compression, headache, or gaze paresis, or hypothalamic symptoms. In those unusual situations with neurological symptoms or signs there is an indication to consider neurosurgical intervention.

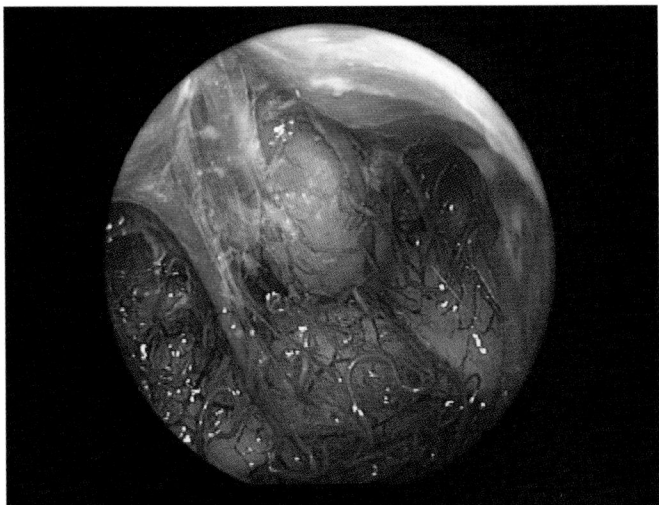

FIGURE 37.2 Endoscopic view using a supracerebellar infratentorial approach demonstrating the pineal gland and the collicular plate. Note the variability of the vascularization; veins injected in blue, arteries in red in a nonfixed human cadaver. *(Courtesy of A. Di-Ieva and M. Tschabitscher, Anatomical Institute, Medical University of Vienna, Austria.)*

FUNCTION

In reptiles, the pineal gland functions as a photoreceptor to change skin color in response to light. In humans, it is involved with hormone secretion for circadian rhythms and is known to have a neurotransmitter secretory function. The pineal gland

FIGURE 37.3 Typical cyst of the pineal region incidentally found in routine magnetic resonance imaging (MRI) scan (40-year-old woman). Sagittal plane (**A**). The cyst is completely unchanged in a follow-up series more than 15 years later (**B**). *(Courtesy of K. Turetschek, Diagnostic Center Favoriten, Vienna.)*

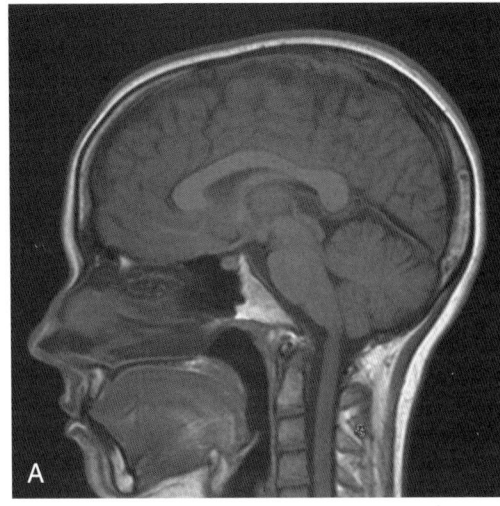
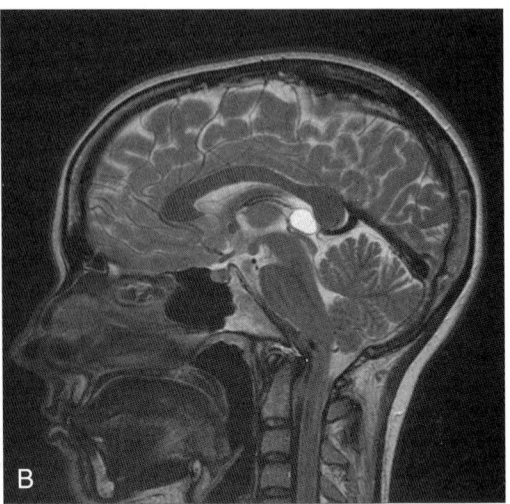

inhibits gonadal development and regulates menstruation, adrenal function, and thyroid function. It is innervated by sympathetic nerves from the superior cervical ganglion that release norepinephrine to increase the pineal gland's melatonin secretion. Light stimuli thereby reach the pineal gland from the retina via a polysynaptic pathway and affect the production of the neuroendocrine substance, melatonin. Melatonin, a derivative of serotonin, is essential in regulating circadian rhythms in endocrine gland activity and produces an antigonadal effect through the hypothalamic-hypophyseal axis. The production of melatonin is inhibited by light. Apparently, in many animals the major function of the pineal gland is to regulate the reproductive cycle; in fall and winter when days are short, more melatonin is produced, causing a gonad-suppressing effect. The exact function of the pineal gland in humans remains unclear. Recent studies could prove a diagnostic value of the melatonin profile in case of tumors of the pineal region. These studies showed a dramatically reduced melatonin rhythm in cases of undifferentiated or invasive tumors as well as the absence of melatonin variation as a consequence of pineal distortion after surgery. Also, the evidence for melatonin deficiency is recognized as a predictive factor to prevent post-pinealectomy syndrome. The absence of production of melatonin, as after pinealectomy, causes a "jet-lag-like" syndrome consisting of a complete disturbance of circadian rhythms.

PATHOLOGY

Pineal region tumors are rare tumors, with an estimated overall incidence of about 1% of all intracranial tumors (ranging from 0.5% to 1.6% in different studies) and are more common in children (3-8%) than in adults (less than 1%). Also, the incidence of pineal region tumors is higher among the Japanese, at 4-6% of all intracranial tumors. A population-based study calculated the incidence of pineal region tumors at 0.06 to 0.07 per 100,000 persons per year. No significant differences in the incidence between races were noted. Other reports describe the incidence in children younger than 20 years of age to be about 0.061 per 100,000 children per year. They are uncommon tumors and occur in a wide variety of different histological types. Furthermore, many tumors are of mixed cell type. The pathological classification depends on the substrate in the pineal region from which the tumor may arise. There are tumors which arise from the pineal glandular tissue itself, such as pinealocytomas (WHO grade I), pineal parenchymal tumors of intermediate differentiation (WHO grades II or III), pinealoblastomas (WHO grade IV), and papillary tumors of the pineal region. Other tumors arise from the glial cells, such as astrocytomas, oligodrendrogliomas, and glial cysts. Arachnoid cells are the basis for pineal-region meningiomas and non-neoplastic arachnoid cysts. Ependymal cells give rise to ependymomas in this region. Sympathetic nerves serve as a substrate for chemodectomas. Germ cell remnants give rise to germ cell tumors such as germinoma, choriocarcinoma, embryonal carcinoma, endodermal sinus tumor (yolk sac tumor), and teratoma. Lastly, the absence of a blood-brain barrier in the pineal gland makes it a suitable site for hematogenous metastases mostly from breast cancer, stomach cancer, renal cancer, or melanomas (Table 37.1).

Several authors have described different classification systems. The most current classification system for pure pineal parenchymal tumors is from the World Health Organization

TABLE 37.1 Types of Pineal Tumors: 2007 WHO Classification of Tumors of the Central Nervous System

Tumor	Origin	Frequency
Germ Cell Tumors	Rest of germ cells	~60%
Germinoma		
Mature Teratoma		
Immature Teratoma		
Teratoma with Malignant Transformation		
Yolk sac tumor (endodermal sinus tumor)		
Embryonal carcinoma		
Choriocarcinoma		
Pineal Parenchymal Tumors	Pineal glandular tissue	~30%
Pineocytoma (WHO grade I)		
Pineal parenchymal tumor of intermediate differentiation (WHO grade II or III)		
Pinealoblastoma (WHO grade IV)		
Papillary tumor of pineal region		
Tumors of Supportive and Adjacent Structures		~10%
Astrocytoma	Glial cells	
Glioma (glioblastoma or oligodendroglioma)		
Medulloepithelioma		
Ependymoma	Ependymal lining	
Choroid plexus papilloma		
Meningioma	Arachnoid cells	
Hemangioma	Vascular cells	
Hemangiopericytoma or blastoma		
Chemodectoma		
Craniopharyngioma		
Non-neoplastic Tumor-like Conditions		<1%
Arachnoid cyst	Arachnoid cells	
Degenerative cysts (pineal cysts)	Glial cells	
Cysticercosis	Parasites	
Arteriovenous malformations	Vascularization	
Cavernomas		
Aneurysms of the vein of Galen		
Metastases	Absence of blood-brain barrier	<0.1%
Lung (most common), breast, stomach, kidney, melanoma		

Louis DN, Cavanee WK, Oghaki H. WHO Classification of Tumours of the Central Nervous System, 4th ed: WHO Classification of Tumours v. 1 (IARC WHO Classification of Tumours), World Health Org; 4th edition (May 2007).

(WHO) Classification of Tumors of the Central Nervous System edited by Louis and associates and published in 2007.

GERM CELL TUMORS

Germ cell tumors derive from pluripotential germ cells and span a wide range of differentiation and malignant characteristics. They constitute a unique class of rare tumors that

FIGURE 37.4 Midline sagittal section through the brain, with gross appearance of a germinoma. The tumor is infiltrating the brainstem at the level of the midbrain (**A**). Frontal section through the brain, gross appearance of a germinoma growing into the ventricle (**B**). Tumor cells of a germinoma in the postoperative cerebrospinal fluid representing a typical large cell with two prominent nucleoli (MGG [May-Grunwald Giemsa], ×600) (**C**). *(Courtesy of Q. Koperek, Neuropathological Institute, Medical University of Vienna.)*

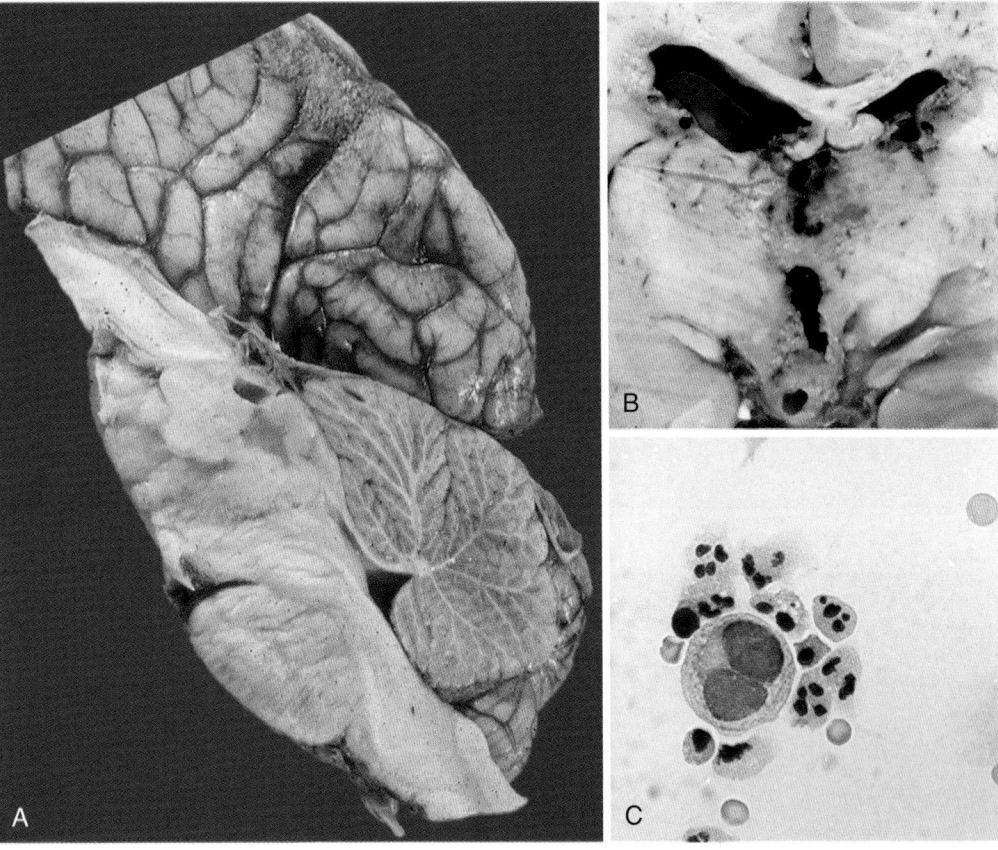

affect mainly children and adolescents. Predominantly they occur in the midline when they arise in the central nervous system (CNS). Intracranial germ cell tumors, in general, account for 0.4% to 3.4% of intracranial neoplasms. Their average incidence is considered to be 0.1 per 100,000 persons per year. Pineal germ cell tumors occur primarily in males. Germ cell tumors in females are more common in the suprasellar region. Most germ cell tumors of the CNS occur in the first three decades (98%) with a peak in the second decade (65%) between 11 and 20 years. The histogenesis of germ cell tumors is a subject of controversy. For a long time, they have been assumed to represent the neoplastic offspring of primordial germ cells. During the last decade, however, a variety of speculative proposals have been published on this topic. As a result of the etiology, certain observations suggest that gonadotropins play a role in the development or progression of CNS germ cell tumors. These include the predilection with Klinefelter syndrome, a condition characterized by chronically elevated serum levels of gonadotropins. Due to the variety of possible origins, the following entities are distinguished: germinoma, embryonal carcinoma, yolk sac tumor (endodermal sinus tumor), choriocarcinoma, mature teratoma, immature teratoma, teratoma with malignant transformation, and mixed germ cell tumors. An accurate histological identification and subclassification of CNS germ cell tumors is critical for current treatment planning and prognostication. In fact, only the germinoma and teratoma are likely to be encountered as pure tumor types.

Germinoma

Pure germinomas (Fig. 37.4A to C) account for 65% to 72% of all intracranial germ cell tumors. These usually occur in the pineal region, although the second most common site is supra- and intrasellar, sometimes also parasellar. Germ cell tumors can be "synchronous," and can be found both in the the suprasellar region and in the pineal region approximately 10% of the time. In fact, the discovery of a synchronous lesion on MRI is indicative of a germ cell tumor. The germ cell tumors are usually poorly circumscribed, light gray, granular, solid neoplasms that destroy the pineal gland and infiltrate the ventricular system and subarachnoid space early in their course. Hemorrhage into the tumor and necrosis or cystic degeneration are not often found. This tumor is composed of uniform cells resembling primitive germ cells, with large, vesicular nuclei, prominent nucleoli, and a clear, glycogen-rich cytoplasm. Additional features include lymphoid or lymphoplasma cellular infiltrates and, less frequently, scattered syncytiotrophoblastic giant cells (Fig. 37.5A and B).

Teratoma

Teratomas (Fig. 37.6A and B) derive from all germ layers and are composed of well-differentiated tissues in an organlike pattern. These tumors in the pineal region most often affect males. They are usually identified within the first two decades of life but occur more often in much younger children than other germ cell tumors (mostly in children

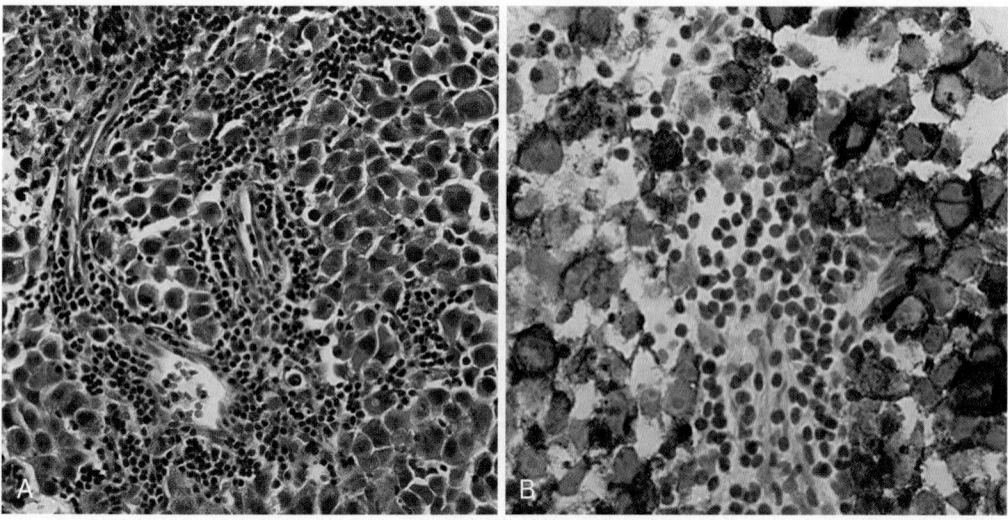

FIGURE 37.5 Histopathological features of a germinoma with typical lymphocytic infiltrates along fibrovascular septae (H&E, ×200) (**A**) and immunohistochemistry staining of the cytoplasm and cytoplasmic membrane with placental alkaline phosphatase (PLAP) (×400) (**B**). *(Courtesy of O. Koperek, Neuropathological Institute, Medical University of Vienna.)*

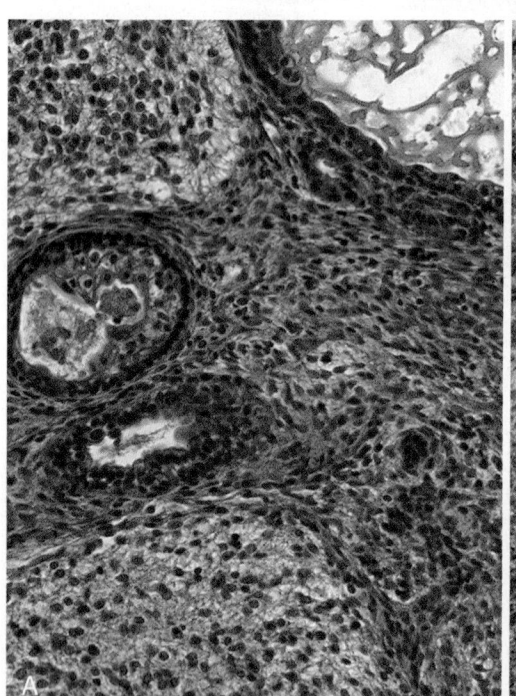 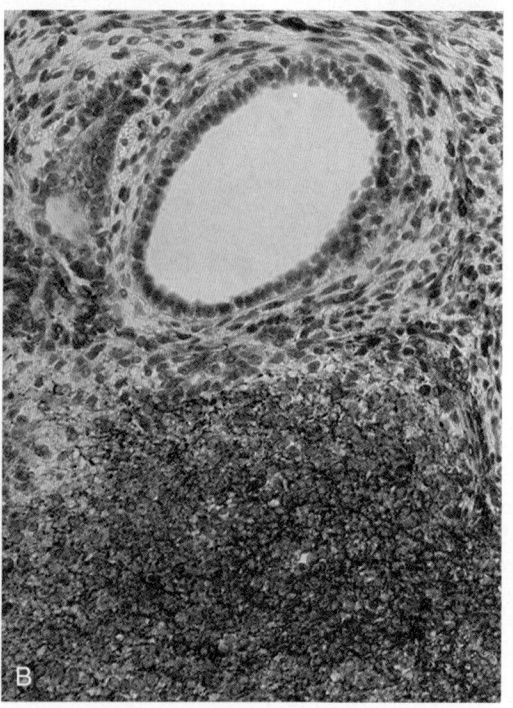

FIGURE 37.6 Histopathological features of a teratoma of the pineal region with fetal-type glands and embryonic mesenchyme–like stroma (H&E, ×200) (**B**). Immunohistochemistry out of (**A**) staining with synaptophysin representing the immature neuronal differentiated appearance (×200) (**B**). *(Courtesy of Q. Koperek, Neuropathological Institute, Medical University of Vienna.)*

younger than 9 years of age; about 20% occur between the ages of 16 and 18). By definition, the term *teratoma* can be used only when tumor elements derive from two or three germ layers. These tumors are usually well circumscribed, round or lobulated, and multicystic and compress the surrounding structures. The cystic component of the tumor may be watery, mucoid, or sebaceous. Sometimes bone, cartilage, hair, or teeth are present. Immature tumors are more frequently associated with a malignant course. Histologically, teratomas differentiate along ectodermal, endodermal, and mesodermal lines (e.g., they recapitulate somatic development from the three embryonic germ layers). Mature and immature variants as well as teratomas with malignant transformation must be distinguished from each other.

Mature Teratoma

Mature teratomas are composed exclusively of fully differentiated, "adult-type" tissue elements that are sometimes arranged in patterns resembling normal tissue relationships. Mitotic activity is low or even absent.

Immature Teratoma

This teratoma variant is composed of incompletely differentiated components resembling fetal tissue. Immature tumors are more frequently associated with a malignant course, but malignant potential may be explained by the presence of other germ cell tumor elements, such as choriocarcinoma or germinoma.

Teratoma with Malignant Transformation

Teratoma with malignant transformation is the generic designation for occasional teratomatous neoplasm that contains as an additional malignant component a cancer of conventional somatic type. Detecting evidence of a malignant transformation within a germ cell tumor should state the specific histological form that this takes.

Yolk Sac Tumor (Endodermal Sinus Tumor)

The histological appearance of endodermal sinus tumors classically features Schiller-Duval bodies, which resemble the yolk sac or endodermal sinus—an extraembryonic endodermal derivative in lower animals. These bodies are composed of a blood vessel invaginating a space, with both being covered by a layer of cuboidal tumor cells with clear cytoplasm, small dark nuclei, and prominent nucleoli set in a loose, variably cellular and often conspicuously myxoid matrix resembling extraembryonic mesoblasts. Eosinophilic hyaline globules, immunoreactive for α-fetoprotein, are a diagnostic feature. Endodermal sinus tumors are usually highly invasive. Sometimes they can occur within the lateral ventricle, although this seems to be very rare.

Embryonal Carcinoma

This type of germ cell tumor is the least frequently reported and is one that represents a primitive neoplasm consisting of pluripotential large cells that proliferate in cohesive nets and sheets. They form abortive papillae or line irregular, gland-like spaces. The tumor may exceptionally replicate the structure of the early embryo, forming "embryoid bodies" replete with germ disks and miniature amniotic cavities. A high mitotic rate and zones of coagulative necrosis complete the histological picture.

Choriocarcinoma

This type rarely arises extragenitally and is characterized by extraembryonic differentiation along trophoblastic lines. These tumors are characterized by two cell types: uniform cytotrophoblastic cells of medium size, with clear cytoplasm, vesicular nucleus, and distinct cell borders, and syncytiotrophoblastic cells, which are larger and multinucleated. The gross appearance of choriocarcinoma is a granular, reddish brown mass, almost always with hemorrhage and necrosis. As for all other tumors of germ cell origin, choriocarcinoma is usually accompanied by elements of either tumor of this group.

PINEAL PARENCHYMAL TUMORS

As described in the previous section, these types of tumors constitute the second major group of pineal region tumors, accounting for 20% to 30% of all neoplasms in this location. They are considered to be the true neoplasm of the parenchyma of the pineal gland and are usually sharply delineated, with some formation of capsule and displacement of surrounding structures such as thalamus and midbrain. As a result of the variety of histological origins, the following entities are distinguished: pinealocytomas (WHO grade I), pineal parenchymal tumors of intermediate differentiation (WHO grades II or III), pinealoblastomas (WHO grade IV), and papillary tumors of the pineal region.

Pinealocytoma (WHO Grade I)

Pinealocytomas are defined as slow-growing pineal parenchymal neoplasms. They represent approximately 45% of all tumors with pineal parenchymal origin and occur throughout life, but most frequently in young adults (25-35 years). There is no sex predilection. Macroscopically, these tumors are well circumscribed with a gray-tan, homogeneous or granular cut surface. Degenerative changes, such as hemorrhage and small cystic cavities, can be present. They may disseminate widely along the CSF pathways. The histological appearance is of a well-differentiated neoplasm composed of small, uniform, mature cells resembling pinealocytes (Fig. 37.7A to C). They grow in sheets, but also feature large pinealocytomatous rosettes composed of abundant, delicate tumor cell processes. Pinealocytomas may contain astrocytic or neuronal components or both (so-called ganglioma of the pineal gland). Such tumors are the most benign of the pineal parenchymal neoplasms.

Pineal Parenchymal Tumor of Intermediate Differentiation (WHO Grade I or II)

This group of true pineal parenchymal tumors represents monomorphous types of lesions characterized by moderately high cellularity, mild nuclear atypia, occasional mitosis, and the absence of large pinealocytomatous rosettes. They occur in approximately 10% of all pineal parenchymal tumors and at all ages with a peak incidence in adulthood. The clinical behavior is variable.

Pinealoblastoma (WHO Grade IV)

This type of tumor (Fig. 37.8A to D) is defined as a highly malignant, primitive embryonal tumor of the pineal gland itself and represents a true primitive neuroectodermal tumor (PNET). Although they are rare intracranial tumors, they constitute approximately 45% of all pineal parenchymal tumors. Usually they occur in the first two decades of life, more often in children, but principally can arise at any age. Some of these tumors may be present during the neonatal period. In larger series, pinealoblastomas are more common in males, with a male-female ratio of 2:1. The tumor usually replaces the tissue of the pineal gland. They are mostly soft, friable, and poorly demarcated and are pink, white, or gray, smooth or granular when cut, sometimes cystic, and frequently hemorrhagic or necrotic. Calcifications are rare and infiltration of the surrounding structures, including the meninges, is common. Constituting the most primitive of pineal parenchymal tumors, pinealoblastomas are composed of patternless sheets of densely packed small cells with round to irregular nuclei and scant cytoplasm. Pinealocytomatous rosettes are lacking, but Homer-Wright and Flexner-Wintersteiner rosettes may be seen. Retinoblastomatous differentiation of pinealoblastomas sometimes occurs and supports the theory of the photoreceptive origin of pineal gland cells. Pinealoblastomas may

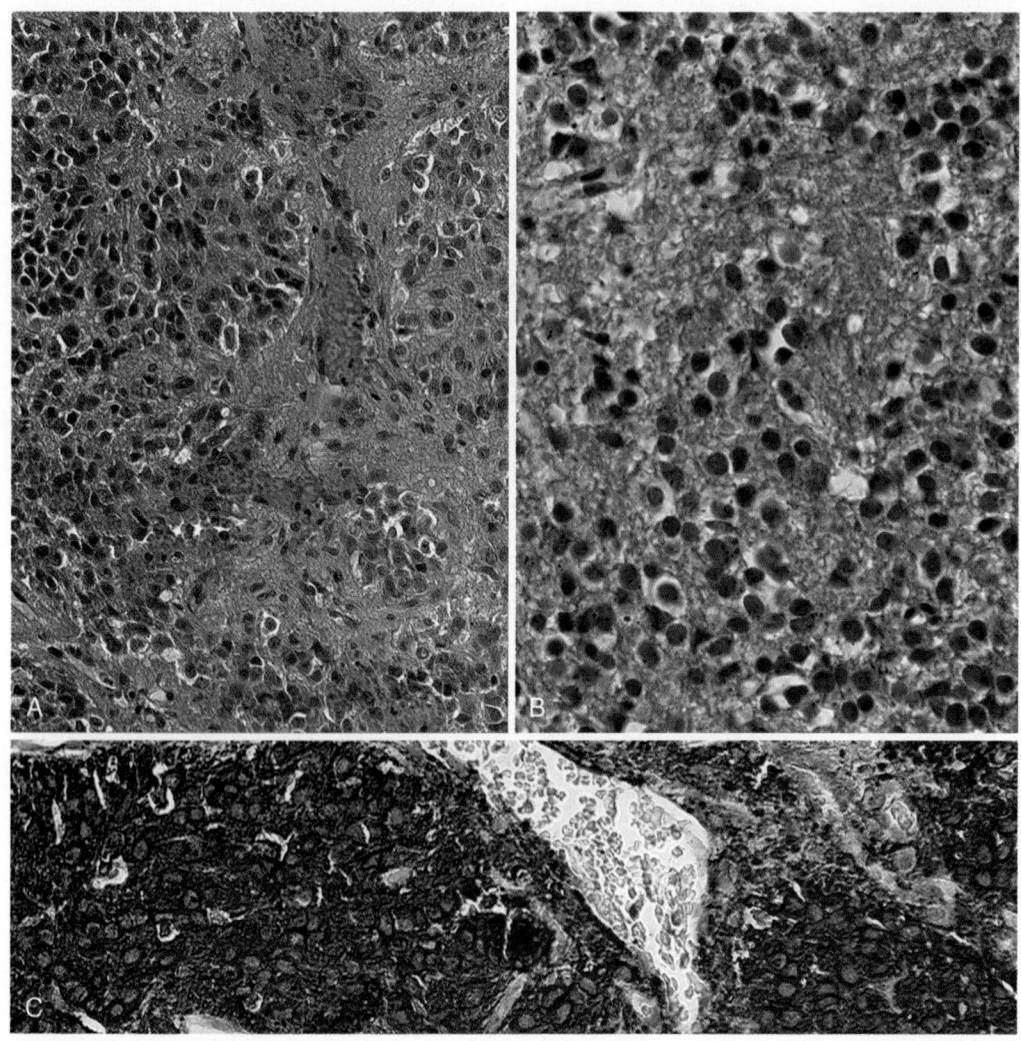

FIGURE 37.7 Histopathological features of a pinealocytoma with characteristic lobular pattern mimicking the structure of the normal pineal gland (H&E, ×200) (**A**), isomorphic cells with small round nuclei and nucleus-free spaces filled with a fine meshwork of cell processes (neuropils) (H&E, ×400) (**B**), and immunohistochemistry intensive diffuse staining with synaptophysin (×200) (**C**). *(Courtesy of Q. Koperek, Neuropathological Institute, Medical University of Vienna.)*

accompany bilateral retinoblastomas, in which case together they are called *trilateral retinoblastoma*. Pinealoblastomas sometimes contain melanin pigment. Because of its infiltrating nature into surrounding structures, dissemination in the CSF is not rare: according to the literature, between 8% and 24%. Metastases to bone, lung, and lymph nodes have been reported.

Papillary Tumors of the Pineal Region (Similar to WHO Grade II or III)

This rather newly defined group consists of rare neuroepithelial tumors in adults characterized by a typical papillary structure and epithelial structure. Their biological behavior is variable and shows a similar course to the one of grade II or III tumors. The first description as a distinct entity goes back to 2003. The origin of that group of tumors is specialized ependymal cells from the subcommissural region. Because of that in later years they have been reported as papillary pineocytomas or pineal parenchymal tumors, choroid plexus tumors, and even as ependymomas or papillary meningiomas. The incidence seems extremely rare and representative data are still not available. Worldwide, no more than 100 cases have reported to date in children as well as

in adults. In this case no sex predilection could be found. In recent studies with a small patient group tumor progression occurred in more than 70%.

Tumors of Supportive and Adjacent Structures

There are several other tumors that can also be considered pineal parenchymal tumors, such as astrocytomas, ependymomas, or less frequently gliomas (glioblastomas or oligodendrogliomas). Glial cell tumors can also occur in the pineal gland, because astrocytes are normally present there, or may arise from the pluripotential pineal parenchymal cells. However, almost all glial tumors may arise from the glial tissue elements intimately surrounding the pineal gland. Real, true astrocytomas of the pineal gland itself are extremely rare. Tumors of other histological types may also occur as a substrate from the surrounding tissue—for example, choroidus plexus papillomas or medulloepitheliomas. Tumors of mesenchymal origin that may occur include meningiomas, hemangiomas, and hemangiopericytomas or blastomas, which arise mostly from the falx and tentorium near their junction or from the velum interpositum at the roof of the third ventricle. Also reported are exceptionally rare cases of chemodectomas and craniopharyngiomas of the pineal region. Another not-so-well-known

FIGURE 37.8 Frontal section of the brain, with gross appearance of a pinealoblastoma. The tumor is infiltrating the third ventricle (**A**). Histopathological features of a pinealoblastoma with Flexner-Wintersteiner rosettes (H&E, ×400) (**B**), typical tumor cells with mitotic activity in the cerebrospinal fluid (MGG, ×600) (**C**), and high cellularity with numerous mitotic figures (H&E, ×400) (**D**). *(Courtesy of D. Koperek, Neuropathological Institute, Medical University of Vienna.)*

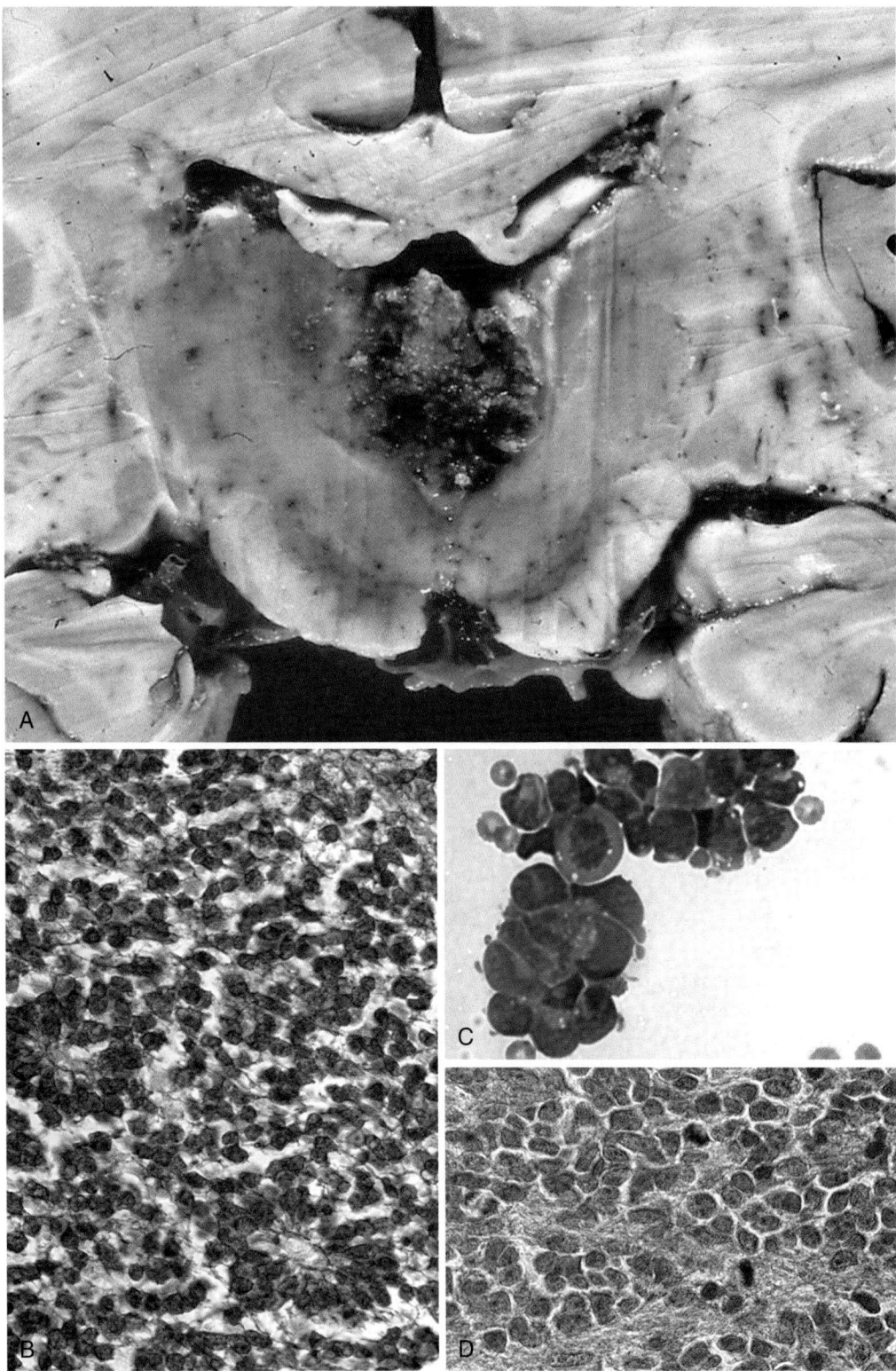

entity is malignant solitary fibrous tumors that also may occur in the pineal gland. Solitary fibrous tumors are rare fibroblastic tumors that most commonly arise in the pleura, sometimes in the orbit. In the CNS in general they are extremely rare with around 100 reports in the literature and just a handful from the pineal region.

NON-NEOPLASTIC TUMOR-LIKE CONDITIONS

Sometimes of neurosurgical importance are non-neoplastic tumor-like malformations, for example, arachnoid cysts arising from the arachnoid cells of that region or "degenerative" cysts lined by fibrillary astrocytes (so-called pineal cysts). They occur in 1.1% to 4.3% but may be seen more often, as proved in autopsy series up to 25% to 40%. Cysticercosis and vascular lesions, such as arteriovenous malformations, cavernomas, and aneurysms of the vein of Galen, can also be included, but are very rare.

METASTASES TO THE PINEAL REGION

The absence of a blood-brain barrier in the pineal gland makes it a susceptible site for hematogenous metastases; however, despite this fact these tumors of the pineal region are surprisingly rare. The most common site of origin for metastases to the pineal region is the lung, followed by the breast and other organs, such as the stomach, kidney, and melanomas.

SIGNS AND SYMPTOMS

The presentation of patients with pineal region tumors relates to the anatomy being affected as well as to the specific tumor histological type. However, the remarkable developments in neuroimaging are helping us to uncover more lesions in the pineal region in patients who have minimal symptoms, and those patients who might not normally be discovered until they became much more symptomatic. If the tumor is large enough to cause clinical symptoms, then these symptoms arise either because of hydrocephalus, local infiltration into surrounding neural structures, or local compression to the adjacent structures.

The most common symptom is Parinaud syndrome. It is present in 50% to 75% of all patients suffering from a pineal region tumor, characterized by its typical ocular movement disorder including paralysis of upward gaze, convergence or retraction nystagmus, and light-near dissociation. Direct pressure of the tumor on the tectum or dilatation of the proximal aqueduct causes the less common sylvian aqueduct syndrome, which includes paralysis of down gaze or horizontal gaze superimposed on Parinaud syndrome. Convergent nystagmus may be present when upward gaze is attempted. The anatomical substrate of these ocular functions is located below the posterior part of the third ventricle and anterior to the aqueduct. Lid retraction (Collier's sign) is quite rare; it is caused by compression of levator inhibitory fibers in the posterior commissure. Pupils are dilated and respond poorly to light, although they may respond to accommodation.

Almost all patients with severe headaches have hydrocephalus by the time of presentation, causing the typical associated signs and symptoms, vomiting, lethargy, and memory impairment. In infants, one typical sign is also an abnormally increasing head circumference and seizures. In the case of large tumors with invasive characteristics, infiltration of the thalamic region or even the internal capsule can cause contralateral hemihypesthesia or paresthesias and sometimes can also be combined with typical thalamic pain syndromes. Depending on the extent of the invasion, extrapyramidal syndromes as well as different types of movement disorders can occur. Sudden presentation of the "sun-setting" phenomenon, caused by hydrocephalus and Parinaud syndrome, together with decreased mental status, especially in children, may be related to hemorrhage into the pineal tumor (pineal apoplexy) or acute hydrocephalus.

A commonly described endocrine disturbance associated with pineal region tumors is precocious puberty, which occurs in 10% of male patients with these lesions, and has been attributed to several potential causes. One hypothesis connects the development of precocious puberty with ectopic secretion of beta human chorionic gonadotropin by choriocarcinoma or germinoma and thus explains the absence of precocious puberty in girls with pineal region tumors. Another hypothesis links precocious puberty with a mass effect or a synchronous lesion in the region of the posterior diencephalon or infundibulum, which blocks its inhibitory effect on the median eminence of the hypothalamus, thereby augmenting secretion of gonadotropins. This hypothesis explains the association of precocious puberty with other symptoms of hypothalamic dysfunction (e.g., diabetes insipidus and polyphagia). According to a third hypothesis, the growth of a tumor in the pineal region causes a decrease in the secretion by the pineal gland of a substance (or substances) with antigonadotropic effect. If a pineal parenchymal tumor causes hypersecretion of such an agent, isolated hypogonadism may occur.

In the case of drop metastases from the CSF, seeding radiculopathy or myelopathy can occur, sometimes from a nonspecific appearance. Signs and symptoms can occur in very rare cases as a result of hematogenous metastases to several structures outside the CNS. The most typical clinical signs and symptoms are summarized in Table 37.2.

DIAGNOSTIC STUDIES

Today, the two most important powerful diagnostic tools are laboratory tests including CSF cytological examination (tumor markers) and neuroradiological examinations using MRI and CT. Both are widely available and have great value.

Imaging

Diagnostic tools such as MRI have revolutionized the management of pineal region tumors (Figs. 37.9 to 37.11). The ability to obtain high-resolution images and multidimensional views makes it possible to show tumor location and extension clearly and accurately. Today, ventriculography and pneumencephalography are primarily of historical value. Skull radiography, formerly an important diagnostic study, has fallen into disuse because of its low sensitivity in detecting tumors. The normal pineal gland is seen on plain films as a calcified mass in 60% of the population over 20 years of age and very rarely in children before the age of 6 years. Any calcified pineal gland that is larger than 1 cm in any dimension should be viewed with suspicion. The appearance of a calcified pineal gland in early childhood is usually abnormal, but can, in fact, be physiologically normal in up to 5% of cases.

CT superseded all other radiological imaging methods for the detection of pineal region tumors in the early 1980s. Currently, high-resolution CT with or without intravenous contrast administration is used to examine the pineal region, but is often more important for planning the appropriate approach than as a diagnostic tool. Carotid and vertebral arteriography are only occasionally required, often in cases in which preoperative embolization may be considered; superselective angiography, in skilled hands, is used in this region for further endovascular treatment when a vascular tumor is encountered. In some institutions, magnetic resonance (MR) angiography or CT angiography

TABLE 37.2 Most Frequent Tumors of the Pineal Region: Typical Characteristics

Tumor Feature	Germinoma	Teratoma	Pinealoblastoma	Pinealocytoma	Glioma	Meningioma
Age	Child	Child	Child	Adult	Child	Adult
Sex predilection	Male	Male	None	None	None	None
Pineal vs. parapineal	Pineal	Pineal	Pineal	Pineal	Parapineal (usually)	Parapineal (usually)
Signal intensity (heterogeneous vs. homogeneous)	Homogeneous (but often hemorrhagic)	Strikingly heterogeneous	Homogeneous (unless hemorrhagic)	Homogeneous	Homogeneous (usually)	Homogeneous
Hemorrhage	Common	Typical	Common	Common	Rare	Rare
Calcification	Rare	Typical	Common	Common	Uncommon	Common
Brain edema or invasion	Common	Variable	Common	Uncommon	Primarily midbrain neoplasm	Occasional
Tendency to metastasize	Yes	Variable	Yes	No	Variable	No
Enhancement	Dense	Variable	Dense	Dense	Variable	Dense
Prognosis with 10-year survival rate, if available	Good with additional therapy: ~85% to >35%	Variable	Poor	Variable	Variable	Excellent

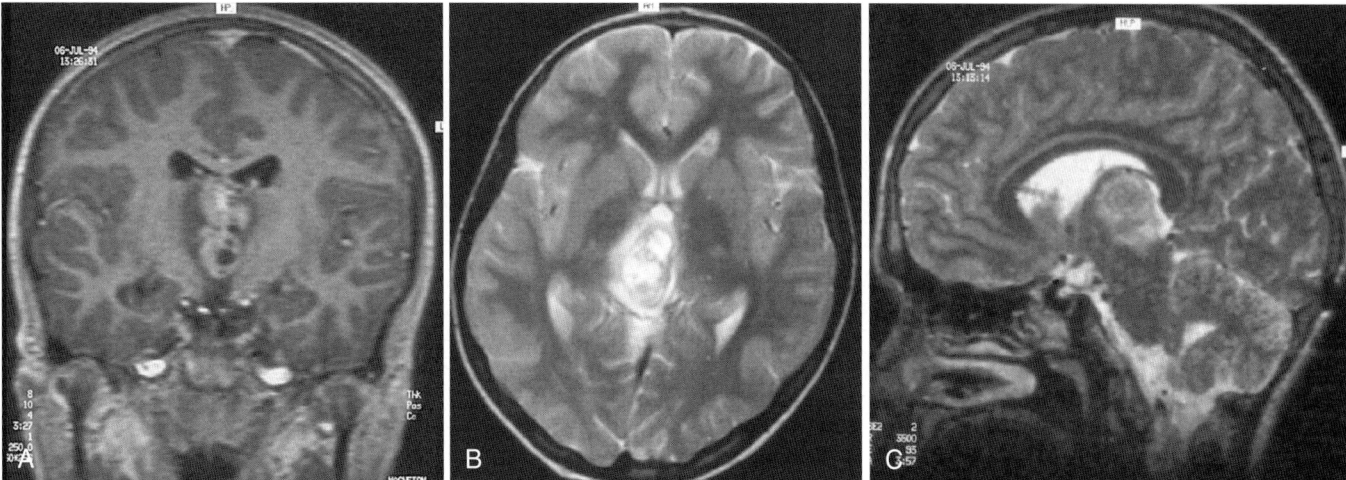

FIGURE 37.9 Coronal T1-weighted gadolinium-enhanced magnetic resonance imaging (MRI) scan demonstrating an enhancing, demarcated mass lesion in the posterior part of the third ventricle representing a pinealoblastoma (**A**). Axial (**B**) and sagittal (**C**) T2-weighted MRI studies of the same patient.

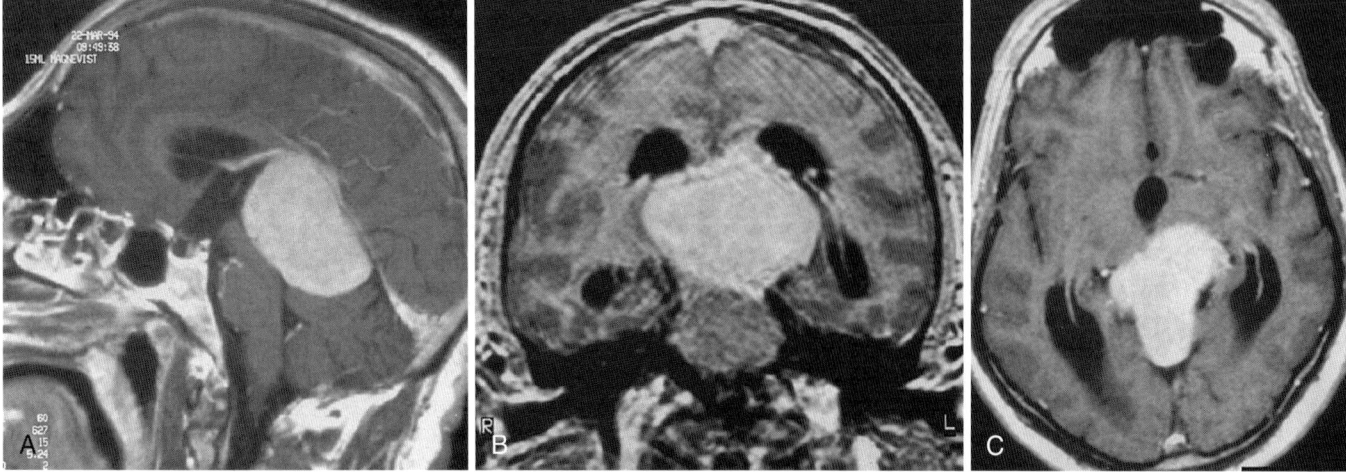

FIGURE 37.10 Infused magnetic resonance imaging (MRI) scans of a patient presenting a typical meningioma in the pineal region. Sagittal T1-weighted (**A**), coronal (**B**), and axial (**C**).

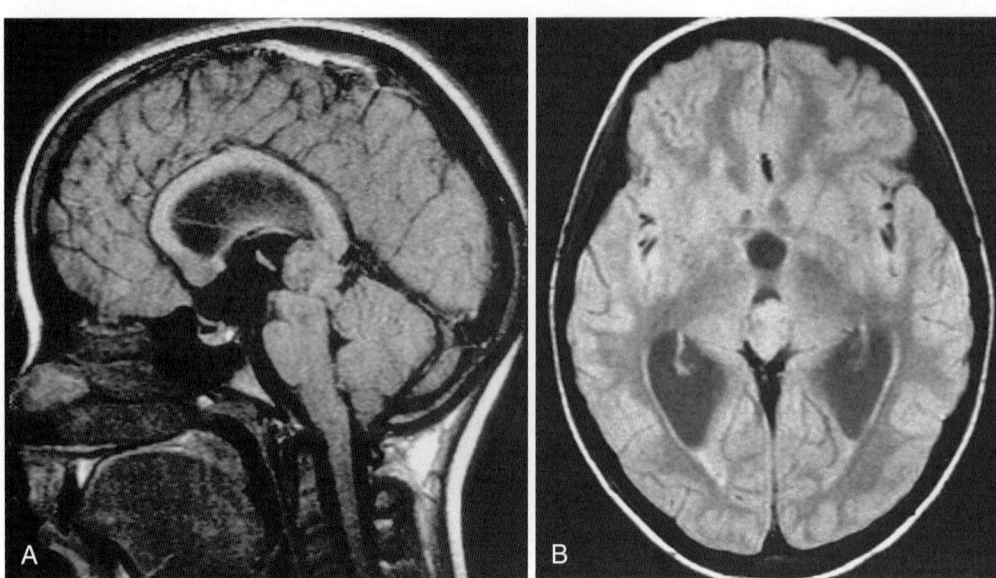

FIGURE 37.11 Infused T1-weighted magnetic resonance imaging (MRI) scans of a germinoma in the sagittal direction (**A**) and axial direction (**B**) compressing the aqueduct, causing obstructive hydrocephalus.

TABLE 37.3	Immunohistochemical Profiles (Tumor Markers) of Tumors of the Pineal Region							
	Alpha Fetoprotein ⊥ (<5ng/mL)	Human Chorionic Gonadotropin ⊥ (<5ng/mL)	Human Placental Lactogen HPL	Placental Alkaline Phosphatase	Cytokeratins (CAM 5.2, AE 1/3)	c-kit (CD 117)	OCT 4	Melatonin
Germinoma	–	+ (<770ng/mL)	–	++	–	+	+	–
Teratoma	+ (<1000ng/mL)	–	–	–	+	+/-	–	–
Yolk sac tumor	+++	–	–	+/-	+	–	–	–
Embryonal carcinoma	++ (<1000ng/mL)	++ (<770ng/mL)	–	+	+	–	+	–
Choriocarcinoma	–	+++ (>2000ng/mL)	++	+/-	+	–	–	–
Pinealocytoma	–	–	–	–	–	–	–	+
Pinealoblastoma	–	–	–	–	–	–	–	++
Papillary tumor	–	–	–	–	++	–	–	–

Modified, with additional data, from Rosenblum et al: In Louis DN, Ohgaki H, Wiestler OD, Cavenee WK: *WHO classification of tumours of the central nervous system,* Lyon, International Agency for Research on Cancer (IARC), 2007.

is the angiographic study of choice for noninvasive evaluation. Both modalities provide accurate information on the anatomy of the arteries and veins in the region for surgical planning. Therefore, the current recommendation is to perform a high-resolution MRI examination, in combination with MR angiography and, when appropriate, in addition, CT scans with and without contrast, respectively, with or without CT angiography. Table 37.3 gives an overview and comparison of the neuroradiological appearance of pineal region tumors in correlation to their pineal versus parapineal appearance, signal intensity (heterogeneous versus homogeneous), appearance of hemorrhage, calcification, brain edema or invasion, and contrast enhancement.

Newer, evolving diagnostic tools can provide additional information. MR spectroscopy provides information of biological behavior or activity, MR chemical shift imaging (CSI) may contribute to a more precise differential diagnosis, tensor diffusion-weighted imaging (DWI) assists with defining the functional anatomy in relation to the lesion, and high-field MRI

(3 tesla up to 7 tesla) can provide a better understanding of the relationship of the tumor with its surrounding anatomy. Intraoperative MRI-guided neuronavigation has been an immensely useful tool in the approach, trajectory, and surgical planning to the pineal region, despite the midline location of this structure. Image fusion modalities make it possible to get all the radiological information integrated so that the surgeon can integrate the anatomical and functional planning during surgery.

Tumor Markers

Certain pineal region tumors manifest tumor markers in the CSF and blood serum. The identification of markers is important not only for diagnostic purposes, when present, but also for monitoring response to treatment and relapse. However, it should be noted that these markers are not uniformly present in all patients with pineal tumors and their absence does not eliminate the diagnosis of a specific tumor.

The most important and useful markers are α-fetoprotein and β-human chorionic gonadotropin (β-hCG). α-Fetoprotein, a glycoprotein, is normally produced by the yolk sac and the fetal liver, and its production stops by the time of birth. An α-fetoprotein value of less than 5 ng/mL in serum and CSF is considered to be normal. The greatest production of α-fetoprotein can be seen in some cases of yolk sac tumors (endodermal sinus tumors). Embryonal carcinomas and immature teratomas produce α-fetoprotein to a lesser extent, less than 1000 ng/mL. β-Human chorionic gonadotropin, also a glycoprotein, is normally produced by the syncytiotrophoblastic giant cells of placental trophoblastic tissue with a normal value in the serum and CSF of less than 5 mIU/mL. Choriocarcinomas normally produce the highest amount, more than 2000 ng/mL. Mild elevations of less than 770 ng/mL can be seen in some patients with germinomas and embryonal carcinomas. The biological half-life is about 5 days for α-fetoprotein, but less than 24 hours for β-hCG. In general, serum titers tend to show higher positivity than do CSF titers, because the tumor should be in direct contact with the CSF for positive markers.

Human placental lactogen (HPL) is well known as a marker in case of choriocarcinoma and other trophoblastic tumors, mostly in the lung or stomach, but also cervix. In recent studies, placental alkaline phosphatase was reported to be a specific marker for primary intracranial germinomas and is measured with an enzyme-linked immunosorbent assay in the serum as well as in the CSF.

Cytokeratin as a marker can be found in teratomas, yolk sac tumors, embryonal carcinomas, and choriocarcinomas but only with lower serum levels. It seems to be more specific in case of papillary tumors of the pineal region. C-kit functions as a tyrosine kinase receptor and represents a target for small molecule kinase inhibitors, found normally in breast or lung cancers. Sometimes it could be found also in germinomas, but is extremely rare in teratomas without significant correlation between c-kit expression and prognosis. OCT4 has some biological functions and clinical applications as a marker of germ cell neoplasia and seems slightly increased in germinomas and embryonal carcinomas but without clinical significance. Melatonin as a tumor marker may be used in cases of tumors that destroy the pineal gland. The absence of melatonin in serum after surgery thereby indicates complete removal of the pineal gland. Elevation of the polyamines putrescine and spermidine in CSF has been reported in malignant brain tumors of childhood, especially PNETs.

Although the levels of markers in serum and CSF, when present, have been found to be extremely useful in assessing the efficacy of various treatment modalities and tumor recurrence, the tumor markers alone do not yield a definitive histological diagnosis. Furthermore, in a large number of patients these tumor markers are simply absent. Table 37.4 gives a brief overview of the serum and CSF levels occurring in pineal region tumors. Advanced neuroimaging (MRI, MRI spectroscopy, CSI and PET, high-resolution CT) and tumor marker evaluation, when present, improve diagnostic accuracy.

CHOICE OF TREATMENTS

Surgical treatment of pineal region tumors has been a topic of debate, controversy, and intellectual innovation for the past 100 years in neurological surgery. In the beginning of

TABLE 37.4 Frequency of Typical Clinical Signs and Symptoms in Pineal Region Tumors

Clinical Sign/Symptom	Frequency
Headache	Common (~80%)
Vomiting	
Lethargy	
Memory disturbance	
Hydrocephalus	
Nystagmus	Common (~60-70%)
Parinaud's sign	Frequent (~50-75%)
Convergence	
Accommodation palsy	
Supranuclear upward glaze	
Lid retraction	Less frequent (~10%)
Setting sun sign (Collier's sign)	
Endocrine disturbance	Less frequent (~10%)
Precocious puberty (in boys)	
Hypothalamic dysfunction	
Diabetes insipidus	
Polyphagia	
Isolated hypogonadism	
Radiculopathy or myelopathy	Rare
Seizures	Rare
Hemihypesthesia/paresthesia	Rare
Thalamic pain	Rare
Extrapyramidal movement disorders	Rare

the twentieth century, the lack of technical, anesthetic, and radiological refinements led to uniformly poor surgical results and a surgical mortality rate close to 90%. For decades, the treatment of these tumors was relegated to CSF diversion followed by radiotherapy. Even until the mid-1970s, the therapy of pineal region tumors consisted of ventricular shunting and radiation therapy, with 5-year survival rates as high as 60% to 80% with some histological types of tumors.

Advanced techniques in microneurosurgery, neuroanesthesiology, neuroimaging, and intensive care medicine have enabled modern neurosurgeons to operate on such lesions with more than acceptable outcomes. This has resulted in a much higher cure rate, decreased surgical mortality and morbidity rates, and increased longevity for those patients who have tumor recurrence after therapy. Today, control of hydrocephalus, which is associated with most of the tumors in this region, is no longer a problem and should be carried out routinely either through a shunting procedure or, more often, via endoscopic third ventriculostomy. Even in the case of nonresectable tumors, a safe and efficient histological identification is advised and worth attempting by endoscopic or stereotactic biopsy. This serves as the basis for further adjuvant radiotherapy and chemotherapy in these nonresectable lesions. There is a subset of tumors that lend themselves to resection despite their size and location. In these tumors a radical resection through a variety of approaches should be attempted by surgeons who are experienced with the technical refinements and surgical anatomy in this challenging region.

Stereotactic Procedures

Stereotactic procedures, frame-base or frameless, have become increasingly more advanced and easy to use as a diagnostic tool for tumors that may not be amenable to resection. Most reports concerning this type of procedure indicate that the risks of intervention are minimal. However, caution is advised because the pineal region is surrounded by an important complex of arteries and veins, as described in the earlier section on anatomy. The vessels may be displaced from their normal position for several reasons, such as tumor mass, or hydrocephalus. Also, some tumors, such as pinealoblastomas or choriocarcinomas, are highly vascular. However, the complication rate in stereotactic biopsy of lesions in this location is low, approximately 1.3% mortality rate and 7% morbidity rate in skilled hands according to a large European series. The diagnostic accuracy and specificity is equivalently high (94%), although stereotactic biopsy may fail to disclose the histological heterogeneity of selected tumors due to sampling error, especially in the case of mixed malignant tumors.

Neuroendoscopy and Hydrocephalus

Recent advances in neuroendoscopic techniques have enabled this technology to become a major component of the treatment strategies of pineal region tumors. In most of the cases, endoscopic biopsy can be performed with more than acceptable results, especially for tumors reaching into the posterior part of the third ventricle. There are now case series of pineal region tumors in which the hydrocephalus is treated by an endoscopic third ventriculostomy followed by a pineal region biopsy. The technique of endoscopic third ventriculostomy has proved to be highly effective and has obviated the need for placement of a permanent shunt. Alternatively, hydrocephalus may be controlled with either tumor mass reduction or a CSF diversion procedure such as a ventriculoperitoneal shunt. Patients presenting acutely with hydrocephalus may be treated using neuroendoscopic third ventriculostomy or, if not available, with external ventricular drainage. The ability of pineal cell tumors to metastasize through a diversionary CSF shunt is rare but has been reported. Certain biopsy-proven germ cell tumors can be reduced in size with concomitant resolution of their associated hydrocephalus within a short time following irradiation or chemotherapy.

SURGICAL APPROACHES

The efficacy of open microsurgery on pineal region tumors is undisputed in the twenty-first century. The main goal is complete tumor removal with minimal morbidity whenever possible. Even if radical resection cannot be achieved for several reasons, histological verification, maximal cytoreduction, and more often, restoration of CSF pathways may be achieved. For the benign pineal region tumor, surgery alone is often curative. Although about 80% of pediatric tumors are malignant, open surgery is recommended in most adult cases and selected pediatric cases in which resection is considered safe based on the appearance of the lesion by MRI. Radical resection is especially helpful in cases of the malignant nongerminoma germ cell tumors, as the extent of resection influences the prognosis of the patient. Because the pineal region is located in the geometric center of the intracranial cavity, operative approaches from

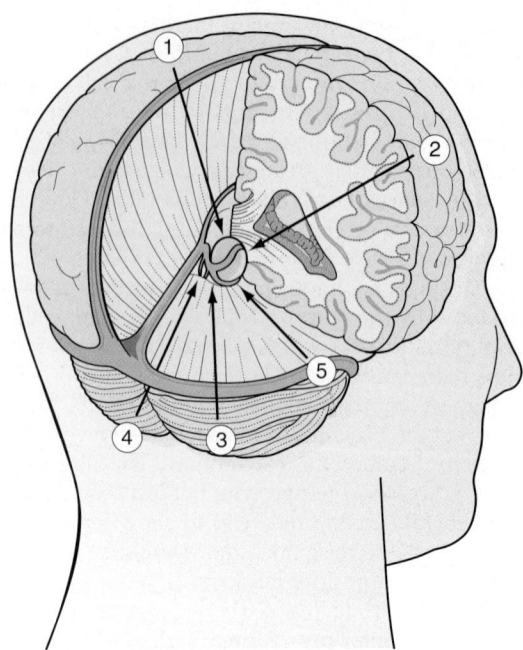

FIGURE 37.12 Schematic drawing of the various operative approaches to the pineal region from every direction. *(Modified from Day JD, Koos WT, Matula C, Lang J, editors. Color Atlas of Microneurosurgical Approaches. Stuttgart: Thieme; 1997.)*

every conceivable angle and direction have been developed (Fig. 37.12). The five most common surgical approaches are as follows:

1. The posterior transcallosal approach pioneered by Dandy
2. The transventricular approach pioneered by Van Wagenen
3. The occipital transtentorial approach pioneered by Foerster and Poppen
4. The infratentorial-supracerebellar approach pioneered by Krause and popularized by Stein
5. The three-quarter prone, operated side down, occipital transtentorial approach described by Ausman

Other approaches include the frontal (anterior) ones in which the pineal region is accessed transcallosally or transcortically. The transcallosal transventricular transvelum-interpositum approach by Sano is useful for large pineal tumors with anterior extension into the third ventricle. An alternative frontal approach to reach the pineal region includes the transcortical, subchoroidal approach.

The Posterior Transcallosal Approach

In 1921, Walter Dandy was one of the first to propose this approach to the pineal region. The primary anatomical structures exposed are the splenium of the corpus callosum, internal cerebral veins, basal vein of Rosenthal, vein of Galen, pineal body, posterior commissure, and quadrigeminal plate. Patient position is similar to the position for the classical anterior transcallosal approach. However, a higher angle is required to provide the appropriate trajectory of about 40 degrees. We prefer a semilunar skin incision over the midline. Craniotomy should include the lambdoid at the posterior margin of the bone flap (Fig. 37.13). A semilunar

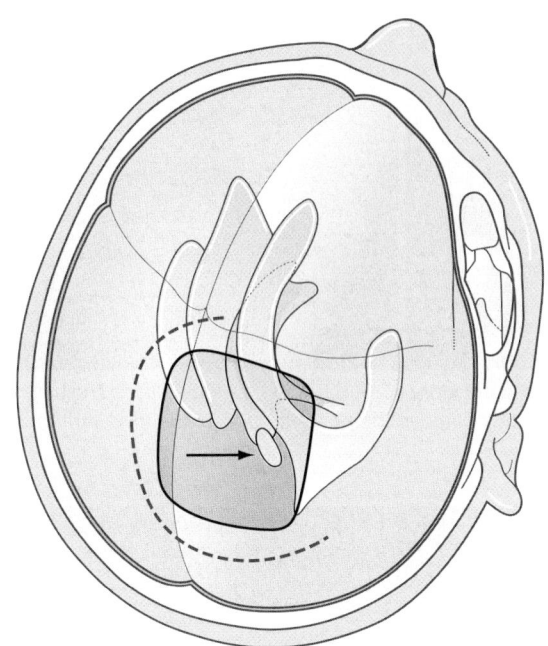

FIGURE 37.13 The posterior transcallosal approach. Direction of the approach, skin incision, and position of craniotomy. *(Modified from Day JD, Koos WT, Matula C, Lang J, editors. Color Atlas of Microneurosurgical Approaches. Stuttgart: Thieme; 1997.)*

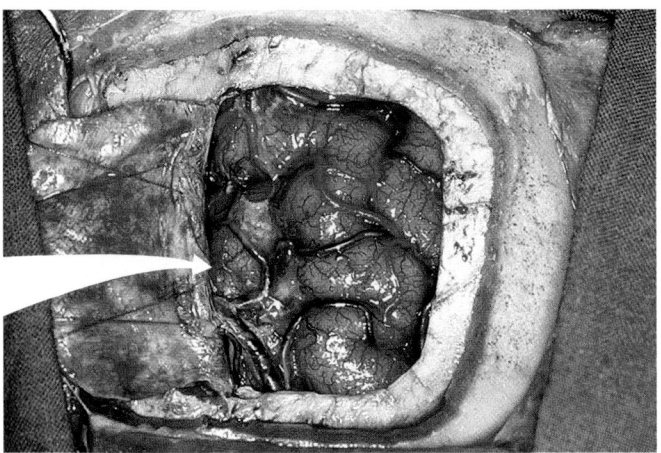

FIGURE 37.14 Dura opening and entrance into the interhemispheric fissure in an anatomical cadaver. *(Modified from Day JD, Koos WT, Matula C, Lang J, editors. Color Atlas of Microneurosurgical Approaches. Stuttgart: Thieme; 1997.)*

dural flap is elevated to expose the cortical surface of the posterior parietal lobe. Entry point is the interhemispheric fissure (Fig. 37.14). Bridging veins are rare posteriorly but should be preserved, whenever possible. Retraction of the mesial parietal lobe exposes the splenium of the corpus callosum and after splitting the splenium, the internal cerebral veins can be seen as they drain into the vein of Galen. The pineal gland is located inferior to the venous complex (Fig. 37.15). The limitations of this approach include difficulty in visualization of the quadrigeminal plate and cerebellum, and laterally the mesial occipital lobe, and the requirement to split the splenium of the corpus callosum and retract the mesial occipital lobe. Advantages of this approach are

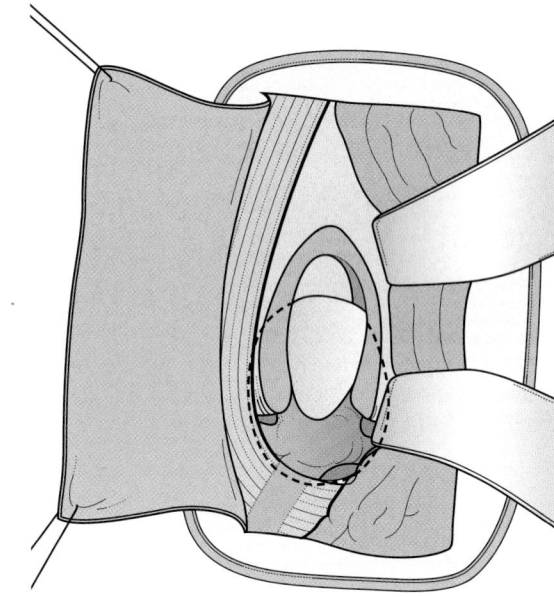

FIGURE 37.15 Approach to pineal region while performing the posterior transcallosal approach, demonstrating the relation from the pineal tumor to the venous system and surrounding structures. *(Modified from Pendl G, editor. Pineal and Midbrain Lesions. Berlin: Springer; 1985.)*

the superior access superior to the venous complex (internal cerebral veins) and the ability to visualize these veins in the velum interpositum so that they are not sacrificed. We recommend this approach for tumors spreading above the venous complex and expanding anteriorly into the third ventricle as well as those extending upward into the corpus callosum (Fig. 37.16A-C). It is an approach that still has indications and should be a part of the surgeon's armamentarium.

The Occipital Transtentorial Approach

This approach was first proposed by Foerster in 1928 and described in detail by Poppen in 1966. Primary anatomical structures exposed are the splenium of the corpus callosum, internal cerebral veins, basal vein of Rosenthal, vein of Galen, precentral cerebellar vermian vein, pineal body, posterior commissure, and quadrigeminal plate. This approach comes from a more lateral direction and we prefer to have the patient in the recumbent, semisitting position with the chin tucked. Skin incision is an inverted L-shaped incision to expose the occipital region. The inion should be clearly exposed and the bone flap is made with its superior margin approximately 1 to 2 cm below the lambdoid suture. The inferior margin is below the inion, thus placing the torcular within the inferior portion of the dural exposure (Fig. 37.17). After opening the dura, the occipital lobe is retracted laterally to expose the posterior incisural edge and its junction with the falx cerebri. After the tentorium is incised, the lateral entry point has been reached and the venous complex can be explored (Fig. 37.18). Sharp dissection of the arachnoid exposes the vein of Galen and the ipsilateral basal vein of

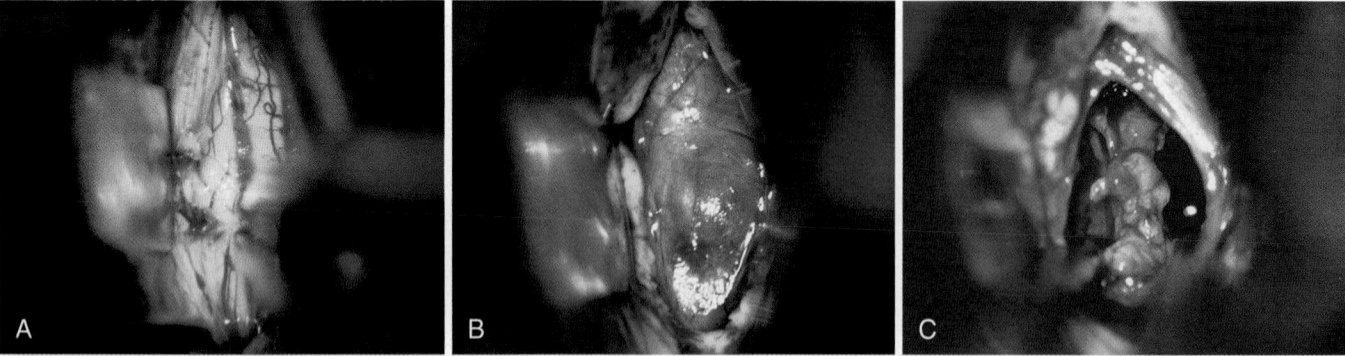

FIGURE 37.16 Intraoperative findings in the case of a pinealoblastoma as presented in Figure 37.6. Situation during splitting the splenium of the corpus callosum using a nonstick bipolar forceps (**A**). Appearance of the tumor located in the posterior part of the third ventricle before resection (**B**) and after complete tumor removal (**C**).

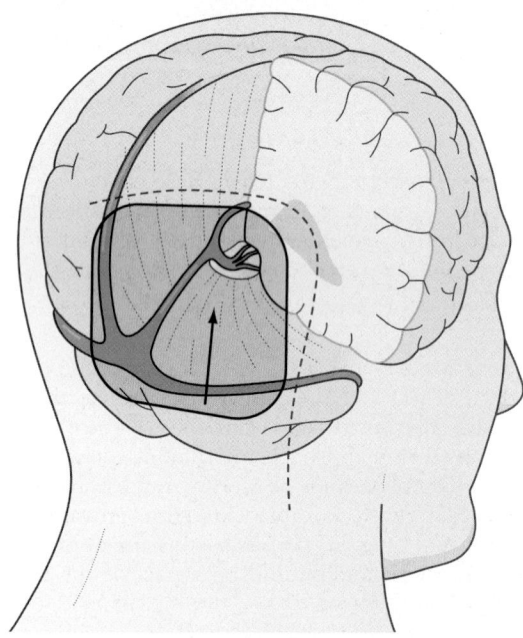

FIGURE 37.17 The occipital transtentorial approach: trajectory of the approach, skin incision, and position of craniotomy. *(Modified from Day JD, Koos WT, Matula C, Lang J, editors. Color Atlas of Microneurosurgical Approaches. Stuttgart: Thieme; 1997.)*

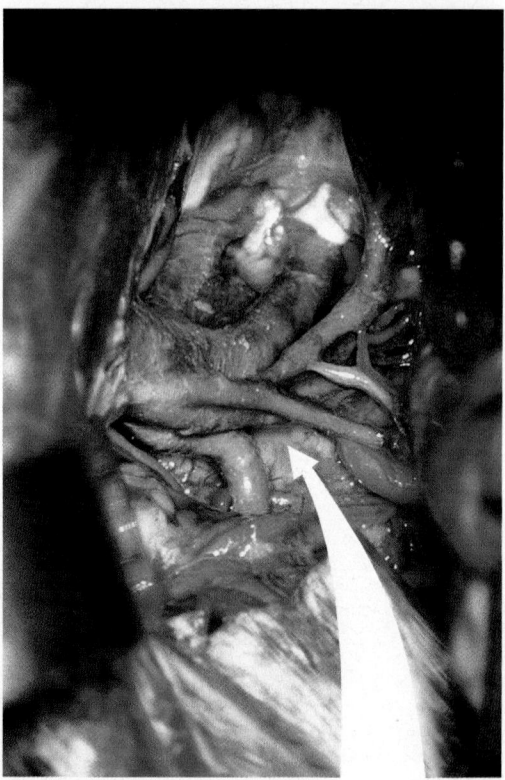

FIGURE 37.18 Dura opening and entrance after incision of the tentorium in an anatomical cadaver. *(Modified from Day JD, Koos WT, Matula C, Lang J, editors. Color Atlas of Microneurosurgical Approaches. Stuttgart: Thieme; 1997.)*

Rosenthal. The pineal gland is most clearly visible inferior to the venous complex (Fig. 37.19).

Limitations of the approach include poor visualization of the internal cerebral veins anteriorly, the quadrigeminal plate inferiorly, the falx cerebri and vein of Galen medially, and the occipital lobe laterally. In addition, it is not uncommon to compress and temporarily affect the visual cortex through the extremes of retraction that are required to lift the occipital lobe. An advantage of this approach is the superb view, both above and below the tentorium. This approach is recommended for tumors growing through the tentorial hiatus with a supra- and infracerebellar extension, and especially in the case of meningiomas (Fig. 37.20A-C). This approach is used in about 20% of the cases in our institution and makes this the second most common approach for dealing with tumors in the pineal region.

The Infratentorial-Supracerebellar Approach

The infratentorial-supracerebellar approach was first described by Krause in 1913 and then modified and popularized by Stein in 1971. Performing this kind of approach in the sitting position means that gravity assists the cerebellum in falling down from the undersurface of the tentorium. Primary anatomical structures exposed are the cerebellum, cerebellar veins, cerebellar vermian veins, internal cerebellar veins, basal veins of Rosenthal, vein of Galen, pineal body, posterior commissure, quadrigeminal plate, splenium of the corpus callosum, and posterior third ventricle. We prefer the patient to be placed

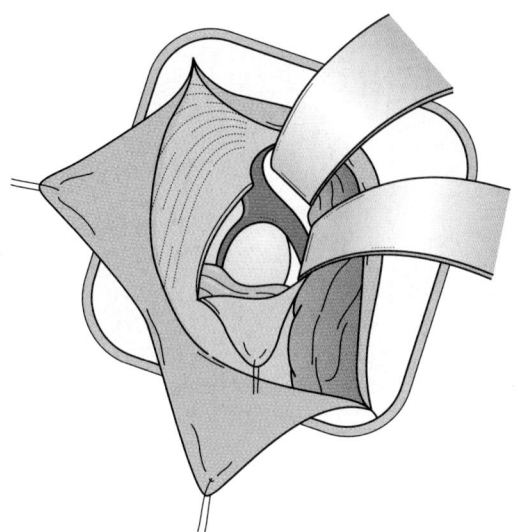

FIGURE 37.19 Pineal region after performing an occipital transtentorial approach presenting the relation of the pineal tumor to the venous system and surrounding structures. *(Modified from Pendl G, editor. Pineal and Midbrain Lesions. Berlin: Springer; 1985.)*

in the sitting position with the head flexed anteriorly. The amount of flexion depends on the relationship of the tumor to the straight sinus. As an alternative position, we recommend the so-called modified concord position that allows the surgeon to sit comfortably behind the patient. One of the main advantages of the concord position is that it decreases the risk of air embolism. One of the disadvantages is that it is sometimes impossible when the tentorium is very steep. The skin incision is made in the midline, and we use either an S-shaped or a straight midline incision. The craniotomy is centered over the external occipital protuberance and includes the torcular herophili at the superior portion of dural exposure (Fig. 37.21). This allows some upward retraction of the sinus complex, decreasing the degree of necessary downward retraction of the cerebellum. In most of the cases it is not necessary to open the foramen magnum to drain the cisterna magnum so that the cerebellum requires very little retraction. The preserved rim of bone inferiorly provides support for the cerebellum, decreasing traction on its superior connecting elements to the brainstem. Arachnoid dissection and division of the superomedial cerebellar bridging veins allow subsequent inferior retraction of the cerebellar hemispheres (Fig. 37.22). In most cases, a very thick arachnoid membrane is found spanning the interval between the cerebellar vermis and the central posterior incisura. After dissection of the arachnoid membrane the venous complex surrounding the pineal gland can be explored (Fig. 37.23). Limitations of the approach are its restriction to the midline and limited extension to the lateral side. The most powerful advantage is the superior access inferior to the venous complex. We recommend this approach in most of the cases (more than 72%) in which the tumors are restricted to the midline and inferior to the venous complex. It also represents a perfect opportunity to use a rigid angled endoscope as an adjuvant during surgery. This so-called endoscope-assisted or endoscope-guided procedure allows not only perfect illumination (which gives the anatomical structures more plasticity), but also enables the surgeon to have a "look around a corner"

without even touching any anatomical structure. This helps the surgeon to detect any residual tumor hiding in the recesses of the pineal region, thus increasing the chance for a radical tumor resection (Fig. 37.24A-D).

Transverse Sinus–Tentorium Splitting Approach

As mentioned previously, depending on the individual situation, it can be very helpful to chose some combination, especially in huge tumors. One of the modifications is the so-called transverse sinus–tentorium splitting approach described by Beck and modified by Sekhar. The key point is the splitting of the transverse sinus and dissection of the tentorium to get the best of both worlds, supratentorial and infratentorial, as schematically drawn in Figure 37.25.

The Transventricular Approach

The transventricular approach, which was first described by Van Wagenen in 1931, is also useful in same select patients. This type of approach is indicated in very rare cases of large, eccentric lesions with ventricular dilatation. The entry point with this approach is usually via a cortical incision in the posterior portion of the superior temporal gyrus. Unfortunately, this exposes the patient to a high risk of visual impairment, seizure, and dominant side language dysfunction. Therefore, this approach is limited to the nondominant hemisphere. In general, the main goal of pineal region microsurgery consists of having a complete tumor resection, combined with no additional neurological deficits. The routine use of transesophageal ultrasound in the sitting position to prevent air embolism, the widespread application of frameless stereotactic neuronavigational systems, and the increasingly common use of endoscopes have helped to refine and increase the safety associated with attempts at radical resection of pineal region tumors.

OTHER THERAPEUTIC MODALITIES

Although in the majority of cases surgical removal is the treatment of choice, some tumors (such as germinomas or nongerminoma germ cell tumors) may require further therapy. These tumors have shown a sensitivity to radiation therapy and chemotherapy, and thus these adjuvant therapies are now established as further therapeutic modalities.

Radiotherapy

Although more than 70% of tumors in the pineal region and the posterior third ventricle are highly radiosensitive, radiation therapy is still a subject of controversy. Select tumors respond to adequate courses of radiation therapy within 3 to 6 months. The current neurosurgical paradigm of the treatment of acute hydrocephalus followed by diagnostic biopsy or radical resection of tumor has obviated the need for preoperative empirical radiation therapy prior to diagnosis. However, it has been clinically proved that germinomas, like seminomas, are highly sensitive to radiation therapy. Radiotherapy is not a benign form of treatment, especially to the developing central nervous system, such as in the pediatric population. Serious consequences of such treatment include

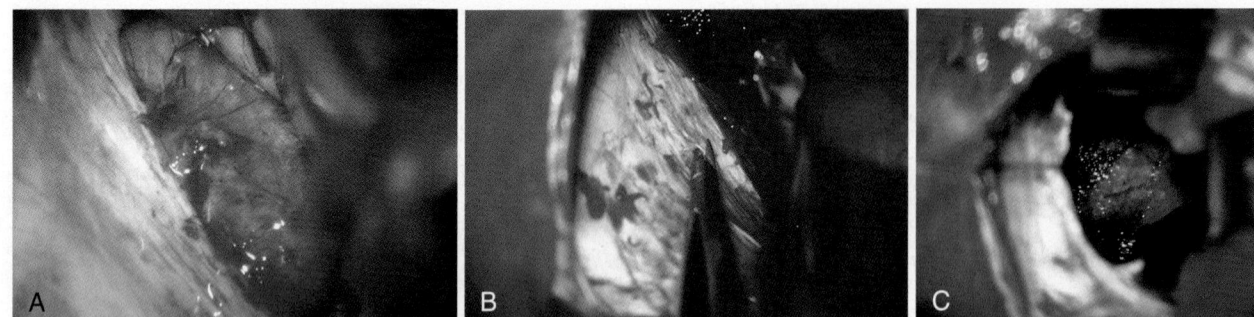

FIGURE 37.20 Intraoperative findings in case of a meningioma as presented in Figure 37.7. Photograph before the incision of the tentorium with the tumor in the background (**A**). Incision of the tentorium, as one of the key steps in performing the approach, (**B**) and the situation after complete tumor removal. The surrounding tissue is covered with Surgicel (**C**).

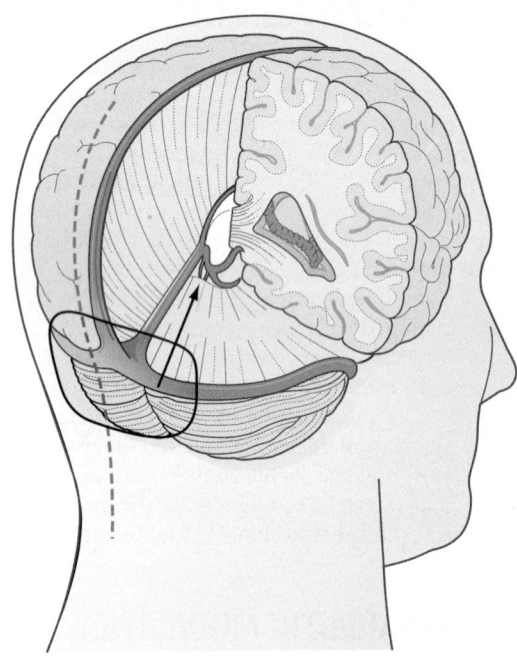

FIGURE 37.21 The infratentorial-supracerebellar approach: trajectory of the approach, skin incision, and position of craniotomy. *(Modified from Day JD, Koos WT, Matula C, Lang J, editors. Color Atlas of Microneurosurgical Approaches. Stuttgart: Thieme; 1997.)*

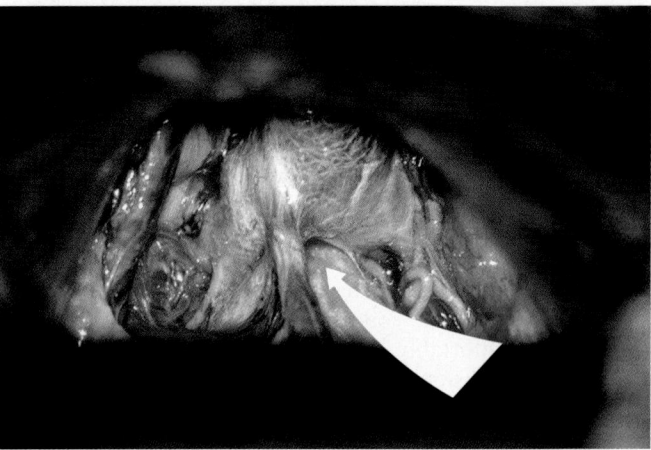

FIGURE 37.22 The infratentorial-supracerebellar entry into the pineal region in an anatomical cadaver. *(Modified from Day JD, Koos WT, Matula C, Lang J, editors. Color Atlas of Microneurosurgical Approaches. Stuttgart: Thieme; 1997.)*

endocrine deficiencies, severe vasculitis, and significant intellectual impairment. All of these risks limit the dosage and modalities used in radiotherapy of pineal region tumors in young children. The application of preradiation chemotherapy and stereotactic radiation techniques such as the linear particle accelerator (linac) and gamma knife radiosurgery may provide some relief from the potential detrimental side effects of radiation on the developing brain. Despite the well-established radiosensitivity of germinomas, about 10% of the patients may experience tumor recurrence. Radiosurgery (linac, gamma knife, or CyberKnife) is increasingly being used to treat tumors in the pineal region, either as an additional therapy after conventional treatments or as a primary treatment. The optimal treatment of huge tumors can be obtained when radiosurgery is used in conjunction with open surgery and conventional radiotherapy.

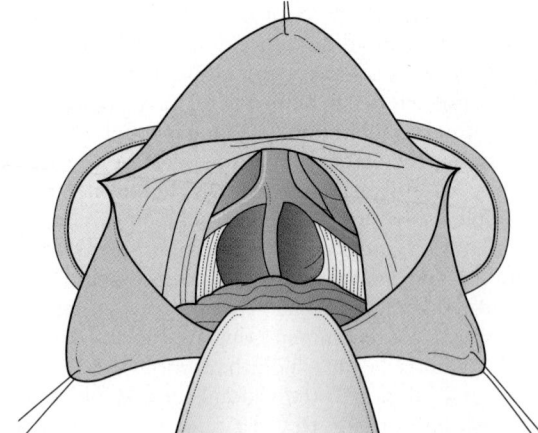

FIGURE 37.23 Pineal region while performing the infratentorial supracerebellar approach presenting the relation of the pineal tumor to the venous system and surrounding structures. *(Modified from Pendl G, editor. Pineal and Midbrain Lesions. Berlin: Springer; 1985.)*

FIGURE 37.24 Intraoperative findings in case of a germinoma as presented in Figure 37.8. Photograph during the opening of the arachnoid membranes in the pineal region with the tumor in the background (**A**). Appearance of the tumor before resection (**B**) and after complete tumor removal (**C**), and endoscope-assisted approach with the view into the third ventricle presenting the intermediate mass, the choroid plexus at the roof, both fornices, and the anterior commissure (**D**).

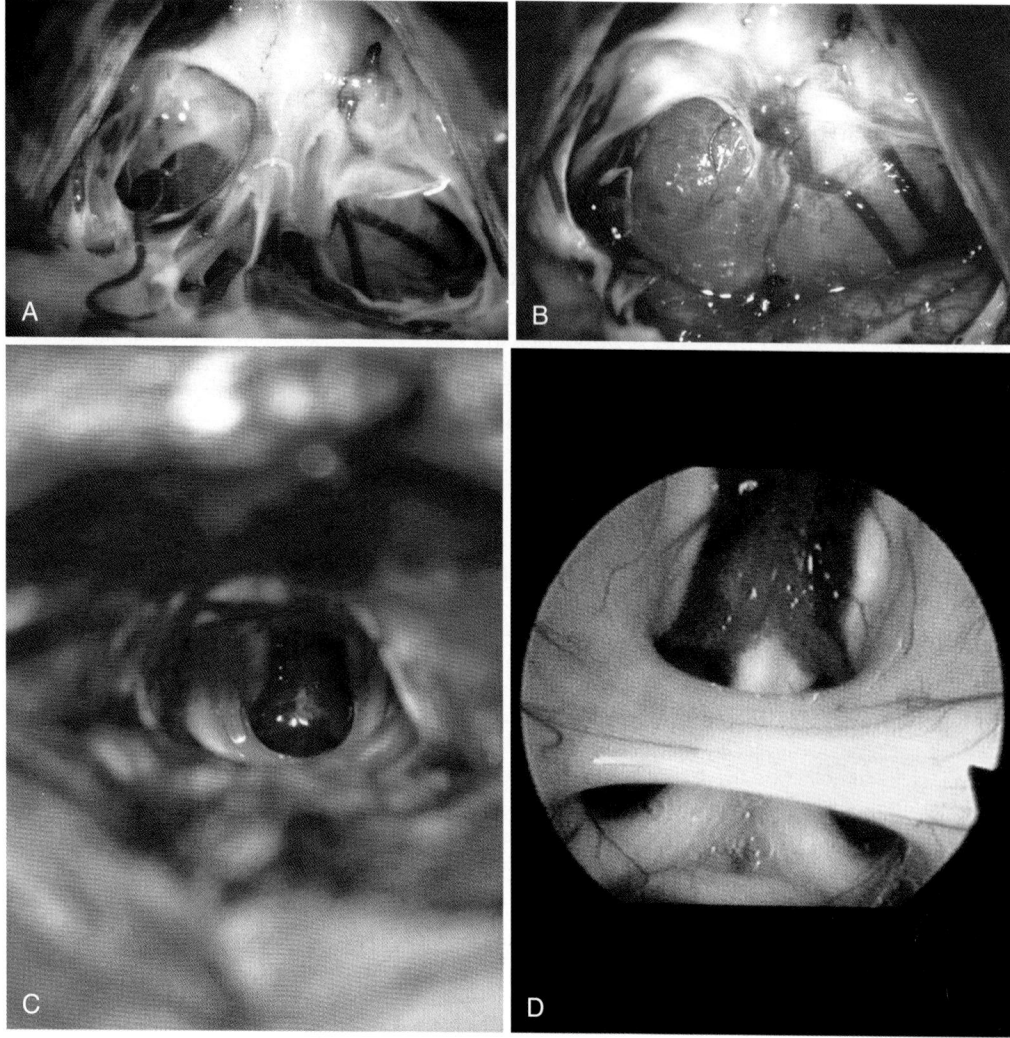

Chemotherapy

Chemotherapy has gained considerable recognition for the treatment especially of malignant germ cell tumors. In 1977, de Tribolet and Barrelet reported the successful use of chemotherapy in a patient with a large pineal tumor. The chemotherapeutic regimen included daunorubicin, vincristine, and bleomycin. Later, the combination of cisplatin, bleomycin, and vincristine (PVB therapy) was employed to treat germ cell tumors in several series with limited success. In 1987, Takakura recommended the use of ACNU (nimustine) and vincristine together with radiotherapy in cases of immature teratomas and PVB therapy after completing the entire course of radiotherapy to prevent recurrence. Responses to chemotherapy are apparent not only on MRI but also from tumor markers. Despite the known toxicity of chemotherapeutic agents, chemotherapy has an accepted role in the treatment of malignant pineal region tumors.

CONCLUSION

In the Western hemisphere, tumors of the pineal region constitute about 1% of all intracranial neoplasms and are more common in children (3-8% of all pediatric brain tumors).

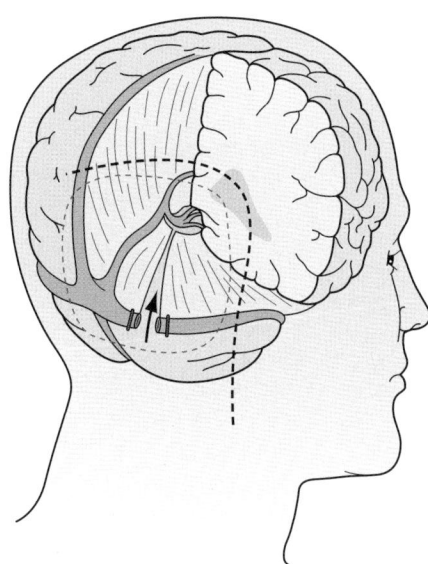

FIGURE 37.25 Combined supra/infratentorial transverse sinus–tentorium splitting approach: trajectory of the approach after dissection of the transverse sinus and splitting of the tentorium.

However, in Japan, pure germ cell tumors are more common for unknown reasons, and pineal region tumors constitute 4% to 7% of all intracranial neoplasms. The author's own data show a predominance of males (67%) to females (33%) in all cases. About 65% of all the cases involve patients who are younger than 20 years of age and about 35% who are aged between 21 and 70. Pathologically, primary tumors of the pineal region can be divided into germ cell tumors (about 60%), pineal parenchymal tumors (about 30%), tumors of supportive and adjacent structures (about 10%), nonneoplastic tumor-like conditions (less than 1%), and metastases (less than 0.1%). Symptoms of tumors in the pineal region are caused either by obstruction of CSF pathways or by local involvement (compression or invasion) of adjacent structures. Characteristic local signs include visual disturbances, the most common being Parinaud syndrome.

The rate of incidental findings of pineal region tumors is currently increasing because of high-resolution imaging modalities. The current initial diagnostic method of choice is MRI, and additional neuroradiological examinations such as MR angiography, MRI spectroscopy, chemical shift imaging (CSI), and positron emission tomography scans may eventually provide more information about the histological morphology and biological behavior. However, even today, imaging techniques cannot provide definitive information about the histological type of tumor. Biopsy (stereotactic or endoscopic), and surgical removal of the lesion represent the best way of establishing the histological diagnosis and definitive treatment. Qualitative and quantitative assessment of tumor markers is nonspecific, and may be negative but is most useful, when present, for following the tumor in terms of response to treatment. It is well documented that the histological types of any pineal tumor can be diverse. The treatment of tumors of the pineal region depends mostly on their histological type and may include a combination of surgery, radiation, and chemotherapy. In the modern microsurgical era, microsurgery for radical resection of pineal region tumors is now increasingly safe with surgical mortality rate generally less than 5% thanks to advances in neuroanesthesia, imaging, and critical care medicine. Patient survival and quality of life can be optimized through the use of multimodal treatment, including surgery, conventional radiation therapy, and radiosurgery, as well as chemotherapy, when applicable. Microsurgical resection requires surgical experience as well as clinical judgment. Management of tumors of the pineal region not only requires technical expertise, it demands multidisciplinary cooperation.

ACKNOWLEDGMENTS

Grateful thanks are given to Mrs R.A. Klim for checking the language, to O. Koperek, Neuropathological Institute (H. Budka), Medical University of Vienna, for arranging and preparing the histopathological figures, to D. Prayer from the neuroradiological department, Medical University of Vienna, for helping with the radiological figures, to A. Di Ieva and M. Tschabitscher, Anatomical Institute, Medical University of Vienna, for preparing the neuroendoscopic figure, and last but not least, to I. Dobsak, our medical illustrator, for her brilliant drawings on which the illustrations in this chapter are based. This chapter contains also text from the first edition, done by Konstantin V. Slavin and James I. Ausman. I am grateful to both for their contribution.

SELECTED KEY REFERENCES

Blakeley JO, Grossman SA. Management of pineal region tumors. *Curr Treat Options Oncol.* 2006;7(6):505-516.

Bruce JN, Ogden AT. Surgical strategies for treating patients with pineal region tumors. *J Neurooncol.* 2004;69(1-3):221-236.

Day JD, Koos WT, Matula C, Lang J, eds. *Color Atlas of Microneurosurgical Approaches. Cranial Base and Intracranial Midline.* Stuttgart: Thieme; 1997.

De Girolami U, Fèvre-Montange M, Seilhean D, Jouvet A. Pathology of tumors of the pineal region. *Rev Neurol (Paris).* 2008;164(11):882-895.

Radovanovic I, Dizdarevic K, de Tribolet N, et al. Pineal region tumors—neurosurgical review. *Med Arh.* 2009;63(3):171-173.

Please go to expertconsult.com to view the complete list of references.

38 Cerebellopontine Angle Tumors

Madjid Samii, Venelin M. Gerganov

CLINICAL PEARLS

- Comprehensive knowledge of the complex anatomy of the cerebellopontine (CP) angle is a prerequisite for achieving good surgical results. The crucial neurovascular structures should be identified as early as possible during surgery, which enables their preservation and guides subsequent operative steps. Whatever the tumor size and extension, the anatomical relationships of the cranial nerves in the area of the fundus of the internal auditory canal and in the brainstem exit/entry zone are constant.

- Most of the CP angle tumors are benign and their complete removal leads to excellent long-term outcomes. The only exception to complete tumor removal is the attempt to preserve function, such as in surgery for vestibular schwannoma in the only hearing ear.

- The major principles of CP angle tumor removal include the following: important neural structures, such as the cochlear and facial nerves, should be identified early; the tumor should be initially debulked; the dissection from the surrounding structures should be performed only after sufficient internal decompression is achieved; the dissection should always be performed in the arachnoid plane; bipolar coagulation, especially in the vicinity of a cranial nerve, should be avoided.

- Our preferred approach is the retrosigmoid approach. It is safe, relatively simple, and provides a panoramic view of the CP angle and petroclival area. Importantly, it is related to a very low procedure-related morbidity rate. The additional removal of the suprameatal tubercle provides access to tumors with extensions into Meckel's cave, into the petroclival area, and even into the posterior cavernous sinus.

HISTORY OF CEREBELLOPONTINE ANGLE SURGERY

Tumors of the cerebellopontine (CP) angle are usually benign and their complete removal leads to the healing of the patient. However, because of the very complex anatomical structure of the area and the severity of the neurological dysfunction in case of iatrogenic damage, surgery in the CP angle has always been a challenge. The first successful complete removal of a CP angle tumor was performed in 1894 by Sir Charles Balance. The tumor was approached via a right posterior fossa craniectomy and removed with the finger inserted in an unsterile fashion between the pons and the tumor. Although the patient had facial anesthesia and complete facial palsy, he recovered from surgery and was alive for at least 18 years.[1] The pathological nature of this tumor is a matter of controversy and the credit for the first removal of a vestibular schwannoma (VS) probably belongs to Thomas Annandale of Edinburgh. In 1895 he removed a tumor "the size of a pigeon's egg" via a unilateral suboccipital craniotomy. Later, major contributions to the surgery of CP angle tumors were made by V. Horsley, von Eiselsberg,

and F. Krause. Krause used for the first time faradic stimulation to differentiate the facial from the audiovestibular nerve.[2] H. Cushing was the first to reduce the complication and mortality rates of VS surgery to an acceptable level by performing intracapsular tumor removal. Expectedly, the tumor recurrence rate in his series was very high. W. Dandy introduced the currently widely accepted concept of VS management. He argued that benign tumors should be removed completely in order to prevent recurrence at a later stage, even at the expense of a somewhat higher perioperative mortality rate. In the following decades, morbidity and mortality rates progressively improved with increased experience and knowledge of the normal and pathological anatomy of the CP angle, earlier detection of such tumors with the introduction of computed tomography (CT) and magnetic resonance imaging (MRI), routine use of intraoperative electrophysiological monitoring, and more reliable and safe anesthetic and operative techniques. Initial efforts at preservation of facial nerve function have expanded to preservation of hearing with increasing success. As a result of these efforts, modern CP angle surgery has been refined to a routine, safe, and low morbidity procedure.

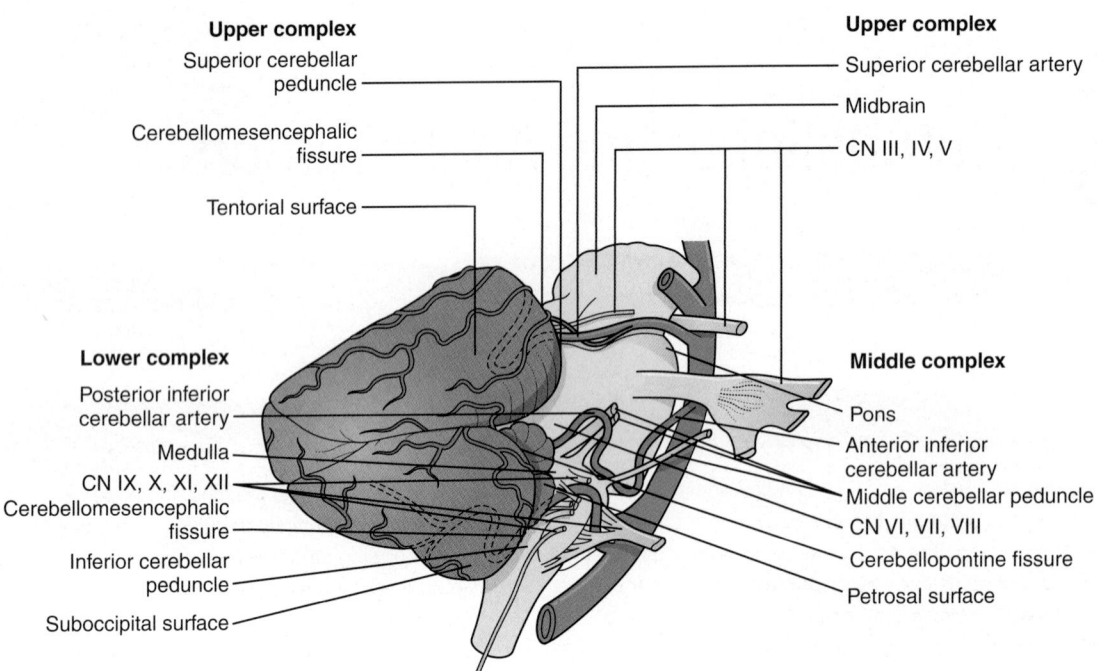

Upper complex
Superior cerebellar peduncle
Cerebellomesencephalic fissure
Tentorial surface

Upper complex
Superior cerebellar artery
Midbrain
CN III, IV, V

Lower complex
Posterior inferior cerebellar artery
Medulla
CN IX, X, XI, XII
Cerebellomesencephalic fissure
Inferior cerebellar peduncle
Suboccipital surface

Middle complex
Pons
Anterior inferior cerebellar artery
Middle cerebellar peduncle
CN VI, VII, VIII
Cerebellopontine fissure
Petrosal surface

FIGURE 38.1 Schematic diagram demonstrating the cerebellopontine angle formed by the superior and inferior limbs of the cerebellopontine fissure with the apex oriented laterally. Also demonstrated are the three neurovascular complexes, the upper, middle, and lower complex and the elements that form each of these complexes. *(Adapted from Rhoton AL Jr. Microsurgical anatomy of posterior fossa cranial nerves. In Barrow DL, editor. Surgery of the Cranial Nerves of the Posterior Fossa, Neurosurgical Topics. Rolling Meadows, IL: American Association of Neurological Surgeons; 1993:1-103.)*

CEREBELLOPONTINE ANGLE ANATOMY

The CP angle is a triangular space located posterior to the pyramid, inferior to the tentorium, lateral to the pons, and ventral to the cerebellum.[3] It is defined by the superior and inferior limbs of the CP fissure (Fig. 38.1).

The CP angle cistern is located between the anterolateral surface of the pons and cerebellum and the posterior surface of the petrous bone and contains the trigeminal, abducent, facial, and vestibulocochlear nerves, the superior cerebellar and anterior inferior cerebellar arteries, a variable number of draining veins, the flocculus of the cerebellum, and the choroid plexus that protrudes through the foramen of Luschka. The facial nerve exits from the brainstem in the lateral part of the pontomedullary sulcus, 1 to 2 mm anterior to the entry zone of the vestibulocochlear nerve. The ninth, tenth, and eleventh cranial nerves are located in the lower part of the CP angle (Fig. 38.2A and B).

Five nerves pass through the internal auditory canal (IAC): the facial, the vestibular (superior and inferior), the cochlear, and the nervus intermedius, accompanied by the labyrinthine artery and occasionally by branches of the anterior inferior cerebellar artery (AICA) or a loop of the AICA itself.[4]

In the area of the fundus of the IAC, the nerves have constant location: the facial nerve occupies the anterosuperior quadrant, the cochlear nerve occupies the anteroinferior quadrant, the superior vestibular nerve is in the posterosuperior quadrant, and the inferior vestibular nerve is in the posteroinferior quadrant (Fig. 38.3). Knowledge of these anatomical relationships is of utmost importance for the surgeon because early identification of the main neurovascular structures is a prerequisite for their preservation.

TUMORS OF THE CEREBELLOPONTINE ANGLE

Tumors of the CP angle account for 5% to 10% of all intracranial neoplasms.[5] VSs are the most common CP angle tumor and account for 80% to 94% of them, followed by meningiomas (3-10% of CP angle tumors) and the epidermoids (2-4%). Much rarer primary tumors are schwannomas of other cranial nerves: of the trigeminal nerve, of the facial nerve, or of the caudal cranial nerves; paragangliomas, chordomas, chordosarcomas, arachnoid or neurenteric cysts, dermoid tumors, and metastases.[6,7] The CP angle could be secondarily involved by tumors extending from the brainstem or fourth ventricle: gliomas, ependymomas, choroid plexus papillomas, medulloblastomas, or lymphomas. Bilateral CP angle tumors are characteristic for neurofibromatosis 2 (NF2) and are typically VSs. Rare bilateral tumors not associated with NF2 are facial nerve schwannomas, plexus papillomas, endolymphatic sac tumors, metastases, or osteomas.[8]

IMAGING

The precise radiological diagnosis of CP angle tumors requires a systematic approach and analysis of the lesions: site of origin, location, shape and margins, density, signal intensity, and contrast enhancement characteristics.[6,9] The enhancing CP

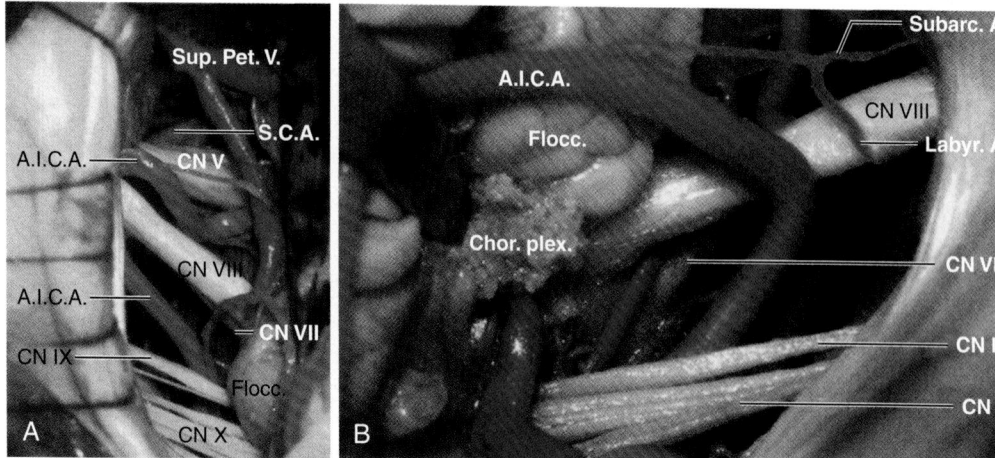

FIGURE 38.2 **A,** The upper neurovascular complex consisting of the trigeminal nerve (CN V, cranial nerve V) contained within the superior cerebellopontine cistern, the superior cerebellar artery (SCA), and the superior petrosal vein (Sup. Pet. V). The trigeminal nerve courses toward the petrous apex anterior to the superior petrosal vein, which is identified by its typical inverted Y configuration at its entrance into the superior petrosal sinus at the tentorial-petrosal dural junction. The superior cerebellar artery usually runs along the superior aspect of the fifth cranial nerve. The middle neurovascular complex consists of the facial nerve (CN VII) and vestibulocochlear nerve (CN VIII), which arise from the lateral part of the pontomedullary sulcus, and the anterior inferior cerebellar artery (AICA). The seventh and eighth cranial nerves course in the cerebellopontine cistern and enter the internal auditory canal. Also seen are the glossopharyngeal nerve (CN IX), vagal nerve (CN X), and the flocculus (Flocc.) of the cerebellum. **B,** Intraoperative view demonstrating the relationship of the anterior inferior cerebellar artery and its two major branches in the CPA, the internal auditory artery (Labyr. A), and the subarcuate artery (Subarc. A). The internal auditory artery travels into the internal auditory canal (IAC) and provides a blood supply to the inner ear and nerves in the IAC. Also demonstrated are the vestibulocochlear nerve (CN VIII), facial nerve (CN VII), the glossopharyngeal nerve (CN IX), vagal nerve (CN X), and the flocculus (Flocc.). *(A from Rhoton AL Jr. The cerebellopontine angle and posterior fossa cranial nerves by the retrosigmoid approach. Neurosurgery 2000;47:S93-S129. B from Rhoton AL Jr. Microsurgical anatomy of posterior fossa cranial nerves. Rhoton's Anatomy–Part 3; October 2003:480, Figure B.)*

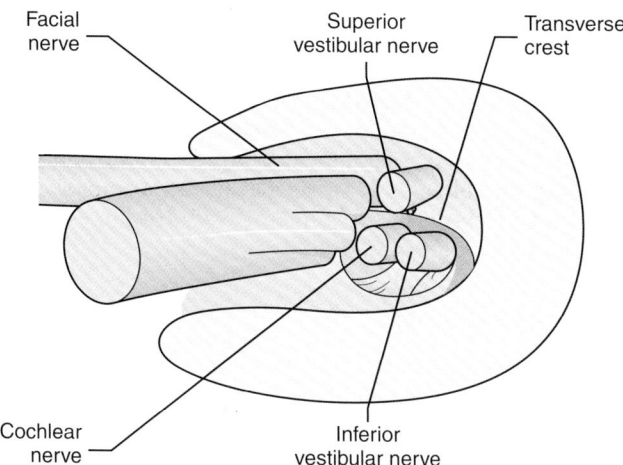

FIGURE 38.3 A schematic diagram of the right internal acoustic meatus demonstrating the facial nerve and cranial nerve VIII dividing into its three parts, the superior vestibular nerve above the transverse crest and the cochlear and inferior vestibular nerves below the crest. *(Adapted from Rhoton AL Jr. The cerebellopontine angle and posterior fossa cranial nerves by the retrosigmoid approach. Neurosurgery 2000;47:S93-S129.)*

angle tumors are most frequently vestibular and nonvestibular schwannomas, meningiomas, metastases and paragangliomas, chondrosarcomas, and chordomas.[7] Nonenhancing extra-axial CP angle lesions may be cystic, such as the epidermoid cysts, the arachnoid cysts, and the neurenteric cyst or may contain fat (dermoid cyst, lipoma). Intrinsic brain tumors with a significant exophytic extension into the CP angle (lymphoma, hemangioblastoma, choroid plexus papilloma, ependymoma, glioma, medulloblastoma, dysembryoplastic neuroepithelial tumor) may be difficult to differentiate from an extra-axial lesion based only on their radiological characteristics.[6]

Bone window thin slice CT shows the bony changes of the pyramid and of the IAC and is essential for surgical planning. Erosion or dilatation of the IAC is seen in 70% to 90% of the patients with VS. Nevertheless, the diagnostic tool of choice for all CP angle tumors is MRI.[7,10,11] On T1-weighted sequences VSs are isointense to slightly hypointense and on T2-weighted sequences they are hyperintense. They enhance intensely and homogeneously after contrast application, with the exception of cystic portions of the tumors. Intrameatal VSs are best visualized with gadolinium enhancement. Meningiomas are most frequently isointense to slightly hypointense to brain parenchyma on T1-weighted MRI studies. On T2-weighted MRI studies they have higher intensity than that of VS and show a homogeneous contrast enhancement. The radiological differential diagnosis between VS and CP angle meningioma is based on several criteria. Meningiomas are centered usually away from the IAC and have broad contact with the petrous bone or the tentorium (Fig. 38.4A and B). The angle between the tumor and the pyramid is obtuse. The IAC is not widened and the tumor very rarely extends into the IAC. Although secondary invasion of the IAC might be observed in 10% to 20%,[12] primarily IAC meningiomas are exceedingly rare.[6,13] Calcification and cystic changes are

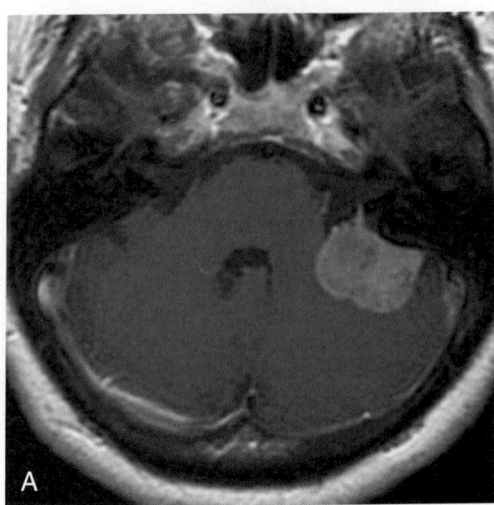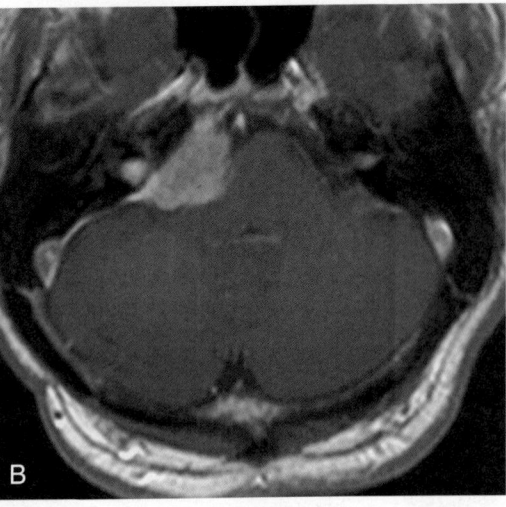

FIGURE 38.4 **A** and **B,** T1-weighted magnetic resonance images following contrast application of a retromeatal (**A**) and a premeatal (**B**) cerebellopontine angle meningioma.

frequent findings. A tail of enhancement along the dura (the dural "tail" sign), although not pathognomonic, is visible in 60% to 72% of meningiomas. VSs are centered at the widened IAC. They form an acute angle with the posterior surface of the petrous bone and almost always extend into the IAC (Fig. 38.5). In VS, calcifications are extremely rarely found.

Epidermoids are hypodense on CT and in up to 25% rim calcification is observed. On T1- and T2-weighted MRI they are usually isointense to cerebrospinal fluid (CSF).[6,11] The signal intensity is related to the contents of the cyst: if cholesterol predominates, the cysts are hyperintense on T1-weighted images and hypointense on T2-weighted images. Fluid-attenuated inversion recovery imaging, diffusion-weighted imaging, and CISS spin-echo MRIs are more precise imaging modalities. Because of their similar characteristics it might be difficult to differentiate epidermoid cysts from arachnoid cysts. Two of the main differences between them are the smaller mass effect caused by the arachnoid cysts and their more homogeneous signal intensity on T2-weighted images.

SURGICAL APPROACHES TO THE CEREBELLOPONTINE ANGLE

The approaches to the CP angle are either posterior (through the posterior cranial fossa) or lateral (through the petrous bone). The most popular approach is retrosigmoid suboccipital, introduced by Fedor Krause (1903) and later modified and refined by many surgeons.[14] The lateral approaches involve removal of a part of the petrous bone either via a subtemporal route (e.g., the middle fossa approach, the extended middle fossa approach, or the Kawase approach) or via the mastoid (the presigmoid approach, the retrolabyrinthine petrosectomy, the translabyrinthine approach (Rudolf Panse, 1904), and the transcochlear approach).[4,14]

Several factors have to be considered when selecting the surgical approach: tumor type, size, and origin; extension in the CP angle or in the IAC; patient's age and general and neurological status, especially hearing level; and surgeon's experience and institutional tradition. The approach should adhere to the following principles: it should provide sufficient exposure of the tumor; it should not be related to significant

morbidity; the neural structures should not be at increased risk; any injury to the venous outflow system should be avoided. Most of the CP angle tumors are benign and their complete removal leads to healing of the patient. The preservation and even the recovery of neurological functions and of the patient's quality of life should always be the first priority. The only exception to complete tumor removal is the attempt to preserve function, such as in surgery for VS in the only hearing ear. Excellent results have been achieved with different operative approaches, which depend more on the individual surgeon's experience than on the advantages or disadvantages of each particular approach. Still, an ever growing amount of evidence suggests that the goals of CP angle surgery are best achieved with the retrosigmoid suboccipital approach (RSA).[3,14-16] It is safe and relatively simple and provides a panoramic view of the whole CP angle and petroclival area. Importantly, it is associated with a very low procedure-related morbidity rate. The additional removal of the suprameatal tubercle—the Samii technique, developed and introduced by the senior author in 1982—provides access to tumor extensions into Meckel's cave, the petroclival area, and even the posterior cavernous sinus.

Retrosigmoid Approach

Each of the possible positions of the patient on the operating table—semisitting, lateral, or supine with the head rotated 90 degrees to the contralateral side—has its advantages and drawbacks in terms of providing sufficient access and avoiding complications. It remains, however, a matter of surgeon's preference and institutional tradition. We prefer the semisitting position that allows the surgeon to work bimanually because there is no need for constant suction. Further, frequent coagulation during tumor removal is evaded thanks to the continuous irrigation of the operative field performed by the assistant. The head is held with a three-point head fixation frame; then it is flexed and rotated approximately 30 degrees to the involved side, avoiding occlusion of venous jugular outflow or hyperflexion of the cervical spine.

A drawback of this patient position is the risk of venous air embolism, paradoxical air embolism, tension pneumocephalus, or circulatory instability. However, in experienced

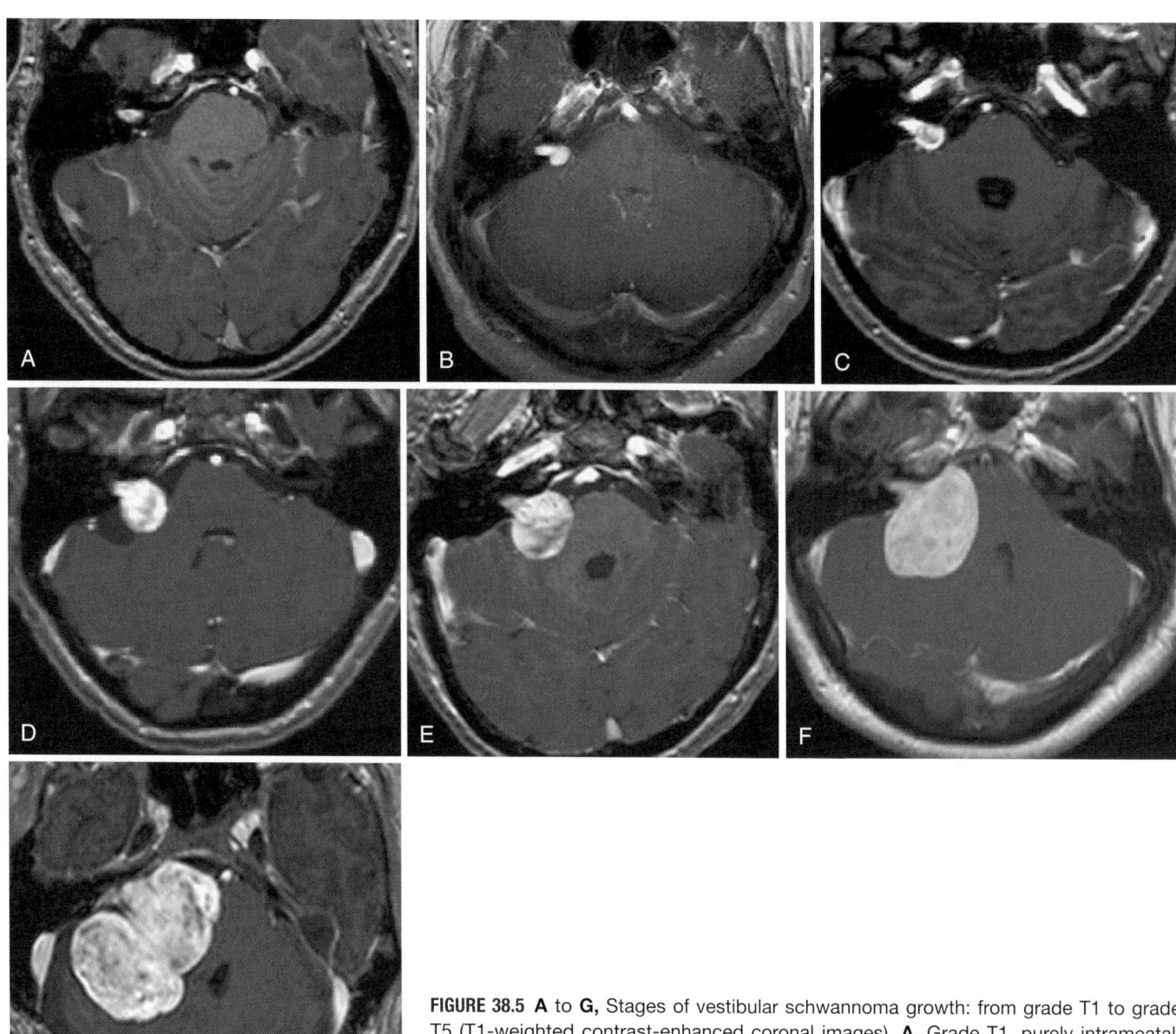

FIGURE 38.5 A to **G,** Stages of vestibular schwannoma growth: from grade T1 to grade T5 (T1-weighted contrast-enhanced coronal images). **A,** Grade T1, purely intrameatal. **B,** Grade T2, intraextrameatal. **C,** Grade T3a, filling the CPA cistern. **D,** Grade T3b, reaching the brainstem. **E,** Grade T4a, compressing the brainstem. **F,** Grade T4b, severe compression and dislocation of the brainstem and fourth ventricle. **G,** Grade T5, giant tumors with extension over the midline. See Table 38.2 for corresponding classification.

hands these effects are not related to any lasting morbidity.[17] Transesophageal echocardiography is the most specific and sensitive method in detection of air embolism but the combined monitoring of end-tidal carbon dioxide and precordial Doppler echocardiography yield similar results. If immediate measures are carried out at the first sign of venous air embolism, the related morbidity is insignificant.

Continuous neurophysiological monitoring should be performed throughout the surgery from the time of positioning of the patient to the skin closure. It includes monitoring of somatosensory evoked potentials (important during patient positioning in order to prevent spinal cord compression); electromyography of the facial nerve; and monitoring of the brainstem auditory evoked potentials in the case of preoperatively available hearing.[18,19] Monitoring of the oculomotor,

trochlear, abducens, and caudal cranial nerves is performed if needed according to the particular tumor extension and clinical presentation.

A slightly curved skin incision approximately 2 cm medial to the mastoid process is performed and the underlying muscles are incised in line with the skin. We make the bur hole approximately 2 to 2.5 cm below the superior nuchal line, two thirds behind and one third in front of the occipitomastoid suture. The asterion is not an absolutely reliable anatomical landmark and is variable both in the cranial-caudal plane and in the anterior-posterior plane.[20] The sigmoid sinus descends along an axis defined by the mastoid tip and the squamosal-parietomastoid suture junction or over the mastoid groove. The course of the transverse sinus is more variable and the superior nuchal line gives a rough orientation of its location.

The issue of whether to make a craniectomy or craniotomy is a matter of individual preference but we avoid making one-piece craniotomy due to the related high risk of injury to the underlying sinuses and the risk of tearing the dura by the craniotome. Excessive traction to the mastoid emissary vein/veins could lead to sinus laceration and increases the risk of venous air embolism. The vein should be skeletonized with a diamond drill until it is free of any bony encasement and can be safely coagulated. The lateral and superior limits of the approach are the borders of the sigmoid and of the transverse sinuses; their edges have to be exposed. Inferiorly, enough bone should be removed in order to provide access to the lateral cerebellomedullary cistern and allow a continuous egress of the CSF or irrigation fluid throughout the surgery.

The dura is incised in a curvilinear manner just 1.5 to 2 mm medial to the sigmoid and inferior to the transverse sinus. This allows for a primary watertight dural closure and avoids the need for using a dural substitute in almost all cases. The lateral cerebellomedullary cistern is then opened and CSF is drained. Thus, the cerebellum relaxes away from the petrous bone and the self-retaining retractor supports and protects the cerebellar hemisphere, instead of compressing it. The further operative steps depend on the pathological tumor type and its extension. However, several general principles should always be followed:

- The important neural structures, such as the cochlear and facial nerves, should be identified early.
- The tumor should be initially debulked.
- The dissection from the surrounding structures should be performed only after sufficient internal decompression is achieved.
- The dissection should always be performed in the arachnoid plane.
- Bipolar coagulation, especially in the vicinity of a cranial nerve, should be avoided.

Following tumor removal, the opened mastoid air cells are sealed with multiple pieces of fat tissue that are fixed with fibrin glue. If necessary, fat pieces are glued on the sutured dura. Bone wax is avoided, except in case of significant bleeding from the bone edges.

Lateral Approaches

The main anatomical obstacle for exposure of the CP angle and of the petroclival area laterally is the petrous bone. Multiple operative techniques, including partial or complete resection of the petrous bone—the so-called transpetrous approaches—have been developed in the past decades. They differ in the approach to the petrous bone—subtemporal or transmastoid, as well as in the amount of bone removal.[21] The advantages of these lateral cranial base approaches include shorter distance to the tumor and surrounding neurovascular structures, improved visualization, and minimized brain retraction.[22] A major drawback is their higher approach-related morbidity rate. Our experience and the evaluation of the long-term outcome, however, prove that simpler and safer approaches lead to better outcome and do not limit the possibility to remove the tumor completely.[14,16,23,24] The complete visualization of both the tumor and of all adjacent structures is not a prerequisite for better outcome.

The middle fossa approach is frequently used in cases of small intrameatal VSs: the tumor is exposed via a temporal craniotomy and removal of the bone overlying the IAC. The adequate access to a larger tumor requires more bone removal, including the resection of the petrous apex behind the horizontal segment of the petrous internal carotid artery medial to the IAC and incision of the tentorium (the extended middle fossa approach and the Kawase approach).[14,22]

Although the terminology used to describe the transmastoid approaches is quite variable,[4] the main categories, in respect to the amount of drilling of the pyramid, are the presigmoid approach, the retrolabyrinthine petrosectomy, the translabyrinthine petrosectomy, and the transcochlear approach or complete petrosectomy. The presigmoid approach combines a supra- and infratentorial exposure with various degrees of petrosectomy. The retrolabyrinthine approach implies removal of the bone between the sigmoid sinus and the semicircular canals and allows hearing preservation. If the semicircular canals and the lateral wall of the IAC are removed, a large exposure both of the intrameatal and extrameatal tumor portions is gained (translabyrinthine approach). The transcochlear approach or complete petrosectomy allows for better visualization of the structures anterior to the IAC and petroclival space. It is used in large tumors in patients with complete hearing loss.

VESTIBULAR SCHWANNOMAS

Vestibular schwannomas are histopathologically benign typically slow-growing neoplasms. They originate most frequently from one of the vestibular nerves in the region of the transition zone between central and peripheral myelin that usually is located in the medial part of the IAC. VSs occur in two different forms: sporadic unilateral (95%) and bilateral, and the latter is associated with NF2 (5%). The patients with sporadic VS usually present in their fifth or sixth decade of life. Patients with NF2 are usually younger and have a predisposition to formation of multiple tumors of the central nervous system, characteristically bilateral VS, meningiomas, ependymomas, and neurofibromas. NF2 is an inherited autosomal dominant disease caused by mutation at the chromosome band 22q12. The mutation affects a gene that encodes the protein schwannomin/merlin. This protein is related to a family of proteins that link actin to the cell membrane molecules and has been implicated in cellular remodeling and growth regulation.

VSs originate within the IAC and gradually fill it; then they expand into the CP angle and occupy the CP angle cistern, displacing the seventh and the eighth cranial nerves, as well as the AICA.

Clinical grading of facial nerve involvement is classified by the House and Brackmann scale (Table 38.1). During its further growth, the tumor reaches and then compresses the brainstem and the cerebellum. Depending on the degree of the tumor's cranial and caudal extension, the fifth and the caudal cranial nerves become involved. The hydrocephalic stage begins with the obstruction of the fourth ventricle and its outlets. Each stage is characterized by specific neurological symptoms. This four-stage concept of growth presents the most frequent development pattern of VS but does not reflect

TABLE 38.1 House and Brackmann Facial Nerve Grading System

Grade	Description/ Deficit	Characteristics
I	Normal	Normal facial function

II	Slight	*Gross*: Slight weakness noted on close inspection, slight synkinesis
		At rest: Normal tone and symmetry
		Motion:
		  Forehead: Moderate to good movement
		  Eye: Complete closure with minimal effort
		  Mouth: Slight asymmetry

III	Moderate	*Gross*: Obvious but not disfiguring asymmetry. Synkinesis noticeable but not severe
		At rest: Normal tone and symmetry
		Motion:
		  Forehead: Slight to moderate movement
		  Eye: Complete closure with effort
		  Mouth: Slight weakness with maximal effort

IV	Moderately severe	*Gross*: Disfiguring asymmetry and/or obvious facial weakness
		At rest: Normal tone and symmetry
		Motion:
		  Forehead: No movement
		  Eye: Incomplete closure
		  Mouth: Asymmetrical with maximal effort

V	Severe	*Gross*: Barely perceptible motion
		At rest: Asymmetrical appearance
		Motion:
		  Forehead: No movement
		  Eye: Incomplete closure
		  Mouth: Trace movement

VI	Total	No facial function

Adapted from House JW, Brackmann DE. Facial nerve grading system. *Otolaryngol Head Neck Surg*1985;93(2):146-147.

TABLE 38.2 INI or (Samii) Classification of Vestibular Schwannoma (VS) Extension

Tumor Grade	Tumor Extension
T1	Purely intrameatal
T2	Intra-, extrameatal
T3a	Filling the CPA cistern
T3b	Reaching the brainstem
T4a	Compressing the brainstem
T4b	Severe compression and dislocation of brainstem and fourth ventricle
T5	Giant tumors (maximal diameter >4 cm), extension over the midline

*In case the VS has been previously treated with radiosurgery, this is designated with an additional "+R"—e.g., Stage "T4a +R."
CPA, cerebellopontine angle; INI, International Neuroscience Institute.

They are commonly divided into five categories: intrameatal, tumors up to 1 cm, from 1 to 2.5 cm, from 2.5 to 4 cm, or larger than 4 cm.[25] Much more important than the size is the extent of the tumor in the CP angle, as well as the presence and severity of brainstem compression.[18] Our classification based on the extent of tumor growth and its relation to the brainstem is presented in Table 38.2 (and Fig. 38.5A-G).

Treatment options of VS include observation, radiation therapy, and microsurgical removal via one of several operative approaches. The conservative approach—observation with regular follow-up MRI examinations and hearing tests—is based upon the assumption that some tumors stop growing or even undergo spontaneous regression.[26] As the natural evolution of VS is still unpredictable, this strategy should be applied only in very carefully selected cases, with strict MRI follow-up (at 6- to 12-month intervals). This management may be applied in case of older or somatically unstable patients with small asymptomatic tumors or tumors causing mild stable symptoms. However, long-term follow-up results indicate that the majority of the tumors enlarge further. In published studies, further tumor growth was observed in 43% to 91% of the cases followed, but tumor involution or "negative growth" is observed in 0% to 18%.[27-29] Another important issue is the loss of serviceable hearing during the follow-up. Charabi and associates[29] reported that from the 28 patients initially classified as candidates for hearing preservation surgery, 75% were unable to have their hearing preserved due to tumor growth and deterioration of hearing following the time delay to surgery.

The goal of radiotherapy of VS, performed either as stereotactic radiosurgery or fractionated stereotactic radiotherapy, is to achieve tumor growth control. Gamma knife radiosurgery is by far the most popular mode: delivery of a single fraction of radiation after a highly conformal dose plan using multiple isocenters. The reduction of dose of radiation in the past few years led to marked reduction in cranial nerve morbidity. The recommended current doses are in the 12- to 14-Gy range and MRI is used for dosimetry planning. Tumor control is achieved in 93% to 98%.[30-32] In 1.1% to 24% of the patients late facial neuropathy appears and the rate of trigeminal dysfunction is 2% to 27%. Hearing preservation is achieved in 40% to 74%. However, in 2% to 7% of the cases tumor enlargement is observed. Importantly, initial

entirely the high variability of these tumors and of the individual anatomy.

Intrameatal tumors present clinically with vestibulocochlear nerve dysfunction: hearing loss, tinnitus, or vestibular dysfunction. Hearing loss is usually of insidious onset and is the most frequent symptom, observed in up to 95% of the patients. Audiograms reveal high-frequency sensorineural hearing loss. Vestibular symptoms frequently are not recognized by the patients, but are always discovered with special testing. During the cisternal stage progressive hearing loss might be observed. A sense of disequilibrium gradually replaces the vertigo. Later on trigeminal symptoms, headache, ataxia, and obstructive hydrocephalus develop. With further brainstem compression, contralateral long tract signs, severe gait disturbance, lower cranial nerve palsies, and signs of intracranial hypertension appear.

VSs are classified either according to their maximal size or according to the degree of their extension into the CP angle.

increase in tumor volume often precedes shrinkage. Additional treatment is indicated only if sustained tumor growth is documented on serial MRI, unless brainstem compression appears, prompting earlier intervention.[32] The appearance of new neurological deficit alone is also not an indication for immediate intervention because it could be a delayed sequence of radiation. As the results of radiosurgical treatment cannot be precisely predicted, a careful follow-up of all patients is mandatory. Every case in which sustained tumor growth is confirmed or the progression of symptoms could be definitely related to tumor enlargement should be subjected to microsurgical removal, before the VS achieves large size. Our continuously increasing experience with surgery of previously irradiated VS shows that it is complicated by the development of postradiation changes. Frequently, the planes of dissection between the tumor and brainstem or cranial nerves are obliterated following radiotherapy, making the likelihood of functional preservation of involved cranial nerves substantially lower.

In large VSs another option is the staged treatment, which includes microsurgical tumor debulking and brainstem decompression at the first stage, followed by radiosurgery of the remnant at a second stage. Although this strategy gains popularity, one should be aware of the additive risk of two different procedures.

The only management option that leads to a definitive healing of the patient is complete surgical extirpation of the tumor. The modern VS surgery is related to a low risk of new morbidity and allows for functional preservation of cranial nerve function in exceedingly higher numbers. Complete tumor removal is achieved in 80% to 99% and the recurrence rates are 0.5% to 5%.[15,18,33-36] The preservation of the anatomical integrity of the facial nerve is a rule today: it is achieved in 93% to 99% of the cases in the large published series.[33,35-37] The main predictor of facial nerve outcome is the tumor size. In our series of VS with extension classes T1 to T3b, the rate of facial nerve preservation was 100%.[33] Excellent or good postoperative facial nerve function (corresponding to House-Brackmann grades I to II) in the large series is achieved in 52% to 93%. In a recent study of 50 patients with giant VS—with maximal extrameatal diameter of 4.4 cm—total removal was possible in 97.6% of the patients. The anatomical integrity of the facial nerve was preserved in 92% in the first follow-up and at last follow-up 75% of the patients had excellent or good facial nerve function, and 19% had fair function.[38] The rate of hearing preservation ranges from 14% to 80%,[39,40] depending on the size of the VS. Although it has been suggested that in tumors larger than 3 cm hearing preservation is not possible and therefore the translabyrinthine approach should be used,[36,41,42] we believe that an attempt for hearing preservation is worthwhile in every patient with useful preoperative hearing and good brainstem auditory evoked responses. Following this concept, we were able to achieve hearing preservation in 29% of the patients with VS extending to and compressing the brainstem (class T4a).[33]

The three most frequently used operative approaches are the (a) middle fossa, (b) the translabyrinthine, and (c) the retrosigmoid suboccipital approaches. The middle fossa approach is a hearing preserving technique that allows direct access to the lateral end of the IAC.[39,43-46] Thus, the most lateral part

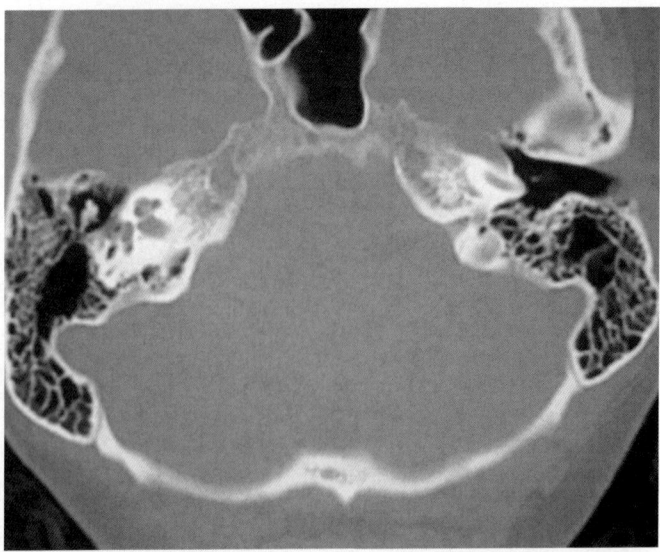

FIGURE 38.6 Postoperative bone window computed tomography (CT) scan demonstrating the degree of internal auditory canal opening and the preservation of semicircular canals. The occipital bone integrity is reconstructed with methylmethacrylate. The epidural Gelfoam piece is visible.

of the tumor could be safely resected, reducing thereby the risk of incomplete removal. The approach is related to low risk of CSF leaks. However, it is applicable to small tumors, necessitates temporal lobe retraction, endangers the vein of Labbé, and offers a restricted access to the CP angle. Using the extended middle fossa approach, VS extending up to 2 cm in the CP angle can be removed.[34,47]

The benefits of the translabyrinthine approach include avoidance of cerebellar retraction, shorter distance to the tumor, and early identification of the facial nerve at the lateral end of the IAC.[5,25,35,36,48] Drawbacks are sacrifice to hearing, restricted access to the CP angle, difficult dissection and hemostasis close to the brainstem, as well as poor visualization and access to the caudal cranial nerves.

The retrosigmoid approach allows for hearing preservation even in large VSs.[3,18,33,39] The approach offers excellent visualization of the whole CP angle and increased safety during dissection from brainstem and lower cranial nerves.[3,5] The facial and cochlear cranial nerves can be identified both in their proximal (close to the brainstem) and lateral part (in the IAC), increasing the chances for their preservation. Potential drawbacks of the approach are the need of cerebellar retraction, the difficulty in visualizing the most lateral part of the IAC without endangering the integrity of the inner ear, as well as the relatively higher rate of postoperative headache. However, a cranioplasty can be performed during closure which may improve the postoperative headache and pain issues (Fig. 38.6). With current neuroanesthesia and modifications of the original retrosigmoid approach and closure, these disadvantages are rather theoretical.[33]

The initial steps of the exposure have been described earlier in the chapter. The intrameatal tumor portion is exposed initially. The dura is stripped off from the posterior lip of the porus and the posterior and superior walls of the internal auditory canal (IAC) are drilled using decreasing sizes of diamond drills under constant irrigation.

FIGURE 38.7 **A** to **D**: **A,** The internal auditory canal (IAC) (3) is opened widely up to its fundus (4) to expose the tumor (1). 2, extrameatal tumor part. **B,** The intrameatal tumor part (1) is mobilized and the facial (3) and cochlear (4) nerves are seen. 4, IAC. **C,** After the intrameatal part has been removed (1), the tumor in the cerebellopontine angle (2) is addressed. **D,** Complete tumor removal with preservation of the facial (1) and cochlear (2) nerves.

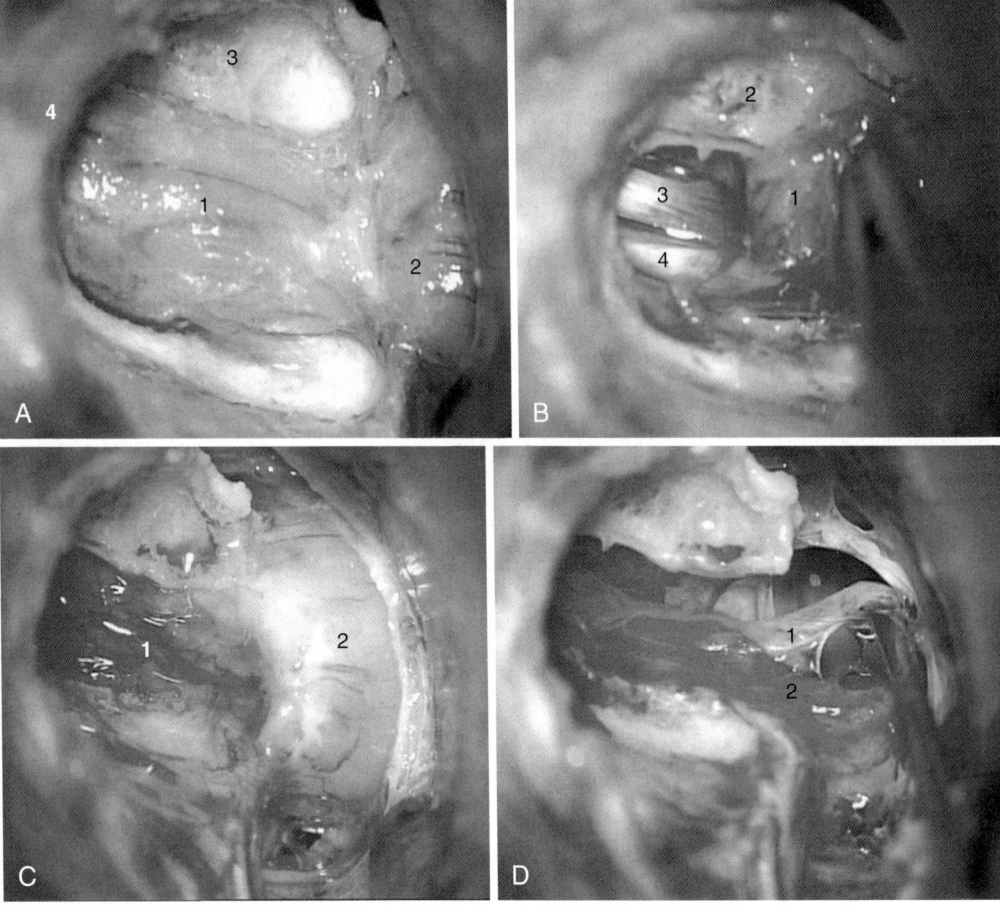

The extent of IAC opening is tailored to the extent of lateral tumor extension (Fig. 38.7A-G). The meatal dura is then incised and the intrameatal tumor portion is carefully mobilized with a microhook or microdissector. The facial and vestibulocochlear nerves are identified and the tumor is removed piecemeal. Then the extrameatal tumor is debulked with the Cavitron ultrasonic aspirator or a platelet-shaped knife. The dissection of the capsule from the surrounding neural structures should begin only after adequate internal decompression is achieved. It is performed by strictly gripping the tumor capsule and dissecting in the level of the arachnoid plane under continuous saline irrigation. Bipolar coagulation is reduced to a minimum and applied only at the end of surgery for final hemostasis. Once complete tumor removal is achieved, the continuity of the facial nerve can be confirmed by its electrical stimulation. In case of nerve discontinuity, immediate nerve reconstruction is performed at the same operation. The opened air cells in the region of the IAC are occluded by placing pieces of fat tissue fixed with fibrin glue.

COMPLICATIONS

Cerebrospinal fluid leaks are one of the most frequent complications and have been reported to occur with a rate of 3% to 26.7%.[49,50] The most common factors associated with such leaks are inadequate dura and wound closure or healing, wound infection, increased intracranial pressure, and opened air petrous air cells that have not been occluded. In our experience the CSF leak is most frequently through the opened air cells during the IAC drilling. The prevention of CSF leaks relies on a watertight dural closure and meticulous sealing of opened air cells. Since we started to use multiple small fat pieces sealed with fibrin glue for plugging of the IAC the leak rate could be further reduced to 2.2% in our recent series.[51] The fat can be harvested from the appropriate subcutaneous layer at the incision site. Further important steps are avoiding raising the intracranial pressure unwillingly during the early postoperative period; early detection of CSF leaks; and adequate treatment. If a CSF leak develops we insert immediately a lumbar drainage and keep it for at least 7 days. If the leak persists despite the drainage or reappears after its removal, surgical revision is required.

From 3% to 15% of the patients with VS have hydrocephalus as a consequence of tumor-induced obstruction at the level of the fourth ventricle and its outlets or due to inadequate resorption of CSF.[52,53] Its optimal management is primarily tumor removal and treatment of the hydrocephalus only if it remains symptomatic thereafter. The insertion of a ventriculoperitoneal (VP) shunt can be avoided in most cases; in our series only 3.8% (5/53) of all patients with hydrocephalus required ultimately a VP shunt. In patients presenting with severe hydrocephalus-related symptoms an external ventricular drainage (EVD) should be inserted before VS surgery. In case of less severe symptoms, the VS is removed initially. The patients should be observed closely after surgery, both radiologically and clinically: if clinical deterioration is seen, correlating with a persisting or increasing widening of the ventricles, an EVD should be inserted and kept at 10 to 12 cm H$_2$O above the level of the external auditory canal for several days. Then it should be elevated progressively, provided the patients showed no signs of intracranial hypertension—the process of gradual weaning from the EVD lasts up to 3 weeks. Only if the weaning fails is a VP shunt placement necessary. If hydrocephalus develops after the VS surgery, it can be managed similarly with a temporary EVD.

The incidence of postoperative symptomatic intracranial hemorrhage is reported to be between 1% and 3%.[15,33,36] This potentially dangerous complication could be prevented by performing a meticulous hemostasis before dural closure. Hidden sources of bleeding should be actively searched for. The compressing of the jugular veins before and after removing the retractor allows for detection of any venous bleeding in the CP angle or from torn supracerebellar bridging veins.

In the past high rates of postoperative occipital headache have been reported and have been attributed to the retrosigmoid approach. Different factors have been implicated: dural adhesions to nuchal muscles or subcutaneous tissues, dural tension in cases of direct dural closure, intradural drilling, and the use of fibrin glue. The reconstruction of the occipital bone with methyl methacrylate (see Fig. 38.3) offers the possibility of achieving good cosmetic result and prevents scar tissue formation between the dura and neck muscles, thus preventing the development of such headaches. The occcurrence of pseudomeningocele is related mainly to the method used for dura and bone reconstruction. Using the above-mentioned techniques we never have experienced such complications.

MENINGIOMAS

Meningiomas located in the CP angle lateral to the trigeminal nerve, regardless of the site of their dural attachment, are defined as *CP angle meningiomas*, and those located medial to the trigeminal nerve are defined as *petroclival meningiomas*.[54] They are the second most common tumor of the CP angle and have similar epidemiological and biological features to other meningiomas:[55] they are slow growing benign lesions that occur most frequently in women, usually in 68% to 92%, in their fifth to sixth decades of life.

CP angle meningiomas arise from groups of arachnoid cells located in high concentrations around the IAC, the lower border of superior petrosal sinus, the lateral border of the inferior petrosal sinus, around the cranial nerve foramina, and in the region of the geniculate ganglion. They are a rather heterogeneous group and have variable attachment sites and extension patterns. Their relation to the surrounding structure and the dislocation of cranial nerves cannot be predicted. In relation to the IAC they are classified as premeatal and retromeatal meningiomas.[54,56] These two types present with distinct clinical features, require different treatment strategy, and have different prognoses. The more medially located the tumor, the greater is the surgical challange and the poorer is the outcome. CP angle meningiomas are further subclassified into premeatal, postmeatal, suprameatal, and inframeatal groups, and those centered at the IAC; however, this subdivision has no major practical significance.[5,16,57]

MRI allows for reliable preoperative differentiation from VS and provides information on their precise location in the CP angle, as well as on their relation to the cochlear and facial nerves. In contrast to VS, in which the differences among patients are a function mainly of tumor size and extent of extrameatal growth, the variety of clinical presentations of CP angle meningiomas is greater. It depends on the size, site of dural attachment, and location of the lesion. The initial complaints are most frequently hearing loss, vertigo, headache, or trigeminal symptoms.[5,16,58] Auditory or vestibular dysfunction is not always the major presenting symptom. At the time of diagnosis hearing loss is observed in 30% to 73% of the cases. Trigeminal nerve signs are found in 13% to 49% of the patients, and cerebellar signs and symptoms are found in in 25% to 52%.[12,59] Tinnitus is noted by 10% to 12% of the patients. Signs of increased intracranial pressure have been reported in 16% to 29% and hydrocephalus in 20% to 31% of the patients in different series. Three percent of the cases of trigeminal neuralgia are due to tumor compression at the root entry zone of the trigeminal nerve and the tumors causing such compression most frequently are meningiomas. Premeatal and retromeatal meningiomas have typical clinical development and symptomatology. Premeatal tumors are diagnosed earlier and consequently are smaller. Their clinical presentation is with trigeminal signs and facial and cochlear nerve signs, whereas retromeatal meningiomas present with cerebellar signs (see Fig. 38.4A and B).

Treatment strategies for CP angle meningiomas are similar to those for VS: observation, surgery, radiotherapy/radiosurgery, or combinations thereof. Total surgical removal is the optimal treatment option but should not be achieved at the expense of new neurological dysfunctions or worsening of quality of life. Different surgical approaches have been successfully used for resection of CP angle meningiomas: the retrosigmoid, the translabyrinthine, the transpetrosal with its multiple modifications, as well as the approaches through the middle cranial fossa.[5,55,59] Still, the principles regarding tumor removal are similar: adequate exposure, interruption of the blood supply along the dural attachment, internal decompression, and cautious dissection of the tumor capsule from the brainstem and cranial nerves at the arachnoid plane. The experience of the senior author has shown that every CP meningioma can be adequately accessed via a retrosigmoid craniotomy. If the tumor is located retromeatally, the pure retrosigmoid approach (RSA) is sufficient; in meningiomas originating anterior to the IAC with propagation into Meckel's cave, petroclival area, or the posterior cavernous sinus, the suprameatal extension of the retrosigmoid approach is required.[14]

The hearing-destructive approaches, such as the transpetrosal and translabyrinthine, have been proposed for patients with severe hearing deficit. Attempts at hearing preservation are proposed to be taken only in retromeatal tumors. On the other hand, hearing loss is usually attributed to compression of the cochlear nerve and hearing restoration has been reported even after removal of large meningiomas.[57] We believe that every attempt should be made to preserve or increase the chances of recovery of neurological functions. The versatility and safety of the retrosigmoid approach makes it the most widely used. It allows removal of both small and large tumors, as well as hearing preservation. With the retrosigmoid approach hearing is preserved in 82% to 90.8% of the patients.[16,55,57]

The outcome of surgery depends mainly on the location and consistency of the tumor, and to a lesser extent on its size. Thus, in the premeatal CP angle meningiomas the preservation of facial and auditory function is less likely than in the retromeatal tumors. The mortality rate in the large series is between 0% and 9%.[12,16,54,59] The percentage of total removal of pure CP meningiomas in experienced hands is 82% to 90% and is limited primarily by the tumor infiltration of the brainstem, cranial nerves, and vessels and the extent of skull base involvement.[12,16,54,59] In the 10% to 20% of the cases in which the pia mater of brainstem or a cranial nerve is infiltrated, part of the capsule should be left to avoid neural damage. Such remnants should be controlled with MRI studies, performed 3 to 6 months after surgery. If they show a growth tendency, radiosurgery/radiotherapy should be considered. Compared to VS, CP angle meningiomas have higher tendency toward recurrence, with a recurrence rate between 0% and 9.5%.

Radiotherapy or radiosurgery has been proposed as a primary treatment option for small meningiomas.[60,61] Surgery may be still required in case of treatment failure or in case a secondary trigeminal neuralgia after the irradiation of a petroclival or Meckel's cave meningioma develops. In case of less than total tumor removal or recurrence, postoperative radiation therapy or radiosurgery has been known to prolong the interval to recurrence and to improve the survival.

EPIDERMOIDS

Epidermoids or epidermoid cysts are the third most common CP angle tumor.[61-63] They are slow growing lesions that extend along the basal cisterns and cause gradual displacement of brainstem and other neural structures. Epidermoids might expand through the tentorial incisura into the middle cranial fossa, grow toward the contralateral CP angle, or extend toward the foramen magnum. These tumors are sometimes densely adherent to the neurovascular structures.

Patients with epidermoids usually present between the third and fifth decades of life with a long-standing history of tinnitus and hearing loss.[63] They cause relatively more frequently trigeminal neuralgia or hemifacial spasm when compared to VS and meningiomas and lead to facial nerve signs much earlier than VS.

The treatment of choice of epidermoids is surgical and the preferred approach is the retrosigmoid.[61,63,64] The endoscope-assisted microsurgical technique has proved to be extremely useful, allowing the surgeon not only to detect hidden tumor parts but also to remove them under endoscopic control. Because of the risk of additional neurological deficits, small remnants of the capsule that are firmly attached to important structures should not be removed. The rates of radical removal range from 50% to 97%. In subtotal resected epidermoids, a late recurrence can develop even after 20 or 30 years, which mandates close follow-up on a long-term basis.

SELECTED KEY REFERENCES

Brackmann DE, Cullen RD, Fisher LM. Facial nerve function after translabyrinthine vestibular schwannoma surgery. *Otolaryngol Head Neck Surg.* 2007;136:773-777.

Lunsford LD, Niranjan A, Flickinger JC, et al. Radiosurgery of vestibular schwannomas: summary of experience in 829 cases. *J Neurosurg.* 2005;102(Suppl):195-199.

Rhoton Jr AL. The cerebellopontine angle and posterior fossa cranial nerves by the retrosigmoid approach. *Neurosurgery.* 2000;47:S93-129.

Samii M, Gerganov V, Samii A. Improved preservation of hearing and facial nerve function in vestibular schwannoma surgery via the retrosigmoid approach in a series of 200 patients. *J Neurosurg.* 2006;105:527-535.

Samii M, Matthies C. Management of 1000 vestibular schwannomas (acoustic neuromas): surgical management and results with an emphasis on complications and how to avoid them. *Neurosurgery.* 1997;40(1):11-21.

Slattery III WH, Brackmann DE, Hitselberger W. Middle fossa approach for hearing preservation with acoustic neuromas. *Am J Otol.* 1997;18(5):596-601.

Yasargil MG, Abernathey CD, Sarioglu AC. Microsurgical treatment of intracranial dermoid and epidermoid tumors. *Neurosurgery.* 1989;24(4):561-567.

Please go to expertconsult.com to view the complete list of references.

Craniopharyngiomas and Suprasellar Tumors

Juraj Šteňo

CLINICAL PEARLS

- Craniopharyngiomas with different points of origin of tumor growth have substantially different topographical relationships with surrounding structures determining their surgical resectability and the outcome of treatment; originally infradiaphragmatic tumors are the most amenable for safe radical removal, which is the best treatment of craniopharyngiomas.

- The majority of craniopharyngiomas growing inside and outside the cavity of the third ventricle have started to grow as intrapial tumors, thus acquiring direct and intimate contact with hypothalamic structures.

- If the floor of the third ventricle cannot be seen directly on preoperative magnetic resonance imaging (MRI)

- scans, the topographical relationship of the tumor with hypothalamic structures may be predicted according to its relation with the chiasm and the presence or absence of hydrocephalus.

- The nature and intensity of the tumor adherence to surrounding structures vary in different cases within each topographical group. Decisions about the optimal extent of tumor removal may thus be made only at surgery.

- The natural history of craniopharyngiomas is unpredictable, the growth potential of the tumor or its residual tumor may differ significantly, and therefore radiotherapy should be indicated in case of tumor progression.

The region above the sella contains anatomical structures of the hypothalamus-pituitary system (hypothalamic structures and infundibulum with its pars compacta named also the pituitary stalk), the structures of the visual pathways (optic chiasm and adjacent portions of the optic nerves and the optic tracts), and important blood vessels. The tumors affecting the suprasellar region may belong to (a) tumors of dysembryogenetic origin (craniopharyngioma, epidermoid cyst, dermoid cyst, hamartoma, germ cell tumors, Rathke's cleft cyst), (b) tumors originating from the tissues of suprasellar structures (gliomas of the visual pathways and hypothalamus, pituicytoma, granular cell tumor of the neurohypophysis, meningioma), (c) tumors extending into the suprasellar space secondarily, most often from the cavity of the sella (pituitary adenoma, Rathke's cleft cyst, and other cysts), and (d) systemic tumors affecting the central nervous system (CNS metastasis, lymphoma, leukemia).[1-3]

The most common tumors of the region are craniopharyngiomas and chiasmatic/hypothalamic gliomas. Differential diagnosis has to be made first of all between the craniopharyngiomas and other cystic tumors and between chiasmatic/hypothalamic gliomas and other solid lesions. The majority of these tumors are presented in this chapter.

The structures of optic pathways and the hypothalamus-pituitary system may be involved also by suprasellar meningiomas or large and giant pituitary adenomas. The latter may

severely displace the floor of the third ventricle upward and may also lead to atrophy of the pia and invade the hypothalamus.[4] Suprasellar meningiomas originating from the lower leaf of the diaphragm can mimic nonfunctioning pituitary adenomas.[5] Extremely rare is a meningioma originating from the pituitary stalk having no connection to surrounding dura.[6]

CRANIOPHARYNGIOMAS

Craniopharyngiomas, benign extra-axial epithelial tumors, often follow an aggressive clinical course resulting in significant morbidity and shortened life expectancy. Incomplete tumor removal is followed by progression of the remnants in virtually all patients. Damage to the structures of utmost functional importance due to repeated tumor recurrences and subsequent therapeutic procedures substantially deteriorates the patient's condition. The most logical treatment seems to be a total tumor removal and thus cure of the patient.

The intention to remove the craniopharyngioma totally whenever technically possible emerged in the past in conjunction with therapeutic and diagnostic improvements: steroid hormone replacement, microsurgery, magnetic resonance imaging.[7-16] Another attitude to management of craniopharyngiomas, namely, intentional incomplete removal and radiotherapy, has been advocated in order to lower the surgical morbidity rate.[17-23] However, radiotherapy cannot prevent recurrences in many instances[24] and causes adverse effects.[16] A compromise solution has been elaborated: radical removal was recommended only for the patients harboring the tumors not involving the hypothalamus.[25] Nevertheless, the definition of "involvement of the hypothalamus" is not clear. Radiological signs of retrochiasmatic growth of the tumor in the direction of the hypothalamus and the impossibility of identifying the latter[26] as a distinct form of the tumor do not indicate whether the hypothalamus is compressed or invaded.[27]

The management of craniopharyngiomas presented in this chapter is based on the results of our morphological studies,[28] the results of the correlation of morphological data with neuroradiological and operative findings,[27] and our clinical experience.

Incidence

Craniopharyngiomas account for 1% to 4.6% of all intracranial tumors and 13% of suprasellar tumors. Their incidence represents 0.5 to 2.5 new cases per 1 million population per year, being more frequent in Nigerian (18% of all CNS tumors) and Japanese children, with an annual incidence of 5.25 cases per 1 million per year. Papillary craniopharyngiomas occur virtually exclusively in adults, at a mean age of 40 to 55 years. A bimodal age distribution of adamantinomatous craniopharyngiomas is observed with peaks in children aged 5 to 15 years and in adults aged 40 to 55 years.[29] In children, craniopharyngiomas account for 2.5% to 13% (average 7.5%) of all tumors and 56% of the sellar-chiasmatic tumors.[30]

Tumor Development

According to the widely accepted embryogenetic theory of Erdheim, craniopharyngiomas take their origin from the remnants of the craniopharyngeal duct or Rathke's pouch. Epithelial cell rests have been reported to occur in the "nests" most frequently along the anterior part of the infundibulum near its origin from the brain and the anterosuperior surface of the adenohypophysis.[29,31] When the cells of the vanishing hypophyseal duct are brought into immediate contact with the infundibular area before the primitive pia mater has developed, they will be intimately adherent to the neuroepithelium and subsequently developed pia mater will incorporate them into the subpial space.[32] Alternatively, when the cell rests do not come into immediate contact with the neuroepithelium they will remain extrapial (Fig. 39.1). On the basis of histological findings, Grekhov[33] distinguished four groups of craniopharyngiomas according to the point of their original growth: infrasellar, intrasellar (intrasellar and suprasellar), pituitary stalk, and infundibular craniopharyngiomas. Intimate contact of the cells of tumor origin with neural elements probably accounts for the manner in which many of these tumors appear to blend with the tuber cinereum, so as to form an intrinsic portion of that structure, or even to replace it.[34] These developmental concepts represent the clue to understanding the topographical variations of craniopharyngiomas.

The metaplastic theory postulates that the nests of squamous epithelium are derived from mature cells of

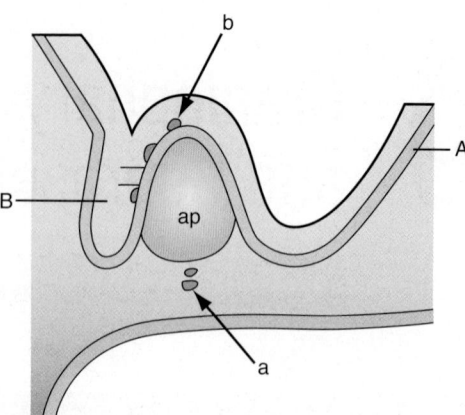

FIGURE 39.1 The remnants of the craniopharyngeal duct. *Arrow a*, below the embryonic base of the anterior pituitary (ap); *arrow b*, below the primitive pia mater (**A**). **B,** embryonic base of the posterior pituitary.

adenohypophysis which undergo metaplasia.[35] However, these nests were not found in persons in their first decade, and rarely in those in the second; according to Kernohan[36] these observations failed to support the origin of craniopharyngiomas from such cells. The theory explains the craniopharyngioma spectrum, attributing the adamantinomatous type (typical for childhood) to embryonic remnants, and the papillary type (common in adult age) to metaplasia.[14]

Pathology and Surgical Anatomy

Microscopic Anatomy

The adamantinomatous craniopharyngioma is a histologically complex epithelial lesion resembling the enamel pulp of developing teeth. A pronounced feature is a palisading of peripheral layer of epithelium. The inner layer often undergoes hydropic vacuolation. This loose stellate reticular zone contains nodules of plump keratinocytes ("wet" keratin) with frequent dystrophic calcification. Areas of cholesterol deposits may be found. Papillary craniopharyngiomas are composed of simple squamous epithelium, which rests on a villous fibrovascular stroma forming papillae.

The brain parenchyma that surrounds both variants of craniopharyngioma is typically gliotic and often shows a profuse number of Rosenthal fibers.[29,34] Tumor tissue, gliosis, and brain parenchyma may form one layer of tissue with a common vascular network. Finger-like protrusions of the tumor into the surrounding gliosis or even into the adjacent brain parenchyma are characteristic of adamantinomatous craniopharyngiomas.[37] On histological sections, these outgrowths appear as isolated islands of epithelium in the zone of intense gliosis.[34,36]

Macroscopic Anatomy

Craniopharyngiomas are solid tumors with a variable, sometimes predominant cystic or multicystic component. The cysts of the adamantinomatous type may contain a cholesterol-rich machine oil–like, thick brownish yellow-green fluid, sometimes with crumbly debris. Calcification may be occasionally

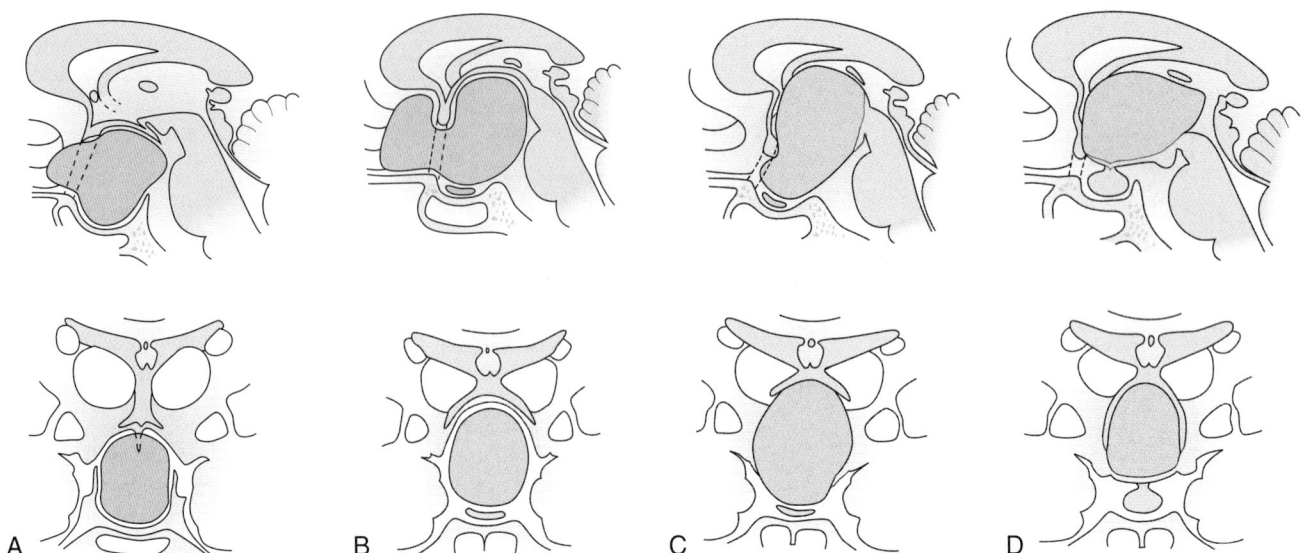

FIGURE 39.2 Schematic representation of the intrasellar and suprasellar (**A**), suprasellar extraventricular (**B**), intraventricular and extraventricular (**C**), and pure intraventricular (**D**) craniopharyngiomas with the sella and the floor of the walls of the third ventricle.

abundant and a part of the tumor may become a stone. The papillary type lacks the cystic component.

Surgical Anatomy

Craniopharyngiomas may start to grow below the sellar diaphragm (*infradiaphragmatic tumors*) or above it (*supradiaphragmatic tumors*). The point of origin of growth of the tumor influences its future relationship with surrounding structures.[28] To a lesser degree the topography of the tumor depends on premorbid anatomy, first of all on the length of the optic nerves and hence the position of the chiasm.

Infradiaphragmatic Craniopharyngiomas

Enlargement of the infradiaphragmatic (i.e., intrasellar) craniopharyngiomas causes upward displacement of the sellar diaphragm and the arachnoid. Such an intrasellar and suprasellar craniopharyngioma grows below the chiasm and gradually compresses and displaces it upward as well as the floor of the third ventricle similar to pituitary adenomas (Fig. 39.2).

Supradiaphragmatic Craniopharyngiomas

The point of original growth of primarily supradiaphragmatic tumors may be in the pituitary stalk or inside the infundibulum (i.e., in the most basal part of the floor of the third ventricle). Tumors starting to grow from the pituitary stalk are located in the subarachnoid space and grow below the chiasm and the floor of the third ventricle (suprasellar extraventricular craniopharyngiomas, SECs). A part of such a tumor almost always extends anteriorly in front of the chiasm between the optic nerves, where it can be reached (see Fig. 39.2). Rare retrochiasmatic location of an entire SEC may be the consequence of premorbid anatomy of short optic nerves and pre-fixed chiasm.

The tumors taking their origin from the infundibulum grow behind the chiasm in the region of its posterior angle between the optic tracts. Growing tumor may disrupt the floor of the third ventricle at an early stage of its development. The

lower part of the tumor then grows in the suprasellar space, and the upper part extends into the cavity of the third ventricle and comes into direct contact not only with the atrophied remnants of the floor of the third ventricle but also with the lateral ventricular walls. Such location of a craniopharyngioma, namely, partially inside and partially outside the cavity of the third ventricle (intraventricular and extraventricular craniopharyngioma, IEVC), is the most common among all the topographical types.

The intraventricular and extraventricular location of the craniopharyngiomas, according to a widespread idea, is a consequence of the disruption of a stretched and thinned-out floor of the third ventricle. This mechanism, which may also be occasionally observed in giant pituitary adenomas,[4] is rather rare. More commonly, it is caused by the mechanism described previously. Our morphological[27,28] and clinical observations showed that the structures of the third ventricular floor undergo atrophy of different degrees. The most affected structure is the tuber: its central part (postinfundibular eminence) is usually absent, and its remnants, the lateral eminences, are located on the lateral or lateral-basal surface of the tumor. The infundibulum (median eminence) is destroyed less frequently, whereas compressed mammillary bodies covering the posterior pole of the tumor can be found in all IEVCs.[27]

The IEVCs are commonly located exclusively behind the optic chiasm. In some cases, presumably with premorbid long optic nerves, a small part of the tumor may occasionally extend below the chiasm or even between the optic nerves.

Some tumors classified in the literature as intraventricular craniopharyngiomas have been described as protruding into the interpeduncular cisterns.[38] We classified such tumors as IEVCs, reserving the term *intraventricular* for rare craniopharyngiomas lying entirely within the ventricular cavity covered from below by the floor of the third ventricle.[39-41] Such a tumor is attached to a partially atrophied floor of the third ventricle while it may only touch its lateral walls (Figs. 39.2 and 39.3). This observation[28] has also been confirmed by others.[42] We have seen only one such tumor in our clinical series.

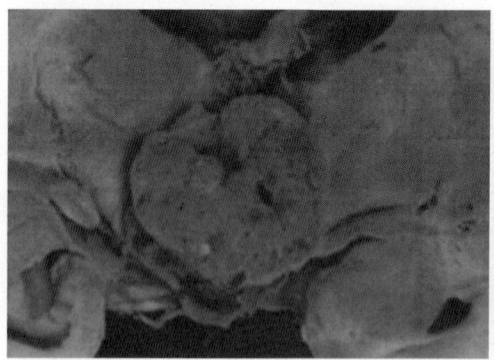 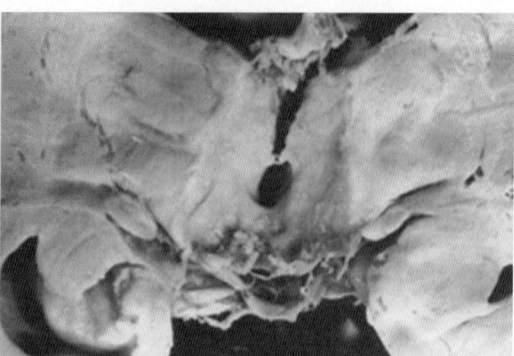

FIGURE 39.3 Anatomical specimen with the intraventricular craniopharyngioma not adhering to the lateral walls of the third ventricle.

Clinical Presentation

The most common signs and symptoms include endocrine deficiencies (over 90%) more frequently in children, and visual disturbances (up to 96%) more frequently in adults. Among hypothalamic disorders in children obesity is prevalent, and mental disorders occur in both age groups.[43] Increased intracranial pressure is the most frequent presenting symptom in children.

Patients with craniopharyngioma generally present late, and visual symptoms are often preceded by a long history of systemic symptoms.[44] Children rarely become aware of visual problems and often present after almost complete visual damage has taken place.[45]

Involvement of the optic pathway manifests itself by the defects of the visual fields and lowering of the visual acuity. Many different varieties of the visual field defects are found, among them bitemporal hemianopia, homonymous hemianopia, concentric contractions of fields, and central or paracentral scotomas.[43] The commonest field defect is asymmetrical bitemporal hemianopia, as a result of the compression of the chiasm, whereas homonymous visual field defects are caused by the tumors located behind the chiasm. The structures of the optic pathway may be compressed not only by the tumor but also by the arteries of the anterior part of the circle of Willis. The tumors growing below the chiasm push the optic structures upward against the anterior cerebral arteries (A1) and the anterior communicating artery (AComA). A strangulation groove may be found on the upper surface of the chiasm or on the terminal portion of the optic nerves. Retrochiasmatic tumors push the chiasm forward and downward below the A1-AComA complex. Strangulation grooves may be found on the most anterior parts of the optic tracts (Figs. 39.4 and 39.5). In the most severe case of our series we observed practically complete amputation of the optic tract from the chiasm.[46] Decompression of the optic pathway in such a case cannot be expected to improve the visual functions. Visual impairment may also be caused by compression of the lower chiasmatic arteries, branches of the internal carotid arteries (ICAs) between the upper surface of the tumor and the stretched chiasm. The decussating fibers in the central chiasm receive their arterial supply solely from this inferior group of vessels.[47,48] Visual defects caused by ischemia may rapidly resolve after surgical decompression.

Long-standing intracranial hypertension causing atrophy of the optic disks may lead to concentric narrowing of the visual fields. Vision may also worsen after the surgery.

Endocrinopathies represented the most common manifestation at diagnosis (68%) in pediatric series of Di Rocco and associates.[16] However, they are rarely the reason for referral. Growth deceleration and diabetes insipidus are often overlooked;[49] gonadotropic deficiency cannot be observed in small children. Delayed puberty in appropriate age was observed in all children with craniopharyngiomas.[49] Adults complain of decreased sexual drive and almost 90% of men complain of impotence, and most women complain of amenorrhea. Growth hormone deficiency in a large group of mostly adult patients was found in 82%.[50] The frequency of presurgery diabetes insipidus varies from 8% to 35%.[16,49,51,52] Compression of the pituitary stalk by a suprasellar mass causes hyperprolactinemia, which can be detected in more than 40% of patients with craniopharyngiomas.[53] Obesity is present in up to 25% of the patients.[51] Its evolution before and after surgery is related to the severity of the involvement of the hypothalamus.[54,55] Growth hormone insufficiency can also lead to increased body fat.[56]

Signs of increased intracranial pressure from obstructive hydrocephalus, headache and vomiting, are more frequent in pediatric patients.[51] This may be explained by the more common occurrence of the IEVCs causing hydrocephalus in children (73%) more frequently than in adults (49%). Extraventricular tumors, even large or giant, usually do not cause complete obstruction of the cerebrospinal fluid (CSF), as can be assumed according to the absence of enlargement of the lateral ventricles.

Cognitive impairment and personality changes occur more often in adults. In a series with the patients over 40 years of age, more than half suffered from impairment of memory.[43] Memory disturbances are attributed to a lesion of the mammillary bodies or of their connections with the hippocampal system, the fornix, and the mammillary-thalamic tract.[57,58]

Radiographic Diagnosis

Infradiaphragmatic craniopharyngiomas (intrasellar, infrasellar, and suprasellar) enlarge the sella similar to pituitary adenomas. Supradiaphragmatic tumors displace the diaphragm and the pituitary downward and the sella is shallow with depressed tuberculum, acquiring a J or a pear shape on plain radiography. Calcifications are present in about 85% of childhood and 40% of adult craniopharyngiomas, and are more readily detected by computed tomography (CT). Calcium deposits are present in most adamantinomatous tumors. Eggshell-like calcification of the wall of a cystic tumor may

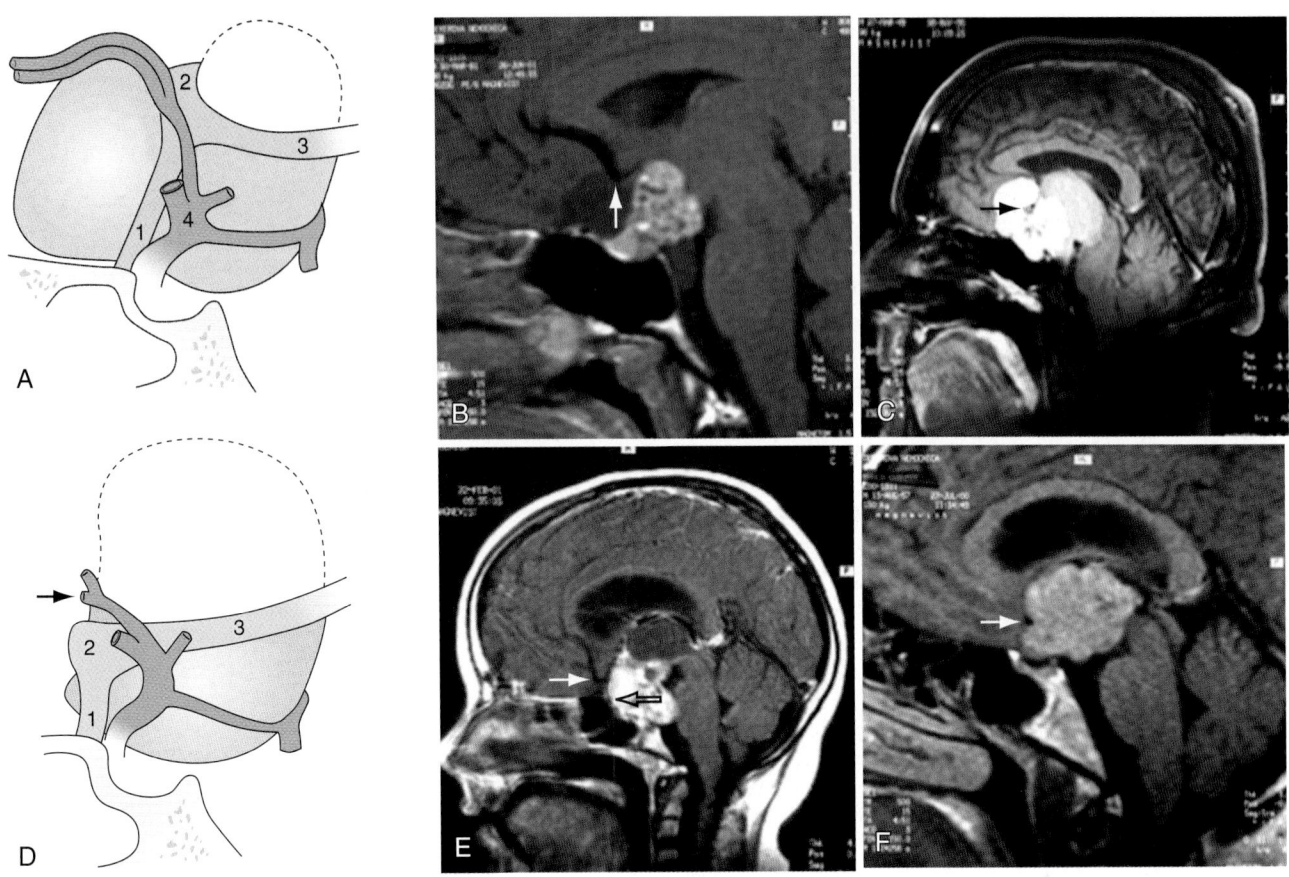

FIGURE 39.4 Relationship of the suprasellar extraventricular (**A** to **C**) and intraventricular and extraventricular (**D** to **F**) craniopharyngiomas with the optic nerves (*1*), chiasm (*2, open arrow*), optic tracts (*3*), internal carotid (*4*), and anterior communicating (*arrows*) arteries.

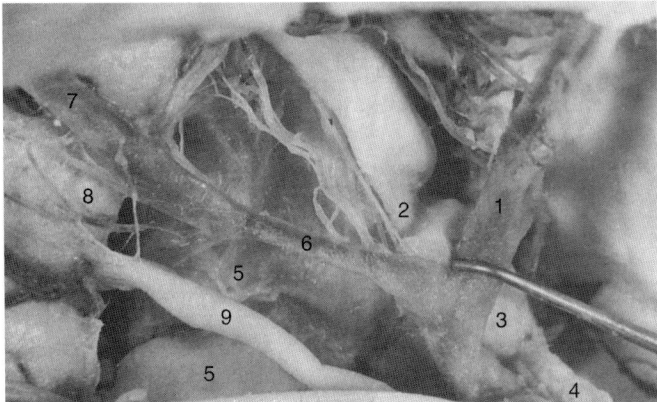

FIGURE 39.5 *1*, Internal carotid artery, displaced anteriorly, strangulating the right optic tract (*2*). *3*, Chiasm; *4*, optic nerve; *5*, extraventricular portion of the tumor (see text); *6*, posterior communicating artery; *7*, posterior cerebral artery; *8*, crus cerebri; *9*, oculomotor nerve.

occasionally delineate the entire lesion (Fig. 39.6). Cyst fluid is usually of low density; however, cystic portions may appear dense or solid if they contain a sufficient quantity of suspended calcium salts (Fig. 39.7). Solid tumor tissue and the cyst walls show contrast enhancement.

The heterogeneous nature of the craniopharyngiomas is best displayed by magnetic resonance imaging (MRI). Solid

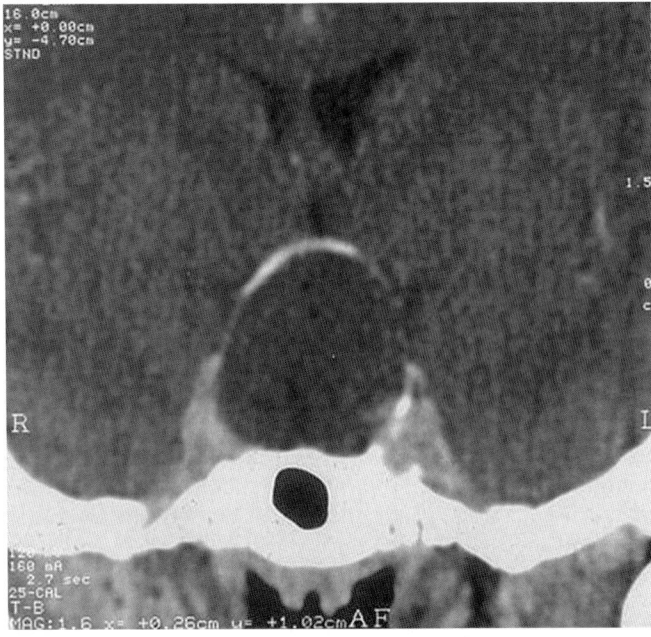

FIGURE 39.6 Eggshell-like calcification of the capsule of intrasellar ane suprasellar craniopharyngioma.

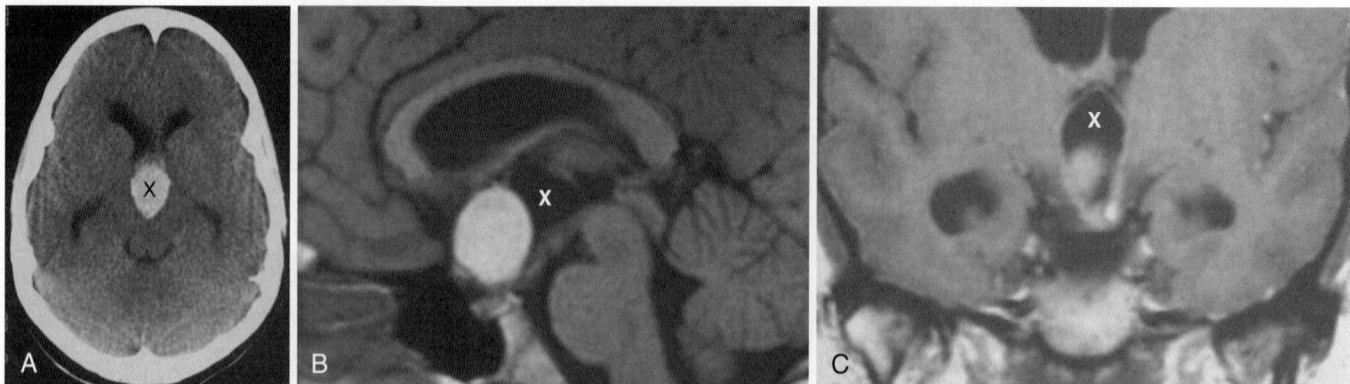

FIGURE 39.7 Computed tomography (CT) (**A**) and magnetic resonance imaging (MRI) (**B** and **C**) scans of predominantly cystic intraventricular craniopharyngiomas with different cysts (see text). X, corresponding part of tumor.

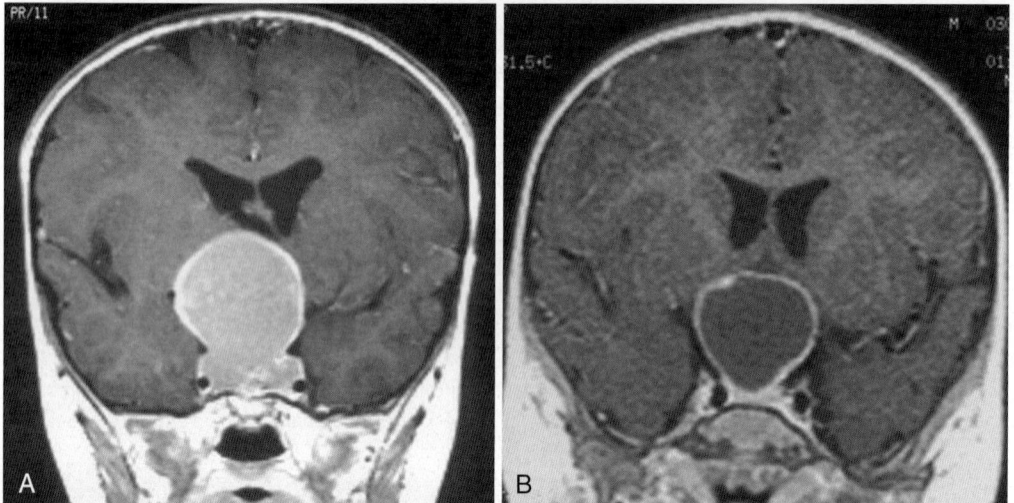

FIGURE 39.8 Intrasellar and suprasellar (**A**), suprasellar extraventricular (**B**), craniopharyngioma on coronal magnetic resonance imaging (MRI) scans.

parts of the tumor are most often isointense on T1-weighted images and show contrast enhancement. Hyperintense ring enhancement of the cyst wall is common. The high signal of the cyst fluid seen on T1 images in some tumors is related to high protein content or blood breakdown products. MRI provides information on the topography essential for planning the surgical approach. A different relation to the sella and its diaphragm may be seen on coronal scans (Fig. 39.8). In a tumor of a large or a giant size, the chiasm and the structures of the floor of the third ventricle often cannot be identified. The position of the chiasm may be detected indirectly as the AComA is always located in its immediate vicinity, most often at its upper posterior surface (see Fig. 39.4). Furthermore, the relation of the tumor with the chiasm and presence or absence of hydrocephalus may indicate the relation of the tumor to the floor and the cavity of the third ventricle with a high degree of probability.[27]

Modalities and Options for Treatment

The benign histological nature and aggressive clinical course of craniopharyngiomas together with technically difficult surgery led to two different attitudes to the initial management of this neoplasm: (a) radical surgical excision or (b) intentional incomplete (subtotal or partial) excision and radiotherapy.

The argument for radical surgery is the recurrence rate, which is considerably lower after complete tumor removal compared to subtotal or partial tumor resection, reaching 0% to 43% and 40% to 100%, respectively, and a worse outcome of secondary surgery.[9,10,12-16,59-63] The authors advocating conservative surgery and subsequent radiotherapy stress lower incidence of endocrine deficit, hypothalamic insufficiency, major disability, and even higher rate of local tumor control after more conservative management.[17-22] There is almost general agreement on decreasing the number of recurrences and progression of residual tumors after radiotherapy. The recurrence rate in children after incomplete removal reaching 44% to 100% lowered to 16% to 37.5% after radiotherapy.[60,64,65] The recurrence-free survival rate representing 38% after partial surgery increased to 77% after radiotherapy.[66] Even a 100% progression-free survival rate after radiotherapy without previous surgery has been reported.[17] Some other studies, however, found no relation between recurrence and adjuvant radiotherapy—neither globally nor in patients with incomplete resection.[24]

There is no agreement concerning the timing of radiation. Lin and colleagues[63] could prevent the recurrence in all cases with radiotherapy applied initially; if radiotherapy was applied at relapse the tumor subsequently recurred in 22%. Some authors therefore recommend routine administration of postoperative radiation.[18,22,67] On the other hand, residual tumor may remain stable for a very long period of time; therefore, others prefer the wait-and-see policy and do not recommend radiotherapy in stable residual tumor.[16]

Irradiation may be applied in fractions as conventional radiation therapy or by means of more advanced techniques: three-dimensional conformal radiation treatment, intensity modulated radiation therapy, or stereotactic radiotherapy. The tolerance of the optic chiasm is 54 Gy in 30 fractions.[17] Gamma Knife stereotactic radiosurgery delivers to a tumor margin a dose from 9.5 to 35 Gy.[68-70] Close tumor relationship to visual pathways, however, is a limiting factor. For targeted single high-dose irradiation the dose to the optic chiasm should not exceed 8 Gy.[69]

Shrinking of a cystic craniopharyngioma may be achieved by means of instillation of the solution of beta particle–emitting radioactive isotopes of yttrium-90, gold-198, or phosphorus-32. Long-term results after yttrium-90 colloid irradiation led to reduction of the initial cyst volume of 79%; in 47 patients in the reduction was more than 80%.[71]

Different modalities of irradiation (conventional external radiation therapy, Gamma Knife or linear accelerator radiosurgery, radioactive yttrium implantation) in our clinical series succeeded in local tumor control in 6 of 11 patients. It failed to prevent the recurrence or progression of residual tumor in another 5 patients, occurring from 6 to 60 months after irradiation.

All modalities of radiotherapy may cause damage to the pituitary, the hypothalamus, and the visual structures, and it may cause moyamoya syndrome, cavernous malformation, and secondary malignant astrocytoma.[16,72-75] Most often affected is the function of the anterior pituitary.[18] Deterioration of vision after instillation of beta wave emitters, attributed to irradiation and as the result of tumor progression, reached 22.5% to 52%.[76,77] New neuro-ophthalmological deficits after yttrium-90 colloid irradiation occurred in 5.8%.[71] The latter was comparable to 6.1% of visual deterioration after radiosurgery.[68] Damage to the carotid was reported after yttrium-90 treatment.[71] In our autopsy series of craniopharyngiomas, the occlusion of the supraclinoid ICA was noted in a 15-year-old boy 6 years after intracystic instillation of 5 mCi of yttrium-90 and 2 years after additional external radiotherapy.

Our policy for the past 20 years is to recommend radiation therapy either by fractionated or a single-dose technique only to progressively growing tumors considered nonremovable at the previous surgery (primary or secondary) performed by us.

Chemotherapy with bleomycin has been used in cystic craniopharyngiomas. It causes thickening of the tumor capsule, and the cyst contracts, pulling away from brain structures, which facilitates cyst removal.[78] However, bleomycin is highly toxic for neural structures if it is allowed to leak from the cyst. In a review of 16 articles[79] at least one severe toxic effect, including visual or hearing impairment, personality changes, seizures, somnolence, or even death, occurred in 19% of patients. A combination of intracystic bleomycin and phosphorus-32 used in nine patients led to an even higher rate of complications.[80]

Other surgical techniques are sometimes used in patients with primary or recurrent craniopharyngiomas. Ventriculoperitoneal shunt or even external ventricular drainage (EVD) may be inserted in cases with severe intracranial hypertension. We have had severe acute intracranial hypertension necessitating EVD in one patient. Some patients have had shunts implanted before referring to us for a tumor removal. Our policy is to restore the patency of the CSF pathways by removal of the tumor. Stereotactic technique is sometimes used for evacuation of a cyst or for instillation of radioisotopes or bleomycin into the tumor cyst.[21,70,81] A repeatedly enlarging large cystic tumor may be treated by the implantation of an Ommaya reservoir, enabling simple evacuation of the cystic contents.

Cyst evacuation, different forms of irradiation, and chemotherapy are recommended mostly as an adjuvant treatment. We believe the best management of craniopharyngiomas is radical tumor removal whenever safely possible. A lower quality of life was observed after radical removal of craniopharyngiomas "involving the hypothalamus."[25,26] However, in cases with "hypothalamus no longer identifiable" on MRI scans the tumor may just compress the floor of the third ventricle and not invade it.[27,28] It may be a good decision to remove the tumor radically in cases of extraventricular craniopharyngiomas and consider it contraindicated when the tumor is intraventricular.[82] Nevertheless, the nature and intensity of the adherence of the tumor to diencephalic structures may differ within any of the topographical groups. Imaging studies do not show directly whether the tumor is simply compressing the hypothalamus or invading it, without a plane of cleavage. Therefore, the final decision about the extent of safe tumor removal cannot be made before the operation.

Surgery

Surgical strategy and tactics are based on the answers to two questions: Where to begin, and when to stop tumor removal? The answer to the first question is related to the choice of the optimal surgical approach. It should respect the topographical relationship of the tumor with the surrounding structures and at the same time it must provide sufficient tumor exposure. The answer to the second question is related to the fact that accessibility of a craniopharyngioma does not mean its resectability. Hypothalamic structures should be avoided during surgical approach and tumor resection (Fig. 39.9). There are two factors limiting preoperative assumption of the tumor–third ventricular floor relationship on rare occasions. First, it may be impossible to find out whether a retrochiasmatic supradiaphragmatic tumor not reaching the foramina of Monro and not causing hydrocephalus lies below the floor of the third ventricle or is embedded inside the infundibulum and the tuber cinereum. Distinction in such an MRI finding is possible only if the structures of the floor of the third ventricle are directly delineated. Second, besides the majority of tumors with expressed topographical features characteristic for one of the described groups, there are transitional types of craniopharyngiomas displaying the features of two topographical groups.

Intrasellar and Intrasellar and Suprasellar Craniopharyngiomas

For intrasellar craniopharyngiomas the only appropriate approach is the transsphenoidal route, which exposes the entire tumor and allows identification of the remnants of the pituitary gland located anterior to the tumor or posterior to it.[83] The transsphenoidal approach is suitable also for the intrasellar and suprasellar craniopharyngiomas, with the exception of giant tumors and the tumors of a dumbbell or multinodular shape, which are rather rare in intrasellar and suprasellar craniopharyngiomas (Fig. 39.10). These tumors can be resected through the extended transsphenoidal approach, which allows removing even supradiaphragmatic craniopharyngiomas.[84,85] In our series of 43 infradiaphragmatic tumors, 4 were intrasellar and 39 extended above the sellar diaphragm. Some of them were large or even giant tumors.

To expose the tumor via the transsphenoidal route we use the unilateral paraseptal, usually sublabial, approach performed under the operative microscope from the first incision. In order to get sufficient exposure of intrasellar contents a large opening of the sphenoid sinus and the sellar floor is mandatory.[83] The anterior wall of the sphenoid sinus and the sellar floor is resected under neuronavigation guidance. In a majority of our cases in which a compressed pituitary

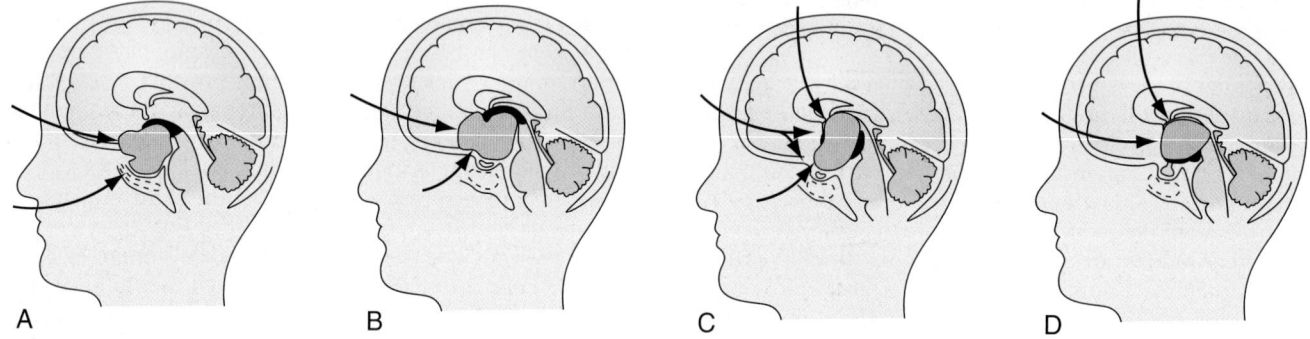

FIGURE 39.9 Schematic representation of the relationship of the intrasellar and suprasellar (**A**), suprasellar extraventricular (**B**), intraventricular and extraventricular (**C**), and intraventricular (**D**) craniopharyngiomas with the floor of the third ventricle (*black*) and surgical approaches (*arrows*) avoiding the hypothalamic structures.

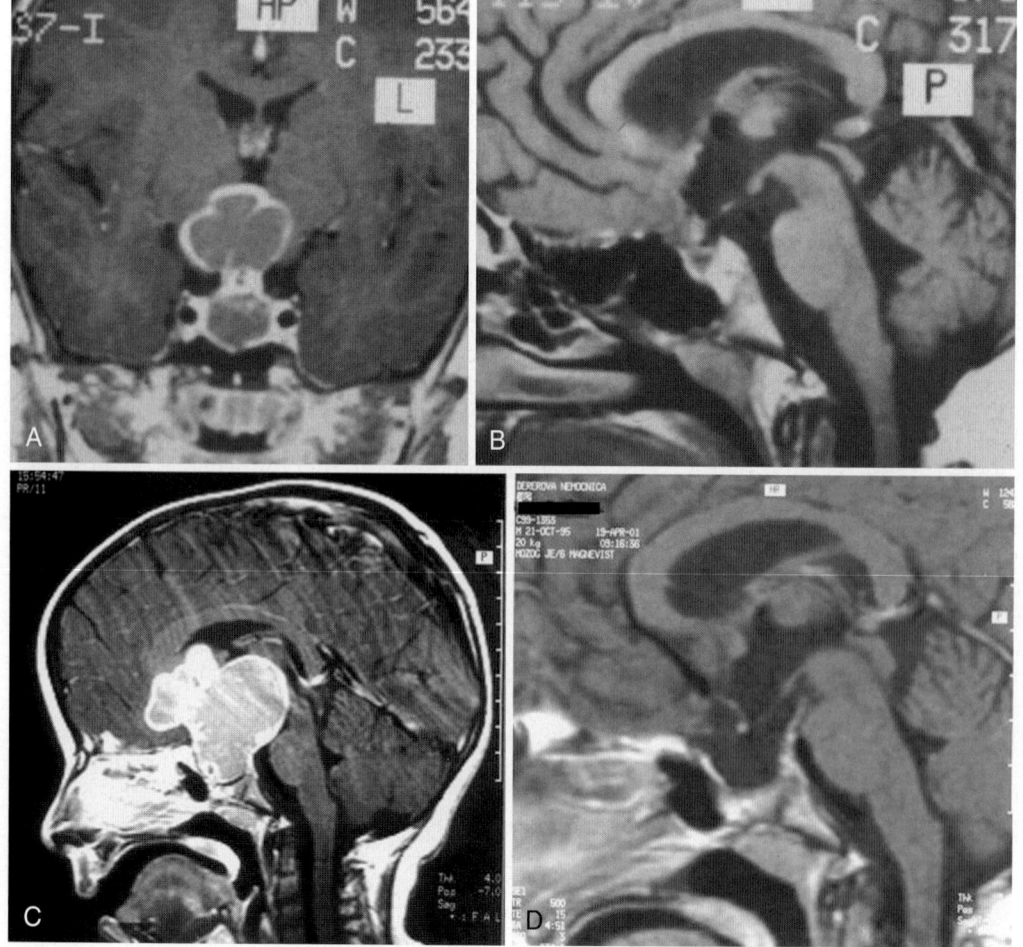

FIGURE 39.10 Intrasellar and suprasellar craniopharyngiomas, dumbbell (**A** and **B**) and multilobulated (**C**, **D**), resected via the subfrontal approach.

gland was found (one third of the intrasellar and suprasellar tumors), it could be detected at the sellar floor immediately after dural incision. The gland, which was identified at the floor of the enlarged sella, was split in the midline and displaced to the side so the tumor capsule could be identified (Fig. 39.11). The capsule always adheres to surrounding dura covering the sellar cavity; nevertheless, the tumor does not invade the cavernous sinus as the pituitary adenomas do. The capsule is separated from the dura by pulling it into the sellar cavity and detaching it by blunt microdissection, although sometimes sharp dissection is necessary. If the capsule is thin and fragile, care must be taken not to lose its continuity as later on it may not be identified and may be unintentionally left in place. On the other hand, if there is a thick firmly adhering capsule, it may not be possible to dissect it free and a part of it may have to be left in place.

The capsule may contain eggshell-like calcification which may be sharp like a blade so that maximum caution is necessary during its removal. Adherence of the capsule to the diaphragm is always extensive, and its removal is sometimes not possible without resection of the diaphragm and transsection of the pituitary stalk. Preservation of the pituitary stalk necessitates leaving the piece of the capsule in some cases.

Suprasellar Extraventricular Craniopharyngiomas

Superior displacement of the chiasm and partial prechiasmatic extension of a great majority of the SECs allow tumor removal through the (1) prechiasmatic space between the optic nerves, anterior angle of the chiasm, and the sellar tubercle; (2) opticocarotid triangle between the lateral margin of the optic nerve and chiasm, supraclinoid carotid artery, and the A1 segment of the anterior cerebral artery; and (3) laterally to the carotid. All these extracerebral routes to the tumor are accessible by the unilateral subfrontal approach, which is our most commonly used craniotomy in craniopharyngiomas (Fig. 39.12).

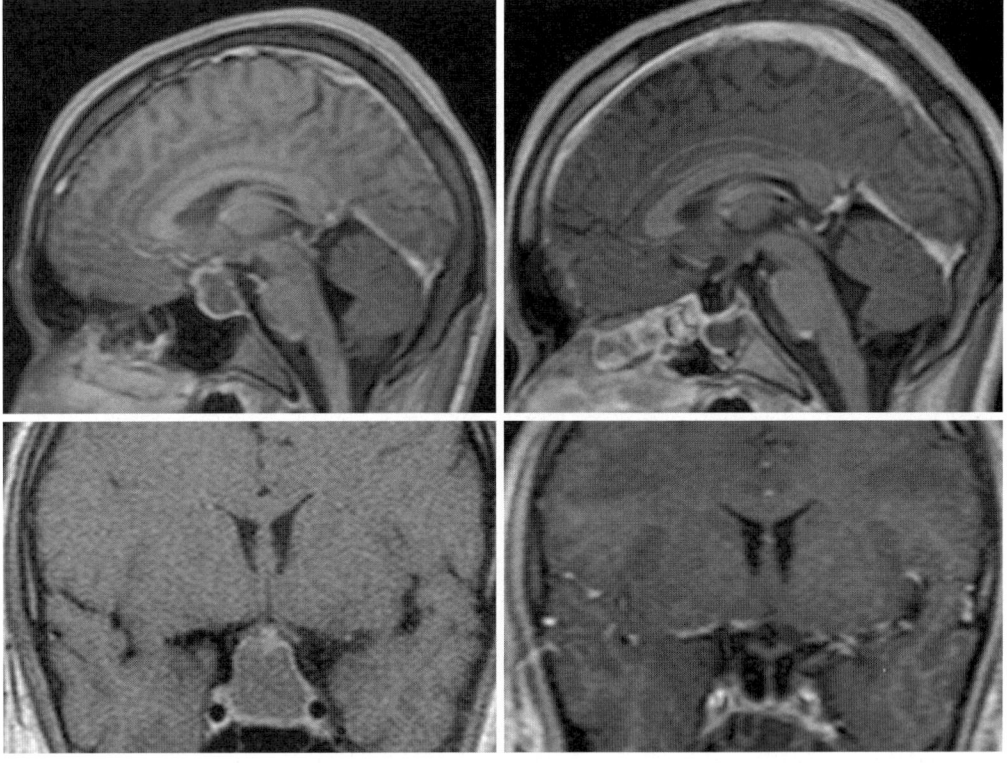

FIGURE 39.11 Intrasellar and suprasellar craniopharyngioma removed transsphenoidally with preservation of the pituitary and no endocrinological deficiency.

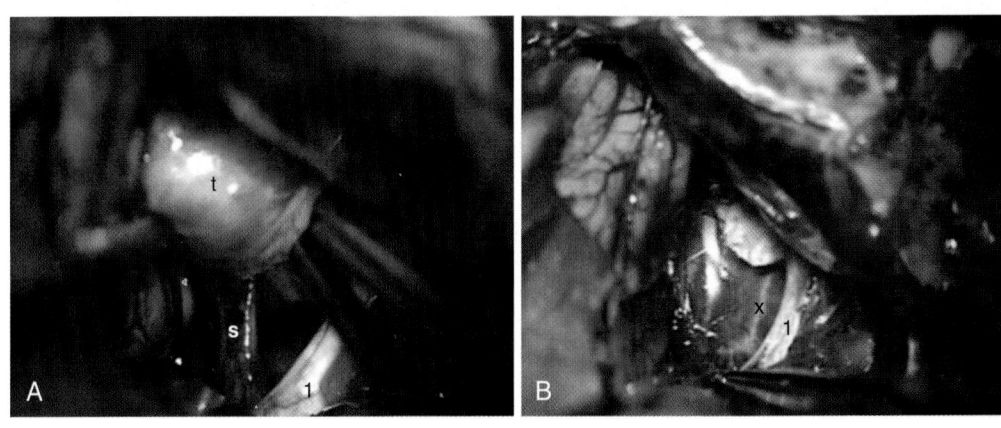

FIGURE 39.12 A, Intraoperative view of a suprasellar extraventricular craniopharyngioma (t) removed via right subfrontal approach (**B**). s, pituitary stalk; x, basilar artery behind the Lilliequist's membrane; 1, right optic nerve.

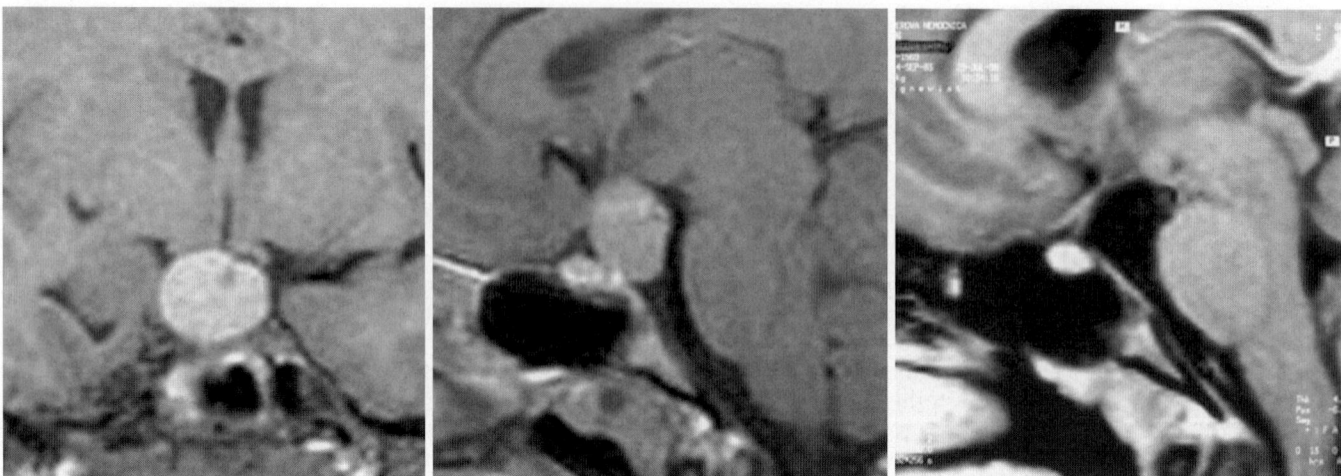

FIGURE 39.13 Retrochiasmatic suprasellar extraventricular craniopharyngioma located behind the pituitary stalk, removed via the frontotemporal approach. Preserved pituitary stalk, no endocrine deficiency.

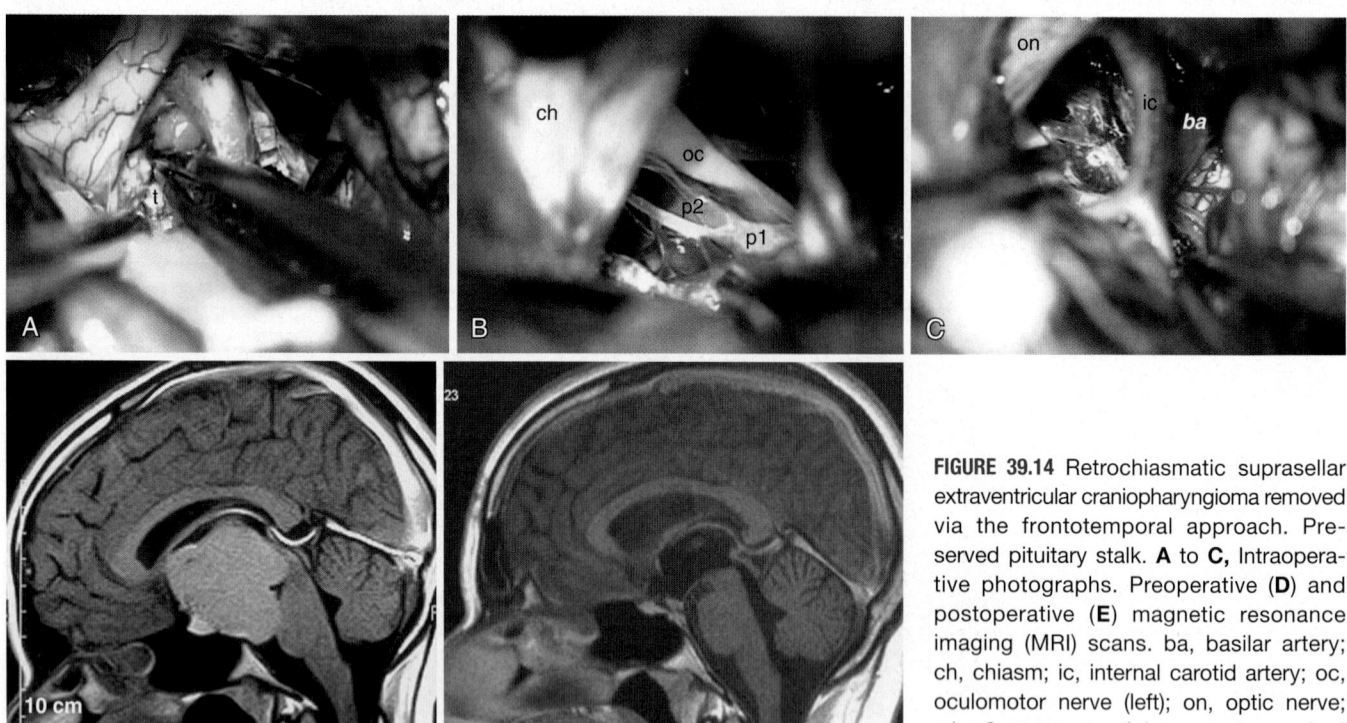

FIGURE 39.14 Retrochiasmatic suprasellar extraventricular craniopharyngioma removed via the frontotemporal approach. Preserved pituitary stalk. **A** to **C,** Intraoperative photographs. Preoperative (**D**) and postoperative (**E**) magnetic resonance imaging (MRI) scans. ba, basilar artery; ch, chiasm; ic, internal carotid artery; oc, oculomotor nerve (left); on, optic nerve; p1, p2, segments of the posterior cerebral artery; t, tumor.

Removal of an extraventricular tumor through the lamina terminalis would jeopardize hypothalamic structures of the floor of the third ventricle covering the upper surface of the tumor. Therefore, with rare SECs growing exclusively behind the optic chiasm we approach below and behind the chiasm through pterional craniotomy (Figs. 39.13 and 39.14). Skull base approaches enabling an approach to the tumor more from below, such as the orbitozygomatic or transpetrosal approach, may be of great help in these cases.[86] In a giant multicystic tumor a bifrontal craniotomy was necessary (Fig. 39.15).

For both subfrontal and pterional approaches we perform frontotemporal skin incision just behind the hair line, beginning from the midline medially and continuing laterally to the zygoma, preferably on the nondominant side. The extent of the bone flap in the subfrontal approach includes the convexity of the frontal bone as its merges with the supraorbital rim at its middle and lateral portions. In cases of a large frontal sinus the latter may be opened and then closed by the periostal flap before opening the dura. After evacuation of the CSF by lumbar drain and opening the dura, the sellar

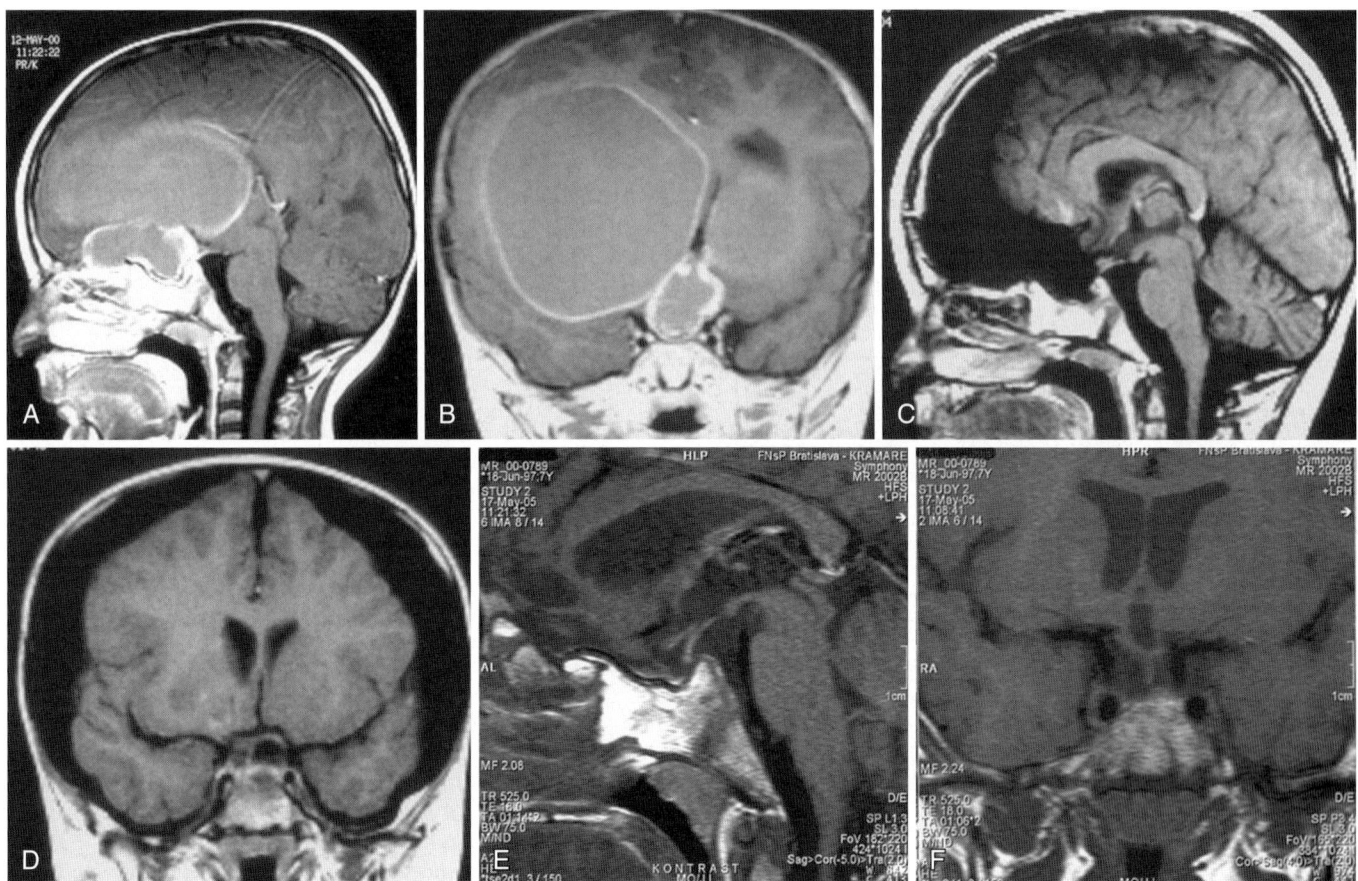

FIGURE 39.15 Giant suprasellar extraventricular craniopharyngioma removed via bifrontal craniotomy (**A** and **B**). Magnetic resonance imaging (MRI) scans 2 days (**C** and **D**) and 5 years (**E** and **F**) after surgery.

region is approached below the frontal lobe with the forceps in one hand and the sucker in the other without a spatula. The carotid and chiasmatic cisterns are opened for more CSF evacuation, and then the medial part of the Sylvian fissure is opened to relieve the pressure on the frontal lobe. Removal of the tumor starts by opening and evacuation of the cyst if visible. The subarachnoid space around the exposed tumor is blocked by cottonoids before opening the cyst to prevent leakage of the cyst contents into the CSF space. A brain spatula is used in later stages of surgery to support the relaxed brain if necessary.

Solid parts of the tumor are removed in a piecemeal fashion. The capsule is then detached from the optic nerves, the optic chiasm, the carotid arteries, and their branches. At this stage the capsule may be dissected from the pituitary stalk located on the posterosuperior tumor surface or displaced by the tumor toward one side. In some cases the dissection of the tumor capsule from the pituitary stalk is relatively easy, whereas in others, its lower part fades into the capsule and cannot be traced down to the sella.

The tumor may adhere to large blood vessels. Intraoperative damage to the internal carotid artery has been reported. Removal of a calcified portion of the tumor from the wall of the carotid in children may be especially dangerous.[8,87] We found such extensive calcifications more commonly in the IEVCs. The SECs could be dissected safely from the adventitia even if they completely envelop the large arteries at the base of the brain. Extreme care must be taken to look for the minute perforating vessels, the branches of the supraclinoid carotid, and the posterior communicating arteries supplying the visual pathways and the hypothalamus. It is important to dissect these tiny vessels from the capsule of the tumor because they often bifurcate, with one branch supplying the tumor and the other continuing to its original destination. The vessel may be occluded only after confirming that it does not supply adjacent neural structures. The branches of the A1 and the AComA come in such close contact only with the tumors growing in front of the chiasm. If the perforators adhere firmly and cannot be safely detached from the tumor surface, a part of the capsule is left attached to the vessels.

A more common cause of an incomplete removal of the SECs is the adherence of the upper pole of the tumor to the pia mater of the superiorly displaced floor of the third ventricle, or more rarely of the chiasm. If the capsule cannot be dissected without disruption of the pial vascular network, then part of it or even a small piece of a tumor tissue has to be left in place. On rare occasions the distended floor of the third ventricle falls down during removal of the upper pole of the tumor. In a majority of the cases we delineate the condition of the ventricular floor by angled endoscope. Unintentionally left tumor remnants may be removed, but those firmly adhering to the pia of the hypothalamus have to be left in place (Fig. 39.16).

Removal of the posterior pole of the tumor usually does not pose a problem as the basilar artery, its branches, and the brainstem are protected by the Liliequist's membrane covering the posterior border of the tumor. In rare cases in which the posterior perforators adhere to the tumor capsule the attachment is rather loose, such that the tumor may be removed without damaging the vessels (see video).

Intraventricular and Extraventricular Craniopharyngiomas

Atrophied hypothalamic structures within the remnants of the floor of the third ventricle in the IEVCs are displaced around

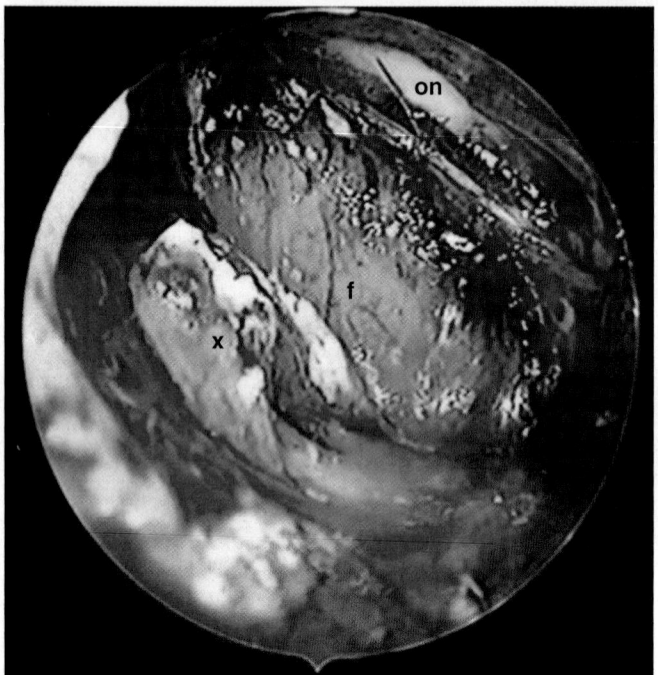

FIGURE 39.16 Endoscopic view of the remnant of a suprasellar extraventricular craniopharyngioma (x) firmly adherent to the pia of the floor of the third ventricle (f). on, left oculomotor nerve.

the "equator" of the tumor. This topographical relationship in principle allows the use of both extracerebral and transventricular approaches to the tumor (Figs. 39.9 and 39.17). However, the retrochiasmatic location of the tumor, common low position of the chiasm, and a slit-like opticocarotid triangle most often preclude extracerebral tumor exposure. The central lower part of the lamina terminalis in the IEVCs is often composed of gliotic tissue and in fact represents the capsule of the anterior pole of the tumor. Its opening between the chiasm and the AComA usually allows good exposure of the anterior and the basal parts of the intraventricular mass and of the entire extraventricular portion of the tumor (Fig. 39.18).

The basal part of the tumor is often calcified; sometimes it turns into a rock-like mass, which has to be broken into pieces by CUSA (Cavitron ultrasonic surgical aspirator). After piecemeal removal of the basal part of the tumor, the pituitary stalk may be seen below the chiasm after pulling the latter upward from the sellar tubercle. The chiasm quite often stays fixed even after complete tumor removal. In some cases the pituitary stalk cannot be identified, or just its lower part can be found at the entrance into the opening of the sellar diaphragm. The rest was already destroyed by the tumor. After removal of the basal part of the tumor, the brainstem comes into view together with the basilar artery and its branches separated from the tumor by Liliequist's membrane. If the mammillary bodies are displaced predominantly basally, they can be seen in front of the brainstem. The remnants of the infundibulum and the tuber, if present, and their supplying blood vessels originating from the posterior communicating artery can be clearly seen and spared. The *condition sine qua non* for the removal of the tumor adhering to the hypothalamus is the identification of the border and the plane of cleavage between the gliotic tumor capsule and the remnants of the third ventricular floor. If this cannot be found, the adhering portions of the tumor capsule or even its parenchyma should be left in place in order to avoid serious damage to the hypothalamus.

The majority of intraventricular and extraventricular craniopharyngiomas may be removed via the trans-lamina

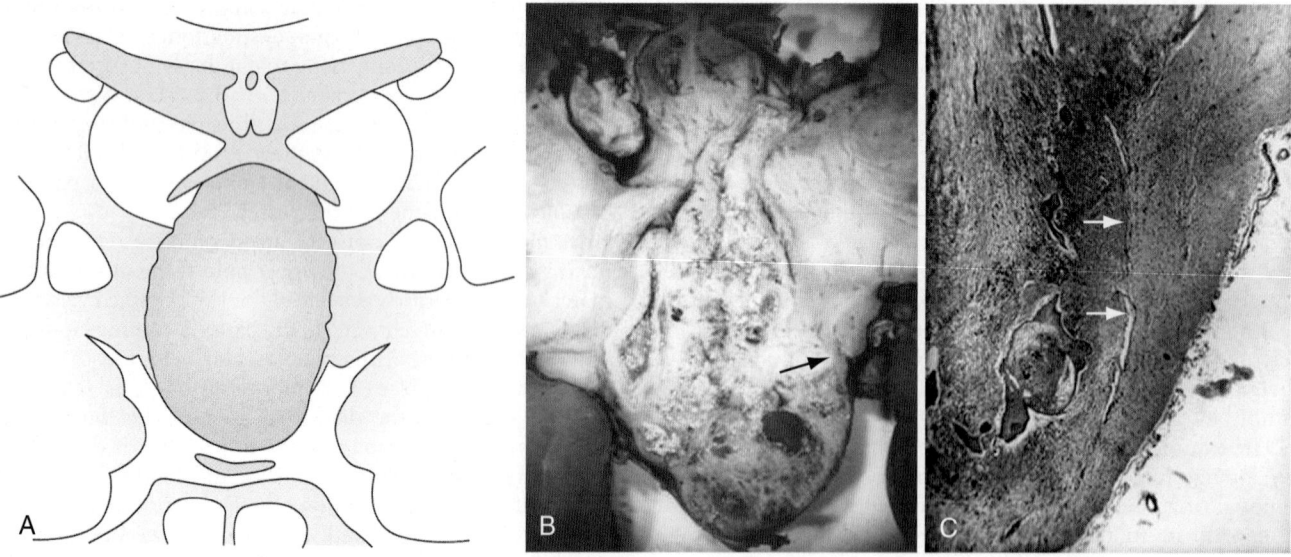

FIGURE 39.17 Relationship of the intraventricular and extraventricular craniopharyngioma with the remnants of the tuber cinereum (*arrows*). **A,** Schematic representation; **B,** anatomical specimen; **C,** microphotograph.

terminalis approach. It provided good access also to the posterior-basal expansion of the tumor into the cerebellopontine angle seen in one patient.

A disadvantage of this approach is an insufficient exposure of the superoposterior part of the third ventricle. The upper limit of the direct visual control of the ventricular cavity is represented by the line connecting the lower limit of the craniotomy and the AComA. The upper part of the tumor hidden above this borderline can thus be seen only after pulling it down to the lower part of the ventricle (Fig. 39.19) or by opening the lamina terminalis also above the AComA.[88] For larger tumors we prefer the transcallosal approach. An advantage of this approach is the possibility of starting tumor removal at its upper pole where it is free from any neural structures at the enlarged foramina of Monro. After evacuation of the cyst following removal of the part of the tumor tissue through a

larger foramen, the larger foramen provides a good access to a whole upper part of the tumor. This part of the tumor only touches and does not invade the fornix and the walls of the third ventricle. It helps to find the border and the plane of cleavage between the cerebral and the tumor tissue as one proceeds farther down to the more basal region where the tumor merges with the hypothalamus. The transcallosal exposure of the tumor eventually may allow removal of the whole tumor, which was the case in two of our patients (Fig. 39.20). If not, evacuation of the CSF from the lateral ventricles and removal of the most of the ventricular portion of the tumor provides a comfortable subsequent subfrontal approach.

The transcallosal approach also has its limitations. The most inferior-anterior part of the tumor may not be exposed sufficiently and has to be approached through the opening of the lamina terminalis. A surgical approach that combines

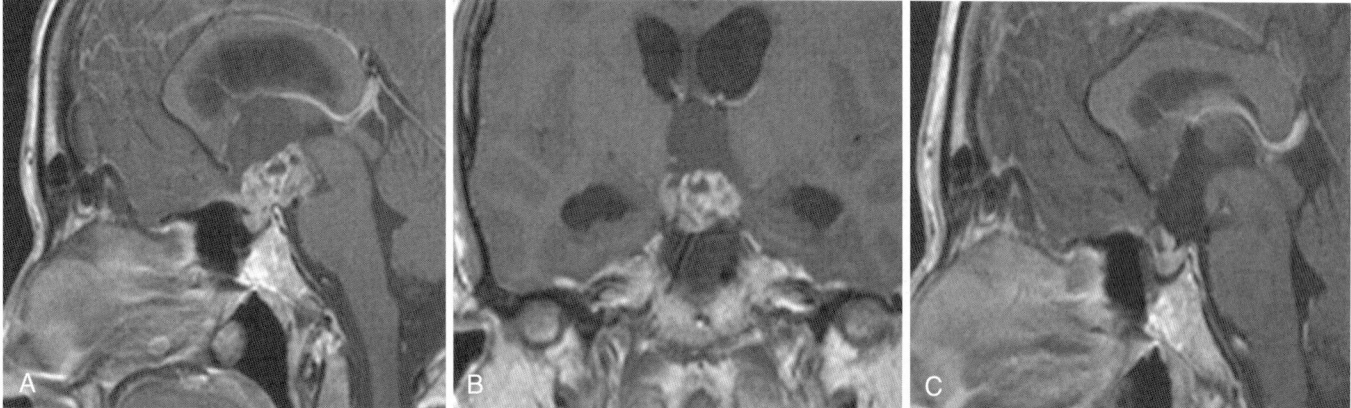

FIGURE 39.18 Intraventricular and extraventricular craniopharyngiomas (**A** and **B**) removed via the trans-lamina terminalis approach. **C** Three months after tumor removal. Note the relatively high position of the anterior communicating artery.

FIGURE 39.19 Intraoperative situation at the exposure of the lamina terminalis (**A**), its opening (**B**), removal of the last portion of the intraventricular and extraventricular craniopharyngioma (x) (**C**), and after tumor removal (**D**). f, Floor of the third ventricle. This is the same patient shown in Figure 39.18.

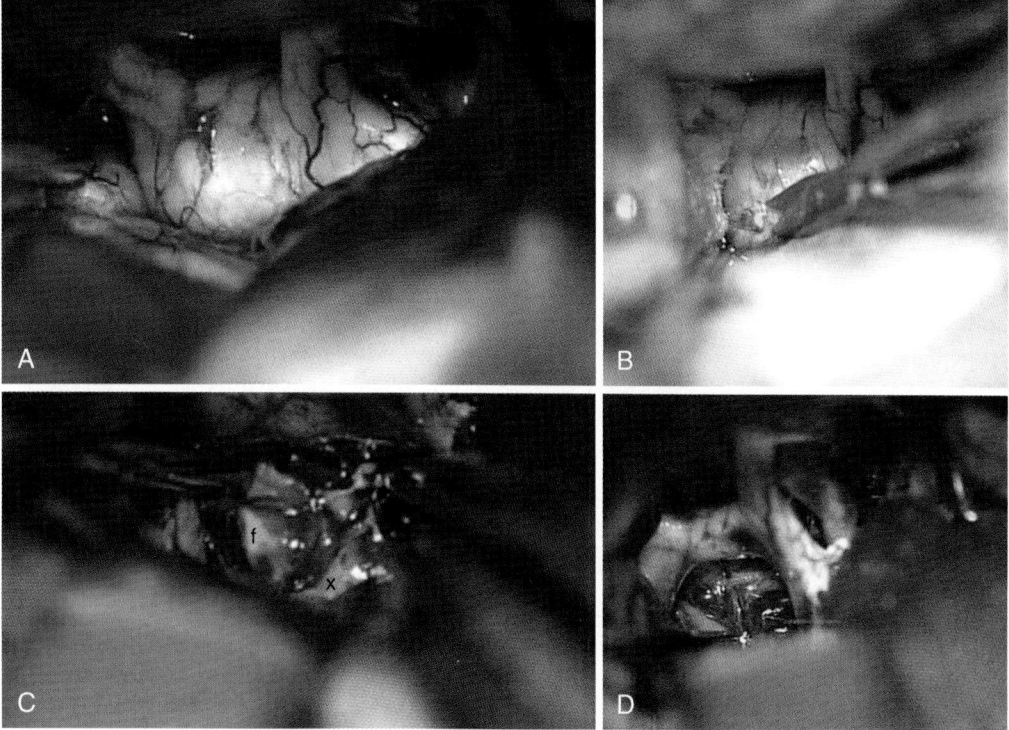

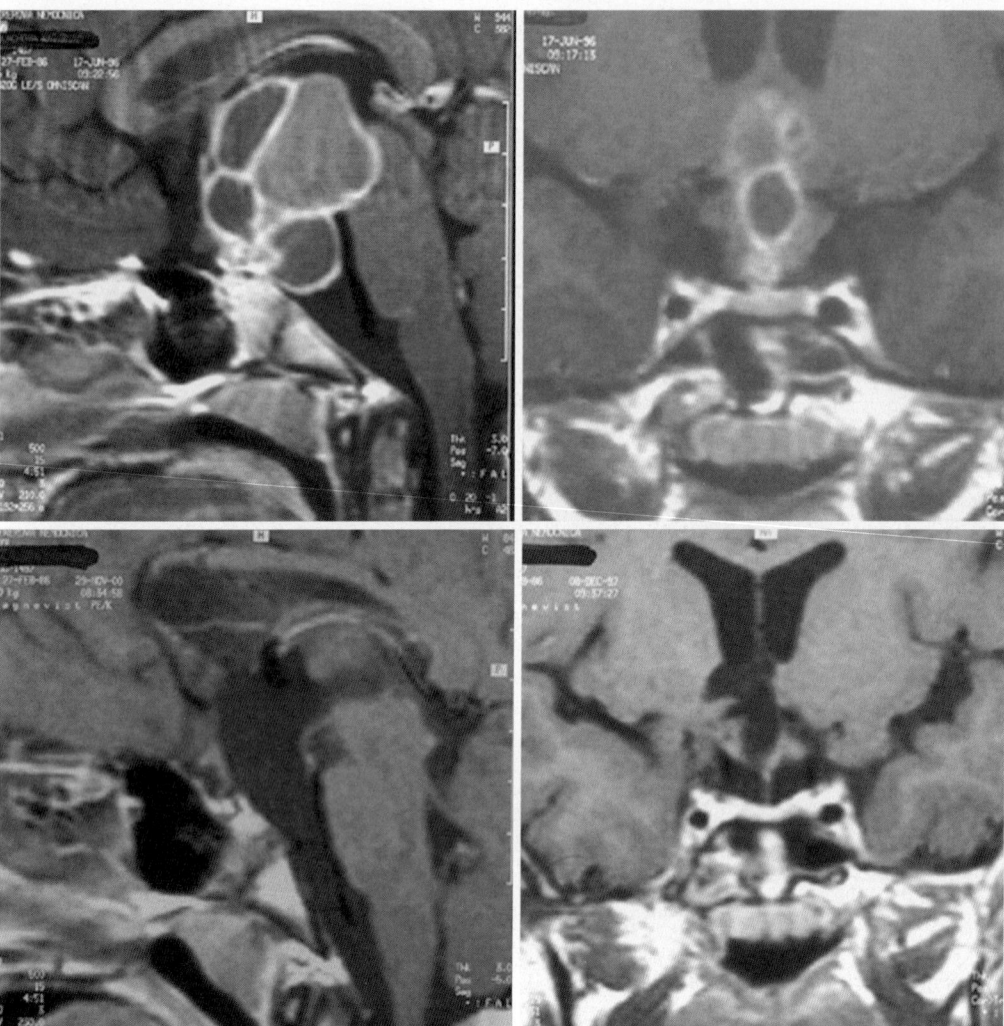

FIGURE 39.20 Intraventricular and extraventricular craniopharyngioma removed radically via the transcallosal approach. Preserved infundibulum and the pituitary stalk seen on magnetic resonance imaging (MRI) 18 months after surgery.

features of both basal and superior exposures is recommended for the suprasellar masses with simultaneous third ventricle involved.[89] Removal of the tumor may be staged[40,83] or performed at one sitting through two separate craniotomies[12] or one larger[60] craniotomy. In large or giant intraventricular and extraventricular craniopharyngiomas located entirely behind the chiasm/AComA reaching the roof of the third ventricle posterior to the foramina of Monro and causing hydrocephalus, we prefer a combined transcallosal and subfrontal approach through one unilateral craniotomy. We perform a large unilateral bone flap beginning at the lateral and the middle thirds of the orbital rim anteriorly, crossing the midline by 1.5 cm medially, and reaching or exceeding by 1 cm the coronal suture posteriorly. An opening of the dura approximately 7 cm long (in anteroposterior diameter) enables combined one-stage transcallosal and subfrontal tumor exposure (Fig. 39.21). One large craniotomy makes sequential or alternating transcallosal and subfrontal exposure easier, if necessary. The exposure of the tumor via a combined approach is as a rule sufficient, and no endoscopic assistance is necessary.

We have abandoned the transfrontal transcortical approach in order to avoid the seizure complications. Our results confirmed the observation of the others that a short

incision up to 2 cm in the anterior part of the corpus callosum behind its genu causes no clinically apparent neuropsychological deficit.[89-92] We have observed severe though transitional short memory disturbances in a single patient with craniopharyngioma in whom the tumor, an intraventricular and extraventricular craniopharyngioma, was removed through the lamina terminalis below and also above the AComA. The cause of memory disturbances lasting for almost 1 year could be a bilateral manipulation of the columnae of the fornix and the anterior commissure.[93] We avoid the manipulation of both parts of the fornix whenever possible. During the transcallosal approach, we try to remove the tumor through one foramen of Monro using the other one for assessing the completeness of tumor removal.

Intraventricular Craniopharyngiomas

Rare purely intraventricular craniopharyngiomas push the floor of the third ventricle downward. An extracerebral approach would jeopardize the hypothalamic structures covering the basal part of the tumor. The tumor may be removed either by opening of the lamina terminalis or through the foramina of Monro. Adherence of the tumor to lateral walls

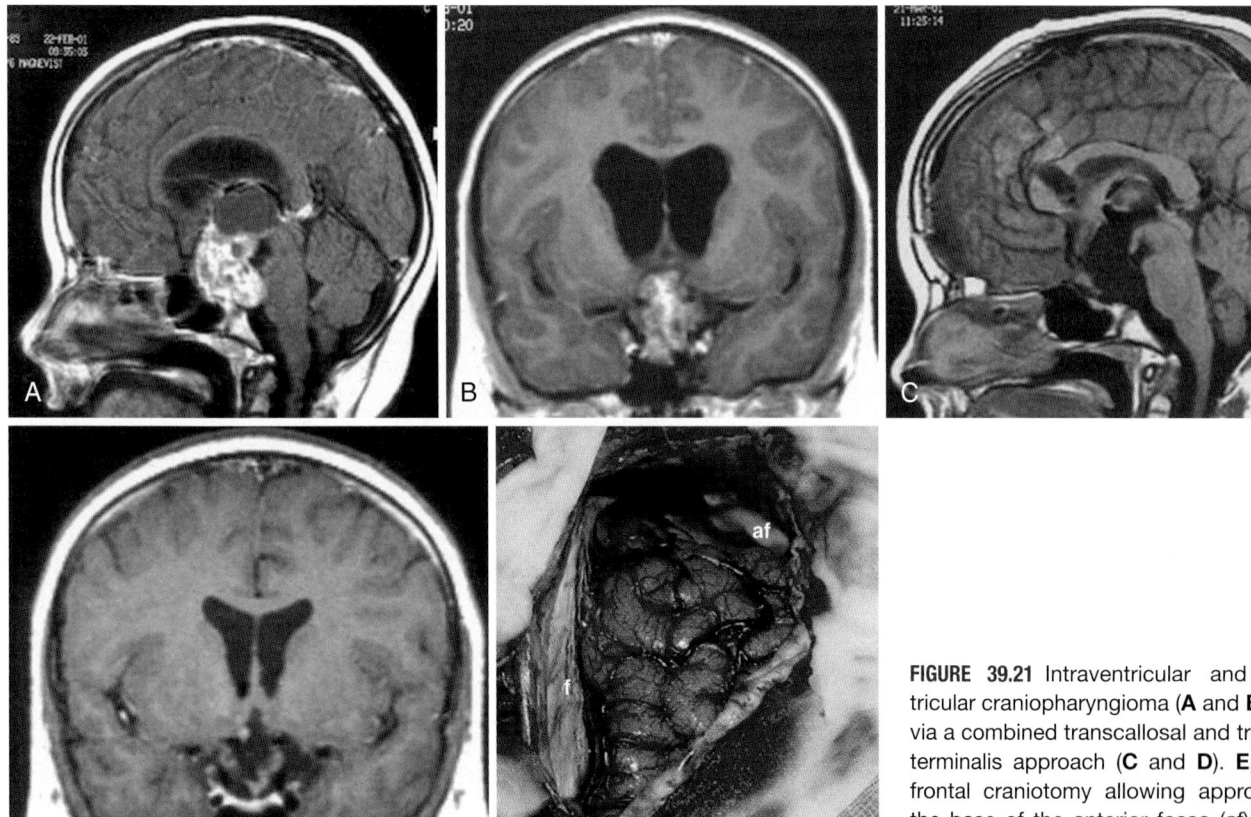

FIGURE 39.21 Intraventricular and extraventricular craniopharyngioma (**A** and **B**) removed via a combined transcallosal and trans-lamina terminalis approach (**C** and **D**). **E,** Unilateral frontal craniotomy allowing approach along the base of the anterior fossa (af) and along the falx (f).

of the third ventricle is less pronounced than in the IEVCs. If the border and the plane of cleavage between the tumor and the hypothalamus can be found, the tumor may be removed radically (see video).

Perioperative Management and Management of Complications

Pituitary insufficiency is common before surgery. Appropriate perioperative hormonal replacement therapy therefore is necessary. The dose of hydrocortisone depends on the location and the extension of the tumor, and the radicality of surgery. In adults with large or giant tumors involving the hypothalamus 400 mg of hydrocortisone is administered during the day of surgery: 100 mg before surgery, 100 mg during tumor removal, and the rest after the operation. In children the dose is calculated according to body weight. The dose is progressively diminished during the next days according to the clinical condition of the patient. If the postoperative course is uneventful, the initial dose is reduced to approximately one fifth on the fifth postoperative day.

Severe acute hypothalamic failure may occur after removal of the tumor adherent to the hypothalamus. Life-threatening complication presents by mineral/water balance disturbances, which may be accompanied by hyperpyrexia, seizures, and decreased levels of consciousness. Careful monitoring and early correction of mineral and water balance disturbances presenting by diabetes insipidus, hypernatremia, and hypokalemia are absolutely mandatory. Such

disturbances may be the consequence of a combination of disruption of pituitary stalk (lack of antidiuretic hormone) and damage of osmoreceptors in anterior hypothalamus (loss of thirst sensation). Disturbances of the fluid and electrolyte balance are treated in the intensive care unit. Detailed measurement of intake of fluid, output of urine, and blood and urine levels of sodium and potassium should start at the day of surgery and continue twice a day afterward. Measurement of osmolality of serum and urine should also be performed twice a day in cases with severe metabolic disturbances. Antidiuretic hormone (ADH) is administered if the diuresis exceeds 1 L in 6 hours and if there is tendency to hypernatremia and hyperosmolality. Hyponatremia and hypo-osmolality may follow after the initial phase of diabetes insipidus.[94] It may be a part of different syndromes, such as syndrome of inappropriate ADH secretion (SIADH), cerebral salt-wasting syndrome (CSWS), and others. Management of the disturbance includes fluid restriction in transient or asymptomatic SIADH and aggressive replacement of urine water losses in CSWS. Sodium replacement is necessary in the advanced stage. These life-threatening metabolic disturbances should be managed by an anesthesiologist experienced in neurointensive care.

Another severe complication is bleeding into the tumor bed, which occurred in two of our patients within 24 hours after surgery. In both of them the hematoma was evacuated through the original surgical approach immediately after it was confirmed by CT. Rarely, a ventriculoperitoneal shunt has to be inserted because of persisting hydrocephalus.

Long-Term Results

Surgical Mortality Rate

The outcome of surgery depends on the location of the tumor, its size, and the extent of surgery. The overall surgical mortality rate reported in most series is below 4%.[15,16,83,87,95] In a large series with 45.7% radical removals the operative mortality rate was 0% after transsphenoidal surgery and 1.1% after primary transcranial surgery. The difference in outcomes of transsphenoidal and transcranial surgery is most probably due to the different topography and the size of the tumors operated by either approach. In another series with over 60% of large and giant tumors in which radical tumor removal was achieved in 90%, the surgical mortality and early postoperative mortality rates together reached 9%. On the other hand, the recurrence rate after such a radical approach was exceptionally low, around 7%.[12] Analysis of our results showed the relation of the outcome to the location of the tumor. In our consecutive series of 105 patients operated since 1991 there were no deaths in 43 infradiaphragmatic tumors (24 transsphenoidal, 19 transcranial) including large and giant tumors with 81% radical removals (90% in primary surgery). Of 62 patients with supradiaphragmatic tumors (76% radical removals) 4 patients died after surgery (6.5%), with the mortality rate in a whole series reaching 3.8%.

Recurrences and Their Management

The extent of resection as seen in the first postoperative MRI is the most important factor concerning the recurrences in craniopharyngiomas.[96] The recurrence rate after subtotal or partial tumor removal is higher than that after radical removal, representing 50% to 100% and 0% to 43%, respectively.[14-16,25,26,59,62,63,65] In the series of Fahlbusch and coworkers[83] the recurrence-free survival rate 10 years after total removal was 81.3%, but 5 years after subtotal and partial removal it reached only 48.8% and 41.5%, respectively. In the group of our patients who were followed for more than 1 year (12-201 months, mean 91 months) the tumor recurred in 19 of 94 patients after primary surgery (20.2%), in 16% after radical removal, and in 40% after incomplete removal.

Removal of recurrent craniopharyngioma is associated with a lower cure rate and a higher risk of complications than primary surgery because of the scarring from previous surgery and adherence of the tumor to surrounding structures. Radiation therapy therefore is recommended as the primary treatment for recurrences.[65] However, some authors stress the possibility of safe resection of recurrent tumors and consider surgery to be the first therapeutic option for recurrent craniopharyngioma.[9,13-15,62,97-100] Radiation therapy should also be considered but only as adjuvant therapy[98] or second-line treatment for subsequent recurrence.[97] Recurrence of craniopharyngioma can be safely managed by using meticulous contemporary microsurgical techniques even without additional radiotherapy.[62] We performed 37 operations in 25 patients with 59.5% radical removals of recurrent tumor and the result comparable with primary surgery. One patient died after removal of a small residual tumor from pulmonary embolism. Permanent morbidity related to surgery occurred in two patients; both experienced visual deterioration in one

eye. We decide to perform repeat surgery as soon as tumor recurrence or progression of the tumor remnant is proved by MRI. Some residual tumors remain stable for years without adjuvant therapy. The presence of a small residual calcification in children without enhancing tumor remnant does not have an impact on the risk of recurrence.[101]

Morbidity Rate

Pituitary hormone deficiency after craniopharyngioma removal occurs often. In a pediatric series some kind of hormonal replacement is necessary in 85% to 100%.[16,51] A high number of multiple pituitary hormone deficiencies was found, regardless of total or partial surgery.[51] After total tumor removal in both children and adults hormone deficits were found in 95%.[102] Growth hormone deficiency is detected in up to 100%, hypogonadism in 65% to 80%, hypothyroidism in 38.5% to 95%, and hypocorticism in 55.2% to 78.1%.[16,51-53,102,103] Diabetes insipidus at postsurgery follow-up is observed in 59.4% to 95% of patients.[16,51,52,94,102,103] A new postsurgical diabetes insipidus in children occurred in 56%.[16] Even if hormone levels seem to be adequate in the short term after treatment, deficiencies may develop over years and these patients need to be monitored closely.[104] Diabetes insipidus may be reversible in some of the patients in whom the stalk was dissected as distally as possible from the tumor although ultimately sacrificed.[105] Such recovery was not observed in another study[103] and in our experience. New diabetes insipidus occurred in 20% of our patients. Permanent hormonal replacement was necessary in 90% of these patients.

Lower quality of life is observed most often after radical removal of retrochiasmatic craniopharyngiomas involving the hypothalamus. Besides the retrochiasmatic tumor location there are other different predictors of postsurgical morbidity: severe hydrocephalus, large size of the tumor, intraoperative adverse events, and young age.[12,74,106-108] Recurrences and additional surgery were also associated with poorer quality of life.[74]

Obesity at follow-up after surgery is found in 58% to 62%.[108-110] Weight gain of different degrees occurred after surgery in 20% of our pediatric patients; in one third of them it was evaluated as the consequence of increased appetite. A risk factor is also familial disposition for obesity.[111] Significantly greater increase of the body mass index was observed in patients with the highest score of postsurgical hypothalamic damage as seen on follow-up MRI scans. Preoperative neuroimaging, however, demonstrated extensive hypothalamic "infiltration" by tumor in most of them.[107] This is in concordance with our experience that the disruption of the third ventricular floor found on MRI scans after removal of IEVCs is most often due to the preoperative damage to the hypothalamus caused by the tumor itself. The postoperative weight gain appears to result from continued impact of preoperative hypothalamic damage.[110] Another cause of obesity may be hypothalamic irradiation with the dose of 51 Gy or more.[112]

The data on mental disorders significantly differ in the literature. Significant school problems after radical tumor removal in children were observed in none[15] to 50%.[108] The neuropsychological outcome in a recent study was more benign than some previous studies have suggested.[113] Satisfactory neuropsychological assessment is reported in almost all pediatric patients.[114] Resolution of the preoperative impairment of cognitive functions in a few weeks in a majority of patients in a large series was reported. New cognitive disorders or personality changes were caused mostly by multiple recurrences treated with surgery and radiotherapy.[95] According to Pierre-Kahn and associates, postoperative academic failure, when present, results more from a behavioral dysfunction than from an understanding incapability.[82] Deleterious behavior (running away, theft, lies, irritability, aggressiveness, and bursts of rage) was observed in all 12 patients with the tumor extending into the third ventricle. Only 2 of their 14 children, both with extraventricular tumors, were attending normal schooling. We have observed mental disturbances much more rarely. The episodes of emotional lability and aggressiveness occurred in 1 child. Another 2 children who were less spontaneous and had less interest in fulfilling daily duties before surgery continued to be the same after the operation. Impaired cognitive functions present before surgery in 2 children improved. Long-lasting temporary memory disturbances occurred in 1 adult. We observed fatigue and worsened physical condition in some of the adult patients after otherwise successful surgical treatment of supradiaphragmatic craniopharyngiomas similar to those reported by others.[115]

Postsurgical behavioral problems may be attributed also to presumed implication of the frontal lobes arising from the surgical approach, which mediates aspects of impulsivity and cognitive flexibility to the hypothalamus which in turn plays an integral role in affect regulation.[74]

Visual functions after tumor removal are stabilized or improved in a majority of patients. Postsurgical visual impairment occurs in 5% to 66%.[12,15,16,60,62,65,83,95,108] A risk factor is prechiasmatic extension of the tumor.[16] In our patients vision improved after surgery in 13% and worsened in 7%. The patient operated on at the age of 11 months with "practical blindness," paradoxical reaction to light, and still recordable visual evoked potentials can read without difficulties, although in one eye only light perception is present.

CYSTS OF THE SUPRASELLAR REGION

In terminology and morphology of the cysts occurring in the suprasellar space a considerable overlap may be found. The term *suprasellar cyst* is sometimes used as a synonym for *craniopharyngioma* or for *arachnoid cyst*.[116] Epidermoid cysts occurring in the suprasellar region are regarded as a variant of craniopharyngioma.[2,117] Rathke's cleft cysts and craniopharyngiomas share a common origin in embryological remnants of the fetal stomodeal cleft. Dumbbell lesions with both types of epithelia—the columnar in the intrasellar part and squamous in the suprasellar part—have been described.[118]

Epidermoid and Dermoid Cysts

Epidermoid cysts and the rarer dermoid cysts arise from the inclusion of ectodermally committed cells at time of closure of the neural groove.[119] Epidermoid cysts account for 1% of all intracranial tumors. About one third of them are situated in some way within the cisterns of the suprasellar region.[2]

Epidermoid cysts tend to occur in older age groups and show a slower natural progression than most craniopharyngiomas. The epidermoid cyst wall is composed of multilayered, keratinized squamous epithelium that rests on an outer layer of collagen. The contents are more likely to be solid, flaky, keratinous rather than the oily fluid typical of craniopharyngiomas. The center of larger cysts sometimes degenerates, the keratin flakes being replaced by greasy brownish fluid containing cholesterol crystals. There is often a patchy chronic inflammatory infiltrate around the outer aspect of the capsule, and adjacent neural tissue almost always shows a dense gliosis with Rosenthal fibers. In the dermoid cyst also the adnexa are found.

Clinical presentation is usually similar to that of craniopharyngiomas, with visual defects and pituitary or hypothalamic dysfunction. Less commonly, episodes of aseptic meningitis occur as a result of leakage of cyst contents into the CSF pathways. On the other hand, even after massive rupture of a suprasellar dermoid cyst excellent recovery could be achieved.[120]

On both T1 and T2 MRI scans epidermoid cysts are slightly more hyperintense compared with CSF-containing arachnoid cysts (Fig. 39.22). With fluid-attenuated inversion recovery (FLAIR) and diffusion-weighted pulse sequences, epidermoid cysts show higher signal intensity than does CSF. The signal intensity of dermoid cysts is usually like that of fat and may be similar to that of lipomas.

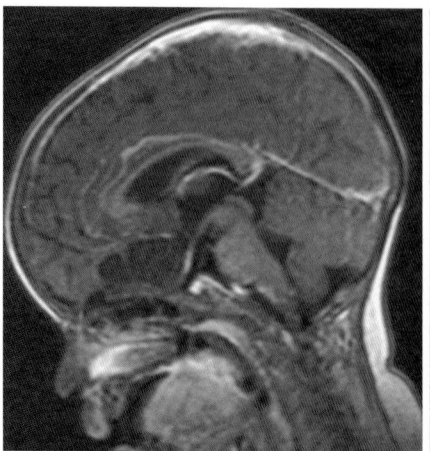 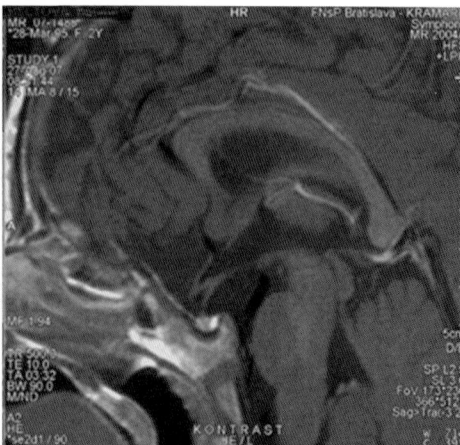 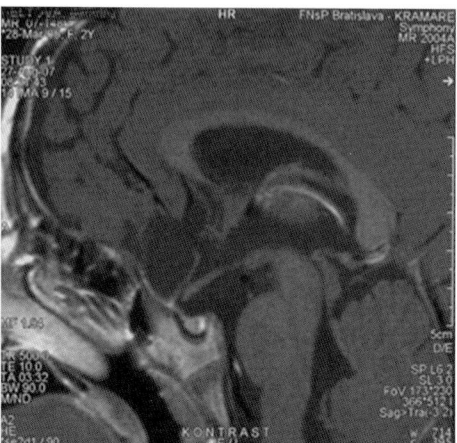

FIGURE 39.22 Suprachiasmatic epidermoid cyst removed via the subfrontal approach.

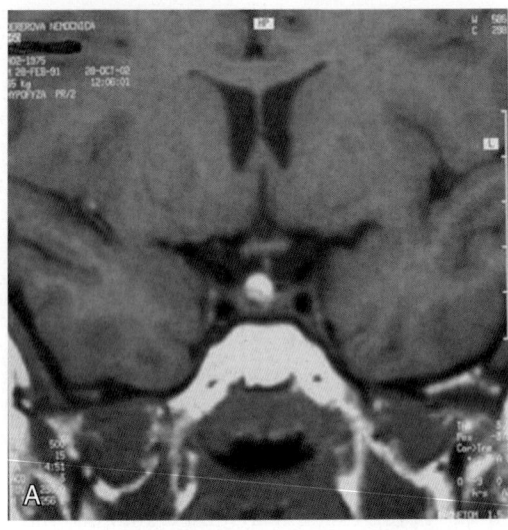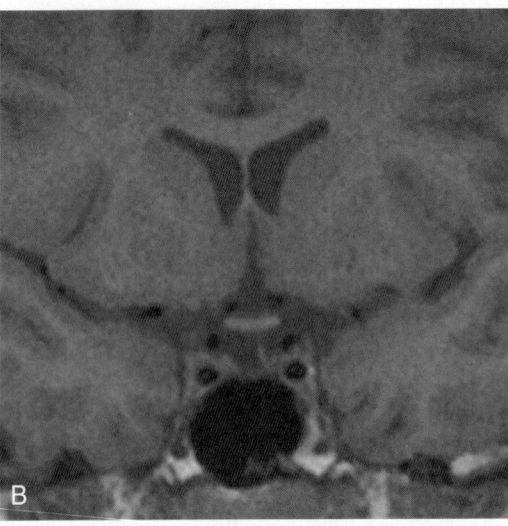

FIGURE   39.23 Suprasellar Rathke's cleft cyst on magnetic resonance imaging (MRI) T1-weighted nonenhanced scan (**A**) removed via the subfrontal approach (**B**).

The ideal treatment is complete surgical removal, but dense adherence of the capsule to adjacent neural and vascular structures may make an attempt at radical resection of the cyst wall hazardous and unwise. If incompletely resected, the epidermoid and dermoid cyst will slowly recur. Chemical meningitis due to leakage of keratin into the CSF pathways during surgery should be prevented by cottonoid blocking of the cisterns and voluminous saline irrigation of the operative field. Local application of steroids is also recommended.

Rathke's Cleft Cyst

Fragments of Rathke's cleft persist in adults as microscopic cysts between the anterior and posterior lobes of the mature pituitary gland. It is presumed the remnants of the cleft persist also above the level of the sellar diaphragm in the pituitary stalk.[117]

The lining epithelium of the Rathke's cleft cyst (RCC) consists of columnar or cuboidal cells with apical cilia, which may be stratified at places. In the suprasellar part of RCCs, the areas of stratified squamous epithelium may be found and occasionally may be very prominent. This has been interpreted as evidence of a close etiological relationship between craniopharyngiomas and RCCs.[117] Keratinization is not seen. Lining epithelium may undergo extensive degeneration, leaving only a collagenous wall in some places.

RCCs are a relatively common incidental finding in otherwise normal adult pituitary glands. Larger symptomatic cysts are very rare. Headache is relatively common. Other symptoms are caused by compression of the pituitary, optic chiasm, or hypothalamus. Recurrent episodes of aseptic meningitis due to cyst leakage into the subarachnoid space may occur. The age at presentation ranges from the second to the eighth decade, with a mean in the fourth decade. Females are more commonly affected than males.

MRI shows a single, uniloculated, round, sharply defined intra- or suprasellar mass that typically lies anterior to the infundibular stalk. The cystic contents may have variable signal intensity: either low signal intensity on T1 images and high signal intensity on T2 images resembling CSF, or high signal intensity on T1 images and variable signal intensity on T2 images owing to a high mucopolysaccharide content. Neither contrast enhancement nor calcifications are usually seen.[3]

Intrasellar and suprasellar Rathke's cleft cysts are approached transsphenoidally. Partial resection of the cyst wall and evacuation of the contents achieved microsurgically or by means of the endoscope is considered the best treatment.[121-123] It allows adequate decompression of the pituitary tissue and the optic chiasm, with possible improvement of preoperative visual and endocrine deficit.[121] Radical resection of the cyst wall may endanger the pituitary stalk. Incomplete removal of the cyst wall, however, leads to recurrences reported in all of the above-mentioned series. Suprasellar lesions are most often exposed through craniotomy.[122,124] Preservation of the pituitary stalk in our patient did not result in improvement of preoperative endocrine deficiency (Fig. 39.23).

GLIOMAS OF THE CHIASM AND HYPOTHALAMUS

Gliomas starting from the optic chiasm may involve the hypothalamus along direct optic fascicles from the lateral chiasm to the anterior hypothalamus.[125] On the other hand, tumors arising within the walls of the third ventricle can infiltrate the chiasm. Usually it is impossible to determine whether the tumor started in the hypothalamus or in the optic chiasm, either clinically or radiologically.[126] The gliomas of the chiasm and hypothalamus are therefore often referred to as a single disease entity named *optic chiasmatic-hypothalamic gliomas,*[125,127,128] *optic pathway/hypothalamic gliomas,*[126] *chiasmal/hypothalamic gliomas,*[129] or *hypothalamic/chiasmatic gliomas.*[130] Konovalov and colleagues[129] distinguish nodular-type and diffuse-type tumors. The nodular type is classified into five groups according to the dominant directions of growth and possible place of origin along the visual pathway: (1) tumors with predominant anterior growth, (2) tumors growing anteriorly and penetrating the third ventricle, (3) tumors with the main part occupying the third ventricle but infiltrating the chiasm as well,

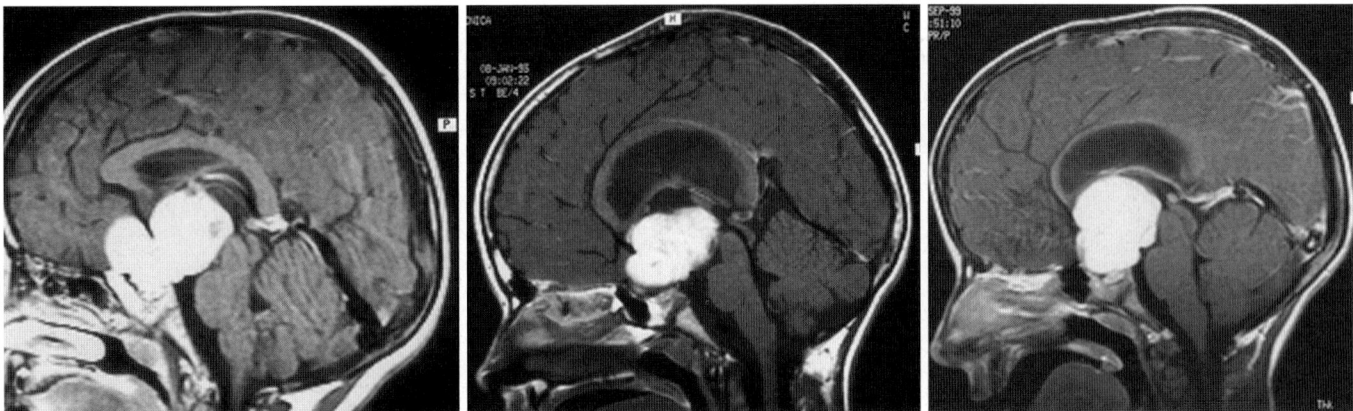

FIGURE 39.24 Variants of the relationship of chiasmatic/hypothalamic gliomas with the anterior communicating artery (see text).

(4) tumors of the optic tract, and (5) gliomas of the floor of the third ventricle. Kornienko and Pronin[131] presented similar classification with the fifth group determined as the tumors of the third ventricle, growing into its lumen and causing occlusion of the CSF pathways.

Almost 90% of the chiasmatic/hypothalamic gliomas (CHGs) are found in the pediatric age group. The usual age of presentation is 2 to 4 years.[132] CHGs in children represent 10% to 18.8% of the tumors of perisellar area.[3,30] In children, the CHGs are typically pilocytic astrocytomas; in general about 40% are fibrillary and 60% are pilocytic in type. Anaplastic astrocytomas are rare (8%) and more often localized in the third ventricle (group 5).[129]

Our surgical experience showed that the gliomas occluding the greater part of or the entire third ventricular chamber may differ in relation to the structures of the optic pathway and the diencephalon. Besides the tumors infiltrating the chiasm or the hypothalamus or both, we found gliomas similar to group 5 of Konovalov and colleagues[129] which infiltrated one lateral wall of the third ventricle and usually only touched the other one and the floor of the ventricle, or was just slightly attached to the latter. According to Yasargil[90] astrocytic tumors of the third ventricle may arise from the ventricular wall as well as from the periventricular region. Fibrillary astrocytomas typically arise from the region of thalamus.[133] We assume these tumors start to grow in the subependymal layer of the lateral wall of the third ventricle, break through it at an early stage of their development, and later grow inside the cavity of the third ventricle.

Differentiation between these two types of gliomas occupying the third ventricle is important from a surgical point of view. To a certain degree this can be assumed according to the relationship of the tumor mass with the AComA. A tumor growing inside the chiasm may expand anterior to the artery. All tumors that did not infiltrate the chiasm or the hypothalamus were located entirely behind the AComA. However, some tumors infiltrating the chiasm were located completely behind the vessel as well (Fig. 39.24). Consequently, in some instances it is not possible to differentiate between these topographic groups on the basis of preoperative MRI scans.

CHGs are almost always hypointense with T1-weighted images and hyperintense with T2-weighted and FLAIR

sequences. Large tumors are heterogeneous with cystic and solid components, with the latter enhancing markedly after contrast material injection.[3]

Clinical Presentation

Progressive loss of vision in tumors of the chiasm is accompanied by slowly developing optic atrophy. Visual fields show less typical hemianopic defects than in craniopharyngiomas.[30] Defects in the temporal half of the visual field of the "better" eye combined with practical blindness in the other eye is typical for chiasmatic gliomas.[129] Association of the visual disturbances with diabetes insipidus, obesity, and genital underdevelopment indicates hypothalamic involvement. Obesity is seen predominantly in adults. Sexual development is nearly normal, but a specific syndrome, precocious puberty, is seen in 8% of children.[129] In CHGs "diencephalic syndrome" is observed in up to 25% of children aged less than 3 years. It is characterized by marked emaciation and loss of subcutaneous fat, which contrasts with normal height and normal (or near-normal) muscle mass. The appetite is normal. The child is alert, vigorous, hyperactive, and may be euphoric.[132] The syndrome is associated with nystagmoid eye movements. Nystagmus is common also independently from the diencephalic syndrome.

Management of Chiasmatic/Hypothalamic Gliomas

The natural course of the CHGs is highly unpredictable. Some tumors remain static and quiescent for many years; others take an aggressive course, increasing rapidly in size and frequently leading to the patient's death. Involution of a pilocytic astrocytoma[134] and fibrillary astrocytoma[135] of the chiasm after partial tumor removal or biopsy has been documented. Others have observed tumor regression only after "substantial" (more than 50%) tumor resection.[126] The natural course is not always in accordance with the histological nature of the tumor. The patterns of malignancy were revealed in some pilocytic astrocytomas: frequent mitoses, pronounced endothelial proliferation, and necrotic foci.[129] The expectation of more aggressive course of fibrillary astrocytomas has not proved to be entirely predictive.[127] There is also disagreement about the

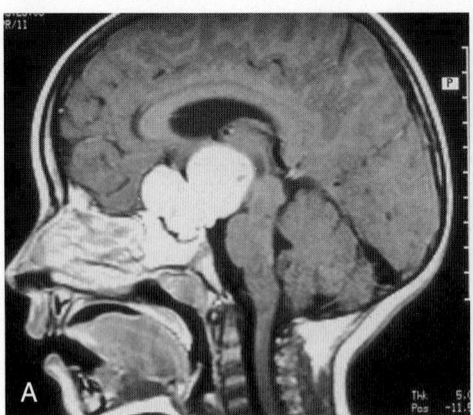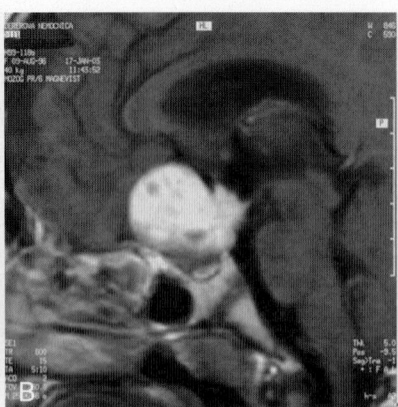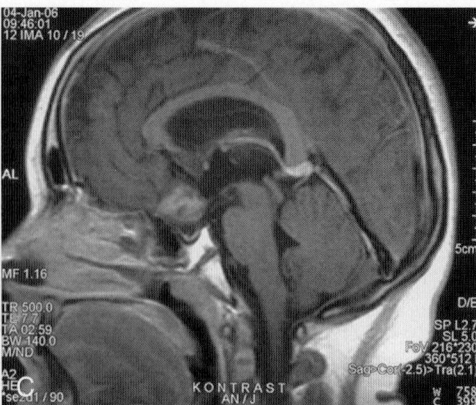

FIGURE 39.25 Chiasmatic/hypothalamic pilocytic astrocytoma (**A**) 41 months after removal of the intraventricular part of the tumor (**B**) and 33 months after external radiotherapy causing tumor regression (**C**).

significance of the association of the tumor with neurofibromatosis 1 (NF1).[132] While some authors have reported better prognosis in these patients,[126] according to others the association with NF1 is prognostically unfavorable[134] and is a predictor of progressive disease.[136]

Prognostic uncertainty led to a divergence of opinion about the management of these tumors.[127] Some authors recommend conservative surgery or biopsy followed by radiation and chemotherapy;[130] others stress the important role of more radical resection.[129,137]

Surgery

The main aim of surgery was to obtain tissue for histological diagnosis and restoration of the patency of the CSF pathways. There is also a trend toward a more radical tumor removal which leads to a much lower recurrence rate and better outcome than partial resection.[129,137,138] The indications for tumor resection are its nodular or exophytic growth without optic tract involvement[136,138] or visual failure.[127,128]

Surgical Approach and the Extent of Tumor Removal

Surgical approaches to CHGs are those commonly used to access the suprasellar region: subfrontal, pterional, subtemporal, anterior interhemispheric, transcallosal, and combined transcallosal-subfrontal and transcallosal-pterional.[127] Our preferred surgical approach to CHGs is subfrontal craniotomy as presented for craniopharyngiomas. The chiasm exposed below the frontal lobe is enlarged and infiltrated by the anterior part of the tumor in the majority of cases and it is not possible to discern the functioning parts of the visual pathway. From the enlarged and infiltrated chiasm we remove only a distinct tumor nodule found in a minority of patients. In cases in which no such nodule can be seen from the surface we enter the tumor through a small incision just below the AComA where the lamina terminalis is expected. From there we proceed posteriorly in the direction of the third ventricle. If an evident tumor is found inside the chiasm we remove only its central portion. In a majority of cases we leave the entire chiasmatic portion of the tumor (Fig. 39.25). This technique allowed us to preserve visual functions in all patients. The most common tumor in this location, the pilocytic astrocytomas, despite its benign nature infiltrates the optic pathways.[139,140]

The posterior part of a CHG often infiltrates the floor of the third ventricle. Gross total tumor removal was achieved in a patient in whom hypothalamic pilocytic astrocytoma did not infiltrate the chiasm and could be distinguished from the floor of the third ventricle (see video). In the great majority of the cases this part of the tumor is also left behind. We usually remove radically only the upper part of the tumor located inside the third ventricle where it is not intimately attached to the lateral walls. Although removal of the tumor from the third ventricular cavity is considered to be the most dangerous part of surgery,[132] our experience showed that this part of the tumor behaves as "exophytic," as also noted by others.[136,138] This "ventricular component of the intraaxial tumor"[89] may be safely removed. However, in a subgroup of the tumors adhering only to one lateral wall of the third ventricle radical resection was possible in more than half of the patients (see Fig. 39.26 and video).

During the translamina terminalis approach the most superoposterior part of a large tumor reaching the roof of the third ventricle may not be exposed.[141] It is hidden behind and above the AComA. The vessel may react even to gentle stretching by spasm. These tumors may be exposed via the transcallosal approach. The interhemispheric approach to the corpus callosum in some patients without previous shunt insertion may require evacuation of the CSF by ventricular puncture. The transcallosal route, however, in some cases does not enable appropriate exposure of the inferoanterior part of the third ventricle. Therefore, a combined transcallosal and translamina terminalis approach may be necessary for the exposure of the entire tumor.[129]

Management of Hydrocephalus

Adequate resection of the upper part of the tumor blocking the foramina of Monro restores the CSF passage. However, after partial tumor removal the reopened CSF pathways may become obstructed again as a result of postoperative edema. In some patients with subtotal or radical tumor removal communicating hydrocephalus may be observed. In these cases shunt insertion after tumor resection may be necessary.

FIGURE 39.26 Fibrillary astrocytoma of the third ventricle with intratumoral bleeding (**A** and **B**) radically removed via the translamina terminalis approach (**C** and **D**).

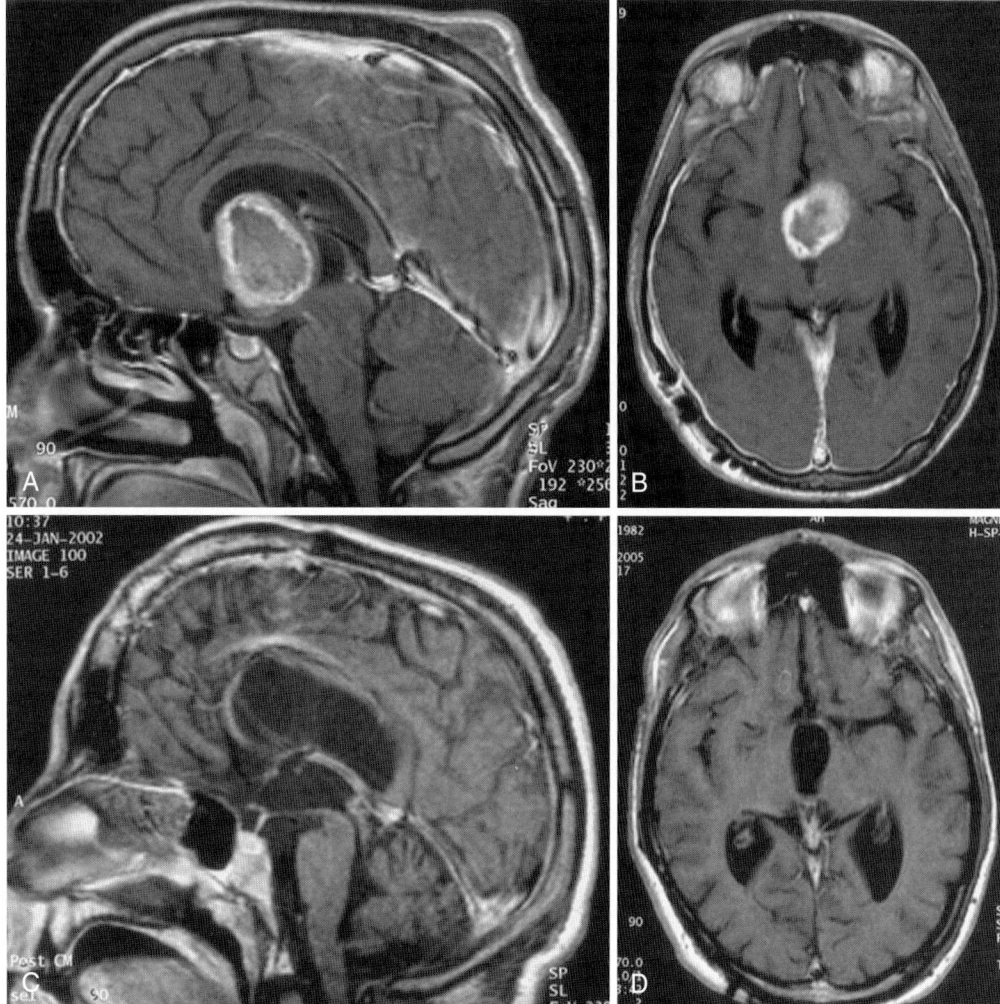

Preoperative CSF diversion may be necessary in acute onset of increased intracranial pressure as an emergency procedure, either as shunt implantation or an external ventricular drainage. We experienced such situations only in gliomas taking their origin from the lateral walls of the ventricle and not in the CHGs.

Adjuvant Therapy

Unlike in the benign gliomas of other locations radiotherapy and chemotherapy are often recommended in CHGs. In general, radiation therapy arrests the tumor growth, although there are reports of irradiated tumors shrinking or completely disappearing.[139] The most utilized dosages range between 45 and 56.6 Gy (median 54 Gy) for chiasmatic gliomas and 55 and 60 Gy for hypothalamic tumors. The efficiency of radiation therapy is reported to be as low as 40% of cases.[132,139] The course of radiation therapy in our series was recommended by medical/radiation oncologists in eight patients with pilocytic and in six others with fibrillary astrocytomas. In eight patients the tumor regressed (five pilocytic, three fibrillary), in five it remained stable (two pilocytic, three fibrillary), and in one (pilocytic) it progressed and had to be reoperated.

Radiation therapy carries a risk of serious adverse effects.[2,16,137] We have observed postradiation complications in two children. MRI performed 11 months after the dose of 50 Gy in a 6-year-old boy showed complete regression of the residual pilocytic astrocytoma and a pathological signal in the right thalamus and the mesencephalon. Afterward the patient lost the sight of both eyes, became obese, and now, 12 years after radiation, he has outbursts of rage. Another patient with residual fibrillary astrocytoma developed diabetes insipidus 2 months after completion of radiation treatment.

Despite their benign nature, most of the CHGs can respond surprisingly well to chemotherapy, allowing for tumor shrinkage and stabilization, or even disappearance in some instances.[130,132,137] Thus, even if radiotherapy is necessary, it can be postponed beyond the age of 5 years to limit its deleterious side effects on intellectual, visual, and endocrine functions.[127,132]

Complications

The most severe complication of early postoperative outcome, acute hypothalamic insufficiency, occurred in two of our patients. We have not seen these disturbances in other patients in whom only the "exophytic" part of the tumor was removed from the third ventricular cavity. Careful monitoring and correction of metabolic disorders as described at craniopharyngiomas were successful in both patients.

Another serious complication is bleeding into the tumor bed, which should be evacuated. Removal of CHGs often results in brain collapse, subdural CSF and blood collection, or tension pneumocephalus, which require additional surgical intervention in 5% of cases. The risk factors are ventriculomegaly and tumor size more than 5 cm.[129] There were no surgical deaths in our series of 34 patients.

Outcome

Radical tumor removal of CHGs may lead to a much better outcome than generally expected. Radicality of surgery dramatically influences the long-term outcome with 5- and 10-year progression-free survival probabilities for the radical, subtotal, and partial surgery of 100%, 74%, and 51%, respectively.[129] In our series including gliomas not infiltrating the chiasm and hypothalamus, after radical tumor removal 14 of 15 (93.3%) patients survived for 46 to 203 (mean 111.6) months; after incomplete removal 13 of 19 (68.4%) patients survived for 42 to 170 (mean 115.6) months. Good clinical condition at the end of follow-up after radical and incomplete removal was achieved in 66.7% and 42.1%, respectively. The cause of death during follow-up was progression of the disease in six patients; one died from pneumonia, and another one died from a nonmedical accident, both after being in good clinical condition.

In the series of Konovalov and colleagues[129] visual functions in the early postoperative period improved in 14% of patients and worsened in 23%. During the follow-up period further improvement was observed; altogether, vision improved in 28%. Deterioration of vision seen at the end of follow-up in 22% was due to recurrence of tumor. Growth retardation and diabetes insipidus (12%) were rare, unlike in craniopharyngiomas, but most patients developed obesity and some precocious puberty (18%).

We avoided postoperative worsening of visual functions by conservative surgery of the anterior portion of the tumor infiltrating the chiasm. Hypopituitarism occurred in three patients, and in one of them obesity and mood instability also occurred. Memory disturbances were observed in one patient. According to the clinical course this morbidity could also be attributed to radiotherapy. Mild intellectual impairment and oculomotor paresis occurred after postoperative bleeding into the third ventricle, tetraparesis after acute subdural hematoma, and meningitis after repeated shunt revisions. There were no severely disabled patients operated on during the past 15 years except for the patient who presented in a comatose state.

GERMINOMAS

Pure germinomas are the most common primary CNS germ cell tumors (GCTs), which account for up to 0.5% of all CNS tumors in general and 3% of CNS tumors in children. Germinoma tissue may also be found in mixed GCTs.[140] The large majority of CNS GCTs occurs about a midline intracranial axis that traverses the third ventricle. Occasionally there is a synchronous pineal and suprasellar region tumor.

It is important to differentiate pure germinomas from those containing an admixture of other GCTs or syncytiotrophoblastic giant cells (STGCs) secreting human chorionic gonadotropin (hCG).[142] Pure germinomas are typically nonsecreting tumors, whereas in nongerminatous GCTs elevation of either α-fetoprotein or human β-hCG in the serum or the CSF is found. "Marker negative" germinomas are prognostically most favorable.

Suprasellar germinomas are infiltrative lesions that tend to involve a variety of structures, including the floor of the third ventricle, pituitary stalk, pituitary gland, and the optic nerves, chiasm, and tracts.[2] Clinical manifestations include visual disturbances, diabetes insipidus, obesity, and pituitary insufficiency. At the time of diagnosis the diabetes insipidus is more frequent and obesity occurs less often than in children with craniopharyngiomas.[143] Precocious puberty almost exclusively occurring in boys may be the consequence of involvement of the hypothalamus[30] and the effect of hCG.[144] Tumors blocking the third ventricle produce the symptoms of increased intracranial pressure.

Most suprasellar germinomas are clearly detected on MRI as homogeneous isointensive or mildly hypointensive on T1-weighted images, and isointensive or hyperintensive on T2-weighted images. On rare occasions they contain small cysts.[3,131] Usually they intensively accumulate contrast medium. Neuroimaging studies may demonstrate CSF-borne metastases along ventricular surfaces or in subarachnoid space.

Germinomas are extremely radiosensitive; therefore, until recently radiotherapy was the cornerstone of treatment. In the past a single fractionated dose has been delivered to the tumor site to assess its radiosensitivity ("biological biopsy"). If a radiographic response was demonstrated, the tumor was considered to have a germinal origin, and high-dose focal radiotherapy was initiated. Because of associated long-term sequelae and morbidity of craniospinal radiotherapy in young children, however, recent strategies have been developed to avoid or reduce the role of radiotherapy in the treatment of germinomas.[140] In our patient, an 18-year-old girl, residual germinoma resolved completely after focal and whole-brain radiation therapy. Seven years after treatment multiple cavernous malformations were found on MRI.

It has become more prevalent to initiate chemotherapy as the primary treatment for patients with CNS GCTs. Pure germinomas demonstrate an 80% complete radiographic response with chemotherapeutic regimens, regardless of the extent of tumor extension. Patients with pure germinomas, included in a good-prognosis group by Matsutani,[145] are treated by three courses of carboplatin-etoposide chemotherapy followed by local radiation dose (24 Gy) delivered to a generous local field. Germinomas with STGC receive 30 Gy to a generous local field and 20 Gy to the tumor site and two additional courses of chemotherapy.

HYPOTHALAMIC HAMARTOMAS

Hamartomas are non-neoplastic nonprogressive congenital malformations that are composed of disordered neurons, glial cells, and myelinated tracts. Hamartomas occurring in the region of the hypothalamus (HH) occur in two general locations: those below the tuber cinereum are usually pedunculated, and those within the third ventricle are sessile.[146,147]

Pedunculated lesions are more likely to be small (less than 2 cm) and to cause precocious puberty but no other neurological symptoms. Etiologically important is a presence of neurons immunolabeling for gonadotropin-releasing factors

FIGURE 39.27 A, Sessile hypothalamic hamartoma subtotally removed via the trans-lamina terminalis approach. **B,** Small remnant of the tumor left because of missing borders with the mammillary bodies.

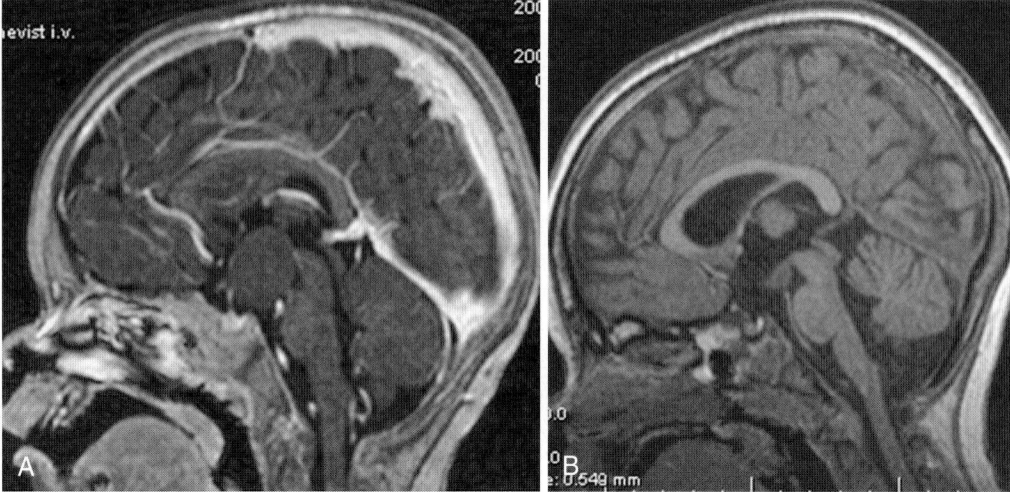

within the hamartoma. Sessile lesions are more often large (2-5 cm) and associated with seizures, particularly gelastic seizures. Subsequently the seizures are of longer duration and develop secondary, generalized epileptic manifestations. Cognitive deterioration ensues and severe behavioral problems commonly develop as well. Approximately two thirds of children with sessile HH have developmental delays, and half also have precocious puberty.[146,147]

Hamartoma is isointense or mildly hypointense on T1-weighted images and isointense to hyperintense on T2-weighted images, with no contrast enhancement, which is helpful in differential diagnosis from other lesions.[3]

Pedunculated HH may be approached via a pterional or subtemporal route. After total removal of the lesion, half of the patients were cured. Subtotal resection rarely leads to clinical and hormonal success.[146] Sessile hamartomas within the third ventricle can be approached through a transcallosal route.[148] After complete or near complete resection via interfornicial route three children were seizure-free, and the seizures in the other two were only occasional, brief, and mild. The children also exhibited marked improvements in behavior, school performance, and quality of life.[148] The main difficulty of surgery seems to be the differentiation between the tissue of hamartoma and normal brain tissue.[146,149] We had the same experience with the sessile HH approached through opening of the lamina terminalis. A small part of the lesion had to be left at the region of the mammillary bodies (Fig. 39.27). Endoscopic removal or disconnection of the hamartoma from the hypothalamus may also lead to clinical improvement.[150]

PITUICYTOMAS (TUMORS OF THE NEUROHYPOPHYSIS)

The tumors of neurohypophysis originate in the pituicytes, modified glial cells of the posterior pituitary gland and

infundibulum. Therefore, they may start to grow within the sella or above it. The term *pituicytoma* was historically also used for other tumors of neurohypophysis (granular cell tumors, pilocytic astrocytomas);[151] the terms *choristoma* and *infundibuloma* were also used.[3] Pituicytoma, a spindle cell neoplasm, is now distinguished from the granular cell tumor of the neurohypophysis composed of nests of large cells with granular, eosinophilic cytoplasm.[152] Both tumors are benign (WHO grade I). Pituicytomas are reported to be extremely rare, occurring only in adults, and granular cell tumors may exceptionally occur also in children.

The clinical presentation in both tumor types resembles that of other slowly expanding lesions of the sellar/suprasellar region. The most common presenting symptom is visual field deficit; other symptoms include various types of hypopituitarism, galactorrhea ("stalk effect"), headache, and diabetes insipidus, which is rather uncommon.[152]

The tumors are very rare, and surgical experience is therefore limited. The firm and vascular nature of the granular cell tumors, sometimes combined with absence of an obvious dissection plane from adjacent brain, may hamper gross total resection.[152] In another case report of a suprasellar granular cell tumor there is no mention about intraoperative bleeding; the gummy, yellowish, slightly glassy tumor could be removed completely.[153] Significant bleeding occurred also in reported cases of pituicytomas; one of them necessitated embolization prior to repeated surgery.[154,155]

The pituicytoma seen in our patient, a 30-year-old woman, presented with diabetes insipidus and hypopituitarism. MRI showed isointense retrochiasmatic infundibular lesion on both T1- and T2-weighted images with significant contrast enhancement. The tumor was removed via the trans-lamina terminalis approach without significant bleeding. Although the pituitary stalk could be preserved (Fig. 39.28), no substantial improvement in endocrinological status was achieved.

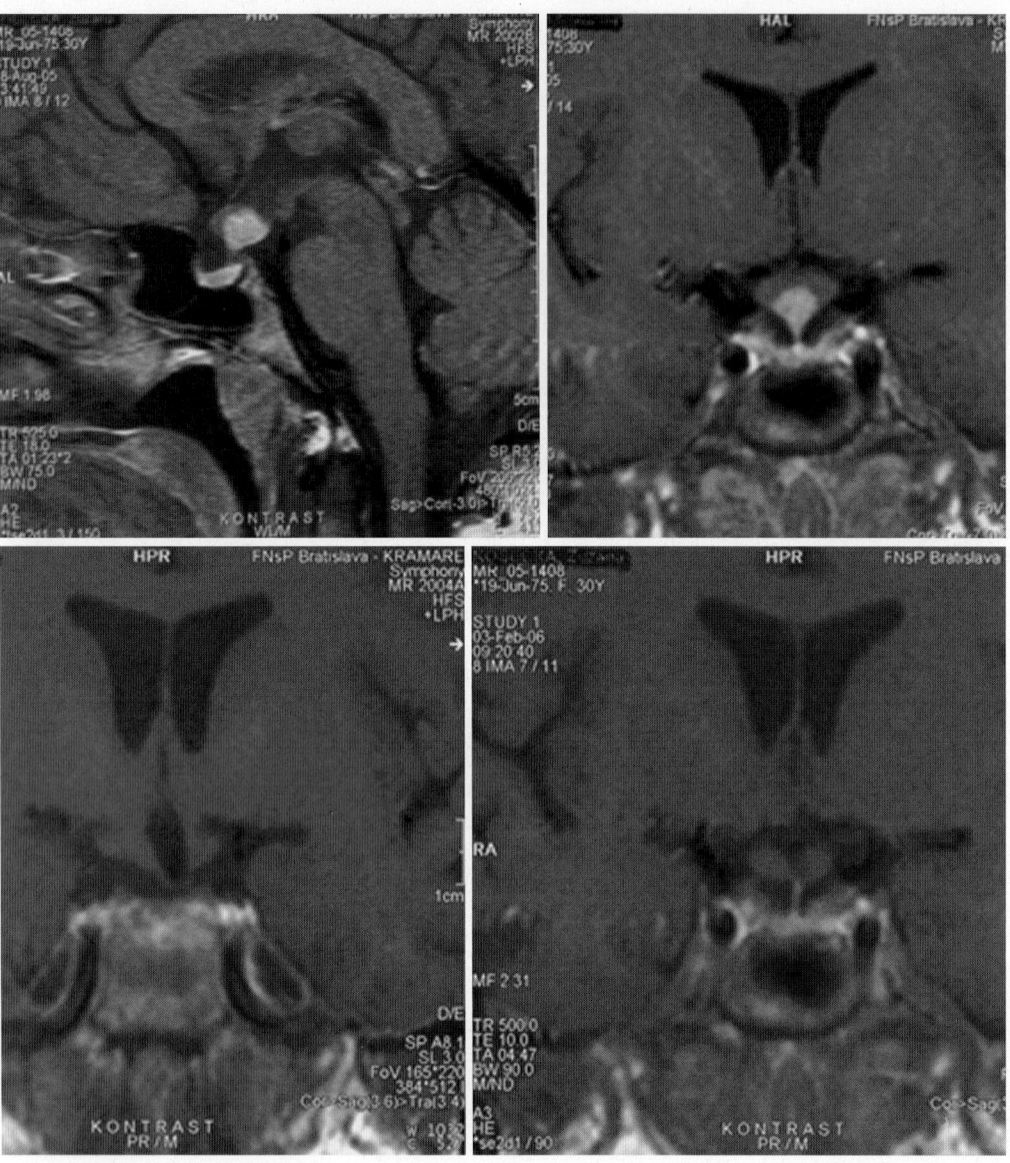

FIGURE 39.28 Pituicytoma radically removed via the translamina terminalis approach with preservation of the pituitary stalk.

SELECTED KEY REFERENCES

Fahlbusch R, Honegger J, Paulus W, Buchfelder M. Surgical treatment of craniopharyngiomas: experience with 168 patients. *J Neurosurg.* 1999;90:237-250.

Konovalov AN. *Operative Management of Craniopharyngiomas. Advances and Technical Standards in Neurosurgery.* Vol. 8, New York: Springer-Verlag; 1981:281-318.

Šteňo J, Maláček M, Bízik I. Tumor-third ventricular relationships in supradiaphragmatic craniopharyngiomas: correlation of morphological, magnetic resonance imaging, and operative findings. *Neurosurgery.* 2004;54:1051-1060.

Šteňo J. Microsurgical topography of craniopharyngiomas. *Acta Neurochir Suppl (Wien).* 1985;35:94-100.

Yasargil MG, Curcic M, Kis M, et al. Total removal of craniopharyngiomas. *J Neurosurg.* 1990;73:3-11.

Please go to expertconsult.com to view the complete list of references.

Pituitary Tumors: Diagnosis and Management

Carrie R. Muh, Nelson M. Oyesiku

CLINICAL PEARLS

- Pituitary tumors present in various ways as a result of excess or deficient secretion of pituitary hormones or extrinsic compression on the pituitary stalk or adjacent structures. Approximately 75% of pituitary adenomas are functioning tumors; of these, half are prolactinomas, less than 25% secrete growth hormone (GH), and the rest secrete adrenocorticotropic hormone (ACTH), follicle-stimulating hormone (FSH), luteinizing hormone (LH), or thyroid-stimulating hormone (TSH).

- Functioning tumors often present with symptoms due to hormone hypersecretion, and nonfunctioning tumors generally present with symptoms due to mass effect.

- Transsphenoidal adenomectomy (TSA) is the first line of treatment for nonfunctioning tumors. Medical therapy is the first line of treatment for prolactinomas. Other functioning

adenomas generally require surgical resection, medical treatment, or radiation therapy. Surgery through the microscopic, extended transsphenoidal, or endoscopic route is safe and effective in experienced hands. Craniotomy may be required for a tumor extending beyond the sellar region.

- Patients with functioning pituitary adenomas require long-term follow-up to assess clinical and laboratory parameters. This is best done at a center that can provide a neurosurgeon, an endocrinologist, a radiation oncologist, and an ophthalmologist. Pituitary hormones should be regularly followed in all these patients; patients with residual tumor after treatment should be monitored with magnetic resonance imaging (MRI) scans, and patients with optic nerve compression require periodic formal visual field testing.

THE PITUITARY GLAND

The pituitary gland regulates the function of numerous other glands, including the thyroid, adrenals, ovaries, and testes. It controls linear growth, lactation, and uterine contractions in labor, and it manages osmolality and intravascular fluid volume via resorption of water in the kidneys. It secretes eight peptide hormones, six from the anterior lobe and two from the posterior lobe (Table 40.1).

The pituitary lies in the sella turcica, a saddle-shaped concavity in the sphenoid bone. Its stalk, which contains the pituitary portal veins and neuronal processes, passes through the diaphragma sella, just above which pass the optic nerves (Fig. 40.1). The cavernous venous sinuses form the lateral borders of the sella, and contain within them the internal carotid arteries, cranial nerves III, IV, and VI, and the ophthalmic and maxillary divisions of cranial nerve V.

In the anterior lobe of the pituitary gland, known as the *adenohypophysis*, five distinct types of cells produce and secrete six different hormones. Lactotroph cells make prolactin (PRL), somatotroph cells produce growth hormone (GH), corticotrophs secrete adrenocorticotropic hormone (ACTH), thyrotrophs make thyroid-stimulating hormone (TSH), and

gonadotrophs produce follicle-stimulating hormone (FSH) and luteinizing hormone (LH). The secretion of these hormones is regulated by the hypothalamus and by inhibitory feedback control by target organ hormone products (Figs. 40.2 and 40.3).

The posterior lobe of the pituitary, the neurohypophysis, secretes antidiuretic hormone (ADH) and oxytocin, which are produced by hypothalamic neurons and released directly from nerve terminals in the posterior pituitary.

The hypothalamus secretes releasing factors to stimulate the production of pituitary hormones. Corticotropin-releasing factor (CRH), thyrotropin-releasing factor (TRH), and gonadotropin-releasing hormone (GnRH) positively regulate the production of ACTH, TSH, and the gonadotropins, LH and FSH. GH secretion is more complicated in that it receives both positive and negative hypothalamic manipulation, via GH-releasing hormone (GHRH) and somatostatin, respectively. Prolactin secretion is primarily inhibited by the hypothalamic release of dopamine, also known as *prolactin-inhibiting factor*. Some of these hypothalamic factors influence the production of more than one anterior pituitary hormone. For instance, TRH, which primarily stimulates TSH production, also has a positive effect on prolactin release.

TABLE 40.1 Summary of Pituitary Functions

| Hypothalamus | PITUITARY | | Organ | END ORGAN | |
	Pituitary Cell	Pituitary Hormone		Hormone	Primary Functions
Anterior Lobe					
Releasing Factors					
Corticotropin-releasing hormone (CRH)	Corticotroph	Adrenocortico-tropic hormone (ACTH)—adre-nocorticotropin, corticotropin	Adrenals	Cortisol	General metabolism; required for physiologic adaptation to stress
Thyrotropin-releasing hormone	Thyrotroph	Thyroid-stimulating hormone (TSH)	Thyroid	Thyroid hormones—T_3, T_4	General metabolism; influences pace of metabolism
Gonadotropin-releasing hormone (GnRH)	Gonadotroph	Follicle-stimulating hormone (FSH)	Ovaries	Estradiol, progesterone	Required for normal female sexual development and fertility
		Luteinizing hormone (LH)	Testes	Testosterone	Required for normal male sexual development and fertility
Growth hormone–releasing hormone (GHRH)	Somatotroph	Growth hormone (GH)—somatotropin	Liver and other tissues	Somatomedin—insulin-like growth factor-I (IGF-I)	Growth, glucose regulation
Inhibiting Factors					
Dopamine—PIF	Lactotroph	Prolactin (PRL)	Breast, gonads	Prolactin	Lactation
Somatostatin	Somatotroph	Growth hormone (GH)	Liver and other tissues	Somatomedin—IGF-I	Growth, glucose regulation
Posterior Lobe					
Antidiuretic hormone (ADH)—vasopressin	ADH produced in hypothalamus stored in posterior pituitary		Kidney	ADH	Resorption of water in the kidney
Oxytocin	Oxytocin produced in hypothalamus; stored in posterior pituitary		Uterus	Oxytocin	Uterine contractions during labor

PIF, prolactin-inhibiting factor; T_3, triiodothyronine; T_4, thyroxine.

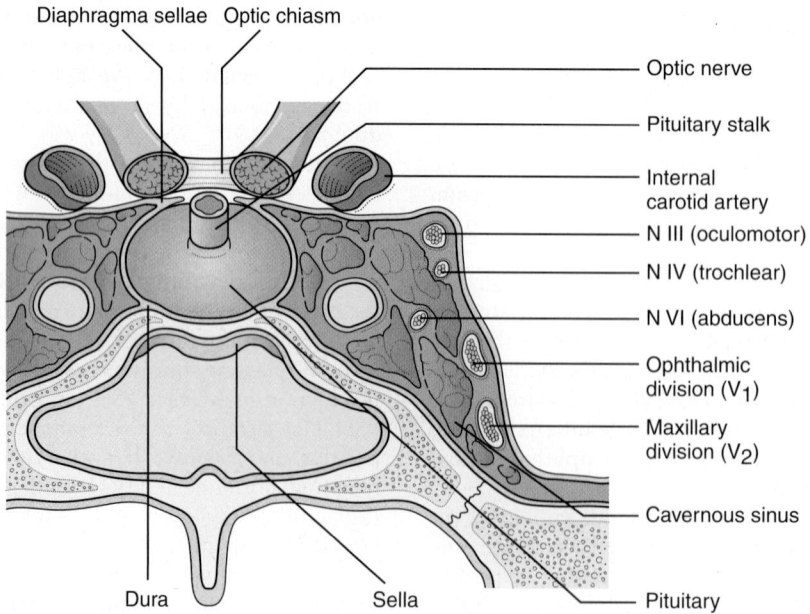

FIGURE 40.1 Anatomical relationships of the pituitary gland. A coronal section through the sella turcica shows the pituitary gland in relation to surrounding structures: the cavernous sinuses, carotid arteries, and cranial nerves II, III, IV, V_1, V_2, and VI.

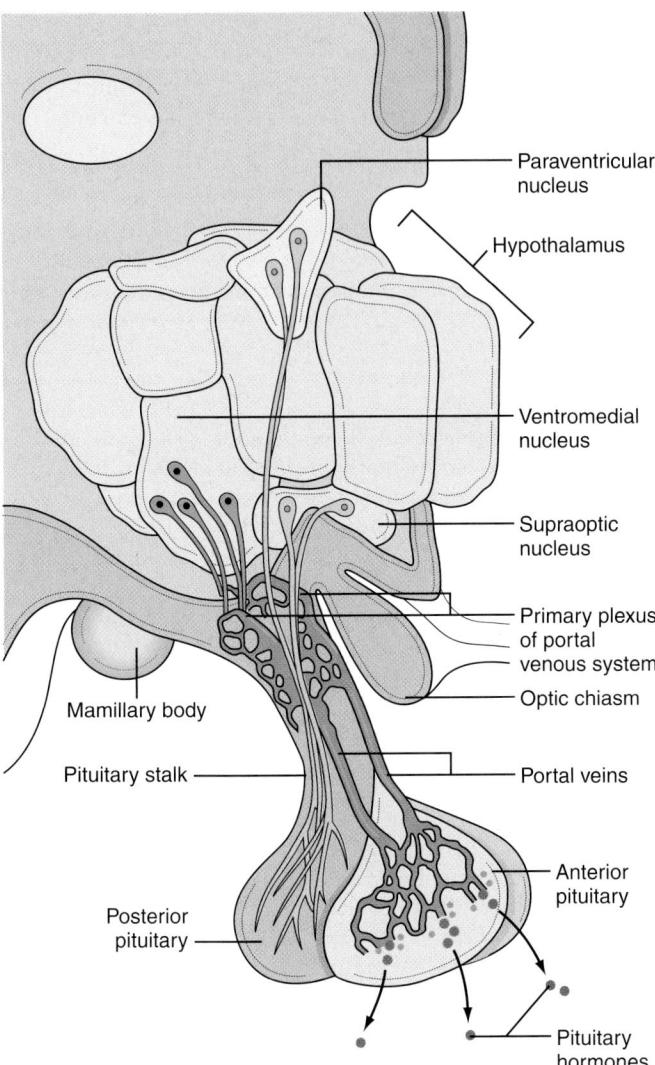

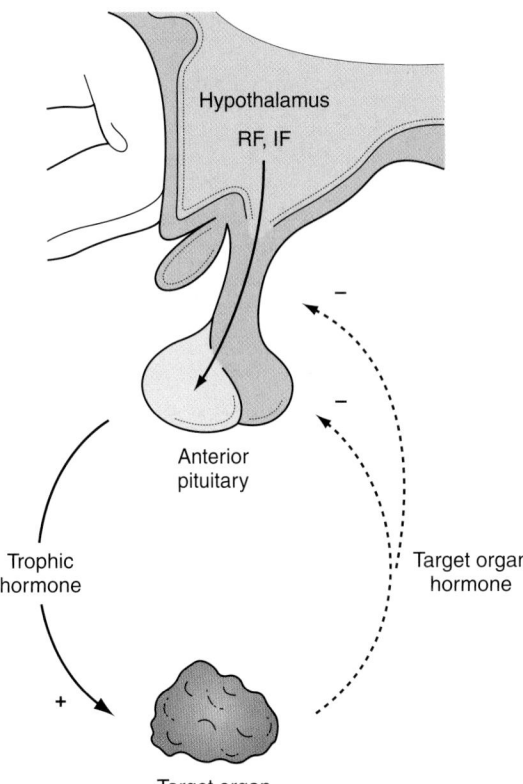

FIGURE 40.3 Negative feedback regulation of the anterior pituitary. The production and secretion of anterior pituitary hormones is inhibited by the hormonal products of the target organs.

FIGURE 40.2 Hypothalamic control of the pituitary. *Anterior pituitary*: The neural processes (*dark green*) of the hypothalamic nuclei terminate on fenestrated vessels of the portal venous system in the median eminence. The portal veins (*blue*) carry releasing and inhibiting factors to the anterior lobe of the pituitary, where they regulate the release of anterior pituitary hormones (*red*). *Posterior pituitary*: The neural processes (*light green*) of the hypothalamic neurons of the supraoptic and paraventricular nuclei (*yellow*) carry the posterior pituitary hormones, antidiuretic hormone, and oxytocin, which are released directly from nerve terminals in the posterior pituitary.

Pituitary adenomas are composed of adenohypophyseal cells, which constitute 10% to 15% of primary intracranial tumors. Among pituitary tumors, the majority are functioning, or hormone-secreting, tumors, while approximately 30% are classified as nonfunctioning adenomas.

Symptoms and signs of disorders affecting the pituitary reflect the function and anatomy of the gland. Because of its diverse array of functions as well as the multiple structures in close proximity to the gland, pituitary tumors present in various ways due to excess or deficient secretion of pituitary hormones or extrinsic compression on the pituitary stalk or adjacent structures.

EPIDEMIOLOGY

Pituitary adenomas have an annual incidence of 25 per 1 million people and account for nearly 10% of all surgically resected brain tumors, with nonfunctioning adenomas and prolactinomas being the most common pituitary tumors.[1,2] Many of these tumors are subclinical and may never present during a patient's lifetime; autopsy studies show an 11% to 27% incidence of occult microadenomas.[3-6] Pituitary tumors are the third most common primary intracranial neoplasm, behind glioma and meningioma,[7] and are more common among African Americans, in whom they account for more than 20% of central nervous system neoplasms.[8]

Microadenomas are most often found in women of childbearing age. Though studies in the 1970s appeared to demonstrate a higher incidence of adenomas among women than men, it is unclear if there is actually a higher prevalence among women or if the effect of a tumor on pituitary function and, therefore, reproduction leads to a higher rate of detection. Autopsy studies show no sex predominance.[2] Men with pituitary tumors more often present with macroadenomas in their fifth and sixth decades of life.[3]

CLASSIFICATION

The major classifications of pituitary tumors are based on their size, secretory abilities, and histological type. Tumors with a diameter of less than 10 mm are microadenomas, and those greater than 10 mm are macroadenomas. Tumors greater than 4 cm are considered giant adenomas.

Functioning adenomas are generally classified by the hormones they secrete. Any of the multiple cell types within the pituitary can lead to a functioning pituitary tumor. Functioning tumors may secrete PRL, GH, ACTH, FSH, LH, or TSH. Nonfunctioning tumors do not secrete clinically relevant levels of hormone. However, even among nonfunctioning tumors, multiple different tumor types are found, including null cell, oncocytoma, silent gonadotropin or glycopeptide-secreting, silent corticotropin-secreting, and silent somatotropin-secreting.[9]

According to the World Health Organization (WHO), tumors with benign histological features are typical pituitary adenomas, but rare invasive tumors with an increased rate of mitosis and extensive p53 nuclear reactivity are classified as atypical adenomas. Pituitary carcinoma is very rare, constituting less than 0.2% of pituitary tumors, and the diagnosis is made only when distant metastases are found.[10,11]

NONFUNCTIONING PITUITARY ADENOMAS

Nonfunctioning adenomas account for 30% of pituitary tumors.[12] The term *nonfunctioning* reflects the fact that these tumors do not cause clinical hormone hypersecretion and so do not cause hypersecretory syndromes.[13] These tumors are heterogeneous with multiple histopathological cell types. Though they do not cause signs of clinical hormone hypersecretion, histopathological evidence of hormone expression is evident in more than 40%.

Pathological specimens of null cell adenomas do not express hormones, but oncocytomas may show focal immunostaining for anterior pituitary hormones and produce hormones in vitro. Silent gonadotropes morphologically resemble glycopeptide-secreting tumors and stain positive for FSH, LH, or the common α-subunit. Silent somatotropes stain positive for GH and silent corticotrophs stain positive for ACTH on pathological specimen, but these tumors do not cause the clinical manifestations of acromegaly or hypercortisolemia, respectively.

Presentation

Nonfunctioning adenomas are benign lesions that are typically large upon presentation and manifest with symptoms of mass effect.[14] Pressure on the pituitary gland can lead to decreased pituitary function, and nearly one third of these patients have hypopituitarism.[15] Gonadotropins are generally the first hormones affected, then GH, followed by TSH and ACTH. Hormone dysfunction may lead to amenorrhea or hypogonadism and decreased libido, or to hypothyroidism with weight gain, depression, fatigue, and mental slowing. These changes develop insidiously as the tumor grows, so the patient may be unaware until the lesion is large.

Parasellar structures may be compressed. Superior enlargement effaces the optic chiasm, causing visual loss. Compression on the inferonasal fibers that decussate at the anterior and inferior aspect of the chiasm leads to superior temporal quadrantanopia, then bitemporal hemianopia. An adenoma may grow laterally into the cavernous sinus, leading to extraocular muscle palsies or deficits to the sympathetic nerves and cranial nerves III, IV, or VI, leading to mydriasis, ptosis, facial pain, or infrequently, diplopia. Headache due to pressure on the dura may occur as well. Once a large tumor has extended out of the sella, it can cause pressure on the temporal or frontal lobes and, rarely, hydrocephalus via obstruction of cerebrospinal fluid (CSF) pathways. Occasionally, large adenomas become suddenly apparent after hemorrhage or infarction known as *pituitary apoplexy*. Pituitary lesions may be discovered incidentally during evaluations for other conditions such as trauma.

Diagnosis

Patients with a pituitary mass should undergo a complete neurological and endocrinological evaluation including a detailed history and physical examination to assess for signs or symptoms of hypersecretory syndromes such as Cushing's disease, hyperprolactinemia, or acromegaly. Endocrinological testing is needed to determine hormonal function. Laboratory studies include prolactin, FSH, LH, GH, insulin-like growth factor 1 (IGF-1), ACTH, cortisol, TSH, thyroxine, estradiol, and testosterone. A mildly elevated prolactin level does not exclude a nonfunctioning tumor as any sellar mass can compress the stalk, interrupting dopaminergic inhibition of PRL and leading to mild hyperprolactinemia up to 150 μg/mL known as the *stalk effect*.

Neuro-ophthalmological examination, including visual field testing and visual acuity, is necessary before and after treatment to document deficits and monitor changes.

Plain radiographs may demonstrate an enlarged, round sella, and the sellar floor may appear doubled due to a thinned, asymmetrically worn lamina dura. High-resolution magnetic resonance imaging (MRI) with cuts through the sellar region is essential for surgical planning, as it will show the precise size and location of the lesion as well as its relationship with the chiasm, cavernous sinus, and other surrounding structures (Fig. 40.4), and a computed tomography (CT) scan will demonstrate the sphenoid sinus anatomy.

The differential diagnosis of a nonfunctioning pituitary adenoma includes multiple other lesions, including functioning pituitary tumors, which can be differentiated by laboratory results. A Rathke's cleft cyst may appear similar to a cystic pituitary adenoma. A tuberculum sellae meningioma may compress the chiasm, but it will generally not cause enlargement of the sella. A craniopharyngioma is more often a suprasellar lesion. Metastasis to the sella will often cause diabetes insipidus or extraocular muscle palsies, which are rarely seen in patients with pituitary adenomas. An internal carotid artery aneurysm may fill the sella; however, a flow void will be visible on MRI. A sarcoid granuloma or a tuberculoma is quite rare.

Treatment Options

Surgery

The first line of treatment for a nonfunctioning pituitary adenoma is transsphenoidal resection of the tumor, which provides immediate relief of mass effect and has a low rate of complications.[16-19] This surgery is generally done as an elective procedure. An extended transsphenoidal approach may

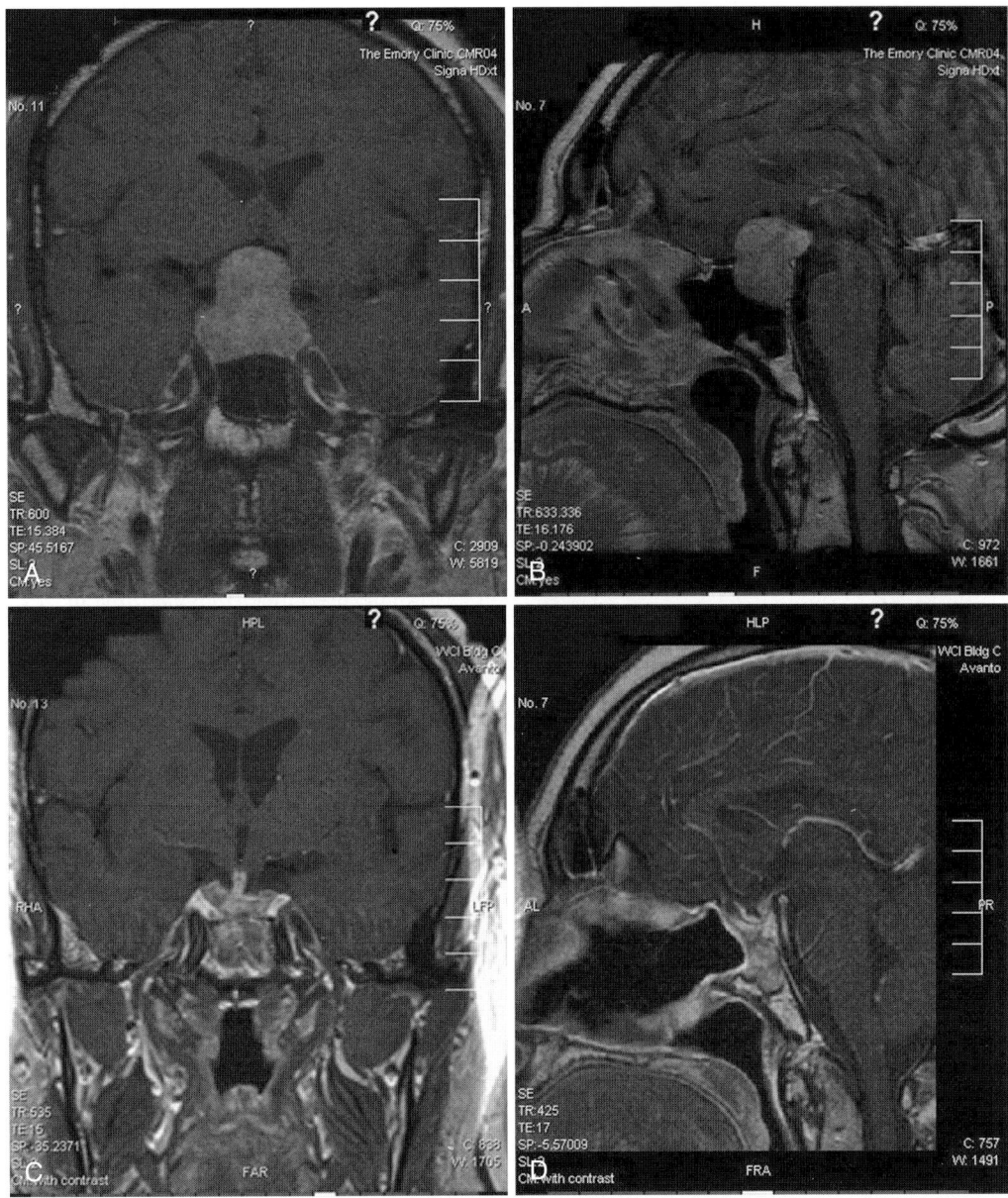

FIGURE 40.4 Magnetic resonance imaging (MRI) of a pituitary tumor. Coronal (**A**) and sagittal (**B**) MRI scans with contrast agent demonstrating a clinically nonfunctioning pituitary macroadenoma prior to treatment. Coronal (**C**) and sagittal (**D**) MRI scans with contrast material of the same patient after surgical resection via a transsphenoidal approach.

be needed when the tumor has reached beyond the sella and a transcranial approach or combined transsphenoidal-transcranial approach may be considered if there is significant supratentorial tumor extension.[20,21]

The goals of surgery are to eliminate mass effect from the pituitary and surrounding structures, to preserve or restore pituitary and visual function, to resect enough of the lesion to prevent recurrence, and to obtain tissue for histopathological analysis.[22]

Hermann Schloffer performed the first transsphenoidal resection of a pituitary tumor in 1907 and Harvey Cushing popularized it in the two decades afterward.[23,24] Neurosurgeons have been trying to perfect the transsphenoidal adenomectomy (TSA) since. The standard methods in use today involve either an endonasal or sublabial approach to the sella.

Endonasal Transsphenoidal Approach

In the endonasal transsphenoidal approach, the patient's head is placed in a Mayfield cranial fixation clamp. The body is placed supine with the neck somewhat extended and the head turned slightly toward the right to face the surgeon, permitting a good view through the nares (Fig. 40.5).

In a direct endonasal approach, the surgeon enters directly into the sphenoid sinus though the ostium. In the microscopic unilateral transseptal approach, a small incision is made in the right nostril mucosa and a submucosal plane is developed along the septum until the anterior wall of the sphenoid sinus is identified. A speculum is inserted and the septum is subluxed and deviated.

The operating microscope is brought into the field and the sphenoid sinus is opened with an osteotome and Kerrison rongeur. The opening is enlarged to allow visualization of the lateral portion of the sella. Some surgeons then obtain fluoroscopic or image-guided confirmation of the sella's position; however, direct visualization is generally sufficient.

An osteotome and up-biting Kerrison rongeur are used to open the sellar floor. The dura is revealed and a midline vertical incision is made with a No. 11 blade. Up-angled scissors are used to enlarge the dural opening and expose the adenoma. The tumor may be debulked intracapsularly, or an extracapsular plane may be developed along the tumor's pseudocapsule. The tumor is extracted piecemeal using ring curets, pituitary rongeurs, gentle suction, and irrigation. Adenoma removal can involve significant bleeding, making adequate suction imperative, as the bleeding often ceases only when the tumor is removed.

After tumor resection, the sellar floor may be repaired with DuraForm, fascia, fat from the patient's abdomen, bone, cartilage, or prosthesis. The sphenoid sinus may be packed with

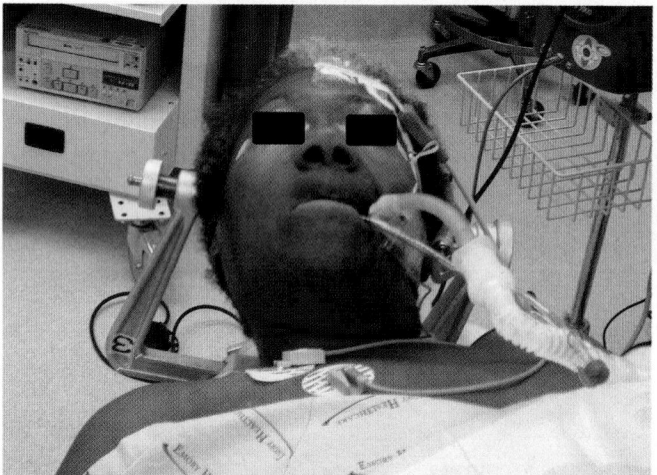

FIGURE 40.5 Intraoperative setup for an endonasal transsphenoidal adenomectomy (TSA). The patient should be supine with the head in a cranial fixation device, such as the Mayfield clamp. The neck is slightly extended and the head is turned gently toward the right to face the surgeon, permitting a good view through the nares. The endotracheal tube should be taped to the left, at the lower lip.

DuraForm, DuraSeal, or fat. The speculum is removed, the septum returned to midline, and the mucosa is sutured shut at the inside edge of the naris with absorbable suture. The patient will have copious mucosal secretions postoperatively, so a nasal trumpet may be placed in the nares overnight.

If a spinal fluid leak occurs through the diaphragm, then a sealant such as DuraSeal or Tisseel can be used to seal the leak and reconstruct the floor of the sella with bone, cartilage, or prosthesis, with or without a free fat graft from the abdomen. A few days of lumbar drainage of CSF may be used as well.

Endoscopy

The endoscope may be used in place of the microscope. When performing an endoscopic TSA, the patient is positioned in a manner similar to that used for the standard microscopic approach. A 4-mm or 2.7-mm endoscope is used to visualize the sphenoethmoid recess. The bilateral sphenoid ostia are entered and widened using a mushroom punch. The posterior nasal septum is incised and resected using a microdébrider and straight through-cutting instruments. The anterior wall of the sphenoid sinus is resected using straight through-cutting instruments and Kerrison punches.

The lesion is removed in the same manner as with the microscopic approach. The endoscope provides a wide field of view and angled scopes permit enhanced inspection of the walls of the sella, as well as the suprasellar, retrosellar, and parasellar regions to search for residual tumor. Three-dimensional endoscopes have been introduced recently and permit a more realistic, nondistorted view of the regional anatomy than do the conventional two-dimensional endoscopes (Fig. 40.6).

After the lesion is removed, DuraForm is placed over the sella. Gelfoam is used to pack the sphenoid sinus, and NasoPore is laid over the bilateral sphenoethmoid recesses. If a CSF leak is present, a mucosal septal flap may be used to assist in closure. A speculum is not needed with this approach.[25,26]

Sublabial Transsphenoidal Approach

Pediatric patients with small nares or patients with large tumors may be treated via a sublabial TSA. The patient's upper lip is retracted and a horizontal incision is made in the gingival

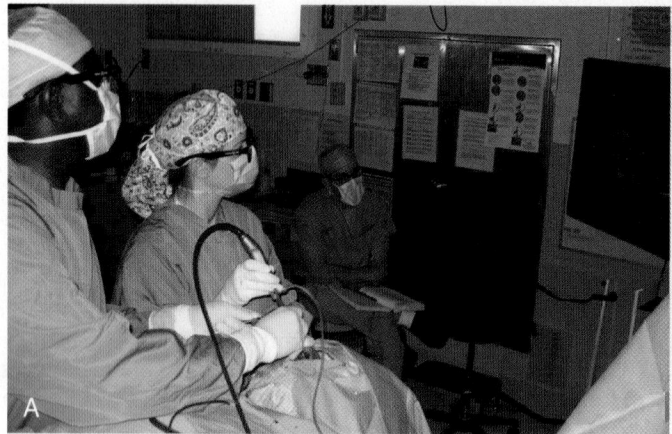
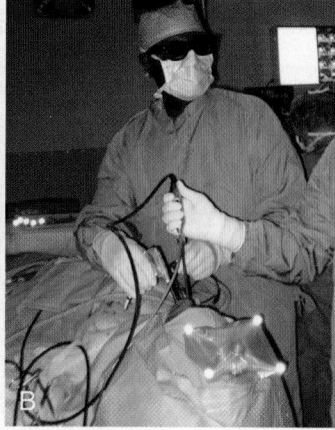

FIGURE 40.6 Using the three-dimensional (3D) endoscope. **A,** The surgeon should use a "three-handed" technique. An assistant drives the endoscope in one naris, while the primary surgeon uses an instrument in each naris. The 3D endoscope, such as the Visionsense, seen here, provides a more realistic view of the anatomy than does the earlier two-dimensional endoscope. **B,** 3D glasses are required.

mucosa. A pathway is followed to the maxilla and floor of the nasal cavity. A vertical incision is made, separating the nasal mucosa from the septum. The anterior septum is subluxed, the speculum is inserted, and the operating microscope or endoscope is brought into the field. The operation continues in a similar fashion to the endonasal approach just described.[27]

Neuronavigation

A TSA may be performed with frameless stereotactic neuronavigation to assist with large lesions that involve the carotid arteries or recurrent lesions where a prior operation has altered the normal anatomy.[28,29] The operation is performed as just described; however, the surgeon is able to check his or her position at any point during the procedure to assess the proximity of surrounding structures or determine when he or she is approaching the limits of the tumor (Fig. 40.7).

Outcomes

Following operative decompression, vision generally improves and endocrine function recovers to a lesser extent, and surgical resection generally halts progressive loss of hormonal function. After TSA, visual field defects will improve in 70% to 89% of patients,[30,31] will not change significantly in 7%, and will worsen in less than 4% of patients.[32]

Approximately 30% of patients with nonfunctioning adenomas have some degree of hypopituitarism prior to surgery.[33] In one quarter of these patients, preoperative pituitary deficiencies will improve after surgery, although 10% of patients have some postoperative worsening of hormone function.[8] Oral hormone replacement is generally sufficient for those patients whose pituitary deficiencies worsen or do not improve.

Complications from transsphenoidal surgery include intracranial hemorrhage, carotid artery injury, ischemic stroke, visual impairment, CSF leak, nasal septal perforation, and epistaxis. The risk of stroke or death is less than 1%, the risk of visual loss is less than 2%, and the risk of CSF rhinorrhea is less than 4%.[34]

After transsphenoidal removal of an adenoma, hormone levels must be closely followed because the patient is at risk for hypopituitarism. Morning cortisol levels are checked for several days, and patients with hypocortisolemia are treated with steroid replacement as needed.

Diabetes insipidus (DI) and the syndrome of inappropriate antidiuretic hormone secretion (SIADH) are common but transient postoperative complications after transsphenoidal surgery. Nearly 18% of patients will develop DI, though this is often temporary.[34] It is imperative to closely monitor fluid balance, serum sodium levels, and urine specific gravity. In a small number of patients, hyponatremia can occur a week or more after the surgery.

Following resection of a giant macroadenoma, when it is likely that some residual tumor may remain, a rare but potentially fatal complication is postoperative apoplexy. This complication must be closely monitored for. In one study of 134 surgically resected giant adenomas, four patients had fatal postoperative pituitary apoplexy.[35]

The mortality rate for patients undergoing transsphenoidal surgery is very low, approximately 0.5%. Among giant macroadenomas, the mortality rate is approximately 1%. After successful surgical resection, 10% to 20% of tumors are reported to recur within 6 years.[30,31] At 10-year follow-up, more than 80% of patients who underwent transsphenoidal resection of a nonfunctioning pituitary adenoma are alive and disease free.[8]

Medical Therapy

Medical therapy is available for functioning tumors, but there are no available effective drug regimens for nonfunctioning pituitary adenomas. Multiple medical therapies have been tested. Dopamine agonists lead to a small reduction in tumor size in less than 10% of patients, and octreotide has improved visual deficits among some patients with macroadenomas.[30,31] However, most patients with nonfunctioning pituitary tumors will gain no clinical or biochemical benefit from medical therapies.

Radiation Therapy

Radiation therapy may be used in patients with recurrent or residual tumor, or in patients who cannot tolerate surgery. Radiotherapy controls tumor growth in 80% to 98% of nonfunctioning tumors.[36]

Conventional radiotherapy calls for fractionated doses of 1.6 to 2 Gy four or five times per week for 5 to 6 weeks, for a maximum dose of 45 to 50 Gy.[9] Tumors respond slowly, with benefits delayed for a year or more.

Stereotactic radiosurgery (SRS) uses only a single session to deliver focused radiation to the lesion with less radiation to surrounding structures. Several forms of SRS are available, including Gamma Knife surgery (GKS), linear accelerator (linac) radiation, and CyberKnife surgery. There is also fractionated stereotactic radiotherapy and proton beam therapy. SRS is generally able to use a higher radiation dose per fraction than is conventional radiation, and usually results in earlier endocrine control. It is not risk-free, however.

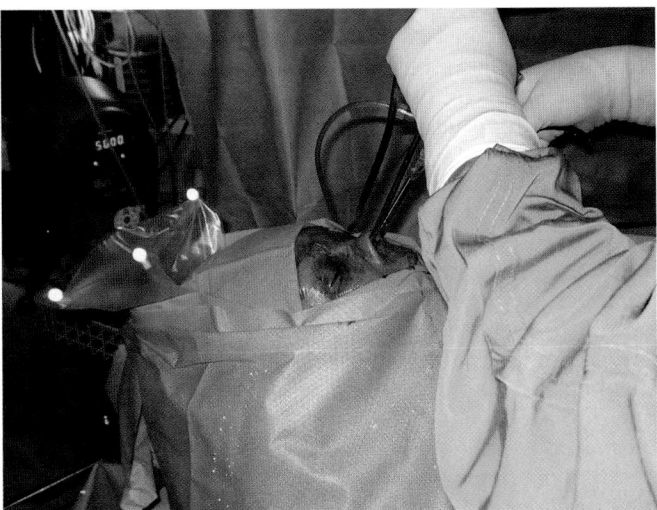

FIGURE 40.7 Using neuronavigation. Large or recurrent tumors may benefit from intraoperative neuronavigation. The headpiece for the Stealth navigation system is attached to the Mayfield cranial fixation clamp. Tegederms are placed on the eyes to protect the corneas while permitting reregistration intraoperatively if the need arises.

The major concern from SRS is radiation damage to the visual pathways, but this can be decreased by limiting the radiation dose to the optic chiasm to less than 10 Gy.[37,38] Patients with adenomas closer than 2 to 5 mm to the optic chiasm or larger than 30 mm in diameter are generally not candidates for SRS, though they may undergo fractionated stereotactic radiotherapy or conventional radiation.[39] The neuronal and vascular structures in the cavernous sinus are less radiosensitive, so an ablative dose may be administered to tumors with lateral invasion or impingement on the cranial nerves. This allows SRS to function as an adjuvant to surgical resection in patients with tumors that have invaded the cavernous sinus.

As with conventional radiotherapy, hormone deficiencies are the most common side effect with an incidence of 13% to 56%.[40-43] The risks of radiation-induced second neoplasm and neuropsychiatric changes are lower with SRS than with conventional radiotherapy. Other side effects are rare. Long-term risk for radiation necrosis is approximately 0.2%. Optic neuropathy occurs in 1.7%, vascular changes in 6.3%, neuropsychological changes in 0.7%, and radiation-induced secondary malignancies in 0.8%.[44] All forms of radiation therapy have delayed benefit, though SRS induces remission more rapidly than does fractionated radiotherapy.[42,45]

Follow-up

Routine postoperative evaluation with MRI and CT should be delayed for at least 4 to 6 weeks after surgery because of the difficulty analyzing the tumor region in the setting of recent surgical changes. Mass effect seen in the early postoperative period usually resolves and can be followed with serial MRI.[46]

Patients with nonfunctioning adenomas should undergo annual MRI or CT, as well as visual and endocrine evaluations, whether or not they have received treatment. If these tumors are not treated, they tend to grow slowly over months or years.

Because of the significant recurrence rate following transsphenoidal resection and the considerable number of patients who develop hypopituitarism after radiation therapy, even successfully treated patients should be followed closely by their medical team.

FUNCTIONING PITUITARY ADENOMAS

Functioning pituitary adenomas secrete excessive quantities of a physiologically active pituitary hormone. They present with clinical syndromes caused by their hormone overproduction.

The majority of pituitary tumors are functioning adenomas. Of these, PRL-secreting tumors, or prolactinomas, account for 40% to 60%, while GH-secreting tumors make up 15% to 25%.[47] Corticotropin-secreting adenomas represent about 5% of functioning adenomas, and gonadotropin- and thyrotropin-secreting tumors account for less than 1%. Neurohypophyseal tumors are very rare.

Prolactinoma

Prolactin Physiology

Lactotrophs secrete prolactin and are unique in that normal cells can proliferate during adulthood. PRL interacts with

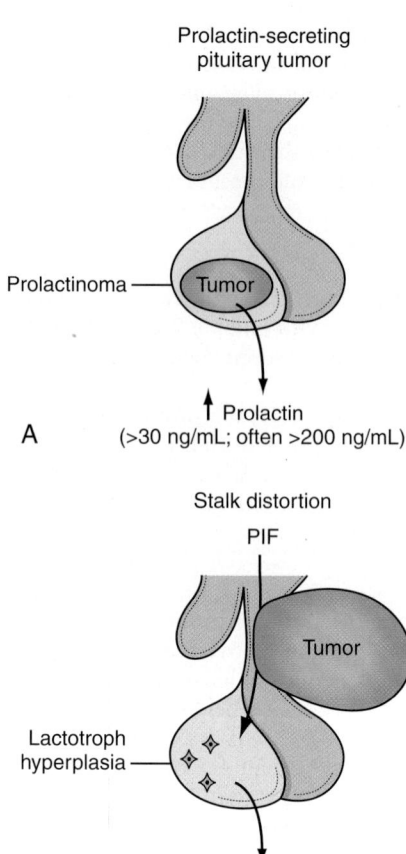

FIGURE 40.8 Abnormal prolactin regulation. **A,** Prolactin-secreting adenomas (prolactinomas) can cause marked elevation of serum prolactin levels. **B,** Distortion of the pituitary stalk by pathological processes, such as tumors arising from the suprasellar region, can cause mild to moderate hyperprolactinemia, known as the *stalk effect.*

receptors in the gonads and acts on breast tissue to initiate and maintain lactation. Hypothalamic moderation of PRL secretion occurs by the release of dopamine into the portal circulation from nerve processes that originate in the arcuate nucleus of the hypothalamus (Fig. 40.8). PRL release is increased by TRH, vasoactive intestinal peptide (VIP), GnRH, peptide histidine methionine, opiates, and estrogen. Pharmacological doses of TRH lead to a rapid release of PRL; however, the physiological role of TRH in PRL production is unclear.

PRL is secreted episodically, with 13 to 14 peaks per day and an interpulse interval of approximately 90 minutes. Small postprandial rises occur secondary to central stimulation from the amino acids in food. Physiological hyperprolactinemia occurs following exercise, psychological and physical stress, sexual intercourse, nipple stimulation, or postpartum breastfeeding, and peak levels occur during the late hours of sleep.

During pregnancy, estrogen stimulates lactotroph hyperplasia and hyperprolactinemia but blocks the action of PRL on the breast, inhibiting lactation until after delivery. Within 4 to 6 months after delivery, basal PRL levels return to normal.

FIGURE 40.9 The hook effect. If there is an exceedingly high amount of prolactin (PRL) in the sample, it will saturate the antibodies and fail to form the antibody sandwich complexes that are required for most radioimmunoassays. Excess hormone will be washed away with the labeled antibody, and the test result will be falsely low. These samples should be diluted to provide a more accurate PRL level.

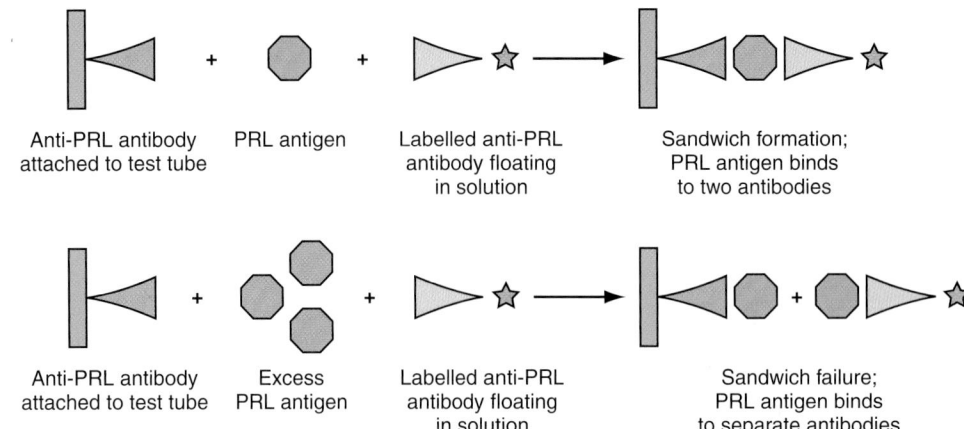

Incidence

Prolactinomas are second only to nonfunctioning adenomas in overall incidence, composing about 30% of all pituitary tumors and more than half of functional pituitary tumors. Hyperprolactinemia from a prolactin-secreting adenoma causes hypogonadism and galactorrhea.[48-50] Women with hyperprolactinemia usually present with amenorrhea, galactorrhea, diminished libido, and infertility. Gonadal dysfunction and decreased estrogen secretion may lead to osteoporosis. In men, hyperprolactinemia manifests as diminished libido, impotence, gynecomastia, or infertility due to a decreased sperm count. Adolescents may present with delay of sexual development. In children and postmenopausal women, signs of hypogonadism may be absent.[50]

In autopsy studies, prolactinomas are found in equal numbers of men and women, but women are four times more likely to become symptomatic. Because they develop symptoms sooner, women more often present with smaller tumors, and men generally present with larger tumors and mass effect. Approximately 5% of women with primary amenorrhea and 52% with secondary amenorrhea not due to pregnancy have a prolactinoma, as do about 2% of men with impotence.[51]

Evaluation

Laboratory testing in patients with suspected hyperprolactinemia includes serial measurements of basal, resting serum PRL levels by radioimmunoassay. Because of the variability in PRL levels over the course of a day, minimally elevated levels should be confirmed with several samples or from a pooled sample.

Normal PRL levels are approximately 5 to 20 ng/mL in men and 5 to 25 ng/mL in nonpregnant women. Any sellar mass can compress the pituitary stalk and interrupt dopaminergic inhibition of PRL. This leads to a "stalk effect," which results in mildly elevated PRL levels, generally 20 to 150 ng/mL, but should not be confused with a true prolactinoma. Serum PRL levels tend to correlate with the size of the prolactinoma, so that microadenomas generally lead to serum prolactin levels of 100 to 250 ng/mL, and macroadenomas may lead to a serum PRL well above 200 ng/mL. Invasive adenomas or giant adenomas may cause a serum PRL to be several thousand to 100,000 ng/mL.[50,52,53] A PRL level more than 200 ng/mL is nearly pathognomonic for a prolactinoma. In patients with

amenorrhea, however, pregnancy must also be excluded, as it is associated with PRL levels of 100 to 250 ng/mL by the third trimester. A PRL level of less than 2 ng/mL is generally associated with hypopituitarism, though this may be due to PRL-lowering medications.

One must be suspicious of the "hook effect," if prolactin values are very low in the presence of a suspected giant prolactinoma.[54,55] If the serum PRL level is extremely high, the amount of prolactin-antigen may saturate the antibodies in the radioimmunoassay, failing to form the antigen plus two-antibody "sandwich" complexes required for accurate measurement, and thus leading to a falsely low value (Fig. 40.9). If a prolactinoma is suspected, the PRL level should be tested with serial dilutions to determine an accurate PRL value.[52,56]

Stimulation of PRL secretion during the TRH-stimulation test suggests the presence of a prolactinoma, but is not diagnostic for this condition. In normal subjects intravenous administration of 200 to 500 µg of TRH stimulates a three- to fivefold rise in serum prolactin levels within an hour. Patients with a prolactinoma, however, usually have a blunted response of less than a twofold increase owing to their limited lactotroph reserve.

Hyperprolactinemia per se is not diagnostic of a prolactinoma, as there are multiple physiological and pathological conditions that can elevate serum PRL. Pregnancy, of course, must be assessed in female patients with hyperprolactinemia. Hyperprolactinemia may also be due to diminished hypothalamic production of dopamine or an interruption of dopamine delivery to the pituitary; interruption of the portal venous system by a sellar tumor or aneurysm compressing the pituitary stalk; previous pituitary irradiation, or the empty sella syndrome; end-stage renal disease, which decreases renal clearance of PRL; and chronic hypothyroidism, which spurs increased TRH secretion stimulating PRL release. Other causes include chest wall or breast lesions, hypoglycemia, hepatic cirrhosis, seizures, polycystic ovary syndrome, or an ectopic site of PRL secretion. Hyperprolactinemia may also occur in up to 40% of patients with acromegaly and has been reported in Cushing's disease.

Dopamine inhibits PRL secretion, so any drug that decreases dopamine levels will increase serum PRL. These drugs include many antidepressants, such as tricyclics, monoamine oxidase inhibitors, and selective serotonin reuptake inhibitors, as well as methyldopa, reserpine, and verapamil.[57] Other medications such as phenothiazines and metoclopramide block dopamine receptors, indirectly leading to increased PRL levels.[57]

When other causes of hyperprolactinemia have been ruled out, an MRI with and without contrast, with thin cuts through the sella, should be obtained to confirm the presence of a prolactinoma.

Medical Treatment

Dopamine agonists are the treatment of choice for prolactinoma.[58] These agents can normalize PRL levels within hours to days, shrink tumors, restore reproductive and sexual function, and allow patients to avoid the potential risks of surgery.

Current dopamine agonists, including bromocriptine, cabergoline, and pergolide, are synthetic derivatives of ergot alkaloids.[59] Bromocriptine is begun orally once daily and increased over several weeks to multiple daily doses. It decreases tumor volume in approximately 85% of patients, and reduces PRL levels to normal in nearly 90%.[50] Bromocriptine works very rapidly, often leading to a decrease in PRL within 1 to 2 hours. More than 10% of tumors are not sensitive to bromocriptine,[60] and 5% to 10% of patients are intolerant of its gastrointestinal side effects, though intravaginal administration may lessen these symptoms.[61]

Cabergoline is more expensive than bromocriptine, but may be better tolerated, and is administered once or twice weekly.[58] It normalizes PRL levels in up to 84% of patients.[62] Studies of cabergoline in women of childbearing age are limited, but bromocriptine has been extensively studied and appears safe in pregnancy. Therefore, if pregnancy is desired, bromocriptine should be used,[63] then discontinued during pregnancy unless symptomatic tumor enlargement occurs.

Medical treatment is generally continued chronically as cessation of either drug may result in recurrent hyperprolactinemia and tumor re-expansion.[64] After initiation of medical therapy, MRI and visual examination should be repeated, and serum PRL levels should be monitored at least annually.[65,66]

One must be cautious with prolonged use of cabergoline and other ergot-derived dopamine agonists, as they may lead to an increased risk of pleural and pericardial fibrosing serositis and valvular heart disease when used in large doses, as they are in patients with Parkinson's disease.[67-69] Patients with prolactinoma receive significantly smaller doses of the drug than do patients receiving the drugs for parkinsonism, and it is unknown if the risk of symptomatic valvular heart disease exists at these low doses. Studies of echocardiograms in patients receiving cabergoline for hyperprolactinemia have reported conflicting results.[70-74] There does not appear to be any statistical increase in incidence of clinically relevant or symptomatic cardiac regurgitation in patients treated with cabergoline. We recommend echocardiographic evaluation of patients who are receiving long-term, high-dose cabergoline.

Surgery

The effectiveness and safety of medical therapy have limited the need for surgery in most patients with prolactinoma. If a patient fails to respond to or is unable to tolerate the side effects of medical treatment, then surgery is recommended, as medication may be more effective after surgical debulking.[75,76] Surgery is also suggested for patients who develop CSF leak while undergoing medical therapy or patients who have a dissociated response to drugs in which their prolactin level falls but the tumor does not shrink. TSA, as described previously, is the surgery of choice.[34,77] An extended transsphenoidal approach may be needed if the tumor is beyond the sella, and craniotomy should be considered if there is significant extension.[20,78]

The higher the PRL level, the lower the chance of surgical cure. Patients with microprolactinomas and serum PRL level below 200 ng/mL have a greater than 90% chance of cure with TSA when performed by experienced pituitary surgeons at high-volume centers, and morbidity and mortality risks are less than 1%.[34,75] However, patients with a preoperative PRL level above 200 ng/mL with large, invasive prolactinomas have a less than 41% surgical cure rate.[76] In patients with giant or invasive prolactinomas, pretreatment with a dopamine agonist may improve the success of surgery; however, long-term pharmacotherapy can alter the tumor's consistency and make surgery more challenging.[79]

Radiation Therapy

Radiation therapy is an option for patients who have failed surgery or medical therapy.[80,81] Though there is a risk of hypopituitarism or damage to the optic nerves, radiation therapy is generally considered safe and effective. Radiotherapy may be combined with medical or surgical management and may be delivered as conventional external beam radiotherapy or SRS.

Conventional radiotherapy regimens use approximately 4500 cGy in 25 to 30 fractions.[82] Tumor growth is controlled in 83% to 100% of patients, and reduction in tumor mass is achieved in 36% to 45% of patients.[83] SRS may provide more rapid endocrine control while permitting the delivery of radiation in a single session with less exposure to surrounding normal tissue.

Dopamine agonists may provide a radioprotective effect on tumors, and preferably should be discontinued during radiosurgery.[80] In a study of 164 patients with prolactinoma who underwent primary treatment with Gamma Knife, tumor growth was controlled in all but two patients, and biochemical cure was attained in more than half.[81]

Growth Hormone–Secreting Adenomas
Growth Hormone Physiology

GH is required for normal human growth; it plays little role in the first year of life, but becomes very important during puberty. GH is required for normal linear growth and is secreted in pulses by the somatotroph cells. Its release is controlled by GHRH and somatostatin, which stimulate and inhibit release, respectively (Fig. 40.10). GH, in turn, stimulates the liver's production of somatomedin-C, also known as *insulin-like growth factor 1* (IGF-1). IGF-1 inhibits GH secretion at the hypothalamus, where it stimulates somatostatin release, and at the pituitary, where it suppresses GHRH-induced GH secretion.

Sleep, stress, exercise, and hypoglycemia increase the release of GH, while obesity, hyperglycemia, and excess glucocorticoids decrease it. GH is anabolic and increases the

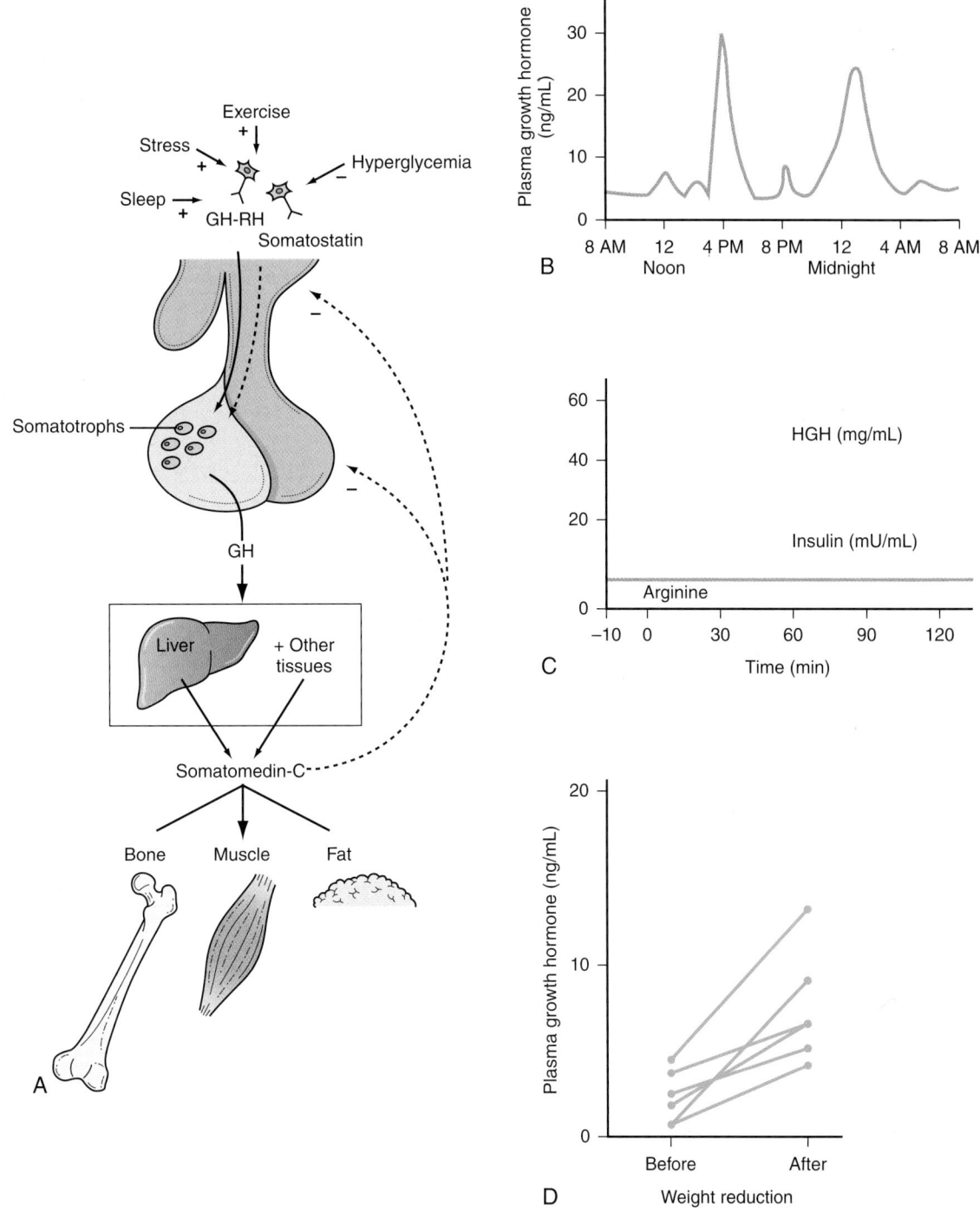

FIGURE 40.10 Regulation of growth hormone (GH) secretion. **A,** Hypothalamic-pituitary axis. Somatotrophs of the anterior pituitary are stimulated to release GH by GH-releasing hormone (GHRH) and are inhibited by somatostatin. Stress, exercise, sleep rhythms, and hyperglycemia alter GH secretion. Somatomedin-C, or insulin-like growth factor 1 (IGF-1), exerts negative feedback on GH release at the pituitary and hypothalamus. **B** to **D,** Plasma GH levels fluctuate during a 24-hour period with peaks related to stress, exercise, and sleep.

uptake of amino acids into tissue; conversely, a rise in amino acids increases GH release in a healthy individual. GH and IGF-1 levels are highest in children and young adults, then decrease with age in normal subjects. In normal subjects, serum GH levels are very low or undetectable for most of the day. GH has a half-life of 20 to 30 minutes and is secreted in short pulses, with two to seven peaks per day, leading to significant fluctuations in levels during the day. Some of these bursts are associated with meals, while others occur during the early stages of sleep. The half-life of IGF-1, on the other hand, is 2 to 18 hours, and serum levels are relatively stable. IGF-1 measurements therefore provide a more reliable indication of the exposure of the body to GH than do GH measurements.

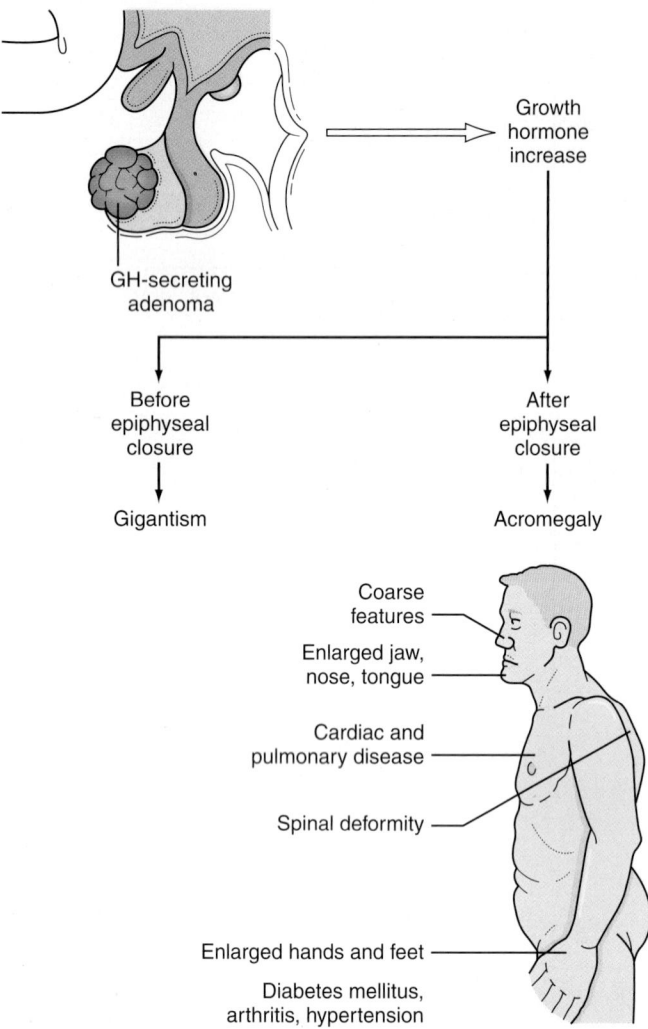

FIGURE 40.11 Clinical manifestations of acromegaly.

Growth Hormone Excess: Acromegaly

Excess GH secretion, which results in excess growth of the soft tissues, bony changes, and multiple biochemical changes, produces the syndromes of acromegaly in adults and gigantism in children who are affected before epiphyseal closure. Characteristics of acromegaly include coarse facial features with prognathism and malocclusion of the teeth, enlargement of the paranasal sinuses with frontal bossing, deepening of the voice, organomegaly, hyperhidrosis, acanthosis nigricans, enlargement of the hands and feet leading to an increase in ring, glove, and shoe size, and headache[84-86] (Fig. 40.11). Insulin resistance can lead to diabetes mellitus. Tongue enlargement produces obstructive sleep apnea. Accumulation of excess soft tissue in the hands results in a wet, doughy handshake and in the feet it produces increased heel-pad thickness on radiographs. Patients with acromegaly also suffer from headache, proximal myopathy, osteoarthritis, carpal tunnel syndrome, cardiomegaly, and hypertension. Metabolic derangements lead to accelerated atherosclerosis and a shortened life expectancy as a result of cardiovascular, cerebrovascular, and respiratory causes. There is also a higher risk of developing other neoplasms, especially colon cancer.[1,87] With

appropriate reduction of GH levels, however, mortality risk decreases and can normalize.[88]

The average annual incidence of acromegaly is approximately 3.3 per million.[88] Ninety-eight percent of patients with acromegaly harbor a GH-secreting pituitary adenoma.[89] From 20% to 50% of these tumors also secrete PRL or other pituitary hormones.[90] Rarely, acromegaly is the result of ectopic GH-producing tumors such as bronchial carcinoid or pancreatic islet cell tumors, a hypothalamic GHRH-releasing tumor, exogenous administration of GH for antiaging treatments, or familial syndromes such as multiple endocrine neoplasia I, McCune-Albright syndrome, or Carney complex.[89]

The disease is generally insidious and presents in the third to fourth decade, and both sexes are equally affected.[91] The average patient with acromegaly has had symptoms for 8 to 10 years before the diagnosis is made, so the majority of GH-secreting adenomas are large at the time of diagnosis.[88] Many compress the optic system and produce loss of visual acuity or bitemporal hemianopia by the time the tumor is recognized.

Evaluation

When acromegaly or gigantism is suspected, endocrine evaluation should include measurement of basal GH and IGF-1 levels and testing to assess suppression of GH secretion by hyperglycemia (an oral glucose tolerance test, OGTT). Because exercise and stress stimulate GH secretion, serum GH levels are ideally obtained in the early morning before the patient arises from bed, or 2 hours after a meal when GH levels would normally be suppressed. In healthy subjects, basal GH levels are usually lower than 5 ng/mL, but more than 90% of acromegalic patients have levels higher than 10 ng/mL. Levels vary widely, however, so some acromegalic patients have normal GH levels. In patients with active acromegaly, the normal pulsatile GH secretory pattern is replaced by a consistent elevation of GH throughout the day. Owing to the short half-life and pulsatile pattern, random GH levels are of limited value and single determinations of GH correlate poorly with severity of disease. Serum GH levels may also be elevated in other conditions including uncontrolled diabetes mellitus, renal failure, malnutrition, and during physical or emotional stress.[90] To confirm the diagnosis of acromegaly, an OGTT can be performed. In an acromegalic, GH will fail to suppress to less than 2 µg/L with glucose loading.

Because serum levels of IGF-1 are more stable than those of GH, measurement of IGF-1 can be used to provide a reliable indicator of the overall exposure of GH on the body. IGF-1 is increased in nearly all patients with acromegaly, even in those whose serum GH levels are within the range of normal. Normal levels of IGF-1 range from 0.45 to 2.2 U/mL in women and from 0.34 to 2.0 U/mL in men.[90] Unlike GH, IGF-1 is not directly affected by stress or exercise, and it is bound to carrier proteins that regulate its function and stabilize its levels. IGF-1 is also a reliable parameter for posttreatment follow-up of acromegaly, because it reflects GH secretion over the prior 24 hours.[85]

TRH stimulation causes at least a 50% rise of GH in untreated acromegaly, whereas normal subjects generally have little change in serum GH in response to TRH injection. Though this finding also occurs in patients with liver disease, renal failure, or depression, it can be highly suggestive of acromegaly in the correct clinical setting. Acromegalic patients who have a positive response to TRH stimulation may respond to bromocriptine therapy. TRH stimulation may also be used to identify those patients who, despite a normal GH level after surgery, have residual GH-secreting tumor and are therefore at risk of tumor recurrence.[92]

An L-dopa test may also be performed. Administration of oral L-dopa to a normal fasting subject will increase GH secretion, but it will paradoxically decrease GH levels in a fasting patient with acromegaly. Likewise, bromocriptine, a dopamine agonist that binds D2 receptors, will raise GH levels in a normal subject, but lower them in the setting of acromegaly. Other dynamic tests include the arginine-stimulation test, insulin-induced hypoglycemia stimulation, somatostatin-stimulation test, and LH-releasing hormone stimulation test. Each of these tests may provide additional information in cases of acromegaly.

Because patients with acromegaly often have large tumors, patients should undergo full endocrine testing for hypopituitarism, formal visual field testing, and a contrast-enhanced MRI with thin cuts through the sella to determine the anatomy of the lesion. Because of the growth of soft tissue structures, sleep studies should be performed to assess for sleep apnea. A colonoscopy is recommended for all patients at diagnosis and, if polyps are found, every 3 to 5 years thereafter.

Rarely, acromegaly is caused by a non-CNS GHRH-secreting tumor. Acromegalic patients who do not have a discrete pituitary tumor on MRI should be evaluated to find another site of a GHRH-secreting tumor. Measurement of plasma GHRH should be used. Ectopic acromegaly such as from a pancreatic islet cell tumor or bronchial carcinoid results in a measurable level of GHRH in the circulation, whereas GHRH is barely detectable when acromegaly is due to a pituitary lesion.[93]

Surgery

Surgical adenomectomy by an experienced neurosurgeon is the first-line treatment for acromegaly.[18,19] A craniotomy may be necessary when there is a large tumor with extensive suprasellar or parasellar extension. Most GH-secreting tumors are sellar or suprasellar lesions that can be removed by the transsphenoidal route using a sublabial, transseptal, or direct endonasal approach with the endoscope or microscope, as described previously. Plasma GH levels may rapidly decrease within hours after surgery, and IGF-1 levels and clinical symptoms decrease over the next several weeks to months.[18,94]

Stringent criteria for a "cure" or remission require a random GH less than 2.5 µg/L, or GH nadir after an oral glucose tolerance test of less than 1 µg/L and a normal age and gender-normalized IGF-1, with no clinical symptoms.[95] Using these strict criteria, a study of 59 patients followed for an average of 13.4 years after transsphenoidal surgery showed that 52% achieved long-term biochemical remission after surgery alone.[96]

About 20% to 25% of GH-secreting tumors are microadenomas, tumors less than 1 cm in diameter, while 75% to 80% are macroadenomas, more than 1 cm in diameter. In a study of 103 patients followed after TSA, remission was obtained postoperatively in 82% of patients with microadenomas, but in 60% of patients with macroadenomas, and only in 24% of

patients with invasive macroadenomas.[96] Several factors are predictive of surgical outcome, including tumor size, invasiveness, extrasellar growth, and secretory activity. Preoperative GH levels have an inverse relationship with the likelihood of biochemical remission following surgery.[18,19,97,98]

GH and IGF-1 levels should be followed 6 weeks postoperatively. If hormone levels are normal at that time, then the patient can be monitored with hormone assays annually, or more often if needed for concomitant conditions such as diabetes mellitus or hypopituitarism. If GH and IGF-1 levels have not normalized, and further treatment is needed, then medical therapy and radiotherapy are options. Reoperation for acromegaly has a lower success rate and higher complication rate than does initial surgery, and should be reserved for patients unresponsive to other forms of treatment or who have progressive visual impairment despite other treatments.[99]

Medical Therapy

Pharmacological options for acromegaly include somatostatin analogs, dopamine-receptor agonists, and GH-receptor (GHR) antagonists.[100]

Somatostatin acts as an endogenous inhibitor of GH secretion.[101] Analogs are indicated for patients awaiting the effects of radiation and patients who are medically unstable for surgery or who have persistent disease after TSA.[102] They can also be offered as primary therapy for patients who refuse surgery or those with severe medical conditions that preclude surgery or who are unlikely to be cured by an operation.[102,103] Poor-risk patients may be reconsidered for surgery if their medical condition improves after several months on octreotide.[104]

Somatostatin analogs reduce GH and IGF-1 levels in 50% to 70% of acromegalic patients and normalize IGF-1 in 30% of patients who have failed pituitary surgery.[105] Up to half of patients attain a decrease in the size of the pituitary tumor as well.[102,104,106,107]

First-generation somatostatin analogs, such as octreotide acetate, have a half-life that is 2 hours longer than that of the native hormone but still require subcutaneous administration multiple times daily.[108,109] The maximum suppression of GH is reached within 2 hours and lasts about 6 hours. Relief of clinical symptoms is often immediate, even preceding the decrease in GH levels. Side effects associated with long-term use of octreotide are relatively minor and include pain at the injection site, abdominal cramps, mild steatorrhea, or impairment of glucose tolerance. Biliary sludge and cholesterol gallstones may occur after long-term treatment due to inhibition of gallbladder emptying.[106,110] As with prolactinomas, discontinuation of medical therapy may result in rebound of pretreatment hormone levels and tumor size.

Newer somatostatin analogs have longer durations of action but similar efficacy and better compliance as compared to the older drugs.[105] These long-acting somatostatin preparations are expensive and require a meticulous reconstitution technique before injection, necessitating long-term medical participation. Slow-release lanreotide (Somatulin SR) has a duration of action of 10 to 14 days, and requires injection two to three times per month, while slow-release depot octreotide (Sandostatin-LAR) requires an intramuscular injection only once every 28 days.[105]

Preoperative treatment with octreotide shrinks macroadenomas by about 40%.[111] It is debatable, however, whether this affects surgical outcome. Two prospective, randomized studies demonstrated no benefit of preoperative octreotide on rate of hormone normalization postoperatively or on duration of hospital stay.[112,113] A retrospective study of other acromegalic patients, on the other hand, found that IGF-1 levels normalized postoperatively in twice as many patients who had been treated with octreotide preoperatively as those who had not.[104] Short-term preoperative octreotide administration decreases surgical risk in patients who have cardiac and metabolic complications of acromegaly.[114] Octreotide should not be used in patients who are undergoing radiation therapy, as it may be radioprotective for some adenomas.[80]

If GH levels remain elevated despite maximized octreotide, then combined therapy with octreotide and dopamine-agonists is recommended.[104] Although dopamine agonists increase GH release in normal subjects, they paradoxically suppress GH secretion in acromegalic patients. Dopamine agents appear to stimulate basal GH production in normal subjects by acting at the level of the hypothalamus, but they inhibit GH release from adenomas via direct action on dopamine receptors on the somatotroph cells.[59]

Bromocriptine is effective in lowering GH and IGF-1 levels in 20% of patients, with 10% achieving normalization.[59,103,115] Bromocriptine should initially be given at a dose of 1.25 mg at bedtime and then increased slowly to a maximum of 20 mg per day in divided doses. Side effects such as nausea, nasal stuffiness, vertigo, and hypotension may result.

Cabergoline and quinagolide are among a newer generation of long-acting D2-receptor agonists that appear to be more effective and better tolerated than bromocriptine.[40,104,116] Cabergoline's serum half-life is 65 hours, requiring once or twice weekly administration. Quinagolide is given once daily. Long-term administration of cabergoline to 64 patients suppressed plasma IGF-1 levels to normal in 39% and achieved modest decreases in another 28%.[40] Dopamine-agonists are most effective in mixed GH- and PRL-secreting tumors, which occur in 30% to 40% of acromegalic patients.[115]

GH receptor (GHR) dimerization is required for GH action. Pegvisomant is a mutated form of the GHR protein that acts as a GHR protein antagonist by binding to the GHR, blocking dimerization and thus inhibiting IGF-1 secretion.[100,117,118] GHR antagonists do not act on the pituitary tumor directly, so a potential risk is an increase in GH secretion and tumor enlargement due to a loss of negative feedback from IGF-1. Studies suggest, however, that while there may be an increase in GH levels, it is not progressive and does not lead to a significant increase in tumor growth in patients followed for up to 2 years.[100,117-120] One should therefore obtain regular MRI scans to monitor tumor size.

Pegvisomant is given as once daily subcutaneous injections and appears to be well tolerated. A randomized, double-blind multicenter trial of pegvisomant in 112 acromegalic patients demonstrated that when patients were treated with pegvisomant in 10-, 15-, and 20-mg doses, normalization of IGF-1 levels was achieved in 54%, 81%, and 89% of patients, respectively.[100] Side effects appear to be minor. Some patients have been found to have asymptomatic hepatocellular injury after initiation of pegvisomant, but hepatic enzyme levels normalized after cessation of the drug.[100,120]

Pegvisomant should be considered in patients in whom surgery and medical therapy with somatostatin or dopamine agonists have proved ineffective or poorly tolerated.[121]

Estrogen receptor modulators are not a standard part of the acromegalic armamentarium, but research suggests that they may be of some benefit to selected patients. Estrogen can lower serum IGF-1 in patients with acromegaly and clinical symptoms of acromegaly often improve during pregnancy.[122] Estrogen may suppress hepatic IGF-1 synthesis and alter GH signaling via its interaction with transcription pathways.[122,123] A study using chronic tamoxifen, a partially competitive estrogen receptor antagonist, led to a transient increase in GH levels, but achieved a lasting decrease in IGF-1 with normalization of IGF-1 levels in 4 of 19 patients.[124] A newer selective-estrogen modulator, raloxifene, was studied in 13 postmenopausal female patients, 9 of whom were resistant to somatostatin analog and dopamine agonist therapies. IGF-1 decreased by more than 30% in 10 patients, and normalized in 7.[125] A study in male acromegalic patients demonstrated that raloxifene could successfully decrease IGF-1 levels; however, there was no change in clinical symptoms with raloxifene in male patients.[126]

Radiation Therapy

Radiotherapy should be considered for patients who are unsuitable for or have failed surgery and in whom medical therapy fails to achieve remission. Conventional radiotherapy is generally delivered in fractionated doses of 1.6 to 1.8 Gy four to five times weekly over 5 to 6 weeks, for a total dose of 45 to 59 Gy.[127] There is a fall in GH levels in the first 2 years, followed by a slow continued decline thereafter.[127-129] GH concentrations higher than 5 µg/L are achieved in 80% of patients within 10 to 15 years, though few patients are ever cured. A study followed acromegalic patients who received conventional external irradiation for an average of 12.8 years after radiotherapy; only one third of these patients achieved normal biochemical parameters.[130]

There are significant risks associated with radiotherapy. Hypopituitarism occurs in 30% to 70% of patients within 10 years after treatment.[42] There are risks of visual changes from radiation effects on the optic nerve or chiasm and cognitive and neurological deficits from radiation necrosis in adjacent brain, and an increased risk for the development of secondary brain tumors such as gliomas.[127,131] There are reports that conventional radiotherapy is associated with an increase in mortality rate from stroke among acromegalic patients.[132]

SRS has lower long-term risks of developing a second neoplasm or cognitive changes than does conventional radiation, and SRS induces remission more rapidly than does fractionated radiotherapy.[42,45] In a report of Gamma Knife radiosurgery (GKS) for GH-secreting adenomas, GKS was used as the primary procedure in 68 of 79 patients. GH levels declined within 6 months in all cases, and GH levels normalized in 96% of the 45 patients who were followed for more than 2 years. Tumors shrank in 52% of patients after 12 months, 87% of patients after 24 months, and 92% of patients after 36 months or more.[45] A small early series using CyberKnife radiosurgery demonstrated that 44% of patients achieved biochemical remission after an average 25 months of follow-up.[43]

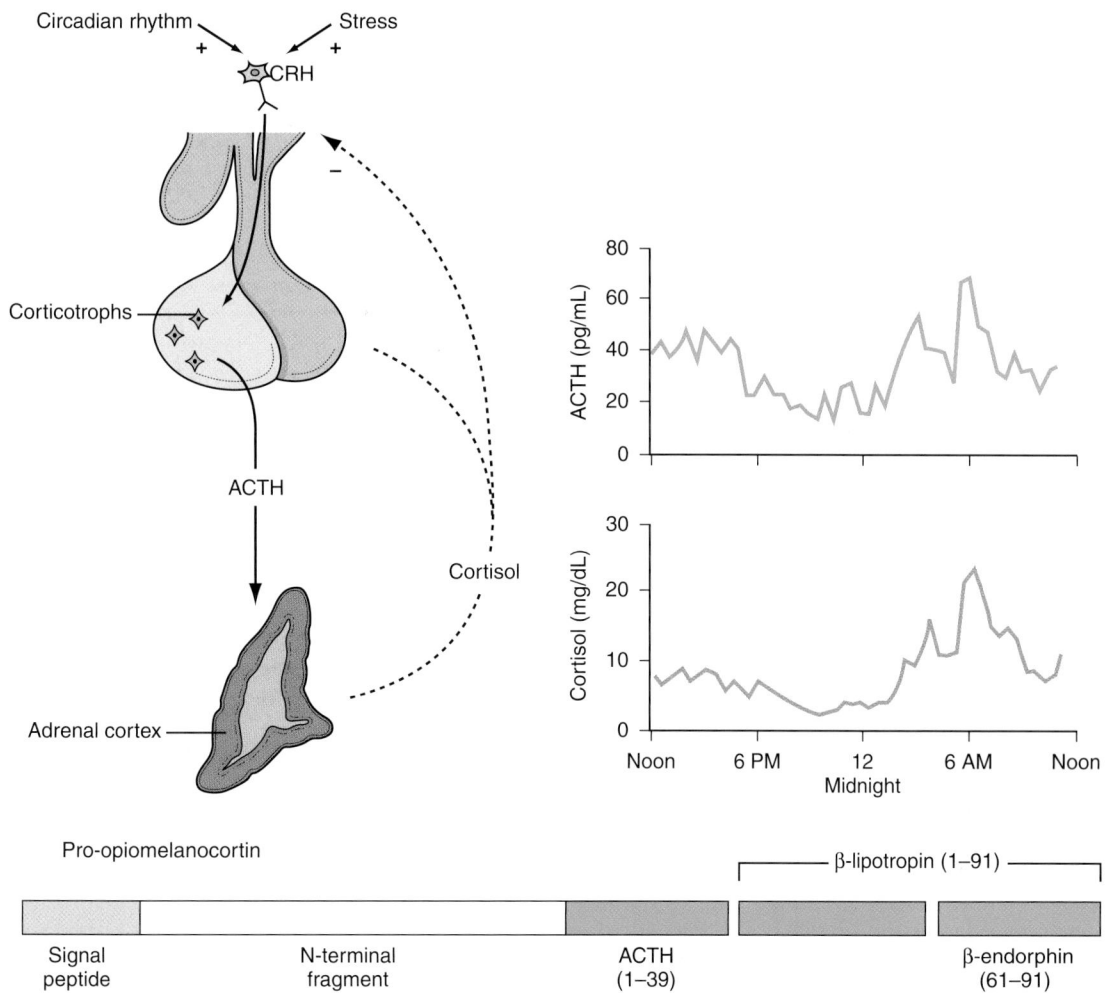

FIGURE 40.12 The hypothalamic-pituitary-adrenal axis. Corticotropin-releasing hormone (CRH) is released by the hypothalamus to stimulate the corticotrophs of the anterior pituitary to secrete adrenocorticotropic hormone (ACTH), which then stimulates cortisol secretion from the adrenal cortex. Cortisol exerts negative feedback at the pituitary and hypothalamus to inhibit further CRH and ACTH release.

Adrenocorticotropic Hormone–Secreting Adenomas

Cortisol Physiology: Hypothalamic-Pituitary-Adrenal Axis

Cortisol is necessary for the maintenance of life and for the homeostatic biochemical and physiological responses to stress. The hypothalamic-pituitary-adrenal (HPA) axis regulates cortisol secretion (Fig. 40.12). Hypothalamic secretion of CRH occurs in response to signals from the brain to produce the circadian variation of plasma cortisol concentrations and in response to emotional, biochemical, and physical stressors. CRH then stimulates pituitary ACTH production and secretion in the corticotrophs. The adrenal glands secrete cortisol in response to ACTH.

ACTH and cortisol have pulsatile secretion patterns. In a normal subject, ACTH peaks in the early morning and then declines to a nadir around midnight. Circadian rhythms affect ACTH secretion, so levels are affected by light and change in time zone. Physical trauma, surgery, fever, and hypoglycemia increase ACTH and cortisol secretion. The half-life of bioactive ACTH is only 4 to 8 minutes, but its immunoreactive half-life is quite variable.

Glucocorticoids increase gluconeogenesis and inhibit glucose uptake and utilization by peripheral tissues. With extended exposure to glucocorticoids, lipolysis is enhanced and body fat redistribution occurs. Glucocorticoids suppress inflammatory responses, lower peripheral lymphocyte counts, and increase the level of circulating granulocytes. They increase osteoclast formation but inhibit osteoblasts and decrease new bone formation. Linear growth is suppressed in children. The catabolic effects of glucocorticoids cause the destruction of muscle proteins and lead to myopathy. Fibroblast proliferation and function are inhibited, as is the synthesis of some extracellular matrix components, leading to impaired wound healing. Glucocorticoids also lead to behavioral changes, including alteration of mood, sleep, and cognition.

Cortisol Excess: Cushing's Syndrome

Chronic exposure to excess cortisol produces Cushing's syndrome. Generally, late evening plasma levels are elevated over the normal values of 5 to 25 ng/mL, and the usual diurnal variation is lost, leading to an elevated mean cortisol level. This chronic hypercortisolemia suppresses hypothalamic CRH

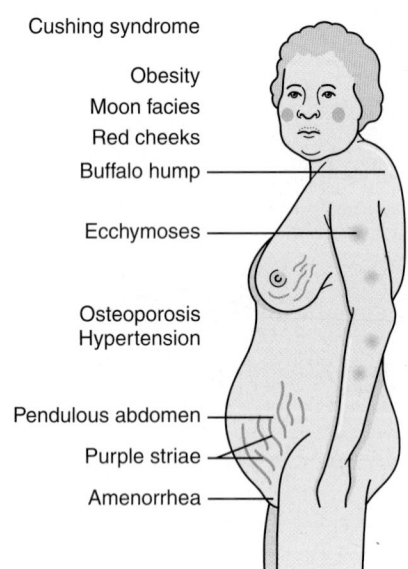

Cushing syndrome
- Obesity
- Moon facies
- Red cheeks
- Buffalo hump
- Ecchymoses
- Osteoporosis
- Hypertension
- Pendulous abdomen
- Purple striae
- Amenorrhea

FIGURE 40.13 Clinical manifestations of Cushing's syndrome.

and pituitary ACTH secretion, and the corticotroph cells atrophy.

Symptoms associated with Cushing's syndrome include centripetal obesity, buffalo hump and supraclavicular fat pad, moon facies due to thickening of facial fat, facial telangiectasias, exophthalmos, hypertension, hyperglycemia or diabetes mellitus, hirsutism, acne, abdominal striae, amenorrhea or hypogonadism, muscle wasting and proximal myopathy, osteoporosis, hyperpigmentation, polyuria, and emotional disturbances including depression or psychosis (Fig. 40.13). Multiple organ systems are affected and, if untreated, the mortality rate is 50% within 5 years.[133] Cardiovascular complications are a major cause of morbidity and death in untreated Cushing's syndrome. Hypertension and congestive heart failure are common.

Cushing's Disease

Cushing's syndrome is a constellation of clinical signs and symptoms that accompany excess serum cortisol, and Cushing's disease is the presence of pituitary corticotroph tumor and accounts for 70% to 80% of all cases of Cushing's syndrome.[133]

Corticotroph cell adenomas fall into two categories: those that secrete ACTH and result in Cushing's disease, and silent tumors, which contain ACTH but do not lead to clinical evidence of ACTH excess. Adenomas in Cushing's disease are generally microadenomas. Macroadenomas are a rare cause of Cushing's disease; they tend to be invasive and are quite difficult to treat. Cushing's disease has a female predilection and usually occurs between the ages of 25 and 45 years. It is gradual in onset and runs a chronic course; most patients have symptoms for 3 to 6 years before diagnosis.[133]

In Cushing's disease, the HPA axis maintains its homeostatic responses, but is altered to respond only to higher than normal glucocorticoid levels. Cushing's syndrome from an ectopic ACTH-secreting tumor, on the other hand, will exhibit autonomous cortisol production and fail to react to any feedback inhibition (Fig. 40.14).

Cushing's disease is unusual in children but does account for about one third of pediatric Cushing's syndrome cases. When it does occur in children, it usually begins after puberty and affects the sexes equally. Cushing's disease in children is manifested by impaired skeletal growth and obesity. Early treatment is imperative because resumption of normal growth can be achieved if patients are treated prior to epiphyseal fusion.[134]

Disease remission criteria have varied over the years, but are currently defined in most studies as a normal 24-hour urinary free cortisol level, a normal or subnormal morning serum cortisol level, regression of clinical stigmata, and cessation of tumor growth. Therapeutic options include microsurgical resection, radiotherapy, medical therapy, and bilateral adrenalectomy. Microsurgical resection remains the first line of care for the majority of patients with Cushing's disease.

A minority of Cushing's syndrome patients have an ectopic, nonpituitary, source of excess ACTH, CRH, or cortisol production. This production is most often due to small cell lung carcinoma, but may be attributable to pancreatic islet cell tumor, pheochromocytoma, medullary thyroid carcinoma, bronchial, thymic or pancreatic carcinoid, adrenal cortisol-secreting tumors, or another neuroendocrine tumor.

Evaluation

When Cushing's syndrome is suspected, one must first establish that there is indeed excess secretion of cortisol. The 24-hour cortisol production must be measured, such as via 24-hour urine collection for free cortisol and 17-hydroxyglucocorticoid excretion. Cortisol urinary excretion products, 24-hour urinary free cortisol levels, are elevated from the normal 20 to 90 μg to more than 150 μg in Cushing's syndrome.

The presence of normal sensitivity of the HPA axis to negative feedback by glucocorticoids should be assessed as well. This can be done with low-dose glucocorticoid tests including the overnight test or the low-dose portion of the 6-day dexamethasone suppression test. Cushing's disease is diagnosed if a patient has (1) increased basal cortisol levels, (2) relative resistance to negative feedback from glucocorticoids, (3) ACTH response to decreased cortisol, (4) ACTH response to CRH or vasopressin, (5) cortisol response to exogenous ACTH, and (6) a pituitary source of the excess ACTH (Table 40.2).

In the overnight dexamethasone suppression test (DST), 0.5 to 1 mg of dexamethasone is given orally at midnight, and serum cortisol is checked at 8:00 AM the next morning, and in the 2-day low-dose DST, 0.5 mg of dexamethasone is given orally every 6 hours for eight doses. In normal subjects, these doses are enough to suppress the HPA axis, leading to serum cortisol levels less than 140 nmol (5 μg/dL), urinary 17-hydroxycorticosteroid (17-OHCS) less than 6.9 μmol (2.5 mg) in 24 hours, and urinary free cortisol less than 55 nmol (20 μg) in 24 hours. Patients with Cushing's syndrome, on the other hand, will not have this HPA axis suppression.

Serum free cortisol filters into saliva and urine, so saliva and urine free cortisol levels are accurate indicators of increased cortisol secretion. Salivary cortisol is easy to use in an outpatient setting and allows for repeated sampling. An 11:00 PM salivary free cortisol greater than 3.6 nmol/L is highly suggestive of Cushing's syndrome.

FIGURE 40.14 Causes of Cushing's syndrome. In ACTH-dependent hypercortisolism, cortisol secretion is excessive in response to adrenocorticotropic hormone (ACTH) secretion by either a corticotroph adenoma or a nonpituitary (ectopic) tumor. In ACTH-independent hypercortisolism, there is autonomous overproduction of cortisol due to an adrenal gland abnormality.

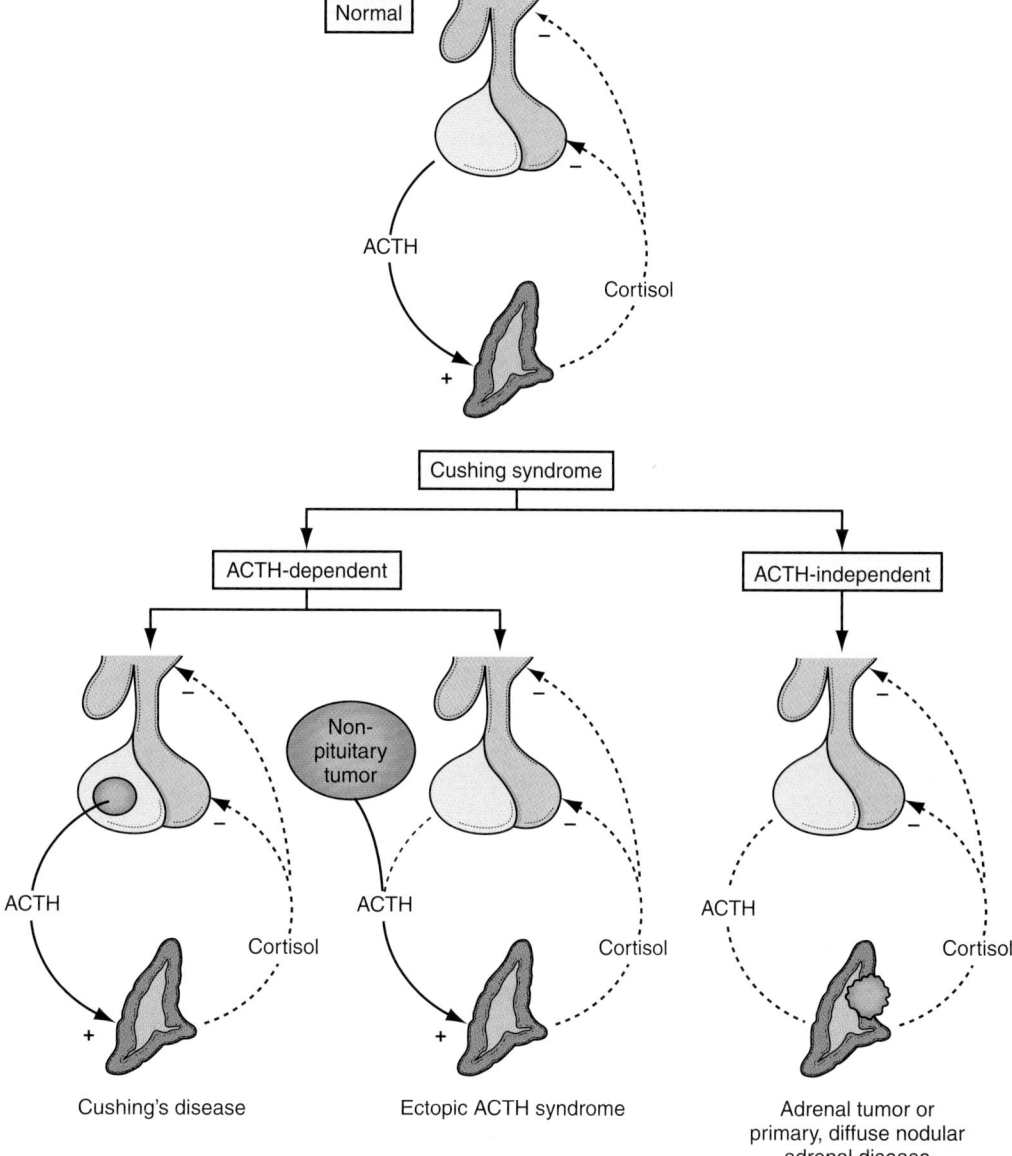

Once it is determined that a patient has Cushing's syndrome, then it must be determined if this is due to Cushing's disease or a nonpituitary source of excess glucocorticoids. Normal ACTH level is less than 10 pg/mL (2 pmol/L). Patients with ACTH-dependent disease have excess cortisol due to excess ACTH, so they will have plasma ACTH levels that are inappropriately elevated for the level of cortisol present. Conversely, the hypothalamic and pituitary portions of the HPA axis are relatively normal in primary adrenal disease, so hypercortisolemia will suppress pituitary ACTH secretion in these patients, and their serum ACTH levels will be undetectable or very low. A simultaneous serum cortisol level must be drawn to properly evaluate the plasma ACTH level.

In nearly all patients with adrenal tumors, the most common form of ACTH-independent Cushing's syndrome, adrenal imaging with MRI or CT scanning identifies an adrenal lesion. Thus, the combined results of the plasma ACTH levels and adrenal imaging are used either to diagnose a primary adrenal disorder or to eliminate primary adrenal disease as the cause.

Many ACTH-secreting pituitary and ectopic tumors are very small and are not easily recognized on radiographic imaging, so diagnosing the cause of Cushing's syndrome may be challenging. Basic endocrinological principles can assist in making the diagnosis. ACTH-secreting pituitary adenomas are well-differentiated tumors that originate from pituitary corticotrophs. They are therefore more likely to respond to glucocorticoids such as dexamethasone or to CRH stimulation than are ectopic ACTH-secreting tumors, which arise from tissues that are not supposed to secrete ACTH, respond to glucocorticoids, or contain receptors for CRH. Therefore, a high-dose, 8-mg overnight dexamethasone suppression test, the high-dose portion of the Liddle test, the CRH or arginine-vasopressin (AVP) stimulation tests, and the metyrapone test may be useful.

Patients with Cushing's disease will generally suppress their levels to 50% of their baseline with the high-dose DST, but patients with ectopic ACTH tumors or adrenal tumors will not have any significant suppression. The Liddle test is

TABLE 40.2 Clinical Approach to Patients Suspected of Having Cushing's Syndrome

Definitive Diagnosis of Cushing's Syndrome
1. Establish hypercortisolism:
- 24-hour urinary free cortisol
or
- 24-hour urinary 17-hydroxysteroid per gram of urinary creatinine
2. Establish resistance to dexamethasone suppression:
- Overnight low-dose (1 mg) dexamethasone suppression test

Differential Diagnosis of Cushing's Syndrome
1. Distinguish between ACTH-independent and ACTH-dependent types of Cushing's syndrome:
- Plasma ACTH
2. For diagnosis of ACTH-independent Cushing's syndrome (adrenal disease):
- Adrenal CT or MRI
3. For diagnosis of ACTH-dependent Cushing's syndrome:
- CRH stimulation test
- High-dose dexamethasone suppression test
  - Overnight high-dose test (8 mg)
or
  - 6-day low-dose, high-dose test (Liddle)
- Bilateral petrosal vein sampling for ACTH (with and without CRH)
4. Confirm diagnosis:
- If tests indicate Cushing's disease: pituitary MRI
- If tests indicate ectopic ACTH secretion: MRI of chest and abdomen

ACTH, adrenocorticotropic hormone; CRH, corticotropin-releasing hormone; MRI, magnetic resonance imaging.

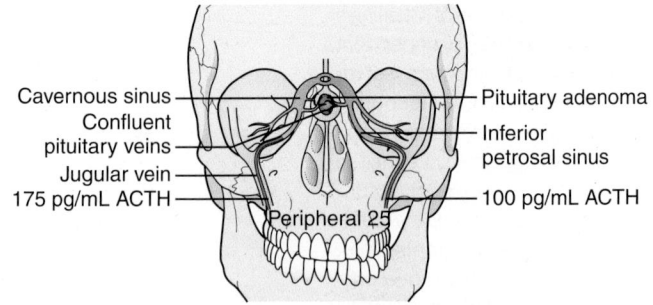

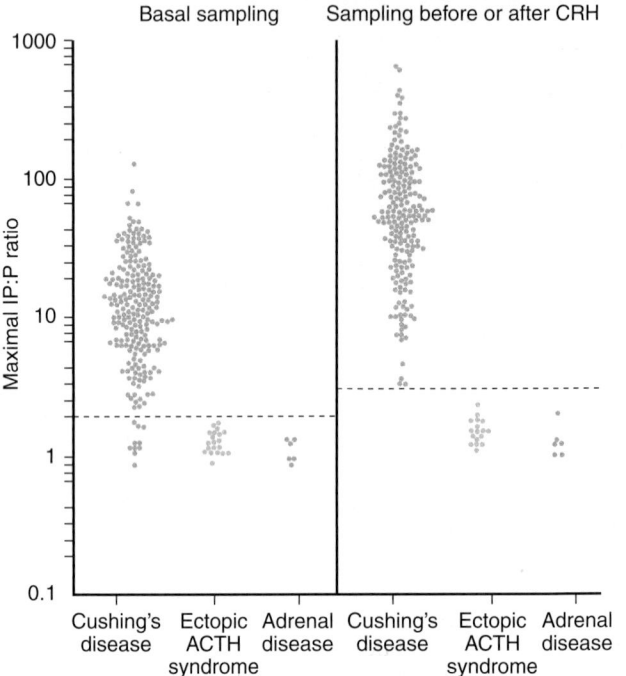

FIGURE 40.15 Inferior petrosal sinus sampling (IPSS). Preoperative lateralization of an adrenocorticotropic hormone (ACTH)-secreting microadenoma may be made by bilateral, simultaneous IPSS. ACTH levels are measured in the peripheral circulation and compared to the levels present in each sinus before and after stimulation of ACTH secretion.

a high-dose 6-day dexamethasone suppression test. A patient undergoes 2 days of baseline urinary 17-hydroxysteroid measurements, then is given 2 days of low-dose dexamethasone, 0.5 mg orally every 6 hours, and finally is given 2 days of high-dose dexamethasone, 2 mg orally every 6 hours. Liddle first observed in 1960 that most patients with a pituitary source of excess ACTH, Cushing's disease, have a more than 50% decrease in 17-OHCS excretion on the second day of high-dose glucocorticoid administration, and that this response was not seen in patients with adrenal tumors.[135]

CRH and AVP are physiological secretagogues to which most pituitary microadenomas will respond. In Cushing's disease, either compound will lead to a significant increase in ACTH, but in cases of ectopic ACTH secretion, ACTH levels will not increase. The metyrapone test is a less commonly used test. Metyrapone is a compound that inhibits cortisol synthesis at several steps, including at the conversion of 11-deoxycortisol to cortisol. As plasma cortisol levels fall, corticotrophs respond by increasing production of ACTH, which can be measured via increased urinary 17-OHCS. For patients with ectopic ACTH production, the hypothalamic and pituitary axis is chronically suppressed and is not reactivated with metyrapone.

When Cushing's disease is suspected, the location of the tumor must be established. If radiographic imaging does not demonstrate a lesion, inferior petrosal sinus sampling (IPSS) can be of assistance. Bilateral catheters are placed via the femoral veins and fed up the internal jugular veins to the inferior petrosal sinuses that drain the pituitary gland. ACTH levels are measured in the peripheral circulation and each sinus both before and after injection of CRH to stimulate ACTH

secretion. Bilateral catheterization allows for simultaneous sampling of the right and left sinuses so that the ACTH concentrations can be compared. A gradient between the sinuses can lateralize the tumor within the pituitary. As spontaneous ACTH release is naturally episodic, CRH stimulation is given to ensure secretion at the time of sampling. An inferior petrosal sinus to peripheral blood (IPS:P) ratio greater than 2.0 in basal samples has up to 95% sensitivity and 100% specificity, while a peak IPS:P ratio greater than 3.0 after CRH administration has been reported to have 100% sensitivity and 100% specificity[136-138] (Fig. 40.15). An intersinus gradient greater than 1.4 predicts the location of the lesion in up to 75% of patients. Cavernous sinus sampling is less commonly used, but can provide slightly more accurate localization.

Mild hyperprolactinemia is present in about one quarter of patients with Cushing's disease, as some of these tumors contain PRL-secreting cells.[139] PRL levels can also be measured as part of the IPSS to assist in localizing the tumor.

Most patients undergo a combination of these tests. It is important to establish that the patient does indeed have Cushing's syndrome before proceeding with tests to determine if the diagnosis is Cushing's disease or an ectopic source. In subjects without Cushing's syndrome, pituitary ACTH secretion is suppressed by dexamethasone and responds to CRH. This result can therefore be erroneously attributed to Cushing's disease, causing a normal patient to undergo unnecessary pituitary surgery.

Surgery

Surgery is the first line of therapy for Cushing's disease, achieving a high cure rate with low levels of morbidity and mortality.[140] The majority of operations done for relief of Cushing's disease are accomplished using a transsphenoidal approach. When a pituitary microadenoma is found intraoperatively and is successfully removed, up to 96% of patients will achieve remission.[141,142] However, clinical recovery often takes 6 months or more. Long-term remission in patients with macroadenomas or tumors that invade parasellar structures is significantly lower, however, at 45% to 65%.[141-143] Recurrence occurs in up to 25% of patients and increases progressively over time.[144,145]

Operative adjuncts include endoscopy, detection of tumors using ultrasonic probes, and IPSS to guide intraoperative exploration. It must be remembered that a small tumor may hide within the posterior lobe, the cavernous sinus dura, the suprasellar region, along the pituitary stalk, or even within the sphenoid bone. Complete exploration of the gland extending to each cavernous sinus and from the tuberculum sellae down to the clivus is imperative. The dura is opened and a subdural dissection should be performed to expose all surfaces of the gland.

If a surface tumor is not uncovered, intraglandular exploration begins with a horizontal incision in the pituitary gland and then external compression is gently applied to the gland surface in the hope that compression will allow the tumor to extrude through the incision.

If unsuccessful in finding a tumor on initial evaluation of the gland, one can explore the gland by vertical incisions in the hemisphere indicated by the IPSS data or along the central mucoid wedge where most corticotrophs reside. If the tumor is still not found, the posterior pituitary should be examined, as some tumors arise at the junction between the anterior and posterior pituitary or in the posterior lobe.

After successful surgery, cortisol will drop to lower than 2 µg/dL or undetectable levels within a day, and the patient may require cortisol replacement until normal corticotroph function is regained. If the patient is not in remission, one should reassess the diagnosis by reviewing all laboratory, radiographic, and pathological results. If it seems certain that a pituitary source is the cause, then re-exploration of the pituitary may be indicated, as this may uncover residual tumor or a previously undetected adenoma.

If the tumor cannot be completely resected, then radiosurgery or radiation therapy may be recommended. In patients who have serious medical problems and cannot be treated effectively by medication, adrenalectomy and radiation therapy to the pituitary should be considered.

Favorable prognostic features for surgery include definitive laboratory data, a visible tumor on preoperative MRI,

and the discovery of an ACTH-staining tumor at surgery.[146] Unfavorable prognostic factors include severe, rapidly progressive Cushing's syndrome, an invasive tumor, and a macroadenoma.

Though the risks of TSA are relatively low, any surgery has associated complications. Some patients benefit from a short course of ketoconazole, a steroidogenesis inhibitor, to assist in stabilizing them prior to surgery. Cushingoid patients generally have multiple medical problems, including chronic hypercortisolemia and diabetes mellitus, which can make wound healing difficult. The risk of diabetes insipidus (DI) is almost 18% following surgery.[34] Patients with Cushing's disease are at increased risk for deep vein thrombosis, and hyponatremia and other electrolyte abnormalities can occur a few days after surgery, especially in patients who develop DI.

Radiation Therapy

Although conventional fractionated radiotherapy is effective in reducing the hypercortisolemia of Cushing's disease, there is a significant delay before the full clinical and biochemical effect occurs. Remission occurs in 50% to 83% and can rise to 90% by 5 years after treatment.[147,148] Though the latent period ranges from 4 to 60 months, remission usually starts after 9 months of treatment, and most patients are in remission within 2 years.[147] A study followed long-term outcomes in 40 patients with Cushing's disease who had failed surgery and were then treated with 45 to 50 Gy of conventional external beam radiotherapy in 25 to 28 fractions. Normalization of cortisol levels was achieved in 28% of patients 1 year after radiation, 73% of patients 3 years after treatment, 78% 5 years after treatment, and 84% 10 years after treatment.[149] In the same study, pituitary hormone deficiencies developed in 62% of patients within 5 years after radiation, and 76% within 10 years.

SRS can be used as primary treatment for patients who are not good surgical candidates, and it can be a useful adjunct to surgery, medical therapy, or fractionated radiotherapy.[150] The peripheral dose ranges from 25 to 40 Gy, and the dose to the optic nerves should not exceed 10 Gy.[38,150,151] It is preferable to have a tumor less than 30 mm in diameter and a distance of at least 2 to 5 mm between the tumor and the optic chiasm.[38,149]

A marked decrease in the serum cortisol level is often obtained within 3 months after SRS; however, achievement of a biochemical cure may be delayed up to 3 years. The most common complication of SRS is hypopituitarism, which has been reported to occur in 16% to 55% of patients within 5 years following GKS.[152] Optic neuropathy has been reported in less than 2% of cases and induction of a secondary neoplasm in less than 1% of cases. The risk of diabetes insipidus appears to be negligible with SRS.[34]

In a series of 90 patients who underwent Gamma Knife radiosurgery with a median marginal dose of 25 Gy, 49 achieved remission as defined by a normal 24-hour urine free cortisol level, with a 13-month mean time to remission.[153] GKS can achieve remission in more than 60% of patients with Cushing's disease who have failed surgery.[154] Another report demonstrated that among 20 patients with Cushing's disease who underwent GKS, there was complete resolution of the tumor on MRI in 30%, and levels of ACTH and cortisol normalized in 35%.[151] Microadenomas appear to have a higher remission rate than do macroadenomas, and complications following SRS are less common in patients with microadenomas than in those with larger tumors.[151,155]

Repeat SRS after a patient has failed to go into remission may increase the risk that the patient will develop visual deficits or cranial nerve palsies, so repeat radiation is reserved only for those patients who are not candidates for surgery or pharmacotherapy.[153]

SRS with proton beam therapy has little damaging effect on tissues surrounding the tumor, can often be given in one session, and does not have the same radiation-induced side effects as does conventional radiotherapy.[156] Proton beam therapy in patients with Cushing's disease generally has a high efficacy, produces high remission rates, is relatively safe, and causes few cases of hypopituitarism. It can be used alone or in combination with unilateral adrenalectomy. In a study of 98 patients who received 80- to 90-Gy proton beam therapy, 90% had normalized hormone values and no clinical signs of disease in 6 to 36 months;[156] 94% of these patients remained in remission 3 to 5 years after radiation.

In fractionated stereotactic radiation therapy (fSRT), a dose of approximately 50 Gy in 1.8 to 2 Gy per fraction is delivered using multiple convergent beams. This process may reduce the risk of damage to the optic chiasm as compared to conventional radiotherapy.[147] In a study of patients with Cushing's disease who had previously failed surgery, complete remission occurred in 9 of 12 patients after a median of 29 months, with partial remission in the remaining patients.[147] Another study compared 48 patients who received fSRT or linac-based SRS. Hormone levels normalized in 33% of the patients who received SRS and in 54% of the patients who received fSRT, after an average latency time of 8.5 months and 18 months, respectively.[157]

Interstitial irradiation, the transsphenoidal implantation of radioactive labeled yttrium-90 (^{90}Y) or gold-198 (^{198}Au) rods into the sella, is also a safe and effective treatment for Cushing's disease. It does not have as long a latency period of external radiation and may induce remission faster than other nonsurgical options.[158] In a study of 86 patients with Cushing's disease who were treated with interstitial irradiation, the 1-year remission rate was 77%. There were no clinical or radiological relapses, though 37% of patients developed hypopituitarism.[158]

Medical Therapy

Pharmacotherapy is reserved for patients who cannot safely undergo surgery or for whom surgery has failed. Medical treatments are also used to transiently control cortisol levels in patients who have undergone radiation therapy and are awaiting the therapeutic effects of the radiation treatment. A major disadvantage of medical therapy is the need for lifelong treatment; in general, recurrence follows discontinuation of treatment, unless radiation therapy has also been received.

Medical options fall into three main categories: steroidogenesis inhibitors that reduce cortisol levels by adrenolytic activity or enzymatic inhibition, neuromodulatory compounds that decrease ACTH release from a pituitary tumor, and glucocorticoid antagonists that block cortisol action at its receptor. Steroidogenesis inhibitors are the medications of choice when pharmacotherapy is being used for Cushing's disease.

Steroidogenesis inhibitors, including ketoconazole, mitotane, and trilostane, decrease cortisol via direct enzymatic inhibition of steroidogenesis. Ketoconazole, a cytochrome P-450 enzyme inhibitor, is the best tolerated of these agents and effectively reduces plasma cortisol levels in about 70% of patients.[159] In general, ACTH levels increase in patients with Cushing's disease during chronic therapy with ketoconazole, suggesting that its major effect in these patients is on the adrenal cortex rather than the corticotrophs. A meta-analysis of 82 patients showed that treatment with ketoconazole alone reduced plasma cortisol levels in 70%. Patients with Cushing's disease respond promptly with resolution of clinical and biochemical manifestations in 4 to 6 weeks; 600 to 800 mg per day total dosage is often required to normalize urinary free cortisol. Side effects include headache, sedation, nausea and vomiting, hepatotoxicity, gynecomastia, decreased libido, and impotence.

Mitotane achieves remission in up to 83% of patients, though only a third sustain remission after discontinuing treatment.[160] Extensive metabolism of the drug is required, so a response may not occur for several months. Side effects include anorexia, diarrhea, ataxia, gynecomastia, hypercholesterolemia, hypouricemia, leukopenia, and arthralgias. Mitotane is relatively contraindicated in women desiring fertility as it may act as a teratogen even years after discontinuation due to gradual release from adipose tissue. Metyrapone is an 11β-hydroxylase inhibitor that may also inhibit ACTH secretion directly at high doses. It can be useful as monotherapy or in combination with radiation. Nausea, dizziness, and rash may limit its use, and it can lead to an increase in androgens and hypertension.

Trilostane is a relatively weak inhibitor of steroidogenesis, which results in some decrease in synthesis of cortisol by the adrenal gland. Side effects include diarrhea, abdominal pain, nausea, flushing, headache, rhinorrhea, decreased libido, and impotence. Aminoglutethimide, an anticonvulsant, blocks the first step in cortisol biosynthesis. It is not useful as monotherapy but can be very effective when given with other agents, usually metyrapone. Side effects include somnolence, headache, goiter, and hypothyroidism, hypoadrenalism, and hypoaldosteronism. Etomidate is given intravenously, so it may be used when patients cannot take medications by mouth. Etomidate is an imidazole anesthetic that blocks 11β-hydroxylation of deoxycortisol and lowers plasma cortisol. It is often used for acute control of hypercortisolemia in hospitalized patients as it significantly decreases cortisol levels within 12 hours. Side effects include fatigue, hypotension, hypertension, and bradycardia.

Neuromodulatory compounds, such as bromocriptine and valproic acid, reduce ACTH release from the tumor. Response rates are poor, but no large-scale placebo-controlled trials have been reported. Approximately 40% of patients in case reports and small series normalized urine or plasma glucocorticoids with chronic bromocriptine therapy.[161] Valproic acid decreased ACTH concentrations in patients receiving the drug to inhibit seizures. However, despite case reports suggesting efficacy, placebo-controlled studies do not support its use as monotherapy.[161]

Mifepristone (RU486) competitively antagonizes glucocorticoid, androgen, and progestin receptors to inhibit the action of endogenous ligands. Its use in Cushing's syndrome has been limited to a few investigations of patients with ectopic ACTH secretion and one patient with Cushing's disease.[162] Rosiglitazone, a thiazolidinedione compound with peroxisome proliferator-activated receptor g (PPARg)–binding affinity, suppresses ACTH secretion in tumors and inhibits tumor cell growth. In patients with Cushing's disease, rosiglitazone reduced cortisol secretion and lowered plasma ACTH; urinary free cortisol levels normalized 30 to 60 days after administration.[163]

Adrenalectomy and Nelson Syndrome

When patients have severe Cushing's disease and have failed multiple prior treatments, bilateral adrenalectomy may be considered. This can be done laparoscopically and is an effective treatment that will definitively treat Cushing's disease

because it removes the source of endogenous cortisol. These patients will, however, require lifelong steroid replacement.

Following bilateral adrenalectomy, the loss of the inhibitory effects of the excess cortisol on a pituitary tumor's ACTH secretion and growth leads to very high levels of plasma ACTH. These levels may suffice to increase skin pigmentation and cause progression of the ACTH-secreting pituitary tumor, which occasionally becomes invasive or even metastatic. This is known as Nelson syndrome and the prevalence after adrenalectomy ranges from 8% to 42%.[164-166] These invasive tumors are unlikely to be cured with TSA; in one study, only 5 of 11 patients with Nelson syndrome achieved remission after surgery.[167] Prior to adrenalectomy, pituitary radiation is often recommended to decrease the risk of developing Nelson syndrome.

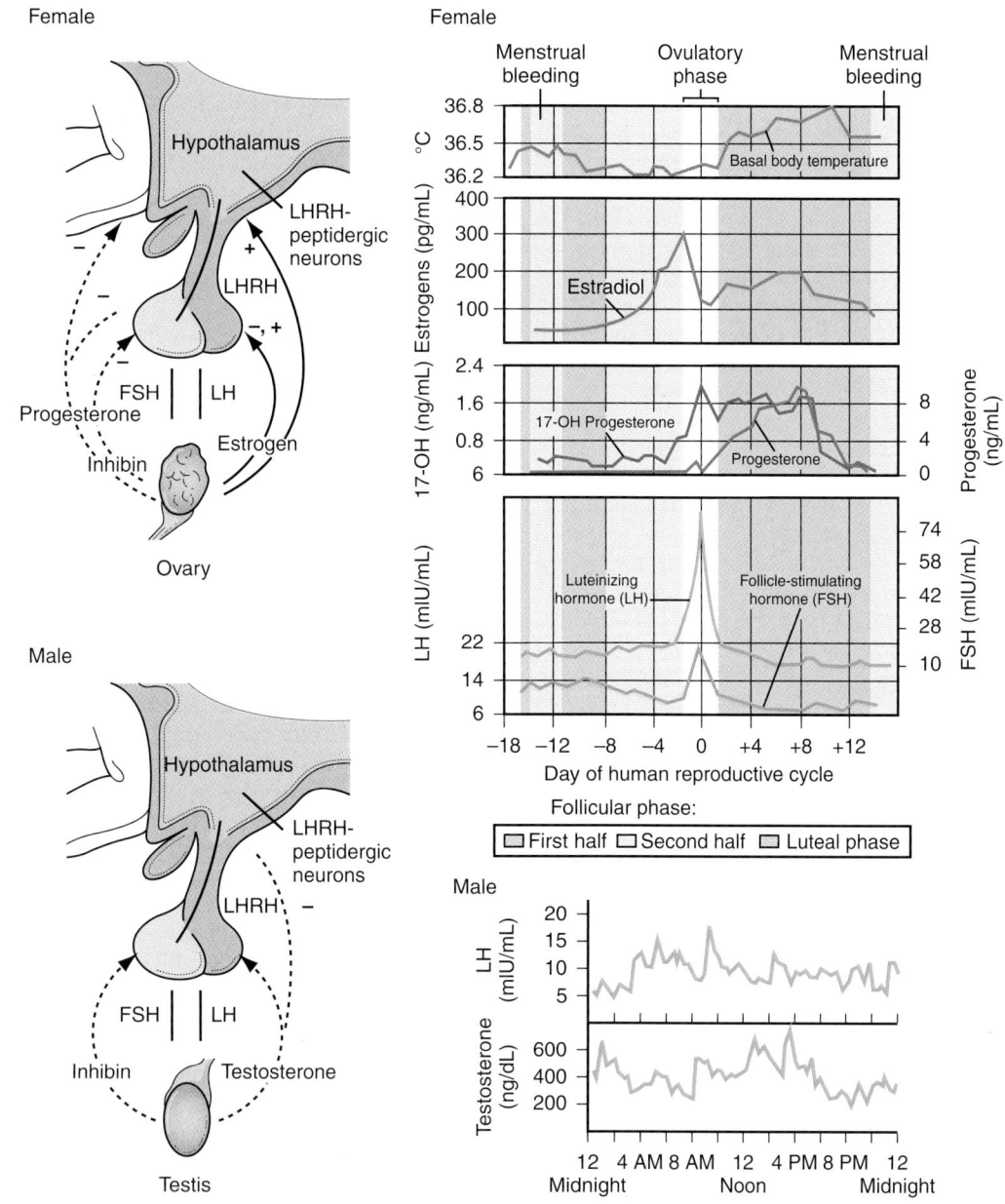

FIGURE 40.16 The hypothalamic-pituitary-gonadal axis. Pulsatile release of gonadotropin-releasing hormone (GnRH) from the hypothalamus stimulates episodic pituitary release of follicle-stimulating hormone (FSH) and luteinizing hormone (LH). Negative feedback regulation is exerted by the sex steroids, estrogen and testosterone, and the peptide inhibin from the ovaries or testes.

Gonadotropin-Secreting Adenomas

Gonadotropin Physiology

FSH and LH are produced and released by the gonadotrophs of the adenohypophysis to regulate ovarian and testicular function (Fig. 40.16). In women, FSH stimulates growth of the granulosa cells of the ovarian follicle and controls their estrogen secretion. At the midpoint of the menstrual cycle, the increasing level of estradiol stimulates a surge of LH secretion, which then triggers ovulation. After ovulation, LH supports the formation of the corpus luteum. Exposure of the ovary to FSH is required for expression of the LH receptors. In men, LH is responsible for the production of testosterone by Leydig cells in the testes. The combined effects of FSH and testosterone on the seminiferous tubule stimulate sperm production.

FSH and LH secretion occur in a pulsatile fashion in response to pulses of secretion of GnRH from the hypothalamus. GnRH is also known as *LH-releasing hormone* (LHRH) because of its potent stimulation of LH secretion. Levels of FSH and LH are regulated by a balance of GnRH stimulation, negative feedback regulation from the inhibin peptide secreted by the ovaries and the testes, and the effect of the sex steroids on the pituitary and the hypothalamus. Appropriate concentrations of FSH and LH are required for normal sexual development and reproductive function in both women and men. LH and FSH circulate in blood predominantly in the monomeric form found in the pituitary. FSH has a half-life of 3 to 5 hours, so serum levels are more stable than are those of LH, which has a half-life of 30 to 60 minutes.

GnRH stimulates gonadotropin secretion from the pituitary for the first few months of life. Then the pituitary becomes unresponsive to GnRH until puberty, when pulsatile secretion of FSH and LH occur in response to pulses of GnRH. At menopause, when gonadal failure occurs, the negative feedback provided by the hormonal products of the gonads is eliminated so serum levels of FSH and LH increase.

Gonadotropin-Secreting Adenomas

Elevated FSH and LH may be seen with polycystic ovary syndrome, paraneoplastic gonadotropin secretion, precocious puberty, and gonadotrope-secreting adenomas. Though FSH- or LH-secreting pituitary adenomas are rarely observed clinically, approximately 5% of pituitary adenomas have immunohistochemical staining for the gonadotropins or their subunits. The glycoprotein pituitary hormones (TSH, FSH, and LH) each comprise two glycopeptide chains, a shared α-chain and a unique β-chain. The most commonly elevated hormone in gonadotrope adenomas is FSH, followed by LH, the α-subunit and the β-subunit of LH. These were the last functioning pituitary tumors to be characterized, likely because of a relative lack of clinical symptoms from the hormone production.

Many tumors previously classified as nonfunctioning are actually gonadotrope adenomas. A majority of clinically inactive, undifferentiated pituitary tumors will demonstrate the α-subunit on immunohistochemical screening. This subunit is frequently secreted along with PRL, ACTH, or GH in other functioning tumors as well.

These tumors are commonly undetected until symptoms occur from mass effect, such as hypopituitarism, headache, and visual problems. Most are found in middle-aged men, and only rarely are these tumors diagnosed in women of reproductive age. Postmenopausal women naturally have elevated LH and FSH levels, so hypersecretion of these hormones cannot be easily detected in these patients. Men with these lesions may have a low testosterone level because normal LH may not be produced, but this rarely affects sexual function.

Thyroid Stimulating Hormone–Secreting Adenomas

Pituitary-Thyroid Axis

Production and secretion of the thyroid hormones thyroxine (T_4) and triiodothyronine (T_3) are regulated via hypothalamic secretion of TRH into the portal venous system. In response to TRH the thyrotropes release TSH, which acts on the thyroid gland to release T_4 and T_3. Both T_3 and T_4 inhibit TRH secretion by the hypothalamus and TSH release by the pituitary (Fig. 40.17). Somatostatin, glucocorticoids, and dopamine also suppress both TRH release and the pituitary response to TRH.

Hyperthyroidism or Hypothyroidism

Symptoms of hyperthyroidism include tremulousness, anxiety, heat intolerance, diarrhea, and changes in mental status. The majority of hyperthyroid patients have a circulating thyroid-stimulating antibody, a thyroid adenoma, or thyroiditis. Hypersecretion of TSH by a pituitary adenoma is quite rare, occurring in less than 1% of hypothyroid patients.

TSH deficiency, which causes secondary hypothyroidism, results from pituitary or hypothalamic disease. It may accompany multihormonal hypopituitarism due to a large pituitary adenoma or suprasellar tumor. Signs and symptoms of hypothyroidism include fatigue, dry skin, cold intolerance, alopecia, and in severe cases, myxedema coma. Most patients with hypothyroidism have primary hypothyroidism due to a disorder of the thyroid gland. Autoimmune Hashimoto's thyroiditis, thyroid destruction after ^{131}I therapy, and surgery for hyperthyroidism are the most common causes of this condition. In primary hypothyroidism, absence of the feedback inhibition of the thyroid hormones on the pituitary and hypothalamus results in elevated TRH and TSH levels. When patients are untreated, the increased TRH secretion stimulates thyrotroph hyperplasia and may lead to pituitary enlargement. As TRH also stimulates PRL secretion, these patients may be misdiagnosed with a PRL-secreting or TSH-secreting tumor.

Hypersecretion of TSH by a pituitary adenoma is a rare cause of hyperthyroidism. Thyrotroph adenomas are the least common adenoma, accounting for less than 1% of all functioning tumors. They occur equally in men and women. The tumors are generally macroadenomas, and though patients usually have hyperthyroidism and a goiter, they often present with symptoms of mass effect.

The production of α- and β-subunits is imbalanced such that excess α-subunit is secreted, which produces a ratio of plasma α-subunit to plasma TSH of more than 1.0. In a

FIGURE 40.17 The hypothalamic-pituitary-thyroid axis. **A,** Release of thyrotropin-releasing hormone (TRH) from the hypothalamus stimulates pituitary release of thyroid-stimulating hormone (TSH). TSH promotes release of triiodothyronine (T$_3$) and thyroxine (T$_4$) from the thyroid gland. The thyroid hormones then inhibit further release of TRH and TSH via negative feedback regulation on the hypothalamus and pituitary. **B,** A thyrotroph adenoma in the pituitary secretes excessive TSH, which stimulates increased T$_3$ and T$_4$ output from the thyroid, leading to secondary hyperthyroidism.

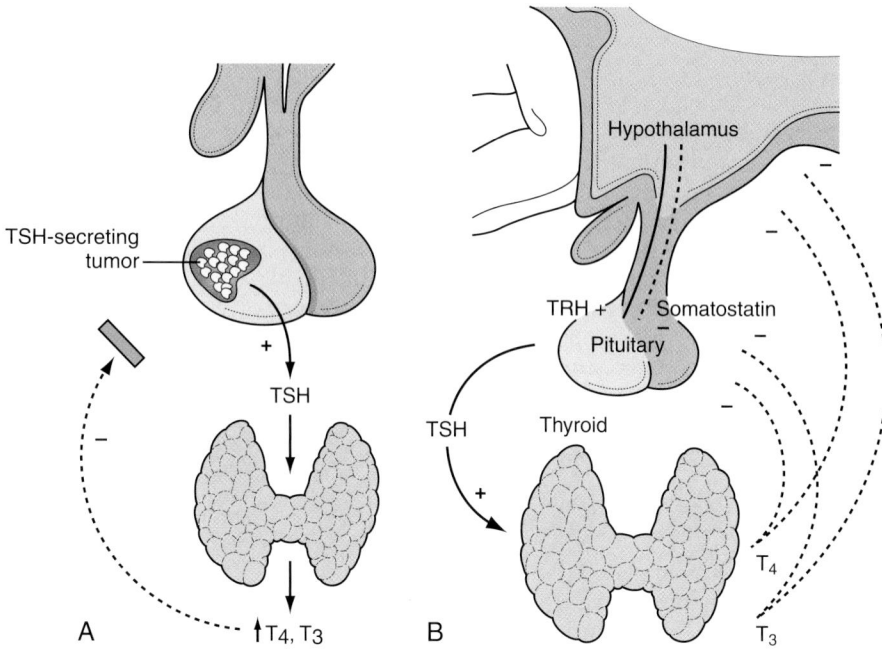

patient with hyperthyroidism, an elevated TSH level combined with an elevated ratio of the molar concentration of α-subunit to TSH indicates the presence of a TSH-secreting pituitary adenoma and calls for further evaluation of the pituitary. Many TSH-secreting pituitary tumors also secrete GH or PRL. These adenomas are chromophobic and stain positively for the α-subunit as well as the β-subunit of TSH.

Treatment

The standard treatment is transsphenoidal adenomectomy. Studies have shown that octreotide may also be used to lower serum levels of TSH, and can be used in patients who cannot tolerate surgery or to shrink the tumor mass prior to surgery.[168-170]

Because hyperthyroidisim is common and TSH-secreting tumors are very rare, many patients with TSH-secreting pituitary tumors are initially misdiagnosed and receive ablative therapy of the thyroid gland. Thus, they may not have hyperthyroidism when the pituitary tumor is discovered. In these patients the high plasma TSH levels do not fully suppress when the patient is given thyroid hormone and the TSH response to TRH is blunted. Because of the delay in diagnosis, TSH-secreting pituitary adenomas are often large, invasive tumors by the time they are recognized. In patients who receive thyroid ablation, the evolution to a large and invasive tumor seems to be analogous to the circumstance that occurs in Nelson syndrome with ACTH-secreting tumors after adrenalectomy.

PITUITARY APOPLEXY

Pituitary apoplexy is a life-threatening condition in which a tumor undergoes sudden hemorrhage or infarction. The lesion rapidly expands, resulting in acute compression of the pituitary gland, optic nerves, and cavernous sinus. Presenting

symptoms include sudden headache, emesis, visual loss, ophthalmoplegia, impaired consciousness, and acute hormonal insufficiency.[35,171]

Acute hypopituitarism can result in life-threatening cortisol deficiency and cardiovascular collapse. Immediate corticosteroid supplementation and careful fluid and electrolyte monitoring may be needed.

Visual field deficits and hormonal abnormalities may be permanent after apoplexy. However, patients who undergo surgery within a few days of the apoplectic event have a significantly higher chance of recovering visual loss than do those in whom surgery is delayed by a week or more.[171,172]

Fortunately this condition is quite rare. Although clinically asymptomatic infarct or hemorrhage has been documented in up to 25% of pituitary adenomas,[173] clinically significant apoplexy is much less common. About 50% of patients with apoplexy have nonfunctioning adenomas.[172] Radiation treatment, endocrine changes, anticoagulation, and severe systemic illness increase the risk of an apoplectic event; however, most cases appear to have no identifiable precipitating cause.[171]

PEDIATRIC ADENOMAS

Pituitary adenomas are rare in the pediatric population, accounting for less than 3% of supratentorial pediatric tumors, and occurring at an incidence of 0.1 per 1 million children.[174] Owing to the location of the gland and the importance of anterior pituitary hormones on puberty, pituitary adenomas can cause significant morbidity including delay in puberty and oligomenorrhea. The majority of pituitary lesions found in pediatric patients are macroadenomas,[175] and tumor size is often proportional to endocrine and neurological dysfunction. Thus, earlier diagnosis may lead to better outcome. Adolescent patients with growth or pubertal abnormalities therefore should undergo evaluation for a possible pituitary lesion.[176]

CONCLUSION

Pituitary tumors may present with an array of neurological symptoms including visual or hormonal abnormalities. Endocrine laboratory testing is necessary to assist in making a diagnosis, and the hormonal nature of the tumor will largely determine the proper surgical or medical management.

Because of the need for close endocrine, visual, and neurological monitoring of patients with pituitary adenomas, it is important to have close collaboration among the multiple physicians involved in each patient's care. The assistance of the endocrinology, neuro-ophthalmology, neuropathology, neuroradiology, and radiosurgery services is invaluable in the management of these patients.

SELECTED KEY REFERENCES

Chandler WF, Barkan AL. Treatment of pituitary tumors: a surgical perspective. *Endocrinol Metab Clin North Am.* 2008;37:51-66.

Ciric I, Ragin A, Baumgartner C, et al. Complications of transsphenoidal surgery: results of a national survey, review of the literature, and personal experience. *Neurosurgery.* 1997;40:225-237.

Jagannathan J, Yen C-P, Pouratian N, et al. Stereotactic radiosurgery for pituitary adenomas: a comprehensive review of indications, techniques and long-term results using the Gamma Knife. *J Neurooncol.* 2009;92:345-356.

Liu JK, Weiss MH, Couldwell WT. Surgical approaches to pituitary tumors. *Neurosurg Clin North Am.* 2003;14:93-107.

Oyesiku N. Multimodality treatment of pituitary adenomas. *Clin Neurosurg.* 2005;52:234-242.

Please go to expertconsult.com to view the complete list of references.

Endoscopic Approaches to Ventricular Tumors and Colloid Cysts

Scott D. Wait, Charles Teo

CLINICAL PEARLS

- It is essential to be knowledgeable about the equipment and practice on a cadaver or under the guidance of an experienced neuroendoscopist.

- Orientation and anatomy are everything. Knowledge of the anatomy will ensure that you know where you are, what you are looking at, and your orientation at all times. If you are not sure, abort the procedure.

- Use the endoscope for its advantages and don't fight its disadvantages. Increase use of angled scopes and increase the size of the visual field.

- Become comfortable with the endoscopic management of hydrocephalus (endoscopic third ventriculostomy) prior to using the endoscope for neuro-oncological applications.

- Endoscopic ventricular applications are not "all or nothing." Some lesions are more safely dealt with from an open microsurgical approach. In these cases use an endoscope-assisted approach to your advantage.

The role of neuroendoscopy in the management of intraventricular tumors and cysts is expanding. In appropriately selected cases it can allow definitive removal, often in a minimally invasive fashion. For many other aspects of neuro-oncology, neuroendoscopy is a useful adjunct. For example, the endoscope can be used to definitively treat hydrocephalus, to biopsy tumors that are best treated with radiation or chemotherapy, and to confirm adequate resection of tumors when the microscopic view is partially obstructed. This chapter will address instrumentation, complication avoidance and management, intraventricular tumor management, intraventricular cyst management, and endoscope-assisted microneurosurgery.

HISTORY

Six major advancements in the use of neuroendoscopy have occurred. A century ago, Lespinasse, a urologist, attempted a choroid plexus coagulation to treat hydrocephalus.[1,2] In the early twentieth century Dandy and Mixter attempted endoscopic third ventriculostomy (ETV).[3] In the 1970s technological advances allowed the production of flexible fiberscopes as well as rigid endoscopes. Throughout the late 1980s and 1990s ETV and decompartmentalization of the ventricular system were popularized, which allowed many neurosurgeons to become familiar with the tools of neuroendoscopy. This familiarity resulted in the fifth and sixth advances. The use of the endoscope for extra-axial lesions was popularized by

pioneers such as Perneczky who championed the keyhole approach to aneurysms. The final and most recent wave of endoscopic enthusiasm has been its application to anterior skull base surgery, especially transsphenoidal and transtubercular surgery. The use of the endoscope for intraventricular neuro-oncological applications including lesion removal, tumor biopsy, and cyst management is also becoming more common, so much so that endoscopic colloid cyst surgery has results that are similar to those of microsurgery, and with a better risk profile.[4-8]

EQUIPMENT

Equipment available for neuroendoscopy is constantly evolving. Basically, there are two types of endoscopes. The rigid endoscope is a fixed-length and fixed-geometry instrument that usually has several viewing angles available (0, 30, and 70 degrees to the long axis of the endoscope). The light source, camera, and shaft of the scope are all in-line and allow for easier orientation when working in the ventricular system.

The flexible fiberscope is maneuverable in three directions with relatively simple controls. The advantage of the flexible scope is that its geometry is not fixed and it may be fashioned to proceed along a curved trajectory such as traversing the foramen of Monro into the posterior third ventricle to biopsy a pineal tumor. This allows a single trajectory to treat hydrocephalus via ETV and sample the tumor (Fig. 41.1A and B). The flexible scope may also be used down the working port of the rigid scope in a "scope-in-scope" technique.[9] The main drawbacks of the flexible scope over the rigid scope are the poorer optical resolution and that the surgeon may inadvertently withdraw the scope in the "bent" configuration with devastating repercussions.

Rigid endoscope-holding arms are available from several manufacturers and allow the scope to be secured rigidly in place. This addresses surgeon fatigue and dependence upon an assistant to hold the endoscope. These rigid arms are generally adjustable in all three planes. However, once set, they all have some degree of "play" or "float" for which the surgeon will need to account when positioning.

Frameless neuronavigation is helpful to guide insertion of the sheath, especially in the absence of ventriculomegaly, and for localizing lesions for biopsy under an intact ependyma.[10] In the instance that the surgeon becomes disoriented or confused by distorted anatomy, stereotaxis can assist in reorientation.

Recently, several potentially important advances in instrumentation available to the endoscopic surgeon have been

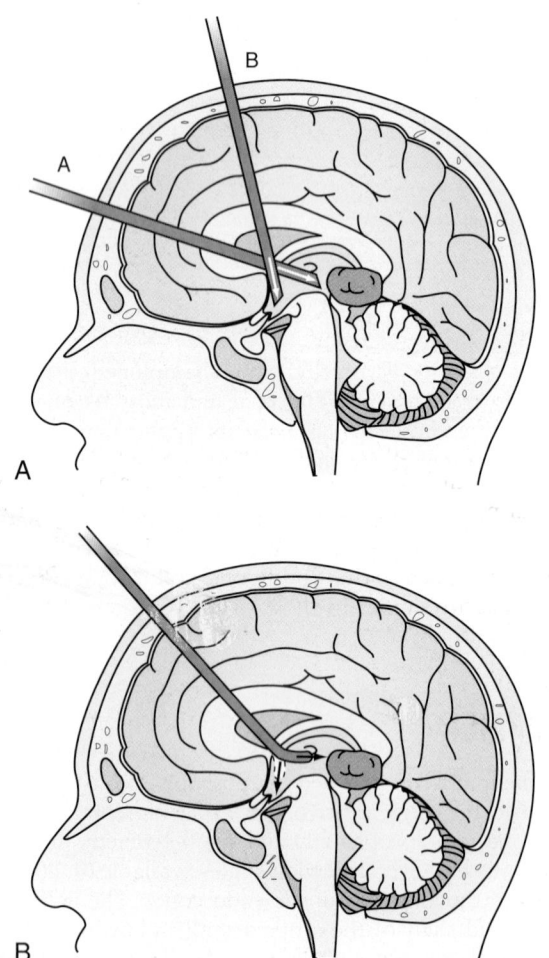

FIGURE 41.1 A, Using a rigid endoscope requires two approaches to perform an endoscopic third ventriculostomy and biopsy a pineal tumor in most cases. **B,** Using a flexible endoscope allows the same maneuvers through the traditional single bur hole approach used for endoscopic third ventriculostomy. *(Adapted with permission from Barrow Neurological Institute; originally published in Winn HR, editor. Youmans Neurological Surgery, 6th ed. Philadelphia: WB Saunders, 2011.)*

reported. The length of time required to aspirate a tumor using a "biopsy after biopsy" approach may be shortened by the use of traditional ultrasonic aspiration with a specialized handpiece down the working port of the endoscope. It has been used successfully on pituitary tumors, intraventricular clot removal, and craniopharyngioma cyst wall removal.[11] Endoneurosonography has been used to supply additional information about the relationship of the tip of the probe and structures orthogonal to it.[12] Water-jet dissection has been reported to be a useful adjunct in the safe perforation of a craniopharyngioma cyst wall, septum pellucidum, or floor of the third ventricle.[13] This may help to decrease the risk of hemorrhage associated with blindly inserting an instrument through a thin structure such as the third ventricle floor.

ENDOSCOPIC PRINCIPLES

Visualization is the key to neurosurgery. If you can't see it you can't safely operate on it. The endoscope offers all the visualization advantages of the microscope and allows them through a minimally invasive approach. This avoids unnecessary morbidity from brain retraction and large openings. Additionally, the magnification and illumination offered are superior to those offered by the microscope. Despite the visualization advantages afforded by the endoscope, the microscope still provides excellent visualization in a straight line and allows more precise, bimanual, three-dimensional microsurgical dissection. Rather than competing methods each method of visualization should be thought of as complementary to the other and both should be mastered to give the patient the best possible surgical treatment.

There are two principal forms of endoscopy: coaxial and extra-axial. Coaxial endoscopic approaches, or "pure" endoscopy, are those in which all components of the endoscopic system (lighting, camera, working channels, irrigant channels, and instruments) are all parallel and enclosed in a single sheath. The instruments are introduced through working channels and are aimed by redirecting the endoscope. The impact to the surrounding brain from removing and reintroducing instruments is minimized because the entire working and visualization area is within the endoscopic sheath. Most intraventricular endoscopic procedures are performed in a coaxial manner.[14]

Extra-axial endoscopic approaches are those in which the endoscope is the mode of visualization and the instruments are introduced alongside the endoscope separately. This generally applies to anterior skull base operations.

During "endoscope-assisted" applications, the microscope is the primary mode of visualization, and the endoscope is used to improve visualization, especially around corners and behind "unmovable" structures.

During "endoscope-controlled" surgery, the endoscope is the sole mode of visualization and surgery is performed using the same techniques and instrumentation as microsurgery, with the addition of curved instruments and suctions that allow the surgeon to operate around corners. In these forms of endoscopy, a substantial learning curve exists because of peripheral distortion, angled view when using non-0 degree endoscopes, and the close proximity of the surgical field to the tip of the endoscope. Once this is overcome, these same "problems" may be used to the surgeon's advantage, resulting in better outcomes.

INTRAVENTRICULAR ENDOSCOPY FOR CYSTS

Colloid Cysts

Colloid cysts of the third ventricle are non-neoplastic masses that typically arise from the roof of the third ventricle. They can occlude the foramen of Monro, causing headache, hydrocephalus, memory disturbances, and sudden death. Colloid cysts have a variable consistency, from mucinous, that are easily aspirated, to a hard and cheesy consistency. Cysts 1 cm or larger and those causing symptoms or hydrocephalus are generally recommended for removal. Other options including shunting and stereotactic drainage are possible but not recommended owing to their poor durability. Microsurgical removal is effective but more invasive than the endoscopic approach.[4,5,15] Therefore, endoscopic removal is recommended in the majority of cases.[16-19] However, when imaging predicts the consistency of the cyst contents to be hard and cheesy the cyst is better removed microsurgically with bimanual dissection. Additionally, cysts larger than 2 cm may compromise or adhere to the fornix and may be more safely removed using microsurgical bimanual dissection.

A single bur hole, approximately 8 cm behind the nasion and 5 to 7 cm lateral to the midline in the nondominant hemisphere (be careful not to injure the caudate head), is sufficient for removal[7,20] (Fig. 41.2). Image guidance helps with the initial ventricular entry. A peel-away sheath is optional. The landmarks of the colloid cyst and foramen of Monro are identified and the overlying choroid plexus is coagulated, avoiding the fornix. The cyst is coagulated and opened and the contents are aspirated. A pediatric endotracheal suction catheter with the end cut to 45 degrees is particularly effective if the consistency is favorable. Alternatively, some endoscope manufacturers have designed rigid endoscopic suction that uses either blunt or beveled tips and works well to suction the mucinous material. One can twist the catheter and use the cut end as a dissector to "morselize" the contents of the cyst

prior to aspiration. If the contents are too dense, forceps may be required to empty the cyst contents. The wall of the cyst is then dissected free of the roof of the third ventricle with generous coagulation. Generally the cyst wall is not densely attached to the fornix and can be removed completely. However, in the case that the wall is so adherent to the internal cerebral veins or the fornix that it cannot be separated using either sharp or blunt dissection it may be prudent to leave a thin "carpet." Under these circumstances, the recurrence rate appears to be low, but we must await reports of long-term outcome.[6,21,22] Symptomatic relief of obstructive hydrocephalus is generally obtained, though mild ventriculomegaly often persists.[21]

Neurocysticercotic Cysts

Neurocysticercosis (NCC) is the neurological manifestation of the parasite *Taenia solium*. This is commonly contracted in underdeveloped countries by hand-to-mouth contamination from unclean water or food. NCC most often presents with seizures but may also present with sudden hydrocephalus due to intraventricular cysts blocking normal cerebrospinal fluid (CSF) pathways. There is a growing body of literature suggesting that neuroendoscopic removal of cysts results in improved patient outcomes and lessens or avoids altogether the need for shunting.[23-25] Recently, pediatric data regarding neuroendoscopic cyst evacuation has been reported. The shunting rate is lower (22%) in the neuroendoscopic group than the traditional medical treatment group (70%) and the Karnofsky performance scale was higher in the endoscopic group (90.0% vs. 85.5%, $p = 0.003$).[23] Two other studies show complete resolution of cysts and no need for shunting with minimal transient morbidity.[24,25]

The procedure is performed either through a single approach with a flexible endoscope or through as many approaches as needed with the rigid endoscope. A disposable plastic sheath is mandatory in order to maintain the transcortical path as sometimes the entire metal sheath needs to be removed with the grabbing forceps in order to maintain the integrity of the cyst wall. If the cyst wall is ruptured and contents spilled into the ventricle, then postoperative steroids will alleviate some of the symptoms of sterile meningitis. Preoperative imaging will determine what CSF spaces need to be explored and the safest way to explore each. The advantages and disadvantages of each type of endoscope have been previously discussed. When using the rigid endoscope, if the ventricle is not drained, firm irrigation can mobilize ipsilateral cysts into view that can be secured with a forceps and removed.

Miscellaneous Cysts

Other cysts, such as arachnoid cysts, occur within the ventricles. Often fenestration of these to normal CSF spaces is desirable. The ease of working in a fluid-filled space makes the endoscope ideal for fenestration. The anatomy is often distorted and the arachnoid surface is often thick and somewhat opaque. Stereotaxis is very helpful in these cases to know what is behind an opaque membrane prior to fenestration. Blunt perforation should be avoided at all costs as pushing against these flimsy membranes may damage important

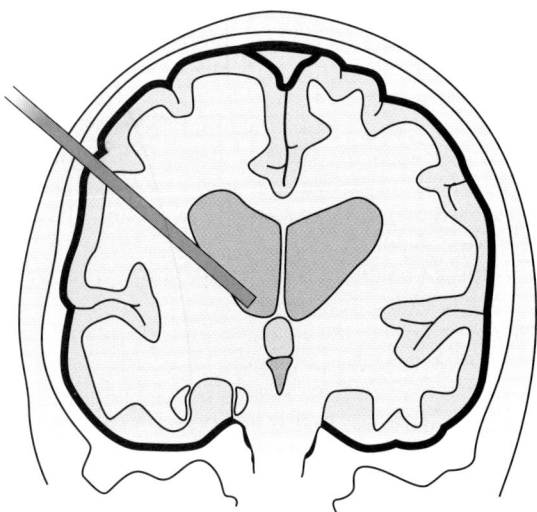

FIGURE 41.2 The suggested approach for endoscopic resection of a colloid cyst is 8 cm posterior to the nasion and 5 to 7 cm right of the midline. The caudate head should be avoided during insertion of the sheath/endoscope.

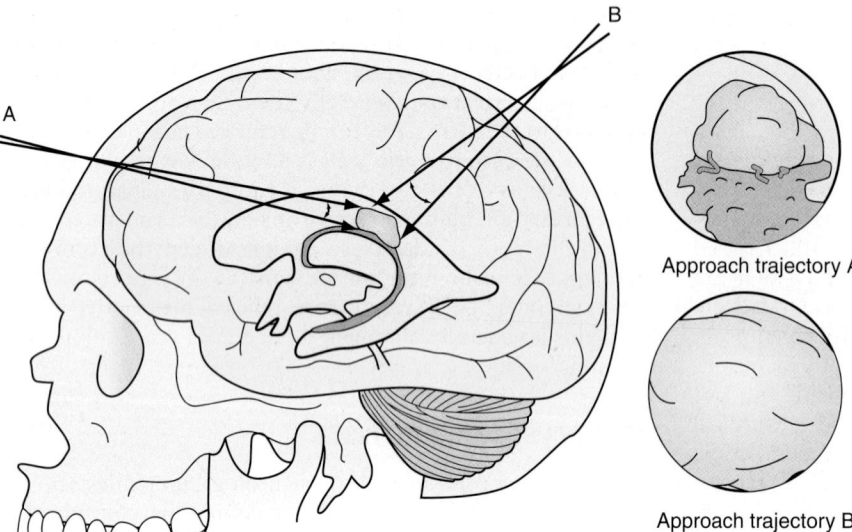

FIGURE 41.3 Choosing an appropriate approach that allows normal ventricle to be traversed prior to encountering the tumor gives a better view of the anatomy of the tumor and surrounding structures. It also allows identification and disconnection of the blood supply. *(Adapted with permission from Barrow Neurological Institute; originally published in Winn HR, editor. Youmans Neurological Surgery, 6th ed. Philadelphia: WB Saunders; 2011.)*

Approach trajectory A

Approach trajectory B

neurovascular structures that lie behind. Enlarging interhemispheric cysts can be fenestrated directly to the ventricle or via cystocisternoventricular fenestration.[26] Fourth ventricular cysts obstructing outflow are also amenable to fenestration.[22]

INTRAVENTRICULAR ENDOSCOPY FOR TUMORS

Endoscopic applications for intraventricular tumors include tumor biopsy, tumor resection, and management of tumor-associated hydrocephalus.[27,28] In general, neuroendoscopy for tumors is a step up in technical difficulty from the endoscopic management of hydrocephalus. The ideal conditions for endoscopic resection of an intraventricular tumor are that it should be small, avascular or with relatively low vascularity, partially or totally cystic, and located in enlarged ventricles. Hydrocephalus creates an ideal working space. However, a normal ventricle is adequate to gain access to a tumor and biopsy it and, for smaller tumors, to resect it safely.[29,30] A recent report even suggests that in experienced hands, operating in a normal-sized ventricle yields the same success/complication rate as operating in large ventricles.

One key to tumor resection within the ventricles is to select a proper working trajectory. Because the brain must be transited in order to reach the ventricles, a single working angle that does not require excessive "windshield wiping" of the endoscope should be chosen.

Considerations when selecting an approach trajectory are to select one which:

1. Enters the ventricle with some normal ventricle between the entry point and the mass
2. Allows access to the blood supply, if vascular
3. Allows access to the point of attachment to the ventricular wall or choroid plexus
4. Does not originate in or traverse eloquent structures
5. Allows management of associated hydrocephalus or trapped CSF spaces

Having some normal ventricle and CSF between the entry point into the ventricle and the tumor allows better visualization of the tumor margin and allows visualized normal structures to aid in orientation (Fig. 41.3). Access to the blood supply and point of attachment may turn a tedious piecemeal tumor resection into a disconnection and en bloc removal. As mentioned above, the use of transendoscope ultrasonic aspirators may speed up tumor removal if en bloc removal is not possible.[11]

Image guidance is particularly valuable for approach planning and execution, and is worthwhile even if it is only used for this step of the procedure.[31-33] Third ventricular tumor resections are particularly dependant on proper approach angle because often the endoscope must traverse the foramen of Monro, putting the fornix, at the anterior border of the foramen, at some risk. Image guidance allows the surgeon to use trajectory views to draw a line from the anterior border of the tumor to the anterior-most border of the foramen of Monro. This line can then be extended to the surface to choose the appropriate entry point and angle. The fornix will not tolerate anterior "windshield wiping" movements of the endoscope while its tip lies in the third ventricle. Posterior movements are tolerated much better; however, the venous structures coalescing at the posterior margin of the foramen of Monro also limit scope excursion. Fortunately, many intraventricular tumors are associated with ventriculomegaly and an enlarged foramen of Monro that allows for larger excursions of the endoscope.

It is worth noting the major source of complications in intraventricular endoscopic approaches for brain tumors is disorientation. Complications can be minimized through appropriate entry point and trajectory choice, prior orientation of the camera, detailed examination of the equipment and video image prior to entry into the brain, a thorough knowledge of normal ventricular anatomy, and a constant self-inquiry into where the endoscope is, what all structures seen represent, and how the endoscope's intrinsic optical distortion is affecting the scene. The use of frameless stereotaxis helps reduce disorientation.

Endoscopic Approaches to Intraventricular Tumors

Details of the diagnosis, pathology, and nonsurgical treatment of intraventricular tumors are discussed in Chapter 42. Certain tumors are more amenable than others for endoscopic removal.[34] When working within the fluid-filled ventricle, bleeding may be difficult to control and obscures the operative field. Therefore, tumors of low vascularity are preferred for purely endoscopic removal. Examples are subependymomas, some ependymomas, the subependymal giant cell astrocytomas associated with tuberous sclerosis, selected neurocytomas, exophytic gliomas (primarily pilocytic or low grade), and hypothalamic hamartomas.[35] Some vascular tumors such as choroid plexus and pedunculated tumors can also be approached endoscopically, because the blood supply is often well defined and easy to coagulate and divide.

The technique of endoscopic tumor removal requires a high level of familiarity with the endoscope and its use, as it represents one of the most technically complex skills in neuroendoscopy. A peel-away sheath is recommended. Its purpose is to avoid buildup of irrigant and increased intracranial pressure, and thus to allow the endoscope to be removed and replaced with ease, especially when the forceps and endoscope are removed together with pieces of tumor that are too large to come up the working channel. The advantage of not using the peel-away sheath is to slightly reduce the size of the track through the brain and to keep some pressure in the ventricle to reduce venous bleeding. The surgeon must communicate effectively with the anesthesiologist during the proceduree. Increased intracranial pressures (ICPs) will generally be manifest by a Cushing's response and will be noted by the anesthesiologist. In this case, one should allow egress of fluid so that the hemodynamic values return to normal.

Piecemeal tumor removal can be very tedious and also lead to tumor spread if fragments are released that float free in the CSF. Removing larger chunks of tumor and drawing them out with the endoscope is more efficient and leads to higher quality specimens.

Prior to placing the peel-away sheath, tapping of the ventricle with a brain needle or a ventriculostomy catheter is recommended. The peel-away sheath can then be placed down the tract using image guidance. The bluntness sometimes also results in the tip deflecting from the ependyma. This problem is overcome when a smaller bore, sharper instrument violates the ependyma.

Most tumors are approached by taking initial biopsy specimens with cup forceps, minimizing coagulation to maintain the quality of the tissue for analysis. Any vessels on the surface of the tumor are then coagulated. Electrocautery (especially monopolar) is capable of generating high CSF temperatures and must be used with caution. Irrigation with warmed lactated Ringer's solution or a spinal fluid substitute solution is used to dissipate this heat.[36] Normal saline is not used because it lacks electrolytes, is acidotic, alters the electrolyte balance in the brain, and leads to postoperative confusion.[37]Again, appropriate egress of irrigant will avoid a dangerous rise in ICP.

Once bleeding is controlled, cautery, blunt dissection, and bites with the forceps or scissors are used to separate the tumor from the normal tissue. The best tumors for neuroendoscopy have a distinct margin and can be gently retracted away from the surrounding tissue. Ideally, a perimeter can be created, the tumor can be isolated as a mass, and it can be removed in one or more large pieces. If the tumor is soft, multiple methods of tumor aspiration are possible. A stainless steel suction cannula or the previously mentioned pediatric endotracheal suction catheter placed down the working channel can be used to morselize and aspirate the tumor.[38] Shortened endovascular catheters can also be used. They have the advantage of a stiffer, thinner wall that can be shaped. The catheter allows a larger inner lumen diameter for more efficient aspiration of appropriate consistency tumors.[39] The gelatinous contents of colloid cysts and some other cystic tumors respond particularly well to this technique. As mentioned previously, the length of time required to aspirate a tumor using a "biopsy after biopsy" approach may be shortened by the use of ultrasonic aspiration with a specialized handpiece down the working port of the endoscope.[11] Regardless of the removal technique, every attempt should be made to avoid dispersion of tumor remnants throughout the ventricles.

After satisfactory tumor removal, attention is paid to hemostasis, usually by irrigation alone. The ventricle is inspected for residual tumor and blood clots, particularly over the foramen of Monro or the aqueduct of Sylvius, where obstruction may occur. The decision about whether or not to leave an external ventricular drain is controversial, and should depend primarily on the risk of obstruction. In cases in which the working trajectory allows it, addition of a septum pellucidotomy or third ventriculostomy may decrease the chance of postoperative symptomatic hydrocephalus.

In some cases tumor biopsy rather than removal may be the goal. Central nervous system (CNS) lymphoma is often periventricular and amenable to endoscopic biopsy for diagnosis. "Nonoperative" gliomas may also be appropriate for this biopsy method. Stereotactic guidance is helpful in locating the tumor. However, identification of the tumor tissue through overlying normal ependyma may be problematic. Recently, the use of 5-ALA (5-aminolevulinic acid) fluorescence to identify and biopsy a midbrain glioma through an intact ependymal layer has been reported.[40]

Complications of tumor biopsy and removal include intraventricular hemorrhage, neurological deficit, tension pneumocephalus, hydrocephalus, and basilar artery injury.[41-43] Tension pneumocephalus results from air being exchanged for CSF during the procedure. To avoid this, the ventricles should be refilled with lactated Ringer's solution. If large quantities of air remain, 100% oxygen administered via face mask will help with dissolution.[44]

Peretta and associates reported an 8.8% complication rate for neuroendoscopic (nonhydrocephalus procedures) in pediatric patients.[45] Hemorrhagic complications of tumor biopsy are reported at 3.5% per patient and 2.4% per procedure.[46] To minimize the incidence of hemorrhagic complications one should never cut or pull any structure without being able to visualize the structure completely.

Hemorrhage is often the rate-limiting step during endoscopic tumor removal. Several techniques can be used to control hemorrhage with the endoscope. The first maneuver is to patiently irrigate. Most bleeding in the ventricle will stop with irrigation alone. The second maneuver is to attempt coagulating the bleeding source, but only if it can be directly visualized. Visualization may be improved by draining the CSF and working in an air-filled ventricle. A third maneuver is to gently tamponade the bleeding point using the endoscope itself or an instrument placed down the working channel. This maneuver is appropriate for larger veins that one is attempting to preserve such as the thalamostriate vein. An external ventricular drain can be left if necessary or as a "safety valve" in the case that tumor or hemorrhage occludes the foramen or aqueduct. The question of whether to leave a drain is not convincingly answered in the literature. We do not routinely leave drains after endoscopic procedures.

Endoscope-Assisted Microsurgical Approaches to Intraventricular Tumors

Many intraventricular tumors cannot be completely removed through a purely endoscopic approach, but endoscopy still maintains an important role. The concept of "endoscope-assisted" refers to a procedure whereby the approach is the traditional microsurgical one and the endoscope is used as an adjunct either through the same opening or through a separate bur hole for better overall visualization.[47] The endoscope allows the surgeon to look around corners and to visualize structures that are not visible by microscopic imaging alone, thus expanding the operating field. Utilizing angled endoscopes can maximize the area of the ventricle visualized. Endoscope-assisted microsurgery has been shown to be useful in 35 patients with traditional microsurgical approaches to the ventricular system done through keyhole craniotomies; 31 of the 35 patients had no morbidity at 6 months and three of the patients with 6-month morbidity had preexisting Parinaud's syndrome that persisted. Seventy-eight percent of patients had complete tumor resections. One procedure was aborted due to hemorrhage and was repeated successfully with gross total removal 2 days later.[48] Another example of endoscope-assisted microsurgery is the transventricular management of craniopharyngioma. This includes gross total removal of intraventricular components, fenestration of cysts as a stand-alone procedure for symptomatic control, and cyst fenestration followed by collapse and subsequent craniotomy for definitive removal of the solid component.[49]

Additionally, diagnostic ventriculoscopy should be performed whenever an endoscope is placed in the ventricle for any reason. With a 30-degree endoscope a wide inspection can often be performed by rotation of the endoscope without any additional brain retraction. For example, ventriculoscopy can identify ependymal tumor deposits that cannot be seen on magnetic resonance imaging (MRI), can confirm whether the septum pellucidum is patent or perforate, and whether the opening of the aqueduct is obstructed or open. In patients undergoing shunting, ventriculoscopy can be performed before the catheter is placed, or through the endoscope with a fiberscope. In most cases, however, endoscopic management of hydrocephalus associated with tumors can be performed and is in fact preferable.

CONCLUSION AND FUTURE DIRECTIONS

Major advances will be directed at allowing neurosurgeons to do microsurgical work "around corners" under the endoscopic view only. Curved instruments that allow microsurgical work to be done in these recesses and instruments that combine the functions of multiple instruments (suction and endoscope or suction and cautery) may facilitate working with the endoscope with a single hand. New tools for endoscopic sharp dissection and control of vascular structures are needed. Finally, every improvement in visualization is welcome. A sharper and brighter picture, the possibility of true three-dimensional endoscopy, flexible endoscopy with a picture equivalent to a rod-lens endoscope, and image injection of frameless stereotactic data into the video image would all be welcome additions to the endoscopic armamentarium.

Advancements will be dependent on instrument development being attractive to commercial vendors. If there is no market to recoup research and development costs, then there will be few advances. Gone are the days when tumor neurosurgeons could divide themselves into neuroendoscopists or microsurgical specialists. To offer the patient the best possible option for management of their intraventricular lesion, one must be able to utilize, expertly, both methods of visualization. As more surgeons are trained to use, become familiar with, and "buy in" to this useful technology, the market for neuroendoscopes and neuroendoscopic tools will grow, as will the technology.

SELECTED KEY REFERENCES

Abdou MS, Cohen AR. Endoscopic treatment of colloid cysts of the third ventricle. Technical note and review of the literature. *J Neurosurg.* 1998;89(6):1062-1068.

Bristol RE, Nakaji P, Smith KA. Endoscopic management of colloid cysts. *Oper Tech Neurosurg.* 2005;8(4):176-178.

Cinalli G, Peretta P, Spennato P, et al. Neuroendoscopic management of interhemispheric cysts in children. *J Neurosurg.* 2006;105(Suppl 3):194-202.

Gaab MR, Schroeder HW. Neuroendoscopic approach to intraventricular lesions. *J Neurosurg.* 1998;88(3):496-505.

Cappabianca P, Cinalli G, Gangemi M, et al. Application of neuroendoscopy to intraventricular lesions. *Neurosurgery.* 2008;62(Suppl 2):575-597:discussion 597-598.

Charalampaki P, Filippi R, Welschehold S, et al. Tumors of the lateral and third ventricle: removal under endoscope-assisted keyhole conditions. *Neurosurgery.* 2005;57(Suppl 4):302-311:discussion 302-311.

Please go to expertconsult.com to view the complete list of references.

CHAPTER 42

Microsurgical Approaches to the Ventricular System

Timothy H. Lucas, II, Richard G. Ellenbogen

CLINICAL PEARLS

- Intraventricular lesions often present with nonspecific symptoms and clinical signs and can affect patients of all ages. They may grow quite large before the diagnosis is secured. Imaging studies, in concert with a detailed knowledge of the surrounding microsurgical anatomy and neural function, permit the surgeon to determine the most effective and safest approach to resection of the lesion.

- The key principles in the microsurgical resection is to approach these deep-seated lesions by the most direct route that provides the least disruption to eloquent cortex and neural function. In addition, the surgical goal includes developing the most favorable trajectory for visualization of the entire lesion, the best proximal control of arterial feeders, least disruption to the venous drainage, and minimal contamination of the cerebrospinal fluid (CSF).

- Transcortical or interhemispheric transcallosal approaches adequately access lesions throughout the entire ventricular system. Transcortical approaches are ideal in patients with hydrocephalus, and interhemispheric approaches work regardless of the ventricle size. Both approaches permit the full range of microsurgical options to enter the third ventricle through the choroidal fissure or between the fornices.

- The midline telovelar approach is a safe and effective approach to resect fourth ventricle lesions extending from the aqueduct of Sylvius to the obex, without having to split the vermis.

- Complete ventricular communication after tumor resection is an important goal. Cystic septations should be removed so that CSF spaces communicate both anatomically and physiologically. Microscopic or endoscopic inspection at the end of the procedure confirms the absence of a blood clot, residual tumor, or septations and ensures that transventricular communication has been achieved.

- Microsurgical approaches are to be tailored to the lesion location, pathological entity, and surgeon's experience. Each approach has distinct technical advantages with associated functional risks. Endoscopic approaches can be used to achieve resection of select intraventricular lesions, most commonly colloid cysts of the third ventricle. Future advances in endoscopic instrumentation, preoperative functional imaging, and fiber tract identification will influence surgical strategies in the coming years.

Microsurgery for ventricular tumors is both challenging for the surgeon and potentially curative for the patient. Accounting for a small percentage of all cerebral lesions,[1] tumors of the ventricles present a unique clinical and elegant microsurgical experience for neurosurgeons. Intraventricular tumors can grow to a very large size, eluding diagnosis until they cause rapid decompensation from hydrocephalus or increased intracranial pressure. Surgical approaches for resection of lateral and third ventricle tumors always require the neurosurgeon to enter through the brain, either the cerebral cortex or corpus callosum. Complete resection of these lesions is often possible through either the transcortical or interhemispheric transcallosal routes. Surgical approaches to the fourth ventricle are different in that splitting of a fissure through a telovelar approach may provide access of the fourth ventricle from the

aqueduct of Sylvius to the obex without sacrifice of any cerebellum (Fig. 42.1).

The age of presentation of intraventricular tumors spans from infancy to the elderly.[2] Preoperative symptoms are often nonspecific; including headache (35%), weakness (25%), sensory loss (25%), nausea and vomiting (22%), dementia (18%), and visual loss (18%).[2-7] Pathological entities range from slow-growing indolent lesions to aggressive malignancies. Tumors arising within the third and lateral ventricles are frequently (but not always) slow-growing and benign,[4,5] whereas lesions arising from the fourth ventricle may be rapidly progressive due to cerebrospinal fluid (CSF) obstruction and brainstem signs and include both benign and malignant pathological types.

Despite these challenges, surgery for intraventricular tumors can be rewarding for the patient. When the symptoms

651

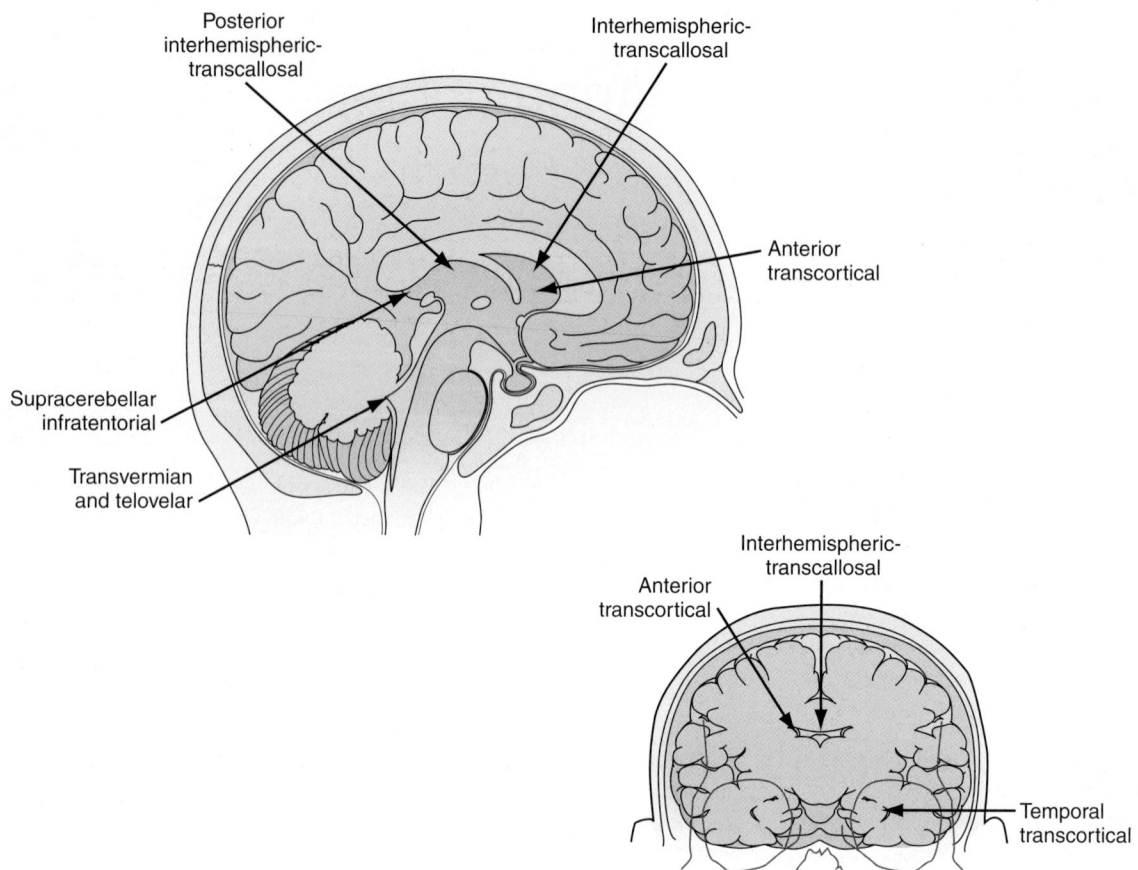

FIGURE 42.1 This sagittal and coronal diagram demonstrates the variety of approaches that may be employed to resect a ventricular lesion based on its location.

are primarily related to the hydrocephalus resulting from the obstructive nature of these tumors, clinical improvement may be immediate. Gross total resections of low-grade lesions may be curative. Finally, the refinements in technique and equipment have improved outcomes substantially since Dandy's first description of surgery for intraventricular tumors in 1922.[8]

The unique challenge in resection of ventricular lesions is to develop a trajectory to these deep-seated lesions that will be cause little morbidity, provide an ample corridor for surgical access, and achieve a radical excision, when possible. The key principles in the microsurgical approach are based on the most direct route that provides the least disruption to eloquent cortex and neural function. In addition, the surgical goal is to develop the most favorable trajectory for visualization and resection of the entire lesion, the best proximal control of arterial feeders, least disruption to the venous drainage, and minimal contamination of the CSF.

In this chapter we consider the major microsurgical approaches to the cerebral ventricles based on our experience, with particular attention to the relevant anatomy and risks versus benefits offered by each approach.

MICROSURGICAL ANATOMY

Mastering the relevant ventricular anatomy is essential in performing microsurgical approaches to the lateral ventricles.

A more detailed review of the anatomy can be found in Professor Albert L. Rhoton's outstanding monograph on the subject, which was produced after years of study in his laboratory and operating room.[9]

The lateral ventricles are paired C-shaped structures that are anchored by each thalamus in the middle of the brain. Each ventricle is divided into five sections. Starting anterior and superior and moving backward they are the (a) anterior horn, (b) body, (c) temporal horn, (d) atrium, and (e) occipital horn (Fig. 42.2). Each of these five sections has a floor, roof, medial wall, and lateral wall and these sections contain structures that are critical to the surgeon for navigation in the ventricles. Specifically, they are structures that either tolerate manipulation to facilitate visual access or, conversely, should not be manipulated. These relationships are important when considering either the transcortical or the transcallosal approach.

If one visualizes the ventricles in a coronal plane, the anatomical relationships are as follows. At the level of the frontal horn of the lateral ventricle, the lateral wall is composed of the oval caudate nucleus, and the medial wall is the diaphanous septum pellucidum that separates the two frontal horns. The roof is made up of the roof of the genu of the corpus callosum, and the floor is composed of the rostrum of the corpus callosum, which wraps around and tucks under the ventricles until it reaches the anterior commissural fibers. At the level of the body of the ventricle, some of the same relationships exist. The corpus callosum makes up the roof, the caudate nucleus

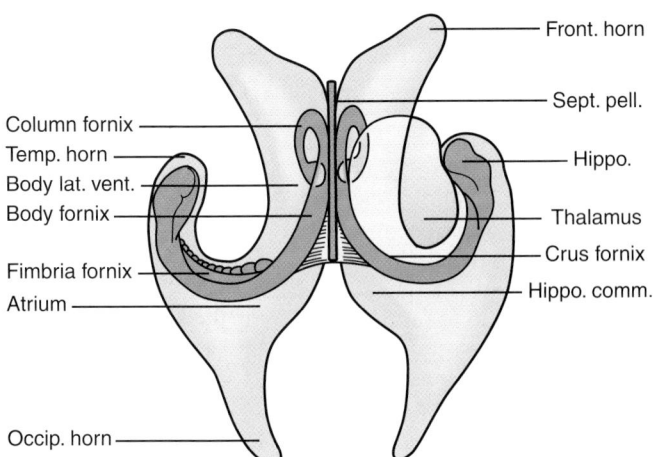

FIGURE 42.2 Each C-shaped lateral ventricle is anchored on the ipsilateral thalamus. The parts of the ventricle include the frontal horn, body, temporal horn, atrium, and occipital horn. The septum pellucidum is in the medial border of the frontal horn and body of the lateral ventricle. The hippocampal formation sits on the floor of the temporal horn. The fornix surrounds the thalamus and runs in the medial part of the temporal horn, atrium, and body. (Adapted from Rhoton Jr AL. The lateral and third ventricles. *Neurosurgery.* 2003;53:S235-S299.)

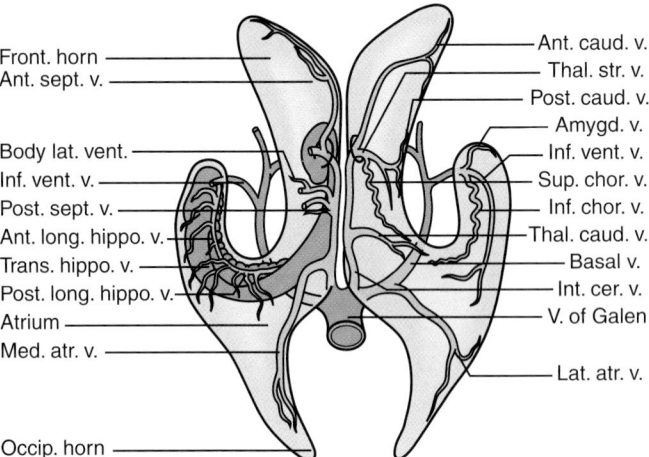

FIGURE 42.3 A drawing with venous relationships of the lateral ventricles in an axial view of the ventricular system. The ventricular veins can be used as navigational guides, once in the ventricle. They are divided into a deep/medial paired system and a paired lateral group of vessels. The medial ventricular veins drain into the internal cerebral vein, which run in the velum interpositum on the roof of the third ventricle. They are joined by the paired basal vein of Rosenthal, as they drain into the great vein of Galen followed by the straight sinus and finally to the torcula. Starting at the frontal horn, the lateral group consists of the anterior caudate vein and anterior septal vein in the frontal horn, which join the thalamostriate vein adjacent to the choroidal fissure. The medial and lateral atrial veins are in the atrium and occipital horn, and the inferior ventricular and amygdalar veins lie in the temporal horn. (Adapted from Rhoton Jr AL. The lateral and third ventricles. *Neurosurgery.* 2003;53:S235-S299.)

the lateral wall, and the medial wall is again separated by the septum pellucidum. Moving posteriorly within the lateral ventricles, the floor is composed of the thalamus. In the midline of the floor lie the columns of the fornix. In the floor of the body of the lateral ventricle, sitting between the fornix and the thalamus, is the choroid plexus, which attaches to the surgically crucial structure called the *choroidal fissure.* Each column of the fornix also forms the curved superior and anterior borders of the foramen of Monro. Moving to the temporal horn, each column of the fornix starts as the fimbria of the hippocampi and starts in the medial wall of the temporal horn. After giving off commissural fibers, these nerve bundles continue in the inferior medial wall of the body as the fornix.[10] The roof of the temporal horn is the tapetum of the corpus callosum, and the floor comprises the folded gyri of the hippocampus. Moving within the ventricle to its posterior limits we find the atrium and the occipital horn. The atrium and occipital horn form a triangular CSF cavity in the occipital lobe. Again, the tapetum of the corpus callosum covers the lateral wall and roof of the atrium. The forceps major, which is a fiber bundle that connects the two occipital lobes through the splenium of the corpus callosum, runs in the superior part of the atrium. The floor is composed of the collateral trigone and the medial wall is the calcar avis of the calcarine cortex.[7]

The primary arteries within the ventricles are the anterior and posterior choroidal arteries,[7,10] branches of which provide the vascular supply to tumors in this region. Understanding the course of the arteries helps the surgeon choose an approach for each lesion and thus permits early proximal control, when possible, of the feeding vessels.

The anterior choroidal artery arises from the internal carotid artery, just a millimeter or so distal to the posterior communicating artery. It exits the anterior incisural space and enters the lateral ventricle through the choroidal fissure, heading

posteriorly to lie near the lateral posterior choroidal artery.[7,10] The anterior choroidal artery generally supplies the choroid plexus in the temporal horn and atrium. Because the choroidal arteries pass through the choroidal fissure, opening this fissure early also facilitates proximal control of the feeding vessels.

The posterior choroidal arteries are grouped into lateral and medial divisions. The lateral posterior choroidal artery is composed of one to six branches, which arise in the ambient and quadrigeminal cisterns, typically from the posterior cerebral aratery (PCA). These branches then pierce the ventricle and pass around the pulvinar and enter through the choroidal fissure at the level of the fimbria/body of the fornix to supply the choroid plexus in the posterior temporal horn, atrium, and body of the ventricles.[7] The medial posterior choroidal arteries arise as one to three branches from the PCA in the interpeduncular and crural cisterns. These arteries circumnavigate the midbrain and move to the pineal gland to enter the roof of the third ventricle and reside in the tela choroidea called the *velum interpositum,* adjacent to the internal cerebral veins. The medial posterior choroidal artery supplies the choroid plexus in the roof of the third ventricle and sometimes the choroid plexus of the lateral ventricle.[10]

The veins are useful as landmarks to help navigate in the body of the ventricle, especially in cases in which hydrocephalus is present (Fig. 42.3). There are many important veins composing the lateral and medial groups, but perhaps the best known for surgical and angiographic orientation is the thalamostriate vein, which helps orient the surgeon toward the foramen of Monro. The thalamostriate vein traverses the lateral wall of the body of the ventricle adjacent to the choroidal fissue between the caudate and thalamus. It then forms the venous angle with an acute posterior turn into the foramen of Monro to empty into the internal cerebral veins traversing the velum interpositum. The veins in the temporal horn drain into the basal vein of Rosenthal (basal vein) as it passes through the ambient cistern on each side. Veins from the atrium and occipital horn drain into the basal internal cerebral veins as well, and finally into the vein of Galen which empties into the straight sinus and torcular herophili.[7]

PATHOLOGICAL ENTITIES

The differential diagnosis of tumors in the lateral ventricle depends on several factors: the age of the patient, location of the tumor, and specific radiological characteristics as described by computed tomography (CT), magnetic resonance imaging (MRI), and cerebral angiography.[11,12] Tumors found in the lateral ventricle of children younger than 5 years of age are often choroid plexus tumors, whereas in older children they tend to be astrocytoma or ependymoma.[11] Choroid plexus tumors are rare lesions with a prevalence of 0.3 per million. They comprise only about 1% of all brain tumors and occur in children with a median age of 3.5 years at the time of presentation.[13,14] Choroid plexus tumors are often quite vascular and demonstrate a tumor blush on CT, MRI, and cerebral angiography. On MRI, they may possess heterogeneous signal characteristics caused by necrosis and calcification and are iso- to hypodense on T1-weighted images relative to the white matter.

The most common hypo- or isodense, nonenhancing tumor in the body or foramen of Monro is a subependymoma. In children with tuberous sclerosis (TS), these lesions are often a subependymal giant cell astrocytoma (SEGA). Roughly 6% of patients with TS develop subependymal giant cell tumors.[15] In this location, they can reach a large size before being diagnosed, sometimes by unilateral ventricular obstruction.[16-18] Astrocytomas can be found in any part of the ventricle as they are surrounded by white matter tracts. Astrocytoma will most frequently arise from the thalamus, where they can infiltrate. Ependymoma, when supratentorial, can be intraventricular as well as intraparenchymal.[11]

In adults older than 30 years of age, tumors in the atrium and trigone are most commonly meningiomas. Intraventricular meningiomas are well-circumscribed, homogeneously enhancing lesions.[19] Meningiomas tend to be isodense to brain on T1-weighted images and brightly enhance with gadolinium administration. Intraventricular masses that engulf the choroid glomus, are calcified, or are demonstrated to have a choroidal artery supply on angiography are usually benign meningiomas.[20,21]

Outside the trigone, tumors in older patients are often either a primary or metastatic malignancy.[11]

Primary or metastatic malignancies present late in life with attachment to the ventricular walls and parenchymal invasion.[11] Malignant intraventricular metastases include renal cell carcinoma, pulmonary adenocarcinoma, gastrointestinal carcinoma, transitional cell carcinoma, and adrenocortical carcinoma.

Central neurocytomas, which occur mostly in adults in the second to fourth decades of life, appear to attach or grow from the septum pellucidum and possess a characteristic imaging appearance.[22] These lesions may be solid with cystic components and flow voids on MRI, and may contain calcifications visualized on CT.[23] These benign World Health Organization (WHO) grade II lesions derive their name from the original description of a well-differentiated neural lesion that was adherent to the septum and ventricle wall.[24] These tumors can be quite large on presentation. Although the natural history and long-term prognosis of these lesions are not completely understood, excision appears to be curative in those patients in whom a gross total resection is achieved. Significant blood loss and a "sticky" connection to the thalamus and third ventricle structures may complicate the attempts at a radical resection.

Cystic lesions include colloid cysts of the third ventricle and infectious lesions such as neurocysticercosis, nocardiosis, and cryptococci. Colloid cysts are covered in another chapter but at our institution they are routinely approached with a single port endoscopic resection. Other non-neoplastic processes such as cysts, sarcoidosis, xanthogranulomas (which appear to be dense on CT scans with flecks of calcification), arteriovenous malformations, and cavernous hemangiomas are also found in the lateral ventricle with geographic variation.[25] In some endemic regions of the world, a new seizure or hydrocephalus associated with cystic intraventricular lesion often indicates neurocysticercosis. In our institution, the history, MRI, and serum or CSF markers may secure the diagnosis of neurocysticercosis, and these patients then receive medical therapy. Endoscopic exploration and resection are used to remove obstructive ventricular neurocysticercosis lesions when indicated by symptoms or examination.

PREOPERATIVE PLANNING AND GENERAL SURGICAL CONSIDERATIONS

A CT scan is often the first radiological study patients undergo simply because of diagnostic ease in the surveillance workup. The presence of calcifications on the CT image may further narrow the differential diagnosis.[26] Calcification may be seen in central neurocytoma, subependymal giant cell tumor, meningioma, and ependymoma.

Subsequent MRI, with and without gadolinium, reveals the precise location and extent of the lesion within the ventricle and, thus, helps guide the surgical approach. At a minimum this should include sagittal, coronal, and axial reconstructions of T1-weighted sequences (with and without gadolinium), T2-weighted images, and fluid-attenuated inversion recovery (FLAIR). These sequences are sufficient to refine the differential diagnosis and begin basic surgical planning. The role of new specialized MRI sequencing is rapidly evolving. Diffusion tensor imaging (DTI) permits reconstruction of large fiber tracts, which may contribute to surgical planning by guiding the surgical trajectory through the least disruptive pathway.[27] Functional MRI (fMRI) has a role in cases in which the approach encroaches on motor or language cortex. Some authors advocate magnetic resonance spectroscopy (MRS) to characterize the chemical composition of the lesion in malignant lesions that may require a biopsy.[28] However, we have found the DTI and fMRI to be more helpful in surgical planning. It is our practice to also obtain magnetic resonance angiography (MRA)and venography (MRV). These images serve several purposes. First, they permit visualization of the blood supply to the lesion. Second, MRV through the vertex allows the surgeon to tailor the placement of the craniotomy based on draining cortical veins. Finally, MRV is helpful when considering choroidal dissection to gain access to the third ventricle.[29]

If increased vascularity of the tumor is noted, when appropriate, we prefer our neurointerventional team to perform an endovascular embolization procedure to decrease the blood flow to the lesion. In cases of successfully preoperatively embolized tumors, the resection is markedly easier, with far less blood loss. We have performed embolization of choroidal vessels with large intraventricular lesions in children as young as 2 years of age. Seemingly small blood loss constitutes a significant blood volume reduction in young children and can cause shock quickly or cause the surgeon to halt or stage an operation. We favor preoperative embolization whenever it is technically feasible in adults as well as children.

Preoperative visual field testing, a neuro-ophthalmological examination, and neuropsychological evaluations are performed for all patients as part of our baseline examination. These examinations often delineate subtle deficits not appreciated on neurological evaluations. The comprehensive neuropsychological examination consists of a thorough assessment of intellectual, academic, sensorimotor, language, spatial, memory, attention, and executive skills. The examination is repeated postoperatively at various intervals to provide data for a more objective assessment of outcomes and a guide for rehabilitation when necessary.

Ventricular communication after tumor resection is an important goal. Septations need to be removed and CSF spaces need to be in communication both anatomically as well as physiologically. Microscopic or endoscopic examination is performed to confirm the absence of blood clot or residual tumor and ensure that intraventricular communication has been achieved. Fenestration of the septum pellucidum to allow bilateral ventricular communication is a maneuver used prior to closure. A saline warmer filled with saline or lactated Ringer's solution is used to ensure that physiological conditions are maintained during the intraventricular irrigation and exploration.

Patients in whom a cortical incision is required receive a loading dose of antiepileptic medicine preoperatively. They are maintained on prophylactic anticonvulsant therapy for approximately 1 week after the procedure, if they have not suffered a preoperative seizure.

A standard external ventricular catheter is placed in the ventricle and run outside the dura through one of the bur holes after surgery. This provides external drainage of proteinaceous material and blood products from the surgery and serves as a convenient ICP monitor.

The beautiful anatomy of the lateral ventricle facilitates a wide variety of surgical approaches. The location and size of the lesion, hemispheric dominance, preoperative deficits, associated hydrocephalus, vascularity of the lesion, and experience of the surgeon all contribute to the ultimate selection of surgical approach. There is simply no class I or II data that dictates one approach is superior to another. The optimal approach facilitates the primary goal of surgery, which is gross total resection of the lesion with minimal trauma to surrounding structures and neural function. At our institution, most lateral ventricle lesions are approached through a transcortical route, a transcallosal route, or in rare cases a combination of the two. As detailed in the following sections, these routes provide excellent access to lesions within the third and lateral ventricles (Fig. 42.4).

CRANIOTOMY FLAP AND CORTICAL INCISIONS

A variety of incisions can be used for ventricular operations, including linear, "zigzag," bicoronal, horseshoe, question mark, and serpentine incisions. Incisions are all performed behind the hairline. "Zigzag" and linear incisions, which heal well, seem to cause slightly less cosmetic hair issues and do not compromise surgical exposure. Regardless of the type of incision, the goal is to provide adequate exposure for a craniotomy that will minimize cortical retraction. For example, for an anterior transcortical approach, the bone flap will have its medial border adjacent to but not over the midline and its anterior border will be above the floor of the anterior fossa. A unicoronal or modified bicoronal incision will best achieve this goal. For the posterior transcortical approaches, the border of the craniotomy should be adjacent to the sagittal and transverse sinuses; linear, serpentine, and horseshoe-shaped incisions all work well. For middle fossa approaches, the craniotomy should be based on the floor of the middle fossa and extend high enough so that all three temporal gyri can be visualized; a standard question mark– or T-shaped incision is sufficient. Interhemispheric incisions can be linear, "zigzag," or box-shaped. The craniotomy is taken across the midline by placing contralateral bur holes and stripping the sagittal sinus prior to passing the craniotome. If the patient does not have hydrocephalus and needs a ventriculostomy, a lumbar drain may be helpful in interhemispheric approaches.

The size and location of the cortical incision are important. The site is chosen based on the topography of the sulci and gyri or location of eloquent cortex based on mapping findings, DTI maps, or directed by frameless navigation. The choice of traversing the sulcus versus gyrus for the cortisectomy in the transcortical approach remains a subject of discussion and primarily is based on surgeon preference. The sulcus incision for the removal of subcortical tumors or arteriovenous malformations works well, although the transcortical gyrus incision, which can be extended, is ideal for the removal of large intraventricular tumors.

To enter the ventricle directly, we employ a simple technique of placing a ventricular catheter by frameless stereotactic guidance, or through a freehand pass to enter the ventricle. Once the trajectory to the ventricle is determined, a small cortical incision is made and followed down to the catheter in the ventricle. The ependyma is opened with nonstick or irrigating bipolar electrocautery, and the ventricle is entered. A cortical aperture is made using flat microinstruments or microsuction to develop a subcortical path to the lesion. Very little of the subcortical white matter is removed, and flat malleable brain retractors or a microsurgical speculum is placed to increase

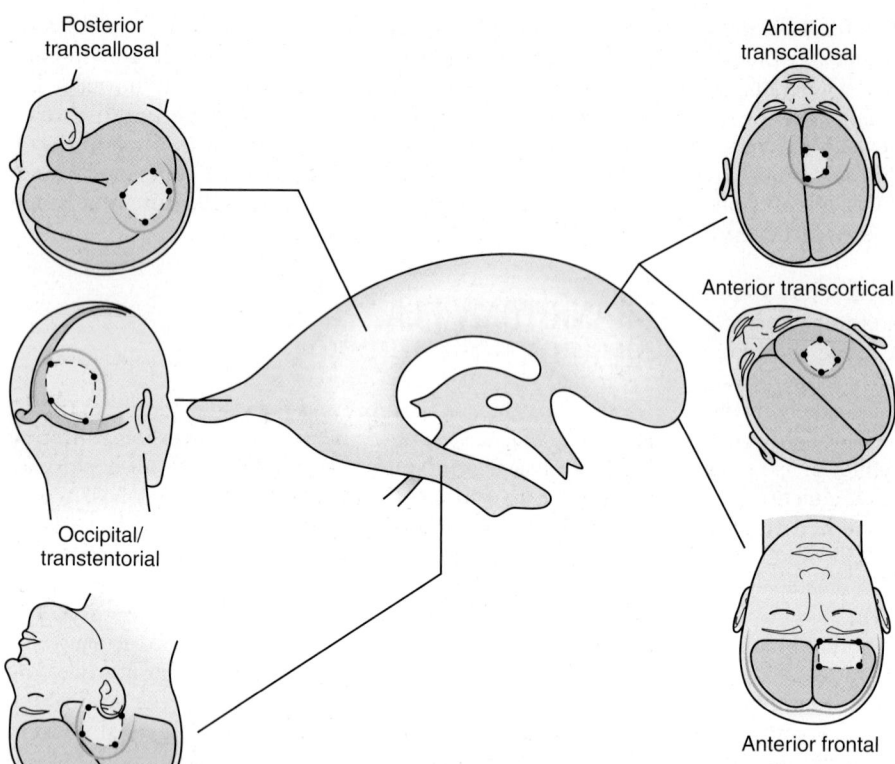

Posterior
transcallosal

Occipital/
transtentorial

Temporal

Anterior
transcallosal

Anterior transcortical

Anterior frontal

FIGURE 42.4 Approaches to the ventricular system. A composite of various approaches to the cerebral ventricles is illustrated. The optimal approach provides the surgeon with a perpendicular line of sight to the lesion within short working distance while minimizing functional deficits from manipulating surrounding structures. The site of the skin incision and the bone flap are shown for each approach to the specific part of the ventricle. (The incisions can be curvilinear as shown, linear, serpentine, or zigzag, depending on surgical preference. The cranial bone flap can be shaped to provide appropriate exposure.)

visibility. The goal is not necessarily to make the smallest cortical incision but to make the most appropriate one. Transcortical surgery has the advantages of wide avenues and a maneuverable microsurgical field.[30]

The anterior transcortical approach is well suited for tumors arising within the lateral ventricle. The principal advantage of the transcortical approach is a direct line of sight to lesions within the lateral ventricle. Isolated lesions in the frontal horn, body, and atrium may be accessed easily. This approach strategy is particularly attractive for lesions that derive their blood supply from the lateral wall of the ventricle, or lesions that are firmly adherent to the structures that constitute the lateral wall of the ventricle. The caudate nucleus, thalamostriate vein, thalamus, and genu of the internal capsule may be identified early in transcortical approaches.

There are limitations to the transcortical approach. This approach may not provide optimal visualization of the contralateral ventricle due to the linear trajectory, which may obscure lesions sitting in a location out of the line of sight of the microscope. The transcortical approach may also predispose the patient to postoperative seizures. The incidence of postoperative seizures ranges in the literature from 5% to 70%,[2,3,31-34] which is higher than in transcallosal approaches when no cortisectomy is performed (0-10%). However, our experience with seizure activity after the transcortical approach parallels that of the transcallosal approach. Specifically, the postoperative seizure rate with very small corticectomy (<15 mm) and prophylactic anticonvulsant treatment for 1 week has successfully lowered the immediate postoperative seizure incidence to the 5% to 7% range.

ANTERIOR TRANSCORTICAL APPROACHES

Tumors in the frontal region are primarily astrocytoma, subependymal giant cell astrocytoma, ependymoma, and central neurocytoma. Tumors of the frontal horn can become very large and cause obstruction of the foramen of Monro with ventricular dilation. The transcortical middle frontal gyrus approach is an excellent route for the excision of tumors in the ipsilateral anterior horn of the lateral ventricle, the anterior body of the lateral ventricle, and the anterior third ventricle. Tumors that extend inferiorly from the lateral ventricle into the third ventricle and require an interforniceal or subchoroidal exposure for removal, can be approached using either a transcortical or a transcallosal route.[10] In patients with small ventricles, tumor in both lateral ventricles, or tumor in the body of the lateral ventricle, the transcallosal approach is employed.

The patient is placed in the supine position with the head elevated 10 to 30 degrees. A free 3 × 4-cm bone flap is placed over the central portion of the middle frontal gyrus. The flap is based on the coronal suture, with the medial border off the midline and the anterior border at least 2 cm anterior to the coronal suture and the posterior border about 2 cm behind. The dura is opened in a cruciate or box-shaped fashion and a ventricular catheter is placed into the frontal horn. This is followed by microsurgical cleavage of the white matter until the ependymal lining is broached. A small ⅜-inch retractor or speculum retractor is used. After the anatomy of the lateral ventricle is visualized through the microscope, regardless of the approach, the anatomy is similar. Once inside the

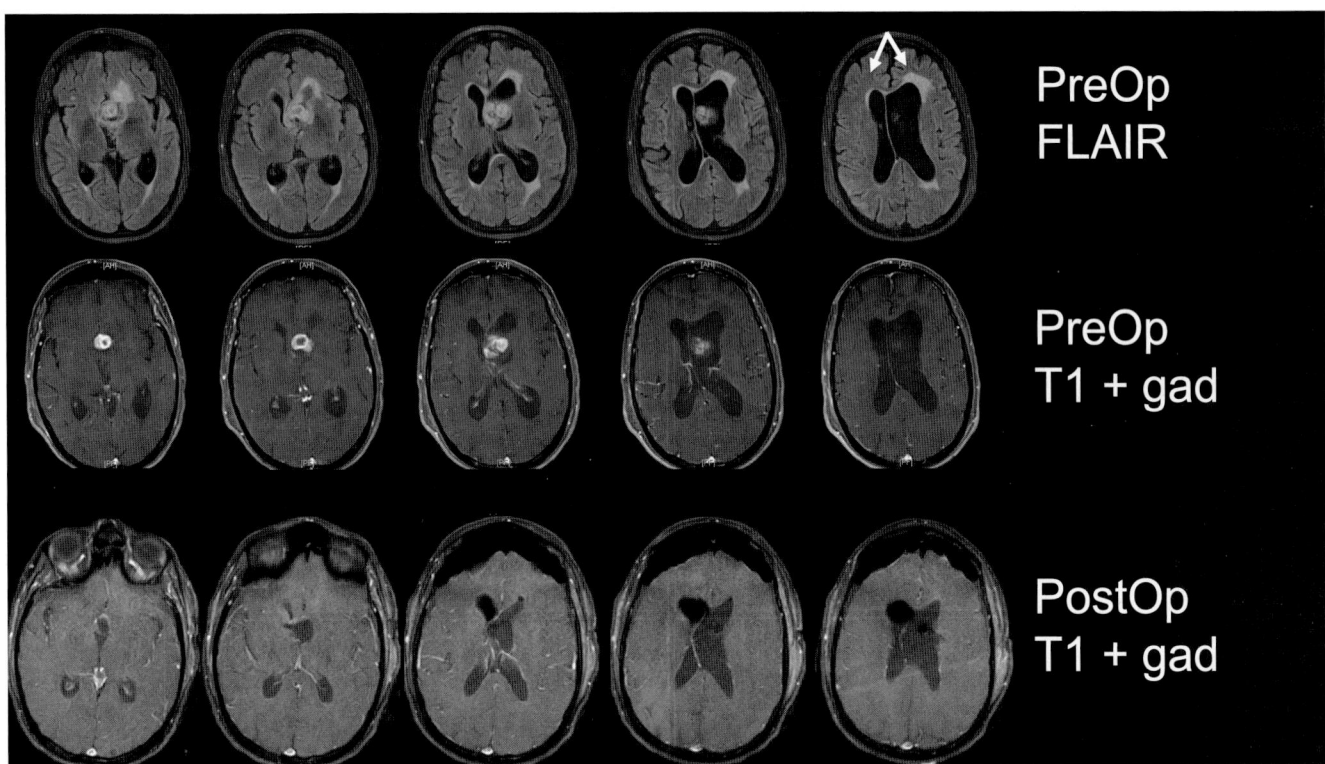

FIGURE 42.5 Adult male patient with no prior neurological history presented with personality changes, memory loss, and headache over several months. The lesion arises from the medial aspect of the floor of the frontal horn of the lateral ventricle, near the septal nuclei. The lesion enhances briskly with gadolinium administration. Fluid-attenuated inversion recovery (FLAIR) imaging reveals asymmetrical transependymal flow, suggesting a trapped left ventricle (*arrows*). This lesion was approached through the transcortical middle frontal gyrus in order to achieve gross total resection and fenestration of the septum pellucidum. The patient returned to baseline premorbid function and his job as an attorney without deficits or seizures. Pathological examination revealed subependymal giant cell astrocytoma (SEGA).

ventricle, surgical landmarks provide orientation. The most important landmarks are the foramen of Monro, the thalamostriate vein, the choroid plexus, and the fornix. Cotton paddies are placed over the foramen and around the lesion to minimize the circulation of blood products and debris during tumor resection.

Lesions within the third ventricle may be accessed from the transcortical approach. If the foramen is enlarged from hydrocephalus or the lesion itself, no additional dissection is necessary. If not, additional access to the third ventricle is made possible by a transchoroidal or suprachoroidal, trans–velum interpositum dissection.[35] To achieve this exposure, the choroidal fissure is opened between the fornix and the thalamus.[36] The suprachoroidal or transchoroidal approach divides the taenia of the fornix between the fornix and choroid plexus. The subchoroidal approach divides the taenia thalami leaf of the tela choroidea between the choroid plexus and the thalamus. The latter approach is more commonly associated with direct injury to the thalamostriate vein and thalamus. Rhoton's elegant lifetime work has been captured in his collected works in *Neurosurgery* and is arguably the most complete work on the subject.[9,37] In his ventricular surgery experience, he has demonstrated that the transchoroidal or suprachoroidal approach, opening the fissure through the taenia fornix, is both safe and effective.[18] Although we have safely opened the fissure through the "subchoroidal" approach on the taenia thalami side, the risk of thalamic

damage is quite real and can be devastating. In contrast, opening on the taenia fornix side in which a unilateral forniceal injury occurs often results in no permanent memory loss (Fig. 42.6). Regardless, these aforementioned considerations are important but must be applied to the specific anatomy at the time of the intraventricular dissection. Complications from injury to the surrounding structures result in hemiparesis, mutism, amnestic syndromes, and confusion.[38] In general, these risks are minimized by a suprachoroidal approach. However, maintaining the integrity of both fornices is important for preservation of memory function. The fornix, which has been reported to carry as many as five times the number of axons as the optic tract,[39] links the hippocampal formation (including the hippocampus proper, dentate gyrus, parahippocampal gyrus, and subiculum) with the septal nuclei, mammillary bodies, hypothalamus, and thalamic nuclei. Visualization of the fornix may be obscured by lesions based on the septum pellucidum, such as central neurocytomas. Patient dissection and meticulous technique here will be rewarded with a favorable postoperative outcome.

Although the precise method of tumor resection is determined on a case-by-case basis, we adhere to certain general principles in all cases. Prior to entering the lesion, attention must be directed first toward any feeding vessels entering the tumor. Once these are coagulated and divided, the tumor capsule itself may be coagulated and incised. The tumor is then internally debulked with ultrasonic aspiration. Early in

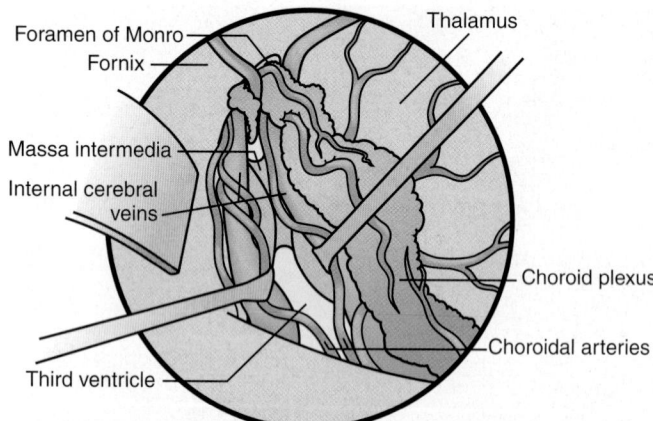

FIGURE 42.6 The third ventricle has been exposed by opening the choroidal fissure along the site of the attachment of the choroid plexus to the fornix. The choroidal fissure can be split on the taenia thalami or taenia fornix side but thalamic injury is avoided if it is opened on the fornix side. This exposes the internal cerebral veins and medial posterior choroidal arteries in the velum interpositum on the roof of the third ventricle.

the dissection, frozen specimens are collected for pathological examination. Care is taken to achieve complete hemostasis at regular intervals. As the excision proceeds, the surgeon may periodically reorient using surrounding anatomical landmarks and neuronavigation. It is critically important to preserve the integrity of the fornices, caudate, thalamus, and normal vascularity to avoid postoperative deficits.

Once the lesion has been removed, the surrounding ventricle surfaces are inspected to ensure that any adherent tumor is resected. Occasionally, direct visualization of all ventricle surfaces is not possible. The 30-degree endoscope or the dental mirror is a helpful aid to visualize the roof of the lateral ventricle and the posterior half of the third ventricle.

Following tumor resection, copious amounts of irrigation cleanse the ventricle of blood and debris. We routinely perform septostomy to facilitate CSF flow between the ventricles. If the endoscope is used, a endoscopic third ventriculostomy may also be performed. The retractors are withdrawn in a graduated fashion to permit hemostasis. Finally, a ventricular catheter is passed through the cortisectomy under direct vision. The dura is closed in watertight fashion. The dura is augmented with pericranium or Duragen and fibrin glue when necessary. The craniotomy is reapproximated with rigid fixation and the ventricular catheter is brought out through a separate posterior stab incision.

APPROACH TO THE TEMPORAL HORN

The transcortical approach is the primary method with which to remove tumors in the temporal horn extending from the temporal tip back to the ambient cistern. The temporal horn, however, is the least likely of the five ventricular regions to harbor a tumor.[6,40]

The scalp incision is performed so that bony landmarks, which include the zygoma, the asterion, and the pterion, can be visualized. A craniotomy to the floor is performed, but care is taken to avoid the middle ear; ear cells that are encountered

need to be occluded.[41] Anatomically, the structures that must be respected during removal of temporal horn tumors include the medial structures such as the hippocampus and its projections, temporal stem, PCA, anterior choroidal artery, and the posterior brainstem. Superiorly, one must avoid the optic tract, Meyer's loop, and arcuate fasciculus.

Three cortical incisions provide access to the temporal horn of the lateral ventricle: (1) the middle temporal gyrus, (2) the lateral temporoparietal junction, and (3) the occipitotemporal gyrus or collateral sulcus incision.

This last cortisectomy[42] may be the safest, especially in the dominant hemisphere. This incision was described by Spencer and Collins[43] in 1982 and was first used in the surgical treatment of epilepsy. It was designed to remove the hippocampus and associated structures and is therefore familiar to many neurosurgeons specializing in the treatment of epilepsy. The approach is also extremely useful for removing large, vascular lesions in either hemisphere, extending back to the brainstem. An incision can also be made in the inferior temporal gyrus as well as the occipitotemporal gyrus or collateral sulcus. Once inside the temporal horn, the choroidal fissure is identified. The fissure can be split by microsurgical technique along the taenia fimbriae, lifting the choroid plexus toward the thalamus, leaving the taeniae thalami and thalamus intact. This step permits visualization of the vascular structures to include anterior and posterior choroidal arteries, basal vein of Rosenthal, and PCA. The fissure can be split as far back as the ambient cistern. There is very little retraction in this approach and this preserves the vein of Labbé and temporal lobe. Early control of the anterior choroidal vessels can be obtained, making tumor or vascular malformation excision slightly less challenging. However, the posterior choroidal artery branches feeding a very large tumor may not be exposed until the bulk of the tumor is removed. Luders and coworkers[44] have described a basal language region in the inferior temporal lobe that is best elicited by cortical stimulation. Its removal does not uniformly lead to a language deficit because it presumably represents ancillary language cortex. Our experience is similar to that of Luders and coworkers. We have also mapped this language area in several patients but have yet to record a postoperative language deficit following a ventricular tumor excision using this approach.[20]

The middle temporal gyrus incision provides a direct route to many middle fossa ventricular lesions. In the nondominant hemisphere, this is a very acceptable route, causing minimal morbidity. In the dominant hemisphere, the danger posed to the language cortex becomes an issue and requires refinement in technique or use of the inferior route through the collateral sulcus as described previously. Ojemann[45] has meticulously detailed the individual variability of language localization to include language encoding in some individuals within 3.5 cm of the temporal tip and in gyri other than the superior temporal gyrus. Thus, in dominant hemisphere lesions, if the middle temporal gyrus approach is used, the risk of causing language deficit is most effectively prevented by cortical stimulation and mapping. Facial apraxia has also been reported in the dominant hemisphere.[40] The middle temporal gyrus approach to the temporal horn of the lateral ventricle has the potential to manipulate the tracts of the visual pathways, resulting in varying degrees of temporary and permanent deficits.[5,18,30,46] The optic tract can be found in the superior medial region of the

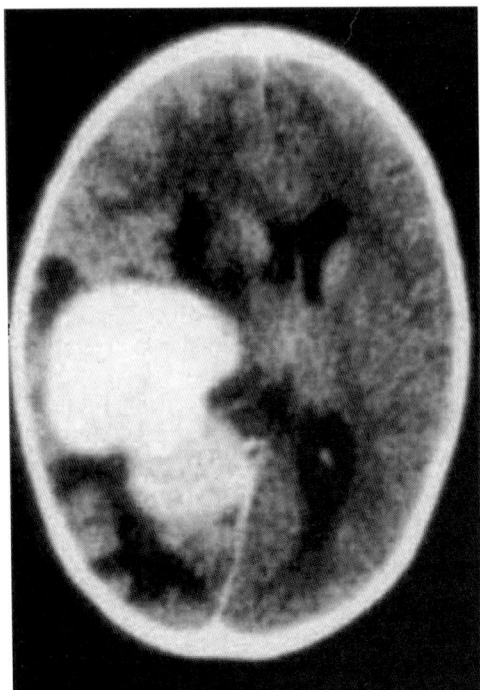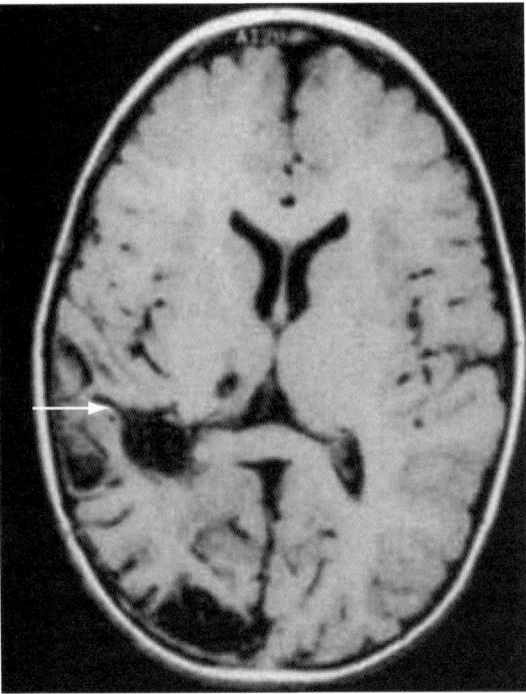

FIGURE 42.7 *Left:* Preoperative computed tomography (CT) scan obtained in a 3-year-old boy harboring a very large choroid plexus carcinoma in the atrium of the left lateral ventricle; he presented with hemiparesis, megacephaly, and malaise. The child required embolization of his posterior lateral choroidal feeding vessels prior to surgery. He then underwent a successful lateral temporoparietal approach for gross total resection of tumor. Despite this being the dominant hemisphere, this was the most direct approach to resect this large tumor and obtain proximal control of the vascular pedicle. Although the embolization was invaluable, rendering this tumor less vascular than most choroid plexus tumors, there was still a vascular pedicle that required ligation. He was neurologically stable without hemiparesis after adjuvant chemotherapy for 5 years. *Right:* The *white arrow* on the postoperative magnetic resonance imaging (MRI) demonstrates the patient's cortisectomy and the surgical approach. *(Adapted from Ellenbogen RG. Transcortical surgery for lateral ventricular tumors. Neurosurg Focus 2001;10:1-13.)*

temporal horn as it courses toward the lateral geniculate body. The optic radiations then head toward the calcarine cortex along the Meyer-Archambault loop in the superior and lateral aspect of the temporal horn and in the tapetum over the roof and lateral aspect of the atrium and occipital horn. Cortical incisions in the middle fossa are best placed parallel to the Meyer-Archambault loop to avoid causing a quadrantanopia or other field deficit.

The lateral temporoparietal junction approach is applicable in patients in which the angular and supramarginal gyri are flattened by a large tumor in the nondominant atrium that lies directly beneath them. In such a case, this is the shortest and most direct route to the tumor. The advantage of this approach is that a small portion of brain needs to be traversed from the cortex to the tumor. The disadvantage of this approach is the potential for significant neuropsychological sequelae, which have been reported when manipulating the angular gyrus. It is useful for very large tumors with overlying attenuated cortex. Regardless of hemisphere, a cortical incision in the temporoparietal junction can result in a visual field deficit caused by the interruption of the optic radiations.[47] A cortisectomy through the angular gyrus in the dominant hemisphere can also cause right-left confusion, digital agnosia, agraphia, and acalculia (i.e., Gerstmann syndrome).[48] In the nondominant hemisphere, visual memory loss and neglect can result, which are also potentially disabling.[47] However, our experience has been only with very large tumors in which

there was extremely attenuated brain with little cortex covering the tumor. In these patients, taking the shortest route with least retraction after DTI analysis of the tracts yielded an improved neuropsychological outcome, perhaps because the patient's function was already compromised and an alternative route would place those fibers at greater risk (Fig. 42.7).

POSTERIOR TRANSCORTICAL APPROACHES

The superior parietal route is one of the best approaches for reaching the collateral trigone, the posterior part of the body, and atrium.[46,49-52] It has been used to reach vascular malformations in the trigone, as well as tumors.[49,53] Postoperative cortical damage manifested by a visual field cut can occur if the medial wall of the atrium adjacent to the calcarine cortex is injured; however, the cortical incision is high enough to avoid the optic radiations in most patients. It is similar to the route taken through the cortex when placing a posterior ventricular catheter for CSF diversion. The superior parietal transcortical approach is riskier in the dominant hemisphere. The potential risks include apraxia, acalculia, visual spatial distortion, and the full-blown Gerstmann syndrome.[6,54] However, this operation can be performed safely in the dominant hemisphere. A large series of the parietal approach has yielded radical tumor resection without neuropsychological sequelae.[55] The vascular supply to the tumor is deep and circumnavigating the tumor may require retraction that can be deleterious to the superior parietal lobule, so preoperative embolization may be helpful in these patients. The patient is placed in the three-quarter prone position with the parietal boss in the most superior position and the face turned toward the floor. The cortical incision is performed on the long axis of the superior parietal lobule with the trajectory directed toward the atrium by frameless navigation. It is made high enough to avoid the optic radiations and posterior enough to avoid language encoded at the junction of the parietal and temporal lobes. The ventricle is entered above the junction of the body, the atrium, and the crus of the ipsilateral fornix. From a coronal plane, one can visualize the choroid plexus and fissure as a navigational landmark. The calcar avis and corpus callosum will make up the medial wall, and the pulvinar will be anterior. The collateral trigone will make up the floor. This is also an excellent approach to resect a thalamic lesion that extends into the atrium. The posterior choroidal artery can be uncovered in the choroidal fissure between the pulvinar and the crus of the fornix.[7] The ventricle atrium is surrounded by subcortical white matter tracts critical for vision. Immediately below the thin layer of tapetal fibers lie the optic radiations, which leave the superior portion of the lateral geniculate nucleus to innervate the superior bank of the calcarine fissure.[56] The inferior bank of the calcarine fissure receives fibers from the inferior portion of the lateral geniculate nucleus which loop forward around the temporal horn of the lateral ventricle. The fibers, which serve vision from the upper visual field, extend through the superior wall of the temporal horn of the lateral ventricle before looping laterally and inferiorly in the atrium.[56] Opening the choroidal fissure at this junction will expose the internal cerebral vein running with the choroidal artery in the velum. One may also visualize the basal vein of Rosenthal or vein of Galen. Within the atrium, the glomus of the choroid plexus receives blood from the anterior and lateral posterior choroidal arteries. Approaches to the ventricle atrium therefore require careful attention to the surrounding anatomy. The atrium may be entered from parieto-occipital transcortical approaches, tailored to the cortical anatomy, draining cortical veins and periventricular white matter tracts.[57] The superior parietal trajectory entails a cortisectomy between the postcentral sulcus and the parieto-occipital sulcus.[54] These approaches are not without morbidity.[58,59] For lesions arising from the medial surface of the atrium, such as the precuneus gyrus, a posterior interhemispheric approach may be preferred to the transcortical route.[27,60] Using this approach, the brain is entered lateral to the splenium through a limited cortisectomy. Obviously, this approach may be complicated by postoperative hemanopia. A more superiorly oriented approach enters the brain lateral to the splenium from a parietal trajectory and is not associated with a high rate of visual loss.[60] A lateral approach enters the trigone through the posterior temporal lobe and parietal lobe.[61]

Interhemispheric Transcallosal and Posterior Third Ventricle Approaches

The anterior and posterior interhemispheric transcallosal approach offers different advantages over the transcortical route. The transcallosal approach does not disrupt the cortex, and is therefore associated with a lower incidence of

postoperative seizures.[62] Also, the functional consequences that may be observed with transcortical approaches are largely absent.[63] Although only a few centimeters of callosal division are necessary to permit ample exposure to the lateral or third ventricle,[27] the anterior two thirds of the corpus callosum may be divided without clinically significant consequences.[64]

The anterior transcallosal approach is best suited for lesions located within the frontal horn of the lateral ventricle, the body of the lateral ventricle, and the anterior third ventricle.[65] Limitations of the transcallosal approach prevent this approach from being utilized in all patients. The extent of lateral exposure within the lateral ventricle may be limited. Complications associated with transcallosal approaches to the third ventricle include hemiparesis, amnesia, and akinetic mutism.[38] Section of the anterior corpus callosum is contraindicated in patients with crossed dominance, that is, patients with language lateralized to one cerebral hemisphere and dominant hand function lateralized to the other.[66,67] Callosal section may result in speech and writing deficits in this patient population.

For standard anterior transcallosal approaches to the lateral ventricle, the patient is positioned supine with the head slightly flexed. For posterior transcallosal approaches the patient is placed in the prone position. Neuronavigation assists the surgeon in defining the extent of the craniotomy based on the intraventricular target. Craniotomy may be performed on either side of the skull because the transcallosal approach permits equal access to both lateral ventricles.[68] However, it is our practice to perform these craniotomies on the right side to minimize the risk of language dysfunction associated with supplementary motor syndrome, which may occur following interhemispheric retraction of the dominant hemisphere.[69] Side of approach is more important when addressing third ventricle lesions to maximize a direct approach through the foramen of Monro to the lesion. We utilize neuronavigation to plan the craniotomy. As with anterior transcortical approaches, we prefer a bicoronal incision because of the wide exposure and cosmetic result.

The craniotomy is necessarily brought past the midline. The dural incision is based medially, to permit visualization down the falx cerebri. Bridging veins and sinus lacunes are carefully protected when more posterior, although some anterior veins can be taken with impunity. A retractor is used in concert with the natural retraction provided by the falx to facilitate the interhemispheric dissection. Below the level of the falx, the cingulate gyrus with its callosal marginal vessels may be densely adherent. Sharp dissection and meticulous microsurgical technique will preserve the pial boundaries. The pericallosal arteries are encountered above the corpus callosum, which is identified by the glistening white surface. The callosum is divided longitudinally. The extent of callosal division is guided by the size and location of the lesion. The usual landmarks are encountered upon entry into the ventricle. If the landmarks are not visible, the approach may have entered a cavum septum pellucidum. Penetration through either septal wall will access the lateral ventricle. Tumor resection and access to the third ventricle then proceed as described previously for transcortical approaches.

This chapter is not intended to review pineal region tumors in detail. A more complete review can be found in Chapter 37. Lesions located in the posterior third ventricle may be difficult

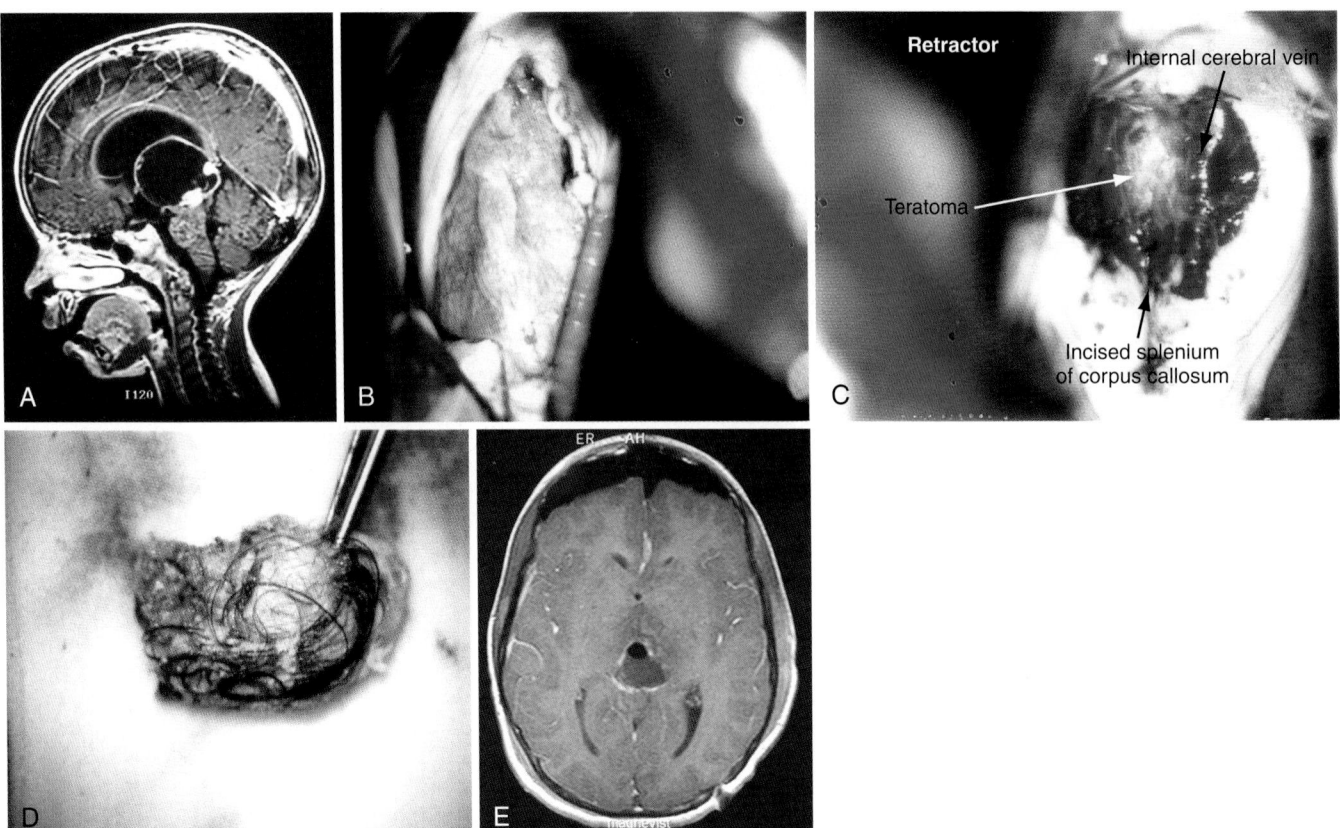

FIGURE 42.8 A, A large posterior third ventricle tumor in a child causing hydrocephalus and neurological decline. This mass is mixed signal containing a variety of components. **B,** A posterior interhemispheric transcallosal approach was undertaken in the prone position. The splenium is split and the velum interpositum is demonstrated. **C,** Once the velum is opened one can see one of the paired internal cerebral veins lying over this large mass arising from the posterior ventricle. **D,** The mass was completely removed and was a teratoma with components including hair, lipoma, and calcium. **E,** Postoperative axial magnetic resonance imaging (MRI) showing complete resection. The patient was neurologically well and performing at grade level 5 years later.

to approach given the complex anatomical relationships. However, the pineal region is the corridor to the posterior third ventricle.

The posterior transcallosal approach through the splenium of the corpus callosum may be used to address a wide spectrum of tumors in the posterior third ventricle.[4,70,71] The posterior interhemispheric route is an ideal approach for large third ventricle lesions that extend into the pineal region. There are many less bridging veins in the posterior approach compared to anterior approach, so the interhemispheric approach to the splenium is often more facile. However, one must be cautious as the trajectory through the splenium takes the surgeon close to deep drainage veins such as the vein of Galen. Despite concern about neuropsychological sequelae with a splenial incision, the patients often tolerate this remarkably well. And, when the splenium is thinned, this approach can be successfully used for both small and large lesions in children and adults (Fig. 42.8A-E).

Yaşargil advocates the median supracerebellar dissection to this region as it takes advantage of the natural corridor between the cerebellum and tentorium.[27] A necessary requirement of this approach is that the angle of the tentorium must not be prohibitively steep. This dissection, also termed the *infratentorial-supracerebellar approach*, permits access to the velum interpositum above the pineal gland and habenular

commissure. Horsley is credited with first attempting this approach for pineal region tumors.[72] The approach begins with a midline occipital and suboccipital craniotomy. Careful protection of the dura overlying the torcular and transverse sinuses is required. The dura is opened below the transverse sinus. The dissection proceeds over the superior surface of the cerebellum. Where possible, lateral veins should be preserved; however, the superior vermian and the precentral cerebellar vein must be sacrificed when they are obstructing the view of the tumor. At the depth of the approach, the quadrigeminal cistern is apparent. Posterior third ventricle tumors originating from the pineal gland often project posteriorly into the quadrigeminal cistern. These lesions are immediately apparent above the quadrigeminal cistern during this dissection. Internal debulking within the tumor capsule will decompress the posterior third ventricle. Lesions within the third ventricle not arising from the pineal gland may be approached above the pineal by developing the potential space in the third ventricle with the velum interpositum being the superior border. However, this is an extremely long and deep reach through a narrow corridor.

The principal limitations to the supracerebellar infratentorial approach is the patient positioning and the deep narrow corridor in which the surgeon must work. The infratentorial supracerebellar approach is often performed in the sitting

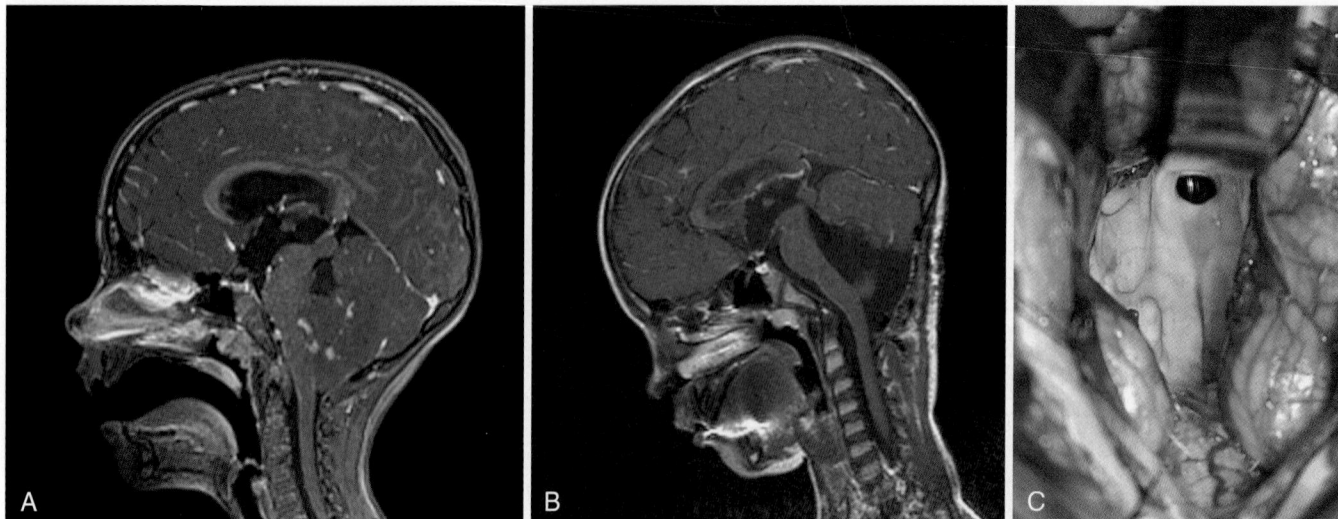

FIGURE 42.9 This child presented with headache, nausea, gait instability, and a new sixth cranial nerve paresis. **A,** The sagittal + gadolinium image demonstrates a large fourth ventricle mass with hydrocephalus. **B,** The postoperative + gadolinium image shows a gross total excision of this tumor through the telovelar approach and resolution of the brainstem compression and ventriculomegaly. **C,** The postresection photograph shows the cerebellar hemisphere elevated without any vermis being sacrificed. The floor is pristine and the view extends as far cranial as the aqueduct of Sylvius. The patient was neurologically improved without postoperative cerebellar mutism.

position to permit the cerebellum to sag for better visualization, although it can be performed in the prone, or Concorde position. Complications related to performing craniotomies in this position are air embolism,[73,74] hemorrhage,[75] tension pneumocephalus,[76] and cervical flexion myelopathy.[77]

The other major approach to this posterior third ventricle region is the occipital transtentorial approach. The occipital transtentorial approach is a powerful route providing a wide 270-degree view of the pineal region to include the major vasculature, brainstem, and third and lateral ventricles. It is best suited for large lesions that occupy supra- and infratentorial space. Patients with a low-lying torcular may have favorable anatomy for transtentorial approaches due to the steep angle of the tentorium. The transtentorial approach can be done in many positions to include the lateral or park-bench position. Frameless navigation is helpful in order to maintain proper orientation when approaching lesions above and below the tentorium.

Broadly considered, pineal region tumors are grouped into three major pathological categories: (1) germ cell tumors, (2) primary pineal cell tumors, and (3) glial cell and all "other" tumors.[73] In selected tumors that have positive markers in the serum or CSF it is worthwhile to follow these values.[73] α-Fetoprotein or β-human chorionic gonadotropin levels, when elevated, can be monitored in patients with malignant germ cell components in the posterior third ventricle to assess their response to adjunctive therapies.

Combined Endoscope-Assisted Microsurgical Approach to the Lateral and Third Ventricles

The use of the neuroendoscope during intraventricular surgery is well described.[78] Neuroendoscopy can be performed through the same approach as microsurgery, or through a separate approach entirely.[79] Minimally invasive techniques are attractive alternatives to conventional microsurgery because

they require little brain retraction. The endoscope offers superior visualization due to the proximity of the camera to the lesion and the high-intensity illumination. Endoscope-assisted resection may achieve gross total resection rates in 80% of selected cases.[80,81] The principal limitations of endoscope-assisted tumor resections relate to technical limitations with the instruments. This subject will be addressed in Chapter 42.

APPROACH TO THE FOURTH VENTRICLE

The most versatile approaches to fourth ventricle tumors are in the midline through the inferior vermis or the telovelar approach, which preserves those structures. The patient is positioned prone. The head is flexed in the Concorde position and the bed angle is adjusted so that the level of the craniotomy is even with the atrium of the heart, thereby reducing the risk of air embolism.[82] A suboccipital craniotomy or craniectomy is performed, depending on surgeon preference. The posterior arch of the C1 lamina is removed after the dura is incised in Y-shaped fashion and reflected superiorly. Opening the cisterna magna affords considerable brain relaxation. Adhesions between the cerebellar tonsils are released with sharp dissection, exposing the vermis in the midline.

The dissection proceeds carefully to identify and protect the floor of the fourth ventricle. Once the floor has been identified under the vermian peg, our preference is to protect it with cotton paddies. Depending on the nature of the fourth ventricle lesion, the tumor may be entered first before arriving at the ventricle proper. Although splitting the vermis may be required, we have avoided that move for most tumors, including large ones, over the past decade. This is frequently the case with medulloblastomas which are midline and arise from the inferior medullary velum.[83] Splitting the vermis is often undesirable in terms of side effects to the patient. The telovelar, or cerebellomedullary, approach permits the surgeon to

TABLE 42.1 Approaches to Microsurgical Resection of Ventricular Lesions: Indications and Risks

Approach	Indication(s)	Potential Complication(s)
Anterior transcortical approach via frontal gyrus	Ipsilateral frontal horn, select bilateral lesions, anterior body lesions and anterior third ventricle, especially for choroidal fissure approaches	Attention deficits in either hemisphere (rare); speech apraxia or abulia in dominant hemisphere; potential collapse of cortex and subdural hygroma, seizure disorder
Transtemporal approach; middle temporal gyrus approach; lateral temporoparietal incision; occipitotemporal gyrus/collateral sulcus or inferior temporal gyrus	Lesions in temporal horn extending as far forward as temporal tip and as far posterior as the ambient and crural cisterns	Language deficits in dominant hemisphere, hemiparesis, safer in nondominant hemisphere, visual field deficit, retraction injury to temporal lobe or vein of Labbé; Gerstmann's syndrome in the dominant hemisphere–angular gyrus injury; neglect and visual field deficit. Injury to vascular structures in choroidal fissure, visual field injury
Anterior interhemispheric transcallosal approach	Bilateral anterior horn and body of lateral ventricles, anterior third ventricle via choroidal fissure or interforniceal approach	Injury to cortical veins, hemiparesis from venous infarct or retraction, injury to pericallosal vessels, seizure disorder
Posterior interhemispheric transcallosal incision	Posterior third ventricle, medial surface of the atrium, and pineal region	Injury to internal cerebral or deep venous system, Gerstmann's syndrome, retraction injury
Posterior transcortical approach	Atrium, occipital horn, posterior and middle portion of the body, collateral trigone, pulvinar, thalamus, corpus callosum, or quadrigeminal cistern	Homonymous field deficit, hemiparesis, neuropsychiatric deficits in dominant hemisphere
Cerebellum/fourth ventricle via vermian or telovelar approach	Fourth ventricle from obex to aqueduct of Sylvius	Cerebellar mutism (less with telovelar approach), cerebellar injury, brainstem or cranial nerve injury, intractable vomiting

Note: This table provides an overview for the various approaches to microsurgical resection of ventricular lesions. Column 2 describes the indications for each approach, and column 3 describes the risks and potential complications.

access the fourth ventricle through the tonsillouveal sulcus.[27] This approach, also performed through suboccipital craniotomy, accesses the ventricle by dividing the tela choroidea and inferior medullary velum along the lateral recess of the vermis.[84] This move permits a wide opening without disturbing the vermis or the tracts from the cerebellum to the thalamus. There are few known deficits that occur from opening the tela and the velum. One can even extend the telar opening toward the foramen of Luschka, thus exposing the lateral recesses of the brainstem and cerebellum. Tumor resection proceeds with a surgical patty on the floor of the fourth ventricle protecting it and ensuring the surgeon can consistently define the plane between the tumor and floor. Once within the ventricle, delivering tumor from the aqueduct of Sylvius above permits the supratentorial ventricular system to communicate with the fourth ventricle, flooding the field with CSF. The lesion is resected with vigilance to preserve the integrity of the floor of the fourth ventricle. Very small and very large vascular tumors can be safely removed from the obex of the brainstem to the aqueduct of Sylvius using this powerful and safe approach (Fig. 42.9A-C).

POSTOPERATIVE DEFICITS AND COMPLICATION AVOIDANCE

The postoperative visual field defect is one of the most common deficits associated with transcortical approaches in the posterior cortical and middle fossa approaches (Table 42.1).

The most common deficit is a homonymous hemianopia or quadrant cut.

The true incidence of cortical incision–related postoperative epilepsy, another known complication, is hard to determine because many factors can contribute to a seizure disorder, including the tumor histological type, presence of preoperative seizures, and many postoperative issues.

Most postoperative weakness is presumably the result of retraction pressure and will resolve. Complication avoidance by using minimal or intermittent retraction, new retractor/speculum systems, avoidance of injury to the vasculature, and DTI MRI guidance has lessened this risk.

Language impairment is a possibility when the tumor is based in the dominant hemisphere. In such cases approximately 10% to 30% of patients will suffer a new speech deficit or worsening of their preoperative deficit.[85] Cognitive deficits and personality disorders are much more difficult to measure objectively, especially if preoperative neuropsychological studies are not conducted. It is wise to leave a small tumor remnant, especially if it is attached to critical structures such as the basal ganglia or fornices, particularly if the lesion is benign. Often, subtotal resections of intraventricular lesions are a result of the tumor histological type and its site of origin, as opposed to the surgical approach.[85-87]

Subdural hygroma formation is a well-recognized problem, especially in patients in whom a large tumor is associated with ventriculomegaly. These subdural fluid collections after significant decompression of the ventricles may occur following either transcortical or transcallosal approaches, with an

PART 6 Tumors

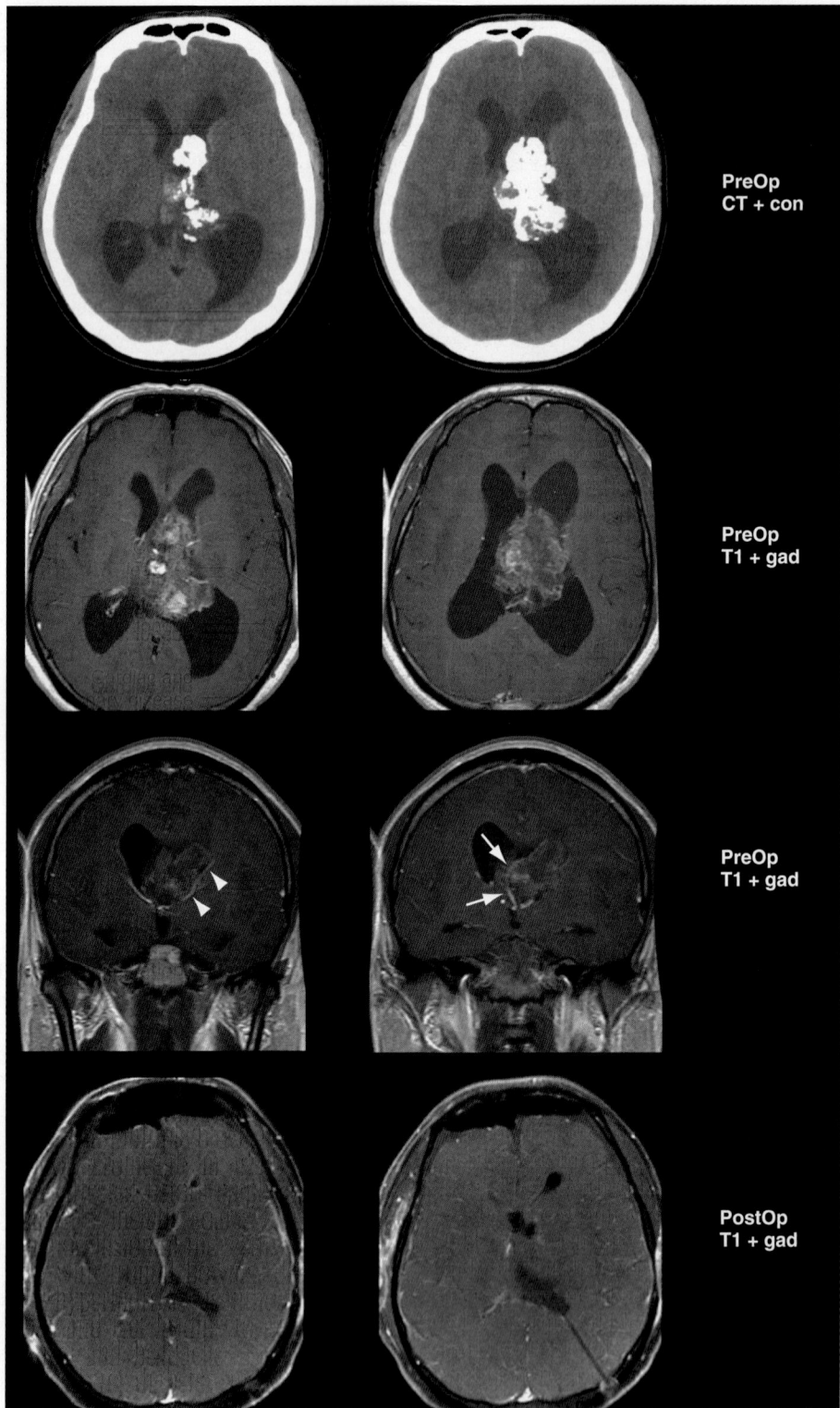

FIGURE 42.10 Adult male presenting with personality changes and headache over the course of several months. On top, the computed tomography (CT) image demonstrates extensive calcifications and hydrocephalus. The lesion was adherent to the ventricle wall superiorly, the caudate and thalamus laterally, the septum pellucidum medially, and the foramen of Monro, thalamus, and choroid plexus inferiorly. Axial magnetic resonance imaging (MRI) reveals a heterogeneous lesion filling the body of the lateral ventricle. −, without gadolinium; +, with gadolinium. Coronal MRI illustrates the relationship of the lesion to surrounding neurovascular structures. The thalamostriate vein is located at the lateral border of the lesion, while enlarged septal veins drain the tumor into the internal cerebral veins. These vessels were readily identifiable at the time of surgery using a combined strategy including both transcortical and transcallosal approaches. Pathological entity was a central neurocytoma. A radical resection was achieved and the patient returned to his baseline function and job within 6 months.

incidence of approximately 5%.[2] The cortical surface may collapse or pull away from the dura and create a hematoma or hygroma, which may eventually require the placement of a shunt. Filling the ventricles with sterile saline or lactated Ringer's solution before the completion of the surgery and leaving both subdural and intraventricular catheters in place may reduce the incidence of hygroma and hydrocephalus. Some surgeons argue that the application of fibrin glue over the cortical surface significantly decreases the rate of subdural fluid collections.[42] We prefer to position the patient with the operated side down for the first 8 hours to lessen the chance that a greater amount of cortex will pull away from the dura and skull. Treatment of this may require subdural taps, external drains, or a subdural shunt. However, most chronic subdural collections are self-limited and require simple observation.

Postoperative ventriculomegaly is common. Not all patients will require placement of a shunt. The precise incidence of shunting after resection is unpredictable and depends on a wide spectrum of parameters such as the tumor type, amount of blood and debris left in the ventricles, and other technical issues.[51] The inability to "wean" a postoperative external ventricular drain or development of a recalcitrant pseudomeningocele may indicate elevated intracranial pressure requiring CSF diversion. All patients may suffer some form of meningeal irritation caused by the presence of blood products and particulate matter in the CSF. This type of chemical meningitis can best be treated by aggressive postoperative ventricular drainage, analgesic agents, and a tapered course of steroids. Occasionally patients will require permanent CSF diversion following all the microsurgical approaches to ventricular tumors. Regardless, external ventricular drainage or external subdural drainage after resection is uniformly beneficial in lessening the chance of shunt-dependent hydrocephalus. Although ventriculitis remains a risk with intraventricular surgery and external ventricular drainage, infection rates of less than 5% are achievable after surgery.[85]

Historically, death was usually secondary to catastrophic postoperative hemorrhage or pulmonary emboli.[17,18,30,46,85-89] Nonetheless, even with our enormous advances in microsurgery, neuroanesthesia, and postoperative technology, a flexible surgical approach is important to lessen risks of morbidity and mortality. Preoperative embolization or a staged removal of a very large vascular lesion via a combined approach is preferable to a single, long, difficult procedure fraught with risks and excessive blood loss.

Postoperative Considerations

Patients are observed in the intensive care unit postoperatively. Ventricular drains, when placed, are set at a height of 10 to 15 cm above the external auditory meatus until the CSF becomes clearer. Drains are weaned gradually thereafter. We routinely perform postoperative MRI to document the extent of the resection within the first 48 hours. Postoperative neuropsychological and ophthalmological evaluations may be performed at a delayed interval to facilitate rehabilitation.

All cases are discussed at multidisciplinary tumor conferences. Adjunctive therapies are considered in cases of malignant disease, although some advocate radiotherapy in cases of subtotal resection of benign lesions, such as central neurocytomas. When applicable, adjunctive therapy may begin as early as 2 weeks following surgery. Patients may experience complications such as delayed hydrocephalus, pseudomeningocele, or subdural fluid collections.[90] Although permanent CSF diversion is a known risk of these operations, we have been successful in managing patients with aggressive ventricular drainage or a lumbar drain.

FUTURE DIRECTIONS

Substantial gains in the treatment of intraventricular tumors have developed since surgery for these lesions was originally described. Early diagnosis, enhanced preoperative imaging, neuronavigation, microsurgical techniques, and endoscopic assistance improve clinical outcomes. Advances along each of these fronts will certainly lead to improved outcome. The greatest advances will likely come in the form of technical improvements in the realm of endoscopic instrumentation and targeted therapies for brain tumors. Flexible and robotic endoscopes, for example, may improve visualization of lesions within the ventricles. Flexible instruments for tumor resection may further reduce the need for brain retraction during transcortical approaches. The ventricular system invites targeted delivery of antineoplastic agents, immunotherapies, and viral vectors, which are under development.[91] Additional advances in preoperative imaging and functional mapping will permit the surgeon to plan approaches around fiber tracts associated with functionally important cortical regions.[37]

CONCLUSION

Intraventricular lesions are rare lesions that require special neurosurgical consideration. Transcortical and transcallosal microsurgical approaches offer different advantages based on lesion location, size, and proximity to surrounding structures. Combined microsurgical approaches are necessary for large lesions when one approach does not permit visualization of critical landmarks (Fig. 42.10). Neuroendoscopic approaches may achieve gross total resection of carefully selected lesions. The future of intraventricular surgery holds improvements in the realm of preoperative functional imaging, DTI, and neuroendoscopy.

SELECTED KEY REFERENCES

Cappabianca P, Cinalli G, Gangemi M, et al. Application of neuroendoscopy to intraventricular lesions. *Neurosurgery*. 2008;62(Suppl 2):575-597:discussion 597-598.

Ellenbogen RG. Transcortical surgery for lateral ventricular tumors. *Neurosurg Focus*. 2001;10:1-13.

Piepmeier JM, Spencer DD, Sass KJ, George TM. Lateral ventricular masses. In Apuzzo MLJ, editor. *Brain Surgery: Complication Avoidance and Management*, New York: 1993:581-599.

Rhoton Jr AL. The lateral and third ventricles. *Neurosurgery*. 2003;53:S235-S299.

Yasargil MG, Abdulrauf SI. Surgery of intraventricular tumors. *Neurosurgery*. 2008;62:SHC1029-SHC1041.

Please go to expertconsult.com to view the complete list of references.

43 Skull Base Approaches

Salvatore Di Maio, Laligam N. Sekhar

CLINICAL PEARLS

- Cranial base approaches are designed to provide greater tumor exposure compared to conventional cranial approaches, while avoiding retraction of normal brain structures. An understanding of the often complex anatomy is key to preserving the critical structures surrounding each approach.

- Selection of an appropriate approach for a specific tumor is determined by the cranial fossa involved and tumor extension, the ability to interrupt the tumor's blood supply early, and relationship of the tumor with surrounding normal structures. For more extensive tumors, either combined approaches or staged operations may be required.

- Complications of skull base approaches include vascular, nerve, or brainstem injury; cosmetic deformity; and cerebrospinal fluid (CSF) leak. In many cases these complications may be avoided by mastery of the surgical anatomy, careful preoperative planning including appropriate structural and vascular imaging, intraoperative monitoring, and meticulous attention to detail during the exposure, osteotomies, and reconstruction.

- The primary indication for the transsphenoidal approach is midline sellar and suprasellar lesions such as pituitary adenomas; this surgical approach can be performed using endoscopic or microsurgical techniques.

- The extended subfrontal approach is excellent for intra- and extradural lesions of the anterior skull base, paranasal sinuses, as well as the sella, and midline clivus down to the foramen magnum. It is excellent for sinonasal malignancies, chordomas, and ethesioneuroblastomas.

- The transmaxillary and extended transmaxillary approaches are best suited for midline extradural lesions centered on the midportion of the clivus, such as chordomas and chondrosarcomas.

- Transoral approaches are excellent for addressing midline lesions of the lower clivus and upper cervical spine from degenerative, congenital, or rheumatic disorders.

- The frontotemporal approach with variations of the orbitozygomatic extension is among the most frequently used skull base approaches. It is applicable to vascular and neoplastic lesions involving the anterior and middle fossa, orbit, orbital apex and cavernous sinus, paraclinoid and parasellar regions, and basilar apex.

- The subtemporal transzygomatic with petrous apex resection is utilized for lesions involving the petrous apex, upper clivus, posterior cavernous sinus, Meckel's cave, and the upper posterior fossa. Typical lesions resected via this approach include trigeminal schwannomas, petrous apex lesions such as cholesterol granulomas, cholesteatomas and chondrosarcomas, meningiomas involving the cavernous sinus and tentorium as well as smaller petroclival meningiomas, and vascular lesions in the region of the basilar artery.

- The preauricular subtemporal-infratemporal approach is an inferior extension of the subtemporal transzygomatic approach, and is better suited for lesions requiring lateral exposure of the mid and lower clivus, such as petroclival chondrosarcomas and cholesterol granulomas.

- Transpetrosal approaches provide an ideal ventral trajectory to the brainstem, particularly for posterior fossa tumors with significant extension above the tentorium, such as petroclival meningiomas.

- The extreme lateral transcondylar approach is well suited for lateral and ventral exposure of the caudal brainstem and upper cervical spinal cord at the level of the foramen magnum.

Skull base approaches were developed in response to a need to expose and maximally treat complex lesions at the base of the skull while minimizing retraction injury to normal neurological structures. As with any surgical approach, modules to the skull base are underpinned by a complete knowledge of the regional anatomy as well as appreciation of an often complex three-dimensional anatomy, supplemented by experience in cadaveric dissection. In many instances, a "skull base" approach implies an extension of classic cranial approaches, whereas in others, the approach is not implicit in typical neurosurgical training. Over the past 30 years, approaches in a circumferential fashion to the entire skull base have been developed and have been subjected to various classification schemes and terminologies. They may, however, be summarized as shown in Box 43.1.

Knowledge and expertise required in these approaches provide the fundamental knowledge for access to virtually every aspect of the base of the skull, and allow for selective implementation of part(s) of specific approaches when indicated by the respective pathology. This chapter provides an overview of approaches to the skull base, and for each module the relevant anatomy, indications, and technical principles with possible surgical pitfalls are discussed. This chapter is a summary that should not replace several extensive references on both the anatomy and surgery of the skull base,[1-5] in addition to practice in the cadaveric laboratory and instruction from experts in cranial base surgery.

PREOPERATIVE DECISION MAKING

Imaging

In most patients, magnetic resonance imaging (MRI) is performed preoperatively to determine the suspected diagnosis, extent of disease, and status of surrounding anatomical structures. Computed tomography (CT) with bone windows is often useful for visualizing the extent of bony skull base involvement by tumor. Major arterial involvement by tumor should prompt diagnostic cerebral angiography with possible test occlusion. For internal carotid artery (ICA) involvement, the contralateral ICA is injected, as are the vertebral arteries to assess collateral supply. For venous sinus involvement, the pattern of venous drainage and patency of venous structures needs to be determined, including any collateralization. If there is arterial involvement with poor collateral supply or a failed occlusion test, preoperative evaluation of donor vessels for likely bypass needs to be performed. Finally, especially for dura-based tumors, preoperative angiography can be performed to embolize feeding vessels.

Selection of Approach

The choice of approach is dependent on the goals of the operation (total versus subtotal resection), the areas of invasion, major arteries involved, and access to the tumor blood supply (tentorium, clinoid carotid, etc.). Previous treatments, including surgery and radiation therapy, can affect the choice of surgical approach from the perspective of wound healing and surgical scar from a certain trajectory. Finally, assistance from other specialties (neuro-otology, plastic surgery) may be required, as is the support of neurointensivists for the immediate postoperative care.

Anesthesia and Intraoperative Monitoring

For cranial base operations, the neuroanesthesiologist maintains blood pressure and oxygenation within normal limits. Arterial line, central venous catheter, and in some cases jugular bulb oximetry are utilized. Brain relaxation is achieved with modest hyperventilation, diuretics, and in some cases, lumbar cerebrospinal fluid (CSF) drainage or ventriculostomy. For prolonged skull base tumor operations, infusions of tranexamic or aminocaproic acid are run to promote hemostasis.

In most cases, transcranial cortically evoked motor evoked potentials (MEPs) and somatosensory evoked potentials (SSEPs) provide information regarding the integrity of the long tracts during the procedure. For this reason, total intravenous anesthetics are often required, consisting typically of propofol and remifentanil. When needed, electrodes are placed in the target muscles of cranial nerves V, VII, IX, X, XI, and XII for intraoperative mapping and assessment of functional continuity.

ANTERIOR SKULL BASE APPROACHES

Anterior skull base approaches are directed to the midline anterior skull base, including the planum sphenoidale, pituitary fossa, and entire rostrocaudal clivus. Typical lesions that arise in this area include planum sphenoidale and tuberculum sellae meningiomas, esthesioneuroblastomas, invasive pituitary adenomas, craniopharyngiomas, clival chordomas, and sinonasal tumors such as squamous cell carcinoma, adenocarcinoma, and adenoid cystic carcinoma.

Transsphenoidal Approach

The primary indication for the transsphenoidal approach is midline sellar and suprasellar lesions, and it is the workhorse approach for most pituitary adenomas. Several authors have reported endonasal techniques of resection of other lesions, such as tuberculum sellae meningiomas and craniopharyngiomas.[6] This approach is limited laterally by the internal carotid arteries; therefore, lesions extending laterally to this point

---

BOX 43.1	Classification of Skull Base Approaches

Anterior Approaches
  Transsphendoidal (open or transnasal endoscopic)
  Extended transbasal approach
  Transmaxillary and extended transmaxillary approach
  Transoral

Anterolateral Approaches
  Frontotemporal orbitozygomatic
  Subtemporal transzygomatic with petrous apex resection
  Preauricular subtemporal-infratemporal

Lateral and Posterolateral Approaches
  Transpetrosal
  Extreme lateral transcondylar

cannot be resected completely. Either the microscope or the endoscope (either as the primary or assistive device) may be used for visualization. Current transsphenoidal instruments remain limited in the ability to apply standard microsurgical techniques of sharp dissection for intradural lesions, and intraoperative complications such as arterial injury are difficult to repair for this reason. Selected intradural lesions, such as tuberculum sellae meningiomas and craniopharyngiomas, may be removed via an extended transsphenoidal approach, provided an adequate arachnoid plane is visualized on preoperative imaging, and the tumor is primarily midline with no lateral extension beyond the carotid arteries or optic nerves. The caveat of an extended approach is an increased risk of postoperative CSF rhinorrhea, given the inherent difficulty of primarily repairing dural or bony openings in a watertight fashion. Dural substitutes, fibrin glue, postoperative lumbar CSF diversion, and nasoseptal mucosal flaps are useful adjuncts to prevent CSF leakage.

The patient is positioned supine with the head elevated above the body to reduce venous pressure and turned slightly to the left for a right-handed surgeon, who operates from the patient's right side. Intraoperative neuronavigation is preferred over C-arm fluoroscopy to assist in localizing the anatomy, particularly the position of the cavernous carotid arteries. Either a sublabial or a purely endonasal approach may be used. For a sublabial approach, the upper gingival mucosa is infiltrated with local anesthetic and incised transversely. A periosteal elevator is used to expose the cartilaginous and then nasal septum, down to the vomer. The cartilaginous septum is fractured from the bony septum, exposing the anterior wall of the sphenoid sinus. The sinus is then opened using Kerrison rongeurs inserted into either sphenoid ostia, or using a microdrill or pituitary rongeurs. At this point, the pituitary fossa and optic and carotid prominences are identified. The bone overlying the pituitary fossa is removed, exposing the sellar dura. For more extensive lesions, bony resection is extended to incorporate the planum and tuberculum sellae.

For a purely endonasal approach, the nasal cavity is first treated with cocaine-soaked cottonoids. The nasal cavity is then entered, with or without the use of a nasal speculum, and the inferior and middle turbinates as well as the choana are used as landmarks until the ipsilateral sphenoid ostium is reached. The middle turbinate is either temporarily outfractured to increase the working space, or resected either with scissors or a microdébrider. If a mucosal flap is not harvested, a small incision is made in the septal mucosa at the junction of the bony and cartilaginous septum, which is outfractured. Submucosal dissection of the contralateral bony septum and vomer is performed, exposing the contralateral sphenoid ostium. Removal of the anterior wall of the sphenoid sinus proceeds as for the sublabial approach described earlier, and the remainder of the surgery proceeds in a similar fashion as well.

For closure, if no CSF leak is apparent, a small piece of Duragen or other dural substitute is tucked under the bony edges of the sellar opening and secured with fibrin glue. The closure may be augmented with Nasopore packing. In cases of intraoperative CSF leak, fat is harvested from the abdomen and placed within the sphenoid sinus to augment the closure, followed by placement of a lumbar drain in the operating room. Occasionally, a Foley catheter may be inflated to secure the nasal packing postoperatively. For larger osteodural

defects, bone substitute such as Medpor (Porex Technologies, Fairburn, GA) may be used, or bony septum harvested from the initial exposure, as well as a mucosal flap, which is rotated on its pedicle to provide vascularized tissue coverage.

Currently, our practice has been to use the endoscopic transsphenoidal approach for most pituitary tumors that appear to have reasonable dissection planes from surrounding neurovascular structures. More invasive tumors with irregular suprasellar involvement or with extensive clival involvement are removed with either a cranial or transmaxillary approach.

Extended Subfrontal Approach

This versatile approach is useful for intra- and extradural lesions of the anterior skull base, paranasal sinuses, as well as the sella, and midline clivus down to the foramen magnum. It is also better suited than the transmaxillary approach for intradural lesions in these areas. Furthermore, it can be adapted for more lateral exposure, including the cavernous sinus and frontotemporal area as needed. As such, it is useful for purely extradural lesions, such as for craniofacial resection of sinonasal malignancies, and for mixed intra- and extradural lesions such as esthesioneuroblastomas, chordomas, and chondrosarcomas (Fig. 43.1).

The patient is positioned supine with the head neutral and the body secured for tilting as required during the procedure for contralateral exposure. Brain relaxation and CSF diversion are facilitated by intraoperative placement of a lumbar drain. A bicoronal incision is performed behind the hairline and reflected anteriorly. A pericranial incision is made from behind the skin incision to maximize the available graft and the pericranium is reflected anteriorly as a separate layer to repair the frontal and ethmoid sinuses as well as the dura at the end of the surgery. Care is taken to preserve the supratrochlear and supraorbital bundles, which may emerge either from a notch or true foramen from above the orbital rim. In the case of a foramen, they are osteotomized with a small straight osteotome and outfractured with the scalp flap. The periorbita is dissected for a distance of approximately 3 cm to allow the orbitofrontal osteotomy to be sufficiently posterior, and the frontonasal suture is also exposed. At this point a low bifrontal craniotomy is performed, taking care not to lacerate the dura or the superior sagittal sinus. The subfrontal dura is mobilized off the orbital roofs bilaterally, sparing the cribriform plate region. A bilateral orbitofrontal osteotomy is then performed using the reciprocating saw, incorporating the orbital bar and through the nasoethmoidal complex in the midline, and circumventing the cribriform plate in order to spare the olfactory dura. The remaining cribriform plate is drilled until the olfactory dural sheath is exposed. Depending on the pathology and the preoperative state of the patient's olfaction, the olfactory nerves can be preserved during this approach, particularly for when the pathology is primarily intradural. Following an osteotomy circumventing the cribriform plate, the dura is opened, and the olfactory tract and sulcus are identified. Arachnoid dissection is used to mobilize the olfactory tracts off their sulci, allowing the basal frontal lobes to relax without transmitting traction on the olfactory tracts. In more extensive primarily extradural lesions, particularly if the patient is anosmic, the entire complex can then be suture-ligated and divided from within the nasal cavity, allowing the

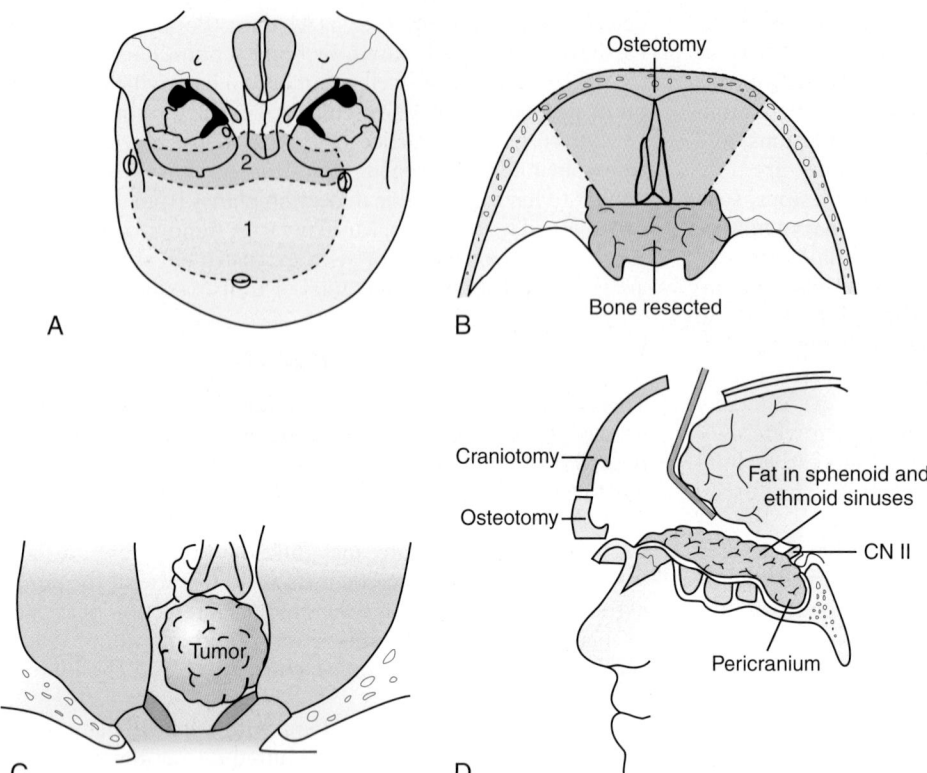

FIGURE 43.1 Extended subfrontal approach. **A,** Craniotomy and orbital osteotomy. **B,** Superior view of osteotomy and area of planum sphenoidale that is removed with a high-speed drill. **C,** View after planum drilled and optic nerves unroofed. Note cavernous carotid arteries bilaterally. **D,** Reconstruction of the anterior cranial base with autologous fat and pericranial grafts.

frontal lobes to relax superiorly. The anterior and posterior ethmoidal arteries are divided.

At this point the optic canals are unroofed using an irrigating microdrilled or ultrasonic curet under microscope visualization. The planum down to the tuberculum sellae is drilled as well, leading into the sphenoid sinus, the pituitary fossa, and the medial cavernous sinus walls bilaterally. Extradural exposure of the cavernous carotid artery is performed if required. Venous bleeding from the cavernous sinus is controlled by filling of the bleeding point with oxidized cellulose followed by fibrin glue, which is very efficacious. From the sphenoid sinus, the sella and clivus are exposed extradurally, and the entire clivus can be drilled if needed down to the foramen magnum, achieving an exposure in this area similar to that obtained with the extended maxillotomy approach. The lateral limits of this clival exposure include the cavernous sinuses, petrous apices, and hypoglossal canals.

Reconstruction involves suturing the pericranial flap to repair all dura defects in a watertight fashion. Mucosal tissue is resected from the exposed sinus and on the craniotomy flap, and the sinus opening and any dead space are obliterated with fat harvested from the abdomen and the pericranial flap as a second layer. The olfactory dural sheaths are also sutured closed in watertight fashion. For larger bony defects along the planum or clivus, structural support is achieved with either a split-thickness bone graft or titanium plate, with screw fixation when possible. The fronto-orbital osteotomy is reaffixed over the pericranial repair and the entire closure is injected with fibrin glue to promote a watertight seal. In occasional cases, a lumbar drain is placed for postoperative CSF diversion. For significant splaying of the eyes secondary to the tumor, a medial orbital canthopexy is performed.

Transmaxillary and Extended Transmaxillary Approaches

This approach is best suited for midline extradural lesions centered on the midportion of the clivus, such as chordomas and chondrosarcomas (Fig. 43.2). The exposure is also well suited for lesions extended superiorly up to the sella turcica. The lateral limits of this exposure include the cavernous sinus and carotid arteries, and the pterygoid space. Depending on the extent of disease, however, the lower clivus, anterior cervical spine, or lateral infratemporal space may be accessed via extended maxillotomy approaches.

We generally prefer a sublabial gingival incision for cosmesis; however, a Weber-Ferguson facial incision or a facial degloving approach may be employed as well. Laterally the maxilla is dissected in a subperiosteal fashion toward the pterygoid plates, as far as the infraorbital foramina and bundles bilaterally. Superiorly, the dissection is carried toward the frontonasal suture and, if required, the periorbital is dissected from the inferomedial orbital walls. A LeFort I osteotomy is planned. Perfect reapposition of the osteotomy is important to prevent malocclusion, hyperphonia, or dysphagia; therefore, plating systems are marked and drilled prior to the osteotomy. The osteotomy is then performed with a reciprocating saw and downfractured.

Following tumor resection, if there is a dural defect it is repaired with an abdominal fascial graft as well as fibrin glue, followed by abdominal fat and, for larger bony defects, the repair is reinforced with titanium mesh, which is secured with screws. The maxillary osteotomy is reapproximated with titanium plates and screws. A lumbar drain is placed for 3 to 5 days postoperatively to promote a watertight dural repair and prevent CSF fistula formation.

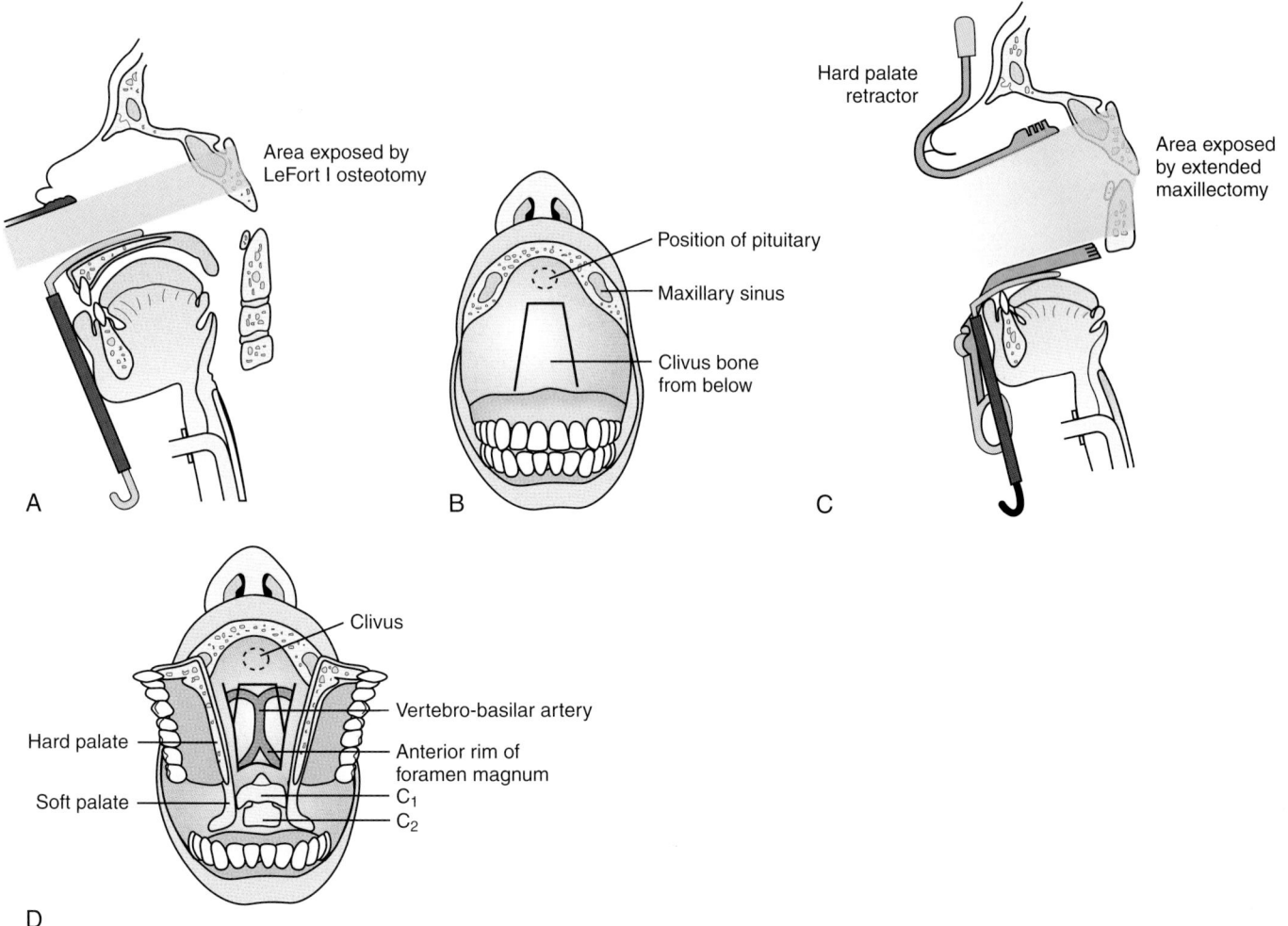

FIGURE 43.2 Transmaxillary and extended transmaxillary approaches. **A** and **B,** Schematic lateral and anterior views, respectively, of the transmaxillary approach, demonstrating the extent of exposure of the sella and mid and upper clivus. **C** and **D,** Exposure is extended caudally down to the upper cervical spine with the extended maxillotomy approach.

For greater exposure extending from the entire clivus to the craniocervical junction, a palatal split may be performed following the LeFort I maxillotomy osteotomy. A horizontal cut is again made similar to the preceding approach, followed by a midline osteotomy in the midline of the hard palate from between the central incisors anteriorly to the junction of the hard and soft palate posteriorly. The maxillary split is then outfractured and swung laterally. A self-retaining transpharyngeal retractor is placed to hold the palate and maxillotomy apart, exposing both the nasopharyngeal space and the longitudinal extent of the clivus. A midline incision in the pharyngeal mucosa along the clivus and between the prevertebral muscles is then performed, and the lesionectomy is performed. Meticulous preparation of the plating system prior to the osteotomies and perfect realignment during reconstruction prevents postoperative palatal dysfunction. Dural repair is performed in a similar manner as described earlier, including postoperative lumbar CSF drainage.

Complications of the maxillotomy and extended maxillotomy approaches include CSF fistula formation, injury to the dental rootlets, and problems related to poor palatal reconstruction such as oronasal fistula, dysphagia and dysphonia, and malocclusion. The majority of these complications are avoided by careful attention to the planning and reconstruction of both the dura and osteotomies intraoperatively, making these approaches long and intricate.

Transoral Approach

The transoral approach is ideally suited for smaller midline lesions of the lower clivus and upper cervical spine; however, more superior exposure is substantially limited by the palate, and more lateral exposure is also restricted compared to maxillectomy and extended subfrontal approaches. This approach is therefore mostly appropriate for degenerative, congenital, or rheumatic disorders of the ventral occipitocervical junction.

Preoperatively, the oral opening must be assessed to be sufficiently mobile and large enough to facilitate the approach. The patient is positioned supine with a variable amount of neck extension depending on the location and nature of the pathology. A self-retaining pharyngeal retractor is placed, and the soft palate is retracted superiorly using a nasally placed rubber cathether. A midline longitudinal incision is then performed along the posterior pharyngeal wall, and the longus

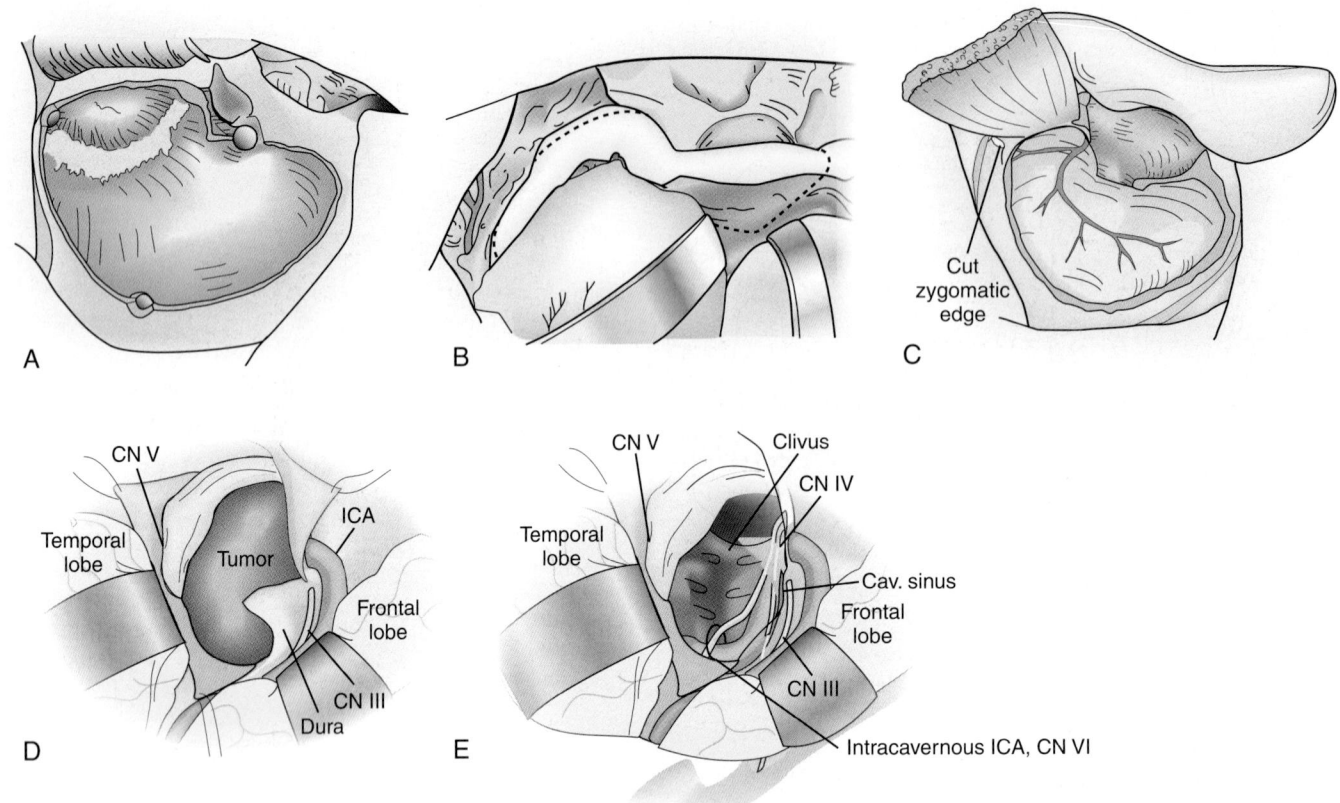

FIGURE 43.3 Frontotemporal orbitozygomatic approach. **A,** Initial exposure and frontotemporal craniotomy. **B,** Cuts for an orbitozygomatic osteotomy. **C,** Final appearance after removal of osteotomy. **D,** Cavernous sinus tumor exposed after splitting the sylvian fissure and the lateral cavernous sinus dura opened. **E,** Following removal of tumor, the upper clivus and cavernous sinus are exposed.

colli and capitis muscles are retracted laterally together with the pharyngeal mucosa. For more exposure superiorly, a midline incision through the soft palate can be performed down to the uvula, and the palate divided in the midline. The anterior tubercle of C1 and the C2 vertebrae are thus exposed. Superiorly, the lower portion of the bony septum may be partially resected to expand the clival exposure. Any compressive osteofibrotic pannus or tumor is resected. Dural penetration is repaired in a similar manner as described in the transmaxillary approach, and the pharyngeal mucosa and muscles as well as the palate are all closed in separate layers. Postoperatively, the patient is kept intubated until oropharyngeal swelling has subsided, and nasogastric tube feeding is continued until the mucosal repair has sufficiently healed.

ANTEROLATERAL SKULL BASE APPROACHES

Frontotemporal Orbitozygomatic Approach

The frontotemporal approach with variations of the orbitozygomatic extension is among the most frequently implemented skull base approaches. Vascular and neoplastic lesions involving the anterior and middle fossae, orbit, orbital apex and cavernous sinus, paraclinoid and parasellar regions, and

basilar apex are accessible with avoidance of brain retraction (Fig. 43.3).

The patient is positioned supine with the head turned 20 to 45 degrees depending on the lesion, with slight extension such that the malar eminence is the highest point. A pterional or modified bicoronal incision is performed behind the patient's hairline, from the skin crease anterior to the tragus of the ear, to the midline or just behind the midline frontal region. The scalp flap is reflected anteriorly, preserving the superficial temporal artery as well as the pericranium and temporalis muscle and fascia. Where the superficial fat pad is encountered laterally, an interfascial or subfascial dissection is required to preserve the frontotemporal branch of the facial nerve. If a supraorbital foramen is encountered, it is outfractured to preserve its neurovascular bundle. Once the orbit and zygomatic root are reached, the dissection is continued in a subperiosteal manner, exposing the entire course of the zygoma. The temporalis muscle is then mobilized, taking care to preserve and avoid cautery injury to the deep temporal fascia, from which the muscle derives its neurovascular supply. Once the muscle is retracted laterally, a frontotemporal craniotomy is done separately from the osteotomy. The medial extent of the craniotomy is usually the supraorbital notch, and laterally it extends to the floor of the middle fossa toward the inferior orbital fissure.

At this point the periorbita and subfrontal dura are carefully dissected off the orbital roof and walls. The temporalis and masseter muscles are sharply freed from the zygomatic arch, and approximately 1 cm of zygoma is exposed to allow placement of a titanium plate. The inferior orbital fissure is palpated from both the intraorbital and cranial compartments. Malleable brain ribbons are used to then protect the globe and frontal lobe, and a reciprocating saw is used to perform the orbitozygomatic osteotomy. The medial cut is made just lateral to the supraorbital notch, angled from lateral to medial and incorporating at least two thirds of the anteroposterior extent of the orbital roof, within safe distance of the superior orbital fissure posteriorly. Too shallow osteotomies after the remaining lesser wing of the sphenoid is rongeured are associated with persistent postoperative pulsatile enophthalmos and should thus be avoided. Laterally, a second cut is made from the inferior orbital fissure to the level of the zygomaticofacial foramen. This is connected to another lateral cut from the anterior, inferior edge of the zygoma, also directed toward the inferior orbital fissure. The final cut is performed obliquely from posterior to anterior at the root of the zygoma and its transition point with the squamosal temporal bone. The osteotomy is completed with gentle fracturing using a small osteotomy and mallet, and removed as a single piece, freeing any remaining attached periorbita or muscle.

Following the osteotomy, the lateral segment of the superior orbital fissure is unroofed, preferably under the operating microscope. The optic canal is then decompressed with a high-speed drill, and a clinoidectomy is performed. The anterior clinoid can be removed extradurally, either en bloc or piecemeal if it is more elongated. After drilling the attachment of the anterior clinoid to the optic canal, optic strut, and superior orbital fissure, it is gently fractured and dissected from its surrounding dural fold, avoiding pressure on the optic nerve. Bleeding from the cavernous sinus is controlled with oxidized cellulose and fibrin glue. The orbitomeningeal dural fold marks the lateral extent of the superior orbital fissure, and may be coagulated and divided to further mobilize the frontal and temporal dura, in order to facilitate the clinoidectomy. For lesions invading the clinoid or in the case of vascular lesions, the anterior clinoid may be removed intradurally. Occasionally, air cells within the clinoid may communicate with the sphenoid sinus, and care should be taken to occlude them with bone wax and occasionally with fibrin glue. Laterally, the superior orbital fissure dura can be incised and an interdural dissection performed, mobilizing the temporal lobe dura from the true dural covering of the superior orbital fissure, maxillary and mandibular branches, as well as the lateral wall of the cavernous sinus and cavernous carotid artery. Finally, for pathology involving the orbital apex, the periorbita is incised beyond the more lateral segment of the superior orbital fissure, which is relatively more devoid of neurovascular structures. The anulus of Zinn, if opened, is sutured after lesion removal.

Subtemporal Transzygomatic Approach with Petrous Apex Resection

This approach is well suited for lesions involving the petrous apex, upper clivus, posterior cavernous sinus and Meckel's cave, including limited extension of pathology into the upper posterior fossa. Typical lesions resected via this approach include trigeminal schwannomas; petrous apex lesions such as cholesterol granulomas, cholesteatomas, and chondrosarcomas;

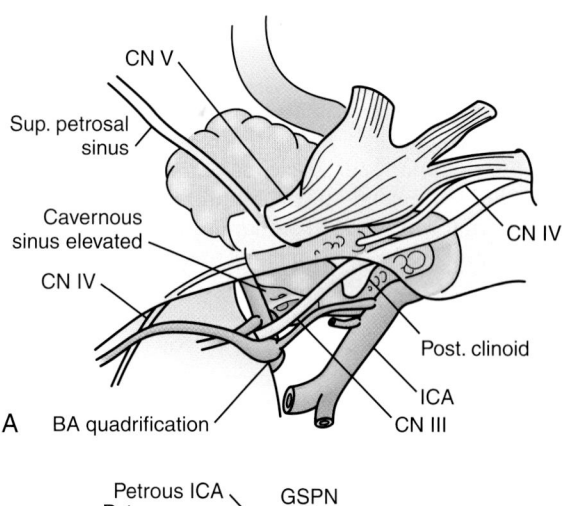

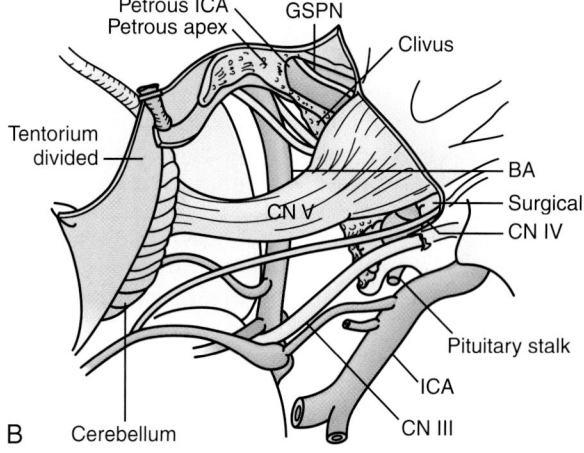

FIGURE 43.4 Subtemporal transzygomatic with petrous apex resection. **A,** Tumor lying in the cavernous sinus and extending to the level of the horizontal petrous internal carotid artery (ICA). **B,** Exposed anatomy after tumor resection with this approach. BA, basilar artery; GSPN, greater superficial petrosal nerve.

meningiomas involving the cavernous sinus and tentorium as well as smaller petroclival meningiomas; and vascular lesions in the region of the basilar apex (Fig. 43.4).

The patient is positioned supine with the head turned 70 degrees to the contralateral side with slight neck extension. Central venous pressures are checked to avoid excessive neck turn. A smaller reverse question mark incision is made in the frontotemporal region, with the inferior limb just anterior to the tragus of the ear. As with the orbitozygomatic approach, the pericranium is preserved for dural reconstruction, and an interfascial dissection of the superficial temporal fascia is performed. The temporalis muscle is mobilized together with its deep fascia to prevent muscle atrophy, and reflected laterally. The zygomatic arch is exposed. If the condylar fossa is included in the zygomatic osteotomy, the temporomandibular joint (TMJ) capsule is carefully dissected from the condylar fossa, and a heavy suture is used to retract the joint inferiorly. Care is taken not to transgress posteriorly into the external auditory canal, and a bony spine serves as a useful landmark between the condylar fossa and ear canal.

A predominantly temporal craniotomy is then performed, and additional temporal bone is craniectomized as necessary to remove obstructing bone from the floor of the middle fossa. The zygomatic osteotomy is then performed, from just lateral to the lateral wall of the orbit, preserving the zygomaticofacial nerve, to the root of the zygoma. If the condylar fossa is included in the osteotomy, the temporal dural vessels are first followed to the foramen spinosum, which is a medial safe landmark for the condylar cuts. An osteotomy that transgresses medial to the foramen spinosum puts the petrous internal artery at risk. Additional cuts are then made from the foramen spinosum medially to the posterior aspect of the condylar fossa and anterior zygomatic cut, laterally. Positioning titanium plates prior to the osteotomy ensures perfect realignment at the end of the surgery to prevent complications related to TMJ dysfunction.

Under microscope visualization, the middle meningeal artery at the foramen spinosum, greater superficial petrosal nerve (GSPN), mandibular portion of the trigeminal nerve and foramen ovale, and the arcuate eminence of the petrous bone are identified. The middle meningeal artery and vein are divided. The GSPN is occasionally divided depending on exposure requirements of the lesion. The dura overlying V2 and V3 is incised and mobilized until sufficient exposure of the petrous apex is achieved. Venous channels around the trigeminal branches are controlled with oxidized cellulose and fibrin glue. Coagulation is avoided to prevent facial numbness and deafferentation. The greater wing of the sphenoid is drilled to further expose the foramina rotundum and ovale, which permits greater mobilization of their respective trigeminal nerve branches. Care is taken not to accidentally expose the mucosa of the sphenoid sinus between V2 and V3.

The petrous segment of the internal carotid artery is situated directly underneath the GSPN and is first identified at the junction of the GSPN and V3 anteriorly. Immediately lateral is the eustachian tube. The carotid artery is then followed posteriorly as far as the posterior genu, and carefully unroofed using a combination of microdrills and small Kerrison rongeurs. At this point the internal carotid artery is gently dissected out of its canal and reflected inferolaterally. Care is taken when drilling posterior to the posterior genu of the ICA due to the vicinity of the cochlea and jugular bulb. Mobilization of the carotid artery facilitates greater exposure of the petrous apex as well as the clivus. An anterior petrosectomy is then performed using a high-speed drill or ultrasonic bone curet.

Once the petrosectomy is completed, the petroclival dura is opened. For lesions extending into the posterior cavernous sinus, it is necessary to split the fascicles of the trigeminal root from within Meckel's cave, reaching the posteromedial border of the cavernous sinus beyond the distal petrous ICA and petrolingual ligament. Alternatively, the trigeminal root may be mobilized superiorly. This is facilitated by opening the temporal lobe dura above the tentorium, and dividing the tentorium and superior petrosal sinus.[7]

Preauricular Subtemporal-Infratemporal Approach

The subtemporal-infratemporal approach is an inferior extension of the subtemporal transzygomatic approach, and is better suited for lesions requiring lateral exposure of the mid and lower clivus, such as petroclival chondrosarcomas and cholesterol granulomas (Fig. 43.5). In addition to an anterior petrosectomy, Glasscock's space is also drilled and the eustachian tube divided, allowing the petrous internal carotid artery to be completed mobilized anteriorly.

As in the subtemporal transzygomatic approach, the middle fossa floor contents are exposed. A zygomatic osteotomy incorporating the condylar fossa is performed as described earlier. The petrous carotid artery is identified, and skeletonization of its vertical segment is achieved once the tensor tympani muscle and eustachian tube are divided. This is performed by packing the anterior end with oxidized cellulose, and the posterior end with a small amount of fat. Each end is then suture-ligated. Toward the entrance to the carotid canal, the thick fibrocartilaginous ligament that surrounds the internal carotid artery must be sharply divided. The remaining bone medial to V3, and lateral to the petrous ICA, is removed, and the petrous and distal cervical internal carotid artery are completely mobilized. Care is taken to avoid the middle ear and facial nerve, which lie superior and posterior to the vertical portion of the petrous ICA, whereas the jugular bulb and lower cranial nerves are posterior and inferior. Inadvertent entry into the jugular bulb is controlled with gentle packing with Gelfoam and occasionally fibrin glue.

The primary concern and potential complication of the subtemporal transzygomatic and preauricular subtemporal infratemporal approaches is injury to the carotid artery. Frequent mapping with the micro-Doppler, neuronavigation, and preparation for possible exposure of the carotid artery in the neck are precautionary measures. CSF rhinorrhea is prevented with definitive closure of the eustachian tube. TMJ complications are avoided by perfect replacement of the condylar fossa osteotomy, which is facilitated by drilling guide holes for screw and plate placement prior to performing the osteotomy. Postoperative TMJ exercises also help maintain pain-free mobility. Other complications include temporal lobe retraction injury or damage to the vein of Labbé, minimized by use of a lumbar drain. Occasionally the dura is opened to drain CSF from the subarachnoid space and relax the temporal lobe.

LATERAL AND POSTEROLATERAL SKULL BASE APPROACHES

Transpetrosal Approaches: Retrolabyrinthine, Partial Labyrinthectomy/Petrous Apicectomy, Translabyrinthine, Transcochlear

These approaches provide a more ventral trajectory to the brainstem, particularly for posterior fossa tumors with significant extension above the tentorium, of which petroclival meningiomas are most typical (Fig. 43.6). Extensive chordomas or chondrosarcomas with brainstem compression from a significant intradural component may also require a transpetrosal approach, as it would allow tumor resection with direct visualization of critical intradural structures. Finally, vascular lesions of the mid and lower basilar arteries, including basilar apex aneurysms in the setting of a low bifurcation, and vertebrobasilar junction lesions may also be better suited with a trajectory from the presigmoid region.

Selection of the type of posterior transpetrosal approach depends on a number of factors, including the preoperative hearing status of the patient, the size and dominance of the

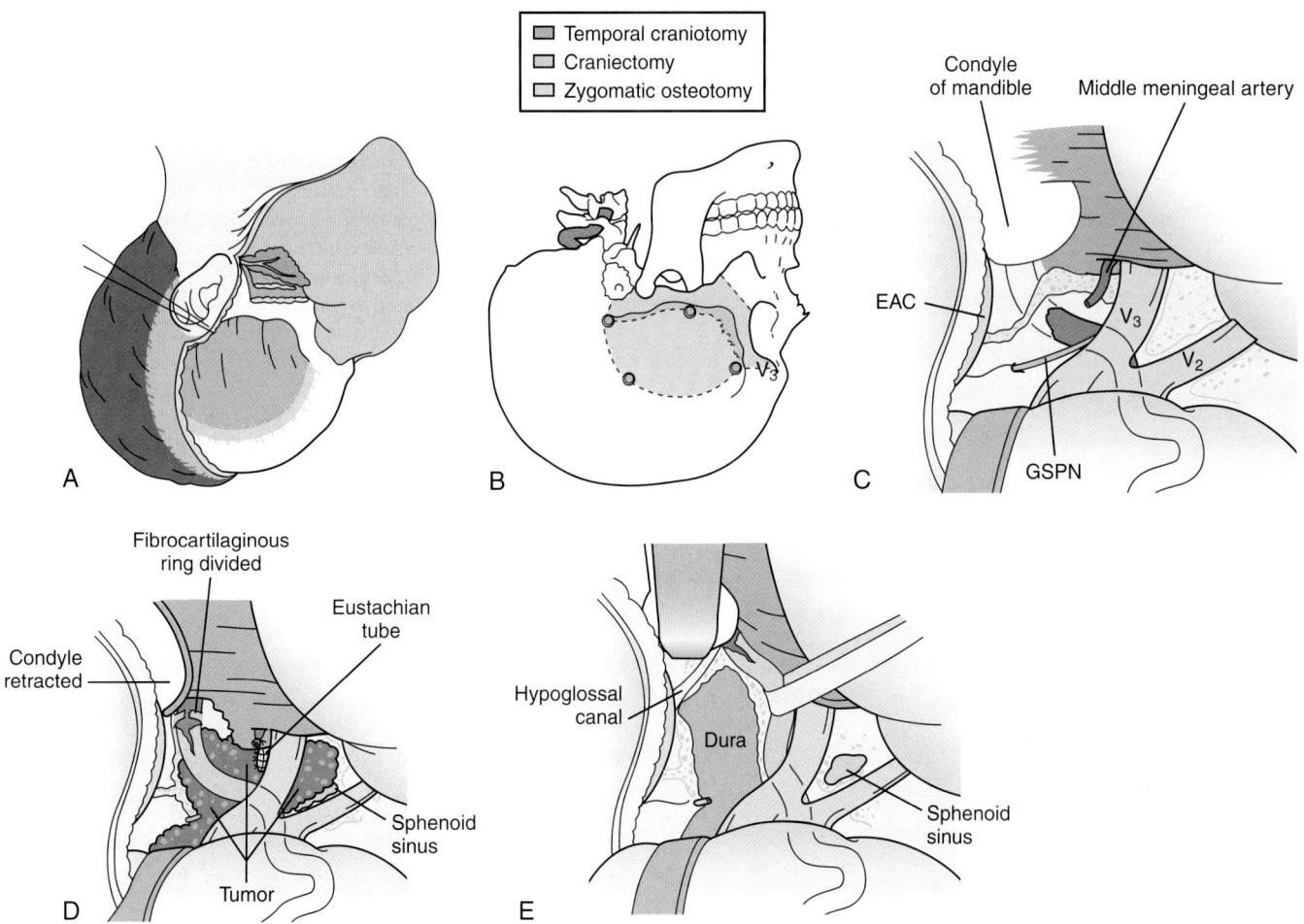

FIGURE 43.5 Preauricular subtemporal-infratemporal approach. **A,** Skin incision. **B,** Temporal craniotomy, area of craniectomy and zygomatic osteotomy. **C,** Temporal lobe dura has been elevated. The middle meningeal artery and greater superficial petrosal nerve (GSPN) have been divided, and the horizontal portion of the petrous internal carotid artery (ICA) has been partially exposed. **D,** The dura propria over the gasserian ganglion and between V2 and V3 has been incised, revealing tumor extending into Meckel's cave and the sphenoid sinus, respectively. **E,** Mobilization of the petrous ICA from the carotid canal after division of the fibrocartilaginous ring.

ipsilateral sigmoid sinus, and extent of disease. Hearing is preserved in the retrolabyrinthine and partial labyrinthectomy approaches. In the partial labyrinthectomy/petrous apicectomy (PLPA), the superior and posterior semicircular canals are waxed as they are opened, in order to prevent leakage of endolymph and hearing loss. Preoperative vascular imaging is carefully reviewed. In cases in which the sigmoid sinus is small, a retrolabyrinthine approach is usually sufficient to have an adequate opening of the presigmoid dura. Otherwise, a more extensive drilling of the labyrinth is performed.

The patient is positioned with the head 70 degrees to the contralateral side, either with the body supine or in a parkbench position, based on the patient's neck mobility. A U-shaped incision is performed from the retromastoid region superiorly to just above the superior temporal line and down toward the zygomatic root. The temporalis muscle and fascia are reflected forward and inferiorly. The posterior third of the temporalis muscle can be rotated inferiorly during reconstruction to provide vascularized tissue to seal the mastoidectomy. The suboccipital muscles are reflected away from the mastoid. A temporal craniotomy is performed superior to the transverse sinus dura and at least 2 cm posterior to the

transverse-sigmoid junction. For the mastoid, different methods of removal are available. A retrosigmoid craniotomy may be performed first, down to the posterior fossa dura, with or without incorporating the bone overlying the transverse sinus dura. Alternatively, a cosmetic osteotomy piece may be cut first, including the outer table of the mastoid and retromastoid bone, and forward to include the superficial bone of the zygomatic root, glenoid fossa, and ear canal. Care is taken not to injure the sigmoid sinus during either exposure.

Under the microscope, the entire mastoid is then decorticated with a larger bur on a microdrill, exposing the mastoid antrum air cells, and skeletonizing the sigmoid sinus dura and middle fossa floor, or tegmen tympani. The bone overlying the lateral semicircular canal is gradually appreciated proceeding through the mastoid air cells. Immediately anteroinferior to the lateral canal is the posterior genu of the facial nerve. The superior and posterior semicircular canals are then skeletonized. For a PLPA approach, the common crus is opened and filled with wax to prevent leakage of endolymph in an effort to preserve hearing, and the superior and posterior semicircular canals are then resected. This step increases the bony exposure of the petrous apex, which is then drilled. In certain cases,

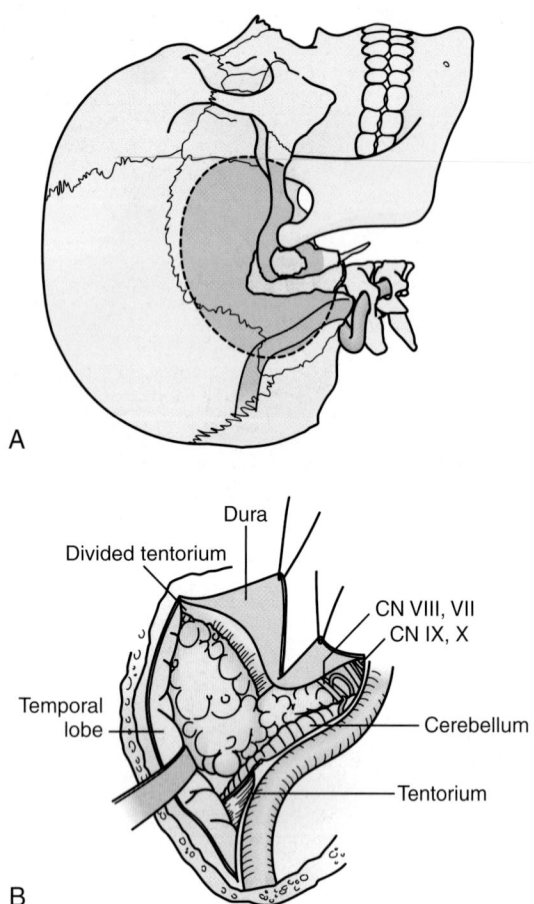

FIGURE 43.6 Posterior transpetrosal approach (partial labyrinthectomy/petrous apicectomy). **A,** Temporal and suboccipital craniotomy with zygomatic osteotomy and posterior transpetrosal approach. **B,** After opening the temporal and presigmoid dura, followed by dividing the superior petrosal sinus and tentorium, the entire craniocaudal extent of tumor above and below the tentorium is exposed.

dural opening and exposing the tentorium. The tentorium is divided, controlling any bleeding with bipolar coagulation or surgical clips. The medial edge of the tentorium is incised, avoiding both the trochlear nerve and superior cerebellar artery. The lateral brainstem is then exposed, from the midbrain to the upper medulla and cranial nerves III through IX, and tumor removal proceeds with minimal cerebellar and brainstem manipulation. If necessary, the dura overlying Meckel's cave can be opened, controlling any venous bleeding with oxidized cellulose and fibrin glue in the usual manner.

For reconstruction, the dura is closed either primarily or with pericranium or synthetic substitute. Any open air cells are carefully waxed off, and the closure is covered with fibrin glue. A pedicled temporalis musculofascial flap (usually the posterior third of the muscle) is rotated down to cover the defect. The bone is replaced, and if required, a titanium mesh is used to reconstruct the mastoid contour.

Complications of the transpetrosal approach include hearing loss or facial nerve weakness, if either the fallopian canal is injured from drill heat or contusion, or if the semicircular canals are injured or not properly waxed. CSF rhinorrhea and otorrhea through either the middle ear passages including the eustachian tube is also a risk. Injury to the trochlear nerve is possible if it is not properly visualized during incision of the tentorium. Also, particularly for left-sided approaches, retraction of the temporal lobe or injury to the vein of Labbé can result in seizures or dysphasia.

Extreme Lateral Approach

This approach is ideally suited for lateral and ventral exposure of the caudal brainstem and upper cervical spinal cord at the level of the foramen magnum. Several variations of this approach have been described, including the retrocondylar approach, the partial transcondylar approach, the transtubercular approach, true transcondylar approach, transjugular approach, and transfacetal approach (Fig. 43.7).[8] For the purpose of this chapter, only the partial and complete transcondylar approaches will be described. Generally, the partial transcondylar approach is sufficient for exposure of ventrally situated intradural lesions at the lower brainstem. A complete transcondylar approach is most frequently indicated for extradural lesions that involve the condyle and lower clivus, such as chordomas.

Preoperative CT or digital subtracted angiography and venography are important to assess the caliber of the ipsilateral and contralateral vertebral arteries, as well as the dominant side of venous drainage of the brain. The course of the vertebral artery is studied as well. In cases of extensive condylar invasion by tumor, a staged surgery must be anticipated and consists of tumor removal followed by an instrumented occipitocervical fusion. Neuronavigation is also useful for guiding resection of tumor within the base of the skull, such as in chordomas.

The patient is placed in a full lateral position with the contralateral arm hung over the edge of the operating table with a sling or arm rest. The head is secured with pin fixation and rotated slightly toward the surgeon, neck flexed and apex dropped slightly toward the floor. Different incisions have been described for this approach. We prefer a C-shaped incision beginning superiorly in the posterior temporal region above the ear down in a curvilinear fashion behind the mastoid

the retrosigmoid bone may be removed as well, allowing the sigmoid sinus to be retracted gently if necessary, and allowing portions of tumor to be resected through a retrosigmoid dural opening. In a translabyrinthine approach, the entire labyrinth is removed to the level of the vestibule, and the bone overlying the internal auditory canal is unroofed. Rarely is a total petrosectomy required for adequate brainstem exposure. In this approach, the entire labyrinth is removed, and the facial nerve is completely skeletonized from the cerebellopontine angle cistern to the fibrous ring at the stylomastoid foramen, allowing it to be mobilized anteriorly after division of the GSPN, albeit with an attendant, at least temporary, postoperative facial weakness. In a manner similar to the preauricular subtemporal-infratemporal approach described previously, the petrous ICA is unroofed and displaced anteriorly. The remaining temporal bone is drilled away, protecting the jugular bulb and lower cranial nerves anteriorly.

The temporal dura parallel to the middle fossa floor and the presigmoid dura parallel to the sigmoid sinus and above the jugular bulb are then opened separately. Care is taken when incising the temporal dura posteriorly to identify and preserve the vein of Labbé. The dura overlying the superior petrosal sinus is suture-ligated and incised, completing the

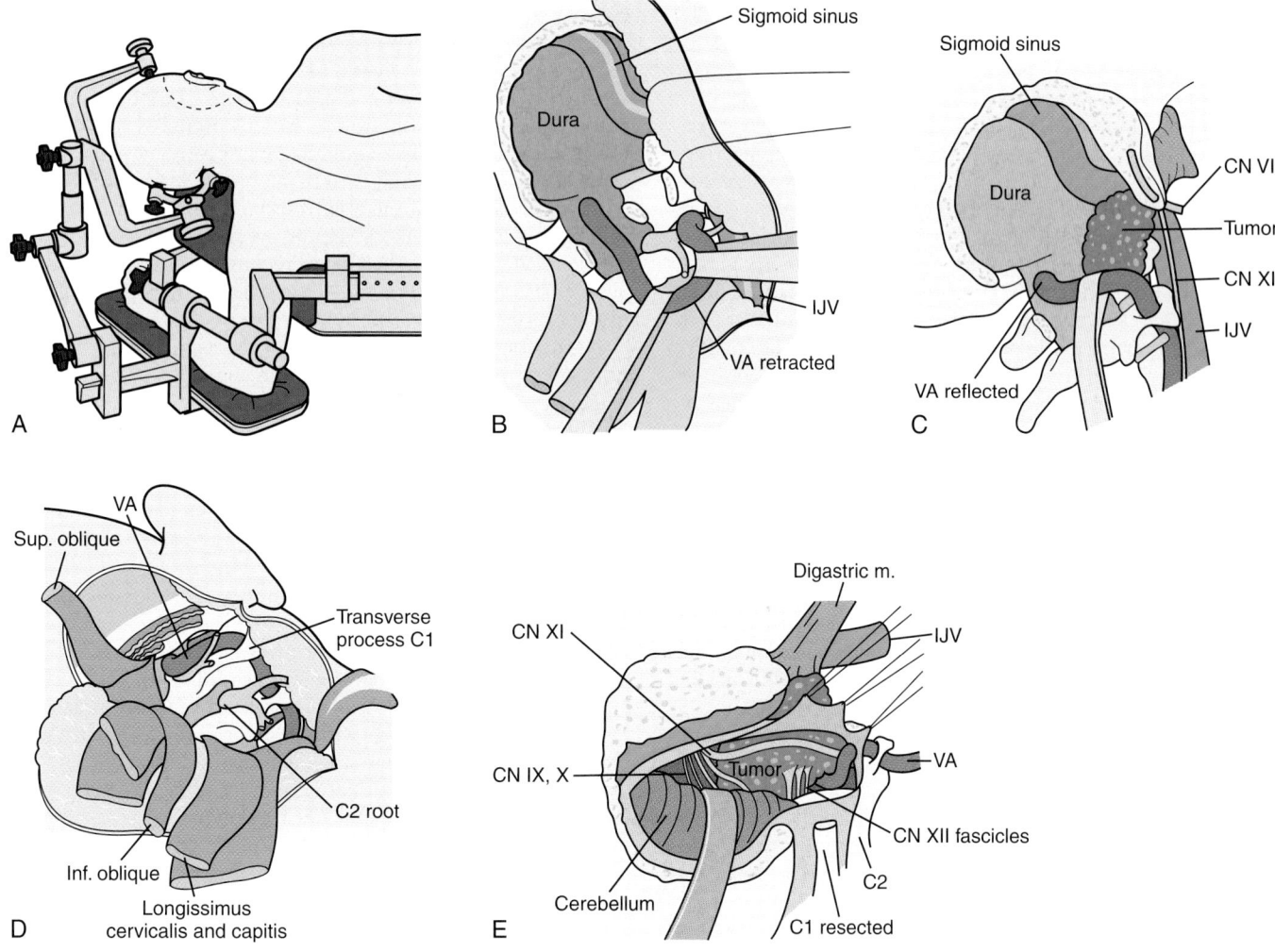

FIGURE 43.7 Extreme lateral partial/complete transcondylar approach. **A,** Patient positioning and incision for a complete transcondylar extreme lateral approach. For cases in which a transcondylar approach is combined with a transpetrosal approach, then the patient is positioned supine with the head turned 45 degrees. **B,** A retrosigmoid craniotomy, including the lateral aspect of the foramen magnum, and C1 laminectomy have been performed. The vertebral artery (VA) has been mobilized medially after unroofing the C1 foramen. The occipital condyle is now accessible and is resected as needed for adequate tumor exposure. **C,** Tumor exposed after drilling the occipital condyle. **D,** Muscular attachments on the transverse process of C1 have been mobilized, illustrating the relationship between the VA, C2 dorsal root, C1 lamina, and occipital condyle. **E,** Extreme lateral partial transcondylar approach for a hypoglossal schwannoma. Intradural exposure shows the relationship of the tumor to the lower cranial nerve and VA. IJV, internal jugular vein.

and toward the posterior border of the sternocleidomastoid muscle. A skin flap is raised, above the muscle but incising the fascial attachment of the sternocleidomastoid such that it is mobilized forward together with this superficial layer, exposing the entire proximal attachment of the splenius capitis muscle. The remaining muscles are elevated in layers. The next muscle is the splenius capitis, which is incised off the mastoid process. At this point the occipital artery is identified in the underlying fascia, superficial to the semispinalis capsis and either below or running through the longissimus capitis. These two muscles are then elevated, exposing the muscles forming the suboccipital triangle, namely, the superior and inferior obliques and rectus capitis muscles.

At this point the key step is to safely identify the vertebral artery, typically the V3 segment first. The microscope is used at this point. Immediately, inferior to the mastoid tip is the transverse process of C1, which is easily palpated.

The attachments of the superior and inferior oblique muscles as well as the levator scapula are identified. The micro-Doppler is used to identify the V3 vertebral artery above the C1 arch and within the suboccipital triangle. The oblique muscles are disconnected from the transverse process of C1 and reflected medially. Subperiosteal dissection on the superior border of the posterior arch of C1 usually exposes the vertebral artery outside its surrounding venous plexus. Venous bleeding is controlled with careful bipolar coagulation and injection with fibrin glue. A fairly consistent muscular branch of the vertebral artery is encountered emerging from the suboccipital triangle; it is coagulated or clipped and divided. The dissection proceeds medially until the vertebral artery curves toward its dural penetration. The fascial tissue medial to this is incised down to the foramen magnum dura. The C1 foramen transversarium is unroofed with a high-speed drill and small Kerrison rongeurs, and the lateral third of the C1 posterior arch is removed. The V3 vertebral artery is now rotated medially, away from the occipital condyle and occipitoatlantal joint.

A small retrosigmoid craniotomy is performed. The thick bone of the lateral foramen magnum is drilled down and the foramen magnum is exposed. A low mastoidectomy is performed posterior to the facial nerve to blue line the postero-inferior edge of the sigmoid sinus and gain further access to the occipital condyle. Bleeding from the condylar vein is controlled with oxidized cellulose and bone wax. Fibrin glue is avoided because of the vicinity to the jugular bulb and possible embolization. The condylar vein serves as a reference point for the hypoglossal canal, which lies immediately inferior to it.

A high-speed microdrill or ultrasonic curet is used to remove the posterior third of the occipital condyle and lateral mass of C1 including the jugular tubercle, unroofing the posterior border of the hypoglossal canal. The hypoglossal canal lies approximately 8 mm deep to the posterior border of the condyle and has a posteromedial to anterolateral trajectory. Adequate bony removal for intradural exposure of intradural tumors is achieved when there is an approximately 1-cm cuff of dura lateral to the entrance of the vertebral artery into the dura mater. The dura is then opened, encircling the vertebral artery. The dentate ligament and C1 rootlets are divided, and tumor removal proceeds with minimal brainstem and lower cranial nerve manipulation.

For reconstruction, pericranium is harvested from the upper incision and a duraplasty is performed. Watertight closure is occasionally difficult and fibrin glue is used to augment the repair. Autologous fat is used to eliminate deadspace, particularly for complete transcondylar approaches. In the setting of complete condyle removal, an occipitocervical fusion is planned, typically around 1 week following tumor resection.

The principal risk of this approach is injury to the vertebral artery. This is avoided by understanding the course of the vertebral artery on preoperative imaging, and by taking the suboccipital muscles down individually and under the microscope. Inadvertent entry into the jugular bulb during bony drilling is possible, and is controlled with oxidized cellulose or Gelfoam. Postoperative occipital pain is prevented by preserving the C2 root under the C1 lamina. Watertight dural closure is difficult, particularly at the cuff of the dura around the vertebral artery, making CSF leak a possible complication.

COMPLICATIONS OF SKULL BASE APPROACHES

Complications related to skull base approaches may be broadly classified as errors in selection of operative approach, patient selection, preoperative planning, and technical intraoperative complications. Surgical complications may be nerve-related, cosmetic, and wound-related, including CSF leakage and vascular complications. The majority of these complications may be avoided by mastery of the surgical anatomy, preoperative planning, including appropriate structural and vascular imaging, intraoperative monitoring, and meticulous attention to detail at every stage of the operation.

Vascular complications are likely the most feared complications of skull base approaches. They may be related to tumor infiltration into circle of Willis vessels, technical error, and inadequate preparation (neuronavigation, micro-Doppler, prepping of graft harvest, etc.). Large tumors related to the base of skull vessels should be evaluated preoperatively with cerebral angiography to assess for collateral circulation and test-occlusion when indicated. For frank tumor invasion into vessels, arterial and venous graft sources should be investigated with ultrasound, and the patient prepared accordingly for bypass. For tumors invading major venous sinuses, the cerebral venous drainage pattern should be assessed. Intraoperatively, occlusion of the involved sinus with temporary clips followed by assessment of venous pressures with manometry can help identify whether sinus reconstruction is necessary. Sinus reconstruction can be performed either primarily or using a fascial graft.

Cosmetic issues have great importance even in larger skull base operations,[9] as they may influence the patient's self-perception and overall satisfaction with care. Keeping cranial incisions behind the hairline or within natural skin creases, preservation of scalp neurovasculature, careful mobilization of musculofascial layers with avoidance of cautery, careful replacement of bone flaps and osteotomy pieces with titanium mesh or bone substitute to restore normal cranial contours, and avoidance of cranial nerve and sensorimotor deficits all contribute to optimizing the cosmetic outcome of the operation.

CSF leakage can occur in almost all cranial base operations where there is entry into the intradural space, as the basal CSF cisterns are usually in communication with the various approaches. Whenever possible, complete watertight closure of the dural opening, with or without a pericranial flap and supplemented by fibrin glue, is the ideal method of avoiding CSF leakage. For anterior skull base approaches, reconstruction of larger bony defects with split-thickness bone or Medpor, and a pedicled pericranial flap in addition to primary dural closure, are necessary adjuncts. Lumbar CSF drainage may also be used. For the lateral and posterior skull base approaches, careful waxing of air cells, suture repair of the eustachian tube if opened, and a pedicled temporalis flap to occlude all opened air cells in the middle ear (e.g., during a posterior petrosectomy approach) have been helpful in our experience in reducing the incidence of CSF otorrhea and rhinorrhea.

The various osteotomies used in skull base approaches must be carefully planned because complications can occur. Orbitozygomatic osteotomies must include at least two thirds of the orbital roof to prevent pulsatile enophthalmos. For inadequate osteotomies or if there is tumor involvement, the orbital wall may require reconstruction with Medpor or split-thickness bone graft. Following replacement of the orbital osteotomy, careful palpation of the orbital space is required to ensure the periorbita is not tethered in the apposition, in order to prevent postoperative restriction of eye movements. Imperfect reposition of the osteotomy can lead to cosmetic defects as well as temporomandibular and palatal complications, and can be prevented by drilling out pilot holes for plate fixation prior to performing the osteotomy.

CONCLUSIONS

Current skull base approaches allow circumferential access to all areas of the skull base; however, sound understanding of the relevant anatomy, fellowship training supplemented by time in the cadaver laboratory, strict attention to detail for all stages of the operation to prevent complications, and ability to treat complications should they occur are all requisites of ensuring a successful outcome.

SELECTED KEY REFERENCES

Cappabianca P, Cavallo LM, Esposito F, et al. Extended endoscopic endonasal approach to the midline skull base: the evolving role of transsphenoidal surgery. *Adv Tech Stand Neurosurg.* 2008;33:151-199.

Rhoton AL. *Rhoton's Cranial Anatomy and Surgical Approaches.* Philadelphia: Lippincott Williams & Wilkins; 2007.

Sekhar L, Fessler R. *Atlas of Neurosurgical Techniques: Brain.* Stuttgart: Thieme; 2006.

Sekhar L, De Oliveira E. *Cranial Microsurgery: Approaches and Techniques.* Stuttgart: Thieme; 1999.

Salas E, Sekhar LN, Ziyal IM, et al. Variations of the extreme-lateral craniocervical approach: anatomical study and clinical analysis of 69 patients. *J Neurosurg.* 1999;90(Suppl 2): 206-219.

Please go to expertconsult.com to view the complete list of references.

CHAPTER 44

Endoscopic Approaches to Skull Base Lesions, Ventricular Tumors, and Cysts

Nancy McLaughlin, Daniel M. Prevedello, Daniel Kelly, Ricardo L. Carrau, Amin B. Kassam, Scott D. Wait, Charles Teo, Aneela Darbar, Sheri K. Palejwala

CLINICAL PEARLS

- Become knowledgeable about the equipment and practice on a cadaver or under the guidance of an experienced neuroendoscopist.

- Orientation and anatomy of the cranial skull base and ventricles are everything! Absolutely know where you are, what you are looking at, and your orientation at all times. In this chapter, the most important neurovascular structures related to the cranial skull base approaches are defined. If you are not sure, abort the procedure.

- Use the endoscope for its advantages and don't fight its disadvantages. Increase your use of angled scopes and increase the size of your visualized field.

- Become comfortable with the endoscopic management of hydrocephalus prior to using the endoscope for neuro-oncological applications.

- Endoscopic ventricular applications are not "all or nothing." Despite being an experienced endoscopist, some lesions are more safely dealt with from a microscopic surgical approach. In these cases use an endoscope-assisted approach to your advantage.

- The transsellar approach is limited to exposing the sella turcica. Because the sella is the epicenter at the crossroads of the sagittal and coronal planes, the transsellar approach is the starting point for most of the expanded endonasal surgical modules.

- All lateral expanded approaches to the middle and posterior fossae require a transpterygoid approach on the ipsilateral side. The vidian nerve is a key anatomical landmark that must be localized and followed back to the anterior genu of the internal carotid artery (ICA) as its petrous portion turns up to form the vertical paraclival ICA.

During the past two decades there has been increased use of neuroendoscopic surgery. Detailed anatomical studies have improved the understanding of endoscopic ventricular and skull base anatomy. This, along with the use of intraoperative image guidance, has enabled surgeons to approach deeply seated lesions through minimally invasive routes. The feasibility and the safety of such extended approaches have been well established in numerous anatomical and clinical studies.[1-11] The endoscope can be used to definitively treat hydrocephalus, to biopsy tumors that are best treated with radiation or chemotherapy, and to confirm adequate resection of tumors when the microscopic view is partially obstructed. On the other hand, the expanded endonasal approach (EEA) can provide access to the anterior, middle, and posterior cranial fossae and is recognized as an important tool in the armamentarium of skull base surgeons.[12,13]

Many surgical advantages have been attributed to EEA in comparison with traditional transcranial approaches including access to deeply seated lesions, a more direct midline exposure, decreased brain parenchyma injury, absent neurovascular

structure manipulation, prompt decompression of visual apparatus when indicated, and early tumor devascularization.[4-6,14] Similar oncological results to those obtained with traditional open approaches have been documented for sinonasal, sellar, and skull base lesions.[1,5,8,9,14-16] From the patient's perspective, decreased surgery time, decreased length of stay, increased patient comfort and lack of external incision are significant advantages to the EEA.[11]

This chapter will address (1) the instrumentation, complication avoidance, and management of intraventricular tumor and intraventricular cyst, and (2) the surgical technique of EEA in a stepwise fashion beginning with the sella and expanding along the sagittal and coronal planes in a set of defined anatomical modules.

HISTORY

Six major advancements in the use of neuroendoscopy have occurred. A century ago, L'Espinasse, a urologist, attempted to perform a choroid plexus coagulation to treat hydrocephalus.[17,18] In the early twentieth century Dandy and Mixter attempted an endoscopic third ventriculostomy (ETV).[19] In the 1970s technological advances allowed the production of flexible fiberscopes as well as rigid endoscopes. Throughout the late 1980s and 1990s ETV and decompartmentalization of the ventricular system because popularized and allowed many neurosurgeons to become familiar with the tools of neuroendoscopy. This familiarity resulted in the fifth and sixth advances. The use of the endoscope for extra-axial lesions was popularized by pioneers such as Perneczky, who championed the keyhole approach to aneurysms. The final and most recent wave of endoscopic enthusiasm has been its application to anterior, middle, and posterior skull base surgery, especially transsellar and transpterygoid approaches. The use of the endoscope for intraventricular neuro-oncological applications including lesion removal, tumor biopsy, and cyst management is also becoming more common, so much so that endoscopic colloid cyst surgery has results that are similar to those achieved with microsurgery and with a better risk profile.[20-24]

EQUIPMENT

Equipment available for neuroendoscopy is constantly evolving. There are basically two types of endoscopes. The rigid endoscope is a fixed-length and fixed-geometry instrument that usually has several viewing angles available (0, 30, and 70 degrees to the long axis of the endoscope). The light source, camera, and shaft of the scope are all in-line and allow for easier orientation when working in the ventricular system and skull base.

The flexible fiberscope is maneuverable in three directions with relatively simple controls. The advantage of the flexible scope is that its geometry is not fixed and it may be fashioned to proceed along a curved trajectory such as a trans–foramen of Monro approach to the posterior third ventricle to biopsy a pineal tumor. This allows a single trajectory to treat hydrocephalus via ETV and sample the tumor; the flexible scope may also be used within the working port of the rigid scope in a "scope-in-scope" technique.[25] The main drawbacks of the flexible scope over the rigid scope are the poorer optical resolution and the risk that the surgeon may inadvertently withdraw the scope in the "bent" configuration with devastating repercussions.

Rigid endoscope-holding arms are available from several manufacturers and allow the scope to be secured rigidly in place. This addresses surgeon fatigue and dependence upon an assistant to hold the endoscope. These rigid arms are generally adjustable in all three planes. However, once set, they all have some degree of "play" or "float" for which the surgeon will need to account when positioning.

Frameless neuronavigation is helpful to guide insertion of the sheath, especially in the absence of ventriculomegaly; for localizing lesions for biopsy under an intact ependyma;[26] and to localize important neurovascular structures during skull base surgery. In the instance that the surgeon becomes disoriented or confused by distorted anatomy, stereotaxis can assist in reorientation.

Recently, several potentially important advances in instrumentation available to the endoscopic surgeon have been

reported. The length of time required to aspirate a tumor using a "biopsy after biopsy" approach may be shortened by the use of traditional ultrasonic aspiration with a specialized handpiece down the working port of the endoscope. It has been used successfully on pituitary tumors, intraventricular clot removal, and craniopharyngioma cyst wall removal.[27] Endoneurosonography has been used to supply additional information about the relationship of the tip of the probe and structures orthogonal to it.[28] Water-jet dissection has been reported to be a useful adjunct in the safe perforation of a craniopharyngioma cyst wall, septum pellucidum, or floor of the third ventricle.[29] This may help to decrease the risk of hemorrhage associated with blindly inserting an instrument through a thin structure such as the third ventricle floor.

ENDOSCOPIC PRINCIPLES

Visualization is the key to neurosurgery. If you can't see it, you can't safely operate on it. The endoscope offers all the visualization advantages of the microscope and allows these through a minimally invasive approach. This avoids unnecessary morbidity from brain retraction and large openings. Additionally, the magnification and illumination offered are superior to those offered by the microscope. Despite the visualization advantages afforded by the endoscope, the microscope still provides excellent visualization in a straight line and allows more precise, bimanual, three-dimensional (3D) microsurgical dissection. Rather than competing methods, each method of visualization should be thought of as complementary to the other and both should be mastered to give the patient the best possible surgical treatment. The recent addition of a 3D endoscope has added yet another tool to the armamentarium of a neuroendoscopist.

There are two principal forms of endoscopy: coaxial and extra-axial. Coaxial endoscopic approaches, or "pure" endoscopy, are those in which all components of the endoscopic system (lighting, camera, working channels, irrigant channels, and instruments) are all parallel and enclosed in a single sheath. The instruments are introduced through working channels and are aimed by redirecting the endoscope. The impact to the surrounding brain from removing and reintroducing instruments is minimized because the entire working and visualization area is within the endoscopic sheath. Most intraventricular endoscopic procedures are performed in a coaxial manner.[30]

Extra-axial endoscopic approaches are those where the endoscope is the mode of visualization and the instruments are introduced alongside the endoscope separately. This generally applies to anterior, middle, and posterior skull base operations and will be discussed further later in this chapter.

During "endoscope-assisted" applications, the microscope is the primary mode of visualization and the endoscope is used to improve visualization, especially around corners and behind "unmovable" structures.

During "endoscope-controlled" surgery, the endoscope is the sole mode of visualization and surgery is performed using the same techniques and instrumentation as microsurgery, with the addition of curved instruments and suctions that allow the surgeon to operate around corners. In these forms of endoscopy a substantial learning curve exists because of peripheral distortion, the view angle when using non–0 degree endoscopes, and the close proximity of the surgical field to the tip of the endoscope. Once this is overcome, these same "problems" may be used to the surgeon's advantage, resulting in better outcomes.

ENDOSCOPIC INTRAVENTRICULAR SURGICAL TECHNIQUES

Cysts

Colloid Cysts

Colloid cysts of the third ventricle are non-neoplastic masses that typically arise from the roof of the third ventricle. They can occlude the foramen of Monro, causing headache, hydrocephalus, memory disturbances, and sudden death. Colloid cysts have a variable consistency, from mucinous, which are easily aspirated, to a hard, cheesy consistency. Cysts 1 cm or larger and those causing symptoms or hydrocephalus are generally recommended for removal. Other options including shunting and stereotactic drainage are possible but not recommended because of their poor durability. Microsurgical removal is effective but more invasive than the endoscopic approach.[20,23,31] Therefore, endoscopic removal is recommended in the majority of cases.[32-35] However, when imaging predicts the consistency of the cyst contents to be hard and cheesy, then the cyst is better removed microsurgically with bimanual dissection. Additionally, cysts larger than 2 cm may compromise or adhere to the fornix and may be more safely removed using microsurgical bimanual dissection.

A single bur hole, approximately 8 cm behind the nasion and 5 to 7 cm lateral to the midline in the nondominant hemisphere (careful not to injure the caudate head), is sufficient for removal.[24,36] Image guidance helps with the initial ventricular entry. A peel-away sheath is optional. The landmarks of the colloid cyst and foramen of Monro are identified and the overlying choroid plexus is coagulated, avoiding the fornix. The cyst is coagulated and opened and the contents are aspirated. A pediatric endotracheal suction catheter with the end cut to 45 degrees is particularly effective if the consistency is favorable. One can twist the catheter and use the cut end as a dissector to "morselize" the contents of the cyst prior to aspiration. If the contents are too dense, forceps may be required to empty the cyst contents. The wall of the cyst is then dissected free of the roof of the third ventricle with generous coagulation. Generally the cyst wall is not densely attached to the fornix and can be removed completely. However, in the case that the wall is so adherent to the internal cerebral veins or the fornix that it cannot be separated using either sharp or blunt dissection it may be prudent to leave a thin "carpet." Under these circumstances, the recurrence rate appears to be low.[21,37,38] Symptomatic relief of obstructive hydrocephalus is generally obtained, though mild ventriculomegaly often persists.[37]

Neurocysticercotic Cysts

Neurocysticercosis (NCC) is the neurological manifestation of the parasite *Taenia solium* and is commonly contracted in underdeveloped countries by hand-to-mouth contamination from unclean water or food. NCC most often presents with seizures but may also present with sudden hydrocephalus due to intraventricular cysts blocking normal cerebrospinal fluid (CSF) pathways. There is a growing body of literature suggesting that neuroendoscopic removal of cysts results in improved patient outcomes and lessens or avoids altogether the need for shunting.[39-41] Recently, pediatric data regarding neuroendoscopic cyst evacuation has been reported. The shunting rate is lower (22%) in the neuroendoscopic group than in the traditional medical treatment group (70%) and the Karnofsky performance scale was higher in the endoscopic group (90.0% vs. 85.5%, $p = 0.003$).[39] Two other studies show complete resolution of cysts and no need for shunting with minimal transient morbidity.[40,41]

The procedure is performed either through a single approach with a flexible endoscope or through as many approaches as needed with the rigid endoscope. A disposable plastic sheath is mandatory in order to maintain the transcortical path because sometimes the entire metal sheath needs to be removed with the grabbing forceps in order to maintain the integrity of the cyst wall. If the cyst wall is ruptured and contents are spilled into the ventricle then postoperative steroids will alleviate some of the symptoms of sterile meningitis. Preoperative imaging will determine what CSF spaces need to be explored and the safest way to explore each. When using the rigid endoscope, if the ventricle is not drained, firm irrigation can mobilize ipsilateral cysts into view that can be secured with a forceps and removed.

Miscellaneous Cysts

Other cysts, such as arachnoid cysts, occur within the ventricles. Often fenestration of these cysts to normal CSF spaces is desirable. The ease of working in a fluid-filled space makes the endoscope ideal for fenestration. The anatomy is often distorted and the arachnoid surface is often thick and somewhat opaque. Stereotaxis is very helpful in these cases to know what is behind an opaque membrane prior to fenestration. Blunt perforation should be avoided at all costs as pushing against these flimsy membranes may damage the important neurovascular structures that lie behind. Enlarging interhemispheric cysts can be fenestrated directly to the ventricle or via cystocisternoventricular fenestration.[42] Fourth ventricular cysts obstructing outflow are also amenable to fenestration.[43]

Tumors

Pure Endoscopic Approaches

Endoscopic applications for intraventricular tumors include tumor biopsy, tumor resection, and management of tumor-associated hydrocephalus.[44,45] In general, neuroendoscopy for tumors is a step up in technical difficulty from the endoscopic management of hydrocephalus. The ideal conditions for endoscopic resection of an intraventricular tumor are that it should be small, avascular or with relatively low vascularity, partially or totally cystic, and located in enlarged ventricles. Hydrocephalus creates an ideal working space. However, a normal ventricle is adequate to gain access to a tumor and biopsy it and, for smaller tumors, to resect it safely.[46] A recent report even suggests that in experienced hands, operating in a normal sized ventricle yields the same success/complication rate as operating in large ventricles.[47]

One key to tumor resection within the ventricles is to select a proper working trajectory. Because brain must be transited in order to reach the ventricles, a single working angle that does not require excessive "windshield wiping" of the endoscope should be chosen.

A proper working trajectory is one that accomplishes the following:

1. Enters the ventricle with some normal ventricle between the entry point and the mass
2. Allows access to the blood supply, if vascular
3. Allows access to the point of attachment to the ventricular wall or choroid plexus
4. Does not originate in or traverse eloquent structures
5. Allows management of associated hydrocephalus or trapped CSF spaces

Having some normal ventricle and CSF between the entry point into the ventricle and the tumor allows better visualization of the tumor margin and allows visualized normal structures to aid in orientation. Access to the blood supply and point of attachment may turn a tedious piecemeal tumor resection into a disconnection and en bloc removal. As mentioned earlier, the use of transendoscope ultrasonic aspirators may speed up tumor removal if en bloc removal is not possible.[27]

Image guidance is particularly valuable for approach planning and execution, and is worthwhile even if it is only used for this step of the procedure.[48-50] Third ventricle tumor resections are particularly dependent on proper approach angle since often the endoscope must traverse the foramen of Monro, putting the fornix, at the anterior border of the foramen, at some risk. Image guidance allows the surgeon to use trajectory views to draw a line from the anterior border of the tumor to the anteriormost border of the foramen of Monro. This line can then be extended to the surface to choose the appropriate entry point and angle. The fornix will not tolerate anterior "windshield wiping" movements of the endoscope while its tip lies in the third ventricle. Posterior movements are tolerated much better; however, the venous structures coalescing at the posterior margin of the foramen of Monro also limit scope excursion. Fortunately, many intraventricular tumors are associated with ventriculomegaly and an enlarged foramen of Monro that allows for larger excursions of the endoscope.

It is worth noting that the major source of complications in intraventricular endoscopic approaches for brain tumors is disorientation. Complications can be minimized through appropriate entry point and trajectory choice, prior orientation of the camera, detailed examination of the equipment and video image prior to entry into the brain, a thorough knowledge of normal ventricular anatomy, and a constant self-inquiry into where the endoscope is, what all structures seen represent, and how the endoscope's intrinsic optical distortion is affecting the scene. The use of frameless stereotaxis helps reduce disorientation.

Certain tumors are more amenable than others for endoscopic removal.[51] When working within the fluid-filled ventricle, bleeding may be difficult to control and obscures the operative field. Therefore, tumors of low vascularity are preferred for purely endoscopic removal. Examples are subependymomas,

ependymomas, the subependymal giant cell astrocytomas associated with tuberous sclerosis, selected neurocytomas, exophytic gliomas (primarily pilocytic or low grade), and hypothalamic hamartomas.[52] Some vascular tumors such as choroid plexus and pedunculated tumors can also be approached endoscopically, because the blood supply is often well defined and easy to coagulate and divide.

The technique of endoscopic tumor removal requires a high level of familiarity with the endoscope and its use, as it represents one of the most technically complex skills in neuroendoscopy. A peel-away sheath is recommended. Its purpose is to avoid buildup of irrigant and increased intracranial pressure and to allow the endoscope to be removed and replaced with ease, especially when the forceps and endoscope are removed together with pieces of tumor that are too large to come up the working channel. The advantage of not using the peel-away sheath is to slightly reduce the size of the track through the brain and to keep some pressure in the ventricle to reduce venous bleeding. The surgeon must communicate effectively with the anesthesiologist during the case. Increased intracranial pressures will generally be manifest by a Cushing's response and will be noted by the anesthesiologist. In this case, one should allow egress of fluid so that the hemodynamic values return to normal.

Piecemeal tumor removal can be very tedious and also lead to tumor spread if fragments are released that float free in the spinal fluid. Removing larger portions of tumor and drawing them out with the endoscope is more efficient and leads to higher quality specimens.

Prior to placing the peel-away sheath, tapping of the ventricle with a brain needle or a ventriculostomy catheter is recommended. The peel-away sheath can then be placed down the tract using image guidance. The bluntness sometimes also results in the tip deflecting from the ependyma. This problem is overcome when a smaller bore, sharper instrument violates the ependyma.

Most tumors are approached by taking initial biopsy specimens with cup forceps, minimizing coagulation to maintain the quality of the tissue for analysis. Any vessels on the surface of the tumor are then coagulated. Electrocautery (especially monopolar) is capable of generating high CSF temperatures and must be used with caution. Irrigation with warmed lactated Ringer's solution or a spinal fluid substitute solution is used to dissipate this heat.[53] Normal saline is not used because it lacks electrolytes, is acidic, alters the electrolyte balance in the brain, and leads to postoperative confusion.[54] Again, appropriate egress of irrigant will avoid a dangerous rise in intracranial pressure.

Once bleeding is controlled, cautery, blunt dissection, and bites with the forceps or scissors are used to separate the tumor from the normal tissue. The best tumors for neuroendoscopy have a distinct margin and can be gently retracted away from the surrounding tissue. Ideally, a perimeter can be created, the tumor can be isolated as a mass, and it can be removed in one or more large pieces. If the tumor is soft, multiple methods of tumor aspiration are possible. A stainless steel suction cannula or the previously mentioned pediatric endotracheal suction catheter placed down the working channel can be used to morselize and aspirate tumor.[47] Shortened endovascular catheters can also be used. They have the advantage of a stiffer, thinner wall that can be shaped. The catheter allows a larger inner lumen diameter for more efficient aspiration of appropriate consistency tumors.[55] The gelatinous contents of colloid cysts and some other cystic tumors respond particularly well to this technique. As mentioned earlier, the length of time required to aspirate a tumor using a "biopsy after biopsy" approach may be shortened by the use of ultrasonic aspiration with a specialized handpiece down the working port of the endoscope.[27] Regardless of the removal technique, every attempt should be made to avoid dispersion of tumor remnants throughout the ventricles.

After satisfactory tumor removal, attention is paid to hemostasis, usually by irrigation alone. The ventricle is inspected for residual tumor and blood clots, particularly over the foramen of Monro or the aqueduct of Sylvius, where obstruction may occur. The decision about whether or not to leave an external ventricular drain is controversial, and should depend primarily on the risk of obstruction. In cases in which the working trajectory allows it, addition of a septum pellucidotomy or third ventriculostomy may decrease the chance of postoperative symptomatic hydrocephalus.

In some cases tumor biopsy rather than removal may be the goal. CNS lymphoma is often periventricular and amenable to endoscopic biopsy for diagnosis. "Nonoperative" gliomas may also be appropriate for this biopsy method. Stereotactic guidance is helpful in locating the tumor. However, identification of the tumor tissue through overlying normal ependyma may be problematic. Recently, the use of 5-aminolevulinic acid (5-ALA) fluorescence to identify and biopsy a midbrain glioma through an intact ependymal layer has been reported.[56]

Complications of tumor biopsy and removal include intraventricular hemorrhage, neurological deficit, tension pneumocephalus, hydrocephalus, and basilar artery injury.[57-59] Tension pneumocephalus results from air being exchanged for CSF during the procedure. To avoid this, the ventricles should be refilled with lactated Ringer's solution. If large quantities of air remain, 100% oxygen administered via facemask will help with dissolution.[60]

Peratta and associates reported an 8.8% complication rate for neuroendoscopic (nonhydrocephalus) procedures in pediatric patients.[61] Hemorrhagic complications of tumor biopsy are reported at 3.5% per patient and 2.4% per procedure.[62] To minimize the incidence of hemorrhagic complications one should never cut or pull any structure without being able to visualize the structure completely.

Hemorrhage is often the rate-limiting step during endoscopic tumor removal. There are several techniques used to control hemorrhage with the endoscope. The first maneuver is to patiently irrigate. Most bleeding in the ventricle will stop with irrigation alone. The second maneuver is to attempt to coagulate the bleeding source, but only if it can be directly visualized. Visualization may be improved by draining the CSF and working in an air-filled ventricle. A third maneuver is to gently tamponade the bleeding point using the endoscope itself or an instrument placed down the working channel. This maneuver is appropriate for larger veins that one is attempting to preserve such as the thalamostriate vein. An external ventricular drain can be left if necessary or as a "safety valve" in the case that tumor or hemorrhage occludes the foramen or aqueduct. The question of whether to leave a drain is not convincingly answered in the literature. We do not routinely leave drains after endoscopic procedures.

Endoscope-Assisted Microsurgical Approaches

Many intraventricular tumors cannot be completely removed through a purely endoscopic approach, but endoscopy still maintains an important role. The concept of "endoscope-assisted" refers to the traditional microsurgical procedure that uses an endoscope as an adjunct either through the same opening or through a separate bur hole for better overall visualization. The endoscope allows the surgeon to look around corners and to visualize structures that are not visible by microscopic imaging alone, thus expanding the operating field. Utilizing angled endoscopes can maximize the area of the ventricle visualized. Charalampaki and colleagues reported that endoscope-assisted microsurgery has been useful in 35 patients with traditional microsurgical approaches to the ventricular system done through keyhole craniotomies. Thirty-one out of 35 patients had no morbidity at 6 months and 3 of the patients with 6-month morbidity had preexisting Perinaud's syndrome that persisted. Seventy-eight percent of patients had complete tumor resections. One procedure was aborted due to hemorrhage and was repeated successfully with gross total removal 2 days later.[63] Another example of endoscope-assisted microsurgery is the transventricular management of craniopharyngioma including gross total removal of intraventricular components, fenestration of cysts as a stand-alone procedure for symptomatic control, and cyst fenestration followed by collapse and subsequent craniotomy for definitive removal of the solid component.[64]

Additionally, diagnostic ventriculoscopy should be performed whenever an endoscope is placed in the ventricle for any reason. With a 30-degree endoscope a wide inspection can often be performed by rotation of the endoscope without any additional brain retraction. For example, ventriculoscopy can identify ependymal tumor deposits that cannot be seen on magnetic resonance imaging (MRI), can confirm whether the septum pellucidum is patent or perforated, and whether the opening of the aqueduct is obstructed or open. In patients undergoing shunting, ventriculoscopy can be performed before the catheter is placed, or through the endoscope with a fiberscope. In most cases, however, hydrocephalus associated with tumors can be managed with the endoscope and is, in fact, preferable.

ENDOSCOPIC ENDONASAL SKULL BASE SURGICAL TECHNIQUE

Endoscopic endonasal approaches have been organized in modules based on anatomical corridors (Box 44.1).[12,13,65,66] The modular approach to learning the various EEAs is based entirely on a thorough understanding of the ventral skull base anatomy as viewed with the endoscope. This is a key principle to avoid complications.

Transsellar Approach[12] (Figs. 44.1 to 44.3)

Exposure

In itself, the transsellar approach is not considered an expanded approach because it is limited to exposing the sella turcica. It is appropriate for the removal of pituitary

Sagittal Plane
Transfrontal
Transcribriform
Transtuberculum/transplanum
Transsellar
Transclival
  Superior third
    Transsellar (intradural)
    Subsellar (extradural)
  Middle third
  Inferior third
  Panclival (combination of three thirds)
Transodontoid and foramen magnum/craniovertebral approach

Coronal Plane
Anterior coronal plane
  Supraorbital
  Transorbital
Middle coronal plane
  Inferior cavernous sinus/quadrangular space
  Superior cavernous sinus
  Infratemporal/temporal fossa approach
Posterior coronal plane
  Medial petrous apex
  Infrapetrous
  Transcondylar/supracondylar
  Foramen jugular

adenomas as well as other intrasellar entities such as Rathke's cleft cysts and craniopharyngiomas with minimal suprasellar extension. However, because the sella is the epicenter at the crossroads of the sagittal and coronal planes, it is the starting point for most of the expanded surgical modules. The sphenoidotomies are widened by exposing the sphenoid lateral recesses and the posterior ethmoidal cells. The planum-tuberculum junction and bilateral lateral opticocarotid recesses (OCR) should be visualized. The floor of the sphenoid is drilled back to the level of the clivus, giving a greater caudorostral trajectory into the suprasellar space. Intrasphenoidal septations are to be drilled down carefully because they may lead directly toward the vertical canal of the internal carotid artery (ICA).[67] The sphenoid mucosa is removed in the areas the bone will be drilled. Once the posterior wall of the sphenoid sinus is completely exposed the following structures are viewed: the sellar prominence in the center, the ventral aspect of the tuberculum sellae covering the superior intercavernous sinus (SIS) above, the clival recess below. The carotid prominences are seen laterally and the optic canals superolaterally and between them the medial OCR and the lateral OCR. Bone removal over the sellar face should extend laterally beyond the medial portions of the cavernous sinus (CS) and expose both superior and inferior intercavernous sinuses (see Fig. 44.2). The medial OCR does not need to be opened unless the lesion has suprasellar and lateral extensions toward the opticocarotid cistern. The most important structures related to this module are the CS, which contains both ICAs and limits the area laterally.

Tumor Removal

The dura mater can be opened in a cruciform fashion or in a half circle with the inferior flap reflected caudally. The tumor resection uses the same techniques as those used in microneurosurgery.

For extremely large tumors, an internal debulking using two suctions is preferred because it enables controlled removal of tumor with less trauma to the normal pituitary, stalk, and cavernous sinus contents. Once the posterolateral tumor dissection is complete (from CS to CS laterally and posteriorly toward the clivus-dorsum junction), the superior part of the dura is opened to pursue superolateral dissection. Grasping and pulling should be avoided. Final inspection is undertaken in a clockwise fashion. Residual gland is often found plastered to the undersurface of the diaphragma sella. If the diaphragma does not descend concentrically, residual tumor in the suprasellar space should be suspected and reviewed. If suprasellar dissection is necessary, the tuberculum sellae must be removed.

In cases of circumscribed pituitary adenomas, particularly for the functional ones, an extracapsular dissection is preferred. In these situations, care must be taken not to enter the pituitary pseudocapsule. A plane between the capsule and the normal gland is encountered and followed all around until the tumor is completely disconnected and removed en bloc.

In the advent of cavernous sinus extension, the medial cavernous wall can be explored from within the sella. Because the carotid siphon is usually displaced anterolaterally, the tumor can be followed inside the medial compartment of the CS safely.

Expanded Endonasal Approaches— Sagittal Plane

The sagittal plane modules extend from the frontal sinus to the second cervical vertebra, enabling access through the crista galli, planum, tuberculum, dorsum sella, clivus, and odontoid process (see Box 44.1).

Transtuberculum/Transplanum Approach[12]

Exposure

The transtuberculum/transplanum approach is indicated for lesions involving both the posterior aspect of the anterior skull base and the suprasellar region. Bony exposure builds on that obtained with the transsellar approach. It is extended rostrally by completing wide bilateral posterior ethmoidectomies. Ethmoidal septations are drilled flush with the anterior cranial base. Anteriorly, bony resection should not continue anterior to the posterior ethmoidal arteries (PEAs) and the rostral margin of the nasal septum is left attached to the skull base. These precautions prevent injury to the olfactory neuroepithelium, preserving olfaction. The planum sphenoidale is drilled eggshell thin. The bone over the sella and the tuberculum sellae over the SIS are removed completely, exposing the dura under the medial OCR (see Fig. 44.2). This enables access to the suprasellar extensions of tumors in the prechiasmatic cisterns with optic nerve and carotid control. The paraclinoid carotid canals can also be opened to allow lateral retraction of soft tissue at that level. Arterial feeders arising from the

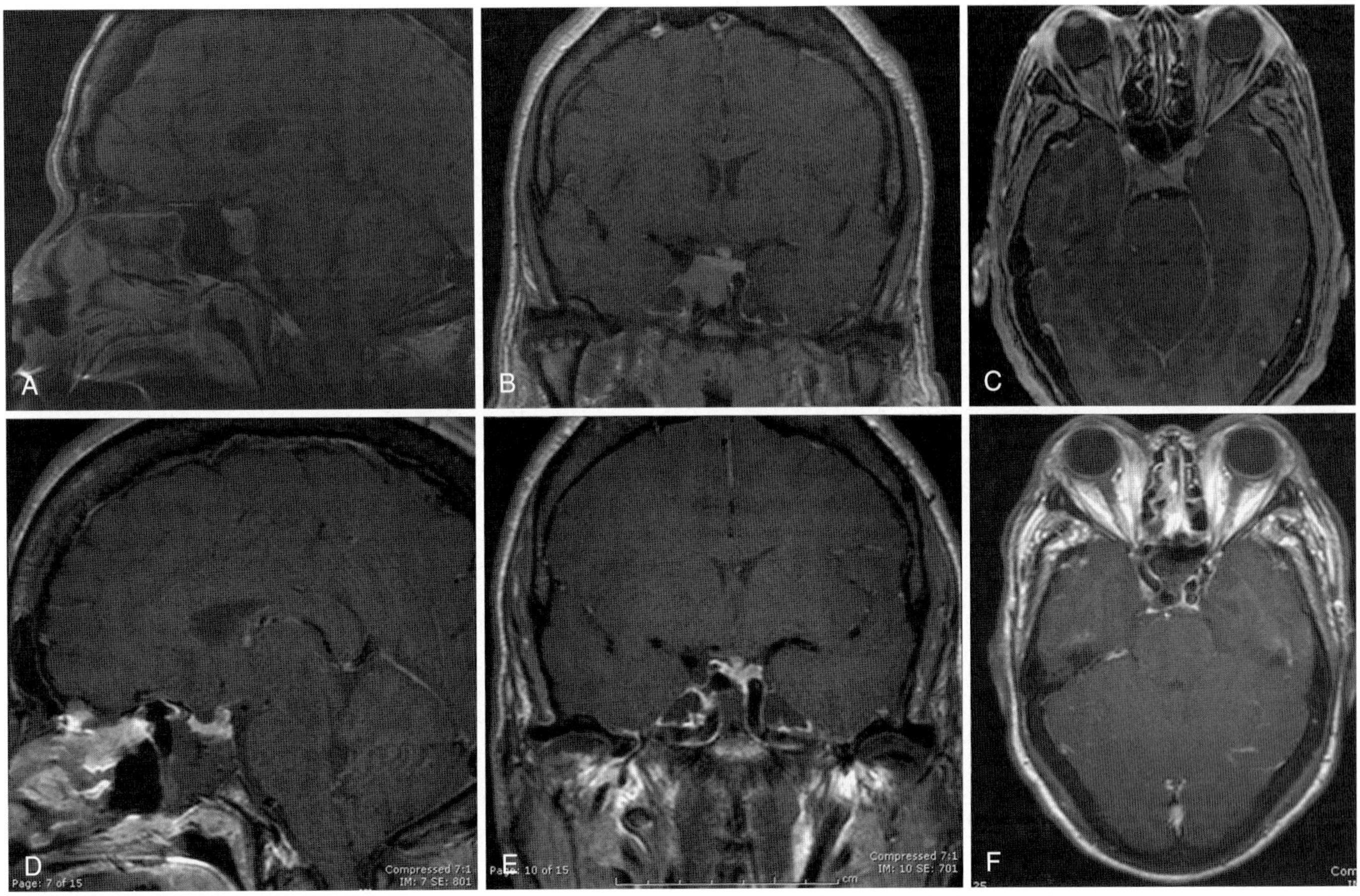

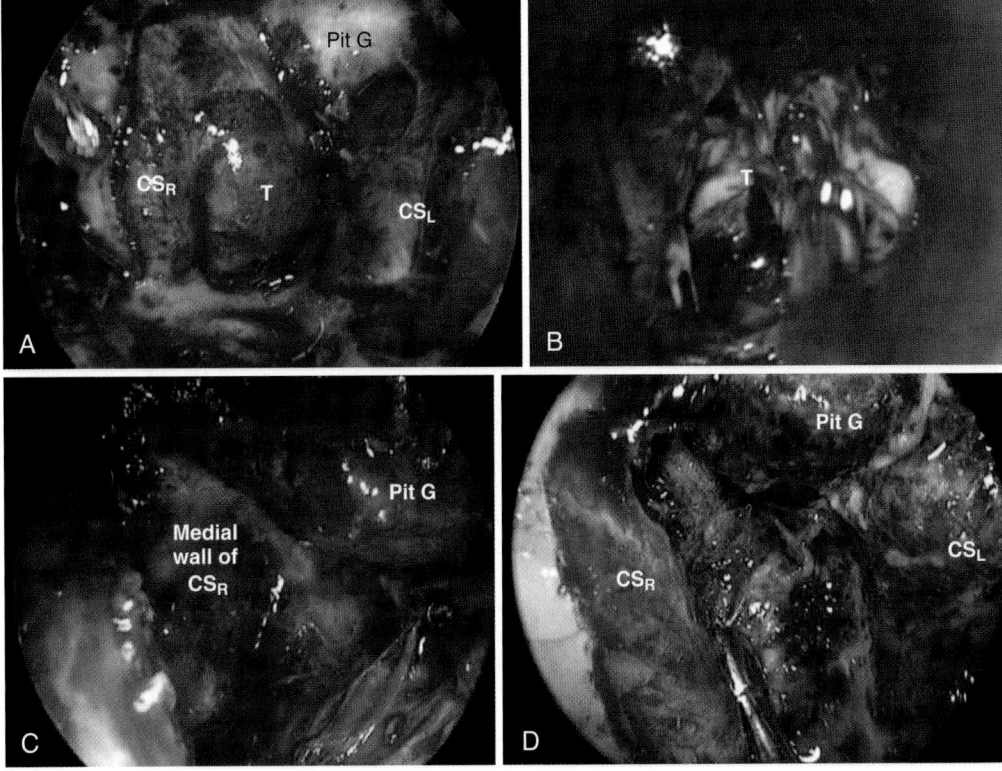

FIGURE 44.1 This 57-year-old female patient presented with characteristic features of acromegaly. Preoperative magnetic resonance imaging (MRI): sagittal (**A**), coronal (**B**), and axial (**C**) views in T1-weighted imaging (WI) postgadolinium scan. Postoperative MRI following transsphenoidal removal of the functional pituitary adenoma: sagittal (**D**), coronal (**E**), and axial (**F**) views in T1-WI postgadolinium scan.

FIGURE 44.2 Intraoperative findings. **A,** View of the tumor prominence between both cavernous sinuses. The pituitary gland is pushed superiorly and toward the left. **B,** Removal of the pituitary macroadenoma. **C,** Careful inspection underneath the internal carotid artery (ICA). **D,** Complete visualization of the medial wall of the right cavernous sinus for evidence of residual tumor or abnormal dura. CS, cavernous sinus; Pit G, pituitary gland; T, tumor.

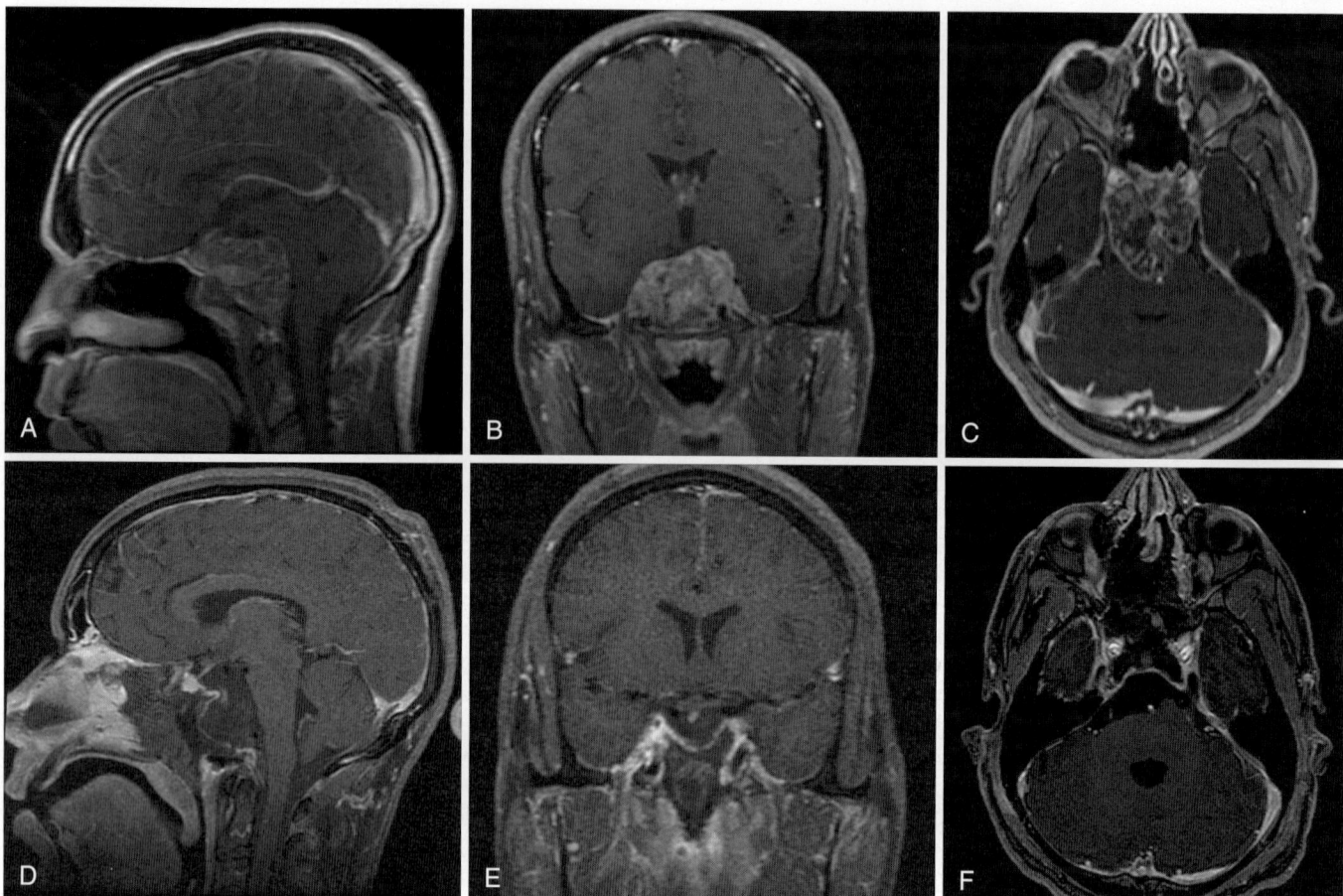

FIGURE 44.3 This 27-year-old man presented with a right side sixth cranial nerve palsy. Magnetic resonance imaging (MRI) performed 3 months after partial resection of a clival chordoma through an endoscopic endonasal approach: sagittal (**A**), coronal (**B**), and axial (**C**) views in T1-weighted imaging (WI) postgadolinium scan. MRI following tumor resection through an expanded endonasal panclival approach: sagittal (**D**), coronal (**E**), and axial (**F**) views in T1-WI postgadolinium scan.

distal portion of the paraclinoid carotid artery at the level of the medial OCR as well as from the PEAs can be hypertrophic in meningiomas and should be identified and coagulated. The SIS is not transected in pure suprasellar tumors such as tuberculum sellae meningiomas. Craniopharyngiomas can occupy sellar and suprasellar compartments and, in these cases, the SIS is coagulated and transected to allow exposure of both locations.

The most important vital structures related to this module are the optic nerves, which mark the lateral limits of the transplanum approach, ICAs, and the anterior cerebral arteries (A1, Huebner's, anterior communicating, and perforators).

Intradural Dissection and Tumor Removal

For extracranial tumors, extracapsular dissection is performed through the parachiasmatic cisterns. Identifying the paraclinoid carotid artery as it emerges intradurally at the level of the medial OCR is essential. When the ICA is followed, it leads to the optic nerves, which are located slightly superiorly. Appropriate debulking is performed in order to further perform extracapsular dissection. At this point the tumor's capsule should be thinned sufficiently and easily pliable, allowing sharp dissection of arachnoid bands in the parachiasmatic cisterns. When working along the superior

surface of the tumor, care should be brought to the anterior communicating artery (AComA) and recurrent artery of Heubner that may be draped over the tumor. Coagulation of the base of the tumor at the tuberculum/sellar junction should only proceed after identification of the stalk, which is often adherent to the posterior margin of the capsule and can easily be damaged during this step. Efforts should be taken to preserve subchiasmatic perforating vessels from the superior hypophyseal arteries (SHA) during the subchiasmatic extracapsular dissection.

Transcribriform Approach[12]

Exposure

This module extends the rostral extension of the previous approach to the level of the crista galli or even the frontal sinus if required. Indeed, the transcribriform approach is commonly combined with a transplanum approach for resection of anterior fossa meningiomas. The attachment of the anterior portion of the nasal septum to the skull base is resected posteriorly, olfaction being most likely already compromised. Complete ethmoidectomies are performed with exposure of the medial orbital walls. The skull base is drilled rostrocaudally starting at the frontoethmoidal recess. The ethmoidal arteries (AEA and PEA) are identified, coagulated, and transected medially, contributing to tumor devascularization. The lamina papyracea can be removed in order to gain lateral exposure, although the periorbital fascia should not be disrupted. After bilateral removal of the cribriform plate, the crista galli is drilled until eggshell thin, fractured, and removed. The ethmoidal arteries represent a risk for retrobulbar hematoma if not well coagulated or clipped before being incised during this approach.

Intradural Dissection

The exposed dura is coagulated and incised individually on both sides of the falx. Tumor is debulked sequentially from each side, exposing the free edge of the falx bilaterally. After coagulation of the falx and any feeding vessels arising from the falcine arteries, it is incised, creating a single intradural working cavity. Tumor debulking is continued closer to midline. Extracapsular dissection is pursued using gentle countertraction and sharp dissection. Subpial invasion may be encountered and requires gentle subpial dissection. Dissection over the superior pole of the tumor proceeds along the interhemispheric fissure, paying attention to A2 and frontopolar arteries that will be draped over the tumor surface. Extracapsular dissection may also proceed toward the parasellar cistern (inferior pole), enabling identification of the optic nerves and the AComA. This provides proximal control of both A2 during dissection along the interhemispheric fissure.

The most important vital structures related to this module are the orbits and the anterior cerebral arteries (A2) and their branches (fronto-orbital, frontopolar).

Transclival Approach[65] (see Fig. 44.3)

The clivus can be divided in three portions along the rostro-caudal direction. The upper third includes the dorsum sella and posterior clinoids down to the level of the sellar floor junction. The middle third extends from the sellar floor junction down to the sphenoid floor junction. The lower third extends from the sphenoid floor junction to the foramen magnum. The transclival approach is frequently used for chordomas and chondrosarcomas involving the clivus. It is also used to access intradural lesions anterior to the brainstem such as meningiomas.

Upper Third of the Clivus

The rostral extension of the superior portion of the clivus is bounded by the dorsum sella in the midline and the posterior clinoids in the paramedian region. These bony structures may be removed either intradurally via a transsellar approach or extradurally via a subsellar approach.

Transsellar exposure (intradural). A transtuberculum/transplanum approach is first performed. Rostral exposure only needs to reach the tuberculum/planum junction. Bone covering the sellar face is removed to expose the SIS, IIS, and the sella-clival junction. Cruciform dural openings are performed over the parachiasmatic cistern and the pituitary gland, taking care not to transgress the pituitary capsule. After ligation and transection of the SIS, both dural openings communicate. If present, the IIS must also be transected. The diaphragma sella is cut in the midline to expose the stalk. The diaphragma sella is

then cut in a paramedian direction to release the stalk circumferentially. The ligaments connecting the pituitary capsule to the medial cavernous sinus wall are systematically cut along the lateral contour of the gland. The gland may be mobilized superiorly, enabling exposure of the posterior sellar dura, which is coagulated and the posterior intercavernous sinus (PIS) is transected, exposing the dorsum sellae and posterior clinoid laterally.[68] These bony structures are then drilled until eggshell thin and are carefully removed, avoiding injury to the ICA and abducent nerve located laterally and posteriorly. Once these structures are drilled, the retroclival dura harboring the basilar plexus is visualized. Transgressing the basilar plexus can generate intense venous bleeding. The surgeons must be prepared to control such bleeding, and hemostatic agents as such as microfibrillar collagen and absorbable gelatin powder with thrombin work very well in this location. Gland transposition enables unobstructed visualization of the posterior wall of the sella.[68]

Subsellar exposure (extradural) (see Fig. 44.3). The subsellar exposure enables removal of the posterior clinoids and dorsum sellae through an extradural route and is indicated especially for midline retrosellar lesions that extend caudally. A transplanum approach is required only if access to a rostral tumor extension is needed. The sellar face, the bone over the SIS and IIS, and the portion of the middle third of the clivus between the vertical carotid canals (paraclival) directly below the sella are removed. The sellar dura is not opened, enabling en bloc elevation of the pituitary fossa. This gives access to drill the posterior clinoids and dorsum sellae.

Once the exposure to the superior clivus is complete, the dura is opened and initial efforts should aim at identifying neurovascular structures within the interpeduncular and prepontine cisterns guarded laterally by the PComA and the third cranial nerve. If the membrane of Liliequist is not violated, efforts should be made to avoid its transgression because it prevents spread of blood to other cisterns.

Middle Third of the Clivus

Isolated removal of this part of the clivus is rarely performed. Its removal is usually undertaken with a portion of the inferior third or as part of a panclival exposure. For didactic reasons we will describe the middle and inferior thirds of the clival approach combined in the panclival approaches.

Panclival Approaches (see Fig. 44.3)

The panclival approach can extend from the dorsum sellae and posterior clinoids to the anterior aspect of the foramen magnum. Modifications of the initial bilateral sphenoid exposure are needed to gain such a caudal access. To gain progressively caudal access, the nasal septum needs to be completely detached from the sphenoid rostrum. Wide sphenoidotomies must be performed as they provide deeper positioning of the scope and enable a direct caudal view. The basopharyngeal fascia is removed from the sphenoid rostrum and clivus face. The sphenoid sinus floor is drilled flush with the clivus. Before drilling the clivus, it is important to identify the vidian nerve because it marks the petrous ICA level. The clivus bone is removed in the midline, between the carotid canals above the level of the vidian nerve. Inferiorly, drilling of the jugular tubercle and petrous bone can be performed laterally bellow the petrous ICA using the vidian canal as the superior limit.[69]

After meticulous coagulation of the underlying dura and basilar venous plexus, the dura is opened segmentally in the midline. Neurophysiological and sixth cranial nerve stimulation should be used to avoid opening on the sixth cranial nerve. Image guidance should also be used under computed tomography angiography (CTA) visualization to determine the vertebrobasilar junction (VBJ). The dural opening should be below the VBJ because the sixth cranial nerve will be above that level.[70]

The most relevant neural structures for the transclival module are the brainstem and cranial nerves, namely, CN II and III for the upper third of clivus with the addition of CN V through X for the panclival approach. Important vascular structures to identify include the vertebral arteries, vertebrobasilar junction, basilar artery, superior cerebellar arteries, posterior cerebral arteries, and respective perforators.

Transodontoid and Foramen Magnum/ Craniovertebral Approach[65,71,72]

This approach can be used for resection of the odontoid process in degenerative or inflammatory disease, or to allow for exposure of the ventral medulla and upper cervical spinal cord. The transodontoid approach is an extension of the transclival approach. However, it can be performed independently with clival preservation because in most cases the disease is isolated in the cervical spine. Furthermore, the sphenoid sinus doesn't need to be exposed in most of these cases. After removing the nasopharyngeal mucosa, the paraspinal muscles and the atlanto-occipital membrane are exposed and partially resected. At this point, the lower clivus as well as the anterior arch of C1 are exposed. Bone removal is guided by the pathological entity and concerns for stability.[73] For foramen magnum exposure, only the superior aspect of the C1 ring needs to be drilled to expose the tip of the odontoid. For transodontoid exposure, the anterior arch of C1 is resected and the odontoid process of C2 is exposed. The anterior cortex of the dens and the trabecular bone are drilled and the posterior cortical shell is removed preferentially by sharp dissection incising the ligaments. After removal of the dens, the normal dura covering the brainstem is exposed or an underlying pannus if surgery is performed in the setting of rheumatoid arthritis.

The most important neurovascular structures for this module are the vertebral arteries, posterior inferior cerebellar arteries (PICAs), brainstem, and lower cranial nerves. The ICAs have to be considered as a risk factor as well because occasionally they can be positioned close to the midline in their parapharyngeal segment under the mucosa.

Expanded Endonasal Approaches— Coronal Plane

Expanded coronal approaches are used for dissections lateral to the midline corridor. The coronal plane approaches are considered in three different levels. The anterior coronal plane has an intimate relationship with the anterior fossa and orbits, the midcoronal plane with the middle fossa and temporal lobe, and the posterior coronal plane with the posterior fossa.

Anterior Coronal Plane: Transorbital and Supraorbital Approaches

The transorbital approach can be divided into intraconal and extraconal approaches. The transorbital extraconal approach is indicated for resection of sinonasal lesions that are invading the medial wall of the orbit as sinonasal malignancies and decompression of the optic nerves in the presence of unresectable intraconal disease. The transorbital intraconal approach is indicated for resection of lesions that are inferior and medial to the optic nerve such as schwannomas, cavernomas, and meningiomas. This module requires at least a unilateral wide resection of the anterior and posterior ethmoid cells in order to expose the lateral wall of the sinonasal cavity. Intraconal access is gained by removal of the lamina papyracea and periorbital opening and by passing between the inferior and medial rectus muscles with preservation of extraocular muscle function. In the supraorbital approach, the medial wall of the orbit is removed and the orbital tissues are displaced to expose the orbital roof.

The most important vital structures related to this module are the optic nerves, the anterior and posterior ethmoidal arteries, and the ophthalmic artery with its central retina artery branch.

Middle and Posterior Coronal Plane[13]

The approaches used to access the middle and posterior coronal plane are grouped on the basis of their relationship to the petrous carotid artery. Infrapetrous approaches give access to the medial petrous apex and the petroclival junction. The suprapetrous approaches give access to the inferior and superior cavernous sinus as well as the infratemporal/middle fossa.

Transpterygoid Approach (Fig. 44.4)

All the modules in the middle and posterior coronal planes begin with a transpterygoid approach. Initially a maxillary antrostomy is performed, providing access to the back wall of the maxillary sinus. The sphenopalatine and posterior nasal arteries are identified and ligated. The soft tissues of the pterygopalatine fossa are mobilized in a medial to lateral direction to expose the base and the medial wedge of the pterygoids. The vidian canal (pterygoid canal) should be identified early because it represents, along with the middle pterygoid plates, critical surgical landmarks for endoscopic approaches to the petrous apex.[69,74] The vidian canal leads directly to the anterior genu of the ICA because its petrous portion turns up to form the vertical paraclival ICA. The medial pterygoid plate (MPP) is drilled medial and inferior to the vidian canal while following it posteriorly, toward the foramen lacerum.

Medial Petrous Apex (Zone 1: Posterior Fossa)

This module adds on the transpterygoid approach and can be conceived as a lateral extension of a transclival approach in its middle third. It is indicated to access lesions in the medial petrous apex such as chondrosarcomas and cholesterol granulomas. Following the transpterygoid approach, drilling of the bone covering the paraclival carotid may be required if the ICA needs to be mobilized laterally.[75] This enables direct access to the petrous apex. Greater access can also be provided by drilling a portion of the lateral clivus at its junction with the petrous apex.

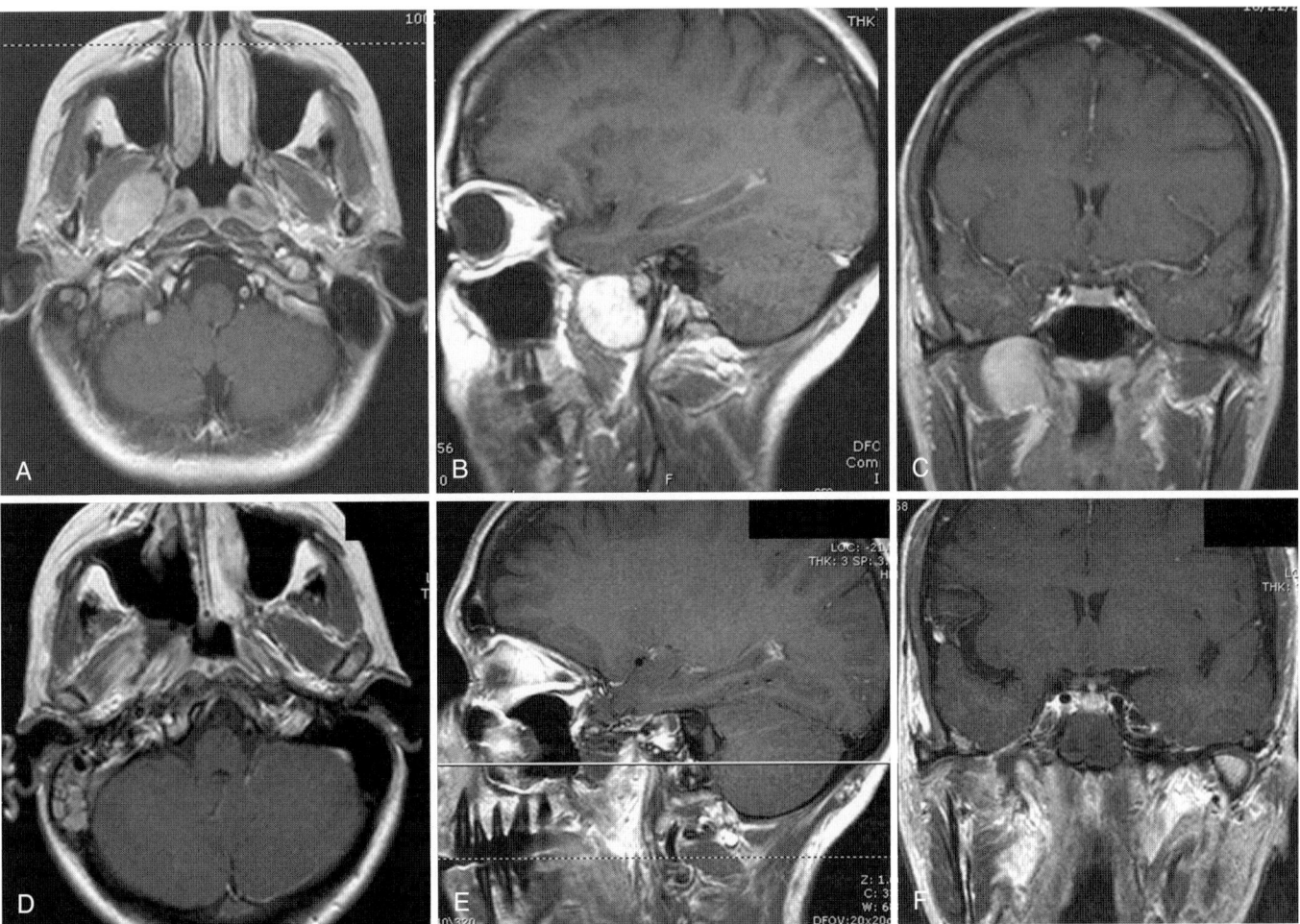

FIGURE 44.4 This 41-year-old female patient reported 6-year right-sided facial pain and numbness, which increased in the recent year. The patient underwent a negative biopsy of her right pterygopalatine fossa mass. Preoperative magnetic resonance imaging (MRI) prior to resection of the lesion through a transpterygoid approach: axial (**A**), sagittal (**B**), and coronal (**C**) views in T1-weighted imaging (WI) post-gadolinium scan. Postoperative MRI following complete resection of her pterygopalatine fossa schwanomma: axial (**D**), sagittal (**E**), and coronal (**F**) views in T1-WI postgadolinium scan.

The most relevant structures are the ICAs and the sixth cranial nerve at Dorello's canal.

Petroclival Approaches (Zone 2: Posterior Fossa)

This module enables access to lesions deeper along the midportion of the petrous bone. This approach can be combined with a medial petrous apex exposure. The bone over the anterior genu of the ICA, the petrous segment (horizontal), and the paraclival segment (vertical) of the ICA is removed to unroof the carotid if lateral displacement is necessary. The cartilaginous fibrous tissue projection from the eustachian tube and basopharyngeal fascia needs to be detached from the undersurface of the foramen lacerum and petroclival synchondrosis in order to expose the bone for drilling. The lateral portion of the clivus at the petroclival junction is drilled laterally followed by petrous bone beneath the petrous (horizontal) segment ICA until the underlying dura of the posterior fossa and venous plexus is identified. The inferior surface of the petrous apex is reached by drilling the bone between the horizontal petrous segment of the ICA and the eustachian tube, medial to V3. The horizontal segment of the petrous carotid and overlying cavernous

sinus represents the superior boundary of this exposure and the middle fossa, the superolateral boundary. If required, the dura deep to the drilled petrous bone can be incised to give access to the paramedian segment of the prepontine cistern.

The important structures related to this module are the vidian nerves and the ICAs.

Inferior Cavernous Sinus/Quadrangular Space (Zone 3: Middle Fossa)[76]

This module is used for resection of Meckel's cave lesions. Pathological entities commonly encountered in this region are invasive adenoid cystic carcinomas, meningiomas, schwannomas, and invasive pituitary adenomas. Removal of the posterior wall of the maxillary antrum is extended laterally until the maxillary branch (V2) of the trigeminal nerve is identified traveling superiorly toward the foramen rotundum. The MPP is drilled inferior and medial to the vidian canal. Next, the bone between the vidian canal and V2 is drilled away, knowing that this bony corridor narrows progressively as it deepens. Removal of this bone gives access to the quadrangular space, which is delimited by the parasellar ICA medially, the V2 and dura of middle fossa laterally, horizontal petrous ICA inferiorly, and the sixth cranial nerve superiorly. Bone covering the horizontal petrous ICA, the anterior genu, and parasellar ICA may need to be removed if mobilization of the carotid is required. The periosteum is opened lateral to the vertical paraclival ICA and medial to V2.

The structures at risk for this approach are exactly its boundaries: ICA, sixth cranial nerve, and trigeminal nerve.[76]

Superior Cavernous Sinus (Zone 4: Middle Fossa)

This module requires the exact same bone removal and ICA exposure as performed for the inferior cavernous sinus module. However, it is rarely used due to the high risk of cranial nerve injury. This approach has mostly served for patients with already established cranial nerve deficits (CN III, IV, VI) such as in apoplectic pituitary adenomas that invade the cavernous sinus or for tumors refractory to medical treatment or radiosurgery.[13] Prior to dural incision, it is advised to identify the medial margin of the ICA in the sella so that it can be protected during dural opening. The dura incision is initiated directly over the superior lateral portion of the cavernous sinus and performed in a medial-to-lateral direction. Often, the cavernous sinus has already thrombosed and little venous bleeding occurs during initial opening. However, profuse bleeding may be encountered once the tumor is removed.

The most important structures related to this approach include cranial nerves III, IV, V, and VI, as well as the ICAs with the associated sympathetic fibers.

Infratemporal Approach/Temporal Fossa (Zone 5: Middle Fossa)

Tumors approached through this route often create a corridor through the pterygomaxillary fissure, extending rostrally in the middle fossa and laterally in the infratemporal fossa. Pathological entities encountered in this region include invasive carcinomas, CSF leaks, encephaloceles, skull base meningiomas, and schwannomas. The vidian canal is identified and the maxillary antrostomy is completed. The MPP is identified and removed flush with the middle cranial fossa and foramen rotundum. The infratemporal module begins once the lateral pterygoid plate (LPP) is isolated and followed posteriorly in the direction of V3. Tumor debulking is begun only after the anterior genu of the ICA and horizontal petrous segment of the ICA are identified. During the lateral dissection, the internal maxillary artery and its branches must be isolated and ligated. The dissection is pursued laterally until the lateral pterygoid plate (LPP) is identified. The LPP is drilled rostrally until flush with the middle fossa and foramen ovale. Venous bleeding from the pterygopalatine venous complex may be profuse enough to require packing and staged resection, allowing the venous complex to thrombose. Because the bony landmarks are often eroded, image guidance is required for these interventions.

The relevant structures in this module are the internal maxillary artery with its branches, the vidian nerve, the trigeminal nerve (V2 and V3) with its branches, and the superior orbital fissure superiorly.

Transcondylar and Supracondylar (Transjugular Tubercle) (Zone 6: Posterior Fossa)[13]

This module builds on the inferior third clivectomy laterally and infrapetrous approach extended caudally. Chondrosarcomas are the commonest pathological entity encountered in this region. The cartilaginous segment of the eustachian tube is resected for about 1 cm.

Once the foramen lacerum is identified, the position of the ICA is secured. The basopharyngeal fascia is elevated from the bone inferiorly exposing the petroclival synchondrosis, which ends in the jugular foramen. Medially the foramen magnum is exposed and followed laterally. The occipital condyle is identified.

Supracondylar (transjugular tubercle) approach. Drilling is performed in the occipital bone above the condyle, preserving the articular capsule medial to the petroclival synchondrosis. The drilling goes in the direction of the jugular tubercle, which is removed, allowing for exposure of the cerebellomedullary junction if the dura is opened.

Transcondylar approach. The medial aspect of the occipital condyle is drilled, allowing for direct visualization of the subarachnoid origin of the vertebral artery, which is essential in order to obtain its proximal control in cases it is needed. Care should be taken as one approaches the hypoglossal canal, which will be located immediately lateral in the superior portion of the condyle emerging from the skull at 2 (left) and 10 o'clock (patient's right).

The vital structures related to this module are the inner ear with the seventh and eighth cranial nerves laterally, the petrous ICA superiorly, and the twelfth cranial nerve inferolaterally.

Jugular Foramen (Zone 7: Posterior Fossa)[3]

This approach is used for resection of invasive carcinomas, paragangliomas, schwannomas, and skull base meningiomas located in this region. The eustachian tube is an important landmark to safely determine the position of the ICA in its ascending parapharyngeal segment at the point it penetrates the carotid canal in the petrous bone. The Rosenmüller fossa is followed laterally. The medial aspect of the occipital condyle is encountered lateral to the foramen magnum and followed laterally. The hypoglossal canal is localized rostrolateral to the condyle and should be navigated carefully. Once the ICA is localized, the jugular foramen is located immediately lateral. The petroclival synchondrosis is followed craniocaudally and ends at the foramen jugularis. Cranial nerves IX, X, and XI are located in between the jugular vein and the ICA.

The most important structures related to this approach are the internal maxillary artery, the ICA (pharyngeal and petrous segments), the trigeminal nerve, the jugular foramen with the jugular vein and lower cranial nerves (IX, X, XI), and the twelfth cranial nerve exiting the hypoglossal canal inferiorly.

COMPLICATION AVOIDANCE DURING THE EXPANDED ENDONASAL APPROACH

The following general principles should prevail during each EEA.

1. The critical neurovascular structures must be located on the perimeter of the lesion, allowing access to the lesion with minimal manipulation of normal neurovascular structures.

2. EEAs must be performed using bimanual and binarial access to allow for a two-surgeon, three/four-hand technique. The bony and soft tissue removal required for dynamic and free movement as well as optimal visualization has been described for each module. A wide surgical corridor enables exposure of key anatomical landmarks, prevents crowding of instruments, minimizes soiling of the lens, and helps maintain an unobstructed view of the surgical field. This step becomes more critical if there is a bleeding complication, so that the surgeons can maintain visualization while controlling the hemorrhage and avoiding injury to adjacent structures.

3. Endoneurosurgical tumor resection uses the same techniques and respects the same principles as microneurosurgery. Specifically, capsular bipolar coagulation, internal debulking, capsular mobilization, extracapsular dissection of neurovascular structures, coagulation, and removal of the capsule are sequentially performed in a bimanual fashion. Grasping and pulling must be avoided.

4. Skull base defect reconstruction is of major importance. The use of vascularized flaps for large dural defects has significantly reduced the incidence of postoperative CSF leaks. Although other materials have been used for closure, we believe the use of a vascularized flap offers the best chance at effective reconstruction following EEAs.

5. EEAs should be performed by an integrated team composed of a neurosurgeon and ear, nose, and throat (ENT) surgeon, both with substantial knowledge in ventral skull base endoscopic anatomy and thorough experience in conventional skull base surgery and expanded endoscopic surgery.

6. Endoscopic cranial base surgery must be learned in an incremental and modular fashion which applies to all endonasal surgeons, irrespective of their specialty (Box 44.2).[66] A level must be fully mastered prior to proceeding to the next because a higher level translates into increased anatomical complexity, technical difficulty, and potential risk of neurovascular injury.

OUTCOME AFTER THE EXPANDED ENDONASAL APPROACH

Numerous series have demonstrated that endoscopic resection of sinonasal, sellar, and various skull base lesions is associated with at least equivalent oncological results to standard transcranial procedures in well-trained hands.[1,5,8,9,14-16] In addition, EEAs have been associated with decreased length of hospital stay, decreased morbidity, increased patient comfort, and lack of external incision.[1,5,8,9,14-16]

Overall, endoscopic skull base surgery shares the same primary goal of oncological surgery as open procedures: to perform the most complete tumor excision. The endoscope provides visualization of tumor limits and margins and enables better assessment of the extent of the tumor. Planning the specific margins of resection is therefore facilitated.[66] Because endoscopic procedures attack lesions from a ventral perspective, the resection of infiltrative skull base tumors may be more extensive considering that bony and dural invasion is more easily addressed through EEAs than through traditional skull base approaches.

BOX 44.2 | Training Program for Endonasal Cranial Base Surgery

Level I (Sinus Surgery) (Not Considered Skull Base Surgery)
Endoscopic sinonasal surgery
Endoscopic sphenoethmoidectomy
Sphenopalatine artery ligation
Endoscopic frontal sinusotomy

Level II
Cerebrospinal fluid leaks
Lateral recess sphenoid
Sella/pituitary

Level III (Extradural)
Medial orbital decompression
Optic nerve decompression
Petrous apex (medial expansion), no internal carotid artery (ICA) manipulation
Transclival approaches (extradural)
Transodontoid approach (extradural)

Level IV (Intradural)
A. Presence of a cortical cuff
   Transplanum approach
   Transcribriform approach
   Preinfundibular lesions
B. Absence of cortical cuff (direct vascular contact)
   Transplanum approach
   Transcribriform approach
   Infundibular and retroinfundibular lesions
   Transclival approach
   Foramen magnum approach

Level V
A. Coronal plane (paramedian)
   ICA manipulation
B. Vascular surgery (aneurysms, arteriovenous malformations)

To date, early outcome data for skull base pathological entities treated by an EEA are promising. The detailed review of these results is beyond the scope of this chapter. Furthermore, the collective experience is currently too brief to describe long-term tumor control following EEA. For some rare skull base tumors, sample sizes are too small, precluding any firm conclusions. Larger series and long-term follow-up studies are required to determine the circumstances in which expanded endonasal procedures are superior to standard open surgery.

CONCLUSION AND FUTURE DIRECTIONS

Endoscopic ventricular and endonasal surgery has significantly evolved over the past two decades. Presently, the entire ventral skull base can be accessed endonasally in the sagittal and coronal planes using purely endoscopic expanded endonasal approaches.

The choice of a specific surgical route should be guided by lesion characteristics, patient comorbidities, and skill and experience of the operating team. Each patient should be evaluated with a 360-degree approach, considering the least destructive route with the fewest complications to achieve the most complete lesion resection. Modular approaches should be combined as mandated by the lesion and its location.[12,13,65] However, when a lesion cannot be completely removed through an EEA, an open route may be considered or a combination of endonasal and open approaches may be used.[1,5,6]

Major advances will be directed at allowing neurosurgeons to do microsurgical work "around corners" under the endoscopic view only. Curved instruments that allow microsurgical work to be done in these recesses and instruments that combine the functions of multiple instruments (suction and endoscope or suction and cautery) may facilitate working with the endoscope with a single hand. New tools for endoscopic sharp dissection and control of vascular structures are needed. Finally, every improvement in visualization is welcome. The possibility of 3D endoscopy has come true, with a sharper and brighter picture. Flexible endoscopy with a picture equivalent to a rod-lens endoscope and image injection of frameless stereotactic data into the video image would be welcome additions to the endoscopic armamentarium.

Advancements will also be dependent on instrument development being attractive to commercial vendors. If there is no market to recoup research and development costs, then there will be few advances. Gone are the days when tumor neurosurgeons could divide themselves into neuroendoscopists or microsurgical specialists. To offer the patient the best possible option for management of the intraventricular lesion, the surgeon must be able to utilize, expertly, both methods of visualization. As more surgeons are trained to use, become familiar with, and "buy in" to this useful technology, the market for neuroendoscopes and neuroendoscopic tools will grow, as will the technology.

SELECTED KEY REFERENCES

Kassam A, Snyderman CH, Mintz A, et al. Expanded endonasal approach: the rostrocaudal axis. Part I. Crista galli to the sella turcica. *Neurosurg Focus.* 2005;19:E3.

Kassam A, Snyderman CH, Mintz A, et al. Expanded endonasal approach: the rostrocaudal axis. Part II. Posterior clinoids to the foramen magnum. *Neurosurg Focus.* 2005;19:E4.

Kassam AB, Gardner P, Snyderman C, et al. Expanded endonasal approach: fully endoscopic, completely transnasal approach to the middle third of the clivus, petrous bone, middle cranial fossa, and infratemporal fossa. *Neurosurg Focus.* 2005;19:E6.

Kassam AB, Prevedello DM, Carrau RL, et al. The front door to Meckel's cave: an anteromedial corridor via expanded endoscopic endonasal approach—technical considerations and clinical series. *Neurosurgery.* 2009;64:71-82.

Kassam AB, Prevedello DM, Thomas A, et al. Endoscopic endonasal pituitary transposition for a transdorsum sellae approach to the interpeduncular cistern. *Neurosurgery.* 2008;62:57-72.

Kassam AB, Vescan AD, Carrau RL, et al. Expanded endonasal approach: vidian canal as a landmark to the petrous internal carotid artery. *J Neurosurg.* 2008;108:177-183.

Please go to expertconsult.com to view the complete list of references.

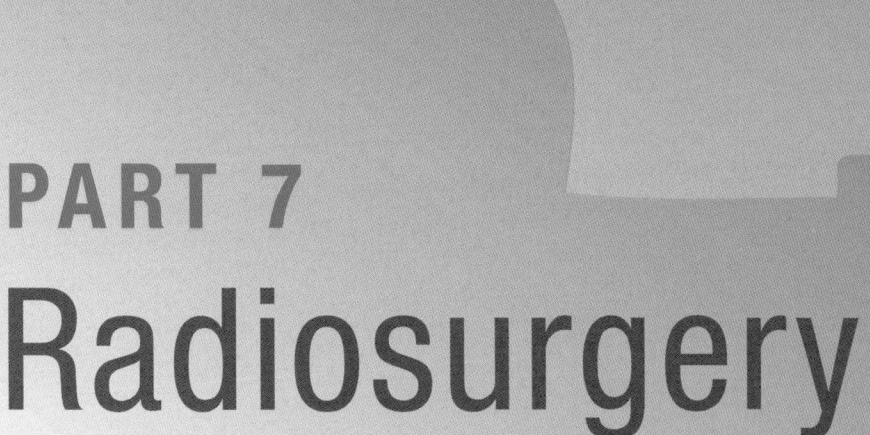

PART 7

Radiosurgery

Application of Current Radiation Delivery Systems and Radiobiology

Jay Loeffler, Helen Shih, Melin Khandekar

CLINICAL PEARLS

- Radiosurgery involves the delivery of a high dose of ionizing radiation to a target in a single or a few fractions.

- Physical properties of high-energy photons or protons used for radiosurgery determine their biological effects.

- The biological consequences of high-dose radiation used for radiosurgery are poorly understood, and may differ from those of conventionally fractionated radiation therapy.

- A number of delivery systems are available for modern radiosurgery, with either photons or protons, each of which has unique characteristics for the patient and the physician.

- In retrospective and prospective studies, there are no data that demonstrate a consistent clinical advantage for one type of radiosurgery device over another.

Radiation therapy has been used for the treatment of benign and malignant central nervous system (CNS) diseases for over 50 years. Ionizing radiation, either from machines known as *linear accelerators* (linacs) or from radioactive sources such as cobalt-60, can be used for either conventional fractionated radiotherapy or single-dose, stereotactic radiosurgery (SRS). Radiosurgery, as defined by both the American Society for Radiation Oncology (ASTRO) and the American Association of Neurologic Surgeons (AANS) is "a distinct discipline that utilizes externally generated ionizing radiation in certain cases to inactivate or eradicate a defined target(s) in the head or spine without the need to make an incision."[1] The definition specifies that radiosurgery is usually delivered in one to five sessions, and uses a stereotactic image guidance system. This definition is in contrast to fractionated stereotactic radiotherapy (fSRT), which uses stereotactic localization and immobilization, but delivers a series of fractions of lower daily dose. This chapter explains the basic physics and biology of radiation therapy, and describes the most common delivery systems used for radiosurgery.

PHYSICS OF RADIOTHERAPY

Radiation therapy takes advantage of the portion of the electromagnetic spectrum known as *ionizing radiation*. Electromagnetic radiation is characterized by sinusoidal electric and magnetic waves that carry energy. By definition, ionizing radiation contains enough energy to result in the removal of electrons from their atoms, and thus leads to the creation of reactive species that cause damage to cells. The energy comes from a source external to the patient, and must pass through a

portion of normal tissue to reach its intended target. Clinical radiation dose, measured in grays (Gy), represents the energy deposited by ionization in material per unit mass of the material. The gray replaced the rad as the unit of radiation dose, with 1 Gy equal to 100 rads. Maximizing the dose of radiation to the target and minimizing the dose to normal tissue is the central goal of any radiotherapy plan.

Photon Radiation

The most common form of ionizing radiation used in radiotherapy is the photon, which is a particle that has no mass, travels at the speed of light, and carries the energy present in microwaves, visible light, ultraviolet light, and x-rays. The nature of the interaction of a photon with matter depends upon the energy of the photon. In the kiloelectron volt (keV) range, which is used in most diagnostic x-ray units, photons interact with matter via the photoelectric effect.[2] A photon interacts with a tightly bound electron, which absorbs most of the energy and is ejected from the atom and is then free to interact with other atoms in the vicinity. This interaction is highly dependent on the atomic number of the material being irradiated. Diagnostic x-ray studies take advantage of this phenomenon, as bone, which is high in calcium, is much more likely to interact with these photons than soft tissue, which is mostly carbon, hydrogen, and oxygen. This differential interaction is the basis of diagnostic x-ray imaging.

At higher energies, which is the energy of most therapeutic radiation, the Compton effect predominates.[2] A high-energy photon in the megaelectron volt (MeV) range interacts with a loosely held orbital electron, which results in ejection of the electron, and scattering of the photon (with a change in

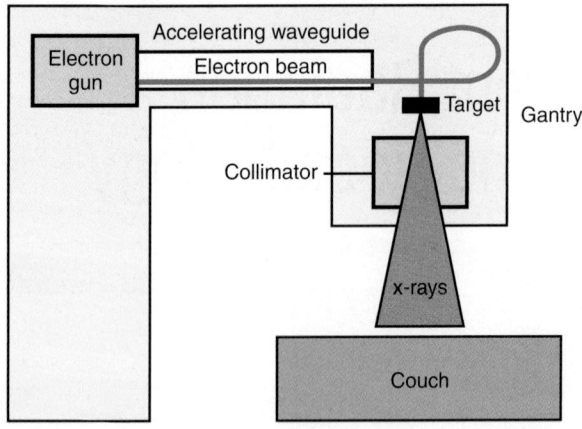
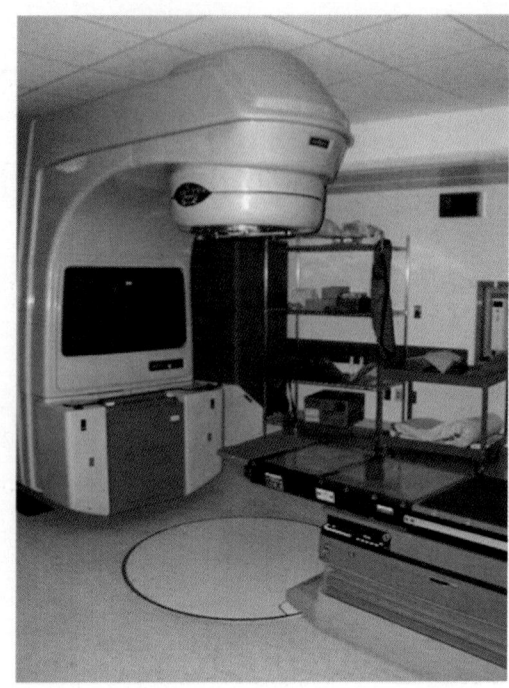

FIGURE 45.1 Linear accelerator diagram. *Left,* A schematic drawing of a linear accelerator. Electrons are generated in the electron gun, and accelerated using microwave energy in the waveguide. The electrons are bent 270 degrees to hit a high-molecular-weight target, which generates high-energy x-rays that are then shaped using the collimator. *Right,* An actual linear accelerator in clinical use. The gantry is capable of 360-degree rotation to deliver radiation from every angle.

energy of the scattered photon). This interaction is independent of the atomic number of the material being irradiated, but it is dependent on electron density. Thus, images generated from therapeutic energy x-rays are less useful for imaging than diagnostic x-rays, as there is little contrast between bone and soft tissue. However, this energy range is useful in radiation therapy, as it is highly penetrating, and is able to interact equally with all tissues.

There are two main sources of high-energy photons used in radiation therapy. The first source is radioactive decay, which is a natural process that occurs in elements with unstable nuclei and results in the emission of energy as the nucleus gains stability. Cobalt-60, the most common element used in radiation therapy units, undergoes a process known as *beta decay* to become nickel-60, which results in the emission of a high-energy photon known as a *gamma ray* (γ-ray). For ^{60}Co, the average energy of the photons generated in the radioactive decay is 1.25 MeV. Radiotherapy devices that take advantage of this phenomenon use a shielded radioactive source, and a small opening or openings result in shaping (known as *collimation*) of the beam to the desired size and shape. As will be discussed later, this is the source of radiation used in devices such as the Gamma Knife.

The other main source of high-energy photons is a linac, which uses microwaves to accelerate electrons to a high energy. These electrons are directed to collide with a high-molecular-weight target, and the resulting interactions between nuclei and electrons result in the production of high-energy photons (X-rays) via a process known as *bremsstrahlung,* or "braking" radiation. The difference between X-rays and γ-rays is simply the site of origin: X-rays are produced by electron interactions but γ-rays are produced by nuclear

decay. Unlike the γ-rays produced by ^{60}Co, the energy of the X-rays generated in a linac is based on the characteristics of the machine, and most commercial units offer multiple energy options. These X-rays are produced in the head of the unit (known as the *gantry*), and can be shaped by a system of controllable leaves, known as a *multileaf collimator* (MLC), placed between the source of the X-rays and the patient (Fig. 45.1).

The physical characteristics of photons determine their biological effects. Photons deposit dose in a characteristic pattern, in which there is an initial buildup of energy after entry into the patient, followed by a steady loss of energy as they pass through the tissue according to the law of exponential decay. The energy of the photon is lost in inverse proportion to the square of the distance traveled. Thus, photons spare the skin to some degree, but deposit the majority of their dose upon entrance into tissue, and continue to deposit decreasing amounts of energy as they exit the body (Fig. 45.2). The shape of this depth-dose curve is dependent on the energy of the photon involved. Higher energy photons exhibit greater skin-sparing effect, but have a slower rate of attenuation as they pass through tissue. In general, photons in the 1- to 6-MeV range are used for SRS, as the desired target depth in the cranium is relatively shallow, and higher energies result in unnecessary increased dose delivered beyond the target point.

Proton Radiation

Another form of ionizing radiation used in SRS involves charged particles, most commonly protons. Proton production starts by stripping the electron from molecular hydrogen gas, and the resulting protons are then accelerated to a

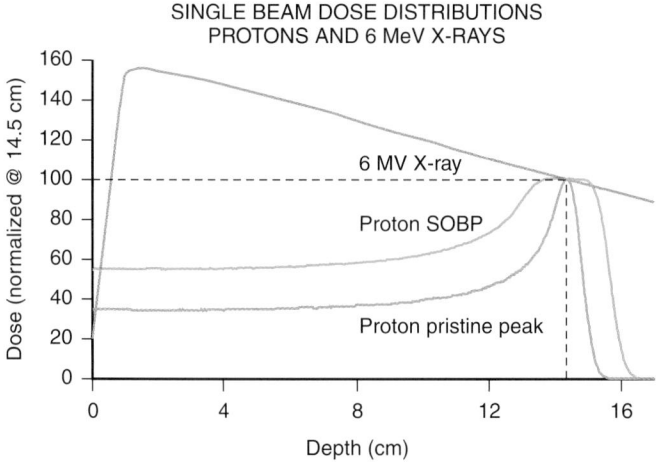

SINGLE BEAM DOSE DISTRIBUTIONS
PROTONS AND 6 MeV X-RAYS

FIGURE 45.2 Depth-dose curve for photons and protons. The x-axis represents depth in tissue, and the y-axis represents the percentage of the total dose delivered (where 100% is the dose at 14.5 cm deep in tissue, a typical depth for cranial radiosurgery). Photon radiation (here shown as a 6-MeV beam) increases upon entrance into tissue until it reaches a maximum, and then decreases in a manner that is inversely proportional to the square of the distance traveled. Proton radiation (pristine proton peak) shows a low entrance dose, and a very sharp buildup known as the Bragg peak. For larger lesions, a spread-out Bragg peak (SOBP) can be used to ensure that the entire target volume is covered by the high-dose region, although this results in higher entrance dose. *(Image courtesy of Marc Bussiere, MSc.)*

therapeutic energy level using alternating magnetic fields in a cyclotron or synchrotron. The physical properties of protons result in a different dose distribution from that of photon radiation. Protons have a defined distance of travel, known as the range, which is dependent on their energy. Protons release their energy primarily at the end of their range, which is known as the *Bragg peak*, after William Henry Bragg, the Nobel Prize–winning physicist. The consequence of the Bragg peak is that protons deposit relatively lower doses of radiation prior to the end of their range compared to photons, and have no exit dose, that is, no dose delivered past their range (see Fig. 45.2). By modulating the energy of protons, a spread-out Bragg peak (SOBP) can be generated to cover wider areas, with the tradeoff of increased entrance dose. Because of their sharp range and lack of exit dose, protons provide a favorable dose profile for use in SRS. The disadvantage of protons is that their availability is limited to a few centers due to the cost and complexity of maintaining such facilities for clinical use.

BIOLOGY OF RADIATION THERAPY

The primary target of ionizing radiation is generally thought to be damage to the DNA of target cells. As described previously, ionizing radiation results in the ejection of electrons from the atoms in the tissue being irradiated. Because most of the cell is water, the photon or proton is most likely to interact with a molecule of water, resulting in the production of superoxide, hydroxyl radicals, and other reactive oxygen species, which damage the DNA and result in replicative failure. Thus,

radiotherapy is believed to be more effective in the presence of oxygen,[3] and it is thought that hypoxic areas of tumors may be less sensitive to the effects of ionizing radiation.[4]

Although many different types of DNA damage can be produced by ionizing radiation, the most critical form of damage in the use of therapeutic radiation is the double strand break. Double strand breaks are more difficult for cells to repair, and the repair process can generate aberrant chromosomes that result in mitotic catastrophe, or mutations that result in reduced replicative fitness.[5] The critical nature of the double strand break is evidenced by the fact that patients with mutations in the ataxia-telangiectasia mutated (*ATM*) gene, one of the key sensors of DNA double strand breaks,[6] and an integral part of double strand break repair, are extremely sensitive to ionizing radiation damage.[7]

The production of double strand breaks is related to the efficiency of the particle in transferring its energy to the surrounding matter. This concept is quantified as the linear energy transfer (LET) of differing radiation modalities, and results in differences in the relative biological effectiveness (RBE) of different types of radiation beams. Photons produced by ^{60}Co are considered to have a low LET and are defined to have an RBE of 1. However, the LET varies with both energy and with the type of particle used in irradiation. For example, neutrons, which are large, noncharged particles, have a very high LET, and produce more double strand breaks for a given dose of radiation, resulting in a higher RBE.[8] Protons at therapeutic energies, although of similar mass to neutrons, do not exhibit a particularly high LET, presumably because their positive charge leads to repulsive forces with atomic nuclei. Protons used in radiotherapy have been calculated to have an RBE of 1.1 compared to photons produced by ^{60}Co.[9] This means that for a given absorbed dose, protons will have a 10% greater biological effect. To avoid confusion, proton therapy doses are typically reported as gray (relative biological effectiveness) (Gy[RBE]), taking this correction factor into account.

Although DNA damage is known to be the primary mechanism of action of radiation, the cellular target of radiotherapy is more controversial. For malignant tumors, which are highly proliferative, and often have impaired DNA repair,[10] the target is thought to be the cancer cells themselves, as they are unable to repair the DNA damage inflicted by ionizing radiation. Furthermore, their rapid progression through the cell cycle results in more potential checkpoints that can trigger cell death. Thus, cancer cells are more sensitive than normal cells to radiation. This effect is seen clinically, as radiation of malignant tissues often causes clinical or radiographic regression of the lesion.

In contrast, for benign disease, the cells are not as proliferative, and may be in resistant phases of the cell cycle. These observations have led some to speculate that benign tumors are relatively radioresistant.[11] However, in clinical practice, radiation appears to induce a quiescent state, which corresponds to radiographic and clinical stability,[12,13] suggesting that benign tumors respond to radiotherapy in some way. It is possible that these tumors undergo DNA damage that limits their replication, but the biology of this process is still unclear.

Although tumor cells have been thought to be the primary target of radiotherapy, many have suggested that radiotherapy has an effect on vascular endothelium, which mediates the primary mode of cell death, especially at the higher doses used in SRS.[14,15] Irradiation of B16 melanoma cell explants in mice with doses of 15 to 20 Gy result in waves of endothelial cell apoptosis 1 to 6 hours after irradiation.[15] The endothelial response was critical to tumor control, as endothelial-specific mutation of *Bax*, a critical regulator of apoptosis, rendered these explants insensitive to doses of 15 Gy. Thus, endothelial cell death may lead to direct hypoxic necrosis of the tumor, or may secrete signaling molecules that may cause tumor death. However, other studies have shown that at even higher radiation doses (>20 Gy), the mode of death in an irradiated gastrointestinal tract appears to become independent of endothelial cell apoptosis,[16] suggesting that the dose response relationship is complex, and may be differentially regulated in different tissues. These differences are the subject of much investigation and may become more important as combination chemotherapy or targeted therapy is considered.

These observations correlate with data from radiosurgical experiments exposing normal rat brain or tumor explants to radiosurgical doses of ionizing radiation. Examination of human acoustic schwannoma xenografts after irradiation with 10 to 40 Gy showed a significant decrease in tumor vascularity, as well as significant intramural vascular hyalinization.[17] Furthermore, irradiation of rat brains with 15 to 30 Gy resulted in changes in local blood flow, leukocyte/endothelial interaction, formation of aneurysmal structures, and thrombus formation.[18] These data suggest that vascular damage by radiosurgery may be an important component of its clinical effect.

Fractionation versus Radiosurgery

Conventional radiotherapy is typically fractionated into daily doses, which is thought to result in reduced effects of radiation on normal tissue. Fractionation allows for DNA repair to occur, which is predicted to favor normal cells that retain the full complement of DNA repair proteins.[19] Furthermore, fractionation allows for reoxygenation of hypoxic areas, resulting in increased sensitivity of malignant cells that were previously hypoxic.[20] Additionally, fractionated therapy allows for reassortment of cells in the cell cycle, as cells are most sensitive to radiation during the G2/M phase of the cell cycle and resistant during the late S phase and G1. Thus, giving radiation in daily fractions allows those cells that are in resistant phases of the cell cycle to move to more sensitive phases of the cell cycle during subsequent fractions.[21] The downside of fractionation is that it allows for repopulation of tumor cells during the therapy. Reoxygenation, reassortment, repair, along with repopulation, are known as the "four Rs" of radiobiology, and explain the radiobiological basis for daily fractionated therapy.

The value of fractionation is more apparent for certain tissues, which typically have high rates of proliferation and show relatively less capability to repair sublethal DNA damage. This concept is quantified as the α/β ratio, which is a radiobiological concept, based on a model of radiation response, that attempts to explain the differential sensitivity of tissues to fractionation.[22] Tissues with a high α/β ratio respond quickly to radiotherapy, and are sensitive to smaller fraction sizes. Examples of these so-called "early" responding tissues include the gastrointestinal tract, lymphocytes, and skin. Tissues with a low α/β ratio respond more slowly to radiation, are typically less proliferative, and show a high capacity for DNA repair. Examples of late responding tissues include neural tissue and the lung.

The α/β ratio can be used to calculate a biologically equivalent dose (BED), which attempts to equalize total doses that are given in different fraction sizes. The equation is BED = (number of fractions * fractional dose) * (1 + (fractional dose/α/β ratio)).[22] Although there is debate over the validity of this model at the high doses used in radiosurgery, it allows one to approximate the effect of doses delivered in fractionated sessions and those given in radiosurgery. For example, if one assumes a tumor to have a high α/β ratio of 10, a dose of 20 Gy in a single fraction is biologically equivalent to a dose of 40 Gy in 8 fractions, or 50 Gy in 25 fractions. However, for normal brain tissue, which has an α/β ratio closer to 3, the schedule 20 Gy × 1 has a BED of 153.3, while 5 Gy × 8 has a BED of 106.7, and 2 Gy × 25 has a BED of 83.3. Thus, the preceding regimens have the same BED for a tissue with a high α/β ratio, but the larger fraction sizes have a much higher BED for tissues with a low α/β ratio. What this means is that although the tumor control would be predicted to be equivalent for 20 Gy in 1 fraction and 50 Gy in 25 fractions, the radiosurgical dose would produce a more profound effect on normal brain tissue. Although the BED is merely an approximation of biological effect and not a real quantity, it can be useful when considering the dose of radiation to be used when the target is close to critical normal structures such as cranial nerves.

Given these advantages to fractionation, the radiobiological rationale for radiosurgery is not immediately obvious. However, proponents of radiosurgery argue that there are some principles that make SRS radiobiologically favorable. First, radiosurgery relies on precise immobilization and localization of the tumor to be treated, with inclusion of minimal margin of normal tissue. The design of the treatment machine, as outlined later in this chapter, creates a high dose of radiation in a very precisely defined space, with a very rapid dose falloff outside the target volume. Thus, even if critical normal structures are very close to the target tissue, the dose received is much lower than that received in the target itself. Thus, the physics of radiosurgery can compensate for suboptimal radiation biology.

Another potential explanation for the excellent clinical effect of radiosurgical doses in malignant disease lies in the possibility that high radiation doses are required to kill radiation-resistant cells. Emerging data suggest that clonogenic cells within tumors may have an intrinsically higher radioresistance due to increased expression of antioxidant genes.[23] It may be that very high radiation doses are able to overcome this effect, resulting in death of those clonogenic cells, and leading to tumor control.

Finally, as described earlier, at high doses of radiation, the primary mode of cell death may be due to endothelial damage, which may explain why the radiobiological rationale of fractionation may not be applicable when considering the observed clinical efficacy of SRS, especially for such targets as arteriovenous malformations. If radiation-induced apoptosis of the endothelium is a response to high dose per fraction, then fractionation may result in less normal tissue toxicity but also less control of the targeted lesion. All of these mechanisms are speculative and remain to be proved in a rigorous scientific fashion.

The radiobiological concerns outlined here suggest some situations when it may be advantageous to choose fractionated treatment over single-fraction radiosurgery. Given that normal neural tissue, including cranial nerves, are late-responding, with an α/β ratio of approximately 3, they will be more sensitive to large radiation doses compared to small ones. If the target to be treated is in close proximity to one of these structures (e.g., optic nerve sheath meningioma[24] or a pituitary tumor very close to the optic chiasm[25]), it may be more prudent to fractionate treatment to reduce the risk of injury to the cranial nerves. Conversely, for hormone-secreting tumors, there is biological evidence that high-dose radiosurgery is associated with more rapid normalization of hormone levels.[26] Thus, the choice between radiosurgery and fractionated treatment must weigh a number of radiobiological and clinical parameters.

HISTORY OF RADIOSURGERY

The development of stereotactic radiosurgery (SRS) can be linked to developments in stereotactic localization for neurosurgical procedures by Spiegel and Wycis in 1947.[27] The concept behind stereotaxy was to attach a fixed external coordinate system to the skull so that every point within the skull could be defined according to the axes present on the external device. The early system of Spiegel and Wycis used axes correlating to the ventricles as seen on pneumoencephalogram, but as imaging techniques advanced, new systems that relied on computed tomography (CT) or magnetic resonance imaging (MRI) were subsequently developed.[28,29] Lars Leksell, a Swedish neurosurgeon at the Karolinska Institute, adapted a similar stereotactic system, and combined this with a variety of types of radiation, ultimately relying on radioactive ^{60}Co to produce multiple small photon beams converging on an intracranial target.[30] This system evolved to become a hospital-based therapy known as the Gamma Knife, the first commercially available radiosurgery system. With further research, conventional linacs were adapted to produce a similar effect through the use of multiple convergent noncoplanar arcs, enabling a wider range of radiotherapy centers to perform SRS.[31-33]

Several investigators, including Dr. Leksell, with his collaborator, radiobiologist Dr. Borje Larsson, began experimenting with protons produced by the cyclotron in Uppsala using a crossfire technique to irradiate the pituitary.[34] At the same time, in 1953, Dr. John Lawrence at the University of California at Berkeley cyclotron began to treat the pituitary using the Bragg peak of a proton beam.[35] Concurrently, Dr. Raymond Kjellberg, a neurosurgeon at the Massachusetts General Hospital, began to experiment with the Harvard Cyclotron in Cambridge, Massachusetts, and began treating patients in 1961. The initial treatments were limited to the pituitary, as the sella turcica was easily visualized on plain film radiography,[36] but he subsequently began to treat arteriovenous malformations based on angiographic images.[37]

CONTEMPORARY RADIATION DELIVERY SYSTEMS

Gamma Knife Radiosurgery

The Gamma Knife was pioneered by Dr. Leksell in the late 1960s, and became the first available commercial radiosurgery unit. The unit, as currently constructed, contains 201 fixed

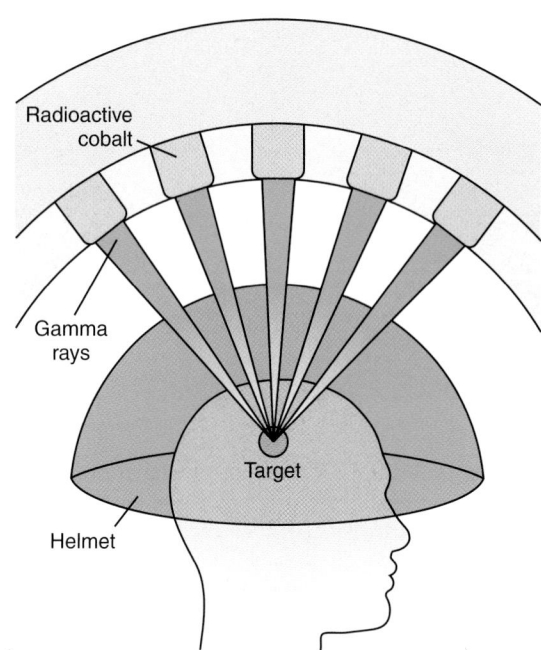

FIGURE 45.3 Schematic depiction of Gamma Knife radiation of an intracranial target. Sources in the primary collimator generate γ-rays, which penetrate through holes in the secondary collimator helmet to converge on a target from multiple directions. This convergence maximizes dose at the isocenter. *(Adapted from National Regulatory Commission file photo.)*

sources of ^{60}Co distributed in a hemisphere, each of which is a thin rod with the long axis oriented along the radius of the sphere, converging on a single point, called the *treatment isocenter* (Fig. 45.3). These sources are surrounded by a primary collimator, which directs the beams. A series of secondary collimators, or "helmets," are available with either 4-, 8-, 14-, or 18-mm diameter holes, which can be chosen based on the desired size of the beams to be produced (Fig. 45.4). This secondary collimation determines the width of the radiation beams at the isocenter. By occluding certain collimator holes, the dose distribution can be altered to produce the desired shape and to protect normal structures. Newer models of the Gamma Knife allow for intensity modulation, which can produce more conformal dose distributions.

For radiosurgery, the Leksell frame is attached to the patient, and then a planning CT scan is performed and is uploaded to the treatment planning software. Once a plan is developed, the frame is attached to the treatment couch. The patient is then inserted into the unit, and the frame is positioned relative to the collimator helmet so that the treatment isocenter is aligned with the planned target isocenter. Because there are no moving parts during treatment, there is a high degree of setup accuracy. The dose to be delivered, along with the activity of the sources, determines the length of the treatment time. If multiple isocenters are used, the patient is repositioned relative to the secondary collimator, and the rest of the isocenters are treated. The half-life of ^{60}Co is 5.3 years, and the sources need to be replaced periodically so that treatment times do not become impractical for patients. Dose rates fall 1% per month with ^{60}Co treatment devices.

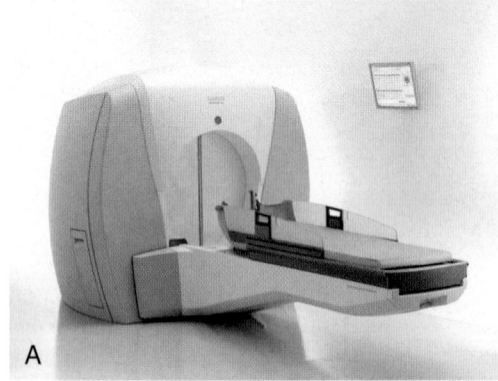
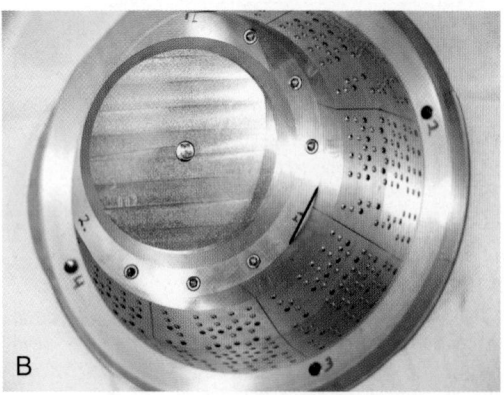

FIGURE 45.4 **A.** The Gamma Knife Perfexion unit. The radioactive sources are contained within the shielded housing. **B.** One of the helmet collimators that is used to create the desired dose distribution. *(Image courtesy of Elekta AB.)*

The Gamma Knife produces a very sharp dose gradient, with the highest dose at the treatment isocenter. Because the prescription dose is at the surface of the volume to be treated, which usually corresponds to the 50% isodose line, the result is that the dose at the treatment isocenter is usually at least 50% higher than the prescription dose. This dose heterogeneity can be helpful if it is present at the center of a malignant lesion, but can be troublesome if there are concerns about tissue necrosis. Although the dose distribution for a single isocenter is spherical, multiple isocenters can be used in an overlapping fashion to create an irregularly shaped volume. The drawback to this approach is that the dose heterogeneity is increased across the lesion.

Linac-Based Radiosurgery

As described earlier, the linac uses microwave energy to accelerate electrons into a therapeutic energy range, and those electrons are used to generate high-energy photons. For radiosurgery, the linac has a secondary collimator attached to the treatment head with a cone-shaped aperture of a specific size, which can be varied based on the size and shape of the lesion to be treated. To produce a dose distribution similar to that of the Gamma Knife, an approach using converging noncoplanar arcs of radiation was adopted[38] (Fig. 45.5).

A stereotactic frame, most commonly the Brown-Roberts-Wells (BRW) frame, is placed on the patient, with four pins securing the frame to the skull. The frame has three orthogonal axes—coronal, lateral, and axial—which intersect at the center of the circular frame. The CT localizer frame has nine fiducial rods, which appear in each axial CT slice, and provide a precise correlation between the axes on the frame and any anatomical point on the CT scan. The frame attaches to the CT simulation couch in a similar manner to the linac treatment couch, so that patient setup is identical in the simulator and the treatment unit. The target is outlined on the CT scan, along with any critical normal structures. MRI scans are often fused with the planning CT scan to facilitate target and normal tissue identification.[39]

Treatment planning software is used to define 3 to 6 arcs converging on the treatment isocenter, which will result in a high dose at the convergence point, with rapid falloff in any given direction away from treatment isocenter (Fig. 45.6). Because arcs are used, the high-dose volume is usually more ellipsoid than a similar sized volume treated by Gamma Knife.

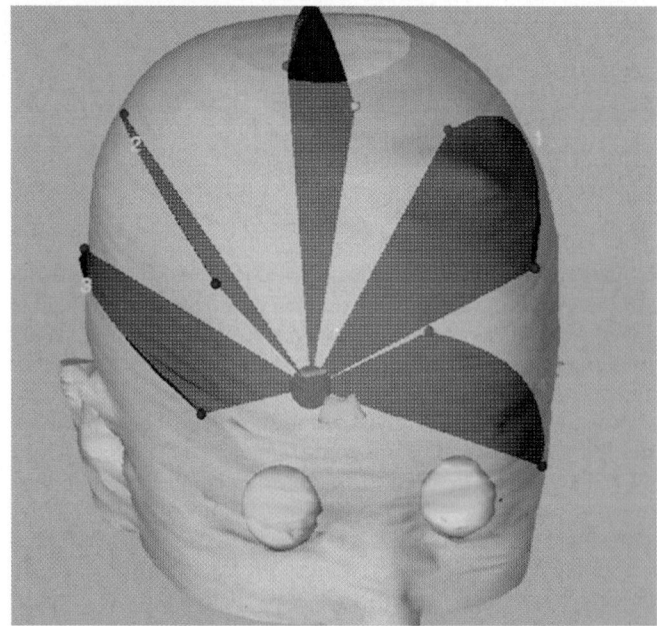

FIGURE 45.5 Example of a linac-based stereotactic radiosurgery (SRS) treatment plan. Five noncoplanar arcs are depicted converging on the treatment isocenter. The eyes and the optic chiasm are also seen as three-dimensional (3D) reconstructed objects so that the treatment planner is aware of these critical normal structures during treatment planning. *(Image courtesy of Kevin Beaudette, MSc.)*

As the number of arcs and the total degrees subtended by each arc increase, the dose to normal tissue decreases, as it is spread out over a larger volume.

When the plan is formed, the patient, with the frame still attached to the skull, is brought to the treatment room, and the frame is attached to the treatment couch. The isocenter of the treatment machine is aligned to the origin of the axes of the stereotactic frame, with an accuracy of less than 1 mm. The treatment isocenter is then aligned with the machine's isocenter. The gantry rotates during the treatment to produce an arc. After the arc is delivered, the couch can be moved and a new arc created. The end result is that multiple arcs converge on a single point. For irregular volumes, multiple isocenters can be used, similar to those used by the Gamma Knife. When all of the planned arcs are treated, the frame is removed, and the patient can usually return home.

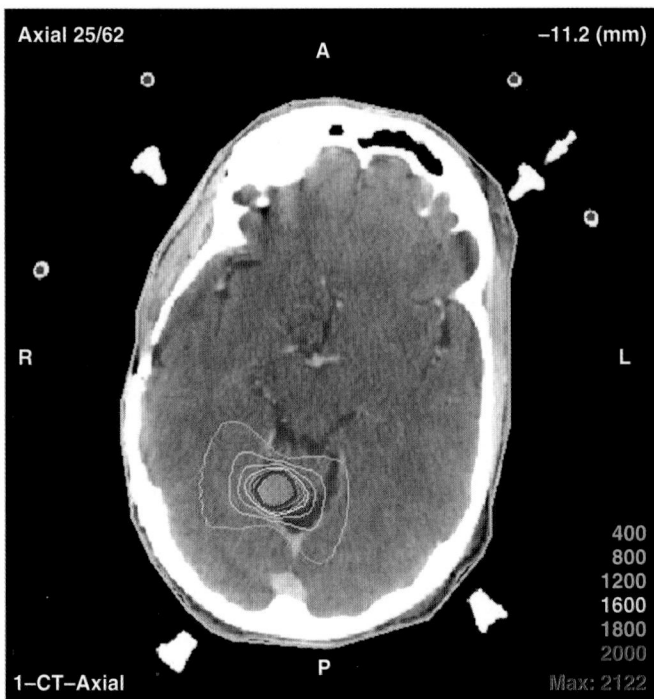

Axial 25/62
A
−11.2 (mm)

R

L

400
800
1200
1600
1800
2000

1−CT−Axial
P
Max: 2122

FIGURE 45.6 Example of linac-based stereotactic radiosurgery (SRS) dosimetry. This image shows a representative axial computed tomography (CT) scan slice with a metastatic lesion in the upper cerebellum. Each colored line, known as an *isodose line*, outlines the area receiving at least the indicated dose. The dose is highest at the center of the target, and falls off rapidly with increasing distance from the isocenter. The directions of less rapid falloff depend on the configuration of the arcs used in the treatment plan. *(Image courtesy of Kevin Beaudette, MSc.)*

One of the more recent advances in SRS is the "frameless" radiosurgery system, which does not require an invasive head frame to be fixed to the patient's cranium. Because conventional SRS required frame placement at the beginning of planning, the patient would often wear the head frame for the entire 5 to 8 hours required for planning and treatment. A number of centers have switched to noninvasive systems that are much more comfortable for the patient, including a thermoplastic mask combined with a dental mold with infrared fiducial markers,[40] or use of orthogonal diagnostic energy x-rays to verify patient setup and positioning. The other advantage of the frameless approach is that the planning and treatment can be done on separate days, which facilitates patient and physician scheduling. These approaches have been adopted at a number of centers, and in some preliminary studies appear to be of similar accuracy and clinical efficacy as conventional radiosurgery.[41] However, there are some concerns that it may not be as accurate as conventional frames, and a planning margin of 1 to 2 mm is sometimes used to ensure target coverage.[42] Thus, this approach has not been universally adopted, and is still under investigation.

Other recent developments in linac-based radiosurgery include the development of special radiosurgical linacs, of which the Novalis Tx is the most common. These linear accelerators can use cone-shaped collimators like conventional linac-based radiosurgery, but also have a multileaf collimator

with small leaf size, allowing for very fine shaping of the radiation beam. These MLCs can be used for intensity-modulated radiation therapy (IMRT), in which the leaves attenuate the radiation beam to varying amounts in different areas of the radiation portal. The radiation is then delivered using a set of static (i.e., not arc) fields, with each field having a different intensity pattern. This technique allows for a much more conformal dose distribution, and can be especially useful in the treatment of irregular lesions. Furthermore, using IMRT, these specialized units can use a single isocenter to treat multiple lesions, which reduces treatment time for the patient. Initial planning studies suggest that the use of IMRT for radiosurgery rather than convergent arcs may allow for increased sparing of normal tissue receiving 50% of the prescription dose, and allows for more precise shaping around critical structures.[43] The downside of the IMRT approach is that there is more low-dose radiation given to normal brain, and the long-term consequences of this low-dose irradiation are still unknown.

Newer technologies for linac-based radiosurgery are on the horizon, including tomotherapy and volumetric arc therapy (VMAT), which deliver radiation in continuous arcs, similar to a CT scan. In these types of radiation therapies, the radiation is delivered in continuous arcs on a slice-by-slice basis as the patient is moved through the unit. Planning studies suggest that both tomotherapy and VMAT offer improved conformal dose delivery, but may result in larger areas of low-dose radiation to normal tissue,[44] although this area is still under investigation.[45]

Robotic Radiosurgery

The last major development in photon radiosurgery is the development of the Cyberknife, in which a miniaturized linac is mounted on a robotic arm with 6 degrees of rotational freedom (Fig. 45.7). The linac produces 6-MeV x-rays, and is equipped with either swappable collimators of specific sizes or with a variable collimator that is adjustable to different sizes during the course of treatment. The linac and robotic arm combination can deliver multiple small beamlets of radiation from many different angles to produce a conformal dose plan. The Cyberknife is combined with an in-room diagnostic x-ray unit that takes images of the patient during the treatment, and can be used to modify the treatment plan in real time if there is any change in patient positioning. Thus, there is no need for an invasive frame, and immobilization with a thermoplastic mask is sufficient to achieve the required accuracy.

The treatment plan is created from a large selection of possible robotic arm positions and possible locations within the tumor. Because the individual beamlets are small, each spot within the tumor can receive a different amount of radiation from each arm position, resulting in a conformality similar to that with IMRT. With a variable collimator, even more treatment options are available from each possible angle. Thus, the Cyberknife offers a very conformal dose plan, but the use of multiple small beams can result in lengthy treatment times for large, irregularly shaped lesions.

Proton Beam Radiosurgery

All of the methods outlined previously use photon radiation, but recently there has been a growing interest in using proton radiotherapy. As discussed earlier, protons provide a dosimetric advantage relative to photons owing to the concentration of energy at the Bragg peak and the lack of exit dose. The result is that the integral dose to the normal brain is lower than that for photon radiosurgery. The early radiosurgical approach adopted by Dr. Leksell in the 1950s used a cross-fire technique, in which opposed beams were directed at the target, but the Bragg peak fell outside the patient.[34] This approach was used because it was felt that the uncertainty of the dose at the Bragg peak could result in failure to provide adequate dose to the target. However, the team at the Harvard Cyclotron Laboratory, led by Dr. Kjellberg, began to perform Bragg peak radiosurgery beginning in 1961.[46] Over the past two decades, there has been a growth in the number of dedicated hospital-based proton therapy sites, beginning with Loma Linda University in 1990, followed by the Massachusetts General Hospital (MGH) in 2001. More recently, a number of centers are opening across the country as interest has increased in proton therapy.

For proton SRS, the immobilization and localization are similar to those used in various other radiosurgical setups. At the MGH, patients receiving proton SRS undergo placement of three radiopaque fiducial markers in the outer table of the skull with local anesthesia as an outpatient procedure. These markers, along with key points of bony anatomy of the skull, create a fixed axis system similar in concept to that created by BRW head frames used in photon radiosurgery.

For treatment planning, if the patient has good dentition, the patient is immobilized in either a modified Gill-Thomas-Cosman (GTC) frame, which consists of a custom occipital headrest and a custom bite block connected by a ring similar to a conventional head frame. If the patient has poor dentition, or has a low-lying tumor, a thermoplastic mask with polyfoam is created for immobilization. This is a marginally less accurate form of immobilization, but pretreatment imaging can correct for initial setup misalignments. With either form of immobilization, a CT scan is obtained with the patient immobilized, and the target and critical normal structures are contoured.

Creation of a proton radiosurgery plan typically uses 1 to 4 conformal portals. Because protons do not have an exit dose, fields can enter the body through a wider range of angles compared to photon arcs (e.g., from the vertex), because the protons will not exit through the rest of the body. The proton range is very sensitive to the tissue density through which the beam passes, and thus attempts are made to avoid sinuses or other air cavities. The energy of the proton beam is modulated to create an SOBP, which can be used to cover targets that are larger than the width of the single Bragg peak. For each field, a custom brass aperture is created to define the field edges, and a Lucite compensator is created to define the distal edge of the Bragg peak (Fig. 45.8).

In the treatment room, the setup and positioning are verified with diagnostic x-rays that confirm the position of the fiducial markers in relation to the bony anatomy of the skull. Some patients are treated using a rotational gantry similar to that of a linac. At the MGH, where one of the treatment rooms has a fixed beamline, some patients are treated in a device known as STAR (stereotactic alignment for radiosurgery), which has greater ability to move and rotate the patient around a fixed beamline (Fig. 45.9). The fixed beam allows for treatment with a slightly higher degree of accuracy as compared to a rotational gantry because the weight of the gantry can result in some positional uncertainty.

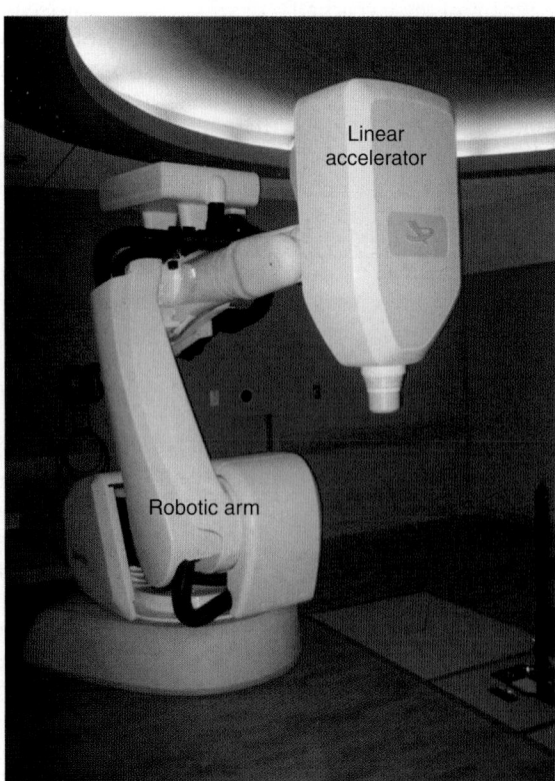

FIGURE 45.7 A Cyberknife robotic radiosurgical unit. The linear accelerator is mounted on a robotic arm, allowing for multiple beam angles.

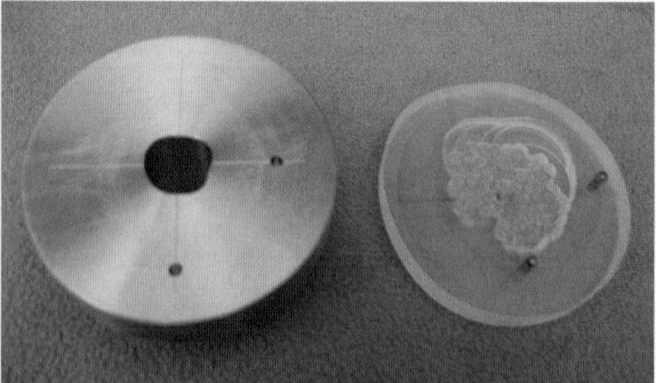

FIGURE 45.8 Brass apertures and Lucite range compensator produced for proton radiotherapy. The brass aperture (on the left) defines the edges of a given stereotactic radiosurgery (SRS) field. The range compensator (on the right) determines the distal edge of the Bragg peak. Custom milling of the compensator creates areas of varying thickness of Lucite. The thicker areas of the compensator result in a Bragg peak closer to the surface, and the thinner areas result in a deeper Brag peak. Thus, the milling pattern determines the shape of the distal edge of the field. *(Image courtesy of Marc Bussiere, MSc.)*

In general, proton radiosurgery results in a very conformal plan, with much less dose inhomogeneity compared to photon-based radiosurgery (Fig. 45.10). These homogeneous plans are desirable for heterogeneous lesions that contain normal tissues such that excessive dose is not wanted. This can be more advantageous than photon plans that produce unacceptable hot spots either within or outside the intended target. The second major advantage of proton radiosurgery is the lack of exit dose, which means that the treatment results in less radiation to the normal brain. Although the risks of low-dose irradiation of normal brain cannot yet be quantified, avoiding this possible complication is desirable.

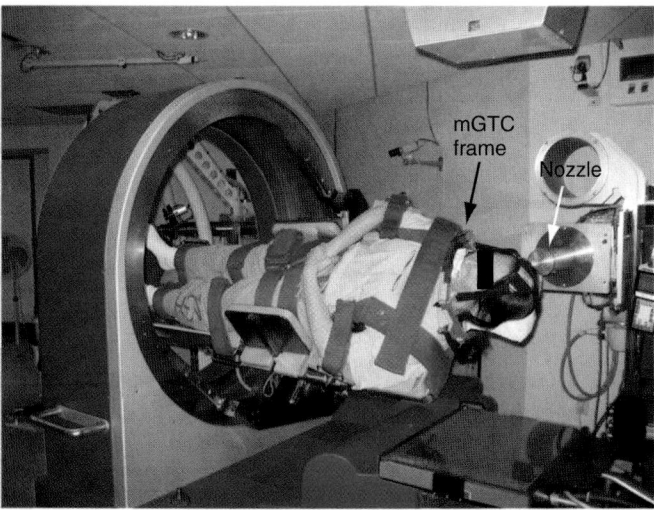

FIGURE 45.9 Stereotactic alignment for radiosurgery (STAR) unit used for proton radiosurgery with a volunteer positioned for treatment. This unit immobilizes and positions the patient, and can be used for stereotactic radiosurgery (SRS) with a fixed proton beamline. The nozzle is the exit point for the protons from the beamline. The modified Gill-Thomas-Cosman (mGTC) frame is used for patient immobilization.

Evaluation and Comparison of Radiosurgery Techniques

The evaluation of radiosurgical plans relies on a few parameters, which have been defined by ASTRO.[47] Key components to evaluate include the ratio between the maximum dose (MD) and the peripheral dose (PD), which gives a sense of the dose homogeneity within the treatment volume. The second key parameter is the ratio between the prescription isodose volume (PIV), which is the total volume that receives at least the prescription dose, and the target volume (TV), which is the volume of the target defined on planning CT scan. This PIV/TV ratio is a measure of target coverage and dose conformality.

Analysis of the Radiation Therapy Oncology Group (RTOG) 90-05 study, a multicenter phase II dose escalation study for SRS of brain metastases, revealed some interesting data regarding both Gamma Knife and linac-based radiosurgery. For Gamma Knife, 94% of the plans had an MD/PD ratio greater than 2, versus only 7% of the linac-based plans.[48] These data suggest that the Gamma Knife plans are less homogeneous and more prone to hot spots at the center of the treatment volume. However, it was noted that increasing the number of isocenters used for a given Gamma Knife treatment plan resulted in MD/PD ratios that were more similar to those with linac-based radiosurgery. Current RTOG protocols use a guideline of an MD/PD ratio of less than 2 to qualify as treatment "per protocol."[49]

In contrast, the results for the PIV/TV ratio were more favorable for Gamma Knife radiosurgery compared to linac-based radiosurgery. Seventy-seven percent of Gamma Knife plans had a PIV/TV ratio between 1 and 2, with no plans less than 1 or greater than 4. Conversely, only 51% of linac plans had a ratio between 1 and 2, and 10% of plans had a ratio less than 1 and 7% had a ratio greater than 4.[48,50] These data suggest that the conformality of plans with Gamma Knife were superior to those produced with linac-based radiosurgery. The RTOG currently recommends a PIV/TV ratio between 1 and 2 as a standard for SRS.[49]

Although there are differences between plan characteristics, it is important to recognize that there do not appear to be

FIGURE 45.10 Representative dose plan of proton stereotactic radiosurgery (SRS) compared to photon SRS. This is a coronal image of a patient with three atypical meningiomas being treated with SRS. The plan on the left shows a proton plan, where one can see that there is no exit dose from the beams used. The plan on the right shows a photon SRS approach, where there is a larger area of low dose given to normal brain tissue. *(Image courtesy of Marc Bussiere, MSc.)*

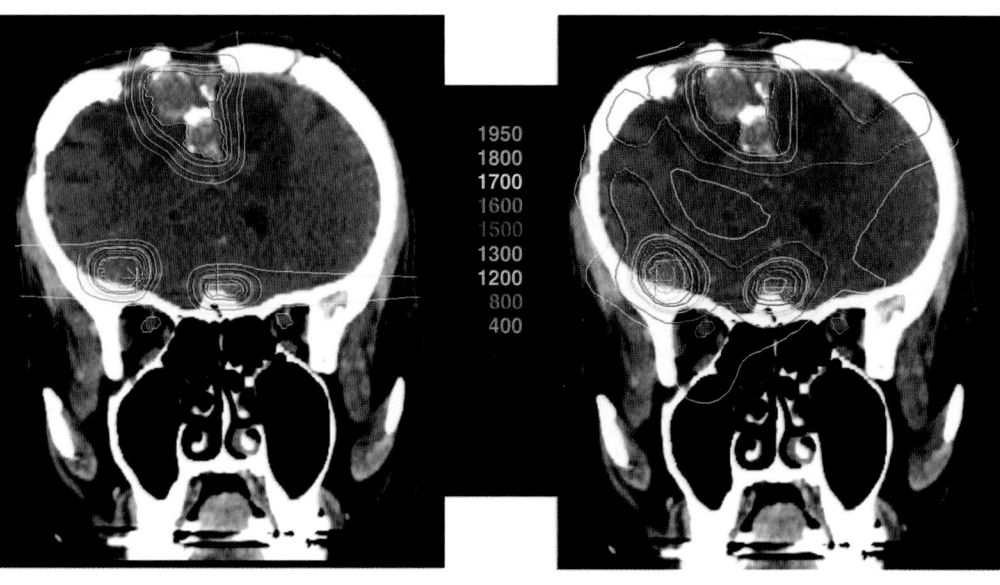

clinical differences in efficacy or toxicity between radiosurgical modalities. Initially, during the development of linac-based radiosurgery, there was some concern that it would prove to be inferior to the Gamma Knife. Multivariate analysis of the RTOG 90-05 study showed that treatment with a linac was associated with an increased risk of local failure, with a hazard ratio of 2.85. The explanation put forward in the paper was that the higher MD/PD ratio and better PIV/TV ratio seen with the Gamma Knife plans resulted in better tumor control compared to linac-based plans. However, proponents of linac-based SRS suggested that this difference could also be due to the fact that Gamma Knife radiosurgery accounted for only 30% of the patients, and was limited to two clinical centers with significant radiosurgical experience, which is difficult to compare to the 70% of treatments performed in 15 institutions with varying degrees of experience with SRS. This hypothesis gained support with data from the RTOG 95-08 study, which randomized patients with one to three brain metastases to receive whole-brain radiotherapy with or without an SRS boost. In this study, there were very few major deviations from the MD/PD and PIV/TV ratios specified by the RTOG with either linac-based radiosurgery or with Gamma Knife, and there was no survival difference based on the type of radiosurgical unit used.[51] Thus, the data suggest that when appropriate radiosurgical guidelines are followed, these two modes of SRS are functionally equivalent.

Fractionated Stereotactic Radiotherapy

Although the radiosurgical literature centers on single fraction radiosurgery for intracranial targets, there has been a growing interest in fractionating therapy based on the radiobiological advantages outlined here. Thus, several groups became interested in applying the immobilization and localization devices used in radiosurgical procedures with fractionated radiation to reduce the risk of late complications. The biggest challenge in fSRT is the reproducibility of positioning the patient daily such that the targeting accuracy is maintained. Most of the immobilization methods described here, especially the fixed head frame, were not suitable for multiday usage, although some groups have tried this approach.[52] One of the most common solutions to this problem was to replace the pins in the head frame with a bite block/dental mold, and an occipital plate to hold the head in position, which became known as the Gill-Thomas-Cosman (GTC) frame.[53] This approach is well tolerated for both children and adults with intracranial tumors.[54] These approaches have been adopted with all of the technologies described earlier, including IMRT, Cyberknife, and proton radiotherapy. However, because of technical challenges, reports of fractionated therapy with Gamma Knife are much rarer.

SUMMARY

Radiation therapy is a noninvasive approach to treatment of benign and malignant intracranial disease, which takes advantage of the high-energy portion of the electromagnetic spectrum to deposit damaging energy within tumors or other malformations in the central nervous system. Radiosurgery involves the administration of a high dose of radiation therapy in a single or a few fractions to result in destruction of the target. Photons or protons can both be adapted for radiosurgical use. Photon radiosurgery is more common, although proton radiosurgery is growing in popularity owing to its favorable dose profile and lower integral dose to the patient. The most common photon radiosurgery devices are the Gamma Knife, the linac, and the Cyberknife, all of which offer similar clinical efficacy, with some differences in dose distribution and patient/physician comfort issues. Proton radiosurgery is increasingly available, and offers similar efficacy as photon radiosurgery, with the potential for lower integral dose to the patient. Fractionated radiotherapy offers the physical advantages of dose localization due to the use of stereotactic techniques, and can combine some of the radiobiological advantage of fractionation, which helps to reduce the risk of late side effects such as cranial neuropathy. Radiosurgery is a constantly evolving field, and the technical aspects of radiation delivery will continue to advance to maximize dose to the intended target, and minimize dose to normal tissue.

SELECTED KEY REFERENCES

Andrews DW, Scott CB, Sperduto PW, et al. Whole brain radiation therapy with or without stereotactic radiosurgery boost for patients with one to three brain metastases: phase III results of the RTOG 9508 randomised trial. *Lancet.* 2004;363:1665-1672.

Khan FM. *The Physics of Radiation Therapy.* 3rd ed. Philadelphia: Lippincott Williams & Wilkins; 2003.

Lutz W, Winston KR, Maleki N. A system for stereotactic radiosurgery with a linear accelerator. *Int J Radiat Oncol Biol Phys.* 1988;14:373-381.

Shaw E, Scott C, Souhami L, et al. Single dose radiosurgical treatment of recurrent previously irradiated primary brain tumors and brain metastases: final report of RTOG protocol 90-05. *Int J Radiat Oncol Biol Phys.* 2000;47:291-298.

Thames HD, Bentzen SM, Turesson I, et al. Fractionation parameters for human tissues and tumors. *Int J Radiat Biol.* 1989;56:701-710.

Please go to expertconsult.com to view the complete list of references.

CHAPTER 46
Radiosurgery of Central Nervous System Tumors

Douglas Kondziolka, Ajay Niranjan, L. Dade Lunsford, John C. Flickinger

CLINICAL PEARLS

- Randomized clinical trials confirm the survival benefit of stereotactic radiosurgery for patients with single brain metastases and the local control benefit for patients with multiple (two to four) tumors.

- Four matched cohort studies (class II evidence) that compare Gamma Knife radiosurgery to resection for patients with acoustic neuromas less than 2.5 cm in diameter show improved outcomes after radiosurgery

- with lower morbidity rate. Indications for microsurgery at institutions with radiosurgery expertise include disabling symptomatic brainstem compression, severe headache, hydrocephalus, trigeminal neuralgia, and patient choice.

- Long-term data are available over the past 10 years from numerous institutions on the value of stereotactic radiosurgery for different benign intracranial tumors.

Stereotactic radiosurgery (SRS) has become one of the most important concepts in the management of patients with central nervous system tumors. The neurosurgeon uses SRS to destroy a tumor using precise, image-guided ionizing irradiation in a single procedure.[1] Over the past two decades, radiosurgery has supplanted fractionated radiation therapy in the care of many tumors, and has forced an evolution of thinking regarding the roles of resection or observation. At a biological level, radiosurgery can halt cell division, cause vascular occlusion, induce apoptosis or necrosis, and affect blood-brain barrier integrity.[2-6]

Radiosurgical devices include the cobalt-60 Gamma Knife, modified linear accelerator systems, and charged particle generators.[7-10] Although initially designed for functional neurosurgery, the use of brain tumor radiosurgery took off in the era of higher-resolution parenchymal brain imaging with magnetic resonance imaging (MRI). Now robotic devices such as the Perfexion or model 4C gamma units or the Cyberknife facilitate dose planning and delivery.[11,12] For use in the brain, accuracy and reliability are crucial. At present no pharmacological agents are used to modify the target response to radiosurgery.[13,14] A listing of indications is shown in Table 46.1.

The first two patients treated with the Gamma Knife in Sweden had tumors (a craniopharyngioma and a pituitary adenoma). Typically, radiosurgery has been used for smaller tumors that do not cause significant disability from mass effect. The question of maximum tumor size is asked commonly. The answer depends not only on the tumor volume, often estimated by tumor diameter, but on the degree of mass effect and any related symptoms. A dose reduction used for a larger tumor may lead to a relatively ineffective total dose.

On the other hand, failure to decrease the dose for larger volumes can lead to an unacceptable risk of adverse radiation effects (ARE).

Not all radiosurgery systems are the same and they differ in both hardware and software. One should seek a system that allows the surgeon to efficiently create highly conformal and selective volumetric dose plans for irregular lesion volumes, because tumors are rarely "spherical."[15] The steep falloff of radiation into the surrounding structures (selectivity) helps to achieve safety. The location of many tumors either within or adjacent to critical brain or nerve makes the requirement for conformal and selective radiosurgery paramount.

RADIOSURGERY OR RADIOTHERAPY?

Fractionated stereotactic irradiation has been used by some centers to treat benign tumors,[16,17] and of course, large-field conventional or whole-brain radiotherapy has been used for decades. Any advantage for the use of fractionated radiotherapy becomes important when large volumes of sensitive surrounding normal tissue need to be included in the treatment volume, such as with the standard 2-cm margin around a malignant glioma. If the volume of normal tissue irradiated inside or outside the target volume is small, then fractionated radiation may be of no additional value. Certain tumors appear to be more resistant to traditional radiotherapy and include meningiomas, schwannomas, and some metastatic tumors such as melanoma, sarcoma, and renal cell carcinoma. The radiobiological response can be addressed with the α/β ratio. A lower number refers to later responding tissue.[18-20]

TABLE 46.1 Applications for Gamma Knife Radiosurgery for Brain Tumors*

Diagnosis	Number of Procedures
Vestibular schwannoma	1439
Trigeminal schwannoma	45
Other schwannomas	65
Meningioma	1377
Pituitary tumor	300
Craniopharyngioma	76
Hemangioblastoma	50
Hemangiopericytoma	41
Glomus tumor	24
Pineocytoma	16
Malignant pineal tumor	13
Chordoma	31
Chondrosarcoma	25
Choroid plexus papilloma	12
Hemangioma	7
Glioblastoma multiforme	349
Anaplastic astrocytoma	134
Fibrillary astrocytoma	43
Mixed glioma	78
Pilocytic astrocytoma	89
Ependymoma	74
Medulloblastoma	24
CNS lymphoma	12
Hypothalamic hamartoma	6
Brain metastasis	3264
Invasive skull base tumor	32
Other tumors	66
Total	7692

*Data from clinical series at the University of Pittsburgh: total procedures = 10,158; total brain tumors = 7692.
CNS, central nervous system.

VESTIBULAR SCHWANNOMAS

The goals of vestibular schwannoma radiosurgery are to prevent tumor growth, preserve cochlear and other cranial nerve function, maintain general function and quality of life, and avoid the risks associated with open surgical resection. Available long-term data have established radiosurgery as an important alternative to resection. Radiosurgery was first offered to patients who were elderly or medically infirm, but with experience, was found ideal for patients of all ages.[21-24] We have found consistent results across age groups.[21,25]

To date we have managed 1397 patients with vestibular schwannomas using Gamma Knife radiosurgery (Fig. 46.1). The mean patient age in our series was 57 years (range, 12 to 95). Eight percent had neurofibromatosis (93 patients). Symptoms before radiosurgery included hearing loss (92%), balance symptoms or ataxia (51%), tinnitus (43%), or other neurological deficit (19.5%). Thirty-four percent of our patients had useful hearing, Gardner-Robertson grade I (speech discrimination score ≥70%; pure tone average ≤30 dB) or grade II (speech discrimination score ≥50%; pure tone average ≤50 dB). Since 1992, the average dose prescribed to the tumor margin was 13 Gy. The 50% isodose line was used in 90% of patients.

Our long-term study documented a 98% clinical tumor control rate (no requirement for surgical intervention) at

5 to 10 years.[21,23] Since the institution of MRI-guided dose planning, there has been a significant reduction in morbidity.[26,27] Currently, the risk for any grade delayed facial nerve dysfunction is below 1%.[26,27] Patients with useful hearing before radiosurgery continue to report an approximate 75% overall rate for maintenance of useful hearing, depending on tumor size, with even better results for intracanalicular tumors.[27-29] In comparison studies, radiosurgery has been shown to be a cost-effective alternative to microsurgery for these patients.

For smaller tumors, it is likely that more patients now receive radiosurgery as primary care. No randomized clinical trials have been conducted, but there are now four matched cohort studies (class II evidence). These studies evaluated patients with similar sized tumors, and evaluated clinical, imaging, and quality of life outcomes. All showed better results after radiosurgery for most clinical measures, similar results for the symptoms of tinnitus and imbalance, and similar freedom from tumor progression rates.[30-33] It is important to tell patients that there can sometimes be a transient expansion of the tumor capsule after radiosurgery and that it usually can be observed without further treatment.[34,35] The value of radiosurgery in neurofibromatosis type 2 has been studied.[36] Based on these data, we believe that there are few remaining indications for surgical resection in a patient with a small to moderate size tumor. These indications include disabling symptomatic brainstem compression, severe headache, hydrocephalus, trigeminal neuralgia, and patient choice. Radiosurgery has also been performed and evaluated for patients with other cranial nerve schwannomas (Fig. 46.2).

MENINGIOMAS

Radiosurgery has transformed the management of intracranial meningiomas, particularly for tumors of the skull base.[37] As for most indications, radiosurgery was first considered for residual or recurrent tumors after prior resection.[38] The steep radiation falloff can be directly conformed to the well-defined tumor margin. The role of aggressive skull base surgery has waned as reports showing excellent clinical outcomes for small basal tumors have been published.[39,40] Larger tumors with mass effect benefit from subtotal resection followed by radiosurgery if complete resection is not feasible. However, because of their more aggressive nature, atypical or anaplastic/malignant meningiomas (WHO [World Health Organization] grade II or III) are best managed with complete resection followed by fractionated radiotherapy because of their tendency to extend beyond the borders seen on imaging.[41] Radiosurgery also is of value in the setting of incomplete resection.

Our 22-year experience includes 1302 intracranial meningiomas. Recently, we published data from 972 patients with 1045 meningiomas (Fig. 46.3).[42] Half of the patients had undergone a prior resection and the average age was 57 years. Tumor locations included middle fossa (351 patients), posterior fossa (307), convexity (126), anterior fossa (88), parasagittal region (113), or other sites (115). Follow-up over the past 5, 7, 10, and 12 years was obtained in 327, 190, 90, and 41 patients, respectively.

The control rate for patients who had radiosurgery for known WHO grade I (benign) meningiomas (after prior

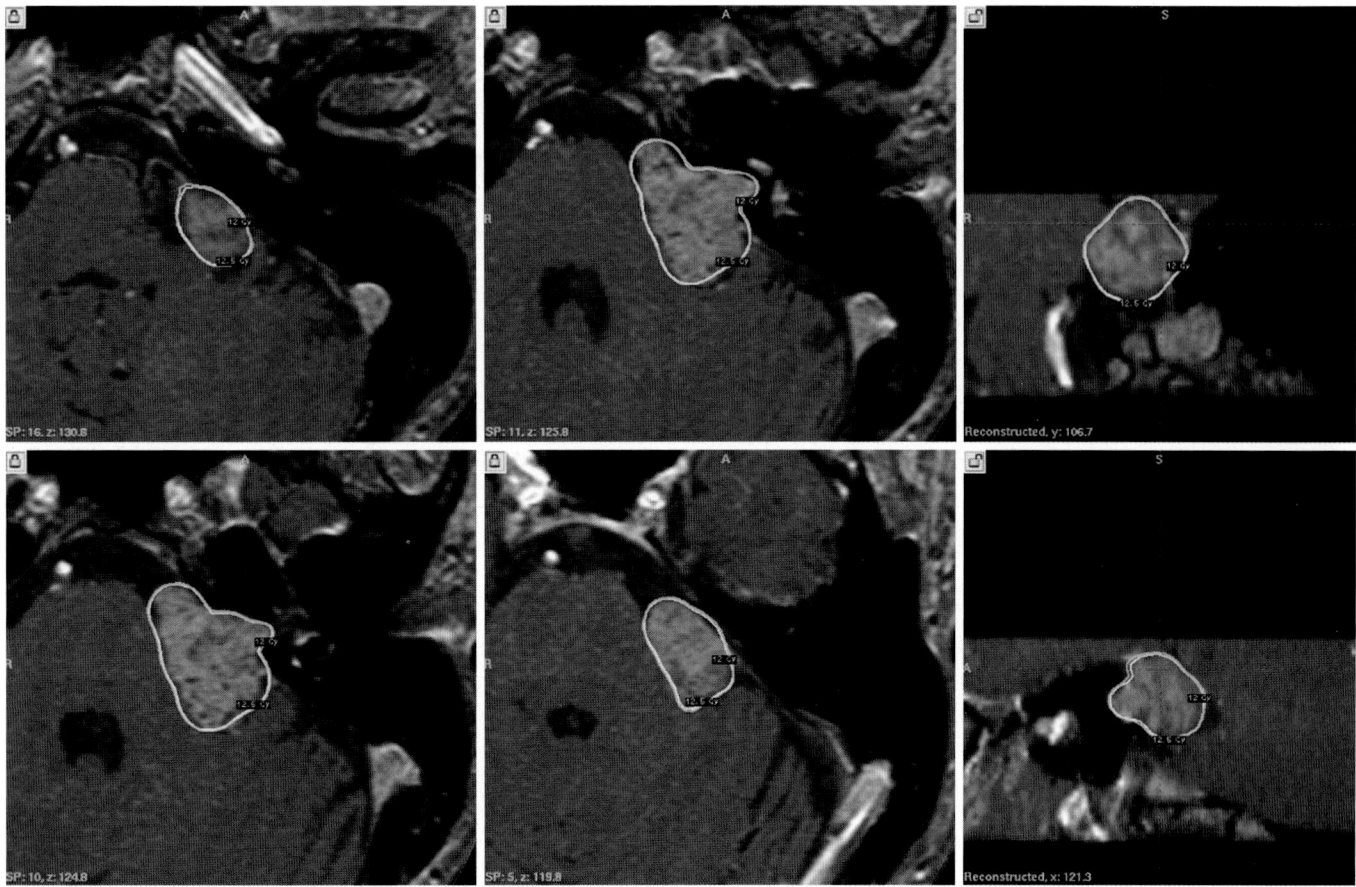

FIGURE 46.1 Magnetic resonance imaging (MRI) showing a Gamma Knife radiosurgery dose plan for a left vestibular schwannoma. The patient received a tumor margin dose of 12.5 Gy.

resection) was 93%. Primary radiosurgery patients (no prior histological confirmation; n = 482), had a tumor control rate of 97%. Adjuvant radiosurgery for patients with WHO grades II and III tumors had tumor control rates of 50% and 17%, respectively. Delayed resection after radiosurgery was performed in 51 patients (5%) at a mean period of 3 years. Additional radiosurgery was performed in 41 patients, usually for new tumors. At 10 years or more, adjuvant grade I tumors were controlled in 91% (n = 53), and primary tumors in 95% (n = 22). There was no case of a subsequent radiation-induced tumor. The morbidity rate was 7.7%. Most centers restrict the dose received by the optic nerve or chiasm to 8 to 9 Gy or less, which should keep the risk for delayed radiation-related optic neuropathy very low.

We believe that SRS has changed meningioma management significantly. Rather than performing a subtotal resection and "following the patient," we now advocate postoperative radiosurgery to reduce the risk of delayed progression.[43-45] We believe this strategy is particularly valuable for younger patients (<75 years). Several longitudinal studies have shown that untreated meningiomas under observation continue to grow over time. We also believe that radiosurgery is the preferred option for a young patient with a critically located small meningioma. No randomized trials comparing radiosurgery to other options have been performed, and all reports represent level 3 evidence.

PITUITARY ADENOMAS

The goal of pituitary adenoma radiosurgery is to arrest the tumor, maintain pituitary and neurological function, and normalize hormonal secretion in case of functional adenomas.[46] We have managed 290 patients with pituitary adenomas. For functional tumor, acromegaly patients typically respond best,[47] with normalization of growth hormone hypersecretion in over 70% of patients, and in approximately half of those with Cushing disease. Follow-up varied from 6 to 102 months (mean 29.5 months); 14 patients had follow-up in excess of 40 months. The mean radiation dose to the tumor margin was 16 Gy.

We found that all patients with microadenomas and 97% of patients with macroadenomas had tumor control after radiosurgery. Gamma Knife radiosurgery was essentially equally effective for control of adenomas with cavernous sinus invasion and suprasellar extension. Endocrine deficits are less common after radiosurgery, although some recent reports with detailed testing show some hormone deficiencies over time. One patient demonstrated tumor growth that resulted in a decline in visual function. A single patient had visual deterioration despite a decrease in tumor size. Advances in dose planning and dose selection facilitated tumor management even when the adenoma was adjacent to the optic apparatus or invaded the cavernous sinus. As for meningiomas, there are

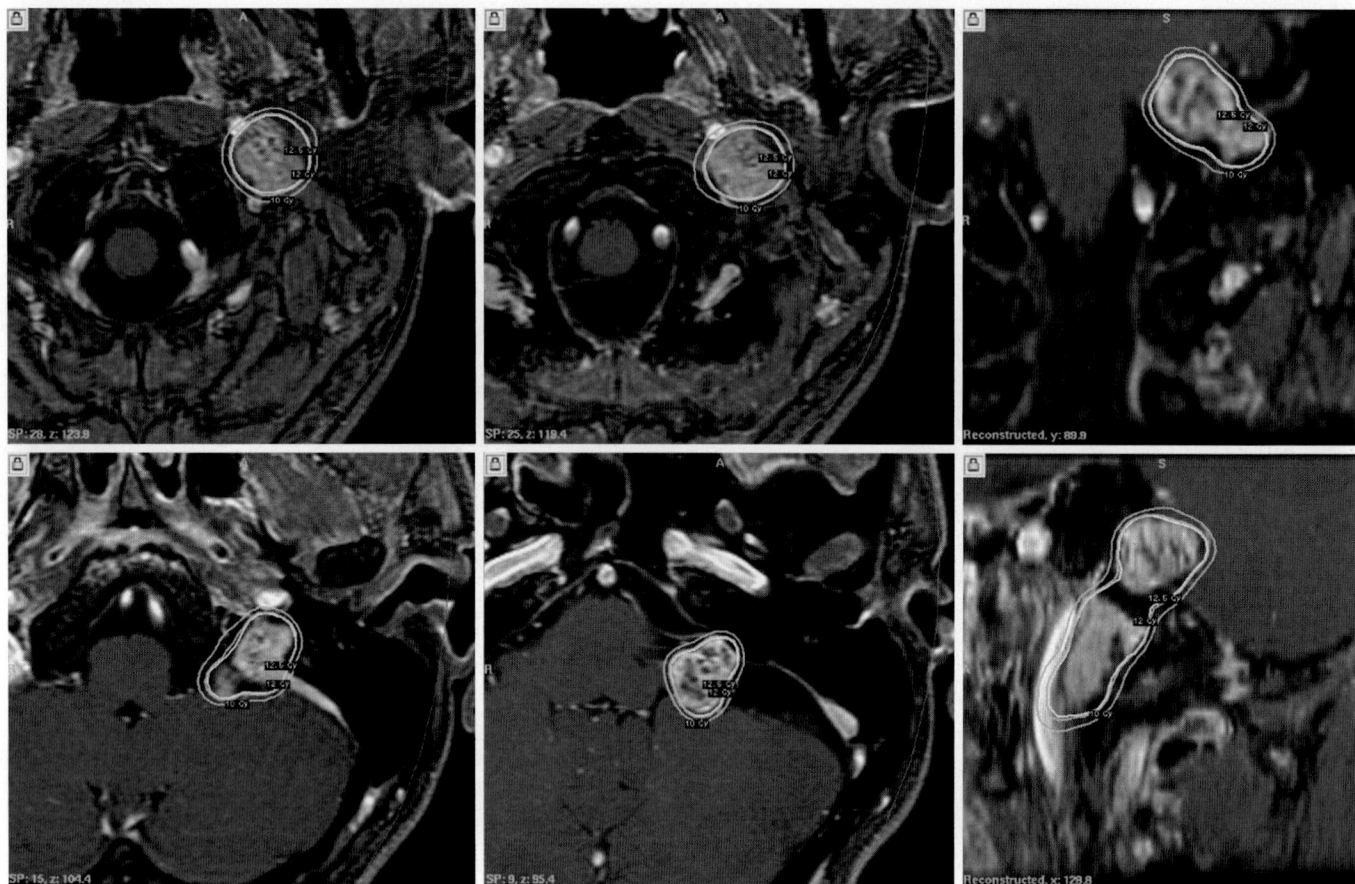

FIGURE 46.2 Magnetic resonance imaging (MRI) at Gamma Knife radiosurgery using the Perfexion unit showing a left jugular foramen schwannoma with intracranial and extracranial extension. The patient presented with mild vocal cord dysfunction. Cranial nerve function was preserved in follow-up.

no class I or II studies. All published reports represent clinical series with class III evidence.

MALIGNANT CRANIAL BASE TUMORS

Malignant tumors of the skull base cause formidable challenges. Such tumors include chordomas, chondrosarcomas, nasopharyngeal carcinomas, or other adenocarcinomas or squamous cell carcinomas from regional structures. To date we have used radiosurgery in 30 patients with chordoma and 22 with chondrosarcoma.[48] In our analysis, the actuarial local tumor control for chondrosarcomas at 5 years was 84.4% ± 10.2%. The overall survival was 84% at a mean of 6.2 years. The actuarial tumor control and survival for chordomas at 10 years was 63.2% ± 10.9%. New techniques in cranial base microsurgery or endoscopic surgery coupled with radiosurgery have improved outcomes.

We also use radiosurgery for residual or recurrent head and neck or metastatic cancers that invade the cranial base. Critical radiosurgical issues include optimal dose planning near the optic apparatus, tumor imaging (sometimes both computed tomography [CT] and MRI may be helpful), and the use of multiple small beam diameters to improve conformality and selectivity. Radiosurgery has important radiobiological advantages over fractionated techniques or brachytherapy

for malignant skull base tumors that can lead to an increased intratumoral cytotoxic effect. Further evaluation will be necessary in larger series of patients to define the response of different tumor histological types. Published reports for these various tumors represent class III or IV evidence.

BRAIN METASTASES

Radiosurgery as the sole approach or as a boost before or after fractionated whole-brain radiotherapy (WBRT) has become a widely practiced treatment for brain metastases (Fig. 46.4). The value of radiosurgery for brain metastases is well reported, including its evaluation in class I studies.[1,49-63] When performed as sole management without WBRT, the goal is tumor control without the potential longer term neurotoxic or cognitive side effects of WBRT.[64] The rationale for radiosurgery used in addition to WBRT is to achieve improved tumor control. For decades, most patients had been managed with WBRT with the goal of simple palliation.[52] Hair loss, fatigue, and delayed cognitive deficits (in longer-term survivors) are noted after WBRT and can adversely impact the patient's quality of life.[65] To achieve better clinical results, neurosurgeons and radiation oncologists have partnered in the evaluation of radiosurgery alone for solitary tumors, or radiosurgery plus WBRT for multiple tumors. In addition, radiosurgery is

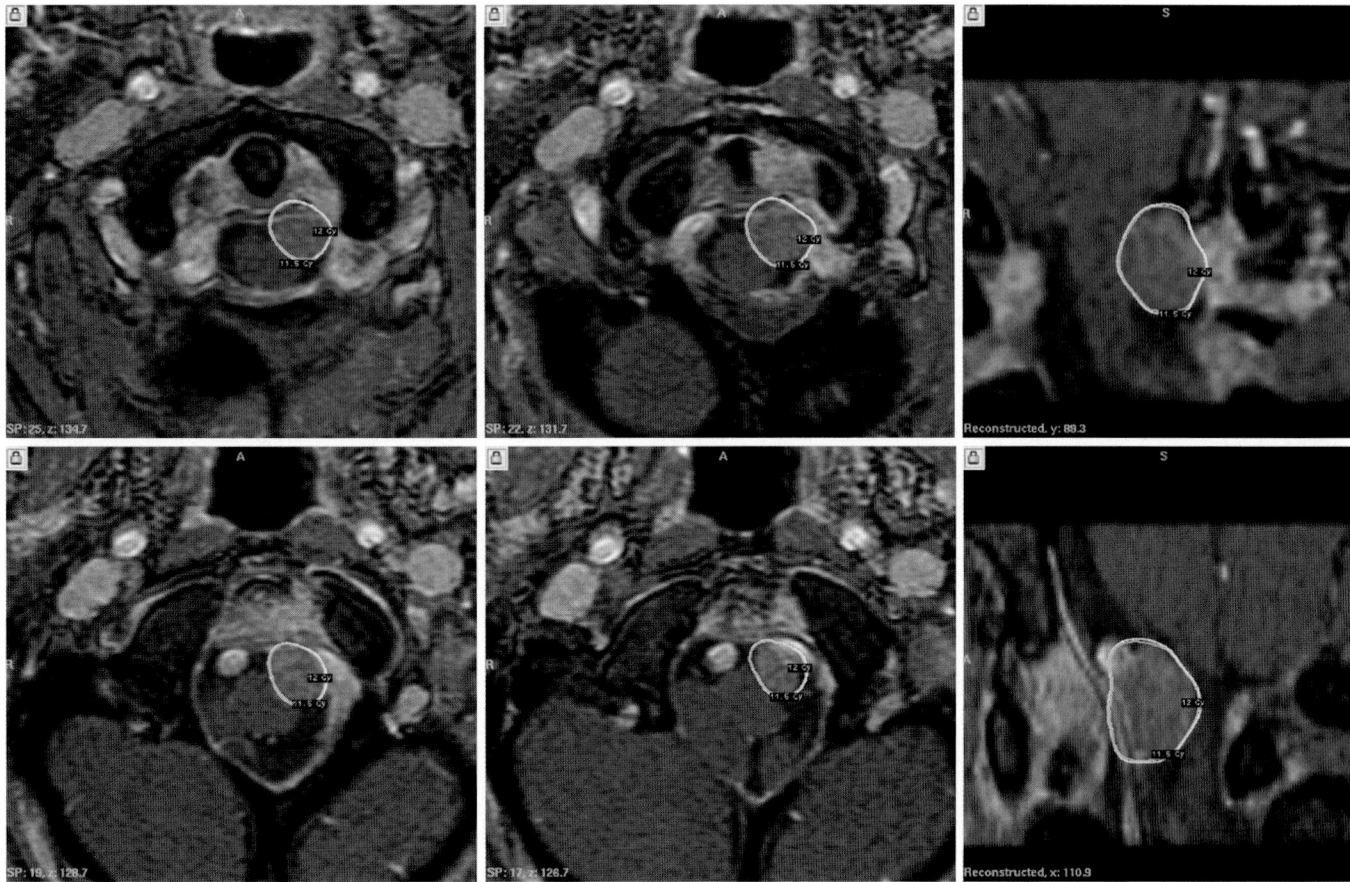

FIGURE 46.3 Magnetic resonance imaging (MRI) during Gamma Knife radiosurgery for a meningioma at the foramen magnum. A margin dose of 11.5 Gy was delivered and led to later tumor regression and no new neurological symptoms.

an attractive concept to medical oncologists because it is effective, is performed as an outpatient, provides excellent local control, palliates symptoms, avoids craniotomy, and can be used in any brain location. To date, the results after radiosurgery plus WBRT appear to be as good as those after surgical resection plus WBRT for "resectable" tumors.[53] Radiosurgery has shown to be more cost effective than any other option. As for other tumor types, patients with large tumors causing mass effect and disabling symptoms should be considered for resection. However, over 50% of brain metastases are now identified in asymptomatic patients, and most are of smaller volume.

We have performed SRS on 3041 patients with brain metastases. Only 10% of these had undergone one or more prior resections. More recently fewer patients have undergone WBRT before referral. Most do not have a disabling neurological deficit and thus the Karnofsky performance score was 100 or 90 in over 90% of patients. The mean tumor volume was 1.7 mL (range 0.1-27 mL). We usually deliver a margin dose of 20 Gy for new tumors and a dose of 16 to 18 Gy for those that had previously been radiated in some way. The tumor margin isodose is selected for the best tumor fit.

Primary tumor locations included lung ($n = 1341$), breast ($n = 563$), melanoma ($n = 502$), kidney ($n = 225$), gastrointestinal tract ($n = 140$), nasopharynx ($n = 30$), sarcoma ($n = 31$), thyroid ($n = 16$), unknown ($n = 72$), and other ($n = 121$). Tumor control rates appear similar across histological types.

The presence of active extracranial cancer activity has become the most important prognostic indicator for survival. The concomitant value of WBRT is minor and does not seem to impact much on survival or local tumor control. However, patients who undergo radiosurgery alone remain at a higher risk for the identification of new small tumors in the initial months of follow-up.

We advocate radiosurgery for patients with multiple brain metastases, whether with active or inactive systemic disease, who remain in good neurological condition. Initially, this paradigm was considered controversial because conventional teaching was that the recognition of more than one metastasis heralded widespread subclinical micrometastases. This concept is no longer valid in the era of double-dose, high-definition MRIs. We conducted a randomized trial that compared radiosurgery plus WBRT to WBRT alone for patients with two to four brain metastases. Improved tumor control was observed when patients received both SRS and WBRT.[65,66] A similar and larger study was conducted by the Radiation Therapy Oncology Group (RTOG).[49] This study and others found that the presence of multiple metastases did not automatically herald the onset of more and more tumors. Thus, patients should continue to be managed aggressively if effective therapies remain for their extracranial cancer.[56] In a recent study, we found that the survival expectation for patients with five to eight tumors was not significantly different from that for patients with two to four tumors, as long as the total tumor

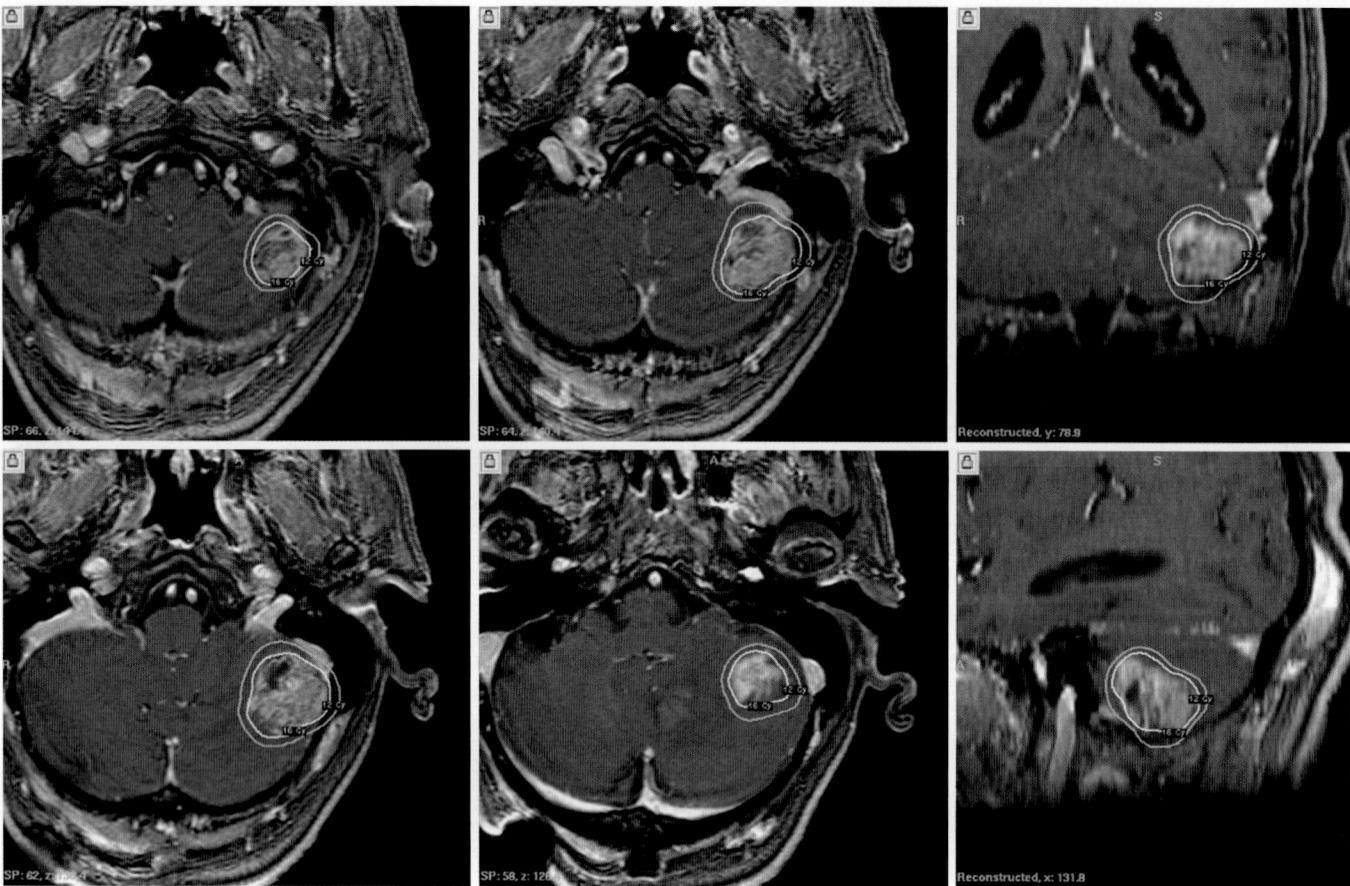

FIGURE 46.4 Magnetic resonance imaging (MRI) during Gamma Knife radiosurgery for a left cerebellar melanoma metastasis. Multiple isocenters were used to deliver a tumor margin dose of 16 Gy. The patient was 20 months from his first radiosurgery procedure for six metastases.

burden was less than 7 mL.[50] Recently, guidelines for the management of brain metastases, including the role of radiosurgery, were published in the *Journal of Neuro-Oncology*.[67] This provides an excellent current summary of the literature regarding radiosurgery, radiotherapy, and resection.

GLIAL NEOPLASMS

For decades, neurosurgeons have tried to maximize the benefits of radiation on glial tumors of the brain.[18,68] Stereotactic brachytherapy with temporary or permanent radioactive isotopes, intracavitary irradiation with colloidal isotopes, and balloon placement of radioactive isotopes have been used. Radiosurgery is a minimally invasive method to boost the radiation effect of fractionated radiotherapy for patients with such tumors.[44,69,70] Radiosurgery has been used mainly for carefully selected patients with residual or deep-seated malignant glial tumors less than 3.5 cm in diameter as part of a multimodality approach. To date, we have performed radiosurgery on 327 patients with glioblastomas and 96 patients with anaplastic astrocytomas. In comparison to patients who received radiotherapy alone, we found that glioblastoma patients had significant prolongation of survival.[66] However, no prospective randomized trial has been completed to study the benefit of boost radiosurgery after radiation therapy for glioblastoma multiforme. There is level one evidence that

evaluated the role of upfront radiosurgery, a concept that was uncommonly practiced. This randomized trial showed no benefit from upfront radiosurgery plus radiotherapy and carmustine, compared to radiotherapy and carmustine alone.[71] We think that radiosurgery is a useful concept for residual or recurrent smaller-volume malignant gliomas after radiation therapy and chemotherapy. It may also be of value at the time of a small volume late recurrence.

The role of radiosurgery for low-grade astrocytomas has been evaluated.[72,73] We have managed 86 patients with pilocytic astrocytomas and 42 with fibrillary astrocytomas. In addition, we cared for 69 patients with mixed gliomas and 19 patients with oligodendrogliomas.[74] Neurocytomas appear to regress impressively after radiosurgery, but the clinical experience is small.[75]

Perhaps the greatest value of glioma radiosurgery so far has been in the management of deep-seated small pilocytic astrocytomas.[76,77] We used SRS in 86 patients whose mean age was 17 years (range, 4-52). Many of these tumors were in the brainstem. Radiosurgery is also used as an alternative to fractionated radiation therapy in the management of patients with residual or recurrent ependymomas, or as additional treatment after tumor recurrence following radiation therapy. To date we have treated 71 patients with ependymomas[78] and 24 patients with medulloblastomas.[79] For all of these tumors, the available literature provides only class III evidence. Table 46.2 summarizes different tumor clinical trials in radiosurgery.

TABLE 46.2 Selected Clinical Trials in Brain Tumor Radiosurgery Treatment

Tumor	Clinical Issue	Evidence Class	Study	Findings
Vestibular schwannoma	Gamma Knife radiosurgery versus resection	2	Pollock et al., 1995[74]	SRS better
Vestibular schwannoma	Gamma Knife radiosurgery versus resection	2	Regis et al., 2002[76]	SRS better
Vestibular schwannoma	Gamma Knife radiosurgery versus resection	2	Myrseth et al., 2005[63]	SRS better
Vestibular schwannoma	Gamma Knife radiosurgery versus resection	2	Pollock et al., 2005[73]	SRS better
Meningioma	Long-term outcomes	3	Kondziolka et al., 2008[37]	Long-term control rates
Metastases	Value in 2-4 tumors	1	Kondziolka et al., 1999[35]	Boost SRS of value
Metastases	Value in 1-4 tumors	1	Andrews et al., 2004[1]	Boost SRS of value for single tumors
Metastases	Value in 1-4 tumors	1	Aoyama et al., 2006[2]	No WBRT survival value
Metastases	Resection or SRS + WBRT	2	Rades et al., 2009[75]	Similar outcomes
Malignant glioma	Upfront radiosurgery	1	Souhami et al., 2004[79]	SRS of no value

SRS, stereotactic radiosurgery; WBRT, whole-brain radiation therapy.

SELECTED KEY REFERENCES

Chan A, Black P, Ojemann R, et al. Stereotactic radiotherapy for vestibular schwannomas: favorable outcome with minimal toxicity. *Neurosurgery*. 2005;57:60-70.

Flickinger J, Kondziolka D. Radiosurgery instead of resection for solitary brain metastases: redefining the gold standard. *Int J Radiat Oncol Biol Phys*. 1996;35:185-186.

Kondziolka D, Mathieu D, Lunsford LD, et al. Radiosurgery as definitive management of meningiomas. *Neurosurgery*. 2008;62:53-60.

Kondziolka D, Patel A, Lunsford LD, et al. Stereotactic radiosurgery plus whole brain radiotherapy versus radiotherapy alone for patients with multiple brain metastases. *Int J Radiat Oncol Biol Phys*. 1999;45:427-434.

Linskey M, Andrews D, Asher A, et al. The role of stereotactic radiosurgery in the management of newly diagnosed brain metastases: a systematic review and evidence-based clinical practice guideline. *J Neurooncol*. 2010;96:45-68.

Please go to expertconsult.com to view the complete list of references.

Stereotactic Radiosurgery of Vascular Malformations

Chun Po Yen, Chris Cifarelli, David Schlesinger, Jason P. Sheehan

CLINICAL PEARLS

- Regardless of modality, radiosurgical devices achieve the desired characteristics of small fields, fast-dose falloff, and highly accurate targeting through the use of two basic principles: superposition of beams and stereotactic targeting.

- The goal of radiosurgery for arteriovenous malformations is to deliver a high absorbed radiation dose to the nidus, while largely sparing the surrounding normal brain tissue. Endothelial damage followed by subendothelial and intimal-medial proliferation of smooth muscle cells and subsequent cellular degeneration and hyaline transformation eventually obliterate the nidus.

- The reported obliteration rate following radiosurgery ranges between 60% and 90%. The outcomes of radiosurgery

- for arteriovenous malformations are dose and volume dependent. The role of preradiosurgical embolization remains to be fully defined.

- Complications associated with radiosurgery for arteriovenous malformations include symptomatic radiation-induced brain damage in 8.7% (permanent in 1.8%), late cyst formation in 1.6%, and radiation-induced tumor within 10 years following radiosurgery in 0.7%.

- Radiosurgery has a smaller role for the treatment of dural arteriovenous fistulas owing to its delayed effects. For patients with cavernous malformations, radiosurgery should be used primarily in compelling cases of repeated hemorrhages from a lesion located in an inoperable site.

Intracranial vascular malformations include arteriovenous malformations (AVMs), dural arteriovenous fistulas (dAVFs), cavernous malformations (CMs), venous malformations, and capillary telangiectasias. Venous malformations and capillary telangiectasias usually have a benign clinical course and rarely hemorrhage; thus, treatment is usually not required. In contrast, AVMs, dAVFs, and CMs might present with hemorrhage, seizure, headache, or neurological deficits that necessitate intervention. Stereotactic radiosurgery, microsurgery, and embolization are important tools in the neurosurgical armamentarium for treating patients with vascular malformations. We will focus on the current role of stereotactic radiosurgery in the management of patients with intracranial AVMs, dAVFs, and CMs.

ARTERIOVENOUS MALFORMATIONS

Management

AVMs are congenital cerebrovascular anomalies consisting of poorly developed vascular channels forming the nidi and shunting arterial blood directly to the venous system. The high blood flow and malformed vascular wall pose the risk of

rupture and intracerebral hemorrhage. Other clinical symptoms patients might experience include seizure, headache, and neurological deficits via the steal phenomenon or from mass effect.

Three management modalities are employed alone or in combination for the management of cerebral AVMs: microsurgery, embolization, and radiosurgery. Several factors should be weighed when choosing the most appropriate choice of treatment. Microsurgery should be used in superficially located nidi because it eliminates the risk of hemorrhage immediately upon a complete total extirpation. Embolization is most commonly used to reduce the size of large AVMs, making them amenable to subsequent microsurgery or radiosurgery. However, new liquid embolization materials (e.g., Onyx) have increased the chance of obliteration solely by embolization.[1,2] Radiosurgery is usually reserved for small to moderate-sized AVMs located in deep or critical areas of the brain.

Role of Radiosurgery

History

The first case of AVM treated with radiotherapy was reported by Magnus.[3] In a patient he operated on with an AVM at the motor cortex, he did not attempt surgical removal because of the high possibility of neurological deficits. After decompressive craniectomy, he treated the patient with radium therapy and reported that the patient was seizure-free 2 years after radiotherapy. No imaging or histological studies were available. Cushing and Bailey reported the first successful surgery on an AVM.[4] Cushing explored a vascular tumor and felt that the lesion could not be attacked without fatal hemorrhage. The patient was treated with radiotherapy. He reexplored the lesion 3 years later and described that the tangle of pulsating vessels previously encountered was largely thrombosed and transformed into a multitude of small bloodless shreds which could be easily separated from the adjacent normal cortex.

There was intense interest in the use of radiation for AVMs following Cushing's discovery, but the initial results were not encouraging. Although some studies[5,6] with small numbers of cases provided evidence of the possible utility of radiation in the treatment of AVMs, most did not provide imaging or histological proof of the efficacy of radiotherapy. This led to an almost unanimous consensus in the assessment of radiation as being worthless in the management of AVMs.

With the introduction of Gamma Knife, the potential value of irradiation in vascular malformations was reassessed. Contributing factors included an increasing body of evidence that the cells constituting the vessel wall were responsive to ionizing radiation. Long-term angiographic follow-up of a small series of AVMs treated with fractionated conventional radiation by Johnson in the 1950s revealed that the AVMs were obliterated in 45% of cases.[7] In 1970, the first radiosurgical treatment for an AVM was performed by Ladislau Steiner and associates at Karolinska Institute in Stockholm. The patient refused surgery, and given the patient's renal insufficiency, the risk of surgery was considered too high. Although the intention was to deliver focused radiation to the nidus, because only small collimators were available, the feeding arteries were targeted and 25 Gy was given as the prescription dose to the 50% isodose line. On angiography 19 months after the treatment, the feeding vessels were obliterated, and the malformation no longer filled. Subsequently, larger collimators were available and could cover the AVM nidi, and more patients were treated successfully. Today more than 50,000 AVM patients have been treated with Gamma Knife radiosurgery, which has been proved to be a safe and effective treatment alternative for AVMs.

Modality

The goal of radiosurgery for AVMs is to deliver a high absorbed radiation dose to the AVM nidus, typically in a single session, while largely sparing the surrounding brain significant dose and thereby minimizing undesirable effects from the treatment. As the number of modalities for delivering radiosurgery have increased over time, so have the numbers that have been applied to the treatment of AVMs. Reports in the literature exist for AVM treatment with various radiosurgical modalities including the Gamma Knife, isocentrically mounted linear accelerators,[8-11] and robotic linear accelerators (CyberKnife).[12] Regardless of modality, radiosurgical devices achieve the desired characteristics of small fields, fast-dose fall-off, and highly accurate targeting through the use of two basic principles: superposition of beams and stereotactic targeting.

Radiosurgery achieves highly conformal dose distributions by spreading the total energy delivered over a targeted volume, either through the superposition of many small beams on the target or through the use of noncoplanar arcs (where each arc can be thought of as a large number of small beams). The energy of any given single beam is too low to cause a significant biological effect. However, the superposition of all the beams at the target delivers a substantial amount of radiation, sufficient to cause biological changes resulting in the occlusion of the AVM nidus.

The details of beam superposition vary by modality. In the case of the Gamma Knife, 192 (or 201, depending on the model of the unit) individual beams are precisely aimed at a focal point, or isocenter, to achieve this effect. The beams are collimated through individual beam channels. In older units, this was achieved with a combination of internal primary and secondary collimation and external "helmet"-based final collimation. In the case of the newer Perfexion model Gamma Knife, the collimator assembly is housed entirely within the main body of the unit.[13]

For early linear accelerators adapted for radiosurgery, finely collimated beams were achieved through the use of circular collimator "cones" that could be attached to the accessory tray of the accelerator.[14] Many currently available accelerators are equipped with micro-multileaf collimators that can achieve irregularly shaped beams that can more precisely conform to the target morphology.[15] Both approaches are often used with a non-coplanar arc technique, which directs the fields at the target while spreading out the overall delivered energy.[16]

The ability to create a focal, high-dose distribution does little good in itself if there is no way to precisely and accurately aim at the target. This problem is elegantly solved using the principles of stereotaxy. Traditionally in intracranial radiosurgery a rigid frame is fixed to the skull. This frame defines a coordinate system by which any point within the brain can be localized. Fiducial markers, which are visible in stereotactic imaging studies as part of the procedure, are directly related to this coordinate system; thus, the target can be visualized and localized in "stereotactic space." Accuracy and precision of treatment are thus guaranteed by the precision and accuracy with which the target can be localized and the assurance that this target will not move during a treatment owing to the rigid head frame. More recent innovations in radiosurgery have included frameless stereotaxy.[17] In these systems image-guidance plays a greater role both before and during the procedure. Less invasive restraint systems such as thermoplastic masks are used in place of the rigid head frame, and periodic imaging is used to track and correct for patient motion.

Histopathology

Several histological studies have described the changes of irradiated vessels with progressive narrowing and obliteration of the lumen.[18] The earliest changes are endothelial damage and endothelial-intimal separation. These are followed by subendothelial and intimal-medial proliferation of smooth muscle cells with elaboration of extracellular matrix components. Cellular degeneration and hyaline transformation of vessel walls follow, and finally the vessels obliterate completely.

The above-mentioned histopathological changes are correlated with time after radiosurgery and tend to occur in smaller vessels.

Gamma Knife Radiosurgery

At the University of Virginia, we perform AVM radiosurgery with the Gamma Knife. Patients are evaluated at least 1 day before the Gamma Knife surgery (GKS). Anticonvulsion medication is used for patients already on these medications and for patients with supratentorial AVMs.

The technique of GKS begins with the placement of the Leksell G-Frame on the patient's head by the neurosurgeon. The Leksell G-Frame consists of a rectangular aluminum base ring to which four aluminum posts are attached. The frame is affixed to the patient through the posts using titanium pins, which are screwed to the outer table of the skull. In our center, we place the frame in the operating room using controlled sedation, local anesthesia, and strict attention to aseptic conditions.

The accuracy of a GKS is ultimately dependent on the visualization of three-dimensional views of the intended target in the brain. Stereotactic biplane angiography is the gold standard for delineating the nidus. Additionally, stereotactic magnetic resonance imaging (MRI) and magnetic resonance angiography source images provide information, especially in the axial plane, which can enhance visualization of the nidus for the purpose of treatment planning.

Treament Planning

Treatment planning is the process of creating a dose distribution that conformally covers the intended target by defining one or more isocenters, or "shots," which each contribute to the total dose distribution. It is an iterative technique requiring detailed knowledge of neuroanatomy, neuroradiology, the biological effect of single-fraction radiosurgery, and the compromises required to create a treatment that will be effective to obliterate the nidus and at the same time tolerable for the surrounding brain structures. Optimal prescription dose has been described by Steiner and associates within the range of 23 to 25 Gy.[19] However, in cases with large nidi or nidi close to critical structures, the dose needed to be adjusted.

Follow-up

The need for adequate and thorough clinical and imaging follow-up cannot be overemphasized. Clinical and imaging responses as well as GKS-related complications and hemorrhage during the latency period should be evaluated following the GKS. We suggest that MRI be performed at 6- to 12-month intervals following radiosurgery until signs of AVM obliteration are evident. When MRI suggests AVM occlusion, follow-up angiography should be performed to confirm complete obliteration of the nidus. Thereafter, patients are advised to have further MRI every 3 to 5 years to rule out delayed adverse effects. To evaluate the outcome and causes of treatment failures, all the images should be analyzed both by neurosurgeons and neuroradiologists interested and experienced in the interpretation of MRI and angiograms.

Outcomes

Following radiosurgery, angiography reveals that hemodynamic changes occur before changes in the size and shape of an AVM.[20] First, the flow rate decreases progressively. This may be related to the changes in the sizes of the feeding arteries and outflow veins. The outcome of an AVM following radiosurgery may be a total, subtotal, or partial obliteration of the nidus.

Total obliteration of the AVM after radiosurgery was defined as "complete absence of former nidus, normalization of afferent and efferent vessels, and a normal circulation time on high-quality rapid serial subtracted angiography."[20] Any remaining nidus, regardless of its size, is considered partial obliteration. Subtotal obliteration of an AVM means the angiographic persistence of an early filling draining veins without demonstrable nidus.[21] The early filling venous drainage suggests that some shunting persists. Our studies have shown that these subtotally obliterated AVMs have very low risk of hemorrhage in spite of the fact that per definition the AVM nidus is still patent as indicated by the shunting. It should be noted that more than 70% of them went on to obliterate completely without further treatment.[21]

The reported obliteration rate following radiosurgery ranged between 30% and 92%.[10,22-24] One should be cautious in terms of the interpretation of the results owing to the biases injected from different cutoff time and imaging modality used to conclude total obliteration. Studies excluding patients with short follow-up, reporting only patients undergoing angiography, or including MRI as an imaging study to conclude obliteration tend to overestimate the success rate of radiosurgery.[23,25,26]

Since 1989, a total of 1023 patients with AVMs treated with GKS at the University of Virginia with follow-up for at least 2 years were analyzed (82 patients completely lost to follow-up and 139 patients with follow-up less than 2 years were excluded; an additional 106 patients with large AVMs undergoing partial treatment will be discussed later). There were 523 males and 500 females with a mean age of 34.2 years (range 4 to 82 years). The presenting symptoms leading to the diagnosis of AVMs was hemorrhage in 529, seizure in 237, headache in 133, and neurological deficits in 94. In 30 patients, the AVMs were incidental findings. The locations of the AVMs were in the cerebral hemispheres in 630, basal ganglion in 96, thalamus in 82, corpus callosum in 38, brainstem in 84, cerebellum in 68, and insula in 25 patients. The Spetzler-Martin grading of the AVMs were grade I in 174 (17%) patients, grade II in 328 (32.1%) patients, grade III in 440 (438%) patients, grade IV in 78 (7.6%) patients, and grade V in 3 (0.3%) patients. One hundred twenty-two patients (11.9%) had previous partial resection of the nidi, and 244 patients (23.9%) underwent preradiosurgical embolization. The nidus volume ranged from 0.1 to 33 cm³ (mean 3.5 cm³). The mean prescription dose was 21.1 Gy (range 5-36 Gy), and the mean maximum dose was 39.0 Gy (range 10-60 Gy). The mean number of isocenters was 2.7 (range 1-22).

The mean follow-up after GKS was 80 months. GKS yielded a total angiographic obliteration in 552 (54%) and subtotal obliteration in 42 (4.1%) patients (Fig. 47.1). In 290 (28.3%) patients, the AVMs remained patent and in 139 patients (13.6%) no flow voids were observed on the MRI. The angiographic total obliteration was achieved in 65.2% of patients with nidus less than 3 cm³; 43.8% between 3 and 8 cm³, and 27.6% with nidus volume larger than 8 cm³. Small nidus volume, high prescription dose, and low number

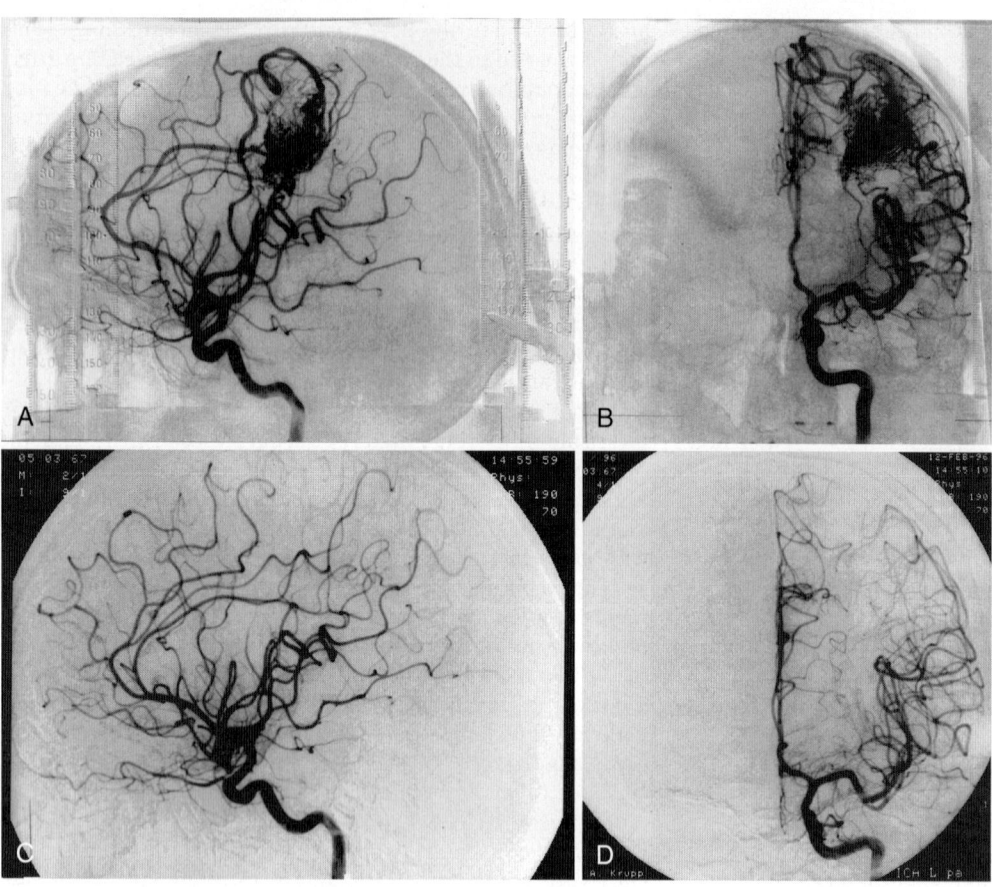

FIGURE 47.1 A 24-year-old man diagnosed with a left-sided arteriovenous malformation (AVM) at left sensorimotor cortex following a hemorrhage. **A** and **B**, Lateral and frontal projections of angiograms. Patient underwent a partial embolization. The nidus obliterated completely 3 years following Gamma Knife surgery (**C** and **D**).

of isocenters are predictive of obliteration. Preradiosurgical embolization has a negative effect on obliteration.

Complications

Early Adverse Effects

Patients might experience headache from frame placement and nausea or vomiting from pain or sedative medications. Few patients developed seizure in the immediate post-GKS period; most who did were those with a prior history of seizure.

Radiation-Induced Changes

Radiation-induced change is an increased T2 signal around the AVM seen on MRI (Fig. 47.2). Radiation damage of glial cells, endothelial cell damage followed by breakdown of blood-brain barrier, excessive generation of free radicals, or release of vascular endothelial growth factors have been proposed to explain this imaging finding. The severity of radiation-induced changes on images and associated neurological deficits varies, ranging from asymptomatic, being only a few millimeters of increased T2 signal surrounding the treated nidus to massive brain edema with symptoms and signs of increased intracranial pressure. From our 1500 Gamma Knife procedures performed for AVM patients with follow-up MRI available for analysis, 34.4% of patients developed radiation-induced changes. Among them, 60% had mild (a few millimeters of increased T2 signal surrounding the nidus), 33% had moderate (compression of ventricle and effacement of sulci),

and 7% had severe (midline shift) radiation-induced changes. The mean time to the development of radiation-induced changes was 13 months after GKS, and the mean duration of the changes was 22 months. Larger nidus volumes, higher prescription doses, history with preradiosurgical embolization, and nidus without previous hemorrhage were associated with higher risk of radiation-induced changes.

One hundred twenty-two (8.7%) patients developed headache, worsening or new seizures, or neurological deficits associated with radiation-induced changes. Patients with severe radiation-induced changes and nidus at eloquent areas were more likely to develop symptoms. Twenty-six patients (1.8%) had permanent neurological deficits.

Cyst Formation

Cyst formation is a rare complication following GKS. Cysts that develop after resolution of previous hemorrhages or fluid cavities from encephalomalacia after surgeries should not be considered as complications related to GKS. Direct radiation injury to the perilesional brain tissue, increased permeability of the blood-brain barrier with accumulation of the exudative fluid, hemodynamic perturbations during gradual obliteration of the nidus with subsequent ischemic tissue damage, and tissue destruction due to subclinical perilesional hemorrhages have been proposed as the possible mechanisms of cyst formation. From our 1272 patients with follow-up MRI available, we found a total of 20 patients (1.6%) developing a cyst after a mean of 8.1 years after GKS. Four cysts were found in 710 patients with follow-up shorter than 5 years, eight cysts

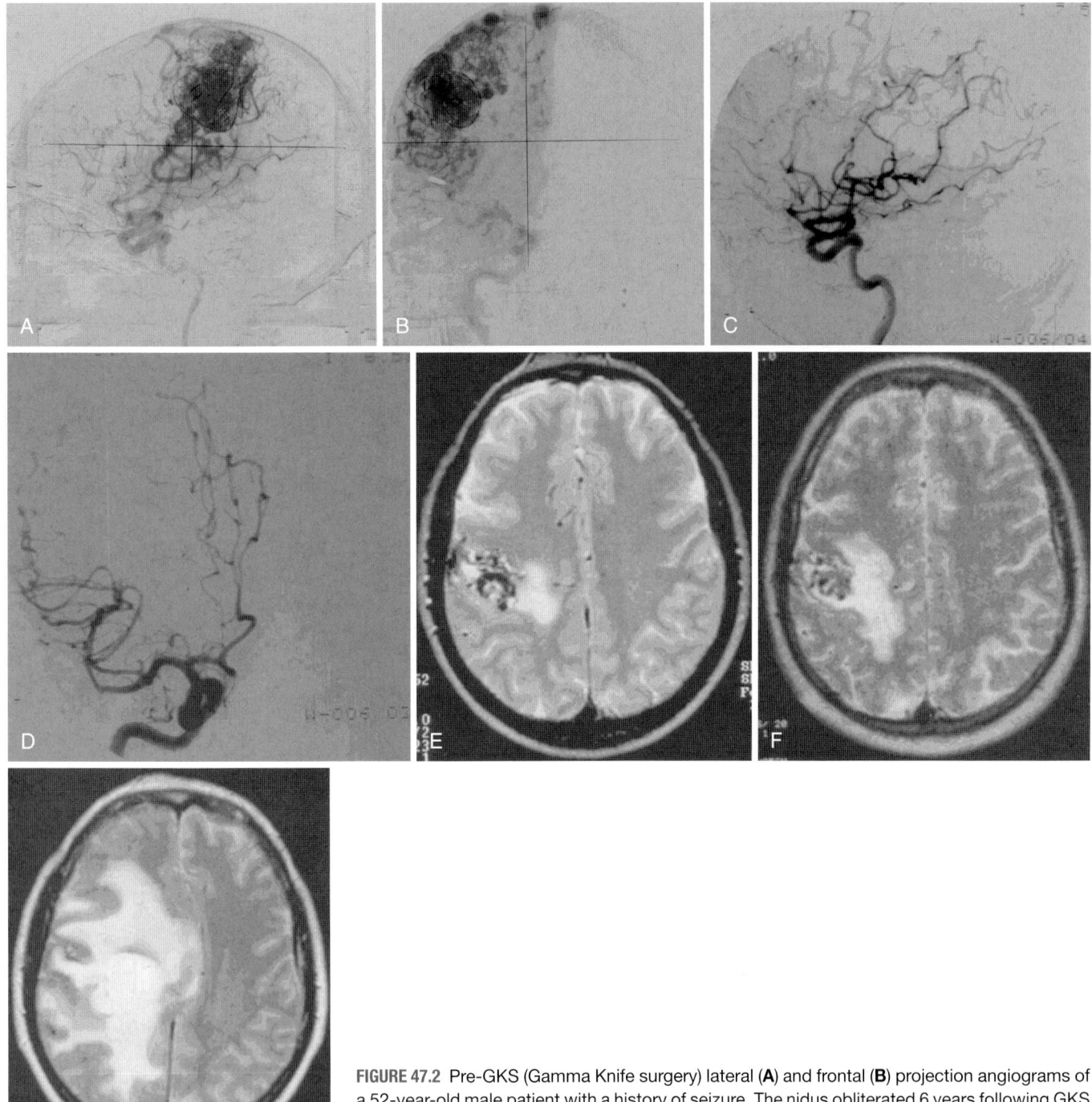

FIGURE 47.2 Pre-GKS (Gamma Knife surgery) lateral (**A**) and frontal (**B**) projection angiograms of a 52-year-old male patient with a history of seizure. The nidus obliterated 6 years following GKS (**C** and **D**). The patient developed radiation-induced changes as shown on the T2-weighted magnetic resonance imaging (MRI) scan 8 months (**E**) and 2 years (**F**) after GKS. A cyst formation with increased T2 signal was seen 6 years after GKS (**G**).

were found in 302 patients with follow-up between 5 and 10 years, and another eight cysts were found in 260 patients with follow-up between 10 and 20 years. Of the 20 patients, 18 had regular MRI follow-up and 14 (78%) of them had radiation-induced changes before the development of cysts. Six patients had large cysts and three of them were symptomatic, requiring surgery. Two patients underwent craniotomy and drainage of the cyst. The cyst wall showed no evidence of neoplasia.

Radiosurgery-Induced Neoplasia

We found two meningiomas from 1333 AVM patients treated with GKS; however, follow-up imaging was performed over a period of at least 10 years in 288 of these patients. If we conservatively estimate that radiosurgery-induced lesions would be evident within a 10-year time interval, then our incidence of radiosurgery-induced neoplasia is 2 in 2880 person-years or 69 in 100,000 person-years. Thus, there is a 0.7% chance that a radiation-induced tumor may develop within 10 years following GKS. This is less than the 1.9% risk detailed by Brada and colleagues,[27] but our results encompass a follow-up period of only 10 years. The long latency and relative rarity of these lesions following radiosurgery may defy a conclusive determination of the true incidence.

Specific Applications of Radiosurgery

Incompletely Obliterated Arteriovenous Malformations

Most reported studies state that the risk of hemorrhage persists as long as the AVM nidus is still patent. These data provided the rationale for re-treatment of still-patent AVMs following the initial GKS.

In our experience, 74 males and 66 females with a mean age of 33 years underwent repeat GKS for still-patent AVM nidi following initial GKS from 1989 to 2007. Causes of initial treatment failure included inaccurate nidus definition in 14, failure to fill part of the nidus due to hemodynamic factors in 16, recanalization of embolized AVM compartments in 6, and suboptimal dose (less than 20 Gy) in 23 patients. Nineteen patients had repeat GKS for subtotal obliteration of AVMs. In 62 patients, the AVM failed to obliterate in spite of correct target definition and adequate dose. At the time of re-treatment, the nidus volume ranged from 0.1 to 6.9 cm³ (mean 1.4 cm³) and the mean prescription dose was 20.3 Gy. Clinical follow-up time ranged from 15 to 220 months with a mean of 84.2 months after repeat GKS.

Repeat GKS yielded a total angiographic obliteration in 77 (55%) and subtotal obliteration in 9 (6.4%) patients. In 38 (27.1%) patients, the AVMs remained patent. In 16 patients (11.4%) no flow voids were observed on the MRI. Higher prescription dose, smaller nidus volume, nidi with only superficial venous drainage, and a negative history of prior embolization were significantly associated with increased rate of AVM obliteration. Clinically, 126 patients improved or remained stable and 14 experienced deterioration (8 due to a rebleed, 2 caused by persistent arteriovenous shunting, and 4 related to radiation-induced changes).

In the early 1990s, angiography was the only imaging modality available for nidus definition and treatment planning during AVM radiosurgery. So far, our treatment planning still depends mainly on angiography and the nidus can be fully appreciated with multiple projections and real-time observation of the hemodynamic changes during the procedure of angiography. However, MRI does sometimes provide extra information for the outlining of the nidi and during the treatment planning less normal brain tissue would be included within the prescribed isodose.

We advise repeat GKS in cases with still-patent nidi 3 to 4 years after initial GKS when open surgery or endovascular procedures were expected to yield higher risk of complications than GKS. Using repeat GKS, we achieved a 55% angiographic cure rate. Although radiation-induced changes were slightly higher (39%) than those in patients undergoing only one GKS procedure, only 4 patients (3.6%) developed permanent neurological deficits. Our experience showed that when repeating GKS a dose of at least 20 Gy led to a higher chance of subsequent nidus obliteration (77% versus 47% with prescription dose less than 20 Gy).

Embolization of Arteriovenous Malformations

The effectiveness of partial embolization followed by GKS in the management of relatively large AVMs remains controversial. Small series of cases managed with this combined approach reported diverse results with obliteration rates ranging between 50% and 76%.[10,28,29] When comparing the outcome in patients treated with Gamma Knife alone to those with combined embolization and Gamma Knife treatment, recent studies reported less favorable outcome in patients with preradiosurgical embolization.[10,30]

Between 1989 and 2007, a total number of 217 AVMs with prior partial embolization were treated with radiosurgery at the University of Virginia. There were 107 males (49%) and 110 females (51%). The mean age at the initial GK treatment was 32.8 years. The presenting symptoms were hemorrhages in 93 (42.9%) patients, seizures in 67 (30.9%) patients, headaches in 27 (12.4%) patients, and neurological deficits in 25 (11.5%) patients. In 5 patients the AVMs were incidental findings. Most of the AVMs were embolized with liquid embolics (59.8%) such as NBCA (N-butyl 2-cyanoacrylate) or ethanol. Other embolic materials used were coils (9.4%), silk (1.6%), Onyx (0.8%), or a combination of them. In 167 patients the nidus was compact after the embolization, whereas the angiogram of 50 patients revealed that the nidus was broken apart after the endovascular procedure. The mean volume of the nidus at the time of GKS was 5.1 cm³ (0.02-24.9 cm³). The mean maximum dose of the GKS was 37.2 Gy (range 20-50 Gy), and the mean prescription dose was 19.6 Gy (range 10-28 Gy).

After GKS an angiographically confirmed total obliteration of the AVMs was achieved in 71 patients (27.1%). A total obliteration on MRI confirmed by the absence of flow voids was observed in 26 patients (9.9%). In 157 patients (59.9%) only a partial obliteration could be obtained after a follow-up period of at least 2 years. Eight patients (3.1%) presented with a subtotal obliteration. Comparing the outcome after GKS between embolized and nonembolized AVM patients (obliteration rate 72%), the Kaplan-Meier curves revealed a significant lower obliteration rate ($p < 0.001$) in patients with pre-GKS embolization.

Twenty-six hemorrhages were recorded during the follow-up period yielding an annual hemorrhage rate of 2.1%. Radiation-induced changes detected on MRI were observed in 94 patients (46%), which were higher than those in patients undergoing GKS alone. Eleven patients developed neurological deficits.

Recanalization of previously embolized parts of the nidus,[31] difficulty in nidus delineation following previous embolization,[10] and attenuation of radiation dose by embolization materials[32] have been proposed to explain the less favorable outcome in patients with pre-GKS embolization. Theoretically, volume reduction following embolization affords a lower chance of GKS-related adverse effect but this expectation was not shown based on our data. Additionally the complications from embolization are not negligible. Therefore, the use of pre-GKS embolization remains problematic and awaits further investigation.

Brainstem Arteriovenous Malformations

Studies have shown that AVMs located in the posterior fossa carry a higher risk of hemorrhage compared to AVMs in other locations.[33,34] Furthermore, owing to the critical location in proximity to vital neuronal pathways and nuclei, there is a high risk of morbidity and mortality once the brainstem AVMs rupture. With the advance of microsurgical techniques, extirpation of the AVMs involving the brainstem is feasible but the associated risks are not negligible. Several surgical series have demonstrated a less favorable obliteration rate with a high risk of complications.[35-37]

Between 1989 and 2007, a total number of 96 patients with AVM nidi mainly located in the brainstem were treated with GKS at our institute. Thirteen cases with a follow-up period shorter than 2 years after GKS were excluded, leaving 83 patients for analysis. There were 53 males and 30 females with a mean age of 33 years (range 6-81 years). The presenting symptoms leading to the diagnosis of AVM were hemorrhage in 53 (63.9%) patients, seizure in 4 (4.8%), headache in 6 (7.2%), cranial nerve palsies in 12 (14.4%), long-tract signs in 3 (3.6%), and hydrocephalus in 2 (2.4%). Three patients were asymptomatic. Nine patients underwent embolization prior to GKS. Incomplete surgical resection was carried out in five patients. One patient had partial resection and embolization before undergoing GKS. The AVMs were located in the midbrain in 43 (51.8%) patients, pons in 29 (34.9%), and medulla oblongata in 11 (13.3%). The maximum diameters of the nidi ranged from 7 to 41 mm (mean 18.6 mm) and the volumes ranged from 0.1 to 8.9 cm^3 (mean 1.9 cm^3). All nidi had deep venous drainage. The mean prescription dose was 19.8 Gy (range 5-32 Gy) and the mean maximum dose 33.8 Gy (range 10-50 Gy).

Following a single GK procedure, 35 (42.2%) patients still had a residual nidus shown on MRI or angiography. In 7 (10.8%) patients, the last MRI revealed absence of flow voids. In 38 (45.8%) patients, total obliteration was confirmed on follow-up angiography. The interval between GKS and angiographic obliteration ranged from 6 to 148 months (mean 38.3 months). Three (3.6%) patients had a subtotal obliteration.

Eighteen patients had a second GKS for still-patent AVM residuals performed at a mean of 4.4 years (range 2.0-10.1 years) after the initial GK procedures. Two patients had the third GK procedures 7 and 16 years after a failed repeat GKS. Of 18 patients undergoing repeat GKS, 11 achieved a total obliteration based on angiography (including 2 patients who underwent a third GK procedure). Two patients obtained nidus obliteration based on MRI. In 5 patients, the nidus remained patent.

Following one or more GKS, angiography follow-up was available in 68 (82%) patients. A total obliteration was confirmed in 49 (59%) and subtotal obliteration in 3 (3.6%). Twenty-two (26.5%) patients still had patent residual nidus. In 9 (10.8%) patients, obliteration was confirmed on MRI only. Prescription dose greater than 20 Gy ($p = 0.037$) was significantly associated with increased rate of obliteration.

The clinical follow-up period ranged from 24 to 264 months (mean 100 months). Following GKS, three patients had two and seven patients had one bleeding. In total, 10 patients experienced 13 episodes of hemorrhage in 457 risk-years, yielding an annual hemorrhagic rate of 2.8%. Of these 10 patients with hemorrhage, six had a complete recovery and four had residual neurological deficits. Two patients with persistent AVMs deteriorated clinically presumably due to mass effect or steal phenomenon. In our series, one patient

died owing to complications of hemorrhage. One patient whose AVM had obliterated died from disease unrelated to the brainstem AVM.

Radiation-induced changes were observed in 33 of 81 (40.7%) patients who had series MRI follow-up. Twenty-three (28.4%) patients were asymptomatic upon the imaging finding of radiation-induced changes, one (1.2%) presented with headache, and nine (11.1%) developed new or aggravated neurological deficits. Among the patients with neurological deficits, four (4.9%) had a full recovery but five (6.2%) patients still had residual neurological deficits at the last follow-up including one who developed a large cyst 6 years following GKS.

Brainstem AVM is a formidable challenge for neurosurgeons because of its high risk of rupture and significant morbidity and mortality rates associated with the hemorrhages. Adding to the conundrum is the fact that none of the treatment modalities available can eliminate the risk of hemorrhage without a significant risk of neurological deteriorations. GKS is a reasonable treatment option, especially if the nidus is located within the parenchyma of the brainstem. In our series, GKS achieves a 59% rate of complete obliteration. However, one should be cautious that the neurological deficits associated with radiation-induced changes are relatively high.

Arteriovenous Malformations in Pediatric Patients

Although AVMs only account for 1.4% of intracerebral hemorrhage in the adult population, they represent the underlying cause of 20% to 50% of cerebral hemorrhage in pediatric patients.[38,39] Studies have shown that pediatric patients have a high cumulative lifetime risk of hemorrhages, and AVMs in the pediatric population also have a high propensity to rupture.[39,40] Radiosurgery has been increasingly used for the management of pediatric AVMs following the success in adult patients.

Between 1989 and 2007, 200 AVM patients under 18 years of age were treated with GKS at the University of Virginia. Fourteen cases with follow-up times shorter than 2 years after GKS were excluded, leaving 186 patients for analysis. There were 98 males and 88 females with a mean age of 12.7 years (range 4-18 years). The presenting symptoms leading to the diagnosis AVMs were hemorrhage in 133 (71.5%) patients, seizure in 29 (15.6%) patients, headache in 11 (5.9%) patients, and neurological deficits in 8 (4.2%) patients. Five (2.7%) patients were asymptomatic and the AVMs were an incidental finding. Thirty-eight patients underwent embolization prior to GKS. Incomplete surgical resection was carried out in 24 patients. Five patients had partial resection and embolization before undergoing GKS. One patient had previous proton beam radiotherapy.

The locations of the AVMs were hemispheric in 101 (54.3%) patients, thalamus in 24 (12.9%), basal ganglia in 23 (12.4%), corpus callosum in 9 (4.8%), brainstem in 18 (9.7%), insula/sylvian fissure in 5 (2.7%), and cerebellum in 6 (3.2%). Five patients had coexistent intranidal aneurysms, and seven had perinidal aneurysms. Three patients had non-flow-directed aneurysms. The nidus volumes ranged from 0.1 to 24 cm^3 (mean 3.2 cm^3). Sixty-two nidi had only superficial venous drainage and 124 had deep venous drainage. The Spetzler-Martin grading at the time of initial GKS was grade I in

23 (12.4%) patients, grade II in 55 (29.6%) patients, grade III in 87 (46.8%) patients, grade IV in 20 (10.8%) patients, and grade V in 1 (0.5%) patient. Forty-one patients had a second GKS for still-patent AVM residuals performed at a mean of 2 to 5 years (range years) after the initial GK procedures. The volumes ranged from 0.2 to 15.9 cm^3 (mean 2.3 cm^3) at the time of repeat GKS.

The treatment parameters at the initial GKS were as follows: mean prescription dose 21.9 Gy (range 7.5-35 Gy); mean maximum dose 40.1 Gy (range 20-50 Gy). The treatment parameters of the second GKS were as follows: mean prescription dose 20.7 Gy (range 4-27.5 Gy); mean maximum dose 39.6 Gy (range 8-50 Gy).

Following a single GKS, 92 (37.1%) patients still had a residual nidus shown on MRI or angiography. In 15 (8.1%) patients, the last MRI revealed absence of flow voids but patients or parents refused to have an angiography to confirm the obliteration of nidus. In 92 (49.5%) patients, total obliteration was confirmed on follow-up angiography. Ten (5.4%) patients had a subtotal obliteration. Of 41 patients undergoing repeat GKS, 17 achieved a total obliteration based on angiography. Three patients obtained nidus obliteration based on MRI. In 16 patients, the nidus remained patent. Five patients had subtotal obliteration of AVMs.

Following one or more GKS, a total obliteration was confirmed in 109 (58.6%) and subtotal obliteration in 9 (4.8%). Forty-nine (26.3%) patients still had patent residual nidus. In 19 (10.2%) patients, obliteration was confirmed on MRI only. The actuarial angiographic obliteration rate was 34% at 2 years, 46% at 3 years, and 51% at 5 years. In general, the imaging outcome of pediatric patients is similar to that observed in the adult population. A negative history of pre-GKS embolization ($p = 0.049$) and a high prescription dose ($p = 0.001$) were significantly associated with increased rate of obliteration.

The clinical follow-up period ranged from 24 to 240 months (mean 98.4 months). Following GKS, seven patients had two bleeding episodes, and 10 patients had one bleeding episode. In total, 17 patients experienced 24 episodes of hemorrhage in 1013 risk-years (assuming patients with completely obliterated AVMs were no longer at risk for hemorrhage), yielding an annual hemorrhagic rate of 2.4%. We do not observe any hemorrhage after angiography concludes a total obliteration. If the 14 patients with follow-up less than 2 years were included, two more hemorrhages in 1016 risk-years yield a hemorrhage rate of 2.6%. The hemorrhage rate was 5.4% per year for the first 2 years and reduced to 0.8% per year from 2 to 5 years after GKS. There were no deaths in our series.

The follow-up MRI period ranged from 6 to 222 months with a mean of 80 months. Radiation-induced changes were observed in 68 of 180 (37.8%) patients who had series MRI follow-up. Fifty-five (30.6%) patients were asymptomatic upon the imaging finding of radiation-induced changes, seven (3.9%) presented with headache, and six (3.3%) developed new or aggravated neurological deficits. Among the patients with neurological deficits, four (2.2%) had a full recovery, but two (1.1%) patients still had residual neurological deficits at the last follow-up. Five patients developed a large cyst following GKS. A 7-year-old boy and a 12-year-old girl each developed a small asymptomatic meningioma 12 and 10 years after GKS.

Only a small series of children went through a systemic psychological test analyzing the cognitive faculties in a long-term follow-up after GKS. However, yearly follow-ups including questioning the parents, the patients, and the referring doctors about the intellectual development and possible cognitive or endocrinological deficits were conducted. According to this information, 95% of the children had normal intellectual development after radiosurgery with satisfactory or good school performance. As adults, they performed from average to excellent and were socially well adjusted. Riva and associates studied patients, ranging in age from 9 to 18 years, treated for AVMs using GKS to record potential effects of radiosurgery on cognitive and neuropsychological performance.[41] Tests for general intelligence, nonverbal intelligence, memory and its components, and attention performance were administered to patients and compared with test results of age-matched siblings or first cousins. No statistically significant difference was found between the performance of patients and control subjects in any of the tests administered.

The reported obliteration rate for pediatric AVMs following radiosurgery ranged between 53% and 86%.[25,42-45] Some studies had proposed that in pediatric patients the response to radiosurgery seems to be less favorable.[25] Hypotheses such as the immature vessels in pediatric patients were more likely to recover from radiation-induced damage and neovascularization in response to radiation have been proposed. Our experience shows comparable result in children compared to adults. Additionally, we observe that radiation-induced damage seems to be more tolerable for kids, suggesting that radiosurgery has a favorable benefit-risk profile in the management of pediatric AVMs. However, the risk of hemorrhage remained in pediatric patients and the development of secondary tumor cannot be overlooked. For pediatric AVMs amenable to surgery, microsurgery should be considered as the first-line treatment.

Large Arteriovenous Malformations

Although satisfactory results in small and moderately sized AVMs following radiosurgery are well documented, reports on the imaging and clinical outcomes in large AVMs are sparse. Few neurosurgeons treated large enough series with appropriate follow-up periods. The main problem with large AVMs is due to the dependence of the obliteration response on dose and volume; this dependency requires a delicate balance in deciding the dose that will be efficient but low enough to avoid adverse neurological deficits.

The following strategies are currently available to treat large AVMs with radiosurgery. First, one can embolize a portion of the AVM and then perform radiosurgery if the nidus shrinks to a size manageable with radiosurgery. However, embolization should effectively shrink the nidus for radiosurgery to achieve good results. Also fragmentation of the nidus into a number of segments should be avoided because that will make the radiosurgical planning difficult and increase the probability of radiosurgery failure. Another strategy involves serial staged radiosurgery to selected volumes of the AVMs. Sirin and associates used staged volumetric radiosurgery in 28 large AVMs.[45a] Of the 21 patients, seven underwent repeat radiosurgery and were eliminated from outcome analysis. Of the remaining 14 patients, 3 had total obliteration on angiograms, and 4 had no flow voids on MRI but had no follow-up angiography. Four patients had hemorrhages after radiosurgery, resulting in two deaths. Worsened neurological deficits occurred in one patient. The third approach is to treat the whole nidus in one session with low-dose radiosurgery. Pan and associates reported an obliteration rate of 25% for AVMs with volume larger than 15 cm³. The obliteration rate increased to 50% at 50 months' follow-up. The morbidity rate was 3.3%. Post-treatment hemorrhage occurred in 9.2%.

For the past 20 years, we evaluated a protocol using combined radiosurgery and microsurgery for the management of large AVMs. Radiosurgery was performed for the deep medullary portion of the AVM as a first step. The second step was planned as microsurgical extirpation of the superficial segment if the goal of the first step, obliteration of the deep segment of the AVM, was achieved. However, this goal was achieved in less than 5% of the patients.

The management of large AVMs demonstrates that every treatment has its limitations. In an effort to solve the problems of the management of large AVMs, a cautious approach is warranted pending the development of new techniques and agents for embolization. In very large AVMs perhaps "wait and see" may occasionally be the best management.

DURAL ARTERIOVENOUS FISTULAS

Intracranial dAVFs comprise a unique subset of vascular malformations from the perspectives of etiology and treatment paradigms. Although dAVFs make up approximately 15% of all intracranial vascular malformations, the precise mechanism of formation remains unknown, with leading theories including adjacent venous sinus stasis as well as alterations in local expression of vasogenic factors, such as vascular endothelial growth factor (VEGF) and fibroblastic growth factor (FGF).[46,47] Unfortunately, the presence of venous occlusion proximal or distal to the dAVFs is not an absolute requirement, complicating the interpretation of its role. Similarly, changes in expression levels of VEGF and FGF have been found in animal models of dAVFs as well as samples of patients treated surgically, but no causative relationship has been shown to exist between these vasogenic substances and dAVF formation.[48-51]

From a treatment standpoint, the experience with dAVFs is distinct from that with AVMs. Whereas size and location of AVMs are correlated with the natural history and optimal treatment protocols, several studies have established that the flow dynamics of dAVFs are the most important indicator of the need to treat and modality of choice, be it endovascular, open microneurosurgical, or radiosurgery.[52-54] Specifically, the current classification systems for dAVFs, excluding those involving the cavernous sinus, have been defined based on the direction of fistulous flow as well as the presence or absence of cortical venous reflux (Box 47.1). In an attempt to validate these classification systems based on a large single institution sample, Davies and co-workers[55] retrospectively analyzed 102 dAVFs in 98 patients focusing on venous anatomy and direction of flow, confirming that the single best predictor of hemorrhage is retrograde leptomeningeal drainage. As the aggressive natural history of lesions with cortical venous reflux differs significantly from lesions without angiographic evidence of

---

BOX 47.1 Classification of Dural Arteriovenous Fistulas

Borden Scale
- Type I – Drainage into dural venous sinus or meningeal vein only
- Type II – Drainage into dural venous sinus or meningeal vein with cortical venous reflux (CVR)
- Type III – CVR only

Cognard Scale
- Type I – Drainage into dural venous sinus only with normal antegrade flow
- Type IIa – Drainage into dural venous sinus only with retrograde flow
- Type IIb – Drainage into dural venous sinus with antegrade flow and CVR
- Type IIa + IIb – Drainage into dural venous sinus with retrograde flow and CVR
- Type III – CVR only without venous ectasia
- Type IV – CVR only with venous ectasia
- Type V – Drainage into spinal perimedullary veins

Adapted from: Borden JA, Wu JK, Shucart WA. A proposed classification for spinal and cranial dural arteriovenous fistulous malformations and implications for treatment. J Neurosurg 1995;82:166-179; Cognard C, Gobin YP, Pierot L, et al. Cerebral dural arteriovenous fistulas: clinical and angiographic correlation with a revised classification of venous drainage. Radiology 1995;194:671-680.

---

cortical venous reflux, early definitive therapy via endovascular procedures or open surgical resection appears to be preferable to radiosurgery as a first-line treatment. Once again, the ionizing radiation delivered via radiosurgery is thought to be an effective agent for decreasing neovascularization in dAVFs, but the time interval needed for the desired effect is too great to justify radiosurgery as a first-line therapy.[48,56]

Given the relatively low incidence of clinically identified lesions with respect to other types of vascular malformations and the percentage of those diagnosed dAVFs treated with radiosurgery, large clinical series are few in number and published studies report the findings of single institutions.[57-60] The long-term analysis of radiosurgery for dAVFs over 25 years at the Karolinska University Hospital in Stockholm, Sweden, included 52 patients treated between 1978 and 2003. The obliteration rate reported in this study was 68% with 16 dAVFs presenting as less aggressive Borden I or Cognard I/IIa lesions. Moreover, 43 of 52 patients received GKS only, with the remaining 9 patients having undergone prior surgical or endovascular treatment.[60] In a similar institutional experience at the University of Virginia between 1989 and 2005, 55 patients with dAVFs were treated with GKS, primarily as an adjunct to surgery or embolization. Obliteration rates measured by angiography at 3 years ranged from 54% to 65%, with the 16 patients classified as Borden I lesions (Fig. 47.3). Unlike the Karolinska study, the majority of patients treated at the University of Virginia received GKS as a secondary therapy, with 41 of the 54 patients receiving surgical or endovascular intervention prior to radiosurgery. Regardless of the difference in utilization of radiosurgery as a primary or secondary treatment modality, the results of these long-term studies indicate that GKS is an effective and safe treatment for intracranial dAVFs. From a purely logistic

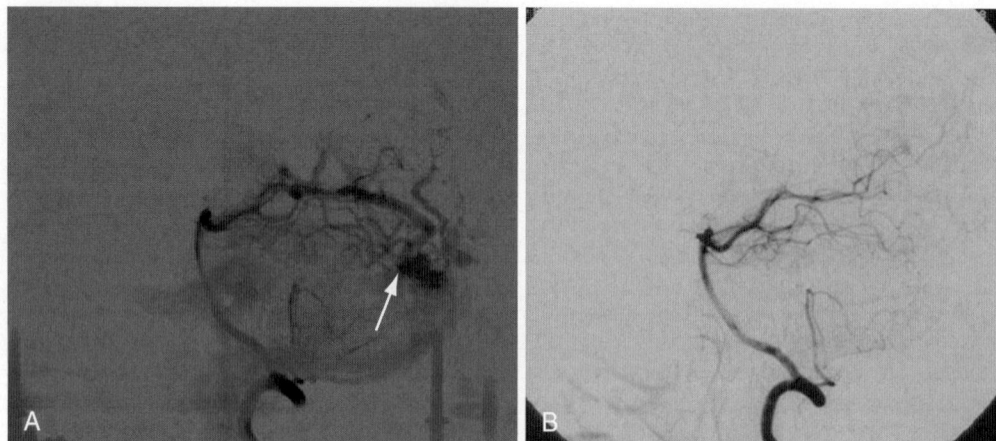

FIGURE 47.3 Lateral view angiogram of a 48-year-old man who presented with sudden onset of severe headache without evidence of intracranial hemorrhage. The patient underwent five neuroendovascular attempts at embolization over the 12 months prior to radiosurgery referral. **A,** Lateral view, right vertebral artery injection. The pretreatment angiogram demonstrated a multihole fistula with sinus drainage involving the torcula (*arrow*). **B,** Lateral view, right vertebral artery injection. The post-treatment angiogram performed at 25 months following radiosurgery documents obliteration of the dural arteriovenous fistula.

standpoint, the role of GKS may remain a second-tier therapy as the majority of lesions are still initially examined via angiography, facilitating treatment at the time of radiographic diagnosis. Of course, radiosurgery may serve as a first-line therapy for deep lesions that are either inaccessible to endovascular treatment given current microcatheter technology or in situations in which there is low risk of intracranial hemorrhage.

CAVERNOUS MALFORMATIONS

Cavernous malformations (CMs) are another type of intracranial vascular malformation. They can also be referred to as *cavernous hemangiomas, angiographically occult vascular malformations,* or *cavernous angiomas.* From a histological standpoint, they are discrete and lobulated lesions composed of dilated sinusoidal vascular channels formed by a single layer of endothelial lining and variable layers of fibrous adventitia. CMs do have a hereditary component and may occur as multiple lesions within the same patient. The proportion of CMs that are developmental anomalies as opposed to acquired malformations and the extent to which the etiology of a cavernous malformation alters its natural history remain the subject of much debate.[61,62] Annual rates of hemorrhage have been reported to be less than 1% to as high as 7% for those with multiple recent hemorrhages.[63,64] Acquired malformations are frequently associated with deep venous anomalies and may point to an underlying pathophysiology associated with venous hypertension.[65,66] Radiosurgery and radiation therapy have even been linked to the formation of CMs.[67,68]

CMs have been associated with headaches, seizures, focal neurological deficits, and intracerebral hemorrhages. In some patients who have symptomatic yet microsurgically inaccessible lesions, radiosurgery has been employed. However, unlike the consensus regarding radiosurgical indications and outcomes for AVMs and dAVFs, opinions vary greatly as to

the risk-to-benefit profile for radiosurgical treatment of CMs. Moreover, few proponents of radiosurgery for CM patients advocate treatment unless there has been at least one if not several prior hemorrhages. In addition, as compared to AVMs or dAVFs, histopathological studies of CMs resected after prior radiosurgery show little in the way of protective changes associated with the treatment.[69]

Proponents of radiosurgery for CMs maintain a reduction in the risk of hemorrhage within 2 years after radiosurgery.[70,71] Less favorable assessments of the benefits of radiosurgery for altering the natural history of hemorrhage associated with CMs have been put forth by others.[24,72,73] It does seem clear that radiosurgery of CMs is associated with a higher rate of complications than for AVMs or dAVFs. This may be related to radiosensitization of surrounding brain parenchyma by iron deposition from repeated clinical and subclinical hemorrhages associated with CMs.[74] If radiosurgery is attempted for a young patient with a surgically inaccessible CM that has repeatedly hemorrhaged (e.g., a deep-seated thalamic lesion or one intrinsic to the brainstem), a lower radiosurgical dose (15 Gy or less) compared to AVMs seems warranted.[24,75,76]

The results in terms of reduction of CM-associated epilepsy following radiosurgery seem a bit more promising.[77] In a randomized, multicenter study of 49 cases, Bartolomei and associates showed that 53% of patients achieved a seizure-free status (Engel's class I) using a mean marginal dose of 19.2 Gy. Two patients in this cohort experienced severe complications.[77] Hsu and colleagues showed Engel's class I seizure control in 64.3% of patients treated with linear accelerator (linac)–based radiosurgery.[78] The improvement in seizures need not be accompanied by a protection from hemorrhage associated with these vascular lesions. Further investigation of the role of radiosurgery for symptomatic CMs in inaccessible or eloquent brain tissue is required. Until then, radiosurgery for CMs must be employed only after careful scrutiny of the risks and benefits likely afforded the patient.

CONCLUSIONS

Radiosurgery for AVMs is associated with a high rate of obliteration and acceptable risk of complications. The treatment outcome is dose and volume dependent; small volume and high prescription dose are associated with high chance of obliteration and low incidence of adverse effects. Unless surgery is medically contraindicated, patients with surgically accessible nidus should be managed with surgery because a complete extirpation of the nidus eliminated the risk of hemorrhage immediately. The management of large AVMs remains a great challenge for neurosurgeons. Although embolization has been used for decades to reduce the size of the nidus and make subsequent radiosurgical procedure feasible, the literature has proved that this approach does not improve the obliteration rate of AVMs treated with radiosurgery.

Radiosurgery has a smaller role for the treatment of dAVFs. For patients with CMs, radiosurgery should be used sparingly and primarily in compelling cases of repeated hemorrhages from a CM located in an inoperable site. A multidisciplinary approach and well-defined treatment plan should be set up before the initiation of each patient's treatment.

SELECTED KEY REFERENCES

Adler Jr JR, Chang SD, Murphy MJ, et al. The Cyberknife: a frameless robotic system for radiosurgery. *Stereotact Funct Neurosurg*. 1997;69:124-128.

Hsu PW, Chang CN, Tseng CK, et al. Treatment of epileptogenic cavernomas: surgery versus radiosurgery. *Cerebrovasc Dis*. 2007;24:116-120.

Karlsson B, Lindquist C, Steiner L. Prediction of obliteration after Gamma Knife surgery for cerebral arteriovenous malformations. *Neurosurgery*. 1997;40:425-430.

Kondziolka D, Lunsford LD, Kestle JR. The natural history of cerebral cavernous malformations. *J Neurosurg*. 1995;83:820-824.

Pan DH, Kuo YH, Guo WY, et al. Gamma Knife surgery for cerebral arteriovenous malformations in children: a 13-year experience. *J Neurosurg Pediatr*. 2008;1:296-304.

Soderman M, Edner G, Ericson K, et al. Gamma Knife surgery for dural arteriovenous shunts: 25 years of experience. *J Neurosurg*. 2006;104:867-875.

Please go to expertconsult.com to view the complete list of references.

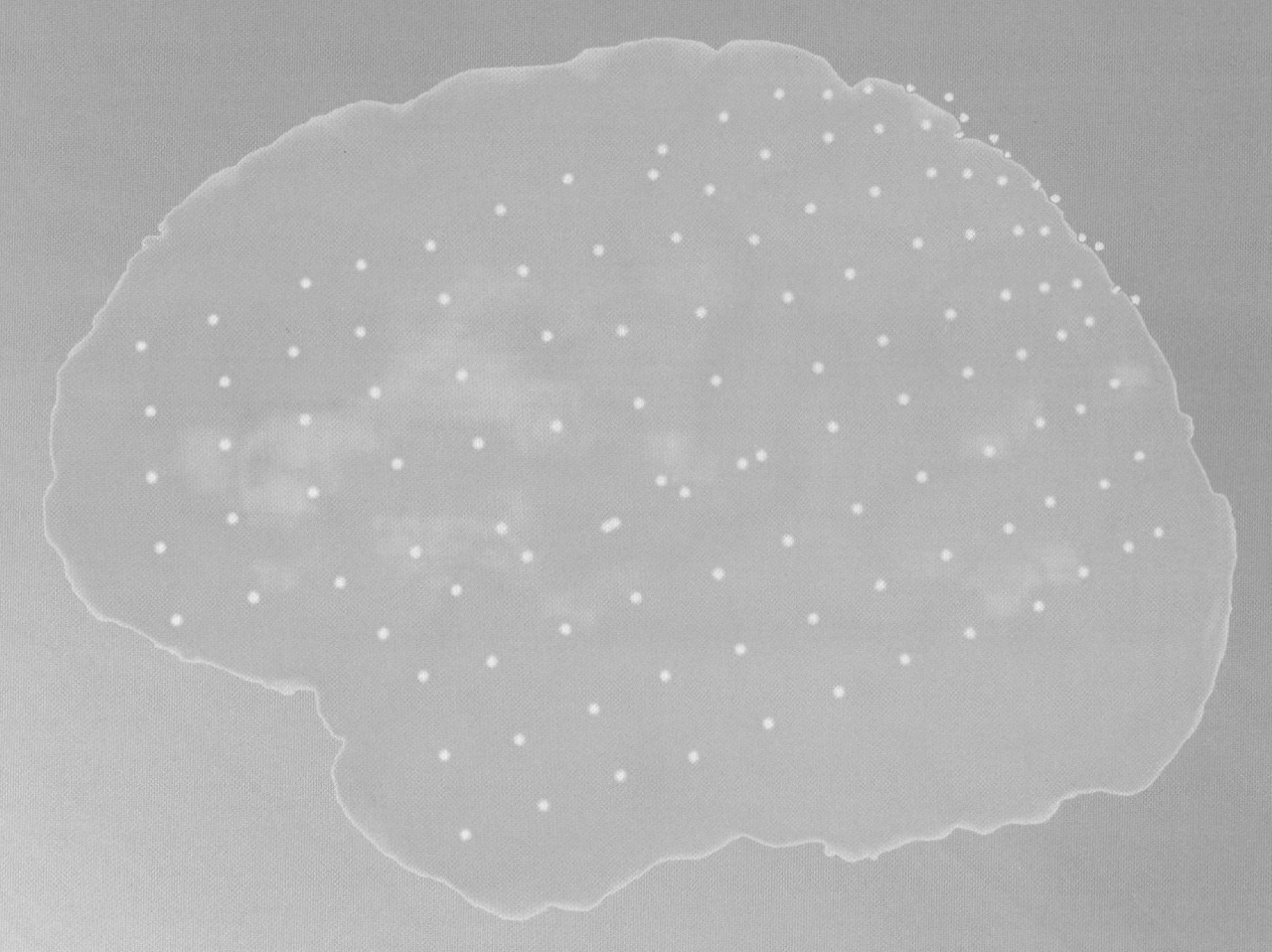

PART 8
Functional/Pain

Trigeminal Neuralgia

Gerald A. Grant, John D. Loeser

CLINICAL PEARLS

- Trigeminal neuralgia is a stereotyped, repetitive, unilateral, electric-shock-like facial pain triggered by non-noxious stimulation with clear pain-free intervals. Tic pain is ordinarily spontaneous in onset, but can frequently be triggered by a non-noxious stimulus.

- Continuous pain without a shock-like quality or a cranial nerve deficit raises the suspicion of diseases other than trigeminal neuralgia. Tic douloureux can be caused by any of a number of conditions affecting the ipsilateral trigeminal system. In the vast majority, the cause seems to be compression of the trigeminal nerve at its exit from the pons by an adjacent artery or vein that has elongated and kinked to become wedged against the nerve. In about 1% to 2% of cases, the pain results from a benign tumor in the cerebellopontine angle, and approximately 1% to 8% of patients with trigeminal neuralgia have multiple sclerosis.

- The diagnosis of tic douloureaux is based on the patient's history of pain as no diagnostic imaging or physiological studies currently available will substitute for the history. Magnetic resonance imaging (MRI) and magnetic resonance angiography (MRA) have improved the sensitivity and specificity of diagnosing neurovascular compression of

the nerve by evaluating the anatomical relationships of the arterial and venous structures with the trigeminal nerve at the root entry zone in the cerebellopontine angle. However, MRI is used primarily as a perioperative adjunct after the clinical diagnosis is made.

- Medical management of tic pain is successful in about 50% of patients and remains the initial approach. The anticonvulsants carbamazepine, phenytoin, and gabapentin appear to be the most effective in controlling the pain of tic douloureux.

- A multimodality approach, including various medical, surgical, or radiosurgical therapies, is most beneficial to patients with tic pain. Gasserian gangliolysis selectively destroys the nocireceptive fibers while preserving the touch fibers. This procedure can be performed using radiofrequency ablation, balloon compression, or glycerol. The success of radiosurgery appears excellent, although long-term recurrence rates are unclear. Of all surgical treatments, microvascular decompression is associated with the lowest rates of recurrence and sensory loss but carries low but significant morbidity rates.

Trigeminal neuralgia, also known as *tic douloureux*, is an excruciatingly painful condition that is most common in people aged 50 to 70 years. It is a stereotyped, repetitive, unilateral, electric-shock-like facial pain triggered by non-noxious stimulation with clear pain-free intervals.[1-5] The incidence of trigeminal neuralgia is 4 to 5 per 100,000 population (median age 67 years).[6] It involves the right side of the face more often than the left side, at a ratio of about 3:2. Women are more often affected than men in a ratio that has varied from 2:1 to 4:3 in reported series.[7]

This is a unique pain syndrome in which the pathogenesis, prognosis, and treatment are not typical of those for other neuropathic conditions.

ETIOLOGY AND PATHOGENESIS

Tic douloureux can be caused by any of a number of conditions affecting the ipsilateral trigeminal system. In the vast majority, the cause seems to be compression of the trigeminal nerve at its exit from the pons by an adjacent artery or vein that has elongated and kinked to become wedged against the nerve. In about 1% to 2% of cases, the pain results from a benign tumor in the cerebellopontine angle, such as a meningioma, epidermoid tumor, or acoustic neuroma, or even an arteriovenous malformation.[8] Other authors have indicated that 1% to 8% of patients with trigeminal neuralgia have multiple sclerosis.[9-13] Very infrequently, trigeminal neuralgia may be the presenting symptom of multiple sclerosis.[14] A variety of other rare etiological associations have been reported, but all of these together probably do not account for more than a low percentage of cases. In a significant number of patients, the cause of the tic douloureux is not apparent.

The pathogenesis of trigeminal neuralgia remains uncertain, as are the mechanisms by which treatments are effective. For example, some authors have postulated that nerve root demyelination resulting from neural compression by a blood vessel or tumor or resulting from multiple sclerosis is an important feature, perhaps permitting ephaptic transmission or ectopic impulse generation between adjacent denuded axons. Both peripheral and central mechanisms are most likely required for the production of tic douloureux. Calvin and colleagues presented a comprehensive theory that utilizes two known physiological mechanisms: the trigeminal dorsal root reflex and repetitive firing of extra action potentials from a focal region of altered axonal size or myelination.[15] Altered

central connectivity and neuronal hyperactivity caused by deafferentation (centralist concept) as well as changes in the trigeminal myelin and axons can lead to altered peripheral sensitivity to chemical and mechanical stimuli (peripheralist concept).[15,16] However, as attractive as such ideas are, no theory has yet been postulated that explains all aspects of tic douloureux, such as the pain-free periods, which may last for months or years early in the course of the condition, the triggering of tic pain by non-noxious stimuli, the separation of the trigger areas from the painful region, and the response to anticonvulsants. Elimination of root compression by adjacent vessels does not take into account the effectiveness of numerous other surgical procedures, most of which injure the root or ganglion, but decompression of the root may relieve pain by facilitating remyelination.

CLINICAL FEATURES

Tic douloureux is diagnosed almost exclusively on the basis of the patient's history (Box 48.1). The International Headache Society defined trigeminal neuralgia as a "sudden, usually unilateral, severe, brief, stabbing, and recurrent pain in the distribution of one or more branches of the fifth cranial nerve."[17,18] The three divisions of the trigeminal nerve are the ophthalmic, maxillary, and mandibular. For the accurate diagnosis of facial pain, a detailed knowledge of the anatomy of the fifth cranial nerve is essential. By definition, the pain of tic douloureux is confined to the distribution of one trigeminal nerve (Fig. 48.1) and more commonly affects the lower part of the face than the upper.[16] The maxillary division of the fifth cranial nerve (V2) is the site of pain alone or in combination with other divisions, most commonly the mandibular division (V3) in 45% of cases. The ophthalmic division (Vl) is least likely to be affected in trigeminal neuralgia (Fig. 48.2). A small number of patients have similar pain

---

BOX 48.1 International Headache Society Criteria for Trigeminal Neuralgia

Paroxysmal attacks of frontal pain last a few seconds to less than 2 minutes.
Pain has at least four of the following characteristics: distribution along one or more divisions of the trigeminal nerve; sudden, intense, sharp, superficial, stabbing or burning in quality; pain intensity severe; precipitation from trigger areas or by certain daily activities such as eating, talking, washing the face or cleaning the teeth; between paroxysms the patient is entirely asymptomatic.
No neurological deficit is found.
Attacks are stereotyped in the individual patient.
Other causes of facial pain are excluded by history, physical examination, and special investigation when necessary.

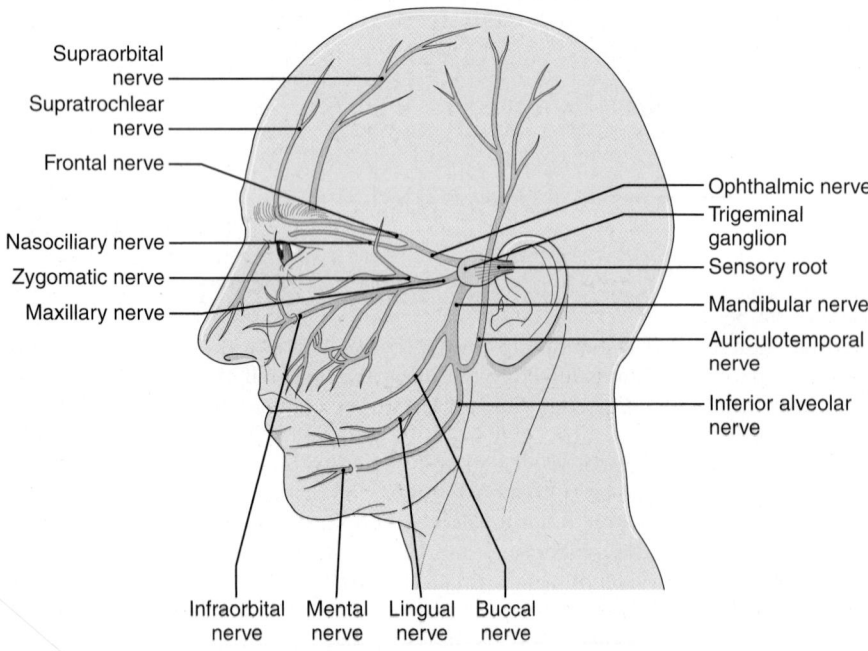

FIGURE 48.1 The peripheral and central aspects of the trigeminal nerve and its branches.

Supraorbital nerve
Supratrochlear nerve
Frontal nerve
Nasociliary nerve
Zygomatic nerve
Maxillary nerve
Infraorbital nerve
Mental nerve
Lingual nerve
Buccal nerve
Ophthalmic nerve
Trigeminal ganglion
Sensory root
Mandibular nerve
Auriculotemporal nerve
Inferior alveolar nerve

syndromes in the territories of the nervus intermedius, glossopharyngeal nerve, or vagus nerve. The pain of untreated tic douloureux occurs unpredictably and is sudden in onset, severe in degree, and short in duration. Often the patient can experience many paroxysms of pain within a single hour, and such bouts may go on for days, with some fluctuation in frequency from hour to hour and day to day. Early in the course of the syndrome, pain-free periods lasting months are common, but as time goes on these natural remissions tend to become less frequent and less prolonged. Although tic pain is ordinarily spontaneous in onset, it can frequently be triggered by a non-noxious stimulus, such as touching the skin on that side of the face, chewing, swallowing, or talking. Some patients are sensitive in certain areas of the face, called *trigger zones*, which when touched cause an attack of pain. Even a gentle breeze can trigger pain in some patients. The pain has been described as lancinating, lightning-like, or electrical in quality, and has been likened to the pain experienced when a dentist drills into the pulp of a tooth.[7] The patient may wince in response to the pain, hence the name *tic douloureux*. A history of bilateral tic pain can be elicited in 3% of patients, although no patient has bilateral tic pain during one episode.[16]

Often the patient who develops tic douloureux sees the dentist first, because lancinating lower facial pain seems to be arising from a certain tooth or teeth. Dentists are often fixated on peripheral lesions as the cause for pain. A diseased tooth in the upper jaw can cause headache on the same side, which may radiate into the orbit or face. A diseased tooth in the lower jaw may cause considerable pain in the distribution of the mandibular division of the nerve, including pain deep in the ear. In addition, dental pain is much more common than tic douloureux. Teeth may be extracted or other dental procedures performed without providing any relief of the pain of tic douloureux. The patient may also consult more than one physician before the correct diagnosis is made. In the majority of patients, the trigeminal neuralgia is idiopathic in that there is no identifiable cause.[8] However, the presence of sensory loss mandates a thorough search for structural pathology. Patients with idiopathic trigeminal neuralgia can develop more atypical features with time in the absence of efficacious therapy.

In all likelihood, this development coincides with ongoing neuropathic injury. Pain that is continuous, lacks a shock-like quality, or is associated with objective evidence of cranial nerve dysfunction should raise the suspicion of diseases other than idiopathic trigeminal neuralgia. However, the most likely cause of this type of pain is a prior ablative procedure that damages the trigeminal nerve. Atypical facial pain is described as deep, burning, and continual. There is no jabbing onset as occurs in tic douloureux. The pain can radiate behind the ear, down onto the neck, or across to the opposite maxillary area. These patients, in contrast, often clutch their face, unlike the patient with tic douloureux who shields her face but is very careful not to actually touch it (Table 48.1). Myofascial pains involving the muscles of mastication and temporomandibular joint pain occur predominantly in the lateral face. They are also described as aching, burning, or cramping pains, and are often associated with tenderness to palpation of the involved muscles.[16]

Deviations from the typical picture of tic douloureux can occur, although the more unusual features the patient manifests, the less likely is a favorable response to either medical or surgical therapies. Furthermore, surgical procedures that damage the trigeminal nerve can produce changes in the findings and in the patient's symptoms. Nerve damage can lead to a burning component of the pain, although these iatrogenically acquired changes in the pain syndrome do not alter the original diagnosis. It is therefore essential to ascertain what the symptoms were prior to any intervention.

DIAGNOSIS

The diagnosis of tic douloureux is based almost exclusively on the history; as this disease consists only of pain, no diagnostic imaging or physiological studies currently available will substitute for the history. The neurological examination is ordinarily normal except for mild sensory changes in a minority of patients in the region of their pain, with the exception that those few patients with multiple sclerosis or a large structural lesion such as a tumor in the cerebellopontine angle usually have altered trigeminal sensation and other evidence that heralds the underlying disorder. Traditionally, diagnostic radiological studies such as computed tomography or magnetic resonance imaging have been normal in the usual patient with tic douloureux, but they have been performed to identify the exceptional patient with a recognizable etiological condition such as those just mentioned.[7] Patients with a Chiari malformation may also develop trigeminal neuralgia, thought to be the result of venous or arterial compression of the cranial nerves along with the tonsillar ectopia. Recent advances in magnetic resonance imaging and magnetic resonance angiography have improved the sensitivity and specificity of diagnosing neurovascular compression of the nerve by evaluating the anatomical relationships of the arterial and venous structures with the trigeminal nerve at the root entry zone in the cerebellopontine angle.[16] However, so far these studies have been more used as a preoperative adjunct than for diagnostic purposes.[19,20] Continued development of MRI is likely to lead to the ability to discern if there is a vascular impingement on the nerve and thereby may influence choice of treatment.

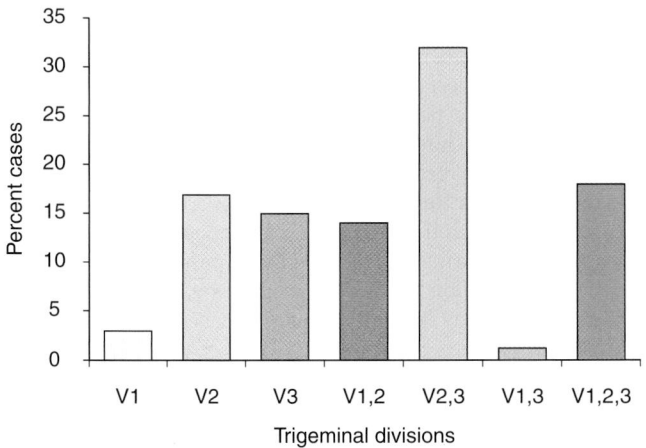

FIGURE 48.2 Distribution of pain among divisions of the trigeminal nerve in patients with tic douloureux *(Data from Loeser J. Tic douloureux. Pain Res Manage 2001;6:156-165.)*

TABLE 48.1 Differential Diagnosis of Facial Pain

Condition/Factor	Trigeminal Neuralgia	Atypical Facial Pain	Migrainous Facial Pain	Acute Herpes Zoster
Age and gender	>50 years, 60% F	30-50 years, 75% F	Typically, age range of 40-50 years; M = F	>70 years, F > M
Site	V2 or V3 most common alone or in combination, but limited to distribution of trigeminal nerve (intraoral or extraoral), unilateral	Deep nonmuscular areas of face, maxillary or whole face, unilateral or bilateral; does not follow nerve distribution	Anywhere in face Deep eye pain, sinus pain or toothache	Herpetic lesions in the distribution of trigeminal nerve; V1 most common Most severe in eyebrow; facial or deep ear pain often precedes vesicular eruption
Character	Sudden severe, brief lancinating, electric-shock-like, no allodynia	Throbbing, deep, diffuse, nagging, aching, burning, cramping; allodynia in some patients	Throbbing or pulsatile, lacrimation or conjunctival injection (cluster headache), no allodynia	Burning, tingling in quality; itching, dysesthesia; allodynia in some patients
Severity	Severe	Moderate to severe	Moderate	Severity varies
Duration	Seconds to minutes	Seconds to minutes or continuous	15 minutes to several hours	Continuous Pain may precede vesicular eruption
Periodicity	Pain-free between attacks, long periods of no pain	Continuous background pain or dysesthesia; complete pain remission less likely, interferes with sleep	Often nocturnal or early morning	Continuous pain until vesicles heal, may then develop as postherpetic neuralgia
Provoking factors	Non-noxious stimulation of discrete trigger zones in face or in buccal mucosa, hot/cold fluids in mouth or chewing	Stress, fatigue	Alcohol, hormone replacement therapy, seasonal, cold, warm	Skin stimulation by clothing or touch

F, female; M, male.

TREATMENT

Despite the relative lack of understanding of pathophysiological mechanisms of trigeminal neuralgia, very effective medical and surgical treatments have been developed. Although generally effective treatments are available for tic douloureux, none is successful in all cases. Few or no randomized trials exist comparing medical, surgical, and interventional techniques, and therefore, treatment decisions for these patients with neuropathic pain can be challenging and are largely empiric. Furthermore, the individual patient frequently requires more than one form of treatment during the course of the disease. The psychosocial and behavioral response patterns of patients with chronic facial pain are similar to those of other patients with chronic pain.

In those few patients with an abnormality along the path of the trigeminal nerve that can be detected radiologically, such as a neoplasm in the cerebellopontine angle, the treatment is directed against the lesion that has been demonstrated. This approach ordinarily will also relieve the tic douloureux. However, the overwhelming majority of patients does not fall into this category and their symptoms must be treated in spite of the absence of structural pathology other than an adjacent blood vessel.

Medication

The initial treatment of patients with trigeminal neuralgia is always pharmacological.[21] Drugs with anticonvulsive properties rather than analgesic ones are most effective. There are a limited number of controlled trials that have studied the pharmacological treatment for trigeminal neuralgia. The anticonvulsants carbamazepine, phenytoin, and gabapentin have been found to reduce or control the pain of tic douloureux.[22] Likewise, oxcarbazepine, lamotrigine, and baclofen are said to have beneficial effects in the treatment of tic douloureux, although the evidence is very limited.

Carbamazepine is considered the first-line treatment for patients with trigeminal neuralgia and is ordinarily begun at a dosage of 200 mg per day, being increased as tolerated to 200 mg three or four times a day, or more. Over 70% of patients report symptomatic improvement, although it is not an analgesic and must be taken regularly to maintain its efficacy. The goal is to reach the smallest dose that provides adequate pain relief. At high doses, the patient may experience the side effects of lethargy, sluggish thinking, and imbalance.[7] Doses higher than 1800 mg have not been more effective.[23] Carbamazepine may also interfere with the production of blood elements and may alter hepatic function. Therefore, a patient being treated with carbamazepine should have periodic complete blood counts and hepatic function studies. Oxcarbazepine is another anticonvulsant that has become popular recently, because it may be dosed less frequently and has fewer side effects than carbamazepine, although it appears to have the same efficacy. When patients have been pain free for several weeks, carbamazepine may be tapered, which should be done very slowly over weeks.

Phenytoin is ordinarily begun at a dosage of 100 mg three times a day. Intravenous phenytoin has been used in some patients for acute exacerbations with frequent, easily triggered, high-intensity pain attacks. Approximately 25% of patients obtain satisfactory pain relief although, unlike epilepsy, relief of tic douloureux pain has been shown to correlate with phenytoin blood levels. Coadministered carbamazepine can raise serum phenytoin concentrations, whereas phenytoin can decrease the half-life of carbamazepine.

Baclofen, a GABA analog, can also be used alone or in combination with phenytoin or carbamazepine. Other agents include clonazepam, valproic acid, lamotrigine, topiramate, and gabapentin. Gabapentin has also shown promise in relieving many forms of neuropathic pain and is well tolerated.[23] There is little or no evidence to support the use of non-antiepileptic drugs in the treatment of tic douloureux.[22]

Any of these three anticonvulsant medicines is used alone at first, and the dose is increased as needed to control the facial pain. With time, a patient may need progressively larger dosages to provide the same degree of relief. The development of toxicity may necessitate a reduction in the dosage, and the occurrence of some other significant side effect may require cessation of the medication altogether and lead patients to consider other forms of treatment. In this case, a second drug may be added to or substituted for the first. At times, it may be necessary to use two or three drugs at once. Approximately two thirds of patients with tic douloureux are adequately managed on antiepileptic drugs, but one third of them cannot tolerate the side effects of these medications. Therefore, about one half of the patients with tic douloureux are candidates for surgery after they have failed medical management

It is important to recognize that opioids are not appropriate medications for the long-term treatment of tic douloureux. This type of neuropathic pain is not likely to respond to opioids. The only exception might be when a patient first experiences tic and time is necessary to establish adequate levels of an anticonvulsant drug. Opioids in such a setting may take the edge off of the patient's pain and anxiety, but they are never an adequate treatment for tic douloureux in isolation or over a long period of time.

Other forms of therapy such as acupuncture, herbs, vitamins, magnets, etc., have no role in the treatment of tic. The bottom line is that either the patient gets good relief with an anticonvulsant or needs to be offered a surgical intervention. Nerve blocks rarely provide pain relief that outlasts the duration of the agent utilized.

Surgical Treatment

Medical management should always precede a surgical procedure and no surgical procedure is warranted unless pharmacological therapy has failed either because of inadequate pain relief or unacceptable side effects. The three primary surgical treatments are gangliolysis, stereotactic radiosurgery, and suboccipital craniectomy with microvascular decompression (Box 48.2).

Gasserian Gangliolysis

Trigeminal gangliolysis avoids the risks of a craniotomy and its objective is to destroy selectively the A-δ and C fibers (nociceptive) while preserving the A-α and β fibers (touch). It can be repeated easily if the pain recurs, and is associated with minimal rate of morbidity. In the gangliolysis procedure, the

BOX 48.2 Surgical Management Options for Trigeminal Neuralgia

Radiofrequency gangliolysis
Balloon gangliolysis
Glycerol gangliolysis
Gamma Knife radiosurgery
Microvascular decompression
Trigeminal rhizotomy
Trigeminal tractotomy

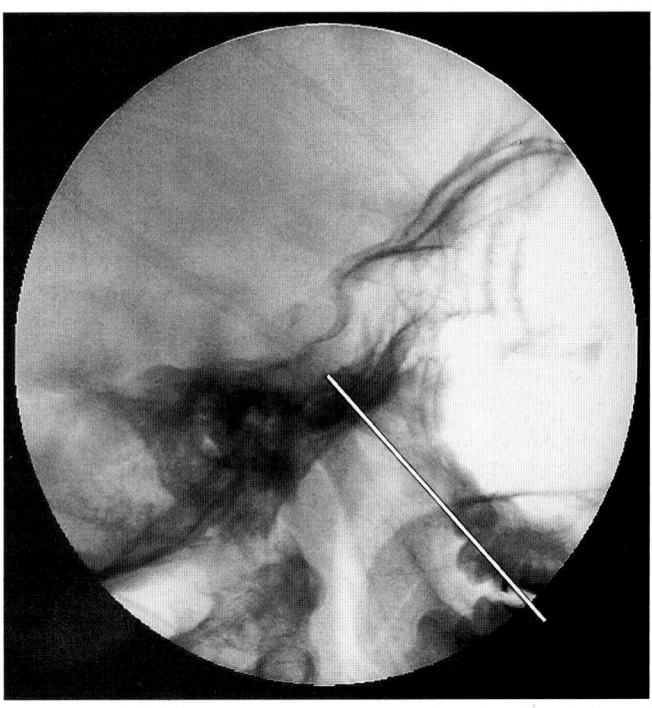

FIGURE 48.3 Percutaneous trigeminal/gasserian rhizolysis. Lateral fluoroscopic skull image shows the needle is inserted through the cheek into the third division of the trigeminal nerve at the foramen ovale and is advanced into the gasserian ganglion and sensory root. The fibers of V3, then V2, and finally V1 are encountered in sequence as the needle is advanced toward the clivus.

gasserian ganglion and adjacent sensory root of the trigeminal nerve are injured, with the expectation that a more permanent effect can be achieved than following a neurectomy because neural regeneration is less likely to occur in these areas than in the peripheral trigeminal branches. In the past, an anterior trigeminal rhizotomy was performed by exposing and dividing or otherwise injuring part or all of the main trigeminal sensory root adjacent to the gasserian ganglion.[4,5] The radiofrequency gangliolysis procedure is performed by inserting a needle through the cheek into the third division of the trigeminal nerve at the foramen ovale, and then advancing the needle under fluoroscopic guidance into the gasserian ganglion and sensory root (Fig. 48.3).[3,22,24-26] The entry point is 2.5 cm lateral to the corner of the mouth in the occlusal plane and the needle is aimed toward the intersection of the coronal plane halfway between the external auditory meatus and the lateral canthus and the sagittal plane centered at the pupil. The needle is advanced through the foramen ovale at the petrosphenoid junction and positioned at the level appropriate for the affected trigeminal branch. The third, second, and first divisions can then be stimulated in sequence by slowly advancing the needle tip. Generally, the mandibular division of the root is encountered 1 cm after penetration of the foramen ovale, V2 is located at 2 cm, and V1 is at 3 cm and at the level of the clivus. Once the needle is ideally situated, the patient is awakened and the relevant nerve root is stimulated to confirm stimulus-provoked cutaneous paresthesia in the painful trigeminal division. Contractions of the masseter and pterygoid muscles can occur at a low stimulation threshold with a medial trajectory. The patient is then reanesthetized and the neural destruction is produced by using a radiofrequency current to create a thermal lesion. Gangliolysis can also be performed under general anesthesia using a Fogarty catheter balloon to damage the ganglion mechanically, or by injecting glycerol into the cistern of the trigeminal ganglion. The goal is to produce the least neurological deficit that will control the patient's pain.

Gangliolysis by any method produces pain relief for a longer period than by the injection or avulsion of a peripheral branch. Radiofrequency gangliolysis offers an 80% chance of 1-year pain relief and a 50% chance of 5-year success.[16,27] Approximately 5% to 10% will not obtain relief initially or will have an early recurrence of pain; during the 5 years after the procedure, about 25% will experience recurrence.[28,29] The complication rate of radiofrequency gangliolysis is 0.5% to 1% and can include meningitis, damage to other cranial nerves, corneal anesthesia, masseter weakness, and anesthesia dolorosa (total sensory loss). Anesthesia dolorosa is the most dreaded complication of ablative lesions of the trigeminal nerve and refers to pain in an anesthetic region. Unfortunately, no pharmacological or ablative surgical treatment is effective for this complication.[22]

Balloon compression is performed under general anesthesia. Using fluoroscopic control, a large 14-gauge guide needle is inserted until it just penetrates the foramen ovale and the balloon is slowly inflated. Balloon compression is technically easier than radiofrequency thermocoagulation; it produces similar results and does not require patient participation. However,

bradycardia should be anticipated during the procedure. For this reason, glycopyrrolate should be administered prior to insertion of the needle when performing any type of gangliolysis. Some authors believe that the risk of corneal hypoesthesia and anesthesia dolorosa is lower with balloon compression and therefore is the procedure of choice in patients with ophthalmic division involvement or in patients who are not good awake surgical candidates for radiofrequency gangliolysis.

Glycerol gangliolysis is less often performed today than the radiofrequency or balloon gangliolysis. Because the location of the glycerol cannot be precisely targeted after injection, the results are somewhat unpredictable; however, overall there is a lower incidence of sensory loss and anesthesia dolorosa than with the radiofrequency lesion. With glycerol gasserian rhizolysis, the long-term results are not quite as good: there is a 5% to 15% incidence of early failure and about a 20% to 30% incidence of later failure.[27,29]

In general, patients are relieved for a longer period after gangliolysis than they are by the injection of alcohol into or avulsion of a peripheral branch. Therefore, peripheral neurectomy is indicated only when gangliolysis has failed and the patient cannot or will not tolerate a suboccipital microvascular decompression. Alternatively, a local anesthetic block into the trigger area or region of pain may provide transient relief until definitive therapy can be undertaken.[2,16,22]

Microvascular Decompression

Vascular compression of the trigeminal nerve at its entrance into the pons is the common etiological factor in trigeminal neuralgia. Jannetta developed an operation to move the offending vessel(s) away from the nerve.[30,31] This procedure is referred to as *microvascular decompression* because it involves an operating microscope and microsurgical technique. The area is exposed through a lateral posterior fossa craniectomy (retromastoid craniectomy), and after the vessel or vessels are separated from the nerve, a material such as a synthetic sponge or Teflon felt is inserted to maintain the separation (Fig. 48.4). The trigeminal nerve must be carefully and circumferentially

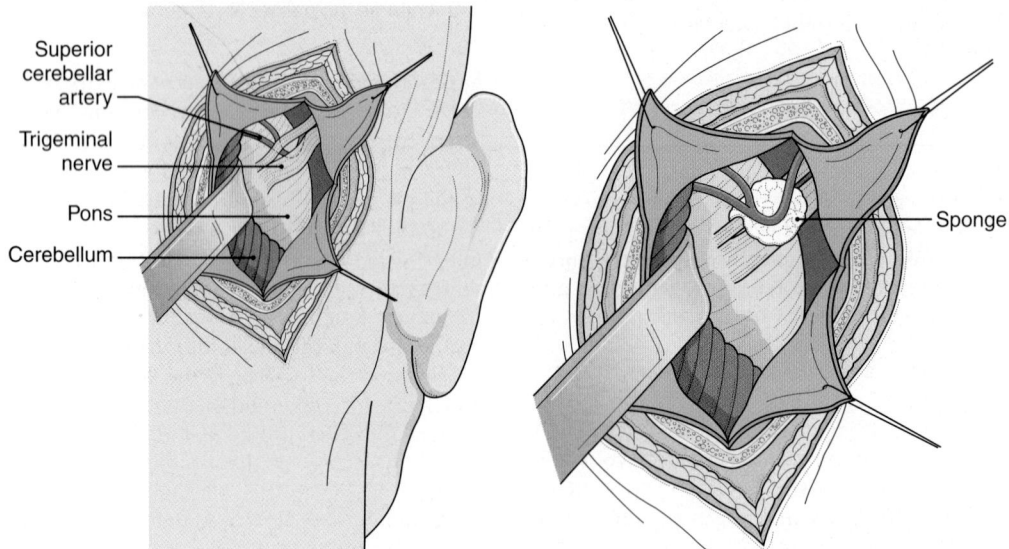

Superior cerebellar artery
Trigeminal nerve
Pons
Cerebellum
Sponge

FIGURE 48.4 Retromastoid craniectomy with microvascular decompression of the trigeminal nerve.

inspected along its entire intracranial course from the root entry zone to its entrance laterally into Meckel's cave. This procedure ordinarily provides pain relief without any facial sensory loss and has a greater potential for producing long-lasting pain relief. It is interesting to note that the tic pain does not always stop immediately following a microvascular decompression, but instead may take several days. Furthermore, nerve manipulation without moving the artery will transiently stop the tic pain although it will soon recur thereafter.

Review of the literature suggests that definite neurovascular compression is found in 88.6% of cases, but an average of 7.5% of explorations reveal no pathology intraoperatively.[19] The results of microvascular decompression are excellent if arterial compression is identified. The superior cerebellar artery is the most common (70-80%) cause of trigeminal neuralgia. When the pain is perceived in V2 or V3 divisions, the usual finding intraoperatively is compression of the rostral and anterior portion of the nerve. The anterior inferior cerebellar artery is the compressive vessel in 10% of cases and occurs in the caudal and posterior portion of the nerve closest to nerve VI. Veins impact the nerve in 5% to 13% of cases.[25] Among 68 personal patients followed for an average of 54 months, 72% had excellent pain relief and 6% had good relief that did not lead to any sensory loss.[21] The initial failure rate for microvascular decompression is in the 5% to 10% range.[23,28,29,32] Subsequently, the rate of pain recurrence averages about 3.5% per year. This procedure is contraindicated in patients with atypical facial pain because of the poor results achieved. Magnetic resonance angiographic imaging effectively excludes secondary causes of trigeminal neuralgia, which warrant nonmicrovascular decompression management. If no significant vascular compression is identified at operation, the main sensory root of the trigeminal nerve can be partially divided adjacent to the pons (posterior trigeminal rhizotomy). This has a similar probability of providing pain relief, but will cause some degree of facial hypoesthesia. The intrinsic somatotopic organization of the nerve tends to spare the superiorly located ophthalmic segment when performing a partial sensory rhizotomy of the lateral two thirds of the nerve.

When compared with other surgical treatments, it is widely accepted that microvascular decompression is associated with the lowest rates of recurrence and sensory loss, although more serious risks of morbidity (5%) and mortality (0.5%) are encountered than after Gamma Knife radiosurgery or gangliolysis. It has the best long-term success rate of any of the available surgical treatments. In the event of a recurrence after microvascular decompression, reexploration of the nerve can be performed, with less rewarding results, but pathological vessel impingement may not be found and a partial rhizotomy still needs to be considered.[33]

Stereotaxic Radiosurgery

Gamma Knife radiosurgery has been advocated as a minimally invasive alternative surgical approach to microvascular decompression or percutaneous surgeries. The short-term results are as good as gangliolysis for tic douloureux, although as is true for all other types of treatments for this disorder, atypical clinical features or a history of prior tic surgery lowers the success rate. Currently there are two types of radiosurgery technologies: linear accelerators (linacs) and Gamma Knife. A 2009 report indicates that over 2800 patients had been treated with the Gamma Knife throughout the world by 1999. From 70% to 80% of patients are pain-free in the short-term, although up to 50% relapse. Doses of 60 to 90 Gy were used in a single session and most of the patients responded to radiosurgery within 6 months of the procedure, with a median of 2 months and a low incidence of complications.[34-38] These results are promising, although the recurrence rate and long-term morbidity rate remain to be seen. In another recent study of 102 patients, despite an 81% early response rate, 56% of patients who experienced initial pain relief suffered treatment failure. Side effects also include facial dysesthesias, corneal irritation, vascular damage, hearing loss, and facial weakness, varying with dose plan and target areas. Oddly, pain relief usually does not occur for 2 to 12 weeks after radiosurgery.[37,38]

Peripheral Neurectomy

Resection or avulsion of a branch of the trigeminal nerve has a long history in the treatment of tic douloureux, but it is rarely a procedure of choice today in countries with developed health care. It produces complete anesthesia in the distribution if the avulsed branch, which can be a significant disability for the patient.[39] Pain relief rarely lasts more than a year or so, and repeating the procedure does not produce as good results as the original. However, if gangliolysis is not available or has failed in a patient who has also failed stereotactic radiosurgery, it could be considered.

Trigeminal Tractotomy

When all other measures have failed, sectioning of the descending trigeminal tract in the medulla produces loss of pain and temperature sensation in the ipsilateral face and pharynx but spares touch. It is carried out through a small suboccipital craniectomy and C1 and C2 laminectomy and requires both anatomical and physiological localization techniques. It is not commonly performed today, although a percutaneous method has also been described.

CONCLUSION

A patient with trigeminal neuralgia who has no discernible mass along the trigeminal pathways should first receive a trial of appropriate pharmacological therapy. Medical management is successful in about one half of patients. If this fails, one of the surgical approaches should then be considered, with the selection based on the location of the pain, the patient's age and health, and the experience and preference of the surgeon. For example, for an elderly patient or one with multiple medical comorbid conditions with medically refractory trigeminal neuralgia Gamma Knife or gangliolysis should be offered as primary surgical procedures. Secondary ablative procedures, such as avulsion of peripheral branches of the trigeminal nerve or trigeminal rhizotomy or trigeminal tractotomy, need to be considered when the three primary procedures have failed.

The patient with trigeminal neuralgia may need different forms of treatment during his or her lifetime. The physician should be aware of the options, selecting the one most likely to help at that particular time, with the least risk.

ACKNOWLEDGMENT

This chapter contains material from the first edition of this text, and we are grateful to the author of that chapter for his contribution.

SELECTED KEY REFERENCES

Barker F, Jannetta P, Bissonette D, et al. Microvascular decompression for typical trigeminal neuralgia: a 20 year experience. *J Neurosurg.* 1994;80:392A.

Burchiel K, Steege T, Howe J, et al. Comparison of percutaneous radiofrequency gangliolysis and microvascular decompression for the surgical management of tic douloureux. *Neurosurgery.* 1981;9:111-119.

Kondziolka D, Lunsford L, Flickinger J. Stereotactic radiosurgery for the treatment of trigeminal neuralgia. *Clin J Pain.* 2002;18:42-47.

Loeser J. Cranial neuralgias. In: Bonica J, ed. *The Management of Pain in Clinical Practice.* 2nd ed. Philadelphia: Lea & Febiger; 1990:676-686.

Sweet W. The treatment of trigeminal neuralgia (tic douloureux). *N Engl J Med.* 1986;315:174-177.

Please go to expertconsult.com to view the complete list of references.

CHAPTER

49 Surgical Therapy for Pain

Giovanni Broggi, Francesco Acerbi, Morgan Broggi, Giuseppe Messina

CLINICAL PEARLS

- Chronic pain syndromes are of two types: cancer-related pain and chronic benign pain.

- In general, the various surgical procedures that are available for the management of the chronic pain syndromes can be categorized into lesional surgery, stimulation procedures, and corrective surgery (microvascular decompression of the trigeminal nerve).

- The efficacy of a number of pain control procedures is difficult to assess from the literature in the absence of class 1 or class 2 evidence. Individual experience and the conjoint services of a pain control program are necessary to evaluate and treat patients with chronic pain.

- Lesional procedures for the control of pain syndromes in order of ascending pain pathway are as follows: peripheral neurectomy, dorsal rhizotomy and dorsol root ganglionectomy, sympathectomy, dorsal root entry zone

leions, anterolateral cordotomy, mesencephalotomy, and cingulotomy.

- Trigeminal neuralgia can be treated by a variety of surgical techniques: peripheral neurectomy, radiofrequency rhizotomy, glycerol injection, balloon compression, microvascular decompression, trigeminal nerve root resection, and radiosurgery. These measures are used when medical treatment has failed.

- Stimulation techniques (neuromodulation procedures) for chronic pain control include deep brain stimulation, motor cortex stimulation, spinal cord stimulation, and peripheral nerve stimulation. The indications for and results of these techniques are different.

- Intrathecal and intraventricular administration of opioid drugs may also be used for pain control in some patients.

Indications to surgical procedures for pain actually depend on the characteristics of the pain, the causative factor(s), and anatomical functional knowledge of circuits subserving the nociceptive transmission. The distinction between chronic malignant and chronic nonmalignant pain is, of course, a first step in the therapeutic decision-making process.

Pain is one of the most common symptoms experienced by cancer patients and probably the one that maximally influences the quality of life. More than 75% of patients with advanced disease complain of severe pain.[1] The majority of these patients can benefit from treatment with oral opioids,[1] probably because of the nociceptive nature of pain in such cases. Other options are rehabilitation techniques, transcutaneous electrical nerve stimulation (TENS), acupuncture, and physical therapies.[2-5] For medically intractable pain from malignant disease, intrathecal administration of drugs can be taken into account, but considering the possible development of addiction and tolerance, which can turn into serious impairment of the overall quality of life,[6] these patients may be considered for neuroablative procedures.[7,8]

Chronic benign pain, on the other hand, can result from a multitude of causes and, despite the individual predominance of nociceptive or neuropathic features, in the majority of cases it is a combination of both, with the significant addition of psychopathological features. For these reasons, chronic pain from nonmalignant disease remains the major challenge to pain doctors and still today there is great uncertainty as to the proper surgical and nonsurgical treatment.[9,10]

Nonmalignant and predominantly nociceptive pain results by definition from non-neural tissue damage (trauma, inflammation, degenerative disease, etc.); conversely, neuropathic pain results from neural tissue damage. In both cases psychological and psychosocial factors, typically coexisting with painful symptoms, make the eventual pre- and postoperative clinical assessment particularly difficult.

For many years, surgical therapy for pain has relied on ablative or "lesional" procedures, consisting of disruption or interruption of anatomical structures and pathways involved in the transmission of painful sensations. However, the rates of complications, pain recurrence, and the development of deafferentation pain due to such procedures were noted to be

737

rather high; over time, these techniques benefited by several improvements, thanks to the introduction of microsurgery and to a more extensive knowledge of the anatomical functional correlations between pain modulative systems.

Although the patients' selection criteria for ablative procedures have become increasingly selective (also with the aid of thermocoagulation and of CO_2 laser), the development of neuromodulation procedures (by means of electrical stimulation or of intrathecal administration of drugs) has led to a decrease in the indications for such surgery.[6]

The recent advancements in the electrophysiological field along with the development of neuronal and axonal network modeling have made possible the explorative instrumental armamentarium now available for functional neurosurgeons, and a large surgical experience has been gained with patients suffering from refractory pain.

LESIONAL SURGERY

Lesional procedures for the treatment of refractory pain have their own rationale in the causative role of a given nuclear or axonal structure in the generation of altered nociceptive information. After the identification of the putative structure responsible for the transmission of established painful symptoms, this structure is ablated or "lesioned" by means of different techniques. It is important to consider neuromodulative procedures before proceeding to ablative techniques, and of course the indication for such surgery strictly depends on the prognosis *quoad vitam* of the individual patient, the previous pharmacological or surgical attempts already administered, the overall medical condition, and the patient's choice. Before considering a patient for an ablative procedure, conservative nonsurgical therapy (or neuromodulation procedures) must have been attempted, maximized, and failed.[11]

Peripheral Neurectomy

Known from the sixteenth century, thanks to Ambroise Paré, neurectomy consists of the resection of a portion or the whole of one or more peripheral nerves. It is an easy and simple procedure, performed under local anesthesia, but its long-term failure rate makes its indications in chronic pain management very limited today.[12] In fact, adjacent intact sensory nerves can reinnervate the anesthetic region, thus causing pain recurrence; a new pain sensation due to the denervation hypersensitivity and painful postoperative neuromas may develop, too.[12,13]

Neurectomy is indicated in those cases in which pain is limited to the nervous distribution of a specific nerve; such cases are rare and it is thus preferable (given the innervation's juxtaposition of different dermatomes) to perform peripheral neurotomies in steps. Painful neuromas following peripheral nerve injuries may benefit from neuroma excision and neurectomy, if conservative nonsurgical treatment has not succeeded.[13,14] Proximal neurectomy in amputee patients with painful stump neuromas can be of benefit, but nonspecific stump pains or phantom limb pains do not respond to nerve resection.[12,15] Chest wall cancer pain and postherpetic neuralgia also do not benefit from neurectomy.

In some rare cases it is possible to perform a trial infiltration of long-acting anesthetic, eventually followed by neurolysis with percutaneous thermocoagulation or with injection of neurodestructive agents, such as phenol or alcohol;[16] potential action sites are the posterior ramus of the second cervical nerve in the case of occipital neuralgia and the posterior rami of the spinal intercostal nerves in the case of drug-refractory intercostal neuralgia.

Dorsal Rhizotomy and Dorsal Root Ganglionectomy

Dorsal rhizotomy implies the sectioning of the dorsal nerve roots. Extradural, percutaneous, and radiofrequency methods have been described as well as partial rhizotomy.[17-20] The procedure was indicated especially in the thoracic and sacral regions for malignant pain,[21] but because of the high rate of pain recurrence[22,23] and development of dysesthesic or deafferentation pain[24] the procedure has been all but abandoned these days.

Performed first in 1966 by Scoville,[25] based on the discovery that a certain number of axons in the ventral root were unmyelinated afferent fibers from the dorsal root ganglion,[26-28] dorsal root ganglionectomy showed some long-term pain relief in the treatment of chest wall pain, known as the *postthoracotomy* syndrome.[11] Some authors suggest it for sciatica, too, but there is some controversy about this indication.

Dorsal Root Entry Zone Lesions

The dorsal root entry zone (DREZ) is an anatomical entity that includes the central portion of dorsal root, the tract of Lissauer (TL), and layers I to V of the dorsal horn, where the afferent fibers synapse with the origins of the sensory pathways.[29] The TL plays an important role in the intersegmental modulation of the nociceptive afferents. It is located dorsolaterally to the dorsal horn and it is divided in two parts: (1) the medial part receives nociceptive afferents directed to the dorsal horn and transmits the excitatory effects of each dorsal root to the adjacent segment;[30,31] (2) the lateral part receives longitudinal endogenous propriospinal fibers interconnecting different levels of substantia gelatinosa (SG) and thus conveying the inhibitory influence of the SG into the neighboring metameres.[31] The SG, through synaptic connections with the dendrites of some neurons of the spinoreticulothalamic (STR) tract, exerts a strong modulating effect on the nociceptive input (Fig. 49.1A). When the large lemniscal afferents in peripheral nerves or dorsal roots are altered, there is reduction of the inhibitory control of the dorsal horn, hence resulting in excessive firing of the dorsal horn neurons and causing deafferentation pain.[32-35]

Following avulsion injuries of the brachial or lumbosacral plexus between 20% and 90% of patients may develop severe deafferentation pain either immediately after injury or delayed until up to 3 months.

The first DREZ open surgery procedure was performed by Sindou in 1972 on a patient with chronic pain due to Pancoast syndrome.[36] Soon after him, in 1974, Nashold started using radiofrequency thermocoagulation.[37,38] Later, DREZ procedures were performed with laser[39,40] and with the use of ultrasound probes.[41,42]

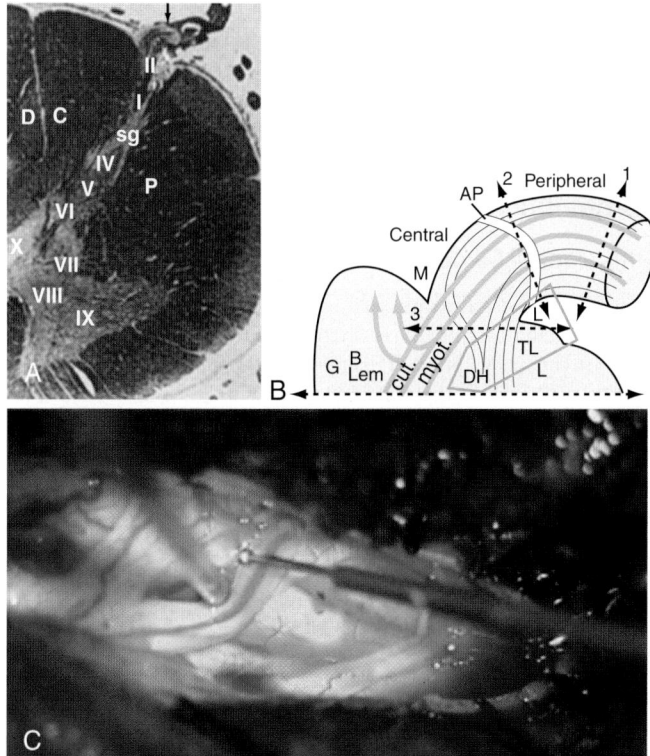

FIGURE 49.1 **A,** Transverse hemisection of the spinal cord at the lower cervical level with myelin stained by luxol-fuchsin showing the myelinated rootlet afferents that reach the dorsal column (DC). *Small arrow:* Pial ring of the dorsal rootlets. *Large arrow:* Microsurgical DREZotomy target. **B,** Scheme of DREZ area and DREZotomy target. The pial ring (AP), located about 1 mm before the penetration of the rootlet into the dorsolateral sulcus, is considered the point of transition from the peripheral to the central segment of the rootlet. Peripherally, the fibers are mixed together, but at the level of the AP, the fine nociceptive fibers run more laterally on the rootlet surface. In the central segment, they group in the ventrolateral portion of the DREZ to enter the dorsal horn (DH) through the tract of Lissauer (TL). The lemniscal fibers (Lem) run dorsomedially in the deeper part of the rootlet, and the myotatic fibers (myot) run in the middle of the DREZ. The black triangle indicates the proposed extent of the surgical lesion. **C,** Intraoperative view during micro-DREZotomy. While the sucker is elevating the dorsal rootlet, the dissector is pointing at the DREZotomy target. DREZ, dorsal root entry zone. *(A modified from Fig. 56.1 in Burchiel KJ, editor. Surgical Management of Pain. New York: Thieme; 2002.)*

The procedure known as *microsurgical DREZotomy* (MDT) was again accomplished by Sindou[29] and involves several segments of the lateral portion of the dorsal horn (where C fibers predominate), meaning the destruction of the LT and laminae I to V of Rexed (Fig. 49.1B and C). By sparing the medial portion of the dorsal horn where large A fibers enter, Sindou tried to avoid complete abolition of tactile and proprioceptive sensation, preserving antinociception and preventing deafferentation.[43] Intraoperative sensory evoked potentials (SEPs) during MDT are recommended for identification of the spinal cord segments and can also be helpful in monitoring the surgical procedure itself.[44-46] Sindou developed special microelectrodes for intraoperative microelectrophysiology

studies and performed microdialysis studies in the dorsal horn as well.[47,48]

MDT has several indications. Some cancer pain patients may benefit from MDT. Good candidates are patients with long life expectancy, sufficient general conditions to undergo surgery and general anesthesia, and topographically delimited pain due to well-localized tumors. MDT from C7 to T2 can be performed for Pancoast syndrome.[49] Malignancies with circumscribed invasion of the thorax, of the abdomen wall, of the perineal floor, or lumbosacral roots or plexus are other indications for MDT. For more extensive cancer, intrathecal opioids or high cervical anterolateral cordotomy is preferable.[29]

Patients with chronic deafferentation pain from plexus avulsion are tremendously difficult to manage for pain doctors. Even if in some cases initial conservative therapy may be of some help, standard analgesics and narcotics are usually ineffective and medical management is limited to antidepressant, sedative, and anticonvulsant medications combined with psychological support.[50] DREZ lesion surgery that is not limited to the avulsed segments but is extended to the adjacent roots is instead recommended for plexus avulsion pain. The results are extremely good, with more than 85% of patients reporting good to excellent pain control after brachial avulsion,[6,36,51-54] although pain relief is fairly lower for conus medullaris root avulsion.[55] Mortality rate is low,[6,51] and morbidity consists of transient sensory deficit and mild weakness.[6] DREZ lesion surgery for lumbosacral avulsion carries less than 10% risks of bladder and sexual dysfunction.[55]

Pain following spinal cord injuries (SCIs) can have a multitude of causes, and hence rigorous patient assessment is mandatory. MDT is indicated for burning pain with radicular distribution at the level of the lesion or for patients complaining mainly of allodynia and electric shock–like border-zone pain. Conversely, pain in the totally or almost totally anesthetic area below the lesion, especially in the perineosacral region, is not favorably influenced by MDT.[29] These patients should be referred to rehabilitation services.

Neurostimulation techniques are the first treatment option for relief of pain due to peripheral nerve injuries and to limb amputation; if these methods fail, DREZ lesion surgery can be considered for both. In peripheral nerve injuries, DREZ surgery may be particularly useful when the predominant component of pain is paroxysmal (electrical shooting pain), associated with allodynia, hyperalgesia, or both.[29] After limb amputation two types of pain may develop and may coexist: pain in the phantom limb and pain in the stump. The former may be reduced by DREZotomy, while the latter is inconstantly influenced.[29]

Finally, MDT can be performed also for severe occipital neuralgia, unbearable laterocervical pain, and postherpetic pain, but the procedure has been performed only in small subgroups of patients and has had a high recurrence rate.[56,57] Based on the fact that muscle tone was decreased in the operated areas after MDT,[36,58] Sindou applied it also for treatment of harmful spasticity with reasonably good results.[59,60-62]

In 1978 Nashold described nucleus caudalis tractotomy/nucleotomy, also known as *caudalis DREZotomy*, in which DREZ lesion surgery is extended to the trigeminothalamic system for treatment of facial deafferentation pain such as trigeminal postherpetic neuralgia and facial anesthesia dolorosa.[10,63] The results are not as good as those for the other major indications of DREZotomy, but almost 50% of patients may obtain pain relief, and it should be considered that these patients are typically not responding to standard narcotic therapies. For patients without prominent allodynia or hyperpathia, on the other hand, neurostimulation procedures are preferred.[6]

Provided that rigorous selection criteria are applied, DREZ surgery can achieve very good pain control in some intractable painful syndromes. Sindou proposed a schematic decision-making process for neuropathic pain.[56] Accurate DREZ surgery requires good knowledge of the radicular innervation and of the surgical anatomy of the spinal cord and roots.[56]

Sympathectomy

Sympathectomy means the interruption of the paravertebral sympathetic ganglion chain at a chosen level. Used since the end of the nineteenth century for several diseases,[64] it is still indicated for the treatment of a wide group of conditions sympathetically maintained and in some cases of vascular diseases.[65-67]

The term *causalgia* ("burning pain") was first introduced by Mitchell in 1864 to describe a syndrome characterized by burning pain following a partial peripheral nerve injury caused by a high-velocity missile. Its classic triad includes burning pain (associated with allodynia and hyperpathia), autonomic dysfunction, and trophic changes.[68] The severe form is known as *major causalgia* and implies always a high-velocity missile injury, and *minor causalgia* is reserved for less severe forms including also some described after nonpenetrating trauma.[69] The median and sciatic nerves and the brachial plexus are most commonly affected.

Reflex sympathetic dystrophy (RDS)[70] consists of many pain syndromes that result from a variety of causes that may or may not include direct nerve trauma. The autonomic nervous system was thought to be implicated, although the "reflexive nature" is still to be demonstrated and the distrophic features are not always present. *Sudek's atrophy* and *Raynaud's syndrome* have been attributed to sympathetically mediated disorders, too.

In order to reduce confusion the term *complex regional pain syndrome* (CPRS) was coined to describe a symptom complex and not a particular syndrome or a medical entity.[71] The expression *sympathetic maintained or mediated pain* embraces a spectrum of conditions in which the main symptom, pain, may be associated with vasospasticity and dystrophic features and can be relieved by interrupting the sympathetic outflow to a body region.[66,72-74]

Upper extremity and upper thoracic sympathectomy implies dividing the chain below the first thoracic ganglion and resecting the T2 ganglion either with open surgery or endoscopically[75,76] or percutaneously by chemical, electrical, or radiofrequency techniques.[77,78]

Lumbar sympathectomy requires the removal of the L2 and L3 sympathetic ganglia (occasionally L1 and T12 to reach the thigh) usually through a retroperitoneal approach.

Open surgical sympathectomy carries high success rates, up to 100%, and low complication rates, between 2.5% and 5%.[6,51,68,79] Pain recurrence is possible, but its rates vary considerably, ranging between 0% and 33% in many series reported.[64,67,68,80] Conversely, it is well recognized that best results are obtained early in the course of the disease before

the development of trophic changes,[64,66,73,74] and therefore, rigorous early assessment by a pain specialist is needed.[10]

Sympathetically maintained pain is one of the few pain syndromes in which the first treatment option may include an ablative procedure rather than conservative therapy.

Cordotomy Procedures

Anterolateral Cordotomy

Anterolateral cordotomy (AC) for the management of pain related to malignancies or chronic pain has been commonly used in the past. Now it is performed much less frequently than it was several decades ago owing to the better results in pain control achieved with the pharmacological approach and the development of neuromodulation devices. However, AC remains a valuable technique for some patients, and it should be part of the armamentarium of any surgeon who is caring for patients with intractable pain.

The basis for AC resides in the neuroanatomy of the ascending pathways transmitting nociceptive information. A detailed description of this anatomy is not the aim of this chapter, and the reader can find more extensive information in other publications.[81,82] Both clinical and experimental observation in the last century provided evidence that the anterolateral quadrant of the spinal cord contained mainly contralateral ascending nociceptive pathways.[83-89] This finding suggested the use of AC for the control of pain. The pathways reaching suprasegmental levels throughout the anterolateral quadrant of the spinal cord are the spinothalamic tract (STT), the spinoreticular tract (SRT), the ventral spinocerebellar pathway, the spino-olivar pathway, and the propriospinal pathways.[90,91] The STT and SRT are the tracts mainly involved in pain transmission. The SRT, also termed *paleospinothalamic tract*, provides indirect connection between the spinal cord and the thalamus,[92] and the STT, also termed the *neospinothalamic tract*, provides a more direct monosynaptic connection mainly to the lateral thalamus.[83] The primary terminations of the SRT are the intralaminar nuclei of the thalamus,[93] thus being primarily related to the aversive and alerting aspect of pain. The STT participates in both the sensory discrimination aspects of pain projecting to the lateral thalamus and in the aversive aspects of pain projecting to the intralaminar thalamus, thus representing the main target of AC. Unfortunately, the STT is not a discrete, separate bundle of fibers, but is diffusely intermixed with other ascending and descending systems (this being responsible for many of the unwanted side effects and complications that can accompany AC). The general organization of the anterolateral quadrant (AQ) ascending sensory system is that lower spinal dermatomes are represented more dorsally and laterally, whereas the higher dermatomes are represented more anteriorly and medially.[90,94,95] The descending spinoreticular pathways are also located in the AQ of the spinal cord, and they mediate myriad automatic functions.

The ideal candidates for AC are cancer patients with unilateral, localized pain. Even unilateral upper body pain, such as that experienced by patients with lung carcinoma, mesothelioma, or Pancoast tumor, can be treated by a cervical percutaneous approach.[96,97] Bilateral cordotomy can be proposed only for cases with bilateral pain in abdominal, pelvic, or lower extremity regions, and pain in the upper trunk or extremity is considered a contraindication because of the high risk of respiratory complications.[96,97] Nonmalignant pain can be treated even if it is probably preferable to use a morphine pump.

Spinothalamic cordotomy aims to interrupt the spinothalamic tract ascending contralaterally to the painful side. The technique of AC has evolved over the past decades in attempts to make the procedure safer and more effective. AC can be performed as an open or percutaneous procedure.

Open Cordotomy

The open approach is done only at high thoracic levels, with the patient in general anesthesia, and with less possibility to control the functional effect of the section of the AQ. This procedure is appropriate only for patients with pain that is lower than the midthoracic level. In addition, there is a discomfort for the patient related to the healing of the thoracic wound. The advantage is related to the ability to destroy the AQ more completely and to avoid the respiratory complications that can attend high cervical cordotomy.

The procedure is performed with the patient in the prone position. Neurophysiological monitoring can be done with electromyography (EMG) activity recorded in the lower extremities during spinal cord stimulation prior to the section.[98] Removal of the spinous processes and the lamina bilaterally at T2-T3 more widely to the side of the AC is performed. The dura is opened under microscopic view. The arachnoid over the lateral spinal cord and associated nerves are dissected carefully in order to identify the dentate ligament, which is divided. The cord is then rotated gently in order to visualize the ventral roots. Using microtechnique, the pia over the AQ is opened at an avascular area from the level of the dentate ligament posteriorly to the level of the ventral roots anteriorly. At this point a cordotomy electrode can be inserted into the white matter of the AQ. Neurophysiological monitoring can be performed to identify the corticospinal tract. Higher frequency of stimulation can be used to activate ascending fibers if the wakeup test is performed, as advocated by some authors.[98] The transverse diameter of the spinal cord is measured, and a right angle probe with blunt extremity that will reach the midline is used to make the incision. The probe is swept anteriorly and a large anterolateral quadrant lesion is completed. The dura is therefore closed in a watertight fashion and the remainder of the wound is closed in a standard fashion.

Percutaneous Cordotomy

Percutaneous AC is superior to conventional open methods. It is performed with the patient under local anesthesia, requires no incision, and allows excellent functional monitoring prior to completion. In addition, with the patient awake in response to neuromodulation, the functional characteristics of the region of the spinal cord to be sectioned can be studied in more detail. It is also more likely to provide pain relief for symptoms above T5 than the open cordotomy. This technique has been pioneered by Mullan and associates,[99] and later modified by the use of radiofrequency, image guidance, and functional mapping.[100-102]

Contrast material should be administered in the subarachnoid space. This could be done preoperatively (20-30 minutes before) by a lumbar puncture (in this case the patient should be maintained in the Trendelenburg position before the procedure) or at the beginning of the procedure by needle insertion at the C1-C2 level. The patient is placed in a supine position in the computed tomography (CT) unit with the head slightly flexed. Under local anesthesia and intravenous sedation if needed, the needle is advanced from the lateral neck into the C1-C2 intradural space. Lateral fluoroscopy allows identification of the appropriate site to start the needle trajectory toward the spinal canal and the final position of the needle (Fig. 49.2A). Once the dura is penetrated, cerebrospinal fluid (CSF) flow will be evident after stylette removal. At this point, an axial scanogram by CT allows the measurement of the spinal cord and is used to better understand intradural needle positioning. The tip diameter of the needle should be guided anterior to the dentate ligament and posterior to the anterior cord (1 mm anterior for lumbar fibers and 2-3 mm anterior for thoracic and cervical fibers). The needle in its ideal position is nearly perpendicular to the spinal cord (Fig. 49.2B). Once the position of the needle is satisfactory, the electrode is passed through the spinal needle into the spinal canal and the spinal cord. Penetration of the pia results in a brief increase in local pain. Correct positioning of the electrode can be performed by CT scan (Fig. 49.2C and D). Now electrical stimulation is performed to adjust the electrode position. Stimulation at low frequency (2-5 Hz) is used to evoke motor responses. Sensory stimulation is done with higher frequency (100 Hz). Placement of the electrode in the STT and SRT area is confirmed by the occurrence of contralateral sensory phenomena, usually a feeling of warmth or cold; with higher stimulus strength, a painful sensation can be evoked.[103] When adequate electrode positioning has been performed, the initial lesion is made by using an electrode with a 2-mm exposed tip applying 30 to 40 mA for 30 to 60 seconds.[101] After this lesion, the patient is examined to evaluate the area of analgesia obtained. Further lesions can be performed in cases of incomplete results in the target area by increasing the time of passing current or advancing the electrode tip in small increments of 0.5, 1 mm. If the procedure is performed satisfactorily, an ipsilateral Horner's syndrome usually occurs.

The results of the cordotomy are variable and mainly related to the investigator who is doing the reporting and the criteria used for determining success.

The more recent literature is almost exclusively related to percutaneous procedures. The results are better for pain related to malignancies. In experienced hands, the initial pain control is achieved in 90% of patients. However, the level of analgesia falls with time, reaching 40% of patients at 2 years.[104]

The complications resulting from AC are related to the damage of the STT and SRT and of all the other adjacent tracts (Fig. 49.2D). Damage to STT and SRT can lead to painful dysesthesias. Damage to nearby structures can result in (a) respiratory failure and death, (b) bowel, bladder, and sexual disfunction, (c) hypotension, (d) ipsilateral weakness, (e) mirror pain, or (f) ataxia. In cervical cordotomies, respiratory dysfunction can be the principal complication. This is particularly true for patients with preexistent respiratory disorders and in cases of bilateral cordotomies. In this last situation, respiratory functions should therefore be carefully observed in the postoperative period. In the past, with the use of open cordotomy, higher rates of complications were observed. Two reasons can be recognized as the cause

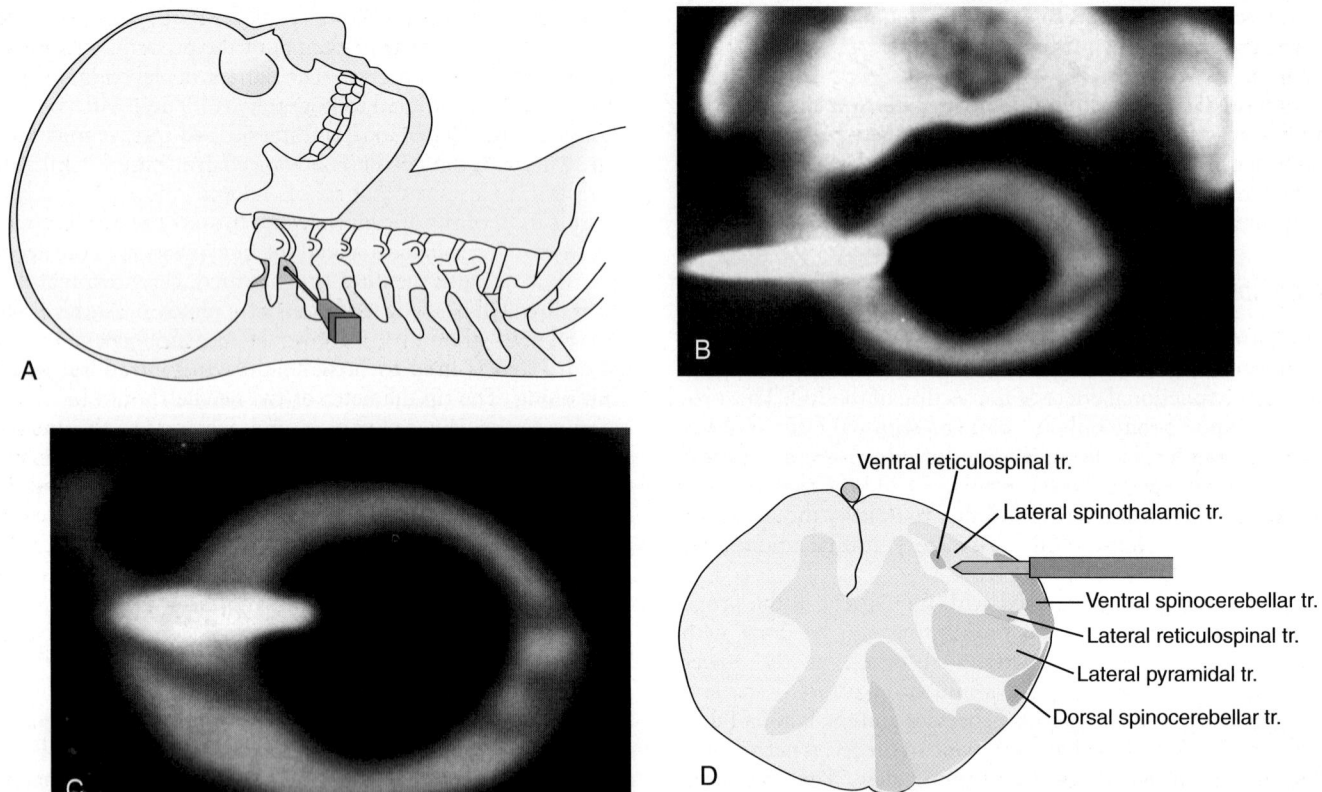

FIGURE 49.2 A, Schematic representation of cordotomy procedure. Insertion of the needle into the C1-C2 level in the supine position (**B**), position of the needle at the right C1-C2 space in the axial computed tomography (CT) image (**C**), and final position of the electrode in the axial CT scan (**D**). Schematic representation shows the final electrode position in the target at the level of the cervical spinal cord and the close anatomical structures. *(Modified from Burchiel KJ, editor. Surgical Management of Pain. New York: Thieme; 2002, Figs. 59.1A (part A), 59.3B (part B), 59.3C (part C), and 59.1C (part D).)*

of complications: (1) needle mislocalization, which is more difficult with the use of CT-guided AC; and (2) involuntary enlargement of the sectioned area, which is less frequent with the use of recently developed electrodes and small thermic lesions. Therefore, percutaneous AC offers a reduction in the percentage of complications.

Percutaneous CT-guided anterolateral cordotomy is an effective method to control pain in cancer patients. It can be used in association with other less invasive methods, such as morphine pumps and neurostimulation, to offer these patients a higher quality of life.

Cingulotomy

Cingulotomy has been successfully used to treat intractable cancer pain.[105-108] The cingulate cortex is a key component of the limbic system, and its anterior cingulate gyrus plays an important role in the integration of nociceptive, motor, affective, and memory functions.[109] Experimental studies on animals and also functional studies in human volunteers demonstrated a role of cingulate gyrus in control of contralateral nociceptive information.[110-115]

Cingulotomy can be considered as an option for patients with intractable cancer pain after failure of antineoplastic and pharmacological treatments and when conservative anesthetic procedures are not available.

Proper pre- and postoperative neuropsychological evaluation should be performed in every case. Magnetic resonance imaging (MRI)-guided stereotactic bilateral cingulotomy is performed.

Results of bilateral cingulotomy are variable. It can assure an improvement of pain control in selected cases.[116] However, even after MRI-guided localization of the cingulate cortex, complications related to behavioral changes or cognitive deficit can occur.[116]

MRI-guided stereotactic cingulotomy, although valuable in selected cases, probably should be reserved for complex and refractory pain problems.

Mesencephalotomy

After the first attempts by Walker[117] and Drake and McKenzie,[118] the procedure was modified by the application of stereotactic technique[119] and avoidance of the medial lemniscus. With these changes, it was possible to reduce the incidence of severe dysesthesia and to reduce the mortality rate.

The first attempts in open surgery were to perform a section of the lateral spinothalamic pathways, but these resulted in unacceptable risks. Stereotactic procedures were therefore applied to interrupt nociceptive pathways with more precision. Looking for an ideal target for pain control, Shieff and Nashold[120,121] elucidated that the procedures worked better and with fewer side effects when the lesion involved the multisynaptic reticulospinal pathways, sparing the spinothalamic tract, which was the original target.

The primary indication for mesencephalotomy is management of cancer pain involving the head, neck, or upper extremities when all other treatments have failed. The most important consideration is patient selection; in fact, this invasive approach can be considered only after an extensive clinical evaluation with a good correlation between the site of cancer involvement and the generation of pain. It can be of particular help when patients report the generation of intense psychological suffering.

Stereotactic procedure is performed to complete the sectioning, following target selection.

Gybels and Sweet[122] reported pain relief in 86% of patients, usually lasting for the remaining part of the patient's life. Mortality rates ranged from 1.8% to 8%, although it can be difficult to attribute deaths to the procedure itself and not to the disease. Oculomotor dysfunction is a relatively frequent complication. Dysesthesia can occur in 15% to 21% of cases.

Mesencephalotomy can be a valuable option for the management of cancer pain in selected cases.

Percutaneous Techniques for Trigeminal (and Glossopharyngeal) Neuralgia

The first clear description of trigeminal neuralgia (TN) was given in 1671.[123] John Fothergill,[124] in a paper published in 1773, described the typical features of TN, including its paroxysmal nature and association with triggering factors such as eating, speaking, or touching the face. In 1756, the French surgeon Nicholas André coined the term *tic douloureux* to describe at least three patients with TN treated by neurectomy.[125-128]

The clinical features of the so-called classic idiopathic TN have been well documented and are now universally recognized. One of the pillars in our understanding of this syndrome is the classification that Eller and colleagues proposed in 2005.[129] These authors classified TN on the basis of two broad categories: the patient's history and seven specific diagnostic criteria. Following Eller's classification, TN type 1 identifies the classic idiopathic form, also known as the typical form of TN, and from now on we will refer to TN as this entity. TN is a chronic pain syndrome whose patients suffer from idiopathic episodes of spontaneous facial pain. This pain, which is experienced in one or more divisions of the trigeminal nerve, expresses itself as paroxysms of brief and excruciatingly intense bouts of stabbing, electrical shocks. These paroxysms of TN can arise spontaneously or in response to gentle tactile stimulation of a trigger point on the face or in the oral cavity. They may also be triggered by such natural activities as chewing, speaking, swallowing, touching the face, or brushing the teeth. TN pain is almost always experienced unilaterally, although there have been some relatively rare reports describing bilateral signs and symptoms.[129] TN type 1 pain typically occurs after conspicuously obvious pain-free intervals that can last for weeks, months, and years. The neurological examination is almost always normal, although cases have been reported in which a slight degree of sensory loss has been described.[130] The diagnosis of TN is always based on the patient's clinical history. In terms of its pathophysiology,

the features of classic TN are currently thought to be related to a compression of the trigeminal nerve root, usually by a blood vessel, at or near the root entry zone of the trigeminal nerve.[131-134]

The incidence of TN is about 2.3 to 4.5 per 100,000 new cases per year.[135] Age at onset is variable, but the incidence increases in the fifth and sixth decades of life.

From the time of its first recognition, TN has been treated in a variety of ways.[136,137] Today several medical and surgical treatments are available.

Medical treatment is mainly based on the use of an anticonvulsant: carbamazepine, phenytoin, and gabapentin are the most frequently recommended. Centrally acting muscle relaxants, such as baclofen, are also used.

Glossopharyngeal neuralgia (GN) is a spasmodic, lancinating, and paroxysmal pain that starts in the posterior throat or base of the tongue and often radiates down the throat and side of the neck. Often pain is triggered by swallowing or yawning. Typically, cocainization of the area reduces pain and has been proposed to confirm diagnosis.[138] Seldom, hypotension, syncope, and cardiac irregularities may accompany GN.[139,140] Isolated GN occurs at a rate of 1 case in every 70 to 100 cases of TN;[141] concurrence of TN and GN is also possible.[142]

Percutaneous Injection of Neurodestructive Substances

In 1912 Hartel proposed the procaine injection, and later in 1914 the alcohol injection, of the gasserian ganglion for TN.[143,144] In 1940 Harris reported a series of 2500 cases treated through this method.[145] However, the high rate of postinjection paresthesia and anesthesia dolorosa and some reported cases of major complications due to the diffusion of alcohol in the posterior fossa, along with a high pain recurrence rate, caused the technique to be abandoned.

Conversely, glycerol injection of the ganglion, first introduced by Hakanson in the 1970s,[146] occasionally is still performed today. The procedure is relatively safe, can be repeated if necessary, and is well tolerated, but it may cause transient sensory loss, corneal anesthesia, and dysesthesia.[147,148] The main drawback is the rate of pain recurrence, which is reported to be up to 10% in the early postoperative period, up to 50% at 3 years, and 90% at 6 years.[147,149,150]

Percutaneous Trigeminal Radiofrequency Thermocoagulation

Even though it had been tried since the beginning of the twentieth century,[151,152] it was not until the mid-1960s, with the modifications of the technique by Sweet, that this procedure became popular. Sweet's modifications consisted of electrophysiological stimulation for precise localization, reliable radiofrequency current for nerve destruction, intermittent patient sedation with short-acting intravenous drugs allowing intraoperative patient assessment, and temperature monitoring to control precisely the configuration of the site.[94,153,154] With these modifications the use of radiofrequency rhizotomy spread widely and it is still commonly used.

The rationale is based on the fact that pain fibers are carried by unmyelinated C-fibers or thinly myelinated Aδ-fibers that are blocked at a lower temperature than those of larger Aα- and β-fibers carrying deep and tactile sensations.[155-157]

Thus, radiofrequency-induced heat will destroy the former fibers, sparing the latter ones.

The procedure is done in the operating room, even though some authors perform it as outpatient surgery in the radiography suite.

The technique consists of the introduction of a needle under fluoroscopy at the level of the gasserian ganglion through the foramen ovale, entering 2.5 cm lateral to the oral commissure and aiming toward the medial aspect of the pupil (Fig. 49.3A and B). Several methods have been described to place the needle into the foramen ovale;[158-160] careful checking under fluoroscopy (Fig. 49.3C) and considerable training and experience are mandatory to avoid internal carotid artery injuries or penetrating the foramina adjacent to the foramen ovale. Once at the target, confirmed by outflow of CSF, the electrode can be inserted.

Electrode placement is guided by fluoroscopy: For V3 pain, the electrode tip lies within 5 mm proximal to the clivus profile and is directed caudal. For V2 pain it should placed at the clivus profile, and for V1 pain the electrode tip lies within 5 mm distal to the clivus profile and is directed cephalad.

The electrode tip should not be advanced more than 8 mm deep to the clivus profile because it can injure the abducens nerve in Dorello's canal or penetrate the temporal lobe. Final placement of the electrode tip is determined by the patient's response to electric stimulation.

With the patient under mild sedation, an average of three lesions at 60 to 70 degrees for 90 seconds are usually done. The goal is analgesia in the primarily affected trigeminal division, hypalgesia in correspondence of trigger points, and mild hypalgesia in the secondarily affected trigeminal divisions. After each lesion, clinical assessment of facial sensitivity, corneal reflex, and strength of the muscles of mastication is mandatory (Fig. 49.3D).

The procedure does not require general anesthesia, can be performed for patients not suitable for open surgery (the elderly, those with comorbid conditions, etc.), and can be repeated if necessary. Immediate pain relief can be obtained in up to 98% of patients,[147,161] but the long-term recurrence rate may be particularly variable: 25% to 37% at 5 years, 25% to 80% after 10 years,[162,163] or 27% overall (early and late recurrence) in a study with an average follow-up period

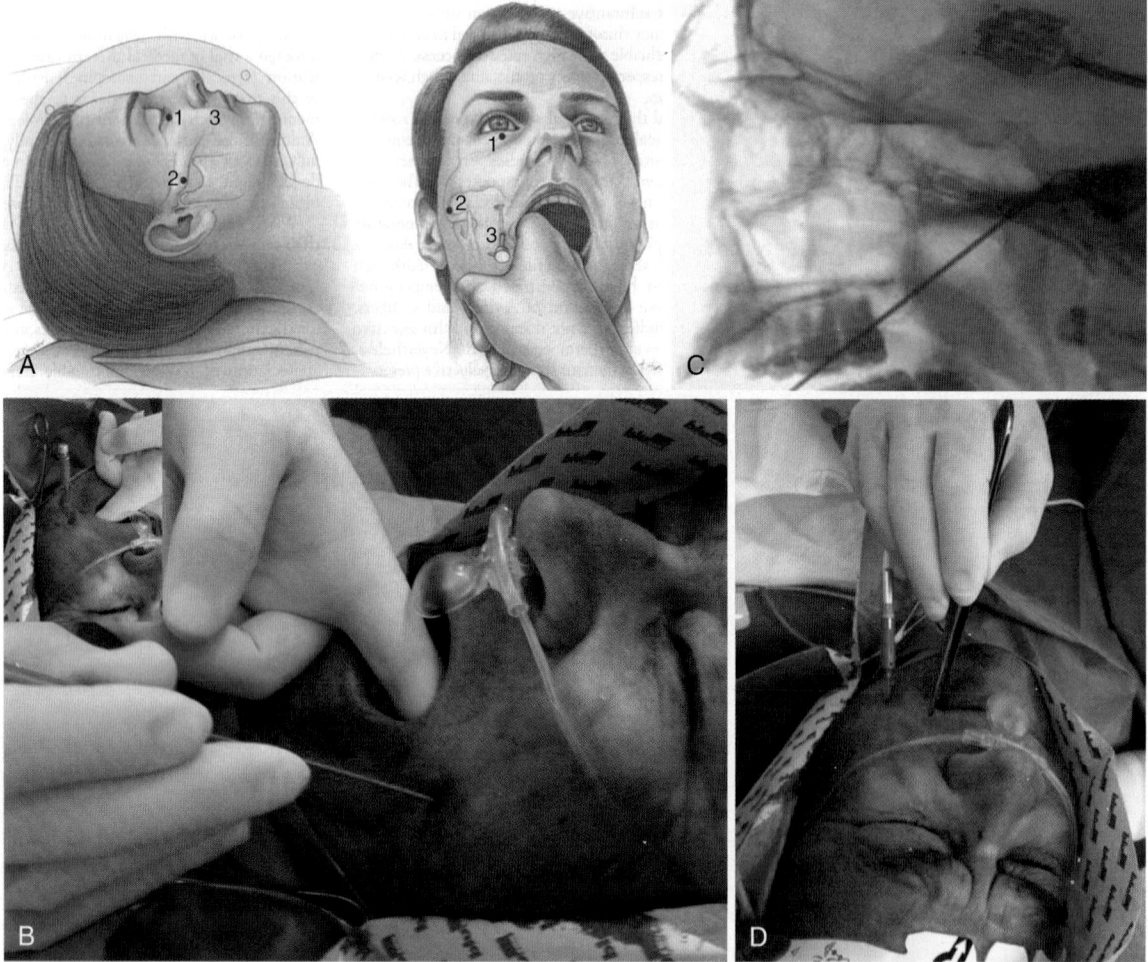

FIGURE 49.3 **A,** Schematic representation of the anatomical landmarks for needle insertion in the foramen ovale, following Hartel's technique. Point 1, medial aspect of the pupil, and point 2, 3 cm anterior to the auditory external meatus, indicate the direction of the foramen; point 3, 3 cm lateral to the oral commissure, defines the point of needle initial penetration. **B,** Intraoperative picture of the needle insertion toward the patient's cheek in the right foramen ovale. **C,** Intraoperative fluoroscopy showing the needle inserted into the left foramen ovale. **D,** Intraoperative clinical assessment of trigeminal functions after thermocoagulation of left trigeminal nerve.

of 9 years.[164] Almost all patients develop numbness in the face after the procedure, but in most cases this is tolerable. The mortality rate is extremely low;[147,165] loss of corneal reflex occurs in 3.5% to 7%; and cheratitis is seen in less than 3%.[147,148] Dysesthesia develops in 6% to 24% of patients, but anesthesia dolorosa occurs in only 0.2% to 4%, with higher risk in more complete or extensive procedures.[147,150,161,164] Trigeminal motor function may be impaired, but most of the time this effect is transient.[164] When patients are asked to rate the procedure and the outcome, the majority of them are usually satisfied.[162,164]

By the same technique, the glossopharyngeal nerve can be reached percutaneously at the foramen lacerum, allowing a postganglionar sectioning of the fibers.[166]

Percutaneous Trigeminal Balloon Compression

The idea of compressing with open surgery the root of the trigeminal nerve to treat TN was first proposed around 1950, but the results were not encouraging.[167,168] Later, Mullan proposed the gasserian ganglion compression through a percutaneus approach, reporting good results.[169-171]

The procedure is performed in the same way as for radiofrequency thermocoagulation until the ganglion is reached. Then a balloon catheter is inserted. A characteristic pear figure appears under fluoroscopy when the balloon is properly inflated with contrast agent in Meckel's cave (Fig. 49.4). The goal is to compress the nerve at 1100 mm Hg or 1.3 to 1.5 atm for 1 minute.

Balloon compression is particularly indicated for first trigeminal division pain, because it carries a lower risk of corneal reflex loss and cheratitis compared to radiofrequency thermocoagulation. Nevertheless, during the procedure the patient may develop bradycardia and hypotension[172] and a pacemaker may be required; the compression is mild and this leads to a higher rate of pain recurrence. The initial rate of pain relief is 92% and the overall recurrence rate is 26%; postoperative numbness and mild to moderate hypesthesia occur in about 50% to 60% of patients; and anesthesia dolorosa and

corneal anesthesia are extremely rare, less than 0.1% of cases. On the other hand, masseter weakness can occur in about 10% of patients.[147]

Microvascular Decompression for Trigeminal (and Glossopharyngeal) Neuralgia

Dandy[173] was the fist to propose that there might be a causal relationship between pain paroxysms and the compression of the trigeminal root. This compression is typically caused by adjacent arterial loops, although on occasion, tumors, arteriovenous malformations, and aneurysms located in this region have been known to cause this kind of compression. Though Dandy was the first to describe the role played by compression in 1929, it was not until the 1950s that any kind of therapeutic relief became obtainable by decompressing the trigeminal nerve in TN patients.[174,175] The notion that a microvascular compression might be causing TN has gained much support from the work of Jannetta,[134,176-178] who was able not only to find a compressing vascular contact in a high percentage of TN patients but also to demonstrate that prolonged pain relief could be obtained by decompressive surgery, without causing any sensory loss. Patients suffering from typical idiopathic TN usually are found to have a blood vessel that is in close contact with the trigeminal root entry zone (TREZ). This finding is typically made during surgery, during the exploration of the cerebellopontine angle (CPA), or radiologically by MRI[176,178-180] (Fig. 49.5).

Microvascular decompression (MVD), also known as *Jannetta's procedure*, is a nondestructive treatment designed to resolve the compressive conflict between the trigeminal nerve and a blood vessel. Today, it is widely recognized as the primary therapeutic option in the treatment of TN.[178,181-184]

The procedure is performed in the operating room under general anesthesia. With the patient in the sitting or lateral position, a small retrosigmoid craniectomy is done, allowing

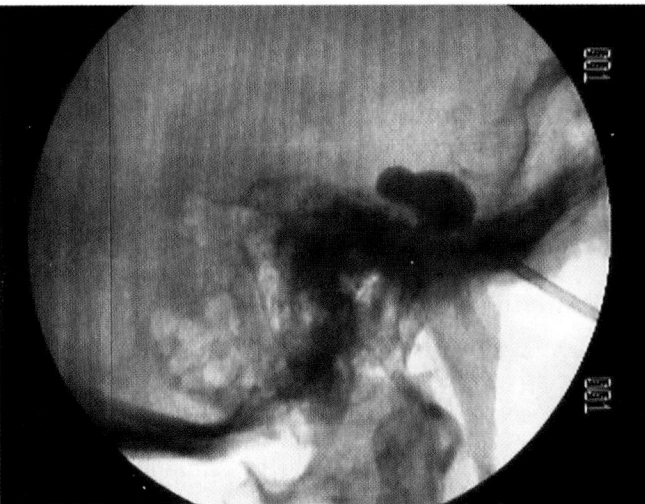

FIGURE 49.4 When the balloon is properly inflated with contrast agent in Meckel's cave, the typical pear-shaped figure appears under fluoroscopy.

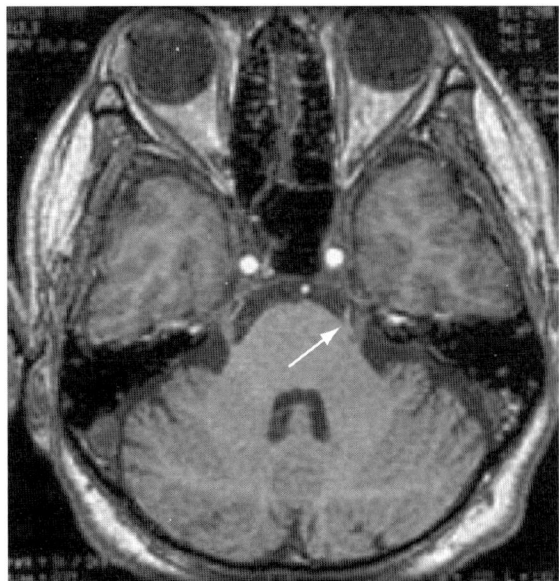

FIGURE 49.5 T1-weighted magnetic resonance imaging (MRI) with intravenous paramagnetic contrast agent showing a neurovascular conflict with the left trigeminal nerve (*white arrow*).

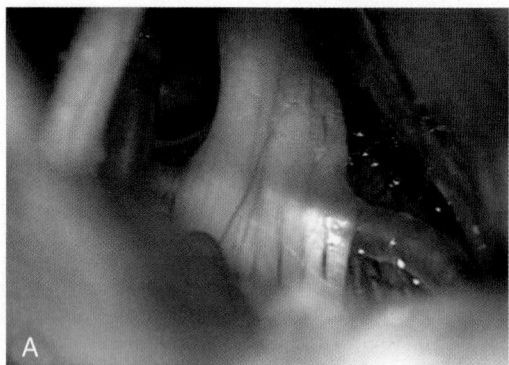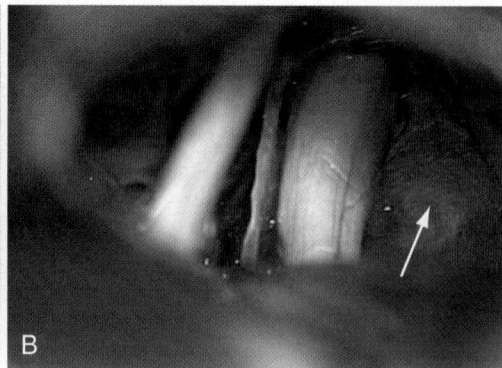

FIGURE 49.6 **A,** Intraoperative view of the neurovascular conflict with the left trigeminal nerve, which is stretched by the artery and is almost flattened. **B,** Intraoperative view showing the resolution of the conflict by noncompressive technique with a small piece of Surgicel (*white arrow*) that keeps the artery away from the nerve.

for exposure of the transverse sinus, the sigmoid sinus, and the junction between the two. Intradurally, by means of opening the CPA cistern, the CSF drainage facilitates a natural cerebellar relaxation, creating a perfect surgical corridor to the fifth cranial nerve and to the seventh to eighth cranial nerve complex. The TREZ is the most common site of vascular compression. It is the locus of transition from central to peripheral myelin and the most vulnerable part of the nerve. After the neurovascular conflict is identified (Fig. 49.6A), a sharp dissection of the arachnoidal bands that fix the artery into its position allows for moving the nerve away from the artery. Many methods have been advocated for keeping the vessel separated from the nerve, including using pieces of muscle, fascia, periosteum, or subcutaneous fat. Our experience is that these strategies usually have little effect. This kind of tissue is usually reabsorbed and favors adhesions, fibrosis, and arachnoiditis, as has been observed during reoperations in patients in whom neuralgia has recurred.[185-189] Most authors dealing with MVD now use synthetic implants, particularly Ivalon sponge,[187,190-192] Dacron knitted material,[189,193] or Teflon felt.[178,193-196] In most of these reports, a small piece of synthetic material has been interposed between the nerve and the vessel. Though they are considered biocompatible, Ivalon, Dacron, and Teflon may, in fact, generate granulomas and carry the consequent risk of distorting or irritating the trigeminal root and, in so doing, producing a recurrence of pain.[197-199] The so-called sling retraction technique[183,193,200,201] has been proposed as an alternative by introducing the concept of a noncompressive technique for MVD (Fig. 49.6B), with good results.[201]

The results with this technique are excellent, with up to 98% of patients reporting immediate pain relief and more than 85% and 80% of patients pain-free without medication at the 5 and 9 years' follow-up, respectively.[150,202] The mortality rate is less than 1%.[150,192,203] The facial numbness rate is only 2%; the rate of dysesthesia, anesthesia dolorosa, corneal anesthesia, and trigeminal motor disfunction approximates 0%. The overall cranial nerve deficit is about 3%;[150,204] fourth and seventh cranial nerve deficit with diplopia and facial weakness may occur, although such effects are usually transient. Deafness has been reported as well. CSF leak, wound infection, and meningitis can occur with an overall rate of 10%,[150] but only a few cases require second surgery or prolonged hospitalization.

Similar results in terms of pain relief and complication rate can be obtained with MVD for GN.[205,206]

Last, when negative or equivocal exploration is encountered during MVD, partial trigeminal rhizotomy can be performed. The technique was first proposed by Dandy.[207] It consists of a partial section of the nerve in the portion adjacent to the brainstem, starting at its posterior inferior margin. This allows the surgeon to spare most of the facial sensibility, corneal reflex, and motor function. Results are rather good, with more than 80% experiencing pain relief, albeit sensory deficit and dysesthesia are obviously higher than with MVD.[208] This procedure can be effective also in patients with demyelinating or neurodegenerative diseases and some consider it the last line of defense for patients who have proved to have a recalcitrant form of TN and have failed all previous treatments.

NEUROMODULATION PROCEDURES

Neuromodulation is the modification of neural electrical activity by means of delivered electrical current or drug administration at the neural interface. Implanted devices are taken into account when conservative treatment has failed to provide clinical benefit to the patient affected by chronic pain. The development and use of modulatory techniques strictly depend on our knowledge of neuronal suprasegmental and segmental electrophysiological characteristics of structures involved in the transmission and control of pain, of the pathological modifications that take place when pain becomes a chronic symptom, and of the psychopathological correlates of the different syndromes.

Deep Brain Stimulation

The first report of deep brain stimulation (DBS) procedures affecting perception of pain dates back to the 1950s, when Pool observed an analgesic effect by stimulating the septum pellucidum and the columns of the fornices during a psychosurgery intervention;[209] subsequently, the same author and Heath reported an antinociceptive effect after the stimulation of the paraseptal regions.[210,211] The first report of thalamic DBS for control of pain was by Mazars in 1960.[212] In the 1970s, Hosobuchi and Richardson were the first to report a case of thalamic and periaqueductal gray (PAG) and periventricular gray (PVG) stimulation.[213-216] According to the gate theory by Melzack and Wall[217] thalamic stimulation induced paresthesias in the pain-affected areas.

Another cerebral region that led to pain alleviation and also paresthesias when stimulated was the posterior limb of the internal capsule.[218] The first report of stimulation of the centromedian nucleus of the thalamus is due to Andy.[219] Although the stimulation of PAG and PVG does not preclude paresthesias, it can lead to "pleasant" sensations in the patient. Another potential target is the centromedianus parafascicular complex of the thalamus, which has been used by Andy for the treatment of dyskinesias.

Many manuscripts discuss the use of DBS in the treatment of drug-refractory pain; nonetheless, an important application of this technique is not possible given the low number of patients considered suitable for it; furthermore, many controversies exist on the optimal target and on the different kinds of pain that could benefit from this therapeutic approach.

The mechanism of action of DBS on pain control depends on the target employed. The thalamus, PAG, and PVG are the most commonly used targets according to the international literature. Some authors believe that the therapeutic effect of PAG/PVG stimulation can be mediated by endogenous opioid substances, on the basis of studies that demonstrate that such an effect can be reversed by administration of naloxone. Other authors instead think that the analgesic effect is due to the activation of several descending suprasegmental systems involved in nociception, included the amine-dependent system.

The analgesic effect of the stimulation of ventralis posterolateralis (VPL) and ventralis posteromedialis (VPM) nuclei, involved in the transmission of sensitive inputs, is, on the contrary, poorly studied and understood. It has been proposed that it can be mediated by the inhibition of neurons of the spinothalamic tract or of the neurons of the dorsal horn. It has also been proposed that a dopamine-mediated mechanism is involved; the most accredited proposal suggests that thalamic stimulation activates the raphe magnus of the rostroventral region of the medulla oblongata, thus leading to the activation of descending inhibitory pathways.

Many clinical observations would tend toward a greater efficacy of the stimulation of PAG/PVG regions in the treatment of nociceptive pain, and of VPL/VPM complexes in the treatment of neuropathic pain; however, as stated earlier, the number of patients treated is still too low, and it is not possible to draw any definitive conclusion without controlled, prospective, and randomized studies. It is also necessary to consider the clinical situations of "mixed" pain (with both nociceptive and neuropathic components) and this once again emphasizes the importance of an accurate patient selection (some authors consider the future use of simultaneous implantation of both thalamic and periventricular electrodes[220]).

Painful syndromes that can be treated with DBS include anesthesia dolorosa, postischemic pain, thalamic pain, brachial plexus avulsion, postherpetic neuralgia, postcordotomy dysesthesia, medullary lesions, failed back surgery syndrome, cancer-related pain, and peripheral neuropathic pain.[221] Other important indications for DBS (the target being in this case the posterior hypothalamic region, pHyp) are refractory trigeminal autonomic cephalalgias (TACs), including chronic cluster headache (CCH). DBS of the pHyp was the first application

in which the choice of target was motivated by neuroimaging functional data. Activation of the pHyp during cluster headache pain attacks was observed during positron emission tomography (PET) studies;[222] this original observation led to the placement of deep brain electrodes within the pHyp to inhibit the pathologically activated neuronal pool in patients with CCH (Fig. 49.7).

Series reported in the literature include 50 patients affected by CCH.[223-229] Five patients affected with TN due to demyelinating disease,[230] two patients affected by short-lasting unilateral neuralgiform headache attacks with conjunctival injection and tearing (SUNCT),[231,232] one patient affected by chronic paroxysmal hemicrania,[233] and four patients affected by neuropathic pain of the face[230] have been reported in the literature.

With regard to CCH, in the Belgian group,[228] whose mean follow-up period was 14.5 months, two out of four patients were pain-free, one patient had a dramatic reduction of pain attacks to less than three per month, and one patient had only transient clinical benefit. In the open-phase period of the study reported by the French multicenter study,[226] the mean weekly attack frequency decreased by 48.4%, and 6 out of 11 patients were considered as "responders" (decrease of at least 50% in the frequency of weekly attacks). In the German group,[223] three out of these six patients were reported to be almost completely attack-free (one mean pain attack per month) after a follow-up period ranging from 9 to 17 months. Of the two patients reported by the British group[233] one patient only reported infrequent pain attacks (seven injections of sumatriptan) at 11 months' follow-up, and the other patient reported a decrease in attack frequency from daily to weekly with "massive reduced severity." In the U.S. group,[229] three out of five patients could be considered responders because of "50% reduction in headache frequency intensity, or both"; the follow-up period ranged from 6 to 12 months in their study. As far as our group is concerned,[227] the mean follow-up time was 4 years; a state of persistent freedom from painful attacks was still present in 10 of 18 patients (62%). Four patients (25%) still required prophylactic drugs to prevent the attacks. In the last 2 years of follow-up, three patients no longer benefited from stimulation despite several changes in parameters. In these three patients, the disease changed from the chronic to the episodic form. Two patients affected by SUNCT who underwent posterior hypothalamic DBS have been reported in the literature to date. The first patient was reported by our group in 2005.[231] The preoperative frequency of pain bouts ranged from 70 to 300 per day; after surgery, a complete and definitive remission of symptoms has been confirmed at the last clinical examination, performed at 5-year follow-up. The second patient with drug-refractory SUNCT treated with hypothalamic DBS was reported by Lyons and co-workers in 2009;[232] a 63% reduction in the mean number of daily attacks (133 attacks per day preoperatively vs. 45 attacks per day) was observed in the first postoperative month; at 12-month follow-up a further improvement was observed, with 80% in reduction in frequency of attacks (25 attacks per day).

Only one patient affected by chronic paroxysmal hemicrania (CPH) submitted to posterior hypothalamic DBS has been reported to date.[233] One of the main criteria for diagnosis of CPH is an absolute response to indomethacin administration; in this patient, however, this drug was discontinued because

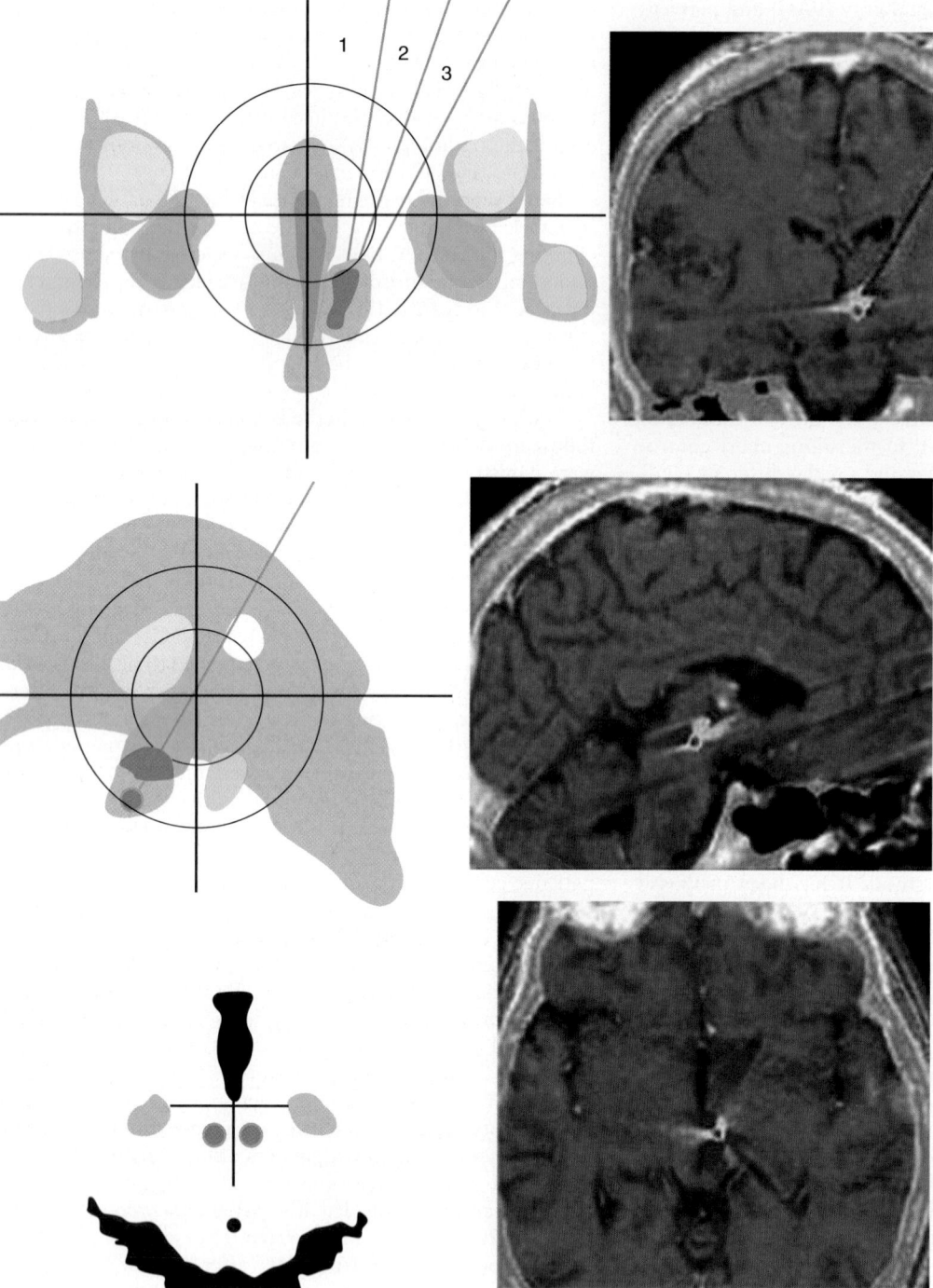

FIGURE 49.7 *Left:* Virtual ventriculographic plates showing the target (pHyp: pink and red) in coronal sagittal and axial sections as part of surgical planning. Different possible trajectories are shown. *Right:* Postoperative computed tomography (CT) images merged with preoperative magnetic resonance imaging (MRI) showing the definitive location of the electrode in coronal sagittal and axial planes.

of the onset of iatrogenic gastritis superimposed on a preexisting Barrett's esophagus; given the refractoriness of symptoms, the patient underwent pHyp DBS. After a 27-month follow-up period she was reported to be symptom-free. At our institute, we implanted with pHyp DBS three patients affected by secondary neuropathic trigeminal pain (the conditions leading to the painful condition were a posterior mandibular carcinoma with subsequent radical transmandibular tumor resection in one patient, a minor dental procedure in the second, and a nasopharyngeal carcinoma in the third patient).[230] None of the three patients had reduction in painful symptoms at the last clinical examination despite several attempts

in modification of stimulation parameters. At our institution five multiple sclerosis (MS) patients affected by refractory TN were submitted to pHyp DBS;[39] three patients had beneficial effects within 24 hours from the procedure; all patients reported a reduction of paroxysmal pain attacks within the ophthalmic branch after surgery. Three patients complained of recurrent pain in the second and in the third branch (but, importantly, not in the first) and underwent further radiofrequency thermorhizotomies.

The other two patients reported relief of pain in all three trigeminal branches by combining stimulation with analgesics and did not necessitate further surgical procedures.

The overall percentage of patients with CCH treated with pHyp considered to be responders is 63%.[234]

Complications of DBS surgery are mainly hemorrhages, infections, failure of the components of the stimulation systems (including breakage of the leads), and stimulation-related side effects, which depend on the target being stimulated (seizures, diplopia, dizziness, paresthesias, cephalalgia).

Motor Cortex Stimulation

The first report about the stimulation of the motor cortex is due to Penfield, who observed some sensitive responses after the stimulation of the motor cortex in a patient previously submitted to postcentral gyrus removal during a surgical procedure for the treatment of epilepsy. Penfield and Jasper subsequently treated refractory hemisomatic neuropathic pain through contralateral postcentral corticectomy; further removal of adjoining precentral gyrus was used to reclaim clinical benefit when a relapse of symptoms occurred.

White and Sweet and Lende performed pre- and postcentral corticectomies for the treatment of cases of hemisomatic and neuropathic facial pain. These reports constitute the background for subsequent employment of motor cortex stimulation (MCS); this research was motivated by the controversial results of DBS and by the progressive refusal of ablative procedures (corticectomy). Although the stimulation of the sensitive, rather than motor, cortex would be in accordance with the "gate" theory of Melzack and Wall, several reports of stimulation of cortical areas different from the main somatosensory area (SI) (such as frontomesial cortex stimulation, performed by Hardy in 1985, which resulted in elevation of the latency of the nociceptive response) allowed an initial understanding of the complexity of the cortical pain modulation mechanisms. It must be remembered that in 1986 Hosobuchi reported the effectiveness of the stimulation of sensitive cortex for the treatment of pain in the lower limbs.

In 1991 Tsubokawa introduced the epidural motor cortex stimulation for the treatment of central deafferentation pain, and his group concluded that sensitive cortex stimulation was not effective for this purpose. He revealed that such technique was able to inhibit burst-like thalamic discharges that had been previously demonstrated to be altered in animal models of deafferentation pain. He also demonstrated the safety of this procedure with particular regard to eventual postoperative development of seizures.[235]

The mechanism of action of MCS is still poorly understood; the comprehension of its physiological effects strictly depends on that of the anatomical connections between the motor cortex and several cortical, subcortical, brainstem, and spinal cord structures. These connections can now be revealed through animal studies and different neuroradiological studies, such as positron emission tomography (PET) and single-photon emission computed tomography (SPECT). Some SPECT studies demonstrated a normalization of the local cortical somatosensory-motor (SI-MI) circuit[236] after MCS; this observation could be in line with Tsubokawa's original view, according to which MCS activates non-nociceptive neurons of primary sensory cortex through both orthodromic and antidromic axonal pathways interconnecting MI and SI, thus leading to activation of surrounding nociceptive inhibition in SI.

Other studies demonstrated that cortical stimulation is able to increase the blood flow to the ipsilateral thalamus, thus modulating the long reverberating thalamocortical loop, and overriding the pathological phenomenon of disrupted oscillation and temporal synchronization.[237]

Interaction of motor cortex with sensory thalamus, perigenual cortex, dorsolateral prefrontal, orbitofrontal cortex, periaqueductal gray matter (PAG) also seems of relevance; it has been suggested that MCS acts through descending inhibitory controls involving the connection between the anterior cingulated cortex (ACC) and PAG; this could in part explain the positive effect of this treatment modality on both the affective and the evoked components of pain (allodynia and hyperalgesia).

Several painful conditions have been treated with MCS up to now, such as thalamic pain (postictal or posthemorrhagic), postischemic bulbar pain which accompanies Wallenberg's syndrome, neuropathic facial (trigeminal) pain, phantom limb pain, deafferentation pain, postherpetic neuralgia, spinal cord injuries, and pain due to avulsion of the brachial plexus. One of the first reports of the efficacy of MCS for treatment of central pain is by Tsubokawa ("good" control of symptoms with MCS in 65% of patients with thalamic and putaminal postischemic and posthemorrhagic pain) and by Katayama who performed MCS in three patients who had been submitted to DBS of the VPL nucleus of the thalamus for pain related to Wallenberg's syndrome; after DBS, these patients reported a worsening of symptoms, but they presented a 60% improvement after MCS. Treatment of facial neuropathic pain has been indicated as the major indication for MCS, in part because of the relatively large cortical representation of the face; and in fact, different authors report a 60% pain improvement after a mean follow-up period of 1 year.[238-242]

MCS can be performed under general or local anesthesia, and implies the positioning of plate-shaped electrodes above the dura mater overlying the motor cortex, although some authors place them subdurally; in some centers the electrode is positioned parallel to the motor strip, and in others it is positioned perpendicular to it, with the most anterior contacts located above the precentral gyrus.

The procedure is carried on after the localization of this structure with neuroradiological methods, intraoperative somatosensory evoked potentials (SSEP), intraoperative stimulation, and implementation of functional MRI in the neuronavigation system, expecially in patients with cerebral ischemia, which could lead to plastic rearrangement of the cortex itself.

Some authors perform MCS by sliding the plate electrode through a simple bur hole centered on the posterior portion of the previously localized precentral gyrus, whereas others perform a craniotomy. Once positioned, the abovementioned integrative methodologies can be used, thus permitting a refinement of the positioning according to the case. In general, it is preferable to position the active contacts just above the area of the motor strip representing the affected part of the body (Fig. 49.8) given that the lower limb representation lies in the medial surface of the hemisphere (anterior portion of the paracentral lobule). MCS is usually performed for facial or upper limb pain; nonetheless, reports exist of placement of the electrode subdurally over the paracentral lobule, or epidurally, very close to the sagittal sinus; in these cases, 6 out of 12 patients with lower limb pain improved by 40% to 50%.[243]

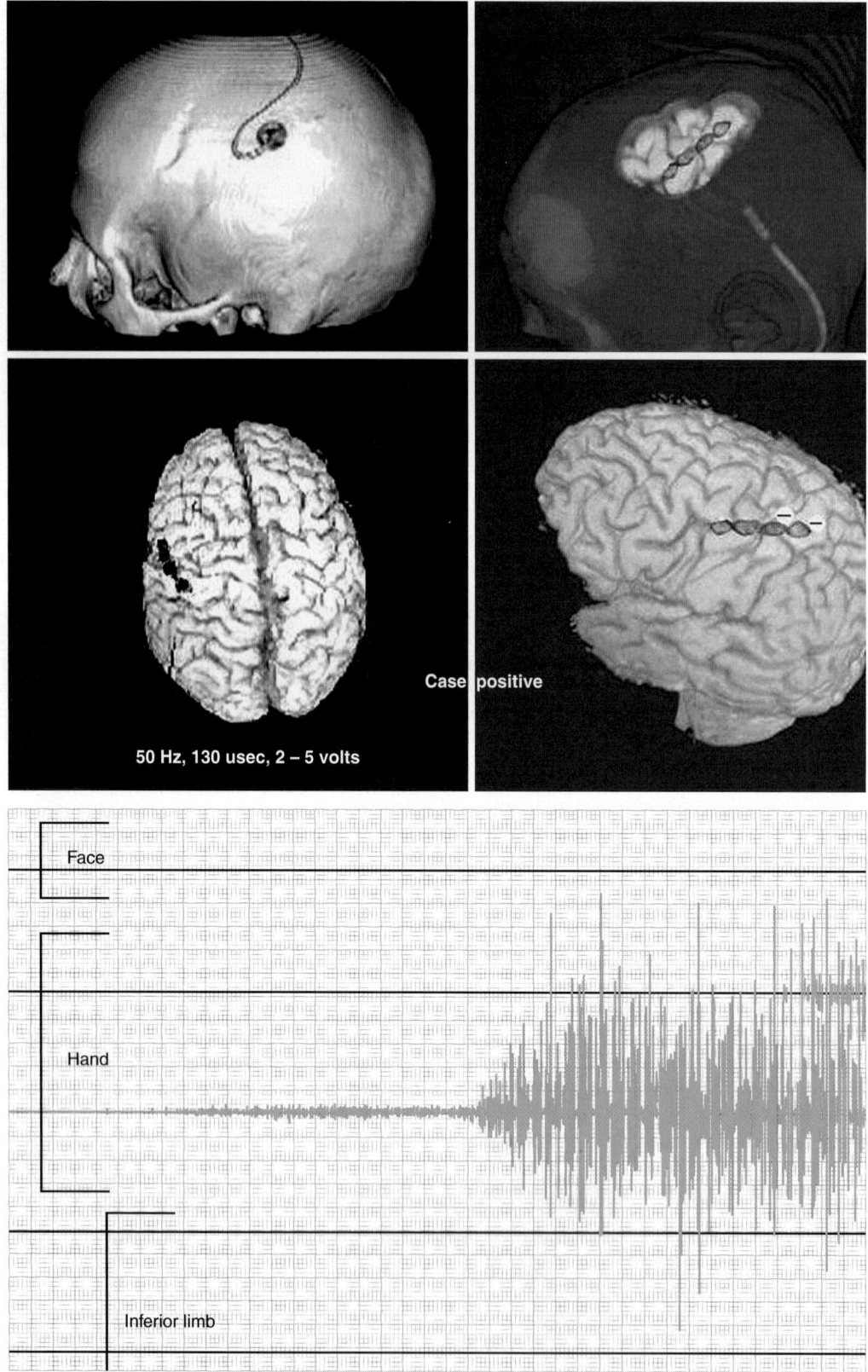

50 Hz, 130 usec, 2 – 5 volts

Case positive

Face

Hand

Inferior limb

FIGURE 49.8 *Upper panel:* Three-dimensional (3D) postoperative reconstruction showing the placement of the chronic leads over the motor cortex. *Lower panel:* Intraoperative stimulation trials evoked electromyography (EMG) response in the abductor pollicis brevis muscle but not in the remaining muscles (from top to bottom: orbicularis oris muscle; brachioradialis m., abductor pollicis brevis m., rectus femori m., anterior tibialis m.).

After the procedure, the implanted pulse generators connected to the intracranial electrodes are activated at various settings, which vary according to the institution, the physician's preferences, and the results obtained. They range from 1 to 5 V, 15 to 130 Hz, 60 to 450 microseconds. The configuration more often used is bipolar rather than monopolar; when in bipolar mode and in those cases of electrodes placed perpendicular to the central sulcus, the most anterior contacts are set as cathodes.[244]

It is difficult to systematically assess the overall results of MCS for chronic pain reported in the literature because of differences among indications, surgical procedures, evaluation scales used, and stimulation parameters. Moreover, only a few studies are prospective or crossover placebo-controlled, even though MCS usually does not induce any perceptible sensations and could thus be ideal for such study design. Some authors consider responders to be patients who report at least 50% pain relief, and others consider a 40% decrease in intensity of pain a responsiveness criterion.

The pain evaluation scales most often employed are the visual analog scale (VAS) and the McGill pain questionnaire, although the majority of authors assess the percentage of pain relief or use indicative terms such as "poor," "fair," "good," or "excellent" when referring to the clinical outcome.

As reported by Fontaine and associates[243] only three studies, comprising 10 patients, reported postoperative CT or MRI for determining the exact location of the electrode;[239,244,245] in seven of these patients, postoperative imaging was obtained to rule out electrode misplacement and in the other three the electrodes were thought to be located in the preoperatively determined target with neuronavigation systems and then assessed with intraoperative stimulation.

Among the abovementioned indications, the best results have been obtained in trigeminal neuropathic pain, phantom limb pain, and spinal cord injury; in this group of patients, at 1-year follow-up 50% were considered responders. Despite the clinical, procedural, and assessment incongruity among the various studies, it could be said that approximately 57% of the treated patients benefited from the procedure (40-50% of pain relief); the most frequent adverse effects were related to the system implanted (infections, hardware failure); less frequently, local pain, subdural or epidural hemorrhage, and intraoperative seizures induced by stimulation were observed. In no case were long-term seizures reported.

Spinal Cord Stimulation

Spinal cord stimulation (SCS) was first introduced (with the name stimulation of the dorsal column of the spine) by Shealy in 1967;[246] initially, though, satisfactory and definitive results were not always achieved, partly because of continuous and indiscriminate use of the method and also because of poor choice of indications.

Better results were obtained beginning in the 1970s, when more accurate patient selection and advancement in technological equipment allowed this technique to gain a wider acceptance.[247]

The procedure consists of the positioning of an electrode (with various shapes, dimensions, and number of contacts) in the epidural spinal space; the site of the implant depends on the site of pain. It is generally placed at the cervical or middle-lower

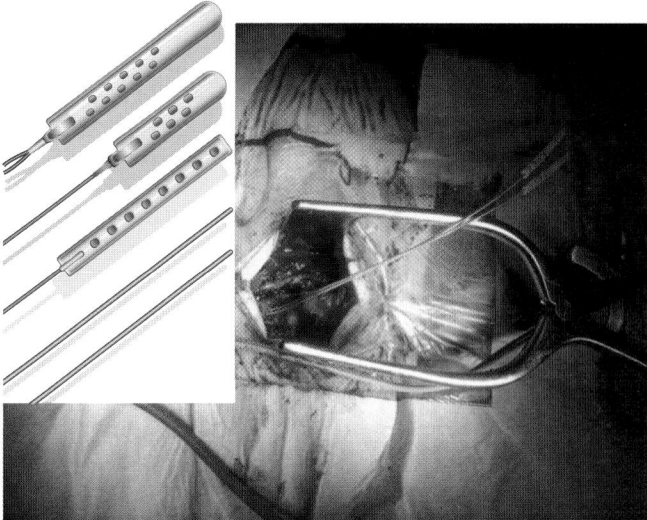

FIGURE 49.9 Intraoperative picture showing the spinal epidural insertion of the electrode for spinal cord stimulation; in the insert, different configurations of leads available for such procedures.

thoracic level (Fig. 49.9). The internal pulse generator (IPG) is positioned in the subcutaneous tissue (generally at the abdominal level) and connected to the electrode through tunneled extension leads.

Stimulation is actually carried out at the level of the posterior funiculi of the spinal cord, where all large-caliber sensitive fibers are grouped. The electrode can be implanted with a laminectomy or with percutaneous technique; in some centers the definitive implant of the system is preceded by a trial stimulation period, during which the clinical efficacy of the device is evaluated with an external stimulator. It is now possible to have programmable devices, which are given to the patient, who can use them for starting or stopping the stimulation with an external magnet that communicates with the IPG. Stimulation parameters employed range from 1 to 5 V as amplitude, 30 to 80 Hz as frequency, and 100 to 300 microseconds as pulse width; in electrodes with complex arrangements of the contacts, the configuration of the electrical field plays a major role in clinical outcome.

SCS is actually employed mostly for neuropathic rather than for nociceptive pain; such pain control does not affect other sensory modalities. Generally after the implantation the patient should perceive paresthesias in the same region of the pain; these paresthesias are due to the stimulation of large myelinated fibers in the dorsal column.

Indications for SCS are failed back surgery syndrome, complex regional pain syndrome (I and II), incomplete avulsion of brachial or lumbar plexus, phantom limb pain, postherpetic neuralgia, pain secondary to spinal cord trauma, peripheral vascular disease in the lower limbs, and angina pectoris. Obviously, all these conditions must be definitively drug refractory to take into consideration SCS as a therapeutic option.

The mechanism of action of SCS is still debated; numerous theories have been proposed, the first of which has obviously been the "gate" theory of Melzack and Wall. New physiological mechanisms have been hypothesized, such as the "orthodromic theory" (the electrical impulses conveyed by the fasciculus gracilis and cuneatus activate suprasegmental centers such as PAG and nucleus of raphe magnum, which exert inhibitory control on pain perception via descending pathways), the "collision current theory" (the current traveling along the dorsal roots enters in collision with orthodromic stimuli traveling through Aδ- and C-fibers, blocking them), and the "inhibitory neurotransmitter" theory, according to which the analgesic effect could be due to the stimulation-induced release of endogenous opioids at the level of the dorsal horns, or to the fact that stimulation leads to an increase of the concentrations of neuroactive substances in CSF such as norepinephrine, GABA, substance P, adenosine, and glycine. In particular, the release of inhibitory amino acids such as GABA and glycine could limit the release of excitatory amino acids such as aspartate and glutamate and could act on their own receptors (especially $GABA_B$ receptors) at various spinal levels, restoring normal GABAergic activity within the spinal cord.

Probably different mechanisms play a role in the analgesic effect of SCS, and as stated by Linderoth[248] the final common effect could be a suppressive effect of current on wide-dynamic range and hyperexcitable neurons located on the dorsal horn of the spinal cord.

As far as ischemic pain is concerned, the analgesic effect of SCS could instead be due to a rebalance between request and contribution of oxygen, increasing oxygen contribution and decreasing its requirement. Furthermore, SCS could lead to peripheral vasodilatation by antidromically activating Aδ fibers traveling in the dorsal roots, with subsequent release of vasoactive substances such as calcitonin-gene-related peptide (CGRP); also, it could inhibit the sympathetic efferent activity, reducing its vasoconstrictive effect both at the level of the lower limbs and at the cardiac level.

Most of the studies report a clinical efficacy of SCS in 50% to 70% of the patients treated (responders: reduction of at least 50% in intensity of pain). SCS has been reported to be superior to surgical reexploration in failed back surgery syndrome in a study by North and co-workers.[249]

The most frequent adverse effects reported in the literature are lead displacement, fractures of the extension leads, infections, CSF leaks, and epidural hematoma. The rate of displacement of cervical leads is largest in cervical electrodes because of the greater motility of the cervical spine.

Peripheral Nerve Stimulation

Whereas large myelinated fibers belonging to nervous structures located upstream from the site of the pain are the target of SCS, regional subcutaneous tissue, where small-caliber fibers run (also called "unnamed fibers"), or single nervous trunks, are the targets of peripheral nerve stimulation (PNS).

Nowadays there is some confusion about this terminology, as in the case of occipital nerve stimulation (ONS), in which the electrode is not just positioned above the nerve but in the proximity of its anatomical course below the inion; this kind of stimulation could be considered an "indirect PNS" rather than subcutaneous stimulation.

The first report of PNS for pain dates back to 1967, when Wall and Sweet inserted an electrode into their own infraorbital foramina and observed a decrease in painful sensitivity during the period of stimulation.[250] In the same period Shelden implanted electrodes around the mandibular nerve in three

patients and delivered electric current through an implanted receiver at a frequency of 14,000 Hz; again, temporary pain decrease was obtained.[251] Weiner and Reed in 1999 described the first percutaneous insertion of an electrode in proximity to the occipital nerves.[252] This report paved the way for the clinical application of ONS, which is now employed for several refractory painful conditions. Slavin and Burchiel subsequently performed the PNS approach for refractory pain in the trigeminal and occipital territories.[253] Subsequently, other reports were published reporting the efficacy and different surgical techniques of this procedure in different syndromes.[254-256]

In general, the relevant teleological difference between the procedures aimed at interacting with the central nervous system interface and PNS consists of the stimulation of areas that are known to be unsatisfactorily controlled by SCS or by major trunk stimulation. In fact, with PNS the electrodes are typically placed above or very close to the area of perceived pain. This procedure is usually performed with cylindrical leads rather than paddle-type leads, in order to resemble a circumferential electrical field.

The basic principle of PNS is the vicinity of the placed electrodes to the area of referred pain. The characteristics of pain should dictate the appropriate placement of the electrode(s); as stated by Barolat,[257] in case of mild allodynia, the implanted electrode or electrodes should be still better placed in the painful area; in cases of severe allodynia, the electrodes should be placed on each side of the allodynic region, so as to "circumvent" it. Barolat states that with this technique allodynic symptoms are likely to be significantly reduced.

The mainstay of the subcutaneous electric stimulation is, as stated previously, to relieve pain in areas that are difficult to reach by SCS or DBS, such as median lumbar pain, median thoracic pain, inguinal pain, or scapular pain, by directly reaching and intercepting the involved peripheral nervous components that generate the aberrant nociceptive discharges. The PNS procedure can be performed under general or local anesthesia, according to the extension of the painful area and compliance of the patient to be treated, and the definitive implant can be preceded by a trial stimulation period by means of external pulse generators delivering appropriate current intensity at established stimulation parameters; in case of satisfactory pain relief in the trial period, the whole system is definitively implanted.

The most frequent indications for PNS are axial lumbar pain (which is typically not well controlled by SCS), thoracic pain, shoulder pain, atypical facial pain, inguinal pain, and more extensively, several headache conditions. According to Barolat[257] the preferred location of the implanted electrodes should be the superficial layer of the subcutaneous tissue, because a more superficial location could lead to lack of perceived paresthesias (considered to be essential, at least as predictive factors, for effective pain relief, also taking into account the "gate control" theory) and a deeper location could lead to undesired muscle contractions (in cases of proximity of the lead to the muscular fascia). The usual preoperative and noninvasive techniques employed before the operation are TENS and anesthetic peripheral nerve block; nonetheless, there is no consensus about the predictive values of such modalities with regard to subsequent PNS.

PNS is a relatively simple technique performed by tunneling a cylindrical electrode through the skin to the affected area of the body and connecting it to an internal pulse generator. The difficulty of the procedure depends on the amount of adipose tissue of the subject and on the extension of the painful area; furthermore, the complexity and the different dysesthetic features of given regions in a given patient can require careful preoperative planning, taking into account bony prominences and possible sites of skin erosion or lead decubitus; different trajectories can in fact be required to address these important operative issues.

Occipital Nerve Stimulation, Peripheral Trigeminal Stimulation, and Vagal Nerve Stimulation

ONS consists of stimulating the great occipital nerve (GON) by means of implanted paddle-type or wire-type electrodes that are positioned in the suboccipital region under the subcutaneous tissue and above the splenium fascial plane. One or two electrodes can be positioned according to the symptoms and to the patient's and clinician's preference. The configuration of such electrodes varies according to the different numbers of contacts and different distance between them. Bilateral implanting procedure implies the use of two symmetrical electrodes positioned about 1 cm below the inion and extending from 1 to 5 cm laterally to the midline, to ensure proper coverage of GONs, which emerge from the splenium muscle's fascia at this level (Fig. 49.10). As for other PNS procedures, the implantation is completed after positioning of the IPGs in the subcutaneous tissue, more often in the infraclavicular or paraumbilical regions. In several centers a trial-stimulation period is performed before definitive implant of the system; during this period, the electrodes, which are sutured to the skin in a sterile fashion, are connected to external pulse generators. Patients reporting more than 50% decrease in pain intensity or painful attack intensity are considered "responders" and recommended for implantation of IPGs.

The main indications for performing ONS are migraine,[258,259] transformed migraine,[260] cluster headache,[261,262] hemicrania continua,[263] cervicogenic headaches,[255] and occipital neuralgia,[264] the latter being the most common so far. Slavin and colleagues[264] reported on 14 consecutive patients with intractable occipital neuralgia treated with ONS. Ten patients were considered responders after the trial stimulation period and proceeded with system internalization. At the last clinical follow-up examinations, seven patients (70%) continued to benefit from the procedure and were able to reduce the daily intake of prophylactic drugs, whereas three patients had their hardware removed because of loss of beneficial effect or occurrence of infection.

Matharu[258] reported results in eight patients submitted to ONS for chronic migraine, who all described the clinical outcome at least as "good," with pain reduction ranging from 75% to 90%.

Popeney and Alo[260] reported on 25 patients with transformed migraine implanted with C1 through C3 peripheral nerve stimulation. The evaluation was carried out using the migraine disability assessment (MIDAS); symptoms had been refractory to conventional treatments for at least 6 months in this series. Prior to stimulation, all patients experienced severe disability (scored as grade IV on the MIDAS). After stimulation, the average improvement in the MIDAS score was 88.7%, and all of the patients reported that their headaches were well controlled after the implantation procedure.

Rodrigo-Royo and associates[255] reported on the results concerning four patients with drug-refractory, long-persistent, and severe pain in the occipital region, who were treated with electrical stimulation of the C1, C2, and C3 peripheral nerves. Results were considered good in all patients; the authors observed the disappearance of continuous pain in all patients and the improvement in intensity and frequency of pain bouts, with subsequent reduction or discontinuation of pharmacological therapy. Burns and colleagues[263] reported on six patients suffering from hemicrania continua submitted for ONS. At

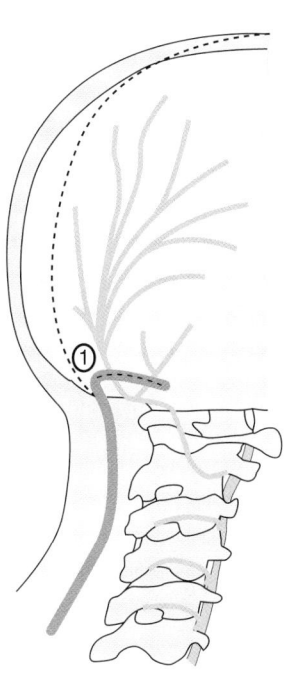
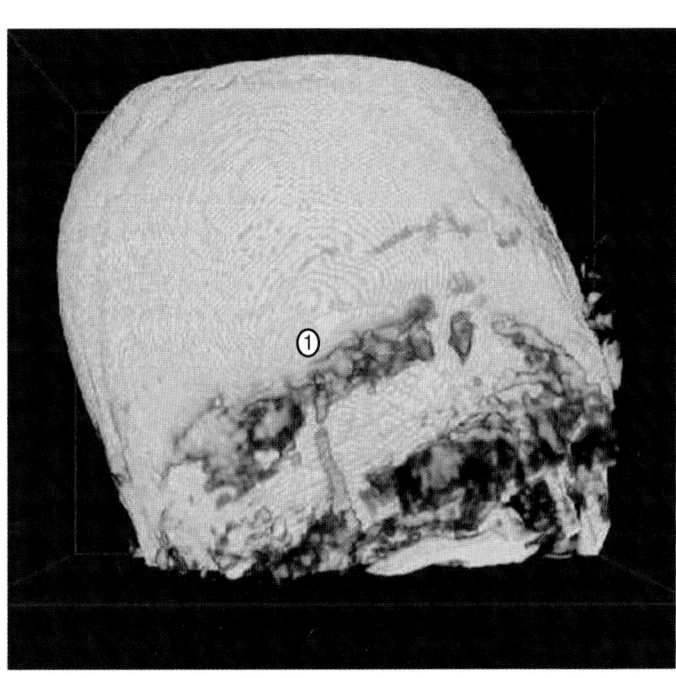

FIGURE 49.10 *Left:* Drawing showing the ideal placement of the occipital lead, from 1 cm to about 5 cm from the inion (midline). *Right:* Postoperative computed tomography (CT) scan of a patient submitted to occipital nerve stimulation (ONS).

long-term follow-up, four of the patients reported 80% to 95% improvement, one patient reported 30% improvement, and one patient reported worsening of symptoms.

Bartsch and Goadsby[265] in 2003 reported that stimulation of nociceptive afferent C-fibers of the dura mater of the rat can lead to a sensitization of second-order cervical spinal neurons. The authors proposed that such a mechanism could be involved in the referral of pain from trigeminal to cervical structures in patients affected by CCH and chronic migraine. Piovesan in 2003[266] highlighted the concept of "trigeminocervical complex," thus hypothesizing the convergence of nociceptive information in trigeminal and cervical territories at the level of the neurons in the trigeminal nucleus caudalis, extending to the C2 spinal segment. Based on this study, Magis and co-workers[261] reported on the results of eight patients with refractory CCH submitted to ONS. Two patients were pain-free after a follow-up period of 16 and 22 months; three patients reported 90% reduction in attack frequency, and two patients reported improvement of about 40%. Switching off the IPGs led to recurrence and increase of attack frequency in all the patients. The mean time elapse from implantation to the onset of beneficial effects was reported to be 2 months.

Burns[263] reported 14 patients with drug-refractory CCH submitted to bilateral implantation of ONS electrodes; the median follow-up period was 17.5 months, and 10 out of 14 patients benefited from the procedure. Three patients reported improvement of 90% or better, three reported a moderate improvement (40% or better), and four reported 20% to 30% improvement. Most of the patients reported relapse of pain attacks when the device was switched off; interestingly in one patient the ONS system helped in aborting acute attacks.

Slavin[267] reported on a case series of 30 patients submitted to a trial period of peripheral nerve stimulation for refractory craniofacial pain, of whom only 22 experienced more than 50% improvement in pain intensity and were subsequently implanted with the complete system. Three patients received infraorbital subcutaneous electrodes, four received supraorbital subcutaneous electrodes, 13 received occipital electrodes, one patient had a combination of infraorbital and occipital stimulation system, and one patient had a combination of supraorbital and occipital stimulation. Follow-up evaluations were carried on for a mean time period of 35 months. At the last clinical examination, the systems had been removed in five patients because of improvement in pain intensity, persistence of symptoms, and infection; 17 patients continued to use the PNS device; three of them had an improvement in pain of less than 50%, whereas 14 reported an improvement of 50% and were considered responders. Reed[268] reported seven patients affected by refractory chronic migraine headaches who received a combined occipital nerve–supraorbital nerve neurostimulation system. In this study, the relative responses to the ONS system alone and to both ONS and supraorbital systems were evaluated. The follow-up period ranged from 1 to 35 months; all patients reported full therapeutic response only to combined supraorbital and occipital neurostimulation, whereas only a partial response was provided by the ONS system alone. The authors conclude that in patients affected by chronic migraine the clinical benefit may be better in those implanted with both systems.

Migraine is often comorbid with a large spectrum of diseases, including epilepsy, stroke, and above all, psychiatric disorders,[269] especially major depression; depressive episodes can influence pain's processing and perception and are associated with a poorer clinical outcome in cephalalgic patients. Given that *vagal nerve stimulation* (VNS), approved by the U.S. Food and Drug Administration as an adjunctive treatment for drug-refractory depressive disorder,[270] has been shown to be effective in controlling episodic migraine,[271,272] our group[273] published preliminary data about the employment of VNS for refractory chronic daily headache (CDH) with comorbid depression.

The vagal nerve stimulation is carried on by wrapping a spiral electrode around the cervical portion of the left vagus nerve. The left nerve is chosen because of the lesser influence on cardiac activity. The IPG is positioned in the left subclavicular region.

In our case four patients were selected for implantation of this device; all of them had a clinical history of CDH lasting at least 2 years, were refractory to conservative treatments for both headache and major depression, and suffered from severe disability on activities of daily living. None of the patients had psychotic features, heart disease, or lung diseases that could contraindicate chronic stimulation of the left vagus nerve. The intensity of stimulation used ranged from 1 to 2.25 mA. Two of the patients showed a significant improvement for both headache and depression after 1 to 3 months from the start of stimulation. The remaining two patients showed limited or no clinical benefit after VNS. Another study by Mauskop[274] reported improvement after VNS in two patients with CCH and in two patients with chronic migraine.

Systems of Spinal Intrathecal Release of Opioids

Intrathecal (IT) delivery of analgesic agents allows for a more focused action of the drugs at the spinal cord level (where respective receptors are present at different locations), thus limiting the adverse side effects of systemic administration. Moreover, in this procedure the dosage needed for the analgesic effect is lower than that of intravenous, intramuscular, or oral administration, and this lower dose also limits the side effects.

The discovery of opioid receptors at the spinal cord level paved the way for this procedure; in 1976 Yaksh and Rudy obtained a reduction of the hind-limb withdrawal reflex in rats exposed to algic stimuli and concomitantly submitted to subarachnoid administration of opioids.[275] The analgesic effect of opioids at the spinal level is thought to be mediated by inhibitory interneurons that act to reduce the nociceptive transmission at higher levels.[276] Intrathecal opioid (morphine chlorhydrate or hydromorphone) therapy is usually performed for pain of nociceptive type, whereas neuropathic pain is sometimes considered a secondary indication, both because of the efficacy of SCS and for the higher opioid concentrations required in this case. Nonetheless, there are reports about the possible efficacy of IT opioids in neuropathic pain.[277] Other types of agents are available for this indication (even if still less studied and tested than morphine).

Classical indications for opioid IT therapy are failed back surgery syndrome, cancer pain, axial spinal pain, complex regional pain syndrome, arachnoiditis, poststroke pain, and spinal cord injury. Other prerequisites are the compliance of the patient and the possibility of performing regular clinical follow-up examinations, which are mandatory for the variation of the daily dosage.

Nonopioid drugs, as mentioned earlier, have been proposed, both alone or in combination with morphine, for IT therapy. They include clonidine, tizanidine, ziconotide, glutamate antagonists, benzodiazepines, tricyclic antidepressants, butamin, and nitric oxide synthetase inhibitors.[221] Most of these drugs have been tested only on experimental models. Hydromorphone can be used in cases of tolerance to morphine, and IT clonidine can be added to IT opioids in cases of tolerance development or if unsatisfactory results are obtained with one drug alone; in particular, two early studies report the safety and efficacy of this combination in noncancer and in cancer pain.[278,279] Baclofen and bupivacaine can be used as a third-line approach, too, alone or in combination to first-line agents.[280]

The implantation procedure can be preceded by a trial bolus of IT morphine (generally 0.5 mg is administered at this stage), after which pain decrease is assessed; if no adverse effects appear in case of absent benefit, the bolus dosage can be slightly increased and the patient evaluated again.

Surgery is performed by first positioning a Tuohy needle in the spinal lumbar subarachnoid space, and through it a silicone catheter is introduced; this catheter is then tunneled subcutaneously and connected to a drug's controlled-release device (pump). The pump is also positioned subcutaneously, and can be externally programmed with a data transferring and receiving device, thus regulating the daily dosage of the administered drug. Different kinds of pumps exist, including pulsatile pumps (hand-operated systems that are activated with tactile stimuli), constant flow pumps (in which case the effective daily dosage of the drug is determined by the concentration of the solution present in the reservoir), and programmable pumps. Programmable pumps are the most versatile devices in that they can be remotely controlled by an external programmer, dictating the daily dosage of the drug according to the concentration of the solution initially present and to the flow rate through the catheter.

For morphine chlorhydrate, initial daily dosage is usually 2 to 3 mg, but it can be varied according to the patient's needs and to the eventual onset of side effects (dosage spectrum is quite wide, ranging from 1 to about 60 mg/day). For clonidine, the recommended dosage range is 10 to 10,000 µg per day.[281] In the current literature, the percentage of pain relief is reported to be 60% to 80% for malignant pain and 60% to 65% for nonmalignant pain.[281]

The most common complications of surgery are hardware failure, infection of the surgical wounds, epidural abscess, and formation of seroma at the tip of the catheter. Drug-related complications with opioids are constipation, urinary dysfunction, nausea, hypogonadism, sweating, weight gain, and respiratory depression. The incidence of respiratory depression (requiring anesthesiological intervention) is estimated to be around 1%. The most common clonidine-related adverse effects are hypotension, decrease in heart rate, and mild sedation.

Systems of Intraventricular Release of Opioids

In local or general anesthesia, after precoronal craniectomy, a right intraventricular catheter is positioned (the exact position may vary) and subsequently connected to a subcutaneous access site (reservoir). At this site, injections of morphine chlorhydrate can be delivered, thus obtaining a powerful and long-lasting antalgic effect, through direct action on the morphinic periventricular receptors. This technique is generally used in cases of diffuse cervical and facial pain, often secondary to neoplastic ear, nose, and throat or stomatological lesions and not well controlled by adequate dosages of oral morphine. Also patients affected from Pancoast-Cuffini syndrome can benefit from the procedure. The initial dosage is inferior to that administered intraspinally (0.5 mg in 24 hours) but in this case it can be increased according to the patient's needs. Despite the central administration, no case of respiratory depression has been reported, thus allowing the drug to act only on the painful symptoms in a selective fashion.

SELECTED KEY REFERENCES

Franzini A, Messina G, Cordella R, et al. Deep brain stimulation of the posteromedial hypothalamus: indications, long-term results, and neurophysiological considerations. *Neurosurg Focus*. 2010;29(2):E13.

Jannetta PJ, McLaughlin MR, Casey KF. Technique of microvascular decompression. Technical note. *Neurosurg Focus*. 2005;18(5):E5.

Linderoth BG, Meyerson BA. Spinal cord stimulation: mechanisms of action. In: Burchiel KJ, ed. *Surgical Management of Pain*. New York: Thieme; 2002:505-526.

Sindou M. Microsurgical DREZotomy. In: Schmidek HH, Sweet WH, eds. *Operative Neurosurgical Techniques*. 3rd ed. Philadelphia: WB Saunders; 1995:1613-1622.

Tasker RR. Percutaneous cordotomy. In: Schmidek HH, Sweet WH, eds. *Operative Neurosurgical Techniques: Indications, Methods and Results*. Orlando: Grune & Stratton; 1995:1595-1611.

Please go to expertconsult.com to view the complete list of references.

Spasticity: Classification, Diagnosis, and Management

Michael R. Levitt, Samuel R. Browd

CLINICAL PEARLS

- Spasticity is velocity-dependent resistance to passive muscle stretch that usually originates from pathological issues with the brain or spinal cord. Symptoms of spasticity include muscle tightness, cramping/pain, and fatigue. Spasticity is primarily due to an imbalance between activation and inhibition of muscle groups.

- Cerebral palsy is the most common cause of spasticity, especially in children. Stroke, multiple sclerosis, and brain or spinal trauma are common causes of spasticity in adults.

- Spasticity results from decreased inhibition of muscle groups and facilitation of hypertonia. The decreased inhibitory input into the motor unit results in coactivation of both agonistic and antagonistic muscle groups during volitional movement, and creates an imbalance of excitatory neurotransmitters in the spinal cord, specifically a lack of the inhibitory substance γ-aminobutyric acid (GABA).

- The Ashworth or Modified Ashworth scales are commonly used to classify the severity of spasticity. The Modified Ashworth scale[1] ranges from 0 (no increase in muscle tone) to 4, in which affected part(s) are rigid in flexion or extension. Management of spasticity is often achieved with a combination of medications and surgical procedures.

- Intrathecal baclofen (ITB) pumps are most effective in pediatric patients older than 3 years when a response to a baclofen "test dose" is observed. ITB is effective in patients with spasticity in all limbs and in dystonia. Baclofen activates $GABA_B$ receptors, and benzodiazepines activate $GABA_A$ receptors; both provide compensatory inhibition in the brain and spinal cord.[2] Spastic patients with intrathecal or oral baclofen withdrawal present with increased tone, pruritus, and anxiety. Severe withdrawal may include fever, seizures, hallucinations, and rarely death. Treatment of withdrawal includes administration of oral baclofen or intravenous benzodiazepines.

- Botulinum toxin injection is useful in treating spasticity of individual muscle groups or extremities.

- Selective dorsal rhizotomy is most effective in the treatment of spastic diplegia, and is more effective than physical therapy alone in selected patients. Cost-effectiveness studies have shown an advantage of selective dorsal rhizotomy (SDR) over ITB in patients with spastic diplegia due to reduced hospital readmissions for pump replacements and complications.

Spasticity is defined as a "velocity-dependent, increased resistance to passive muscle stretch."[3] It is distinguished from other common hypertonic movement disorders (such as dystonia) by quantifying the amount of abnormal movement: Spasticity is isokinetic (abnormal but not increased movements), while dystonia and other movement disorders are hyperkinetic (abnormal and increased movements).[4] It is often associated with muscle tightness, cramping/pain, and fatigue, and its severity may range from mild to disabling. Even though spasticity is considered a diagnosis unto itself, it is always related to an underlying injury to the brain or spinal cord. The treatment of spasticity involves a combination of medical and surgical management.

CAUSES

Spasticity is typically defined by the causative diagnosis. The most common causes are cerebral palsy (CP),[5] traumatic injury (including injuries to either the brain[6,7] or spine[8]), stroke,[9] and multiple sclerosis (MS);[10] other inherited disorders (e.g., Wilson's disease, Hallervorden-Spatz disease) are rare causes.

Cerebral Palsy

Cerebral palsy is the most commonly encountered spastic disorder, occurring in 2.4 per 1000 children and accounting for up to 75% of affected patients.[11,12] Cerebral palsy is usually described as "a range of nonprogressive syndromes of posture and motor impairment that results from an insult to the developing central nervous system."[13] One or both of the following signs are required for diagnosis, according to the task force for pediatric hypertonia: (1) an increase in resistance to externally applied movement in the same direction as joint movement; and (2) a rapid rise in resistance to externally applied movement above a threshold speed or joint angle.[5]

Brain or Spinal Trauma

Injuries to either the brain or spinal cord can result in spasticity.[6,7,14,15] These injuries include involvement of any of the following: basal ganglia, cerebellum, motor cortices, and spinal cord. It is estimated that up to 25% of patients with moderate or severe trauma develop spasticity symptoms.[7]

Stroke

Similar to traumatic spasticity, stroke-related spasticity is commonly encountered after lesions to either upper motor neurons or descending inhibitory systems (see later discussion). Approximately 15% to 40% of patients develop clinical spasticity disorders after major stroke.[9,16,17]

Multiple Sclerosis

Multiple sclerosis is a demyelinating disease often affecting upper motor neuron areas of the brain and spinal cord. A substantial proportion of MS patients develop spastic symptoms; one major study found that 84% of a large database of MS patients suffered from at least minimal spasticity during the disease course, with 34% reporting moderate to severe or disabling symptoms.[10]

CLASSIFICATION

Many practitioners further classify spasticity within the following anatomical categories, first described for CP:[18]

- Quadriparesis/tetraplegia—involving all four extremities
- Paraparesis/diplegia—involving the bilateral lower extremities
- Hemiparesis—involving ipsilateral upper and lower extremities
- Monoparesis—involving one extremity
- Truncal/cervical—involving axial, postural, or neck muscles

This classification is the most important aspect of spasticity for the practicing neurosurgeon, as the anatomical location (as well as severity) influences treatment strategy.

PATHOPHYSIOLOGY

Understanding the neurophysiology of spasticity requires detailed knowledge of the control and regulation of movement and posture in the central nervous system. In normal conditions, a balance exists between alpha motor neurons in the spinal cord (activated by descending corticospinal tracts) and the descending inhibition created by the basal ganglia,

cerebellum, and reticular activating system. These inhibitory systems exert their control on the spinal cord via descending input from the reticulospinal and other tracts, which synapse on the motor neurons or interneurons of the spinal cord. This system maintains baseline muscle tone and posture, as well as facilitates the complementary deactivation of antagonistic muscle groups via Ia and Ib afferents in the dorsal root of the motor unit. For example, flexion of the thigh is facilitated by positive input from the corticospinal tracts in conjunction with deactivation of extensors via descending inhibitory tracts.[19,20]

Spasticity results from decreased inhibition or facilitation of hypertonia.[19,20] The decreased inhibitory input into the motor unit results in coactivation of both agonistic and antagonistic muscle groups during volitional movement, and creates an imbalance of excitatory neurotransmitters in the spinal cord (in particular, a lack of the inhibitory substance γ-aminobutyric acid [GABA]). Chronic spasticity may lead to denervation supersensitivity, and ultimately permanent soft tissue contractures requiring surgical release, especially in the ankle joint and Achilles tendon.[21]

DIAGNOSIS

A careful history and physical examination is imperative for the diagnosis of both the cause and classification of spasticity. In pediatric patients with CP-related spasticity, a failure to meet motor system and other developmental milestones is often apparent by age 1 to 2 years, and is most severe by age 3.[13] Often, symptoms of CP will decline over childhood, with one major study describing 66% of patients with spastic diplegia and 50% with CP of any kind "outgrowing" their symptoms by age 7.[22] Older patients with alternative causes of spastic disorder will complain of characteristic muscle tightness, cramping, pain in the affected extremities, and generalized as well as focal fatigue.

Physical examination findings are often linked with the location of injury. Patients with CP often manifest with di- or tetraplegia of varying severity, often with disproportionate involvement of flexors, adductors, and internal rotators.[4] In patients with cervical spinal cord injury, both flexor muscles in the arms and extensors in the leg (so-called antigravity muscles) are often affected, but lesions in the thoracic or lumbar spine typically affect only leg extensors. Cortical spasticity from stroke or trauma is often related to the laterality of injury, with contralateral extremities or a single extremity affected.[23] Multiple sclerosis patients are heterogeneous in presentation depending on the areas of demyelination, but often present with leg adductor and extensor imbalance.

Resistance to passive muscle stretch correlating with the speed of the stretch is the hallmark of the physical examination in affected muscle groups in patients with spasticity. Several clinical scales have been developed to determine the severity of symptoms. The Ashworth scale grades spasticity as follows: 0 = normal muscle tone; 1 = slight increase in muscle tone, "catch" when limb moved; 2 = more marked increase in muscle tone, but limb easily flexed; 3 = considerable increase in muscle tone; and 4 = limb rigid in flexion or extension.[24] The Modified Ashworth scale[1] provides further precision, especially in patients with hemiplegia: 0 = no increase in muscle tone; 1 = slight increase in muscle tone, manifested by a catch and release or by minimal resistance at the end of the range of motion (ROM); 1+ = slight increase in muscle tone, manifested by a catch, followed by minimal resistance throughout the remainder (less than half) of the ROM; 2 = more marked increase in muscle tone through most of the ROM, but affected part(s) easily moved; 3 = considerable increase in muscle tone, passive movement difficult; 4 = affected part(s) rigid in flexion or extension. Most studies of the diagnosis and treatment of spasticity employ these scales, as well as other indices of motor function and dexterity, to grade the physical findings of individual patients.

TREATMENT

The treatment of spasticity almost always involves multidimensional or multimodality therapy that may include physiotherapy, medical therapy (oral medications, percutaneous injections), neurosurgical therapy (surgical implantation of intrathecal infusion pumps, permanent selective denervation procedures such as selective dorsal rhizotomy), and orthopedic procedures.[25]

Medical Therapy

The most common oral medications used in the treatment of spasticity include baclofen, benzodiazepines, tizanidine, dantrolene, gabapentin, and pregabalin. A summary of these medications is found in Table 50.1. They rely on two common mechanisms to reduce spastic symptoms throughout the body, often in combination: (1) compensating for reduced GABA or other inhibitory neurotransmitters in the brain or spinal cord, or (2) reducing the amount of excitatory neurotransmitters through direct inhibition or activation of inhibitory interneurons. The common mechanism of action of these medications also results in a similar side effect profile, including most commonly somnolence, ataxia, and muscle weakness.[15,26]

Baclofen, the most common oral medication in the treatment of spasticity, binds to $GABA_B$ receptors in Rexed laminae I to IV of the spinal cord.[27] Activation of these metabotropic

receptors leads to increased cell permeability of K^+, causing cation efflux and resultant hyperpolarization of the cell membrane.[12] This hyperpolarization leads to a reduction in the release of excitatory neurotransmitters (such as glutamate and aspartate), as well as substance P. Important side effects of baclofen include orthostatic hypotension and withdrawal symptoms such as seizures, fever, hallucinations, and rebound spasticity. One drawback of oral baclofen is poor penetration of the blood-brain barrier with cerebrospinal fluid (CSF) drug levels 10-fold lower than serum concentrations. It is common that oral dose escalation leads to side effects before full therapeutic efficacy is reached. Intrathecal delivery of baclofen is highly effective and is the favored modality of drug delivery when patients are unable to tolerate increased doses of oral baclofen (see later discussion).

Benzodiazepines facilitate the binding of existing GABA to the $GABA_A$ receptor,[28] found in high concentrations in the reticular formation and polysynaptic spinal tracts. In contrast to the $GABA_B$ receptor, the $GABA_A$ receptor is ionotropic. Its activation results in the increase in cell permeability of Cl^-, causing anion influx and hyperpolarization. This hyperpolarization increases presynaptic inhibition and reduces monosynaptic and polysynaptic reflexes throughout the spinal cord. A variety of different benzodiazepine compounds are available including oral, intravenous, and rectal routes of administration, with different durations due to the rate of metabolism. The most important (and often dose-limiting) side effect of this medication class is sedation. Rapid reversal of benzodiazepine toxicity can be achieved with the administration of flumazenil. Additionally, habituation and tolerance may develop, and prolonged use is associated with addiction.

Tizanidine and related medications (such as clonidine) provide an alternative mechanism to the preceding medications via the reduction of excitatory neurotransmitters. Tizanidine is an α_2-adrenergic agonist that acts throughout the central nervous system (CNS) to reduce excitatory amino acid release from spinal interneurons.[29,30] Tizanidine is particularly effective in adult spasticity from spinal disease or multiple sclerosis.[31] Important adverse effects include nausea and vomiting, hypotension (clonidine), and sedation (tizanidine).

TABLE 50.1 Oral Medications in the Treatment of Spasticity			
Drug	**Mechanism of Action**	**Effect(s)**	**Additional Adverse Effects***
Baclofen	Binds $GABA_B$ receptors, increasing K^+ efflux	Reduces release of excitatory NTs and substance P	Orthostatic hypotension Withdrawal may cause seizures, hallucinations, rebound spasticity, fever
Benzodiazepines	Increases existing GABA affinity for $GABA_A$ receptors, increasing Cl^- influx	Increases presynaptic inhibition, reduces monosynaptic and polysynaptic reflexes	Hypotension, significant sedation Withdrawal may cause seizures
Tizanidine	α_2-Adrenergic agonist	Reduces excitatory NT release from spinal interneurons	Potential hepatotoxicity
Dantrolene	Binds ryanodine receptor in skeletal muscle, decreasing intracellular calcium concentration by sequestering Ca^{2+} in sarcoplasmic reticulum	Excitation-contraction decoupler in skeletal muscle	Weakness may include respiratory muscles Potential hepatotoxicity
Gabapentin Pregabalin	Binds to α_2-δ subunit of voltage-gated calcium channels	Reduces excitatory NTs in brain and spinal cord	Well tolerated and less sedating Isolated cases of myopathy

*All medications can cause various degrees of sedation, ataxia, muscle weakness, and fatigue.
GABA, γ-aminobutyric acid; NT, neurotransmitter.

Dantrolene is unique among oral medications in the treatment of spasticity due to its effects on skeletal muscle. Dantrolene binds to skeletal muscle ryanodine receptors, preventing the release of calcium into the cytosol from its sequestration in the sarcoplasmic reticulum during motor unit activation. Thus, its action is defined as an "excitation-contraction decoupler" in skeletal muscle.[32-34] It is also used in the emergency treatment of malignant hyperthermia and neuroleptic malignant syndrome. Although it is less sedative than other antispasticity agents, its effect on skeletal muscle may result in significant weakness of both volitional and (in severe cases) respiratory muscles.[35] Another important side effect is the approximately 1.8% risk of hepatotoxicity, which is increased with coadministration of other agents (i.e., valproate, tizanidine).[36] Some clinicians recommend routine surveillance of liver function tests in patients taking dantrolene.

Two newer medications, gabapentin and pregabalin, were originally developed as anticonvulsants but have found utility in the management of spasm and other disorders such as neuropathic pain. Both medications work in a similar fashion as GABA analogs that bind to the $\alpha_2\delta$-subunit of voltage-gated calcium channels, inhibiting calcium influx. This mechanism reduces the concentration of excitatory neurotransmitters such as glutamate and aspartate in the CNS.[37,38] Gabapentin is a well-established therapy for the treatment of spasticity of spinal origin[39,40] and in the management of MS.[41] Pregabalin is emerging as an alternative agent with similar properties.[42] Both medications are well tolerated with minimal side effects, such as sedation, even after significant titration. Gabapentin has been associated with myopathy, especially in patients with renal failure, as it is renally excreted,[43] and pregabalin is somewhat more sedating and may cause dose-limiting ataxia.[44]

Recent advances have been made in the treatment of spasticity of focal hypertonia using percutaneous injection of botulinum neurotoxin (BoNT), often in conjunction with the general effects of oral medications or surgical treatments,[45] or as monotherapy for isolated limb spasticity.[46-48] BoNT is derived from *Clostridium botulinum* exotoxin, and acts by cleaving polypeptides required for exocytosis, such as synaptosomal-associated protein (SNAP)-25, vesicle-associated membrane protein (VAMP), and syntaxin, within the cytosol of motor neurons.[49,50] Cleavage of these peptides prevents the release of acetylcholine into the neuromuscular junction, relieving focal muscle hypertonia. Additional indirect beneficial effects on muscle tone, such as the suppression of other excitatory neurotransmitters and reduced autonomic activity, may occur. A single treatment remains effective for 2 to 4 months at a time,[26] providing a useful adjunct treatment for persistent symptoms involving a single muscle group, such as the calf, upper extremity, leg adductor, or cervical musculature.

There are three main adverse effects of BoNT injection.[45] First, inhibition of acetylcholine release may spread to neighboring nerve endings, including respiratory muscles. This has led to a black-box warning for all BoNT formulations regarding the risk of potentially life-threatening respiratory failure. Second, sustained or repeated administration to a single anatomical area may produce effects similar to denervation, such as muscle atrophy. Third, the patient's host response may generate antibodies to the BoNT protein, leading to

immunoresistance that prevents its association with neuronal membranes.[51] These antibodies may lead to a habituation to BoNT injections over time.

Surgical Therapy

Intrathecal delivery of baclofen (ITB) has been shown to be safe, efficacious, and cost effective in the long-term treatment of both spasticity and dystonia.[52-55] Patients report subjective improvement in spasticity symptoms in 60% to 85% of cases, and improvement in motor function in 20% to 33%; Ashworth scores are typically reduced by 1 to 1.8 points.[56-60] Compared to oral baclofen administration, ITB delivers approximately four times the concentration of medication to the spinal cord with minimal systemic side effects, as plasma levels of intrathecal baclofen are undetectable.[61,62] Most neurosurgeons advocate a screening protocol prior to pump implantation to predict clinical benefit.[63] Baclofen is administered via lumbar puncture at a dose of 25 µg for children less than 40 lb and 50 µg for children or adults more than 40 lb. Postinfusion evaluations of spasticity are performed every 2 hours for 6 to 8 hours after injection, and patients with an improvement of one point or greater in the Ashworth score are considered candidates for pump implantation. A temporary intrathecal catheter connected to an external pump may be used for more prolonged evaluation, especially in adults or patients with dystonia in which a higher test dose is required.[56]

Pump implantation techniques have been thoroughly documented in the neurosurgery literature.[64,65] The patient is placed in the lateral decubitus position to give clear access to the lumbar spine and abdomen. Meticulous sterile prep and draping are performed, and preoperative antibiotics administered. A 2-cm midline incision is made at the L4-L5 interspace, through the lumbosacral fascia. The thecal sac is accessed with a large-bore Tuohy needle, and the catheter is placed through the needle and advanced cephalad under fluoroscopy. Final catheter placement is based on the patient's underlying disorder: for patients with spastic paraparesis, T10-T11; spastic quadraparesis, C6-T2; generalized secondary dystonia, C1-C4.[64] The needle is removed, and the catheter is secured to the lumbosacral fascia with care to avoid kinking.

Following intrathecal placement, a subfascial pocket is made in the abdominal wall via an oblique subcostal incision. A pump is chosen from the available sizes based on patient weight and drug reservoir volume; proper selection is essential to prevent pressure on the wound. The pump reservoir is filled with baclofen, and sometimes placed in a Gore-Tex pouch before insertion into the subfascial pocket, to prevent pump rotation or malposition. A tunneling device is used to pass the catheter from the lumbar spine to the abdominal pocket, where it is connected to the pump. Careful irrigation and multilayered wound closure are performed at both surgical sites. Postoperative radiographs assess the position of the pump in the abdomen and the catheter in the spinal canal (Fig. 50.1A and B). The typical initial ITB dose is 100 µg per day, and may be titrated in the postoperative period to reach maximum clinical benefit. The pump reservoir is refilled by percutaneous injection, at an interval determined by the patient's individual concentration and dosage needs. Pump battery life is usually 5 to 7 years.

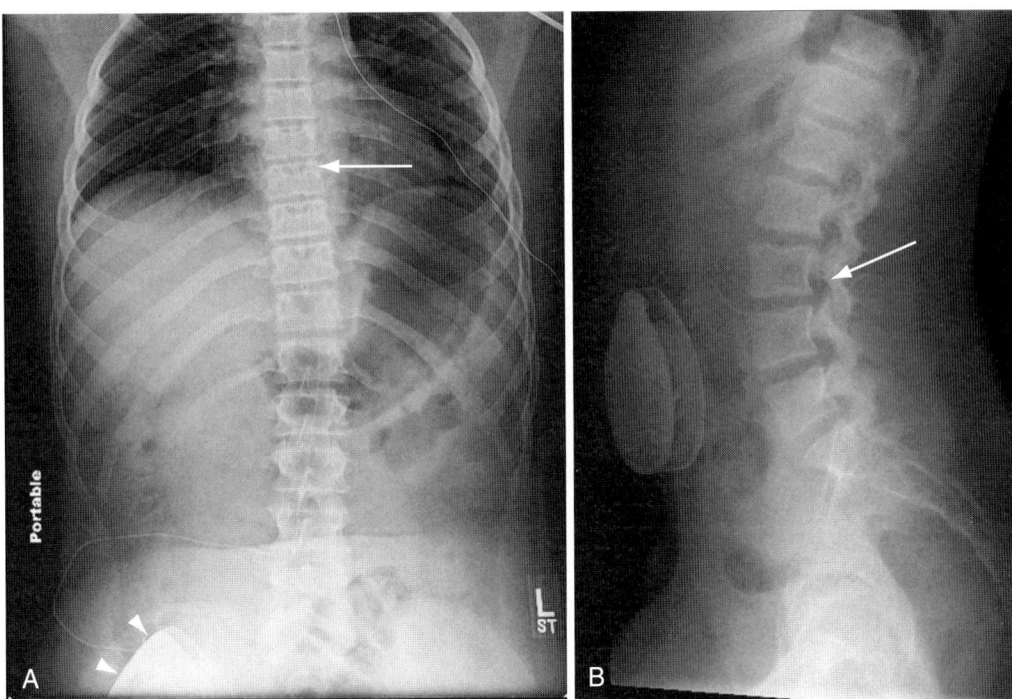

FIGURE 50.1 Postoperative radiographs after intrathecal baclofen pump implantation. **A,** Anteroposterior view demonstrates the cranial extent of the intrathecal catheter, terminating at the level of T8 in this case (*arrow*). The pump is partially visible in the right lower quadrant (*arrowheads*). **B,** Lateral view demonstrates the entry of the catheter into the intrathecal space (*arrow*).

Side Effects and Complications of Intrathecal Baclofen Therapy

The most common presenting sign of pump malfunction is baclofen withdrawal.[2] Patients present with increased tone, pruritus, and anxiety. Severe withdrawal effects are similar to those with oral baclofen and may include fever, seizures, hallucinations, and rarely death.[66,67] Treatment of withdrawal includes oral baclofen, intravenous benzodiazepines, or immediate pump revision. In contrast, ITB overdose results in hypotonia, sedation, cardiorespiratory depression, and coma; the most common cause of ITB overdose is improper pump programming. Treatment for overdose includes supportive care and resetting or deactivating the pump.

The technique for pump implantation is optimized to reduce the most common complications such as infection (3-15% overall; approximately 1% per year), catheter obstruction or disconnection (2-16%), and CSF leak (5-9%).[68-71] Patients must be of adequate weight to permit subcutaneous abdominal pump implantation, usually age older than 3 years. Immediate, transient postoperative urinary retention is common for up to 72 hours after pump implantation, and resolves without intervention.[56]

The most common organism found in infected pump systems is *Staphylococcus aureus*; most infections occur within 6 to 8 weeks of implantation.[68-71] Treatment involves removal of the pump and catheter, followed by long-term antibiotics and oral baclofen supplementation. Reimplantation may be considered at 8 to 12 weeks, and may occur in the same pump location.

Catheter failure is usually the result of disconnection or retraction.[56,68-70] Disconnection is the most common catheter-related complication, typically at the point of connection to the pump. Catheter retraction is caused by movement of the pump within its pocket, or by normal patient growth. The intrathecal end of the catheter may back out of the thecal sac and coil in the subcutaneous space (Fig. 50.2), or retract completely into the pump pocket. These failures occur early (within 3 months of implantation) and require surgical revision. For cases in which catheter malfunction is unclear, percutaneous injection of radiopaque contrast agent into the pump's side port, followed by radiography or computed tomography (CT), can aid in the diagnosis.

CSF leaks occur around the intrathecal catheter entry site, and are more common after revision surgery or when multiple attempts are made to access the thecal sac during implantation. Treatment options for CSF leak include bed rest, pressure dressings, lumbar drain placement below the ITB catheter, epidural blood patch, or open revision. It is important to assess the patient for untreated hydrocephalus in the setting of persistent CSF leak.[56]

Selective Denervation Procedures

Foerster first reported transection of the posterior lumbar and sacral nerve roots as a treatment for spasticity in 1913;[72] the procedure has since evolved to selective dorsal rhizotomy (SDR), the most common neurosurgical denervation procedure for spasticity. The lack of descending inhibition in spastic patients causes increased activation of antagonistic muscle groups via Ia and Ib reflexive afferents. By sectioning a portion of each dorsal root, SDR decreases the output of these Ia and Ib reflexive afferents, reducing spasticity.

Careful patient selection is necessary to determine which patients will derive maximum benefit from SDR. The optimal

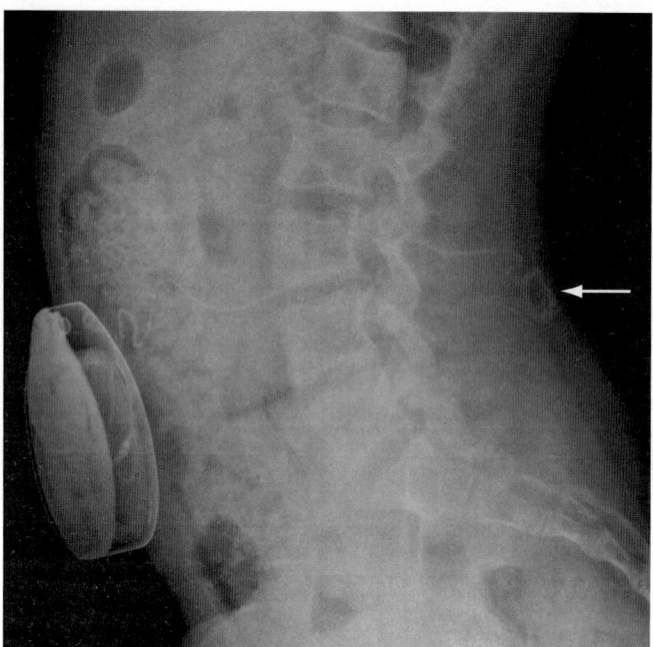

FIGURE 50.2 Disconnection and retraction of an intrathecal baclofen pump. Lateral radiographs demonstrate the intrathecal catheter coiled in the subcutaneous space (*arrow*). The patient required catheter revision.

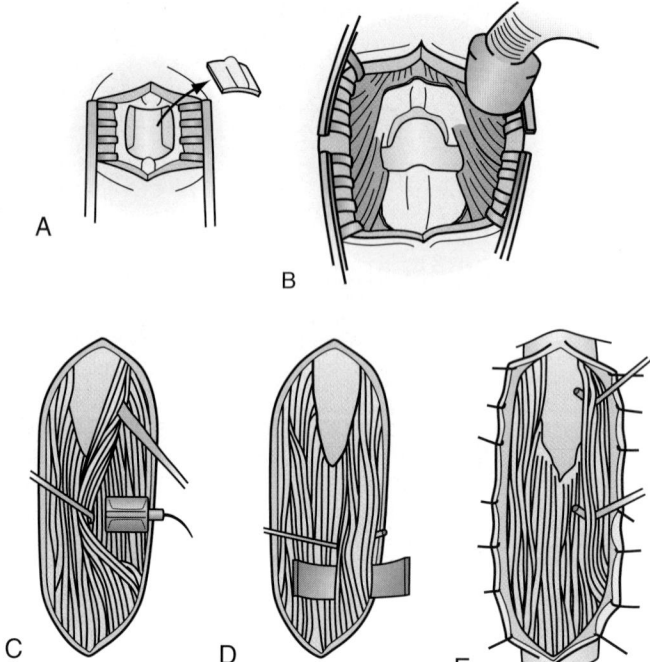

FIGURE 50.3 Selective dorsal rhizotomy: surgical technique. **A,** Single-level laminectomy just below the level of the conus medullaris. **B,** Ultrasound localization of the conus medullaris after laminectomy. **C,** Initial separation of ventral versus dorsal nerve roots. **D,** Placement of Silastic sheet to separate dorsal and ventral roots. **E,** Nerve root stimulation to determine electromyography (EMG) response.

candidates are children older than 2 years of age with spastic diplegia, though some benefit is also seen in patients with spastic quadriplegia. Several randomized trials have demonstrated an advantage of SDR with physical therapy over physical therapy alone in appropriate patients. Ashworth scores may improve by 0.5 to 1.5 with SDR.[73-75] Contraindications to SDR include severe muscle weakness; orthopedic deformity; and increased muscle tone secondary to hydrocephalus, intracranial infection, or traumatic brain injury.[76]

The SDR procedure has been refined over several decades, and requires coordination between neuroanesthesia, neurophysiology, and neurosurgery personnel.[4,76] Once intubated, the patient is placed prone with the bed in a slight Trendelenburg position to reduce CSF loss. Neurophysiological monitoring is established and baseline measurements are taken. The level of the conus medullaris, having been identified on preoperative magnetic resonance imaging (MRI), is identified with interoperative fluoroscopy, typically between T12 and L3. A midline incision is made and a single-level laminectomy is performed (Fig. 50.3). The conus medullaris and cauda equina are usually identified with interoperative ultrasound prior to opening the dura.

Using the operative microscope, the dura is opened and the dorsal and ventral nerve roots are separated by following them back to their origins on the conus medullaris. A silastic sheet is inserted between the dorsal and ventral roots to prevent comingling of the roots during the procedure. First, each dorsal root is stimulated using a curved electromyographic (EMG) stimulation probe at increasing intensity until a reflex response is seen. Each dorsal root is then bluntly subdivided into three to five smaller rootlet fascicles, and the individual EMG reflex threshold of each rootlet is recorded. Once the reflex threshold is known, a tetanic stimulus is applied and the

TABLE 50.2 Grading Scale for EMG Response in Selective Dorsal Rhizotomy

Grade	EMG Response
0	Unsustained or single discharge to a train of stimuli
1	Sustained discharges from muscles innervated through the segment simulated in the ipsilateral lower extremity
2	Sustained discharges from muscles innervated through the stimulated and immediately adjacent segments
3	Sustained discharges from segmentally innervated muscles and muscles innervated through segments distant from the one stimulated
4	Sustained discharges from contralateral muscles with or without sustained discharges from the ipsilateral muscles

EMG, electromyography.
Adapted from Park TS, Johnston JM. Surgical techniques of selective dorsal rhizotomy for spastic cerebral palsy. Technical note. *Neurosurg Focus* 2006;21:e7.

EMG response is graded on a scale from 0 to 4 (Table 50.2).[76] A score of 0 indicates an unsustained or single discharge, and scores of 3 and 4 indicate sustained discharge with segmental spread and discharge from contralateral muscle, respectively.

The rootlets at each spinal level are sectioned according to the following criteria: All rootlets with a 0 response are left intact, all with a 4 response are cut, and a number of rootlets with intermediate responses (grades 2 or 3) are also cut; the total number of rootlets sectioned is approximately 60%. To prevent complete sensory loss, at least one rootlet at each level is left unsectioned regardless of EMG response. The procedure is performed bilaterally on each dorsal root from L2-S2. Some authors section 50% of the L1 dorsal root, regardless of EMG response, to obtain reduced spasticity in the hip flexors.

After sectioning is complete, intradural analgesics may be injected, and a watertight dural closure is performed, followed by a multilayer wound closure to prevent CSF leak. Bed rest is maintained for approximately 72 hours, and may require continuous analgesic infusion in young patients. Once mobilized, intensive physical therapy begins immediately.

Complications of Selective Dorsal Rhizotomy

Complications of SDR include paraplegia, sensory loss, hypesthesia, bowel or bladder incontinence, CSF leak, and infection.[73-75,77,78] The most common complications include self-limiting urinary incontinence (4.4%) and dysesthesia/hypesthesia (8.9%) in the perioperative period. Permanent sensory changes and neurogenic bowel/bladder complications are found in 4% and 5.1% of patients, respectively.[77] Cost-effectiveness studies have shown an advantage of SDR over ITB in patients with spastic diplegia owing to reduced hospital readmissions for pump replacements and complications.[79]

CONCLUSIONS

The management of spasticity is complex, requiring an interdisciplinary team of primary care physicians, neurologists, neurosurgeons, physiatrists, and orthopedic surgeons. Although a variety of oral agents are available, surgical treatment options often become the treatment of choice for patients with moderate to severe spasticity. Baclofen pumps provide known benefit and are cost effective compared to oral medications, but have an appreciable complication rate. Selective dorsal rhizotomy provides proven benefit in patients with spastic diplegia with long-term cost savings over ITB. Future research into new surgical procedures and medications will continue to improve the quality of life of patients affected with this disorder.

SELECTED KEY REFERENCES

Albright AL, Barron WB, Fasick MP, et al. Continuous intrathecal baclofen infusion for spasticity of cerebral origin. *JAMA.* 1993;270:2475-2477.

Albright AL, Turner M, Pattisapu JV. Best-practice surgical techniques for intrathecal baclofen therapy. *J Neurosurg.* 2006;104:233-239.

Gooch JL, Oberg WA, Grams B, et al. Complications of intrathecal baclofen pumps in children. *Pediatr Neurosurg.* 2003;39:1-6.

Park TS, Johnston JM. Surgical techniques of selective dorsal rhizotomy for spastic cerebral palsy. Technical note. *Neurosurg Focus.* 2006;21:e7.

Steinbok P, Daneshvar H, Evans D, Kestle JR. Cost analysis of continuous intrathecal baclofen versus selective functional posterior rhizotomy in the treatment of spastic quadriplegia associated with cerebral palsy. *Pediatr Neurosurg.* 1995;22:255-264:discussion 265.

Please go to expertconsult.com to view the complete list of references.

51 Surgery for Temporal Lobe Epilepsy

Jeffrey G. Ojemann, Carlo Giussani, Carlo Marras

CLINICAL PEARLS

- The most common medically intractable epilepsy appropriate for epilepsy surgery has a temporal lobe origin.

- Mesial temporal lobe epilepsy (MTLE) represents a large percentage of all localization-related epilepsy and has a strong association with an early injury before the age of 4 years. The seizures arise in the hippocampal and parahippocampal areas and in the amygdala. MTLE also presents common diagnostic features including unilateral interictal and ictal electroencephalography (EEG) and magnetic resonance imaging (MRI) features showing sclerosis of the mesial structures, resistance to medical therapy, and responsiveness to selective resection. The pathogenesis of this syndrome represents a special substrate: the so-called mesial temporal sclerosis (MTS).

- Lesional temporal lobe epilepsy may be seen in the presence of many different histopathological entities such as tumors (astrocytoma, dysembryoplastic neuroepithelial tumor, ganglioglioma) (see Fig. 51.1), vascular malformations, and developmental lesions (cortical dysplasia, neuronal heterotopias, and others).

- Cognitive impairment in cases of pharmacoresistant epilepsy of early onset is not uncommon, and is related to different overlapping factors: the electrophysiological abnormalities of continuous seizures on a developing brain, the constant need for anticonvulsant drugs, and the presence of multiple medication regimens.

GENERAL FEATURES

When epilepsy is uncontrolled by traditional anticonvulsant therapy, surgical resection of the epileptogenic region may be performed. The most common uncontrolled epilepsy eligible for epilepsy surgery has temporal lobe origin. In fact, the temporal lobe neocortex and the amygdalohippocampal complex are highly prone to seizure-induced brain injury. The efficacy of temporal lobe resection for the treatment of epilepsy in children was reported over 40 years ago by Davidson and Falconer.[1]

Natural History

The natural history of medically intractable epilepsy has demonstrated the prognosis to be poor,[2] especially as children with temporal lobe epilepsy of early onset can be affected in all areas of cognitive functions and intelligence as well as behavior and psychosocial skills. The cognitive impairment of pharmacoresistant epilepsy of early onset is postulated to be related not only to the continuous seizures and their electrophysiological abnormalities on a developing brain but also to different overlapping factors. These factors include the constant need for anticonvulsant drugs, the presence of multiple medication regimens, and the use of near-toxic doses in case

of status epilepticus, as demonstrated in animals models.[3,4] An onset of uncontrolled seizures under the age of 3 carries the worst prognosis, with a low IQ and motor delays with tonic and myoclonic features and spasms.[5] Other adverse prognostic factors are the presence of daily complex partial seizures, at least five episodes of grand mal, at least one episode of status epilepticus, and a long duration of seizures prior to control.[6]

Classification of Temporal Lobe Epilepsy

The most recent classification of the International League Against Epilepsy reports mesial temporal lobe epilepsy (MTLE) with hippocampal sclerosis as a specific electrophysiological syndrome.[7] MTLE represents a large percentage of all localization-related epilepsy and has a strong association with an early injury before the age of 4 years, particularly febrile seizure, which may be present in 40% of cases. The seizures arise in the hippocampal and parahippocampal areas and in the amygdala. MTLE also presents common diagnostic features including unilateral interictal and ictal electroencephalography (EEG) and magnetic resonance imaging (MRI) features showing sclerosis of the mesial structures, resistance to medical therapy, and responsiveness to selective resection.

The pathogenesis of this syndrome represents a special substrate: the so-called mesial temporal sclerosis (MTS).

The cause of MTS is unclear. An association with a history of febrile seizures has been proposed[8] and it is suggested to be associated with complex features of febrile seizures.[9] However, this connection has been questioned.[10] Instead of being the consequence of recurrent temporal lobe seizures the MTS is frequently associated with a history of unusual febrile seizures in childhood with a later development of complex partial seizures. From a histopathological point of view the mesial structures show a loss of neurons with gliosis in the hippocampus associated with a modification of the normal gray matter architecture. Especially there is an involvement of the Sommer's sector, the end folium, and the CA3 regions.[11] MTS tends to be more common in adults than children but occurs frequently in association with cortical dysplasia in these patients, accounting for the early onset of epilepsy in this group.[12,13] Despite the multitude of clinical and basic science studies on MTS the cause and maintenance mechanisms of epileptogenicity are not fully understood.

Lesional temporal lobe epilepsy may be seen in the presence of many different histopathological entities such as tumors (astrocytoma, dysembryoplastic neuroepithelial tumor, ganglioglioma) (Fig. 51.1), vascular malformations, and developmental lesions (cortical dysplasia, neuronal heterotopias and others). Even in patients with long-lasting histories of seizures when the hippocampus has been resected, the neuronal loss is small (up to 25%) and there is no architectural reorganization (see Fig. 51.1).[14,15]

Seizure Semiology

Temporal lobe seizures may originate in hippocampal and immediately adjacent structures or arise from extrahippocampal neocortical regions. The clinical differentiation of hippocampal and extrahippocampal temporal lobe epilepsy may help guide the extent of resection.[16] The presence of an aura with experiential phenomena, such as a feeling of depersonalization or familiarity, or visual or auditory illusions is associated with a neocortical temporal ictal origin. In 70% of cases the epigastric aura occurs in the setting of mesial temporal lobe epilepsy; however, this rate significantly increases (98% of cases) if the abdominal aura evolves into an automotor seizure.[17] Fearful and olfactory auras are commonly associated with involvement of the amygdala, whereas gustatory auras may occur in the hippocampal region or arise from extrahippocampal neocortical regions.[18] The "déjà vu" onset needs a concomitant activation of hippocampus and temporal neocortex and it is not specific for the activation of hippocampus or neocortex.

Usually the ictal behavior shows different patterns including behavioral arrest and motionless staring that are described as typical symptoms of mesial temporal origin. Oral automatisms (chewing, lip smacking, tongue protruding, and lip pursing) and manual automatisms (manual exploratory behavior, grabbing, and rubbing) are both associated with temporal lobe epilepsy (TLE).[19] The early onset of automatisms is frequently associated with a primary involvement of the mesial temporal lobe; moreover, the association of ipsilateral hand automatism with simultaneous contralateral dystonic posturing allows a correct lateralization. Contralateral head rotation just before seizures and secondarily generalized and unilateral tonic and dystonic posturing can be of value in localization, but they

are not always accurate.[20] A variety of autonomic symptoms, including elevated blood pressure, tachycardia, skin pallor, pilomotor erection, and mydriasis, have been reported in the course of MTLE seizures.[21] Ictal speech and postictal dysphasia has been demonstrated to be consistent with seizure onset in the dominant hemisphere; in addition, active testing of postictal reading ability indicated a seizure focus in the language-dominant hemisphere. It has been reported that early postictal nose wiping is a reliable lateralizing sign pointing to the ipsilateral hemisphere.[22]

Temporal lobe seizures are more likely to occur during wakefulness, whereas frontal lobe seizures have a greater chance of occurring during sleep, implying that sleep has distinct effects on seizure threshold in different brain regions.[23] Furthermore, sleep can influence the extent of seizure spread, such that seizures in temporal lobe epilepsy are more likely to secondarily generalize during sleep than during wakefulness.[24,25]

EVALUATION FOR SURGERY

Presence of mesial temporal lobe sclerosis resistant to pharmacotherapy is the most common indication for surgery in adults, accounting for 75% in adult surgical series.[26,27] The major indication for TLE surgery in children is a lateral neocortical alteration, frequently cortical dysplasia alone, or eventually in combination with MTS and lesion-related TLE, especially gangliogliomas and dysembryoplastic neuroepithelial tumors (DNET).

The correlation between electroclinical data and hippocampal sclerosis in MTLE has been known for over half a century.[8,28-30] To examine the evidence base for surgery for uncontrolled seizures, the Quality Standards Subcommittee of the AAN (American Academy of Neurology) performed a systematic review of the efficacy and safety of anterior temporal lobe resections.[31] Based on one randomized trial and observational studies, they found that anterior temporal lobe resection reduced the occurrence of disabling seizures and improved patients' quality of life. Furthermore, they speculated that the "greater potential for achieving freedom from disabling seizures offered by surgical treatment, as opposed to continuing pharmacotherapy, may reduce the risks of long-term mortality." Moreover, pharmacoresistant epilepsy has been associated with decreased survival,[32,33] and in the appropriate candidate, temporal lobectomy has actuarial benefit on life expectancy.[34]

Noninvasive Evaluation

The semiology, interictal and ictal scalp video-EEG, and imaging (anatomical, metabolic, and functional) as well as neurocognitive evaluation, represent the armamentarium of evaluation for surgical candidacy in the patient with pharmacoresistant epilepsy. Most evaluations would include interictal scalp recordings and inpatient video-EEG to capture typical seizures. However, the best outcomes are found in patients with concordant MRI and interictal scalp EEG concordant for unilateral MTLE.[35] In fact, lack of concordance with interictal EEG and other studies is a worse predictor of surgical outcome than ictal disconcordance. However, in all but the most

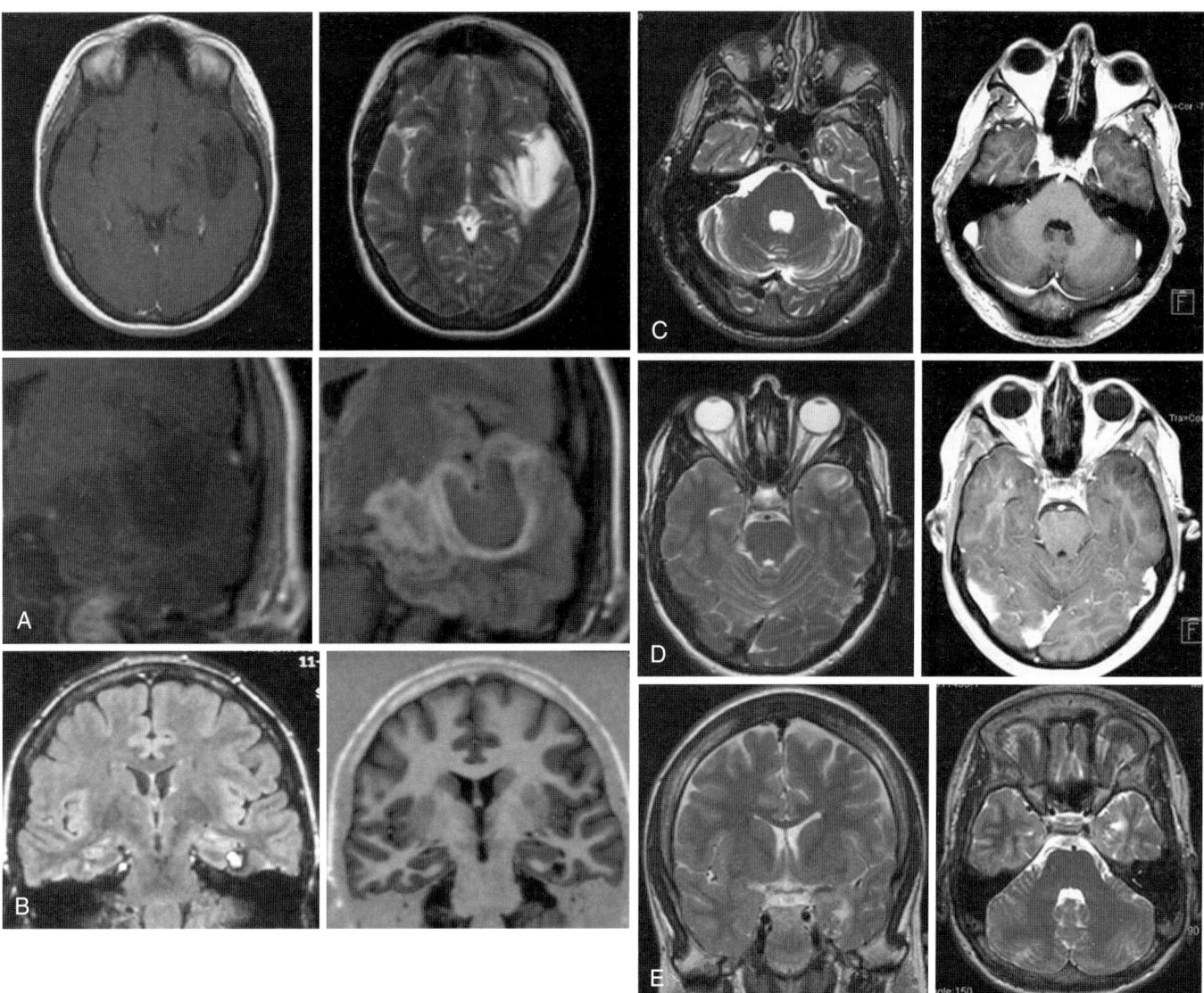

FIGURE 51.1 Magnetic resonance imaging (MRI) of lesional temporal lobe epilepsy cases. **A,** MRI of a 24-year-old woman who had seizures since the age of 14 years. Seizures were characterized by bilateral auditory illusions, loss of consciousness, oral automatisms, skin pallor, left mydriasis, and tonic posture of the right upper limb. Duration was typically about 2 minutes, followed by postictal anomia. Frequency was one seizure a week. MRI showed an anterior left temporal lesion (*top left:* axial T1-weighted with gadolinium image; *below left:* coronal T1-weighted with gadolinium image; *top right:* axial T2-weighted image; *below right:* coronal fluid-attenuated inversion recovery [FLAIR] image) extended to the insula and mesencephalon. Interictal and ictal activity was left temporal. The patient underwent anterior temporal lobectomy including the lesion and the mesial structures (uncus, amygdala, and hippocampus). She is seizure-free 30 months after surgery. Pathological examination revealed a dysembryoplastic neuroepithelial tumor (DNET). **B,** A 41-year-old man with seizures since the age of 36 developed drug-resistant epilepsy symptomatic of left temporal cavernoma (*left:* coronal FLAIR image; *right:* coronal inversion recovery [IR] image). Seizures were always the same and consisted of epigastric aura, loss of contact, oral automatisms, and dystonic postures of the right hand. Patient underwent lesionectomy, and 4 years afterward continues to have seizures (Engel IIc). **C,** MRI of 39-year-old man who developed seizures at the age of 19 years after head injury. Seizure semiology never changed; the patient had left blinking and motionless staring, appearing as if petrified. After seizure onset he was never seizure-free. Video-electroencephalography (EEG) and stereo EEG showed interictal and ictal acitvity involving the anterior temporal lobe. MRI showed an anterior and mesial lesion of the left temporal lobe (*left:* axial T2-weighted image; *right:* axial T1-weighted image with gadolinium). The patient submitted to an anterior temporal lobectomy including the lesion, the uncus, and the amygdala. Three years after surgery the patient is seizure-free. The pathological examination showed a fibrillary astrocytoma (WHO [World Health Organization] grade II). **D,** A 26-year-old woman developed nocturnal generalized tonic-clonic seizures at the age of 14 years with monthly frequency. The MRI scan showed an anterior left temporal lobe lesion (*left:* axial T2-weighted image; *right:* axial T1-weighted image with gadolinium). The video-EEG during sleep showed two seizures characterized left version, dystonic posture of the right hand, and delayed automatisms. The ictal EEG showed a fast activity of low amplitude on the left anterior temporal lobe, spreading to the posterior temporal lobe and then to the ipsilateral suprasylvian region. The patient underwent a left anterior temporal lobectomy including the lesion, the uncus, and the amygdala. Pathological examination revealed an oligodendroglioma (grade II WHO). Forty months after surgery the patient is seizure-free. **E,** MRI of a 19-year-old woman with seizure characterized by epigastric aura, behavioral arrest, right version of the head and eyes, pallor, and oral automatisms. Sometimes the patient had secondary generalized tonic-clonic seizure. Seizures began at age 9. Duration of attack was about 30 seconds with a daily frequency (3-4 episodes). MRI scans (*left:* coronal T2-weighted image; *right:* axial T2-weighted image) showed a left mesial temporal lesion, with calcification, involving the parahippocampus, gyrus, and uncus. The patient underwent a left anterior temporal lobectomy including the lesion, the uncus, the amygdala, the head, and the anterior third of the hippocampus body. For 2 years the patient has been seizure-free. *(Courtesy of Dr. Roberto Spreafico and Dr. Flavio Villani, Division of Epilettologia Clinica e Neurofisiologia sperimentale, Fondazione Istituto Neurologico Carlo Besta, Milan, Italy.)*

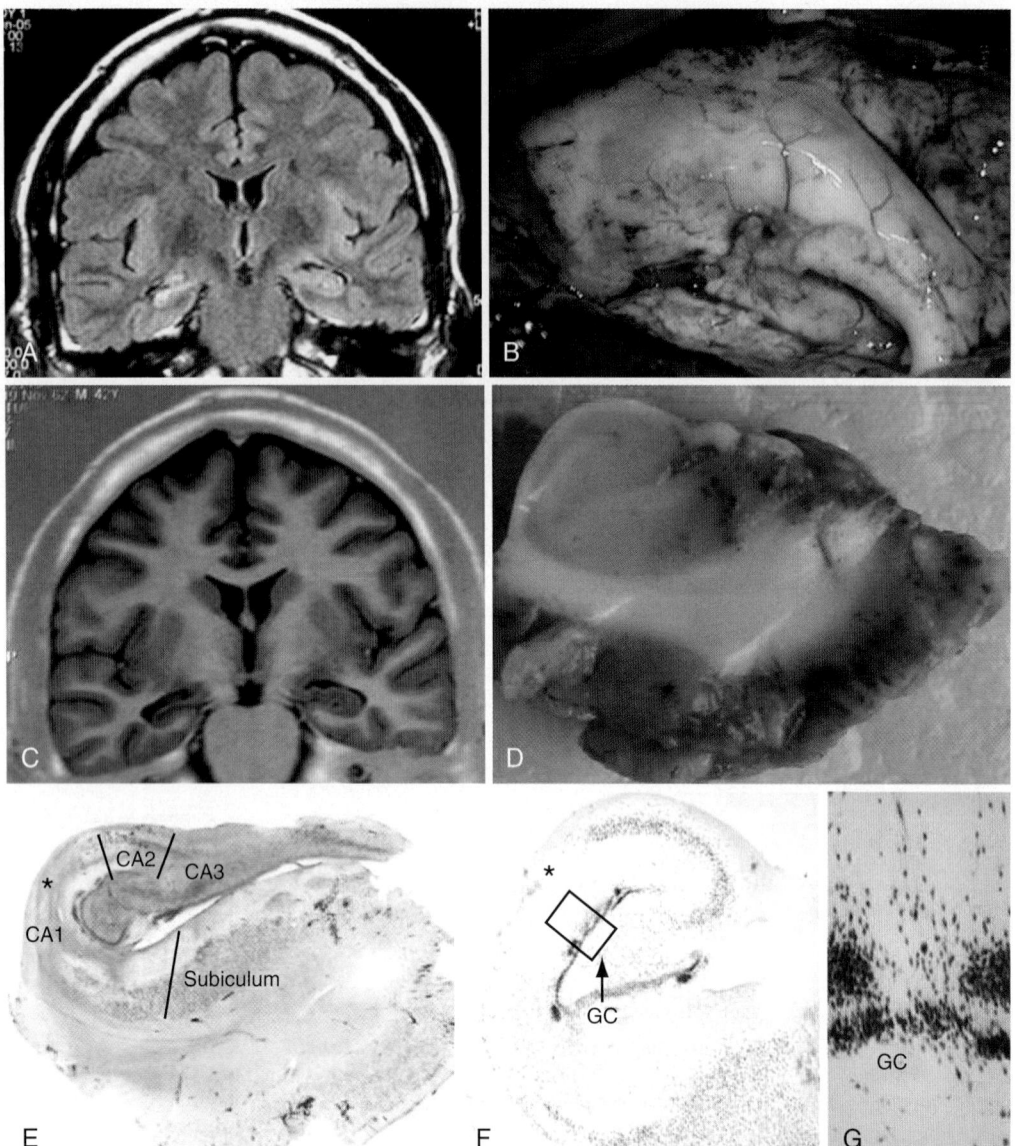

FIGURE 51.2 Right hippocampus sclerosis. Magnetic resonance imaging (MRI) coronal fluid-attenuated inversion recovery (FLAIR) image (**A**) showed a hyperintensity of the right hippocampus that also appeared smaller than on the contralateral side. Intraoperative picture (**B**) showing the head and the anterior third of the right hippocampus. At the MRI coronal inverson recovery (IR) image (**C**) the right hippocampus appeared small with an enlargement of the temporal horn. Sections of the hippocampus, shown in **D**, stained, respectively, with thionin (**E**) for cytoarchitectonic control, and with anti-NeuN (**F** and **G**) to detect neuronal nuclei (NeuN). Note the evident neuronal cell loss in the pyramidal cell layer of CA1 (indicated by asterisks in E and F) visible both in thionin- and NeuN-stained sections. The granule cell layer (GC) appears bilaminated, and dispersed (*arrow* in F), and significant loss of granule cells can be observed in the higher magnification (G). *(Courtesy of Dr. Roberto Spreafico and Dr. Flavio Villani, Division of Epilettologia Clinica e Neurofisiologia sperimentale, Fondazione Istituto Neurologico Carlo Besta, Milan, Italy.)*

straightforward of cases, several typical clinical spells are usually of value to be recorded by inpatient EEG.

Imaging of MTLE by MRI has made the diagnosis of hippocampal sclerosis much more straightforward, in addition to a variety of evolving imaging tools.[36] Fine-cut coronal sequences perpendicular to the axis of the hippocampus are particularly useful. Coronal fluid-attenuated inversion recovery (FLAIR) sequences suppress the cerebrospinal fluid signal and enhance the increased tissue free-water signal characteristic of mesial temporal sclerosis. Volumetric hippocampal MRI studies through serial thin-cut coronal images permit a comparison of the volumes of both hippocampi, unmasking

eventual differences in volume between the normal and the affected mesial structure (Fig. 51.2A and B).[37] Recent advances in high-field MRI have been particularly helpful in identifying subtle abnormalities in hippocampal or neighboring mesial temporal structures.[38,39]

Magnetic resonance spectroscopy (MRS) can also detect abnormalities in various metabolites using the proton signal.[40,41] Nuclear medicine studies are also employed, primarily interictal positron emission tomography (PET) and ictal/interictal single-photon emission computed tomography (SPECT). Fluorodeoxyglucose (FDG) PET looks for interical hypometabolism. It can be helpful in identifying surgical candidates in the setting of normal MRI scans, and also may detect those with bilateral disease with poorer outlook for seizure freedom.[42] However, the area of hypometabolism demonstrated by FDG PET often shows greater extent than foci demonstrated by EEG or MRI. Although PET is a sensitive diagnostic method, it provides only approximate localization of the epileptic zone and may not be adequate for precise localization, though it may be useful for differentiating between TLE of mesial or lateral origin.[43]

SPECT studies require injection very soon after seizure onset for maximal accuracy. The use of SPECT image registration to subtract an ictal from interictal injection, when coregistered with the anatomical MRI, can result in useful ictal localization information, even with a normal MRI scan.[44]

Invasive Evaluation

When noninvasive methods do not indicate the seizure focus, invasive diagnostic recordings can be used. When bilateral MTLE is of concern, bitemporal electrodes can be used. The two strategies most often employed are depth electrodes that penetrate the brain structures, or subdural electrodes that are passed subtemporally and medially toward mesial structures. Though these methods are typically used on a less favorable group of patients, good outcomes can be achieved in this subset and are generally well tolerated.[45] Invasive monitoring indications and interpretation can be more challenging in the pediatric population because of the frequent temporal and extratemporal neocortex involvement.[46]

Neuropsychology

A thorough neuropsychological evaluation is part of the presurgical assessment for medically intractable seizures.[47] Neuropsychological testing can help lateralize the seizure focus[48,49] because dominant temporal lobe epilepsy is typically associated with verbal memory deficits as a predominant factor. Excessive speech difficulties, global memory problems, or extensive difficulties in other domains should raise concerns as to the localization of medial temporal lobe epilepsy.

Neuropsychological testing is also critical to assess for the emotional, behavioral, and psychiatric disorders that are very common in this population.[50] Depression in particular can be quite significant, and many preoperative factors and expectations can impact surgical decision making, perceived benefit from surgery, and quality of life outcomes.[51]

Testing is also important to establish language dominance and define memory risks preoperatively. The cerebral amytal test has long been used to determine dominance and assess the effect on memory of anesthetizing one hemisphere through intracarotid injection.[52] The test is invasive and there is variability in its use. Because right-handed patients with right-sided lesions have a very small chance of being dominant,[53] some of these patients, for example, may not require extensive study of dominance through intracarotid amytal testing. Functional MRI can make assessment of dominance and memory, but the exact tests and their reliability are still a subject of debate.[54] The precise language test to be used in functional MRI is unknown, but some batteries have been quite successful in establishing dominance.[55,56] Memory in particular is difficult to assess by either method.[57]

SURGICAL TECHNIQUES

Different surgical techniques have been proposed over the years for the treatment of TLE. From a purely technical point of view the differences between the surgical techniques are primarily related to the extent of the lateral resection and to the anatomical approaches to the mesial temporal structures. Approaches that are tailored to the specific pre- or intraoperative electrophysiology are also a reasonable option.

The "classic" or "standard" anterior temporal lobectomy includes resection of anterior neocortex and the mesial temporal structures. This technique is used historically in case of MTS, and also addresses seizures of lateral neocortical origin (in those cases when mesial structures are to be included in the resection). The resection would typically involve the anterior 4 cm of dominant, and 6 cm of nondominant temporal lobe.[58]

Smaller lateral resections are typically used; most techniques begin with a resection of the anterior T2 and T3 gyri with the subpial resection taken deep, with care not to drift posteriorly or superiorly, until the lateral aspects of the temporal horn is unroofed. After the unroofing of the temporal horn, the amygdala and the head of the hippocampus and its tail are resected anteroposteriorly, sparing the mesial arachnoid as a barrier that helps avoid damage to the branches of the choroidal and the posterior cerebral artery (PCA), as well as the third cranial nerve and the brainstem. The extent of hippocampal resection is not proscribed, but typically goes back to at least the posterior brainstem.

A variant of this approach involves alternative entries to the ventricle, including a stereotactic entry through the middle temporal gyrus to the ventricle, subtemporal entry through the basal temporal lobe, and the sylvian fissure approach that requires entry of the hippocampal structures medially. Selective approaches may have advantages in cognitive outcome over the larger "standard" approaches.[59]

The selective amygdalohippocampectomy has been advocated by Yasargil and associates for nonlesional temporal lobe epilepsy and for MTS without lateral neocortex contribution.[60,61] The amygdalohippocampal complex is resected, avoiding passage through the lateral neocortex by a transsylvian arachnoid splitting approach. Specifically, the surgeon exposes the middle cerebral artery branches by splitting the sylvian fissure arachnoid and identifies the limen insulae. The ventricle is entered through the superior aspect of the temporal stem that is mesial to the superior temporal gyrus and posterior to the limen insulae, by a transcortical approach. A longitudinal corticectomy is made in the depth of the first temporal sulcus reaching the lateral aspects of the temporal horn. Alternatively, a subtemporal approach is performed reaching the inferolateral aspects of the temporal horn through a small corticectomy in the depth of the collateral sulcus between the third and the fourth temporal gyri.[62,63]

None of these techniques is truly selective owing to the fact that each of them violates the gray matter of the lateral/ventral temporal lobe cortex or the white matter fibers of the temporal stem as the fasciculus uncinatus that harbor important associative functions. However, the subtemporal amygdalohippocampectomy has a direct trajectory through the collateral sulcus to the temporal horn. As an alternative strategy, the degree of resection can be guided by patient-specific factors, including intraoperative interictal electrocorticography (ECoG). Intraoperative ECoG permits the surgeon to map the electrical abnormalities. The language is mapped in the dominant hemisphere of an awake patient by direct electrocortical stimulation administering language tasks to the patient during surgery. The hippocampus is resected on the basis of the intraoperative ECoG findings by the use of a strip electrode that is introduced in the temporal horn and slides posteriorly. The extent of the posterior margin of resection of the hippocampus tail can be guided based on the intraoperative ECoG.[64,65] Resection of the lateral temporal lobe on the dominant side can also be tailored to the subject's own language anatomy[66] in attempts to minimize cognitive deficits. Comparisons of "selective" anatomical studies have not been directly compared to the tailored methods in epilepsy outcome studies.

Radiosurgery

Despite this high success rate of resective epilepsy surgery, novel surgical therapies for MTLE are being evaluated,[64] and radiosurgery poses an attractive alternative in this respect. The use of radiosurgery to successfully treat various types of epilepsy as arteriovenous malformation or cavernomas related to epilepsy has been reported.[67,68]

A multicenter study on the use of radiosurgery for the treatment of MTLE has shown promising initial results with 85% of patients who received 24 Gy to the 50% isodose line becoming seizure-free.[69] Moreover the data coming from the Marseilles group is encouraging in terms of neuropsychological improvements and outcome. From the authors' perspective the long-term safety and efficacy of radiosurgery for MTLE is comparable to surgical resection, but radiosurgery has the advantage of sparing verbal memory in patients treated by Gamma Knife (GK) on the dominant side.[70]

However, other authors have reported less positive outcomes in the treatment of MTLE with radiosurgery. In these papers radiosurgery did not lead consistently to seizure control and sometimes led to transient seizure worsening associated with the risk of brain edema and intracranial hypertension.[71-73] All the authors agree with the strategy of surgery resection of the amygdalohippocampus complex in patients who demonstrate radiosurgery treatment failure.

Deep Brain Stimulation and Neuromodulation

Patients with complex partial seizures arising from the hippocampus who undergo resective surgery of the epileptic focus have a good outcome. Nevertheless, there are a number of candidates in whom it is not advisable to perform temporal lobectomy or hippocampectomy because of the risk of memory deficit,[74] or even severe amnesia.[75] This appears to be more likely to occur in patients with bilateral hippocampal surgery.[76] Therefore, patients with bilateral mesial temporal epilepsy are either excluded from resective procedures, or surgery is performed after extensive counseling in which the risks include incomplete epileptic foci resections and residual seizures. Consequently, there is a current need to develop nonresective alternative therapies. Neuromodulation has been proposed in these patients. Several neuroanatomical targets have been suggested and stimulated, including the centromedian thalamic nucleus,[77] vagal nerve,[78] and a variety of cerebellar targets.[79]

All these targets have improved secondary seizure generalization, but have shown inconsistent results regarding complex partial seizures. The neuromodulation of the hippocampal epileptic foci has been proposed by Velasco and co-workers. In surgical series of patients with bilateral mesial temporal epilepsy and normal MRI, the chronic stimulation of bilateral or unilateral hippocampus at long-term follow-up has demonstrated a seizure reduction of between 95% and 50%. No patient had neuropsychological deterioration, nor did any patient show side effects.[80] Similar results were collected by Boon and co-workers, who reported a series of 12 patients requiring invasive monitoring to exclude bitemporal epilepsy. After a follow-up of more than 12 months, 9 out of 10 patients receiving stimulation of both hippocampi had a seizure frequency reduction higher than 50%, and 1 patient was seizure-free.[81]

RESULTS

Postoperative Outcome

After temporal lobe resection, usually including uncus, amygdala, sclerotic hippocampus, and the lateral temporal lobe, 48% to 84% of patients are seizure-free (Table 51.1). The short-term (<5 years) rate of seizure-free patients is around 70%.[31,51,82,83]

Positive predictive factors for seizure-free outcome after temporal lobe resection include preoperative hippocampal sclerosis (unilateral), focal localization of interictal epileptiform discharges, absence of preoperative generalized seizures, tumor etiology, and complete resection of the lesion with or without medial structures.[84-86]

Younger age at surgery or at onset of epilepsy and absence of seizures in the first postoperative week often predict good seizure outcome after temporal lobe resection.[87,88] Long-term follow-up (>5 years) studies show that 41% to 79% of patients remain seizure-free after temporal lobe resection[89-92] and that 15% to 20% of patients have relapses after initial seizure freedom at 5 to 10 years after surgery. Although potential explanations for this phenomenon, such as contralateral mesial temporal pathology or dual pathology, have been suggested, the only uniform predictor for late relapse is failure to enter remission immediately after surgery.[93,94]

TABLE 51.1 Evidence-Based Medicine Evidence Class for Preoperative Features, Postoperative Factors, and Surgical Techniques as Predictors of Seizure-Free Outcome in Drug-Resistant Temporal Lobe Epilepsy

Evidence Factor	Class
Febrile seizure	IIb
Effectiveness of surgery versus medication	Ia
Effectiveness of temporal lobectomy versus selective amygdalohippocampectomy	IIIa
MTLE versus MTLE with neocortical dysplasia	IIIa
Postoperative result after 6 months	IIb

MTLE, mesial temporal lobe epilepsy.

Longitudinal studies of patients with anterior temporal lobe resections have shown that the seizure status at 1 year after surgery does not remain stable over subsequent follow-up. Some studies provide long-term data of seizure control (up to 10 years) status after anterior temporal lobe resection.[95-99] Among patients seizure-free at the end of year 1 following surgery, the annual probability of seizure relapse between years 1 and 5 is 5.6%, and beyond year 5 the probability is 4.2%.[97-99] In contrast, Kelley and Theodore found that the likelihood of further relapse for patients seizure-free at year 10 was 0%.[97] Among patients with persistent seizures at the end of year 1 after surgery, the annual probability of becoming seizure-free between years 1 and 5 is only 5.9% and the probability of becoming seizure-free after year 5 is a mere 2.0%.[95,97] So far Choi and colleagues, applying the same relative risk reduction used by other authors, predicted that the probability for seizure-free outcome falls to 1.6% beyond year 5.[34]

Factors that predict good seizure outcome include presence of a discrete lesion on MRI, complete resection of the lesion, localized scalp EEG ictal onset, concordant hypometabolism on FDG-PET, longer duration of epilepsy, and lack of febrile seizures.[26,31,100]

Some studies include both adult and pediatric patients and a mixture of seizure etiology, to include mesial temporal sclerosis (dual pathology). In recent surgical series, 1% to 11% of patients had reoperation for surgical failure, which is most common after neocortical resections. Causes of surgical failures include incomplete resection of lesions, erroneous identification of epileptogenic regions, generation of new epileptogenic zones, and limited resections due to the risk of functional impairment. Surgical resections are usually done in the same region as the previous surgery. After reoperation, 39% to 57% of patients are seizure-free. Siegel and colleagues[100] found that a duration of epilepsy of 5 years or less and preoperative focal interictal epileptiform discharges predicted good outcome.

Complications, Cognitive, and Psychosocial Outcomes

Any surgical procedure, including temporal lobectomy, carries both general surgical and specific inherent risks. Although the overall risk of morbidity is quite low, there are significant complications associated with this operation.[101] Reported complications include infection, cerebrospinal fluid leak, and damage to the perforating arteries that can lead to hemiparesis, hemianopia, sensory loss, and aphasia on the dominant side.

Varying degrees of deficits have to be expected in mesial temporal lobe surgery. Visual field deficits from damage to Meyer's loop can be present even in selective approaches.[102] Advances in the application of techniques of MRI tractography may help reduce this risk;[103] however, the vulnerable location of these visual field fibers is an anatomical reality.

Cognitive deficits can be found after basal temporal resection. Memory deficits can be potentially seen in the presurgical setting, and these can worsen postoperatively, especially in the setting of normal MRI and better presurgical memory.[104] Word-finding deficits, especially of specific items such as faces and landmarks, are common after dominant TLE. Recognition deficits can also follow lobectomy for nondominant TLE.[105] Favorable neuropsychological and social outcomes are seen in temporal lobectomy, especially when seizure freedom is achieved.[101]

FUTURE PERSPECTIVES

The surgical treatment of temporal lobe epilepsy is frequently performed when psychological and social rehabilitation for intractable epilepsy is unlikely. New insights into the role of MTLE in humans and in animal models have unravelled specific events related to seizures.[106] Recent pathophysiology and technology advances contributed to our understanding of mesial temporal lobe epilepsy and promoted early identification of surgically remediable epilepsy as soon as the seizure disorder becomes progressive and pharmacoresistant.

The high-frequency (250-500 Hz) interictal epileptiform EEG activity is recorded in the hippocampus of patients with mesial temporal lobe or neocortical epilepsy. This EEG abnormality, named *fast ripples*, could identify the epileptogenic region, and even predict the development of epilepsy.[107-109] So far the possibility to record fast ripples by magnetoencephalography or by specific spike-associated blood flow patterns of scalp EEG coupled with functional MRI could be practically useful to define the epileptogenesis noninvasively.[110]

Neuroimaging studies offer an interesting perspective in the presurgical stage. MRI mapping of structural patterns of the hippocampi could predict the development of epilepsy after prolonged febrile seizures in children with hippocampal abnormalities, and may predict disease progression and pharmacoresistance.[111,112] Moreover, there is evidence that α-methyltryptophan (AMT) uptake is identified with the epileptogenic tuber in patients with tuberous sclerosis, and in other forms of epilepsy.[113,114] Other radionuclide tracers, such as flumazenil PET, may also provide additional information on localization for temporal lobe epilepsy ^{11}C-flumazenil PET in temporal lobe epilepsy with unilateral and bilateral hippocampal sclerosis.[115] Finally, magnetic resonance spectroscopy studies allow the detection of neuroprogenitor cells and is able to measure neurogenesis in vivo in mesial temporal lobe epilepsy with hippocampal sclerosis.[116]

It is possible that advances of transcranial magnetic stimulation (TMS), particularly with the development of TMS-EEG,[117] will identify changes associated with epileptogenesis in neocortical areas accessible to this technique.

CONCLUSION

Temporal lobectomy is a highly effective treatment for epilepsy in the appropriate population. Advances in diagnosis through novel radiological/anatomical and physiological techniques may expand the population who may benefit from surgical treatment strategies. The only caveat is that outcomes as favorable as those seen in mesial temporal sclerosis with concordant electrophysiology are not to be expected. Cognitive, neuropsychological, and social outcomes are not perfect, and the ideal surgical approaches to mitigate the deleterious effects of epilepsy surgery are still evolving.

ACKNOWLEDGMENT

For their constant help in the development of the knowledge about epilepsy we thank the Associazione per le Neuroscienze Paolo Zorzi, Milan, Italy.

SELECTED KEY REFERENCES

Berg AT, Berkovic SF, Brodie JM, et al. Revised terminology and concepts for organization of seizures and epilepsies: report of the ILAE Commission on Classification and Terminology, 2005-2009. *Epilepsia*. 2010;51(4):676-685:(Epub 2010 Feb 26).

Bien CG, Kurthern M, Baron K, et al. Long-term seizure outcome and antiepileptic drug treatment in surgically treated temporal lobe epilepsy patients: a controlled study. *Epilepsia*. 2001;42:1416-1421.

González-Martínez JA, Srikijvilaikul T, Nair D, Bingaman WE. Long-term seizure outcome in reoperation after failure of epilepsy surgery. *Neurosurgery*. 2007;60:873-880.

Marks Jr WJ, Laxer KD. Semiology of temporal lobe seizures: value in lateralizing the seizure focus. *Epilepsia*. 1998;39:721-772.

Schramm J. Temporal lobe epilepsy and the quest for optimal extent of resection: a review. *Epilepsia*. 2008;49:1296-1307.

Uijl SG, Leijten FS, Arends JB, et al. Decision-making in temporal lobe epilepsy surgery: the contribution of basic non-invasive tests. *Seizure*. 2008;17:364-373.

Wiebe S, Blume WT, Girvin JP, et al. For the effectiveness and efficiency of Surgery for Temporal Lobe Epilepsy Study Group. A randomized controlled trial of surgery for temporal lobe epilepsy. *N Engl J Med*. 2001;345:311-318.

Please go to expertconsult.com to view the complete list of references.

CHAPTER 52

Extratemporal Procedures and Hemispherectomy for Epilepsy

Gwyneth Hughes, William Bingaman

CLINICAL PEARLS

- Intractable disabling epilepsy, a localizable epileptogenic zone, and a low risk of postoperative deficits are considered the three basic tenets that must be met before a patient can be considered a candidate for epilepsy surgery.

- One should apply surgical technique for extratemporal resections to match the underlying cause.

- Patients with hemimegalencephaly and intractable seizure disorder benefit from more tissue resection, and anatomical hemispherectomy is an excellent choice.

- Patients with encephalomalacia and large ventricles benefit from less tissue removal, and hemispherotomy is an excellent choice.

- Frontal lobe resections convey the lowest chance for successful postoperative results. Patients with a circumscribed lesion on preoperative magnetic resonance imaging (MRI) fared significantly better. Posterior cortex epilepsy resections convey a slightly higher chance of favorable outcome.

Epilepsy represents a broad spectrum of disease processes sharing the common characteristic of unwanted synchronous electrical activity. The majority of patients with epilepsy will be successfully managed with anticonvulsant therapy. The remainder is left searching for alternative treatment strategies, often leading to an evaluation for a potential surgical management option.

Wilder Penfield performed the first temporal lobe resection for epilepsy in 1936. Mesial temporal sclerosis has since become the most common indication for epilepsy surgery in adult patients. As a result, Penfield's temporal lobectomy, or a variation thereof, has become the flagship procedure of epilepsy surgery in adults and is the only procedure for which class I medical evidence demonstrates a favorable outcome after surgery compared with medical management.[1] However, a significant number of epilepsy patients do not have underlying temporal disease, but rather an epileptogenic zone extending into the regions outside the temporal lobe. These so-called extratemporal lobe epilepsy (ETLE) patients present unique management challenges. As the characteristics of ETLE have become better understood, the distinctive management challenges have become better defined. The result has been the development of new concepts of epileptogenesis, new diagnostic technologies, and from a neurosurgical perspective, the development and refinement of surgical techniques.

UNIQUE CHALLENGES IN EXTRATEMPORAL LOBE EPILEPSY

ETLE refers to epilepsy arising outside the temporal lobe and may result from a variety of causes including neoplasms, vascular malformations, malformations of cortical development, and encephalomalacias related to prior ischemic or traumatic events (Fig. 52.1). In addition to a variety of causes, the epilepsy may arise in the frontal, parietal, or occipital lobes and rapidly spread to involve large regions of cortex. These unique factors result in a broad spectrum of imaging findings, complex seizure semiology, and potentially diffuse electroencephalography (EEG) data.

Seizure semiology in ETLE may be complex depending on the site of seizure origin. The nature of ETLE lends itself to areas of ictal onset that may not necessarily result in clinical manifestations until the symptomatogenic zone becomes activated. With extratemporal areas of ictal onset, the location that is suggested by semiology has a greater propensity to be a result of secondary spread, resulting in potential diagnostic confusion. Similarly, EEG data may be particularly difficult to interpret because of rapid spread and artifact from muscle movement during the seizure. Deep cortical areas such as the interhemispheric and insular regions are particularly difficult to record epileptic activity from on-scalp EEG. Patients whose seizures start in these areas can present a particular challenge,

773

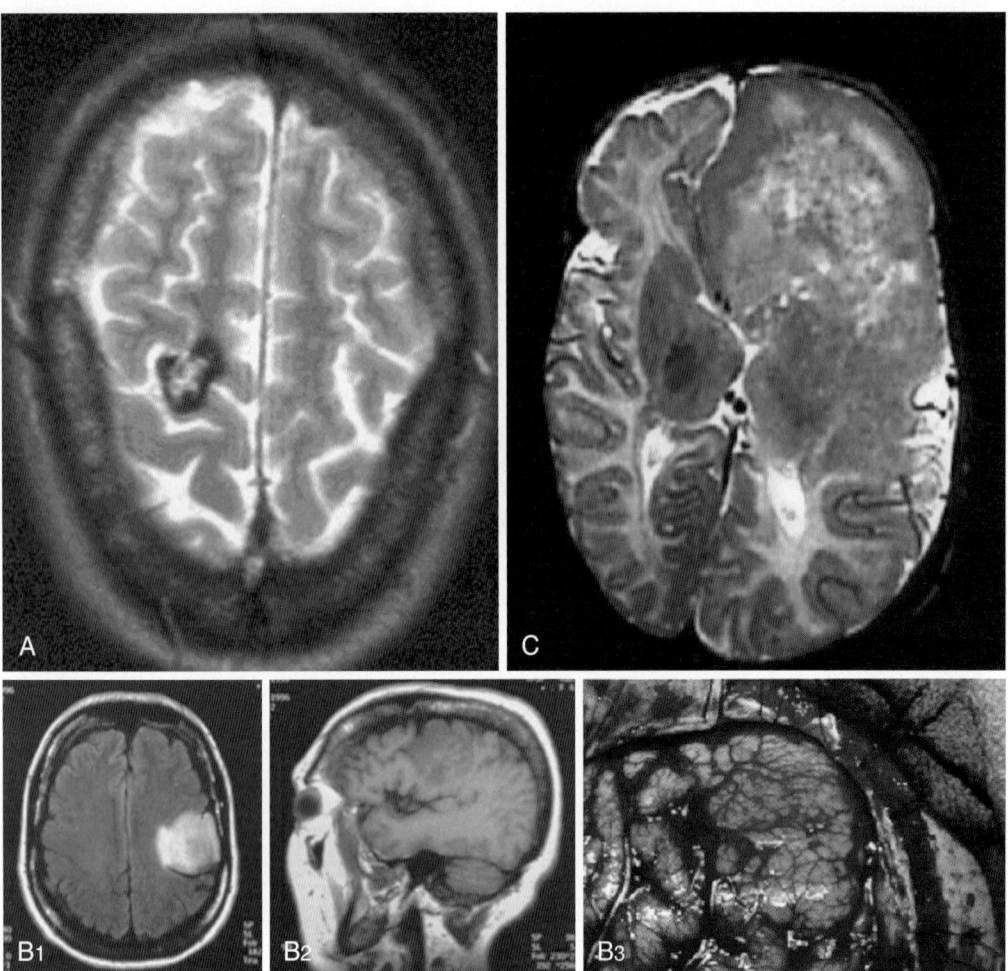

FIGURE 52.1 **A,** T2-weighted magnetic resonance imaging (MRI) scan demonstrating right frontal cavernous angioma. **B,** Preoperative MRI and intraoperative photo of left perirolandic oligodendroglioma. **C,** T2-weighted MRI of left hemimegalencephaly.

as electrical seizure activity may be absent on standard EEG arrays, or it may falsely localize as originating in another area entirely.

Magnetic resonance imaging (MRI) findings in ETLE are generally broken down into nonlesional and lesional categories. The goal of MRI evaluation is to identify and characterize any potentially epileptogenic lesion(s). For those patients without MRI lesions, defining a potential area for surgical resection is inherently more challenging, often necessitating the use of adjuvant investigative techniques. Although the radiographic presence of a lesion may prognosticate a better outcome after surgery, more information is usually necessary prior to surgical removal. The lesion's location and its relationship to functional cortex must be defined in a hypothesis that agrees with the semiology and EEG data.

SURGICAL INDICATIONS

Intractable disabling epilepsy, a localizable epileptogenic zone (defined as the area of tissue that must be removed to prevent further seizures), and a low risk of postoperative deficits are considered the three basic tenets that must be met before a patient can be considered a candidate for epilepsy surgery.[2] It is important to recognize that medical intractability makes a patient a candidate for further investigation regarding the appropriateness to undergo surgery for epilepsy, but it does not guarantee that surgical management should ultimately be offered. Although no clear definition of medical intractability exists, recent reports in the literature suggest that successful treatment with anticonvulsant therapy is unlikely once two different medicines fail to control seizures.[3] The optimal surgical patient will be highly motivated with a social support system in place, and additional coexisting psychiatric illness will be well controlled. Neurocognitive risks must be assessed and discussed with each patient, and risks should be deemed acceptable from both the perspective of the patient and the treatment team. A high probability of improving a patient's overall quality of life must be confirmed before undertaking the procedure.[4]

Preoperative Evaluation

The starting point for any patient evaluation should include a detailed history and physical examination, with special focus on seizure semiology. Lateralizing and localizing signs, such as ictal eye movements, motor or sensory features, presence or absence of ictal speech, and the presence or absence of aura, should be noted. Video-electroencephalography (VEEG) data allow correlation of a patient's behavior during a seizure with the changes recorded on scalp EEG. It allows for confirmation of the epilepsy and may provide helpful lateralization/localization to aid in the surgical hypothesis.

FIGURE 52.2 Example of left temporoparietal and bitemporal hypometabolism seen on [¹⁸F]-fluorodeoxyglucose (FDG) positron emission tomography (PET) scanning.

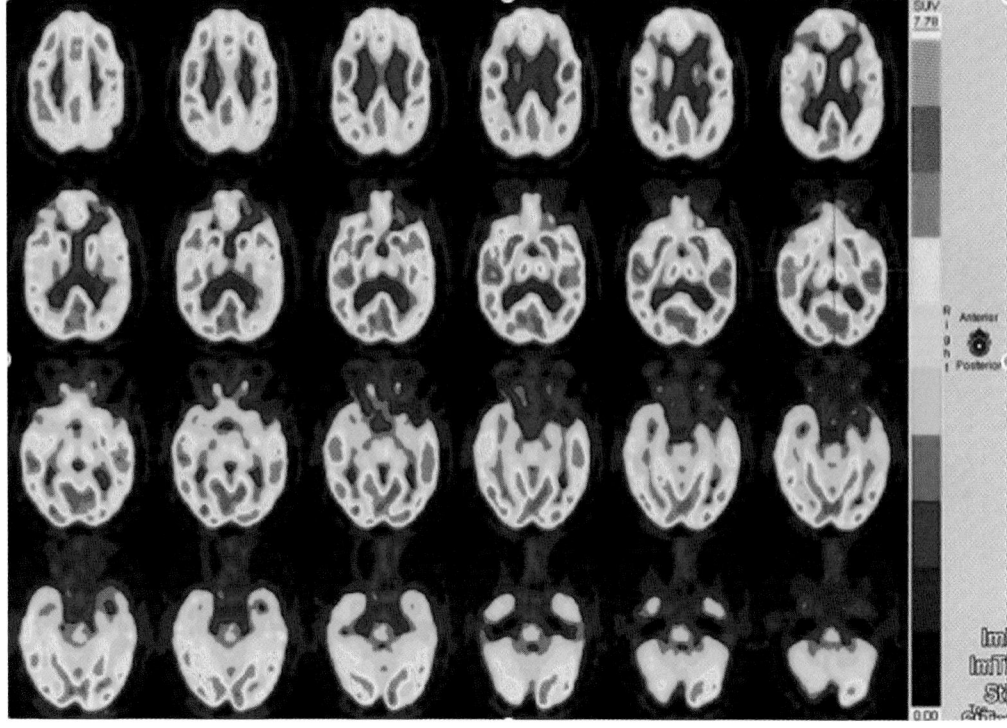

MRI studies for patients with suspected extratemporal lesions should include axial T2 sequences, axial and coronal fluid-attenuated inversion recovery (FLAIR) sequences, a sagittal T1 sequence, and a high-resolution (thin-cut) coronal magnetization prepared rapid gradient echo (MPRAGE) sequence.[5] Although 1.5-tesla magnet strength is considered acceptable, 3-tesla or higher machines and the use of surface coils over the region of interest may add to the diagnostic yield. Additional studies such as subtraction single-photon emission computed tomography (SPECT), [¹⁸F]-fluorodeoxyglucose (FDG), positron emission tomography (PET), or magnetoencephalography (MEG) provide complementary information and may help to formulate the surgical hypothesis (Fig. 52.2). These studies may also be used as an adjunct in patients with multilobar lesions or discordant data.[6] Functional MRI (fMRI), MEG, or intracarotid sodium amytal testing may be performed for localization of language and sensorimotor cortex (Fig. 52.3). After review of all available data, a likely cause should be determined for the patient's seizures; an underlying cause has been correlated with the probability of postoperative seizure freedom across a number of surgical case series.[7,8]

The goal of the presurgical evaluation is the creation of an individualized surgical hypothesis. This is best done by a multidisciplinary team skilled in the treatment of epilepsy. All the data gathered should be presented to the epileptologist, neurosurgeon, neuropsychologist, psychiatrist, social worker, and neuroradiologist on the team. Initially, each available diagnostic study is analyzed independently of the other investigative modalities. No single study can measure the epileptogenic zone and so all data must be considered together with the video-EEG data, seizure semiology, and MRI, which is perhaps the most important. Adjuvant testing such as PET, SPECT, MEG, neuropsychological testing, and fMRI help to round out the surgical strategy.

PREDOMINANTLY LEFT SIDED LANGUAGE LATERALIZATION

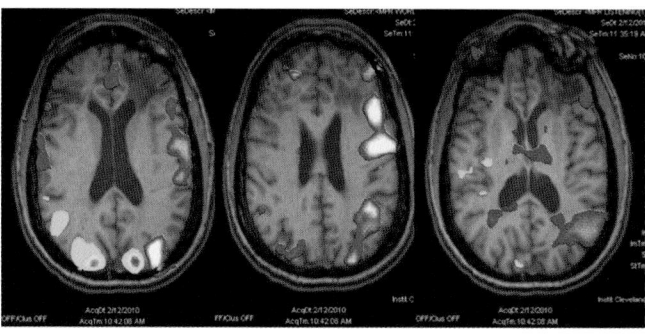

Rhyming   Word generation   Listening

FIGURE 52.3 Left hemispheric language dominance documented by word generation, listening, and rhyming tasks during functional magnetic resonance imaging (fMRI).

The strongest hypothesis is formed when the localization predicted by individual studies is concordant. Any discrepancies must be evaluated and resolved in relation to surgical planning. Discrepancies between semiology, EEG, or MRI are considered the most troubling. If localization differs based on these studies, or if the MRI is nonlesional, then potentially clarifying information should be sought with either FDG-PET or ictal SPECT. When discrepancies cannot be resolved, additional methods of strengthening the working surgical hypothesis should be considered. Chronic extraoperative intracranial recordings may provide critical information in such patients (Fig. 52.4). These may also be used when noninvasive evaluation leads to a hypothesis involving a large cortical area and further delineation of the epileptogenic zone is desired. A working hypothesis of the ictal onset zone based on

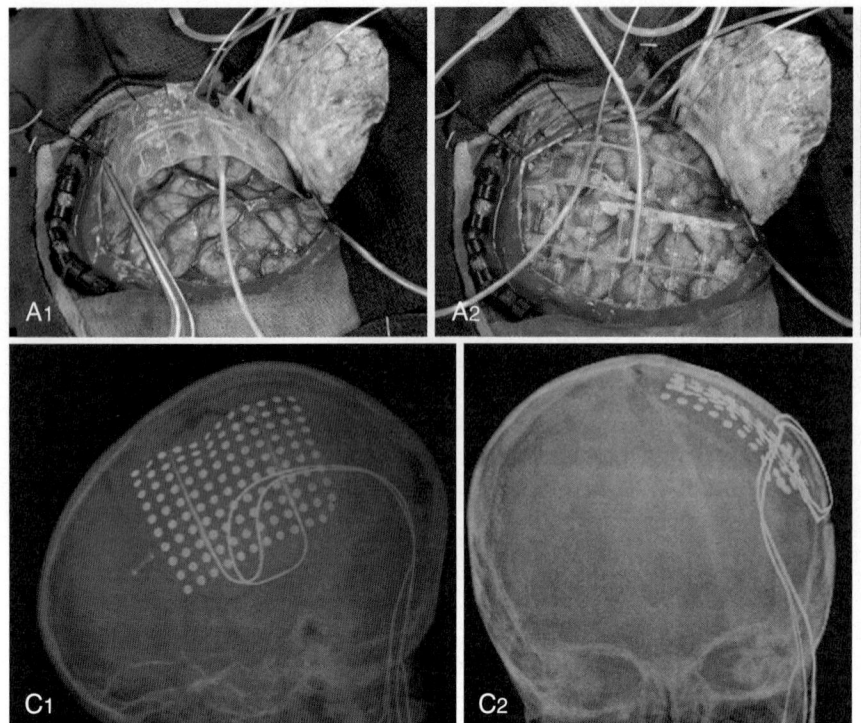

FIGURE 52.4 **A,** Example of subdural grid electrode insertion over left hemisphere. **B,** Sagittal magnetic resonance imaging (MRI) reconstruction with electrode colocalization. **C,** Anteroposterior (AP) and lateral skull film localization of subdural electrodes.

noninvasive data helps guide the placement of the intracranial electrodes in an effort to confirm it prior to surgical resection.

Invasive intracranial electrodes also have a distinct advantage in mapping functional cortex. Consequently, their placement should be considered when epilepsy is thought to arise from within or near eloquent cortex. They are especially useful for localizing functional cortex in those patients unable to tolerate awake craniotomy (Fig. 52.5).

It is also not uncommon that after a full noninvasive presurgical evaluation, the concordance of data results in a hypothesis that would preclude the patient from undergoing surgical treatment. Even though the patient may still have intractable disabling epilepsy, there is no longer a localizable epileptogenic zone, or the localized epileptogenic zone may confer a high risk of unacceptable postoperative deficit. This possibility should be introduced and discussed with the patient at the onset, not the conclusion, of the surgical evaluation.

SURGICAL PROCEDURES

There is a broad range of surgical techniques for the treatment of extratemporal epilepsy. These procedures can be loosely divided into resective techniques and palliative techniques.[9] Resective techniques include lesionectomy, tailored focal resection (a "lesionectomy plus" approach), lobectomy, multilobar resections, and hemispherectomy and its variants. Palliative techniques include corpus callosotomy, multiple subpial transections, and vagal nerve stimulation. Other stimulation techniques currently under investigation include thalamic targeted deep brain stimulation, responsive cortical stimulation, and transcranial stimulation. Intraoperative techniques include stereotactic neuronavigation, ultrasound,

intraoperative neuromonitoring with somatosensory evoked potentials (SSEPs) or electrocorticography (ECoG), and intraoperative MRI.

The surgical approach depends not only on surgical and functional anatomy, but also on age of the patient, medical comorbid conditions, and anticipated underlying disease. In particular, certain types of focal cortical dysplasias, neoplasms, and cavernomas can often be resected with pure lesionectomy, typically resulting in good surgical outcome (Fig. 52.6).[10-12] The general tenet is focal resections for focal disease, and progressively larger areas of resection for more diffuse or for multifocal disease. The extension of a resection beyond the area of visible lesion may be performed with the assistance of intraoperative ECoG, SSEPs, or extraoperative recording with the use of implanted intracranial electrodes. The use of such techniques may be more important in cases of cortical dysplasia where the epileptogenic zone often extends beyond the margins of the radiographic lesion.

Hemispherectomy, and related procedures, tend to be limited primarily to the pediatric population. Anatomical hemispherectomy and disconnective hemispherectomy procedures are the available techniques.[7,13] To be considered for hemispherectomy, the ideal patient should have epilepsy arising from a single affected hemisphere. The underlying disease should be unilateral and most patients considered for these procedures will have preexisting neurological deficits, including homonymous hemianopia and contralateral hemiparesis with absence of functional fine motor movements of the hand. If they do not, counseling regarding these anticipated deficits should be extensive, including the likelihood that the patient will not drive due to the visual field defect.

Anatomical hemispherectomy remains in use for selected pathological processes such as hemimegalencephaly and diffuse

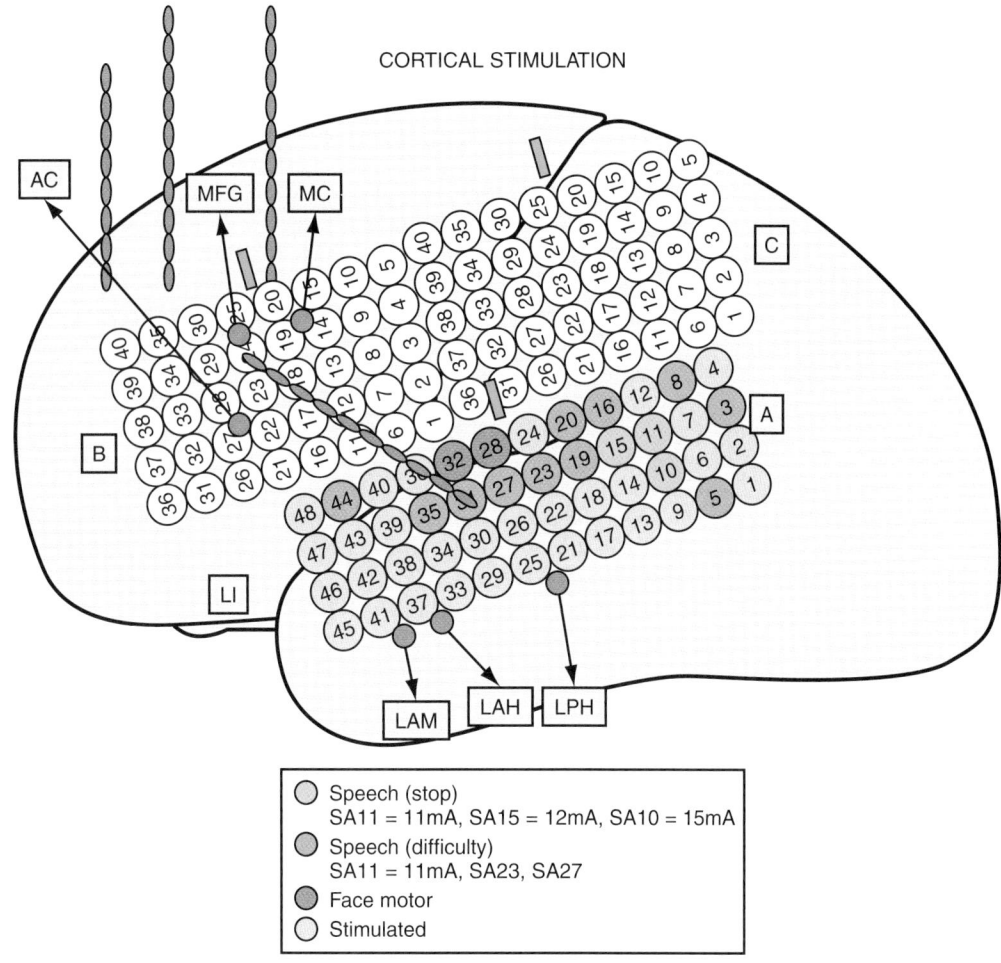

CORTICAL STIMULATION

O Speech (stop)
SA11 = 11mA, SA15 = 12mA, SA10 = 15mA
O Speech (difficulty)
SA11 = 11mA, SA23, SA27
O Face motor
O Stimulated

FIGURE 52.5 Example of cortical stimulation map displaying stimulation identified language and face motor sites.

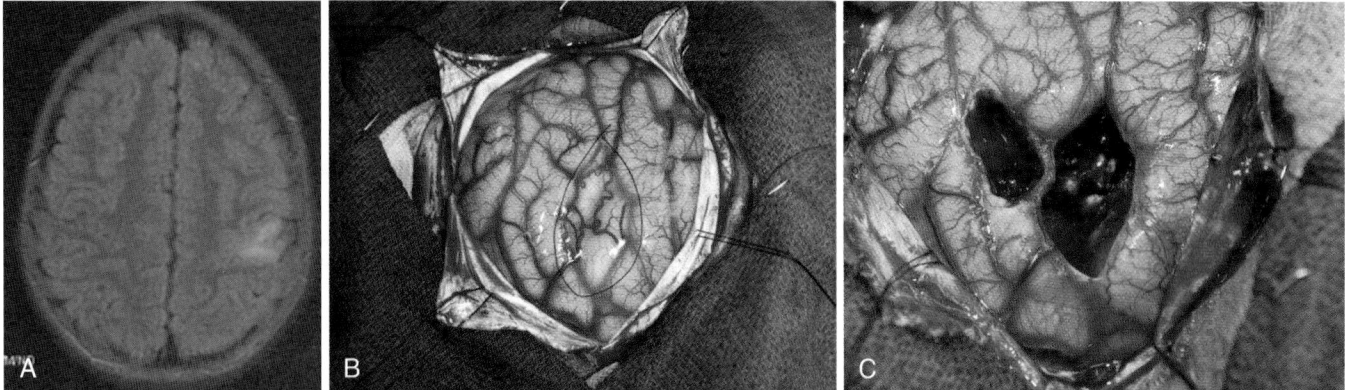

FIGURE 52.6 **A,** Fluid-attenuated inversion recovery (FLAIR) axial magnetic resonance imaging (MRI) demonstrating balloon cell dysplasia in left perirolandic region. **B,** Intraoperative photograph demonstrating same balloon cell dysplasia (encircled by suture). Ictal onset localized on grid recordings to the borders of the lesion. **C,** Photograph taken after lesionectomy plus ictal onset zone in adjacent cortex

malformations of cortical development. It is also commonly utilized when patients have failed prior disconnective hemispherectomy techniques.[14] Disconnective hemispherectomy techniques are usually considered in those patients with perinatal stroke, Sturge-Weber syndrome, or Rasmussen's encephalitis.[7] The goal of these less extensive procedures is isolation of the hemispheric cortex while reducing the perioperative

risks that are more prevalent with the anatomical technique (blood loss and hydrocephalus). From a practical standpoint, this translates to disconnection of the horizontal frontal fibers, mesial temporal structures, corpus callosum, and the internal capsule and corona radiata (see video).[15] The completeness of disconnection, in addition to seizure etiology, relates directly to surgical outcome.[16]

Functional hemispherectomy as described by Rasmussen implies removal of the temporal lobe (including mesial structures) followed by a limited central resection of frontoparietal tissue.[17] This limited resection allows access to the lateral ventricle, facilitating the disconnection of the remaining hemisphere through the ventricular space. The majority of the disconnected hemisphere is then left in situ in an attempt to reduce perioperative morbidity (blood loss, hydrocephalus) and the long-term risk of superficial cerebral hemosiderosis.

The Rasmussen technique, initially reported in 1973, has since undergone a number of modifications. The resulting evolution has yielded both the hemispherotomy and hemispherical deafferentation techniques.[18,19] The main variation among these procedures is the amount of tissue resected as the surgeon enters the ventricular space, with more recent refinements of technique focusing on reducing the amount of tissue resected. The smaller resection window of hemispherotomy and hemispherical deafferentation is ideally suited for those patients with anatomical variations that make the process of disconnection straightforward, such as large ventricles or encephalomalacia.

Each hemispherectomy technique has unique advantages and disadvantages, with selection of technique individualized to the patient's anatomy and underlying disease. For those patients with malformations of cortical development including hemimegalencephaly, anatomical hemispherectomy is the most direct way to completely remove the malformed tissue. These patients often have small ventricles and no clearly defined gray/white interface, producing a situation that makes complete disconnection via a less invasive hemispherectomy technique almost impossible. The disadvantage to the anatomical technique is a slightly higher risk of perioperative morbidity and a higher incidence of postoperative hydrocephalus. The theoretical risk of superficial hemosiderosis is often quoted when discussing anatomical hemispherectomy, but this complication has not been reported in the neurosurgical literature since the 1960s.

The functional technique is well suited to those patients with Rasmussen's encephalitis where the normal gray/white anatomy is preserved. Removal of the temporal lobe and peri-insular frontoparietal operculum facilitates removal of the insula and may lead to a better outcome in this unique group of patients. Finally, those patients afflicted with perinatal vascular events are ideal candidates for peri-insular hemispherotomy as the surgeon can utilize the encephalomalacia to access the ventricle and disconnect the hemisphere. Advantages to these less invasive techniques include reduced blood loss and risk of hydrocephalus. The one real disadvantage is the higher reoperation rate when seizures persist postoperatively and there is cortical tissue left in place.

Surgical Technique: Anatomical Hemispherectomy

The patient is positioned either on a rigid fixation device or resting on a head support. The head is turned 90 degrees and elevated above the level of the heart to assist with venous return. An ipsilateral shoulder support is placed. A T incision is then marked such that it consists of one line at least 0.5 cm from midline and another perpendicular line extending from the zygomatic root just anterior to the tragus. The midline incision should extend from hairline to 4 to 5 cm above the inion (Fig. 52.7). The incision is infiltrated with a local anesthetic and the skin is incised, taking care not to injure the sagittal sinus in the area of an open anterior fontanelle. Careful attention is paid to hemostasis throughout the procedure, with all bleeding points controlled with bipolar coagulation and hemostatic agents. The temporalis muscle is incised and reflected inferiorly to allow adequate exposure of the temporal lobe. Bur holes are then placed just above the zygomatic arch, the keyhole, and along the parasagittal area to allow an exposure of the entire hemisphere. High-speed air craniotome is then used to remove the craniotomy flap. Dural tack-up sutures are then placed and the dura is opened in an H-fashion. The surface of the cortex is examined, the sylvian fissure identified, and venous drainage patterns noted (see Fig. 52.7). Major draining veins to the sagittal sinus are carefully protected to avoid potentially devastating hemorrhage. Initial dissection is performed to open the sylvian fissure (see Fig. 52.7). The middle cerebral artery (MCA) is exposed at a point just distal to the lenticulostriate branches. The inferior and superior circular sulci of the insula are then exposed (see Fig. 52.7) and the MCA is ligated with bipolar cautery and surgical clips, if necessary.

Infrasylvian dissection and ventricular access is then performed. Disconnection of the temporoparietal white matter proceeds through the inferior circular sulcus, facilitating access to the temporal horn of the lateral ventricle. The ventricle is opened anteriorly to the amygdala and then posteriorly so that the temporal horn is exposed from its anterior aspect to the trigonal region. The lateral ventricular sulcus of the temporal horn is then opened and the collateral sulcus is followed to the tentorial edge and mesial temporal pia. The parahippocampal gyrus is aspirated, exposing the tentorial edge, and the pia is coagulated and divided from the temporal pole to the trigonal region. The posterior cerebral artery branches are encountered and ligated as they course over the tentorial edge on their way to the temporo-occipital cortex.

Attention is then turned to the suprasylvian dissection. The superior circular sulcus is opened to divide the corona radiata and expose the lateral ventricle longitudinally. The ipsilateral foramen of Monro is occluded with a cotton ball to prevent blood entering the dependent hemisphere. Both the choroid and basal ganglia are protected in order to minimize bleeding. Hemostatic agents applied to the surface of the basal ganglia are effective in controlling surface bleeding. The frontoparietal white matter is aspirated to open the entire ventricular system, connecting to the posterior temporal disconnection from the infrasylvian dissection. The middle cerebral artery branches in the posterior aspect of the sylvian fissure are coagulated and divided.

Mesial frontoparietal disconnection and corpus callosotomy are then performed. Identification of the corpus callosum is facilitated by careful aspiration of the roof of the lateral ventricle just above its intersection with the septum pellucidum. The gray matter of the cingulate is easily identified. Aspiration of a portion of the cingulate allows clear visualization of the pericallosal arteries and corpus callosum. During this portion of the procedure the surgeon must be careful to avoid injuring either pericallosal artery, as it is difficult to ascertain which branch supplies the contralateral hemisphere. The cingulate

FIGURE 52.7 A, The T incision for exposure of the cerebral hemisphere. **B,** The right cerebral hemisphere exposure needed for anatomical removal. **C,** The right sylvian fissure is opened and the circular sulci exposed (not shown). **D,** An example of a "split sylvian fissure" with exposure of the middle cerebral artery (MCA) vessels and circular sulci. **E,** Surgeon's line drawing demonstrating ligation of anterior circulation branches above the corpus callosum. **F,** Postoperative anatomical hemispherectomy cavity.

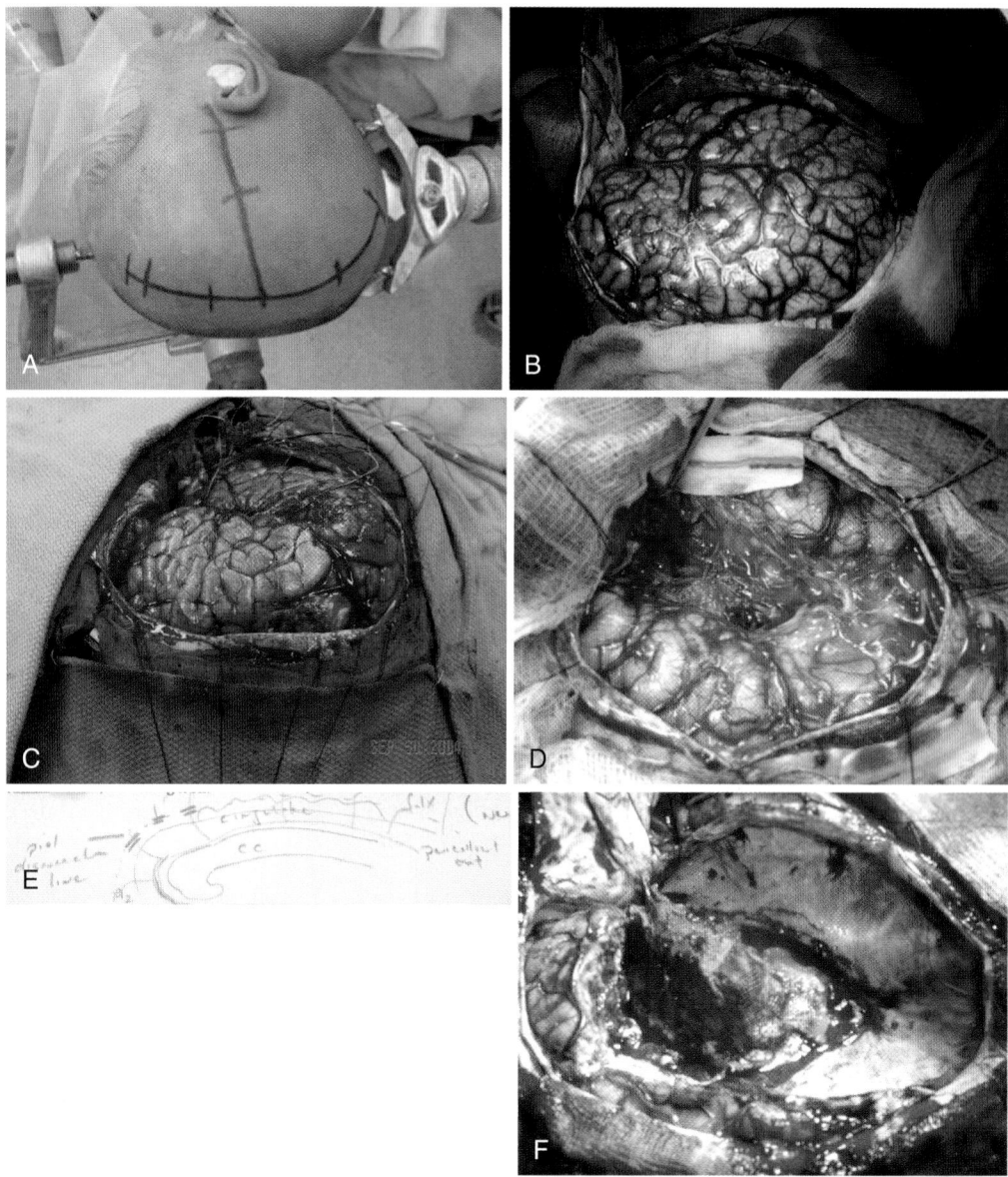

and corpus callosum are then aspirated to achieve complete disconnection, being careful to avoid injury to the contralateral frontal lobe. The ipsilateral fornix is then interrupted by aspiration just anterior to the splenium in the posterior aspect of the lateral ventricle.

The anterior callosal dissection is continued, dividing the pia of the mesial frontal lobe and any branches from the anterior circulation, until the olfactory nerve is reached. The falx and pericallosal arteries provide an excellent anatomical reference to ensure complete frontal disconnection (see Fig. 52.7). The mesial frontoparietal pia and anterior circulation branches should be coagulated and divided above the inferior aspect of the falx to ensure that the contralateral frontal lobe is not injured. Posterior dissection is then performed along the falx until it transitions to the tentorium, effectively connecting to the infrasylvian basal temporal disconnection.

At this point, the only remaining connection is that of the basal orbitofrontal surface. The remaining orbitofrontal tissue, extending from the anterior sylvian fissure to the

posterior basal frontal lobe is aspirated and the orbitofrontal pia divided. The gyrus rectus is aspirated and care should be taken to protect the contralateral frontal lobe. The lateral aspect of the pia along the olfactory nerve is divided to avoid injury to the olfactory nerve. The residual basal frontal lobe is removed with a posterior limit of the internal carotid artery.

Once the entire mesial pia has been divided, the draining veins to the sinuses are coagulated and divided sequentially. During this portion of the procedure it is common to have bleeding from the dura around the sagittal sinus. Packing the bleeding areas with a combination of hemostatic agents and cotton balls works well to avoid excessive blood loss. Once the draining veins have been ligated, the entire hemisphere has been disconnected and can be carefully removed. Finally, removal of the temporal mesial structures and insula is performed and the cavity irrigated and hemostasis achieved (see Fig. 52.7). A ventricular drain is placed in the cavity and the dura is closed in a watertight fashion. The bone flap is replaced and the wound is closed in anatomical layers.

COMPLICATION AVOIDANCE

Complications of epilepsy surgery can be analyzed from a number of different perspectives: immediate versus delayed, minor versus major, general complications of craniotomy versus those specific to a given procedure, and neurological versus surgical. These divisions can be further broken down into expected versus unexpected and may depend on the location of the resection. If a postoperative deficit is anticipated as an unavoidable consequence of the procedure, and the patient receives counseling in light of this expectation, the resulting deficit is typically not considered a complication.

Tanreverdi and associates, in 2009, published an analysis of postoperative epilepsy surgery morbidity rates in 1905 patients over the course of 2449 epilepsy surgery procedures. Of these 1905 patients, 517 underwent extratemporal procedures consisting either of lobectomy or multilobar resections. Morbidity was subdivided by frontal, central, parietal, occipital, or multilobar resection location, resulting in major neurological morbidity rates of 0.7%, 1.4%, 0%, 5.1%, and 2.6%, and minor morbidity rates of 5.2%, 5.9%, 0%, 2.5%, and 12%, respectively. When surgical morbidity was analyzed across the same subdivisions of frontal, central, parietal, occipital, or multilobar resection, rates of complication were 5.6%, 1.5%, 14%, 0%, and 4%, respectively. Whereas parietal resections had the lowest neurological morbidity rate, they had the highest surgical morbidity rate of any reported group. Infection was the most common surgical complication, occurring in 2.1% of extratemporal procedures, followed by hematoma at 1.5%. Only one patient developed hydrocephalus.[20]

With extratemporal resections, the most common neurological complications are those secondary to working in or near areas of eloquent cortex. Parieto-occipital resections, for example, are reported to have visual field deficits as their most common postoperative complication. This is followed by new or worsening hemiparesis, hemisensory loss, and aphasia.[8] Resections in or near the dominant parietal lobe may result in a characteristic pattern of deficit. The most common complication of frontal lobe surgery is hemiparesis; however, aphasia is also a potential complication when operating in or near the dominant frontal operculum.[21] The use of invasive monitoring to delineate eloquent cortex prior to resection aids in preventing and predicting postoperative neurological deficits. When surgical planning involves resection in or near functional cortex the relationship of the epileptogenic zone to eloquent cortex may limit the potential for seizure-free outcome.

Hemispherectomy and multilobar resection patients are at increased risk of specific complications, including hemorrhage, infarction, hydrocephalus, coagulopathy, anemia, and aseptic meningitis, when compared to those patients who undergo lobar resections.[14] These risks are elevated in both the acute and delayed postoperative setting. In addition, disconnective hemispherectomy can be complicated by postoperative hemispheric cerebral edema or infarct, with resultant intracranial hypertension and death.[22]

Complication avoidance is performed through a combination of both surgical and medical management techniques. Placement of intraventricular drains, subgaleal drains, peri- and postoperative dexamethasone, and admission to an intensive care unit are all utilized as part of complication avoidance. Routine monitoring of coagulation panel, platelets, and hematocrit every 6 hours for the first 48 hours postoperatively is performed for hemispherectomy patients, with early and aggressive correction of anemia and coagulopathy. Routine postoperative MRI is performed within the first 24 hours, assessing for extent of resection, presence of hemorrhage, and postoperative ventricular size. All hemispherectomy patients have computed tomographic imaging at a 6-week follow-up.

CONCLUSION

Patients with ETLE compose a significant portion of medically intractable epilepsy. Surgical management provides an effective therapeutic option for many of these patients. Success rates vary by location, pathology, and extent of resection. Despite the team-based approach for preoperative evaluation of the epilepsy patient, the primary responsibility for selection of surgical approach remains with the neurosurgeon. The importance of this decision is underscored by the fact that, in recent surgical series, 1% to 11% of epilepsy patients underwent reoperation due to surgical failure.[23-25]

Surgical failure has been noted to be more common in neocortical resections. Possible reasons for this include incomplete resection of the lesion and the epileptogenic zone. Jehi and colleagues remark in a review of outcomes in 57 patients who underwent posterior cortex epilepsy surgery, resection was felt to be complete in 67% of patients. Within this cohort, at 6-month routine EEG follow-up, 56% of patients with incomplete resection of their MRI lesion had spiking on their EEG versus 27% of those patients who had complete resections.[8]

Frontal lobe resections convey the lowest chance for successful postoperative results. Overall seizure-free outcome for a combined series of both lesional and nonlesional frontal lobe epilepsy patients was 56% at 1 year, 45% at 3 years, and 30% at 5 years. Patients with a circumscribed lesion on MRI preoperatively fared significantly better, having a 79% seizure-free rate at 5 years.[21]

Posterior cortex epilepsy resections convey a slightly higher chance of favorable outcome. In parietal, occipital, and parieto-occipital resections in a series of 57 patients, 5-year seizure-free rates were 52%, 89%, and 93%, respectively. The overall 5-year seizure-free rate for the posterior cortex cohort was 54%.[8]

Older single institution series of hemispherectomy patients report rates of seizure freedom from 53% to 67%, with malformative lesions having the worst prognosis. The more recent University of California at Los Angeles series of 141 pediatric patients reports a seizure-free rate of 83% for all hemispherectomies performed after 1997.[26] Outcomes are certainly not perfect for patients undergoing surgery for management of their ETLE; however, for patients who are deemed surgical candidates, these percentages of seizure freedom far exceed those offered by any other treatment strategy.

SELECTED KEY REFERENCES

Gonzalez-Martinez J, Srikijvilaikul T, Nair D, Bingaman WE. Longterm seizure outcome in reoperation after failure of epilepsysurgery. *Neurosurgery*. 2007;60:873-880.

Marras CE, Granata T, Franzini A, et al. Hemispherotomy and functional hemispherectomy: indications and outcome. *Epilepsy Res.* 2010;89(1):104-112.

Rasmussen T, Villemure JG. Cerebral hemispherectomy for seizures with hemiplegia. *Cleve Clin J Med.* 1983;56:S62-S68.

Schramm J, Clusmann H. The surgery of epilepsy. *Neurosurgery.* 2008;62:463-481.

Wiebe S, Blume WT, Girvin JP, et al. A randomized, controlled trial of surgery for temporal lobe epilepsy. *N Engl J Med.* 2001;345:311-318.

Please go to expertconsult.com to view the complete list of references.

Basic Principles of Deep Brain Stimulation for Movement Disorders, Neuropsychiatric Disorders, and New Frontiers

Alexander S. Taghva, Chima O. Oluigbo, Ali R. Rezai

CLINICAL PEARLS

- The spectrum of movement disorders treated with deep brain stimulation (DBS) includes Parkinson's disease (PD), essential tremor, and dystonia. The cardinal features of PD are resting tremor, bradykinesia, rigidity, and postural instability. Replacement of dopamine via dopamine agonists and L-dopa is the mainstay of medical treatment. DBS is the neurosurgical therapy of choice for movement disorders. DBS can improve motor symptoms, decrease medication usage, and decrease on/off motor fluctuations in patients with good response to L-dopa.

- In choosing an appropriate target for neuromodulation by DBS, it is important to note that multiple targets can be efficacious for a single disease. For example, Parkinson's disease responds well to DBS of the globus pallidus interna (GPi) and subthalamic nucleus (STN).

- Deep brain stimulation of the ventralis intermedius nucleus of the thalamus can be used to treat patients with disabling essential tremor. Extremity tremors are more reliably treated than axial tremors.

- Primary generalized and focal dystonias can be treated with deep brain stimulation of the GPi. Some secondary dystonias may respond to deep brain stimulation; however, this is a heterogeneous group of disorders and response to deep brain stimulation may be the exception rather than the rule.

- Deep brain stimulation of the ventral capsule/ventral striatum is approved under a Food and Drug Administration

- (FDA) humanitarian device exemption for the treatment of severe, treatment-refractory obsessive-compulsive disorder. Active investigation of deep brain stimulation for neuropsychiatric disorders, pain, epilepsy, and others is currently ongoing.

- The pharmacological therapies available for dystonia are limited; therefore, surgical alternatives have been developed. These include intrathecal baclofen pumps, botulinum toxin injections, ablative procedures such as thalamotomy, and neuromodulation procedures such as DBS. The GPi is the DBS "target of choice" for "primary generalized dystonia."

- Careful selection of appropriate patients is critical to good outcomes in DBS procedures.

- DBS for movement and neuropsychiatric disorders should be performed in the context of a multidisciplinary team.

- In common movement disorders, surgical targets are the STN and GPi for Parkinson's disease, ventralis intermedius nucleus of the thalamus for essential tremor, GPi for dystonia, and the ventral capsule/ventral striatum (VC/VS) target for neuropsychiatric disorders such as depression and obsessive-compulsive disorder (OCD).

- Targeting of subcortical nuclei in DBS is based on stereotactic principles.

HISTORICAL BACKGROUND

Deep brain stimulation (DBS) is now considered the neurosurgical therapy of choice for movement disorders, with over 80,000 patients having undergone DBS worldwide.[1] DBS works through the delivery of therapeutic electrical energy to highly specific targets in the brain. The safety and efficacy of DBS have been validated in many high-quality studies in over 20 years of use. DBS is also the subject of intense intellectual study; a recent PubMed search for "deep brain stimulation" returned over 3500 published studies.[2] A particularly exciting aspect of the ongoing research in DBS is evaluation of expanding indications for the therapy, which span neuropsychiatric disorders, epilepsy, and disorders of consciousness, among others. This chapter reviews the historical underpinnings of DBS, indications for use, and future horizons. Additionally, a brief description of DBS components and purported mechanisms of action will be provided.

Historical Beginnings

The modern era of deep brain stimulation has its historical roots in the development of stereotactic surgery, which has its own origins in the work of the French mathematician and philosopher René Descartes. In part II of his 1637 work, *Discourse on the Method*, Descartes describes a method for specifying the location of a point based on its relationship to two intersecting axes.[3] (Of note, this work is best known for its famous quotation, *"Je pense, donc je suis"* [I think, therefore I am], which occurs in part IV.) This method, known as the Cartesian coordinate system, facilitated the development of calculus by Isaac Newton and Gottfried Wilhelm Leibniz as well as modern stereotactic neurosurgery.

The happy marriage of the fields of stereotaxy, movement disorder surgery, and psychosurgery gave rise to the underlying principles of modern DBS surgery. On the movement disorders front, much work had been done on cortical resections and subcortical lesioning to palliate these disorders. In 1909, Sir Victor Horsley, who described the first stereotactic apparatus in animals, relieved hemiathetosis in a 15-year-old boy by removing the precentral gyrus somatotopically associated with the upper extremity.[4] In 1931, Bucy performed the same procedure for seizure relief and relieved the patient's choreoathetosis in the process.[5] He later, in 1937, performed this procedure with Theodore Case for the treatment of post-traumatic tremor.[6] These patients had postoperative hemiparesis and dyspraxia that resolved to a great extent postoperatively.[7] In 1931, Putnam began sectioning of the extrapyramidal tracts in the high cervical cord, with good results for choreoathetosis but not with parkinsonian tremor.[8,9] Given that cortical ablation would relieve tremor, but extrapyramidal ablation would not, he reasoned that impulses in the pyramidal tract were responsible for the production of parkinsonian tremor, and in 1940, he reported the results of lateral pyramidotomy in the high cervical region in seven patients.[10] Again, these patients had postoperative improvement of tremor but some resultant hemiplegia.

The search for a suitable procedure to maximize tremor control yet minimize postoperative morbidity led to cerebral pedunculotomy by Walker;[11] open, transcortical, transventricular removal of portions of the basal ganglia by Meyers;[12] and anterior choroidal artery ligation by Cooper.[13-15] (As an aside, Cooper's procedure was discovered accidentally when he tore the anterior choroidal artery during an aborted cerebral pedunculotomy.) These procedures, while therapeutic, were both variable in their outcomes and suffered from high perioperative morbidity rates, thereby necessitating more precise and less invasive targeting.

Furthermore, proponents of psychosurgery wanted a means for performing controlled prefrontal lobotomy.[16] In the 1940s, there was concern among neurosurgeons regarding the high morbidity and mortality rates associated with open psychosurgical procedures including prefrontal leucotomy as introduced by Egas Moniz and prefrontal lobotomy as introduced by Walther Freeman and James Watts.[17] There was a general feeling that the principles of psychosurgery were sound, but smaller and more specific structures should be targeted to achieve optimal therapeutic benefit while avoiding unnecessary morbidity and unwanted neurological deficit.

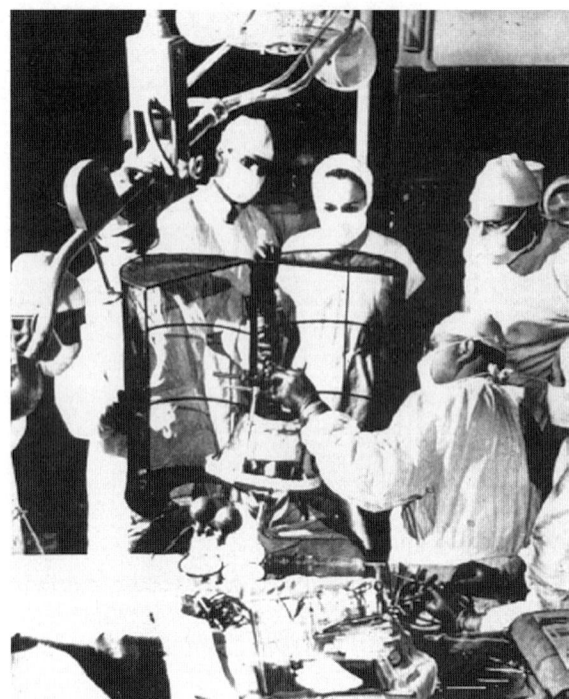

FIGURE 53.1 Spiegel (on left of shielding cage) and Wycis (standing) in the operating room, using their stereotactic apparatus. The cage seen is a grounded copper cage to shield electrode recording from ambient interference.

Initial attempts of stereotactic surgery began in the late nineteenth and early twentieth centuries. In 1889, D.N. Zernov, a Russian surgeon in Moscow, used a navigation system (called an *encephalometer*) based on polar coordinates and referenced to external landmarks to drain a cerebral abscess.[18,19] The first truly modern stereotactic apparatus based on Cartesian coordinates and based on internal cerebral landmarks was first described in animals in the early part of the twentieth century by Sir Victor Horsley and Robert Clarke. In 1908, they described a stereotactic apparatus that could introduce a probe into subcortical structures defined in a Cartesian coordinate system.[20]

The first device developed for inserting an electrode accurately into a chosen structure in the human brain was described by Ernest A. Spiegel, Henry T. Wycis, and others in 1947[21] (Fig. 53.1). At that time, cerebral anatomical structures were targeted based on location relative to the third ventricle using ventriculogram x-rays. Electrode position in the apparatus of Spiegel and Wycis was adjusted by sliding the carrier along a base plate in the anteroposterior and lateral directions, with vertical adjustments made by a microdrive. Leksell introduced a semicircular arc apparatus in 1949, allowing for the introduction of an electrode to a target along any trajectory, because the target now would lie in the center of the arc[22] (Fig. 53.2).

The first lesioning procedures performed by Spiegel and Wycis were in the dorsomedial thalamic nucleus for agitation and psychosis, the medial thalamus for epilepsy, and mesencephalic pain pathways for intractable pain.[7,23] With the advent of stereotactic lesioning procedures, many new techniques were developed for the management of psychiatric and movement disorders. These included pallidotomy and thalamotomy for

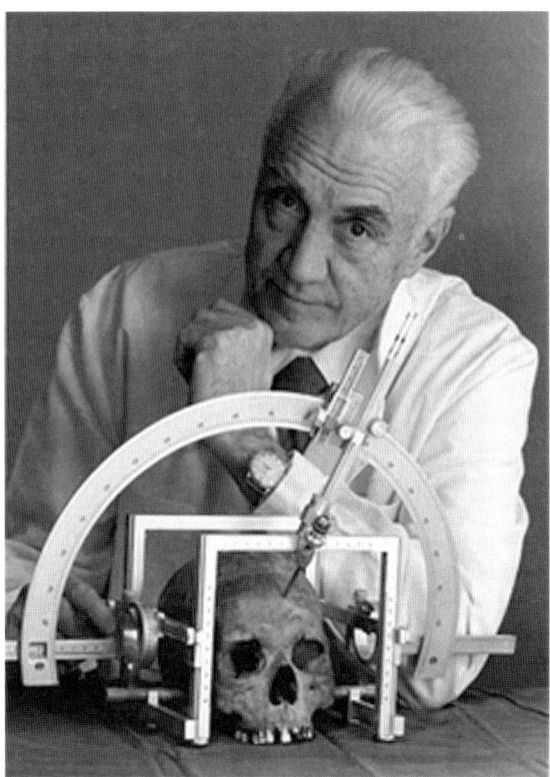

FIGURE 53.2 Lars Leksell with his stereotactic arc. With this system, the target can be approached from any angle because it uses a center-of-arc principle. The basic components are the Cartesian coordinate frame, which is attached to the patient's head using four pins, and the semicircular arc. *(Reproduced with permission of Elekta AB, Stockholm, Sweden.)*

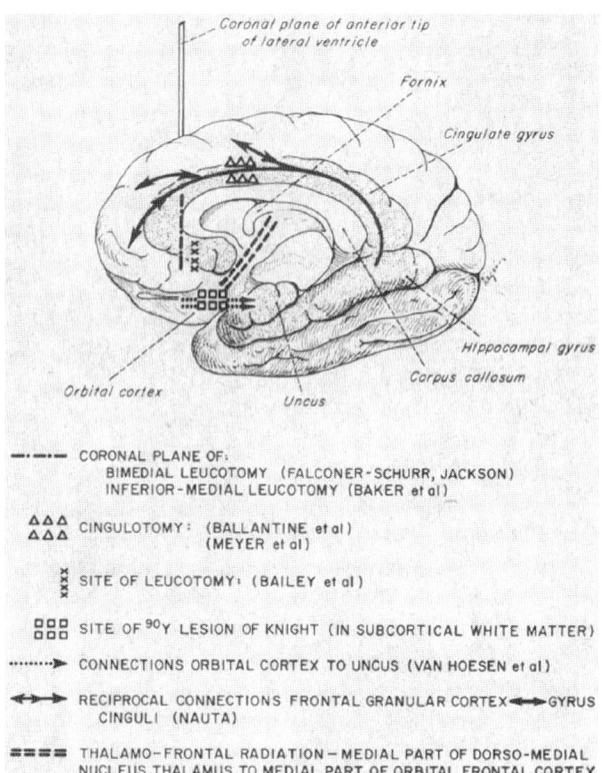

FIGURE 53.3 Classical drawing depicting locations of stereotactic lesioning procedures for psychosurgery. *(Reprinted from Sweet WH. Treatment of medically intractable mental disease by limited frontal leucotomy—justifiable? N Engl J Med. 1973;289(21):1117-1125; used with permission of the Massachusetts Medical Society.)*

the relief of Parkinson's disease (PD)–associated tremor,[24-29] as well as anterior cingulotomy,[30,31] anterior capsulotomy,[32] subcaudate tractotomy,[33] and limbic leucotomy[34] in the treatment of affective disorders[7,17,35,36] (Fig. 53.3). However, with the advent of L-dopa in the 1960s for PD, there was a steep decrease in surgery for PD.[37] Similarly, the introduction of lithium in the late 1940s and the antipsychotic drug chlorpromazine in the mid-1950s led to a nonsurgical bend in the management of psychiatric disorders.[17,36,38] Therefore, the next paradigm shift in the treatment of these disorders did not come until the limitations of these medications with their side effects and lack of sustained benefits were realized, and DBS provided a safer, nondestructive, reversible, and adjustable approach for the treatment of these disorders.

In 1809, Rolando first demonstrated that electrical impulses could modify the function of brain regions, and prior to that, Aldini attempted stimulation of the brains of criminals immediately following their executions.[37,39] Hassler found, during stereotactic exploration of the brain for pallidotomy, that low-frequency stimulation would worsen tremor and high-frequency stimulation would ameliorate it.[37,40] This was first put into practice in 1967 by Bechtereva and associates with chronic DBS of the thalamus, striatum, and pallidum for the treatment of movement disorders.[41]

It was not until the 1970s and 1980s, however, that the modern era of chronic stimulation was ushered in. Hosobuchi and co-workers reported on stimulation of the VPM

thalamus for the control of facial anesthesia dolorosa following rhizotomy for trigeminal neuralgia in 1973.[42] DBS of ventral periaqueductal gray matter in the midbrain for the treatment of cancer pain was reported by Richardson and Akil in the mid-1970s.[43] Chronic DBS for the management of movement disorders was utilized by several groups including Benabid and colleagues,[44,45] Blond and Siegfried,[46] Siegfried and Shulman,[47] and Brice and McLellan.[48] DBS has similar efficacy to its corresponding lesioning procedures, but with an improved safety profile, inherent reversibility, and adjustment of the stimulation parameters over time to accommodate the patient's needs. These factors have led to DBS being adopted as the neurosurgical standard of care for movement disorders as well as the expansion of DBS to the treatment of epilepsy, psychiatric disorders including obsessive-compulsive disorder (OCD) and depression, as well as chronic pain, Tourette's syndrome, and even disorders of consciousness and addiction.

Basic Neurocircuitry Principles

Parallel cortico-striato-pallido-thalamo-cortical (CSPTC) circuits exist for limbic, associative, and motor function.[49] The motor loop is the most commonly described loop and is important in the pathogenesis of PD and the therapeutic efficacy of DBS in this condition.[37] Limbic and associative circuits have been implicated in the pathogenesis of neuropsychiatric conditions including OCD and major depressive disorder (MDD), which respond to DBS of critical nodes along the circuit, including the ventral

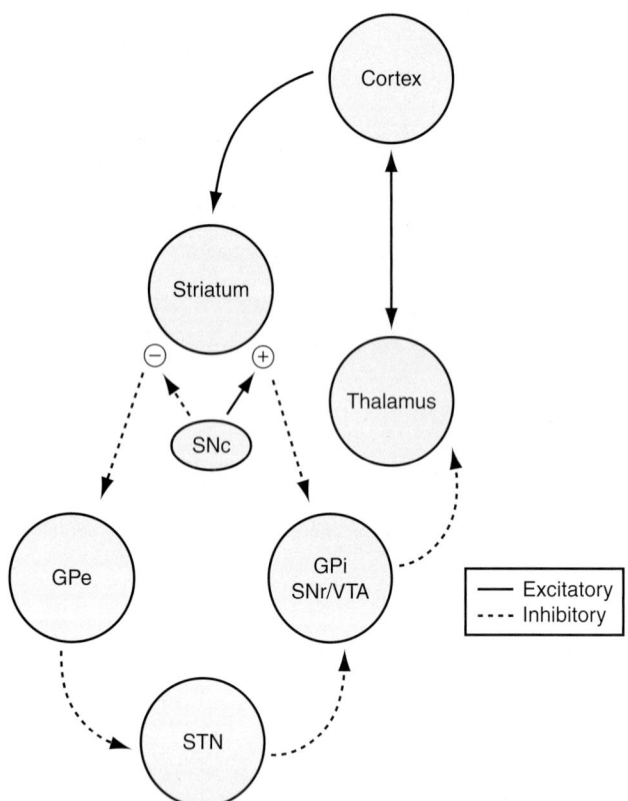

FIGURE 53.4 Schematic of relevant cortico-striato-pallido-thalamo-cortical (CSPTC) neural circuitry.

capsule/ventral striatum (VC/VS), anterior limb of the internal capsule (ALIC), nucleus accumbens (NAc), subgenual cingulate cortex (SCC), and inferior thalamic peduncle.[49-61] These circuits maintain some degree of topographic segregation, with motor circuitry more dorsolateral, limbic circuitry ventromedial, and associative circuitry in between.[62]

These circuits are not strictly "parallel." Haber and associates demonstrated some interface between these circuits in primates with the more medial limbic circuits ultimately influencing more dorsolateral motor circuits.[62] This unique arrangement allows for a link between emotion and motivation (limbic circuits) with cognition and planning (associative circuits), which finally manifests with a motor output and behavior (motor circuits).

Both direct and indirect loops exist for the associative and limbic circuits, as they do for the motor circuits.[49] The direct loops connect from the striatum to the globus pallidus pars interna (GPi), substantia nigra pars reticulata (SNr), and ventral tegmental area (VTA). From there, the projections head to the thalamus. Indirect loops connect from the striatum to the globus pallidus pars externa (GPe), and then head to the subthalamic nucleus (STN) before going to the GPi, SNr, and VTA (Fig. 53.4).

In choosing an appropriate target for neuromodulation by DBS, it is important to note that multiple targets can be efficacious for a single disease. For example, we know that PD responds well to DBS of the GPi and subthalamic nucleus.[37,63] In psychosurgery, multiple targets have been used, for example, in OCD including the ALIC,[52,59] VC/VS and NAc,[51,57] inferior thalamic peduncle,[56] and subthalamic

nucleus.[58] This is likely secondary to the rich connectivity of the modulated circuits and the mechanism of action of DBS. High-frequency stimulation (HFS) has a net inhibitory effect and low-frequency stimulation (LFS) has a net excitatory effect; however, the mechanism of DBS (high-frequency) is likely more complex with activation of nearby axons and suppression of abnormal impulses through the circuits involved.[37]

DEEP BRAIN STIMULATION SURGERY: INDICATIONS, TARGET, AND OUTCOMES

DBS surgery for movement and other disorders should be planned and managed in the context of a multidisciplinary team consisting of the neurosurgeon, movement disorder neurologist, psychiatrist, neuropsychologist, neurophysiologist, and physician extenders such as nurse practitioners and physician assistants. Accurate diagnosis of the specific movement disorder or neuropsychiatric disorder by a movement disorder neurologist or a psychiatrist, respectively, is an essential first step, because success of the procedure significantly depends upon selecting the appropriate patient. Following accurate diagnosis, risk-benefit analysis of intervention for each individual patient should be performed. In general, patients to be considered for DBS should have significant disability in the performance of activities of daily living, despite adequate maximal medical therapy and, in the case of neurobehavioral disorders, adequate cognitive therapy.

Candidates for DBS should be healthy enough to undergo surgery and should be optimized with respect to other medical conditions including any heart disease, hypertension, or diabetes. Patients receiving anticoagulation should be able to tolerate stoppage of these medications for a period before and after surgery. Patients should also have the mental fortitude and physical stamina to undergo a lengthy procedure awake and immobilized in a stereotactic frame while providing feedback during microstimulation during the DBS procedure. Mental agility and physical stamina are also important in the postoperative period as stimulator programming may require prolonged sessions.

From a social standpoint, the patient must be able to tolerate the psychosocial demands of surgery, be compliant with medication changes and postoperative care, and have a strong support network in place. These patients need to be willing to commit time and personal resources for medication and programming adjustments. In addition, patients need to understand the risks and benefits, and have realistic expectations of surgery. Importantly, patients and families need to understand that DBS is not a curative procedure but rather one aimed at improving quality of life.

All patients should undergo detailed neuropsychological assessment. The aim is to identify patients who have underlying cognitive deficits or psychiatric conditions that may be worsened by DBS. Severe dementia or cognitive impairment is generally a contraindication to DBS, and patients with even mild deficits in frontal executive function or cognition need especially strong social support following surgery. Psychiatric conditions as depression, mania, and anxiety should be identified and optimized preoperatively, and patients with psychosis or personality disorders should generally be excluded from

TABLE 53.1 General Principles of Patient Selection in Deep Brain Stimulation Surgery: Predictors of Successful Outcome

- Accurate diagnosis of the specific movement disorder or neuropsychiatric disorder by a movement disorder neurologist or a psychiatrist
- In Parkinson's disease, evidence of levodopa responsiveness: 30% improvement of the Unified Parkinson's Disease Rating Scale (Part III) except in tremor-predominant disease)
- Absence of underlying cognitive deficits or psychiatric conditions that may be worsened by deep brain stimulation
- Realistic expectations from patient, family, and caregivers
- Strong social support networks from patient's family and caregivers

TABLE 53.2 Deep Brain Stimulation Surgery: Targets, Indications, and Relationship to Anterior Commissure–Posterior Commissure (AC-PC) Line

Target	Indication	Anatomical Coordinates*
STN	Parkinson's disease	11-13 mm lateral to midline 4-5 mm ventral to the AC-PC plane 3-4 mm posterior to the MCP
GPi	Dystonia	19-21 mm lateral to the midline 2-3 mm anterior to the MCP 4-5 mm ventral to the AC-PC plane
VIM	Essential tremor	11-12 mm lateral to the wall of the third ventricle At the level of the AC-PC plane Between $2/12$ and $3/12$ of the AC-PC distance anterior to the PC

*Relationship to AC-PC line and MCP.
GPi, globus pallidus interna; MCP, midcommissural point; STN, subthalamic nucleus; VIM, ventralis intermedius nucleus of the thalamus.

surgical intervention.[37] These factors underscore the importance of a multidisciplinary team devoted to the care of DBS patients. (Selection criteria are summarized in Table 53.1.)

The relevance of age to outcomes following DBS is still debated. However, advanced age is associated with higher incidence of postoperative cognitive changes and higher overall risk of surgical complications. An age cutoff point for patients, however, is not recommended, and decisions should be individualized. Older patients may benefit from staged procedures to maximize recovery. Finally, patients benefit from a strong social support network from their family and caregivers. The patient and family need to have realistic expectations about surgical outcome, potential complications, and the multiple steps involved in the preoperative assessments, surgery, and perioperative and follow-up care, including stimulator programming.

SURGICAL TECHNIQUE

Preoperative Imaging and Planning

The specific steps in the surgical technique for DBS vary depending on local practices. However, stereotactic principles firmly underlie each approach. The main aspects of the DBS placement are stereotactic anatomical targeting, physiological verification of the target, implantation of the DBS lead, and implantable pulse generator (IPG) placement. The various components may be performed in the same operative session or may be staged.

Stereotactic anatomical targeting may be by indirect or direct methods. Indirect targeting utilizes stereotactic atlases based on cadaveric sections. Known distances of the different nuclei from the midcommissural point (MCP), the halfway distance between the anterior commissure (AC) and posterior commissure (PC), are used in determining the position of the anatomical target. Typical anatomical coordinates for the common targets are as follows: STN (10-13 mm lateral to midline, 3-5 mm ventral to the AC-PC plane, and 2-4 mm posterior to the MCP), the GPi (19-21 mm lateral to the midline, 2-3 mm anterior to the MCP, and 4-5 mm ventral to the AC-PC plane), the ventralis intermedius (VIM) (11-12 mm lateral to the wall of the third ventricle, at the level of the AC-PC plane and between $2/12$ and $3/12$ of the AC-PC distance anterior to the PC). Table 53.2 shows the typical stereotactic

targets for different indications as well as their stereotactic locations with reference to the AC, PC, and MCP.

Direct targeting involves direct visualization of the deep nuclei using magnetic resonance imaging (MRI). Although computed tomography (CT) can be used in stereotactic targeting, it is difficult to visualize the various target nuclei or the AC and PC using CT alone. On the other hand, MRI offers multiplanar imaging capabilities with excellent anatomical delineation. The AC and PC can be identified on T1-weighted images while the STN can be identified on T2-weighted images (Fig. 53.5). The MRI studies may then be merged with stereotactically acquired CT images. The evident advantage of direct targeting is that discrete anatomical variation between individuals is taken into account because it is based on the individual's anatomy as obtained from imaging. Generally, a combination of indirect and direct targeting methods is used. Following the targeting, localization of the target within the stereotactic space may be performed by frame-based or frameless systems.

A variety of stereotactic head frames are available. Figure 53.2 shows the Leksell stereotactic head frame (Elekta, Stockholm, Sweden) that is used in our institution, and Figure 53.6 shows a frameless system. The accuracy of the various systems has been demonstrated in previous studies, and the use of any system depends on surgeon preference, familiarity, and what is available in a particular institution. In addition to stereotactic anatomical targeting, imaging is also used to plan an entry point and trajectory to the target. The entry point and trajectory are chosen with the aim of avoiding cortical, subcortical, and periventricular blood vessels, thus reducing the risk of hemorrhagic complications. Contrast-enhanced T1-weighted MRI or contrast-enhanced CT scans help to delineate vessels along the electrode path and assist with vessel avoidance during planning.

Surgical Procedure

The stereotactic frame is placed (Fig. 53.7) and the patient is positioned supine with the stereotactic head frame fixed to the operating room table after acquisition of a stereotactic

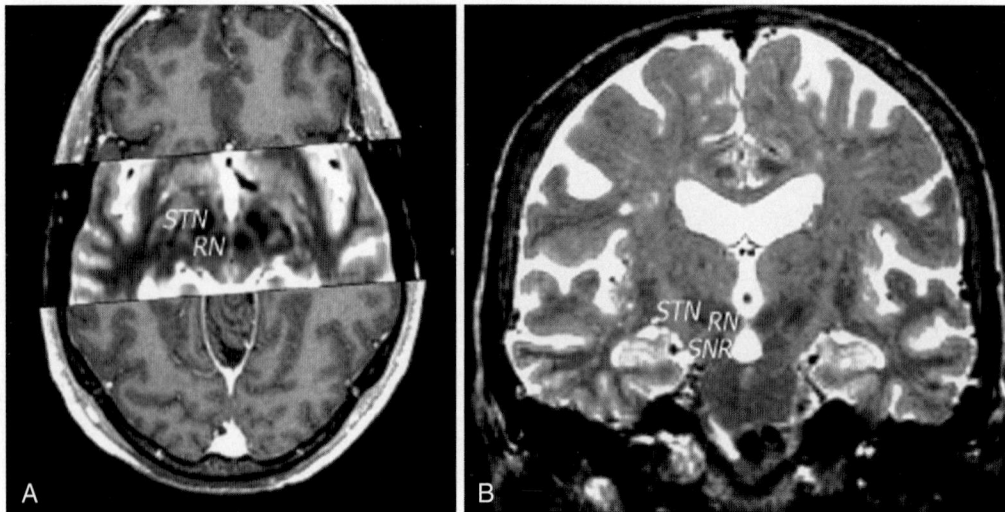

FIGURE 53.5 Subthalamic nucleus (STN) on magnetic resonance imaging (MRI). High-resolution axial (**A**) and coronal (**B**) T2-weighted MRI scans. The STN is located anterosuperolateral to the substantia nigra pars reticulata (SNR) and red nucleus (RN). *(Reprinted with permission from Rezai AR, Machado AG, Deogaonkar M, et al. Surgery for movement disorders. Neurosurgery 2008;62(Suppl 2):809-838.)*

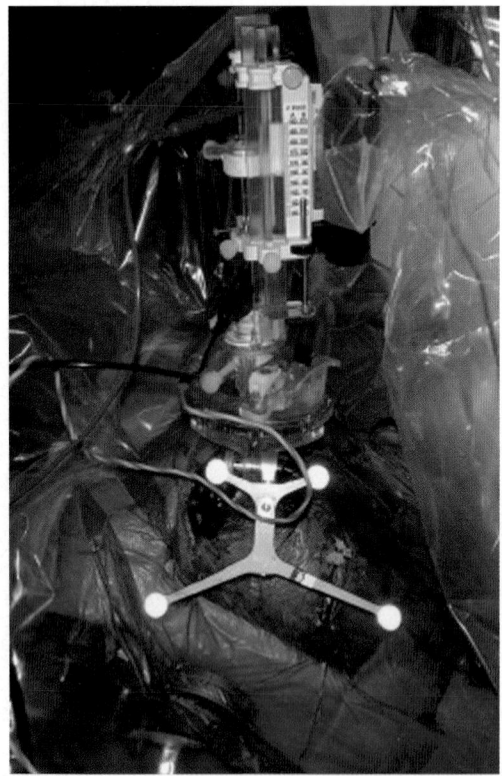

FIGURE 53.6 Intraoperative image of frameless stereotactic systems. Depicted are the Nexframe and Nexdrive (Medtronic, Minneapolis, MN). Nexframe is a disposable device that fits over the Navigus Stimloc base (Medtronic) and allows deep brain stimulation (DBS) procedures to be performed without a stereotactic head frame. Once Nexframe is aligned with the intended trajectory using image guidance software, it functions as a stable cranium-mounted guide for the introduction of the DBS lead. On the top is a disposable microdrive that also acts as a simplified interface for microelectrode recording (MER) and is used for MER and final implantation of DBS electrodes. *(Reprinted with permission from Rezai AR, Machado AG, Deogaonkar M, et al. Surgery for movement disorders. Neurosurgery 2008;62(Suppl 2):809-838.)*

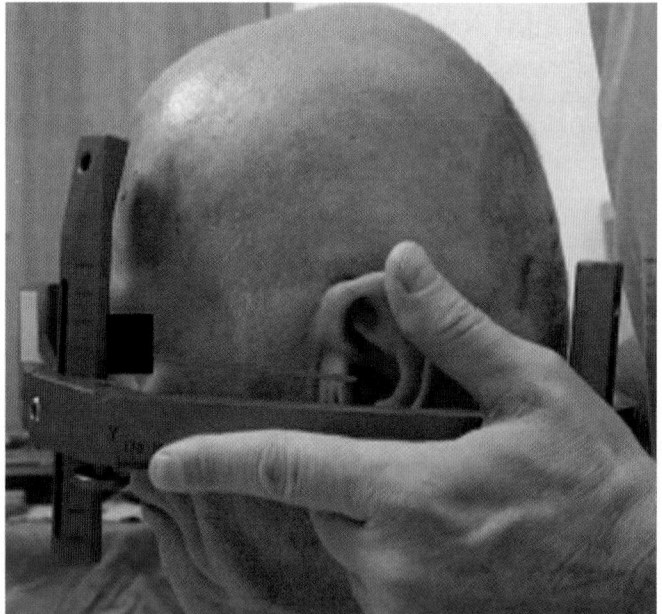

FIGURE 53.7 Method for stereotactic head frame placement. The frame placement is performed under local anesthesia with sedation with the patient in the sitting position. The frame should be placed parallel to a line extending from the lateral canthus to the tragus (orbitomeatal line depicted in red) to approximate the plane of the anterior commissure-posterior commissure (AC-PC) line. *(Reprinted with permission from Rezai AR, Machado AG, Deogaonkar M, et al. Surgery for movement disorders. Neurosurgery 2008;62(Suppl 2):809-838.)*

CT scan. Typically, the stereotactic CT scan is then merged with the previously acquired MRI scan and the stereotactic coordinates are obtained. The stereotactic coordinates are set on the frame and used to determine the site for skin incision and bur hole based on earlier entry point and trajectory planning. Generally in the planning, a bur hole and entry point anterior to the coronal suture are chosen. After the bur hole is performed, the dura is opened and pia coagulated for corticotomy. The microelectrodes are then inserted with the tip of the

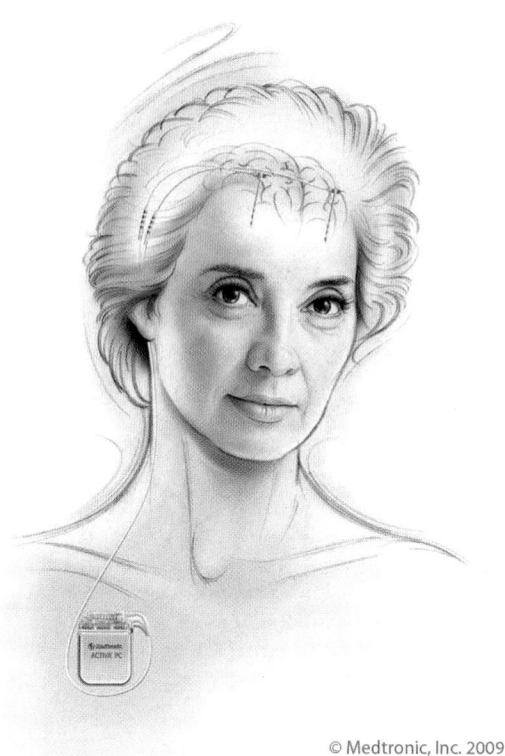

© Medtronic, Inc. 2009

FIGURE 53.8 Depiction of a patient with two intracranial electrodes and a single dual-channel implantable pulse generator (IPG). *(Reproduced with permission of Medtronic, Minneapolis, MN.)*

electrode placed at a defined offset above the target. At this time microelectrode recording (MER) is commenced as the electrodes are advanced in sub-millimeter steps. All sedation should be stopped before the commencement of microelectrode recording as the sedation may affect the electrophysiological mapping. MER allows for definition and verification of the physiological target. The frequency and pattern of activity of the various nuclei and white matter tracts encountered in the path to the physiological target are noted and may help determine the relationship of the trajectory to the target. These characteristic electrophysiological signatures of the targeted nuclei help confirm the physiological target. Macrostimulation is then performed to determine benefits and side effects of the stimulation.

The main components of the DBS system are an intracranial electrode and an implantable pulse generator, by an extension wire (Fig. 53.8). After the physiological target is confirmed, the electrode is implanted at the target. The two currently available electrodes are the Medtronic 3389, which spans 7.5 mm, and the 3387, which spans 10.5 mm (each model has four contacts which are 1.5 mm in height with 0.5-mm spacing between the contacts in the 3389 and 1.5-mm spacing in the 3387 model) (Fig. 53.9). The implantation can be confirmed by fluoroscopy. After the implantation, intraoperative stimulation is then performed with the DBS lead to assess for clinical improvements and side effects of stimulation.

Following implantation of the DBS electrode, it is affixed to the skull using anchoring devices such as the Navigus Stimloc device or the Medtronic bur hole ring and cap. Other institutions use bone cement or plates to secure the electrode. The distal tip of the electrode is covered by a connector or plug

to protect the contacts and the electrode wire is buried in the subgaleal space for use at the time of the implantation of the pulse generator.

The implantation of the pulse generator can be performed on the same day of the implantation of the DBS lead or at a later date. The patient is placed supine and the head is turned to the side opposite the intended side of the pulse generator implantation. An infraclavicular incision is made and a subcutaneous pocket is fashioned. Occasionally, a pocket is created below the pectoralis fascia and the IPG is buried in this pocket. The advantage of this latter site is that there is less chance of downward migration and drift of the IPG with time compared to locations within a subcutaneous pocket. Other locations may be used for the placement of the IPG to accommodate variations in body habitus and for cosmetic reasons. Available IPGs include single-channel, dual-channel, rechargeable, and nonrechargeable devices. These devices can be programmed transcutaneously with a handheld module. Typical parameters that can be adjusted include voltage, pulse width, frequency, and electrode polarity.

Complications

Complications associated with DBS may be related to the surgical implantation process, related to the hardware/device, or linked to stimulation. The most serious potential complication associated with DBS electrode implantation is intracranial hemorrhage (ICH), which may result in profound neurological deficits and even death (see Fig. 53.9). ICH is reported to occur between 0.2% and 12.5% of the time.[37] Asymptomatic hemorrhage is more common than symptomatic cases and is detected only incidentally on postoperative brain CT imaging. In any case, intracerebral hemorrhage is usually related to direct damage to an arterial blood vessel. Occasionally, it may be due to injury to a cortical draining vein when it may present in a delayed manner with venous infarction. Careful preoperative planning of the entry point and trajectory of approach to the target that avoids evident cortical, subcortical, or periventricular blood vessels on a contrast-enhanced brain MRI scan is a first step in avoiding hemorrhagic complications. Other strategies to prevent intracerebral hemorrhagic complications include tight intraprocedural blood pressure control (maintenance of systolic blood pressure below 130 mm Hg), prevention of entry of large amounts of intracranial air by filling the subdural space with saline and occluding the bur hole with Gelfoam and tissue glue during microelectrode recording, avoiding repeated coughing or sneezing during the procedure, and avoiding the coagulation of cortical veins. There may also be increased risk of hemorrhage based on the choice of target. For example, the GPi is reported to have higher hemorrhage rates than the STN. Binder and co-workers showed a 7% risk of hemorrhage in targeting the GPi versus a 2.2% risk in targeting the STN.[64] The DBS study group reported a 9.8% risk of hemorrhage in the GPi versus 2.9% risk in the STN.[65]

Elderly patients may develop transient episodes of confusion and agitation following DBS, especially with procedures. Staging of bilateral DBS procedures in these elderly patients may reduce the incidence of this complication. Infection of the hardware is an ever-present risk in these procedures. Risk of infection ranges between 1% and 15% in published studies, and most commonly affects the site of

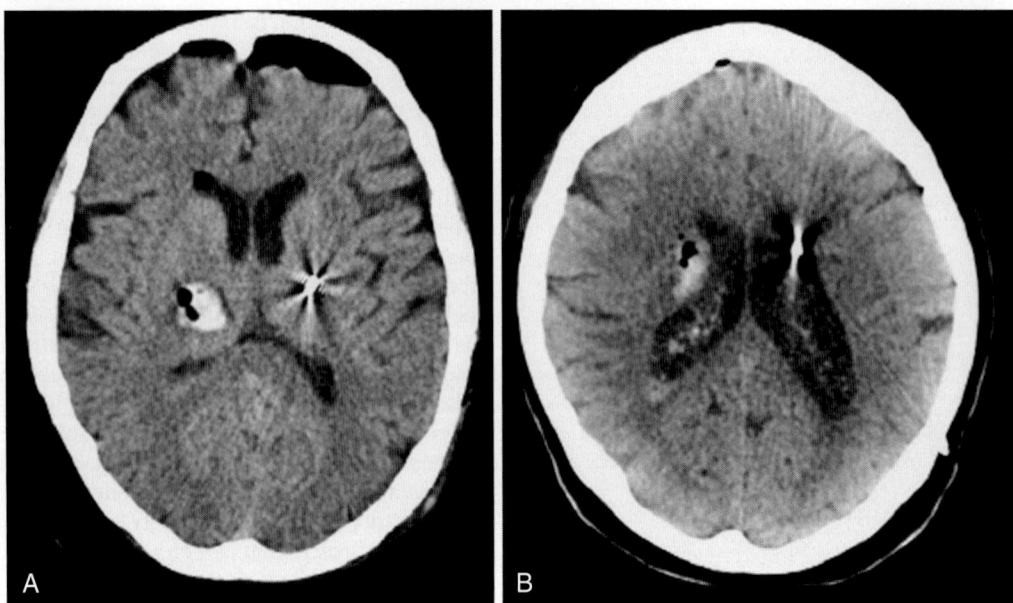

FIGURE 53.9 Axial noncontrast computed tomography (CT) scans showing intracerebral hemorrhage following placement of a deep brain stimulation (DBS) electrode. **A,** Thalamic hemorrhage at the target site. **B,** Periventricular hemorrhage with intraventricular extension. *(Reprinted with permission from Rezai AR, Machado AG, Deogaonkar M, et al. Surgery for movement disorders. Neurosurgery 2008;62(Suppl 2):809-838.)*

the IPG.[37] The risk of infection may be reduced by adhering strictly to aseptic principles during the procedure as well as the judicious use of prophylactic antibiotics. Treatment of the infection may require removal of the DBS hardware and use of appropriate antibiotics. For superficial incisional site infections in which there is no evidence of direct hardware involvement, the patient may be treated only with the exhibition of appropriate antibiotics without the need for hardware removal.

The hardware-related complications have an incidence between 2.7% and 5%, may develop over the long term, and include lead fractures, lead migration, and hardware erosion.[37] Lead migration and fracture may be prevented by placing the junction of the distal end of the DBS electrode wire and the proximal end of the extension wire (the connector) under the scalp and not in the cervical area where excessive motility of the head on the neck can tug and torque the leads and the connector, resulting in fractures. Wire fracture can usually be diagnosed with the use of x-rays. Hardware erosion may be prevented by utilizing low-profile hardware.

Complications related to stimulation are frequently reported, are usually transient, and may include paresthesias; manifestations of capsular stimulation include muscular contractions, dysphasias, and conjugate and disconjugate eye movements. These complications are linked to the target, surrounding structures, stimulation amplitude, and relative location of the electrode within the structure. For example, electrodes placed near the lateral border of the STN may stimulate the nearby internal capsule, leading to contralateral contractions. Emotional lability including acute onset of depression, euphoria, and bouts of laughter have been reported. Accurate location of the DBS electrodes and intraoperative macrostimulation to detect side effects is essential to reduce the incidence of these side effects and avoid the need for revision surgeries.

SPECIFIC DISORDERS: INDICATIONS AND EFFICACY

Movement Disorders

Parkinson's Disease

The spectrum of movement disorders treated with DBS includes PD, essential tremor, and dystonia. PD is a progressive neurodegenerative disorder classically described as loss of dopaminergic neurons in the substantia nigra. The cardinal features of PD are resting tremor, bradykinesia, rigidity, and postural instability. Replacement of dopamine via dopamine agonists and L-dopa is the mainstay of medical treatment. Patients over time tend to require escalating doses of dopamine equivalents to achieve therapeutic response, and these dose increases can be associated with motor fluctuations (on/off periods) as well as dyskinesias.[37,66-68] The circuitry implicated in the pathogenesis of PD is the direct and indirect dopaminergic pathways that begin with dopamine release in the substantia nigra and have downstream effects on the striatum, globus pallidus, subthalamic nucleus, and thalamocortical projections. The net result is hypokinesis resulting from a paucity of glutamatergic excitation from thalamocortical projections.

DBS can improve symptoms, especially those involving the extremities. In addition, DBS, of the STN in particular, can decrease the need for oral dopaminergic replacement, consequently improving dyskinesias.[65,69-72] A recent, randomized study showed that in patients under 75 years old with severe motor complications from advanced PD, STN DBS was more effective than medical management alone.[73] GPi stimulation is also effective in alleviating some of the motor symptoms of PD, and although some evidence suggests superiority of STN stimulation, other recent evidence suggests the results may be equivalent.[63] In 2010, a multicenter study of 299 patients suggested that the primary motor outcome following GPi or STN DBS was equivalent; however, patients undergoing STN stimulation had worse visuomotor processing scores and depression ratings than those undergoing GPi stimulation. However, there was a trend toward increased ICH in the GPi group, and this has been suggested by other studies, as described previously.[64,65]

With this in mind, there are several key points in determining if a patient with PD is a candidate for DBS. These determinants can be classified as factors related to ensuring a patient can tolerate surgery and improving the chances that a patient will achieve maximal therapeutic benefit from the procedure. The factors related to patient tolerance are both psychosocial and medical.

Regarding patient selection criteria, patients with classical PD, and not those with atypical parkinsonism, are candidates for DBS. Patients with progressive supranuclear palsy, Lewy body disease, and others do not respond well to and may even worsen after surgery.[74] A corollary to this is that positive response of symptoms to L-dopa predicts outcome and benefit from stereotactic procedures including DBS, according to most authors,[37,75,76] and this relationship was originally demonstrated in patients undergoing stereotactic pallidotomy.[77] A 30% improvement of the Unified Parkinson's Disease Rating Scale (Part III) score is a good indication of L-dopa responsiveness and is used as a cutoff point at our institution. An important exception to this is patients with tremor-predominant PD who still obtain good tremor control with STN DBS in spite of L-dopa unresponsiveness. Furthermore, surgical candidates tend to have one or more of the following features: troublesome dyskinesias and motor fluctuations despite optimal therapy, medication resistance, disabling tremor, freezing or rigidity, dystonia, or bradykinesia.

Surgery is more likely to improve symptoms involving the extremities than it does axial symptoms involving posture, balance, speech, and gait.[37]

Tremor

Essential tremor is a benign, common movement disorder with an estimated prevalence ranging from 0.4% to 5%.[78] It is characterized by a 4- to 12-Hz tremor that is generally postural or intention associated and disappears at rest. It is often familial, exacerbated by anxiety, and commonly improved with alcohol intake. Generally, tremor can be managed medically with propranolol, a β-adrenergic blocker, or primidone, an anticonvulsant.[79] In cases of disabling tremor despite optimal medical management, DBS of the VIM nucleus of the thalamus is a treatment option. Patients with distal, resting, or postural tremors of the upper extremities benefit most from surgery. Patients with intention tremor or tremors of the head, neck, voice, or lower extremities are more difficult to treat.[80] In general, distal tremors respond better than proximal tremors. Furthermore, patients with axial, head, voice, or neck tremors are more challenging to manage and often require bilateral DBS.[37] DBS for upper extremity tremor has excellent success rates, with reported ranges of 70% up to 90% of patients having significant resolution of the tremor.[79] In a prospective single-blind, randomized trial, DBS of the VIM nucleus of the thalamus was as effective for the suppression of drug-resistant tremor with fewer adverse effects than thalamotomy.[81] Again, DBS results are equivalent to those of lesioning procedures but with inherent reversibility of the side effect profile.

Dystonia

Dystonia represents a heterogeneous group of disorders characterized by sustained muscle contractions leading to twisting or repetitive movements and abnormal postures. Dystonias can be broadly categorized into four groups: primary dystonias, secondary dystonias, dystonia plus syndromes, and those associated with other degenerative neurological disorders (heredodegenerative dystonia).

Primary dystonias are syndromes in which no clear etiological factor is responsible for its onset, and the dystonia is the only clinical sign. These patients have normal brain imaging, no history of brain injury, and normal cerebrospinal fluid and other laboratory results. A subset of these patients have a mutation denoted *DYT-1*, which encodes the *TorsinA* gene. *TorsinA* is a member of the AAA family of adenosine triphosphatases (ATPases) and related to the CLP protease/heat shock protein family. It has been localized to the 9q34 locus and is expressed prominently in the substantia nigra pars compacta.[82] It is the most common mutation leading to childhood-onset primary dystonia, and although other mutations have been identified, they remain rare.[83]

Secondary dystonias represent a large, heterogeneous group of disorders in which the cause of the dystonia is secondary to other insults including drugs, stroke, tumors, trauma, perinatal anoxic injury, and infections. Dystonia plus syndromes are neurochemical, nondegenerative disorders associated with another movement disorder. These include dopa-responsive dystonia (Segawa syndrome), rapid onset dystonia-parkinsonism, and myoclonus dystonia syndrome. Finally, dystonias may be a part of a neurodegenerative disorder. These disorders include autosomal dominant disorders such as Huntington's disease, autosomal recessive disorders such as Wilson's disease and pantothenate kinase–associated neurodegeneration (PKAN), and other metabolic disorders including mitochondrial diseases and the X-linked recessive disorder Lesch-Nyhan syndrome.[83]

In addition, dysonias can be classified according to the distribution of affected body parts. Generalized dystonia, as the name implies, affects most body parts. Focal dystonia affects a single region of the body, as is the case in blepharospasm (eyes), writer's cramp, laryngeal or spasmodic dystonia, cranial dystonia (Meige syndrome), and cervical dystonia or torticollis. In segmental dystonia, two or more adjacent body parts are affected, such as in cranial-cervical dystonia, crural dystonia, or brachial dystonia.

The pharmacological therapies available for dystonia are somewhat limited; therefore, surgical alternatives have been developed that include both peripheral procedures including intrathecal baclofen pumps, botulinum toxin injections, and denervation procedures as well as central procedures including thalamotomy and DBS. Historically, thalamotomy was the surgical treatment of choice for dystonia; however, results are variable and DBS, as mentioned before, provides a reversible, controlled therapy relative to ablative procedures.[83]

Bilateral DBS of the GPi is the surgical treatment of choice for generalized dystonia, of both *DYT-1* and non-*DYT-1* subtypes.[37,83] Improvements in the 40% to 80% range of motor and disability scores of the Burke-Fahn-Marsden Dystonia Rating Scale (BFMRS) have been reported.[84-90] In 2005, the French Stimulation du Pallidum Interne dans la Dystonie

(SPIDY) Study Group published a study of 22 patients undergoing bilateral GPi DBS for primary, generalized dystonia. The BFMRS movement subscore improved from a mean 46.3 before surgery to 21.0 at 12 months. The disability subscore improved from 11.6 before surgery to 6.5 at 12 months. Similar results have been described in segmental dystonia as well.[83,85,90-93] A 2006 study from the Deep Brain Stimulation for Dystonia Study Group evaluated 40 patients with primary generalized or segmental dystonia undergoing GPi DBS, and these patients had an average 15.8-point improvement in the movement subscore of the BFMRS.

In generalized dystonias, predictors of good outcome include age of onset older than 5 years and lack of multiple orthopedic deformities.[94] Additionally, appendicular symptoms tend to be more responsive than axial symptoms.[95] Regarding focal dystonias, bilateral and unilateral GPi DBS has also shown some efficacy in the management of cervical dystonia, with improvements on the Toronto Western Spasmodic Rating Scale (TWSTRS) ranging from 40% to 60%.[88,95-97]

Clinical results in secondary dystonia are more disappointing. Tardive dystonia, however, is the exception to this rule, and these patients do derive benefit from DBS.[97-100] There is also a suggestion of benefit in postanoxic dystonia.[83] Finally, data are sparse, but DBS may have some role in the palliation of dystonia in neurodegenerative disorders including Lesch-Nyhan syndrome, PKAN, Hallervorden-Spatz disease, and Huntington's disease.[101-106]

Epilepsy

Despite advances in the medical management of epilepsy, a significant portion of patients remain refractory to maximal therapy. It is estimated that approximately 40% of newly diagnosed epilepsies are pharmacotherapy resistant. That is, approximately 47% of patients become seizure-free (no seizures for 1 year) after initiating a single antiepileptic drug (AED), and only an additional 13% become seizure-free after use of an additional agent.[107] This leaves approximately 40% of patients that may benefit from surgical evaluation. Traditionally, surgical management of epilepsy has centered on lesional or seizure focus resection, but in difficult-to-manage cases, neuromodulation therapies are finding a promising role. These therapies include cerebellar cortex stimulation, vagal nerve stimulation, and DBS of targets including the anterior nucleus (AN) of the thalamus, centromedian (CM) thalamus, STN, and hippocampus.

There is evidence that thalamocortical interactions are important in the development and propagation in various types of seizures.[108-112] Furthermore, the dorsomedian (DM) nucleus of the thalamus has been shown to be important in the propagation and maintenance of seizures, particularly in limbic epilepsy.[113,114] The AN, as part of the Papez circuit and limbic system, has afferent connections from the hippocampus and mammillary bodies via the mammillothalamic tract and has efferent projections to the cingulate cortex and parahippocampal cortex, which in turn connect widely to the neocortex.[115,116] Bilateral DBS of the AN recently was studied as a therapy for refractory epilepsy in the SANTE (stimulation of the anterior nucleus of the thalamus for epilepsy) trial.[117] In this multicenter, double-blind, sham-controlled, randomized

trial of 110 patients, subjects receiving stimulation experienced a median reduction in seizures of 56% at 2 years. A 50% responder rate was achieved in 54% of patients, and approximately one quarter of patients receiving stimulation were seizure-free. As a cautionary note, significant side effects of depression, confusion, and memory impairment were seen more commonly in the stimulation group.

Another intracranial stimulation paradigm, where electrical stimulation is automatically delivered to seizure foci, may also prove useful in the management of epilepsy. The NeuroPace RNS system is one such closed-loop system in which electrographic recordings from a patient's brain are continuously monitored, and stimulation is applied to seizure foci when they are detected. The results of a randomized, double-blind, sham-controlled trial of 191 patients indicated a mean reduction in disabling seizures of 29% compared to 14% in the sham group.[118]

CM thalamic nucleus stimulation has shown some promise in the management of refractory epilepsy as well. Results currently seem most promising in the management of Lennox-Gastaut syndrome, where an 80% seizure reduction was seen.[119] Chkhenkeli and colleagues reported a 40% to 80% reduction of seizure frequency with CM stimulation in patients with mesiotemporal epilepsy.[120] Other groups report mixed results. Fisher and co-workers, in a study with blinded and open trial arms, did not demonstrate a overall reduction in seizure frequency, except in generalized, tonic-clonic seizures, in a trial of CM thalamus stimulation.[121] Complications including lethargy, confusion, and anxiety have been reported,[122] and the safety profile of CM stimulation in large numbers of patients has yet to be established.[116]

Hippocampal stimulation seems to be an obvious option, and early results from several groups seem promising in the management of temporal lobe onset epilepsy, especially those without mesiotemporal sclerosis.[123-125] Stimulation of the STN is an appealing option because of its widespread use in the management of PD and its connections to the limbic system via the modulation of the substantia nigra, but results in open-label human trials have been mixed.[126,127]

Neuropsychiatric Disorders

Perhaps the most exciting new frontier of DBS is the management of neuropsychiatric disorders, namely, OCD and MDD. OCD and MDD are increasingly being considered as circuit-based or "network" problems, and therefore, attempts to modulate these networks have been the surgical goal in treatment of refractory cases. Although still in its early stages, DBS for OCD and MDD has made major advances in the past 15 years. Preliminary results suggest that DBS will become a mainstay in the management of treatment-resistant cases of these disorders in the near future.

Obsessive-Compulsive Disorder

OCD is characterized by intrusive thoughts (obsessions) and repetitive behaviors (compulsions) that significantly impact the lives of those afflicted. These obsessions and compulsions become time-consuming and impairing, leading patients to go to great lengths to avoid situations that provoke them. These behaviors are not desired or enjoyed by the patients, and are deleterious to social, scholastic, and occupational functioning. The prevalence in Western countries is approximately 2% of the population,[128] and OCD is initially managed with pharmacotherapy and cognitive behavioral therapy. OCD is managed with selective serotonin reuptake inhibitors (SSRIs) as a first line, then clomipramine, a tricyclic antidepressant (TCA), as a second line, and finally atypical antipsychotics to augment therapy.[129] Despite good response to pharmacotherapy in many patients, approximately 7% of patients are refractory to treatment.[130]

Although the details of the neurobiological basis of OCD have yet to be fully elucidated, much neuroimaging work has focused on the cortico-striato-thalamo-cortical circuitry. More specifically, some evidence points to dysfunction in the loops involving the orbitofrontal cortex (OFC), anterior cingulate cortex (ACC), and basal ganglia.[129] Specifically, the anterior limb of the internal capsule is the most widely used target for stimulation, and this consists of fiber tracts connecting the thalamus, frontal cortex, and basal ganglia.[131] In movement disorder physiology, the cortico-subcortical loop connects the dorsal basal ganglia to the ventrolateral thalamus. However, as described earlier, a parallel loop involving ventral striatopallidal structures to the mediodorsal thalamus is believed to be the key structure that links motor function to motivational and emotional inputs, and this is further suggested by the presence of limbic cortical inputs to the striatum.[62,132-134]

Historically, attempts to modulate or disrupt this aberrant circuitry have consisted of lesioning procedures including subcaudate tractotomy, anterior cingulotomy, limbic leucotomy, and anterior capsulotomy (see Fig. 53.3). Geoffrey Knight first introduced the subcaudate tractotomy in the treatment of movement disorders in the early 1960s,[135] and clinical improvement in about half of patients has been reported.[136,137] Ballantine reported on the use of anterior cingulotomy in the 1980s, with improvements in the range of 25% to 50%.[31,138] Limbic leucotomy was introduced by Kelly, which was in essence, a combination of anterior cingulotomy and subcaudate tractotomy. At 16 months in a series of 66, he reported significant improvements in 89% of patients.[139,140] Anterior capsulotomy was introduced by Talairach[32] and popularized by Leksell,[22] and large series indicate that nearly half of patients achieve at least a 50% reduction of symptoms, with most others having at least a 33% improvement in symptoms as determined on the Yale-Brown obsessive-compulsive scale (YBOCS).[141] Adverse effects for these procedures have similar profiles, with lethargy, confusion, transient incontinence, and personality changes being most common.[129]

The advent of DBS provides a reversible, nondestructive method to modulate these circuits. A series of patients undergoing bilateral stimulation of the ALIC was originally described by Nuttin and associates[52] in *The Lancet* in 1999. Six patients received stimulation with quadripolar electrodes, and four patients continued with stimulation for 21 months; three of the four patients achieved significant improvement of symptoms. Three-year follow-up of a multicenter study of eight patients with OCD demonstrated significant improvement in 75% of patients.[51] Hypomania was reported as an adverse event as was relapse of OCD symptoms with battery failure. STN stimulation has been attempted as well, and a 10-month, double-blind, crossover study published in 2008

demonstrated a mean reduction of symptoms of approximately 32% with active stimulation.[58] Transient psychiatric and motor symptoms as well as one parenchymal brain hemorrhage were reported as adverse events.

Major Depressive Disorder

MDD is a common, debilitating psychiatric disorder with an estimated lifetime prevalence of approximately 9.5%.[142] The primary medical treatment for MDD is SSRI medication, with other second-line antidepressant medications including monoamine oxidase (MAO) inhibitors, TCAs, and dual serotonin and norepinephrine reuptake inhibitors (SNRIs); however, up to a third of patients do not respond to any of these medications.[143] The current neurocircuitry model of depression is based on neuroimaging studies that demonstrate abnormalities in regional metabolic brain activity that normalizes with successful treatment. Frontal abnormalities are most reproducibly found, including abnormalities in metabolism of the dorsolateral and ventrolateral prefrontal cortex, orbitofrontal cortex, and ventromedial frontal cortex. Anterior and subgenual cortical changes are also seen, in particular, changes in Brodmann areas (BA) 24 and 25.[144]

Similar to OCD, limbic leucotomy, anterior capsulotomy, cingulotomy, and subcaudate tractotomy have all been used to treat depression. Results were promising, with initial responder rates of around 67% for the procedures.[145] Again, DBS provides an attractive option due to its nondestructive, reversible nature. Stimulation of the SCC has been described originally by Mayberg and co-workers in six patients,[55] and then in a larger study of 20 patients out of Toronto.[54] Approximately two thirds of patients in these studies had improvement of their MDD symptoms, and 35% of patients in the Toronto study have had resolution of symptoms.

Stimulation of the ALIC has also improved depressive symptoms in patients with comorbid OCD, as described by Greenberg and colleagues, who reported that four of the eight patients with comorbid MDD experienced improvements in mood and affect.[51] The ventral striatum and nucleus accumbens target may also prove to be valuable. The nucleus accumbens projects to the limbic brain areas including the SCC, and as we will describe later, there may be farther-reaching, expanding indications with stimulation of this target in the management of addiction and disorders of brain reward circuitry. A recent study of 15 patients with stimulation of the VC/VS by Malone and colleagues demonstrated a 50% responder rate and 20% remission rate.[61]

EMERGING INDICATIONS

Tourette's Syndrome

The inherent ability of DBS to modulate neurobehavioral circuitry has opened the door for treatment of a number of otherwise intractable disorders. Tourette's syndrome (TS) is characterized by chronic vocal and motor tics that have their onset typically in early school age and is often comorbid with attention-deficit hyperactivity disorder or OCD. TS is thought to affect 0.7% to 4.2% of individuals, though symptom severity typically lessens in adulthood.[146]

Vocal tics include coughing, clearing one's throat, and coprolalia. Motor tics include blinking, grimacing, snapping, or movements of the face. These movements or gestures tend to resemble coordinated or repetitive fragments of normal behaviors. Tics are exacerbated by stress, fatigue, and boredom and are often present during sleep.[146] Owing to the nature of tics, they can be disabling from a social, occupational, and overall functioning standpoint if they do not abate in adulthood.

It is thought that disruptions in CSPTC circuits mediate the behavioral disturbances in TS.[147-149] Neuroimaging studies suggest abnormalities in the metabolism of the ventral striatum in TS.[150] With this in mind, DBS may have efficacy in treatment of TS. Several reports indicate that both thalamic stimulation and stimulation of the GPi are effective in the reduction of tics.[151-166]

Disorders of Consciousness and Cognition

In 2007, Schiff and associates reported on the use of bilateral thalamic DBS in the management of a 38-year-old patient in a minimally conscious state (MCS).[167] This patient had a severe traumatic brain injury (TBI) leading to inability to communicate or follow commands consistently over 6 years following his injury; however, MRI demonstrated preservation of bihemispheric language networks, but thalamic and midbrain injury. Bilateral DBS was targeted to the anterior interlaminar thalamic nuclei and paralaminar regions of the association nuclei, as these regions had maximal concentrations of calbindin-positive neurons that have projections to supragranular cortical regions and are believed to play a role in arousal. The patient had significant improvements in arousal, limb control, and oral feeding in the DBS on versus off state. Some results in larger trials have been mixed, however. For example, circa 1990, Medtronic initiated a trial for implantation of DBS into vegetative state (VS) patients. These patients received bilateral CM thalamus or cervical spinal cord dorsal columns in patients in a VS. Although some centers reported significant functional improvement,[168,169] this result was not consistently identified.[168,170,171] Some of the reasons for the mixed results may be that the group of patients enrolled were heterogeneous in terms of their injuries; that is, patients with widespread cortical or subcortical damage may have less potential for recovery than patients with intact networks and central arousal deficits.[172] Clearly, careful patient selection and further trials must be done to determine the role in patients with TBI and disorders of consciousness.

DBS may find a role in the near future in the management of dementias. The group of Lozano reported on a patient who, during stimulation of the hypothalamus for obesity, began having autobiographical memories.[173] This finding led to a phase 1 trial evaluating forniceal/hypothalamic DBS in the treatment of Alzheimer's disease. The study suggested the potential slowing of cognitive decline in their cohort,[174] opening the door to more research in this realm.

Addiction and Eating Disorders

Dysfunction in the reward circuitry underlying eating disorders and addiction is quickly becoming a target for DBS. Over 30 years ago, Quaade and co-workers stereotactically

TABLE 53.3 Evidence-Based Medicine Summary of Clinical Results for Deep Brain Stimulation (DBS) Surgery

Evidence Class	Findings
1	DBS of the STN and GPi is effective in the management of the motor symptoms of PD.[63,65,73] Bilateral GPi stimulation is effective in the treatment of primary generalized or segmental dystonia.[84,85] DBS of the VIM nucleus of the thalamus is effective for the suppression of drug-resistant tremor with fewer adverse effects than with thalamotomy.[81] Bilateral DBS of the AN of the thalamus reduces seizure frequency in medically resistant epilepsy.[117]
2	DBS of the ALIC, VC/VS, NAc ameliorates the symptoms of OCD.[50,51,184,185] DBS of the STN treats the symptoms of OCD.[58] DBS of the subgenual cingulate gyrus can reduce the symptoms of treatment-resistant depression.[54,55] DBS of the VC/VS can be effective in the management of treatment-resistant depression.[61]
3	DBS of the bilateral thalamus reduces motor and sonic tics in treatment-refractory Tourette's syndrome.[158,162]

ALIC, anterior limb of the internal capsule; AN, anterior nucleus; GPi, globus pallidus interna; MCP, midcommissural point; NAc, nucleus accumbens; OCD, obsessive-compulsive disorder; PD, Parkinson's disease; STN, subthalamic nucleus; VC/VS, ventral capsule/ventral striatum; VIM, ventralis intermedius.

electrocoagulated portions of the lateral hypothalamus and safely achieved some weight reduction in three patients.[175] Furthermore, animal studies have identified the lateral hypothalamus (LH), ventromedial hypothalamus (VMH), and NAc as potential targets for managing obesity.[176] The NAc has overlaps in circuitry with the lateral hypothalamus and may be involved in food reward circuitry. Furthermore, the central role of the NAc in reward circuitry makes it an attractive target in treating addiction. Rat studies suggest that DBS of the NAc may ameliorate cocaine addiction.[177] Preliminary studies in humans undergoing DBS of the NAc for other disorders (including Tourette's syndrome and OCD) indicate that smoking cessation may be more feasible with NAc stimulation.[178] A group from the Netherlands recently reported NAc stimulation in a single patient leading to both smoking cessation and weight loss.[179] DBS of the bilateral NAc was also reported to reduce alcohol dependency in a patient undergoing the procedure for an anxiety disorder.[180] On the flip side, DBS of the NAc/ventral striatum or subgenual cingulate cortex may show promise in the management of anorexia nervosa.[181,182] With regard to eating disorders, some early results suggest DBS may be effective in the management of anorexia nervosa.[181,182]

CONCLUSION (TABLE 53.3)

DBS has transformed the management of more than 80,000 advanced and medication refractory patients with movement disorders. DBS is now being explored for the emerging indications in the management of neurobehavioral and neuropsychiatric disorders,[183-185] epilepsy, obesity, Alzheimer's disease, anorexia, traumatic brain injury, and disorders of consciousness. These emerging indications are enhanced by the intrinsic advantages of reversibility and adjustability of DBS, compared to stereotactic lesioning procedures. Efforts at expanding the clinical utility of DBS must, however, be tempered by ethical considerations and the need for rigorous scientific and evidence-based evaluations of these interventions.

SELECTED KEY REFERENCES

Deuschl G, Schade-Brittinger C, Krack P, et al. A randomized trial of deep-brain stimulation for Parkinson's disease. *N Engl J Med.* 2006;355(9):896-908.

Follett KA, Weaver FM, Stern M, et al. Pallidal versus subthalamic deep-brain stimulation for Parkinson's disease. *N Engl J Med.* 2010;362:2077-2091.

Greenberg BD, Gabriels LA, Malone Jr DA, et al. Deep brain stimulation of the ventral internal capsule/ventral striatum for obsessive-compulsive disorder: worldwide experience. *Mol Psychiatry.* 2008.

Kopell BH, Greenberg BD. Anatomy and physiology of the basal ganglia: implications for DBS in psychiatry. *Neurosci Biobehav Rev.* 2008;32(3):408-422.

Lozano AM, Mayberg HS, Giacobbe P, et al. Subcallosal cingulate gyrus deep brain stimulation for treatment-resistant depression. *Biol Psychiatry.* 2008;64(6):461-467.

Rezai AR, Machado AG, Deogaonkar M, et al. Surgery for movement disorders. *Neurosurgery.* 2008;62(Suppl 2):809-838:discussion 809-838.

Schuurman PR, Bosch DA, Bossuyt PM, et al. A comparison of continuous thalamic stimulation and thalamotomy for suppression of severe tremor. *N Engl J Med.* 2000;342:461-468.

Vidailhet M, Vercueil L, Houeto JL, et al. Bilateral deep-brain stimulation of the globus pallidus in primary generalized dystonia. *N Engl J Med.* 2005;352:459-467.

Please go to expertconsult.com to view the complete list of references.

Index

A

A (plateau) waves, 315–316, 316f
AAD. *See* Atlantoaxial dislocation
Abbas, Haly, 9–10
Abdominal cutaneous reflex, 39–40
Abducens nerve (cranial nerve VI), 41–43
Abernethy, John, 24
The Abnormal Encephalogram (Davidoff and Epstein), 34
Acetazolamide, 115
Acetylcholine, 510
Achondroplasias, 3, 5f
Acoustic nerve (cranial nerve VIII), 44, 586, 587f
ACR Appropriateness Criteria, 53
Acromegaly, 632–634, 632f
Addiction, 794
Adenohyposeal cells, 623
Adenomas, pituitary
  adrenocorticotropic hormone-secreting, 635f–637f, 635, 638t
  anterior skull base approach for, 668–669
  classification of, 623–624
  epidemiology of, 623
  functioning, 628–643, 628f–629f
  glycoprotein-secreting, 641f, 642
  growth hormone-secreting, 630–634, 631f–632f
  nonfunctioning, 624–628, 625f
  overview, 623, 644
  pediatric, 643
  pituitary apoplexy and, 643
  stereotactic radiosurgery for, 709–710
Adenomectomy, 621, 625–626, 626f, 633, 643
Adie's pupil, 41–42
Adjuvant therapy, for low-grade gliomas, 532
Adrenalectomy, 641
Adrenocorticotropic hormone-secreting adenomas, 621, 635, 635f–637f, 638t
Adult spinal deformity (ASD)
  alignment goals in treatment of, 505–506
  classification of, 504–505, 506t
  overview of, 503, 507
  predicting surgical outcomes and, 506–507, 507t
  radiographic evaluation of, 503–504, 504f, 505t
Africanus, Constantinus, 11, 12f
Airway management, 332, 373
ALARA (as low as reasonably achievable) principle, 55
Albucasis, 10–11, 11f
Alcohol consumption, hemorrhagic stroke and, 259
Alcohol injection, 743
American College of Radiology (ACR), 53
Aminoglutethimide, 640
Amygdalohippocampectomy, selective, 769
Analgesics, 344, 443, 754–755

Anatomiae (Dryander), 15–16
Ancillary diagnostic tests, 49–51, 50t
Anderson and D'Alonzo classification, 405–407, 406t, 407f
Anesthesia, history of neurosurgery and, 25
Aneurysm coils, 276–284
Aneurysms. *See also* Giant transitional internal carotid artery aneurysms; Subarachnoid hemorrhage
  arteriovenous malformations and, 239
  headaches and, 51
  hemorrhagic stroke and, 259–261, 260f
  intracranial
    clinical presentation of, 212–214, 212f
    endovascular neurosurgery for, 276–284
    epidemiology of, 210, 210t
    natural history of, 211–212, 212b
    overview of, 209, 228
    pathogenesis of, 210–211, 211f
    treatment of, 215–228, 276–284
  intranidal, 239
ANG. *See* Angiopoietins
Angiogenesis, 235, 235t
Angiography. *See also* Computed tomographic angiography
  for arteriovenous malformations, 231
  cerebral, 199–200, 200f
  cerebral tumors and, 51
  contrast-enhanced, 56
  digital subtraction, 54, 199–200
  magnetic resonance, 55, 67–70, 71f
  for meningiomas, 542
  moyamoya syndrome and, 191
  overview of, 50
  for penetrating brain injuries, 359–360, 362b, 362f–363f
  phase contrast, 55–56
  for subarachnoid hemorrhage, 215–216, 216f
  time-of-flight magnetic resonance, 67, 69–70, 71f
  traumatic brain injury and, 337
Angioplasty, carotid with stenting, 274–276
Angiopoietins (ANG), 236
Antagonism, da Vinci and, 14
Antegrade flow, 516
Anterior chiasmatic syndrome of Traquair, 49, 49f
Anterior clinoidal meningiomas, 551–552
Anterior communicating artery aneurysms, 223–224, 224f
Anterior cord syndrome, 452–453, 452f
Anterior plagiocephaly, 150–152, 150f–151f
Anterior sacral meningocele, overview of, 100, 100f–101f
Anterior spinal artery syndrome, 45
Anterolateral cordotomy (AC), overview, 740–741
Anticoagulation therapy, hemorrhagic stroke and, 259, 263
Anticonvulsants, 344, 732–733
Antiplatelet therapy, 201–202, 266
Antisepsis, history of neurosurgery and, 25

Page numbers followed by "*b*" indicate boxes; "*f*" figures; "*t*" tables.

797

Decompression *(Continued)*
    for syringomyelia, 466–467, 469
    transoral, 479, 483
    for trigeminal neuralgia, 734–735, 734f, 745–746
Decompressive hemicraniotomy, 318–319, 319f
Deep brain stimulation (DBS)
    for addiction and eating disorders, 794
    for disorders of consciousness and cognition, 794
    for dystonias, 791–792
    for epilepsy, 792
    for essential tremor, 791
    history of, 783–786, 784f–785f
    for major depressive disorder, 793
    for mesial temporal lobe epilepsy, 770
    for obsessive-compulsive disorder, 792–793
    overview of, 746–749, 748f, 794–795, 794t
    for Parkinson's disease, 790–791
    principles of, 785–786, 786f
    sitting position and, 83
    surgery
        complications of, 789–790
        indications, target, and outcomes of, 786–787, 787t
        preoperative imaging and planning for, 787, 787t
        procedure overview, 787–789
    for Tourette's syndrome, 793–794
Deep venous thrombosis (DVT), 214, 342–343
Degenerative arthritis, 481–483
Degenerative spine disease. *See* Spine, degenerative disease of
Delayed ischemic neurological deficit, 286–287
Della Torre, Marcantonio, 14
Demyelination, 448
Denis three-column classification system, 415–416, 415f
Dermoid cysts
    overview of, 599f, 613–614
    of posterior fossa, 131–134, 132f–133f, 169, 180–181
Descartes, René, 784
Dexamethasone suppression tests (DST), 636–638
Diabetes, 517, 627
Diastematomyelia, 98–100, 99f, 455–456, 459f
Dickman modification to Jefferson classification system, 405, 406f
Diffuse (axonal) brain injuries, 328, 329f, 330
Diffuse intrinsic pontine gliomas (DIPG), 170, 182–183
Diffusion tensor imaging, 73, 654–655
Diffusion-weighted imaging (DWI)
    of low-grade gliomas, 530
    of metastatic brain tumors, 536
    overview of, 67
    of posterior fossa and brainstem tumors, 171
Digital subtraction angiography (DSA), 54, 199–200
Dilantin, 344, 732–733
DIPG. *See* Diffuse intrinsic pontine gliomas
Diplopia, clinical evaluation of, 49
Direct feeders, arteriovenous malformations and, 231–232
Diskectomy, 492–493, 493f
Diskography, 490–491
Disks, degeneration of, 488
Distraction osteogenesis, 143
DNET. *See* Dysembryoplastic neuroepithelial tumors
Dolichocephaly (sagittal synostosis), 138f, 146–150, 147f–149f
Dopamine, 629–630
Dopamine agonists, 630, 634

Dorsal decompression, 413, 418
Dorsal rhizotomy, selective, 738, 757, 761–763, 762f, 762t
Dorsal root entry zone (DREZ), lesions of, 738–740, 739f
Dorsally exophytic brainstem tumors, 184
Double crush syndrome, 517
Double insurance method of atlantoaxial fixation, 473f, 475
Double strand breaks, 699
Drag, 354
Drainage, venous, 232–233
DREZ. *See* Dorsal root entry zone
Drug use, stroke and, 189, 259
Dryander, Johannes, 15–16, 16f
DSA. *See* Digital subtraction angiography
DST. *See* Dexamethasone suppression tests
DTI tractography. *See* Tractography
Dural arteriovenous fistulas (dAVF)
    classification of, 723b
    embolization of, 286–287
    overview of, 229–230, 244–246, 245t, 246f
    stereotactic radiosurgery for, 723–724
Duraplasty grafts, 465
DWI. *See* Diffusion-weighted imaging
Dyke, Cornelius, 34
Dynamic contrast-enhanced (DCE) magnetic resonance perfusion, 70
Dynamic susceptibility contrast (DSC) method, 70
Dysdiadochokinesia, cerebellar dysfunction and, 44–45
Dysembryoplastic neuroepithelial tumors (DNET), 766
Dyslipoproteinemias, pediatric ischemic stroke and, 188
Dysmetria, cerebellar dysfunction and, 44–45
Dysnomia center, 38
Dysphasias, 38, 39t
Dystonias, 791–792

E

Eating disorders, 794
Ebers papyrus, 3–4
EC-IC bypass. *See* Extracranial-intracranial bypass
Edema, cerebral, 59–60, 320–321, 320t
EDH. *See* Epidural hemorrhage
Edwin Smith papyrus, 3–4, 5f
Effendi classification, 407–408, 407f
Egypt, history of neurosurgery and, 3–4
Eichmann, Johann, 15–16, 16f
Eisenhardt, Louise, 541
Elastance, overview of, 311
Electrocorticography, intraoperative, 769–770
Electromyography (EMG), 50–51, 463
Elsberg, Charles, 33–34, 34f
EMA staining. *See* Epithelial membrane antigen staining
Embolic agents, 240–241, 287
Embolic protection devices, 268
Embolism, stroke and, 260
Embolization
    for arteriovenous malformations, 240–242, 285–287
    of arteriovenous malformations, 720–721
    balloon-assisted coil, 276–277, 277f, 279–280
    balloon-assisted onyx, 267, 277–278
    preoperative in meningioma treatment, 544–545
    of tumors, 287–288
Embryonal carcinoma, 571
Embryonic period, 3–4

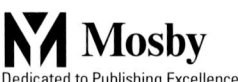
Mosby
Dedicated to Publishing Excellence

Editor: Laurel Craven
Developmental Editor: Dana Battaglia
Project Manager: Linda Clarke
Project Supervisor: Vicki Hoenigke
Interior Design: Sheilah Barrett
Cover Design: Annette Melvin

Printed in the United States of America
Composition by the Clarinda Company
Printing/binding by Walsworth

Mosby–Year Book, Inc.
11830 Westline Industrial Drive
St. Louis, MO 63146

ISBN 0-8151-7513-2

95 96 97 98 99 / 9 8 7 6 5 4 3 2 1

Corneal Laser Surgery

Editor

James J. Salz, M.D.
Clinical Professor of Ophthalmology
University of Southern California
Beverly Hills Eye Medical Group, Inc.
Los Angeles, California

Associate Editors

Peter J. McDonnell, M.D.
Associate Professor of Ophthalmology
University of Southern California
School of Medicine
Doheny Eye Institute
Los Angeles, California

Marguerite B. McDonald, M.D., F.A.C.S.
Director of the Refractive Surgery Center of the South,
at the Eye, Ear, Nose, and Throat Hospital
Clinical Professor of Ophthalmology
Tulane University
New Orleans, Louisiana

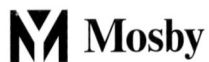 Mosby

St. Louis Baltimore Berlin Boston Carlsbad Chicago London Madrid

Naples New York Philadelphia Sydney Tokyo Toronto

To my loving wife Judy and my children, Jim, Mark, Heather, and Elisabeth for their constant encouragement despite my frequent absences related to refractive surgery.

And also to my loyal friends and colleagues in the International Society of Refractive Keratoplasty, especially Rick Villasenor, Perry Binder, Cas Swinger, Miles Friedlander, Larry Rich, Dick Lindstrom, George Waring, Jeff Robin, Ted Werblin, Peter McDonnell, and Marguerite McDonald who have all supported and inspired me over the past 14 years.

Preface

Marguerite McDonald's honorary Barraquer lecture at the Annual International Society of Refractive Keratoplasty section during the 1993 American Academy of Ophthalmology meeting in Chicago was entitled, "Refractive Surgery Comes of Age." During the 1980s we witnessed tremendous improvements in the technique of cataract surgery. These improvements were the results of a fortuitous combination of individual surgeon's ingenuity (capsulorehexis, nuclear fracture techniques) combined with dramatic improvements in instrumentation (phacoemulsification machines with exquisite control capabilities), and improvements in intraocular lens designs (foldables and one-piece lenses).

The 1980s was truly the decade of cataract surgery. While cataract surgery was maturing, refractive surgery was struggling for acceptance. The concept of operating on a perfectly normal cornea merely to eliminate the need for glasses was considered by many to be irresponsible. For the most part, refractive surgery in the 1980s was radial keratotomy, performed by a small percentage of ophthalmologists under heavy criticism by the majority. There were only minimal improvements in instrumentation and technique and the procedure never really captured the attention of the general public because it was always felt to be "controversial."

All this is about to change because of the determined efforts of Herbert Kaufman, M.D., Marguerite McDonald, M.D., at LSU, Theo Seiler, M.D., in Germany, and John Marshall, M.D., in England and their loyal, hard-working colleagues. The idea of safely changing corneal curvature with the unique laser envisioned by Stephen Trokel, M.D., Francis L'Esperance, M.D., and Charles Munnerlyn, Ph.D., has become a reality. The concept of precisely changing the curvature with laser energy has captured the imagination of both ophthalmologists and the general public throughout the world.

Despite the disadvantages of dealing with an extremely complicated and expensive technology, it is estimated that over 100,000 patients have undergone Excimer laser photorefractive keratectomy at over 500 worldwide sites. There are now at least six companies manufacturing excimer lasers (Summit, Medetec, Nidek, VISX, Technolos, and Schwind): in addition, several other companies are developing alternative laser systems for both surface ablations and intrastromal procedures. These include Sunrise, Intelligent Laser Systems, Lasersight, Novatec, and the Summit Holmium module. The 1990s are expected to be the "Decade of Refractive Surgery."

The purpose of this book is to assemble the latest information about the rapidly evolving field of corneal laser surgery from a worldwide panel of pioneers in the field. By providing an authorative textbook, a teaching set of 35-mm slides, and an informational video to be used for patient education, the publishers and contributors to this collaborative effort hope to enable ophthalmologists to become knowledgeable about corneal laser surgery and to allow them to educate their patients about what may prove to be one of the most exciting developments in the history of ophthalmology.

I would like to take this opportunity to thank all of the contributors to this textbook for their efforts and for their timely adherence to the tight publishing deadlines.

James J. Salz, M.D.

Foreword

Dr. James J. Salz's idea of publishing this excellent book on the ablative applications of laser beam to the cornea comes just at the right moment. Given the broad base of experience acquired by a substantial number of researchers, there is an increased demand by patients and ophthalmologists to provide surgical treatment for ametropias in order to curtail physical and psychological impairment in those individuals who do not tolerate prosthetic correction.

This text will also serve to instruct new ophthalmologists, not only concerning the physics and tissue interactions of laser, but also in mathematical and pathophysiological principles of subtraction lamellar refractive surgery, "Keratomileusis," and algorithms for controlling the ablative emission, and the non-empirical calculation of the resection required for correcting any given ametropia. This knowledge will make new ophthalmologists masters in the area and not merely technicians who push buttons to perform the operation.

In 1948, while performing a lamellar keratoplasty of 11 mm in diameter in a patient with a large keratoconus, I observed the change in curvature throughout the corneal surface as well as the resultant change in refraction. Several similar experiences led me to establish the concept of corneal flattening to correct myopia and of corneal steepening to correct hypermetropia.

In 1949 I published a paper under the title of Refractive Keratoplasty explaining the concept of surgical correction of spherical ametropias and several methods to achieve this goal. I suppose I attached some importance and significance to the idea, since the paper was published in English, French, Spanish, and German. Although the original idea initially flashed through my mind, it took me 13 years of experimentation with various animal models before developing the concept of Keratomileusis and the Law of Thickness.

Today, this Law continues to apply to all subtraction laminar techniques, whether they are performed using a lathe, a microkeratome, a laser beam or any other method yet to be developed. Thus, the Law is applied in all instances of myopic or hypermetropic corrections, either superficial or intrastromal.

It is worth noting that, today, the modification of the corneal power is accomplished only in the central zone (Zo). This may give rise, and occasionally does, to visual distortions, especially in night vision. The ideal technique would be to modify the entire corneal surface as I proposed initially, possibly using methods which failed years ago (Ring Resection for myopia and Keratomiosis for hypermetropia).

I hope that the collaborative effort of many ophthalmologists will eventually bring about the degree of perfection that we all desire for our patients.

Prof. Jose I. Barraquer, M.D.

Contributors

Adrian A. Abarca, MD
Monterrey, Mexico

Dimitri T. Azar, MD
Assistant Professor
Department of Ophthalmology
Wilmer Institute
Johns Hopkins University Hospital
Baltimore, Maryland

Michael J. Berry, MD
Sunrise Technologies
Fremont, California

Perry S. Binder, MD
President, National Vision Research Institute
Associate Clinical Professor
Department of Ophthalmology
University of California, San Diego
San Diego, California

Stephen Brint, MD
Clinical Faculty
Tulane Medical Center
Department of Ophthalmology
Eye Surgery Center of Louisiana
New Orleans, Louisiana

Mauros Campos, MD
Professor
Department of Ophthalmology
Baulista School of Medicine
San Paolo, Brazil

Timothy B. Cavanaugh, MD
Director Corneal Services
Ophthalmology
Hunkeler Eye Clinic
Kansas City, Missouri

Jan Daniel, MD
Emory University School of Medicine
Atlanta, Georgia

Dieter Dausch, MD
Professor
Department of Ophthalmology
Marienhospital Amberg
Amberg, Germany

Daniel S. Durrie, MD
Director, Refractive Surgery Program
Hunkeler Eye Clinic
Kansas City, Missouri

Akef El-Maghraby, MD
President and Medical Director
El-Maghraby Eye Hospital
Jeddah, Saudi Arabia

Daniel Epstein, MD, PhD
Department of Ophthalmology
University Hospital
Uppsala, Sweden

Per Fagerholm, MD
St. Eriks Eye Hospital
Karolinska Institute
Stockholm, Sweden

Bradley D. Fouraker, MD
Assistant Professor of Ophthalmology
Department of Ophthalmology/Corneal and
    External Diseases and Refractive Surgery
University of South Florida
Tampa, Florida

Howard V. Gimbel, MD, HPH, FRCSC, FAAO
Chief Surgeon and Medical Director
Gimbel Eye Centre
Assistant Clinical Professor
University of Calgary, Alberta
Calgary, Alberta, Canada

David T. Gubman, OD
Hunkeler Eye Clinic
4321 Washington, Suite 6000
Kansas City, Missouri 64111

Elizabeth A. Haft, BS
Baylor College of Medicine
Houston, Texas

Helen Hamberg-Nystrom, MD
St. Eriks Eye Hospital
Karolinska Institute
Stockholm, Sweden

David R. Hardten, MD
Attending Surgeon
Phillips Eye Institute
Clinical Instructor of Ophthalmology
University of Minnesota
Minneapolis, Minnesota
Staff Physician
Department of Ophthalmology
St. Paul-Ramsey Medical Center
St. Paul, Minnesota

Joy Heitzman, PhD
Mericos Eye Institute
Scripps Memorial Hospital
La Jolla, California

Sandeep Jain, MD
Cornea Fellow
The Wilmer Ophthalmological Institute
The Johns Hopkins University
Baltimore, Maryland

Barry Kassar, MD, FACS
Medical Director
Mericos Eye Institute
Scripps Memorial Hospital
La Jolla, California

Shigeru Kinoshita, MD
Professor and Chairman
Department of Ophthalmology
Kyoto Prefectural University of Medicine
Kyoto, Japan

Craig Kliger, MD
Cornea Fellow
Jules Stein Eye Institute
University of California, Los Angeles
Los Angeles, California

Steven D. Klyce, MD
Professor of Ophthalmology
Louisiana State University School of Medicine
New Orleans, Louisiana

Douglas D. Koch, MD
Associate Professor of Ophthalmology
Director, Residency Training Program
Department of Ophthalmology
Cullen Eye Institute
Baylor College of Medicine
Houston, Texas

Ronald R. Krueger, MD
Assistant Professor of Ophthalmology
Anheuser-Busch Eye Institute
St. Louis University School of Medicine
St. Louis, Missouri

Shui T. Lai, MD
President, Novatec Laser Systems, Inc.
Carlsbad, California

Monika Landesz, MD
Department of Ophthalmology
University Hospital
University of Groningen
Groningen, The Netherlands

Richard L. Lindstrom, MD
Medical Director
Phillips Eye Institute Center for Teaching and
    Research
Minneapolis, Minnesota

Jeffery J. Machat, MD, FRCS(C), DABO
Medical Director
The Laser Center
Windsor, Ontario, Canada

Jonathan I. Macy, MD
Assistant Clinical Professor
Department of Ophthalmology
University of California, Los Angeles
Assistant Clinical Professor
Department of Ophthalmology
University of Southern California School of
    Medicine
Los Angeles, California

Ezra Maguen, MD, FACS, FICS
Senior Research Associate
Ophthalmology
Research Laboratories
Cedars Sinai Medical Center
Associate Clinical Professor of Ophthalmology
Jules Stein Eye Institute
University of California, Los Angeles School of
    Medicine
Los Angeles, California

Robert K. Maloney, MD
Assistant Professor
Department of Ophthalmology
Jules Stein Eye Institute
University of California, Los Angeles
Los Angeles, California

Marguerite B. McDonald, MD, FACS
Director of the Refractive Surgery Center of
   the South, at the Eye, Ear, Nose and Throat
   Hospital
Clinical Professor of Ophthalmology
Tulane University
New Orleans, Louisiana

Peter J. McDonnell, MD
Associate Professor of Ophthalmology
University of Southern California School of
   Medicine
Doheny Eye Institute
Los Angeles, California

Anthony B. Nesburn, MD, FACS
Clinical Professor of Ophthalmology
Ophthalmology Research/Surgery
Cedars-Sinai Medical Center
Los Angeles, California

J. James Rowsey, MD
Professor and Chairman
Department of Ophthalmology
University of South Florida
Tampa, Florida

Luis Ruiz, MD
Director Centro Oftalmologico Colombiano
Centro Oftalmologico Colombiano
Santa Fe de Fofota, D.C. Colombia

Tarek Salah, MD
Refractive Surgery
Refractive Surgery Consultant
El-Maghraby Eye Hospital
Jeddah, Saudi Arabia

James J. Salz, MD
Clinical Professor of Ophthalmology
University of Southern California
Beverly Hills Eye Medical Group, Inc.
Los Angeles, California

Donald R. Sanders, M.D.
Associate Professor
Department of Ophthalmology
University of Illinois at Chicago
Chicago, Illinois

Heike Schmidt-Peterson, MD
Oberarztin
Universitatsaugenklinik
Tu Dresden, Medizinische Fakultat
Dresden, Germany

D. James Schumer, MD
Corneal Refractive Surgery
Ohio Eye Associates
Mansfield, Ohio

Theo Seiler, MD, PhD
Universitatsaugenklinik
Tu Dresden, Medizinische Fakultat
Dresden, Germany

Neal A. Sher, MD, FACS
Attending Surgeon
Phillips Eye Institute
Clinical Associate Professor
Department of Ophthalmology
University of Minnesota Medical School
Minneapolis, Minnesota

Stephen G. Slade, MD
Clinical Faculty
University of Texas Medical Center-Houston
Hermann Eye Center
Houston, Texas

Walter Stark, MD
Professor
Department of Ophthalmology
The Wilmer Eye Institute
John Hopkins University
Baltimore, Maryland

Roger F. Steinert, MD
Assistant Clinical Professor
Harvard Medical School
Associate Surgeon
Massachusetts Eye & Ear Infirmary
Boston, Massachusetts

Scott X. Stevens, MD
Associate Professor of Ophthalmology
Department of Ophthalmology
University of South Florida
Tampa, Florida

R. Doyle Stulting, MD
Professor of Ophthalmology
Emory University School of Medicine
Atlanta, Georgia

Casimir A. Swinger, MD
Assistant Clinical Professor of Ophthalmology
Mount Sinai School of Medicine
Associate Attending Surgeon
Manhattan Eye, Ear and Throat Hospital
New York, New York

Jonathan H. Talamo, MD
Acting Director, Cornea Service
Director, Keratorefractive Surgery Unit
Massachusetts Eye and Ear Infirmary
Harvard Medical School
Boston, Massachusetts

Björn Tengroth, MD
St. Eriks Eye Hospital
Karolinska Institute
Stockholm, Sweden

Keith P. Thompson, MD
Assistant Professor of Ophthalmology
Emory University School of Medicine
Atlanta, Georgia

Vance Thompson, MD
Associate Professor of Ophthalmology
University of South Dakota School of Medicine
Director of Refractive Surgery
Department of Ophthalmology
Sioux Valley Hospital
Sioux Falls, South Dakota

Stephen J. Trokel, MD
Professor of Clinical Ophthalmology
Columbia University
New York, New York

Stephen Updegraff, MD
Clinical Fellow
Ophthalmology
Hermann Eye Center
University of Texas Medical Center-Houston
Houston, Texas

Arthur Vassiliadis, MD
Sunrise Technologies
Fremont, California

Rogelio Villarreal, MD
Monterrey, Mexico

George O. Waring, III, MD, FACS
Professor of Ophthalmology
Director, Refractive Surgery
Emory University School of Medicine
Atlanta, Georgia

John A. van Westenbrugge, MD, FRCSC, Dip.ABO
Senior Surgeon
Gimbel Eye Centre
Calgary, Alberta, Canada

Josef Wollensak, MD
Professor and Chairman
Universitatsaugenklinik
FU Berlin, UKRV
Berlin, Germany

Kristin Woods
Research Assistant
Corneal Wound Lab
The Wilmer Eye Institute
Johns Hopkins University
Baltimore, Maryland

Contents

Corneal Laser Surgery

1

History and Mechanism of Action of Excimer Laser Corneal Surgery

Stephen Trokel

HISTORY

"Excimer" describes a recently developed class of lasers with output in the ultraviolet (UV) range of the electromagnetic spectrum. The possibility that this type of laser could be built was first suggested in 1975 when xenon atoms (Xe) were found to react with halogens (X) to produce an unstable noble gas–halide compound, XeX*. These compounds, XeX*, were found to rapidly dissociate to the ground state with the release of an energetic ultraviolet (UV) photon. This pattern of excitation and dissociation led to the observation that ". . . these . . . emissions have considerable potential as ultraviolet laser systems for mixtures of xenon (or other rare gases) and halogen containing compounds."[1] Shortly after this report, four molecules, xenon fluoride (XeF), xenon chloride (XeCl), xenon bromide (XeBr), and krypton fluoride (KrF), were observed[2-4] to lase when excited in an electron beam, and laser action at 193.3 nm from the argon fluoride (ArF) molecule was reported[5] in May 1976.

Different names are being used for these UV lasers. The short-lived, excited complex molecule at the heart of the laser's action has come to be known as an "excimer," short for an "excited dimer," and has given rise to the most popular name for the series of lasers based on this class of compounds. This word *excimer*, first used by photochemists in 1960,[6] was originally coined to describe an energized molecule with two identical components. Because it was first theorized that the rare gas molecules in these new UV lasers formed an excited dimer with two identical components during its excitation, the descriptive name *excimer* was applied to the active medium. This term has

persisted even though the lasing medium is now known to be a combination of two different elements, the rare gas and the halide, and is most accurately described as an "excited molecular complex." The term *excimer* is widely used as a generic name for this class of lasers and coexists with more accurate alternative names which include "rare gas-halide lasers" as a general descriptive term, and "argon-fluoride laser," to describe the specific system based on the mixture (Table 1-1) of the noble gas argon and the halogen fluorine.

The first laboratory excimer lasers were cumbersome because the molecule at the heart of the laser action, the halogen and noble gas combination, requires input of a large amount of energy to excite. This large amount of energy was obtained for the first demonstrations of excimer action by using a linear accelerator as the energy source to create the excited ArF molecule. This system was of limited practical use for biological experiments. Laser action was subsequently shown to be possible[7] in a relatively compact device using a transverse electrical discharge, a system adapted from that used in carbon dioxide lasers. This was the basis of the laser systems which led to the development of practical commercial UV lasers. After the demonstration of UV laser action, there was a great deal of discussion in the optical, electronic, and scientific literature, as well as the popular press,[8-12] about potential applications and unusual hazards. By 1979, excimer lasers suitable for limited laboratory use became available, and by late 1981 laser designs were sufficiently reliable and had enough output to make them suitable for general laboratory use.

Table 1-1.

Excimer laser type	Abbreviation	Wavelength (nm)	Photon energy (eV)
Fluorine	F_2	155	7.90
Argon fluoride	ArF	193	6.42
Krypton chloride	KrCl	222	5.59
Krypton fluoride	KrF	248	4.99
Xenon chloride	XeCl	308	4.03
Nitrogen	N_2	337	3.68
Xenon fluoride	XeF	351	3.53

HOW THE EXCIMER LASER WORKS

The unstable diatomic molecules that serve as the active laser medium and emit the UV photons are formed by applying a high-voltage discharge across a chamber (Fig. 1-1) containing the rare gas–halide mixture. This ionizes the mixture and produces the reaction:

$$A + X \rightarrow AX^* \rightarrow A + X + h\nu \qquad (1)$$

where A is a rare gas, i.e., argon, xenon, krypton X is a halide, i.e., fluorine, chlorine $h\nu$ = ultraviolet photon energy, which is dependent upon A and X (see Table 1-1)

The excited molecule AX* immediately dissociates to its ground state and emits an energetic photon of UV light whose emission wavelength and photon energy are determined by the gas mixture in the laser cavity as listed in Table 1-1. Lasing action will also occur for pure fluorine or nitrogen gases in the cavity.

Only ArF, KrF, XeCl, and XeF have sufficient energy in their outputs for practical surgical applications. Of these, only ArF and XeCl have found medical applications, the former for corneal surgery and the latter for fiber-delivered tissue ablation. The UV laser light is emitted in an individual pulse of photons which lasts about 10 to 50 ns. This pulse duration, the energy it contains, and the rapidity with which it can be repeated, vary with the design of the laser cavity. Typically, repetition rates to 100 Hz, and energies to 1 J per pulse are available.

DESIGN

A cross section of a typical excimer cavity is diagrammed in Fig. 1-1. The diagrammed plane is perpendicular to the laser beam's path. The laser cavity at the right is adjacent to a large gas reservoir which makes up the bulk of the laser volume. The electrode pair which creates the excited dimer (6 in Fig. 1-1) bounds the length of the laser cavity (1 in Fig. 1-1). The gas mixture contained in the reservoir (2) is circulated across the electrodes (6) by a fan (3) contained within the reservoir. Water cooling (4) may be used when high output is required to maintain temperature

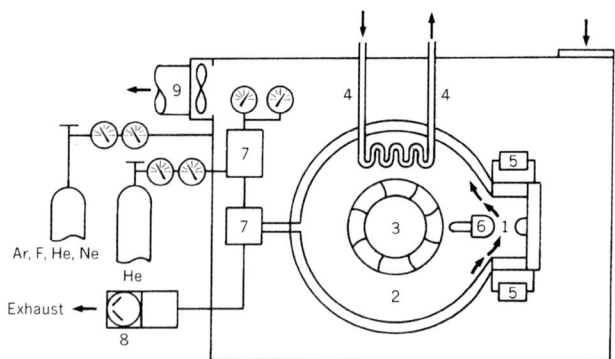

Fig. 1-1. Elements of an excimer laser cavity. A cross section of a typical excimer cavity shows the internal structural elements of the cylindrically shaped excimer laser in a plane oriented perpendicular to the laser beam path. Water cooling (4) may be necessary to maintain sustained high output. The laser gas is circulated into the laser channel by the fan (3). The exciting energy is an electrical discharge across the electrodes (6) which creates the ArF-excited molecule. Mirrors which bound the cavity create the laser action.

stability. The gas is ionized by a separate set of electrodes (not shown) just before a high-voltage (about 30,000 eV) electric pulse is discharged across the gas-filled space separating the electrodes. The supply of gas is automatically controlled in medical laser systems, which place all laser operations under computer control. Because the laser action degrades with contaminants, the gas mixture must be maintained in an extremely pure state within the laser. To maintain this purity, the gas must be either constantly cleaned or frequently replaced to maintain the stability of the laser output since the fluorine gas interacts with contaminants from the internal components of the laser cavity which are released by the laser action. Cleansing of the gas requires a liquid nitrogen cryogenic device which precipitates contaminants that appear within the laser cavity and the reservoir. The alternative to cryogenic purification is to flush the cavity periodically which exchanges the used gas with fresh gas from the attached cylinder. Both these approaches have been used in existing medical laser systems. Improvements in the materials used in laser construction have reduced the contamination that arises from within the cavity. This has reduced the need for cryogenic gas purification and prolonged the lifetime of a single gas fill.

MECHANISMS OF ACTION
Ablation of Organic Materials

The mechanism of tissue ablation produced by the ArF excimer laser appears to be substantially different from tissue ablation produced by conventional surgical lasers, which ablate by a process described as photothermal ablation. Conventional surgical lasers ablate because temperature elevation of exposed tissues occurs when the laser energy is absorbed by water or other tissue chromophores. This temperature elevation becomes high enough to burn away the laser-exposed tissue volume, with associated residual thermal damage extending into adjacent unexposed tissues that are distorted both at an ultrastructural and gross morphologic level.

The mechanism of ablation by laser light at 193 nm is different because the high photon energy of the ArF excimer laser appears to ablate tissue by a process which is photochemical in nature. This process is called photochemical ablation or ablative photodecomposition to distinguish it from the thermal ablation processes induced by the CO_2 and other surgical lasers. The theory which explains the highly localized tissue interaction is based on the fact that each photon produced by the ArF excimer laser has 6.4 eV of energy. This high photon energy is adequate to break covalent bonds. Only the more energetic fluorine laser (F_2), which has 7.9 eV of energy at 155-nm output, has been shown to produce a similar interaction with biological tissues. However, the energy of the F_2 laser is limited and it can be transmitted and processed only with great difficulty. All systems currently developed for corneal surgery use the substantial output of the ArF laser, which can be reasonably transmitted by existing high-quality optical elements. The prevailing view[13] of the action of the ArF laser on biological tissues is that the intramolecular bonds of exposed organic macromolecules are broken when a large number of high-energy 193-nm photons are absorbed in a short time. The breakage of the intramolecular bonds creates molecular fragments that occupy a larger volume than the original tissue. These fragments rapidly expand and are ejected from the exposed surface at supersonic velocities. Using high-speed photography, investigators[14] have photographed these ejected tissue components and have shown (Fig. 1-2) a highly directional plume. This mechanism explains the observation that only the irradiated organic materials are affected and adjacent areas are not, which offers an understanding of why the boundaries of exposed ablated areas are so sharply defined and smooth.

EXCIMER LASER INTERACTION WITH THE EYE

The laser effects laboratory at the United States Air Force (USAF) School of Aerospace Medicine first investigated the interactions of these new lasers with the eye. They reported[15] that rabbit corneal epithelium exposed to the KrF[15] laser's 248-nm emissions either became opacified or developed fluorescein staining which took the shape of the laser beam distribution. A subsequent study[16] exposed the cornea to a 0.1-cm^2 rectangular beam of 193-nm light from an ArF laser

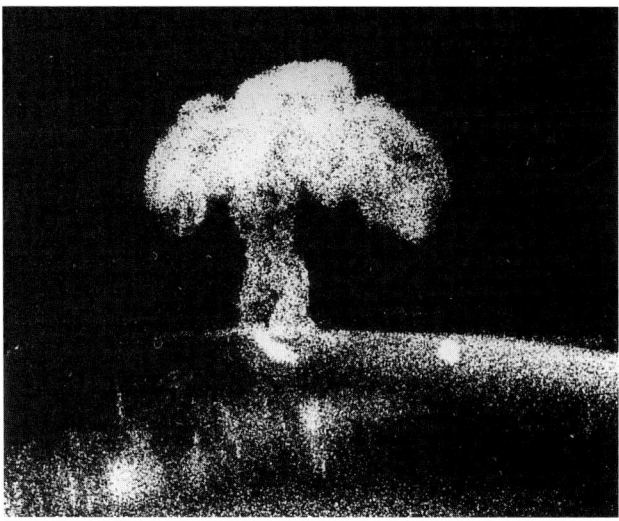

Fig. 1-2. High-speed photograph of ejected tissue components after laser ablation. The *vertical column* indicates the restricted spatial distribution of the ejected materials. As the velocity slows, there is lateral spread of the material. The entire column is dissipated in a small fraction of a second. (With permission from Puliafito CA et al: High-speed photography of excimer laser ablation of the cornea, *Arch Ophthalmol* 105:1255-1259, 1987.)

operating at low energies. A search was made for damage similar to that found after exposure of the cornea to the KrF beam. They noted the appearance of the cornea which after exposure to the higher irradiance of 27.5 mJ/cm^2 showed an immediate indentation of the corneal surface which took the shape of the beam. One hour later, the surface indentation would fill in. The authors postulated that the far-UV light was resonantly captured in random electromagnetic cavities formed by the microprojections of the anterior epithelial cell layer which caused a preferential temperature jump in this thin layer of tissue. The observation of an "indentation" without report of transparency loss within adjacent epithelium or stroma suggested that tissue was being removed, and stimulated studies of this phenomenon.

In June 1983 Srinivasan, at the International Business Machines (IBM) T.J. Watson Laboratory, described interaction of 193-nm laser radiation with organic materials that included creating grooves in strands of human hair. The grooves seen in the scanning electron micrograph (SEM) in Fig. 1-3 are a dramatic illustration of the precision of the ablation technique. In a paper[13] describing the effect of 193-nm light on plastic, Srinivasan noted that, "A threshold . . . for ablative photodecomposition . . . was measured at 10 mJ/cm^2. Thus, one pulse at 16 mJ/cm^2 gave an etch mark that was clearly visible in reflection, whereas 50 pulses at 4 mJ/cm^2/pulse did not leave any etch mark. . . ."[13] This seemed to explain the previous observation of the corneal epithelial in-

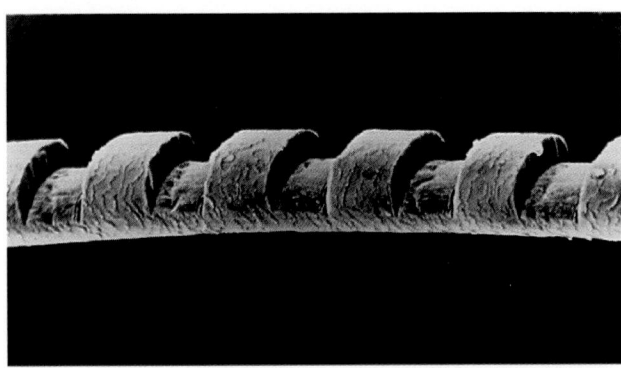

Fig. 1-3. Grooves cut in human hair. The accuracy with which tissue can be ablated becomes apparent in these sections partway through a human hair.

dentation, and the creation of grooves in a human hair demonstrated the precision that could be obtained. These observations pointed to the possibility of optical control of the corneal surface by tissue removal, and provided impetus for further studies.

EXCIMER LASER INTERACTION WITH THE CORNEA
Thresholds and Ablation Rates

Measurements of the quantitative aspect of the excimer UV interaction showed (Fig. 1-4, *A*) a threshold for ablation that increased with wavelength and appeared to be independent of laser firing rate at the 193-nm wavelength. The threshold for this effect was

about 50 ± 20 mJ/cm^2 for 193-nm photons. The amount of corneal stroma removed per pulse was extremely small (Fig. 1-4, *B*), measuring a fraction of a wavelength of light per pulse. The amount of stroma at twice threshold was about 0.1 μm per pulse, increasing[17] to about 0.2 μm per pulse at 160 mJ/cm^2. These findings supported a surgical potential because they implied that the corneal stromal surface could be exposed to laser radiation and reshaped to a smoothness better than one third to half the wavelength of visible light, which covers the visible range from 0.4 to 0.8 μm.

Observations[18] of the morphology of the ablated surface also supported the corneal surgical potential for this laser system (Fig. 1-5). Many laser pulses exposed to the cornea produced crisply edged grooves in the corneal tissue, which became deeper as the number of pulses increased. The figure shows no collateral damage in adjacent stroma, and a smooth ablated surface that was unique in contrast to other[19] known laser interactions with the cornea. Fig. 1-6 shows the healed surface of a large field ablated into a rabbit stroma by a 3.5-mm beam from the ArF laser and allowed to heal for 6 weeks. These observations demonstrated the essential elements of the interaction of ArF excimer laser radiation with the cornea which continues to reinforce the view that it had serious surgical potential as a method to alter the corneal curve.

The quantitative studies of excimer action demonstrated a threshold phenomenon for ablation at all ex-

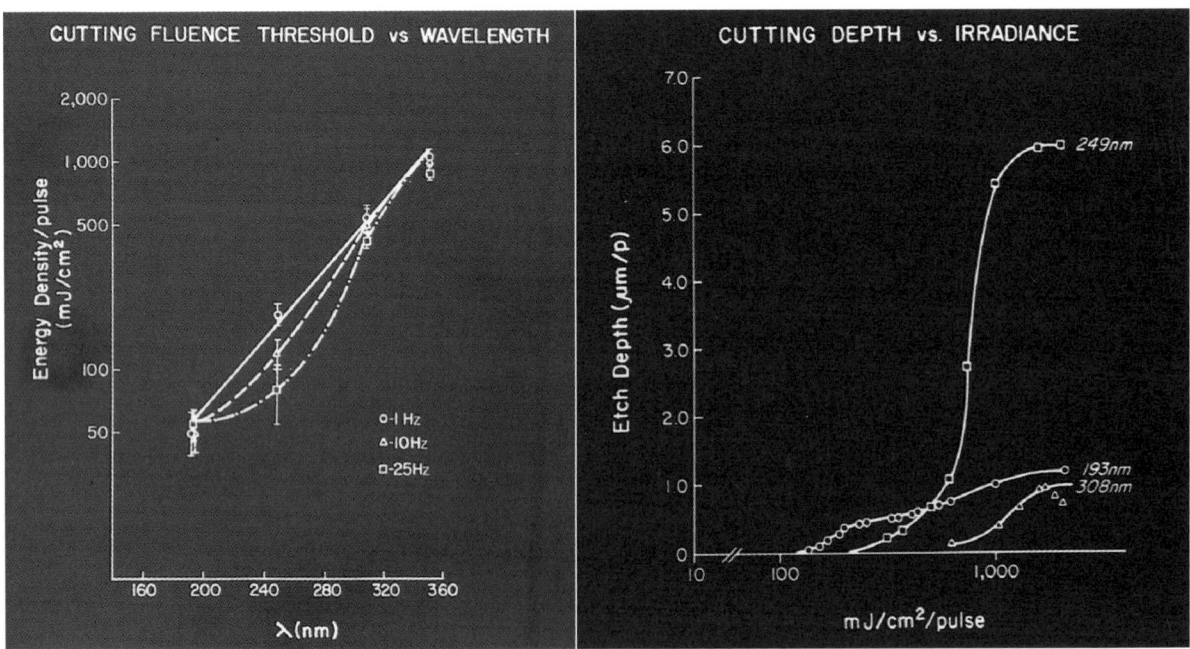

Fig. 1-4. Ablation threshold and ablation rates. **A,** The threshold is a nonlinear phenomenon and varies with laser photon energy. For the ArF laser, the threshold is about 50 ± 20 mJ/cm^2, and independent of the laser firing rate. **B,** The amount of tissue removed for each pulse increases with increasing energy. At several times the threshold, the ablation rates are a small fraction of the wavelength of light.

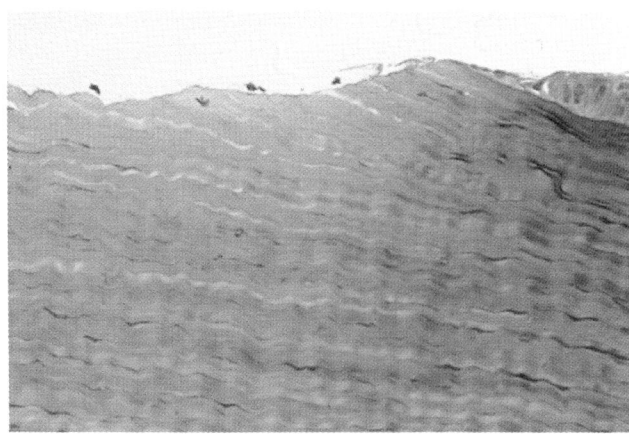

Fig. 1-5. Histology of acute ablation. The lack of damage adjacent to the smooth and regular surface was impressive and unique in evaluating laser-cornea interactions. The smooth regular surface created by this ablation was the finding that suggested that recontouring the cornea would be feasible.

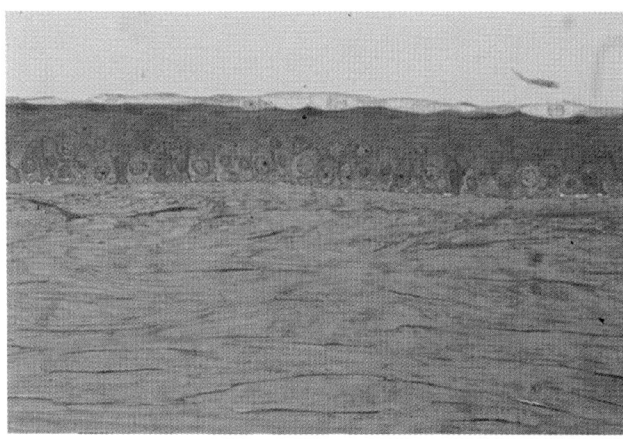

Fig. 1-6. Analysis of the healed corneal surface. The clarity after healing encouraged further studies. The smoothness of the surface seen after epithelialization was evidence that the tissue had been removed to standards of optical precision.

cimer wavelengths, the threshold increasing with the wavelength (see Fig. 1-4, *A*), and a fraction of a micron of corneal tissue being removed (see Fig. 1-4, *B*) with each pulse of laser light. The studies of the morphology showed that the resulting surfaces were extremely smooth and uniform and there was no collateral damage to the adjacent unirradiated tissues. Furthermore, the shape and pattern of tissue removed were adjusted by controlling the shape and irradiance of the incident beam.

Possible surgical applications of the ArF laser to remove either narrow strips of tissue which would resemble an incision or large areas of tissue to form a controlled laser lamellar keratectomy were suggested in the first paper to describe corneal ablation using the ArF laser: "The laser can be used to reshape the corneal curvature in a manner similar to keratomileusis

. . . excising more tissue either centrally or peripherally. The net effect would be to flatten or steepen the cornea." Conventional wisdom made a strong presumption that Bowman's layer was essential to maintain corneal transparency. This assumption was based on unsuccessful attempts to directly alter the corneal refractive power by direct tissue removal[20,21] using conventional surgical technology. These attempts failed probably because it had never been possible to form a new corneal surface that was smooth to optical standards prior to the advent of the excimer laser.

Studies of Animal Corneas

The implications of these initial observations were confirmed by higher-resolution SEM and transmission electron microscope (TEM) studies[22-28] which showed that damage was restricted, and SEM showed the surface to be smooth and featureless. It was found that circular ablations performed on a primate cornea healed with remarkable clarity. SEM analysis of rabbit corneas that had 3.5-mm circular ablations showed smoothness of the freshly ablated surface with the healed, reepithelialized surface appearing similar to the adjacent unablated surface. TEM studies showed that the damage zone was limited to less than 100 nm with a uniform-appearing surface (Fig. 1-7). These studies increased the interest in direct surface recontouring. The quantitative relationships associated with

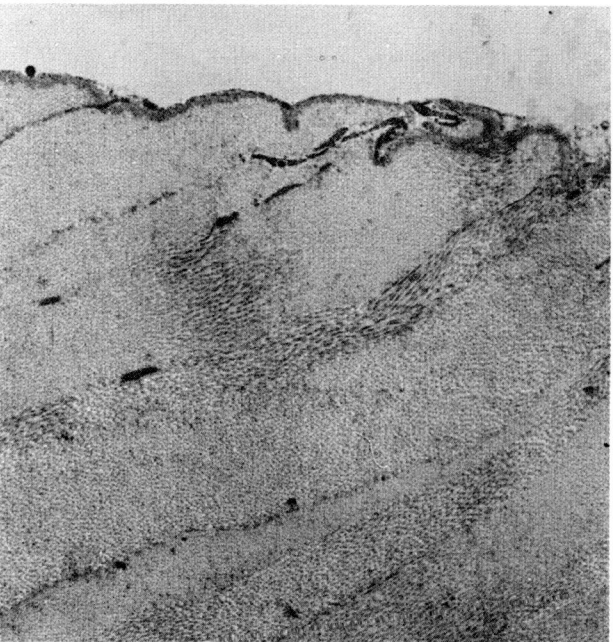

Fig. 1-7. Transmission electron microscopy of freshly ablated surface. The damage is restricted to a uniform 100-nm zone at the ablated surface. This layer has been called a pseudomembrane because of its uniform characteristics. Collagen adjacent to this layer shows no disruption or thermal damage.

removing central corneal tissue from the anterior surface were derived as early as 1984[29] and showed that only 5 μm of tissue had to be removed to lower the corneal refractive power of a 4-mm optical zone by 1 D. The term *photorefractive keratectomy* was coined in this paper that was not published until 4 years later because it was deemed too "speculative and of no practical value" by several editors. Further research quantitated the histologic nature[30,31] of the interaction for the broad range of excimer wavelengths available. Early attempts to perform therapeutic keratectomy showed[31] that the ablated surface would heal without scarring.

REFRACTIVE SURGERY

Refractive surgeons were very interested in improving the precision of corneal surgical technology, which led to intense interest in the excimer laser because of its precise and localized tissue interaction. The basis of this interest was the hope that the laser's increased surgical precision could be translated into more accurate refractive surgery.

Excimer Surgical System Design

The first prototype excimer systems that had integrated delivery systems were developed by Seiler in Germany and Puliafito in the United States, the former using an operating microscope and the latter a slit-lamp delivery system. These instruments were used largely for laboratory investigations, although the first[33] investigative clinical work was done with the Seiler prototype for therapeutic excision of diseased tissue, and subsequently for creating relaxing keratotomies. The first commercial system was developed by Meditec G.m.b.H. and was soon followed by a system developed by the Ophthalmic Laser Division of Cooper-Vision Inc. The Meditec effort sought to develop a practical clinical laser system that could create linear keratotomies and the Cooper-Vision system developed equipment to deliver a circular pattern of laser light to the cornea that would selectively remove tissue to create a flatter new corneal contour.

The idea of selective tissue removal from the cornea stroma was not new. Efforts to achieve this were reported in the late nineteenth and early twentieth centuries.[34,35] Recent interest dates to Barraquer's[36] work in 1949 when he devised a procedure in which the corneal curve is altered by creating a lamellar keratectomy, freezing the lamellae, removing tissue from its posterior surface using a cryolathe, and then suturing the altered corneal lamellar button back onto its original bed. The term he coined to describe this surgical procedure is *keratomileusis*.

A number of surgical procedures have been devised to induce refractive change in the cornea. These include radial keratotomy (RK), and relaxing incisions placed in the corneal periphery. The radial incisions placed in the peripheral corneal stroma during RK will cause the peripheral cornea to bulge and the central cornea to flatten, thereby reducing the refractive power of the eye. Relaxing incisions placed in the corneal periphery at a right angle to a steep meridian will reduce refractive astigmatism.

Thermal keratoplasty has also been of continuing interest. Heat has been applied to the corneal stroma to steepen the central optics by placing peripheral thermal lesions which flatten the peripheral and steepen the central corneal optical zones. Conversely, a smaller concentric ring of thermal lesions has been shown to flatten the central cornea. Heat has been applied on the surface of the cornea with hot probes, within the surface of the cornea using heated wires, and at all levels of the cornea using a variety of infrared[37] lasers.

Use of the excimer laser to directly recontour the cornea became possible only when the belief was overcome that preservation of Bowman's layer is essential to preserve regular corneal topography and clarity. The importance of Bowman's layer was probably overemphasized because prior to the excimer laser, all available surgical technology created a rough, uneven surface following lamellar keratectomy. Barraquer's surgical procedure removed tissue from the stromal side of a lamellar section because he used the superficial lamellar cap to smooth the resultant surface. The excimer laser changed this because it made a surface that was smooth to optical standards. Each laser pulse removes about 0.2 μm of tissue, which is less than half the wavelength of light. This means the newly ablated corneal surface is smooth to optical standards. Animal studies proved that the corneas would heal with their unimpaired transparency and maintain a smooth optical surface.

ABLATION PATTERNS—LARGE VS. SMALL AREA ABLATIONS

Two approaches have been advocated to prepare these new surfaces, one using a small laser beam which is rapidly scanned over the corneal surface and the other using a large beam of laser light which can simultaneously remove tissue from the entire area that is to be ablated. The time required to alter the corneal surface will be minimized when a large area of the cornea is simultaneously irradiated. This is the simplest way to quickly alter the cornea in the shortest time compared to systems which scan a small beam over the corneal surface.

Tissue can be removed from a large area in two ways. Either the cornea can be irradiated with a number of laser pulses, each of which has a varied energy distribution or the eye can be irradiated with a series of laser pulses of uniform irradiance but varying geometry. In Fig. 1-8, the center of the laser beam contains the highest concentration of energy which decreases toward the beam periphery. This beam will remove more tissue centrally than peripherally with each pulse, which flattens the cornea. If the irradiance were made greater in the periphery, more tissue would be removed from the edges than from the center, which would steepen the cornea. In principle, any contour can be transferred to the cornea by controlling the energy distribution within the beam. The same effect can be achieved by exposing onto the corneal surface a series of circular laser beams of uniform energy density but increasing diameter. The result of this is that the center of the cornea receives more laser pulses, and has more tissue removed. The greater removal of tissue from the center will cause the cornea to become flatter. The amount of flattening and the resulting dioptric change can be controlled by changing the diameter, size, and number of exposures of laser light, all under control of a computer algorithm.

A scanning system can be similarly configured to reshape the corneal contour. The main advantage of a scanning system is that it requires a less powerful laser and each exposure produces a minimal shock wave. The disadvantage of a scanning system is that there is a substantial increase in the laser exposure time with increased difficulties in stabilization and alignment of the scanning beam during exposure. Attempts are being made to incorporate tracking systems into the systems to guide the scanner and improve alignment during the entire exposure.

Currently, there are substantial clinical investigations underway testing excimer laser systems that use

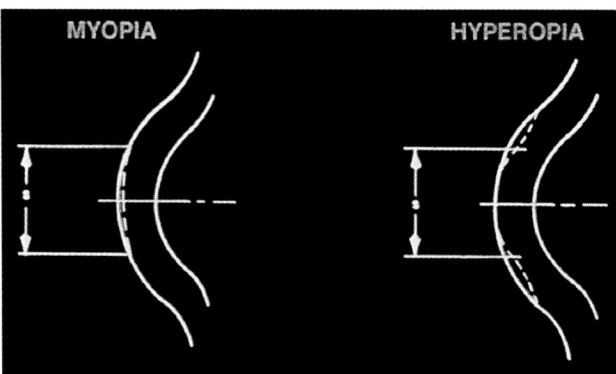

Fig. 1-8. Patterns of tissue removal. A laser beam that is more intense at the center than at the edge will remove more stromal tissue centrally than peripherally with each pulse. Increasing the number of pulses increases the dioptric effect. The same effect can be achieved by using a closing iris diaphragm to expose the cornea to circles of laser light of progressing decreasing diameter. The number of laser pulses at each diameter determines the amount of central corneal flattening and the dioptric change. The iris diameter and number of laser pulses are under computer control.

large areas (VISX, Summit, Technolas, Schwind), and those that scan (Meditec, Nidek, Lasersite, Autonomous Technologies). Some systems (VISX, Technolas) have combined scanning elements with large beam areas in an attempt to develop maximum flexibility in their scanning programs. The appendix contains a table summarizing the features of many of the currently available excimer laser systems.

OPTICS

All current commercial excimer lasers use an operating microscope to align the laser and deliver the energy to that portion of the cornea which surrounds the entrance pupil of the eye. The patient is supine, which appears to facilitate stability and fixation during the procedure. Important design elements that have been recognized include the necessity for achieving beam homogenization, accurate transport of the laser beam from the cavity to the eye, computer-controlled shaping of the beam, and coaxial delivery with the operating microscope. Fig. 1-9 shows one manufacturer's approach to creating an optical train to perform these functions. The rectangular output of the laser cavity is folded, passed through homogenizing optics, and rotated to produce radial symmetry. An iris diaphragm and adjustable slit are computer-controlled to adjust the distribution of light on the corneal surface. Each commercial system has a unique engineering approach and clear-cut advantages for one over another have not been definitively demonstrated at this time. There is stated surgeon preference for coaxial delivery systems, and theoretical arguments have been made in favor of achieving as uniform a corneal ablation as possible to facilitate postoperative healing and minimize irregular astigmatism. Different systems have never been compared in any prospective manner. It is not clear which approach has produced clinical results which show the most accuracy, precision, and clearest corneas. The comparison is further complicated by associated surgical and pharmacologic regimens which appear to affect the clinical course and vary among different laser system users.

EXCIMER SYSTEMS

With the perception that excimer systems can be successfully applied to a large range of refractive errors, there has been increasing commercial interest in the development of this technology. Listed in Table 1-2 is a summary of excimer systems in some state of commercial development.

All of the systems described above are currently being evaluated and refined for commercial applications. Substantial clinical experience has been obtained with excimer systems manufactured by the Meditec, Summit, and VISX companies. Complete excimer laser systems include a protective housing for

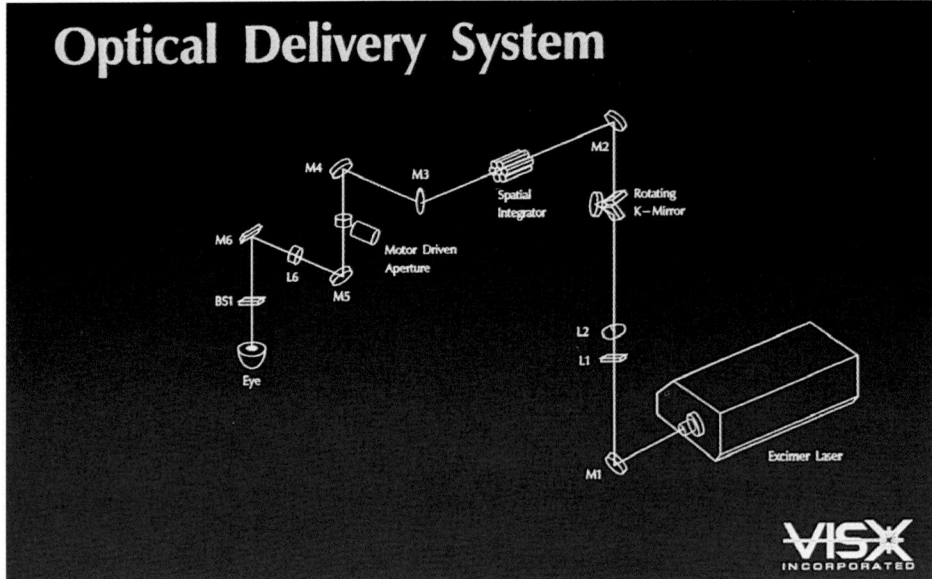

Fig. 1-9. Laser optical elements. The optical elements of the laser are outlined in this picture. The laser beam is folded, and rotated by optical elements before it is projected onto the eye. The diameter of the iris diaphragm is regulated by a computer which controls the distribution of laser light on the corneal surface.

laser gases and an operating microscope delivery system. The entire operation of the laser system is automated and under computer control. The shape of the ablated curve is created by the computer which regulates the number of laser pulses falling on the cornea for each diameter of the iris or slit aperture setting. The amount of tissue removed depends on the diameter of the area ablated and the irradiance (energy per unit area) of the laser beam.

A large number of patients have been treated with the scanning excimer system manufactured by Meditec. This system scans a narrow 1-mm beam firing at 20 Hz across a progressively closing iris diaphragm or other beam-shaping element held and centered over the entrance pupil of the eye.

LASER CALIBRATION

Calibration of the laser system is essential to achieve the accuracy that is believed to be inherent in this technique. Different approaches have been taken to calibrate the laser because direct measurement of the energy is difficult. Meters are notoriously unreliable and have an accuracy no better than ±20% at this wavelength. Some form of measured ablation is used by all system users to calibrate the laser output. If the laser output is too high, the laser will remove more tissue than desired and an overcorrection will occur. If the laser output is too low, than the laser will ablate less tissue and the patient will be undercorrected.

One calibration approach tests the output of the laser by ablating a test refraction onto a piece of plastic. The lens so formed, shown in Fig. 1-10, can be used

to assess the fluence of the laser as well as its alignment and the action of the mechanical elements which shape the beam. The power of the lens so created is measured with a lensometer which confirms that the laser is properly adjusted and calibrated. The appearance of the lens may indicate distortion which suggests some defect on the distribution of light within the laser beam.

Another approach adjusts the laser energy until a plastic Wratten filter of known thickness is perforated by a given number of pulses. The number of pulses required to ablate a defined plastic gives a direct measure of the ablating power of the laser beam. The uni-

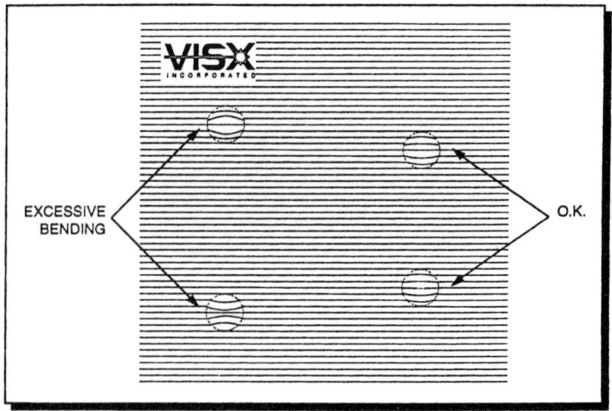

Fig. 1-10. Plastic test lens against a quality screen. This test allows assessment of laser function as well as the mechanical elements within the delivery system and the operation of the computer control software.

Table 1-2. Excimer laser systems

Laser system	Beam shape	Pattern shaper	Fixation
Meditec	Scanning 1- × 7-mm slit	Mask held against cornea	Held
VISX	7.0-mm circle	Iris, parallel leaves, scanning	Self/held
Summit	6.5-mm circle	Iris, ablatable mask	Self
Nidek	Scanning, rotating slit	Iris	Self
Technolas	6.0-mm circle	Scanning mirror	Self
Schwind	6.0-mm circle	Template and zoom	Self
LaserSite	Submillimeter element	Scanning system	Self
Mikof (Russian)	6.0-mm circle	Variable irradiance, with lens-shaped filter	Self
Autonomous	Submillimeter element	Scanning	Tracker
Lions Research	6.0-mm circle	Iris	Self

formity of the beam is assessed by adjusting the laser pulses to penetrate only 90% of the plastic. The quality of light transmission through the resulting plastic is assessed for uniformity and "hot spots." In a similar manner, the quality of the ablated plastic lens may be viewed directly and assessed by the quality of the image of the mires in the lensometer.

INITIAL CLINICAL STUDIES

Clinical experience with these laser systems shows that the animal studies correctly predicted preservation of the cornea's optical properties following ablation with both scanning and large area exposure patterns.[28,31] The transparency and modified surface optical properties that were created on the healed surfaces of primate eyes were similarly found in human corneas. In the first clinical applications, the excimer was used to excise superficial areas of diseased and scarred corneal tissue that were interfering with vision. The first refractive applications[33] copied diamond knife function to create relaxing incisions in the corneal stroma to relieve corneal astigmatism. The first sighted patient to have a successful photorefractive keratectomy was operated on by McDonald and colleagues[38] in June 1988. Since that time, clinical studies throughout the world have treated several hundred thousand patients. The lasers used in these procedures have been progressively refined, as have the algorithms and surgical techniques used to ablate tissues.

CONCLUSIONS

The intense interest in clinical applications of the excimer laser systems increased dramatically after their clinical feasibility was demonstrated. Unfortunately, the successful clinical applications diverted attention away from the laboratory where important issues remain to be studied. This is disturbing, as the questions that remain unanswered and require investigation are not trivial. For example, What is the best way to achieve the ablation pattern which recontours the optical surface of the cornea? What is the optimal irradiance and laser firing rate that should be used? What shape should be ablated onto the corneal surface? Is the shape of the newly ablated corneal surface critical? What are the factors which trigger formation of new collagen? What should be the shape of the blend or junction zone where the ablated and normal areas of the cornea meet? What postoperative care should be offered?

Calibration studies are difficult because there is a 3-month delay between the surgery and a reasonable estimate of the result. Therefore, any change in laser factors or surgical techniques from those that have been developed with care and difficulty must be made with a great deal of caution.

We hope that clinical and laboratory studies will continue to address these issues so that the clinical promise of this laser can be fully met.

REFERENCES

1. Velazco JE, Setser DW: Bound-free emission spectra of diatomic xenon halides, *J Chem Phys* 62:1990-1991, 1975.
2. Searles SK, Hart GA: *Appl Phys Lett* 27:243, 1975.
3. Ewing JJ, Brau CA: *Appl Phys Lett* 27:350, 1975.
4. Brau CA, Ewing JJ: *Appl Phys Lett* 27:435, 1975.
5. Hoffman JM, Hays AK, Tisone GC: High-power UV noble-gas-halide lasers, *Appl Phys Lett* 28:538-539, 1976.
6. Stevens B, Hutton E: Radiative lifetime of the pyrene dimer and the possible role of excited dimers in energy transfer processes, *Nature* 186:1045-1046, 1960.
7. Burnham R, Djeu N: Ultraviolet-preionized discharge-pumped lasers in XeF, KrF, and ArF, *Appl Phys Lett* 29:707-709, 1976.
8. Short-wavelength output at Optical Society of America, a meeting report from Tucson, *Laser Focus,* 15-18, 1977.
9. Eden G, Burnham R, Champagne LF, et al: Visible and UV lasers: problems and promises, *IEEE Spect* 16:50, 1979.
10. Huestis DL: The excimer age: lasing with the new breed, *Optical Spectra* 13:51, 1979.
11. Rhodes CK, editor: *Excimer lasers: topics in applied physics,* vol 30, New York, 1979, Springer-Verlag.
12. Ruderman W: Excimer laser in photochemistry, *Laser Focus* 15:68, 1979.
13. Srinivasan R: Kinetics of the ablative photodecomposition of organic polymers in the far ultraviolet (193 nm), *J Vac Sci Technol Bull* 4:923-926, 1983.
14. Puliafito CA, Stern D, Krueger RR, et al: High-speed photography of excimer laser ablation of the cornea, *Arch Ophthalmol* 105:1255-1259, 1987.

15. Taboada J, Mikesell GW, Reed RD: Response of the corneal epithelium to KrF excimer laser pulses, *Health Phys* 40:677-683, 1981.

16. Taboada J, Archibald CJ: An extreme sensitivity in the corneal epithelium to far UV ArF excimer laser pulses, Proceedings of the Scientific Program of the Aerospace Medical Association, San Antonio, 1981.

17. Krueger RR, Trokel SL: Quantitation of corneal ablation by ultraviolet laser light, *Arch Ophthalmol* 103:1741-1742, 1985.

18. Trokel SL, Srinivasan R, Braren B: Excimer laser surgery of the cornea, *Am J Ophthalmol* 96:710-715, 1983.

19. Keates RH, Pedrotti L, Weider H, et al: Carbon dioxide laser beam control for corneal surgery, *Ophthalmic Surg* 12:117, 1981.

20. Mueller OF, O'Neill P: Some experiments on corneal grinding, *Exp Eye Res* 6:42-47, 1967.

21. Olson RJ, Kaufman HE, Rheinstrom SD: Reshaping the cat corneal anterior surface using high speed diamond fraise, *Ophthalmic Surg* 11:784-786, 1980.

22. Marshall J, Trokel SL, Rothery S, et al: An ultrastructural study of corneal incisions induced by an excimer laser at 193 nm. *Ophthalmology* 92:749-758, 1985.

23. Puliafito CA, Steinert RF, Deutsch TF, et al: Excimer laser ablation of the cornea and lens, *Ophthalmology* 92:741-748, 1985.

24. Marshall J, Trokel S, Rothery S, et al: Photoablative reprofiling of the cornea using an excimer laser, photorefractive keratectomy. *Lasers Ophthalmol* 1:21-48, 1986.

25. Marshall J, Trokel SL, Rothery S, et al: A comparative study of corneal incisions induced by diamond and steel knives and two ultraviolet radiations from an excimer laser. *Br J Ophthalmol* 70:482-501, 1986.

26. Krauss JM, Puliafito CA, Steinert RF: Laser interactions with the cornea, *Surv Ophthalmol* 31:37-53, 1986.

27. Kerr-Muir MG, Trokel SL, Marshall J, et al: Ultrastructural comparison of conventional surgical and argon fluoride excimer laser keratectomy, *Am J Ophthalmol* 103(part II):448-453, 1987.

28. Marshall J, Trokel SL, Rothery S, et al: Long term healing of the central cornea after photorefractive keratectomy using an excimer laser, *Ophthalmology* 95:1411-1421, 1988.

29. Munnerlyn CR, Koons SJ, Marshall J: Photorefractive keratectomy: a technique for laser refractive surgery, *J Cataract Refract Surg* 14:46-52, 1988.

30. Krueger RR, Trokel SL, Schubert HD: Interaction of ultraviolet laser light with the cornea, *Invest Ophthalmol Vis Sci* 26:1455-1464, 1985.

31. Trokel SL: The cornea and ultraviolet laser light, *Laser in der Ophthalmologie, vol 113, Bücherei des Augenarztes,* Stuttgart, 1988, Ferdinand Enke Verlag.

32. Serdarevic O, Darrell RW, Krueger RR, et al: Excimer laser therapy for experimental *Candida* keratitis, *Am J Ophthalmol* 99:534-538, 1985.

33. Seiler T, Bende T, Trokel S, et al: Excimer laser keratectomy for correction of astigmatism, *Am J Ophthalmol* 105:117-124, 1988.

34. Lans LJ: Experimentelle Untersuchungen über Entstehung von Astigmatismus durch nicht perforierende Corneawunden, *Graefes Arch Clin Exp Ophthalmol* 44:117-152, 1898.

35. Weiner M: Meier's method of peeling of the cornea, *Ophthalmol Year Book* 52, 1917.

36. Barraquer JI: Queratoplastia refractiva, *Est Inform Oftal* 2:10, 1949.

37. Kanoda AN, Sorokin AS: Laser correction of hypermetropic refraction. In Fyodorov SN, editor: *Microsurgery of the eye,* Moscow, 1987, Mir Publishers.

38. McDonald M, Kaufman HE, Frantz JM, et al: Excimer laser ablation in a human eye, *Arch Ophthalmol* 107:641-642, 1989.

2

The Effects of Excimer Laser Photoablation on the Cornea

Ronald R. Krueger, Perry S. Binder, Peter J. McDonnell

The development of the ultraviolet (UV) excimer laser and introduction of the process of ablative photodecomposition created a new form of laser surgery of the cornea. Excimer laser photoablation of the cornea represents a landmark development in ophthalmology and has spawned a resurgence of interest in keratorefractive surgery. How many ophthalmologists 10 years ago would have anticipated the ability to alter the anterior corneal curvature with a shallow superficial ablation to correct myopia? Who would have believed that it would be feasible to excise Bowman's membrane without introducing a corneal scar sufficient to permanently reduce visual acuity? The introduction of this technology has opened a new understanding of laser-tissue interaction and laser refractive surgery of the cornea. The science behind excimer laser photoablation of the cornea, however, can be considered only after first addressing other types of laser interaction in comparison with that of the excimer laser. This chapter also goes into the scientific detail on both the corneal biophysics and biological response of this unique mechanism of laser interaction.

LASER INTERACTION WITH THE CORNEA
Corneal Photocoagulation

Argon laser photocoagulation has been useful in treating retinal disease and glaucoma because of the unique ability of its energy to be absorbed by a chromophore within the ocular tissue. The two greatest chromophores to argon laser photocoagulation are blood and melanin. Argon laser photocoagulation of retinal vascular disease has made use of blood as a chromophore while panretinal photocoagulation and argon laser trabeculoplasty have used the high absorptivity of melanin to achieve their tissue effects. Since the cornea is largely a transparent structure to visible light and has no naturally occurring chromophore, photocoagulation has minimal relevance to the cornea. However, certain diseases and conditions associated with introduction of pigment into the cornea can be treated with visible light lasers, including corneal neovascularization and retrocorneal pigmented plaques.

In 1973, Cherry et al.[1] reported the use of an argon laser in their treatment of corneal neovascularization in humans. These investigators found that the application of hundreds of small argon laser pulses eliminated the neovascularization, but the effect was usually transient. Only one of the four treated patients achieved permanent vessel closure, and it was observed that removal of the stimulus for neovascularization was an important factor in preventing regrowth of new vessels. Argon laser photocoagulation can also be used to treat feeder vessels in patients with lipid keratopathy. Secondary lipid deposition is commonly seen in patients with chronic inflammatory disease. In a study by Marsh and Marshall,[2] 20 eyes were treated with argon laser photocoagulation of the feeder vessel and followed for 1 year. Although the visual acuity only improved in six patients (30%), 50% had a diminished density and extent of lipid deposition. In 1982, Bahn et al.[3] reported the use of argon laser photocoagulation to lyse a vitreous adhesion to the corneal wound after trauma. This was possible because of pigmentation of the vitreous band by hemoglobin from a vitreous hemorrhage. The argon laser can also be used to photocoagulate retrocorneal pigmented plaques[4] and iridocorneal adhesions in patients whose trabeculectomies for open-angle glaucoma have been complicated by transient postoperative flat anterior chambers.[5] Recently, Baer and Foster[6] used a yellow dye laser at 577 nm for the photocoagulation of corneal neovascularization. This was found to be efficacious only in a group of patients with active graft rejection, resulting in diminished extent of neovascularization and resolution of graft rejection in five out of five patients.

Although photocoagulation using a visible light laser source shows some efficacy in treating corneal disease, the normal cornea is largely transparent to visible light and these lasers have no therapeutic effect in the absence of pigmentation or vascularization. Even when these chromophores are present, corneal photocoagulation results in the loss of corneal transparency which would have little potential benefit in refractive surgery, even if these chromophores were present. In addition, the high corneal transmissibility of visible light lasers could lead to damage of intraocular structures if the laser light is not completely absorbed by the artificially placed chromophore.

Photovaporization

Another type of laser-tissue interaction which allows for precise cutting of corneal collagen lamellae is corneal photovaporization. This effect is produced by the longer infrared laser light sources including the carbon dioxide and erbium:yttrium-aluminum-garnet (Er:YAG) lasers. These wavelengths are strongly absorbed by water, making them of potential use in any water-containing tissue, including the cornea. Early work by Fine et al.[7] using a continuous-wave CO_2 laser demonstrated that at sufficiently high energy levels the laser was capable of perforating the cornea. However, surrounding this ulceration was a white ring of charred corneal tissue with collagen lamellae fused into a structureless mass. The authors later established that the degree of corneal damage was linearly proportional to the amount of energy used.[8]

In 1971, Beckman et al.[9] suggested that using a pulsed CO_2 laser might significantly reduce the thermal damage to surrounding tissue by allowing less time for heat conduction. The authors performed penetrating circular keratectomies simulating corneal trephination using microsecond pulses at up to 300-Hz repetition rate. This resulted in a conical-shaped crater with less thermal damage than continuous-wave CO_2 laser vaporization, but there was still a 0.12-mm zone of charred tissue around the incision site with edges less sharp than they would have been with mechanical trephination. Ten years later, Keates et al.[10] went one step further, reducing the exposure duration to 500-ns pulses using a Q-switched CO_2 laser. This

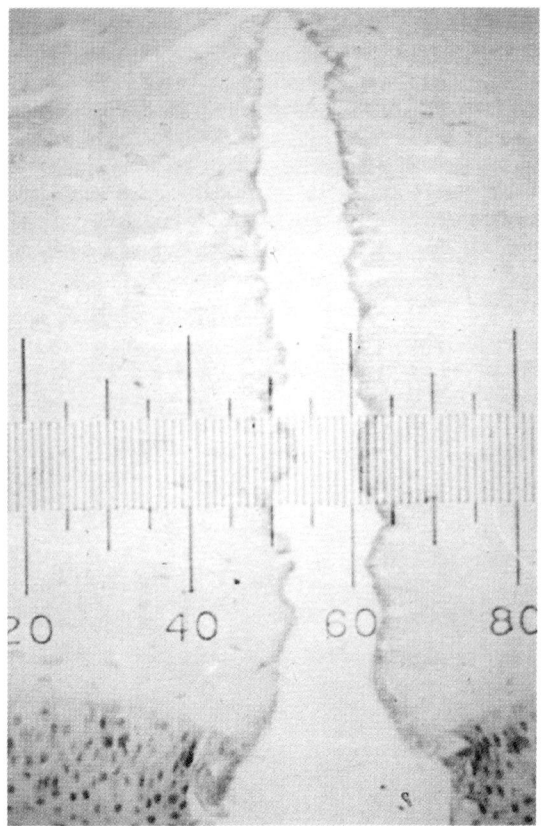

Fig. 2-1. Histologic section of an incision made by a short-pulse carbon dioxide laser on bovine cornea. The excision is approximately 50 μm in width and demonstrates a small, 5-μm zone of adjacent thermal damage. LM 100× magnification. (With permission from Keates RH et al, Carbon dioxide laser beam control for corneal surgery, *Ophthalmic Surg* 12:117-122, 1981.)

approach produced more uniform and reproducible lesions (Fig. 2-1).

The CO_2 laser, however, is not the only infrared laser that can produce a photovaporization effect in the cornea. The Er:YAG laser and other lasers in the 3-μm wavelength range can produce lesions with even greater precision and less thermal damage.[11-15] The absorption coefficient of the CO_2 laser is 950 cm^{-1}.[16] This corresponds to a penetration depth of 63% of the laser energy into 20 μm of tissue. In comparison, when using an Er:YAG laser or hydrogen fluoride laser at 2.9-μm wavelength, the absorption coefficient is significantly higher, nearly 8000 cm^{-1}, and the penetration depth is correspondingly smaller, being only 1.3 μm for 63% of the laser energy[16] (Fig. 2-2). This penetration depth is even smaller than that found when using the excimer laser in corneal tissue, which is measured at approximately 4 μm.

Corneal vaporization using a hydrogen fluoride laser emitting infrared wavelengths near 2.9 μm shows a fine corneal cut with a narrow zone of thermal damage ranging from 10 to 15 μm in width near the surface and 1 to 2 μm wide deep within the incision.[17,18]

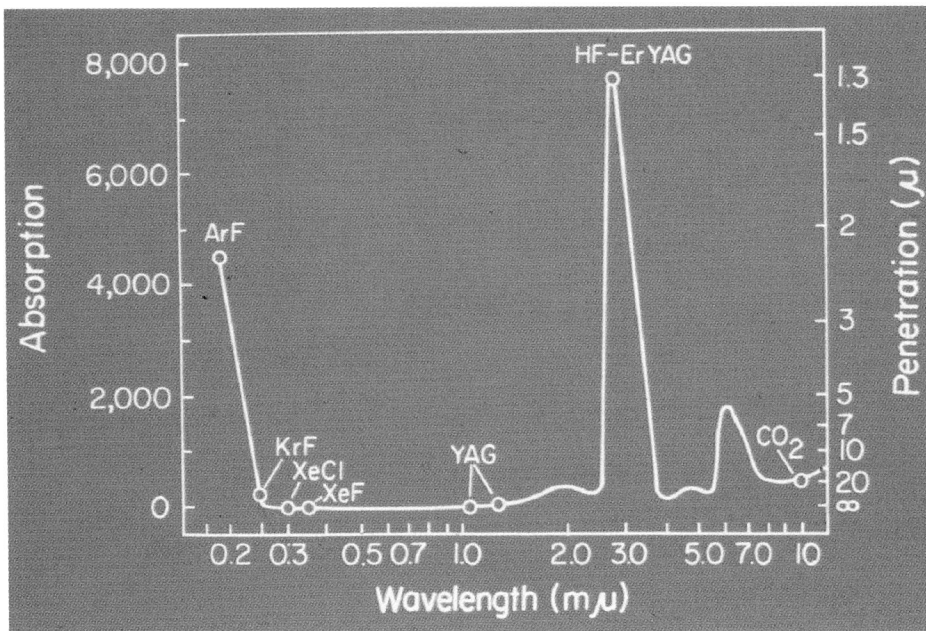

Fig. 2-2. Wavelength spectrum of the absorption coefficient in corneal stromal tissue and anticipated corneal penetration depth of 63% of laser energy. Also indicated are the various laser sources that supply the laser energy at the corresponding wavelengths. (Modified with permission from Loertscher H et al, Preliminary report on corneal incisions created by a hydrogen fluoride laser, *AJO* 102:217-221, 1986.)

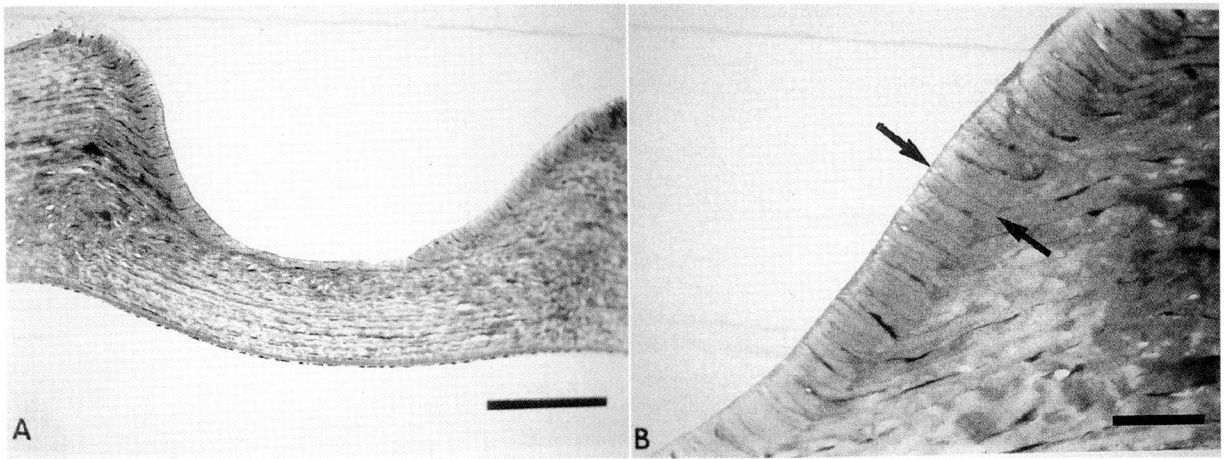

Fig. 2-3. A, Light micrograph of a wide area ablation of rabbit cornea, with an Er:YAG laser at 300 mJ cm^2 showing a greater zone of thermal damage along the excision edge than at the base of the excision. Bar = 200μm. **B,** Higher magnification view of the excision edge demonstrating 40-μm zone of thermally altered tissue. The laser pulse width is 200 microseconds, allowing for the larger zone of thermal damage. Bar = 50 μm. (With permission from Peyman GA et al: Corneal ablation with infrared laser, *Ophthalmology* 96:1160-1170, 1989.)

A Raman-shifted neodynium:YAG (Nd:YAG) laser can also be used to achieve this wavelength range, and at 2.8 μm with a short pulse duration of 8 ns, smooth slitlike incisions can be made with thermal denaturation zones ranging from 1.5 μm at lower fluences to as much as 10 μm at the higher fluences.[19]

The Er:YAG laser at 2.94 μm can be used to perform precise linear corneal excisions[11] as well as wide-area surface ablations.[14,15] When performing lamellar excisions similar to those of photorefractive keratectomy, a 16- to 40-μm zone of thermal damage was noted with few underlying vacuoles[14] (Fig. 2-3, *A* and

B). These eyes were then followed postoperatively for a period of 2 to 6 months, noting a very faint haze similar to that of excimer laser ablation and with an increased population of keratocytes and mild disorganization of the lamellae. Bende et al.[12] also showed a similar effect in the corneal photoablation and, more recently, Seiler and Wollensak[20] reported on preclinical studies using a high-energy Er:YAG laser in the fundamental mode, such that the spatial distribution of energy with each pulse corresponds exactly to that required to produce a myopic ablation pattern. This would allow for slit-lamp delivery of the Er:YAG laser energy with no additional need for focusing optics or a mechanical iris aperture.

Corneal Photodisruption

Laser-induced optical breakdown or plasma formation is another type of laser interaction in ocular tissue which has also been implemented in the cornea. Over 20 years ago, Krasnov[21-23] showed the feasibility of optical breakdown of transparent nonpigmented media by a high-powered pulsed ruby laser. Further work by Aron-Rosa[24,25] and Fankhauser[26,27] and colleagues demonstrated the clinical utility of an Nd:YAG laser in a broad range of anterior segment laser procedures. Of greatest interest with this new method of tissue photodisruption was posterior capsulotomy following cataract extraction.

These early photodisrupters and many still used today achieve their high-peak powers by a method known as optical Q-switching. A typical Q-switched pulse has a duration between 2 and 30 ns (a billionth of a second), allowing for high-peak powers sufficient to produce optical breakdown.[16,28] Further shortening of the pulse duration can be achieved by a method called mode-locking.[16,29] Mode-locking results in a series of 7 to 10 pulses each of 20 to 60 ps (a trillionth of a second) duration spread over a total envelope of approximately 35 to 50 ns. Thus, an average individual mode-locked pulse is 500 times shorter than a typical Q-switched pulse and consequently has much higher peak power.

The significance of these extremely short pulse disruptions in terms of corneal surgery is that recently a new picosecond photodisrupter has been designed for intrastromal photorefractive keratectomy.[30-33] The advantage of the picosecond pulsing is that optical breakdown can be achieved at much lower pulse energies, allowing for less thermal and acoustic damage to the surrounding tissue.[29,34] The tissue effects of photodisruption are generated by the dynamic processes which accompany laser-induced optical breakdown. When the laser pulse interacts with tissue it first generates a laser-induced plasma that is a localized high-temperature ionized gas generated by the high-energy absorption.[16,28] This plasma causes an increased absorption and scattering of the incident laser energy which gives rise to a plasma shielding effect and further expansion of the plasma.[28,35] The high temperatures associated with plasma formation result in localized heating of the tissue, generating a shock wave which propagates radially from the site of optical breakdown.[16,28,29] The heating of the tissue also produces a gas-liquid phase change which gives rise to a cavitation or gas bubble formation.[28] The gas bubble expands rapidly for several microseconds before it finally collapses, resulting in a secondary shock wave.[29,36] Basically, optical breakdown is character-

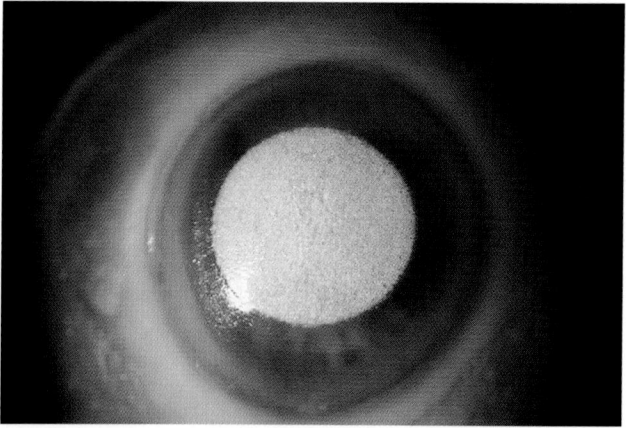

Fig. 2-4. Surface view of cavitation bubbles within the cornea immediately following Nd:YLF laser intrastromal photodisruption (intrastromal PRK). The gaseous by-products diffuse out of the cornea over a 24-hour period following treatment

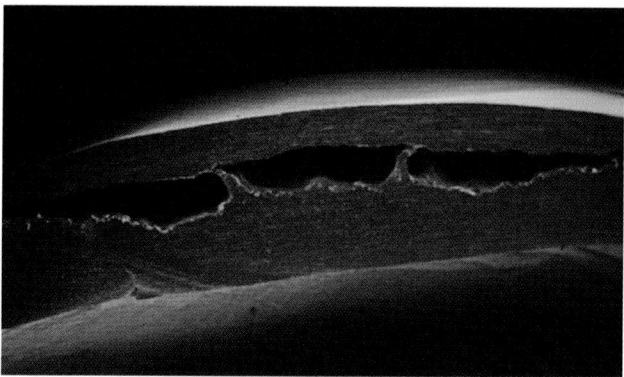

Fig. 2-5. Scanning electron micrograph of cavitation site immediately following intrastromal PRK, demonstrating the precision of picosecond photodisruption

ized by three major events: (1) plasma formation, (2) shock wave generation, and (3) gas bubble cavitation.

The effect of optical breakdown within the corneal stroma can be seen in Figs. 2-4, 2-5, and 2-6. Fig. 2-4 shows the immediate postoperative slit-lamp view of intrastromal photorefractive keratectomy (PRK). A myriad of tiny gas bubbles are generated by the plasma cavitation effect. Fig. 2-4 shows a scanning electron micrograph of the cavitation site immediately following intrastromal PRK. One can see that the optical breakdown vaporizes the collagen lamellae and results in cavitation due to bubble formation. The histopathology of intrastromal PRK in Fig. 2-5 shows very little thermal damage of tissue adjacent to the site of vaporization. Mass spectroscopy analysis of the cavitation bubbles reveals a mixture of CO_2, water vapor, and carbon monoxide.[37] These gaseous byproducts are then diffused out of the intact cornea, allowing the area of cavitation to collapse within 24 hours, resulting in thinning of the cornea.

The resultant refractive change of the pattern seen in Fig. 2-5 is corneal flattening or reduction of myopia. Multiple layered spiral patterns of 6 mm diameter with an energy of 25 to 80 μJ per pulse and spot separation of 15 μm has resulted in central corneal thinning of 10 to 120 μm and corresponding topographic flattening of 2 to 13 D in experimental cat eyes.[38] A mild subepithelial haze seen following resolution of the gas bubbles at 1 month is no longer visible at 2 months for the low-energy intrastromal ablations. Corneal endothelial damage due to the acoustic shock waves was not seen in any eye in which intrastromal ablation was limited to the anterior half of the corneal stroma,[39] and even in physiologic saline endothelial damage could not be seen for picosecond optical breakdown outside of 200 μm from the corneal epithelium.[29]

These studies suggest that intrastromal PRK using a picosecond neodynium: yttrium lithium fluoride (Nd:YLF) photodisrupter may prove to be a useful refractive surgical modality with potential advantages over excimer laser corneal surface ablation by avoiding disruption of Bowman's membrane, postoperative pain, and surface irregularities due to the ablation environment. However, the potential disadvantages include initial confinement of the ablation byproducts to within the corneal stroma as well as uncertainty of the refractive effect in human subjects whose Bowman's membrane remains intact. Further studies using this picosecond plasma-mediated intrastromal photodisruption are ongoing and, at the time of this writing, phase I Food and Drug Administration (FDA) clinical trials are being performed in blind eyes. Photodisruption and intrastromal PRK are also being evaluated with a Q-switched frequency-doubled YAG laser at 9-ns pulse width and is discussed in detail in Chapter 19.

Photothermal Tissue Shrinkage

Over 100 years ago Lans[40] first described a method of correcting corneal astigmatism by shrinking corneal collagen, a technique now known as thermokeratoplasty. Attempts to perfect the procedure continued in the mid-1970s using thermal probes to produce the desired corneal shrinkage effect.[41-44] The thermal probes are heated to temperatures of 90° to 120° C and have been shown to result in corneal ulceration with heated ring applications of as low as 98° C.[44] Additionally, much of the refractive effect induced by the application regressed over time. Corneal stromal collagen has been shown to shrink to approximately one third of its original length when heated to temperatures of 60° to 70° C, being 30° C over the ambient corneal temperature.[45-47]

The use of a CO_2 laser to induce thermal changes in the cornea was examined by Peyman et al.[48] in 1980 but was shown not to be effective in modifying corneal curvature because of the shallow penetration depth of the laser. Recently, a cobalt-magnesium fluoride laser and holmium laser were shown to induce stable refractive change in rabbit and human subjects, respectively.[49,50] Both these systems used a contact probe application of the laser energy. In the study by Seiler et al.,[50] holmium laser light was delivered through a 400-μm fiber handpiece with a pulse duration of 200 μs and energy of 25 to 35 mJ per pulse. Eight circumferential spot applications were applied at various clear zone diameters showing that a hyperopic correction is achievable and is negatively related to the distance of the coagulations from the center of the cornea.[50]

The holmium laser has also been shown to cause tissue shrinkage and induce corneal steepening by noncontact slit-lamp delivery of the laser energy, as shown in Fig. 2-7.[51] The eight spots are simultaneously delivered by projecting the light through an eight-faceted polyprismatic lens mounted to the slit lamp. Fig. 2-8 shows a scanning electron micrograph of the

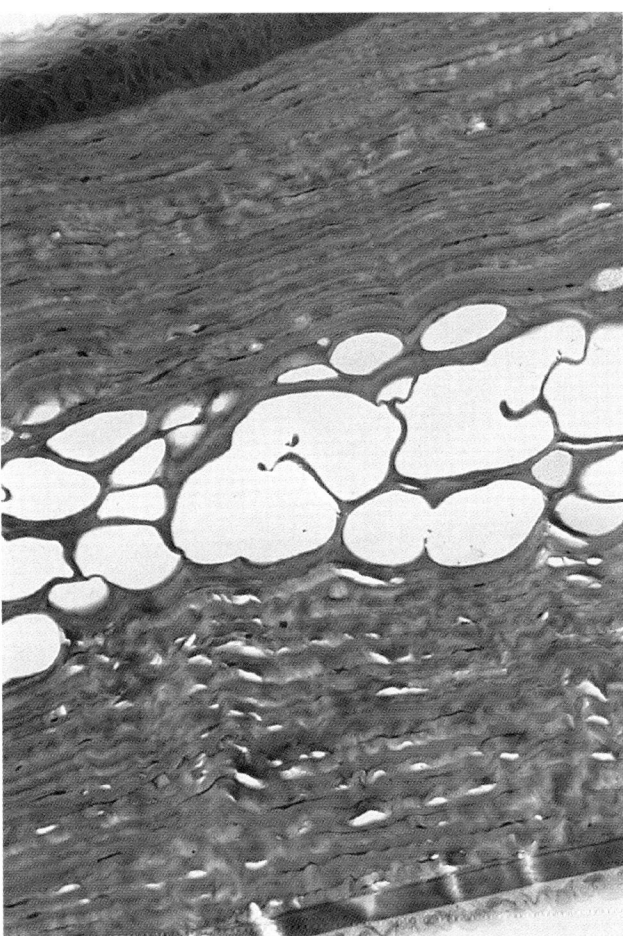

Fig. 2-6. Histologic view of picosecond Nd:YLF laser intrastromal photodisruption demonstrating cavitation with no perceptible zone of adjacent tissue damage. LM 20 × magnification

corneal surface following multiple spot applications of sufficient energy to induce corneal tissue shrinkage without thermal necrosis. The multiple laser spots result in a circular band of tissue shrinkage with central corneal steepening. Fig. 2-9 shows the histologic findings in a rabbit cornea 4 weeks following holmium laser thermal keratoplasty. The immediate effect is swelling of the surrounding stroma with some loss of the stromal lamellar pattern. At 4 weeks, however, the

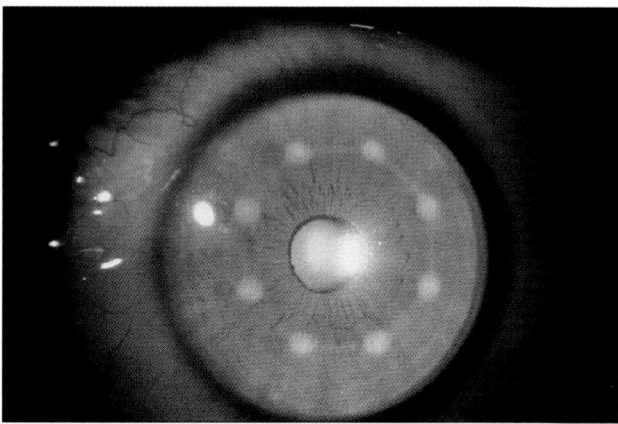

Fig. 2-7. Clinical slit-lamp photo of a circular pattern of 8 Ho laser thermokeratoplasty spots applied simultaneously with a noncontact slit-lamp delivery system.

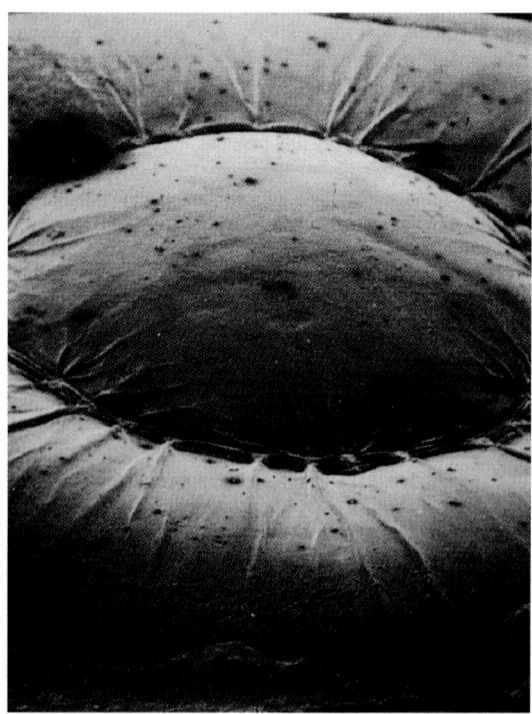

Fig. 2-8. Scanning electron micrograph demonstrating a circular pattern of tissue shrinkage with central steepening following application of 32 Ho laser thermokeratoplasty spots. (With permission from Moreira H et al, Holmium laser thermokeratoplasty, *Ophthalmology* 100:752-761, 1993.)

wedge-shaped area shows clear shrinkage of the irradiated corneal collagen.

In a recent review of noncontact holmium laser keratoplasty, Koch presented his experimental and clinical work with the laser (the Binkhorst Lecture, American Academy of Ophthalmology, Chicago, November 16, 1993). Using a wavelength of 2.12 μm and a pulse duration of 250 μs, he treated 19 sighted eyes with an eight-spot pattern at both 6- and 7-mm diameters, firing ten pulses within each spot for a total of 2-second treatments. He demonstrated that with low enough energy density he was able to achieve collagen shrinkage at 55° C while avoiding relaxation of the collagen, which occurs at 78° C. This resulted in a net steepening effect in the central cornea. The eyes were slightly overtreated and there was some early regression, but stability was seen later over a 7-month follow-up period. This information suggests that holmium laser thermal keratoplasty may be a viable option in the future for correction of hyperopia and astigmatism. This topic is covered in more detail in Chapter 17.

Corneal Photoablation

The final type of laser-tissue interaction and the subject of focus of this book is that of corneal photoablation. Initial introduction of laser photoablation to the field of ophthalmology was made by Stephen Trokel in 1983 when he and his co-workers[52] demonstrated that the laser could remove corneal tissue with precision on the order of a wavelength of light, resulting in a smooth ablation surface without any thermal damaging effects. The precise nature of this new laser-tissue interaction was cleavage of intermolecular bonds by the highly energetic photons of UV laser light. The resulting tissue removal avoids the convection of heat seen with longer-wavelength lasers, result-

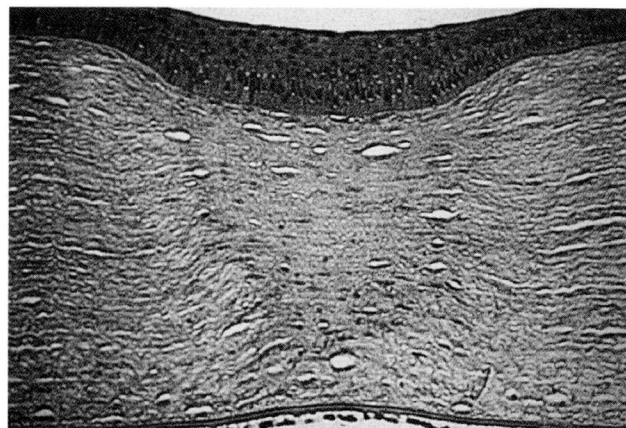

Fig. 2-9. Histologic view of noncontact holmium laser thermokeratoplasty spot demonstrating collagen tissue shrinkage. LM 16X magnification. (With permission from Moreira H et al, Holmium laser thermokeratoplasty, *Ophthalmology* 100:752-761, 1993.)

ing in adjacent tissue damage. The spectrum of UV laser photoablation was demonstrated by one of us (R.R.K.) by comparing the tissue effects of the four major wavelengths produced by the excimer laser.[53] Each of these wavelengths was generated by varying the type of excited gas in the laser cavity. An argon fluoride (ArF) gas mixture is used to generate the 193-nm wavelength that is currently used clinically. The smoothness and precision of this wavelength in ablating corneal tissue is shown in Fig. 2-10. The border of the incision shows a fresh edge of the cleaved corneal collagen lamellae with no apparent thermal tissue damage. This is in comparison to the ablation with the krypton fluoride (KrF) gas mixture, producing a wavelength of 248 nm, in which the incision shows thermal charring and vacuolization (Fig. 2-11).

As longer wavelengths within the UV range are examined, greater amounts of thermal interaction are associated with photoablation. Figure 2-12 shows the tissue effect of the 308-nm wavelength, produced by a xenon chloride (XeCl) gas mixture, where thermal charring is present in addition to shrinkage of the bordering collagen lamellae. Finally, when one uses a xe-

non fluoride (XeFl) gas mixture at 351 nm, considerable thermal damage and destruction is seen (Fig. 2-13).

When one views the ultrastructure of excisions produced with the 193-nm wavelength, one can see a narrow zone of increased electron density measuring approximately 70 nm in width with a lightly staining zone of similar thickness along the edge of the ablated tissue (Fig. 2-14).[54-57] This narrow zone behaves as a pseudomembrane as discussed later in the chapter. A comparison of the ultrastructure of ablations with the 193-nm wavelength and that of a diamond knife incision reveals marked similarity, whereas the 248-nm excimer laser excisions and steel knife incisions showed greater tissue irregularity.[57]

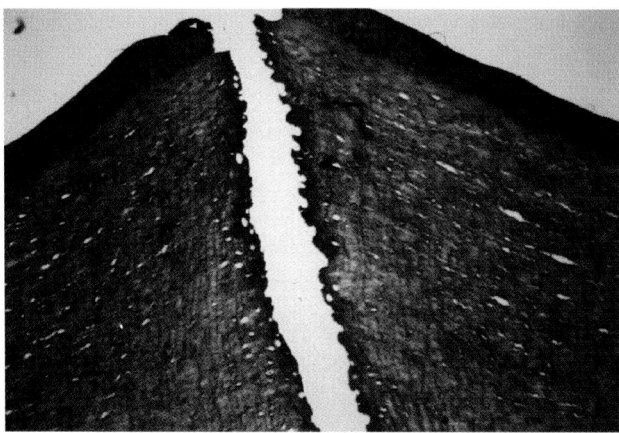

Fig. 2-11. Histologic view of a linear excision using KrF excimer laser light at 248-nm wavelength. Note the jagged excision edge with cavitation vacuoles and small 10-μm zone of thermal damage. LM 24× magnification. (With permission from Krueger RR et al: Interaction of ultraviolet laser light with the cornea, *Invest Ophthalmol Vis Sci* 26:1455-1464, 1985.)

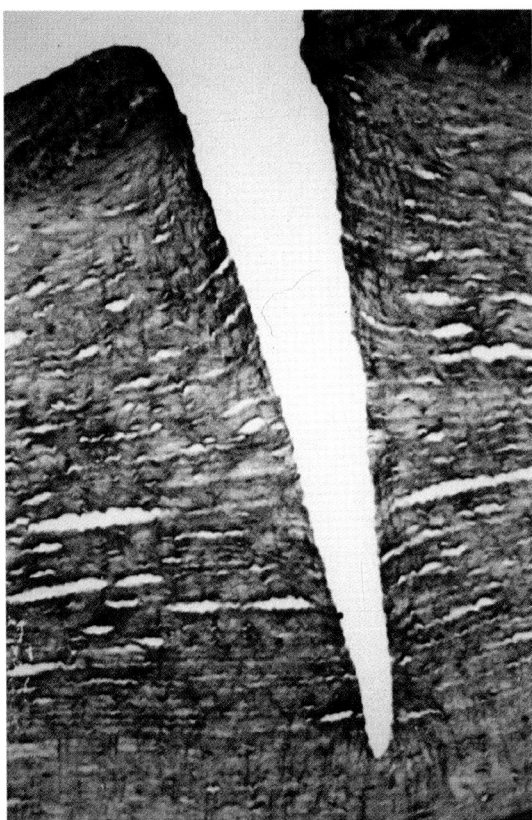

Fig. 2-10. Histologic view of a linear excision using ArF excimer laser light at 193-nm wavelength. Note the smooth ablation edge without apparent adjacent tissue damage. LM 24× magnification. (With permission from Krueger RR et al: Interaction of ultraviolet laser light with the cornea, *Invest Ophthalmol Vis Sci* 26:1455-1464, 1985).

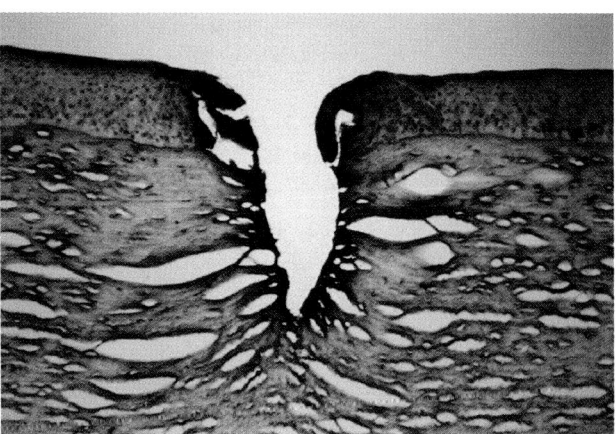

Fig. 2-12. Histologic view of a linear excision using XeCl excimer laser light at 308-nm wavelength. Note the 10- to 20-μm zone of adjacent thermal damage with localized tissue shrinkage. LM 24× magnification. (With permission from Krueger RR et al: Interaction of ultraviolet laser light with the cornea, *Invest Ophthalmol Vis Sci* 26:1455-1464, 1985.)

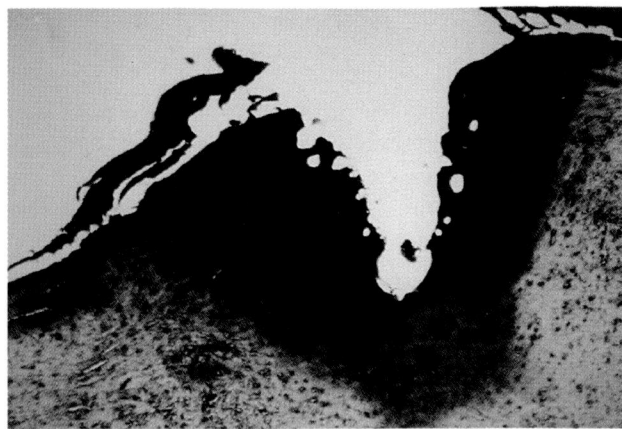

Fig. 2-13. Histologic view of a small square excision using XeF excimer laser light at 351-nm wavelength. Note the large zone of thermal denaturization exceeding the thickness of actual tissue ablation. LM 24× magnification. (With permission from Krueger RR et al: *Invest Ophthalmol Vis Sci* 26:1455-1464, 1985.)

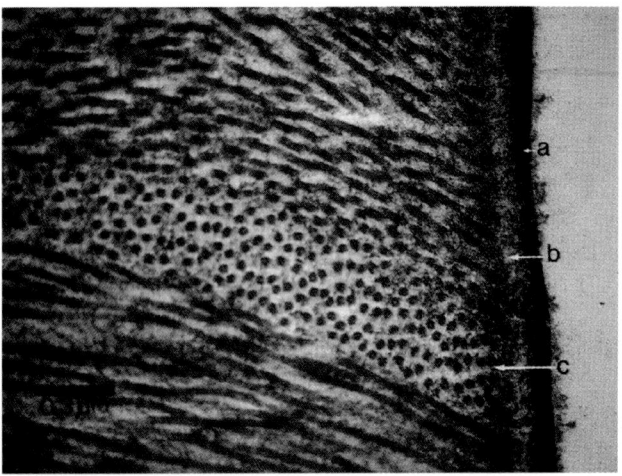

Fig. 2-14. Ultrastructural view of 193-nm excimer laser corneal ablation. Note the zone of abnormality consists of an outer densely staining region **(A),** middle lightly staining region **(B),** and an inner region **(C)** showing some increased staining in the area where the fine structure of the collagen is preserved. Each zone measures approximately 70 nm. TEM 66,000× magnification. (With permission from Puliafito CA et al: Excimen laser ablation of the cornea and lens: experimental studies, *Ophthalmology* 92:741-748, 1985.)

Recently, other solid-state UV laser sources have attempted to replace the excimer by eliminating the need for using an expensive and space-occupying gas laser. Similar precision of corneal ablation has been demonstrated by Ren and colleagues[58] using a frequency-quintupled pulsed Nd:YAG laser coupled to a computer-controlled optical scanning delivery system. The Q-switched Nd:YAG laser produces a wavelength of 1064 nm, which when modified with nonlinear optical crystals, can emit 213 nm by capturing the fifth harmonic frequency. This wavelength is slightly longer than the 193-nm wavelength but is of

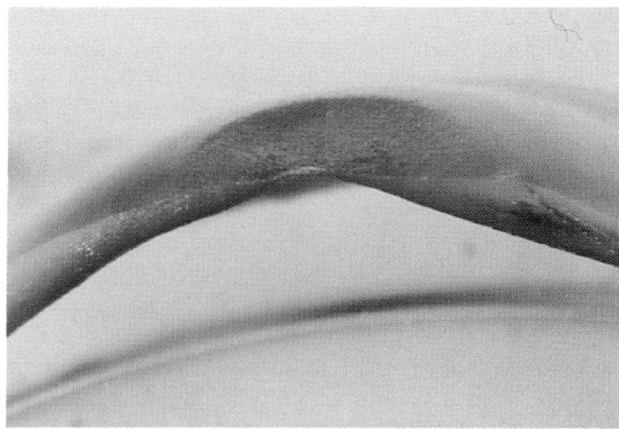

Fig. 2-15. Sectioned profile view of frequency quintupled Nd:YAG laser corneal ablation (213 nm). Note the relatively smooth ablation crater and profile of corneal thinning. (Courtesy of Quishi Ren, Ph.D., UC Irvine, Irvine, CA).

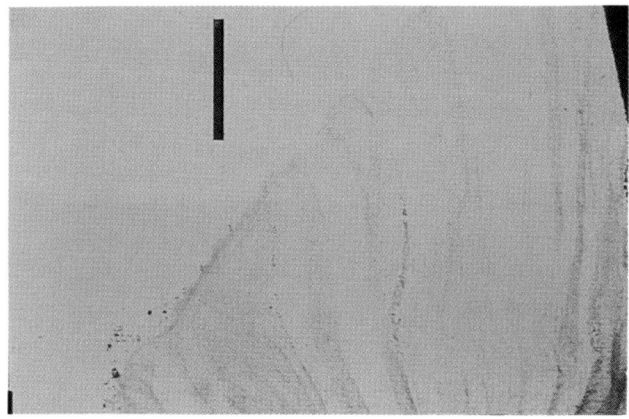

Fig. 2-16. Ultrastructural view of 213-nm ultraviolet laser corneal ablation. Note the outer densely staining zone with an inner lightly staining region similar to that of 193-nm ablation; however, the total width of the zone of abnormality "pseudomembrane" is up to 600 nm, being at least three times that seen with 193-nm ablation. TEM: bar marker = 5 μm. (Courtesy of Quishi Ren, Ph.D., UC Irvine, Irvine, CA.)

similar pulse width (10 ns). It produces a grossly similar type of refractive tissue removal (Fig. 2-15). Ultrastructural analysis of an excision with this laser reveals a similar smooth surface profile with a slightly thicker pseudomembrane being up to 0.6 μm in width (Fig. 2-16). Although this laser has been used in experimental studies, it has not yet been used clinically in the United States.

Another solid-state laser source utilizing the fifth harmonic frequency is the picosecond Nd:YLF laser at 1053 nm which is frequency-quintupled to 211 nm. This solid-state UV laser source is similar to the previously mentioned laser, except that it is mode-locked and omits picosecond pulses.[59] It has the advantage of UV laser photoablation combined with picosecond photodisruption and produces precision excisions (Fig. 2-17) with an ultrastructural border zone similar

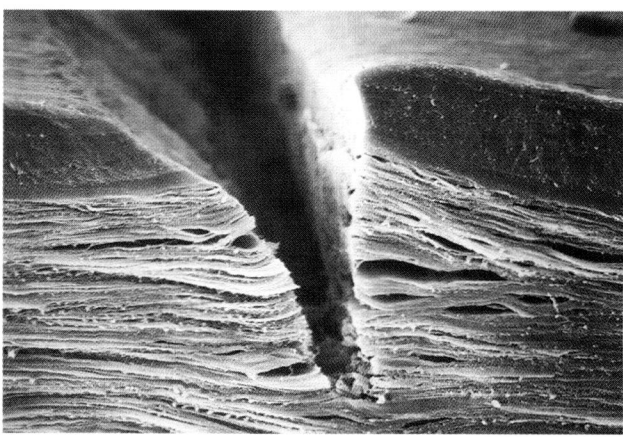

Fig. 2-17. Scanning electron micrograph of human cornea ablated with a frequency quintupled picosecond Nd:YLF laser (211 nm). Note the sharply defined excision edge. SEM 550× magnification. (Courtesy of Xin-Hua Hu, Ph.D., UC Irvine, Irvine, CA.)

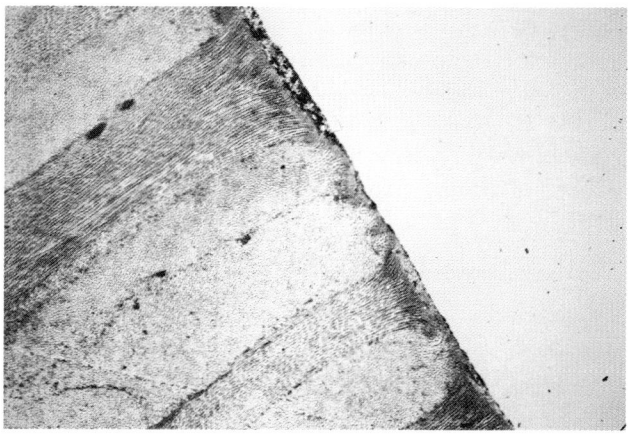

Fig. 2-18. Ultrastructural view of picosecond 211-nm ultraviolet laser corneal ablation. Note the similar pseudomembrane seen with other UV laser ablation, here varying from 100 to 600 nm. TEM 6750× magnification. (Courtesy of Xin-Hua Hu, Ph.D., UC Irvine, Irvine, CA.)

to that of excimer laser photoablation (Fig. 2-18). The picosecond pulses have a shorter thermal relaxation time, allowing use of a higher pulse frequency, up to 1000 Hz, and, consequently, faster ablation.

Finally, a solid-state UV laser source which achieves corneal photoablation at approximately 205-nm wavelength is being investigated.[60] At present, the details of this laser system remain undisclosed. A thorough review of this laser is presented in Chapter 18.

BIOPHYSICS OF EXCIMER LASER CORNEAL ABLATION
Theory of Ablative Photodecomposition

The excimer laser is unique from other lasers used in corneal refractive surgery by virtue of the mechanism of tissue interaction. All other wavelengths besides those in the far-UV range require a cumulative application of laser energy in order to break molecular bonds and remove corneal tissue. "Photocoagulation" using visible light, "photothermokeratoplasty" using near-infrared light, and "photovaporization" using far-infrared light, all achieve their desired effect with some local heating of the adjacent corneal tissue as the accumulated laser energy undergoes thermal diffusion.[16] Thermal diffusion is minimized by shortening the laser pulse in comparison with the thermal relaxation time of the irradiated tissue. The beneficial effect of shortening the laser pulse is accentuated in picosecond photodisruption, where peak powers sufficient to produce optical breakdown and plasma formation are achieved. With this type of tissue interaction it is possible for even the cornea, which is transparent to visible light, to be surgically altered intrastromally.

The uniqueness of UV laser corneal ablation is that the individual photons of light energy are of sufficiently high energy to cleave individual molecular bonds.[61-63] The photon energy of 193-nm laser light is 6.4 eV, which is appreciably greater than the energy required to break molecular bonds.[62] When the concentration of photons or energy density of laser light exceeds a critical value, the broken bonds no longer recombine but the material decomposes ablatively, hence the name *ablative photodecomposition*.[61] The driving forces for this phenomenon are twofold. First, there is a large increase in the required volume for the fragments as compared to the polymer chains they replace. Second, the energy of the photon in excess of that required to break the bond serves to excite the fragments and helps to provide the kinetic energy for ejection from the surface, signifying the onset of ablation.[61] Fig. 2-19 pictorially demonstrates the process of ablative photodecomposition. Photons are initially absorbed into the tissue sample, leading to the bond-breaking phenomena and subsequent ablation. The precision of this type of tissue removal is far superior to that of both photovaporization with a CO_2 laser and photodisruption with an Nd:YAG laser, as shown in the ablation of polymethylmethacrylate plastic in Fig. 2-20.

Characterization of Corneal Ablation

Ablation threshold. The irradiance, or energy density of ablation, is a measure of the amount of laser light energy per unit area projected onto the target tissue. This has often been incorrectly termed *fluence,* which actually is a measure of energy per unit volume. *Irradiance* is a function of the output energy and beam diameter of the laser, and reflects the density of photons striking the cornea with each laser pulse.

At low irradiance levels, the cornea remains grossly unaffected by the laser energy. As irradiance of the laser exposure progressively increases, a faint clouding of the exposed corneal tissue occurs, ranging from a faint discoloration at 193 and 249 nm to a penetrating stromal clouding at 308 and 351 nm.[53] With further increases, coagulative changes are seen at all excimer wavelengths except 193 nm. At this wavelength, tis-

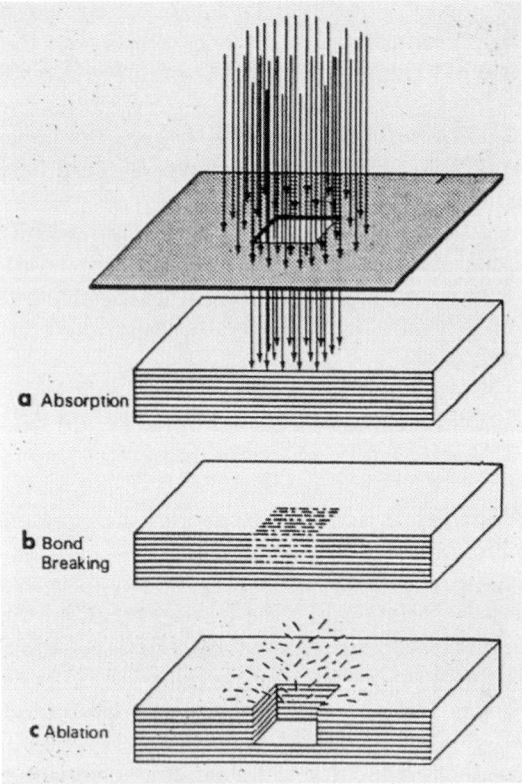

Fig. 2-19. Pictorial demonstration of ablative photo decomposition. The photons are first absorbed leading to bond breaking without reformation. Subsequent ablation occurs as the fragments assume a larger volume and are ejected from the surface. (With permission from Srinivasan R et al, Kinetics of the ablative photodecomposition of organic polymers in the far ultraviolet (193 nm). *J Vac Sci Technol* B1:923-926, 1983.)

sue ablation occurs with no intervening tissue coagulation, suggesting the absence of a thermal component. The threshold for ablation at 193 nm is ~50 mJ/cm², and is the lowest among the excimer laser wavelengths that have been tested.[53] With longer UV wavelength, the ablation threshold increases logarithmically, as shown in Fig. 2-21. Although the threshold for ablation of 193 nm remains the same with a more rapid pulse frequency, this semilogarithmic relationship breaks down as the frequency of pulses increases owing to the rapid accumulation of energy. This suggests that 193-nm ablation is purely photochemical, while a thermal component exists for the other UV wavelengths.

Other studies of ablation threshold suggest a difference in threshold irradiance with different ocular tissue and species type. Puliafito and colleagues[56] show a lower 193-nm ablation threshold for bovine cornea of 20 mJ/cm², while human corneas were ablated at a threshold of 46 mJ/cm².

Kermani and colleagues[64] used the rapid rise in intensity of mass spectroscopy to indicate the threshold energy for ablation of human cadaver eyes at 40 mJ/cm². These values are slightly lower than those reported by Krueger et al.[53] and suggest a transition zone of ablation threshold outside of which there is either no corneal ablation or clearly perceptible ablation.

Ablation Depth (Ablation Rate)

As energy density increases above the ablation threshold, each pulse of laser light removes a precise quantity of corneal tissue of uniform depth. This corneal ablation depth is dependent on the amount of energy striking the cornea, and follows a roughly sigmoidal curve with increasing pulse irradiance. Fig. 2-22 depicts the ablation depth as a function of irradi-

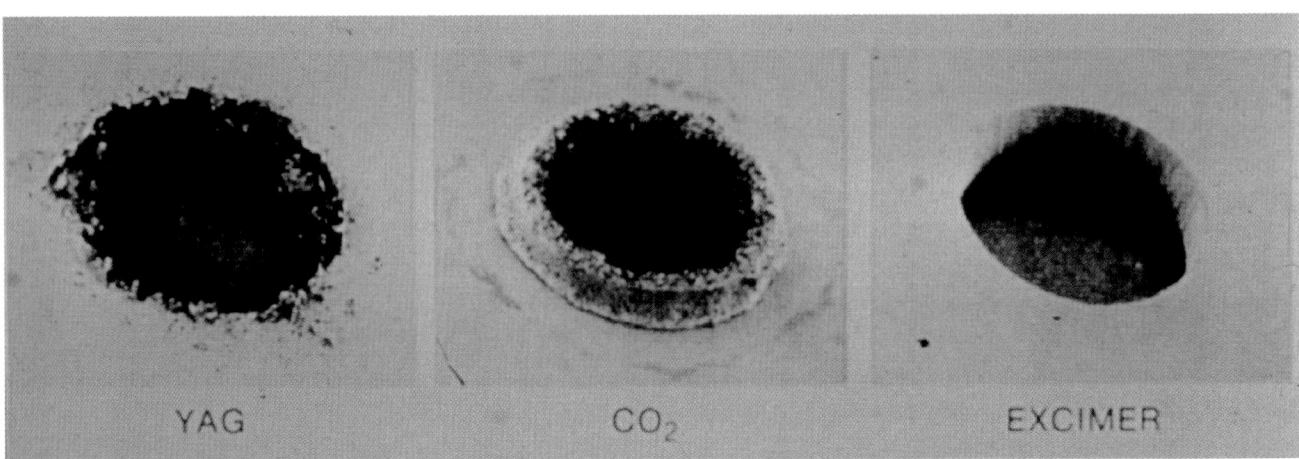

Fig. 2-20. Comparison of the differences in polymer ablation when using a CO_2 laser, Nd:YAG laser and ArF excimer laser. The excimer ablation shows a much smoother border.

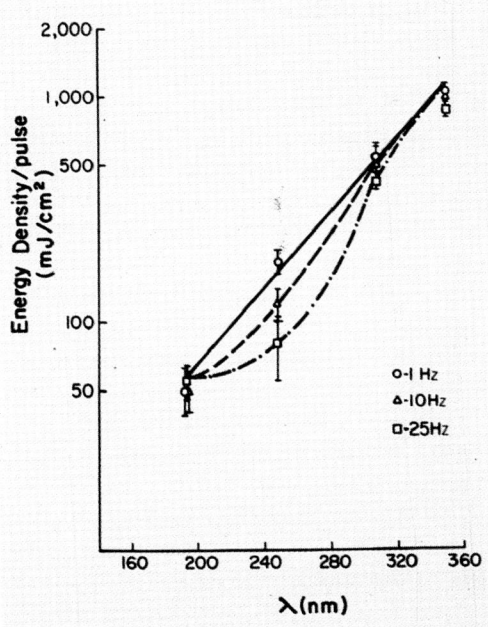

Fig. 2-21. Threshold for ultraviolet laser corneal ablation, as tested for the four major wavelengths produced by the excimer laser. There is a semilogarithmic relationship of threshold with increasing wavelength at 1 Hz. The departure from the logarithmic relationship with lowering of the threshold at the 248-nm wavelength, when pulsing the laser at a higher repetition rate, implies a thermal component of the laser tissue interaction not seen with the 193-nm wavelength. (With permission Krueger RR et al, *Invest Ophthalmol Vis Sci* 26:1455-1464, 1985.)

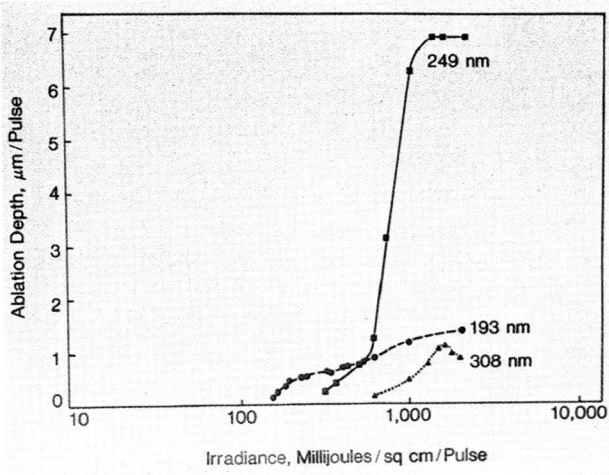

Fig. 2-22. Corneal ablation depth as a function of pulse radiance for three of the major wavelengths produced by the excimer laser. The depth increases in a roughly sigmoidal relationship with energy density with a much greater amount of tissue removed by the 248-nm wavelength, suggesting, in part, a photovaporization process due to absorption by proteins at this wavelength. (With permission from Krueger RR et al, Quantitation of corneal ablation by ultraviolet laser light, *Arch Ophthalmol* 103:1741-1742, 1985.)

ance for three UV laser wavelengths, and shows a large difference in the pulse ablation depth between wavelengths.[65] At 193 nm, the energy density varies from 0.13 μm at 150 mJ/cm² to 0.45 μm at 200 mJ/cm², and gradually increases thereafter. This is in contrast to the ablation depth at 249 nm, which is as high as 6.25 μm per pulse. The smaller ablation depth at 193 nm allows for greater precision in tissue ablation, with a smoother ablation surface than at 249 nm. When one considers the total amount of energy (radiant exposure) to remove 100 μm of corneal tissue, the most efficient energy density for ablation is 200 mJ/cm² at 193 nm.[65] This irradiance requires the least amount of total energy to remove a given amount of tissue, leaving less expenditure of energy for interactions other than ablation.

Since this first study of ablation depth in 1985, experiments by other investigators have sought to verify these findings and more carefully explore the factors affecting the ablation rate. In 1987, Puliafito and colleagues[56] repeated the ablation rate studies, demonstrating reproducible curves; however, they concluded that 600 mJ/cm² would be the best energy density of ablation, since it represented an area in the curve with minimum variation (minimum slope). Van Saarloos

and Constable[66] also repeated the study in 1990, but with greater precision, yet found their results to be within ±50% of the previous two studies. They also demonstrated that the ablation efficiency was greatest over a range of 150 to 400 mJ/cm², rather than at just a single value.

In the same year, Seiler and colleagues[67,68] went a step further and determined the ablation rate for epithelium, Bowman's layer, and the stroma in human eyes, instead of bovine eyes as studied previously. They showed that at 205 mJ/cm², the ablation rate in stroma (0.55 ± 0.1 μm per pulse) was higher than that in Bowman's layer (0.38 ± 0.05 μm per pulse) and lower than that in epithelium (0.68 ± 0.15 μm per pulse). At the same time, Terry and colleagues[69] studied living rabbit eyes and found that in a range of 120 to 180 mJ/cm², the ablation rate was 0.266 ± 0.86 μm per pulse, and that intraoperative stromal drying could lead to 12% stromal thinning, affecting the ablation rate.

With all these factors to consider, clinical studies began using an empirical value for ablation depth which was altered by trial and error to compensate for the healing response. For eyes treated with 160 to 180 mJ/cm², an ablation rate of between 0.21 and 0.27 μm per pulse (VISX laser) and ~0.26 μm per pulse (Summit laser) is used to achieve the optimal refractive outcome.[70,71] When nitrogen gas blowing is used, the corneal tissue is dehydrated and the ablation rate increases, being as high as 0.27 μm per pulse.[70] Finally, Seiler et al.[71] photographed the corneal curvature be fore and immediately after PRK, and determined this change to be nearly identical to the attempted refractive change. This verified the clinical ablation rate (0.26 μm per pulse at 180 mJ/cm^2) to be a real physical constant, and not just a "fudge factor."[71] A pulse ablation depth around this value should be used during PRK, but care should be taken during phototherapeutic keratectomy (PTK), since corneal scars can have a much lower ablation rate and may even be resistant to ablation.[72]

Ultraviolet fluorescence. A laser-induced fluorescence occurs as the excimer laser light strikes the cornea, creating a photochemical transition, and emitting a broad spectral band of UV light of longer wavelength. This longer-wavelength UV light may pass through the cornea, affecting intraocular structures or producing alterations in the adjacent corneal tissue and cells. Knowing that UV wavelengths between 295 and 400 nm are partially transmitted by the cornea and absorbed by the lens, a significant concern is addressed as to whether excimer laser radiation may lead to the formation of cataracts.

Several investigators have studied the luminance associated with excimer laser corneal ablation and have shown the spectral pattern of fluorescence to cover a broad range of wavelengths from as low as 260 to over 500 nm.[73-76] The peak wavelength for laser-induced fluorescence of human epithelium is 460 nm, while that for human cornea stroma is 310 to 320 nm[75]

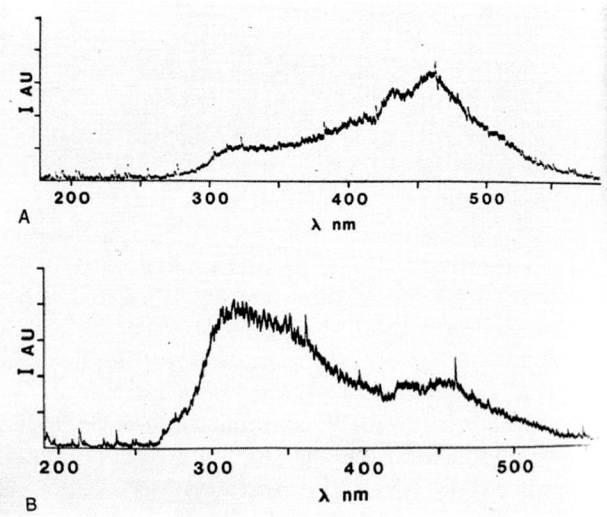

Fig. 2-23. Fluorescence spectra for human cornea irradiated with an ArF excimer laser using a lucite filter to remove scattered laser radiation in epithelium **(A)** and stroma **(B)**. The visible light fluorescence peak in epithelium at 460 nm is evident visually in contrast to that of stroma and explains a loss of characteristic fluorescence color of epithelium as it is removed by ablation. (With permission from Tuft S et al, Characterization of the fluorescence spectra produced by excimer laser irradiation of the cornea, *Invest Ophthalmol Vis Sci* 31:1512-1518, 1990.)

(Fig. 2-23). This difference between stromal and epithelial tissue explains the observation that differences in the color of fluorescence may be used to monitor the removal of the epithelium.[77]

The actual percentage of excimer laser radiant energy converted into fluorescent light of longer UV wavelengths is calculated as 0.001%.[75] If one considers 400 pulses at 200 mJ/cm^2, and the partial absorption of the cornea of longer UV wavelengths, the dose of fluorescent energy delivered to the lens through a 4-mm pupil would be on the order of 10 μJ.[75] An actual measured value using the same number of pulses is ~80 μJ/cm^2.[76] These values are 2000 to 10,000 times lower than the threshold for generating lens opacities in rabbits,[78] and the minimum average annual exposure of solar UVB, respectively.[79]

Finally, UVB radiation can lead to photokeratitis, similar to sunburn of the skin. The wavelength spectrum of threshold for photokeratitis is lowest for wavelengths between 220 and 310 nm, ranging from 5 to 100 mJ/cm^2.[80] With subablative 193-nm excimer laser irradiation, the measured threshold for photokeratitis is 10 mJ/cm^2,[80] which can be explained by the fluorescence in the UVB range. If only 0.001% of the incident excimer laser energy is converted to UVB fluorescence,[75] then the amount of fluorescent energy emitted during clinical PRK would be several times smaller than that required to produce photokeratitis, making the use of protective goggles unnecessary.

Mutagenesis. Since the highly energetic UV light can result in mutations of DNA, some concern over the potential mutagenesis of 193-nm excimer laser radiation has been raised. A number of experimental studies have been performed to address this issue, and each one has shown that 193-nm radiation does not result in cytotoxic damage to DNA and mutagenicity.[81-85] One way of measuring mutagenic damage to DNA is by monitoring the amount of unscheduled DNA synthesis. It is known that UV radiation at wavelengths below 280 nm produces cyclobutyl pyrimidine dimers in DNA.[86] Excision repair appears to be the most important mechanism for removing the damaged DNA, and this can, in turn, be monitored by the amount of unscheduled DNA synthesis. This unscheduled DNA synthesis was studied at the edge of ablated human skin[81] and rabbit cornea,[82] showing no replacement of damaged DNA with 193-nm radiation, but significant replacement when the tissue was irradiated with a germicidal lamp at 254 nm or with a 248-nm excimer laser. Fig. 2-24 shows the amount of sparsely labeled cells indicating unscheduled DNA synthesis in corneal tissue irradiated with the above-mentioned wavelengths. The 193-nm wavelength results in little damage to DNA in comparison with the 248- and 254-nm wavelengths, and this is comparable to unir-

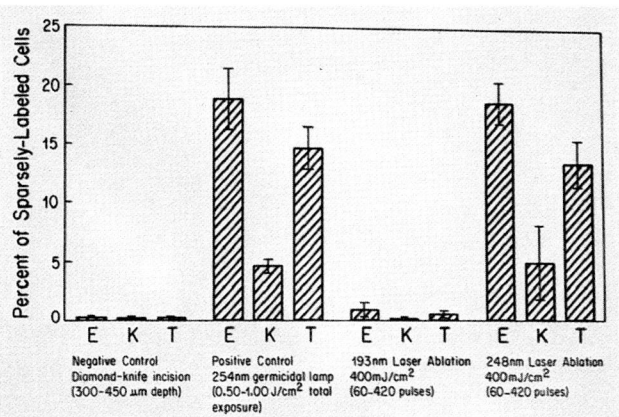

Fig. 2-24. Percentage of sparsely labeled cells indicating unscheduled DNA synthesis in corneal tissue irradiated with 193-nm and 248-nm excimer laser wavelength and a positive and negative control. The 193-nm wavelength produces a similar low percentage of sparsely labeled cells, as with a diamond knife, in comparison with a large percentage seen with the 248-nm wavelength and positive control. (With permission from Nuss RC et al, Unscheduled DNA synthesis following excimer laser ablation of the cornea in vivo, *Invest Ophthalmol Vis Sci* 28:287-294, 1987.)

radiated corneal tissue.[82] The reason proposed for this lack of damage to DNA at 193 nm is the high absorbtivity of this laser wavelength by that of protein structures in the cell. Ninety percent of 193-nm radiation is absorbed by 1 μm of cytoplasm. The distance between the cell wall and the nucleus in a corneal epithelial cell is about 1.5 to 3.0 μm.[83] Therefore, the cellular constituents—cell membrane and cytoplasm—shield the nuclear material from the incident energy. Although some feel that the replacement of damaged DNA may be inhibited by thermal effects created by the laser wavelength,[81] this is not the case since the excision repair process was seen with the 248-nm wavelength which has an even greater thermal component. When performing in vitro mutagenesis experiments with a smaller cell line of yeast cells, a significant amount of DNA repair was noted after exposure to the 193-nm radiation.[87] This can be explained by the asymmetric shape and eccentric nuclei seen in yeast cells leaving the nuclear material unprotected by the cellular constituents. Finally, Gebhardt et al.[88] examined the laser's oncogenic potential in corneal tissue by irradiating mouse cornea and keratocytes which were then implanted subcutaneously in syngeneic recipients, showing no evidence of tumor growth after many months. Even though the 193-nm wavelength appears to be safe regarding mutagenesis, one might think that the secondary UV fluorescence could lead to DNA damage, but as was already mentioned in the previous section this level of exposure is 10,000 times lower than the minimum average annual exposure of solar UVB radiation.[79]

Integrity of corneal strength. One of the major concerns with incisional keratotomy is the strength of the corneal wound and its resistance to rupture due to blunt trauma. Although several reports conclude that these eyes are resistant to rupture,[89-91] others demonstrate that globe rupture does occur even in eyes following prolonged healing.[92,93] Although there are no known reports of corneal rupture following excimer laser corneal ablation, a question of the integrity of corneal strength following PRK in comparison to radial keratotomy (RK) has been addressed.

In a study by Campos et al.,[94] the ocular integrity after refractive surgery was examined in porcine eyes undergoing RK, PRK (10-D myopic correction), or PTK at various depths. They found that upon globe compression, the eyes undergoing RK all ruptured at the site of the incision, whereas eyes undergoing PRK ruptured along the sclera, as did normal, unoperated eyes. After PTK, corneal rupture occurred when ablations were about 40% depth or greater.

Although the refractive effect following PTK is that of a hyperopic shift (corneal flattening),[95,96] corneal steepening has been observed in eye bank eyes for ablations of 150-μm depth or greater.[97] Although this corneal steepening may represent the formation of steep central islands,[98,99] it may also reflect a weakening of the structural integrity of the stromal lamellae with deeper ablations. This latter consideration has been verified with finite element computer modeling, showing that corneal curvature starts to increase rapidly after an ablation depth of 40%[100] (Fig. 2-25). This depth of ablation interestingly correlates the onset of corneal steepening with corneal rupture under compression, further suggesting that structural weakening of the cornea is responsible.

Few cases of PTK have gone beyond 40% ablation depth,[95,96] yet with RK we know that incisions are near full thickness. Visual fluctuations are a common side effect following RK, and clearly represent weakening of the structural integrity of the cornea.

Excimer Laser Surface Phenomena

Shock wave and particulate ejection. In 1987, Puliafito and colleagues[101] used high-speed photography to investigate excimer laser ablation and found that a plume of particulate material was ejected from the cornea on a time scale ranging from 500 ns to 150 μs. Fig. 2-26 shows the ablation plume at 193 nm, which resembles a mushroom cloud of smoke similar to that seen after an atomic bomb explosion. The individual particles were too small to optically resolve, but traveled at velocities on the order of several hundred meters per second. Using mass spectroscopy, the majority of ejected material was of smaller molecular weight, being H_2O radicals and other simple carbons and hydrocarbons,[64] but several larger-molecular-

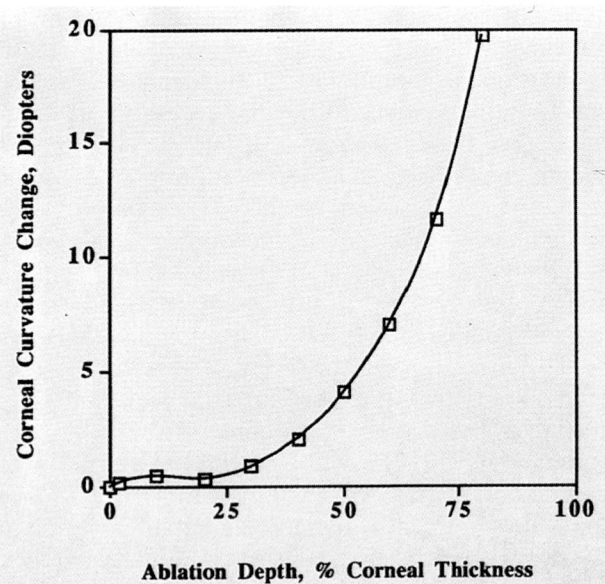

Fig. 2-25. Computer-generated line graph showing the exponential increase in central corneal steepening with excimer laser ablation depth in excess of 40% of the corneal thickness. The results are based on a mathematical (finite element) model of the cornea and sclera, assuming a Young's modulus of 3.0×10^4 dynes/mm^2 (corneal stroma) and 7.0×10^4 dynes/mm^2 (sclera and Bowman's layer) and a Poisson's ration = 0.45. Successive layers of elements were removed over the central 6 mm to simulate ablation with a 6-mm treatment zone. (Courtesy of Michael Bryant, Ph.D., Doheny Eye Institute, Los Angeles, CA.)

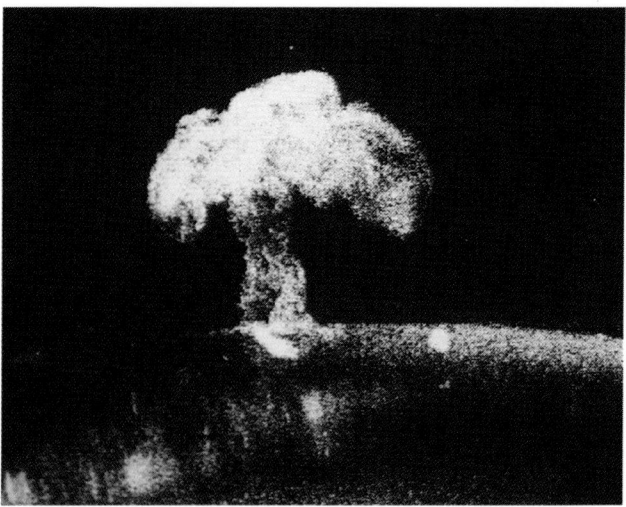

Fig. 2-26. Photograph of the ejection plume of 193-nm excimer laser corneal ablation at 50 μs following pulse impact. The plume resembles a mushroom cloud of smoke similar to that seen after an atomic bomb explosion. (With permission from Puliafito CA et al: High-speed photography of excimer laser ablation of the cornea, *Arch Ophthalmol* 105:1255-1259, 1987.)

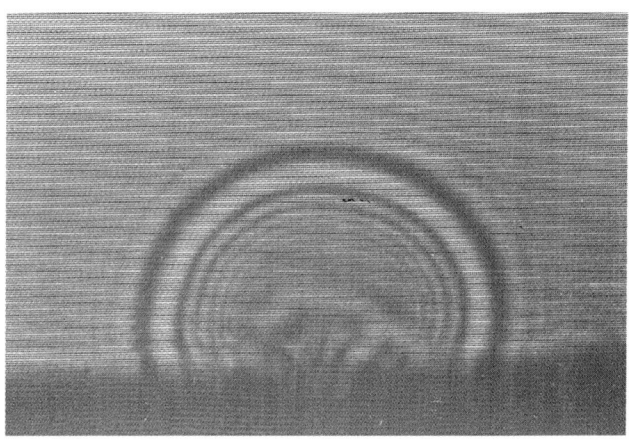

Fig. 2-27. Shadow photograph of the shock wave in air created during excimer laser photoablation. The shock wave is captured 240 ns following impact of the excimer laser pulse, being seen at a much shorter time lag than that of the ejection plume.

weight compounds, mostly alkanes, have also been observed.[102]

The particles are ejected in the direction of the next oncoming laser pulse, and it has been suggested that they may interfere with the uniformity of the energy profile. One manufacturer designed an effluent remover and fixation ring with nitrogen blower to eliminate the gaseous and particulate debris. The effluent remover aids in removing the ablation by-products, but also removes toxic ozone produced when the excimer laser reacts with oxygen. The nitrogen gas blower, however, was noticed to produce an undesirable effect and was discontinued from use.

Prior to particulate ejection, the impact of the excimer laser pulse with the cornea results in an acoustic shock wave, creating an audible snap. The shock wave has been photographed in the air above the eye[103-105] (Fig. 2-27) and recorded posteriorly underneath the cornea using a piezoelectric transducer.[106] In each case the velocity of the leading edge of the shock wave is a function of the material through which it propagates. In air the velocity is ~3 to 4 km/sec,[103-105] in helium it is ~6 km/sec,[103] and passing through the cornea it travels at the speed of sound (~1.6 km/sec).[106] The laser-induced shock wave has been shown to generate a pressure of ~100 atm, resulting in mechanical

stress to the cornea. This may lead to structural damage to adjacent collagen layers or cellular alterations in keratocytes or endothelial cells, or both.[106]

The high-velocity particles and gases of the plume are ejected as the potential energy of molecular bond formation is released and converted to kinetic energy. The recoil of the plume ejection results in a surface wave which emanates from the point of laser impact[104,105] (Fig. 2-28). This surface wave has an initial amplitude as high as 0.15 to 0.40 mm, and propagates along the surface at several meters per second. The significance of this surface wave is that it represents a significant displacement of corneal tissue which can

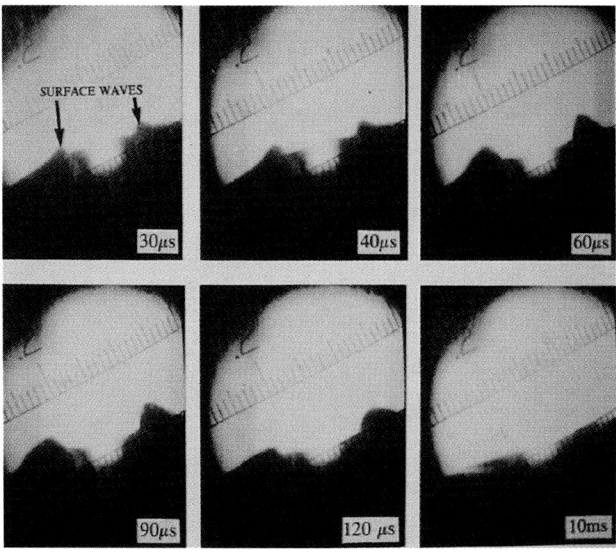

Fig. 2-28. Photograph of the surface waves seen during excimer laser corneal ablation. The surface wave is caused by the recoil forces of the plume ejection and is seen immediately following the ablation plume. Depending upon the energy density of ablation, the amplitude of this wave can be as high as 0.15 to 0.40 mm. (With permission from Bor Z et al, Plume emission, shock wave and surface wave formation during excimer laser ablation of the cornea, *Refract Corneal Surg* 9:S111-S115, 1993.)

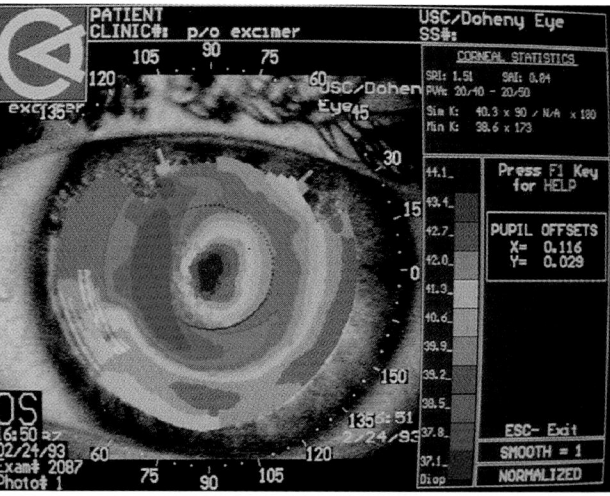

Fig. 2-29. Topographic central zone of corneal steepening seen following excimer laser photorefractive keratectomy, referred to as a "topographic steep central island."

damage or tear the layers of the cornea,[105] yet these effects have not been clearly seen histopathologically. Both the shock wave or later-occurring surface wave may result in the production of surface fluid from within the cornea, leading to attenuation of corneal ablation centrally and topographic steep central island formation[98,99,107] (Fig. 2-29).

Surface heating. Although excimer laser photoablation is predominantly a nonthermal process, the release of energy as molecular bonds break does give rise to temperature changes on the surface. In 1988, Bende and colleagues[108] showed a temperature increase of approximately 10° to 20° C in the stromal tissue adjacent to the laser-ablated area. Berns et al.[109] verified this using a thermal camera, again showing an average corneal temperature increase of 20° C. With pulsed laser energy, it is obvious that higher temperature spikes are excited on the surface. Although these temperature spikes may not be sufficient to denature the surface corneal collagen, they may affect keratocyte activation and corneal wound healing. Recently attempts have been made in Japan to reduce surface heating by cooling the cornea during the procedure (presented by Kazuo Tsubota, M.D., at the Japanese Society of Ophthalmic Surgeons Meeting, Yokohama).

Another way corneal surface heating may be minimized is by reducing the excimer laser pulse width. In 1987, Srinivasan and Sutcliffe[63] presented a model whereby the ejection of ablation by-products began

within the time span of the laser pulse. Since then, another study has suggested that the leading edge of the excimer laser pulse creates a surface plasma on the cornea, which shields the transmission of laser light at the end of the pulse.[110] This plasma shielding sequesters further energy at the surface which may lead to heating of adjacent tissue. By shortening the excimer laser pulse, one might eliminate the potential interaction with ablation by-products and the plasma shielding effect, thereby minimizing surface heating. Although this has not been clinically or histologically substantiated, it is being investigated and deserves mention.

Effect of hydration and dehydration. One of the most important environmental factors in excimer laser ablation is tissue hydration. Upon removal of the corneal epithelium, the corneal stroma can swell, while at the same time the light of the operating microscope can promote superficial dehydration. As previously mentioned, the ablation rate of the excimer laser depends strongly on the level of tissue hydration, with deeper ablations occurring when the tissue is dehydrated.[69,70]

In early clinical studies with the nitrogen gas blower, tissue dehydration resulted in good predictability of refractive outcome, but with a reticular corneal haze.[111] An animal study was then performed examining the effects of the nitrogen gas blower, and demonstrated a greater surface roughening and greater corneal haze with nitrogen blowing than when no blowing was used.[112] Fig. 2-30, *A* and *B* shows the relative smoothness of the corneal surface with no gas blowing in comparison to the gas-blowing surface as seen by scanning electron microscopy. As a result of this finding, clinical use of the nitrogen gas blower

Fig. 2-30. Scanning electron micrographs of corneal surface following excimer laser ablation comparing the surface with no gas blowing *(a)* to that of gas blowing *(b)* during a procedure. Nitrogen gas blowing results in greater surface roughening and subsequently greater corneal haze. (With permission from Krueger RR et al, Corneal surface morphology following excimer laser ablation with humidified gases, *Arch Ophthalmol* 111:1131-1137, 1993.)

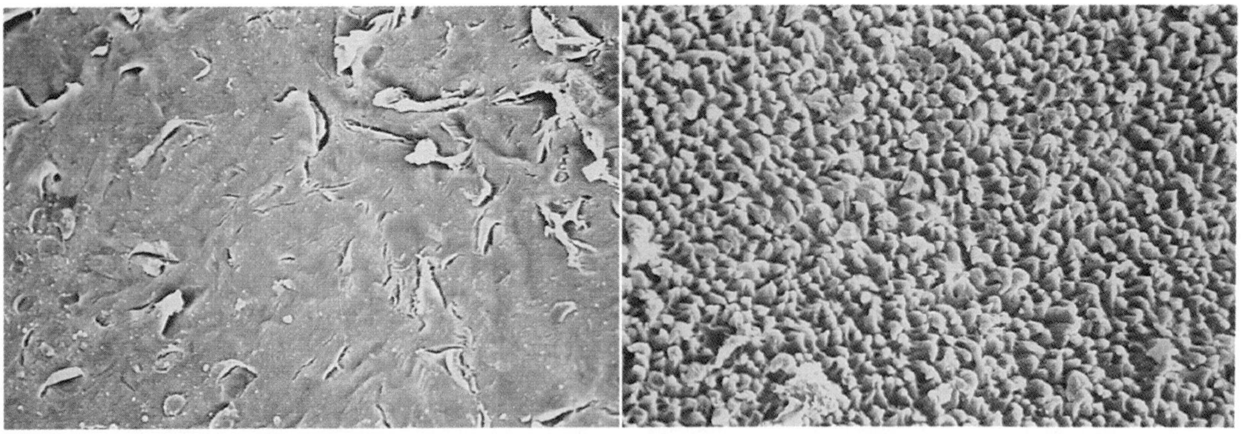

was discontinued, and subsequent clinical analysis has demonstrated less corneal haze and improved refractive results over those that are seen with the gas blower.[70]

With the nitrogen gas blower no longer in use, the question regarding the adequate removal of the ablation by-products was reintroduced. The formation of topographic steep central islands was now being seen with some frequency,[98,99] and there was some thought that a vortex plume existed near the corneal surface, resulting in island formation. A subsequent animal study was then performed comparing the effects of blowing both dry and humidified gas over the corneal surface during PRK.[113] The results showed that corneas ablated using humidified gas were smooth and equivalent to those ablated under ambient conditions, whereas those ablated using dry gas blowing again showed surface irregularity.

Humidified gas blowing may be helpful during excimer PRK, but what seems most important is to maintain a constant level of corneal hydration. If the cause of topographic steep central island formation is central surface fluid due to a shock wave,[99,114] then removal of ablation by-products using humidified gas blowing may not be necessary, unless it can restore a uniform level of hydration. When using an ablatable mask[115] or slit mask,[116] gas blowing must be used since the ablation by-products will deposit on the undersurface of the mask and interfere with passage of the laser light. In this case, humidified gas blowing would probably be best, and its use has been reported.[117]

Pseudomembrane formation. The formation of a pseudomembrane in association with excimer laser photoablation was first described in 1986, when Marshall and colleagues[57] noted that some epithelial cells

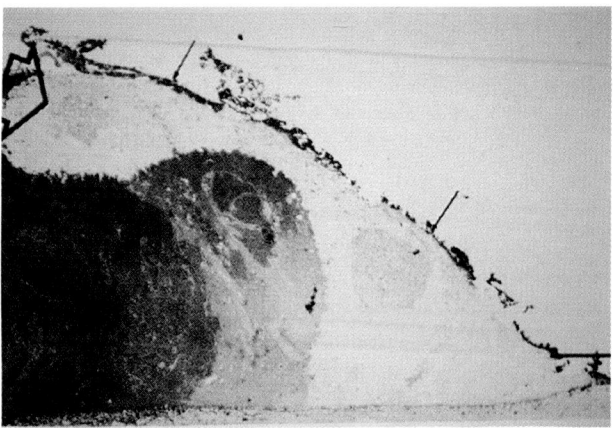

Fig. 2-31. Pale-staining epithelial cell cleaved by the excimer laser and maintained by an electron dense condensation with membrane-like properties, "pseudomembrane." (With permission from Marshall J et al, An ultra structural study of corneal incisions induced by an excimer laser at 193 nm, *Ophthalmology* 92:749-758, 1985.)

immediately adjacent to the ablated area had a pale-staining cytoplasm. On closer examination, these pale-staining cells had no cell membrane along the border adjacent to the ablated area, but had actually been cleaved by the photoablation process (Fig. 2-31). The severed edge was bounded by an electron-dense condensation of less than 100-nm thickness which seemed to maintain the integrity of the cell, suggesting a "membrane-like" function; hence the term *pseudomembrane.*

This pseudomembrane bordering the cells and collagen stroma actually has two components: (1) an electron-dense outer layer, and (2) a less dense inner layer of up to 200-nm thickness.[118] Along the ablation edge, individual collagen fibers cleaved by the laser seem to converge and are pinched together as if the

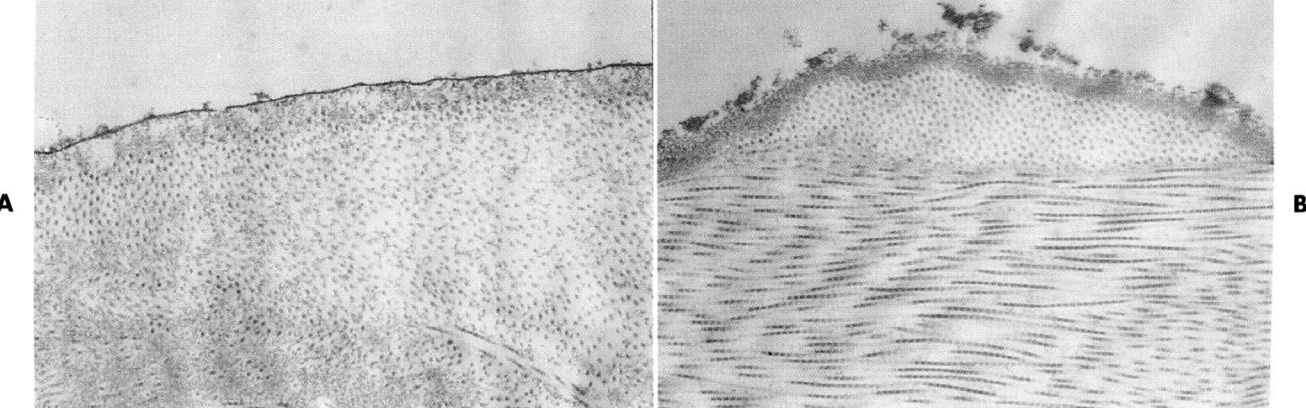

Fig. 2-32. Transmission electron micrographs of pseudomembranes following excimer laser corneal ablation with dry nitrogen gas blowing *(a)* and humidified gas blowing *(b)*. Dry gas blowing results in a thicker pseudomembrane with frequent surface discontinuities and detached fragments due to corneal dehydration. This is in contrast to humidified gas blowing (as well as no gas blowing), where hydration at physiologic levels keeps the pseudomembrane thin and uniform. (With permission from Krueger RR et al, Corneal surface morphology following excimer laser ablation with humidified gases, *Arch Ophthalmol* 111:1131-1137, 1993.)

ends had been sealed.[119] The greater the energy density of ablation, the greater the thickness of the pseudomembrane, ranging nearly linearly from 50 to 250 nm for energies from 100 to 180 mJ/cm^2.[120] Although the cause of pseudomembrane formation is unknown, some believe that it is formed from uncoupled organic double bonds created during photoablation, while others contend that we are observing a thermal effect.[119] The differences in pseudomembrane appearance and thickness under different hydration conditions suggest a possible thermal mechanism, but even if this is so there is no conductive damage adjacent to the pseudomembrane.

When nitrogen gas blowing is used, the pseudomembranes appear thicker, less dense, and with frequent surface discontinuities and detached fragments, while those with humidified blowing or no blowing have thin, flat, highly electron-dense layers[113] (Fig. 2-32, *A* and *B*). Corneal dehydration seems to have a detrimental effect on the pseudomembrane, while hydration at physiologic levels keeps it thin and uniform. Perhaps the water in the cornea helps to dissipate any heat generated during the procedure.

Whatever the cause of pseudomembrane formation, its membranelike properties appear to have a beneficial effect. Like true membranes, its structural integrity allows it to wrinkle during critical point drying prior to scanning electron microscopy.[119] It maintains integrity of sectioned cells, at least temporarily, and its smooth, uniform surface appears to serve as a template for reepithelialization during healing. Finally, the pseudomembrane serves as a barrier to water transportation, and prevents significant corneal swelling after photorefractive keratectomy, as compared to conventional lamellar keratectomy.[117]

Surface smoothness and uniformity. As was already mentioned, excimer laser photoablation results in precise etching of corneal tissue, leading to a smooth, uniform surface bordered by a pseudomembrane. The smoothness and uniformity that one achieves seems to be related to a maintenance of corneal transparency and absence of significant scar formation. It had been a long-held axiom and clinical observation that violation of Bowman's layer would lead to scar formation, and that one should avoid operating on the visual axis of the cornea. Prior to excimer laser photoablation this was true, as lamellar keratectomy could only be performed within the corneal stroma and required replacement of Bowman's layer. Now with excimer laser photoablation, a smooth enough surface is achieved which allows one to operate in the visual axis, and remove Bowman's layer.

One of the most important factors in surface smoothness and uniformity is homogeneity of the beam. The excimer laser beam profile as it exits the laser cavity is rectangular and has a gaussian distribution along its short axis. Additionally, there are often energy spikes of higher intensity, "hot spots," which could lead to focal areas of greater ablation. The beam energy must be redistributed into a homogeneous pattern before exiting the clinical laser system. If the beam profile is not homogeneous, then corneal ablation will not be uniform, but will mimic the spatial intensity pattern of the laser beam.

Several methods of beam reshaping have been used to achieve a uniform beam profile and uniform corneal ablation. These include, in addition to a series of lenses and mirrors, a rotating dove prism,[121,122] rotating slit beam,[123] prismatic integrator with telescopic

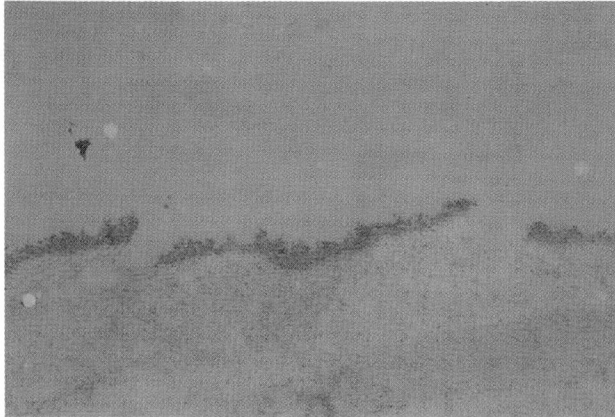

Fig. 2-33. Surface discontinuities in the pseudomembrane seen with excimer laser PRK using a contracting iris diaphragm. Switching to an expanding aperture eliminates the discontinuities seen with the former method. (With permission from Sinbawy A et al, Surface ultrastructure after excimer laser ablation: expanding vs. contracting apertures, *Arch Ophthalmol* 109:1531-1533, 1991.)

zoom,[124] and an absorbing cell system.[125] Once a uniform "top hat" energy configuration is achieved, a myopic ablation pattern can be sequentially projected onto the cornea using either a mechanical iris aperture,[126,127] a series of circular apertures,[124,128] or an ablatable mask.[129] The mechanical iris aperture is most commonly used for clinical PRK. The greater the number of steps as the iris opens and closes, the greater the surface smoothness and the greater the rate of successful healing.[130]

When performing PRK using the iris diaphragm system, the VISX laser initially used a contracting iris diaphragm, but later changed to an expanding aperture because of discontinuities in the pseudomembrane with the former method[126,127] (Fig. 2-33). These discontinuities resulted as the edge of the laser beam profile was projected onto the corneal surface without a subsequently larger-diameter beam smoothing over the previous edge. Even with an expanding aperture system, stepped edges can sometimes be seen acutely after excimer PRK, which are not seen after PRK using an ablatable mask.[129] These steps can be seen more easily in ablated plastic, and can be minimized by defocusing the image of the aperture[131] (Fig. 2-34). The defocused image of the edge of the iris diaphragm allows for a smoother transition of the incident energy. Whether this leads to any benefit in the optical or refractive outcome is unknown.

Finally, smoothness and uniformity depend on the hydration of the cornea and uniform moisture of the ablation environment. Differential hydration changes can lead to nonuniform ablation rates and result in topographic irregularities, such as topographic steep central islands.[98,99]

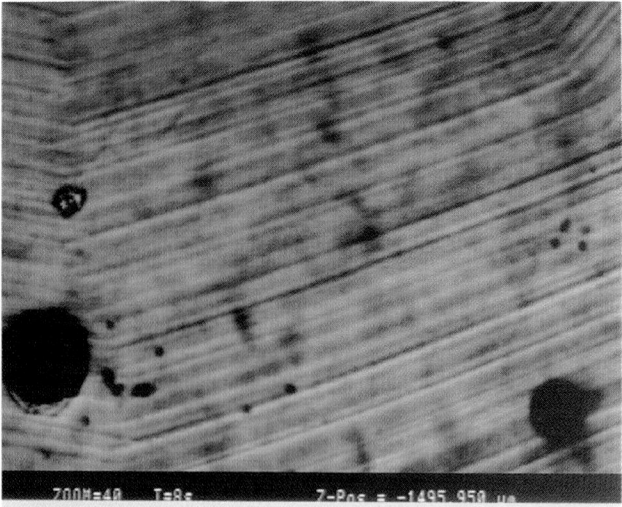

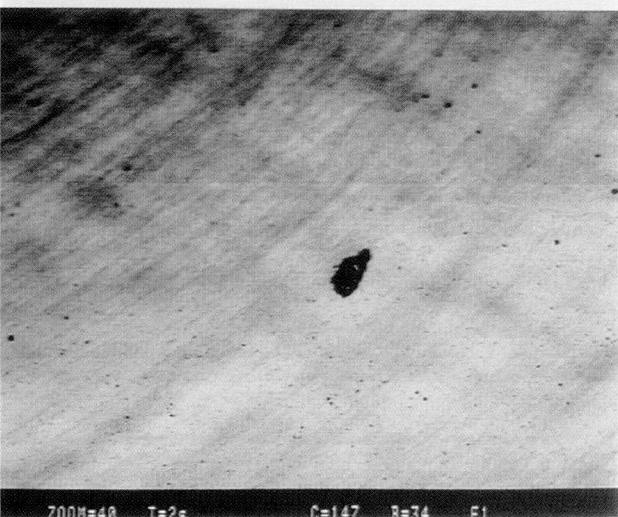

Fig. 2-34. Stepped edges of excimer laser PRK with an expanding aperture, as seen in plastic. Defocusing the image of the edge of the iris diaphragm results in a smoother ablation *(below)* with less prominent stepped edges.

BIOLOGICAL RESPONSE OF EXCIMER LASER CORNEAL ABLATION
Excimer-Induced Changes in Corneal Morphology

Epithelial response to excimer laser photoablation. Following the initial excision of superficial layers of the cornea with a 193-nm ArF excimer laser, the primary response of the cornea is to cover the ablated surface with epithelium.[77] Clinical studies have shown that reepithelialization occurs within the first 3 to 5 days,[132-134] and the initial epithelial thickness consists of three to five cells. Over the following 6 to 18 months, the epithelium thickens primarily at the deepest part of the ablation site.[127,135-146] Currently we are unsure of the stimulus for epithelial thickening.

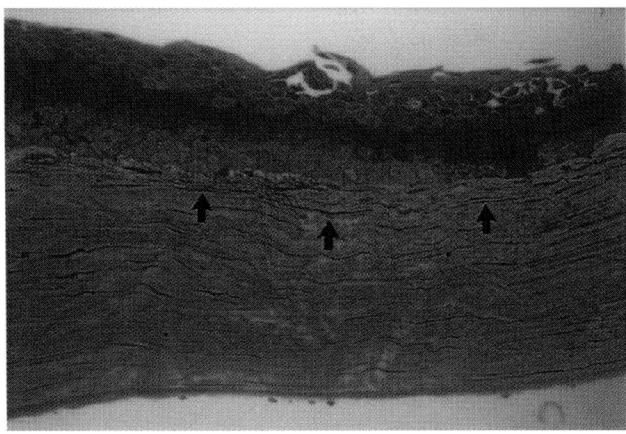

Fig. 2-35. Histologic view of epithelial hyperplasia in a human cornea 6 months following excimer laser PRK. Epithelial hyperplasia up to 12 cells thick is seen over the ablation site *(arrows)* but not in the adjacent untreated stroma; human, corneal trichrome stain. LM 50× magnification. (Courtesy of Robert Lambert, Ph.D., and Janet Anderson, Ph.D., National Vision Research Institute, San Diego, CA.)

One theory suggests that the tear film thickness stimulates epithelial hyperplasia.[147] Others have suggested that the shape of the excised tissue (excision profile) determines the degree of epithelial hyperplasia with smaller-diameter ablations (<5 mm) or single-profile excisions theoretically stimulating a greater hyperplastic response compared to larger-diameter excisions or multiple-profile excisions, i.e., ablations at 4-mm, 5-mm, and 6-mm diameter.[148] The clinical impact of epithelial hyperplasia is thought to be the regression of refractive effect.

Since the epithelial response is acute, one may assume the refractive changes documented in the first 3 to 6 months are associated with this response. Increasing corneal power, increasing corneal thickness, decreasing the diameter of the ablation site as measured by corneal topography, and associated loss of refractive error (refractive regression) are all common events. Since the stromal wound healing response is much slower compared to the epithelial response, these early changes are most likely due to epithelial hyperplasia. Rabbit,* nonhuman primates,[136,140] and human pathologic studies[138,150-153] have confirmed epithelial hyperplasia within the ablation site in the postoperative period up to 6 months after surgery (Fig. 2-35). Studies of nonhuman primates and of human pathologic specimens obtained up to 18 months after surgery have also documented significant epithelial hyperplasia.[154,155] Clinical studies have confirmed continued regression of refractive effect between

months 12 and 18, but not between months 18 and 24.[156] Since epithelial hyperplasia occurs early and persists, the late changes in refractive error are due, most likely, to stromal remodeling (new collagen, or proteoglycan production, or both).

One of the early concerns of excimer laser photoablation is the possibility of recurrent epithelial erosions caused by abnormalities in the adhesion of the epithelium to bare stroma.[145] Morphologic studies of the epithelium† have documented completely normal-appearing cells. Sophisticated morphologic and immunohistochemical studies have confirmed the production of normal epithelial attachment complexes[155,158-160] as evidenced by the presence of type III collagen (anchoring fibrils), beta$_4$-integrin (epithelial hemidesmosomes), and type IV collagen (basement membrane), as shown in Fig. 2-36, *A-C*.

Recent studies of human specimens that were excised following failed PTK procedures have documented the absence of PAS (periodic acid–Schiff) staining (which normally stains the epithelial basement membrane) under the normal-appearing epithelium,[155] even though the same area appeared to have morphologic and immunohistochemical evidence of normal epithelial attachment complexes. This finding suggests incomplete re-formation of normal anatomy months after excimer laser surgery. Recurrent epithelial erosions following excimer laser photoablation are rare occurrences,[161,162] and, in fact, the excimer laser has been used as a treatment for recurrent corneal erosions.[163,164]

Bowman's layer response to excimer laser photoablation. Destruction of Bowman's layer has previously been associated with permanent corneal scarring in the area of its removal either by infection or following freehand lamellar dissection.[165,166] Acute and short-term studies of cornea excised after excimer laser photoablation have demonstrated a smooth, but sharply defined excision of Bowman's layer in the periphery of the ablation site.[67,135,143,167,168] Rarely, following planned superficial ablations, remnants of Bowman's layer have been found within the ablation site[155] (Fig. 2-37). The absence of Bowman's layer may not be necessary for maintenance of permanent corneal clarity based on a lack of recurrent erosions following laser treatment, the presence of normal clarity in animals whose corneas lack a Bowman's layer, rare reports of cases of congenital absence of Bowman's layer maintaining corneal clarity, and excellent morphologic recovery of normal epithelial enhancement complexes.

*References 110, 136, 139, 142, 144, 146, 149.

†References 77, 112, 127, 146, 155, 157, 158.

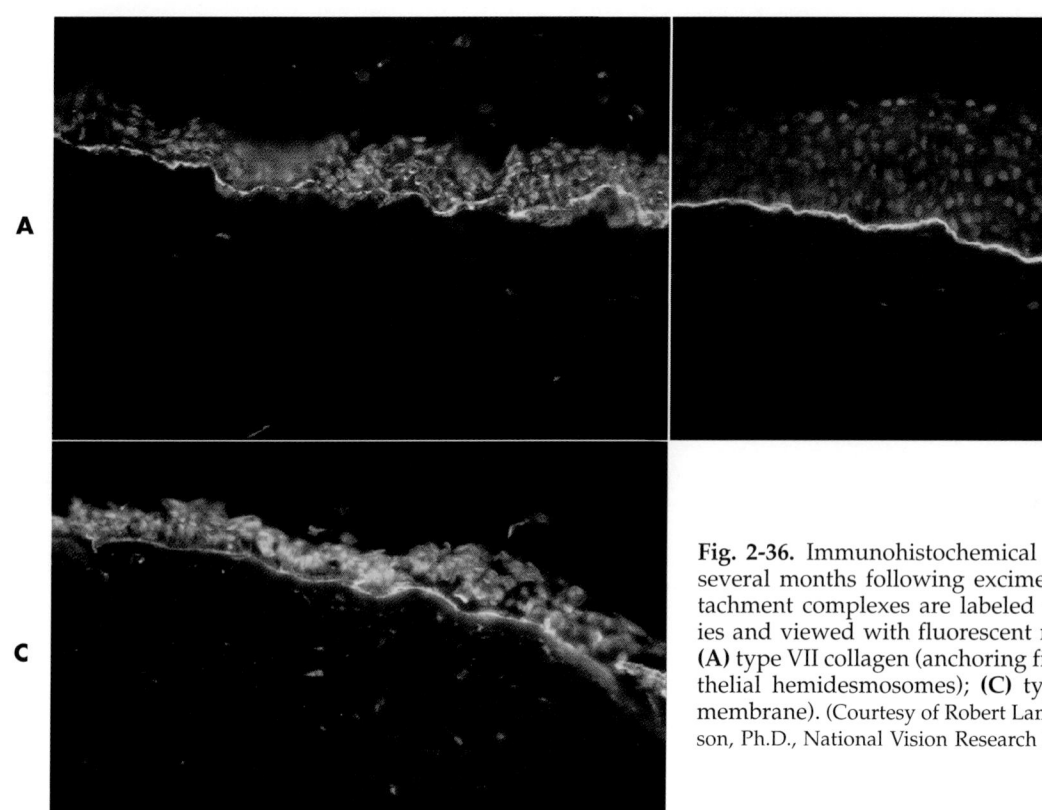

Fig. 2-36. Immunohistochemical staining of human cornea several months following excimer laser PRK. Epithelial attachment complexes are labeled with monoclonal antibodies and viewed with fluorescent microscopy demonstrating (A) type VII collagen (anchoring fibrils); (B) β 4 integrin (epithelial hemidesmosomes); (C) type IV collagen (basement membrane). (Courtesy of Robert Lambert, Ph.D., and Janet Anderson, Ph.D., National Vision Research Institute, San Diego, CA.)

Corneal stromal response to excimer laser photoablation. Acute morphologic studies after PRK demonstrate the presence of a thin pseudomembrane over the ablated surface; normal collagen fibers at their edges are present immediately underlying the pseudomembrane. As the cornea responds to the laser injury, new collagen and proteoglycans are produced, and the pseudomembrane disappears. The thickness of newly modeled corneal tissue varies, depending upon multiple factors, many of which are poorly understood. Morphologic studies of the scar tissue demonstrate the presence of disorganized collagen.[138,155] Immunohistochemical studies suggest that the newly formed collagen could be type III collagen.[160,169] Proteoglycans are also produced in response to injury, with most studies suggesting keratin sulfate as the major compound produced.[160,169,170]

The stromal events leading up to the production of new collagen and proteoglycans may be due, in part, to the absence of epithelium overlying the freshly ablated corneal collagen. Within the first 24 hours after excimer PRK, stromal wound healing begins, as inflammatory cells invade the corneal stroma from the tear film.[171,172] Ingress of polymorphonuclear leukocytes (PMNs) can be seen after deepithelialization alone, but the number is significantly greater after PRK[171] (Fig. 2-38). Tear film plasmin levels are also markedly elevated during the postoperative period and signify involvement of the plasminogen activator system which facilitates degradation, removal, and repair of damaged collagen and extracellular matrix.[173,174] Immediately following PRK, keratocytes in the anteriormost collagen layers have vacuolated cytoplasm with ruptured cell membranes.[175] Within the first 3 days, both the PMNs and anterior stromal keratocytes disappear.[175] The marked decrease in keratocytes can also be seen following deepithelialization without stromal ablation, and repopulation occurs over a 2-week period. Following excimer laser PRK, the fibrocytes not only repopulate but also increase in density, being seen in over three times their normal number by the third postoperative week.[136,141,175]

These activated keratocytes are responsible for the formation of new collagen and proteoglycan matrix. The new collagen and vacuoles filled with proteoglycan debris are responsible, in part, for a high level of light scatter resulting in corneal haze.[144,176-178] Experimentally, corneal haze is correlated with new collagen formation which can be seen as early as 1 week following treatment, and appears to achieve its maximum thickness at 1 month.[77] The use of fluorescent dye, dichlorotriazinyl aminofluorescein (DTAF), applied experimentally immediately following excimer PRK demonstrates fluorescence of the underlying normal stroma with a lack of fluorescence in the new col-

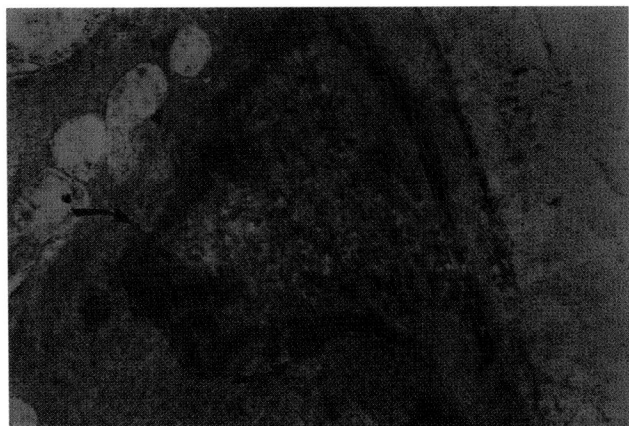

Fig. 2-37. Ultrastructural view of anterior corneal tissue 16 months following clinical excimer laser PTK demonstrating remnants of Bowman's layer, 2.9-μm thick within the ablation site. TEM 24,000× magnification. (Courtesy of Robert Lambert, Ph.D., and Janet Anderson, Ph.D., National Vision Research Institute, San Diego, CA.)

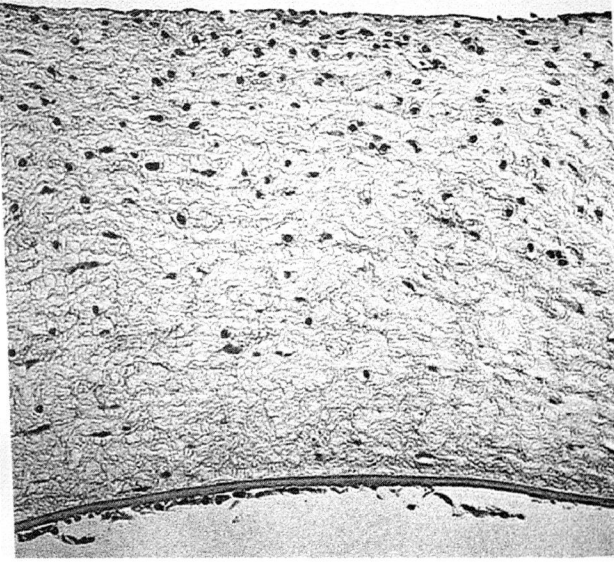

Fig. 2-38. Large numbers of polymorphonuclear leukocytes invading the anterior corneal stroma 10 hours following photorefractive keratectomy in a rabbit cornea. LM 25× magnification. (With permission from Phillips AF et al: *Arch Ophthalmol* 111:1273-1278, 1993.)

lagen layer.[77,146,179,180] (Fig. 2-39, *A* and *B*).

The histologic use of DTAF is particularly useful following PTK where there is difficulty distinguishing the primary host pathologic changes from the corneal wound-healing response to the laser. This is especially true for cases of herpes simplex keratitis and other causes of scarring of the anterior 25% of the corneal stroma. In a recent study of human subjects without use of the dye, it was difficult to tell where the excimer laser wound response ended and the primary host scarring began in three cases following PTK for scarring associated with herpes simplex virus.[155] The analysis of 14 human specimens obtained following PTK suggested the mechanisms of failure of the procedure to eliminate opacity was most likely due to differential rates of ablation in scar tissue compared to healthy tissue. Other causes of failure appear to be inappropriate planned excision parameters, i.e., the abnormality was deeper than the intended depth of ablation.

Since the cornea mounts a wound-healing response following excimer PRK in the form of fibroblast activation,* and since it has previously been demonstrated that corticosteroids inhibit fibroblast proliferation,[186,187] it was logical to treat corneas with topical steroids following excimer photoablation.[185,188-196] Although experimental studies have demonstrated the effectiveness of steroids at reducing new collagen for

mation and hyaluronic acid formation, morphologic studies have demonstrated the persistence of activated keratocytes up to 18 months postoperatively in nonhuman primates[154] and humans,[155] suggesting that short-term use of steroids is inadequate.[197] Corneal wound-healing modulation with topical steroids and other agents is discussed at the end of this chapter.

Descemet's membrane response to excimer laser photoablation. Acute and chronic morphologic studies of Descemet's membrane following PRK have demonstrated an unusual fibrillar response in the mid- to anterior one third in the rabbit[139,175] (Fig. 2-40). Only one human specimen has been found to have a similar change.[141] The ultrastructure of this change has not been studied, and its cause is unknown. Although one might assume that acoustic damage from the laser must play a role, this change has also been seen following manual lamellar keratectomy.[175]

Endothelial response to excimer laser photoablation. A concern about operating on normal, healthy corneas for refractive purposes has been the potential for endothelial cell damage, especially considering the history of late-onset corneal edema following radial keratotomy performed in Japan.[198] Acute morphologic studies of the endothelium in animals and humans have failed to demonstrate endothelial changes, unless the excimer laser beam approaches Descemet's membrane.[57,199-201] Following

---

*References 112, 135-137, 139, 141, 144, 146, 151, 154, 155, 167, 169, 170, 179, 181-186.

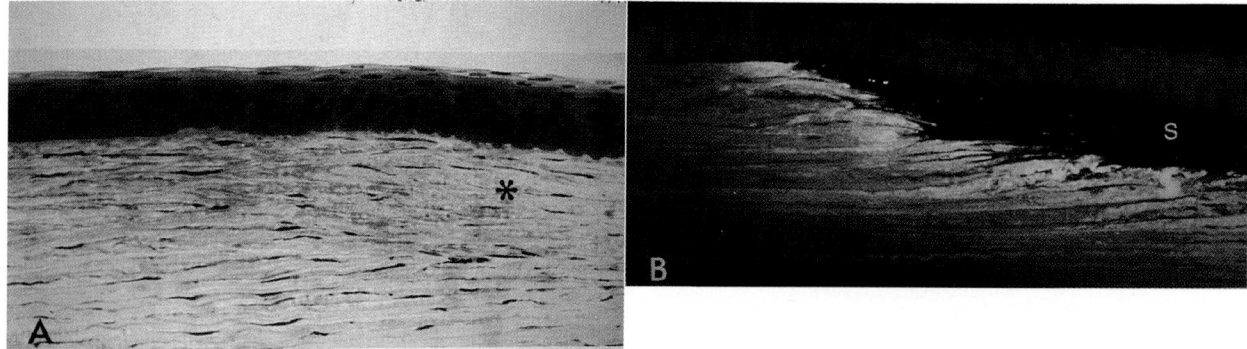

Fig. 2-39. Histologic view of corneal remodeling 3 months following excimer laser keratectomy of 75 μm depth **(A)** The light micrograph demonstrated generated collagen fibers with an altered orientation suggestive of scar tissue (*), **(B)** fluorescent microscopy really demonstrates the unlabeled connective tissue scar *(S)* in contrast to the native collagen as labeled with DTAF fluorescent dye. LM 100× magnification. (With permission from Tuft SJ et al: Corneal repair following keratectomy: A comparison between conventional surgery and laser photoblation, *Invest Ophthalmol Vis Sci* 30:1769-1777, 1989.)

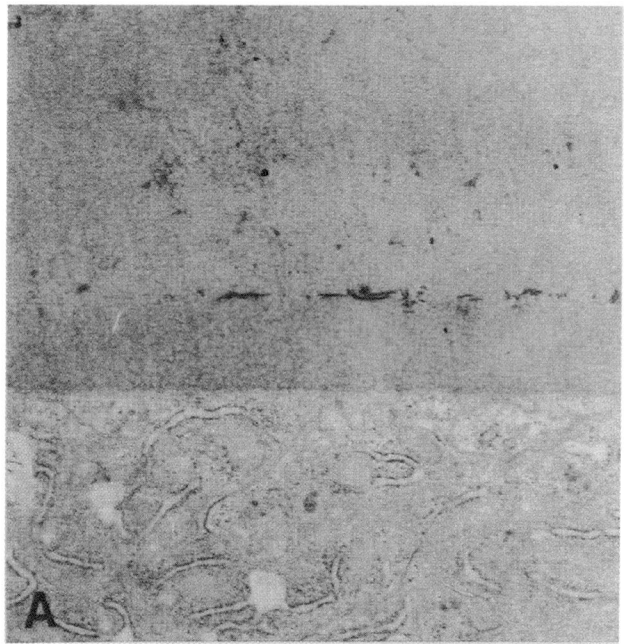

Fig. 2-40. Transmission electron micrograph of Descemet's membrane 3 weeks after photoablation of a rabbit cornea to 80% depth. Note the densely staining fibrillar material within Descemet's membrane. TEM 10,800× magnification. (Courtesy of Robert Lambert, Ph.D., and Janet Anderson, Ph.D., National Vision Research Institute, San Diego, CA.)

large area ablations in bovine eyes, Zabel et al.[202] described endothelial changes being correlated with depth area and energy density of ablation. Clinically, however, little information has been recorded suggesting significant endothelial cell loss. Carones et al.[203] reported 2% and 3% cell loss at 2 months and 1 year, respectively, following PRK on 76 eyes treated for up to −13.5 D (98-μm depth). Stephen Trokel verified these findings by stating that there is an overall 3% cell loss for eyes treated with the VISX

excimer laser (University of California, San Francisco, Update Meeting, December 1993). A more significant endothelial cell loss was initially reported up to 1 year following PRK in 19 eyes by Beldavs and co-workers,[204] but when they completed a thorough analysis of all eyes in their series, they found that significant cell loss (13%) was limited to the cornea periphery and was proportional to the preoperative myopic error (Thompson, personal communication). Another study in 26 eyes demonstrates no endothelial cell loss at 1 month and 1 year following excimer PRK.[205]

Because of the potential acoustic damage associated with the excimer laser,[103-106,206,207] Binder and co-workers[208] performed an analysis of the effects of excimer laser photoablation by looking at cultured cells from a treated human cadaver eye and its untreated mate (Fig. 2-41). They found that cell damage was associated with attempted depth of ablation and was significant for deeper ablation patterns. The findings of cell loss in the eye bank model and the apparent absence of cell loss in clinical studies suggest that the eye bank model is more sensitive to cell damage, the energy delivered in PTK mode was excessive, or the in vivo endothelium may be able to repair any acoustic damage, or any combination of these.

Functional effects and pharmacologic modulation of excimer laser corneal ablation
Pain and corneal sensitivity. One of the major concerns associated with clinical PRK is that of postoperative pain. In the early investigational trials in the United States, as well as the initial treatments of patients internationally, severe postoperative pain was a significant complication of excimer laser PRK. Neurophysiologic studies of corneal nerves in rabbits following excimer laser PRK have demonstrated an exagger-

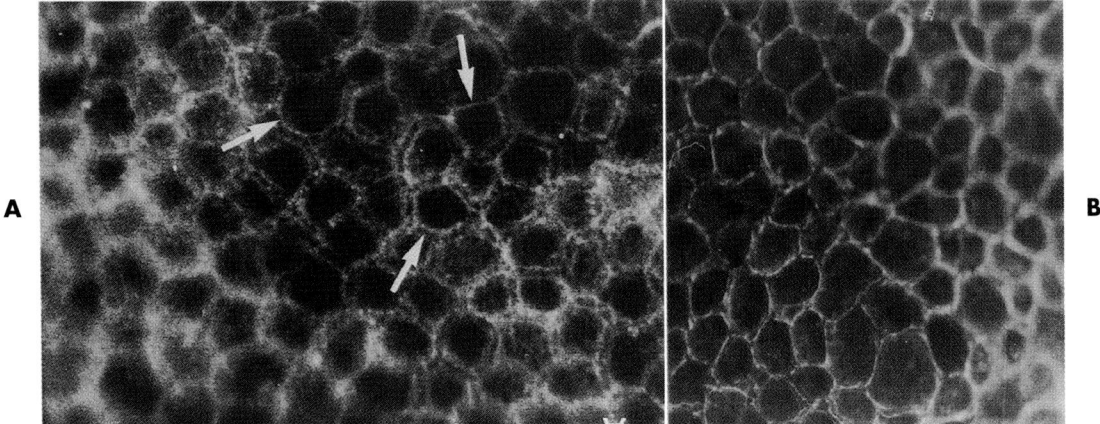

Fig. 2-41. Endothelial flat mount of cultured human corneas 7 days after excimer laser keratectomy of 150-μm depth. **(A)** The endothelial cells of the untreated mate cornea are uniformly hexagonal and show a cortical distribution of F-actin *(arrows)*. (Cell density = 2401 cells/mm², 420×). **(B)** The endothelial cells of the laser-treated cornea are less uniform in size and shape than in the central cornea. (Density = 1952 cells/mm², 420×) The difference in cell density was statistically significant ($P < 0.05$). (Courtesy of Robert Lambert, Ph.D., and Janet Anderson, Ph.D., National Vision Research Institute, San Diego, CA.)

ated neural response to stimulation with return to baseline more slowly after PRK than after keratectomy wounds.[209] Severe pain was experienced by the majority of patients in the first 12 to 36 hours following excimer laser PRK and required large doses of pain medication for relief.

Recently, a topical nonsteroidal anti-inflammatory drug, 0.1% diclofenac sodium, was used following excimer PRK with dramatic improvement in postoperative pain.[210] The topical medication is used immediately after surgery and the four times per day for several days until reepithelialization occurs. Subsequent clinical studies comparing the degree of pain and discomfort of patients undergoing bilateral PRK with one eye treated with fluoromethalone 0.1%, cycloplegics, and a contact lens, and the other with the same regimen plus diclofenac sodium 0.1%, reveal markedly less pain in the diclofenac-treated eye.[211,212]

Recent experimental evidence of arachidonic acid metabolism after excimer laser surgery has shown a rapid and sustained increase in prostaglandin E_2 production following PRK.[172] Prostaglandin E_2, a product of the cyclooxygenase pathway of arachidonic acid metabolism, is a potent sensitizer of pain fibers, and this increase in prostaglandin E_2 might explain the severe pain experienced by some patients after the procedure. The spiking concentration of prostaglandin E_2 within the corneal tissue appears to be at least partially related to the mechanism of tissue removal, as elevation in corneal levels of this metabolite were much less after mechanical keratectomy with a microkeratome (Peter McDonnell, M.D., unpublished data, January 1993). Treatment with topical diclofenac sodium immediately after laser ablation significantly de-

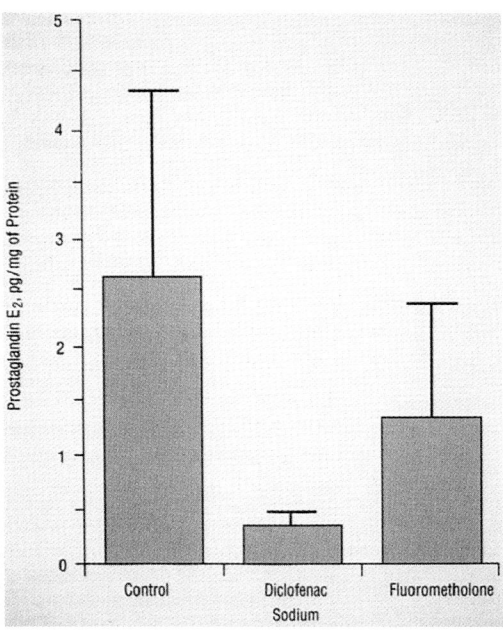

Fig. 2-42. Reduction of prostaglandin E_2 production in a rabbit cornea 10 hours following photorefractive keratectomy when treated with diclofenac sodium in comparison with fluoromethalone and vehicle control. (With permission from Phillips AF et al: Arachidonic acid metabolites after excimer laser corneal surgery, *Arch Ophthalmol* 111:1273-1278, 1993.)

creased the elevation of prostaglandin E_2 concentration.[172] Pretreatment with diclofenac sodium did not produce any additional effect on suppression of prostaglandin E_2 levels.[213]

Fluorometholone treatment is not particularly effective at reducing the rise in prostaglandin E_2 in comparison to diclofenac sodium (Fig. 2-42). It does, however, significantly reduce the number of PMNs during the early postoperative period, while topical diclofenac sodium actually increases the number (Fig. 2-43).[210] Although fluorometholone helps in reducing postoperative inflammation, it has no significant effect in reducing postoperative pain.[211,212] These results favor the use of a topical, nonsteroidal anti-inflammatory drug or, perhaps a systemic nonsteroidal anti-inflammatory drug, in the control of pain following PTK and PRK.

Care should be taken not to overuse or exclusively use these topical NSAIDs since recent reports from Canada have shown an unexpected complication of sterile stromal infiltrates in one out of 250 PRK treated eyes receiving topical diclofenac sodium or kelorolac without concomitant topical steroids use.

This complication can be attributed to the experimental increase in number of polymorphonuclear leukocytes in response to topical diclofenac sodium.[210] Consequently, the authors recommend using topical nonsteroidal anti-inflammatory drugs not more than four times per day for the first several days following excimer laser PRK, and together with the concomitant use of topical steroids.[213a] Longer-term use of topical NSAIDs and corticosteroids for the purpose of altering refractive outcome and modifying corneal haze is the subject of considerable debate and studies looking at the role of these agents are currently in progress.

Following the heightened pain response and increase in prostaglandin E_2 levels, PRK is associated with a transient reduction in corneal sensitivity. After surgery to correct moderate to high (-11 to -22 D) myopia, a decrease in corneal sensitivity of up to 50% can be measured within the first postoperative month. By 3 months postoperatively, corneal sensitivity has returned to normal in almost all cases. No loss of epithelial integrity or other problems seem to occur related to this temporary loss of sensitivity.[214]

Histologically, this loss of sensitivity is correlated with removal of the subepithelial nerve plexus immediately following ablation. Reappearance of the subepithelial plexus occurs at 1 month, being morphologically disorganized, with further regeneration continuing up to 4 months following treatment.[215]

Loss of optical clarity. Following PRK, the optical clarity of the cornea can be altered by at least one of two different means: opacifying haze or irregular astigmatism. As mentioned previously, corneal haze develops as part of the wound-healing response when activated keratocytes lay down new collagen and proteoglycan matrix. Almost every cornea exhibits some form of haze following treatment with the excimer laser. L'Esperance et al.[152] were the first to describe the most common response as a reticular haze. Since that initial report, several centers have studied the wound-

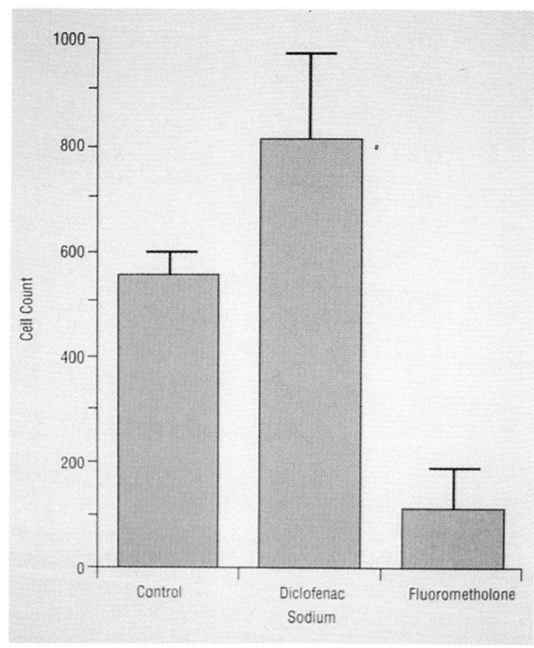

Fig. 2-43. Reduction of polymorphonuclear leukocyte cell count per section 10 hours after photorefractive keratectomy when treated with topical fluoromethalone, in comparison with diclofenac sodium and vehicle control. (With permission from Phillips AF et al: Arachidonic acid metabolites after excimer laser corneal surgery, *Arch Ophthalmol* 111:1273-1278, 1993.)

healing response in animals* and clinically using the slit lamp,† the opacity lensometer,[221] high-frequency ultrasound,[222] the confocal microscope,[184,223,224] or using the Scheimpflug principle.[71,225] This last utilized a Nidek NAS 2000 camera in which photographs can be manipulated using computer analysis and the depth and width of the scar semiquantitated. Subjective evaluation of haze using a slit lamp is the most practical way of rating the level of haze following excimer PRK. Several authors[136,178,226,227] have subjectively classified haze according to the following grading scale: grade 0 = totally clear cornea; grade 0.5 = barely perceptible haze, as seen only by indirect broad tangential illumination; grade 1 = trace haze of minimal density seen with direct and diffuse illumination; grade 2 = mild haze, easily visible with direct focal slit illumination; grade 3 = moderate haze that partially obscures iris details; and grade 4 = severe haze that completely obscures iris details. The clinical time course of subjectively perceptible haze is illustrated in Fig. 2-44, seen in a study of 285 patients with 1 to 10 D of myopic correction over an 18-month follow-up period and is expressed in terms of mean and standard deviation. Clinically, stromal haze is initially apparent at approximately 1 month following excimer la-

---

*References 77, 112, 127, 139, 140, 144, 146, 154, 167, 169, 170, 179, 181-183, 216-218.
†References 132, 174, 177, 179, 189, 219, 220.

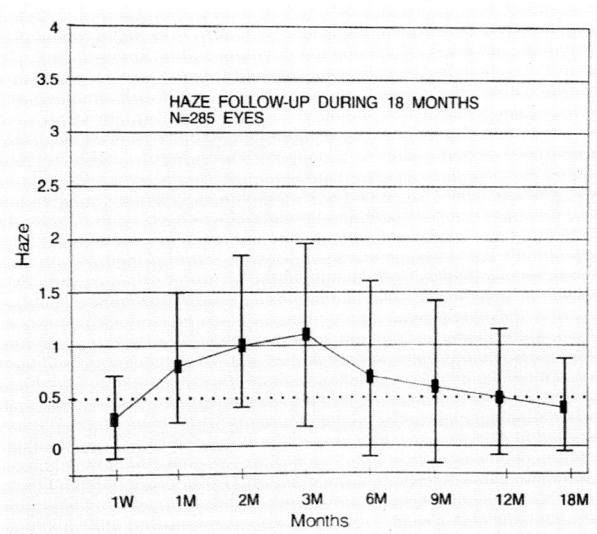

Fig. 2-44. Clinical time course of subepithelial haze after photorefractive keratectomy showing mean and standard deviation according to a grading scale as defined in the text. Note that subepithelial haze is maximum at 3 months and thereafter gradually dissolves. (With permission from Caubet E et al: Efficacy of corticosteroids in reversing regression after myopic photorefractive keratectomy, *Refract Corneal Surg* 9:S65-S70, 1993.)

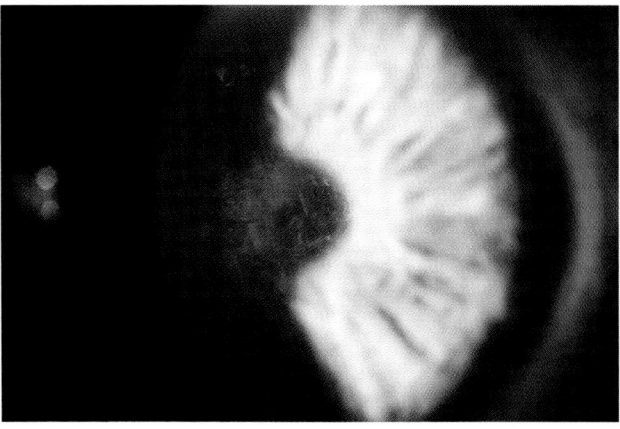

Fig. 2-45. Slit-lamp photograph of grade 1.5 to 2 haze seen following excimer laser PRK for high myopia. This patient experienced one line loss of best corrected visual acuity.

ser PRK and achieves a maximum at 3 months with a gradual decrease in magnitude thereafter as anterior stromal remodeling ensues.[178,226,227] In a nonhuman primate animal model, the maximum level of haze is seen slightly earlier at 2 months and decreases to relative corneal clarity more rapidly in about 6 to 9 months.[137,154,177,228]

The loss of transparency of the cornea as viewed by the observer is not a true measure of haze, but rather corresponds to the amount of reflected light from the corneal stroma. Haze is a subjective phenomenon experienced by the patient viewing through a light-scattering medium. Lohmann and colleagues[229] objectively determined the true level of haze by developing a polarizing system which measured and discriminated between reflected and scattered light. They showed good correlation between the signal generated by scattered light and the reduction in the contrast visual acuity performance, whereas the signal of reflected light was poorly correlated with this value. These disturbances in low-contrast visual performance were only significant during the first 3 to 4 postoperative months, returning thereafter to their normal preoperative value as clinically perceptible haze began to dissipate.

Although true haze is that experienced by the patient as scattered light, visually significant haze can be roughly assessed at the slit lamp when the density of opacification exceeds that of grade 1.5 to 2 on the classification scale. Often haze at this level (Fig. 2-45) or

greater is associated with loss of at least one line of best corrected visual acuity.[132,162,230] Visually significant haze can be seen in approximately 3% to 11% of patients overall[132,178] and in 10% to 40% with higher diopter corrections.[148,162,178] The factors which appear to be correlated with greater levels of haze are multiple and difficult to ascertain, yet several studies have determined that higher levels of correction,[132,148,162,230] smaller ablation diameter (>4.5 mm),[178] male subjects,[178] and noncompliance with postoperative steroid medication[132,178] are positively correlated with greater haze.

This brings up the issue of the role of pharmacologic modulation in reducing the loss of corneal clarity. As mentioned earlier in the chapter, corticosteroids have a role in inhibiting fibroblast proliferation and may be useful in inhibiting the formation of corneal haze following excimer laser PRK. Early experimental studies have demonstrated the effectiveness of topical steroids in reducing corneal haze[77,144] (Fig. 2-46, *A* and *B*) and retrospective clinical experience has verified this finding.[132,134,162,178] Most of these patients had begun proper use of topical steroids, but for some reason topical steroid use was discontinued. In a prospective double-blind trial to determine the efficacy of topical steroids in reducing stromal haze, topical steroid use was shown to have no statistically significant difference on anterior stromal haze in comparison to placebo control.[189] It was recommended that topical steroids not be used after PRK; however, others suggest that there exists a significant haze risk group in which the absence or discontinuation of topical steroids will lead to significant haze.[132,178] Continued research regarding the efficacy of other pharmacologic modulators in reducing corneal haze is ongoing and includes antifibrotic agents such as mitomycin,[185,195] interferon-alfa-2b,[231] pirenzepine (a

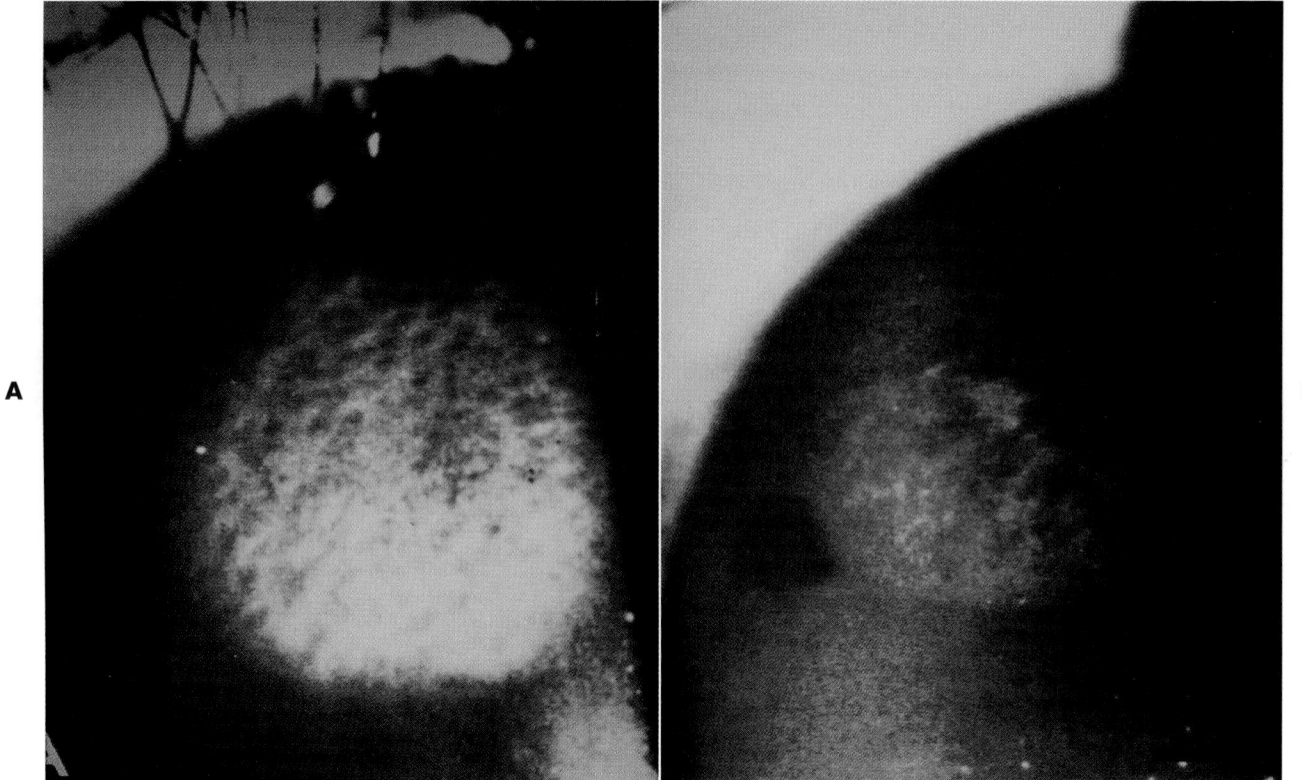

Fig. 2-46. (A) External photograph of white subepithelial haze in a rabbit cornea 3 months after excimer laser keratectomy. (B) Postoperative treatment with topical steroids markedly reduced the intensity of this haze over a similar follow-up period. (With permission from Tuft SJ et al: A comparison between conventional surgery and laser photoablation, *Invest Ophthalmol Vis Sci* 30:1769-1777, 1989.)

muscarinic antagonist),[218] protease inhibitors such as aprotinin (plasmin inhibitor).[173,174]

Irregular astigmatism can also result in loss of optical clarity and can be seen following decentered excimer laser ablation or in the form of topographic steep central islands following excimer laser PRK. Gross eccentricities of the ablation zone (1.0-1.5 mm) can diminish optical clarity and result in loss of one or two lines of best corrected visual acuity.[133] The incidence of significant decentration occurs in approximately one to two cases per series, ranging from 0.3% to 3.0%, depending on the number of patients treated.[133,162]

Irregular astigmatism in the form of topographic steep central islands is a more frequent phenomenon, occurring in 16% to 50% of patients 1 month following excimer laser PRK.[98,99] In a study by Krueger et al.,[99] 72% of patients with topographic steep central islands at 1 and 3 months had loss of best corrected visual acuity, whereas only 12% without central island formation had equivalent visual loss during the same period. This association implies that central island formation is, at least in part, responsible for the loss of optical clarity during the postoperative period. Fortunately, 80% of patients with central island formation at 1 month and resolution of islands at 3 months had return of their best corrected visual acuity at 3 months when the central island was no longer present.[99]

Finally, corneal light scattering and visual performance in patients with excimer laser PRK were compared with other myopic patients receiving spectacles or contact lenses.[232] Patients with excimer laser PRK had the greatest amount of corneal light scattering and loss of low-contrast visual acuity at 3 months postoperatively, but with marked improvement in both parameters at 1 year, being significantly better than hard and soft contact lens wear and comparable to those of spectacles.

Corneal curvature changes. The principle of excimer laser PRK for the correction of myopia is based on a graded removal of tissue resulting in a decreased corneal radius of curvature. The ablation process is analogous to the removal of a biologic contact lens from the central corneal surface, as shown in Fig. 2-47.[122] Here the thickness of this biologic contact lens (t_o) depends upon the diameter of tissue removal (S), as well as the desired amount of myopic correction (D), and can be expressed by the equation $t_o = -S^2D/8(n - 1)$

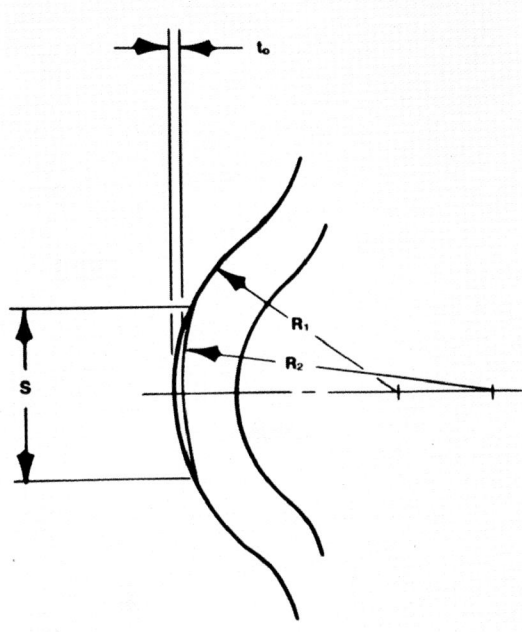

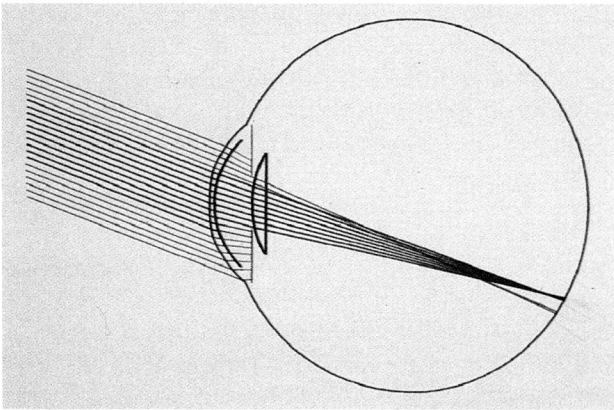

Fig. 2-49. Ray tracing of peripheral light through a cornea following excimer laser PRK with an ablation diameter equal to the pupil size. Note that a substantial portion of the peripheral light passes through the unablated cornea and is not focused on the retinal creating glare. (Courtesy of Charles J. Koester, Ph.D., Harkness Eye Institute, New York, NY.)

Fig. 2-47. Geometric relationship of forming a new radius of corneal curvature. Note that increasing the optical zone diameter correspondingly increases the depth of tissue removal. (With permission from Munnerlyn CR et al: Photorefractive keratectomy: A technique for laser refractive surgery, *J Cateract Refract Surg* 14:46-52, 1988.)

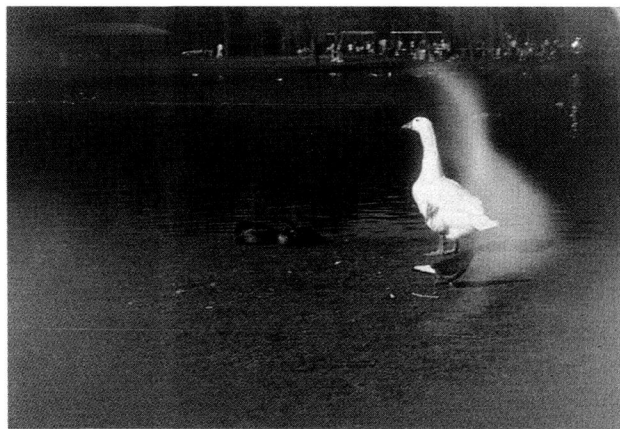

Fig. 2-50. Photographic simulation of excimer laser PRK with ablation zone diameter equal to the pupillary diameter. The central objects in the photo are clearly focused, whereas the peripheral images create glare and ghost images as can be seen by the "ghost goose." (Courtesy of Charles J. Koester, Ph.D., Harkness Eye Institute, New York, NY.)

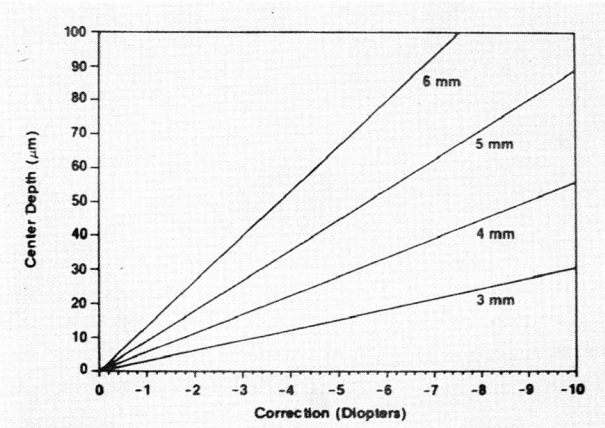

Fig. 2-48. Line graph illustrating the maximum depth of tissue removal required to correct a given myopic refractive error at various ablation zone diameters. The relationship can be described by the equation: $t_o = -S^2D/3$. (With permission from Munnerlyn CR et al: Photorefractive keratectomy: A technique for laser refractive surgery, *J Cateract Refract Surg* 14:46-52, 1988.)

Although the maximum depth of tissue removal can be minimized by reducing the diameter of the ablation zone, optical zones less than or equal to the pupil diameter can result in significant glare and halos due to light refraction through the peripheral, uncorrected zone[132,226,233] (Fig. 2-49). This can have disturbing consequences, especially in younger people who have a greater pupillary diameter in both dim and bright light.

The simulated effect of an ablation zone diameter equal to that of the pupillary diameter is shown in Fig. 2-50. Here the photograph is taken with a camera that has a negative lens placed over the camera lens, and the iris diaphragm of the camera is opened to approximately the same diameter as the negative lens. It is

or, more simply, $-S^2D/3$. Thus, for a given amount of myopic correction, the maximum central depth of ablation increases in proportion to the square of the ablation diameter. The relationship is shown pictorially in Fig. 2-48.[122]

clear that a sufficiently large ablation zone diameter is required for asymptomatic excimer laser PRK, and reports suggest that 6 mm is sufficient to reduce postoperative glare, whereas 5.0 and 5.5 mm is associated with 37% and 5.5% of patients reporting significant glare, respectively.[234]

After creating a new corneal curvature with the excimer laser, the refractive power undergoes an initial maximal change with progressive lessening of effect or regression over time. As was previously mentioned early in this chapter, refractive regression due to epithelial hyperplasia has been demonstrated in rabbit,[112,139,144,146,149] nonhuman primate,[136] and human pathologic studies[138,150-153] at 6 months following PRK and persisting for up to 18 months in both primate and human specimens.[154,155] Additionally, new collagen and proteoglycan production also contributes to regression, with clinical changes in refraction occasionally continuing up to 18 months following PRK and finally stabilizing thereafter.[156] Although it was initially believed that a smaller ablation diameter would be associated with a shallower maximum depth and, consequently, less wound healing, reduction of ablation zone diameter with higher dioptric corrections actually results in greater regression and undercorrection than larger ablation diameters.[148,210]

As with corneal haze, the role of corneal wound-healing modulators has been addressed in attempting to control refractive regression. The same prospective double-blind study evaluating the effectiveness of topical steroids following excimer PRK also commented on refractive outcome.[189] Six weeks following treatment in 113 patients with placebo or topical dexamethasone, the mean change in refraction was significantly greater in the steroid-treated group than in the placebo-treated controls. However, when corticosteroids were discontinued at 3 months, this significant difference became statistically insignificant. Since long-term use of corticosteroids to maintain the initial beneficial effect on refraction would be unacceptable, the authors of that study concluded that topical corticosteroids should not be used after excimer PRK.[189]

Another group, however, performing a similar study with a larger group of patients, has shown significantly less regression in eyes treated with topical dexamethasone for 3 months over eyes treated for only 5 weeks.[192] Hearing the initial group's findings, the second group stopped the use of dexamethasone on subsequent patients and noticed myopic regression within the first postoperative month, increasing to levels greater than those seen in their earlier experience. As a result, at 3 months, they felt it was impossible to avoid steroid use in these patients. Upon reinstituting use of topical steroids,

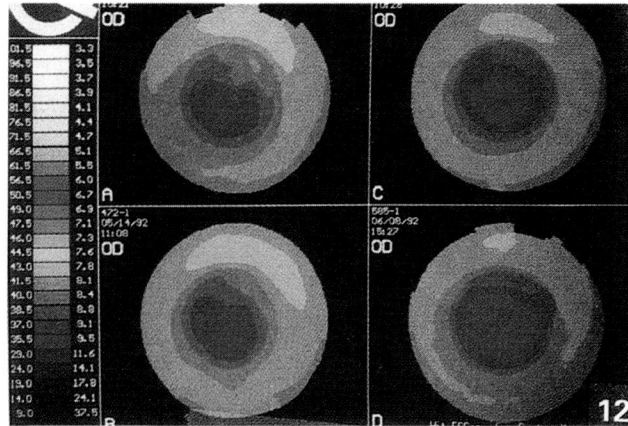

Fig. 2-51. Corneal topographic images of a patient with refractive regression (**A**) demonstrating a topographic reversal of myopic regression at 2 days (**B**), 4 days (**C**), and 1 month (**D**) following the onset of retreatment with topical dexamethasone. (With permission from Carones F et al: Efficacy of corticosteroids in reversing regression after myopic photorefractive keratectomy, *Refract Corneal Surg* 9:S52-S56, 1993.)

they saw reversal of the myopic shift with actual restoration to emmetropia or even slight hyperopia in a number of cases.[194] They concluded that topical steroids were active and necessary during the healing phase following excimer laser PRK. Other authors have had similar experiences of an increase in myopic regression upon discontinuing topical steroids with a complete or near-complete reversal of the regression after reinstituting the medication[193,235,236] (Fig. 2-51).

It seems clear that topical steroids do play a role in the pharmacologic modulation of refractive results, in at least some eyes, following excimer PRK. Yet controversy still exists as to how much and how long topical steroids should be instituted or reinstituted. A comparison of topical fluorometholone 0.1% and topical dexamethasone 0.1% in identical twins revealed no difference in refractive result, suggesting that fluorometholone may be adequate and preferable since it is associated with fewer side effects with long-term use.[237]

In conclusion, the effects of excimer laser photoablation on the cornea have been compared with those of other laser refractive surgical procedures. The biophysical, biological, and functional effects of excimer laser PRK have been carefully reviewed considering the present state of excimer laser development. Overall, the corneal photoablation appears to be an efficacious and safe way of changing the corneal curvature. Further study of the effects of excimer laser on the cornea and the potential pharmacologic modulation of the wound-healing response will no doubt continue and, it is hoped, further perfect this revolutionary technology.

REFERENCES

1. Cherry PM, Faulkner JD, Shaver RP, et al: Argon laser treatment of corneal neovascularization, *Ann Ophthalmol* 5:911-920, 1973.

2. Marsh RJ, Marshall J: Treatment of lipid keratopathy with the argon laser, *Br J Ophthalmol* 66:127-135, 1982.

3. Bahn CF, Vine AK, Wolter JR, et al: Argon laser photocoagulation of a vitreo-corneal adhesion after trauma, *Ophthalmic Surg* 13:53-55, 1982.

4. Sugar J, Jampol LM: Photocoagulation therapy of a pigmented retrocorneal plaque, *Ophthalmic Surg* 13:562-563, 1982.

5. Gross JG, Robin AL: Argon laser iridocorneal adhesiolysis, *Am J Ophthalmol* 100:330-331, 1985.

6. Baer JC, Foster CS: Corneal laser photocoagulation for treatment of neovascularization. Efficacy of 577 nm yellow dye laser, *Ophthalmology* 99:173-179, 1992.

7. Fine BS, Fine S, Peacock GR, et al: Preliminary observations on ocular effects of high-power, continuous CO_2 laser irradiation, *Am J Ophthalmol* 64:209-222, 1967.

8. Fine BS, Fine S, Feigen L, et al: Corneal injury threshold to carbon dioxide laser irradiation, *Am J Ophthalmol* 66:1118-1131, 1968.

9. Beckman H, Rota A, Barraco R: Limbectomies, keratectomies, and keratostomies performed with a rapid-pulsed carbon dioxide laser, *Am J Ophthalmol* 71:1277-1283, 1971.

10. Keates RH, Pedrotti LS, Weichel H, et al: Carbon dioxide laser beam control for corneal surgery, *Ophthalmic Surg* 12:117-122, 1981.

11. Wolbarsht ML, Foulks GN, Esterowitz L, et al: Corneal surgery with an Er:YAG laser at 2.94 μm, *Invest Ophthal Vis Sci* 27(suppl):93, 1986.

12. Bende T, Kriegerowski M, Seiler T: Photoablation in different ocular tissues performed with an Er:YAG laser, *Lasers Light Ophthalmol* 2:263-269, 1989.

13. Lasser T, Ludwig K, Lukashev A, et al: Photoablation on bovine cornea with a Q-switch Er:YAG laser. In Parel JM, Katzir A, editors: *Ophthalmic technologies II,* Bellingham, Wash, 1992, SPIE.

14. Peyman GA, Badaro RM, Khoobehi B: Corneal ablation in rabbits using an infrared (2.9 μm) erbium-YAG laser, *Ophthalmology* 96:1160-1170, 1989.

15. Peyman GA, Beyer C, Kuszak J, et al: Long-term effect of erbium-YAG laser (2.9 μm) on the primate cornea, *Int Ophthalmol* 15:249-258, 1991.

16. Lin CP. Laser-tissue interactions: Basic principles, *Ophthalmol Clin North Am* 6:381-391, 1993.

17. Seiler T, Marshall J, Rothery S, et al: The potential of an infrared hydrogen fluoride (HF) laser (3.0 μm) for corneal surgery, *Lasers Ophthalmol* 1:49-60, 1986.

18. Loertscher H, Mandelbaum S, Parrish RK II, et al: Preliminary report on corneal incisions created by a hydrogen fluoride laser, *Am J Ophthalmol* 102:217-221, 1986.

19. Stern D, Puliafito CA, Dobi ET, et al: Infrared laser surgery of the cornea: studies with a Raman-shifted neodymium: YAG laser at 2.80 and 2.92 micron, *Ophthalmology* 95:1434-1441, 1988.

20. Seiler T, Wollensak J: Fundamental mode photoablation of the cornea for myopic correction. I. Theoretical background, *Lasers Light Ophthalmol* 5:199-203, 1993.

21. Krasnov MM. Laser puncture of the anterior chamber angle in glaucoma, *Am J Ophthalmol* 75:674-678, 1973.

22. Krasnov MM. Q-switched laser goniopuncture, *Arch Ophthalmol* 92:37-41, 1974.

23. Krasnov MM. Laser phakopuncture in the treatment of soft cataracts, *Br J Ophthalmol* 59:96-98, 1975.

24. Aron Rosa D, Aron JJ, Griesemann J, et al: Use of the neodymium YAG laser to open the posterior capsule after lens implant surgery: a preliminary report, *J Am Intraocul Implant Soc* 6:352-354, 1980.

25. Aron Rosa D: Use of a pulsed neodymium-YAG laser for anterior capsulotomy before extracapsular extraction, *J Am Intraocul Implant Soc* 6:352-354, 1981.

26. Fankhauser F, Roussel P, Steffen J, et al: Clinical studies on the efficacy of high power laser radiation upon some structures of the anterior segment of the eye, *Int Ophthalmol* 3:129-139, 1981.

27. Fankhauser F, Loertscher HP, Van der Zypen E: Clinical studies on high and low power laser irradiation upon some structures of the anterior and posterior segments of the eye, *Int Ophthalmol* 5:15-32, 1982.

28. Fujimoto JG, Lin WZ, Ippen EP, et al: Time-resolved studies of Nd:YAG laser-induced breakdown: plasma formation, acoustic wave generation, and cavitation, *Invest Ophthalmol Vis Sci* 26:1771-1777, 1985.

29. Zysset B, Fujimoto JG, Puliafito CA, et al: Picosecond optical breakdown: tissue effects and reduction of collateral damage, *Lasers Surg Med* 9:193, 1989.

30. Niemz MH, Kancnik EG, Bille JF: Plasma-mediated ablation of corneal tissue at 1053 nm using a Nd:YAG oscillator/regenerative amplifier laser, *Lasers Surg Med* 11:426-431, 1991.

31. Freuh BE, Bille JF, Brown SI: Intrastromal relaxing excisions in rabbits with a picosecond infrared laser, *Lasers Light Ophthalmol* 4:165-168, 1992.

32. Remmel RM, Dardenne CM, Bille JF: Intrastromal tissue removal using an infrared picosecond Nd:YLF ophthalmic laser operating at 1053 nm, *Lasers Light Ophthalmol* 4:169-173, 1992.

33. Niemz MH, Hoppeler TP, Juhasz T, et al: Intrastromal ablations for refractive corneal surgery using picosecond infrared laser pulses, *Lasers Light Ophthalmol* 5:149-155, 1993.

34. Stern D, Schoenlein RW, Puliafito CA, et al: Corneal ablation by nanosecond, picosecond and femtosecond lasers at 532 and 625 nm, *Arch Ophthalmol* 107:587-592, 1989.

35. Steinert RF, Puliafito CA, Trokel SL: Plasma formation and shielding by three ophthalmic neodymium-YAG lasers, *Am J Ophthalmol* 96:427-434, 1983.

36. Juhasz T, Hu XH, Tufi L, et al: Dynamics of shock waves and cavitations generated by picosecond laser pulses in corneal tissue and water, *Lasers Light Ophthalmol,* in press.

37. Kaiser R, Habib MS, Speaker MG, et al: Mass spectrometry analysis of cavitation bubbles generated by intrastromal ablation with the Nd:YLF picosecond laser, *Invest Ophthalmol Vis Sci* 35(suppl):2026, 1994.

38. Juhasz T, Speaker MG, Habib MS, et al: Refractive effects of myopic intrastromal ablation of the cat cornea with the Nd:YLF picosecond laser, *Invest Ophthalmol Vis Sci* 35(suppl): 2026, 1994.

39. Habib MS, Speaker MG, McCormick, SA, et al: Acute effects of intrastromal ablation on the corneal endothelium of the cat with the Nd:YLF picosecond laser, *Invest Ophthalmol Vis Sci* 35(suppl):2026, 1994.

40. Lans LJ: Experimentelle Untersuchungen über Entstehung von Astigmatismus durch nicht perforierende Corneawunden, *Graefes Arch Clin Exp Ophthalmol* 44:117-152, 1889.

41. Gasset A, Shaw E, Kaufman H, et al: Thermokeratoplasty, *Trans Am Acad Ophthalmol Otolaryngol* 77:441-454, 1973.

42. Aquavella J: Thermokeratoplasty, *Ophthalmic Surg* 4:39-48, 1974.

43. Keates R, Dingle J: Thermokeratoplasty for keratoconus, *Ophthalmic Surg* 6:89-92, 1975.

44. Gruenberg P, Manning W, Miller D, et al: Increase in rabbit corneal curvature by heated ring application, *Ann Ophthalmol* 13:67-70, 1981.

45. Stringer H, Parr J: Shrinkage temperature of eye collagen, *Nature* 204:307, 1964.

46. Mapstone R. Measurement of corneal temperature, *Exp Eye Res* 7:237-243, 1968.

47. Shaw EL, Gasset AR. Thermokeratoplasty (TKP) temperature profile, *Invest Ophthalmol* 13:181-186, 1974.

48. Peyman GA, Larson B, Raichand M, et al: Modification of rabbit corneal curvature with use of carbon dioxide laser burns, *Ophthalmic Surg* 11:325-329, 1980.

49. Horn G, Spears KG, Lopez O, et al: New refractive method for laser thermal keratoplasty with the Co:MgF2 laser, *J Cataract Refract Surg* 16:611-616, 1990.

50. Seiler T, Matallana M, Bende T: Laser thermokeratoplasty by means of a pulsed holmium:YAG laser for hyperopic correction, *Refract Corneal Surg* 6:355-359, 1990.

51. Moreira H, Campos M, Sawusch MR, et al: Holmium laser thermokeratoplasty. *Ophthalmology* 100:752-761, 1993.

52. Trokel SL, Srinivasan R, Braren B: Excimer laser surgery of the cornea, *Am J Ophthalmol* 96:710, 1983.

53. Krueger RR, Trokel SL, Schubert HD: Interaction of ultraviolet laser light with the cornea, *Invest Ophthalmol Vis Sci* 26:1455-1464, 1985.

54. Puliafito CA, Steinert RF, Deutsch TF, et al: Excimer laser ablation of the cornea and lens: experimental studies, *Ophthalmology* 92:749-758, 1985.

55. Marshall J, Trokel S, Rothery S, et al: An ultrastructural study of corneal incisions induced by an excimer laser at 193 nm, *Ophthalmology* 92:749-758, 1985.

56. Puliafito CA, Wong K, Steinert RF: Quantitative and ultrastructural studies of excimer laser ablation of the cornea at 193 and 248 nanometers, *Lasers Surg Med* 7:155-159, 1987.

57. Marshall J, Trokel S, Rothery S, et al: A comparative study of corneal incisions induced by diamond and steel knives and two ultraviolet radiations from an excimer laser, *Br J Ophthalmol* 70:482-501, 1986.

58. Ren Q, Simon G, Parel JM: Ultraviolet solid-state laser (213-nm) photorefractive keratectomy: in vitro study, *Ophthalmology* 100:1828-1834, 1993.

59. Hu X, Juhasz T: Experimental study of corneal ablation with picosecond laser pulses at 211 and 263 nanometers. In Parel JM, editor: *Ophthalmic technologies IV*. Bellingham, Wash, 1994, SPIE.

60. Swinger CA, Lai ST, Binder PS, et al: Surface ablation in non-human primates using solid state laser with scanning delivery system. Presented at ISRK–Pre-American Academy of Ophthalmology Meeting, Chicago, Nov 13, 1993.

61. Srinivasan R: Kinetics of the ablative photodecomposition of organic polymers in the far ultraviolet (193 nm), *J Vac Sci Technol B* 1:923-926, 1983.

62. Garrison BJ, Srinivasan R: Laser ablation of organic polymers: microscopic models for photochemical and thermal processes, *J Appl Phys* 57:2909-2913, 1985.

63. Srinivasan R. Sutcliffe E: Dynamics of the ultraviolet laser ablation of corneal tissue, *Am J Ophthalmol* 103:470-471, 1987.

64. Kermani O, Koort HJ, Roth E, et al: Mass spectroscopic analysis of excimer laser ablated material from human corneal tissue, *J Cataract Refract Surg* 14:638-641, 1988.

65. Krueger RR, Trokel SL: Quantitation of corneal ablation by ultraviolet laser light, *Arch Ophthalmol* 103:1741-1742, 1985.

66. Van Saarloos PP, Constable IJ: Bovine corneal stroma ablation rate with 193-nm excimer laser radiation: Quantitative measurement, *Refract Corneal Surg* 6:424-429, 1990.

67. Seiler T, Kriegerowski M, Schnoy N, et al: Ablation rate of human corneal epithelium and Bowman's layer with the excimer laser (193 nm), *Refract Corneal Surg* 6:99-102, 1990.

68. Kriegerowski M, Bende T, Seiler T, et al: Ablationsverhalten verschiedener Hornhautschichten. *Fortschr Ophthalmol* 87:11-13, 1990.

69. Terry MA, Stevens SX, Scoper SV, et al: Excimer laser stromal ablation rate. *Invest Ophthalmol Vis Sci* 31(suppl):245, 1990.

70. Salz JJ, Maguen E, Nesburn AB, et al: A two-year experience with excimer laser photorefractive keratectomy for myopia, *Ophthalmology* 100:873-882, 1992.

71. Seiler T, Hubscher J, Genth U: Corneal curvature change immediately after PRK as detected by scheimpflug photography, *Invest Ophthalmol Vis Sci* 34(suppl):703, 1993.

72. McDonnell JM, Garbus JJ, McDonnell PJ: Unsuccessful excimer laser phototherapeutic keratectomy: clinicopathologic correlation, *Arch Ophthalmol* 110:977-979, 1992.

73. Loree TR, Johnson TM, Birmingham BS, et al: Fluorescence spectra of corneal tissue under excimer laser irradiation, *Proc SPIE* 908:65, 1988.

74. Muller-Stolzenburg NW, Schrunder S, Buchwald HJ, et al: UV exposure of the lens during 193 nm excimer laser corneal surgery, *Arch Ophthalmol* 108:915-916, 1990.

75. Tuft S, Al-Dhahir R, Dyer P, et al: Characterization of the fluorescence spectra produced by excimer laser irradiation of the cornea, *Invest Ophthalmol Vis Sci* 31:1512-1518, 1990.

76. Ediger MN: Excimer-laser–induced fluorescence of rabbit cornea: radiometric measurement through the cornea, *Lasers Surg Med* 11:93-98, 1991.

77. Tuft SJ, Zabel RW, Marshall J: Corneal repair following keratectomy. A comparison between conventional surgery and laser photoablation, *Invest Ophthalmol Vis Sci* 30:1769-1777, 1989.

78. Pitts DG, Cameron LL, Hose JG, et al: Optical radiation and cataracts. In Waxler M, Hitchins VM, editors: *Optical radiation and visual health*. Boca Raton, Fla, 1986, CRC Press.

79. Taylor HR, West SK, Rosenthal FS, et al: Effect of ultraviolet radiation on cataract formation, *N Engl J Med* 319:1429, 1988.

80. Krueger RR, Sliney D, Trokel S: Photokeratitis from subablative 193 nm excimer laser radiation, *Refract Corneal Surg* 8:274-279, 1992.

81. Green H, Margolis R, Boll J, et al: Unscheduled DNA synthesis in human skin after in vitro UV-excimer laser ablation, *J Invest Dermatol* 89:201-204, 1987.

82. Nuss RC, Puliafito CA, Dehm E: Unscheduled DNA synthesis following excimer laser ablation of the cornea in vivo, *Invest Ophthalmol Vis Sci* 28:287-294, 1987.

83. Trentacoste J, Thompson K, Parrish RK, et al: Mutagenic potential of a 193-nm excimer laser on fibroblasts in tissue culture, *Ophthalmology* 94:125-129, 1987.

84. Van Mellaert CE, Missotten L: On the safety of 193-nanometer excimer laser refractive corneal surgery, *Refract Corneal Surg* 8:235-239, 1992.

85. Kochevar IE: Cytotoxicity and mutagenicity of excimer laser radiation. *Lasers Surg Med* 9:440-445, 1989.

86. Sutherland B, Harber L, Kochevar F: Pyrimidine dimer formation and repair in human skin, *Cancer Res* 42:3181-3185, 1980.

87. Seiler T, Bende T, Winckler K, et al: Side effects in excimer corneal surgery: DNA damage as a result of 193 nm excimer laser radiation, *Graefes Arch Clin Exp Ophthalmol* 226:273-276, 1988.

88. Gebhardt B, Salmeron B, McDonald M: Effect of excimer laser on energy growth potential of corneal keratocytes, *Cornea* 9:250-210, 1990.

89. John ME Jr, Schmitt TE: Traumatic hyphema after radial keratotomy, *Ann Ophthalmol* 15:930-932, 1983.

90. Spivack L: Case report: radial keratotomy incisions remain intact despite facial trauma from plane crash, *J Refract Surg* 3:59-60, 1987.

91. Forstot SL, Damiano RE: Trauma after radial keratotomy, *Ophthalmology* 95:833-835, 1988.

92. Pearlstein ES, Agapitos PJ, Cantirll HL, et al: Ruptured globe after radial keratotomy, *Am J Ophthalmol* 106:755-756, 1988.

93. Bloom HR, Sands J, Schneider D: Corneal rupture from blunt

trauma 22 months after radial keratotomy, *Refract Corneal Surg* 6:197-199, 1990.

94. Campos M, Lee M, McDonnell PJ: Ocular integrity after refractive surgery: effects of photorefractive keratectomy, phototherapeutic keratectomy, and radial keratotomy, *Ophthalmic Surg* 23:598-602, 1992.

95. Sher NA, Bowers RA, Zabel RW, et al: Clinical use of the 193 nm excimer laser in the treatment of corneal scars, *Arch Ophthalmol* 109:491-498, 1991.

96. Campos M, Nielsen S, Szerenyi K, et al: Clinical follow-up of phototherapeutic keratectomy for treatment of corneal opacities, *Am J Ophthalmol* 115:443-440, 1993.

97. Litwin KL, Moreira H, Ohadi C, et al: Changes in corneal curvature at different excimer laser ablative depths, *Am J Ophthalmol* 111:382-384, 1991.

98. Parker PJ, Klyce SD, Ryan BL, et al: Central topographic islands following photorefractive keratectomy, *Invest Ophthalmol Vis Sci* 34(suppl):803, 1993.

99. Krueger RR, Saedy NF, McDonnell PJ: Topographic steep central islands following excimer laser photorefractive keratectomy (PRK), *Refract Corneal Surg* in press.

100. Bryant MR, Frederiks DJ, Campos M, et al: Finite element analysis of corneal topographic change after excimer laser phototherapeutic keratectomy, *Invest Ophthalmol Vis Sci* 34 (suppl):804, 1993.

101. Puliafito CA, Stern D, Krueger RR, et al: High-speed photography of excimer laser ablation of the cornea, *Arch Ophthalmol* 105:1255-1259, 1987.

102. Kahle G, Stadter H, Seiler T, et al: Gas chromatographic and mass spectroscopic analysis of excimer and erbium:yttrium aluminum garnet laser–ablated human cornea. *Invest Ophthalmol Vis Sci* 33:2180-2184, 1992.

103. Krueger RR, Krasinski JS, Radzewicz C, et al: Photography of shock waves during excimer laser ablation of the cornea: effect of helium gas on propagation velocity, *Cornea* 12:330-334, 1993.

104. Bor Z, Hopp B, Racz B, et al: Plume emission, shock wave and surface wave formation during excimer laser ablation of the cornea, *Refract Corneal Surg* 9(suppl):S111-S115, 1993.

105. Bor Z, Hopp B, Racz B, et al: Physical problems of excimer laser corneal ablation, *Opt Eng* 32:2481-2486, 1993.

106. Kermani O, Lubatschowski H: Struktur und Dynamik photoakustischer Schockwellen bei der 193 nm Excimer Laserphotoablation der Hornhaut, 88:748-753, 1991.

107. Lin DTC, Sutton HF, Berman M: Corneal topography following excimer photorefractive keratectomy for myopia, *J Cataract Refract Surg* 19:149-154, 1993.

108. Bende T, Seiler T, Wollensak J: Side effects in excimer corneal surgery: corneal thermal gradients, *Graefes Arch Clin Exp Ophthalmol* 226:277-280, 1988.

109. Berns MW, Liaw LH, Oliva A, et al: An acute light and electron microscopic study of ultraviolet 193-nm excimer laser corneal incisions. *Ophthalmology* 95:1422-1433, 1988.

110. Krasinski JS, Krueger RR, Radzewicz C: Characterization of a surface plasma created during excimer laser photoablation. In Pirel JM, editor: *Ophthalmic technologies III,* Bellingham, Wash, 1993, SPIE.

111. Salz JJ, Maguer E, Macy JI, et al: One-year results of excimer laser photorefractive keratectomy for myopia, *Refract Corneal Surg* 8:269-273, 1992.

112. Campos M, Cuevas K, Garbus J, et al: Corneal wound healing after excimer laser ablation: effects of nitrogen gas blower, *Ophthalmology* 99:893-897, 1992.

113. Krueger RR, Campos M, Wang X, et al: Corneal surface morphology following excimer laser ablation with humidified gases, *Arch Ophthalmol* 111:1131-1137, 1993.

114. Colin J, Cochener B, Gallinaro C: Central steep islands immediately following excimer photorefractive keratectomy for myopia, *Refract Corneal Surg* 9:395-396, 1993.

115. Waring GO: Development of a system for excimer laser corneal surgery, *Trans Am Ophthalmol Soc* 86:854-983, 1989.

116. Schroder E, Dardenne MU, Neuhann T, et al: An ophthalmic excimer laser for corneal surgery, *Am J Ophthalmol* 103:472-473, 1987.

117. Gordon M, Brint SF, Durrie DS, et al: Photorefractive keratectomy at 193 nm using an erodible mask. In Parel JM, editor: *Ophthalmic technologies II,* Bellingham, Wash, 1992, SPIE.

118. Marshall J, Trokel S, Rothery S, et al: Photoablative reprofiling of the cornea using an excimer laser: photorefractive keratectomy, 1:21-48, 1986.

119. Trokel S: Evolution of excimer laser corneal surgery, *J Cataract Refract Surg* 15:373-383, 1989.

120. Campos M, Wang X, Hertzog L, et al: Ablation rates and surface ultrastructure of 193 nm excimer laser keratectomies, *Invest Ophthalmol Vis Sci* 34:2493-2500, 1993.

121. Mandel ER, Krueger RR, Puliafito CA, et al: Excimer laser large area ablation of the cornea, *Invest Ophthalmol Vis Sci* 28(suppl):275, 1987.

122. Munnerly CR, Koons SJ, Marshall J: Photorefractive keratectomy: a technique for laser refractive surgery, *J Cataract Refractive Surg* 14:46-52, 1988.

123. Hanna K, Chastang JC, Pouliquen Y, et al: A rotating slit delivery system for excimer laser refractive keratoplasty, *Am J Ophthalmol* 103:474, 1987.

124. Forster W, Beck R, Busse H: Design and development of a new 193-nanometer excimer laser surgical system, *Refract Corneal Surg* 9:293-299, 1993.

125. Fyodorov SN, Semyonav AD, Magaramov JA, et al: PRK using an absorbing cell delivery system for correction of myopia from 4 to 26 D in 3251 eyes, *Refract Corneal Surg* 9(suppl):123-124, 1993.

126. Sinbawy A, McDonnell PJ, Moreira H: Surface ultrastructure after excimer laser ablation: expanding vs contracting apertures, *Arch Ophthalmol* 109:1531-1533, 1991.

127. Campos M, Cuevas K, Shieh E, et al: Corneal wound healing after excimer laser ablation in rabbits: expanding versus contracting apertures, *Refract Corneal Surg* 8:378-381, 1992.

128. L'Esperance FA, Warner JW, Telfair WB, et al: Excimer laser instrumentation and technique for human corneal surgery, *Arch Ophthalmol* 107:131-139, 1988.

129. Maloney RK, Friedman M, Harmon T, et al: A prototype erodible mask delivery system for the excimer laser, *Ophthalmology* 100:542-549, 1993.

130. McDonald MB, Beuerman R, Falzoni W, et al: Refractive surgery with the excimer laser, *Am J Ophthalmol* 103:469, 1987.

131. Krueger RR, Wang X, Rudisill M, et al: Diffractive smoothing of excimer laser ablation using a defocused beam, *J Refract Corneal Surg* 10:20-26, 1994.

132. Seiler T, Wollensak J: Myopic photorefractive keratectomy with the excimer laser. One-year follow-up, *Ophthalmology* 98:1156-1163, 1991.

133. McDonald MB, Liu JC, Byrd TJ, et al: Central photorefractive keratectomy for myopia. Paritally sighted and normally sighted eyes, *Ophthalmology* 98:1327-1337, 1991.

134. Sher NA, Chen V, Bowers RA, et al: The use of the 193-nm excimer laser for myopic photorefractive keratectomy in sighted eyes. A multicenter study, *Arch Ophthalmol* 109:1525-1530, 1991.

135. Renard G, Hanna K, Saragoussi JJ, et al: Excimer laser experimental keratectomy: ultrastructural study, *Cornea* 6:269-272, 1987.

136. Fantes F, Hanna D, Waring GO III, et al: Wound healing after excimer laser keratomileusis (photorefractive keratectomy) in monkeys, *Arch Ophthalmol* 108:665-675, 1990.

137. Del Pero R, Gigstad J, Roberts A, et al: A refractive and histopathologic study of excimer laser keratectomy in primates, *Am J Ophthalmol* 109:419-429, 1990.

138. Taylor D, L'Esperance F Jr, Del Pero R, et al: Human excimer laser lamellar keratectomy: a clinical study, *Ophthalmology* 96:654-664, 1989.

139. Gaster RN, Binder PS, Coalwell K, et al: Corneal surface ablation by 193 nm excimer laser and wound healing in rabbits, *Invest Ophthalmol Vis Sci* 30:90-98, 1989.

140. Fantes F, Hanna K, Waring GO III: Myopic laser keratomileusis on monkeys. Clinical microscopic and ultrastructural observations, *Invest Ophthalmol Vis Sci* 30(suppl):217, 1989.

141. Wu WCS, Stark WJ, Green WR: Corneal wound healing after 193-nm excimer laser keratectomy, *Arch Ophthalmol* 109:1426-1432, 1991.

142. Burstein N, Gaster R, Binder P: *Corneal healing after excimer surface ablation,* Bellingham, Wash, 1988, SPIE.

143. Ozler SA, Liaw L-HL, Neev J, et al: Acute ultrastructural changes of cornea after excimer laser ablation, *Invest Ophthalmol Vis Sci* 33:540-546, 1992.

144. Rawe I, Zabel R, Tuft S: A morphological study of rabbit corneas after laser keratectomy, *Eye* 6:637-642, 1992.

145. Gipson I: Corneal epithelial and stromal reactions to excimer laser photorefractive keratectomy. I. Concerns regarding the response of the corneal epithelium to excimer laser ablation, *Arch Ophthalmol* 108:1539, 1990.

146. Shieh E, Moreira M, D'Arcy J, et al: Quantitative analysis of wound healing after cylindrical and spherical excimer laser ablations, *Ophthalmology* 99:1050-1055, 1992.

147. Dierick H, Missotten L: Is the corneal contour influenced by a tension in the superficial epithelial cells? A new hypothesis, *Refract Corneal Surg* 8:54-60, 1992.

148. Heitzman J, Binder P, Kassar B, et al: The correction of high myopia with the excimer laser, *Arch Ophthalmol* 111:1627-1634, 1993.

149. Seiler T, Woolensak J: In vivo experiments with excimer laser: technical parameters and healing processes, *Ophthalmologica* 192:65-70, 1986.

150. Aron-Rosa D, Boerner C, Gross M, et al: Wound healing following laser radial keratotomy, *J Cataract Refract Surg* 14:173-179, 1988.

151. Aron-Rosa D, Boerner C, Bath P, et al: Corneal wound healing after excimer laser keratectomy in a human eye, *Am J Ophthalmol* 103:454-464, 1987.

152. L'Esperance FA, Taylor DM, Warner JW: Human excimer laser keratectomy: short-term history, *J Refract Surg* 4:118-124, 1988.

153. Binder P, Anderson J, Rock M, et al: The morphologic features of human excimer laser photoablation (abstract), *Ophthalmology* 99:142, 1992.

154. Hanna K, Pouliquen Y, Savoldelli M, et al: Corneal wound healing in monkeys 18 months after excimer laser photorefractive keratectomy, *Refract Corneal Surg* 6:340-345, 1990.

155. Binder PS, Anderson J, Rock M, et al: The morphologic features of human excimer laser photoablation, *Ophthalmology* 101:6, 979-989, 1994.

156. Epstein D, Tergroth B, Fagerholm P, et al: Excimer PRK for myopia, *Ophthalmology* 100:1605-1606, 1993.

157. Amano S, Shimizu K, Tsubotoa K: Corneal epithelial morphology following excimer laser photorefractive keratectomy (abstract), *Ophthalmology* 99:123, 1992.

158. Ahmad O, Green R, Stark W, et al: Excimer laser keratectomy: morphometric analysis of epithelial basement membrane and hemidesmosome reformation, *Invest Ophthalmol Vis Sci* 34(suppl):703, 1993.

159. Paallysaho T, Tervo K, Van Setten G, et al: Distribution of integrins α6 and β4 in the rabbit corneal epithelium after anterior keratectomy. *Cornea* 11:523-528, 1992.

160. Binder P, Rock M, Anderson J: Immunohistochemical analysis of healing after excimer laser keratectomy in human corneas, *Invest Ophthalmol Vis Sci* 34(suppl):703, 1993.

161. Vrabec MP, McDonald MB, Chase DS, et al: Traumatic corneal abrasions after excimer laser keratectomy, *Am J Ophthalmol* 116:101-102, 1993.

162. Seiler T, Wollensak J: Komplikationen der Laserkeratomileusis mit dem Excimerlaser (193 nm). *Klin Monatsbl Augenkeilkd* 200:648-653, 1992.

163. McDonnell PJ, Seiler T: Phototherapeutic keratectomy with excimer laser for Reis-Buckler's corneal dystrophy, *Refract Corneal Surg* 8:306-310, 1992.

164. Hahn T, Woo J, Kim J: Phototherapeutic keratectomy in nine eyes with superficial corneal diseases, *Refract Corneal Surg* 9(suppl):S115-S118, 1993.

165. Binder P, Wickham M, Zavala E, et al: Corneal anatomy and wound healing. In *Symposium on the cornea. Transactions of the New Orleans Academy of Ophthalmology,* St Louis, 1980, Mosby–Year Book.

166. Binder PS: What we have learned about corneal wound healing from refractive surgery, *J Refract Corneal Surg* 5:98-120, 1989.

167. Kerr-Muir M, Trokel S, Marshall J: Ultrastructural comparison of conventional surgical and argon fluoride excimer laser keratectomy, *Am J Ophthalmol* 103:448-453, 1987.

168. Altmann J, Grabner G, Husinsky W, et al: Corneal lathing using the excimer laser and a computer-controlled positioning system: Part I—lasting of epikeratoplasty lenticules, *Refract Corneal Surg* 7:377-384, 1991.

169. Sundar RAj N, Geiss M III, Fantes F, et al: Healing of excimer laser ablated monkey corneas: an immunohistochemical evaluation, *Arch Ophthalmol* 108:1604-1610, 1990.

170. Malley D, Steiner R, Puliafito C, et al: Immunofluorescence study of corneal wound healing after excimer laser anterior keratectomy in the monkey eye, *Arch Ophthalmol* 108:1316-1322, 1990.

171. Campos M, Abed HM, McDonnell PJ: Topical fluorometholone reduces stromal inflammation after photorefractive keratectomy, *Ophthalmic Surg* 24:654-657, 1993.

172. Phillips AF, Szerenyi K, Campos M, et al: Arachidonic acid metabolites after excimer laser corneal surgery, *Arch Ophthalmol* 11:1273-1278, 1993.

173. Lohmann CP, Marshall J: Plasmin- and plasminogen-activator inhibitors after excimer laser photorefractive keratectomy: new concept in prevention of postoeperative myopic regression and haze, *Refract Corneal Surg* 9:300-302, 1993.

174. Lohmann CP, Obart D, Patmore A, et al: Plasmin-inhibitors and plasminogen-activator inhibitors after excimer laser PRK: new concept in prevention of myopic regression and haze, *Invest Ophthalmol Vis Sci* 34(suppl):705, 1993.

175. Hanna KD, Pouliquen Y, Waring GO, et al: Corneal stromal wound healing in rabbits after 193-nm excimer laser surface ablation, *Arch Ophthalmol* 107:895-901, 1989.

176. Lohmann C, Gartry D, Kerr-Muir M, et al: Haze in photorefractive keratectomy: its origins and consequences, *Lasers Light Ophthalmol* 4:15-34, 1991.

177. Marshall J, Trokel SL, Rothery S, et al: Long-term healing of the central cornea after photorefractive keratectomy using an excimer laser, *Ophthalmology* 95:1411-1421, 1988.

178. Caubert E: Cause of subepithelial corneal haze over 18 months after photorefractive keratectomy for myopia, *Refract Corneal Surg* 9(suppl):S65-S70, 1993.

179. Tuft S, Marshall J, Rothery S: Stromal remodeling following photorefractive keratectomy, *Lasers Ophthalmol* 1:177-183, 1987.

180. Goodman G, Trokel SL, Stark WJ, et al: Corneal healing fol-

lowing laser refractive keratectomy, *Arch Ophthalmol* 107:1799-1803, 1989.

181. Hanna K, Pouliquen Y, Fantes F, et al: Long term corneal wound healing in monkeys after initial repeated excimer laser keratomileusis, *Invest Ophthalmol Vis Sci* 31(suppl):478, 1990.

182. Hanna K, Pouliquen Y, Waring GO III, et al: Corneal wound healing in monkeys after repeted excimer laser photorefractive keratectomy, *Arch Ophthalmol* 110:1286-1291, 1992.

183. Reidy J, Kemp J, Apple D: Histopathology of an excimer laser phototherapeutic keratectomy for HSV stromal keratitis two years post laser, *Invest Ophthalmol Vis Sci* 34(suppl):1245, 1993.

184. Rajpal R, Essepian J, Rapuano C, et al: Evaluation of human corneal wound healing with confocal microscopy after excimer laser keratectomy, *Ophthalmology* 99:126, 1992.

185. Talamo J, Gollamudi S, Green W, et al: Modulation of corneal wound healing after excimer laser keratomileusis using topical mitomycin C and steroids, *Arch Ophthalmol* 109:1141-1146, 1991.

186. Fitzsimmons TD, Fagerholm P, Harfstrand A, et al: Hyaluronic acid in the rabbit cornea after excimer laser superficial keratectomy, *Invest Ophthalmol Vis Sci* 33:3011-3016, 1992.

187. Basu P, Avaria M, Jankie R: Effect of hydrocortisone on the mobilization of leukocytes in corneal wounds, *Br J Ophthalmol* 65:694-698, 1981.

188. McDonald T, Borgman A, Roberts M, et al: Corneal wound healing: inhibition of stromal wound healing by three dexamethasone derivatives, *Invest Ophthalmol Vis Sci* 9:703-709, 1970.

189. Gartry D, Kerr-Muir M, Lohmann C, et al: The effect of topical corticosteroids on refractive outcome and corneal haze afterr photorefractive keratectomy, *Arch Ophthalmol* 110:944-952, 1992.

190. Piebenga LW, Deitz MR, Matta CS, et al: Excimer photorefractive keratectomy for myopia, *Ophthalmology* 100:1335-1345, 1993.

191. Brancata R, Tavola A, Carones F, et al: Excimer laser photorefractive keratectomy for myopia: results in 1165 eyes, *Refract Corneal Surg* 9:95-104, 1993.

192. Tengroth B, Epstein D, Fagerholm P, et al: Excimer laser photorefractive keratectomy for myopia (clinical results in sighted eyes), *Ophthalmology* 100:739-745, 1993.

193. Carones F, Brancato B, Venturi E, et al: Efficacy of corticosteroids in reversing regression after myopic photorefractive keratectomy, *Refract Corneal Surg* 9(suppl):S52-S60, 1993.

194. Tengroth B, Fagerholm P, Doderberg P, et al: Effect of corticosteroids in postoperative care following photorefractive keratectomies, *Refract Corneal Surg* 9(suppl):S61-S64, 1993.

195. Fitzsimmons T, Fagerholm P, Harfstrand A, et al: Steroids after excimer surgery decrease corneal hydraulic acid content, *Invest Ophthalmol Vis Sci* 33(suppl):766, 1992.

196. Liu J, Steinemann T, McDonald M, et al: Effects of corticosteroids and mitomycin C on corneal remodeling after excimer laser photorefractive keratectomy (PRK), *Invest Ophthalmol Vis Sci* 32(suppl):1248-1991, 1991.

197. Aquavella J, Gasset A, Dohlmann C: Corticosteroids in corneal wound healing, *Am J Ophthalmol* 58:621-626, 1964.

198. Yamaguchi T, Kanai A, Tanaka M, et al: Bullous keratopathy after anterior-posterior radial keratotomy for myopia and myopic astigmatism, *Am J Ophthalmol* 93:600-606, 1982.

199. Cowden T, Tran T, Cowden J, et al: Scanning electron microscopy (SEM) of the cornea following deep stromal excimer laser photoablation of alkali scarred rabbit corneas, *Invest Ophthalmol Vis Sci* 34(suppl):798, 1993.

200. Koch J, Lang G, Naumann G: Endothelial reaction to perforating and non-perforating excimer laser excisions in rabbits, *Refract Corneal Surg* 7:214-222, 1991.

201. Dehm EJ, Puliafito CA, Adler CM, et al: Corneal endothelial injury in rabbits following excimer laser ablation at 193 and 248 nm, *Arch Ophthalmol* 104:1364-1368, 1986.

202. Zabel R, Tuft S, Marshall J: Excimer laser photorefractive keratectomy: endothelial morphology following area ablation of the cornea, *Invest Ophthalmol Vis Sci* 29(suppl):390, 1988.

203. Carones F, Brancato R, Venturi E, et al: The corneal endothelium after myopic excimer laser photorefractive keratectomy, *Invest Ophthalmol Vis Sci* 34(suppl):804, 1993.

204. Beldavs R, Thompson K, Waring GO III, et al: Quantitative specular microscopy after PRK (abstract), *Ophthalmology* 99:125, 1992.

205. Amano S, Shimizu K: Corneal endothelial changes after excimer laser photorefractive keratectomy, *Am J Ophthalmol* 116:692-694, 1993.

206. Yashima Y, McAuliffe D, Jacques S, et al: Laser induced photoacoustic injury of the skin: effect of inertial confinement, *Lasers Surg Med* 11:62-68, 1991.

207. Lubatschowski H, Kerman O, Ertmer W: Characterization of acoustic effects in corneal photoablation and its possible use for on-line control of cutting depths (abstract), *Refract Corneal Surg* 8(102):1992.

208. Binder P, Anderson J, Lambert R, et al: Endothelial cell loss associated with excimer laser, *Ophthalmology* 97:107, 1993.

209. Beuerman RW, McDonald MB, Varnell RJ, et al: Neurophysiological evaluation of corneal nerves in rabbit following excimer PRK, *Invest Ophthalmol Vis Sci* 34(suppl):704, 1993.

210. Sher NA, Barak M, Daya S, et al: Excimer laser photorefractive keratectomy in high myopia, *Arch Ophthalmol* 110:935-943, 1992.

211. Eiferman RA, Hoffman RS, Sher NA: Topical diclofenac reduces pain following photorefractive keratectomy, *Arch Ophthalmol* 111:1022, 1993.

212. Sher NA, Frantz JM, Talley A, et al: Topical diclofenac in the treatment of ocular pain after excimer photorefractive keratectomy, *Refract Corneal Surg* 9:425-436, 1993.

213. Szerenyi K, Wang X, Lee M, et al: Topical diclofenac treatment prior to excimer laser photorefractive keratectomy in rabbits, *Refract Corneal Surg* 9:437-442, 1993.

213a. Sher NA, Krueger RR, Teal P, et al: The role of topical steroidal and nonsteroidal anti-inflammatory drugs in the etiology of stromal infiltrates after excimer photorefractive keratotomy, *J Refract Corneal Surg* (in press).

214. Campos M, Hertzog L, Grabus JJ, et al: Corneal sensitivity after photorefractive keratectomy, *Am J Ophthalmol* 114:51-54, 1992.

215. Trabucchi G, Brancato R, Verdi M, et al: Corneal nerve damage and regeneration after excimer laser photorefractive keratectomy in rabbit eyes, *Invest Ophthalmol Vis Sci* 35:229-235, 1994.

216. Keates RH, Bloom RT, Ren Q, et al: Fibronectin on excimer laser and diamond knife incisions, *J Cataract Refract Surg* 15:404-408, 1989.

217. David T, Serdarevic O, Salvodelli M, et al: Comparison of the effects of steroidal and nonsteroidal antiinflammatory agents on corneal wound healing after photrefractive keratectomy (PRK) for moderate myopia, *Invest Ophthalmol Vis Sci* 34(suppl):705, 1993.

218. Lam D, Chew S, McDonald M, et al: Modulation of corneal wound healing after excimer laser keratoplasty with muscarinic and histamine receptor antagonists, *Invest Ophthalmol Vis Sci* 34(suppl):705, 1993.

219. Lohmann CP, Gartry DS, Kerr Muir M, et al: Corneal haze after excimer laser refractive surgery: objective measurements and functional implications, *Eur J Ophthalmol* 1:173-180, 1991.

220. Flicker L, Steele A, Kirkness C, et al: Excimer laser photore-

fractive keratoplasty for myopia (abstract), *Ophthalmology* (9A): 127, 1992.

221. Angotti-Andrade H, McDonald M, Liu J, et al: Evaluation of an opacity lensometer for determining corneal clarity following excimer laser photoablation, *Refract Corneal Surg* 6:346-351, 1990.

222. Ediger M, Pettit G, Weiblinge R: Noninvasive monitoring of excimer laser abaltion by time resoloved reflectometry, *Refract Corneal Surg* 9:268-275, 1993.

223. Kriegerowski M, Bende T, Bachmann W, et al: Corneal silicone case in vivo and in vitro for photorefractive keratectomy, *Invest Ophthalmol Vis Sci* 34(suppl):1251, 1993.

224. Haight D, Auran J, Koeste C, et al: In vivo confocal scanning slit microscopy of the human cornea after excimer laser photorefractive keratectomy, *Invest Ophthalmol Vis Sci* 34:703, 1993.

225. Bosem M, Weinreb R, Binder P: Corneal wound healing after excimer laser photoablation, *Refract Corneal Surg* 1994, in press.

226. Gartry DS, Kerr Muir M, Marshall J: Excimer laser photorefractive keratectomy: 18 month follow-up, *Ophthalmology* 8:1209-1219, 1992.

227. Seiler T, Kahle G, Kriegerowski M: Excimer laser (193 nm) myopic keratomileusis in sighted and blind human eyes, *Refract Corneal Surg* 6:165-173, 1990.

228. McDonald MB, Frantz JM, Klyce SD, et al: One-year refractive results of central photorefractive keratectomy for myopia in the nonhuman primate cornea, *Arch Ophthalmol* 108:40-47, 1990.

229. Lohmann CP, Timberlake GT, Fitzke FW, et al: Corneal light scattering after excimer laser photorefractive keratectomy: the

objective measurements of haze, *Refract Corneal Surg* 8:114-121, 1992.

230. Liu JC, McDonald MB, Varnell R, et al: Myopic excimer laser photorefractive keratectomy; an analysis of clinical correlations, *Refract Corneal Surg* 6:321-328, 1990.

231. Morlet N, Gillies MC, Crouch R, et al: Effect of topical interferon-alpha 2b on corneal haze after excimer laser photorefractive keratectomy in rabbits, *Refract Corneal Surg* 9:443-451, 1993.

232. Lohmann CP, Fitzke F, O'Brart D, et al: Corneal light scattering and visual performance in myopic individuals with spectacles, contact lenses, or excimer laser photorefractive keratectomy, *Am J Ophthalmol* 115:444-453, 1993.

233. Roberts CW, Koester CJ: Optical zone diameters for photorefractive corneal surgery, *Invest Ophthalmol Vis Sci* 34:2275-2281, 1993.

234. Dello Russo J: Night glare and excimer laser ablation diameter, *J Cataract Refract Surg* 19:565, 1993.

235. Brancato R, Carones F, Venturi E, et al: Corticosteroids vs. diclofenac in the treatment of delayed regression after myopic photorefractive keratectomy, *Refract Corneal Surg* 9:376-378, 1993.

236. Fitzsimmons TD, Fagerholm P, Tengroth B: Steroid treatment of myopic regression: acute refractive and topographic changes in excimer photorefractive keratectomy patients, *Cornea* 12:358-361, 1993.

237. Machat JJ: Double-blind corticosteroid trial in identical twins following photorefractive keratectomy, *Refract Corneal Surg* 9(suppl):S105-S107, 1993.

3

Myopic Photorefractive Keratectomy: The Experience in the United States with the VISX Excimer Laser

Marguerite B. McDonald, Jonathan H. Talamo

The use of the 193-nm argon fluoride excimer laser for the treatment of myopia has undergone rapid evolution during the past 10 years. The earliest investigators were scientists in Silicone Valley who used the excimer laser for the ablation of various polymers. Taboada and colleagues[1,2] noted an extreme sensitivity in the corneal epithelium to excimer laser pulses, and Srinivasan[3,4] noted the action of far-ultraviolet light on various organic polymer films during his application of excimer laser to semiconductor technology. In 1983, Stephen Trokel and co-workers published their landmark paper, during which the authors noted the high degree of precision of excimer laser photoablation of the cornea, and the lack of thermal damage to adjacent tissue. In this publication, it was noted that the excimer laser could be used for corneal surgery, and refractive surgery in particular. Subsequently, there was an outburst of investigative activity worldwide,[6-12] with the publication of many studies in which investigators attempted to use the excimer laser to perform radial keratotomy.[6-8,13-16] When this effort failed, investigators attempted wide-area ablation (otherwise known as corneal sculpting, central corneal sculpting, or photorefractive keratectomy, PRK).[9-12,17-21] It had been demonstrated that submicron amounts of corneal tissue could be precisely removed within a relatively wide area without thermal damage to surrounding structures, resulting in a change in the corneal curvature and refractive properties of the eye.[17,22-23] In 1988, Munnerlyn, Koons, and Marshall[24] published a computer-generated algorithm relating diameter and depth of the ablation to the required dioptric change. This algorithm was used in the earliest investigations in nonhuman primate eyes, demonstrating stable changes in dioptric power of the cornea with an acceptable healing response and long-term clarity of the cornea following PRK. In 1987, the first superficial keratectomies on human subjects were performed by excimer laser photoablation in the United States on blind eyes or eyes destined for enucleation; the surgeries were performed by McDonald and colleagues at Louisiana State University (LSU) Eye Center and by L'Esperance and colleagues[25] at Columbia University. Histopathologic examination showed that the epithelium was slightly hyperplastic, but there was no evidence of inflammation or abnormal keratocyte activity.

The first excimer PRK for myopia on a "normally sighted" human eye was performed at the LSU Eye Center in July 1987, by McDonald and colleagues. That same year, the Food and Drug Administration (FDA) allowed VISX to enter phase I of the PRK study, which entailed central PRKs for myopia on nine legally blind eyes.[26,27] Good results in this "blind-eye study" encouraged the FDA to allow ten LSU patients who were "partially sighted" (20/50 or worse best corrected) to have excimer PRK under the phase I protocol. These results also indicated that PRK had an acceptable risk-benefit ratio.[28]

The FDA allowed phase Ia of the PRK study for the correction of myopia to begin on June 13, 1989. The study included 40 patients who were considered to be "normally sighted," as they were correctable to 20/50 or better. These operations were performed by McDonald at the LSU Eye Center, and by Deitz and Piebenga at University of Missouri in Kansas City. The results were good, with no sight-threatening complications, and once again the FDA allowed VISX to proceed to phase IIb, the clinical trial. Phase IIb began in September 1990, and was expanded to include five investigational sites and 80 fully sighted patients. The phase IIb results were excellent, and once again no sight-threatening complications were found. Simultaneous with these PRK studies were several studies investigating the use of the excimer laser for the removal of corneal scars and corneal surface irregularities (phototherapeutic keratectomy, or PTK). The last phase of the FDA study, PRK III, began in the spring of 1991; three United States ophthalmic excimer laser manufacturers were allowed to enter this study: Summit Technology of Watertown, Mass., VISX of Sunnyvale, Calif., and Taunton Technologies of Monroe, Conn. VISX and Taunton have since merged as VISX, headquartered in Santa Clara, Calif. Seven hundred patients at a maximum of ten laser sites were enrolled throughout the country for each of the three laser companies. A total of 2100 patients are involved in the PRK III studies at the three companies. The follow-up examinations extend through 2 years. This is the last phase of the study prior to FDA approval, which optimists expect in 1995, and pessimists expect in 1996 or 1997. The 1-year results of the phase PRK III VISX study are presented later in this chapter; they are extremely encouraging, with good uncorrected visual acuity, stability, and lack of significant vision-threatening complications. In the past several years, the excimer laser has been used extensively outside the United States, and an enormous amount of worldwide experience is now available.[29-36] The results from abroad are also encouraging, although extremely rigorous FDA-style multicenter studies have not been conducted outside the United States.

PATIENT SELECTION

Patient selection and education are extremely important in any form of refractive surgery, but particularly with a technique that is still considered investigational. The patient should understand all the preoperative evaluations and necessary tests, the details of the operative procedure itself, and the postoperative evaluations that are required. It is important to use videotapes and printed information in educating patients; the last step in a full informed consent is a discussion between the patient and the surgeon, during which the patient must be given an opportunity to ask questions.

The patient must understand that early postoperative vision is often poor, especially for older patients who cannot accommodate during their hyperopic stage (which lasts longer than in a younger patient). The patient must understand that there is a period of haze and glare, which is most marked at months 2 and 3, but that this will gradually resolve over time. The risks of undercorrection, overcorrection, and regression must be pointed out to the patient, as well as the risk of an exuberant haze ("scar") that may take months or years to fade. The early postoperative complication of corneal ulceration, and later postoperative problems, such as those associated with steroid response (if steroids are used), should be mentioned to the patient as well. Patients in their later thirties and early forties should be introduced to the notion of monovision. They should clearly understand that, if they choose to have both eyes corrected for distance vision, they will need glasses to see near objects and read small print. They should be given a full explanation, and possibly a demonstration, of monovision prior to operating on the first eye.

Patients in the United States understand that, under present FDA guidelines, there will be a delay of treatment of 6 months before the second eye can be treated. During that time, they may need to depend on a contact lens in the untreated eye, or allow for spectacles correction with a blank lens over the first (treated) eye. It is critical that patients understand the need for the follow-up examinations and be willing to return on the FDA-required schedule. This is particularly important if the patients have been placed on steroids, so that a potential steroid regimen can be modified in the event of steroid response. The inclusion criteria for PRK phase III study patients are such that the patients must be 18 years old, with −1.00- to −6.00-D spherical equivalent at the corneal plane. They must have a best corrected visual acuity of 20/40 or better in both eyes; this group of patients is limited to those with an astigmatic component of the manifest refraction of less than or equal to 1.00 D. Contact lens wearers must remove their soft or hard gas-permeable contact lenses at least 2 weeks prior to baseline measurements, and at LSU we require 3 weeks for gas-permeable lenses. Though it is not required, we often attempt to demonstrate that there are two consecutive measurements that do not differ by more than 0.5 D in either the spherical or astigmatic component after the lenses have been removed.

These FDA guidelines are actually a bare minimum, since corneal topographic changes have been noted in patients who are "unwarping" after contact lens removal for much longer than has been previously described. Of course, for non-contact lens wearers, the spherical or cylindrical portions of the manifest refraction cannot change by an amount greater than 0.5 D between the baseline examination and time of surgery. There are many contact lens–intolerant patients who will seek excimer laser surgery; they may have underlying conditions, such as marginal (and undertreated) dry eyes, allergies, or giant papillary conjunctivitis. Others may have lagophthalmos or other lid conditions that make contact lens wear difficult. There is, of course, a large group of patients who might benefit from excimer PRK because of the occupational need to have excellent uncorrected vision. Compared with radial keratotomy, excimer laser surgery offers at least the theoretical advantage of no significant weakening of the globe, which would be an added benefit for pilots and law enforcement officers.

Surgeons who are not obliged to follow FDA guidelines should carefully exclude those patients who have a high likelihood of postoperative complications or poor visual results. It is advisable to perform this procedure only on patients who are 18 years of age or older, since there is less likelihood of further change in their refractions. It is also important to allow any patient to have at least a trial of contact lens wear. In *any* patient, but particularly those under 25 years old, it is critical to show evidence of stability of refraction; this can be done with old records, or by measuring old pairs of glasses or contact lenses.

In any patient demonstrating progressive myopia, early keratoconus should be considered. Keratoconus is, at this writing, considered an absolute contraindication to excimer PRK, as it is believed that this corneal-thinning abnormality will be exacerbated by a tissue-subtracting procedure. Since undetected keratoconus occurs in anywhere from 6% to 15% of the patients presenting for keratorefractive surgery, it is critical to look for the early signs with retinoscopy, slit-lamp examination, and (most of all) with corneal topography. Contact lens warpage can also be detected with preoperative corneal topography, and the affected corneas can be monitored until the warpage disappears, or at least stabilizes; most laser experts believe that corneal warpage cases can be treated once they have completely unwarped or at least stabilized, and that this cautious approach will enhance the predictability of the dioptric results in these patients.

Other contraindications to excimer PRK include marked uveitis, advanced keratitis sicca, severe lagophthalmos, or severe blepharitis that has not been or cannot be adequately treated. Patients taking systemic medications that would inhibit wound healing, or who are immunocompromised by disease, are also poor laser candidates. In addition, moderate or advanced corneal neovascularization within a millime-

ter of the planned treatment zone would reduce the evenness of the ablation and the dioptric accuracy in a patient having myopic PRK; the resulting irregular astigmatism would decrease spectacles acuity. Lastly, patients with systemic connective tissue disorders, such as rheumatoid arthritis or lid abnormalities affecting epithelialization, should first be diagnosed and treated for their condition before PRK is scheduled. If the treatment of these patients is not considered effective enough to avoid problems with reepithelialization after PRK, the patients should not be scheduled.

PREOPERATIVE EVALUATION

The preoperative evaluation should be performed as close to the date of surgery as possible. Currently, the FDA requires that our PRK phase III patients have a preoperative examination within 45 days of the scheduled surgery. We stress that all previously evaluated contact lens–wearing patients must discontinue their use at least 2 weeks prior to their presurgical evaluation in the case of soft or rigid gas-permeable contact lenses, and 3 weeks in the case of polymethylmethacrylate (PMMA) lenses. It is desirable, as we have stated previously, that at least two identical K-readings and baseline refractions be obtained prior to the procedure in the case of all contact lens wearers, particularly those who have been wearing PMMA lenses.

Of course, preoperative evaluation should include a complete ophthalmic examination of *both* eyes. An extremely careful uncorrected best corrected visual acuity measurement should be taken, along with both manifest and cycloplegic refractions, no matter what the patient's age may be. The cornea should be carefully scrutinized for any signs of pathologic conditions that might affect the surgical outcome.

The PRK III study requires numerous other measurements that are not part of the routine ophthalmic examination, including pachymetry, glare testing, evaluation of visual fields, corneal sensitivity, and endothelial cell counts (some are conducted in substudies only). Of course, most of these measurements will not be required for the normal preoperative and postoperative examinations once PRK III has been completed and the FDA has, it is hoped, granted premarketing approval for the treatment of myopia. Most centers now routinely obtain corneal topography measurements at baseline, and at least one more time postoperatively (usually at 6 or 12 months). During the preoperative evaluation, the informed consent form can be presented to the patient and discussed as needed (see Appendix for sample of written informed consent suggested by VISX and then modified, according to desires of local institutional review board [IRB]). At this point, we routinely give our patients their prescriptions for both preoperative and postoperative medications, as well as a copy of their informed consent form. We routinely give an information sheet outlining the date and time of surgery, and the necessary preoperative preparations. Our patients are instructed to have a very light meal on the day of the procedure, if they are scheduled after 10 o'clock in the morning, and to take one 5-mg tablet of diazepam (Valium) prior to arrival in the laser unit. Our patients are asked to come with a friend or relative, since they will be medicated. If we have obtained a poor refractive endpoint during previous evaluations, or there has been a disparity between previous manifest refractions, we often repeat the manifest refraction on the day of surgery prior to sedating the patient. Indeed, the accuracy of the manifest refraction cannot be overemphasized; it should correspond very closely to the cycloplegic refraction, and it is by far the most important measurement taken prior to undergoing excimer PRK.

SURGICAL TECHNIQUE

Once the patients have arrived at the treatment center, they should be given a wristband with their names and medical record numbers and the operative eye indicated. It has been reported that sedated patients will often answer to the wrong name when called into the surgical suite, and a busy laser team may not catch this mistake. The patient is also given two acetaminophen and codeine tablets (Tylenol no. 3), as well as another 10 to 15 mg of diazepam, depending upon body weight. In some cases, 25 to 50 mg of dimenhydrinate (Dramamine) is given 20 to 30 minutes prior to surgery, in the case of very anxious patients. Once the patient has been sedated, he or she is walked into the laser room with assistance and positioned in the chair which is directly connected to the VISX laser (Fig. 3-1). Prior to the patient's entry into the laser suite, many tasks have been performed by the laser team. The laser technician, without question the most important member of the support staff, has arrived 2 hours prior to the first surgery, and has prepared the laser and readied the instrumentation. There is a checklist that includes a laser energy reading and beam alignment, as well as a check on the uniformity and diameter of the beam with PMMA test blocks. Before each surgical procedure, one or more test ablations are performed in PMMA blocks, and are read in a lensometer to be certain that the amount of ablation is consistent with that wanted for the individual patient. When the PMMA test lens is consistent with the desired correction, a calibration table supplied by the laser company is checked to be sure that the appropriate depth per pulse is used for entry into the computer. The television monitor and video setup is double-checked to be certain that the ablation will be recorded, as part of the patient's medical record and as a way for the laser team to check their performance or review a surgical case in the event of a problem. The patient's name, the date, eye to be treated, and study or protocol designation are recorded on the videotape. The eyepieces of the operating microscope are adjusted to the proper pupillary distance for the surgeon, and the prescription is dialed into the eyepiece,

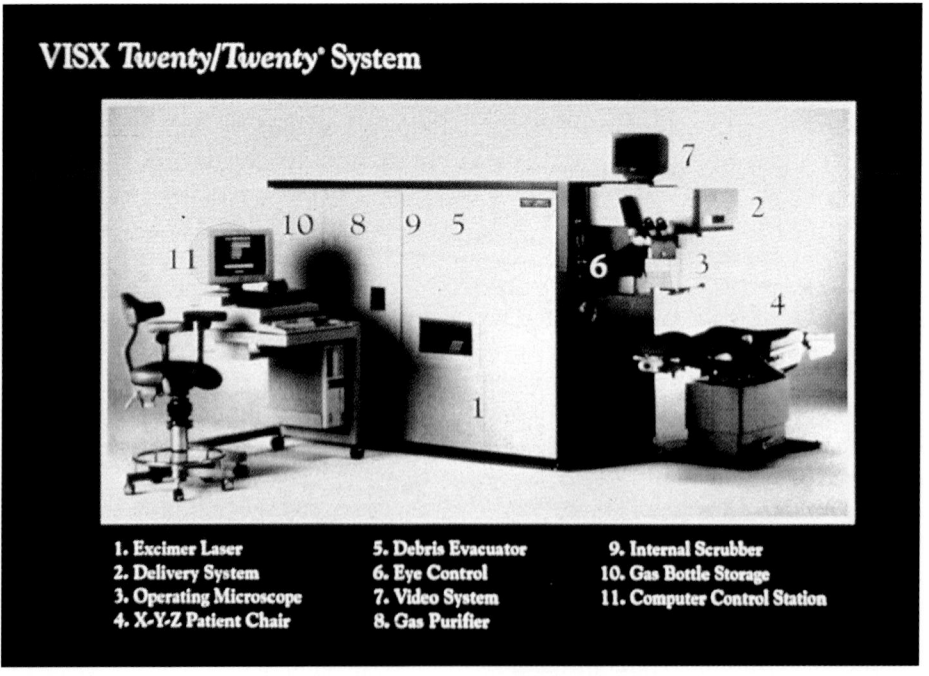

Fig. 3-1. VISX 20/20 excimer laser system.

unless the surgeon intends to wear his or her correction during surgery.

The preoperative keratometry readings and refraction are entered into the computer that controls the laser, and the patient is seated in the chair or gurney, so that the eye to be treated will be directly under the operating microscope. A surgical head bonnet is used by many investigators to prevent hair from suddenly appearing in the surgical field. The patient's armrests are adjusted for comfort, and a vacuum is pulled on the "beanbag headrest," so that the patient's head is comfortably immobilized. A drop of proparacaine is placed in each eye, and the nontreated eye is patched so that the patient cannot cross-fixate during the procedure.

A lid speculum is placed between the upper and lower lids, and an annular sponge, soaked in proparacaine, is dropped onto the limbus. The patient is asked to look directly at the fixation light, which is coaxial with the laser beam in the VISX and Summit lasers, and a Sinskey hook is used to mark the center of the pupil. Some investigators do this under three different levels of room illumination, in order to be absolutely certain that the center of the pupil has been located correctly.

Though some surgeons choose to skip the aforementioned visual axis marking with a Sinskey hook, *all* surgeons perform the next step: creation of a circular optical zone mark with a large radial keratotomy (RK) optical zone (OZ) marker. Some surgeons use a marker that is exactly the same size as the intended ablation zone, while others use a marker 0.5 to 1.0 mm larger. In addition, some surgeons choose to press the RK marker into a sterile pad of gentian violet, particularly when making a teaching film or for documentation for medical records.

Currently, we are using a 6.5-mm OZ marker; the crosshairs on the RK OZ marker are placed over the mark in the epithelium that had been made with the Sinskey hook. Next, the central epithelium within the mark is removed with a Paton spatula.

It is important that stromal hydration be uniform just prior to ablation; some investigators believe that a quick wipe with a cellulose sponge is all that is needed, while others feel that artificial tears, followed by a "squeegee" maneuver with a blunt instrument, such as a cyclodialysis spatula, suffices. At LSU, it is believed that stromal hydration is best maintained in a uniform fashion by simply removing the epithelium quickly and completely, and starting the ablation.

Many surgeons are now using patient self-fixation, though some, such as those at LSU, continue to use the surgeon-held fixation handpiece. This handpiece was designed as a modification of the original Barraquer suction handpiece from the original keratophakia-keratomileusis set by Steinway. The inferior surface, which contacts the limbus, has a soft sterilizable silicone ring with holds and, when hooked to a suction unit, will maintain steady and firm fixation of the globe. The device allows the surgeon to completely control the position of the patient's eye during PRK. As of this writing, studies are underway to determine whether patient self-fixation or surgeon fixation is superior for optimal centration of the ablation. It is possible that the handpiece may eventually be used only for PTK procedures.

With the VISX microscope, a magnification setting of 12/14 is needed for the ablation to be aligned properly with the reticle of the eyepiece (in the right ocular of the operating microscope). At this magnification, if a 6.0-mm RK OZ marker was used to make the gentian violet mark, it can be aligned perfectly with a 6.0-mm ring of the reticle in the right eyepiece.

The large debris aspirator is attached to the VISX 20/20 unit so that it hovers over the patient's lower lid, in a position to remove debris effectively; the tip is 1.5 in. higher than the corneal plane, and 0.75 in. from the laser beam itself. Next, the position of the patient's iris plane is checked to be certain that it is parallel to the floor and therefore perpendicular to the path of the laser beam. The position of the iris is verified by two surgical assistants, one on each side of the surgeon.

A thorough dress rehearsal will acclimate the patient to the sound of the debris aspiration device, and the startup noises of the laser. For a second or two, it is possible to initiate the procedure without actually engaging the laser, and it is most assuring to the patient to have at least one dress rehearsal before the actual treatment. Most ablations take approximately 11 to 45 seconds for the treatment of 1- to 6-D myopia; it is important that the surgeon concentrate to maintain the position of the eye with the fixation device, or to stop the ablation if, during patient self-fixation, the surgeon notices that the eye is beginning to drift. If a "drifting" ablation is performed, irregular astigmatism and unpredictable diopter outcome can result.

At the completion of the ablation, the assistant irrigates the eye and postoperative medications are instilled. Many surgeons use one drop of homatropine 5%, and a drop of ciprofloxacin (Ciloxan). A semipressure patch is applied to the eye, or, as more recently, a bandage contact lens. Many surgeons also instill a drop of diclofenac sodium (Voltaren); researchers at LSU and in Minnesota have demonstrated that diclofenac is effective for the control of postoperative pain with excimer laser surgery.

The patient can be supported while leaving the room, and is brought to a waiting area where the postoperative instructions are reviewed with the patient and his or her family.

At the end of the PRK, the VISX laser system generates a printout for the patient's chart, including all the laser parameters, the attempted change in diopters, the depth per pulse in the stroma, and the number of shots at each step in the opening of the iris diaphragm.

POSTOPERATIVE EVALUATION

Follow-up examinations are scheduled at 24-hour intervals until reepithelialization is documented. Patients using a bandage contact lens can instill medication directly into their own eyes (generally an antibiotic, a dilating agent, and diclofenac are applied); if the patient is being patched, the surgeon instills the medications once a day at the time of the examination. Reepithelialization usually is complete within 3 to 5 days, after which the patient is placed on an artificial-tear regimen. Unpreserved artificial tears are best for the delicate new epithelial layer that has just covered the ablated area; in addition, many of these patients have dry eyes and require extra lubrication to prevent recurrent epithelial defects.

As the result of a recent study conducted at the LSU Eye Center, patients no longer routinely receive a topical steroid; this regimen is reserved only for those patients who appear to be regressing rapidly.

It is important to prepare the patient for a moderate amount of postoperative pain; at LSU, two prescriptions for pain are given—acetaminophen with codeine (Tylenol no. 3) and meperidine-promethazine (Mepergan Fortis). Patients taking Tylenol no. 3 are instructed that if they cannot obtain adequate pain control, they should move up to the stronger medication, Mepergan Fortis.

After reepithelialization is complete, the patient can be discharged from daily care; at present, the FDA protocol requires that the patient return for a 1-month visit. It should be explained, however, that the eye will be quite blurry, somewhere between 20/200 and 20/50, for the first 1 to 2 postoperative weeks, but that it is possible for the patient to resume all normal physical activities and a normal work schedule (except swimming, which is best delayed for at least 3 weeks postoperatively until the epithelial layer is of normal thickness, to protect against invasive microorganisms that may be found in swimming pools).

Overcorrection is extremely common in the first few weeks; if one is attempting to achieve full distance correction, it is desirable. People near 40 years of age will notice decreased distance vision and near vision for the ensuing weeks or months; the length of their poor vision is age-dependent and outcome-dependent (in other words, patients with higher dioptric corrections) and patients will take longer to come out of their hyperopic stage. We instruct the patients that driving a care with good vision in the other eye is not a prob-

lem and, if spectacles are worn, a blank lens can be placed over the treated eye.

At present, a 6-month interval is required by the FDA before the second eye can have excimer PRK; in addition, patients must return for visits at 1, 3, 6, and 12 months, as well as a 24-month visit. When premarketing approval is granted, the surgeon may schedule postoperative visits at his or her discretion, though at least 1-, 3-, and 6-month postoperative visits are recommended for mild to moderately myopic patients.

RESULTS OF PHOTOREFRACTIVE KERATECTOMY STUDIES

The first clinical application of the excimer laser to a human—creating transverse incisions for the correction of astigmatism—was performed in Germany in April 1985 by Theo Seiler and his associates;[10] central sculpting, or wide-area ablation (PRK) was first performed on a normally sighted myopic eye in June 1988 by McDonald and associates[37] at LSU in New Orleans. This patient has maintained 20/20 uncorrected vision and her 4.5-D correction for 7 years, as of this writing. This patient demonstrated for the first time that the subepithelial haze in an early postoperative period does not generally interfere with Snellen acuity, and is almost completely resolved in most patients by 4 to 6 months.

Nine patients underwent PRK for myopia at LSU with attempted corrections from 2 to 11 D, as part of the blind-eye study which began in July 1988.[26,27] Significant flattening of the cornea was observed with no clinically significant increase in keratometric or refractive astigmatism; there was, however, some regression of the initial effect noted at 6 months. It was also noted, for the first time, that the amount of regression appeared to be proportional to the amount of dioptric correction attempted.

With the demonstration of long-term clarity and stability in these corneas, LSU was allowed to treat ten partially sighted eyes as part of PRK phase I, and 19 normally sighted eyes as part of PRK phase IIa.[28] In both partially sighted and normally sighted studies, the patients with greater than 5 D of attempted correction were much more likely to experience undercorrection than patients receiving 5 D or less of attempted correction. In the normally sighted eyes, 44% achieved uncorrected visual acuities of 20/40 or better; this result climbed to 86% in those patients with attempted corrections of 5 D or less, but dropped to only 18% in the higher myopic group with attempted corrections greater than 5 D. The best corrected visual acuity in the normally sighted eyes maintained an average of 20/20 from before laser surgery to the end of the study. Corneal clarity was well maintained, and there appeared to be no relation between the haze and the depth of the ablation. In addition, this group of patients was free of medical complications—there were no recurrent erosions, corneal ulcers, or nonhealing epithelial defects. These patients were overcorrected at 1 month and experienced a regression toward myopia by 6 months, after which the refractions were stable. The LSU investigators theorized that deeper stromal ablations could possibly incite a greater wound-healing response; Seiler and his co-workers experienced similar results with the Summit laser, treating 10 blind and 13 sighted eyes; they also found a difference in dioptric predictability, with lower degrees of attempted correction experiencing a higher degree of dioptric accuracy, and higher attempted corrections resulting in a tendency toward undercorrection.

Sher and co-workers used a Taunton laser to perform PRK in phase IIa as part of a multicenter study on sighted eyes.[38] Thirty-one sighted myopic eyes were entered into the study, with preoperative refractive errors ranging from −3.75 to −12.00 D. At 6 months post operation, 67% of the moderate myopia group (−3.12-−6.00 D) had a postoperative spherical equivalent refraction of plano to −1.00 D. In contrast, only 16% of the high myopia group (−6.12-−12.00 D) had a spherical equivalent refraction of plano to −1.00 D, and 26% had a refraction of −1.12 to −2.00 D. The authors noted, as had previous investigators, subepithelial haze in a reticular pattern which peaked at 3 weeks and diminished over the next 3 to 4 months; the Minnesota group felt that this was not visually significant. The authors also noted no statistically significant change in endothelial cell counts, corneal sensation, astigmatism, or contrast sensitivity. The authors also used the Perspective Evaluation of Radial Keratotomy (PERK) study for comparison, and determined that these two surgical methods (RK and PRK) were comparable in correcting myopic refractive errors.[38]

Liu and co-workers[39] at LSU performed a retrospective study with analysis of clinical correlations of excimer PRK for myopia, looking for significant clinical correlations that might predict clinical outcome. Blind, partially sighted, and normally sighted eyes were included in the study (phases I and IIa). This analysis found that larger attempted corrections resulted in lower dioptric predictability and poorer uncorrected visual acuity, and that the relationship between the amount of attempted correction or depth of ablation in corneal clarity was very weak (not statistically significant). This study also documented that corneal haze was not statistically significant in affecting visual acuity. Older patients tended to have better postoperative results than younger patients, regardless of the amount of attempted correction or the depth of abla-

tion.[39] More recently, investigators have noted that older patients tend to be more hyperopic postoperatively, and to stay in that stage longer than younger patients, i.e., the rate of regression is slower. Contrast sensitivity has been studied extensively in PRK patients; Hogan and co-workers[40] at LSU evaluated contrast sensitivity in 17 PRK patients from phases IIa and IIb using the Vistech MCT 8000. The results indicated that contrast sensitivity of eyes undergoing PRK for myopia with the VISX system was depressed temporarily at 6 months postoperatively, but was fully recovered by 12 months with no statistically significant difference in preoperative values.

Diurnal fluctuations were studied by Parker et al.[41] by performing manifest refractions and keratometry measurements at two time periods during the same day. In this six-patient study, preoperative myopia ranged from −5.00 to −8.25 D. There was minimal regression from the third week to the 1-year follow-up, and no diurnal fluctuation of visual acuity or refraction was noted during the entire study.

Corneal topography of PRK patients has been studied extensively by Klyce and co-workers,[42-44] Wilson and co-workers,[45,46] and others.[47-51] Wilson and co-workers[46] studied decentration in a series of 17 normally sighted phase IIa patients 1 year after PRK for myopia; the majority (10) showed decentration of 0.5 to 1.0 mm. There were three eyes that were decentered from 1.0 to 1.5 mm, and one badly decentered eye that was 2.1 mm from the center of the pupil. Since that time, the surgical technique has evolved such that badly decentered ablations are a rare event.

The most recent and last phase of FDA studies for PRK is phase III, in which each of the laser companies are allowed to treat 700 patients with −1 to −6 D of myopia, divided among ten treatment centers. Two years of follow-up on at least 500 patients is required for premarket approval. The VISX 1-year results were presented at the American Academy of Ophthalmology in 1993, and are summarized here. The principal investigators, locations, and number of eyes treated in the Phase III VISX photorefractive keratectomy trial are: Jerald Tennant, M.D.—Dallas Eye Institute, Dallas, TX, 142 eyes; Joseph Dello Russo, M.D.—New Jersey Eye Center, Berengfield, NJ, 128 eyes; James Salz, M.D.—Cedars-Sinai Medical Center, Los Angeles, CA, 105 eyes; Larry Peibenga, M.D.—Eye Foundation of Kansas City, Kansas City, MO, 87 eyes; Marguerite McDonald, M.D.—Louisiana State University, New Orleans, LA, 59 eyes; David Haight, M.D.—Manhattan EET Hospital, New York, NY, 41 eyes; Barry Kassar—Mericos Eye Center, San Diego, CA, 40 eyes; Manus Kraff, M.D.—Kraff Eye Institute, Chicago, IL, 32 eyes; Frank O'Donnell, M.D., O'Donnell Eye Foundation, St. Louis, MO, 32 eyes; and James

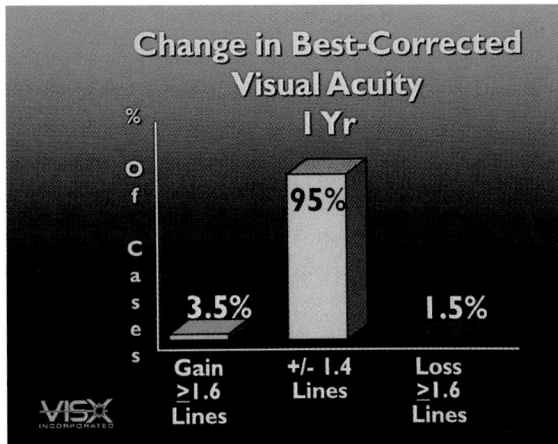

Fig. 3-2. Change in best corrected visual acuity at 1 year; the vast majority have no cjange of any clinical significance.

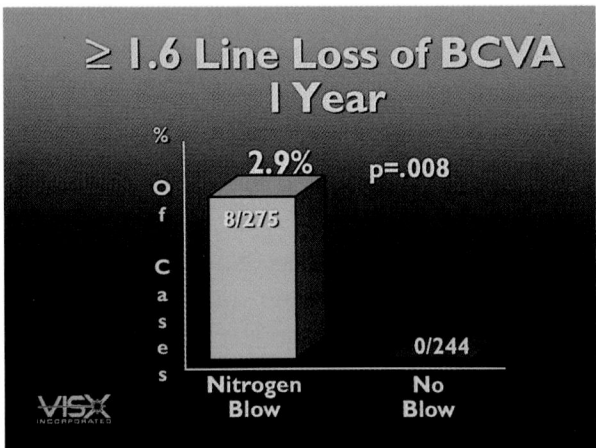

Fig. 3-3. Greater than or equal to 1.6 lines of best corrected visual acuity lost at 1 year; all patients were in the group utilizing the earlier surgical technique that was employed in the first half of the PRK (photorefractive keratectomy) III study, i.e., vigorous purging of the ablated surface to remove effluent so that the next shot could strike the cornea unimpeded by debris.

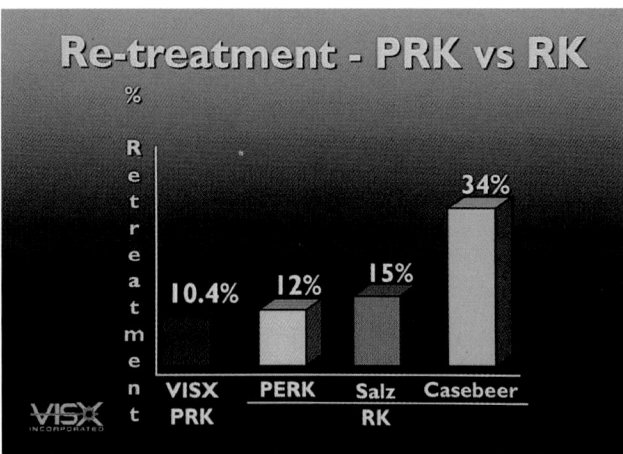

Fig. 3-4. Re-treatment rates comparing photorefractive keratectomy (PRK) and radial keratotomy (RK); PRK is lower than in three well-known RK series: (the Perspective Evaluation of Radial Keratotomy [PERK] study, and two single-surgeon series by prominent RK experts).

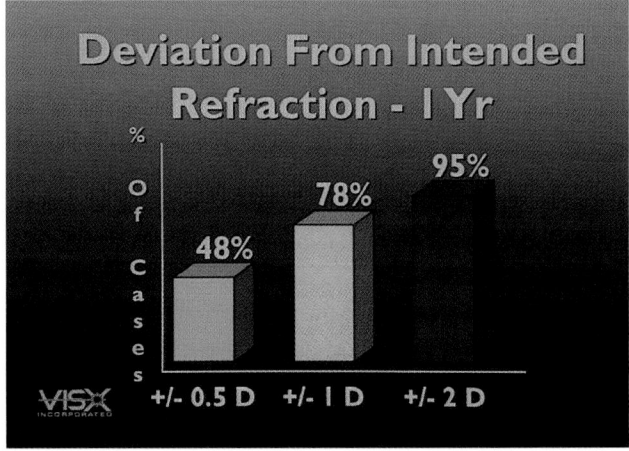

Fig. 3-5. Deviation from intended refraction at 1 year; roughly half of the patients were within ±0.5 D of intended correction at 1 year.

Aquavella, M.D., Rochester Eye Foundation, Rochester, NY.

Five hundred twenty-one patients reported for a 1-year follow-up out of a 691-patient study population. The entry criteria included myopia of −1.0 to −6.0 D, and less than or equal to 1.0 D of astigmatism in the manifest refraction. The myopia had to be stable, and patients had to be 18 years or older.

The patients were scheduled for study visits daily until reepithelialized, and then at 1, 3, 6, 12, 18, and 24 months. The patients had no incidents of serious first reactions: corneal decompensation, corneal edema, recurrent erosions, bacterial keratitis, hypopyon, cataract, and corneal perforation.

An ETDRS vision chart was used at each center. There are five letters on each line of this chart, and, as with the PERK study, up to seven letters of loss (1.4 lines) was considered within the "noise" of the measurement.

At 1 year (Fig. 3-2), 95% of the patients had no change in best corrected visual acuity (i.e., 1.4 lines of loss or less), 1.5% had a loss of greater than or equal to 1.6 lines, and 3.5% gained greater than or equal to 1.6 lines of acuity. The loss of best corrected acuity of greater than or equal to 1.6 lines was not as dramatic as it first appears (Fig. 3-3); two patients fell from 20/12.5 to 20/20, three regained by 18 months what they had lost earlier, two lost eight letters of vision, and one lost nine letters of vision. It is interesting to note that all cases of clinically significant visual loss at 1 year were in the group of patients in the first half of the study, who had nitrogen blowing across their cornea during the ablation. The surgical technique was changed midway through the study, and the "no-blow" cohort had no patients with greater than 1.6 lines of loss of best corrected visual acuity at 1 year.

The re-treatment rate was 10.4% at 1 year; 70 of the cases were re-treated for undercorrection or for haze and undercorrection. One patient was re-treated twice in the same eye.

Re-treatment is less for VISX PRK than for three well-known RK studies (Fig. 3-4): the incidence in PERK was 12%; in a recent Salz study, 15%; and in a very recent Casebeer system study, 34%.

The deviation from intended refraction at 1 year was quite good (Fig. 3-5): 78% of the patients were ±1 D at 1 year. Forty-eight percent were ±0.5 D at 1 year, and 95% of the patients were ±2 D at 1 year. Once again, PRK compares favorably with RK in this regard (Fig. 3-6). The percentage of patients who were within ±0.5 D at 1 year was 48% for PRK and 36% for PERK, and the percentage of patients within ±1 D was 78% for PRK and 64% for PERK (using only those PERK patients who were between 1 and 6 D preoperatively).

It is reassuring to know that no patient lost uncorrected visual acuity: 94.6% had gained five or more lines at 1 year, and 75.2% had gained nine or more lines at 1 year. The mean improvement at 1 year was 8.7 lines of acuity.

When comparing uncorrected visual acuity at 1 year to published data from RK studies (Fig. 3-7) the results are comparable. Fifty percent of the PRK patients were 20/20 or better uncorrected at 1 year vs. 47% for PERK and 47% for a recent Deitz study. When those data are widened to 20/40 or better uncorrected acuity (Fig. 3-8) the groups are still comparable: 88% for PRK vs. 81% for PERK (the 1- to 6-D group), and 88% for Dietz.

At 1 year, only 1% of the eyes were assigned a haze score greater than 1 (mild haze not effecting refraction). A haze score of 1.5 indicated mild haze with slight effect on refraction. A score of 2.0 means moderate haze, refraction possible, but difficult. No eyes were scored higher than 2.0. Fig. 3-9 illustrates grade

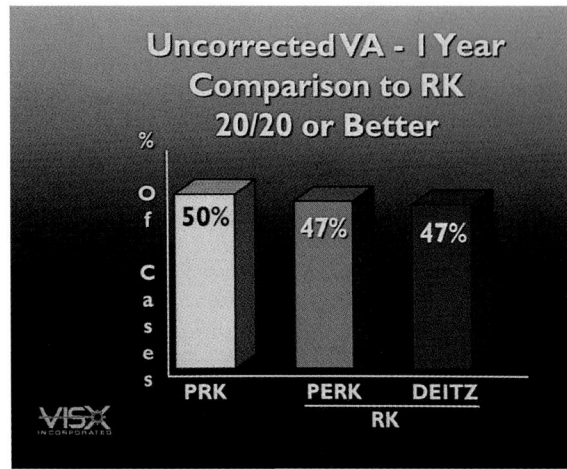

Fig. 3-7. Uncorrected visual acuity at 1 year: comparison of PRK to RK (percentage of patients 20/20 or better); PRK is comparable to RK as performed in the PERK study and in the single-surgeon Deitz study.

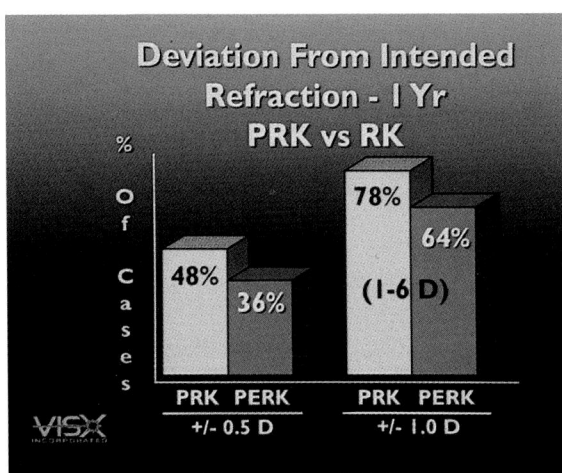

Fig. 3-6. Deviation from intended refraction at 1 year: PRK compared to RK; although the PERK technique reflects a study designed from the early 1980s, PRK outperforms PERK RK at both the 0.5-D and 1.0-D gates.

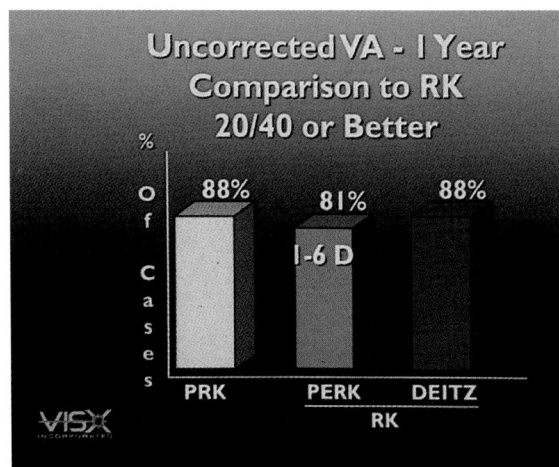

Fig. 3-8. Uncorrected visual acuity at 1 year: comparison to RK (percentage of patients 20/40 or better); once again, PRK is comparable to RK as performed in the PERK and Deitz studies.

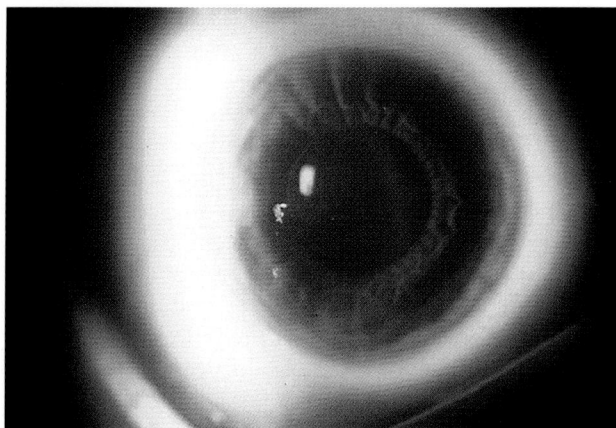

Fig. 3-9. A 3-month postoperative photograph of a typical patient from the PRK III study; the mild to moderate anterior subepithelial haze is typical; though most patients have a diffuse haze (as seen above), some patients exhibit a more reticular pattern.

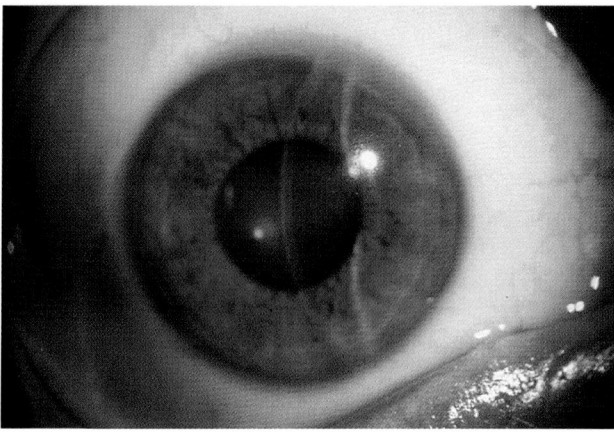

Fig. 3-10. The same patient as in Fig. 3-9 seen now 6 months postoperatively, with a marked reduction in the anterior subepithelial haze.

1 haze at 3 months and Fig. 3-10 shows the same eye at 6 months with a significant reduction in haze to grade 0.5.

It is clear that, based on the 1-year results, PRK is safe with a low complication rate, and little or no visual loss. It is efficacious in that it decreases myopia, and the predictability and stability are superior to RK.

Talamo et al., and the VISX Moderate Myopia Study Group[52] analyzed their initial results with excimer PRK for moderate myopia. They performed PRK in 89 eyes of 80 patients with moderate myopia (between 6 and 8 D, with a mean preoperative spherical equivalent of −6.98 ±0.90 D) at nine investigational sites. Sixty of the eyes received single-zone 6.0-mm ablations and 29 eyes received two-zone ablations; follow-up ranged from 1 month (n = 89) to 6 months (n = 46), and all patients were treated with the VISX laser using standard settings.

At 1 month, 49% of the eyes had an uncorrected visual acuity of 20/40 or better, and 66% of the eyes were within ±1 D of the intended correction. By 3 months, the patients had improved further: 75% of the eyes had best-corrected acuities of 20/40 or better, and 78% of the eyes were within ±1 D of the intended correction. The percentage of patients who had lost two or more lines of best-corrected acuity had dropped from 33% at 1 month to 9% at 3 months. By 6 months, only 2% (1/46) had lost two lines of best corrected visual acuity, 74% of the eyes were 20/40 or better without correction, and 67% of the eyes were within ±1 D of the intended correction.

These results are encouraging; they suggest that PRK for moderate myopia is safe and reproducible with large-diameter ablation zones, providing more predictable results than have been reported in the past using smaller ablation zone diameters. Though it is well acknowledged that higher myopic corrections require longer to stabilize, more definitive data regarding recovery of best corrected visual acuity, stability, effects of postoperative steroid therapy, and single- vs. double-zone ablations will be obtained as this group is followed for an additional 1 to 2 years.

REFERENCES

1. Taboada J, Archibald CJ: An extreme sensitivity in the corneal epithelium to far UV ArF excimer laser pulses. In Proceedings of Scientific Progress in Aerospace Medical Association, San Antonio, 1981.
2. Taboada J, Mikesell GW Jr, Reed RD: Response of the corneal epithelium to KrF excimer laser pulses, *Health Phys* 40:677-683, 1981.
3. Srinivasan R: Action of far-ultraviolet light on organic polymer films: applications to semiconductor technology, *J Radiat Curing* Oct 12-15, 1983.
4. Srinivasan R: Kinetics of the ablative photodecomposition of organic polymers in the far ultraviolet (193 nm), *J Vac Sci Technol B* 1:923-926, 1983.
5. Trokel SL, Srinivasan R, Braren B: Excimer laser surgery of the cornea, *Am J Ophthalmol* 96:710-715, 1983.
6. Aron-Rosa D, Carre F, Cassiani P, et al: Keratorefractive surgery with the excimer laser (letter), *Am J Ophthalmol* 100:741-742, 1985.
7. Marshall J, Trokel S, Rothery S, et al: An ultrastructural study of corneal incisions induced by an excimer laser at 193 nm, *Ophthalmology* 92:749-758, 1985.
8. Puliafito CA, Steinert RF, Deutsch TF, et al: Excimer laser ablation of the cornea and lens: experimental studies, *Ophthalmology* 92:741-748, 1985.
9. Aron-Rosa DS, Boulnoy JL, Carrè F, et al: Excimer laser surgery of the cornea: qualitative and quantitative aspects of photoablation according to the energy density, *J Cataract Refract Surg* 12:27-33, 1986.
10. Seiler T, Wollensak J: In vivo experiments with the excimer laser—technical parameters and healing processes, *Ophthalmologica* 192:65-70, 1986.
11. Seiler T, Marshall J, Rothery S, et al: The potential of an infrared hydrogen fluoride (HF) laser (3.0 μm) for corneal surgery, *Lasers Ophthalmol* 1:49-60, 1986.
12. Marshall J, Trokel S, Rothery S, et al: Photoablative reprofiling of the cornea using an excimer laser: photorefractive keratectomy, *Lasers Ophthalmol* 1:21-48, 1986.

13. Cotliar AM, Schubert HD, Mandel ER, et al: Excimer laser radial keratotomy, *Ophthalmology* 92:206-208, 1985.
14. Loertscher H, Mandelbaum S, Parrish RK II, et al: Preliminary report on corneal incisions created by a hydrogen fluoride laser, *Am J Ophthalmol* 102:217-221, 1986.
15. Marshall J, Trokel S, Rothery S, et al: A comparative study of corneal incisions induced by diamond and steel knives and two ultraviolet radiations from an excimer laser, *Br J Ophthalmol* 70:482-501, 1986.
16. Gaster RN, Berns MW, Burstein NL: Excimer laser interaction with the cornea (ARVO abstract), *Invest Ophthalmol Vis Sci* 27(suppl):92, 1986.
17. Krueger RR, Trokel SL: Quantitation of corneal ablation by ultraviolet laser light, *Arch Ophthalmol* 103:1741-1742, 1985.
18. McDonald MB, Beuerman R, Falzoni W, et al: Refractive surgery with the excimer laser, *Am J Ophthalmol* 103 (3, II):469, 1987.
19. Tuft S, Marshall J, Rothery S: Stromal remodelling following photorefractive keratectomy. *Lasers Ophthalmol* 1:177-185, 1987.
20. Berns, MW, Liaw LH, Oliva A, et al: An acute light and electron microscopic study of ultraviolet 193-nm excimer laser corneal incisions, *Ophthalmology* 95:1422-1433, 1988.
21. Marshall J, Trokel SL, Rothery S, et al: Long-term healing of the central cornea after photorefractive keratectomy using an excimer laser, *Ophthalmology* 95:1411-1421, 1988.
22. Srinivasan R: Ablation of polymers and biological tissue by ultraviolet lasers, *Science* 234:559-565, 1986.
23. Srinivasan R, Sutcliffe E: Dynamics of the ultraviolet laser ablation of the cornea, *Am J Ophthalmol* 103:470-471, 1987.
24. Munnerlyn CR, Koons SJ, Marshall J: Photorefractive keratectomy: a technique for laser refractive surgery, *J Cataract Refract Surg* 14:46-52, 1988.
25. L'Esperance FA Jr, Taylor DM, Warner JW: Human excimer laser keratectomy: short-term histopathology, *J Refract Surg* 4:118-124, 1988.
26. McDonald M, Shofner S, Klyce S, et al: Clinical results of central photorefractive keratectomy (PRK) with the 193 NM excimer laser for the treatment of myopia: the blind eye study, *Invest Ophthalmol Vis Sci* 30(suppl):216, 1989.
27. McDonald MB, Frantz JM, Klyce SD, et al: Central photorefractive keratectomy for myopia: the blind eye study, *Arch Ophthalmol* 108:799-808, 1990.
28. McDonald MB, Liu JC, Byrd TJ, et al: Central photorefractive keratectomy for myopia: partially sighted and normally sighted eyes, *Ophthalmology* 98:1327-1337, 1991.
29. Lohmann CP, Gartry DS, Muir MK, et al: Korneale Trübung nach photorefraktiver keratektomie mit einem Excimer Laser: Ursache, objecktive Messungen und funktionelle Konsequenzen, *Ophthalmologe* 89:498-504, 1992.
30. Cho YS, Kim CG, Kim WB, et al: Multistep photorefractive keratectomy for high myopia, *Refract Corneal Surg* 9(suppl):S37-S41, 1993.
31. Förster W, Grewe S, Busse H: Clinical use of the excimer laser for the treatment of superficial corneal opacities: therapeutic strategy and case reports, *Klin Monatsbl Augenheilk* 202:126-129, 1993.
32. Brancato R, Tavola A, Carones F, et al: Excimer laser photorefractive keratectomy for myopia: results in 1165 eyes, *Refract Corneal Surg* 9:95-104, 1993.
33. Unkroth A, Kleinschmidt J, Ziegler W, et al: Ablation of the cornea by using a low-energy excimer laser, *Graefe's Arch Clin Exp Ophthalmol* 231:303-307, 1993.
34. Siganos DS, Papatzanaki ME, Makridakis GS, et al: Corneal topography changes following myopic excimer laser photorefractive keratectomy, *Ophthalmologia* 5:28-33, 1993.
35. Rogers C, Lawless M, Cohen P: Excimer laser keratectomy (letter), *Aust N Z J Ophthalmol* 20:271, 1992.
36. Lawless MA, Rogers C, Cohen P: Excimer laser photorefractive keratectomy: 12 months followup, *Med J Aust* 159:535, 1993.
37. McDonald MB, Kaufman HE, Frantz JM, et al: Excimer laser ablation in a human eye, *Arch Ophthalmol* 107:641-642, 1989.
38. Sher NA, Chen V, Bowers RA, et al: The use of the 193-nm excimer laser for myopic photorefractive keratectomy in sighted eyes: a multicenter study, *Arch Ophthalmol* 109:1525-1530, 1991.
39. Liu JC, McDonald MB, Varnell R, et al: Myopic excimer laser photorefractive keratectomy: an analysis of clinical correlations, *Refract Corneal Surg* 6:321-328, 1990.
40. Hogan C, McDonald M, Byrd T, et al: Effect of excimer laser photorefractive keratectomy on contrast sensitivity (ARVO abstract), *Invest Ophthalmol Vis Sci* 32(suppl):721, 1991.
41. Parker P, Chen V, Lindstrom RL, et al: Stability of correction after excimer photorefractive keratectomy (ARVO abstract), *Invest Ophthalmol Vis Sci* 32(suppl):721, 1991.
42. Klyce S: Corneal topography in refractive keratectomy. In Thompson FB, McDonnell PJ, editors: *Color atlas/text of excimer laser surgery. The cornea.* New York, 1992, Igakv-Shoin.
43. Klyce SD, Smolek MK: Corneal topography of excimer laser photorefractive keratectomy, *J Cataract Refract Surg* 19(suppl):122-130, 1993.
44. Klyce SD, Updegraff SA, Smolek MK, et al: Predictability in keratorefractive surgery, *Invest Ophthalmol Vis Sci* 34:801, 1993.
45. Wilson SE: Excimer laser (193 nm) myopic keratomileusis: differential stability in lower and higher myopes (letter), *Refract Corneal Surg* 6:383-385, 1990.
46. Wilson SE, Klyce SD, McDonald MB, et al: Changes in corneal topography after excimer laser photorefractive keratectomy for myopia, *Ophthalmology* 98:1338-1347, 1991.
47. Cantera E, Cantera I, Olivieri L: Corneal topographic analysis of photorefractive keratectomy in 175 myopic eyes, *Refract Corneal Surg* 9(suppl):19-22, 1993.
48. Spadea L, Sabetti L, Balestrazzi E: Effect of centering excimer laser PRK on refractive results: a corneal topography study, *Refract Corneal Surg* 9(suppl):22-25, 1993.
49. Maloney RK: Corneal topography and optical zone location in photorefractive keratectomy, *Refract Corneal Surg* 5:363-371, 1990.
50. Parker P, Zabel RW, Maguire LJ, et al: Computed topographic analysis following myopic excimer laser photorefractive keratectomy, *Invest Ophthalmol Vis Sci* 31(suppl):480, 1990.
51. Siganos DS, Papatzanaki ME, Makridakis GS, et al: Corneal topography changes following myopic excimer laser photorefractive keratectomy, *Ophthalmologia* 5:28-33, 1993.
52. Talamo JH, Siebert K, Wagoner MD, et al, and the VISX Moderate Myopia Study Group: Excimer photorefractive keratectomy for moderate myopia: initial results, in preparation.

4

Photorefractive Keratectomy with the Summit Excimer Laser: The Phase III U.S. Results

Keith P. Thompson, Roger F. Steinert, Jan Daniel, R. Doyle Stulting

Photorefractive keratectomy (PRK) performed by the 193-nm excimer laser is receiving increasing acceptance in the correction of low to moderate myopia.[1-3] We estimate that over 100,000 eyes have been treated worldwide. The excimer laser was introduced to ophthalmology in 1983 with Trokel's observation that the 193-nm wavelength could precisely etch and contour corneal tissue.[4] This technique has evolved through basic science and animal studies, and human clinical trials with blind and sighted eyes (Fig. 4-1).

The Food and Drug Administration (FDA) has issued stringent guidelines for the clinical evaluation of this new technique in the United States. Two manufacturers of delivery systems, VISX (Santa Clara, Calif.) and Summit Technology (Waltham, Mass.), have completed patient enrollment in phase III clinical trials.

This study reports the 1-year follow-up of 585 of 701 eyes enrolled in the phase III clinical trial for PRK with the Summit UV-200 LA excimer laser system.

PHASE III STUDY DESIGN

Seven hundred one treated eyes of 701 patients were entered in the study at the sites shown in Table 4-1. Follow-up data on 585 eyes were available at 1 year. Attempted correction ranged from 1.5 to 6.0 D of spherical equivalent myopia with a mean of 4.07 D. All patients had a complete ophthalmologic examina-

tion to verify absence of any ocular or systemic disease affecting the eyes. Patients whose manifest refraction revealed more than 1.00 D of astigmatism were excluded from the study.

Preoperatively, 94.3% of the patients had a best corrected spectacle visual acuity of 20/20 or better, and 5.7% had spectacle corrected best acuities of 20/25 to 20/40. Like other patients seeking refractive surgery, most patients who sought excimer laser PRK were motivated to decrease their dependence on corrective eyewear.[5] Many had tried and failed contact lenses in the past.

For measuring uncorrected and best corrected visual acuity, back-illuminated EDTRS charts were used at a testing distance of 4 ms. Manifest refractions were performed using a fogging technique. Testing for glare disability was performed with the clinical Brightness Acuity Tester (Mentor, Santa Barbara, Calif.) using the brightest light. To determine cycloplegic refraction, one drop of 1% cyclopentolate was instilled 30 minutes prior to examination. Contact lens wearers were instructed to discontinue lens wear 2 weeks prior to their preoperative examination.

Contrast sensitivity was measured with the CSV-1000 (Vector Vision Inc., Dayton, Ohio) at 3, 6, 12, and 18 cycles per degree with undilated and dilated pupils at a testing distance of 2.4 ms. The box on p. 58 lists the preoperative examinations performed.

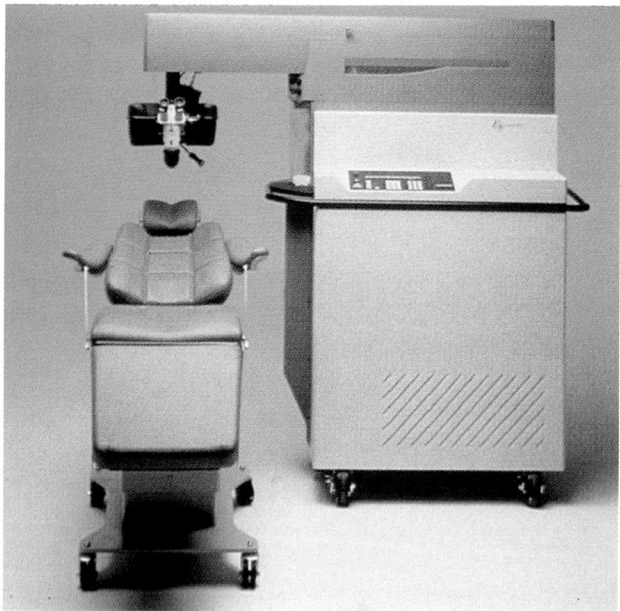

Fig. 4-1. Summit Technology Omnimed Excimer Laser System in current use.

Clinical Examination prior to and after Photorefractive Keratectomy

Uncorrected visual acuity
Manifest refraction
Cycloplegic refraction
Best corrected visual acuity (BCVA)
    BCVA with undilated pupil
    BCVA with dilated pupil
    BCVA with glare
Contrast sensitivity (undilated and dilated)
Applanation tonometry
Slit lamp examination
Manual keratometry
Computer-assisted videokeratography
Specular endothelial microscopy
Dilated fundoscopic examination
Pupillary examination

Table 4-1. Clinical centers enrolled in the Summit Phase III FDA protocol

Investigators	Location	No. of eyes
Brint	New Orleans	104
Durrie, Hunkeler, Cavanaugh	Kansas City	136
Galusha	Tulsa	54
Pepose	St. Louis	36
Gold, Milstein	Galveston	68
Gordon	San Diego	89
Michelson, Owen	Birmingham	58
Steinert, Puliafito	Boston	39
Wright	Colorado Springs	67
Waring, Stulting, Thompson	Atlanta	50

To determine the size of the ablation zone, the diameter of the pupil was measured under ambient lighting of 21 lux. Patients with pupil sizes 5 mm or greater were designated to receive 5.0-mm ablation zones; patients with pupils less than 5 mm in diameter received 4.5-mm ablation zones.

A complete written informed consent approved by the local institutional review board was obtained from all patients.

A subset of 142 patients underwent corneal endothelial specular microscopy. In each patient photographs of the endothelium were taken in the central, paracentral, and peripheral cornea. All photographs were numbered, masked, and the endothelial cells were counted at the Emory Eye Center (Atlanta). Digitization and analysis of the endothelial cell content represented by the photographic print were accomplished by a computer-assisted morphometric analysis described previously.[6,7] Cell density and the size of endothelial cells were measured and the percentage of hexagonal cells and the coefficient of variation were calculated in the involved eyes.

SURGICAL PROCEDURE

Several drops of 1% proparacaine or tetracaine were instilled, and a lid speculum was inserted. In order to familiarize the patient with the sensation of photoablation, a small amount of 1% methylcellulose was placed on the corneal epithelium and the patient was instructed to fixate his or her eye upon a green-colored light-emitting diode located coaxial to the excimer la-

ser beam delivery aperture. Several trains of laser pulses were then delivered to the methylcellulose-protected cornea until the patient demonstrated the ability to maintain stable fixation.

The methylcellulose was removed with a sponge and 25 laser pulses were administered to the patient's epithelium again to establish the patient's ability to maintain fixation. A 6 or 7 mm optical zone marker was then used to mark the epithelium over the entrance pupil, and the corneal epithelium within this zone was debrided with a no. 69 Beaver blade. The surface of the cornea was carefully cleaned of debris. A very thin coat of 1% methylcellulose was applied with a cellulose sponge. The Excimed UV 200 LA excimer laser programmed by input of the spectacles manifest refraction spherical equivalent was activated by the surgeon's foot pedal. The radiant exposure of the laser at the corneal surface was 180 mJ/cm^2. The repetition rate was 10 Hz, and the ablation rate was assumed to be 0.25 μm per pulse. In early phase III all patients received a 4.5-mm optical zone. This was subsequently expanded to 5.0 mm. Ultimately 58% of the eyes received a 5.0-mm ablation zone and 42% received a 4.5-mm ablation zone.

The number of pulses used ranged from 70 to 246 with an average of 163 pulses, requiring slightly more than 16 seconds of ablation time.

Postoperatively, the lid speculum was removed, Tobradex (dexamethasone-tobramycin) ointment was instilled in the eye, and the eye was patched overnight. Oral narcotic analgesic pain medication was prescribed for the first postoperative day. The patient was seen back on the first postoperative day and the patch was removed.

The patients were then treated with Tobradex ointment 5 times daily and optional patching until the corneal epithelium healed. Patients were then placed on fluoromethalone alcohol 2.5% drops five times daily for the first month; fluoromethalone 1.0% drops four times daily for the second month, three times daily for the third month, and then further tapered at the surgeon's discretion so that steroids were fully discontinued by the sixth postoperative month.

On their postoperative follow-up visits, patients underwent the examinations listed in the box on p. 58. Subepithelial corneal haze was graded clinically on a scale of clear, trace, mild, moderate, or marked, as described elsewhere.[8-11]

RESULTS

Corneal reepithelialization of the ablated area was complete in 91% of eyes before 72 hours and in all eyes at 1 week. There were no reports of corneal erosions or corneal infections.

Best Corrected Visual Acuity

The change in best corrected visual acuity for the 585 eyes is shown in Table 4-2. Initially, the best spectacles-corrected visual acuity of 20/20 or better dropped from a preoperative rate of 94.3% to 82.1%

at 1 month postoperatively. At 3 months the best corrected visual acuity reached the preoperative level, and exceeded this level at all further follow-up examinations.

Thirteen eyes were found to have lost two lines of best corrected visual acuity and five eyes lost more than two lines. Table 4-3 lists these patients. Most of these patients had preoperative visual acuity better than 20/20 and postoperative visual acuity of 20/20 or 20/25. The one patient with 20/80 postoperative visual acuity at 1 year had received an eccentric ablation. He subsequently has recieved a second ablation with a return of visual acuity to 20/25.

Uncorrected Vision

Table 4-4 summarizes uncorrected visual acuity following PRK. Compared with 0.1% preoperatively, 90.7% of the patients achieved an uncorrected visual acuity of 20/40 or better 1 year postoperatively; 66.4% of the patients had an uncorrected visual acuity of 20/20 or better at the 1 year follow up examination.

Refractive Predictability

Table 4-5 shows the refractive predictability at 1 year in this patient group: 77.7% of the patients had a manifest refraction spherical equivalent within 1.00 D of emmetropia at the 1-year follow-up examination compared with 0.0% preoperatively.

The correlation between predictability and attempted diopters of correction is provided in Table 4-6. Eighty percent of the patient subgroup with an attempted correction of 1.50 to 2.90 D reached an uncorrected visual acuity of 20/20 or better, but in the subgroup with desired correction of 5.00 to 5.90 D, the portion with uncorrected visual acuity of 20/20 dropped to 58.9%.

Corneal Haze

Figs. 4-2 and 4-3 show the prevalence of anterior stromal reticular haze graded by slit-lamp examination 3 and 12 months postoperatively. Twelve months after surgery 89.3% of all patients were free of clinically significant haze, and no eyes suffered from

Table 4-2. Best corrected spectacles visual acuity

Visual acuity	Preoperative n (%)	1 mo n (%)	3 mo n (%)	6 mo n (%)	12 mo n (%)
20/20 or better	660 (94.3)	562 (82.1)	623 (93.8)	643 (96.4)	576 (96.0)
20/25-20/40	40 (5.7)	120 (17.6)	41 (6.2)	22 (3.4)	23 (3.8)
20/50-20/80	0 (0.0)	2 (0.3)	0 (0.0)	1 (0.2)	1 (0.2)
20/100-20/160	0 (0.0)	0 (0.0)	0 (0.0)	0 (0.0)	0 (0.0)
20/200 or worse	0 (0.0)	0 (0.0)	0 (0.0)	0 (0.0)	0 (0.0)

Table 4-3. PRK Phase III: BCVA loss 2 lines or greater

Patient	Preop	Postop	Loss/Gain
No. 1	20/20	20/80	−6
No. 2	20/12	20/32	−4
No. 3	20/12	20/25	−3
No. 4	20/12	20/25	−3
No. 5	20/12	20/25	−3
No. 6	20/12	20/20	−2
No. 7	20/12	20/20	−2
No. 8	20/20	20/32	−2
No. 9	20/12	20/20	−2
No. 10	20/12	20/20	−2
No. 11	20.12.5	20/20	−2
No. 12	20/16	20/25	−2
No. 13	20/10	20/16	−2
No. 14	20/16	20/25	−2
No. 15	20/12	20/20	−2
No. 16	20/10	20/16	−2
No. 17	20/16	20/25	−2
No. 18	20/12	20/20	−2

Table 4-4. Uncorrected visual acuity after photoreactive keratectomy

Visual acuity	Preoperative n (%)	1 mo n (%)	3 mo n (%)	6 mo n (%)	12 mo n (%)
20/20 or better	0 (0.0)	195 (28.2)	365 (54.8)	413 (61.6)	399 (66.4)
20/25-20/40	1 (0.1)	272 (39.3)	218 (32.8)	203 (30.3)	145 (24.3)
20/50-20/80	28 (4.0)	175 (25.3)	61 (9.2)	39 (5.8)	36 (6.1)
20/100-20/160	105 (14.9)	35 (5.1)	17 (2.7)	9 (1.5)	11 (1.9)
20/200 or worse	567 (81.0)	14 (2.1)	3 (0.5)	5 (0.8)	8 (1.3)

Table 4-5. Manifest refraction spherical equivalent prior to and after photorefractive keratectomy

	Preoperative n (%)	1 mo n (%)	3 mo n (%)	6 mo n (%)	12 mo n (%)
±0.50 D	0 (0.0)	137 (19.9)	256 (38.2)	345 (51.4)	351 (58.5)
±1.00 D	0 (0.0)	234 (34.0)	413 (61.9)	512 (76.4)	466 (77.7)
±2.00 D	39 (5.6)	467 (67.8)	604 (90.7)	623 (93.1)	563 (93.9)

marked haze. The tendency for early postoperative haze to clear is apparent.

Contrast Sensitivity

The preoperative dilated and undilated contrast sensitivity log means were used as the baseline contrast sensitivity measurement ±1 SD.[12] At the 3-, 6-, and 12-month postoperative visits, the undilated and dilated contrast sensitivity log means for all spatial frequencies were within 1 SD. These minimal changes are not considered to have a clinically significant effect.

Specular Microscopy

In comparison to the preoperative values, central corneal endothelial cell density, size, and pleomorphism showed no statistically significant changes at either 3 or 12 months after PRK.

In the peripheral cornea the endothelial cell density was decreased 4.5% ($P = .01$) 3 months and 6.4% ($P = .001$) 12 months postoperatively. Changes in pleomorphism and polymegethism were found to be statistically insignificant at 3 and 12 months after PRK as compared to preoperatively.

CONCLUSIONS

The primary motivation of patients undergoing refractive surgery is to decrease their dependence on corrective eyewear.[13] The achievement of this goal depends on the patient's daily visual needs. Most patients who achieve 20/25 or better vision can function independently without corrective eyewear. In this series, 77% of patients achieved an uncorrected Snellen acuity of 20/25 or better, and 92% achieved 20/40 or better. These percentages compare favorably with published series detailing the results of radial keratotomy (RK). Consequently, PRK appears to be highly effective in achieving its stated objective, although the technique is still not as accurate or as predictable as correcting myopia with contact lenses or spectacles, which have a virtually 100% chance of achieving 20/20 or better vision in a healthy eye.

Assessing the dioptric refractive outcome following PRK is less meaningful than the uncorrected visual acuity because corneal asphericity caused by PRK results in visual acuity that is better than expected based on the refractive outcome. For this reason, uncorrected visual acuity (and other measures of visual performance such as contrast sensitivity) should be the primary parameters used when assessing the efficacy of refractive surgical procedures. Nevertheless, 77% of patients were found to be within 1 D of emmetropia at 1 year. The refractive outcome appeared to stabilize by the sixth month after surgery for most patients except the higher myopes, and by the ninth month for all patients, as shown in Fig. 4-4.

The vast majority of patients maintained or improved their best corrected visual acuity. Improving best corrected visual acuity following PRK is explained by appreciating the increase in image magnification that results when the correction occurs at the corneal plane instead of the spectacle plane.

Because PRK involves treating the central cornea, considerable attention has been given to the subepithelial corneal haze resulting from the procedure. Multiple studies have shown that the haze is most likely due to abnormal glycosaminoglycans or nonlamellar collagen, or both, deposited in the anterior stroma as a consequence of epithelial-stromal wound healing.[8,14-16] This study does not investigate whether postoperative topical corticosteroids are needed to manage corneal wound healing. Wound healing is documented to cause a regression of refractive effect. The requirement for postoperative steroids to modulate wound healing remains controversial and studies

Table 4-6. Correlation between predictability and attempted correction in diopters

Visual acuity	1.5-2.9 D n (%)	3.0-3.9 D n (%)	4.0-4.9 D n (%)	5.0-5.9 D n (%)	6.0-6.9 D n (%)
20/20 or better	92 (80.0)	102 (68.4)	101 (69.2)	73 (58.9)	4 (6.1)
20/25-20/40	19 (16.5)	39 (26.2)	31 (21.2)	34 (27.2)	22 (34.0)
20/50-20/80	3 (2.6)	6 (4.0)	11 (7.5)	11 (8.9)	5 (7.7)
20/100-20/160	0 (0.0)	1 (0.7)	3 (2.1)	4 (3.2)	3 (4.6)
20/200 or worse	1 (0.9)	1 (0.7)	0 (0.0)	2 (1.6)	5 (7.7)

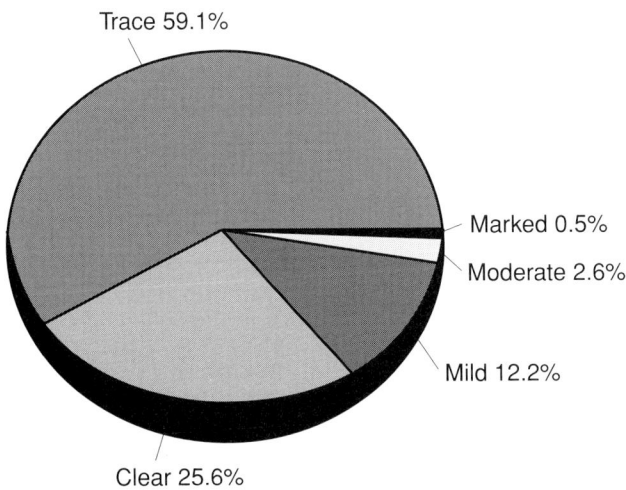

Fig. 4-2. Anterior stromal haze grading 3 months after photorefractive keratectomy.

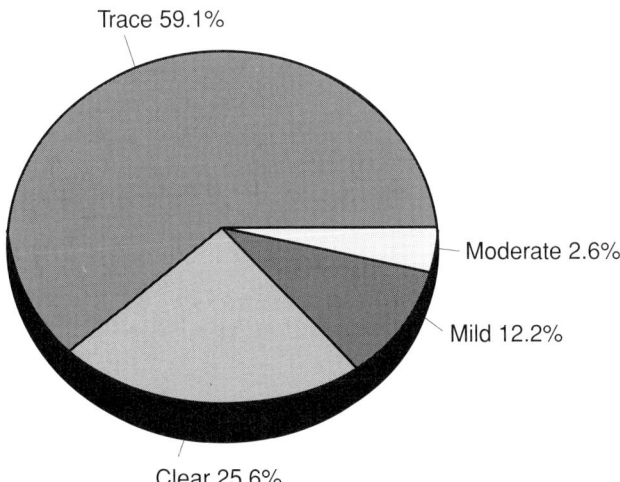

Fig. 4-3. Anterior stromal haze grading 12 months after photorefractive keratectomy.

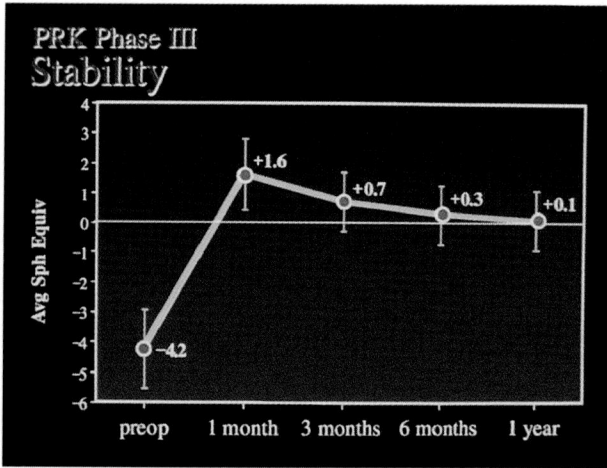

Fig. 4-4. Mean refractive error over 12 months following photorefractive keratectomy.

have shown contradictory results.[17-20] Further evaluation of this issue with large randomized double-blind studies are needed.

Complications of PRK in this study were quite minor. There were no incidences of infection, recurrent erosion, or any sight-threatening events. An evaluation of the corneal endothelium by specular microscopy showed a 6.4% decrease in peripheral endothelial cell density and no change in central cell density or morphology at 12 months compared with preoperative values. This represents a very small cell loss and is probably comparable to or less than the loss occurring after RK.[21-23] The reason for cell loss peripherally but not centrally is unclear.

A number of patients report optical aberrations including ghost images and halos following PRK. These complaints seem to be exacerbated at night and are most prevalent in young myopic females with large pupillary diameters. These symptoms most likely are caused by an effective optical zone that is smaller than the entrance pupil under conditions of dim illumination. In general, a larger, more uniform, and well-centered optical zone will provide the patient with better quality of vision, especially at night. Complaints of halos at night were fewer in patients with the 5.0-mm optical zone compared to those with the 4.5-mm optical zone. Increased depth of ablation does not appear to result in clinically important problems, and therefore Summit has further expanded its treatment zone size up to 6.5 mm in post-phase III trials.

SUMMARY

Photorefractive keratectomy is a safe, effective, and relatively predictable means of correcting low to moderate myopia. The procedure offers several advantages over RK from a patient's perspective. The cornea is not weakened and thus the risk to the eye from blunt trauma is not increased. There is no diurnal variation as is encountered frequently following RK.[24-27] Resuming soft contact lens wear following PRK should not be a problem, whereas soft contact lens wear following RK can be associated with multiple complications.[28,29] The need for contact lenses after PRK is quite low, however. The primary disadvantage of PRK compared to RK for low to moderate myopia appears to be the length of time required for visual recovery. Many patients have excellent uncorrected visual acuity on the first postoperative day following RK, allowing them to return quickly to their normal functions. Because the central corneal surface must first reepithelialize and then become regular, many patients have degraded vision for several weeks following PRK. Patients over 40 years old have the additional problem of becoming hyperopic (without the ability to accommodate) during the first 1 to 3 months following PRK. If only one eye has been treated, it is very useful for the patient to be able to wear a contact lens in the untreated eye during this interval; otherwise, the anisometropia may be troublesome.

Despite these drawbacks, patient acceptance of PRK is very high. Further improvements in technique, such as improvement in the contour of the ablated zone, less performance on pharmacologic manipulation of wound healing, and more effective postoperative pain control should lead to even greater acceptance of PRK for the treatment of myopia.

REFERENCES

1. Salz JJ: Radial keratotomy versus photorefractive keratectomy. In Thompson FB, McDonnell PJ editors: *Color atlas/text of excimer laser surgery: the cornea,* New York, 1993, Igako-Shoin.
2. Thompson KP: Photorefractive keratectomy, *Ophthalmol Clin North Am* 5:745-751, 1992.
3. Brancato R, Tavola A, Carones, et al: Excimer laser photorefractive keratectomy for myopia: results in 1165 eyes, *Refract Corneal Surg* 9(suppl):95-104, 1993.
4. Trokel SL, Srinivasan R, Braren BA: Excimer laser surgery of the cornea, *Am J Ophthalmol* 96:710-715, 1983.
5. Gimbel HV, Van Westenbrugge JA, Johnson WA, et al: Visual, refractive, and patient satisfaction results following bilateral photorefractive keratectomy for myopia, *Refract Corneal Surg* 9(suppl):5-10, 1993.
6. Inaba M, Matsuda M, Shiozaki Y, et al: Morphologic analysis of human corneal endothelium, *Invest Ophthalmol Vis Sci* 25(suppl):240, 1984.
7. Yee RW, Matsuda M, Schultz RO, et al: Changes in the normal endothelial cellular pattern as a function of age, *Curr Eye Res,* 6:671-678, 1985.
8. Fantes FE, Hanna KD, Waring GO, et al: Wound healing after excimer laser keratomileusis (photorefractive keratectomy) in monkeys, *Arch Ophthalmol* 108:665-675, 1990.
9. Anrade HA, McDonald MB, Liu JC, et al: Evaluation of an opacity lensometer for determining corneal clarity following excimer laser photoablation, *Refract Corneal Surg* 6:346-351, 1990.
10. Lohmann C, Fitzke F, Timberlake G, et al: Corneal transparency after excimer laser photorefractive keratectomy: a new technique for objective measurement of haze, *Refract Corneal Surg* 8:15-21, 1992.

11. Lohmann C, Gartry D, Kerr Muir M, et al: Haze in photorefractive keratectomy: its origins and consequences, *Lasers Light Ophthalmol* 4:15-34, 1991.
12. Adams AJ, Heron G, Husted R: Clinical measures of central vision function in glaucoma and ocular hypertension, *Arch Ophthalmol* 105:782-787, 1987.
13. Bourque LB, Rubenstein R, Cosand BB, et al: Phsychosocial characteristics of candidates for the Perspective Evaluation of Radial Keratotomy (PERK) study, *Arch Ophthalmol* 102:1187-1192, 1984.
14. Malley DS, Steinert RF, Puliafito CA, et al: Immunofluorescence study of corneal wound healing after excimer laser anterior keratectomy in the monkey eye, *Arch Ophthalmol* 108:1316-1322, 1990.
15. Hanna KD, Pouliquen YM, Waring GO, et al: Corneal wound healing in monkeys after repeated excimer laser photorefractive keratectomy, *Arch Ophthalmol* 109:1296-1301, 1992.
16. Hanna KD, Pouliquen YM, Salvodelli M, et al: Corneal wound healing in monkeys 18 months after excimer laser photorefractive keratectomy, *Refract Corneal Surg* 6:340-345, 1990.
17. Fagerholm P, Tengroth B: The effect of postoperative topical steroids on the refractive outcome of excimer laser photorefractive keratectomy for myopia. Presented at American Academy of Ophthalmology meeting, Chicago, November 1993.
18. Tengroth B, Fagerholm P, Soderberg H, et al: Effect of corticosteroids in postoperative care following photorefractive keratectomies, *Refract Corneal Surg* 9(suppl):61-64, 1993.
19. Gartry D, Kerr Muir M, Lohmann C, et al: The effect of topical corticosteroids on refractive outcome and corneal haze after refractive keratectomy, *Arch Ophthalmol* 110:944-952, 1992.
20. Carones F, Brancato R, Venturi E, et al: Efficacy of corticosteroids in reversing the regression after myopic photorefractive keratectomy, *Refract Corneal Surg* 9(suppl):52-56, 1993.
21. Huang JT: Radial keratotomy for the treatment of myopia, *Chung Hua Yen Ko Tsa Chih* 28:328-330, 1992.
22. Bergmann L, Hartmann C, Renard G, et al: Damage to the corneal endothelium caused by radial keratotomy, *Fortschr Ophthalmol* 88:368-373, 1991.
23. Hoffer KJ, Darin JJ, Pettit TH, et al: Three years experience with radial keratotomy: the UCLA study, *Ophthalmology* 90:627-636, 1983.
24. Seiler T, Hell K, Wollensak J: Diurnal variation in refraction after excimer laser photorefractive keratectomy, *Graefer Arch Clin Exp Ophthalmol* 1:19-21, 1992.
25. Kwitko S, Gritz DC, Garbus JJ, et al: Diurnal variation of corneal topography after radial keratotomy, *Arch Ophthalmol* 110:351-356, 1992.
26. McDonnell PJ, Fish LA, Garbus J: Persistence of diurnal fluctuation after radial keratotomy, *Refract Corneal Surg* 5:89-93, 1989.
27. McDonnell PJ, McClusky DJ, Garbus JJ: Corneal topography and fluctuating visual acuity after radial keratotomy, *Ophthalmology* 96:665-670, 1989.
28. Marmer RH: Radial keratotomy complications, *Ann Ophthalmol* 19:409-411, 1987.
29. Shivitz IA, Arrowsmith PN, Russel BM: Contact lenses in the treatment of patients with overcorrected radial keratotomy, *Ophthalmology* 94:899-903, 1987.

Photorefractive Keratectomy for Astigmatism

Mauro Campos, Peter J. McDonnell

Astigmatism, both naturally occurring and postoperative, has challenged ophthalmic surgeons for decades. Recent advances in cataract surgical techniques, including the use of multifocal intraocular lenses and corneal arcuate incisions at the time of the cataract extraction, have stimulated interest in minimizing early postoperative astigmatism and maximizing postoperative unaided acuity. Similarly, there has been renewed emphasis on identifying those surgical variables (e.g., trephination technique, suture placement) that contribute to postkeratoplasty astigmatism, which is a major limitation of keratoplasty surgery.

Although the pathogenesis of congenital astigmatism remains unclear, postoperative astigmatism is the consequence of asymmetric corneal deformation by the surgery. The spherical cornea has radially symmetric topography with a single keratometric endpoint in all meridians, circular photokeratoscope images, and excellent acuity when corrected with spherical lenses. With computer-assisted topographic analysis, the most "spherical" corneas are actually seen to be aspheric, with the cornea being steepest centrally and gradually flattening toward the limbus. With the astigmatic cornea, the refractive power of the eye varies with the orientation of incident light rays. Astigmatism is said to be regular when two principal or major meridians are identifiable by refraction and keratometry, the meridians are 90 degrees apart, the endpoint of keratometry is distinct, the photokeratoscope mires are regular circles or ovals, and when excellent acuity is achievable with spectacle correction. With computer-assisted topographic analysis, regular astigmatism typically has a figure-of-eight pattern that is symmetric about the two principal meridians, which are oriented 90 degrees apart. Astigmatism is irregular if the principal meridians are separated by an angle other than 90 degrees, the endpoint of keratometry is indistinct, the circular mires of the photokeratoscope are distorted, and when excellent acuity is not achievable with spectacle correction, but refraction over a hard or gas-permeable contact lens does result in excellent acuity. With computer-assisted topographic analysis, the topography is seen to not be symmetrically distributed about the corneal apex. The two steep hemimeridians, which should be oriented 180 degrees apart, may be separated by 170 degrees, 160 degrees, or even less. Also, the amount of steepening in the two hemimeridians may not be symmetric about the center of the corneal apex, with one steep hemimeridian being substantially steeper than the opposite steep hemimeridian. Similarly, the flat hemimeridians may be separated by an angle other than 180 degrees and exhibit asymmetry about the corneal apex. Occasionally seen in unoperated astigmatic corneas, this irregular astigmatism is typical after trauma or penetrating keratoplasty. Initially after cataract surgery in which astigmatism is induced, the astigmatism is usually irregular, with a peripheral wedge-shaped zone of steepening or flattening in the quadrant of the incision. Months after the surgery, however, the topography typically resembles that of regular, naturally occurring astigmatism. Appreciation of the sometimes complex topography of astigmatic corneas has been a recent phenomenon. Of the papers that describe surgery for astigmatism, almost all describe nomograms involving a "cookbook" approach based entirely on refraction; few have considered the preoperative topography when planning the placement of incisions or sutures. The next major advance in the field of refractive surgery for astigmatism will likely involve the use of topography in a direct way for the preoperative planning of surgery for astigmatism.

A BRIEF HISTORY OF SURGICAL CORRECTION OF ASTIGMATISM

Many surgical procedures, including relaxing incisions (radial, transverse, and arcuate), trapezoidal astigmatic keratotomy (Ruiz procedure), wedge resection, and toric epikeratophakia have been described for the correction of naturally occurring and postoperative astigmatism.[1-13] The number and variety of techniques reflect the inability of any particular approach to predictably eliminate astigmatism in all patients, and substantial variability in outcome is reported in most series.[14-17] These techniques are based on the possibility of inducing changes in the corneal curvature by incising the paracentral and peripheral cornea. Presumably, interindividual variability in corneal wound healing and a possible asymmetric corneal response to the mechanical stress induced by the surgery play a role in the variability of the final results.

In the case of intersecting corneal incisions, touted at one time for the correction of astigmatism, poor healing, epithelial ingrowth into the stroma at the site of intersection, and excessive corneal scarring typically result in irregular astigmatism with loss of best corrected spectacles acuity. The optical rehabilitation of the irregular corneas is quite challenging. In our experience, success with suturing these incisions closed is limited by irregular astigmatism and a tendency for the sutures to erode and degrade with time. Most of these patients seen in our referral practice are fitted with rigid gas-permeable contact lenses. Incisional procedures will continue to have limited predictability until we discover a method for in vivo measurement of the biomechanical properties of the corneal tissue layers and the distribution of stress and stress-induced strain within the individual human cornea preoperatively.

Initially, the excimer laser was used in an attempt to correct corneal astigmatism by creating straight or arcuate linear excisions into the corneal stroma. The guiding concept for this approach was that unpredictable outcomes after astigmatic keratotomy were due to variation in incision geometry (depth and length), and that the excimer laser could be used to create linear ablations of corneal tissue of precisely known dimensions. This technique involved the use of a mask placed over the cornea, into which had been cut the appropriate curved or straight slit, so that the desired excision was created. Despite initial enthusiasm for this procedure, experience showed that it did not, in most hands, represent a substantial improvement over the diamond knife in terms of accuracy or wound healing, and this approach has been abandoned.

In early 1990, we initiated studies using the excimer laser to perform toric ablations of the cornea. Just as myopic photorefractive keratectomy differs from radial keratotomy in that the former procedure does not involve creation of deep stromal incisions, our approach to astigmatism using the excimer laser has been to correct the refractive error by performing a superficial ablation of tissue in the shape of a cylindrical lens, rather than creating deep incisions (or excisions) into the stroma. Based on the ability of the laser to induce flattening of the central cornea to eliminate myopic refractive errors,[18] we developed a nonradially symmetric approach to tissue ablation, with selective flattening of the steep meridian.[19] An expanding slit was created, with no refractive change intended parallel to the slit opening, and central flattening was induced in the meridian in which the slit was expanded. After encouraging experimental results in polymethylmethacrylate blocks, plastic corneas, and rabbit corneas,[19] we investigated this cylindrical ablation technique in human clinical trials.[20] Later, a modification on the diaphragm was introduced to allow ablations with an elliptic shape so as to achieve a more gradual transition from the astigmatic ablation to the circular ablation, necessary for correction of associated spherical errors.[21] As with superficial ablations for myopia, these represent new approaches to the surgical correction of astigmatism, one that does not rely on creation of deep corneal incisions, excisions, or compression sutures.

PREOPERATIVE PREPARATION
Selection of patients

As discussed elsewhere in this text, careful selection of patients is crucial to identify those individuals who are appropriate candidates for refractive surgery in general, and for excimer laser photorefractive keratectomy in particular. Fortunately, in the management of patients with astigmatism, we have found that a "perfect" result is not usually required for postoperative patient satisfaction. For example, a patient with between 2.5 and 3.0 D of astigmatism preoperatively is typically delighted with a reduction in cylinder to 1.25 D; this allows for reasonably good uncorrected visual acuity (20/25-20/30) at distance and reasonably good uncorrected acuity at near as well, due to the multifocal effect from the refractive astigmatism.

Patient expectations are determined early in the patient selection process. A patient whose goal is to obtain sufficient uncorrected visual acuity to allow him or her to perform many of the activities of daily living without corrective lenses is an appropriate candidate. Such a person accepts the fact that glasses may be needed for selected activities (e.g., driving, attending the theater). A perfectionist, the so-called type A personality, who demands perfect 20/20 or 20/15 postoperative acuity without correction, and who demands around-the-clock spectacles independence, is currently not an appropriate candidate for excimer laser photorefractive keratectomy or, in our opinion, any other refractive surgical procedure.

Candidates for photorefractive keratectomy for astigmatism should have healthy corneas and stable refractive errors. We have operated on patients who have had naturally occurring astigmatism and on patients who had postoperative (after keratoplasty and cataract extraction) astigmatism. Patients with postsurgical astigmatism should have had all sutures removed, with stable topography and refraction documented by repeat examinations performed at least 1 month apart. Our patients are primarily young adults who lead active lives, but no restrictions have been placed on their activities or participation in sports following surgery. Just as with photorefractive keratectomy for myopia, underlying eye diseases, such as dry eye or chronic blepharitis, are contraindications to the surgery and should be looked for carefully and treated preoperatively. The preoperative examination consists of measurement of visual acuity with and without correction, refraction, keratometry, biomicroscopic evaluation, pachometry, funduscopy, tonometry, measurement of pupil diameter, and computer-assisted corneal topographic analysis. Despite their protestations, patients who initially present with contact lenses in place should be required to return for repeat examination, as both soft and rigid contact lenses (especially the latter) can substantially alter the corneal topography and measured refractive error. Be wary of patients wearing hard or rigid lenses who state they were given these lenses because they could not obtain adequate visual correction with spectacles or soft contact lenses; this history suggests the possibility of keratoconus. The amount of time required for the cornea to return to its "native" topography is highly variable, and the changes that occur probably take longer and are of greater magnitude with rigid compared to soft contact lenses. The refraction and topography should be followed until they are stable. Patients who start out with asymmetric inferior steepening that is replaced by a more spherical and symmetric cornea probably have contact lens-induced corneal warpage. Patients who develop progressively greater inferior corneal steepening may have mild keratoconus, and should be examined repeatedly and carefully before deciding to do surgery. We currently decline to operate on patients with even mild keratoconus that can be appreciated only by topographic examination.[22,23]

Informed Consent

All patients are informed fully about the nature of excimer laser surgery of the eye, and of the risks and alternatives to this procedure. At the time this chapter is being written, the excimer laser is investigational in the United States, and patients are informed that the proposed surgery will be carried out under an investigational protocol approved by the Food and Drug Administration (FDA). We carefully differentiate this procedure from radial keratotomy, and review the potential implications of superficial ablations vs. deep incisions.[24]

Planning the Surgery

The amount of correction desired is based on the patient's preoperative refraction. The computer is programmed to perform cylindrical or elliptic ablations designed to correct the patient's cylindrical error, and the desired refractive change is programmed into the computer in minus cylinder form. If the patient has compound myopic astigmatism, we can correct the myopia and astigmatism sequentially by performing a cylindrical ablation (for astigmatism) and a spherical ablation (for myopia), or we can correct them simultaneously with an elliptic ablation. In general, we err on the side of undercorrecting any coexisting myopia, with the understanding that residual myopia can be addressed, if necessary, with a subsequent spherical ablation. This approach is analogous to the "enhancement" approach that is becoming increasingly popular with radial keratotomy, in which every effort is made to avoid rendering a patient hyperopic. As we have gained experience with the refractive changes following sequential and simultaneous ablations for astigmatism, however, we are better able to anticipate the change in spherical equivalent.

Interpreting the Surgical Outcome

Changes in astigmatism after surgery are most appropriately reported in terms of vector-corrected changes in astigmatism. Briefly, such an approach to data analysis takes into account the fact that astigmatism is a vector and not a scalar quantity, and simply reporting magnitude of the final refractive cylinder does not convey information about possible shifts in cylinder axis or cylindrical overcorrections. The reader is referred to several papers, that discuss this topic in detail and that describe the mathematical formulas used for this analysis.[14,25-28]

DESCRIPTION OF THE PROCEDURE AND SURGICAL TECHNIQUE
Laser Operation

We use a 193-nm argon fluoride excimer laser (Twenty-Twenty Excimer Laser, VISX Corp., Santa Clara, Calif). To correct myopia, this laser uses a computer-controlled iris diaphragm to vary the diameter of the ablation beam so as to ablate more tissue centrally than peripherally, thereby flattening the cornea.

Cylindrical ablation (Figs.5-1, 5-2, and 5-3). To correct astigmatism, the large-diameter excimer beam is passed through a set of parallel blades. The separation of the blades is under computer control, and the resultant variable slit is used to control the laser delivery much as the iris diaphragm used for myopia ablations.[29] In the case of the slit, however, the cornea should be flattened only in the meridian perpendicular to the long axis of the slit (termed the *mechanical axis*); no refractive change is intended along the mechanical axis (long axis of the slit). Thus, if the mechanical axis is oriented horizontally (in the 180-degree meridian), a flattening of the cornea will occur in the vertical (90-degree) meridian. Primarily, this technique is designed to eliminate myopic astigmatism. The slit mechanism can be rotated, also under computer control, such that the mechanical axis can be aligned with the astigmatic axis of the patient. The blades are oriented by the computer to be parallel to the axis of refractive cylinder, expressed in minus cylinder form, thereby flattening the cornea in the appropriate (steep) meridian. With this approach, a vertical "wall" equal to the astigmatic ablation depth would

appear at the two ends of the resultant rectangular ablation, along the mechanical axis. For this reason, a "transition zone" of 0.3 mm is generated at the ends of the slit to form a sigmoidal transition between unoperated and ablated cornea.

Elliptic ablation (Figs. 5-4 and 5-5). A modification of the diaphragm hardware allows production of an elliptical area of ablation. The flattening of the cornea will occur along the meridian of the slit expansion, as described for the cylindrical ablations. In myopia surgery, a series of concentric circular ablations is performed, while this technique for astigmatism creates a series of concentric elliptic ablations. This technique can be used when the magnitude of the cylindrical error is less than or equal to the magnitude of the spherical myopia, when the refractive error is expressed in minus cylinder form. The width of the narrow dimension of the ellipse is dependent on the ratio of the spherical error to the cylindrical error. When the cylindrical error is small compared to the spherical error, the ellipse is nearly circular. When the cylindrical refractive error approaches the magnitude of the spherical component of the refractive error, the nar-

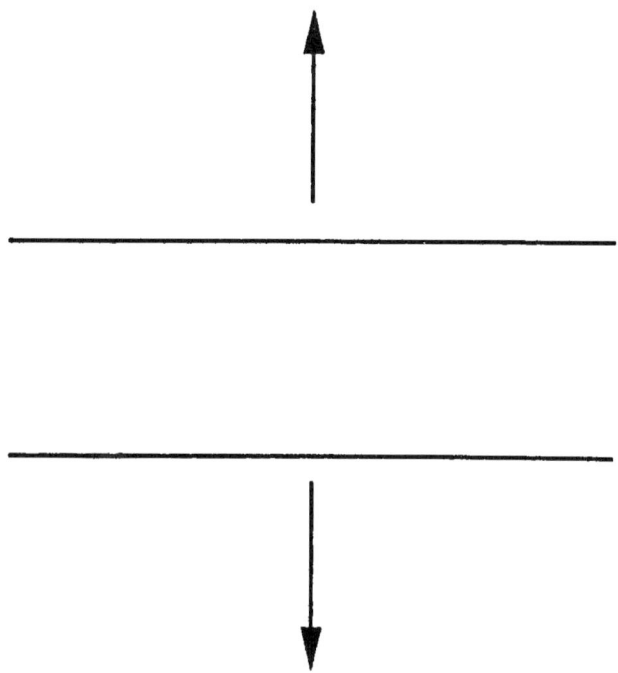

Fig. 5-1. Schematic illustration of the method of creating toric ablations by progressively widening the separation between blades during the ablation. Variables that can be controlled include depth of ablation, width of ablation zone, and orientation of the slit. With blades oriented as shown, the cornea would be preferentially flattened in the horizontal meridian (with-the-rule astigmatism).

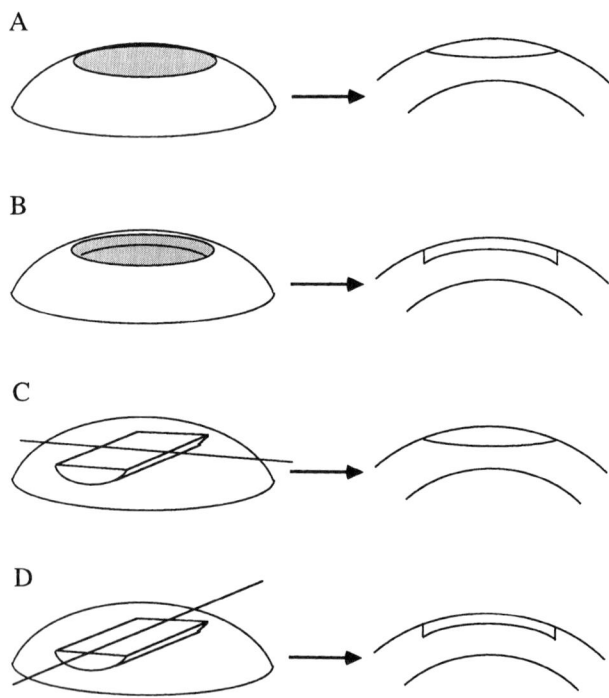

Fig. 5-2. Comparison of myopic ablation (A), in which the greatest amount of tissue is removed centrally and progressively less toward the periphery; phototherapeutic keratectomy (B), in which a uniform amount of tissue is ablated; and cylindrical ablation (C and D) for correction of against-the-rule astigmatism. Cross section through the steep horizontal meridian (C) is identical to myopic ablation (A), while cross section through the flat meridian (D), in which no refractive change is intended, is identical to phototherapeutic keratectomy (B).

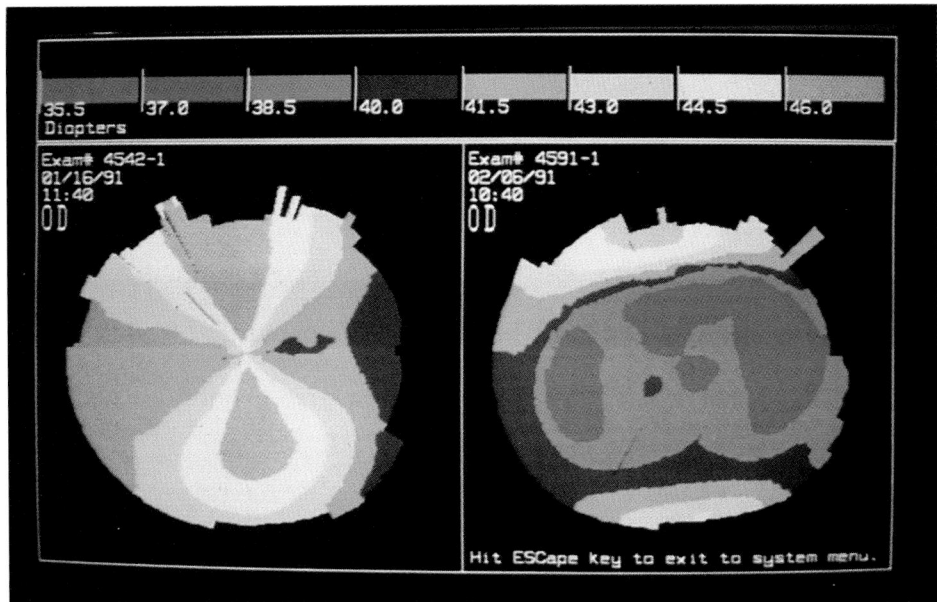

Fig. 5-3. Topography of patient before *(left)* and after *(right)* toric ablation for high congenital astigmatism. Preoperative refraction was −1.00-5.50 × 7, uncorrected visual acuity was 20/80, and acuity with spectacles was 20/30. Postoperatively, refraction at 3 years was +0.50-1.00 × 176, uncorrected visual acuity was 20/40, and acuity with spectacles was 20/20. (From McDonnell PJ, Moreira H, Clapham TN, et al: *Arch Ophthalmol* 109:1370-1373, 1991. Used by permission.)

row dimension of the ellipse becomes progressively shorter, with the smallest acceptable width being to 4.8 mm. The elliptic ablation has the theoretical advantages of producing a transition at the edge of the ablation in the flat meridian of the cornea, and it produces simultaneous correction of the spherical refractive error, thereby shortening the duration of the procedure and consequently the likelihood that the corneal surface will become dry or that the patient will lose fixation during the surgery.

Preparation of the Patient

As described for spherical myopic photorefractive keratectomy, the patient is placed under the excimer laser and topical proparacaine hydrochloride 0.5% is instilled into the eye. The patient is instructed to fix with the operative eye on the red coaxial fixation light, and the surgeon centers the laser over the entrance pupil. Because of the possibility of cyclotorsion of the globe, the orientation of the patient's cylinder is confirmed immediately prior to surgery using the Axis measurement device (VISX, Inc.) The VISX Axis measurement system projects a parallel line pattern through the camera port of the microscope onto the patient's eye. The patient's spherical error is first corrected by a slides lens to focus the line pattern at the patient's far point. Then the pattern is rotated by the patient until the lines are as sharp as possible. This identifies the axis of the myopic cylinder (negative notation) of the patient to within a few degrees. The dis-

tinctness and accuracy of the endpoint is better for larger amounts of refractive cylinder. This is repeated several times to get an average and to test consistency before treatment.

In our series of patients treated with this technique, we have found little evidence to date of cyclotorsion. In addition, we have photographically searched for evidence of cyclotorsion in subjects who assume a reclining position, but have not been able to document this phenomenon, which suggests that it is relatively uncommon. A few pulses of laser energy are then applied with the slit maximally narrowed in order to confirm proper orientation of the slit relative to the corneal cylinder and to acquaint the patient with visual, auditory, and olfactory (!) sensations associated with the laser ablation. The patient's preoperative topographic corneal map is placed upside down above the oculars of the operating microscope, matching the surgeon's view, so that the surgeon can readily double-check that the laser slit is properly oriented. The corneal epithelium is then removed with a blunt spatula, or by performing a 6.0-mm-diameter ablation through the epithelium, and then using the blunt spatula to make certain that no residual islands of epithelium remain on Bowman's layer. This latter technique minimizes the time required for epithelial removal, and thus the likelihood of dehydration of the corneal surface. Centration of the laser over the entrance pupil is confirmed while the patient fixates on the flashing centration light.[30] We do not mark the cen-

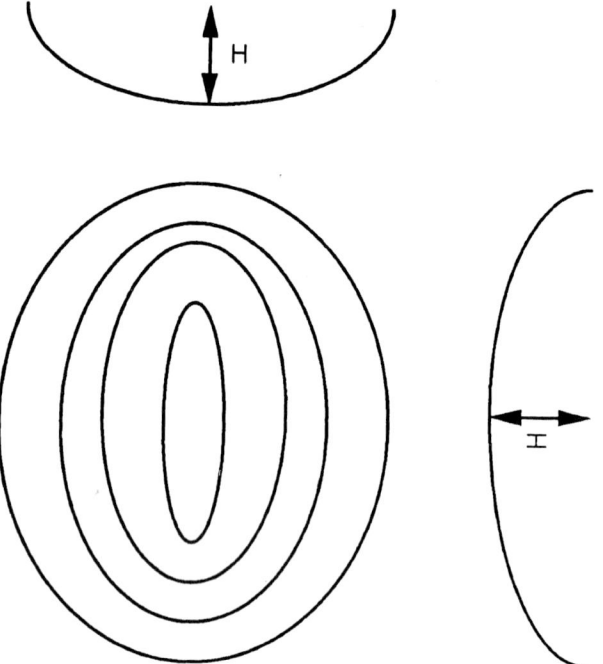

Fig. 5-4. Schematic illustration of elliptic ablation for simultaneous correction of myopia and against-the-rule astigmatism. Unlike the concentric circular ablations for spherical myopia, a series of concentric elliptic ablations are created. The narrowest width of the ellipse is oriented parallel to the preoperatively steep meridian. Cross section through the horizontal meridian *(top)* shows greater removal of tissue per cross-sectional area than does cross section through the vertical meridian *(right)*. Because the central depth *(H)* is identical, greater corneal flattening is achieved in the horizontal meridian.

ter of the entrance pupil with any instrument, and we do not hold the globe during the procedure.

We attempt to avoid intraoperative corneal hydration changes by minimizing the interval between epithelial removal and corneal ablation. This is because our previous studies in vitro and in living animal eyes suggested that maintaining corneal hydration during the procedure leads to a smoother corneal surface and to less superficial corneal haze postoperatively.[16,31,32] Because we use no pharmacologic sedation as part of our surgical routine, we attempt to put the patient at ease before and during the procedure by maintaining surgeon-patient physical contact, by explaining the steps of the procedure as they are performed, and by desensitizing the patient to the noises and other sensations associated with laser treatment. Failure to adequately calm the patient or to acquaint him or her with the procedure will invariably result in sudden movement in response to the first few laser pulses. Only when the patient is adequately prepared is laser treatment begun. Should the patient make any movements during the procedure that result in loss of

proper centration, the procedure is immediately interrupted, centration is reestablished, the patient is reassured, and the procedure completed.

Intraoperative Considerations

The patient fixates on the fixation light during the entire procedure. The surgical assistant reports the number of pulses remaining to be delivered. The surgery can be stopped by the surgeon, if necessary, at any time during the procedure. We have had no intraoperative complications to date. If the surgeon does hold the eye with a forceps or a fixation ring, care must be taken to not tilt or rotate the eye during the procedure. An axial error of only 10 degrees can induce an astigmatic undercorrection of nearly 40%, which emphasizes the need to avoid rotating the globe during the surgery. Tilting or rotation of the globe to this degree could easily result from inadvertent movement of the surgeon's hand, and would not be discernible through the operating microscope. Deviations from precise axial alignment can arise also from angular measurement errors in the preoperative refraction, misalignment of the patient's head on the table, misalignment of the laser beam, and angular motion during the surgery.

POSTOPERATIVE CONSIDERATIONS
Postoperative Care and Follow-Up

We no longer patch eyes postoperatively, but instead instill one drop each of a nonsteroidal anti-inflammatory agent and a combination antibiotic-steroid in the eye, followed by placement of a therapeutic soft contact lens. The nonsteroidal anti-inflammatory drug dramatically reduces patient discomfort postoperatively, apparently by blunting the increase in prostaglandin E_2 levels within the cornea.[33] Patients are examined daily or every other day until reepithelialization is complete. The nonsteroidal anti-inflammatory agent is used four times daily for the first 24 hours, during which time patient discomfort is maximal, and is then decreased to twice daily to minimize any possible toxicity. As soon as the epithelium covers the treated cornea, we remove the contact lens. Because of the possibility that the inflammation associated with the surgery might stimulate an allograft reaction, we treat patients with postkeratoplasty astigmatism with a penetrating corticosteroid (1% prednisolone acetate) every 2 to 3 hours for 2 days after the epithelium is healed, and then decrease the frequency to four times daily. Patients with naturally occurring astigmatism are given fluorometholone acetate four times daily for 2 weeks, three times daily for 4 weeks, and then twice daily for the following 4 weeks. The value, if any, of this steroid therapy, for minimizing corneal haze and refractive regression is uncertain. We perform refraction, keratometry, and

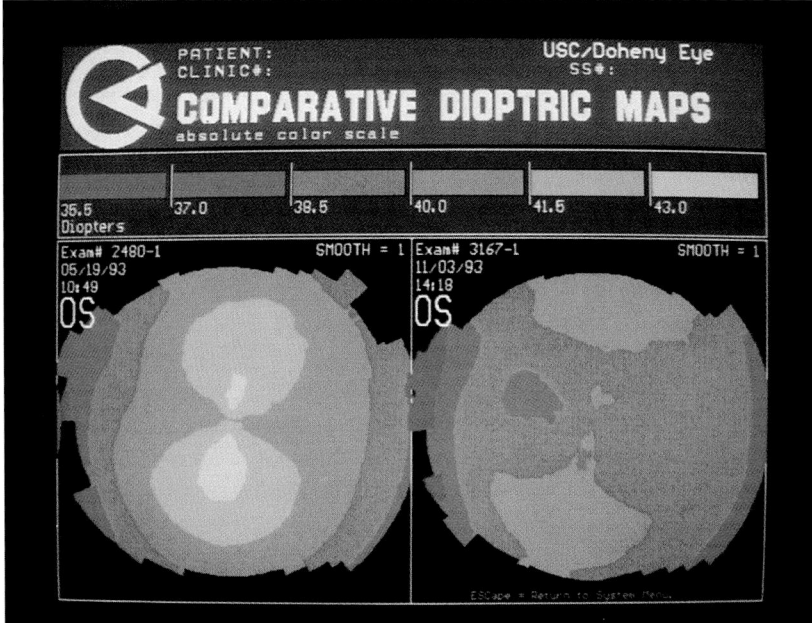

Fig. 5-5. Pre- and postoperative corneal topographies of a 35-year-old man after elliptic ablation for naturally occurring compound myopic astigmatism. The dimensions of the elliptic ablation were 6.0 × 4.2 mm. Preoperative refractive error was −2.50-2.25 × 176, and refractive error 6 months after surgery was stable at −0.75-1.00 × 173. Uncorrected visual acuity improved from 20/400 preoperatively to 20/25 +2 postoperatively.

computer-assisted corneal topographic analysis as early as 2 weeks after the procedure. Patients are seen 1, 3, 4, 6, and 12 months after surgery and thereafter on a yearly basis.

Because we have observed reactivation of herpetic dendritic keratitis in an eye that underwent laser treatment for postkeratoplasty astigmatism,[25] we now prophylactically guard against such recurrences with oral acyclovir (Zovirax), 200 mg orally four times daily. Studies in rabbits have shown that latent herpesvirus can reactivate after excimer photorefractive keratectomy, which should not be surprising because ultraviolet light exposure is known to have the potential to cause such recurrences in the clinical situation.[34]

Wound Healing and Complications

Corneal reepithelialization is usually complete within 3 days after treatment. We have, however, had two patients operated on for correction of postkeratoplasty astigmatism who had delayed reepithelialization, requiring about 2 weeks to close the epithelial defect. One of these patients had originally undergone corneal grafting for an alkali burn, and the slow epithelial healing was presumably a consequence of residual effects from the chemical injury. The other patient was a man is his mid-thirties who had undergone corneal grafting for keratoconus, and the explanation for his delayed epithelial healing remained

elusive. Both of these patients also had greater than average postoperative corneal haze.

In general, patients who undergo surgery for postkeratoplasty astigmatism experience less discomfort and pain than do patients operated on for correction of naturally occurring astigmatism. Although we usually provide patients with oral analgesics (acetaminophen and codeine) in the event that they experience significant discomfort, it is unusual for more than one of these tablets to be needed.

A mild corneal haze develops at about 1 month after surgery, but this usually decreases markedly within 6 months postoperatively. The intensity of the corneal haze after photorefractive keratectomy for compound myopic astigmatism does not appear to differ from that observed after photorefractive keratectomy for spherical myopia. What is different in these patients, however, is that the wound healing intensity may differ between the flat and steep corneal meridians. In animals, we have shown that the wound-healing response of the cylindrical ablation varies according to the corneal meridian.[35] This is something that we have observed clinically as well, and is probably related to the different wound edge profiles, with a less tapered edge in what was the flat meridian preoperatively. None of our patients have experienced disturbances in visual acuity that we could attribute to the corneal haze. We have not observed other wound-healing complications, recurrent epithelial erosions, or episodes of corneal graft rejection. We specifically warn all patients operated on for postkeratoplasty ametropia of the risk of allograft reactions, but have seen no such events, perhaps because of the relatively intensive course of topical prednisolone acetate administered once the graft has reepithelialized. Furthermore, we have observed that corneal sensitivity after excimer laser corneal surgery for astigmatism is mildly compromised for a short period of time, but returns to normal within the first 3 months after surgery.[17]

Computer-assisted corneal topographic analysis has demonstrated that an unintended variable flattening of the flattest meridian may occur concomitant with the flattening of the steepest meridian. We do not consider this to be an adverse effect in patients who have compound myopic astigmatism, and in whom an associated treatment for the myopic component of the refractive error is desired.

RESULTS
Naturally Occurring Astigmatism

Both the sequential (two separate ablations, one cylindrical and one myopic) and elliptic ablations have proved successful at treating compound myopic astigmatism.

United States experience. Phases IIa and IIb of the FDA-supervised clinical trials have been completed. This technique has proved successful at reducing myopic spherical and cylindrical error. As with myopic photorefractive keratectomy, the success rate is partially dependent on the amount of preoperative refractive error. When we began treating these patients at our institution, we programmed undercorrections of the spherical error because of concern that the treatment of astigmatism might produce a greater than anticipated overall corneal flattening, and hence a spherical overcorrection. In patients treated at the Doheny Eye Institute for myopic astigmatism of from 1.00 to 7.00 D, and for whom follow-up of 6 months or longer is available, about 70% of patients have a postoperative spherical equivalent within 1 D of emmetropia, and the average vector-corrected reduction of corneal cylinder is about 60%. Because of the tendency to undercorrection of cylindrical refractive error, we now program the computer to achieve a correction 20% greater than the measured refractive cylinder.

Similar to photorefractive keratectomy for myopia, postoperative corneal haze has been minimal, with the number of patients with substantial haze increasing as the preoperative myopic spherical equivalent increases.

Proper alignment of the ablation relative to the patient's cylinder has not proved difficult. Failure to align the narrower dimension of the elliptic or cylindrical ablation in the steep corneal meridian should result in two undesired outcomes: (1) undercorrection of the astigmatism and (2) a shift of the axis of the astigmatism. Rarely have we observed a significant (> 5 degrees) shift of cylinder axis, with most of the postoperative cylinder axes being equal to the preoperative axes (within the error of measurement of cylinder axis with refraction).

Although both sequential and elliptic ablation techniques have proved successful, the elliptic technique, because it is quicker and therefore easier on the patient, has come to be preferred. We found that the delay between the cylindrical and spherical ablations, owing to the necessity of reprogramming the computer for the second ablation, sometimes caused patients to become uncomfortable. In addition, the superficial corneal dehydration that can occur during this prolonged period might result in greater postoperative haze.

Experience Outside the United States. Taylor and colleagues have reported on their results with correction of myopic astigmatism using the VISX Twenty-Twenty laser at the University of Melbourne.[35a] Their experience is of particular interest in that it involved a very large group of 25 surgeons, and thus might better reflect the results to be achieved by groups of surgeons each of whom performs relatively small numbers of these procedures. They compared the results of 139 consecutive eyes that had photoastigmatic refractive keratectomy for myopic astigmatism (myopia $\leq$ −15.0 D with astigmatism $\leq$ −6.0 D) with results in 107 consecutive and concurrent eyes that received photorefractive keratectomy for spherical myopia ($\leq$ 15.0 D). They reported uncorrected visual acuities of 20/40 or better in 72% of astigmatism patients and in 90% of spherical patients at 6 months, while the percentages of eyes with postoperative spherical equivalents within 1 D of emmetropia were 68% and 77% for astigmatic and spherical eyes, respectively. They found the results with sequential (cylindrical and spherical ablations) and simultaneous (elliptic) ablations to be comparable in terms of refractive correction.

Kim and colleagues in Seoul, Korea (personal communication, August 1993), presented results of elliptic ablation in addition to spherical ablation on 168 eyes with compound myopic astigmatism. The mean preoperative astigmatism in their series of 1.51 $\pm$ 0.81 D (range, 0.5-4.25 D) was reduced to 0.70 $\pm$ 0.58 D at 3 months postoperatively, and to 0.67 0.60 D 6 months after the surgery. When analyzed according to the amount of preoperative astigmatism, patients with less than 1 D of astigmatism had a reduction of 48%, patients with between 1 and 2 D of astigmatism achieved 53.5% reduction, patients with between 2 and 3 D achieved 59.1% reduction, and those with more than 3 D of preoperative astigmatism achieved 68.8% reduction of the preexisting astigmatism. Of interest in these 168 treated eyes is that more than half of the patients had more than 10 degrees of axis change after the surgery.

Postkeratoplasty Astigmatism

While maintaining graft clarity after penetrating keratoplasty is relatively straightforward, disabling astigmatism is common after this procedure. In most series, average postkeratoplasty astigmatism is 3 D or more, with many patients having cylindrical errors far beyond those correctable with spectacles. After keratoplasty for keratoconus, up to one half of patients may require visual rehabilitation because of postoperative refractive errors. This group of contact lens–intolerant patients with postkeratoplasty astigmatism is therefore one for whom excimer photorefractive keratectomy offers the possibility of restoring functional vision.[36]

We have operated on over 30 patients with disabling postkeratoplasty astigmatism. All patients were contact lens–intolerant and were unable to tolerate the high cylindrical prescription in their glasses. Surgery was performed based on the refractive cylinder corrected to the corneal plane. An overall reduction of 58% of the preoperative cylindrical error was achieved at 6 months after surgery. The spherical equivalent revealed a hyperopic shift within the first 16 weeks after surgery, with a slight reduction of the effect thereafter. Uncorrected visual acuity was improved by at least one Snellen line in all but two patients. Fifteen patients had improvement in best corrected visual acuity by at least two Snellen lines. One patient had delayed epithelial healing related to his underlying disease (chemical burn), and another patient who underwent corneal grafting for keratoconus had delayed epithelial healing for unknown reasons. The amount of haze detected in these two patients was greater than in the other patients treated for postkeratoplasty astigmatism, while the haze in this group of patients overall was slightly more intense than we have seen in our naturally occurring astigmatism patients. One patient had an easily detectable haze that did not interfere with retinoscopy or visual acuity. This group of patients had less postoperative pain than did the naturally occurring astigmatism patients, presumably due to incomplete reinnervation of the grafts.[37] In our experience, regression has been more common in these postkeratoplasty patients than in the patients treated for naturally occurring astigmatism. The regression also seems to appear earlier in the postoperative period, but is not usually accompanied by substantial haze. We have re-treated a few patients who experienced regression of effect after the initial surgery, but the outcomes in these eyes have not been encouraging.

CONCLUSIONS

Naturally occurring astigmatism and postoperative astigmatism are common problems in general ophthalmic practice. The extensive list of different approaches described in the literature indicates that the optimal means for surgical correction of astigmatism remains to be determined. Incisional procedures have limited precision but are technically simple and the instrumentation is relatively inexpensive. Excimer laser surgery of the cornea, by contrast, is an expensive and technology-intensive procedure with unknown long-term complications.

The technique described here was designed for regular astigmatism, with symmetric steepening in the two steep hemimeridians. We know, however, that not all astigmatism is regular. Irregular astigmatism is frequently encountered after penetrating keratoplasty,[38] refractive surgical procedures such as epikeratophakia,[39] with intersecting corneal incisions,[40] or even in corneas unoperated on.[11] Thus, patients with substantial irregular astigmatism will have limitation of uncorrected or spectacles-corrected acuity after reduction of the regular astigmatism with the technique described here. Recently, Trokel and colleagues (personal communication, February 1993) have developed techniques for dealing with the irregular component of the astigmatism by performing multiple small ablations to make an irregular corneal refractive surface smoother and with less irregular astigmatism. We have also investigated the possibility of using a collagen gel, molded into a smooth spherical surface, to aid in the smoothing of irregular corneas and also to treat irregular corneal astigmatism.[41]

The ideal patient for this technique has a myopic spherical refractive error in addition to the myopic astigmatism. In our studies to date, we have utilized a conservative approach when programming the amount of desired correction in almost all patients so as to avoid rendering them hyperopic. We did, in fact, leave most of our patients undercorrected (i.e., with residual myopia). Using this conservative approach we did not observe a progressive effect of the surgery in flattening the cornea, even with the greater corrections performed on postkeratoplasty patients. Thus, we avoided a hyperopic shift in these patients. With the excimer laser, a subsequent myopic photorefractive keratectomy can be performed to treat residual myopic refractive errors. Currently, studies are underway to evaluate the ability of the VISX Twenty-Twenty laser to steepen the cornea and correct hyperopia. If successful, this approach should allow for the selective steepening of the flat corneal meridian, thereby providing treatment for hyperopic astigmatism.

Although we substantially undercorrected the astigmatism in many of our early patients using a conservative approach, we have been impressed by patient satisfaction and good improvement in unaided visual acuity. It would appear that the requirement for correction of nearly all refractive error, typical with surgery for myopia, may not apply as much in surgery to correct myopic astigmatism. For example a patient with 3 D of myopia would likely be disappointed with a 50% correction, while we have many patients who are delighted with the 50% reduction of this amount of astigmatism.

To date, targeted astigmatism correction is usually equal to the magnitude of the preoperative astigmatism. However, small degrees of residual astigmatism may actually be desirable, as argued by Sawusch and Guyton[42] owing to an increase in the depth of focus. This may be desirable when considering surgery on presbyopic patients. Also, techniques of vector analysis of astigmatism designed specifically for photoablative surgery, and real-time topographic analysis may improve predictability of excimer laser correction of astigmatism.

Another approach to the correction of astigmatism with the excimer laser is the use of a premanufactured "ablatable mask" that has a toric geometry.[43] The laser is used to ablate through the mask, with the underlying cornea subsequently being ablated when the laser breaks entirely through the mask. In this fashion, the underlying cornea is differentially ablated according to the thickness of the mask material overlying each portion of the cornea. The use of this approach is described in greater detail elsewhere in this book.

SUMMARY

It is clear at this point that the excimer laser can successfully treat corneal astigmatism by ablating superficial stroma in the shape of a cylindrical lens. The problems of interindividual variability in wound healing and correction of irregular astigmatism remain.

REFERENCES

1. Arciniegas A, Amaya LE: Corneal curvature modification by scleral surgery: preliminary results, *Ann Ophthalmol* 17:221-226, 1985.
2. Duffey RJ, Jain VN, Tchah H, et al: Paired arcuate keratotomy: a surgical approach to mixed and myopic astigmatism, *Arch Ophthalmol* 106:1130-1135, 1988.
3. Franks JB, Binder PS: Keratotomy procedures for the correction of astigmatism, *J Refract Surg* 1:11-17, 1985.
4. Krachmer JH, Fenzl RE: Surgical correction of high postkeratoplasty astigmatism: relaxing incisions vs wedge resection, *Arch Ophthalmol* 98:1400-1402, 1980.
5. Lavery GW, Lindstrom RL: Clinical results of trapezoidal astigmatic keratectomy, *J Refract Surg* 1:70-74, 1985.
6. Lavery GW, Lindstrom RL, Hofer LA, et al: The surgical management of corneal astigmatism after penetrating keratoplasty, *Ophthalmic Surg* 16:165-169, 1985.
7. Lindstrom RL, Lindquist TD: Surgical correction of postoperative astigmatism, *Cornea* 7:138-148, 1988.
8. McCluskey DJ, Villaseñor R, McDonnell PJ: Prospective topographic analysis in peripheral arcuate keratotomy for astigmatism, *Ophthalmic Surg* 21:464-471, 1990.
9. Rowsey JJ: Review: current concepts in astigmatic surgery, *J Refract Surg* 2:85-94, 1986.
10. Sugar J, Kirk AK: Relaxing keratotomy for postkeratoplasty high astigmatism, *Ophthalmic Surg* 14:156-158, 1983.
11. Troutman RC: Corneal wedge resections and relaxing incisions for postkeratoplasty astigmatism, *Int Ophthalmol Clin* 23:161-168, 1983.
12. Troutman RC, Swinger C: Relaxing incision for control of postoperative astigmatism following keratoplasty, *Ophthalmic Surg* 11:117-120, 1980.
13. Villaseñor RA, Stimac GR: Clinical results and complications of trapezoidal keratotomy, *J Refract Surg* 4:125-131, 1988.
14. Alpins NA: A new method of analyzing vectors for changes in astigmatism, *J Cataract Refract Surg* 19:524-533, 1993.
15. Bogan SJ, Waring GO III, Ibrahim O, et al: Classification of normal corneal topography based on computer-assisted videokeratography, *Arch Ophthalmol* 108:945-949, 1990.
16. Campos M, Cuevas K, Garbus J, et al: Corneal wound healing after excimer laser ablation: effects of nitrogen gas blower, *Ophthalmology* 99:893-897, 1992.
17. Campos M, Hetzog L, Garbus JJ, et al: Corneal sensitivity after photorefractive keratectomy, *Am J Ophthalmol* 114:51-54, 1992.
18. McDonald MB, Frantz JM, Klyce SD, et al: Central photorefractive keratectomy for myopia: the blind eye study, *Arch Ophthalmol* 108:799-808, 1990.
19. McDonnell PJ, Moreira H, Garbus J, et al: Photorefractive keratectomy to create toric ablations for correction of astigmatism, *Arch Ophthalmol* 109:710-713, 1991.
20. McDonnell PJ, Moreira H, Clapham TN, et al: Photorefractive keratectomy for astigmatism: initial clinical results, *Arch Ophthalmol* 109:1370-1373, 1991.
21. McDonnell PJ, Campos M, Hertzog L et al: Photorefraktive Keratektomie zur Korrektur von myopem Astigmatismus, *Klin Monatsbl Augenheilkd* 202:238-244, 1993.
22. Maguire LJ, Bourne WM: Corneal topography of early keratoconus, *Am J Ophthalmol* 108:107-112, 1989.
23. Rabinowitz YS, Garbus J, McDonnell PJ: Computer-assisted corneal topography in family members of patients with keratoconus, *Arch Ophthalmol* 108:365-371, 1990.
24. Campos M, Lee M, McDonnell PJ: Ocular integrity after refractive surgery: effects of photorefractive keratectomy, phototherapeutic keratectomy, and radial keratotomy, *Ophthalmic Surg* 23:598-602, 1992.
25. Cravy TV: Calculation of the change in corneal astigmatism following cataract extraction, *Ophthalmic Surg* 10(1):38-49, 1979.
26. Hall GW, Campion M, Sorenson CM, et al: Reduction of corneal astigmatism at cataract surgery, *J Cataract Refract Surg* 17:407-414, 1991.
27. Holladay JT, Cravy TV, Koch DD: Calculating the surgically induced refractive change following ocular surgery, *J Cataract Refract Surg* 18:429-443, 1992.
28. Retzlaff J, Paden PY, Ferrell L: Vector analysis of astigmatism: adding and subtracting spherocylinders, *J Cataract Refract Surg* 19:393-398, 1993.
29. Marshall J, Trokel S, Rothery S, et al: Photoablative reprofiling of the cornea using an excimer laser: photorefractive keratectomy, *Lasers Ophthalmol* 1:21-48, 1986.
30. Uozato H, Guyton DL: Centering corneal surgical procedures, *Am J Ophthalmol* 103: 264-275, 1987.

31. Campos M, Trokel SL, McDonnell PJ: Surface morphology following photorefractive keratectomy, *Ophthalmic Surg* 24:822-825, 1993.

32. Krueger RR, Campos M, Wang XW: Corneal surface morphology following excimer laser ablation with humidified gases, *Arch Ophthalmol* 111:1131-1137, 1993.

33. Phillips AF, Szerenyi K, Campos M, et al: Arachidonic acid metabolites after excimer laser corneal surgery, *Arch Ophthalmol* 111:1273-1278, 1993.

34. Laycock KA, Lee SF, Brady RH, et al: Characterization of a murine model of recurrent herpes simplex viral keratitis induced by ultraviolet β radiation, *Invest Ophthalmol Vis Sci* 32:2741-2746, 1991.

35. Shieh E, Moreira H, D'Arcy J, et al: Quantitative analysis of wound healing after cylindrical and spherical excimer laser ablations, *Ophthalmology* 99:1050-1055, 1992.

35a. Taylor HR, Guest CS, Kelly P, Alpins NA: Excimer Laser and Research Group. Comparison of excimer laser treatment of astigmatism and myopla, *Arch Opthalmol* 111:1621-1626, 1993.

36. Campos M, Hertzog L, Garbus J, et al: Photorefractive keratectomy for severe postkeratoplasty astigmatism, *Am J Ophthalmol* 114:429-436, 1992.

37. Rao GN, John T, Ishida N, et al: Recovery of corneal sensitivity in grafts following penetrating keratoplasty, *Ophthalmology* 92:1408-1411,1985.

38. Maguire LJ, Bourne WM: Corneal topography of transverse keratotomies for astigmatism after penetrating keratoplasty, *Am J Ophthalmol* 107:323-330, 1989.

39. Reidy JJ, McDonald MB, Klyce SD: The corneal topography of epikeratophakia, *Refract Corneal Surg* 6:26-31, 1990.

40. McDonnell PJ, Caroline PJ, Salz J: Irregular astigmatism after radial and astigmatic keratotomy, *Am J Ophthalmol* 107:42-46, 1989.

41. Englanoff JS, Kolahdouz-Isfahani AH, Moreira H, et al: In situ collagen gel mold as an aid in excimer laser superficial keratectomy, *Ophthalmology* 99:1201-1208, 1992.

42. Sawusch MR, Guyton DL: Optimal astigmatism to enhance depth of focus after cataract surgery, *Ophthalmology* 98:1025-1029, 1991.

43. Seiler T: Photorefractive keratectomy: European experience. In Thompson FB, McDonnell PJ, editors: *Color atlas/text of excimer laser surgery. The cornea,* New York, 1993, Igaku-Shoin Medical Publishers.

6

Correction of High Myopia with the Excimer Laser: VISX 2015, VISX 2020, and the Summit Experience

VISX 2015:

David R. Hardten, Neal A. Sher, Richard L. Lindstrom

VISX 2020:

Barry Kassar, Joy Heitzman

Summit:

Daniel S. Durrie, D. James Schumer, Timothy B. Cavanaugh, David T. Gubman

This chapter is divided into three sections each having been contributed by a separate group of authors. The Phillips Eye Institute and the U.S. VISX 2015 results are presented by David R. Hardten, Neal A. Sher, and Richard L. Lindstrom. The results of the VISX 2020 U.S. study are presented by Barry Kassar and Joy Heitzmann. The last section on the Summit Laser experience is contributed by Daniel S. Durrie, D. James Schumer, Timothy B. Cavanaugh and David T. Gubman.

The VISX 2015 Excimer Laser

David R. Hardten, Neal A. Sher, Richard L. Lindstrom

Photorefractive keratectomy (PRK) with the 193-nm excimer laser has the potential to eliminate or reduce myopia in a brief surgical procedure under topical anesthesia. Patients with myopia greater than 8 D represent a small portion of the millions of myopic patients (<5%), although these highly nearsighted patients are significantly visually disabled without correction, and are highly motivated to seek surgical correction of their refractive error. Results of excimer laser PRK for low to moderate myopia have been excellent, with over 90% of eyes achieving uncorrected visual acuity better than 20/40.[1-4] The results in high myopia have been promising, but do not achieve the same level of correction as those eyes with low to moderate myopia.[5-10] This section addresses correction of high myopia with the VISX 2015 laser, presenting the Phillips Eye Institute and the United States VISX 2015 results.

HISTORY

In the early clinical studies of PRK, experience treating high myopia lagged behind that for low myopia because of the belief that the deeper ablations that were needed for large corrections would cause unacceptable corneal haze and scarring.[11,12] Smaller amounts of corneal tissue can be removed to achieve a given correction when a small optical zone is used. A larger optical zone requires that an increased amount of corneal tissue be removed.[13] Early attempts at high myopia correction therefore involved small ablation diameters. Significant regression and increased corneal haze were seen in high myopia treatment in comparison to eyes undergoing PRK where the correction attempted was less than 6 D.[11,12,14] The configuration of these cuts was such that there were steep edges at the transition zones, and the cornea appeared to generate a healing response in which the stroma and epithelium filled in the ablation as though it were an incision.[14]

Larger ablation zones, such as the 5.0-mm ablation zone used in the Phillips Eye Institute phase II study of eyes with myopia ranging from −5.5 to −12.0 D gave more favorable results.[15] Heavy topical corticosteroids were used in this study, and less serious haze and regression were found than in the earlier studies. This was believed to be due to the use of a larger ablation zone, which allowed a more gradual transition zone.

High myopia treatment with the excimer laser continues to develop, and several studies of PRK and higher myopia have been published.[5-9,16,17] There continues to be considerable variation in the results, under- and overcorrections, haze, and regression continue to be present, but overall the results are improving.

Most of these studies have used ablation diameters of 5.0 mm. Most of the studies have also been single treatment zones. Some new studies suggest that the use of multiple treatment zones may be beneficial, with improved predictability and reduced haze.[5,7,10]

PHILLIPS EYE INSTITUTE STUDY

The laser used at the Phillips Eye Institute was the VISX/Taunton model 2015 (VISX, Santa Clara, Calif.). This laser uses an argon fluoride gas mixture to produce a 193-nm wavelength at 10 Hz which is adjusted to deliver a fluence of 100 to 120 mJ/cm^2.[9]

Sixty-five eyes of 56 patients with myopia between −8.00 and −15.00 D were treated with excimer PRK. The mean preoperative spherical equivalent was −10.0 ±2.1 D. The mean age of the patients was 45 years. Fifty-six eyes have at least 6 months of follow-up and 33 eyes have at least 12 months of follow-up.

In all cases, the epithelium was removed before treatment. The laser energy was delivered through a rotating series of 15 apertures of diminishing size, with a maximum beam diameter of 5.0 to 6.2 mm. Following the ablation, tobramycin-dexamethasone suspension drops (Tobradex) and in some cases 5% homatropine hydrobromide were instilled, and a disposable soft contact lens (Vistakon Acuvue, Johnson & Johnson, Claremont, Calif.) was placed. In some cases, diclofenac sodium solution (Voltaren) was used for pain control. A 0.3% solution of tobramycin (Tobrex) was administered four times per day until the epithelium was healed. The contact lens was removed on the third postoperative day, after the epithelium had healed. Fluorometholone 0.1% (FML Forte) was used every 2 hours for the first week, four times a day for 1 month, three times a day for 1 month, twice a day for the third month, and then once daily for the fourth through sixth months.

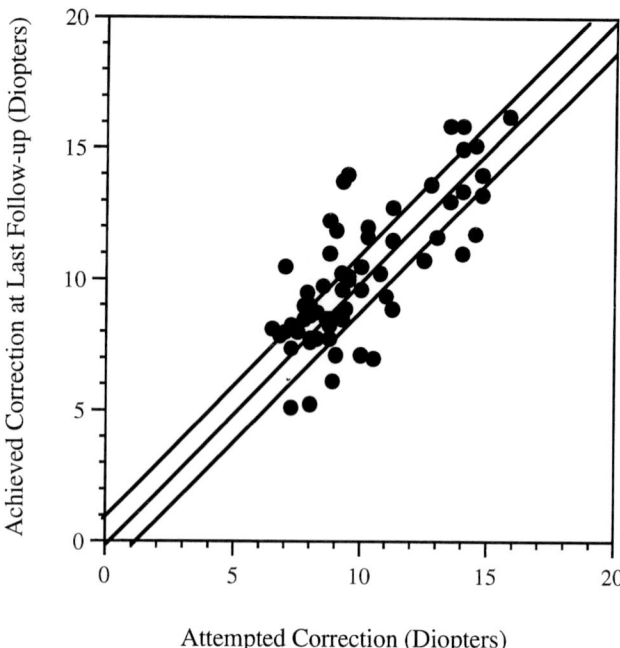

Fig. 6-1. Attempted vs. achieved correction in 65 highly myopic eyes treated at the Phillips Eye Institute at the patients' most recent follow-up visit after excimer PRK, without re-treatments taken into account. All refractions are manifest refractions in diopters.

Results

At 6 months after surgery, correction within 1 D of attempted was achieved in 47% of eyes. Seventy-nine percent of eyes achieved correction within 2 D of that attempted. At the follow-up visit before any retreatment, 54% and 77% of eyes were corrected within 1 and 2 D of attempted correction, respectively. Fig. 6-1 shows the attempted vs. achieved correction for the 65 eyes at the last examination.

Four patients were re-treated after 12 months postoperatively for undercorrections of more than 2 D. With re-treatment taken into account, 58% and 79% of eyes were corrected within 1 and 2 D of attempted correction, respectively.

At the 6-month visit, 20 of 56 eyes (36%) had uncorrected visual acuity of 20/25 or better, while 40 of 56 eyes (76%) had 20/40 or better vision uncorrected. Twelve months postoperatively, 10 of 33 eyes (30%) had 20/25 or better uncorrected visual acuity (UCVA), and 26 of 33 eyes (79%) were 20/40 or better uncorrected.

There is an early overcorrection, followed by some regression up to 12 months (Fig. 6-2). This is similar to the typical time course seen in PRK on eyes with lower degrees of myopia. No regression was seen in this group of patients between 12 months and 18 months.

Three eyes (10%) had a haze score of 2 or more at 6 months. This was slightly higher than the haze ob-

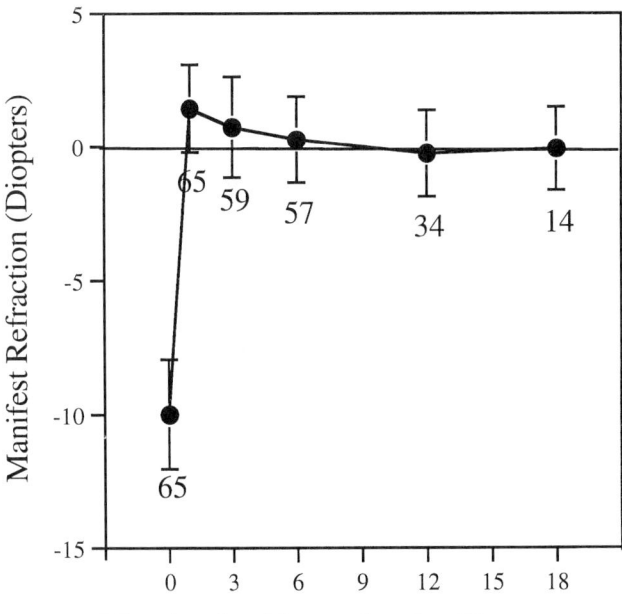

Fig. 6-2. Mean manifest refraction in diopters plus or minus standard deviation at various time intervals after excimer PRK in high myopia. The numbers adjacent to points represent the number of eyes at each data point.

served in PRK eyes with low myopia. One patient had a haze score of 2 or more at last follow-up (haze, 2.0; 18 months).

At 12 months, four eyes (12%) lost two lines of best corrected visual acuity (BCVA), and 28 eyes (85%) had no change in BCVA or lost or gained one line. One eye (3%) gained two lines in BCVA. The visual loss was attributed to a combination of irregular astigmatism, confirmed by corneal topography, and corneal haze.

Complications

There were no cases of recurrent corneal erosions, delayed epithelial healing, or infectious keratitis. One ablation was significantly decentered from the entrance pupil by 2.4 mm. This patient lost one line of BCVA and noted halos at night. Three other eyes had decentration from the pupillary center of 1.0 to 1.5 mm. One of these patients complained of significant night glare, shadows, and ghosting.

Computed corneal topography was performed preoperatively and postoperatively at various intervals using the computed anatomy system, model TMS-1 (Tomey Technology Co, Cambridge, Mass.). Using subtraction maps, corneal topographic elevated areas surrounded by depressed areas, termed *central islands,* were defined as areas of elevation greater than 1.0 mm in diameter and greater than 1 D steeper than the surrounding cornea at 6 months or later. There were three eyes which demonstrated central islands. None of

these eyes lost any lines of BCVA or described any significant visual complaints.

NATIONAL VISX 2015 STUDY

The VISX model 2015 laser was used in five sites in the United States to perform excimer PRK in high myopia. The current series includes 45 eyes of 29 patients. The mean age of these patients is 39.4 years. The mean refractive error is −10.4 ±1.6 D.

The average follow-up after the initial treatment before any re-treatments was 12.4 months. Thirteen eyes were re-treated for undercorrection at least 12 months after the initial procedure. The average residual refractive error in these patients was −3.9 ±1.9 D. Laser treatment was performed as described in the Phillips Eye Institute experience. Following the ablation, antibiotic and steroid drops were used, as well as a disposable soft contact lens in selected patients. In some cases, diclofenac sodium solution was used for pain control. The postoperative regimen was the same as that used in the Phillips Eye Institute series.

Results

Nineteen of 45 eyes (42%) achieved correction within 1 D of attempted correction with one treatment. Twenty-eight of 45 eyes (62%) achieved correction within 2 D of attempted. Thirteen eyes were re-treated postoperatively for undercorrections of more than 2 D. With re-treatment taken into account, 53% and 67% of eyes were corrected within 1 and 2 D of attempted correction, respectively.

Three patients (7%) had a corneal haze score of 2 or more at last follow-up. This was slightly higher than the haze observed in the PRK eyes with low myopia.

At last follow-up, 10 eyes (22%) had lost two lines of BCVA, and 35 eyes (78%) had no change in BCVA or lost or gained one line. The visual loss was attributed to a combination of irregular astigmatism confirmed on corneal topography, decentration of the ablation zone, or corneal haze.

Complications

There were no cases of recurrent erosion, delayed epithelial healing, or infectious keratitis in this series.

DISCUSSION

Excimer PRK for high myopia is a promising technique in its early stages of development. Several difficult problems must be solved to increase the acceptance of this technique for correction of high myopia. Certainly corneal haze, regression, and under- and overcorrections need to be minimized.

The predictability of PRK for high myopia presented in these results was less than PRK for lower degrees of myopia.[1,4,11] In the latest series of almost 300 eyes at the Phillips Eye Institute using the same methods, 93% of eyes with −1.0 to −6.0 D of myopia achieved vision better than 20/40. Diminished reproducibility in high myopia is probably due to a combination of increased ablation depth and an increased contribution of wound healing to the final result. Therefore, more regression is seen in these highly myopic eyes.

A multizone approach using 20% or correction at a 6-mm optical zone, 30% of correction at a 5-mm optical zone, and 50% of correction at a 4-mm optical zone offers some theoretical advantages. Three patients have been treated with the VISX 2015 laser in this manner. The results are still preliminary and the optimal algorithms are still being elucidated. This may provide a more tapered transition zone and reduce the ablation depth by 30% to 40%. Some of the theoretical disadvantages of a multizone approach include increased corneal haze at the transition zones, greater potential regression which has been seen in some patients, and greater undercorrection. Other investigators have tried multiple tapered transition zones and shown some encouraging results.[5,7,17]

Loss of BCVA in eyes with high myopia treated with excimer PRK is considerably greater than PRK in the lower myope. In low myopia, excimer PRK loss of more than one line of BCVA after excimer PRK is extremely rare. This may be due to subtle topographic changes and haze which can affect the quality of vision. Most of the eyes in the higher myopic ablations had a decrease from 20/15 to 20/20 without subjective complaints. Further study is needed to determine whether the topographic abnormalities and the haze persist. Better control of the collagen remodeling process, improved ablation homogeneity, and improved methods of centration will be needed to maximize effectiveness and safety.

Topical corticosteroids were used in the studies presented here. The use of topical corticosteroids after excimer PRK has been controversial. New collagen deposition after experimental PRK can be reduced through the use of corticosteroids.[18] Corneal haze and refractive error differences appear to be minimally affected by corticosteroid use. In some patients in the current series regression of effect and increased haze developed when the topical corticosteroids were tapered. Several of these eyes responded with decreased haze and less regression when topical corticosteroids were reinstituted. If no effect is seen in the first few weeks after the corticosteroids are reinstituted, then retreatment with the excimer laser may be necessary.

The postoperative pain and photophobia have been significantly reduced from the early studies. Currently, diclofenac and a bandage soft contact lens are used to reduce postoperative discomfort.[19] These patients should be monitored closely for the development of infectious or sterile keratitis.

The surgical treatment of high myopia still faces many challenges. Further advances in laser technology and pharmacologic modification of wound healing will improve future results. Carefully controlled studies are necessary to determine the optimal protocol for the treatment of high myopia.

REFERENCES

1. Salz JJ, Maguen E, Nesburn AB, et al: A two-year experience with excimer laser photorefractive keratectomy for myopia, *Ophthalmology* 100:873-882, 1993.
2. Tengroth B, Epstein D, Fagerholm P, et al: Excimer laser photorefractive keratectomy for myopia: clinical results in sighted eyes, *Ophthalmology* 100:739-745, 1993.
3. Gartry DS, Kerr Muir MG, Marshall J: Excimer laser photorefractive keratectomy: 18 month follow-up, *Ophthalmology* 99:1209-1219, 1992.
4. Talley AR, Hardten DR, Sher, NA, et al: The use of the 193-nm excimer laser for photorefractive keratectomy in low to moderate myopia: one year results, *Am J Ophthalmol* (in press).
5. Kim JH, Hahn TW, Lee YC, Sah WJ: Clinical experience of two-step photorefractive keratectomy in 19 eyes with high myopia, *Refract Corneal Surg* 9 (suppl):s44-s47, 1993.
6. Buratto L, Ferrari M: Photorefractive keratectomy for myopia from 6.00 D to 10.00 D, *Refract Corneal Surg* 9 (suppl): s34-s36, 1993.
7. Cho YS, Kim CG, Kim WB, Kim CW: Multistep photorefractive keratectomy for high myopia, *Refract Corneal Surg* 9 (suppl):s37-s41, 1993.
8. Ehlers N, Hjortdal JO.: Excimer laser refractive keratectomy for high myopia: 6-month follow-up of patients treated bilaterally, *Acta Ophthalmol* 70:578-586, 1992.
9. Sher NA, Barak M, Daya S, et al: Excimer laser photorefractive keratectomy in high myopia: a multicenter study, *Arch Ophthalmol* 110:935-943, 1992.
10. Dausch D, Klein R, Schroder E, et al: Excimer laser photorefractive keratectomy with tapered transition zone for high myopia: a preliminary report of six cases, *J Cataract Refract Surg* 19:590-594, 1993.
11. Seiler T, Wollensak J: Myopic photorefractive keratectomy with the excimer laser: one year follow-up, *Ophthalmology* 98:1156-1163, 1991.
12. Gartry DS, Kerr Muir MG, Marshall J.: Photorefractive keratectomy with an argon fluoride excimer laser: a clinical study, *Refract Corneal Surg* 7:420-435, 1991.
13. Munnerlyn CR, Koons SJ, Marshall J: Photorefractive keratectomy: a technique for laser refractive surgery, *J Cataract Refract Surg* 14:46-52, 1988.
14. McDonald MB, Liu JC, Byrd TJ, et al: Central photorefractive keratectomy for myopia: partially sighted and normally sighted eyes, *Ophthalmology* 98:1327-1337, 1991.
15. Sher NA, Chen V, Bowers RA, et al: The use of the 193-nm excimer laser for myopic photorefractive keratectomy in sighted eyes: a multicenter study, *Arch Ophthalmol* 109:1525-1530, 1991.
16. Lavery FL: Photorefractive keratectomy in 472 eyes, *Refract Corneal Surg* 9 (suppl):s98-s100, 1993.
17. Brancato R, Tavola A, Carones F, et al: Excimer laser photorefractive keratectomy (PRK): first report from the Italian study group, *Ital J Ophthalmol* 3:189-195, 1991.
18. Tuft SJ, Zabel RW, Marshall J: Corneal repair following keratectomy, *Invest Ophthalmol Vis Sci* 30:1769-1777, 1989.
19. Sher NA, Frantz JM, Talley A, et al: Topical diclofenac in treatment of ocular pain after excimer photorefractive keratectomy, *Refract Corneal Surg* (in press).

The VISX 2020, Excimer Laser
Barry Kassar, Joy Heitzmann

The excimer laser has been shown to effectively correct myopia. Clinical and refractive results reported by several authors with different lasers and surgical techniques show similar results in the lower (2-6 D) range of myopia.[1-8] For myopia exceeding 6 D, different surgical approaches have been attempted with variable results.[9] Poor predictability or complications associated with corneal wound healing[10] have been noted.

This chapter addresses the correction of high myopia in excess of 8 D, by excimer laser photokeratectomy. The results obtained by three surgeons (Barry S. Kassar, Perry S. Binder, and Lee T. Nordan) using the VISX 2020 excimer laser at one center (Mericos Eye Institute, Scripps Memorial Hospital, La Jolla, Calif.), and the combined results of the work at four United States centers using the VISX 2020 for high myopia treatment are reviewed.

Within the Food and Drug Administration (FDA) phase IIa study of high myopia, we have treated 19 eyes with −8.00 to −19.50 D of myopia. Within the FDA PTK (phototherapeutic keratectomy) II protocol, we have treated 4 eyes with myopia greater than −8.00 D for anisometropia or residual myopia after refractive surgery. The surgical procedure, pre- and postoperative care, and initial results, including detailed 6-month follow-up data for 18 of these 23 eyes, have been published by us in the *Archives of Ophthalmology* in December 1993.[11]

Around the United States, VISX sponsored four sites doing excimer laser photokeratectomy for high myopia. VISX submitted data to the FDA in February 1994. The report was based on 25 patients followed for 1 year, and is summarized later in this chapter.

MATERIALS AND METHODS

The VISX 2020 excimer laser (VISX, Santa Clara, Calif.) at the Mericos Eye Institute was used for all treatments. Laser fluence was 160 mJ/cm^2 with a repetition rate of 5 Hz.

Twenty-three eyes of 18 patients with myopia between −8.00 and −19.50 D were treated.[11] The mean preoperative spherical equivalent was −11.83 ±2.92 D. The mean attempted ablation depth for all treatments was 93 μm. All 23 eyes have at least 12 months of follow-up.

The epithelium was removed manually prior to laser photoablation. Multizone ablations (4.0, 5.0, 6.0 mm) were performed to reduce the ablation depth characteristic of single-zone treatments. Fifty percent of the refractive error was ablated at the smallest optical zone, 30% at midzone, and 20% at the largest optical zone diameter. Nitrogen was not blown across the ocular surface. A fixation handpiece was used for all procedures.

Following treatment the ocular surface was flushed with an antibiotic drop. Postoperative regimens varied but usually included a cycloplegic, a steroid-antibiotic, and in some cases, diclofenac sodium solution (Voltaren). After the surface epithelium healed, eyes were treated with fluorometholone every 2 hours for week 1, four times a day for month 1, three times a day for month 2, and twice a day for month 3. Eyes received one drop of fluorometholone daily for months 4, 5, and 6.

RESULTS

The Mericos Eye Institute data for 23 eyes at 1 year following excimer PRK are as follows: three eyes were re-treated for undercorrection or haze at about 9 months postoperatively (Figs. 6-1 and 6-2); one eye underwent a secondary radial keratotomy (RK) at 6 months postlaser treatment (Figs. 6-3 and 6-4, *A, B,* and *C*). All subsequent data include re-treatment results.

One year after laser surgery, 39% (9 of 23) of eyes were within 1 D of attempted correction; 74% (17 of 23) of eyes were within 2 D of attempted correction. The mean spherical equivalent refraction was −1.39 ±1.94 D.

Preoperatively, all 23 eyes had count fingers UCVA. At 1 year, 13 eyes (57%) had UCVA of 20/40 or better; 10 eyes (43%) were worse than 20/40. Four eyes (17%) had uncorrected visual acuity of 20/25 or better.

Two eyes lost one Snellen line of BCVA at 1 year postoperatively. In contrast, 11 eyes (48%) gained one Snellen line and 2 eyes gained two Snellen lines of BCVA. Eight eyes (35%) had no change in BCVA. One year after laser surgery, corneal haze scores of 1.5 or greater were reported for 30% of eyes (7 eyes). Most eyes with significant corneal haze also exhibited regression of refractive effect and loss of UCVA

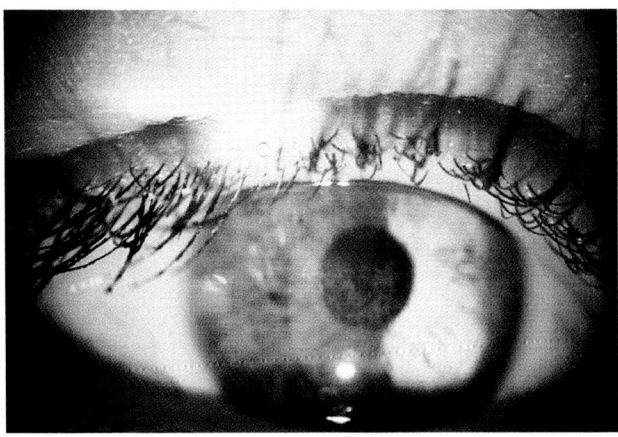

Fig. 6-3. Significant haze in a cornea several months post PRK.

(six cases). One year after treatment, 22% of eyes had a stable refraction; 44% exhibited mild regression of refractive effect, and 30% exhibited significant regression (change of 1.75 D or more between follow-up visits at least once during the follow-up period).

A majority of patients (14 of 19) reported problems with night vision, experiencing halos or starburst 1 year following laser treatment. Despite this, overall patient satisfaction with the outcome has been positive.

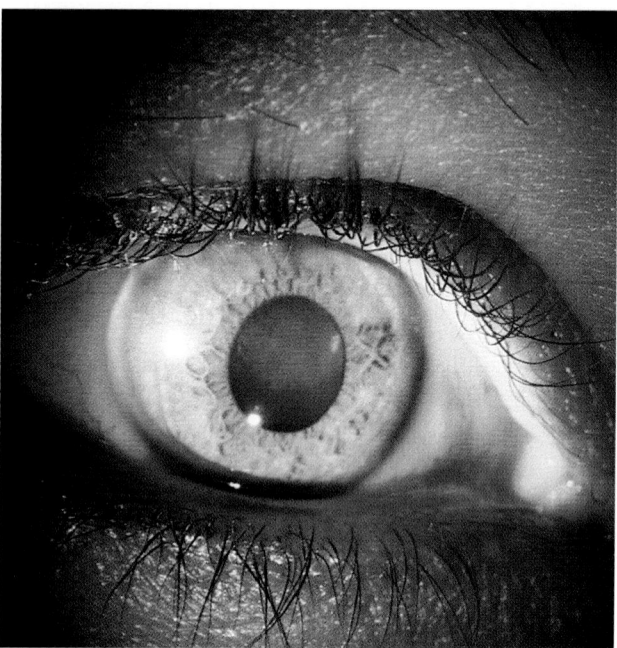

Fig. 6-4. Reduction in corneal haze in the same eye as Fig. 6-3, several months following corneal re-treatment by excimer laser.

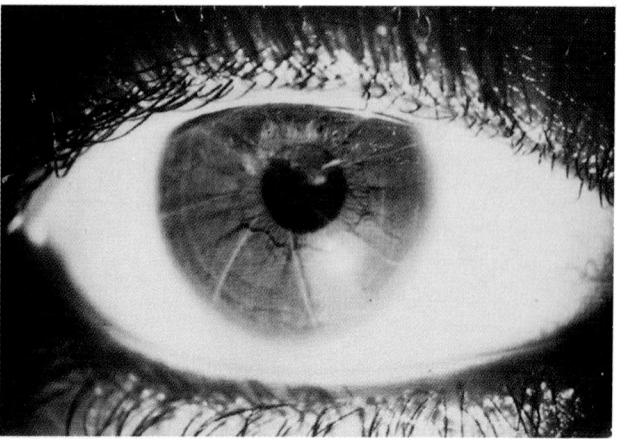

Fig. 6-5. Radial kerotomy incisions 9 months out, done 6 months following excimer laser PRK for high myopia.

The combined United States–VISX experience is reported in 25 patients treated at these four centers, under the direction of the named principal investigators.

Center	n (%)
Mericos Eye Institute San Diego, CA (Barry Kassar)	15 (60%)
Doheny Eye Institute Los Angeles, CA (Peter McDonnell)	4 (16%)
Massachusets Eye Infirmary Boston, MA (Micheal Wagoner)	4 (16%)
Louisiana State University New Orleans, LA (Marguerite McDonald)	2 (8%)

Data extracted from this report reflect the outcomes from these four centers, and reasonably mirror the data presented from our center only.

Twenty-five patients were enrolled in the study nationwide. During the first year, one patient underwent RK and five patients were re-treated by excimer laser. These six patients, who were excluded from the 12-month data, had spherical equivalent refractions ranging from −4.50 D to −9.25 D at 6 months. One patient was not examined at the 12-month gate. The 12-month data therefore pertain to 18 patients.

No patient in this series is reported to have developed any adverse effects from the excimer laser treatment. There appears to be a progressive reduction in mean corneal haze between 6 and 12 months. The mean keratometry readings at 6 months were 40.00 ±2.61; at 12 months, these were 40.07 ±2.84. These appear to reflect a stable corneal curvature, on average, between 6 and 12 months. Five patients have lost more than one line of BCVA at 6 months; one additional patient lost more than one line of BCVA at 12 months. Of these original five, two patients regained lines at 12 months, and three were re-treated by excimer. Excluding those who underwent re-treatment, 28% of eyes are within ±0.5 D of intended correction; and a total of 50% are within 2.0 D of intended correction at the 12-month mark.

Of those 6 patients who underwent excimer re-treatment, five were re-treated for assorted degrees of regression and haze; at the last reported visit, at varying times after re-treatment, these eyes have UCVA of 20/60 (two), 20/50, and 20/40 (two); these eyes also have BCVA of 20/50, 20/40, 20/30 (two); and 20/25. One patient was re-treated for undercorrection only at the sixteenth month, and had UCVA of 20/32 and BCVA of 20/20 at the last visit. Overall, at 1 year following excimer PRK for high myopia, this states-wide VISX group demonstrated UCVA of 20/20 in 5.6%; 20/40 or better in 38.9%; and 20/160 or better in 72.2%.

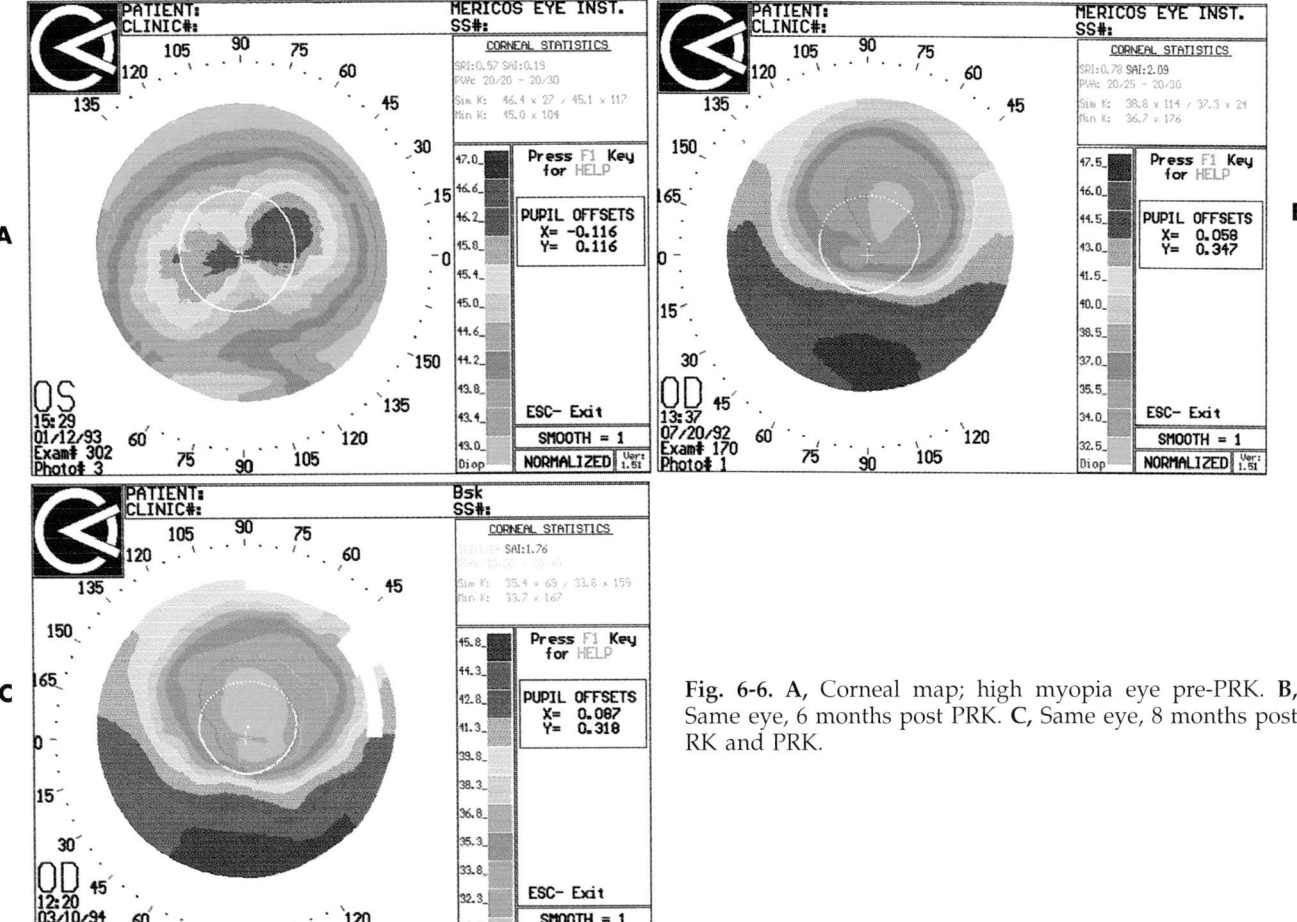

Fig. 6-6. A, Corneal map; high myopia eye pre-PRK. **B,** Same eye, 6 months post PRK. **C,** Same eye, 8 months post RK and PRK.

DISCUSSION

We find excimer photoablation for the treatment of high myopia (> 8.0 D) to be less predictable or efficient than excimer photoablation for the treatment of low myopia. There is a higher incidence of regression of refractive effect, corneal haze, and decreased quality of vision (halos, etc.) in the high myopia group of patients. Although not statistically significant, it appears that younger, generally female patients, requiring deeper ablations, may be at risk for developing corneal haze and regression. Individual healing variability may also play an important role.

Limiting the ablation depth by a multizone technique does not appear to prevent the incidence of corneal haze for high myopia excimer patients. The resulting smaller functional optical zone diameter may be associated with increased incidence of regression of refractive effect. We observed no difference in patient response to changing from 4.0-, 5.0-, or 6.0-mm (iris diaphragm opening) treatments to 4.5-, 5.0-, or 6.0-mm (iris diaphragm closing) treatments. We have patients with significant corneal haze without regres-

sion, and patients with refractive regression without haze. Three patients at our center requiring repeat PRK procedure had significant corneal haze and regression together.

Effective excimer treatment of high myopia may require correcting the myopia in stages, rather than at one session. One approach incorporates successive treatments with the excimer laser. Another approach may combine procedures, such as RK and excimer laser keratectomy; in this group, RK may precede or follow the excimer laser procedure.

Continued follow-up of high myopia patients as well as modifications in treatment protocols and postoperative regimens are critical to developing the full potential of excimer photoablation as an effective procedure to correct high myopia. Controlled studies comparing alternative "combined procedures" will provide important insight into the true utility of the excimer laser in the treatment of high myopia.

In the VISX multicenter data, (excluding re-treated eyes), 40% of these highly myopic patients achieved

UCVA of 20/40 or better. This is a substantial improvement in UCVA and refraction. Even those who are unable to dispense with their eyeglasses entirely enjoy a marked improvement in overall vision, and a significant reduction in the strength of required optical correction.

REFERENCES

1. McDonald MB, Frantz JM, Klyce SD, et al: One-year refractive results of central photorefractive keratectomy for myopia in the nonhuman primate cornea, *Arch Ophthalmol* 108:40-47, 1990.
2. Gartry D, Kerr Muir M, Marshall J: Excimer laser photorefractive keratectomy, *Ophthalmology* 99:1209-1219, 1992.
3. McDonald M, Leach D, Ahmed S, et al: Photorefractive keratectomy (PRK) phase III (abstract), 99:106, 1992.
4. Piebenga L, Deitz M, Irvine J, et al: The effectiveness of excimer photorefractive keratectomy for myopia (abstract), *Ophthalmology* 99:106, 1992.
5. Waring G III, Maloney R, Hagen K, et al: Refractive and visual results of a multicenter trial of excimer laser photorefractive keratectomy (abstract), *Ophthalmology* 99:106, 1992.
6. Seiler T, Wollensak J, Jean B: Complications of myopic photorefractive keratectomy (PRK) with the excimer laser (abstract), *Ophthalmology* 99:107, 1992.
7. Flicker L, Steele A, Kirkness C, et al: Excimer laser photorefractive keratoplasty for myopia (abstract), *Ophthalmology* 99:127, 1992.
8. Salz J, Maguen E, Macy J, et al: One-year results of excimer laser photorefractive keratectomy for myopia, *Refract Corneal Surg* 8:269-272, 1992.
9. Sher NA, Barak M, Daya S, et al: Excimer laser photorefractive keratectomy in high myopia, *Arch Ophthalmol* 110:935-943, 1992.
10. Binder PS: What we have learned about corneal wound healing from refractive surgery, *J Refract Corneal Surg* 5:98-120, 1992.
11. Heitzmann J, Binder PS, Kassar BS, et al: The correction of high myopia using the excimer laser, *Arch Ophthalmol* 111:1627-1634, 1993.
12. VISX Study Report: High myopia phase 11-A: 12 month follow-up, Santa Clara, Calif, Feb 11, 1994, VISX Corp.

The Summit Experience

Daniel S. Durrie, D. James Schumer, Timothy B. Cavanaugh, and David T. Gubman

Photorefractive keratectomy for the treatment of myopia has shown significant promise based on the precision of corneal ablation obtained using excimer laser technology. However, as a refractive procedure it is essential to determine the accuracy, predictability, and stability of the ultimate correction. Experience from other refractive procedures, primarily RK, has demonstrated that the magnitude of myopia has implication for the ultimate visual outcome. Most recent studies confirm that the predictability of RK is better for lower levels of myopia (< 4 D).[1] PRK requires similar investigation into the efficacy and predictability of high myopic correction.

THE GARTRY ET AL. STUDY—EXCIMER PHOTOREACTIVE KERATECTOMY

Recently, a study by Gartry et al.[2] reports data on 18-month follow-up after excimer PRK. This report examined PRK outcomes for patients receiving treatment between 2 and 7 D of attempted myopic correction. The results indicate a decreasing accuracy with increasing magnitude of attempted correction. Attempted corrections of 3.00 D resulted in 70% of eyes within ±1.00 D of intended correction at 1 year. The treatment group that received 7.00 D of attempted correction obtained a result within ±1.00 D in only 20% of eyes at 1 year. Burrato and Ferrari[3] found similar results for PRK in patients with myopic refractive errors between 6 and 10 D. Their data found 35% of eyes achieved an intended correction within ±1.00 D. These studies include a fixed regimen of postoperative topical steroid therapy regardless of postoperative refractive error or observed corneal haze.

Several possible factors have been proposed for these results, including a treatment algorithm error more pronounced at higher corrections. Also, variations in the edges of ablation zones may have differing effects for differing levels of correction. Deeper ablation depths for higher levels of myopic correction show steeper slopes at the edge of the ablation site than are found in lower corrections. An additional and important factor may be an increased corneal wound-healing effect with increased ablation depth.

PHOTOREFRACTIVE KERATECTOMY USING THE SUMMIT LASER

The following data and discussion seek to evaluate the accuracy, predictability, and safety of PRK using the Summit laser for −6.00 to −10.00 D of myopia with postoperative steroid therapy adjusted to the individual healing response as evidenced by slit-lamp findings and manifest refraction. In addition, these results are compared to results in a second group of patients who have undergone PTK for residual myopia following RK. This second patient group also had an original level of myopia between −6.00 and −10.00 D prior to RK.

All PRK procedures were performed using the Summit ExciMed UV200 (Summit Technology, Waltham, Mass.). Patient selection and treatment protocol were standardized according to the FDA criteria for phase III of the excimer laser clinical trial and preoperative refractive error was limited to a maximum of 10 D of myopia. Ten eyes of 10 patients underwent PRK only for high myopia. The average preprocedural spherical equivalent refractive error was −7.13 D with a range of −6.00 to −9.00 D. As a comparison, 20 eyes of 17 patients underwent PRK for residual myopia following RK at a single trial site (Hunkeler Eye Clinic, Kansas City). This group had an original spherical

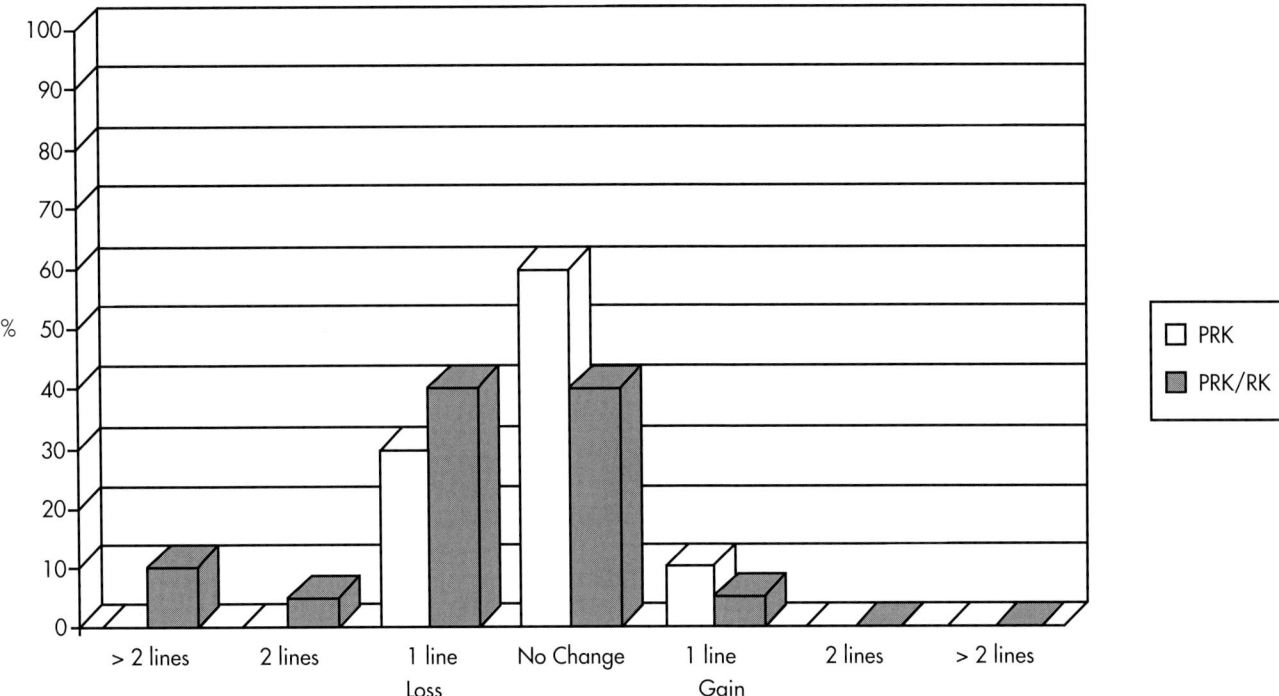

Fig. 6-7. Best corrected visual acuity at 1 year comparing PRK alone with PRK after RK.

equivalent refraction of −8.43 D and a range of −6.13 to −10.50 D. The average post-RK–pre-PRK spherical equivalent refractive error was −4.12 D with a range of −2.00 to −6.88 D.

Safety

One measure of the safety of any refractive correction is the preservation of best acuity. Fig. 6-7 indicates the BCVA at 1 year comparing PRK alone with PRK after RK. Seventy percent of patients receiving only PRK had either no change or an increase in BCVA compared with 45% for those receiving PRK after RK. Three of ten (30%) eyes receiving PRK only showed a one-line loss in best corrected acuity. Two of these three eyes went from 20/15 to 20/20 recorded acuity. The remaining eye showed a one-line loss from 20/20 to 20/25. Of the 20 eyes that underwent PRK after RK, 11 (55%) eyes showed a loss in best corrected acuity and 1 eye showed a gain in acuity from 20/20 to 20/15. Seven (35%) of those eyes showed an acuity change from 20/15 to 20/20. The remaining 3 eyes (15%) showed greater than a one-line loss in best corrected acuity.

Efficacy

The efficacy of a corneal refractive procedure is usually evaluated in terms of visual acuity following the procedure without the aid of additional optical lenses (uncorrected). Fig. 6-8 shows the UCVA results following the corneal refractive procedure obtained at 1 year. One hundred percent of the PRK-only group achieved

20/40 uncorrected acuity compared to 65% of the PRK-after-RK group. UCVA of 20/20 was attained by 50% of the PRK-only group compared to 15% of the PRK-after-RK group.

Accuracy and Predictability

Deviation from intended correction describes the accuracy and predictability of the refractive procedure. The intended refractive correction was not always plano for each eye. Rather, a monovision correction was most often desired whereby the dominant eye is refracted near plano while the nondominant eye is intentionally left with approximately 1.00 D of myopia. This allows a most versatile visual system in order to achieve clear distance vision as well as functional near vision, particularly considering the inevitable onset of presbyopia. Monovision is a well-established refractive concept which is used successfully in contact lens fitting for presbyopia.[4] Fig. 6-9 summarizes the refraction predictability outcome at 1 year. Both groups show comparable accuracy of myopic correction with 60% and 80% within ±1.00 D of intended correction for eyes undergoing PRK and PRK after RK, respectively. This percentage difference is reversed when looking at the ±1.50-D range. Here, 100% of the PRK-only group and 95% of the PRK-after-RK group showed correction within ±1.50 D. The small sample sizes of 10 eyes in the PRK-only group and 20 eyes in the PRK-after-RK group must be taken into account when interpreting these results.

The excimer laser ablation study described here

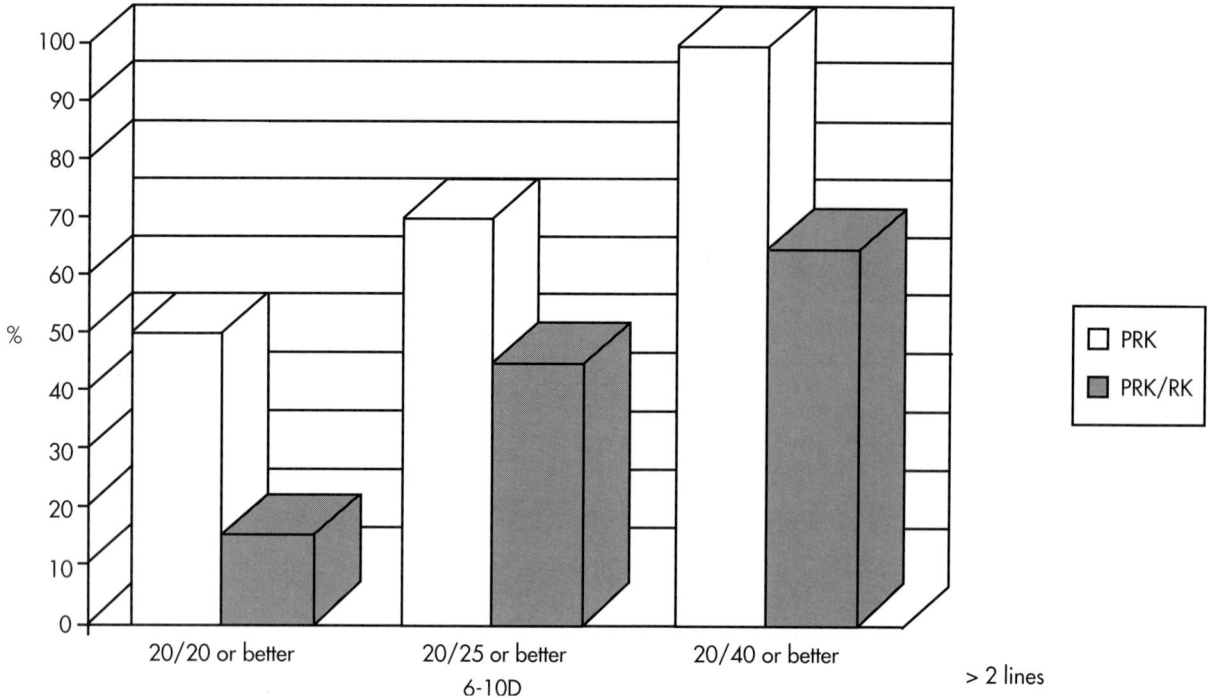

Fig. 6-8. Uncorrected visual acuity results following the corneal refractive procedure, obtained at 1 year.

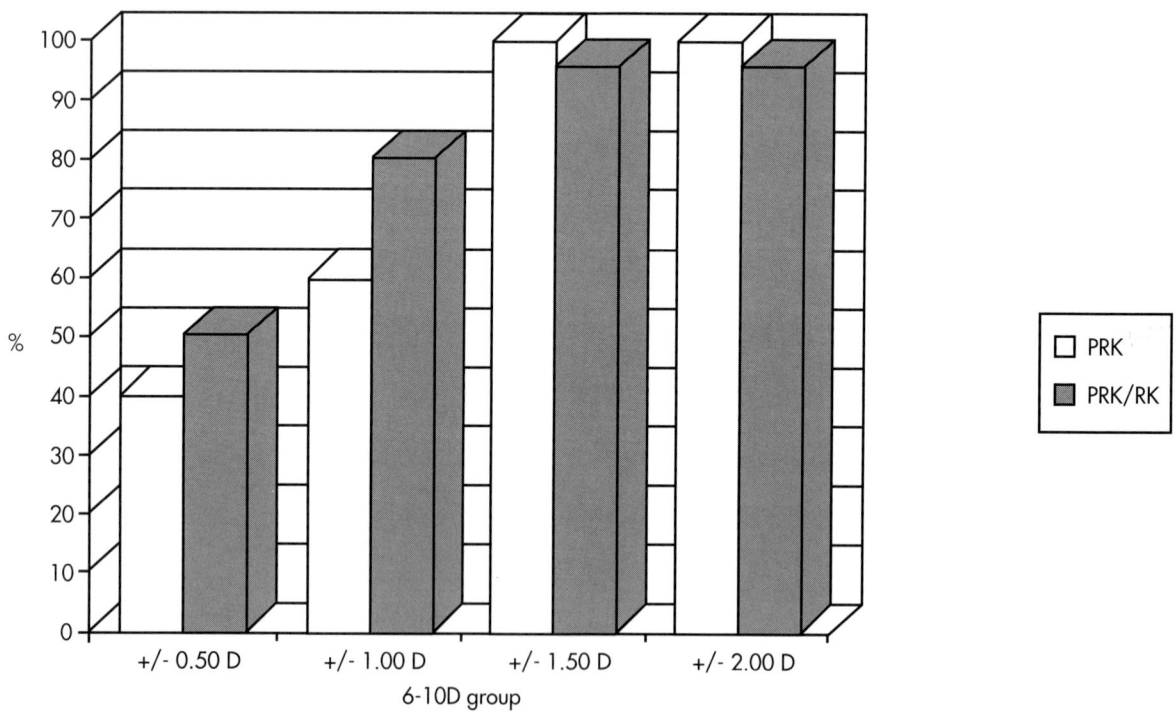

Fig. 6-9. The accuracy and predictability outcome after 1 year in the PRK-only and PRK-after-RK groups.

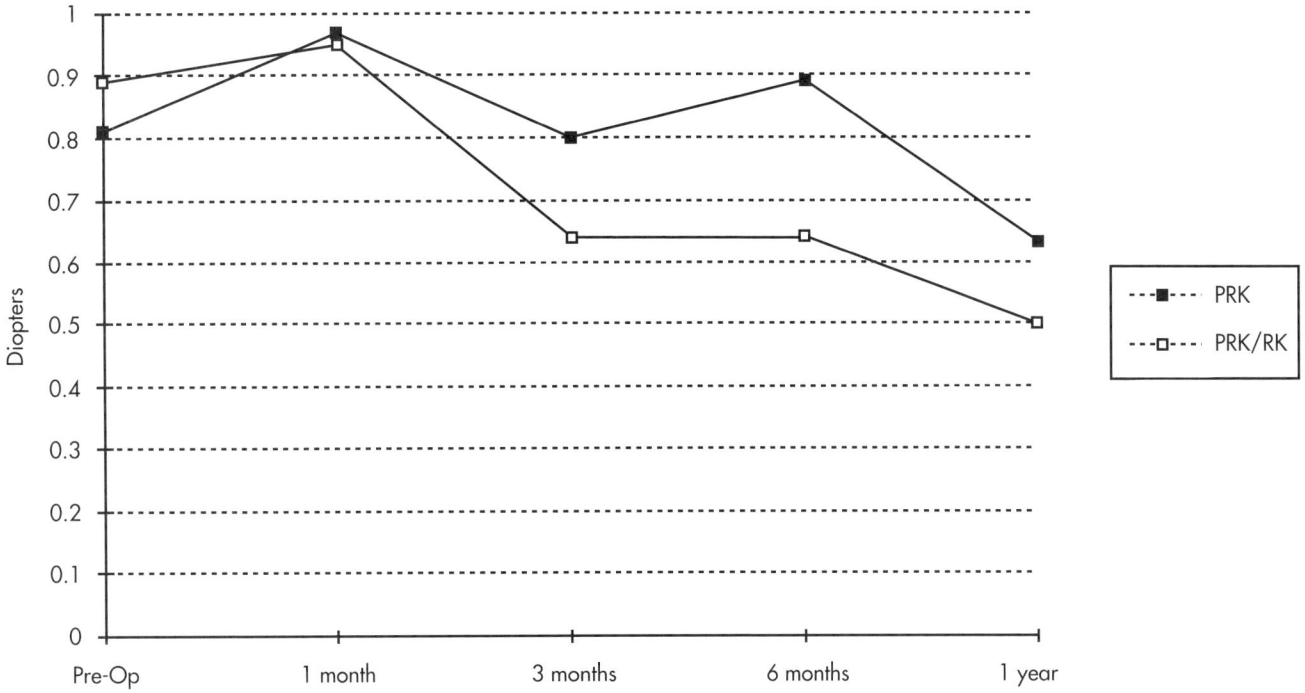

Fig. 6-10. Results 1 year after the excimer laser ablation study.

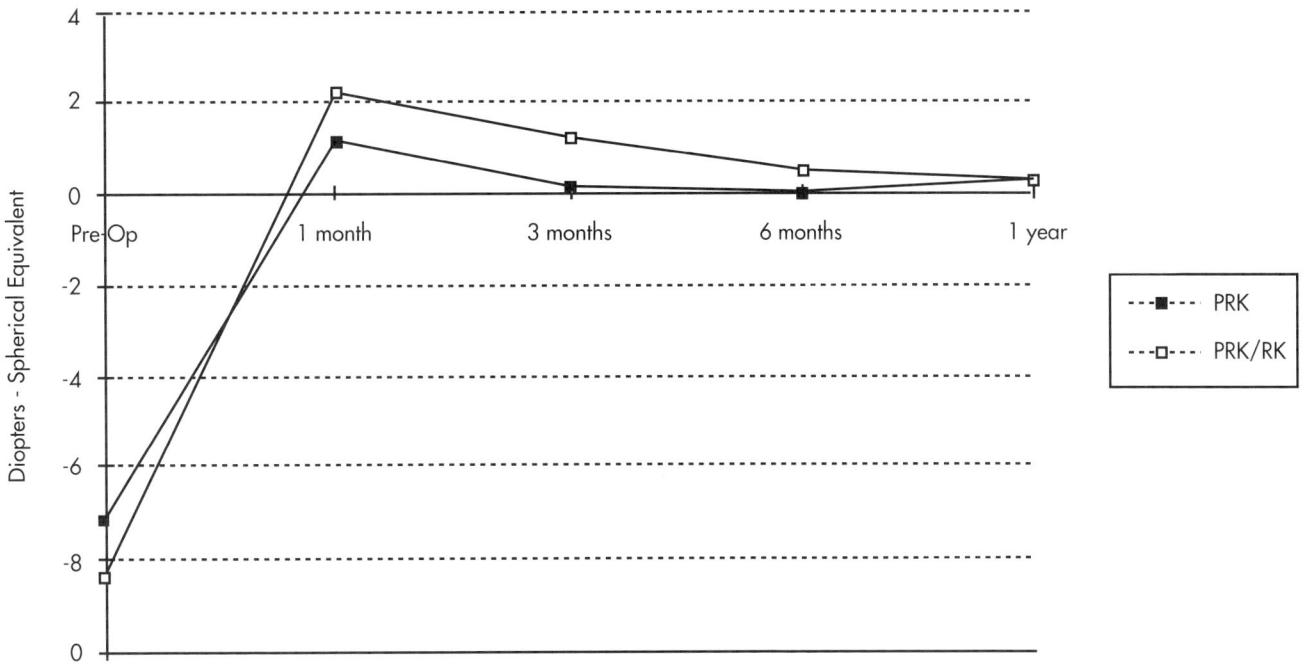

Fig. 6-11. The stability of correction over time.

was not designed to treat astigmatism created by corneal toricity. Neither procedure induced additional astigmatism and there is an overall slight mean decrease in corneal cylinder compared to preprocedure levels. Fig. 6-10 summarizes the 1-year results.

Fig. 6-11 indicates the stability of correction over time. Again, each group shows approximately equal

stability after 1 year with the characteristic initial overcorrection and subsequent regression toward the intended correction observed with the Summit excimer laser.

Fig. 6-12 displays corneal topography 3 months and 12 months after PRK. The original spherical equivalent refractive error was −9.00 D. The early topogra-

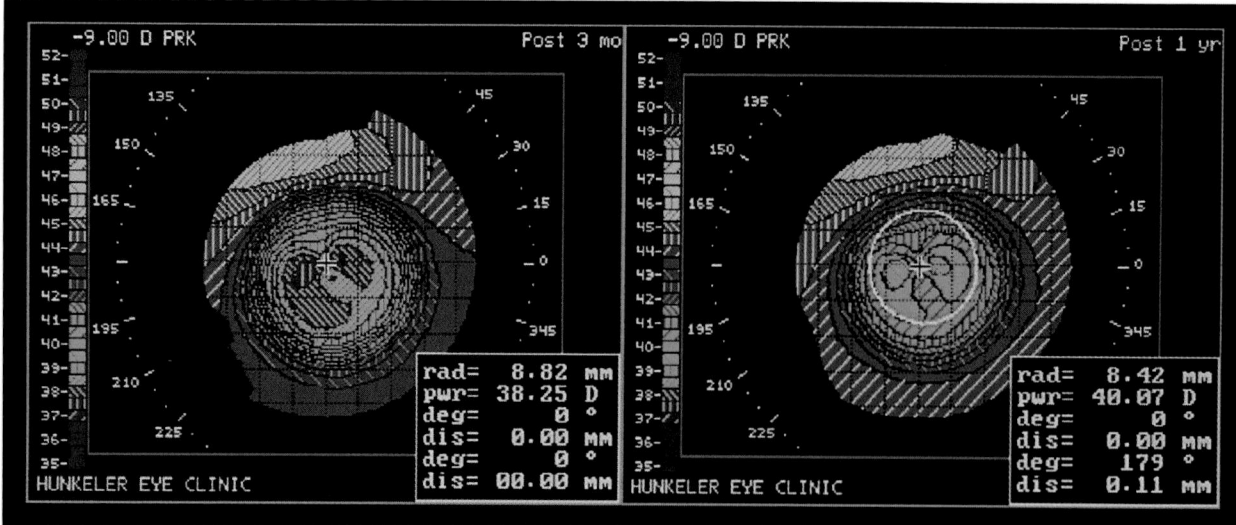

Fig. 6-12. Corneal topography 3 months and 1 year after PRK.

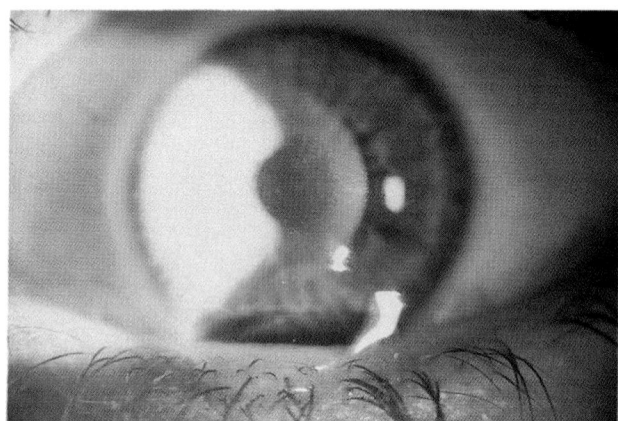

Fig. 6-13. The cornea at 3 months with a slight central reticular appearance graded at 1/8 trace haze.

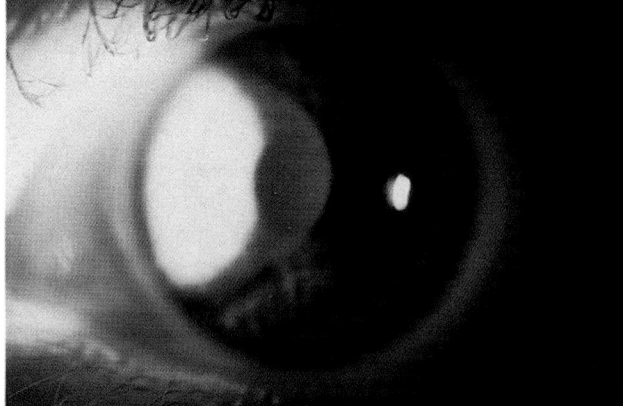

Fig. 6-14. The cornea in Fig. 6-13 after 1 year, with the haze resolved.

phy shows a darker central blue zone with a corresponding dioptric curvature of 38.25 D. The subsequent late topography at 12 months shows a mild steepening to 40.07 D. These values correspond well with the manual keratometry measurements taken at the same visits. Fig. 6-13 shows the clinical picture of the cornea at 3 months with a slight central reticular appearance graded as 1/8 trace haze. Fig. 6-14 shows this haze to be resolved at the 1-year visit. This healing pattern is considered typical and the most common clinical course following PRK. UCVA was 20/15 with a cycloplegic refractive measurement of plano.

Fig. 6-15 shows the topography for another patient with a more aggressive type of healing response. The original spherical equivalent was also −9.00 D for comparison purposes. Included in this figure is the topographic video image from which the color maps are processed. Fig. 6-16 shows a greater reticular appear-

ance than Fig. 6-13 and was graded as 1/2 trace haze. This haze had increased by 6 months and the patient was started on a short course of fluorometholone (FML Forte) and diclofenac sodium (Voltaren) four times daily. Fig. 6-17 shows that by 12 months the haze is dissipating, breaking up inferiorly more quickly than superiorly. At 1 year, the uncorrected visual acuity was 20/25, with a cycloplegic refractive error of −0.25-0.75 × 015 20/20.

Fig. 6-18 shows the topography of a PRK at 4 and 18 months performed subsequent to a previous RK with residual myopia. The original spherical equivalent refractive error prior to RK was −9.00 D. Fifteen months following RK the residual myopia was −2.50 D. The patient underwent PRK and Figs. 6-19 and 6-20 show the corneal picture at 4 and 18 months. It is apparent that the reticular haze is more diffuse early and becomes more densely coalesced into discrete clumps

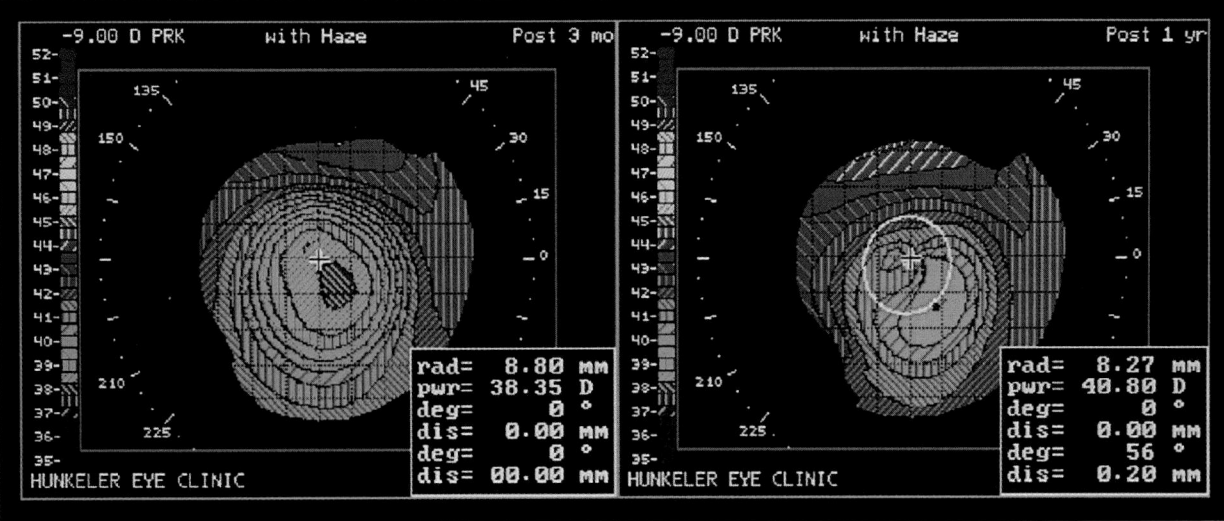

Fig. 6-15. Topography of a patient with an aggressive type of healing response.

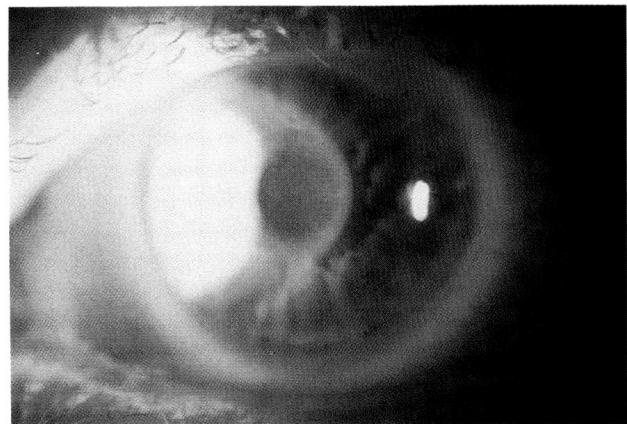

Fig. 6-16. Greater reticular appearance than in Fig. 6-14 with 1/2 trace haze.

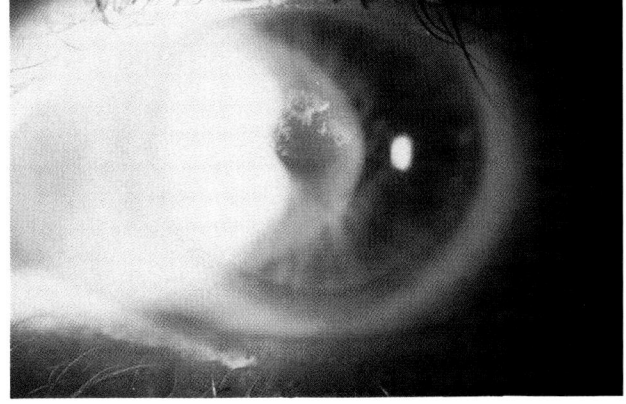

Fig. 6-17. At 12 months the haze shown in Fig. 6-16 is dissipating, breaking up inferiorly more quickly than superiorly.

with clear spaces in between. UCVA was 20/25, with a cycloplegic refractive error of −0.50 sphere 20/20.

RK is currently the most common procedure employed in altering corneal curvature to reduce myopic refractive error. However, the downside risk of additional incisions, increasing incision depth, and smaller clear zone diameters limit the magnitude of safe and effective myopic correction. The argon fluoride excimer laser may permit a more precise and controlled method than can be achieved with a surgical blade.

Topical steroid therapy adjustment in the postoperative period can be important to the ultimate refractive outcome. Regression and corneal haze can be significantly affected by changes in topical anti-inflammatory drugs. At the 1-month visit, patients are classified according to their healing response as average, inadequate, or aggressive. Patients judged as ag-

gressive healers display corneal haze that is increased in both density and confluence. Manifest refraction in aggressive healers also shows more rapid regression of the initial hyperopic overcorrection. Increased steroid therapy in these patients in effective in moderating the healing response and preserving the desired refractive result. By contrast, inadequate healers tend to show clear corneas and display minimal regression, thereby retaining the initial postoperative hyperopic refraction. Decreasing or removal of steroid therapy allows a more active corneal healing response and subsequent refractive regression toward the intended correction.

In a recent article, Heitzmann and co-workers[5] report PRK results in 23 highly myopic eyes with a mean refractive error of −11.83 D (±2.92 D) and a range of −8.00 to −19.50 D. They found 12 eyes (52%) attained 20/40 or better uncorrected acuity and 9 eyes (39%)

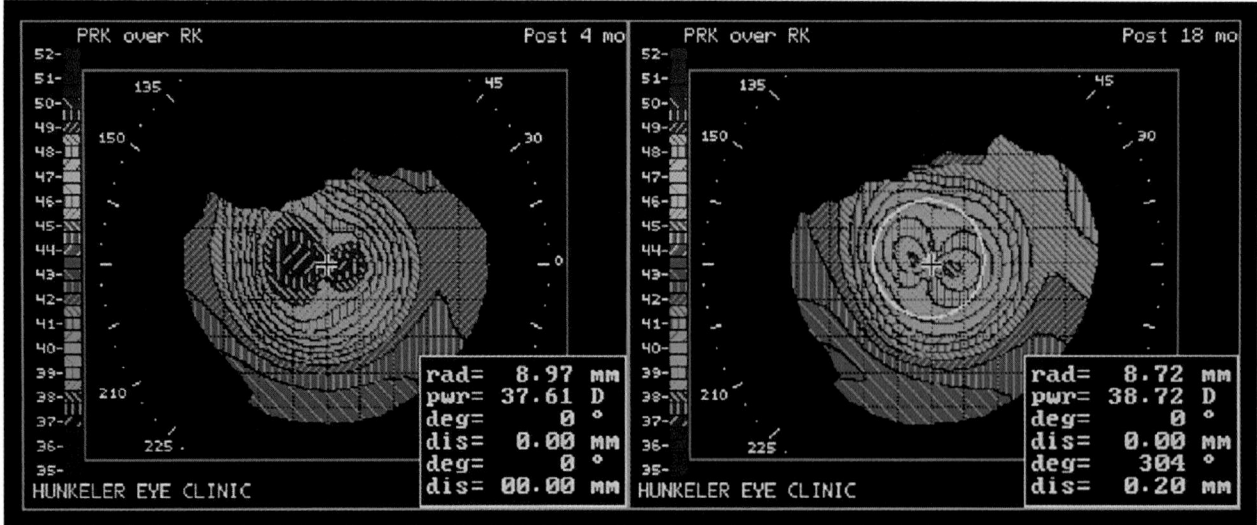

Fig. 6-18. Topography of a PRK at 4 and 18 months performed subsequent to a previous RK with residual myopia.

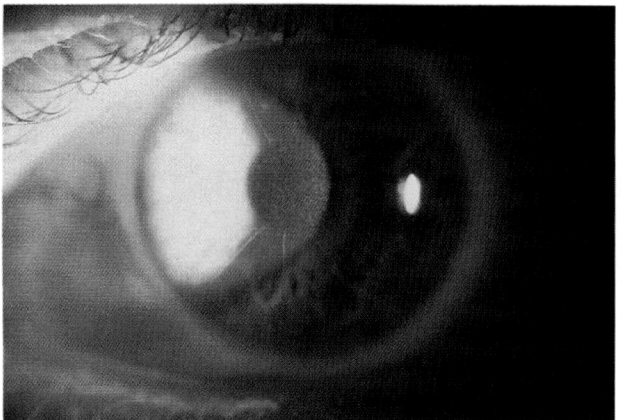

Fig. 6-19. PRK corneal picture at 4 months.

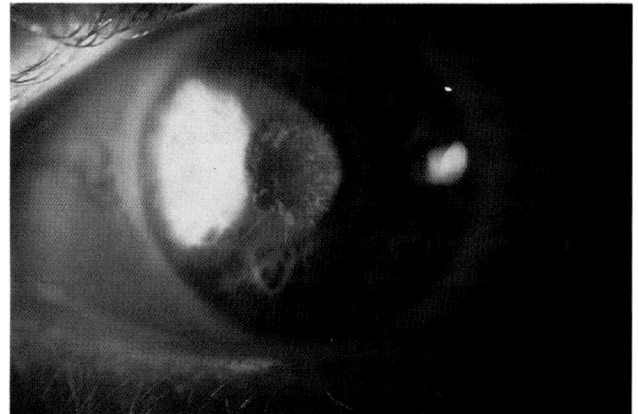

Fig. 6-20. PRK corneal picture at 18 months.

measured a refraction within ±1.00 D of intended correction. Fig. 6-21 summarizes the visual and refractive outcomes for highly myopic PRK procedures (>6.00 D). It is apparent from these results that steroid therapy manipulation tailored according to individual healing response by observable biomicroscopic and refractive findings may increase the effectiveness in achieving the intended correction in highly myopic eyes.

The high level of accuracy and safety in treating low myopia (<5.00 D) with RK or excimer laser[6,7] have led some to conclude that high myopia correction should be performed with a combination of procedures such as RK and PRK to achieve the higher corrections. However, the BCVA data reported here indicate that the PRK procedure is safer alone than when combined with RK, with fewer patients showing a decrease in best corrected vision. For the PRK-only

group, 2 of 10 patients showed a decrease in correctable acuity from 20/15 to 20/20 and 1 (10%) of 10 patients lost acuity from 20/20 to 20/25. One-line variation in best corrected vision may result from varying testing conditions and measurement error, but it may also indicate the lingering visual effects of remaining corneal haze. In the PRK-after-RK group, however, 11 of 20 (55%) eyes showed a decrease in best corrected acuity and of those, 3 eyes (15%) had a decrease in vision of two lines or greater.

Given these successful PRK results for highly myopic eyes we recommend a single treatment procedure with postoperative follow-up tailored according to the variable clinical response. This approach is further supported by the results indicating better safety of the single PRK procedure in comparison to those undergoing RK and subsequent PRK as estimated by loss in BCVA. Certainly PRK after RK provides a reason-

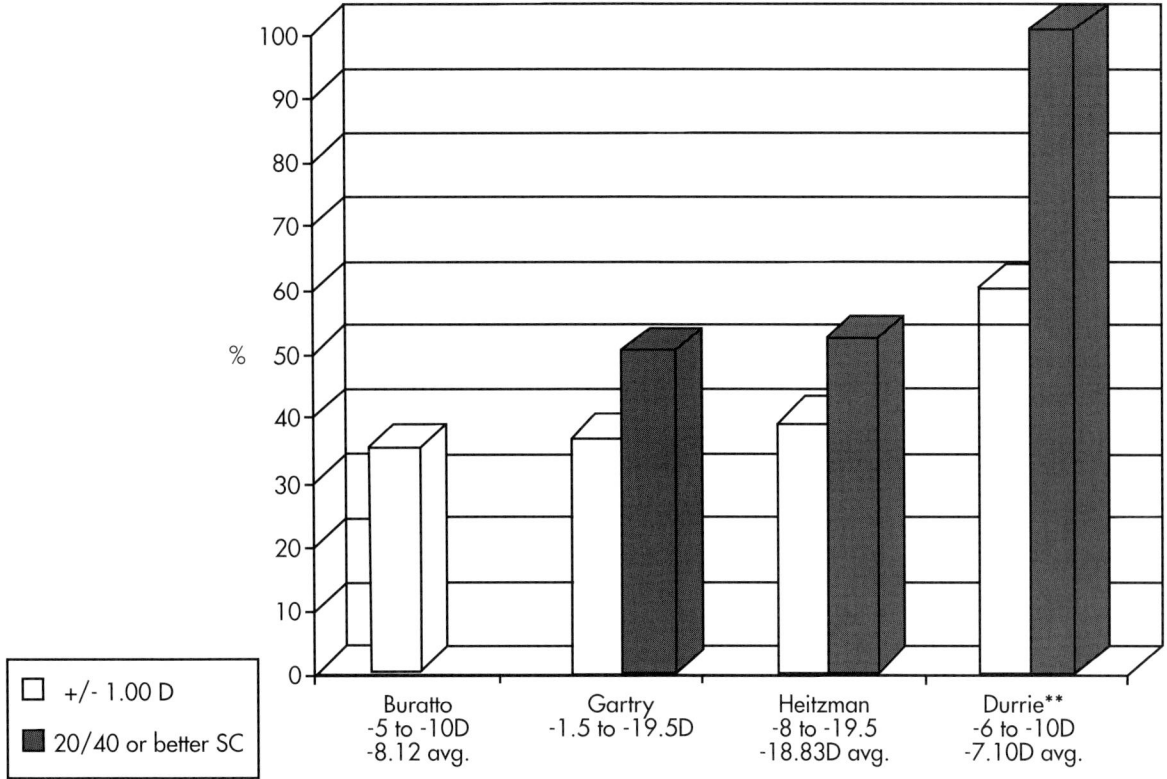

Fig. 6-21. The visual and refractive outcomes for highly myopic PRK procedures (>6.00 D). (Data from Buratto and Ferrari,[3] Gartry et al.,[2] Heitzmann et al.,[5] and Durrie.)

able alternative for residual myopic correction when necessary. However, it is suggested that as an initial surgical plan for high myopic correction, the ultimate efficacy and safety favor the single PRK procedure.

REFERENCES

1. Waring GO, Lynn MJ, Nizam A, et al: Results of the prospective evaluation of radial keratotomy (PERK) study five years after surgery, *Ophthalmology* 98:1164-1176, 1991.
2. Gartry D, Kerr Muir M, Marshall J: Excimer laser photorefractive keratectomy, *Ophthalmology* 99:1209-1219, 1992.
3. Buratto L, Ferrari M: Photorefractive keratectomy for myopia from 6.00 D to 10.00 D, *Refract Corneal Surg* 9:S34-S36, 1993.
4. Erikson P: The potential range of clear vision in monovision, *J Am Optom Assoc* 59:203-205, 1985.
5. Heitzmann J, Binder P, Kassar B, et al: Correction of high myopia using the excimer laser, *Arch Ophthalmol* 11:1627-1634, 1993.
6. Salz J, Maguen E, Macy J, et al: One-year results of excimer laser photorefractive-keratectomy for myopia, *Refract Corneal Surg* 8:269-272, 1992.
7. Seiler T, Wollensak J: Myopic photorefractive keratectomy with the excimer laser: one-year follow-up, *Ophthalmology* 98:1156-1163, 1991.

7

Computerized Corneal Topography of Surface Ablations with the Tomey (TMS-1)

Stephen D. Klyce and Marguerite B. McDonald

The next generation in keratorefractive surgery has arrived with the use of the excimer laser for photorefractive keratectomy (PRK).[1-7] While radial keratotomy can and has achieved remarkable success in the hands of skilled refractive surgeons, there is no incisional technique known today that can compete with the theoretical precision of tissue removal made with the area ablation method of the excimer. The ability of the excimer laser to remove a uniform disk of tissue 0.3 μm per application far exceeds the precision that can be achieved by mechanical means. In this chapter we review data provided by the Tomey/ Computed Anatomy Topography Modeling System (TMS-1) videokeratoscope, with caveats on the use of PRK for myopia.

The outcome of keratorefractive surgery is judged by the final refractive status of the eye, and the predictability of a procedure is measured from the correspondence between induced and attempted change in refraction. While it is necessary to measure the change in refraction, changes in axial length or accommodation with time can confound interpretation. Additionally, change in refraction provides no information on the uniformity of the curvature change, the size of the optical zone, or the position of the treated area relative to the center of the pupil. These are all factors that may influence contrast sensitivity and produce glare or ghost images without altering the refractive status of the eye. Since keratorefractive surgery aims to modify corneal curvature, evaluation of the result would be most objectively accomplished by measuring its alteration directly. It is becoming apparent that keratometry is unable to faithfully represent central corneal curvature after refractive surgery because keratometer mires do not always fall within the treated area.[8] Therefore, an objective evaluation of a keratorefractive procedure, particularly when it is in the investigational phase, should include the full measurement of corneal topography using videokeratography.

THE TOMEY/COMPUTED ANATOMY TMS-1 VIDEOKERATOSCOPE

Placido disk photokeratoscopy was the origin of modern videokeratoscopy, but a number of important advances were made to adapt this technology for the automatic analysis of corneal contour over a fairly broad region of the surface.[9-17] Early efforts to computerize corneal topography analysis relied on manual digitization of keratoscope photographs,[9,10] an expensive and labor-intensive process, which demonstrated feasibility and utility, but required automation for widespread use. Such automation was first developed commercially by Computed Anatomy, Inc., New York, NY. who introduced video image capture, automatic mire acquisition, and a novel placido disk cone that projects mires onto a large area of the corneal surface without interference from the nose or orbital ridge.[12,13] The original Corneal Modeling System (CMS) measured topography plus corneal thickness profiles, but was streamlined into a much less expensive and compact unit, the TMS-1, which is shown in Figs. 7-1 and 7-2. The TMS-1 measures up to 6400 (25 rings) or 7680 (30 rings) points from the corneal surface depending on whether the interchangeable standard cone or the contact lens cone is being used. The standard cone makes measurements of its mire diameters on the corneal surface from 0.3 mm to 9.0 mm, while the contact lens cone measures an area 10.5 mm or more in diameter (these numbers are approximate since precise mire diameter is a function of corneal power). The accuracy and reproducibility of the TMS-1 has been measured independently[18,19] and its clinical usefulness and validity has been verified in hundreds of publications.

The primary method the TMS-1 uses for data presentation is the color-coded contour map of corneal surface power developed at LSU (Louisiana State University) Eye Center in New Orleans.[11] The raw data provided by the TMS-1 are the three-dimensional coordinates of the reconstructed corneal surface, which are used to calculate corneal curvature. Because of the large number of data points, graphical representation was necessary for clinical utility. Because the original clinical audience for this technology consisted of ophthalmologists, the curvature was expressed as power in diopters. The color-coded map employs two principles useful for diagnosis: (1) color association, where cool colors represent lower-than-normal powers, greens and yellows represent powers associated with the normal cornea, and warm colors represent higher-than-normal powers; and (2) pattern recognition, where, e.g., bow ties connote regular astigmatism, central flat areas connote myopic refractive surgery, and localized areas of corneal steepening connote keratoconus.

With this rationale, the color-coded map was first commercially implemented with the so-called *international standard* or *absolute scale,* which spanned corneal power ranges of 9 to over 100 D. Recently, Wilson and co-workers[20] have introduced a more practical scale (the *Klyce-Wilson Scale,* Fig. 7-3) ranging in equal 1.5-D intervals from 28.0 to 65.5 D. While it has been argued that a 1.5-D interval between contours is wide enough to mask irregularities in corneal topography, clinical study[20] showed that this interval provided sufficient sensitivity to make the correct topographic interpretation in 100% of the study cases, and, in addition, provided a range broad enough to cover all but advanced or unusual corneal abnormalities (advanced keratoconus, abnormally steep corneal grafts). While the TMS-1 has a very high radial spatial resolution (0.17-mm spacing between rings), the routine use of a fixed standard scale showing only adequate detail and not redundant information or extraneous (noise) data is essential to efficient and accurate clinical interpre-

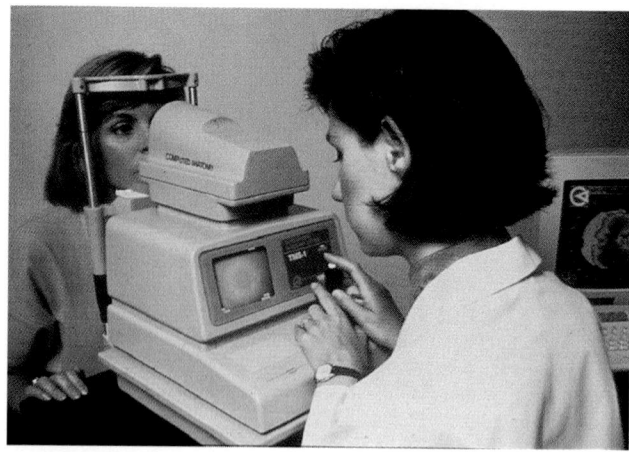

Fig. 7-1. The Tomey/Computed Anatomy Topography Modeling System (TMS-1).

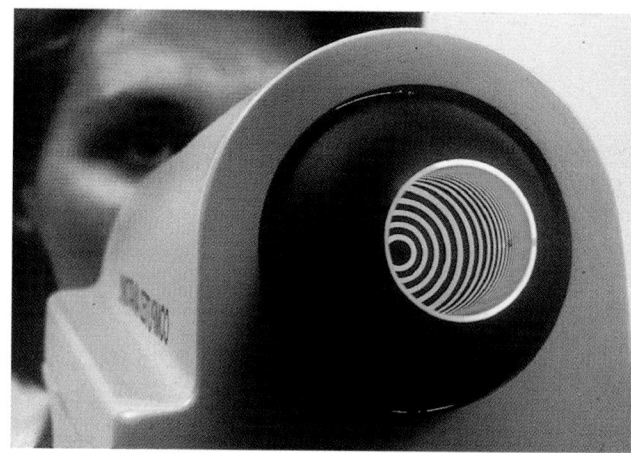

Fig. 7-2. The TMS-1 cone-shaped placido illuminator. The small size of the cone prevents peripheral corneal data loss that occurs with a standard faceplate keratoscope.

tation. A finer, higher-resolution contour interval can be selected; doing so will often reveal topographic features that are not of consequence to visual acuity, but their depiction may be used, e.g., to inspect the details of a refractive procedure. Nevertheless, in this chapter, videokeratograph illustrations are prepared with the same Klyce-Wilson Scale.

The color-coded map is a qualitative diagnostic aid in the sense that it masks information unnecessary for interpretation between the contour intervals. Therefore, to provide a quantitative adjunct to videokeratography, it is necessary to develop and present useful statistical indices from the entire processed data set. A variety of indices have been created, from simple values that simulate standard clinical keratometry (SimK values) to those which correlate the topography to the potential visual acuity of the eye.[21-23] In this way, objective characteristics of surgical procedures can be obtained; this objectivity is necessary in

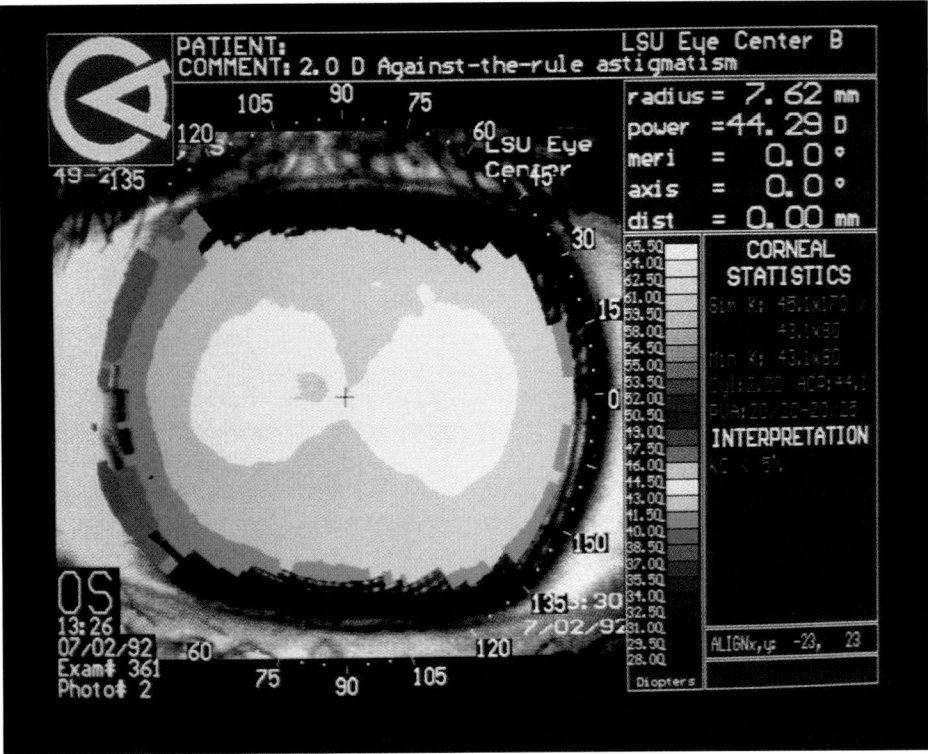

Fig. 7-3. The topography of a normal cornea illustrating the use of the Klyce-Wilson Standard Scale.[20] Note that this patient has 2.0 D of against-the-rule keratometric cylinder, and that this information is qualitatively evident in the videokeratograph. Quantitative values from corneal topography are obtained from statistics drawing their data from the raw numbers. Alternatively, a cursor is provided so that the power at any number of points on the cornea can be read directly.

order to use videokeratography scientifically in clinical research.

PREOPERATIVE SCREENING OF REFRACTIVE SURGICAL PATIENTS WITH TOPOGRAPHIC ANALYSIS

At LSU every keratorefractive surgical candidate undergoes preoperative screening with videokeratography as a routine element of the qualifying clinical tests. Originally, this screening was performed primarily because there was a need, during the early development phase of the excimer laser, to compare the quality of the excimer laser corneal ablation to current procedures used in keratorefractive surgical practice. During the succeeding clinical trials of phases IIA, IIB, and III, we continued screening candidates for PRK with videokeratography because PRK was an investigational procedure that needed preoperative data so that the change in corneal topography with time could be accurately ascertained. In the midst of these trials, we found a compelling reason for routine preoperative videokeratography screening for all refractive surgery candidates. During a training visit to a new excimer laser site abroad, we found that 8 of the 22 corneas presented as candidates for PRK at that site had

the topographic characteristics associated either with early keratoconus (with the attendant subtle clinical signs) or with keratoconus suspect (S.D. Klyce and M.B. McDonald, unpublished observation, 1991).

Subsequently, reports have appeared in the literature[24,25] that confirm the observation that a high percentage of candidates for keratorefractive surgery have clinical keratoconus. Whereas in the general population the incidence of keratoconus is quite small (1 in 2000, or 0.05%, has been reported[26]), in the patient population presenting for keratorefractive surgery, the incidence is orders of magnitude higher—as much as 6% to 12%. We hypothesize that patients with keratoconus, even those with preclinical keratoconus, select themselves into alternative forms of refractive correction, because even with subtle shape changes, often they are not satisfied with the vision they can achieve with spectacles, nor, perhaps, are they best candidates for contact lenses because an adequate fit to these corneas is not easily achieved.

Our grounds for excluding patients with clinical or preclinical keratoconus from keratorefractive surgery are straightforward. In addition to normal neural function and clear ocular media, good vision requires that the topography of the cornea be radially symmetric and free of irregular astigmatism, particularly those central areas of the cornea over the entrance pupil. Keratorefractive surgery achieves its success through the uniform flattening of the central cornea. When a surgical procedure produces irregular astigmatism (lamellar and full-thickness keratoplasties are good examples), the best achieved spectacles visual acuity is suboptimal. To achieve a good visual result, radial keratotomy relies upon the existence of a stable stromal thickness that is radially uniform. Performing radial keratotomy on an eye with keratoconus risks perforation in areas of stromal thinning and can induce or accelerate the onset of irregular corneal astigmatism. Performing excimer laser PRK on an eye with keratoconus has little risk of perforation, but the cornea can end with marked irregular astigmatism from progression of the keratoconus. Even though the same progression of keratoconus and irregular astigmatism could have occurred without the surgery, when the patient has been properly diagnosed and informed, the chances for disappointment to both surgeon and patient diminish. There have been indications in the literature, largely in articles lacking peer review, reporting successes with radial keratotomy on corneas with the topographic irregular astigmatisms associated with keratoconus. Such clinical judgment seems pre-

mature in the absence of a carefully controlled clinical trial.

An interesting hypothesis has been put forward[27] suggesting that the progressive hyperopia noted in 24% of the Prospective Evaluation of Radial Keratomy (PERK) study patients[28] might be due to the fact that PERK patients were not screened preoperatively with videokeratography. It will be interesting to observe the topography of the PERK patients during their 10-year postoperative follow-up to see if there is in fact any association between changes seen in patients with progressive hyperopia and topographic changes suggestive of progressive keratoconus.

Keratoconus suspects are most easily detected with videokeratography which is the most sensitive means for screening, irrespective of ongoing controversy.[29] Using the standard 1.5-D interval scale, keratoconus-suspect patients are easily found (Fig. 7-4) by looking for a local area of corneal steepening. Since many refractive surgeons have been taught to use different fixed or even variable dioptric scales, it may be difficult for them to learn what specific topographic alterations are consistent with keratoconus. Hence, automatic keratoconus detection schemes have been devised and validated for the TMS-1 to strengthen clinical opinion.[30]

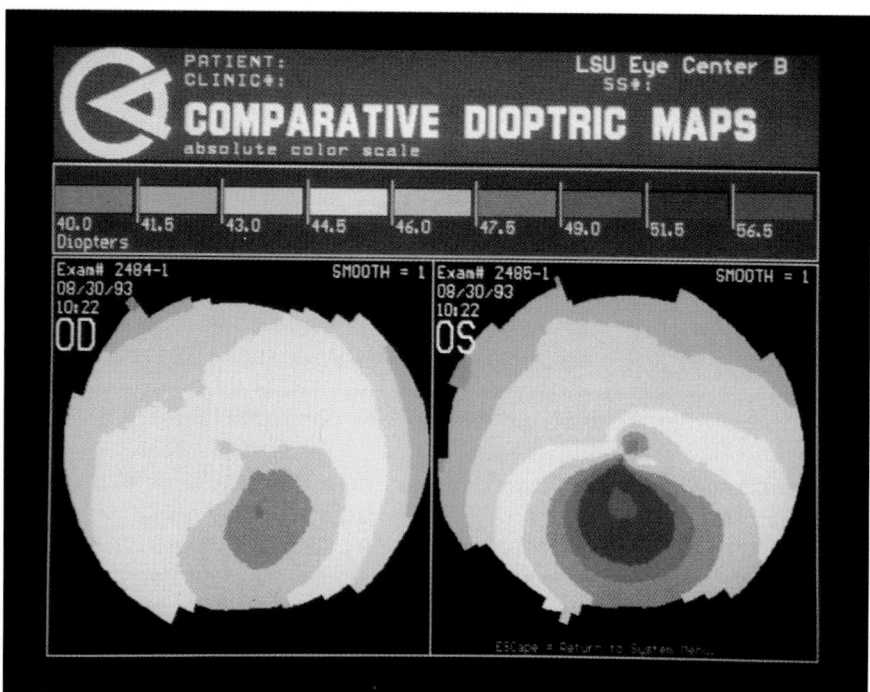

Fig. 7-4. Videokeratographs of the eyes of a keratoconus patient. The right eye has no accompanying usual clinical signs, while the topography indicates keratoconus suspect from the local area of corneal steepening. The left eye shows the topography consistent with early keratoconus and this eye does have signs of clinical keratoconus. Note that the 1.5-D scale has a resolution adequate to reliably detect the earliest keratoconic changes—a higher resolution scale is not necessary for this.

However, whenever the interpretation of keratoconus suspect is made from videokeratography (local area of corneal steepening, generally in the inferior half of the cornea), the possibility of pseudokeratoconus must also be considered. One form of pseudokeratoconus is found often in contact lens wearers who have with-the-rule corneal astigmatism and who have worn decentered contact lenses. This combination of factors can flatten the area of the cornea in the semimeridian under which the contact lens is displaced; the result can resemble keratoconus and can be topographically indistinguishable.[31] Such a case is presented in Fig. 7-5.

Contact lens warpage is a concern in the preoperative screening of refractive surgical patients, not only because warpage can resemble keratoconus but also because contact lens warpage can destabilize the refraction of the eye. While corneal curvature or more specifically, keratometry readings, are inputted to excimer laser computers to calculate the sequence for obtaining a given dioptric corrective, the keratometry readings themselves alter the calculations in a minor way. However, it has been established that contact lenses, both rigid and soft, can alter corneal curvature such that weeks must pass after discontinuance of contact lens wear before a stable refraction is achieved. For example, the average length of time for corneal curvature to stabilize in patients with rigid contact lens warpage was 15 weeks.[32] The change in corneal power was often over 1 D and there were examples of both flattening and steepening. Hence, to maximize predictability in a refractive surgical procedure, it is clear from this finding that, for patients with contact lens wear history, one should obtain repeated refractions, or better still, repeated videokeratographs, until stabilization has been achieved.

In summary, the screening of refractive surgery candidates for corneal ectatic disorders and other shape anomalies has been used routinely at the LSU Eye Center since 1984. Doing so, we have excluded a large number of patients with shape anomalies from receiving refractive surgery, because it was our opinion that neither the expectations of the surgeon nor those of the patient would be satisfied with this modality for attaining suitably long-term functional visual correction. Additionally, as part of the patient workup, patients who have a recent history of contact lens wear must discontinue lens wear and have two topographic examinations, 3 or 4 weeks apart, to confirm that the topography is both normal and stable.

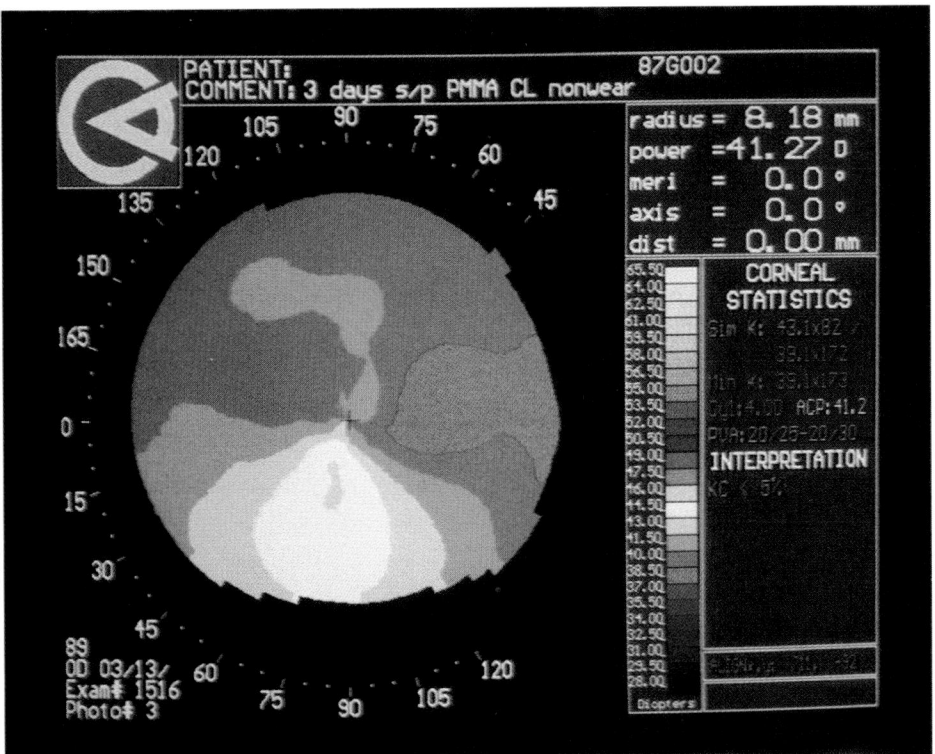

Fig. 7-5. The right eye of a patient with contact lens warpage, 3 days after not wearing a polymethylemthacrylate rigid contact lens. Note the local area of steepening which is also characteristic of keratoconus; this pattern can be differentiated from keratoconus by discontinuing lens wear and repeating examinations until the topography is stable. This patient's eye relaxed to a vertical bow-tie pattern (with-the-rule corneal astigmatism) in 4 months' time.

TOPOGRAPHIC ANALYSIS OF EXCIMER LASER PHOTOREFRACTIVE KERATECTOMY FOR MYOPIA

While we were not able to obtain reliable topography from initial excimer ablations with the rabbit eye,[33] subsequent efforts with monkey eyes[34] lent themselves to topographic analysis with our research topography system.[10,11] The early success with animal research enabled the five series or groups of patients treated with the excimer at the LSU Eye Center (blind eye series, n = 9; partially sighted series, n = 10; phase IIA sighted eyes, n = 19; phase IIB sighted eyes, n = 19; and phase III sighted eyes, n = 150; in 100 patients as of Feb. 11, 1994). Both corneas of every patient in these series were examined with the TMS-1 videokeratoscope or its earlier prototypes preoperatively and at 1-month and 3-month postoperative visits, and at 6-month intervals thereafter. In each series, significant new information was collected with the topographic data which led to refinements in both surgical approach as well as laser technology.

The LSU Blind Eye Series

For the earliest human studies, a prototype of the modern VISX Twenty-Twenty excimer laser was used, one that lacked the power capabilities and beam uniformly of the current-generation machine. The nine eyes that were included in the LSU Blind Eye study[3]

had attempted corrections as high as −11 D, but with ablation diameters as small as 4.25 mm to avoid removing more than the initial criterion of 50 μm of depth. While good alignment of the cornea during subsequent topographic analysis in these eyes was not possible, repeated examinations could be used to confirm the reliability of the measurements. These examinations could not be used to characterize certain topographic features such as adequacy of centration of the ablation. A few of these first corneas underwent vigorous remodeling with complete disappearance of the ablation within 13 weeks in one case, tempting speculation as to whether the addition of surface material was due to epithelial hyperplasia or to stromal remodeling.[3] However, stromal keratocytes are a considerably more dynamic cell population than had been known; they hastily depopulate the anterior stroma after epithelial removal and subsequently repopulate the stroma in pace with the epithelium as it re-covers the surface.[35]

While a certain amount of regression seemed to characterize some of the initial blind eye corneas, it is this series that has the longest follow-up, providing valuable information about stability. Fig. 7-6 shows an example of the time course of the topographic variation measured in the center of the ablation from an eye treated for the correction of −11 D. For 16 postoperative weeks, the eye sustained its full −11-D in-

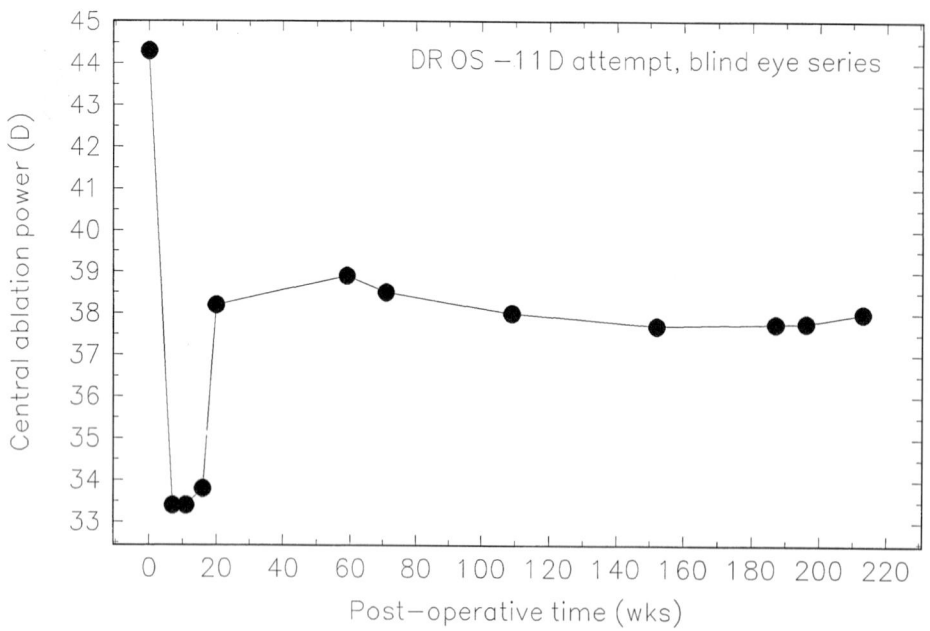

Fig. 7-6. Stability of corneal power measured with videokeratography. In the early blind eye series, powers of −11D were attempted. After the regression that occurred just before the 5-month examination topography remained stable beyond 4 years.

tended correction with central ablation power hovering near 33.5 D. Between weeks 16 and 20, a period of only 1 month, there was a 5-D regression such that at 5 months the central ablation power rose to 38.25 D. All but one of the subsequent central power readings with topography were within 0.25 D of the latter value out to the last examination on record, which occurred just over 4 years postoperatively. These data support the potential long-term stability of the excimer laser ablation as well as validate the reproducibility of the videokeratography equipment used to collect it.

The Initial LSU Sighted Eye Studies: Phases IIA and IIB

In the LSU phase IIA series, 19 eyes underwent myopic PRK for myopia with attempted corrections (at the corneal plane) ranging from −2.25 to −8.00 D.[6] Seventeen of these eyes were available for follow-up with the TMS-1.[36] In the LSU phase IIB Sighted Eye study, an additional 19 eyes were treated with attempted corrections ranging from −1.71 to −8.00 D. With the sighted eye series, it became possible to have reliable patient fixation during topographic examinations permitting quantitative and objective assessment of additional aspects of ablation topography. Corneal topography generally underwent a transition during the postoperative period from an early, 2- to 4-week

marked change in central corneal curvature through a gradual abatement to a stable level at 6 months (Fig. 7-7). The characteristics of the changes in the ablations with time were assessed by recording and plotting the power of the ablation centers postoperatively.[36] Importantly, the mean change in corneal surface powers at the center of the ablations closely matched the changes in manifest refractions for these patients, which provides an independent, objective verification of the clinical data, eliminating the possibility that progressive increases in axial length might be interpreted as a loss of effect. The characteristic decline from the initial overcorrection appears to have been greater for those eyes where the attempted correction was larger than −5.0 D.

Most, if not all, of the initial overcorrection could arise from the nature of epithelial regrowth. While the epithelium covers the corneal stroma after excimer laser ablation in 3 to 6 days, the central epithelium could remain thinner than normal for a period of time. A 20% reduction in central epithelial thickness for a 5-mm ablation is equal to a hyperopic shift of over 1 D.[37] However, it is also certain that in some, if not all, eyes, stromal wound healing can come into play with some tissue addition being associated with anterior stromal haze.

Once good patient fixation could be achieved with the initiation of the sighted eye series, it became pos-

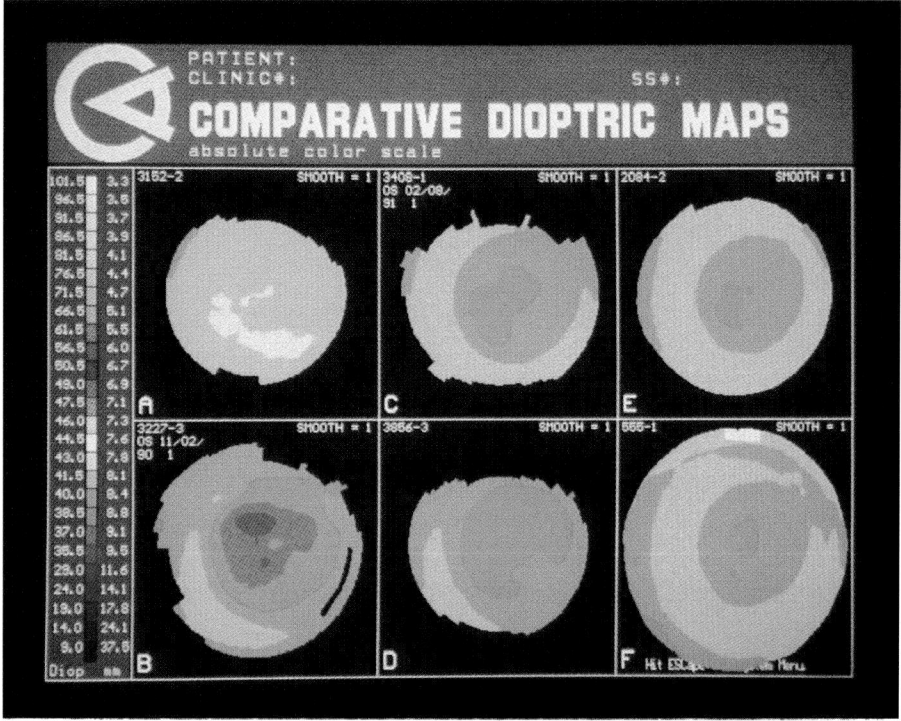

Fig. 7-7. An eye in the PRK phase IIB series is shown to illustrate the early hyperopic shift followed by stabilization. **A,** Preoperative examination. **B,** After 3 weeks. **C,** After 2 months. **D,** After 10 months. **E,** After 15 months. **F,** After 21 months.

sible to examine the issue of the centration of the treated area or optical zone. The optimal keratorefractive surgical procedure might be one that predictably alters the curvature of the entire cornea from limbus to limbus. Even radial keratotomy, which is often believed to achieve large area effective zones, cannot achieve this ideal and encroachment on the paracentral stroma produces the starburst visual complaint. With the excimer laser, the amount of energy required to perform area photoablation increases with the square of the radius of the treated zone; a small increase in ablation diameter results in a large increase in the required energy that can reach the technical limitations of available excimer laser sources and their associated delivery systems. Additionally, in order to treat high myopia, it is necessary either to greatly reduce the size of the optical zone or to remove tissue beyond the initial conservation ablation depth in the stroma of 50 μm.

Refractive surgical procedures were initially centered over the line of sight; however, it is now generally accepted that the optical zone should be centered over the entrance pupil, as rigorously demonstrated by Uozato and Guyton.[38] Maloney[39] emphasized that keratorefractive surgical procedures should be centered on the virtual pupil while the patient is fixating coaxilly with the surgeon. He predicted that a small or decentered optical zone could decrease visual acuity, reduce contrast sensitivity scores, or produce glare phenomena. With a 4-mm effective optical zone, Maloney calculated that 16% of the incident rays would fall outside of the pupil with just 0.5 mm of decentration.[39]

Several measurements of excimer ablation centration have appeared in the literature. In the LSU phase IIA series,[36] ablation decentration was found to average 0.88 ±0.11 mm from the line of sight and 0.79

±0.11 mm from the center of the pupil (Fig. 7-8, *A*). Decentration was less than 0.5 mm in three eyes, 0.5 to 1.0 mm in ten eyes, 1.0 to 1.5 mm in three eyes, and 2.1 mm in one eye. There were no systematic decentration errors detectable from the average values of decentration that could implicate a procedural bias or equipment misalignment. Additionally, in this early series there was no learning curve with the associated reduction in decentration with surgeon experience.[40] However, when these data were examined retrospectively with vector analysis, an apparent alignment overcompensation was found in the direction of the pupil center from the line of sight[41] (Fig. 7-9). In another early series of five eyes, Maguire and associates[42] reported an average decentration of 1.14 mm from the center of the pupil.

A great deal of additional attention was subsequently given to alignment during the LSU phase IIB series (19 eyes were followed with topographic analysis) with a marked improvement in ablation alignment (Fig. 7-8, *B*). For the LSU phase IIB eyes, the average distance of the ablation centers was 0.47 ±0.06 mm from the center of the pupil. Others using the TMS-1 report similar alignment averages for recent PRK series. Cavanaugh and associates[43] report an average decentration from the line of sight of 0.52 mm in 110 patients treated with the Summit Technology excimer laser, which, when translated to distance from the pupil, would amount to an estimate of 0.43 mm. Lin and associates[44] report average decentration of 0.36 ±0.25 (mean ±SD; n=97). When the latter investigators analyzed their data on the basis of including only the last 20 eyes, the results improved to 0.20 ±0.15 mm. These excellent results were obtained with voluntary patient fixation (after the first 13 eyes) and the VISX excimer laser. Hence, it appears that with careful attention to procedure and detail, excellent centration of the exci-

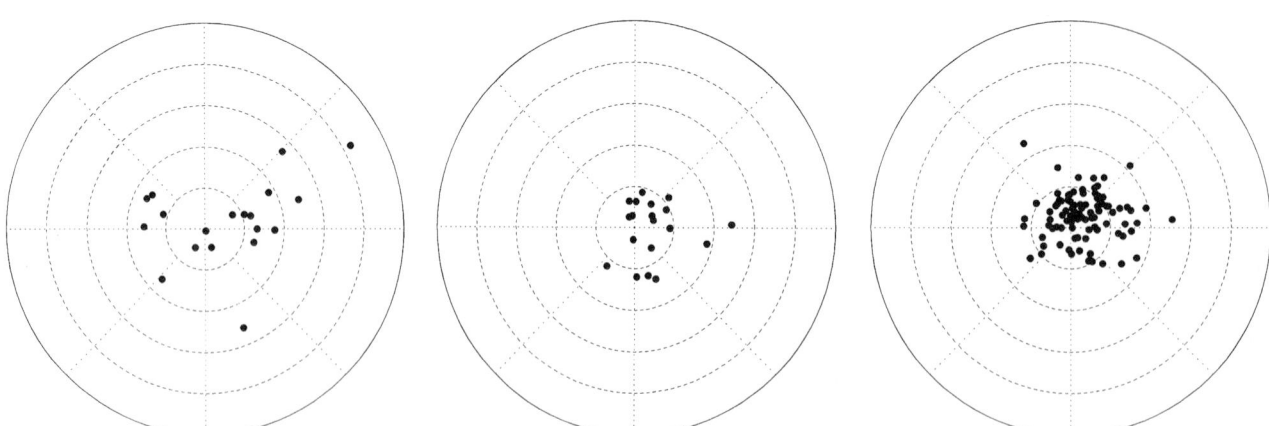

Fig. 7-8. Polar plots of the center of ablations relative to the center of the entrance pupil measured with the TMS-1. **A,** PRK phase IIA. **B,** PRK phase IIB. **C,** PRK phase III. The grids are spaced 0.5 mm apart on all three graphs. Note the improvement in centration between each series. No consistent offset was found.

mer laser ablation can be achieved. However, even with the greatest preparation and skill, ablations that are more than 1 mm from the center of the pupil still occur.

All of the patients at LSU were treated with the use of the VISX handpiece to align the eye during surgery (surgeon fixation), while other centers most often employed patient voluntary alignment during treatment (patient fixation). There has been considerable controversy regarding the merits of each approach, much of it based on anecdotal information. While it can be shown that the differences between some of the decentration averages presented above are statistically significant, this information cannot be used to judge which type of fixation might be superior. There are differences in lasers and in alignment techniques among investigators, in addition to fixation technique. However, with attention paid to the centration issue, it appears that the earlier large amounts of decentration are avoidable with either technique.

The extent of decentration is probably a combination of technique and a lower boundary of achievable alignment. It is clear from the second-generation results of the most skillful surgeons, that better alignment aids and techniques would be welcomed by future apprentices to this procedure. In our preliminary data analysis of centration while following our ongoing phase III patients, it is interesting to note that there may be a tendency for the left-handed surgeon to achieve better centration on left eyes than on right eyes (Fig. 7-10). In measurements made from 38 left

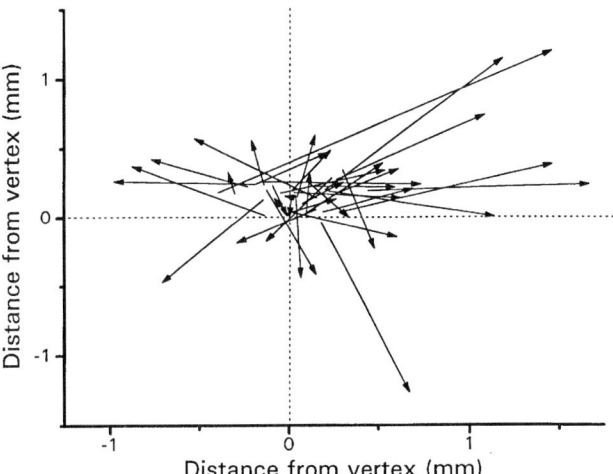

Fig. 7-9. *Arrows* are used to indicate the position of the pupil center *(tail)* and the position of the ablation center *(head)* for PRK phase IIA and IIB patients. The graph origin lies on the vertex normal, the point at which keratoscopes are aligned. The data indicate bias in alignment leading to overcompensation for pupil offset (P = .0023). (Data from Gardner, Klyce, Thompson, et al: Centration of photorefractive keratectomy: topographic assessment, *Invest Ophthalmol Vis Sci* 34:803, 1993.)

eyes, decentration from the pupil averaged 0.37 ±0.21 mm, whereas in 56 right eyes, decentration averaged 0.49 ±0.25 mm. The difference between the means was statistically significant (P = .017).

With either fixation approach there will be a small, but potentially significant amount of translational motion (vibration or jiggle). With patient fixation, there will be the inevitable microsaccadic eye movements, with excursions of 0.1 to 0.2 mm or more. These should, however, average out to a very small number. Likewise, with surgeon fixation there will be some translational error as the eye is maintained in position against patient motion and vibration (in males, the heart beat is often strong enough to produce periodic oscillations during surgery). Hence, with either technique for stabilizing the eye during surgery, the minor motions or vibrations should average out. These might result in a minor smoothing effect, similar to that proposed by Krueger and associates,[45] that would occur by blurring the focus of the laser at the plane of the iris diaphragm to achieve a smoother cut.

As noted above, decentration of the treated zone can be expected to have visual consequences. A reduction in visual acuity could well occur, especially if a large portion of the entrance pupil were rendered multifocal by decentration. However, we[40] found no correlation between the LSU PRK phase IIA centration data and the best corrected spectacles visual acuity of the patients. In fact, one patient with the greatest decentration of 2.1 mm had an acuity of 20/20 at 6 months and 1 year postoperatively. This finding is consistent with the results of Lin and colleagues.[44] Cavanaugh and associates[43] claim there is a decrease in visual acuity with decentration, but in the absence of any supporting statistical evidence, their contention must be considered hypothetical.

One can propose a reasonable hypothesis why decentration may not degrade Snellen acuity. Decentration will produce a narrow band of multifocal power across the pupil, plus, with a large amount of decentration, a more peripheral region of native corneal power from the area beyond the ablation. We have found in our studies[46] that with irregular astigmatism, the visual acuity of the eye will correlate with the regularity of those parts of the corneal topography within the entrance pupil of the eye that are within 1 D of the most frequently occurring power. Hence, for this application one might predict that a 4-mm ablation decentered from the pupil by 2 mm would result in bifocal vision with no loss of visual acuity (high-frequency components of contrast sensitivity), but a reduction in middle-frequency contrast sensitivity, plus, in the specific case of a bifocal cornea, ghost images and halos. As pointed out by Baron and Munnerlyn[47] halos and ghost images cannot be assessed

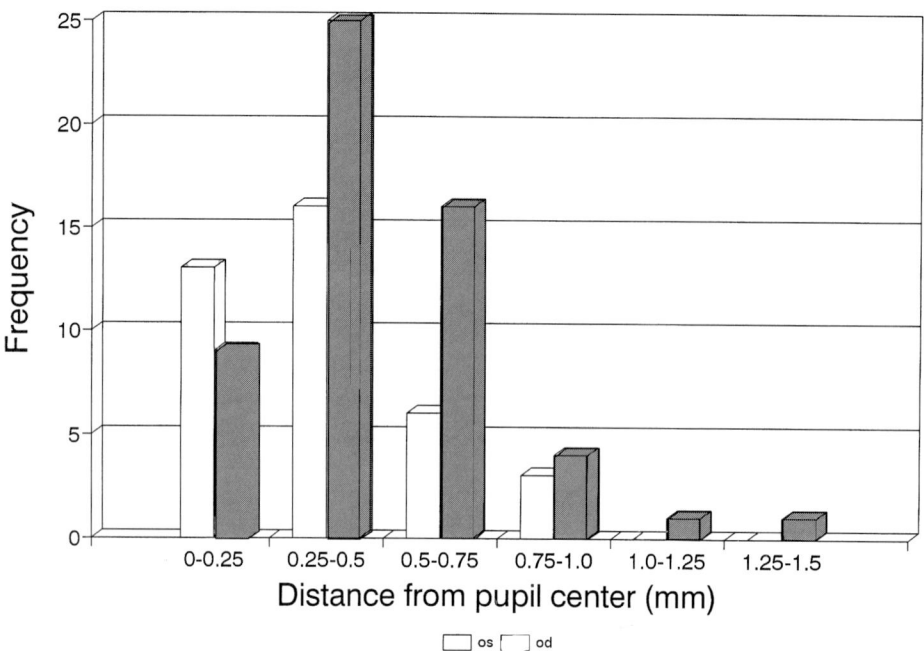

PRK III Decentration
Frequency Distribution

Fig. 7-10. The PRK phase III patients exhibited a small difference in the average centration between the left and right eyes. Centration appeared to be better for the left eye with manual fixation; the surgeon is left-handed.

with acuity or contrast sensitivity tests. Maguire[48] asserts that the characteristics of the optical aberrations that may be produced in keratorefractive surgery must be measured with more sensitive and appropriate indicators; perhaps this task will be accomplished with new quantitative parameters drawn from videokeratography.

The effects of a small optical zone and decentration have varied psychophysical interpretations. A clinical trial with the Summit Technology UV200 excimer laser performed in the United Kingdom used 4-mm-diameter optical zones.[49] Under ordinary daytime conditions, the adult human pupil will average 4 to 5 mm in diameter and the healing process itself will often reduce the size of the effective optical zone below that of the intended. In this study 78% of the patients reported a halo effect at night. This halo occurrence is not a diffraction phenomenon, as is Sattler's veil, which is caused by epithelial edema,[50] but is said to result from the refraction of light from untreated areas of the cornea that overlie the entrance pupil of the eye. This particular type of halo was thought to occur anytime the ablation diameter was smaller than the active pupil or with marked decentration of the laser procedure. The halo experience diminished with time, which probably was related to neural adaptation. Corneal topographic assessment of this series was not pro-

vided; this objective correlate would have been a powerful tool with which to support the concluding hypothetical origin of the psychometric evaluation.

The LSU Sighted Eye Study: Phase III

In the LSU phase III series, 152 eyes from 108 patients had been treated at the time that data were collected for this chapter. As with phases IIA and IIB, centration of the ablations has been measured in all treated eyes where possible. The average distance from the center of the pupil in 94 eyes of phase III patients was 0.44 ±0.23 mm (Fig. 7-8, C), not significantly different from the 0.47-mm average reported for phase IIB.

Phase III excimer patient topography was uneventful for a number of months. Centration was less of an issue and attention turned toward the stromal haze issue and the possible association of the haze with regression. To search for possible correlations between haze, keratocyte activation, and subsequent stromal remodeling, we examined the ultrastructure of the ablated stromal surface, with and without the N$_2$ purge gas, which is used with the original VISX eye fixation handpiece. We found that the corneal stromal surface of rabbit eyes, ablated with the normal high flow of N$_2$ purge gas, exhibited a periodic spicular appearance with anatomic dimensions on the order of 2 to 4

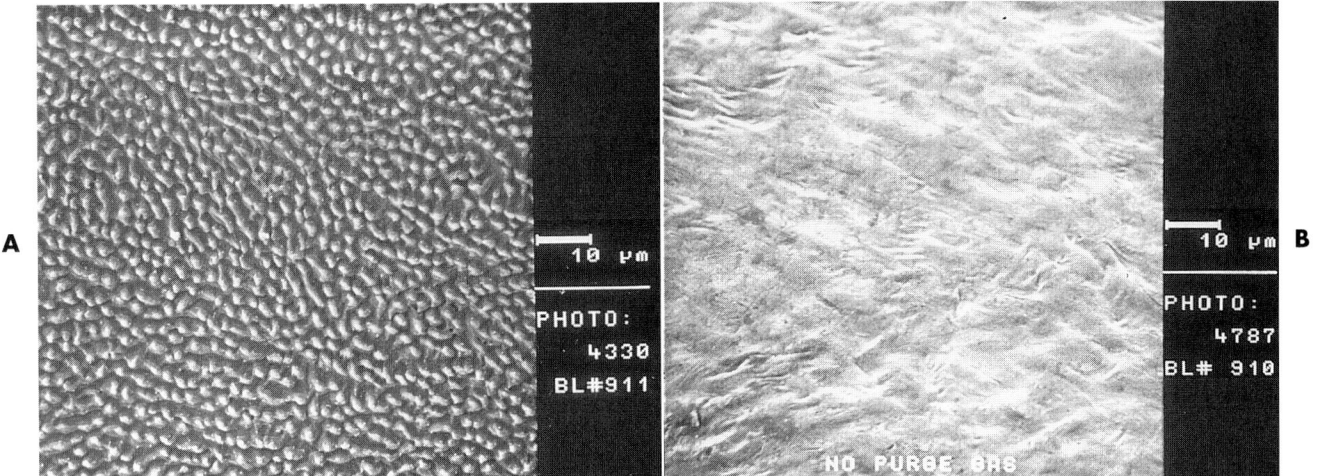

Fig. 7-11. Scanning electron microscopy of the rabbit corneal stroma after excimer laser ablation. **A,** The stromal surface with N_2 purging at 10 cfm through the handpiece. The spicules are related to drying of the surface while ablating, apparently a material property of the connective tissue. **B,** A second rabbit eye treated with the laser, but without purge gas.

μm (Fig. 7-11, *A*). Features of these dimensions are sufficient by themselves to cause light scatter and haze, although the normal reepithelialization process leads to their disappearance. When the rabbit corneal stroma was ablated without purge gas, there was a smooth surface, absent of the spicules (Fig. 11, *B*). As a result of this observation, a number of treatments were done without the steady N_2 purge. However, irregular astigmatism in the form of a nearly central elevation in corneal power was noted in a substantial number of eyes treated without purge gas; this feature was termed a *central island.*[51] These observations are not singular; Lin and his colleagues[44] have published excellent examples of central islands. Whereas phase IIA, IIB, and early phase III ablations were characterized by topographically uniform ablations (Fig. 7-12), when no purge gas was used to evacuate the plume of ejecta from the stromal surface and to provide a uniform atmosphere over the corneal surface, irregular astigmatism appeared in the form of contiguous elevations of corneal power within the treated zone of the cornea. A typical example of this anomaly is shown in Fig. 7-13.

In our attempt to determine the cause of the central island, we examined its appearance within the LSU phase III patients in a serial fashion using difference maps of the change in topography before and after treatment provided by the TMS-1. Using the criterion of a contiguous feature being present that was 1 D or greater than the surrounding stroma and more than 1 mm in diameter on the cornea, we found a positive correlation between the presence and absence of the purge gas (Table 7-1). We have also examined the occurrence sequence of the islands (Fig. 7-14), with the observation that for a given set of conditions, their presence or absence was apparently random. Within

a single treatment group on a single day, there were some patients with notable irregular astigmatism and others with high uniformity, which argues against there being a failure of the laser optics, at least in the LSU patients. With no purge gas flow, we have observed the formation of a vortex of ejected material rising randomly and sporadically from the corneal surface which one can liken to a tornadic condition. The presence of a contained vortex of material would possibly be centrally located and would therefore reduce laser efficiency in that region. The fixation handpiece might be suspected, but others using the VISX laser treat patients without the handpiece and find central islands. Other hypotheses have been proposed such as the excimer occasionally firing in a different mode—this would fit the random character of the islands. Machat (personal communication) theorizes that the shock wave from successive pulses causes pooling of fluid centrally, but it is hard to reconcile this notion with the random character of central island formation. A novel and unpredictable wound healing of the epithelium could occur, but how would blowing vigorously on the surface eliminate this biological response? As a result, we have returned to using purge gas at a low flow rate as a compromise between potential haze formation and central island formation. However, as one can see from Fig. 7-14, there is still a bothersome occurrence of central islands that frustrates comprehension.

Central islands of sufficient size can contribute to irregular astigmatism and a reduction in the achieved dioptric correction. It is important to note, however, that when these observations first came before the keratorefractive surgical community, many examples of irregular astigmatism in ablations from corneal to-

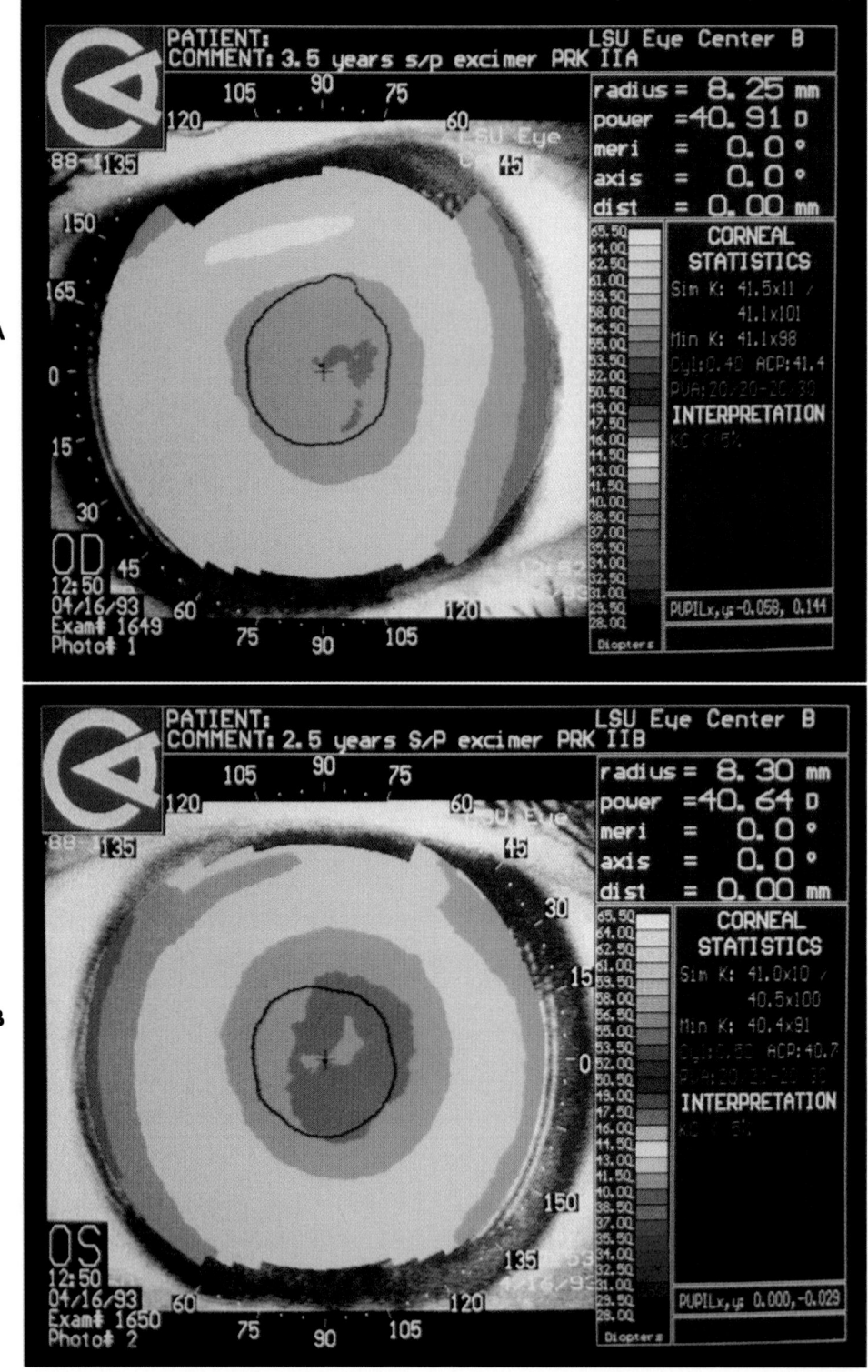

Fig. 7-12. Examples of the ideal result with the excimer laser. The ablations are well centered over the pupil and are uniform. Note that the statistics are all green, which means that the values obtained are +2 SD from normals. **A,** The right eye 3½ years postoperatively from PRK phase IIA. **B,** The left eye of the same patient 2½ years postoperatively from phase IIB.

pographic analysis were brought to our attention. A majority of those cases presented with low contour interval scales of 1.0 D or less. It is important to note that topographic irregularities observed with contour intervals less than 1.5 D will often not be of clinical significance or of consequence to visual acuity.[20] Hence, additional studies are needed to analyze the amount of irregular astigmatism within the treated zone and to correlate this with predictability, visual acuity, contrast sensitivity, and psychophysical phenomena (halos) in order to understand the impact of central islands.

PREDICTIONS FOR THE FUTURE AND CONCLUSIONS

From the perspective of corneal topography analysis with the TMS-1, it is clear that excimer laser area ablation has enormous potential for becoming the

standard keratorefractive surgical procedure for the correction of low to moderate amounts of myopia. One can forecast that procedures or medication will be discovered to inhibit stromal remodeling or perhaps even encourage it in a controlled fashion to tune up overcorrections. And with this ability, investigators would be encouraged to be more adventurous in developing methods for the stable correction of high myopia.

What are the limitations to the correction of high myopia with tissue subtraction techniques? Can one ablate 250 μm of Bowman's membrane plus stroma and avoid the slow appearance of corneal ectasia due to a reorganization of the stromal lamellae? These questions await resolution and a careful vigil with the TMS-1 is in order.

The ablation centration problem needs to be resolved to enable productive skills transfer. Epikeratophakia for the correction of myopia had enormous success among a small number of highly talented surgeons. The excimer laser procedure needs a simple and effective alignment aid to be developed for ease of learning.

What of the central irregular astigmatism that has intruded on the previously uniform curvature of the corneal stroma? One cannot ignore the fact that the LSU incidence of central islands was virtually nonex-

Table 7-1. Central islands in photorefractive keratectomy*

Purge	−	±	+
On (n = 57)	46 (81%)	11 (19%)	0 (0%)
Off (n = 22)	4 (18%)	12 (55%)	6 (27%)
Low (n = 40)	33 (83%)	5 (12%)	2 (5%)

*+ = island; ± = minor irregularity; − = uniform ablation.

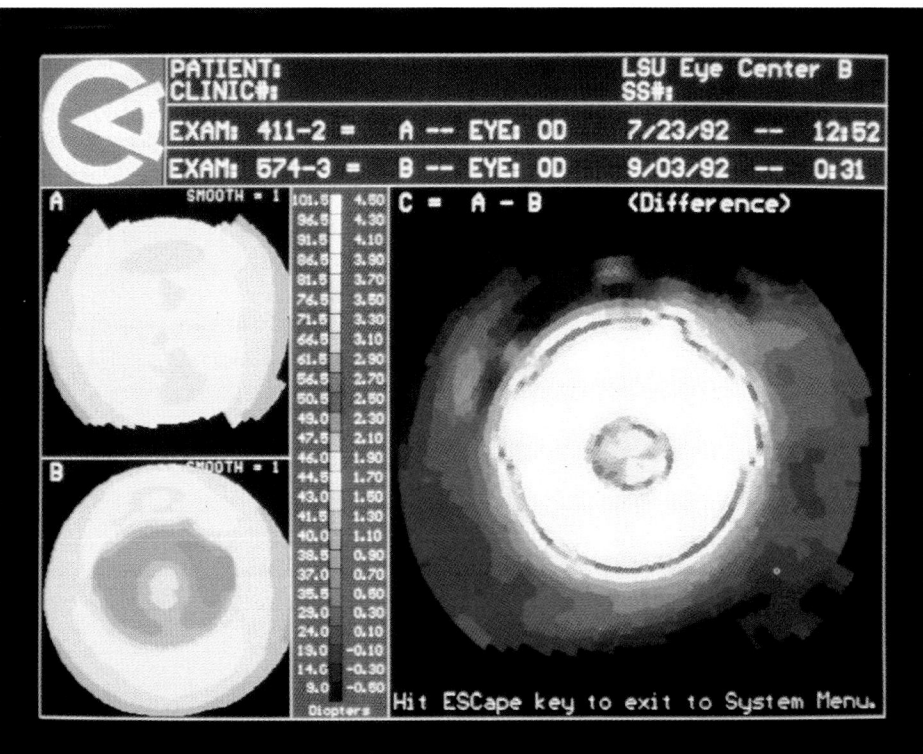

Fig. 7-13. Difference plot of patient from PRK phase III with a notable central island. **A,** Preoperative topography. **B,** Same eye 5 weeks postoperatively. **C,** A–B from a point by subtraction.

istent until the N_2 purge gas was eliminated or reduced. We can predict that this problem will be resolved; doing so is necessitated by the quest for a predictable, crisp visual result.

Real-time corneal topographic analysis may find its way to the operating room to guarantee the accuracy of laser sculpting, although in our experience with the calibration modalities available with the VISX system, this added control should not be necessary. On the other hand, there are other laser systems being used and developed which do not produce test blocks smooth enough for immediate preoperative evaluation and equipment calibration, and for these machines intraoperative topographic assessment is recommended for safety and assurance of efficacy.

Quantitative descriptors of corneal optical performance, such as the Surface Regularity Index (SRI), will be strengthened by incorporation of pupil size and relative ablation location considerations. New funda-

mental aspects of visual function could result from the development of spatially resolved refractometry and comparison to corneal topography.[52] The ray tracing model provided by Maguire and colleagues[42] could be refined and implemented on topography equipment so that patient vision can be simulated in the clinic, which will be particularly valuable for diagnosis and evaluation when visual anomalies such as diplopia are experienced.

The excimer laser procedure developed for the correction of myopia has a resolution of 0.3 μm per cut. What other knife could the ophthalmologist control that would offer such precision? The potential of the excimer laser for PRK has been carefully evaluated and scrutinized with the most powerful and sensitive tool available: videokeratography. Topographic evidence suggests that PRK for myopia provides as good or better optical quality than radial keratotomy. There is no other keratorefractive surgical procedure available today that has undergone such scrutiny. Corneal

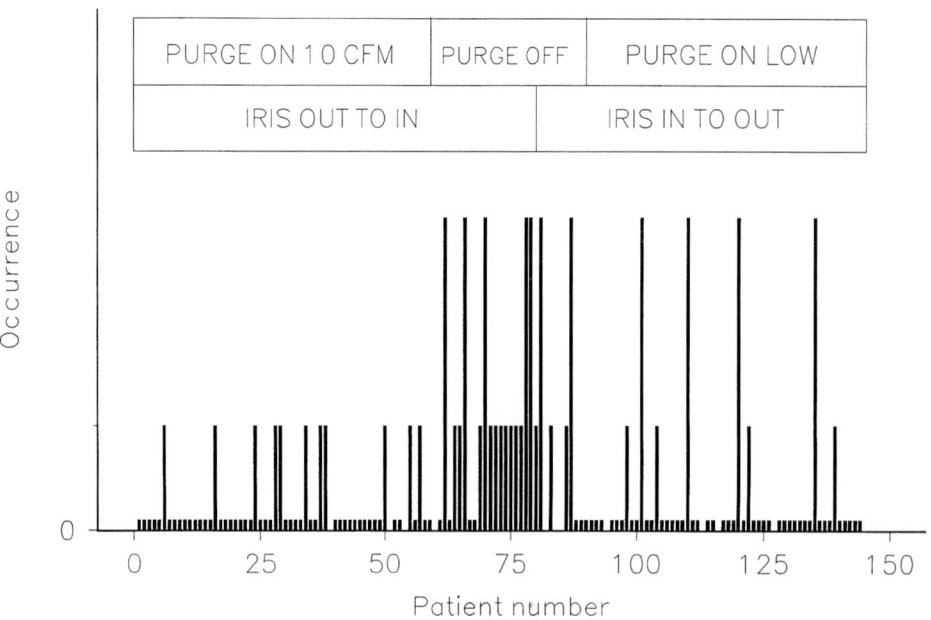

Fig. 7-14. The occurrence sequence of central islands from the PRK phase III eyes. All patients were examined at 1 to 3 months postoperatively with difference maps of the type shown in Fig. 7-13. About halfway through this series, VISX upgraded the laser and changed the iris diaphragm program from closure to opening. The *tall bars* indicate the presence of a contiguous topographic feature (island or, rarely, peninsula) within the ablation zone more than 1 D higher than the surround and greater than 1 mm in diameter. The *intermediate-sized bars* represent those corneas with a moderate amount of irregular astigmatism within the treated zone, and the *short bars* represent ablations that were highly uniform. Note that this is a subjective evaluation, and that a 1-D island, 1 mm in diameter, may not have a visual consequence. Nevertheless, the phenomenon needs resolution.

topographic analysis has achieved for radial keratotomy and PRK its intended goal: improving refractive surgery for the benefit of our patients.

REFERECNES

1. L'Esperance FA, Taylor DM, Warner JW: Human excimer laser lamellar keratectomy: short-term histopathology, *J Refract Surg* 4:118-124, 1988.
2. Taylor DM, L'Esperance FA, Del Pero RA, et al: Human excimer laser lamellar keratectomy: a clinical study, *Ophthalmology* 96:654-664, 1989.
3. McDonald MB, Frantz JM, Klyce SD, et al: Central photorefractive keratectomy for myopia. The blind eye study, *Arch Ophthalmol* 108:799-808, 1990.
4. Seiler T, Kahle G, Kriegerowski M: Excimer laser (193 nm) myopic keratomileusis in sighted and blind human eyes, *Refract Corneal Surg* 6:165-173, 1990.
5. Gartry DS, Muir MGK, Marshall J: Photorefractive keratectomy with an argon fluoride excimer laser: a clinical study, *Refract Corneal Surg* 7:420-435, 1991.
6. McDonald MB, Liu JC, Byrd TJ, et al: Central photorefractive keratectomy for myopia: partially sighted and normally sighted eyes, *Ophthalmology* 98:1327-1337, 1991.
7. Zabel RW, Sher NA, Ostrov CS, et al: Myopic excimer laser keratectomy: a preliminary report, *Refract Corneal Surg* 6:329-334, 1990.
8. Cantera E, Cantera I, Olivieri L: Corneal topographic analysis of photorefractive keratectomy in 175 myopic eyes, *Refract Corneal Surg* 9(suppl):S19-22, 1993.
9. Doss JD, Hutson RL, Rowsey JJ, et al: Method for the calculation of corneal profile and power distribution, *Arch Ophthalmol* 99:1261-1265, 1981.
10. Klyce SD: Computer-assisted corneal topography: high resolution graphical presentation and analysis of keratoscopy, *Invest Ophthalmol Vis Sci* 25:1426-1435, 1984.
11. Maguire LJ, Singer DE, Klyce SD: Graphic presentation of computer-analyzed keratoscope photographs, *Arch Ophthalmol* 105:223-230, 1987.
12. Gormley DJ, Gersten M, Koplin RS, et al: Corneal modeling, *Cornea* 7:30-35, 1988.
13. Mammone RJ, Gersten M, Gormley DJ, et al: 3-D corneal modeling system, *IEEE Trans Biomed Eng* 37:66-72, 1990.
14. Arffa RC, Warnicki JW, Rehkopf PG: Corneal topography using rasterstereography, *Refract Corneal Surg* 5:414-417, 1989.
15. Belin MW, Litoff D, Strods, SJ, et al: The PAR technology corneal topography system. *Refract Corneal Surg* 8:88-96, 1992.
16. El Hage SG: A computerized corneal topographer for use in refractive surgery, *Refract Corneal Surg* 5:418-423, 1989.
17. Koch DD, Foulks GN, Moran CT, et al: The Corneal EyeSys System: accuracy analysis and reproducibility of first generation prototype, *Refract Corneal Surg* 5:424-429, 1989.
18. Hannush SB, Crawford SL, Waring GO, et al: Accuracy and precision of keratometry, photokeratoscopy, and corneal modeling on calibrated steel balls, *Arch Ophthalmol* 107:1235-1239, 1989.
19. Wilson SE, Verity SM, Conger DL: Accuracy and precision of the corneal analysis system and the topographical analysis system, *Cornea* 11:28-35, 1992.
20. Wilson SE, Klyce SD, Husseini ZM: Standardized color-coded maps for corneal topography, *Ophthalmology* 100:1723-1727, 1993.
21. Dingeldein SA, Klyce SD, Wilson SE: Quantitative descriptors of corneal shape derived from computer-assisted analysis of photokeratographs, *Refract Corneal Surg* 5:372-378, 1989.
22. Wilson SE, Klyce SD: Quantitative descriptors of corneal topography: a clinical study, *Arch Ophthalmol* 109:349-353, 1991.
23. Maeda N, Klyce SD, Hamano H: Alteration of corneal asphericity in RGP contact lens-induced warpage, *CLAO J* 20:27-31, 1994.
24. Nesburn AB, Bahri S, Berlin M, et al: Computer assisted corneal topography (CACT) to detect mild keratoconus (KC) in candidates for photorefractive keratectomy, *Invest Ophthalmol Vis Sci* 33(suppl):995, 1992.
25. Wilson SE, Klyce SD: Screening for corneal topographic abnormalities prior to refractive surgery, *Ophthalmology* 101:147-152, 1994.
26. Kennedy RH, Bourne WM, Dyer JA: A 48-year clinical and epidemiologic study of keratoconus, *Am J Ophthalmol* 101:267-273, 1986.
27. Saragoussi JJ, Pouliquen YJM: Does the progressive increasing effect of radial keratotomy (hyperopic shift) correlate with undetected early keratoconus?, *Refract Corneal Surg* 10:45-48, 1994.
28. Waring GO, Lynn MJ, Kutner MH: Stability of refraction after refractive keratotomy. In Waring GO, editor: *Refractive keratotomy for myopia and astigmatism,* St Louis, 1992, Mosby–Year Book.
29. Rabinowitz YS, Klyce SD, Krachmer J, et al: Opinions. Keratoconus, videokeratography, and refractive surgery, *Refract Corneal Surg* 8:403-407, 1992.
30. Maeda N, Klyce SD, Smolek MK, Thompson HW: Automated keratoconus screening with corneal topography analysis. *Invest Ophthalmol Vis Sci* (in press).
31. Wilson SE, Lin DTC, Klyce SD, et al: Rigid contact lens decentration–a risk factor for corneal warpage, *CLAO J* 16:177-182, 1990.
32. Wilson SE, Lin DTC, Klyce SD, et al: Topographic changes in contact lens-induced corneal warpage, *Ophthalmology* 97:734-744, 1990.
33. McDonald MB, Beuerman R, Falzoni W, et al: Refractive surgery with the excimer laser, *Am J Ophthalmol* 103:469, 1987.
34. McDonald MB, Frantz JM, Klyce SD, et al: One year refractive results of central photorefractive keratectomy for myopia in the nonhuman primate cornea, *Arch Ophthalmol* 108:40-47, 1990.
35. Crosson CE: Cellular changes following epithelial abrasion. In Beuerman RW, Crosson CE, Kaufman HE, editors: *Healing processes in the cornea.* Woodlands, 1989, Portfolio, 3-14.
36. Wilson SE, Klyce SD, McDonald MB, et al: Changes in corneal topography after excimer laser photorefractive keratectomy for myopia, *Ophthalmology* 98:1338-1347, 1991.
37. Colliac JP, Shammas HJ, Bart DJ: Photorefractive keratectomy for the correction of myopia and astigmatism, *Am J Ophthalmol* 117:369-380, 1994.
38. Uozato H, Guyton DL: Centering corneal surgical procedures, *Am J Ophthalmol* 103:264-275, 1987.
39. Maloney RK: Corneal topography and optical zone location in photorefractive keratectomy, *Refract Corneal Surg* 6:363-371, 1990.
40. Klyce SD, Smolek MK: Corneal topography of the excimer photorefractive keratectomy, *J Cataract Refract Surg* 19(suppl):122-130, 1993.
41. Gardner BP, Klyce SD, Thompson HW, et al: Centration of photorefractive keratectomy: topographic assessment, *Invest Ophthalmol Vis Sci* 34:803, 1993.
42. Maguire LJ, Zabel RW, Parker P, et al: Topography and raytracing analysis of patients with excellent visual acuity 3 months after excimer laser photorefractive keratectomy for myopia, *Refract Corneal Surg* 7:122-128, 1991.
43. Cavanaugh TB, Durrie DS, Riedel SM, et al: Centration of exci-

mer laser photorefractive keratectomy relative to the pupil, *J Cataract Refract Surg* 19(suppl):144-148, 1993.

44. Lin DT, Sutton HF, Berman M: Corneal topography following excimer photorefractive keratectomy for myopia, *J Cataract Refract Surg* 19(suppl):149-154, 1993.

45. Krueger RR, Wang XW, Rudisill M, et al: Diffractive smoothing of excimer laser ablation using a defocused beam, *Refract Corneal Surg* 10:20-26, 1994.

46. Wilson SE, Klyce SD: Quantitative descriptors of corneal topography: a clinical study, *Arch Ophthalmol* 109:349-353, 1991.

47. Baron WS, Munnerlyn C: Predicting visual performance following excimer photorefractive keratectomy, *Refract Corneal Surg* 8:355-362, 1992.

48. Maguire LJ: Keratorefractive surgery, success, and the public health, *Am J Ophthalmol* 117:394-398, 1994.

49. Gartry DS, Muir MGK, Marshall J: Photorefractive keratectomy with an argon fluoride excimer laser: a clinical study, *Refract Corneal Surg* 7:420-435, 1991.

50. Lambert SR, Klyce SD: The origins of Sattler's veil, *Am J Ophthalmol* 91:51-56, 1981.

51. Parker PJ, Klyce SD, Ryan BL, et al: Central topographic islands following photorefractive keratectomy, *Invest Ophthalmol Vis Sci* 34:803, 1993.

52. Webb R, Penney CM, Thompson KP: Measurement of ocular local wave front distortion with a spatially resolved refractometer, *Appl Optics* 31:3678-3686, 1992.

8

Computerized Corneal Topography of Surface Ablations with the EyeSys System

Daniel S. Durrie, Donald R. Sanders, D. James Schumer

EyeSys HARDWARE AND SOFTWARE

Corneal topography is now considered essential in the evaluation and management of the excimer photoablation patient. This chapter outlines our experience using the Corneal Mapping System, or CMS (EyeSys Technologies, Houston, Texas). Fig. 8-1, *A* demonstrates the Model 2 on which all of our work is based. It has been replaced with the Model 3 shown in Fig. 1, *B,* which is actually a family of units starting with the relatively inexpensive EyeCon system which has a user-friendly icon-based software interface and requires minimal computer skills to operate. The EyeCon system also allows for the capture of screen images in order to produce slides. The EyeSys Windows Workstation utilizes the more advanced graphical interface of Microsoft Windows. The windows system has a networkable patient database and the capability to archive millions of patient files to an optical mass storage device.

Both systems have a 16-ring (8 light and 8 dark rings) conical placido disc that is positioned 92 mm in front of the cornea, and a chinrest for patient examination (Fig. 8-2, *A*). The patient examination portion of the procedure typically takes 2 minutes for both eyes. Within the housing of the corneoscope is a CCD camera for image capture. The computer system digitizes or converts the data obtained from the video output into a form that can be analyzed. A typical corneoscopic image obtained by the instrument is shown in Fig. 8-2, *B.*

For a 42.5-D cornea, the diameter of the measured region is 0.9 to 9.2 mm. An edge detection program identifies the white-to-black *(yellow dotted lines)* and black-to-white *(red dotted lines)* interfaces of the corneoscopic pattern (Fig. 8-3, *A*). Each of the 16 interfaces is measured at 1-degree intervals for 360 degrees for a total of 5760 points. Simple observation of the alternating yellow- and red-line pattern will verify if the edges were appropriately detected. Since the human brain is markedly superior as a pattern recognition system to any computer, the EyeSys unit allows the operator to edit the computer's pattern recognition findings. Also, special image subtraction and enhancement techniques are used to find the patient's pupil (Fig. 8-3, *B*). This feature has been found to be critical for detecting proper centration of excimer procedures.

Once the ring edges and the pupil have been properly identified, a number of highly sophisticated programs convert the data into a series of user-selectable color graphics displays. The best known and possibly the most useful is the normalized scale color-coded map which differentiates 15 colors. For each cornea, the computer software calculates the average dioptric power. The color of the midrange dioptric power is always dark green. The hot colors, such as red and yellow, are used to denote the steeper areas of the cornea, whereas the cool colors, i.e., shades of blue, are used to denote flatter areas of the cornea. The software may adjust the dioptric power increments associated

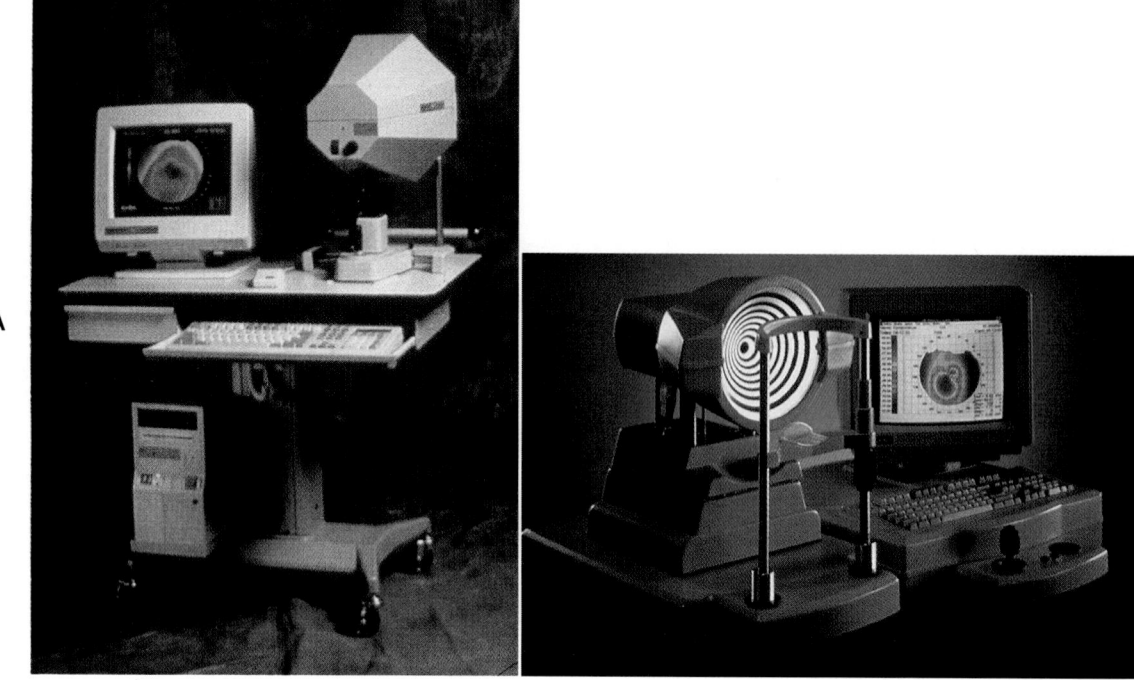

Fig. 8-1. A, The Model 2 corneal topography unit from EyeSys Technologies. All of the work described in this chapter is based on this first-generation unit. **B,** The newer Model 3 from EyeSys which is available in both disk operating system (EyeCon) and Windows environments (Windows Workstation).

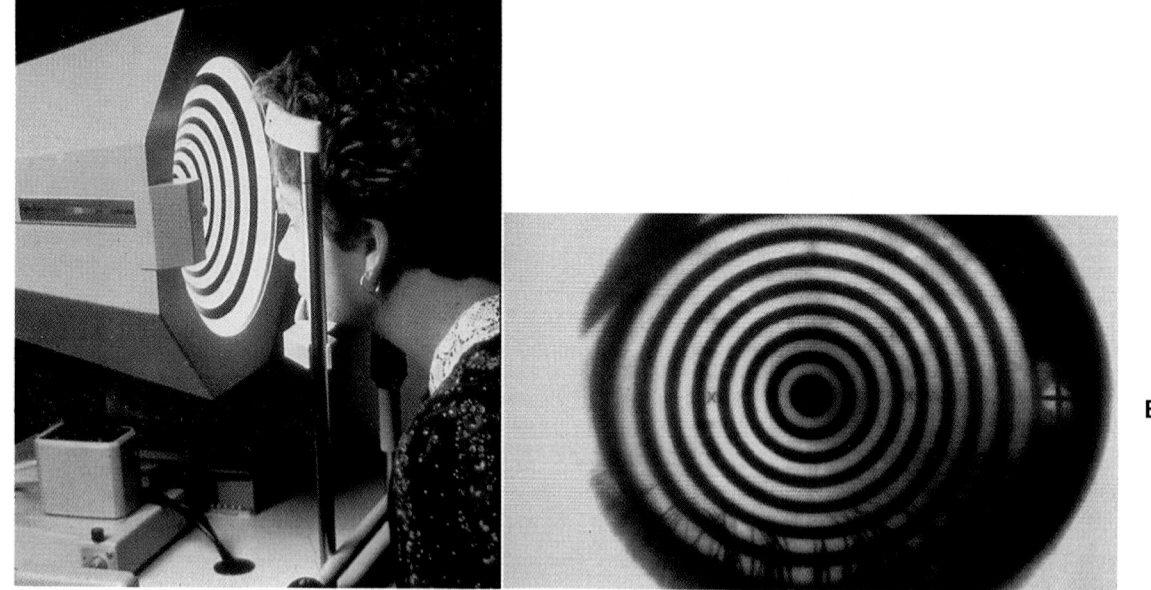

Fig. 8-2. A, The corneoscope projects a pattern of 16 concentric rings onto the corneal surface. **B,** Typical corneoscopic or "eye" image. Measurement along the 8 light and 8 dark rings at 1-degree intervals yields 5760 bits of information.

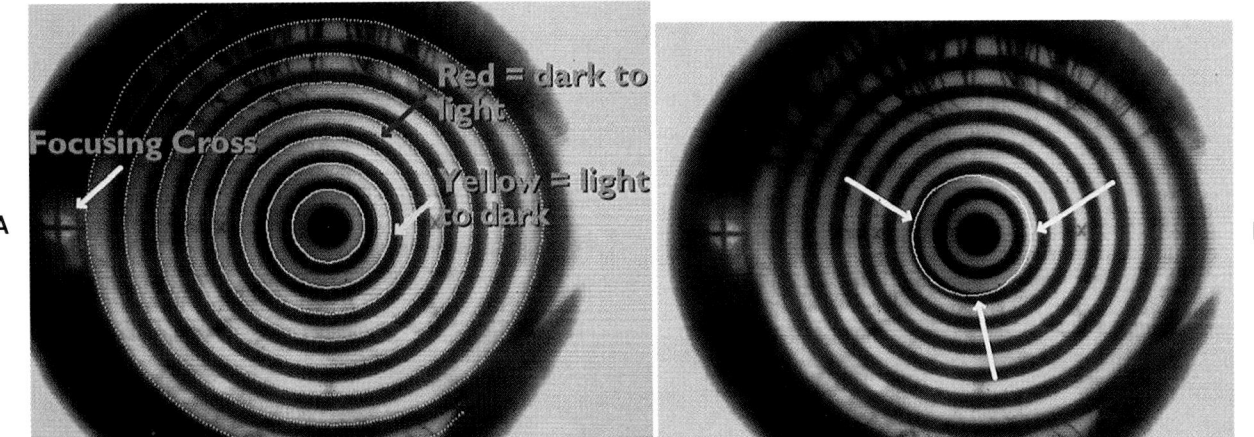

Fig. 8-3. A, The edge detection program identifies the light-to-dark *(yellow rings)* and dark-to-light *(red rings)* transitions of the corneoscopic image. The EyeSys unit allows for editing of the computer-determined transition rings to ensure correspondence to the actual corneoscopic image and thereby eliminate artifacts. **B,** Pupil detection program identifies the pupillary edge.

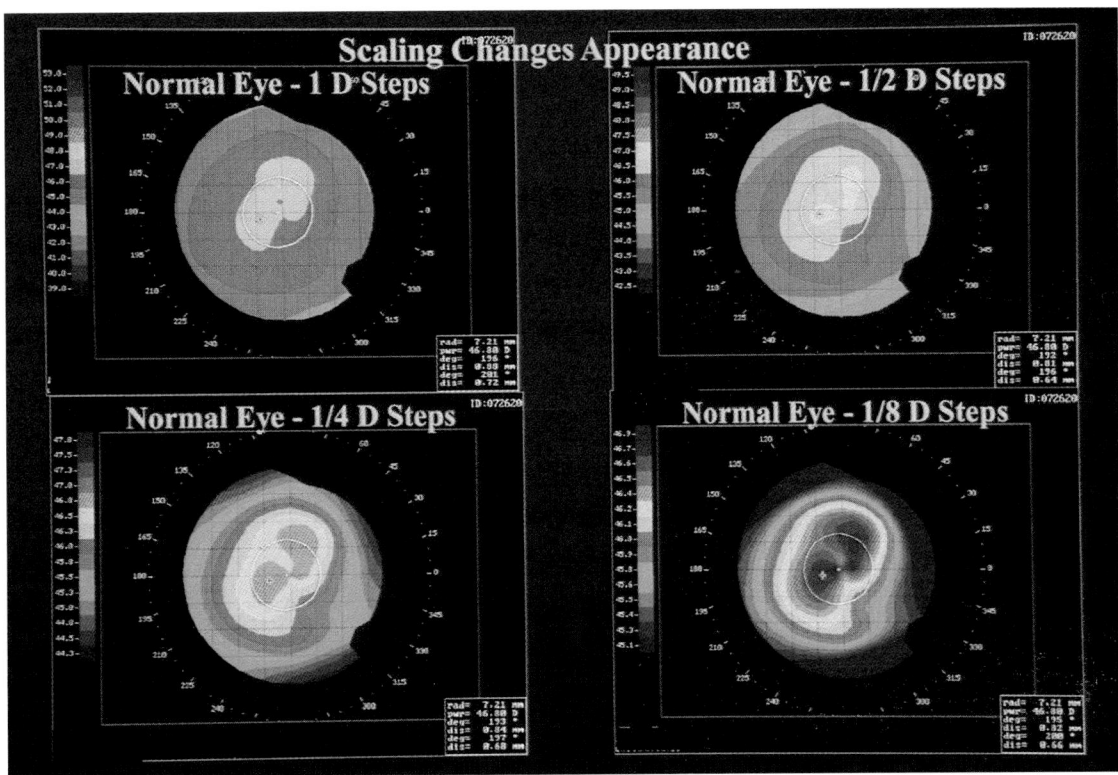

Fig. 8-4. Examples that detail the effect of changing the scale from 1.0-D *(upper right)* to 0.125-D *(lower left)* increments on the visual appearance of the color map. The 0.5-D scale is the scale most frequently used throughout this chapter.

with the color changes. By default, the normalized scale will be in 0.5- or 1.0-D increments, spanning a 7.5- to 15.0-D range, depending on the range of power in the cornea. The user can adjust the increments to higher or lower values. The normalized scale will be used to demonstrate most of the important findings with excimer laser use (Fig. 8-4).

Each topography image has a data box associated with it which appears in the lower right-hand corner. The information contained in this box is a function of the cursor position and includes radius of curvature and corresponding corneal power, the distance (in millimeters) and orientation (in degrees) of the cursor from the center of the image or "vertex normal," and the distance and orientation of the cursor from the center of the pupil. Each of these elements of the data box will be further discussed in detail.

Another key element of corneal topography is the change map, also called the difference or delta map, which is a point-for-point subtraction of one map from another. This feature allows the user to take maps from two different visits and display the corneal changes which have occurred between examinations. The change map is particularly useful in evaluating the effects of surgical or laser procedures or therapeutic interventions by subtracting a preoperative or pre-intervention image from a postoperative or postintervention image. For the change map, dark green is used to specify areas of no change in dioptric power, while reds and yellows denote areas of the cornea which have steepened, and shades of blue denote areas of the cornea which have flattened.

PREOPERATIVE EVALUATION

It is clear that corneal topography is a necessary tool for preoperative screening of prospective excimer laser patients to detect undiagnosed keratoconus and other unusual corneal curvature. Rabinowitz and McDonnell[1] found three quantitative parameters of corneal topography to be highly correlated with clinical keratoconus. (1) A central corneal curvature greater than 46.6 D, (2) a difference between eyes in central keratometry greater than 0.8 D, and (3) an inferior-superior keratometry ratio greater than 1.6 D (indicative of inferior steepening) were characteristics of eyes with definite keratoconus as compared to normal eyes.

Maguire and Bourne,[2] in their investigation of the usefulness of corneal topography in keratoconus suspects, discovered the existence of large amounts of corneal distortion despite excellent corrected acuity, little distortion of keratometry mires, and no slit-lamp evidence of keratoconus. They studied nine eyes of seven patients with no slit-lamp evidence of keratoconus. Six of these eyes had no distortion of keratometry mires. However, using corneal topography, seven eyes were documented to have keratoconus.[2] More recently, Waring[3] has suggested that the term *keratoconus suspect* be used to designate a cornea with inferior steepening determined by corneal topography. As keratoconus has generally been considered a contraindication to refractive surgery, preoperative videokeratographic evaluations are of great importance.[4-7]

In a videokeratopographic evaluation of 100 consecutive eyes presenting for radial keratometry, Dr. Robert G. Martin (personal communication, 1993) observed abnormal corneas in 6% of eyes, where "abnormal" included keratoconus suspects and cases with unusual areas of steepness or irregular patterns which were not detectable during clinical evaluation or with keratometry. Further, 32% of eyes presented with

asymmetric astigmatism. In fact, substantial variability in corneal topography even in normal eyes has been observed and may affect the predictability of surgical procedures designed to alter the shape of the cornea.[8]

The other major value of obtaining preoperative topography is to allow one to produce a difference or change map which subtracts the preoperative power map from the postoperative map and thus allows exact visualization of procedure-induced changes. The value of change maps will be documented with clinical examples in the appropriate sections.

EARLY POSTOPERATIVE EVALUATION
Preoperative vs. Postoperative Treatment

Fig. 8-5 *(top, left)* shows the topographic appearance of a normal cornea. Note that the central cornea is steeper compared to the peripheral cornea. This prolate shape is termed *positive asphericity* and is the natural state of the cornea. Theoretically, a prolate cornea reduces spherical aberrations which would otherwise be present when the pupil widely dilates. The resultant central flattening that occurs with photorefractive keratectomy (PRK) on the same cornea is shown in Fig. 8-5 *(top, right)*. There is marked central flattening with loss of positive asphericity. In fact, an oblate shape or *negative asphericity* results after myopic PRK, leaving the peripheral cornea steeper than the central cornea. This shape can potentially increase spherical aberrations that may become clinically significant when the pupil dilates beyond the central treatment zone.

A myopic PRK performed with the use of an expanding computer-controlled diaphragm results in a spherical ablation. Fig. 8-6 *(top, left)* shows the pre-PRK topography of a cornea with symmetric with-the-rule astigmatism. After a myopic PRK, there is no significant change in astigmatism (i.e., the cornea remains flatter in the horizontal meridian) even though the cornea is obviously flatter (Fig. 8-6, *top, right*). The change map (Fig. 8-6, *bottom*) is completely spherical, also demonstrating no astigmatism correction.

Decentration

Decentration of refractive corneal procedures can result in blurred images, glare, ghost images, poor visual acuity, or poor contrast sensitivity.[9,10] Various methods of centering surgical corneal refractive procedures have been described.[11,12] Walsh and Guyton,[10] Uozato and Guyton,[9] and Maloney[13] believe that proper centering of excimer procedures requires the patient to fixate on a point that is coaxial with the surgeon's sighting eye and the cornea is marked at the point in line with the center of the patient's entrance pupil, ignoring the corneal light reflex. Besides the optical arguments for using the entrance pupil, the Stiles-

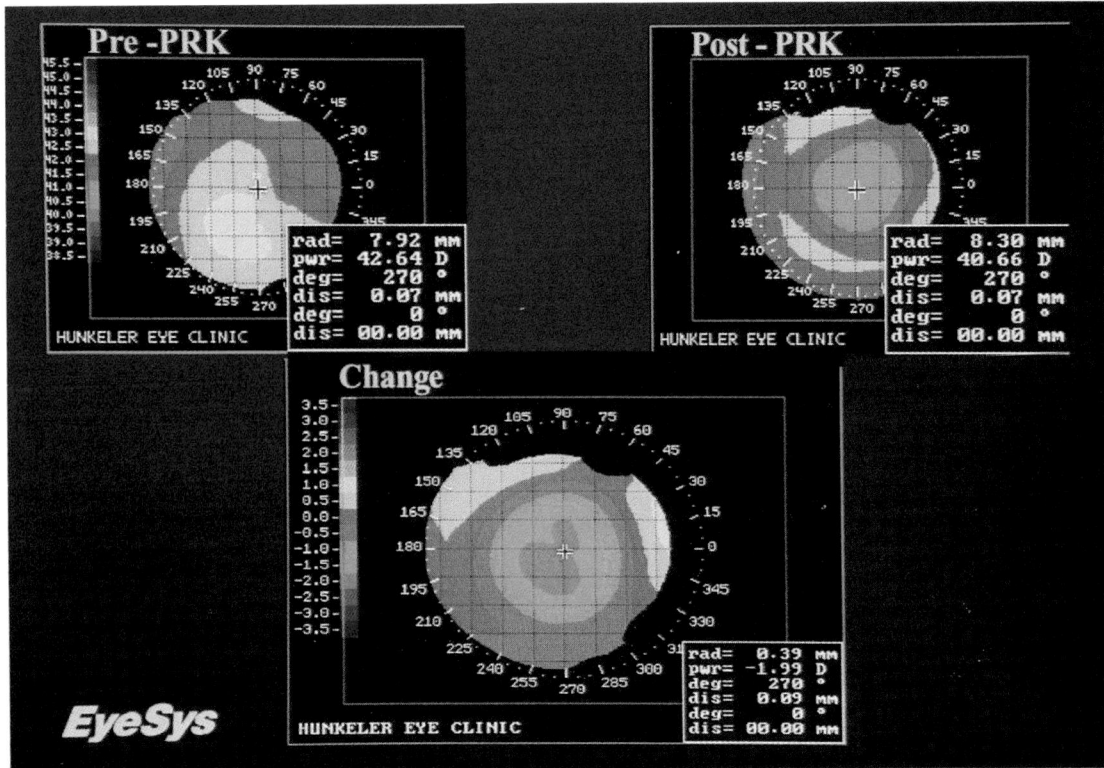

Fig. 8-5. Pre-PRK *(upper right)*, post-PRK *(upper left)*, and change maps *(bottom)*. The change map shows approximately 2 D of central flattening.

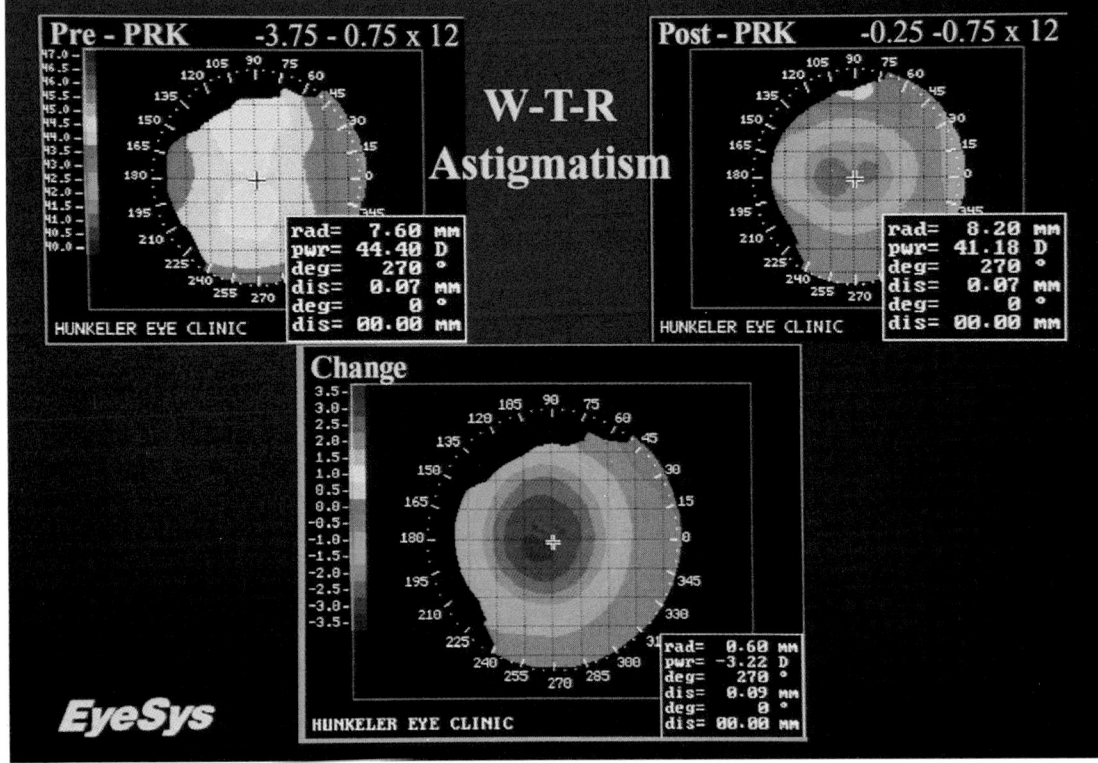

Fig. 8-6. Pre-PRK *(upper right)*, post-PRK *(upper left)*, and change maps *(bottom)* in the eye with 0.75 D of preexisting with-the-rule astigmatism. Despite the preexisting astigmatism, the change map shows approximately 3.0 D of symmetric flattening of the central cornea.

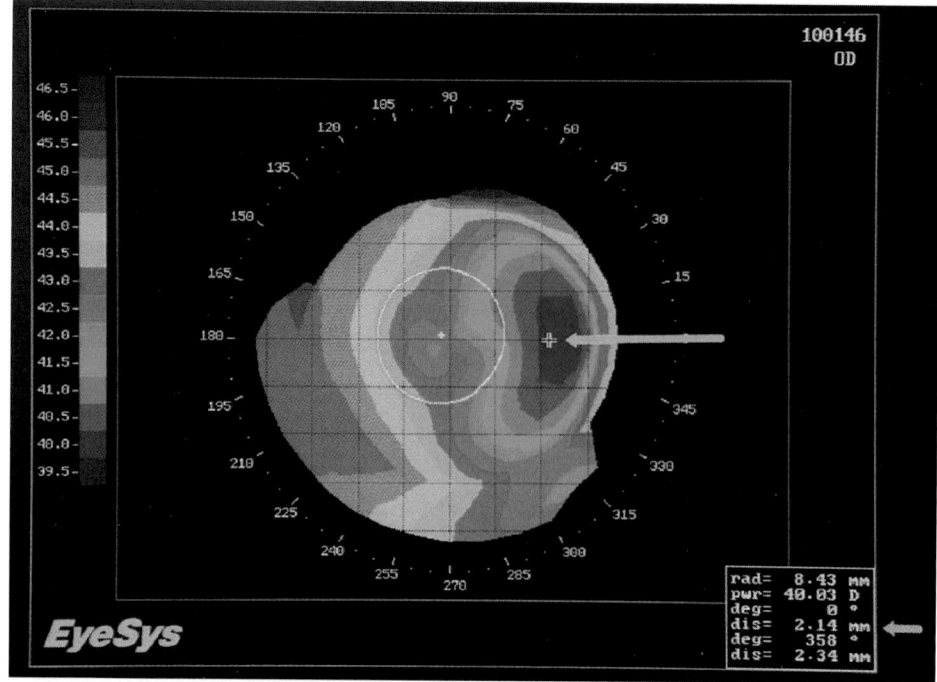

Fig. 8-10. Post-PRK map showing substantially decentered ablation. The center of the ablation zone is 2.14 mm from the vertex normal and 2.34 mm from the pupil center. This patient, however, was asymptomatic at 1 year post PRK with corrected and uncorrected acuities of 20/20 and 20/25 respectively. (Courtesy of Eye Foundation of Kansas City, Kansas City, MO.)

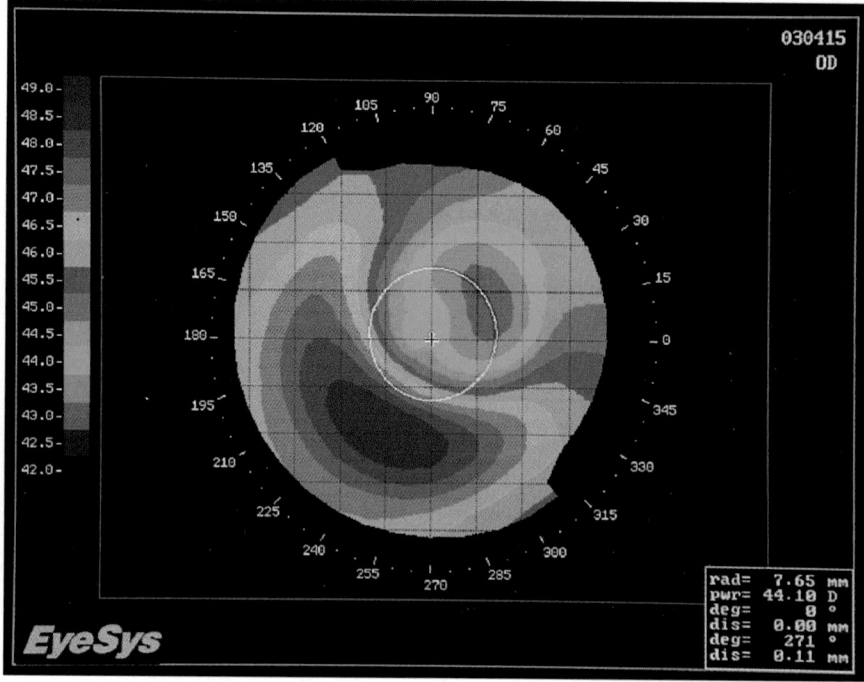

Fig. 8-11. Post-PRK map showing moderately decentered ablation that is 1.26 mm from the pupillary center. This patient was symptomatic, complaining of multiple images. (Courtesy of EyeSys Technologies, Houston, TX.)

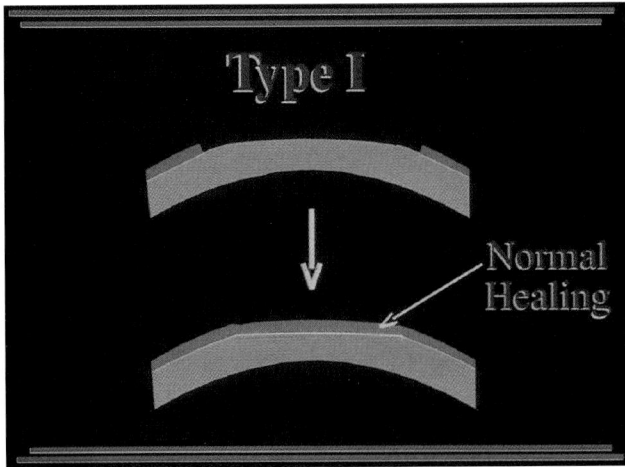

Fig. 8-12. Schematic detailing the mechanics of type I healing following myopic PRK with the Summit laser. This is the most common healing pattern observed and is characterized by slight hyperopia at the 1-month visit with subepithelial reticular haze. Typically, the haze resolves between 3 and 6 months post PRK with gradual corneal steepening leaving a persistent refractive change.

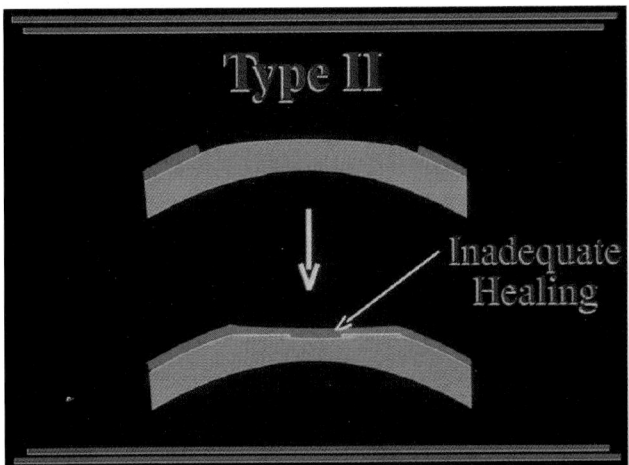

Fig. 8-13. Schematic detailing the mechanics of type II healing following myopic PRK with the Summit laser which is characterized by hyperopia and lack of expected subepithelial haze at 1-month post PRK. Discontinuation of normal steroid regimen or contact lens usage is usually sufficient to stimulate these eyes into a typical healing pattern.

While the three healing processes to be described appear to occur with all excimer lasers, their relative proportions are variable depending on the specific laser used. They have only been quantitated in our hands with the Summit excimer system so that relative proportions of healing types refer to that laser system. The most typical response seen in 85% of patients is termed *type I healing*. At the 1-month visit the patient is slightly hyperopic (+1–+2 D) with a faint reticular haze appearing in the subepithelial region of the treatment site. With the appearance of haze,

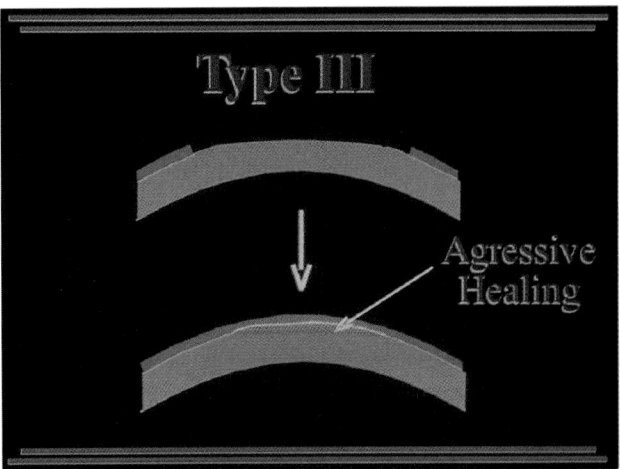

Fig. 8-14. Schematic detailing the mechanics of type III healing following myopic PRK with the Summit laser which is characterized by the appearance of a dense reticular subepithelial haze with progressive myopia. Use of fluorometholone and diclofenac sodium 0.1% can lead to reversal of corneal steepening.

gradual central corneal steepening ensues as the hyperopia resolves. This is consistently measured by keratometry, refraction, and topography between the 1- and 4-month visits. Throughout this time period the patient is on a tapered dose of 0.1% fluorometholone. Fig. 8-15 shows the slit-lamp appearance, refraction, keratometry, and corneal topography of a *type I healing* response. This demonstrates that the cornea steepens as a slight subepithelial haze develops. Typically, the haze resolves between the 3- and 6-month visits, leaving a persistent refractive change.

Type II healing is characterized at the 1-month visit by hyperopia and lack of the expected subepithelial haze. If the patient has been continued on topical steroids, the clear cornea and hyperopia persist indefinitely (Fig. 8-16). As these patients are identified, the topical steroids are discontinued. This alone stimulates most of the patients into a typical healing pattern. If after 1 month there is no corneal haze formation or decrease in hyperopia, a soft disposable contact lens is placed. The patient is instructed to wear the lens continuously and return for weekly visits. Through either a mechanical or hypoxic stimulus, the contact lens induces proper healing in the majority of patients. The contact lens is discontinued as corneal haze formation and regression of hyperopia are noted. A few patients have not responded to an aggressive trial with a contact lens. If no evidence of haze formation is noted and the patient remains hyperopic, an epithelial debridement is performed. A no. 64 Beaver blade is used to remove the central corneal epithelium over the PRK treatment zone. The patient is followed with appropriate topical antibiotics but no anti-inflammatory drug is used. Within several weeks, cor-

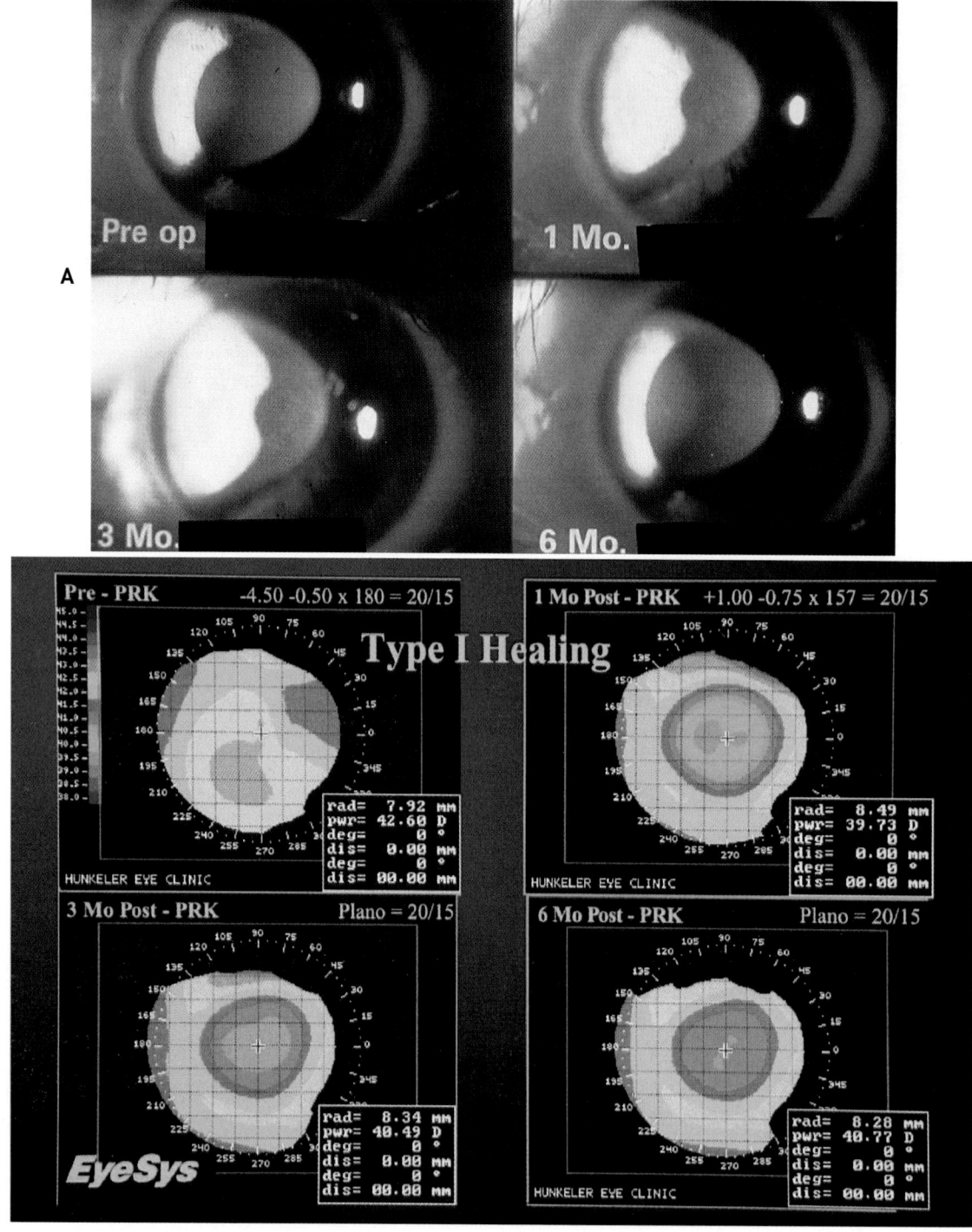

Fig. 8-15. A, Slit-lamp photographs pre- and 1, 3, and 6 months post PRK (Summit) demonstrating a type I healing response. **B,** Corresponding corneal topography and residual refractive correction. As the subepithelial haze develops there is gradual corneal steepening. When the haze resolves a stable refractive change results.

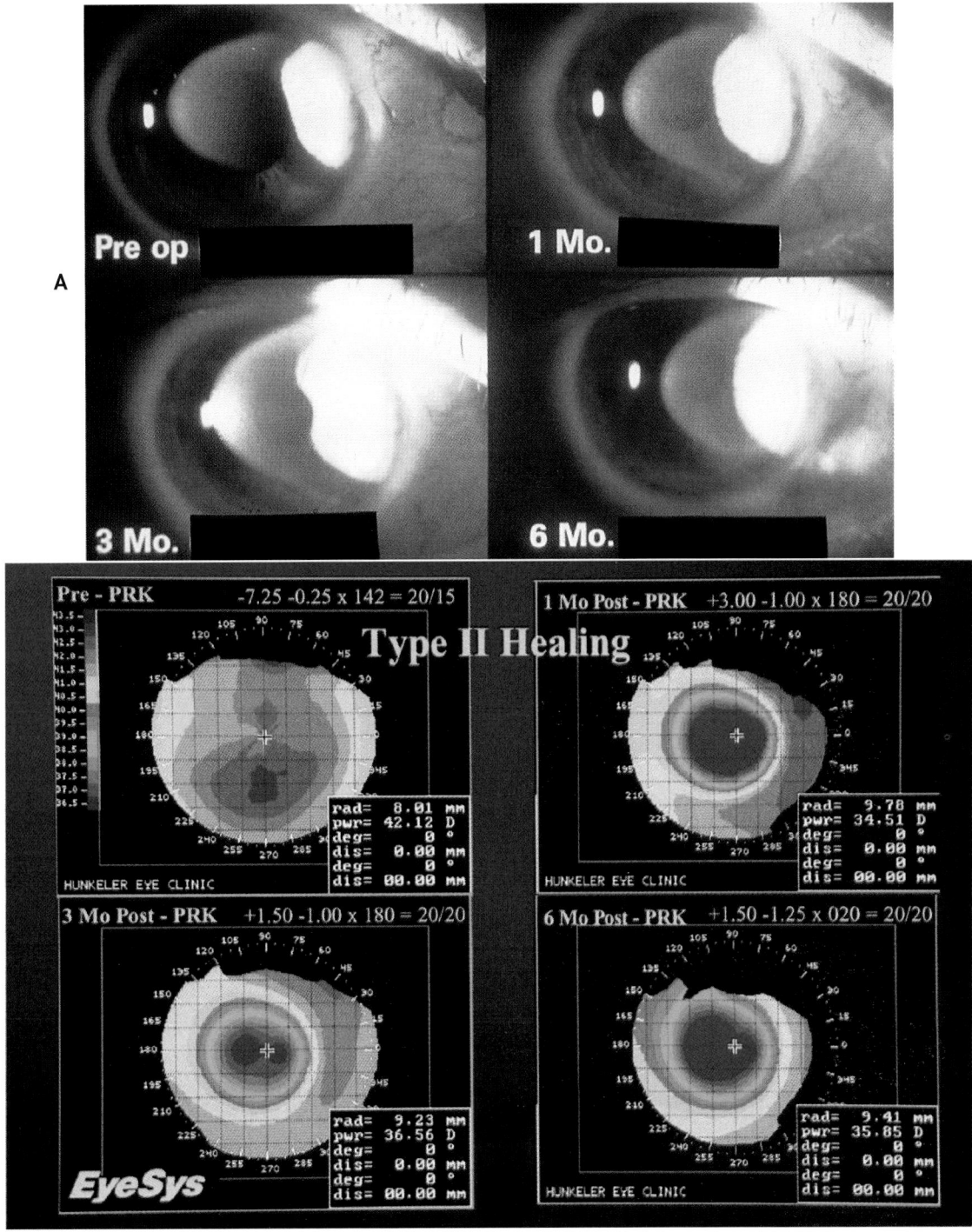

Fig. 8-16. A, Slit-lamp photographs pre- and 1, 3, and 6 months post PRK (Summit) demonstrating a type II healing response. **B,** Corresponding corneal topography and residual refractive correction. If the patient is continued on topical steroids, the clear cornea and hyperopia may persist indefinitely.

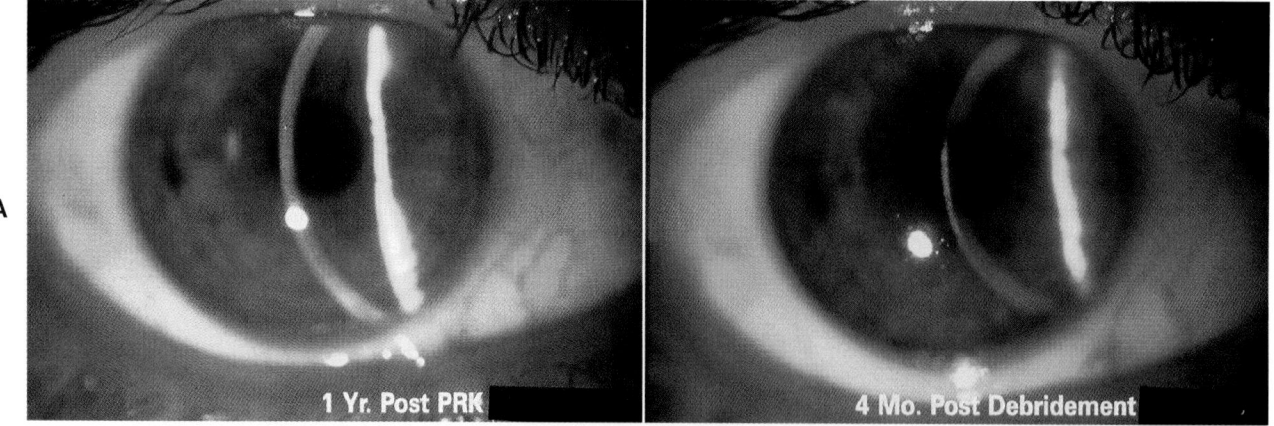

Fig. 8-17. An example of type II healing that was unresponsive to cessation of steroid treatment and an aggressive trial with a contact lens following PRK (Summit). An epithelial debridement was performed. Slit-lamp photographs **(A)** pre-debridement (1 year post PRK) and **(B)** 4 months following debridement. Note the appearance of subepithelial haze with steepening of the central cornea following debridement.

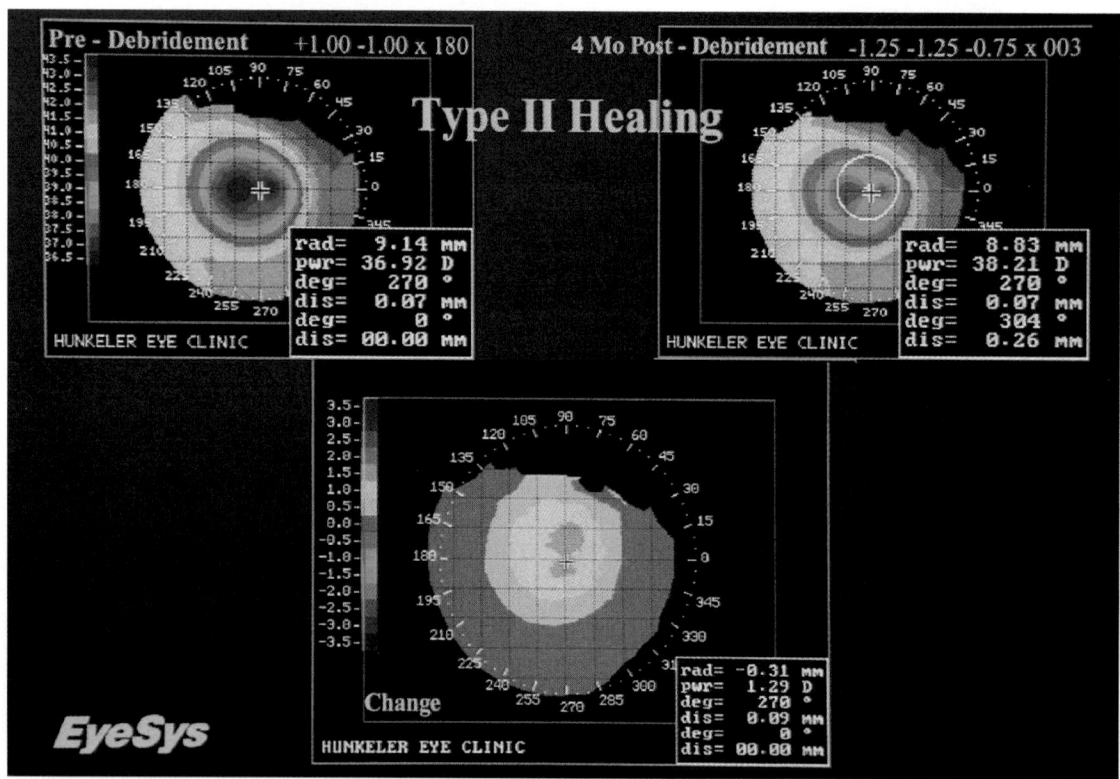

Fig. 8-18. Corneal topography of the type II healing response depicted in Fig. 8-17. The change map demonstrates approximately 1.25 D of central steepening as a result of epithelial debridement.

neal haze and steepening develop with regression of hyperopia (Figs. 8-17 and 8-18).

Type III healing is recognized by the appearance of a dense reticular subepithelial haze. This typically decreases the best corrected vision while producing a progressive myopic shift. Corneal steepening results and can be confirmed by keratometry or topography (Fig. 8-19). Once identified, fluorometholone (FML Forte) and diclofenac sodium 0.1% (Voltaren) are used four times a day. Reversal of corneal steepening can result as soon as 1 week after instituting this topical regimen. Such a quick response was unexplainable until the corneal haze was identified. Marshall has determined that the post-PRK subepithelial haze is

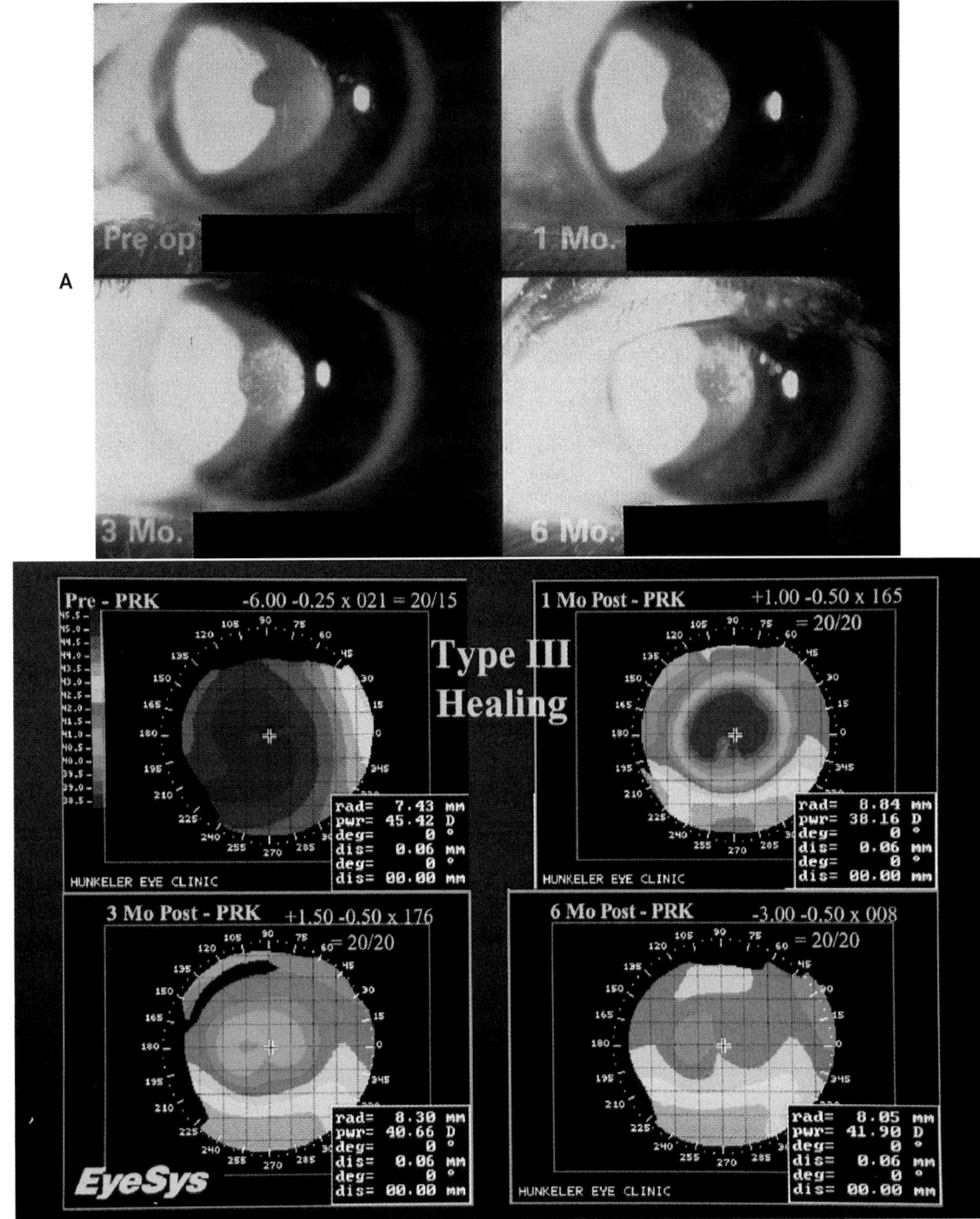

Fig. 8-19. A, Slit-lamp photographs pre- and 1, 3, and 6 months post PRK (Summit) of a type III healing response. **B,** Corresponding corneal topography and residual refractive correction demonstrating the progressive myopic shift.

caused by mucopolysaccharide. This extracellular material appears to respond to topical anti-inflammatory medications, causing the cornea to flatten as the haze resolves. Subsequently, the myopia may resolve, eliminating the need for further surgery. Figs. 8-20 and 8-21 demonstrate the clinical and topographic data of a type III healer. The topography and refraction show a

dramatic response over 1 month to topical fluorometholone and diclofenac sodium. The value of the change map is especially obvious here. In this case, as shown in Fig. 8-21, a 1-month course of topical steroidal and nonsteroidal agents resulted in 2.6 D of central flattening due to a reversal of postlaser regression of effect.

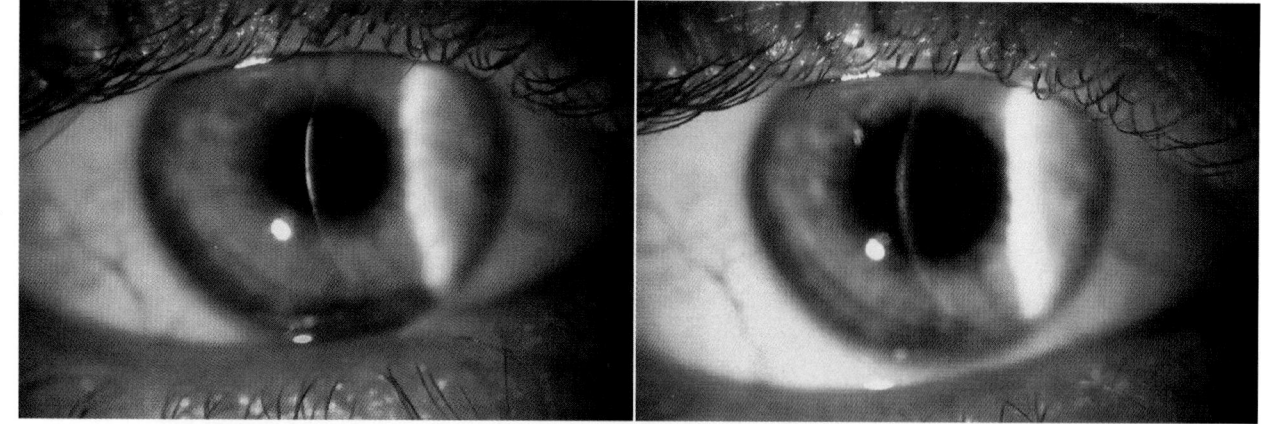

A   B

Fig. 8-20. Slit-lamp photographs of the type III healing response shown in Fig. 8-19 which was controlled with topical medical therapy. **A,** Before medical therapy (6 months post PRK). **B,** 6 months following initiation of medical therapy. Note that the dense haze has resolved.

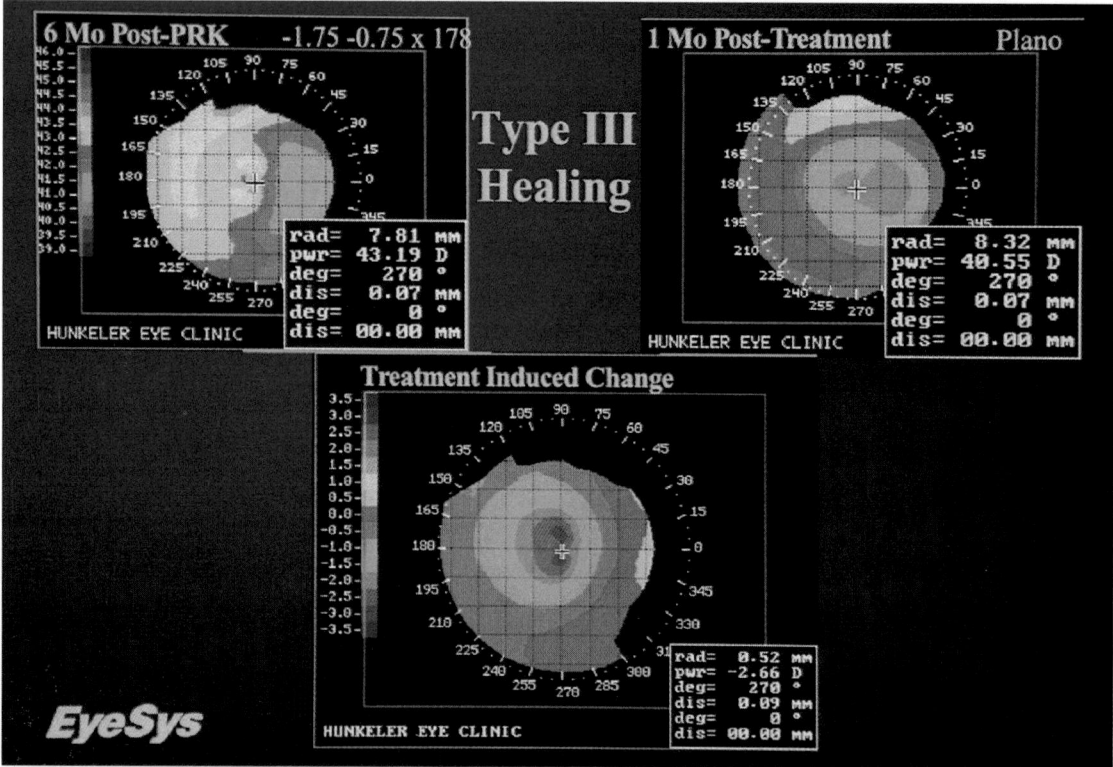

Fig. 8-21. Corresponding corneal topography of the type III healing response shown in Fig. 8-20 which was controlled with topical medical therapy. **A,** Before medical therapy (6 months post PRK). **B,** 6 months following initiation of medical therapy. The change map *(bottom)* indicates approximately 2.6 D of central flattening resulting from medical therapy.

Here is an example of a case treated with the VISX laser which demonstrated typical type III healing characteristics. This patient had a pre-PRK spherical equivalent of −5.25 D and a 6-month post-PRK refraction of −2.50 D. Fig. 8-22, *A* shows the pre- and 6-month post-PRK topography, and the change or difference map indicating 2.6 D of residual myopia cor-

rection centrally. The patient began intensive topical steroid treatment. Fig. 8-22, *B* demonstrates the topography prior to and 2 weeks after steroid treatment, and the difference map demonstrating an additional 1.28 D of flattening caused by the steroid regimen. Another case documenting the efficacy of topical steroid treatment on excessive regression of excimer effect is

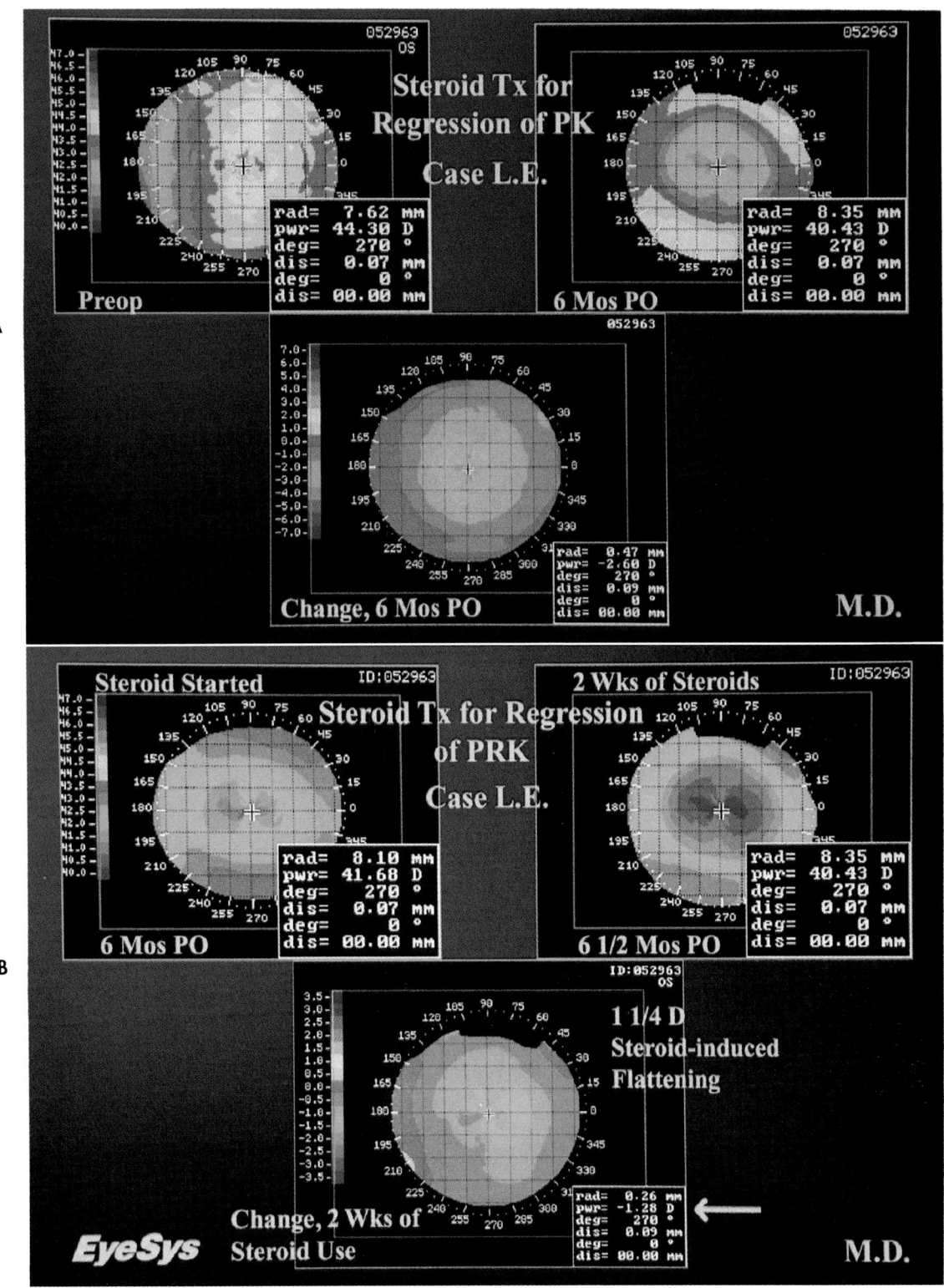

Fig. 8-22. Corneal topography of a type III healing response following PRK (VISX). **A,** Pre- and 6 months post PRK with change map. **B,** Before and 2 weeks after initiation of steroid treatment and with change map showing approximately 1.25 D of central flattening resulting from the steroid regimen. (Courtesy of Eye Foundation of Kansas City, Kansas City, MO.)

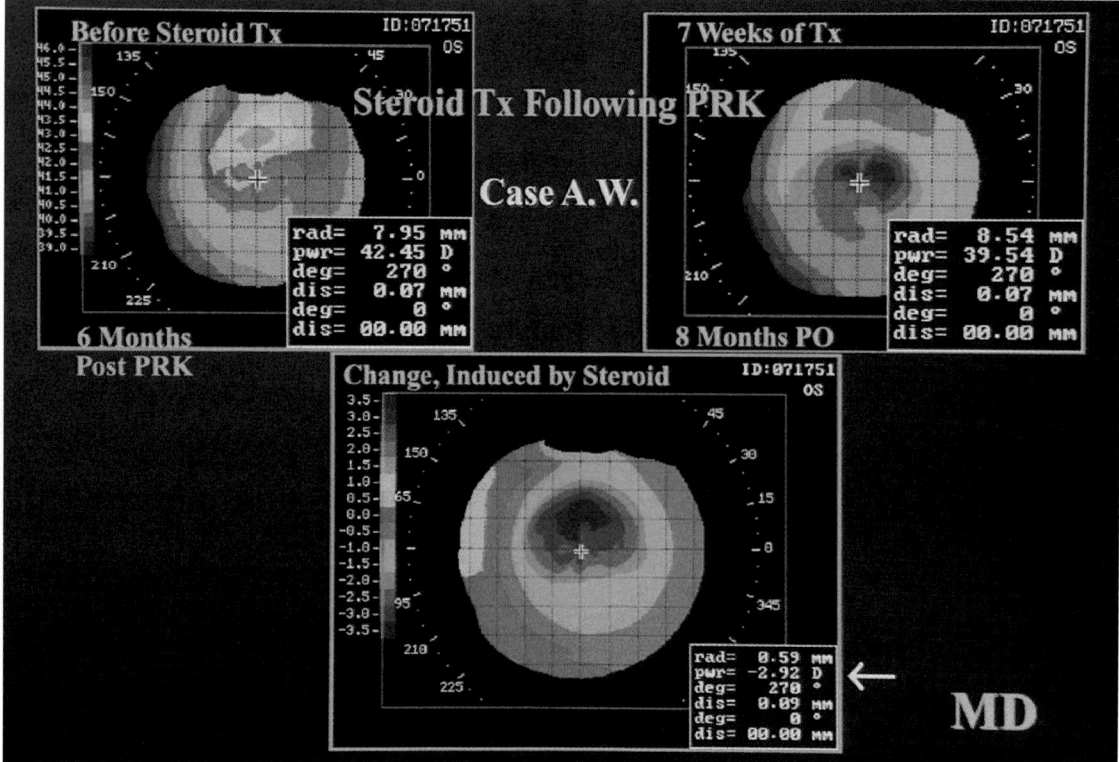

Fig. 8-23. Corneal topography of another type III healing response following PRK (VISX). After 7 weeks following initiation of steroid therapy, an additional 3 D of central flattening is observed. (Courtesy of Eye Foundation of Kansas City, Kansas City, MO.)

shown in Fig. 8-23. After 7 weeks of topical steroids the typical central flattening seen with excimer treatment has returned *(upper right)* and the change map documents an additional 3 D of corneal flattening.

It would appear from the clinical data that prior to collagen deposition this extracellular mucopolysaccharide haze can respond to topical treatment, thereby flattening the cornea. Obviously, once stromal collagen is laid down, topical medications will become ineffective and re-treatment is the only alternative.

Central Islands and Central Hot Spots

Photorefractive keratotomy involves the transformation of the corneal surface from one spherical surface to another, of slightly different radius of curvature, by removing tissue in a highly controlled fashion with the application of laser energy. Depending on the algorithm used to control the size of the aperture that limits the laser beam, the uniformity of the laser beam, and the uniformity of the ablation of corneal tissue, deviations from an absolutely spherical surface are likely to occur. Such deviations can be measured with a videokeratoscope.

The videokeratoscope produces a map of the cornea which shows the radius of curvature, expressed as dioptric power, of a number of points on the cornea. It should be emphasized that, because the

changes in radius of curvature are expressed in terms of dioptric power, two areas of different size which show the same dioptric change do not represent equal physical deviations from a spherical surface. Table 8-1 shows the relationship of the overall diameter of an irregular feature to the "height" of the feature relative to the surrounding topography. Thus, although the color changes on the topographic map may appear to represent large changes in corneal structure, the actual physical dimensions of these irregular areas are, in fact, quite small and generally optically insignificant. As a matter of perspective, the magnitude of such changes should be compared to the thickness of the normal corneal epithelium, which averages 50 μm. During the first months following treatment the epithelium covers the ablated area by thinning down to

Table 8-1. Central islands: physical height of surface irregularities of varying size (in microns)

Diameter (mm)	1 D	2 D	3 D
1.0	0.33	0.66	0.99
1.5	0.75	1.50	2.25
2.0	1.30	2.60	3.90
2.5	2.10	4.20	6.30
3.0	3.10	6.20	9.30

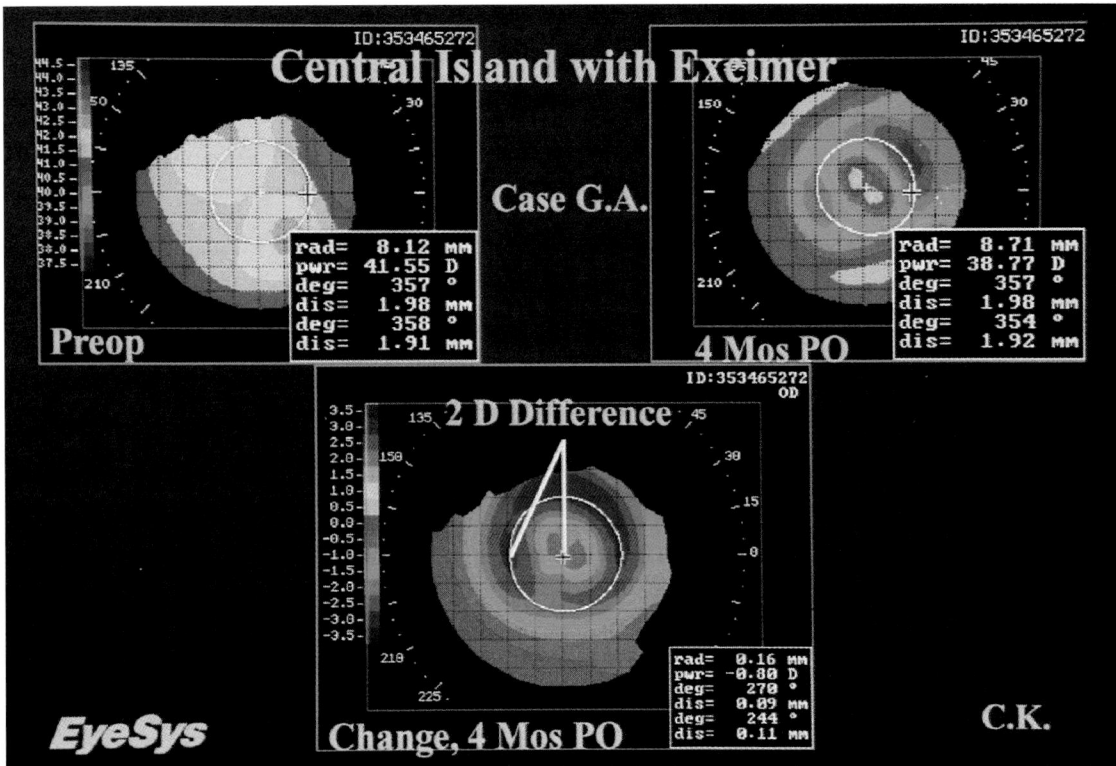

Fig. 8-24. A central island at 4 months post PRK (VISX). The change map shows a 2-D difference in induced flattening between the central and peripheral regions of the ablation zone. (Courtesy of Colman Kraff, M.D., Chicago.)

approximately one cell in thickness (approximately 10 μm) and sliding over the surface, slowly regaining its normal thickness and thus reducing the effect of any nonspherical ablation. Figs. 8-24 and 8-25 demonstrate two cases in which there is a 2.0- to 2.5-D difference in flattening induced between the center of the ablation zone and the region surrounding it. Since keratometry does not characterize the center of the cornea, it could not have picked up this phenomenon. Only corneal topography, with its ability to characterize the entire cornea, could detect this anomaly.

The change or difference map must be used to document these islands since any irregularities or asymmetries in preoperative topography may simulate or mask an island in the postoperative map. Since, as previously mentioned, the change map is a point-for-point subtraction of the pretreatment from post-treatment topography, it will reflect a true treatment-induced change.

Some investigators[16] have reported the occurrence of areas of relative central steepness, or underablation. They showed a decline in the incidence of the central areas from 11% at 1 month to 2.6% at 6 months to 1.2% at 1 year posttreatment. Thus, the typical natural course for these central islands is to resolve, becoming flatter over time, as shown in Fig. 8-26. It is atypical for this phenomenon to progress, as shown in Fig.

8-27. In the rare case in which the islands progress, the cause may be an abnormal wound-healing process and may not be related to the original ablation characteristics.

In the case of the VISX system, any increase in the occurrence of relative central underablation has been associated with the smoother corneal surfaces produced when the use of nitrogen flow across the cornea during treatment was discontinued, which may have had the effect of reducing corneal hydration. The variation in the hydration of the cornea may be the primary contributor to variations in the corneal profile following ablation. However, when the PRK group treated without nitrogen flow is compared with the group treated using flow, the optical results are superior in the absence of nitrogen flow despite the presence of this topographic anomaly. Interestingly, Colman Kraff (personal communication, February 1994) has reported that with a new ablation program developed by VISX, the central island phenomenon has disappeared in his last 40 consecutive cases with 3-month follow-up. The significance of central island is, in any case, unknown. McDonald and Klyce have found no loss of best corrected visual acuity or contrast sensitivity in those cases with central islands present (see Chapter 3).

Results from studies with the Summit laser,[17] which

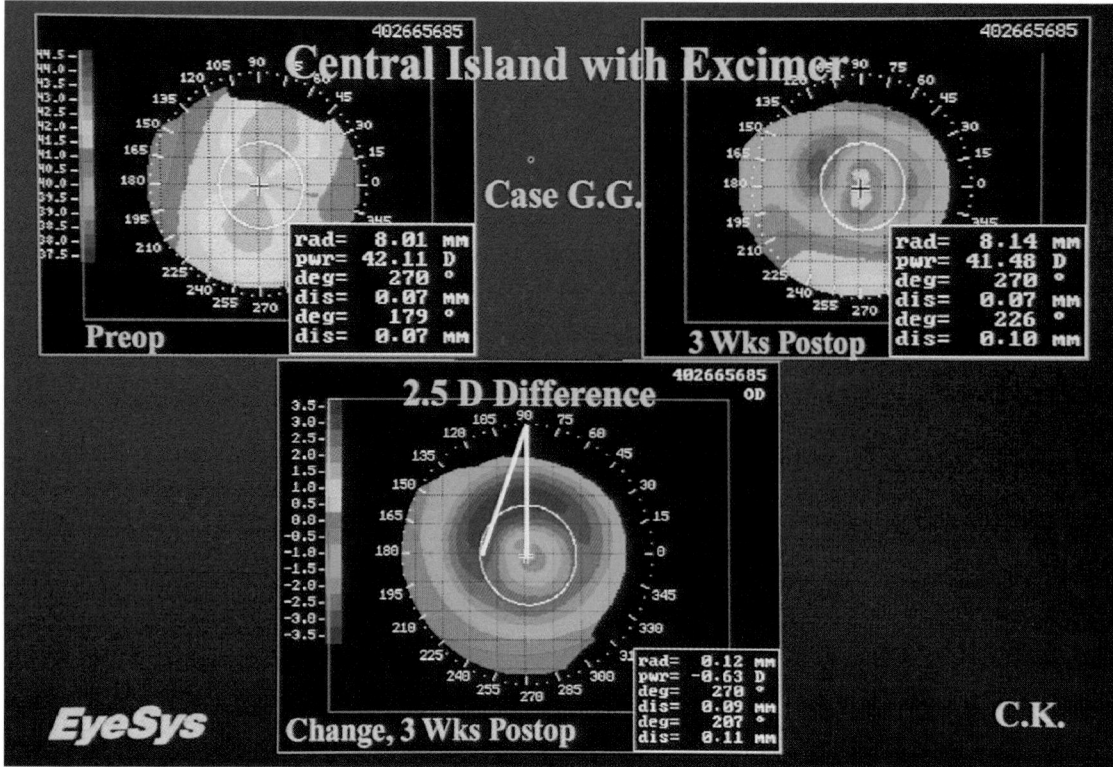

Fig. 8-25. A central island at 3 weeks following PRK (VISX). The change map shows a 2-D difference in induced flattening between the central and peripheral regions of the ablation zone. (Courtesy of Colman Kraff, M.D., Chicago.)

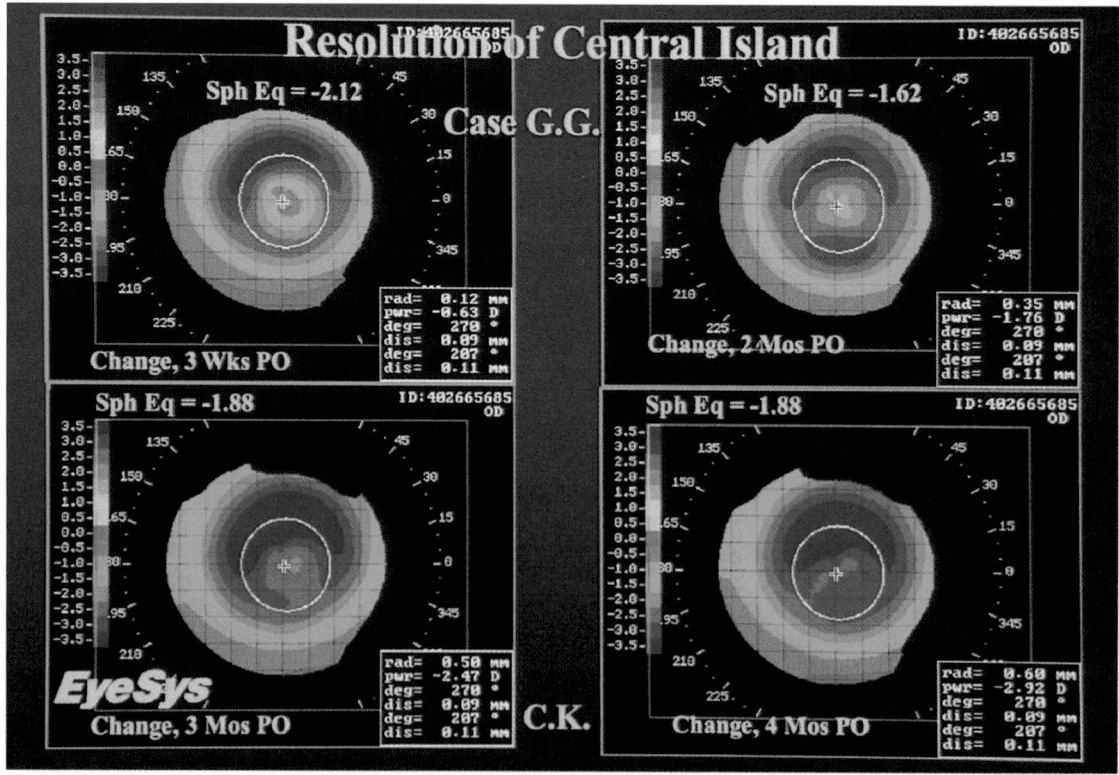

Fig. 8-26. Progressive resolution of central islands is the typical course. By 4 months post PRK (VISX) the change map is devoid of any signs of an island. (Courtesy of Colman Kraff, M.D., Chicago.)

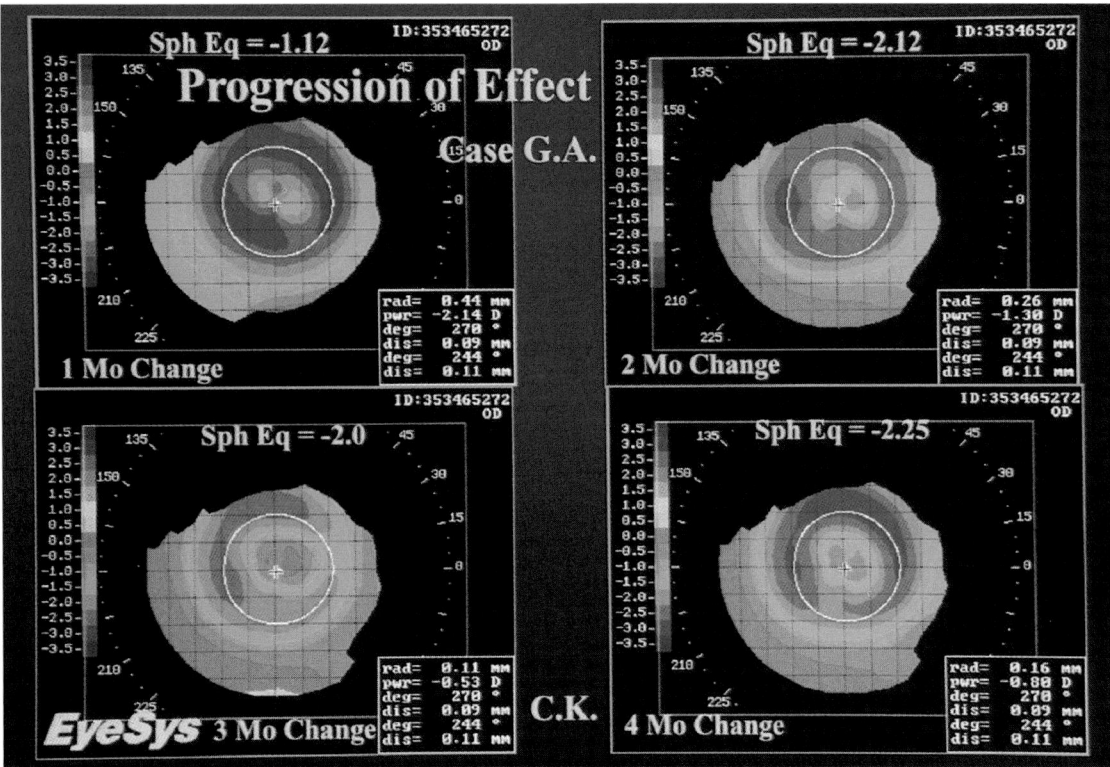

Fig. 8-27. Progressive worsening of central islands is atypical. In these rare cases, the cause may be an abnormal healing process rather than characteristics of the original ablation. (Courtesy of Colman Kraff, M.D., Chicago.)

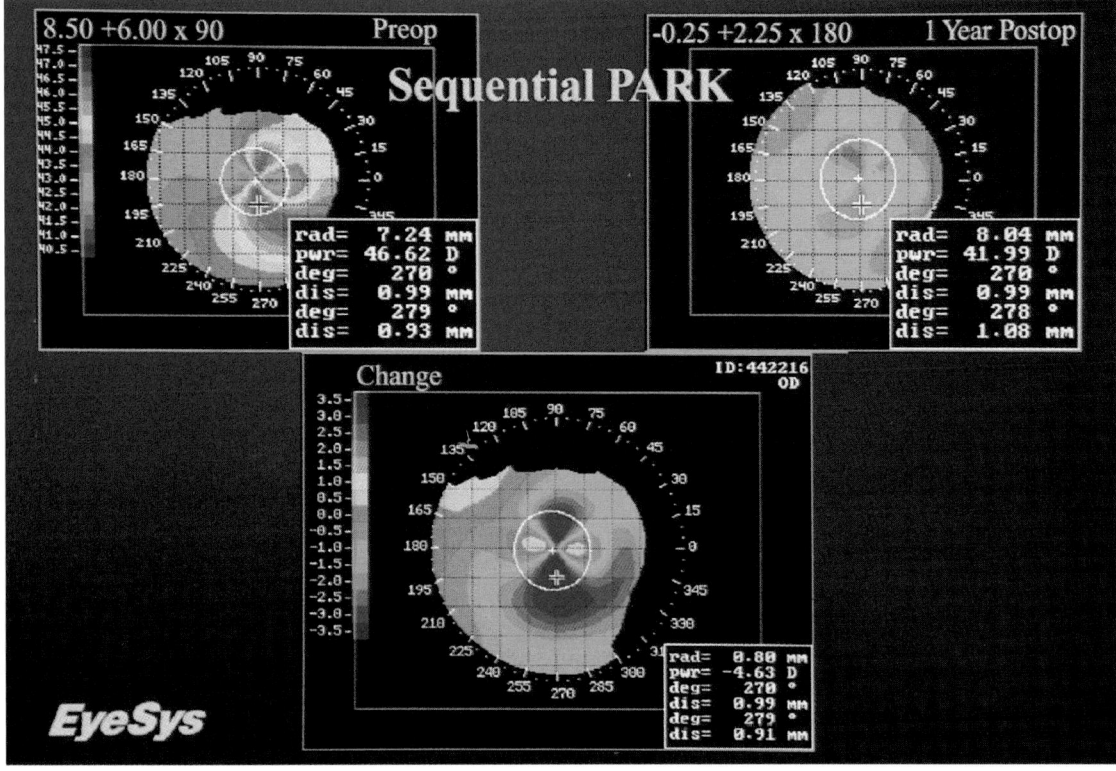

Fig. 8-28. Corneal topography of excimer treatment of astigmatism (VISX). The change map clearly demonstrates neutralization of 6 D of preexisting cylinder. (Courtesy of Colman Kraff, M.D., Chicago.)

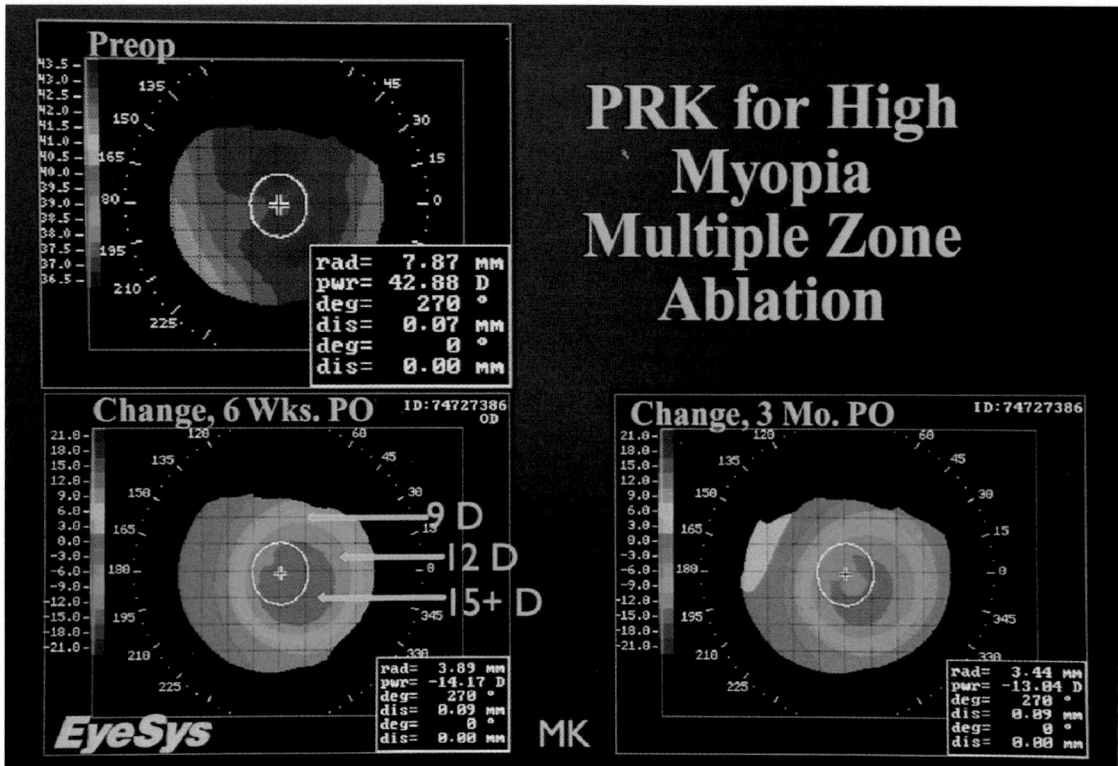

Fig. 8-29. Corneal topography of excimer treatment of high myopia (VISX). The change map demonstrates approximately 13.6 D of central flattening with a multiple zone ablation technique. (Courtesy of Manus Kraff, M.D., Chicago.)

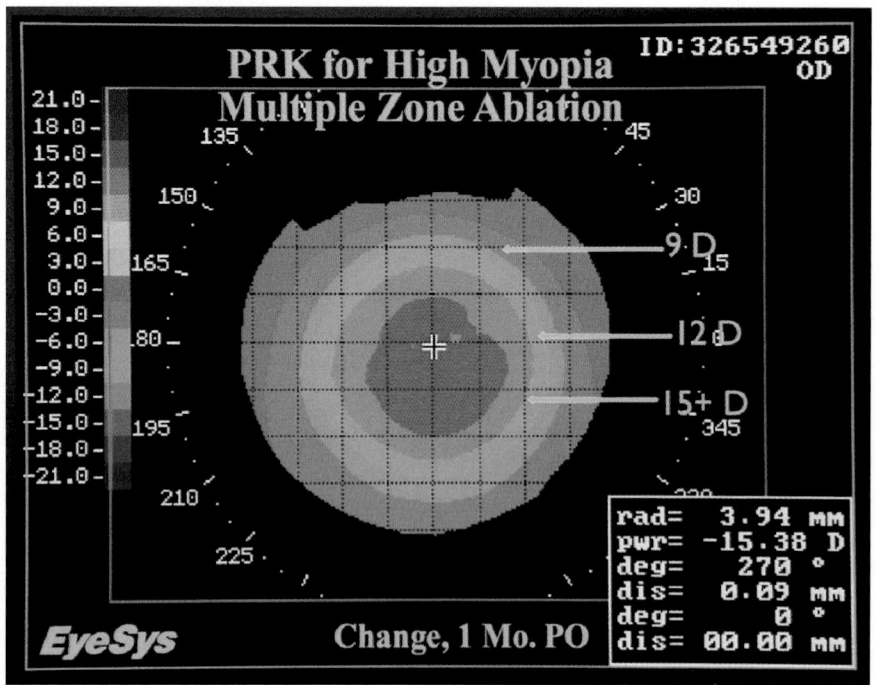

Fig. 8-30. Change map of another case of excimer treatment of high myopia. The details of the multiple zone ablation are clearly visible. (Courtesy of Manus Kraff, M.D., Chicago.)

has a beam profile known to be more intense in the center, show an overablation in the central cornea with a diameter of 2.4 mm and a difference of several diopters, which regresses by 2.7 D between 4 and 37 weeks. While a central "island" or elevation would be expected to transiently produce less ablative effect, this hot spot would produce more. This is precisely what is seen with the Summit laser. Thus, it may be that the original overcorrection seen with the Summit laser is a manifestation of a phenomenon (central hot spot of divot) similar to the central island seen with other systems.

SPECIAL APPLICATIONS
Treatment of Astigmatism

Corneal topography is especially useful for documenting the efficacy of astigmatic correction. Fig. 8-28 presents a case which had a penetrating injury with a repaired corneal laceration leaving 6 D of induced astigmatism and a best corrected acuity of 20/60. Postexcimer treatment, this patient had no refractive cylinder and a best corrected acuity of 20/20. The change map demonstrates flattening which is virtually superimposable on the preoperative area of steepening.

Treatment of High Myopia

The sensitivity and reliability of the EyeSys system in evaluating excimer laser procedures is well demonstrated in cases undergoing PRK for high myopia using multiple zone ablation techniques. Figs. 8-29 and 8-30 demonstrate change or difference maps in two cases receiving multiple zone ablation to treat 15 D of myopia. With multiple zone ablation techniques, progressively smaller apertures are used to create greater effect centrally. The transition zones, having progressively greater effect as one moves centrally, can be observed directly on the change maps with the peripheral portion of the ablation demonstrating 9 D of effect, the paracentral portion 12 D of effect, and the central portion 15 D of effect.

REFERENCES

1. Rabinowitz YS, McDonnell PJ: Computer-assisted corneal topography in keratoconus, *Refract Corneal Surg* 5:400-408, 1989.
2. Maguire LJ, Bourne WM: Corneal topography of early keratoconus, *Am J Ophthalmol* 108:107–112, 1989.
3. Waring GO: Nomenclature for keratoconus suspects, *Refract Corneal Surg* 9:219–222, 1993.
4. Ellis W: Radial keratotomy in a patient with keratoconus, *J Cataract Refract Surg* 18:406–409, 1992.
5. Mamalis N, Montgomery S, Anderson C, et al: Radial keratotomy in a patient with keratoconus, *Refract Corneal Surg* 7:374–376, 1991.
6. Schachar RA, Black TD, Huang T: *Understanding radial keratotomy,* Denison, Tex; 1981, CLA Publishing.
7. Binder PS, Nayak SK, Deg JK, et al: An ultrastructural and histochemical study of long-term wound healing after radial keratotomy, *Am J Ophthalmol* 108:107–112, 1989.
8. Dingeldein SA, Klyce SD: The topography of normal corneas, *Arch Ophthalmol* 107:512–518, 1989.
9. Uozato H, Guyton DL: Centering corneal surgical procedures, *Am J Ophthalmol* 103:264–275, 1987.
10. Walsh PM, Guyton DL: Comparison of two methods of marking the visual axis on the cornea during radial keratotomy (letter), *Am J Ophthalmol* 97:660, 1984.
11. Steinberg EB, Waring GO, III: Comparison of two methods of marking the visual axis on the cornea during radial keratotomy, *Am J Ophthalmol* 96:605, 1983.
12. Thornton SP: Surgical armamentarium. In Sanders DR, Hofmann RF, Salz JJ editors: *Refractive corneal surgery,* Thorofare, NJ, 1986, Slack Inc.
13. Maloney RK: Corneal topography and optical zone location in photorefractive keratectomy, *Refract Corneal Surg* 6:363–371, 1990.
14. Enoch JM, Laties AM: An analysis of retinal receptor orientation. II. Prediction for psychophysical tests, *Invest Ophthalmol Vis Sci* 10:959, 1971.
15. Bonds AB, MacLeod DIA: A displaced Stiles-Crawford effect associated with an eccentric pupil, *Invest Ophthalmol Vis Sci* 17:754, 1978.
16. Sutton HG, Lin DT, Berman MD: Photorefractive keratectomy for myopia. Presented at American Academy of Ophthalmology Annual Meeting, Nov 14–18, 1993.
17. Kawesch GM, Maloney RK, Derse M, et al: Contour ablation zone after photorefractive keratectomy, *Invest Ophthalmol Vis Sci* 33:1105, 1992.

9

Complications After Myopic Photorefractive Keratectomy, Primarily with the Summit Excimer Laser

Theo Seiler, Heike Schmidt-Petersen, Josef Wollensak

Keratorefractive surgery has to be considered as elective surgery because in the majority of myopia cases optical correction is available. Although modern ophthalmic surgery in general aims toward minimizing the risk of complications, efforts to increase the benefit-risk ratio are absolutely mandatory in keratorefractive surgery. A first step in this direction is to define the complications and, in a second phase, establish strategies to anticipate, prevent, and manage them.

Regarding myopic photorefractive keratectomy (PRK), a procedure that has been in clinical use for only 4 years, we are still in the first phase of collecting all possible complications. During the last 2 years we have begun the second phase—searching for solutions to avoid and handle complications. Therefore, this discussion is a "work-in-progress" report and it may well be that with an increasing number of treatments new but very rare complications will be found, or that unknown long-term complications will appear. Also and even more important, any change in laser parameters or in the procedure itself may result in new types of complications. For example, the so-called central islands occurred when VISX investigators moved on to larger ablation zones or changed the technique of plume removal.[1]

There are two ways to document the safety of a keratorefractive procedure: (1) in order to estimate the rate of vision-threatening complications, the incidence of eyes with substantial visual loss may be enumerated; (2) specific complications may be described as well as their consequences for the refractive and visual results. Providing both sets of information about complications is the appropriate way to draw a complete picture of the safety of a refractive procedure.

ESTIMATION OF THE OVERALL COMPLICATION RATE

As mentioned before, the safety of a kertorefractive procedure may be defined by the rate of treated eyes that suffer postoperatively form substantial visual loss. There is some ongoing discussion about the term "substantial loss" since visual acuity and refraction show considerable natural variation from examination to examination. We believe today that only changes of more than one Snellen line may be considered as clinically significant.[2,3] Also, the time interval after the visual loss is documented is of concern. At least, we should wait until refraction and the corneal surface modeling process have reached a kind of steady state. In the case of PRK for myopia correction, such a steady state is obtained not earlier than 6 months after surgery and there is increasing agreement that 1 year after surgery is an appropriate time to approximate the final result in most treated eyes (except in high myopia).

Such substantial visual loss estimations after keratorefractive surgery have to be enumerated in prospective studies. However, PRK for myopia correction has been the subject of only two published studies outside the United States that included 100 or more treated eyes: an English trial[4,5] and the Berlin prospective study for evaluation of myopic PRK.[6,7] As a consequence, we refer here mostly to the results of these two clinical trials. In both studies, Summit excimer laser (Summit Technology, Waltham, Mass.) was used; however, the laser parameters were different. Whereas we used a system that was calibrated clinically in a pilot study and included ablation zones of 4.5 mm to 5.0 mm in diameter, the English study group used only 4.0-mm ablation zones including a preliminary algorithm that was not calibrated for optimal refractive outcome. Therefore, it was logical that the refractive results achieved in the English study would be suboptimal, but except for refractive complications the documented complication rates are reliable and descriptive. Other European studies were either not designed as prospective studies with a strict protocol or were published inappropriately.[8,9]

In the Berlin study, 193 eyes were included and in 91.2% of these eyes the 1-year follow-up was completed. Reoperations of undercorrected eyes and of those that developed scars were included.[7,10] After 1 year, two eyes suffered from a loss in best corrected spectacle visual acuity of two lines: one patient had an ablation 1.4 mm eccentric from the center of the pupil and another patient developed between postoperative months 3 and 6 a dense corneal scar that was not reoperated on at 1 year after surgery because of occupational reasons. Therefore, the incidence of postoperative "substantial visual loss" at 1 year after surgery was 1.1%. On the other hand, 3.6% of the patients gained two lines, which may be explained by the optical magnification of the retinal image achieved by the operation. It is worthwhile to note that the patient with the scar was reoperated on at 14 months after primary PRK with no signs of recurrence of the scar at 24 months after surgery. At 2 years, the best corrected spectacles visual acuity was identical to the preoperative activity (20/20).

Gartry and co-workers[4] reported on 3 eyes out of 120 eyes treated with PRK that lost two lines of Snellen acuity. These three patients had undergone −6-D or −7-D procedures, but no clinical cause for the visual loss was reported. Also, reoperations were not scheduled owing to the protocol of the prospective study. Therefore, the incidence of substantial visual loss in the English study was 2.5%, not including reoperations.

An Italian multicenter study,[8] although not strictly prospective, reports on 8 eyes with visual loss out of 1236 myopic eyes (2.4%) treated with the Summit excimer laser. Clinical explanations were: subretinal macular neovascularization (3 eyes) and cataract (1 eye). Eccentric ablations may have been missed in this study because corneal topography was not performed in all centers. The incidence of visual loss might be higher than 2.4% since the follow-up of 1 year was not completed in all 1236 treated eyes. On the other hand, reoperations were also not included in this study.

In summary, visual loss after myopic PRK may occur in 1% to 3% of treated eyes, but this rather high number can be reduced by reoperations.

SPECIFIC COMPLICATIONS
Refractive Complications

Overcorrection. In general, myopic patients seem to accept undercorrection better than overcorrection. This is more evident in presbyopic or nearly presbyopic patients. Patients in their twenties, however, easily adjust to an overcorrection +0.5 D. However, if an overcorrection of more than +1.0 D occurs, there is a demand for increased accommodation with accompanying accommodation-convergence of the near reflex which creates a stress on the vergence system. The patient experiences monocular vision or even double images. Because of this symptom complex, we consider overcorrection of more than +1.0 D as a real complication.

Significant overcorrection mostly results in patients with a minimal healing reaction which is frequently accompanied by an increased steroid response.[11,22] This type of healing response occurs in about 10% of our patient population. At the 1 month follow-up examination, such eyes do not show the regular subepithelial haze, but the cornea is perfectly clear. Usually the intraocular pressure (IOP) is elevated by 5 to 10 mm Hg compared to the preoperative pressure. Immediate cessation of steroid therapy promptly reduces the IOP and some regression of the overcorrection may take place during the following months.

At 1 year, the incidence of overcorrection greater than +1.0 D was 0% in the low myopia group (baseline, up to −3.0 D), 3.5% in the middle myopia group (baseline, −3.1 D−6.0 D), and 3.7% in the high myopia group (baseline, −6.1 D−9.0 D).[12] No such information was available from the Italian[9] or English studies.[6]

If the eye is still overcorrected at 9 to 12 months we recommend a manual abrasion of the epithelium with no postoperative steroid medication. Corneal healing cascades are initiated a second time and during the following months a regression of another 1 to 3 D will take place.

In cases that do not respond to this treatment (in our patient population 5 out of more than 2000 treated eyes) a third intervention will be necessary, either holmium:yttrium-aluminum-garnet (Ho:YAG) thermokeratoplasty or even a hyperopic mask PRK. In four of our five overcorrected patients this treatment was successful. In one eye, the hyperopic mask treatment was eccentric by 1.5 mm, which created irregular astigmatism and reduction of best corrected spectacles visual acuity by two lines.

Undercorrection. Although eyes undercorrected after PRK can be re-treated, and even though myopic patients are accustomed to being myopic and have the option of wearing glasses or contact lenses after PRK, undercorrected patients are often very disappointed.

The incidence of undercorrection is directly related to the attempted refractive change: in the low myopia group (baseline, up to −3.0 D) 2.4% of the treated eyes were undercorrected by more than 1.0 D; in the middle myopia group (baseline, −3.1 D-−6.0D), 4.7%; and in the high myopia group (baseline, −6.1 D-D-−9.0D), 52%. These numbers compare favorably with those of the English study where the incidence of undercorrection was much higher.[4,5] However, since a different algorithm was used during the laser treatment, the attempted corrections did not aim toward emmetropia.

On the other hand, undercorrected eyes can be re-treated with good results. In a series of 30 undercorrected eyes, two thirds of the patients were successfully re-treated with refractions within 1.0 D of emmetropia at 6 months post re-treatment.[10] During the re-treatment, we used laser photoablation for removal of the corneal epithelium, but manual abrasion seems to be a possible alternative (Björn Tengroth, personal communication, August 1993).

In some cases, the undercorrection is caused by corneal scarring (see Scarring, below). During the re-treatment for undercorrection caused by manifest scars, the scar tissue is removed either by laser ablation or manually. We recommend a postoperative corticosteroid treatment of dexamethasone 0.1% four times daily for at least 2 months, tapering during the following months according to the healing response of the re-treated cornea. However, we saw several cases where the scar recurred which have not been re-treated a second time.

Re-treatment of undercorrected eyes with ablation zones larger than those of the initial PRK (e.g., 6.5-mm reablation of corneas that were originally treated with a 5.0-mm beam) bears an additional risk. Because the epithelium is thicker in the center of the treatment zone, laser removal of the epithelium creates a kind of hyperopic correction (Fig. 9-1) which results in additional undercorrection. Having this in mind, you will have to add another 1.0 to 1.5 D to your intended correction!

Astigmatism. The increase of regular corneal astigmatism or the induction of irregular astigmatism is not uncommon after conventional refractive procedures, but it is a rare complication after PRK. Changes in refractive astigmatism may be considered as clinically meaningful if the cylinder power increases or decreases by more than 0.5 D.

In our prospective study, at 1 year after surgery in 5.6% of the treated eyes a significant increase in cylindrical power was detected ranging from 0.75 D to 1.5 D, whereas in 1.1% the refractive cylinder decreased by 0.75 D. The axis of the astigmatism was not changed in any of these cases. At 2 years, a persistent increase in astigmatism was found in only 3 of these patients (0.75 D, 1.0 D, 1.0 D), whereas the astigmatism was permanently lowered in one eye by 0.75 D. Therefore, a significant surgically induced astigmatism occurs in 1.7% of the eyes treated by myopic PRK; all other changes must be interpreted as refraction fluctuations.[12] The English prospective study could not find any statistically significant change in astigmatism between the preoperative and 6-month values.[4] However, the authors did not specify single cases with permanent increase in cylinder power nor were pairwise statistics reported. These numbers compare favorably with those after radial keratotomy (RK), where an induction of astigmatism of 1.0 to 3.0 D occurs in 2% to 10% of the eyes operated on.[13]

Most probably the induction of astigmatism after PRK is due to a slightly eccentric ablation, one of the most important intraoperative complications (see Eccentric Ablation, below). On the other hand, inhomogeneity of the beam or incomplete removal of the corneal epithelium is also a possible source. We want to emphasize that eccentric ablations may occur during the learning curve but should be extremely rare with experienced refractive surgeons using the no-touch technique. However, with mask techniques such as handheld rotating (Meditec) or erodible masks (Summit) positioned near the patient's eye, the risk of eccentric ablation increases. Using such techniques en-

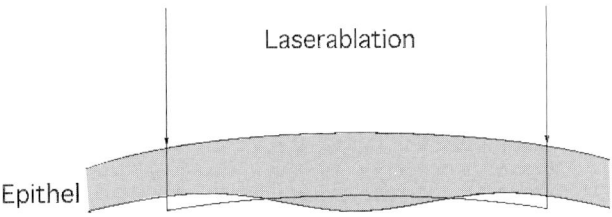

Fig. 9-1. By performing a simple phototherapeutic keratectomy (PTK) procedure for reoperation, a hyperopic PRK effect may occur. Since the epithelium is thicker in the center of the cornea than paracentrally, during the PTK ablation paracentral stromal tissue is removed resulting in an undercorrection of up to 1.5 D.

hances the rate of eccentric ablations by more than 1 mm to typically 5% to 10%.

Stability of refraction. Two types of instability of the refraction are of concern after refractive surgery: long-term instabilities (regression or progressive hyperopia) and short-term instabilities (diurnal fluctuations). When comparing refractions that are obtained 1 year apart we have to be reminded that the measurement "examination of refraction" is plagued by measurement errors, as is any test. During the Prospective Evaluation of Radial Keretotomy (PERK) study, 156 patients with one eye not operated on were examined preoperatively and 1 year after surgery by the same clinical coordinator both times and under conditions as standardized as possible. The change in refraction during this year was 0.25 D or less in 44%, and 0.5 to 0.89 D in 56% of the eyes. None changed 1.0 D or more. Changes in the direction of increasing minus power were similar to changes in the direction of decreasing minus power, indicating a lack of a trend consistent with random variation.[14] Nizam and coworkers[3] recommend 1.0 D as a meaningful cutoff for stability of refraction.

Based on the 137 eyes that had the 2-year examination in the Berlin prospective study (71%) we can estimate the long-term stability of refraction after PRK.[12] At 2 years, none of these eyes showed a refraction that was 1.0 D more hyperopic or less myopic than at the 1-year examination. These data indicate that "progressive hyperopia" either does not exist or is very rare after PRK. In contrast, regression of the refractive effect is dependent upon the attempted refractive change during the second year after surgery, as shown in Table 9-1. Eyes reoperated on were excluded from this analysis. Differences in refraction at 1 and 2 years were statistically significant only in the group with higher baseline myopia (−6.1 D–−9.0 D). Continued regression of more than 1.0 D during the second year was not detected in eyes with a baseline refraction of up to −3.0 D, but it was observed in 8.6% of the eyes with a baseline refraction between −3.1 D and −6.0 D, and in 20% of the eyes with baseline refractions between −6.1 D and −9.0 D. This relation of regression to attempted correction indicates stronger and longer-lasting healing processes in higher corrections.

Diurnal fluctuations of vision (or refraction) are not a common complaint of patients operated on by PRK. We investigated ten patients who reported such fluctuations for as long as 6 months after PRK.[15] None of the treated eyes revealed a refraction shift toward myopia as the day went by, but some, specifically those that were still hyperopic, showed a diurnal shift toward hyperopia. This is quite in contrast to patient reports after radial keratotomy where undercorrected patients see better in the morning than in the evening

because the cornea progressively steepens.[16] A possible explanation for our findings is accommodation that decreases over the day.

Glare problems. A major concern about refractive surgery has been that the residual corneal scars would scatter light and thus increase glare after both RK and PRK. Since most of the eyes treated by PRK showed more or less subepithelial haze, it was logical to relate glare problems to this haze. However, a number of patients with virtually clear corneas also complained about problems with night driving (Fig. 9-2) which made us believe that corneal scars may not be the only reason for glare problems. In a retrospective evaluation of 15 eyes with clear corneas after PRK,[17] the subjective reports of glare of halos and loss of glare vision were significantly correlated only with the effective spherical aberration of the centrally flattened cornea (Table 9-2). Increased effective spherical aberration of the postoperative cornea seems to be directly responsible for the degradation of the retinal image and this degradation becomes worse as the pupil dilates under night lighting conditions. Therefore, except in

Table 9-1. Regression of the refractive effect during the second year after photorefractive keratectomy (reoperations not included)*

Baseline refraction	Change in refraction (D)
≤−3.0 D	−0.03 ±0.43 D
−3.1 D–−6.0 D	−0.29 ±0.59 D
−6.1 D–−9.0 D	−0.48 ±0.64 D†
≥9.1 D	−2.63 ±1.68 D

*Data from Seilert, Holschbach A, Derse M, et al: *Ophthalmology* 101:153-160, 1994.
†Statistically significant (*P* < .02).

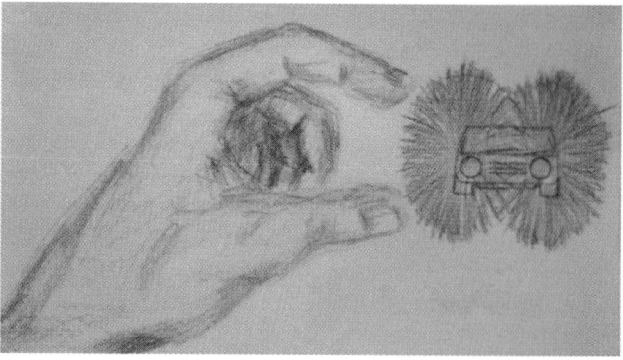

Fig. 9-2. This patient's drawing demonstrates the subjective experience of the halo effect. The refraction was +0.5 D 3 months after a 5.5-D correction (5-mm ablation zone). Uncorrected visual acuity was 20/16 −2; however, visual acuity under glare condition was only 20/30. The cornea was totally clear.

those cases with central manifest scars we consider increased glare and halos an optical-refractive complication rather than a consequence of a reduced transparency of the cornea.

In the English prospective study, 6 to 12 months after surgery, 78% of the patients experienced some halo effect based on direct questions about their night vision, and 10% considered this a significant problem.[4] It is worthy of note that throughout the English study the beam diameter was fixed at 4 mm. In a later report, less than 3% of patients treated by a 5-mm PRK complained about significant halos.[18] This is in agreement with our experience that less than 1% of the patients treated with ablation zones of 6 mm and more in diameter experience halos 1 year after PRK (unpublished data).

The loss of more than two lines of visual acuity un-

der glare conditions 1 year after PRK was clearly related to attempted correction in patients treated with 4.5- to 5.0-mm ablation zones.[8] Such a loss in glare vision was detected in from 0% to 19% of patients (Fig. 9-3). Again, since most of these eyes had clear corneas, the glare effect has to be interpreted not as a consequence of reduced corneal clarity but of the reduced optical homogeneity of the postoperative cornea. The effective optical zone (OZ) is smaller and the transition zone wider in higher corrections, as demonstrated by corneal topography. Enlargement of the ablation zone as well as aspherical algorithms may further help to reduce or eliminate the glare problems.[19]

Intraoperative Complications

In principle, many mistakes can occur during PRK surgery, but in our clinical experience only three types

Table 9-2. Statistical significance of the correlation of subjective halo and glare and some surgery parameters*

	Effective spherical aberration	Attempted correction	Loss in glare visual acuity	Eccentricity of optical zone
Subjective halo and glare	Highly significant	Highly significant	Significant	Not significant
Loss in glare visual acuity	Highly significant	Significant		Not significant
Eccentricity of optical zone	Significant	Not significant	Not significant	

*Significant = $P < .05$; highly significant = $P < .01$.

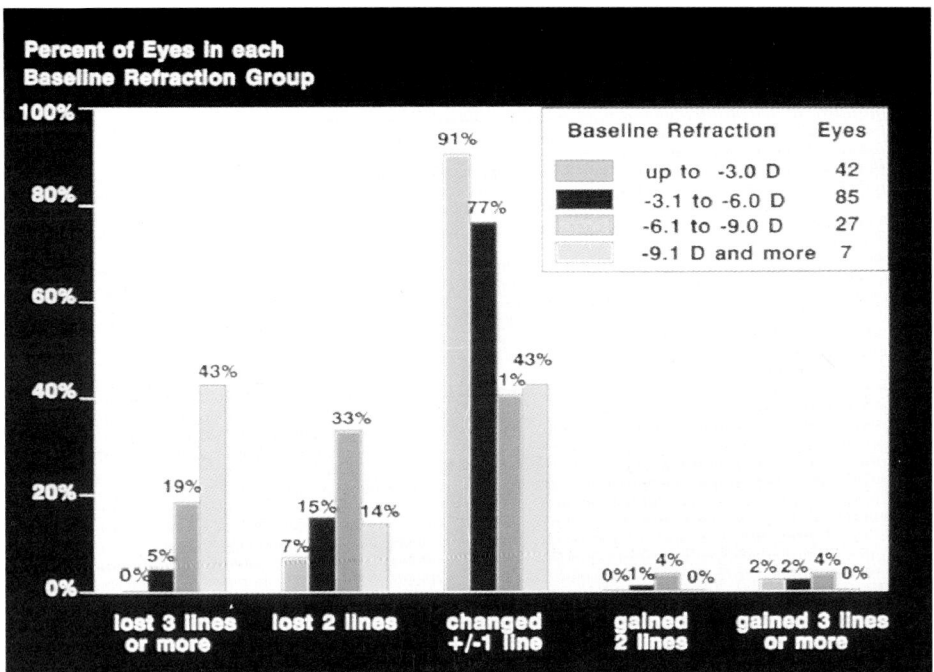

Fig. 9-3. Change in visual acuity under glare conditions 1 year after PRK compared to preoperatively. The losses in glare vision are clearly related to the attempted correction.

of errors are likely: (1) laser failure, inappropriate laser programming, or inappropriate laser adjustment; (2) incomplete removal of the epithelium; and (3) eccentric ablation.

Laser failure. Once the training procedures are completed, the epithelium is removed, and Bowman's layer is cleaned, it may happen that the laser does not test properly (because of low energy output, etc.) or the laser shuts down due to an electrical breakdown. Changing gases or starting the laser again takes at least 5 minutes and the surgeon must decide whether to continue the procedure. Since the ablation rate of corneal tissue is related to the hydration of the cornea we have to assume that waiting another 5 minutes or more may interfere with the precision of the depth of ablation and the refractive change. To our best knowledge, there are no reliable data available in the literature as to whether dehydration by evaporation, or increased hydration by repeated rinsing of the denuded cornea, influences the refractive outcome of PRK. Until such data are available, we recommend that the procedure be stopped and attempted again 10 days or so later. Although the patient will be disappointed, this is the safest way to avoid further complications.

As in any type of surgery using high-tech instrumentation, the instrument is only as intelligent as the operator. If the laser is programmed inappropriately (wrong OZ, wrong attempted refractive change) the surgeon may not recognize this mistake until after surgery. On the other hand, after completion of the iris position calculations, the laser terminal displays the final data such as OZ and attempted refractive change and the operator can compare the parameters with the patient file one last time. It may also be helpful if the operator read aloud the displayed data so that the surgeon can approve it.

The laser beam and the aiming system (the crossed helium-neon lasers and the blinking green fixation light) may be misaligned because of several reasons. Also, the homogeneity of the excimer laser beam may be incorrect because of degradation of the optics or mechanical shocks. It is therefore mandatory to control the centration of the aiming system and the homogeneity of the beam prior to surgery according to the specifications of Summit. It may not be necessary to perform these controls prior to every treatment but controls should be performed at least at the beginning and the end of a session.

Epithelial removal. Especially in eyes with a long history of contact lens wear, the epithelium adheres strongly to Bowman's layer and it may be difficult to remove all epithelial cells. In addition, in older prototypes of the Summit excimer laser with noncoaxial illumination and noncoaxial view, tiny islands of epithelium may be missed. If the photoablation starts from such an irregular surface, the irregularity will be reproduced on a lower level in the stroma and irregular astigmatism may result. Although we have not found such an irregular astigmatism in our patients we had the opportunity to observe localized paracentral areas of undercorrection in patients treated with PRK and referred to our hospital because of postoperative visual loss. Such localized spots are highly suspicious for incompletely removed epithelium. Since all newer Summit systems include coaxial illumination, irregular reflections of the surface can be detected easily and an incomplete removal of epithelial cells should not occur.

Sometimes shallow defects of Bowman's layer become obvious during epithelial removal (e.g., resulting from corneal foreign bodies) that were missed preoperatively by slit-lamp inspection. However, such shallow irregularities have not had any impact on the postoperative corneal surface regularity in our clinical experience.

Eccentric ablation. As in any refractive surgical procedure. PRK requires proper centration on the cornea. Eccentric PRK results in a typical kind of irregular astigmatism depending on the amount of eccentricity and the diameter of the ablation zone (Fig. 9-4). Today, most refractive surgeons believe that the optical zone should be centered around the center of the entrance pupil[20] rather than around the abstract and poorly defined visual axis. This is easily obtained by centering the entrance pupil between the two projection spots of the crossed helium-neon lasers on the iris. If the surgeon has binocular sight the corneal light reflection of the green fixation target (first Purkinje image) is then coincident with the merged red spots on the corneal surface. However, this assumes a concentric constriction of the pupil which might not be the case in high myopes. Therefore, we recommend only mild preoperative miosis obtained by one or two drops of pilocarpine 1%.

Since the Summit system uses the no-touch technique, involuntary movements of the patient's eye may occur. In the English prospective study, 1 patient of 120 patients "moved bodily slightly down the operating table during the treatment."[4] The ablation, eccentric by approximately 1 mm, resulted in an astigmatism of 2.0 D at 1 month, regressing to 0.75 D at 4 months, and an asymmetric halo effect.[4] In our study, 1.1% of the ablation zones were decentered by more than 1 mm (1.2 and 1.4 mm). The refractive astigmatism increased to 1.25 D and 1.5 D at 1 year and decreased to 1.0 D at 2 years accompanied by an undercorrection of approximately 1.0 D. In another 23% of the treated eyes the eccentricity of the ablation zone was between 0.5 and 1.0 mm with no impact on best corrected visual acuity or refractive astigmatism. In general, eyes with eccentric ablation zones had worse visual acuity under glare conditions.

In order to avoid eccentric ablation, the surgeon should be trained to interrupt the procedure as soon as he or she recognizes a systematic movement of the eye to be treated. Small irregular movements can be tolerated. If the surgeon has discontinued the photoablation, after a few seconds the patient can be asked to fixate the green light again. The software of the system is configured in a way that the procedure will continue at the point where the surgeon has stopped.

Once an eccentric ablation is noticed postoperatively and the patient complains about asymmetric halos during the night, a decision has to be made about re-treatment. Such re-treatments can be performed with good success by means of a second PRK, eccentric by the identical distance to the center of the pupil but opposite to the initial PRK. The attempted refractive change of this second PRK should amount to the local undercorrection at the center of the pupil as deduced from a corneal map. The epithelium inside the area of the second ablation has to be removed with

the eximer laser. This procedure may leave some residual regular astigmatism of up to 1 D but the asymmetric halos and the undercorrection improve significantly (Fig. 9-5).

Ptosis and anisocoria. We found a unilateral blepharoptosis of more than 1 mm in 1% of our cases at 1 month after surgery. At 6 months, the condition had significantly improved. Blepharoptosis has also been reported after RK with unknown pathogenesis.[21]

In approximately 5% of the unilaterally treated patients we found a larger pupil in the treated eye that persisted up to 1 year. This side effect is presumably caused by an individually prolonged reaction to the postoperative dilation of the pupil by homatropine.

Early Postoperative Complications

The following complications may occur during the early postoperative period of approximately 3 months: (1) delayed epithelial healing and related disorders, (2) corticosteroid-induced increase of IOP, and (3) hemorrhages from preexisting subretinal neovascularizations.

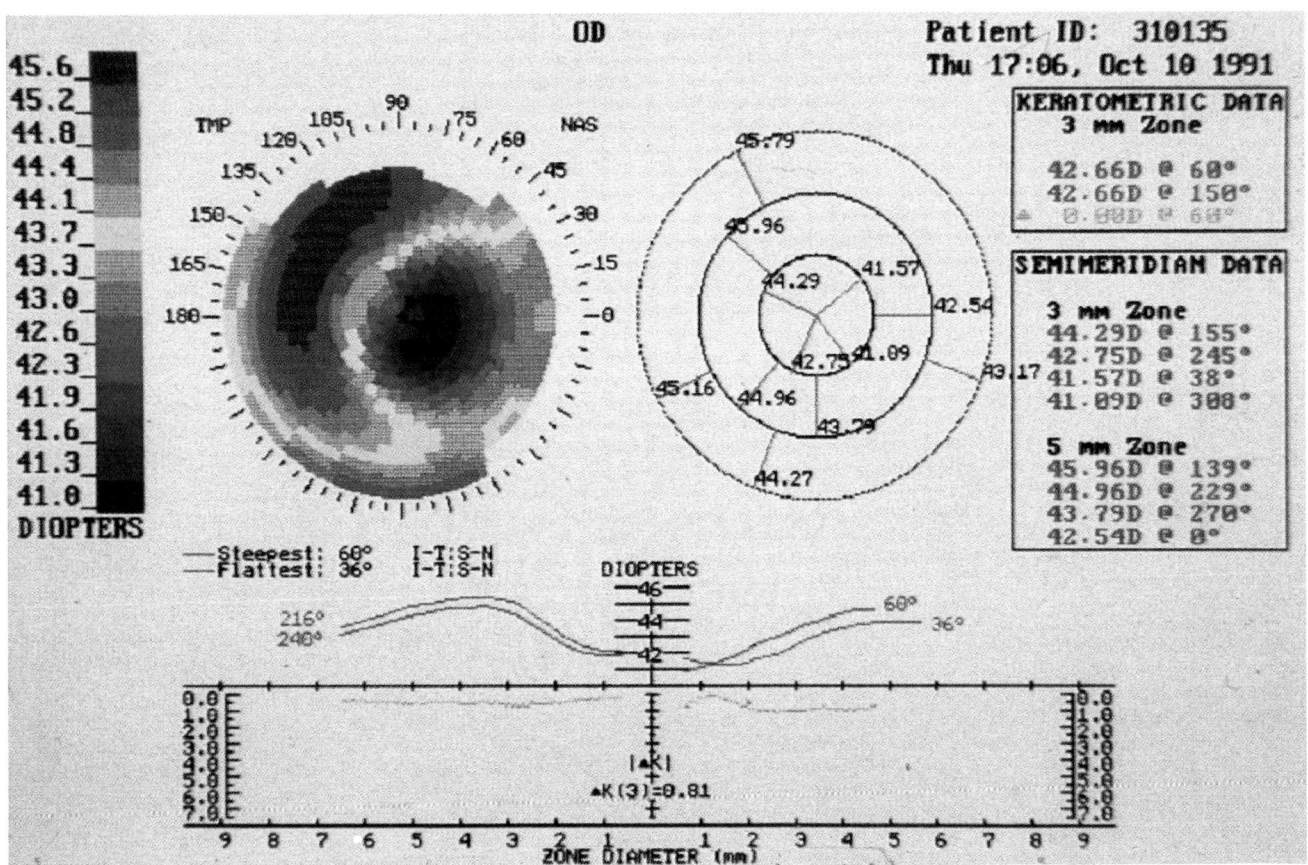

Fig. 9-4. Corneal topography of a cornea after eccentric PRK (−6.5-D correction, 4.5-mm ablation zone). The flattened area is 1.4 mm eccentric compared to the center of the entrance pupil. The patient reported asymmetric halos and had an induced astigmatism of 1.0 D 1 year after PRK.

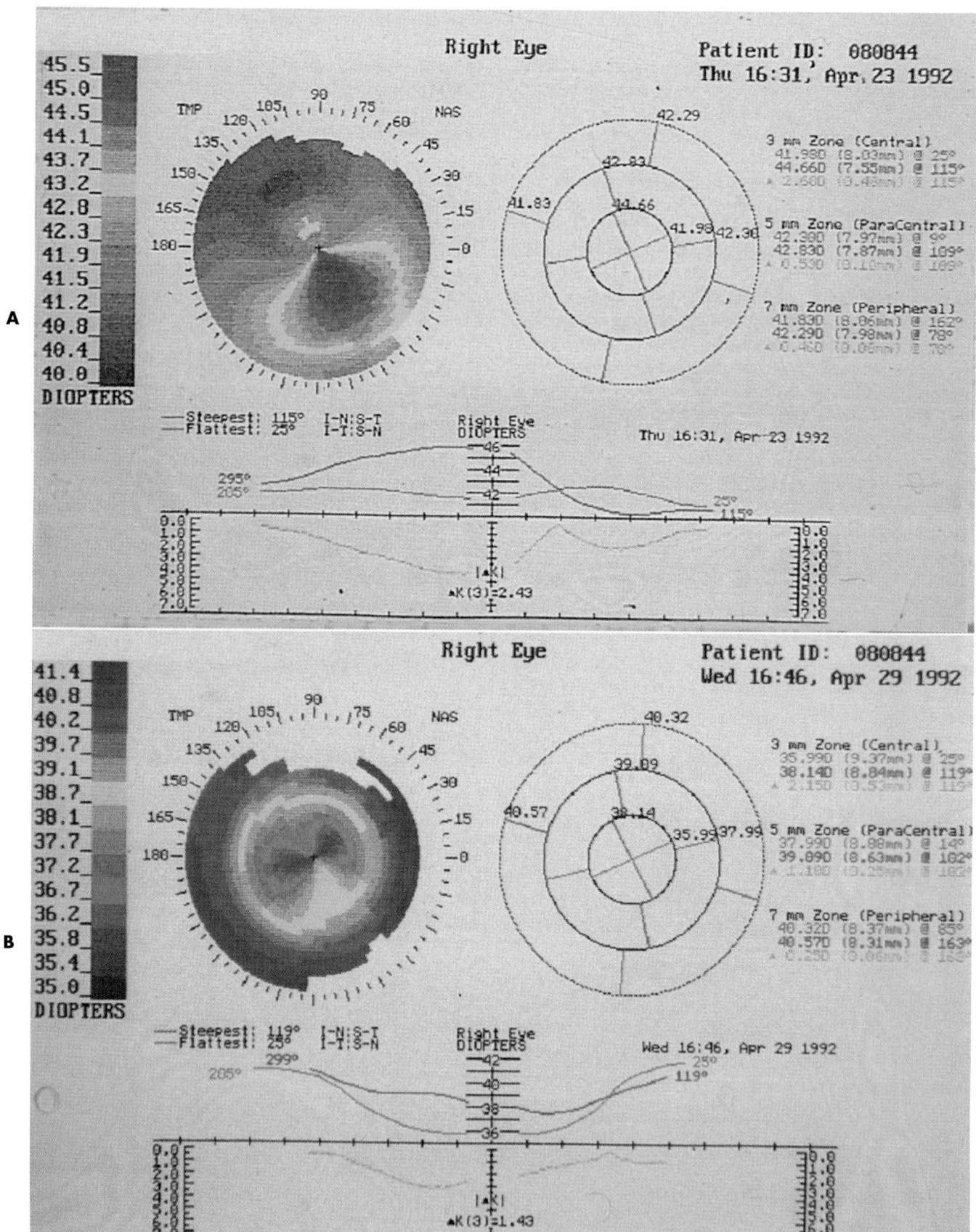

Fig. 9-5. Corneal maps of an eye before **(A)** and after reoperation **(B)**. During the initial PRK, the patient's head moved downward. One year after initial PRK, best corrected visual acuity was 20/50. Already 1 week after reoperation, uncorrected visual acuity was 20/30.

Epithelial disorders. In the vast majority of cases the epithelium is closed within 4 days after surgery and during the following weeks the epithelium adhesion complex is restored. During this period, up to 20% of the patients report slight foreign body sensations.[4] Epithelial healing, however, may be delayed by the early use of topical corticosteroids. We therefore recommend that only antibiotic ointments be used until the epithelium has closed. Some patients also report that the treated eye is tender to touch over the first couple of months. Painful epithelial instability episodes are rare. We had 1 patient out of 2000 who had recurrent erosions that constantly needed to be treated by ointment.

A severe complication occurred when a patient suffering from undiagnosed lupus erythematosus developed an ulcer 30 days after PRK (Fig. 9-6). It was a painless noninfectious ulcer that required penetrating keratoplasty.[6] In some connective tissue and autoimmune diseases even microtrauma can induce melting of corneal tissue. Therefore, we consider such diseases an absolute contraindication to keratorefractive surgery and we recommend investigation of any history of rheumatic disease prior to PRK.

Corticosteroid-induced increase of intraocular pressure. There is an ongoing discussion about whether corticosteroids should be used to modulate corneal healing after PRK. Starting from the very first PRKs, the postoperative management included steroids[22] to prevent scarring or as a method to titrate the refractive effect.[6] This approach was based on animal studies that showed that haze was minimized by topical corticosteroids.[23] However, the only clinical double-blind trial comparing refractive results and corneal clarity in eyes with and without such medication found no important role for steroids.[24] On the other hand, others believe that the regression of the refractive effect after PRK is attributable to stromal production of hyaluronic acid by keratocytes, which can be inhibited by topical steroids. These authors conclude that corticosteroids are "active and necessary during the healing phase" after PRK.[25]

Corticosteroid-induced IOP elevation occurs in up to 30% of myopic patients depending on the definition of significant IOP increase. Independent of baseline refraction up to −9.0 D, the incidence of steroid responders ranged from 26% to 32% in the different refraction groups.[26] It is worth noting that five of the six overcorrected eyes in the Berlin prospective trial showed a corticosteroid-induced increase in IOP. In order to avoid the overcorrection due to steroid response it may be beneficial to test the patients for corticosteroid-induced IOP elevation prior to surgery (Werner Förster, Münster, personal communication, November 1992).

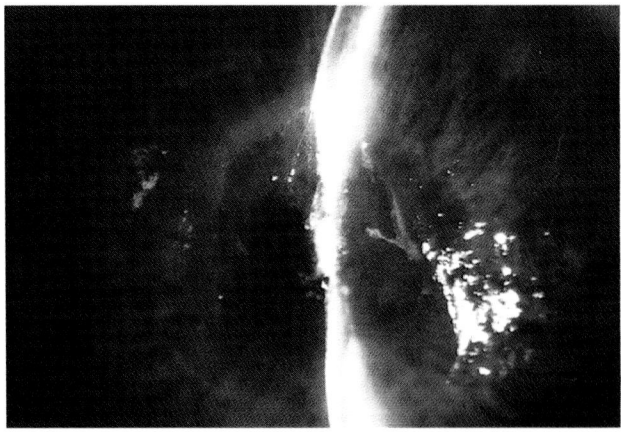

Fig. 9-6. Perforated ulcer 30 days after a 10-D PRK. The patient suffered from undiagnosed systemic lupus erythematosus.

In any case, close monitoring of the IOP is mandatory after PRK in patients receiving steroids for postoperative medication. If the IOP increase is detected at 1 month after surgery, cessation or at least significant reduction of the steroid dose and the administration of β blockers led to normal pressures within 1 or 2 weeks. Nevertheless, the healing response may stay depressed for several more months and the eye may remain overcorrected (for management of overcorrection, see above).

Subretinal hemorrhages. In the Italian study, 3 out of 1236 treated eyes suffered from severe visual loss due to subretinal hemorrhage during the postoperative period.[8] Unfortunately, the authors did not mention at what time after surgery the bleeding occurred. Another case of ours, a 52-year-old woman received an 8-D PRK and developed a subretinal hemorrhage 2 months after surgery. The fellow eye showed subretinal vessels also, as detected by fluorescein angiography. Whether the incidence of subretinal hemorrhage is a consequence of the myopia correction by PRK is not proven, but during PRK mechanical shock waves with an amplitude of more than 100 bar travel through the eye and may irritate the fragile vessels of the subretinal neovascularization.

Inspection of the fundus clearly belongs in a thorough preoperative examination and besides the retinal periphery the posterior pole also merits attention. The possibility of a subretinal hemorrhage has to be discussed with the patient prior to surgery.

Late Postoperative Complications

Besides the above-mentioned steroid glaucoma and the one case of perforated ulcer, there is no specific intraocular complication after PRK reported in the literature. We have seen cataracts after PRK, but since the cataracts developed more or less symmetrically in both eyes or some incipient cataract was recorded pre-operatively, we consider them as naturally occurring, presumably unrelated to the procedure. On the other hand, prolonged topical corticosteroid use may cause cataract formation.

After RK, bacterial and fungal keratitis may occur late, after 1 to 3 years, probably because of continued remodeling of the corneal epithelium. In principle, such a late infection seems also to be possible after PRK, although to date there is no report of such a case in the literature.

Recurrent herpes simplex keratitis can be stimulated by numerous exogenous insults to the eye, including the trauma of PRK. Indeed, two working groups reported herpes keratitis after phototherapeutic keratectomy (PTK).[27,28] However, in another study of PTK the incidence of recurrence was not increased compared to the natural development.[29] So far, only one case of herpes simplex keratitis after PRK has been reported (Peter McDonnell, presented at a symposium on refractive surgery, Houston, January 29, 1994). Nevertheless, corneal sensitivity testing should be part of every ophthalmic examination prior to keratorefractive surgery to rule out patients with a history of herpes keratitis.

Scarring. The formation of manifest central scars interfering with best spectacle corrected visual acuity is probably the only late postoperative complication after PRK. Approximately 50% of the scars develop during the first 3 months after surgery, but we have also seen scars that occurred as late as 1 year after PRK. These scars should be differentiated from the subepithelial haze that is transient and, on clinical assessment, maximal at about 3 months. Also, the subepithelial haze never interferes with best corrected spectacle (see above) visual acuity and since it occurs in vitually any cornea after PRK it should be considered a normal healing reaction.

The incidence of scars is strongly dependent on the attempted refractive change[7]: in the Berlin prospective study we found ten eyes at 1 year that developed scars (Table 9-3) and in corrections greater than 6.0 D, scar formation was significantly more likely than after corrections up to −6.0 D (17.3% vs. 0.7 $P < .001$). The development of manifest scars was believed to be caused by the depth of the keratectomy, but high myopia corrections using wider ablation zones resulted in an identical incidence or even fewer scars although the keratectomies were substantially deeper.[30] Alternatively, one can speculate that the high myopia population includes a genetic subentity that shows a corneal healing pattern different from the normal population. This assumption is supported by other genetically determined pathologic reactions that occur more frequently in the high myopia population (e.g., glaucoma, steroid response).

We had the opportunity to follow a cornea for 4 years that responded to PRK with a manifest dense central scar 6 months after surgery. The scar faded gradually year by year and after 4 years it was hardly detectable by slit-lamp inspection. The reduction in optical density of the scars is also a common finding in patients with shorter follow-up and we can extrapolate that most of the scars will disappear after a few years. However, scar formation always is accompanied by excessive regression of the refractive effect and, therefore, most of the eyes with scars end up undercorrected.

Clinically, we can differentiate two types of scars after PRK. The more frequent type includes many trabeculae and has a honeycomb appearance (Fig. 9-7), whereas the other type includes a homogeneous milky plaque comparable to Salzmann-like degenerations. With time, some of the honeycomb scars transform gradually into milky scars and in some eyes both types coexist. Whether these clinically different scar types are caused by different healing mechanisms is not clear.

Table 9-3. Incidence of manifest scars during 2 years after photorefractive keratectomy (study population: 193 eyes)*

Baseline refraction	Incidence of manifest scars
≤−3.0 D	0%
−3.1 D-−6.0 D	1.1%
−6.1 D-−9.0 D	17.5%
≥ −9.1 D	16.7%

*Data from Seiler T, Holschbach A, Derse M, et al: *Ophthalmology* 101:153-160, 1994.

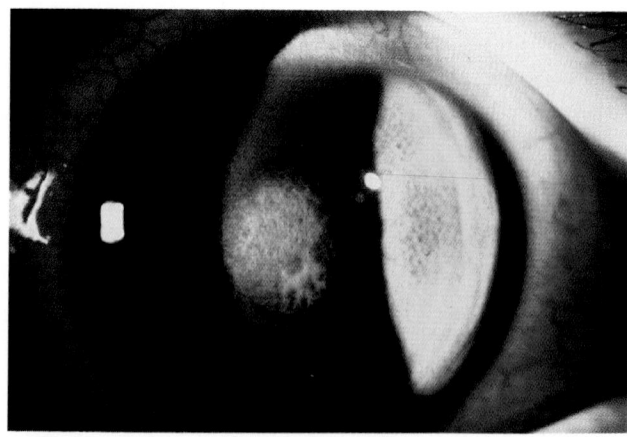

Fig. 9-7. Manifest scar after PRK. The trabeculated structure is easily visible. Some scars transform into a Salzmann-like milky-white plaque.

Even eyes with dense scars have a surprisingly good visual acuity, often as good as 20/25, although there is a significant decrease in the quality of vision because of glare. Since most of the eyes with scars are undercorrected, the demand for reoperation is brought up frequently by patients. Since the undercorrection is a consequence of the scar formation, any removal of the scar should also resolve the refractive error. In some cases, the epithelium adheres strongly to the underlying scar and, therefore, we recommend removing the epithelium and scar by photoablation. During ablation of the epithelium (PTK mode of the laser), the surgeon may observe a blue fluorescent disk as long as the laser beam hits the epithelium. As soon as the keratectomy penetrates to the scar tissue, the fluorescence vanishes and black spots appear within the blue disk. As the epithelium is thicker in the center than paracentrally, the black spots usually are observed in the periphery of the blue disk and the ablation should be discontinued as soon as these spots form a black ring. After that, a standard PRK should follow with an attempted correction of the actual undercorrection plus 1.0 D. Using this technique, in most cases the scar is totally removed. The postoperative medication consists of dexamethasone 0.1% four times a day for 2 months, tapering during postoperative months 3 and 4.

We were surprised by the results of such retreatment, which should not be performed earlier than 6 months after the initial PRK. In only 4 out of 21 eyes re-treated because of manifest scars did the scar recur. In another three patients the corneas developed significantly less dense scars. So far, a second retreatment has not been undertaken.

CLOSING REMARKS

Our subject was an estimation of the safety of PRK for myopia correction. Significant complications such as overcorrection, significant loss of visual acuity under glare conditions, scarring, and eccentric ablation are rare and can be managed in most cases. Comparing these complications with the efficacy of the procedure for myopic corrections of up to −6.0 D makes PRK one of the most powerful and promising tools in refractive surgery.

It was this high benefit-risk ratio that convinced the German Ophthalmological Society in September 1993 to approve PRK for corrections of myopia up to −6.0 D. However, in spite of all the advantages of PRK, we still believe that PRK be considered only as an alternative after spectacles and contact lenses.

REFERENCES

1. Lin DT, Sutton HF, Berman M: Corneal topography following excimer photorefractive keratectomy for myopia, *J Cataract Refract Surg* 19:149-154, 1993.
2. Kremer FB, Marks RG: Radial keratotomy: prospective evaluation of safety and efficacy, *Ophthalmic Surg* 14:925-930, 1983.
3. Nizam A, Waring GO, Lynn MJ, et al: Stability of refraction and visual acuity during 5 years with simple myopia, *Refract Corneal Surg* 8:439-477, 1992.
4. Gartry DS, Kerr Muir MG, Marshall J: Photorefractive keratectomy with an argon fluoride excimer laser: a clinical study, *Refract Corneal Surg* 7:420-435, 1991.
5. Gartry DS, Kerr Muir MG, Marshall J: Excimer laser photorefractive keratectomy: 18 months follow-up, *Ophthalmology* 99:1209-1219, 1992.
6. Seiler T, Wollensak J: Myopic photorefractive keratectomy with the excimer laser: one year follow-up, *Ophthalmology* 98:1156-1163, 1991.
7. Seiler T, Wollensak J: Results of a prospective evaluation of photorefractive keratectomy at one year after surgery, *German J Ophthalmol* 2:135-142, 1993.
8. Brancato R, Tavola A, Caronas F, et al: Excimer laser photorefractive keratectomy for myopia: results in 1165 eyes, *Refract Corneal Surg* 9:95-104, 1993.
9. Tengroth B, Epstein D, Fagerholm P, et al: Excimer laser photorefractive keratectomy for myopia. Clinical results in sighted eyes, *Ophthalmology* 100:739-745, 1993.
10. Seiler T, Derse M, Pham T: Repeated excimer laser treatement after photorefractive keratectomy, *Arch Ophthalmol* 110:1230-1233, 1992.
11. Durrie DS, Lesher MP, Cavanaugh TB: Classification of variable clinical response after myopia photorefractive keratectomy. In Selser RE, editor: *Medical cornea—corneal and refractive surgery*, Amsterdam, 1994, Kugler.
12. Seiler T, Holschbach A, Derse M, et al: Complications of myopic photorefractive keratectomy with the excimer laser, *Ophthalmology* 101:153-160, 1994.
13. Waring GO, et al: Radial keratotomy for myopia. Statement of the AAO, *Ophthalmology* 96:671-687, 1989.
14. Lynn MJ, Waring GO, et al: Stability of refraction after radial keratotomy compared with unoperated eyes in the PERK study, *Invest Ophthalmol Vis Sci* 28(suppl):223, 1987.
15. Seiler T, Hell K, Wollensak J: Diurnal variation in refraction after excimer laser refractive keratectomy, *German J Ophthalmol* 1:19-21, 1992.
16. Schanzlin DJ, Santos VR, Waring GO, et al: Diurnal change in refraction, corneal curvature, visual acuity, and intraocular pressure after radial keratotomy in the PERK study. *Ophthalmology* 93:167-175, 1986.
17. Seiler T, Reckmann W, Maloney RK: Effective spherical aberration of the cornea as a quantitative descriptor in corneal topography, *J Cataract Refract Surg* 19(suppl):155-165, 1993.
18. Lohmann CP, Fitzke FW, O'Brart D, et al: Halos—a problem for all myopes?, *Refract Corneal Surg* 9(suppl):S72-S75, 1993.
19. Seiler T, Genth U, Holschbach A, et al: Aspheric photorefractive keratectomy with the excimer laser, *Refract Corneal Surg* 9:166-172, 1993.
20. Uozato H, Guyton DL, Waring GO: Centering corneal surgical procedures. In Waring GO, editor: *Refractive keratotomy*, St Louis, 1992, Mosby-Year Book.
21. Caroll RP, Lindstrom RL: Blepharoptosis after radial keratotomy, *Am J Ophthalmol* 102:800-801, 1986.
22. Seiler T, Kahle G, Kriegerowski M: Excimer laser (193 nm) myopic keratomileusis in sighted and blind human eyes, *Refract Corneal Surg* 6:165-173, 1990.
23. Tuft SJ, Zabel RW, Marshall J: Corneal repair following keratotomy: a comparison between conventional surgery and laser photoablation, *Invest Ophthalmol Vis Sci* 30:1769-1777, 1989.
24. Gartry DS, Kerr Muir MG, Lohmann CP, et al: The effect of topical corticosteroids on refractive outcome and corneal haze after photorefractive keratectomy, *Arch Ophthalmol* 110:944-952, 1992.

25. Tengroth B, Fagerholm P, Söderberg P, et al. Effect of corticosteroids in postoperative care following photorefractive keratectomy *Refract Corneal Surg* 9(suppl):S61-S64, 1993.

26. Seiler T, Wollensak J: Komplikationen der Laserkeratomileusis mit dem Excimerlaser, *Klin Monatsbl Augenheilk* 200:648-653, 1992.

27. Pepose JS, Laycock KA, Miller JK, et al: Reactivation of latent herpes simplex virus by excimer laser photokeratectomy, *Am J Ophthalmol* 114:45-50, 1992.

28. Vrabec MP, Durrie DS, Chase DS: Recurrence of herpes simplex after excimer laser keratectomy, *Am J Ophthalmol* 116:101-102, 1992.

29. Fagerholm P, Öhman L, Örndahl M: Phototherapeutic keratectomy in herpes simplex keratitis, *Acta Ophthalmol* 1994, in press.

30. Sher NA, Barak M, Sheraz D, et al: Excimer laser photorefractive keratectomy in high myopia, *Arch Ophthalmol* 110:935-943, 1992.

10

Complications of Photorefractive Keratectomy, Primarily with the VISX Excimer Laser

Ezra Maguen, Jeffrey J. Machat

Photorefractive keratectomy (PRK) has proved successful for the correction of low to moderate myopia. Many of the complications encountered in PRK patients such as undercorrections and overcorrections are similar to those experienced by RK patients. Other complications such as corneal haze and central islands, however, are specific to the excimer laser. It is extremely rare to obtain a final result that is the same or worse than the preoperative refraction and no reports of lost vision or lost eyes have been published. Anecdotal reports of the need to perform corneal transplants following PRK have come from Europe, yet no such occurrence has been reported in the United States under the Food and Drug Administration (FDA)–guided long-term evaluation of PRK.

The most common complications of PRK did not significantly affect either vision or any other function of the eyes operated on. At the same time, it is important to evaluate these complications and to attempt to uncover their causes, thereby making PRK a safer and more successful procedure.

We discuss complications of PRK from the following sources: a series of 240 procedures performed by five surgeons at Cedars-Sinai Medical Center in Los Angeles during the past 3 years; the nationwide results of phase III of the FDA-guided VISX clinical trials at 1 year postoperatively; a review of the literature; and a series of over 1000 procedures performed by one of us (J.J.M.) using the Summit, VISX, Summit, and Technolas excimer lasers (The Laser Center Inc., Windsor, Canada).

COMPLICATIONS RELATED TO UNPLANNED DEVIATIONS FROM INTENDED CORRECTION
Overcorrection, Undercorrection, and Induced Astigmatism

The accepted standard of accuracy of the final optical correction in refractive surgery is a maximal deviation of ± 1.00 D of the intended correction. In a series performed with the VISX (VISX Inc., Santa Clara, Calif.) model Twenty-Twenty excimer laser[1] at Cedars-Sinai, the optical correction stabilized between 3 and 6 months postoperatively. At 6 months following surgery, 88% of a sample of 124 eyes were corrected within 1.00 D of the intended correction. The amount of undercorrections was significantly larger than that of overcorrection. This was due in part to the discontinuation of nitrogen flow which provided better short-term rehabilitation following PRK,[2] but induced a mean undercorrection of 0.8 D at 18 months postoperatively.[3]

A significant number of overcorrections were reported by users of the Summit Technologies ExciMed UV-200 excimer laser. Gimbel et al.[4] reported on the need to reduce the amount of correction by 25% in order to neutralize the tendency toward overcorrection in their hands. Both the risk of overcorrection and the symptoms produced are substantially greater in patients over 40 years of age.

Undercorrections are more easily managed than overcorrections. Significant undercorrections can be managed by re-treatment of the undercorrected eye with the excimer laser (see Chapter 11). The multi-center data of PRK with the VISX Twenty-Twenty laser shows an incidence of 10.4% of re-treatments (72 of 691 eyes), with 70 of the 72 eyes re-treated for undercorrections. Uncorrected visual acuity was 20/40 or better in 79% of retreated eyes. Incisional keratotomy following PRK should be undertaken with caution as the nomograms available may not be accurate. At the present time, there is no effective and safe treatment for overcorrection. If high doses of topical steroids are used on an overcorrected eye, the medication should be tapered down quickly, with, it is hoped, a decrease in hyperopia. Overcorrected eyes not responsive to withdrawal of topical steroids may be fitted with an extended-wear contact lens in an attempt to produce a hypoxic state of the cornea, thereby promoting regression. As a final attempt the epithelium may be debrided to enhance the wound-healing process.

Regular and irregular astigmatism may be induced following PRK. In the Cedars-Sinai series, 4% of 240 eyes showed induced regular astigmatism of 1.00 D or greater at 12 months postoperatively.[1] Astigmatism increased more than 1.00 D in 6.1% of the 521 patients of the national VISX series. We have successfully treated 3 patients with peripheral arcuate incisions made peripheral to the ablation zone for regular astigmatism of 1.50 to 2.5 D following PRK.

Irregular astigmatism is often evident early in the healing period following excimer laser ablation, reducing best corrected spectacle visual acuity. Nitrogen flow produced a greater incidence of irregular astigmatism, which resolved over weeks to months with the smoothing of the epithelium.

Severe Regression

Severe regression of most or all the correction obtained after PRK is rare. In our series, 2 of 240 patients showed severe regression. One case, previously described (Figs. 10-1 and 10-2), was associated with severe corneal haze, whereas the second patient had a clear cornea. The possible causes of regression are unknown. Gartry et al.[5] found a "good correlation" between corneal haze and regression. The combined incidence of regression and haze was more frequent in patients with preoperative high myopia.[6] Wilson et al.[7] found regression to be more common and more pronounced in eyes with intended correction of more than 5.00 D. Tengroth et al.[8] report the occurrence of regression following discontinuation of topical steroids and the ability to reverse regression with the same medication. Carones et al.[9] report the same findings in six eyes. There are several anecdotal reports of significant myopic regression following intense ultraviolet light exposure during the first few months of

healing. It is surmised that eyes which have undergone PRK may be more sensitized to ultraviolet exposure and that further exposure can retrigger or accelerate the healing process. A series of six female patients who became pregnant in the immediate postoperative period following PRK is reported (Machat, verbal communication). All eyes experienced myopic regression, two associated with severe haze. There appeared to be a definite correlation between hormonal imbalance and regression, with the most severe cases experiencing severe morning sickness. The least affected patient had the least problems with her pregnancy and another nonpregnant patient being treated for a hormonal imbalance found her vision fluctuating dramatically. Her refraction changed by 1.00 D and vision fluctuated between 20/20 and 20/50 whenever her hormonal fluctuation peaked over her monthly cycle.

Because of the low incidence of severe regression in human eyes and the lack of experimental models,

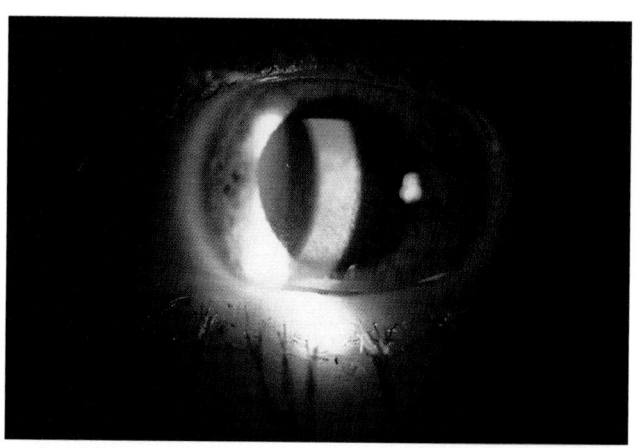

Fig. 10-1. Severe corneal haze, one year postoperatively.

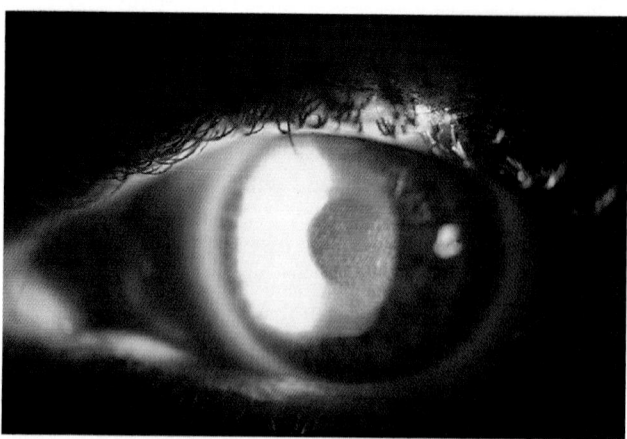

Fig. 10-2. Same patient as in Fig. 1, 18 months after retreatment for severe corneal haze.

it is impossible at this point to have a good understanding of this process and to prevent it. One may propose two possible mechanisms: (1) the overproduction of collagen or fibrous tissue, or both, and (2) epithelial hyperplasia filling the defect created by ablation. Treatment essentially consists of starting or increasing the frequency or potency of topical steroids. Regressions associated with haze could be re-treated with the excimer laser in a transepithelial fashion along with stromal ablation in the amount necessary to correct the present myopia (PRK protocol). Caution should be exercised in treating clear corneas with the excimer laser and one may consider transepithelial treatment with minimal stromal ablation (PTK protocol) if epithelial hyperplasia can be demonstrated with high power slit-lamp observation. Clinically, multizone techniques utilizing larger optical zones to blend in the new contour have reduced the risk of regression when correcting cases of high myopia. A multizone technique algorithm to maximize optical zone (OZ) diameter to 7 mm while minimizing depth of ablation for all degrees of correction was developed at The Laser Center.

COMPLICATIONS RELATED TO POSTOPERATIVE MEDICATIONS AND THERAPEUTIC CONTACT LENSES
Steroid-Induced Complications

Increase in intraocular pressure (steroid response). In the initial stages of the FDA guided investigation of PRK, high doses of steroids were used such as prednisolone sodium acetate (Pred Forte) eye drops four times daily to the operated eye.[10] Later, because of steroid response and other concerns, fluorometholone 0.25% (FML Forte) was used in an attempt to decrease the incidence of steroid-induced increase in intraocular pressure (IOP). The Cedars-Sinai series showed an incidence of 1.7% of operated eyes on which an IOP equal to or higher than 25 mm Hg was measured at any time postoperatively. The same incidence was noted in the national VISX series. Other reports showed incidences ranging between 3.1% and 25.3%.[11] In series where higher incidences of steroid response were reported, higher-potency topical steroids were used such as dexamethasone 0.1%. Management of steroid response associated with PRK consists of the control of IOP with topical antiglaucoma medications while the topical steroid is continued. At times it may be necessary to reduce the potency of the topical steroid to achieve better IOP control. Fluorometholone 0.5% (FML Forte®) eye drops may be an adequate substitute. In all cases, IOP reverted to normal values upon discontinuation of topical steroids in our series, and no reports of persistent increased IOP exist in the literature.

Steroid-induced ocular herpes simplex keratitis. The use of topical steroids may induce ocular herpes simplex virus (HSV) keratitis. At the same time, the immediate tissue response after PRK is an acute photokeratitis. This acute inflammatory response may in itself cause shedding of HSV, thereby inducing the viral keratitis. Indeed, such cases have been described[12] and such a case was treated in our series of PTK with success (M. Mannis, verbal communication, 1993). Management consists of discontinuation of topical steroids and the use of trifluorothimidine eye drops every 2 hours initially along with systemic acyclovir 200 mg, one tablet five times a day. We screen all candidates for PRK for possible HSV dermatitis (cold sores or "fever blisters") and treat these patients prophylactically with the same dose of acyclovir starting from 1 week preoperatively and continuing until the acute keratitis has subsided and the epithelium has regenerated over the treatment area. One might also consider a shorter-term regimen of topical steroids; while this medication is used, it should be covered by a topical antiviral agent.

Ptosis. Steroid-induced ptosis is more common in young females. It is minimal and measures usually 1 to 2 mm. It worsens as the day progresses, improves with decreasing frequency and potency of the topical steroid used, usually resolves with discontinuation of topical steroids, but can be permanent. Ptosis may also occur as a result of stretching Muller's muscle with a lid speculum. One case occurred in the Cedars-Sinai series and was corrected with a Muller muscle–conjunctival resection.

Posterior subcapsular cataracts. Three posterior subcapsular cataracts following use of dexamethasone phosphate 0.1% were observed by one of us (J.J.M.) (Fig. 10-3). All patients were treated by other surgeons. The duration and frequency of steroid use varied from four times daily for 3 months to every 2 hours for 8 months to control regression. All cases underwent PRK with the Summit ExciMed laser. No such cases were reported with the use of fluorometholone.

Superficial Keratopathy

A large variety of topical medications are used in conjunction with PRK. These include topical antibiotics, nonsteroidal anti-inflammatory drugs (NSAID), topical steroids, artificial tears, and on occasion, antiglaucoma medications. It is therefore not surprising that on occasion we have encountered superficial keratopathy related to either the preservatives or the topical medications themselves. Treatment consists of trying to identify the responsible medication and replacing it with an equivalent containing a different preservative. If this is not feasible, nonpreserved medication should be used. A nonspecific keratitis may develop in patients 1 week following excimer ablation lasting 1 to 3 weeks. The superficial punctate staining may be associated with an increase in clinical haze. These findings may reflect a UV photokeratitis related to underlying stromal inflammation. Treatment similarly consists of lubrication.

COMPLICATIONS RELATED TO THERAPEUTIC CONTACT LENSES
Sterile Paracentral Corneal Infiltrate and Infectious Corneal Ulcers

In the Cedars-Sinai series, we have encountered one episode of a paracentral sterile corneal infiltrate following PRK. Because of the lack of pathogens in the corneal scraping, it is unclear whether this was an infectious corneal ulcer or a corneal infiltrate associated with the use of disposable extended-wear lenses as described by Serdahl et al.[13] One should always assume

that such keratitis is infectious and treat it intensively. If the epithelium is intact, one may consider not scraping the cornea and follow the patient closely. One of us (J.J.M.) has treated a total of six corneal ulcers out of a total of 3000 patients evaluated in relation to PRK (Figs. 10-4, 10-5, and 10-6). The incidence of corneal ulcers in this series is 0.1%. All eyes were treated with postoperative contact lenses. All resolved with fortified topical antibiotics. Two ulcers grew *Staphylococcus epidermidis* on cultures.

Other Contact Lens–Related Complications

Disposable extended-wear contact lenses are now used in the majority of PRK procedures performed, along with topical NSAID to control postoperative pain. At times, these lenses may become dislocated, mostly because of a loose fit. In order to avoid infection, our patients are instructed to patch the eye that was operated on and to not reinsert the lens if such an event occurs. Systemic pain medication may then be used as needed and a lens can be reinserted with a

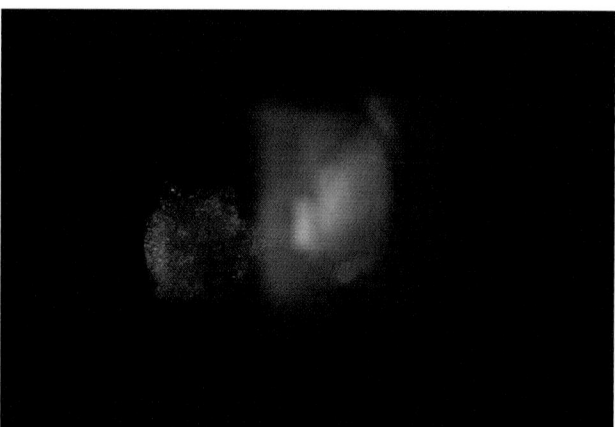

Fig. 10-3. Posterior subcapsular cataract occurring following PRK, associated with long-term postoperative treatment with dexamethazone eye drops.

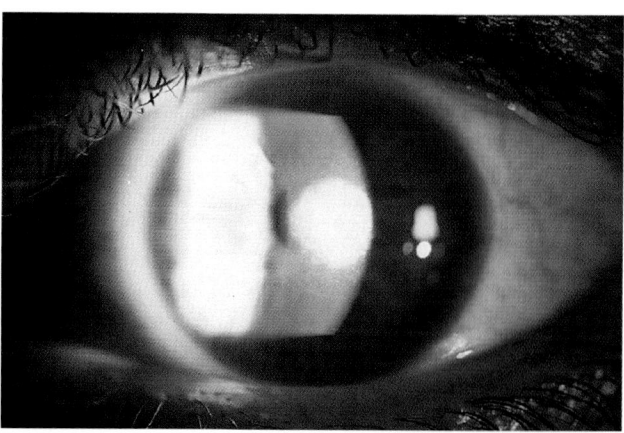

Fig. 10-5. Healed central corneal ulcer following PRK with central scar.

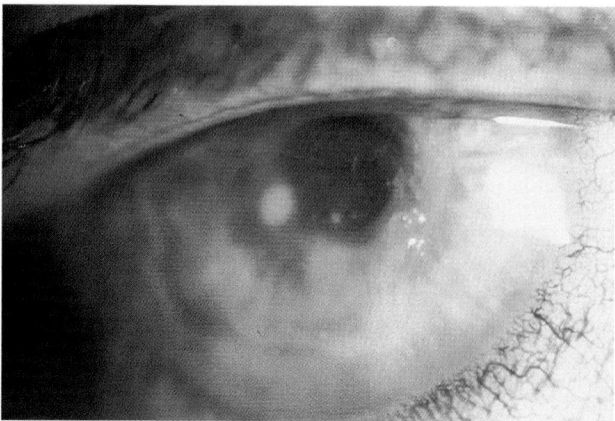

Fig. 10-4. Corneal infiltrates which occurred following PRK and application of therapeutic contact lens.

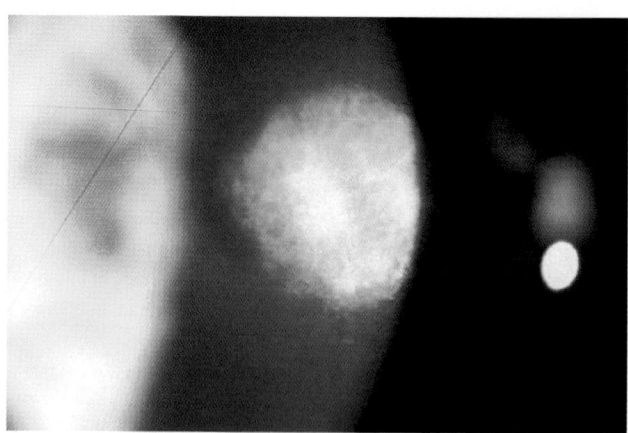

Fig. 10-6. Magnified view of Fig. 5.

sterile technique as soon as feasible.[14] Lenses that are fitted too tightly may cause a variant of the "tight lens syndrome,"[15] which manifests itself by a red painful eye, chemosis, a tightly fitting lens, and in the extreme, corneal edema. In most cases, replacing the lens with a flatter curve will provide relief. Disposable lenses appear to undergo spoilage quickly and, in our experience, 72 hours postoperatively patients complain of foreign body sensation and tearing which are relieved by the removal of the lens if the epithelium is intact, or its replacement if the epithelium needs further healing.

COMPLICATIONS RELATED TO CORNEAL WOUND HEALING
Superficial Stromal Opacification of the Cornea (Haze)

The appearance of superficial stromal opacification of the cornea following PRK is extremely common and reflects a biological healing response to PRK. Malley et al.[16] found with immunofluorescence in the monkey eye that the patterns produced during wound healing by excimer laser ablation and mechanical keratectomy were qualitatively identical. They concluded that corneal opacity associated with wound healing may be due to the following factors: deposition of type III collagen, absence of sulfated keratan sulfate from the extracellular matrix, and the absence of Bowman's layer and of an orderly array of collagen fibers. Fibronectin and laminin were also found in high quantities, associated with an increase in size and number of keratocytes adjacent to the treatment area. Hanna et al.[17] describe early histochemical postoperative changes in the rabbit including the presence of marked staining for type IV collagen, proteoglycans, fibronectin, and laminin. These changes reflect an effort to reepithelialize the ablated area.

Fantes et al.[18] described the histologic changes associated with the presence of corneal haze following PRK in primates' eyes. At 10 to 12 weeks postoperatively, the authors wrote, ". . . the histopathologic distinction between corneas with denser clinical haze (grades 1 to 2) and trace haze (grade 0.5) were more marked. In the corneas with greater amount of haze, there were more dark basal epithelial cells, greater amounts of vacuolization at the epithelial-stromal junction, more fragmentation of the newly secreted basement membrane, larger numbers of activated fibrocytes in the anterior stroma and larger amounts of extracellular matrix deposits, both amorphous and fibrillar."[18]

There was no evidence of large-diameter collagen fibrils or disorganized cicatricial tissue suggestive of subepithelial fibrosis. Marshall et al.[19] described essentially the same histologic changes and both Fantes et al. and Marshall et al. described near-normal corneal morphology by 8 to 9 months postoperatively.

Clinically, the development of reticulated corneal

haze is a normal part of the healing process and appears during the first postoperative month. Its incidence peaks between 1-3 months postoperatively and gradually decreases over the first year. The haze scores obtained nationwide with the VISX laser are described in Fig. 10-7. The density of the haze was scored in up to 3 subjective units whereby a 1+ score was deemed functionally significant. Corneal haze of 2+ or more occurred in 2.3% of eyes at 3 months and decreased to 0.4% at 12 months postoperatively (Fig. 10-8). The hallmark of clinically significant haze is confluence. Confluent haze, whether focal or diffuse, arcuate or circular, is associated with a higher risk of: (1) immediate and long-term regression and (2) loss of best corrected visual acuity related to irregular

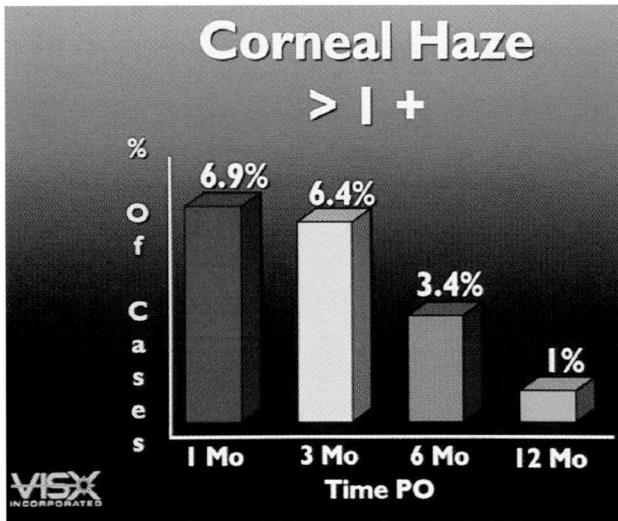

Fig. 10-7. Distribution of corneal haze of more than one unit at different postoperative times, national VISX series.

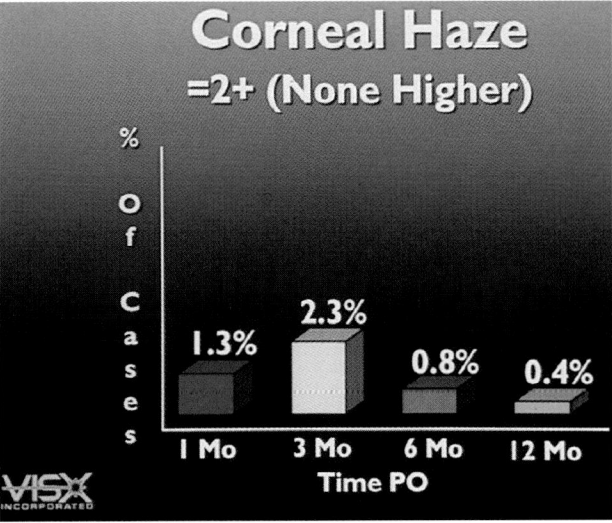

Fig. 10-8. Distribution of corneal haze of 2+ units at different postoperative times, national VISX series.

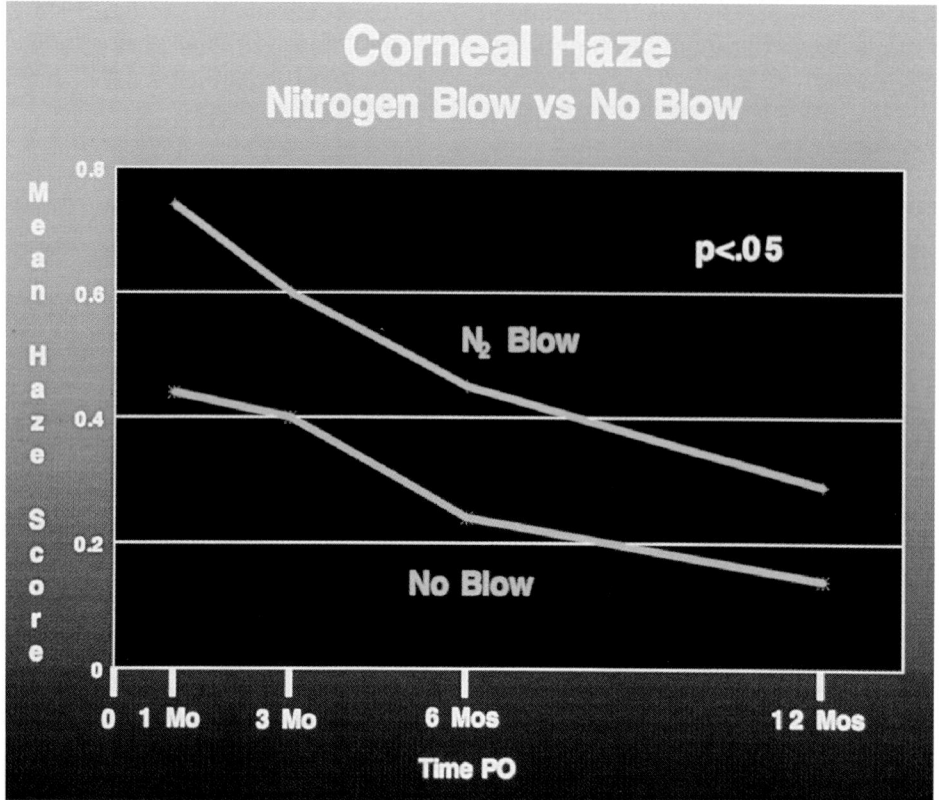

Fig. 10-9. Distribution of mean corneal haze scores with and without nitrogen flow over one year, national VISX study. The mean haze scores are significantly greater with nitrogen flow.

astigmatism or abnormal topography. Corneal haze is not only related to depth of ablation but to steep wound contours, intraoperative stromal hydration, and patient variability. Corneal haze appears to have significantly decreased with the discontinuation of nitrogen flow during surgery (Fig. 10-9) and its scores are higher when the preoperative myopia is higher (Fig. 10-10).

Corneal haze may be observed with the slit lamp by sclerotic scatter. The opacities are located in the superficial stroma immediately beneath the epithelium covering the ablation zone. They may assume several appearances: thin granules, coarse clumps, or a confluent opacity involving part or all of the ablation zone (see Figs. 10-10). Over time, most opacities fade and in several cases, it is difficult to detect any opacification at all. Associated symptoms may include: blurred vision with a decrease in uncorrected and best corrected visual acuity, and symptoms related to light scattering such as a starburst effect when viewing oncoming lights in evening traffic.

Another school of thought associates night glare with spherical aberration alone and not haze directly. Indeed, a cornea may show dense haze with no glare and clear corenas may be associated with severe glare. The method by which haze affects glare is by induc-

ing myopia through steepening the corneal curvature and affecting topography, reducing the effective OZ. In the nationwide VISX data, glare testing with the BAT device in conjunction with the CSV 1000 contrast sensitivity device showed that 3.7% of 150 eyes had an abnormal response and 0.7% had such a response at 12 months postoperatively. Seventeen percent of 521 patients reported being sensitive to light preoperatively. Thirty percent were sensitive to light at 12 months postoperatively. This compares favorably with similar testing in the PERK study where 56 patients were sensitive to light at 12 months postoperatively.

One case in our series demonstrated severe opacification along with regression of correction and irregular astigmatism (see Fig. 10-1). This eye was re-treated (see Fig. 10-2) with a resultant decrease in haze and with best corrected spectacles vision of 20/40, and best corrected vision of 20/30 with a gas-permeable contact lens (preoperative corrected vision was 20/30).

Management of corneal haze usually consists of waiting until the opacity fades spontaneously. When corneal haze is dense or if subepithelial fibrosis appears, topical steroids may be started or increased. In severe cases, potential topical steroids such as dexamethasone or prednisolone acetate may be used. If no improvement can be obtained, one may consider re-

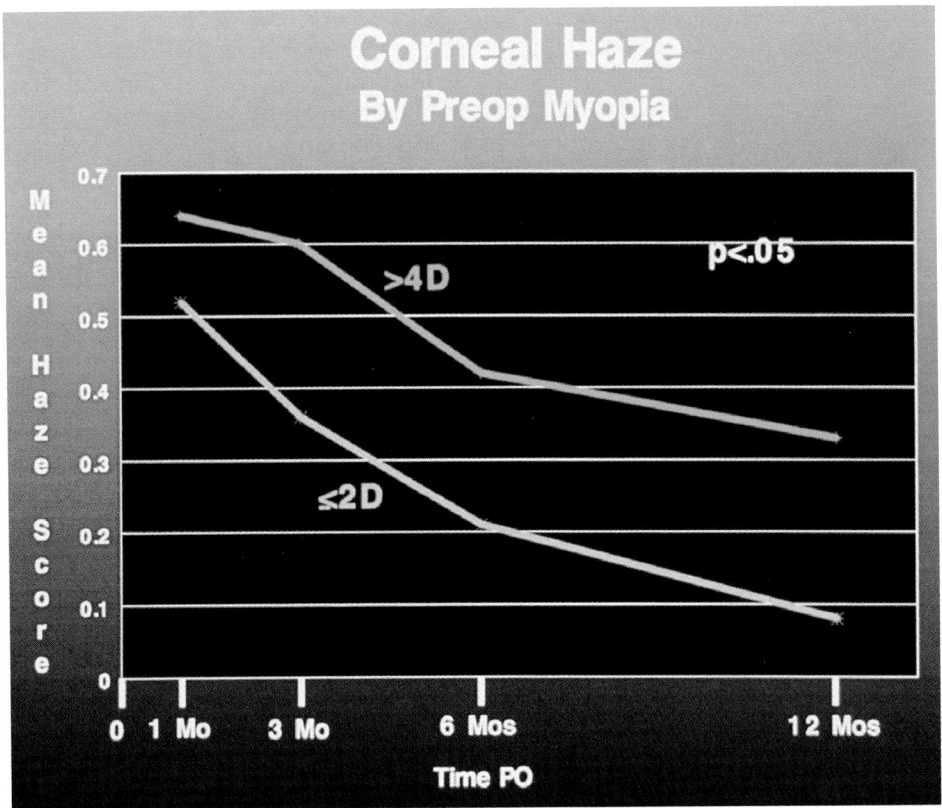

Fig. 10-10. Distribution of corneal haze correlated with preoperative myopia over one year period, national VISX study. The mean scores of haze are significantly greater in myopes of 4.00D or more.

treating the cornea with the excimer laser. Further experience demonstrates that re-treatment is an effective alternative to long-term use of topical steroids and it prevents subjecting the patient to steroid-induced complications. It has become obvious at this point that in order to obtain significantly better postoperative results, the biological response to PRK should be controlled and modulated. More time and further research will, it is hoped, provide refractive surgeons with this capability.

Plaque Formation

Lindstrom (verbal communication, 1992) described one case of epithelial plaque formation in an eye which previously underwent myopic epikeratoplasty to correct high myopia. The correction regressed and PRK was performed. A dense epithelial plaque formed with a significant decrease in visual acuity. The plaque was debrided manually. The cornea cleared but the correction obtained totally regressed. No similar findings were reported in normal corneas prior to surgery.

Recurrent Corneal Erosions

Four cases of recurrent corneal erosions (RCE) occurred following PRK in the Cedars-Sinai series. Several patients were also seen in The Laser Center se-

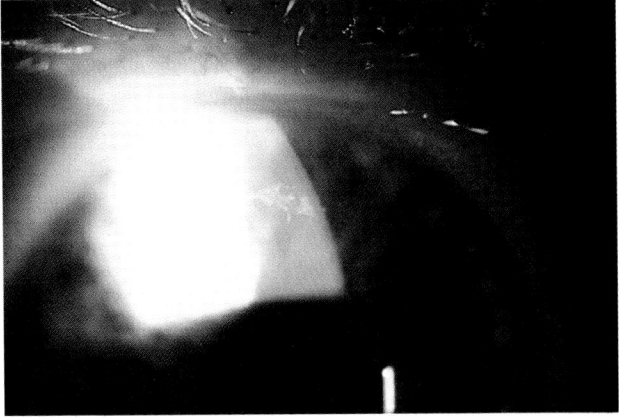

Fig. 10-11. Recurring corneal erosion following PRK which occurred outside the ablation zone but within the area of epithelial debridement.

ries (Fig. 10-11). All patients were screened for ophthalmic diseases prior to surgery and no evidence of corneal dystrophy was found. Two cases (one bilateral) display both the clinical signs and symptoms of RCE. One patient has intraepithelial cysts and is asymptomatic. One case shows the symptoms of RCE but has not displayed the clinical signs of this syndrome.

Table 10-1. Recurrent corneal erosions following photorefractive keratectomy: some surgical variables*

Case	Preoperative spherical equivalent (D)	Postoperative interval (Mo)	Nitrogen flow†
1R	−6.00	9	F
1L	−6.00	14	NF
3	−1.75	1	F
4	−1.75	29	F
5	−5.62	5	NF

*Data from Cedars-Sinai Medical Center, Los Angeles.
†NF = no flow; F = flow.

Table 10-1 shows that there is no pattern in the following variables that might explain the occurrence of RCE: preoperative refraction, time elapsed between surgery and onset of symptoms, and whether nitrogen flow was or was not used during surgery.

The incidence of RCE in the Cedars-Sinai series was 2.1%, a figure extremely close to the incidence reported in the general population.[20] In addition, the clinical features of this dystrophy may be absent even though the patient may develop them later. Also, the area of dystrophy was seen both within and away from the ablation zone. Therefore, one cannot rule out the possibility that epithelial dystrophy preexisted in these eyes. Only time and more reports of this phenomenon will tell if this observation is of concern. The lack of pattern in several variables suggests perhaps multiple causes for this finding: the frequent use of topical anesthetic and the physical force applied to the epithelial sheath during debridement with a blunt instrument—either could have an impact. It is a widely accepted observation among surgeons performing PRK that some epithelia can be debrided much easier than others. This may occur because the hemidesmosomal attachments are sometimes weaker and the added trauma of frequent topical anesthetics, the debridement, and perhaps in some way the photoablation, contribute to the occurrence of this finding.

Treatment of RCEs under these circumstances is similar to that of RCE not associated with PRK. All symptomatic patients found relief with the use of hypertonic saline and one patient was successfully treated with PTK in The Laser Center series.

COMPLICATIONS RELATED TO MECHANICAL FACTORS
Halos

Patients undergoing PRK complain sometimes of seeing halos around lights with or without a starburst effect. These phenomena are related to light scattering, mostly due to surface irregularity and corneal haze, or to spherical aberrations, as described above. In addition, the relation between the ablation zone diameter and the diameter of the pupil, especially in dim light, is important. Gimbel et al.[4] report 50% of the surveyed patients complaining of rings or halos and 45.2% of a "haze effect" 8 months postoperatively with ablation zones between 4.5 and 5.0 mm. Other studies report an incidence between 10% and 78% of eyes operated on, depending on the time interval between surgery and the report of the symptom.[5,21,22] The Laser Center series correlates this symptom mainly with the OZ size utilized. Incidences of 75% to 80% night glare were found with 4-mm OZ ablations, 35% to 40% night glare with 4.5-mm OZ ablations, 20% night glare with 5-mm OZ ablations, less than 5% night glare with 6-mm OZ ablations, and less than 0.5% night glare with 7-mm OZ ablations. The nationwide VISX data show that 30% of patients surveyed 1 year postoperatively complain of sensitivity to bright lights compared to 17% who had the same complaint preoperatively.

Roberts and Koester[23] provide the theoretical framework to explain these symptoms by generating a ray tracing defining the edge of the OZ for any given pupil size. They concluded that OZ diameters in PRK must be at least as large as the entrance pupil diameter to prevent foveal glare and larger than the entrance pupil diameter to prevent parafoveal glare. In addition, the postoperative corneal curvature also plays a role as it determines magnification of the pupil. Clinically, in The Laser Center series, a 7-mm OZ ablation seems to be adequate for 9- or 10-mm pupil dilation in dim light. Indeed, measurement of the pupillary diameter in dim light prior to surgery is extremely important and patients with very wide pupils should be advised preoperatively of this possible complication and in extreme cases, discouraged from having refractive surgery.

Management of halos and the starbursting effect should address the probable cause of the symptoms. If corneal haze is the cause, treatment should be undertaken as described above. In those instances where OZs are less than 5.5 mm and there is a disparity between pupil size and the edge of the zone, one may attempt enlargement of the OZ in a transepithelial fashion with blending of the peripheral edge when residual myopia is present. If the symptomatic eye is emmetropic or hyperopic, peripheral re-treatment should not be attempted. Low concentrations of pilocarpine were used anecdotally to remedy this symptom. We believe that the risk of chronic use of pilocarpine in myopic eyes precludes this medication as an alternative. Indeed, in our experience, this medication was not generally well tolerated as it induced in the younger population undergoing this surgery a va-

Table 10-2. Decentration of the ablation zone in photorefractive keratectomy

Amount of decentration (mm)	Percentage of light rays falling on the retina that miss the optical zone
0	0
0.5	16
1.0	31
2.0	61
3.0	86
4.0	100

From Maloney RK: Corneal topography and optical zone location in photorefractive keratectomy, *Refract Corneal Surg* 6:363-371, 1990.

riety of symptoms such as blurred vision, headaches, dimming of light, and others.

Decentration of ablation zone

Decentration of the ablation zone may occur because of inadequate fixation by the patient and because of an inadequate method of marking the optical center during PRK. Maloney[24] calculated the percentage of light rays falling on the retina that miss the OZ (Table 10-2) assuming a 4-mm OZ and entrance pupil. Indeed, according to this author, a 1-mm decentration would result in a blurred ghost image and monocular diplopia. The Stiles-Crawford effect may reduce the intensity of this phenomenon. Several authors[4,25,26] clinically documented this finding and the presence of decreased uncorrected and best corrected visual acuity in decentrations exceeding 1 mm. An extreme case is described whereby uncorrected vision was 20/12 in bright light and less than 20/200 in dim light owing to decentration of the ablation zone. The amount of decentration was not documented.[26]

Treatment of significant decentration is difficult. If significant undercorrection is associated, one may attempt re-treatment after thoroughly evaluating the topography of the affected cornea. When residual myopia is present, one may attempt to treat it with a larger OZ to include the decentered area. At the same time, no reported cases of re-treatment under these circumstances have been published. Small amounts of decentration should not be treated; they rarely induce symptoms.

Central Islands

Various topographic abnormalities have been described following excimer ablation. Lin et al.[27] identified four topographic patterns: (1) a uniform circular ablation (44%-45%); (2) a central island of steepened cornea within the ablative zone (10%-26%); (3) a keyhole ablative pattern (12%); and (4) a semicircular ablative pattern (18%-33%). Both the keyhole pattern and the semicircular patterns demonstrated inad-

equate inferior ablations predominantly. Visual acuity was still excellent with best corrected visual acuity often maintained.[27] The most significant topographic abnormality observed with respect to patient symptoms was the central island.

The definition of a *central island* is a central or pericentral steepening of (1) at least 1 to 3 D in height; (2) a diameter of at least 1 to 3 mm; (3) measured at least 1 month postoperatively; and (4) associated with clinical symptoms of monocular diplopia, ghosting of images, or qualitative visual changes. Factors increasing central islands include (1) lasers with homogeneous or flat energy beam profiles; (2) single-zone techniques; (3) large OZs; (4) moderate or severe degrees of myopia; and (5) moist corneas intraoperatively.

There are four main theories as to the cause of central islands: (1) focal central epithelial hyperplasia; (2) the vortex plume theory; (3) degradation of laser optics; and (4) the acoustic shock wave theory. Central island formation is likely multifactorial.

Cases of focal epithelial hyperplasia have been documented in patients with central islands with corneal topography, but these islands invariably are short-lived and are clinically different. Patients do not have the classic ghosting of images commonly associated with central island formation. There is also no explanation as to why the epithelium would heal differently after myopic ablation with the Summit ExciMed laser. The epithelium appears clinically normal in almost all cases of central islands. A diagnosis of central island formation is made from the association of clinical symptoms described by the patient and the corneal topography, not by slit-lamp examination.

The vortex plume theory proposed that the emitted plume of ablative debris forms a random vortex centrally blocking successive pulses. This theory was advanced by Stephen Klyce based upon his observation that central islands were detected once nitrogen flow was discontinued.[28] However, this theory fails to explain why central islands, although observed with the VISX, Taunton, and Technolas lasers, were essentially nonexistent with the Summit ExciMed UV-200 unit. The Summit ExciMed had no vacuum aspiration system and the pulse repetition rate was twice that of the VISX, allowing half the time for plume dissipation prior to the next pulse, which, according to the Vortex plume theory, should have resulted in a higher incidence of central islands.

Lin et al.[27] and other investigators have proposed that degradation of the beam optics centrally would result in less ablative effect centrally. Central islands, however, have been observed with normal calibration test plastics, following replacement of optics, as well as on new laser systems. In addition, nitrogen flow or the method of epithelial removal should have no effect on the incidence of central islands if the primary

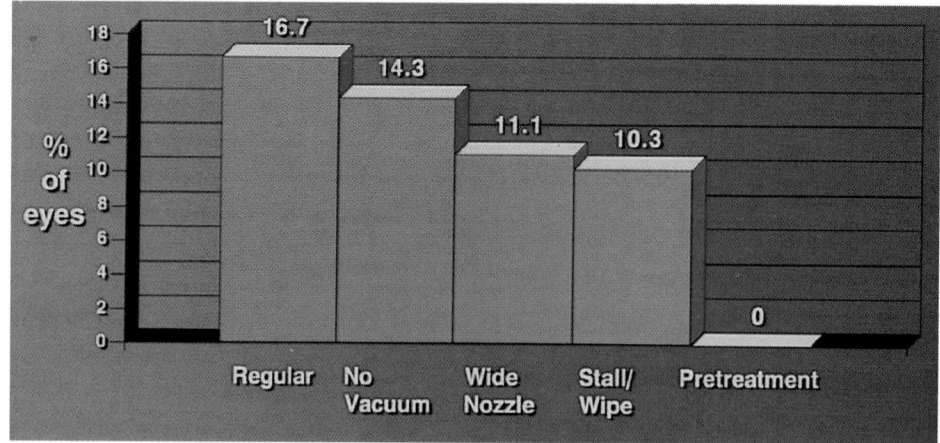

Fig. 10-12. Incidence of central islands with 4 different techniques of ablation.

cause is a defect within the optical pathway, which has been clinically noted to be the case.

The theory which seems to have gained acceptance is the acoustic shock wave model (J.J. Machat, verbal communication, April 1993). This model is based on clinical impressions obtained while using both the Summit ExciMed UV-200 and the VISX Twenty-Twenty excimer lasers. In over 1500 cases, no central islands were seen with the Summit ExciMed. However, a 17% incidence of central islands was noted with the VISX Twenty-Twenty.

In a study of 167 eyes of 97 consecutive patients, aged 20 to 58 years, of whom 68 (70%) were male, five operative techniques were studied prospectively for the incidence of central islands. Preoperative myopia ranged from −1.00 to −12.75 D with up to −3.50 D of cylinder. The first three techniques were designed to look at the role of the VISX vacuum aspiration system on the incidence of central islands. The latter two techniques examined the effect of the central fluid accumulation. The basic technique involved blunt epithelial debridement followed by a no-flow PRK technique with patient self-fixation. A multizone technique was utilized for procedures above −6.00 D, and a 6-mm OZ was utilized for all single-zone treatments.

The incidence of central islands in the first three subgroups ranged from 16.7% to 11.1% as the vacuum aspiration system was turned off, then modified to have a wide nozzle reducing air turbulence (Fig. 10-12). The fourth subgroup was treated with a stall-and-wipe technique, whereby the central stromal fluid was wiped clear with a blunt spatula every few seconds intraoperatively or allowed to evaporate with the low vacuum aspiration. The incidence of central islands was reduced in group IV to 10.3% at 3 months.

Based on differences in the intraoperative hydration pattern observed while performing procedures with the Summit ExciMed UV-200 and the VISX Twenty-Twenty systems, it was postulated that the al-

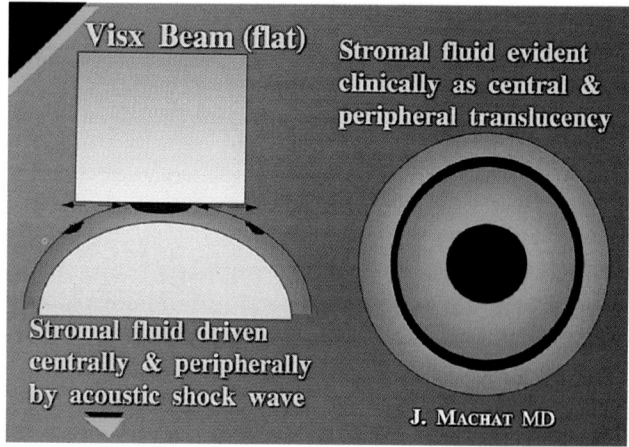

Fig. 10-13. Fluid dynamics during ablation with the VISX laser, as observed clinically, explaining the formation of a central island.

tered hydration pattern was the cause of central islands. The corneal stroma in the Summit laser subgroup appeared uniformly moist intraoperatively. Whereas the stroma in the VISX subgroup become moist centrally, appearing as an area of increased translucency with the midperiphery remaining relatively dry intraoperatively, the periphery was somewhat moist, thus creating a target pattern (Fig. 10-13). It was estimated that half the pulses were being blocked by the stromal fluid centrally and therefore were being rendered ineffective. That is, the pulse energy centrally was removing fluid rather than stromal tissue, or the stroma became more hydrated and less compact centrally.

Based on these observations, a "pretreatment technique" was developed, treating the central 2 to 3 mm of the cornea prior to PRK. The pretreatment consists of an ablation of 1 μm per diopter of correction for single-zone ablations of up to 6.00 D, and 0.6 μm per diopter of correction for multizone ablations above

6.00 D. There was a dramatic improvement in both the qualitative and quantitative visual results with the elimination of central islands in the final treatment group of 43 eyes. An additional 120 procedures were performed utilizing Machat's modified formula with no occurrence of central islands. Uncorrected visual acuities for each study subgroup are noted in Fig. 10-14, with a breakdown of the visual acuity results in pretreatment study group V. Figs. 10-15 and 10-16 show that 97.7% of eyes in the pretreatment study group achieved uncorrected vision of 20/40 or better at 6 months postoperatively. These patients also noted

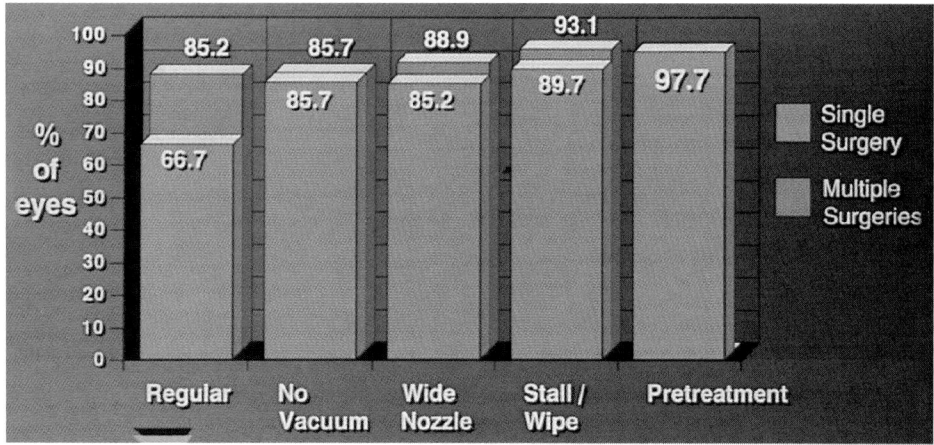

Fig. 10-14. Uncorrected visual acuity of 20/40 or better as obtained with the different techniques in eyes treated once and in retreated eyes. Uncorrected vision is best after pretreatment.

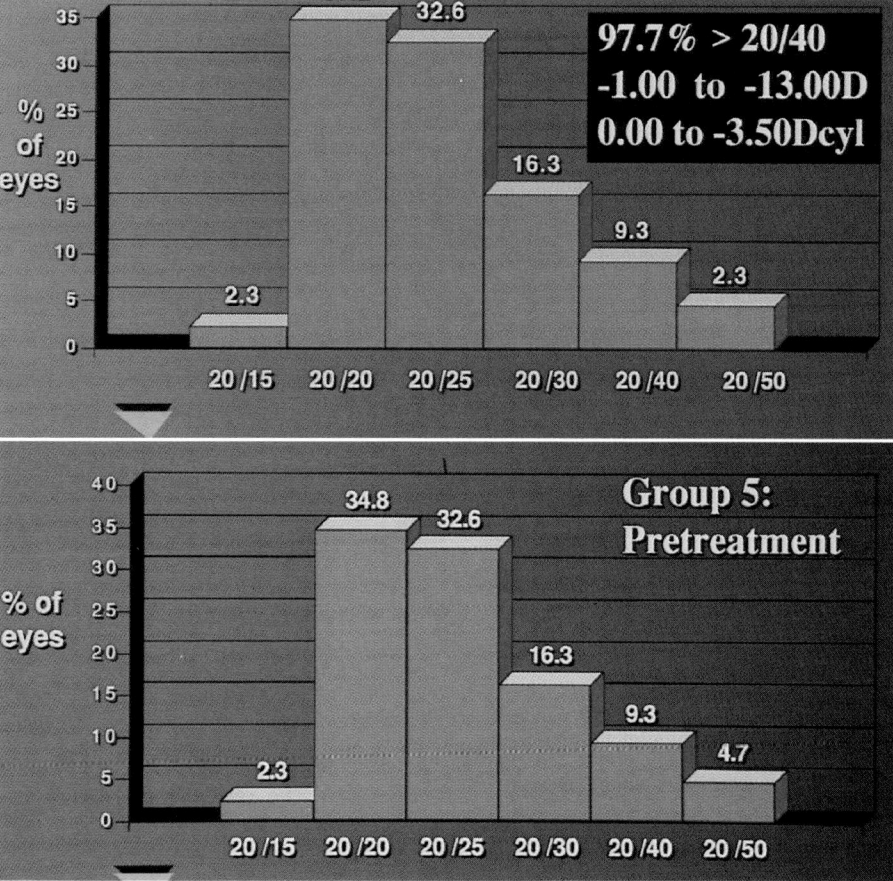

Fig. 10-15 and 10-16. Distribution of uncorrected visual acuity in pretreated eyes, 6 months postoperatively.

qualitative subjective improvement in their vision often relative to their fellow eye, which was not pretreated but had no central island. Refractive predictability was improved with three fourths of pretreated patients being within 0.50 D of emmetropia (Fig. 10-17). Leaving a moist cornea helped preserve corneal clarity, with three fourths of pretreated eyes graded as trace haze or clear, with no cases of clinically significant or confluent haze observed (Fig. 10-18).

According to the model, each pulse produces an acoustic shock wave, the pattern of which is related to the energy beam profile of the laser. Intraoperative stromal hydration patterns are determined by the acoustic shock wave pattern. Flat or homogeneous energy beam profiles produce central fluid accumulation intraoperatively which result in reduced ablation centrally. Based on the acoustic shock wave model, blowing nitrogen would reduce islands by drying this central fluid pocket. Since excessive drying produces increased corneal haze, some investigators have utilized humidified gases with success.[29] Removal of the epi-

thelium with alcohol was found to reduce the incidence of central islands by altering the stromal fluid dynamics. Larger OZs would be at greater risk of inducing islands owing both to the larger shock wave amplitude, and the tendency of the beam energy to drop centrally as the diameter is increased. One can use the analogy of a tent to understand: as the tent poles are spread apart, the tent begins to sag centrally. This is why there is an increased beam edge effect creating circular shock waves. Donald Johnson performed PRK on a series of patients with the VISX Twenty-Twenty with a reduced fluence of 120 mJ/cm^2 from the VISX standard of 160 mJ/cm^2 and found an incidence of central islands greater than 90%. The effect of reduced fluence is to increase pulse-to-pulse variability resulting in a less homogeneous beam profile exacerbating the beam edge effect. This dramatic increase in central island formation is best explained with this model. Single-zone techniques for moderate myopia utilized the greatest number of successive pulses and therefore had the highest frequency of cen-

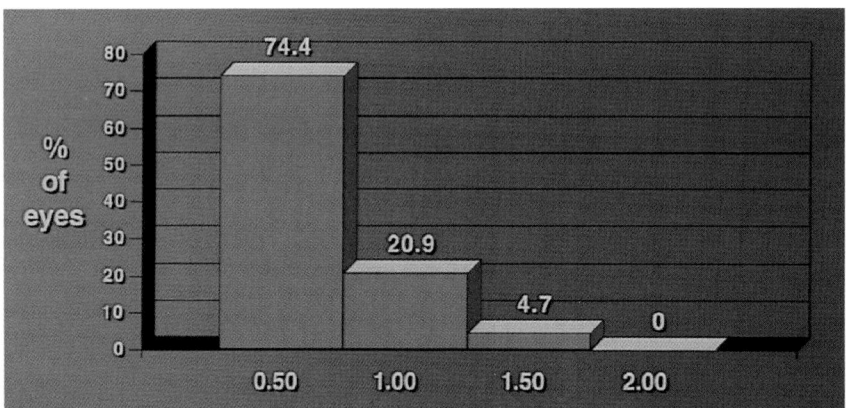

Fig. 10-17. Refractive outcome 6 months postoperatively in pretreated eyes. 74% of all eyes were within ±0.50D of emmetropia.

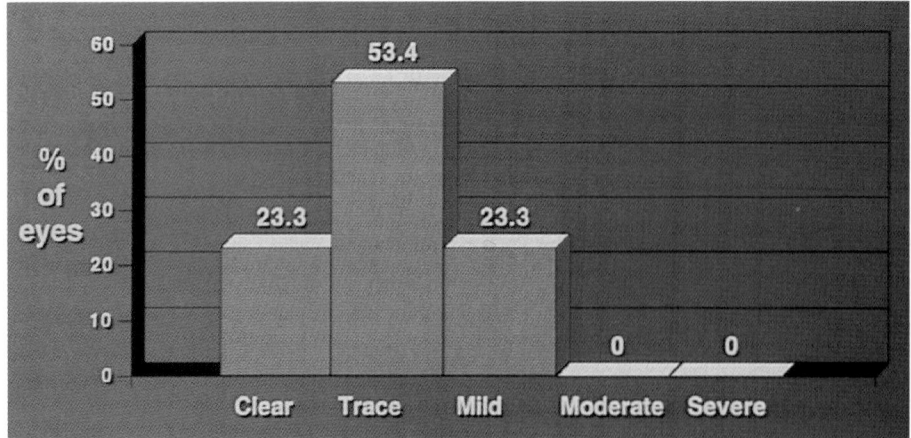

Fig. 10-18. Grading of corneal haze in pretreated eyes, 6 months postoperatively. 87% of eyes were clear or had trace haze 6 months postoperative.

tral islands in the study. Multizone techniques allow the stroma to dry between steps, and by starting each zone centrally, alter the stromal hydration pattern, driving fluid peripherally. Rapid procedures with moist corneas and low vacuum aspiration rates would increase the risk of central island formation.

All lasers with a flat-top energy beam profile produce central islands but improved stability with little regression of effect. The Summit ExciMed UV-200 laser has a gaussian energy beam profile with a higher energy density centrally, preventing central islands but resulting in a greater regression of effect. There-

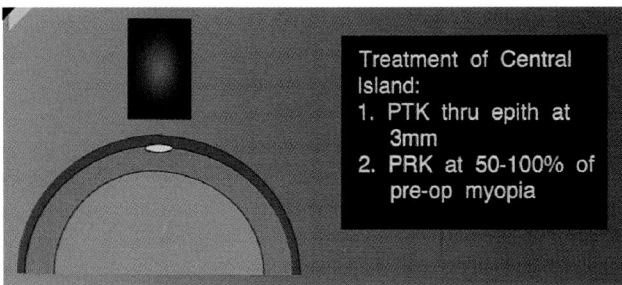

Fig. 10-19. Treatment of central islands in a transepithelial fashion (Machat).

fore, the Summit ExciMed algorithm is set higher to account for the regression of effect, such that immediate postoperative hyperopia is greater than +2.00 D, more than double that of other lasers. The gaussian beam profile acts as a wedge to drive fluid peripherally. Also, the largest OZ obtained with the Summit ExciMed UV-200 was limited to 5.0 mm.

Intraoperative stromal hydration, although increasing the incidence of central islands, improves patient fixation and reduces both corneal haze and irregular astigmatism, helping preserve best corrected visual acuity. Therefore, techniques which leave the cornea moist are advocated. However, software modification must be made to apply additional pulses centrally in order to compensate for the accumulated moisture.

It is important to understand excimer ablation dynamics based on the corneal stroma as a fluid model rather than a plastic test target. The Munnerlyn formula determining the amount of ablation in the VISX excimer laser for a given correction is based upon creating a myopic excision pattern in solid polymethylmethacrylate (PMMA). When one assesses clinical results, many patients have central islands, but only 15% manifest them clinically with respect to both symptoms and topographic changes. It must be realized

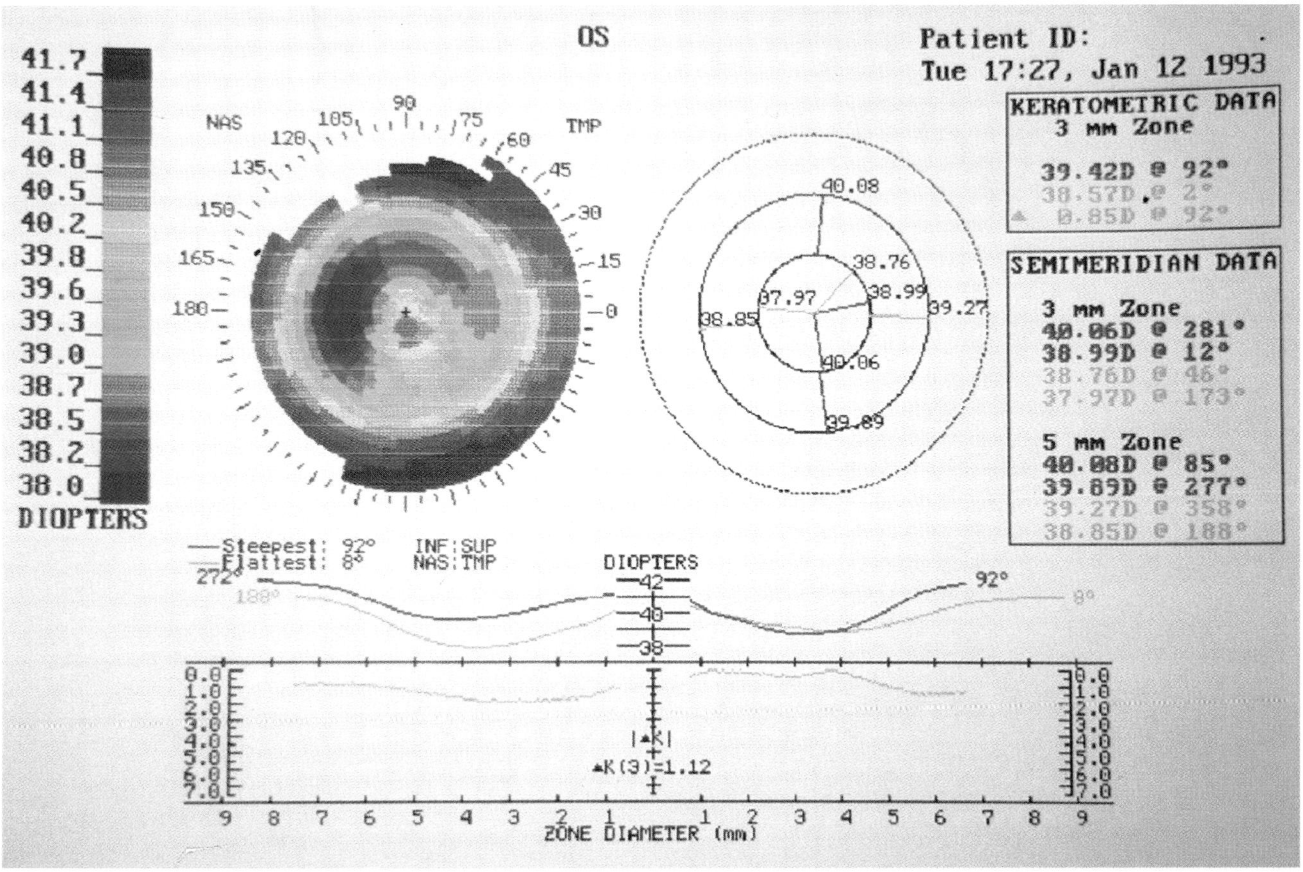

Fig. 10-20. Topographic corneal map of a central island.

that the reported incidence of central islands varies considerably between centers and surgeons (10%-26%) and at which postoperative examination the eye is checked: 60% to 85% at 2 weeks and 2% to 10% at 6 months[27,28] (J.J. Machat, Aron-Rosa, ASCRS April 1993, oral communications). One fundamental concern of VISX was that pretreating all patients may leave a facet with a reverse island effect. The study, however, demonstrated that the eye tolerates a facet much better than a bump. Also, pretreatment only removes tissue that the procedure algorithm was calculated to remove but did not because it did not account for the acoustic shock wave altering the fluid dynamics of the cornea. In fact, most patients find qualitative vision improved because the topography is improved, even in those patients who would not have manifested a central island. The VISX software was based upon treating PMMA and not a fluid cornea and therefore was deficient in treating the central 2 to 3 mm, which the Machat modification compensated for. Following this modification, VISX altered its algorithm and developed a central island factor software to add additional pulses centrally.

A transepithelial approach is advocated for the treatment of central islands and involves applying 50% of the original myopic correction to the central 2 to 3 mm with a PRK approach (Machat). In treating 40 patients with central islands, no residual central island remained. Similar findings were reported by other investigators. Johnson recommends programming the laser with 100% of the preoperative myopic correction and has not induced a reverse central island effect. The risks of excessive treatment include central haze due to sharp wound edges with deeper ablations and hyperopic overcorrection.

MISCELLANEOUS COMPLICATIONS

Seiler and Wollensak[27] described a single case of central corneal ulceration and perforation secondary to a persistent epithelial defect. It was associated with "rheumatic attacks" and positive rheumatoid factor and antinuclear antibodies. A penetrating keratoplasty was necessary to restore vision and ocular integrity. The authors concluded that autoimmune diseases constitute a contraindication to PRK.

A case of toxic keratopathy secondary to the use of paraformaldehyde for disinfection of the laser iris cone was described in three patients.[28] Intense kerati-

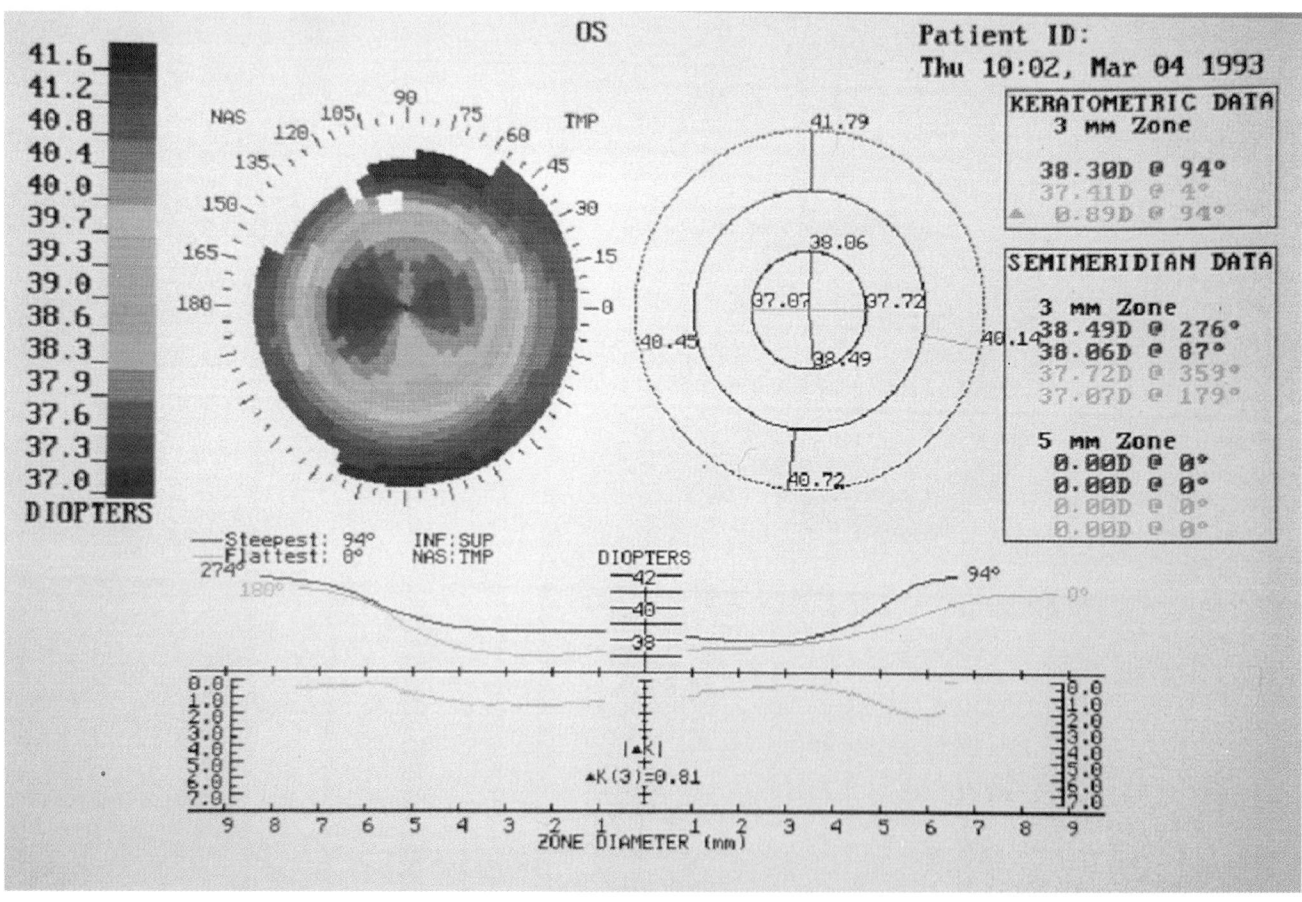

Fig. 10-21. Topographic corneal map of the same eye as in Fig. 20, following treatment of the central island.

tis developed along with corneal opacification which resolved with treatment over 4½ to 6 months.

Monocular diplopia[4,26] was described in association with corneal haze and decentration of the ablation zone. In some instances, the patient reported seeing multiple images. An additional possible cause may be the presence of irregular astigmatism. Binocular diplopia is also possible in phoric patients who lost fusion because of the anisometropia induced after performing PRK on the first eye.

Anisocoria was reported[11] in one series of 1165 eyes in 97 patients (9%). This phenomenon was observed during the first postoperative month and disappeared in time whereby no anisocoria was seen at 12 months postoperatively. The authors suggest that the cause of this transient phenomenon may be the intraocular release of anticholinergic factors, but they admit there is no conclusive explanation for this finding. The Laser Center series documented 1 case out of 2500 cases examined, lasting over 6 months following PRK with the Summit laser. The cause remains unknown.

"Fluctuation of vision"[21,29] was described in both moderately myopic and highly myopic eyes undergoing PRK. It is unclear whether this phenomenon was transient, or whether it was similar to that occurring following radial keratotomy. One possible cause for concern may be the possibility that deep ablations may decrease the stability of the cornea, thereby inducing changes in curvature. Another cause may be that patients accommodate better in the morning hours and experience spherical aberration with reduced visual quality in the later hours of the day. Further such reports and attempts to better explain this symptom will provide better insight into this phenomenon.

An episode of corneal graft rejection was induced following PTK[32] in an eye with recurrent lattice corneal dystrophy. The episode was successfully controlled with hourly doses of 1% prednisolone acetate along with high doses of systemic and subconjunctival steroids. The keratitis induced by the intense use of short UV laser light may indeed cause such a rejection episode. One might consider some form of pretreatment with steroid treatment of eyes with corneal transplants prior to PRK or PTK along with appropriate antibiotic coverage. Such patients should be closely followed until the keratitis has subsided and the corneal epithelium has regrown.

Two patients were seen at The Laser Center with frank iritis following PRK. One had a history of previous iritis and was HLA-B27-positive. The iritis occurred in both eyes postoperatively and resolved with the instillation of topical steroids within 2 to 3 days. The second patient had no history of iritis and no other medical history. It similarly resolved within 48 hours of starting topical steroids, with no recurrence.

A number of patients were reported complaining of ocular tenderness following PRK lasting indefinitely. The pain may only occur in one eye of a patient treated bilaterally and is more common in patients who have been patched rather than those that received a bandage contact lens with a topical NSAID. It may be related to dry eye or more likely corneal nerve ending damage, or it may represent symptomatic cases of RCE in which the corneal changes were not documented.

REFERENCES

1. Salz JJ, Maguen E, Nesburn AB, et al: A two year experience with excimer laser photorefractive keratectomy, *Ophthalmology* 100:873-882, 1993.
2. Maguen E, Nesburn AB, Papaioannou T, et al: 193 nm excimer laesr photorefractive keratectomy: short term visual rehabilitation with and without nitrogen flow, *Refract Corneal Surg,* in press.
3. Maguen E, Salz JJ, Newburn AB, et al: Results of excimer laser photorefractive keratectomy for the correction of myopia at Cedars-Sinai Medical Center—1993, (in press).
4. Gimbel HV, Van Westenbrugge JA, Johnson WH: Visual, refractive, and patient satisfaction results following bilateral photorefractive keratectomy, *Refract Corneal Surg* 9(suppl):S5-S10.
5. Gartry DS, Kerr Muir MG, Marshall J: Excimer laser photorefractive keratectomy. 18-month follow-up, *Ophthalmology* 99:1209-1219. 1992.
6. Heitzmann J, Binder PS, Kassar B, et al: The correction of high myopia using the excimer laser, *Arch Ophthalmol* 111:1627-1634, 1993.
7. Wilson SE, Klyce SD, McDonald MB, et al: Changes in corneal topography after excimer laser photorefractive keratectomy for myopia, *Ophthalmology* 90:1338-1347, 1991.
8. Tengroth B, Fagerholm P, Soderberg H, et al: Effects of corticosteroids in postoperative care following photorefractive keratectomies, *Refract Corneal Surg* 9(suppl):S61-S64, 1993.
9. Carones F, Brancato R, Venturi E: Efficacy of corticosteroids in reversing regression after myopic photorefractive keratectomy, *Refract Corneal Surg* 9(suppl):S52-S56, 1993.
10. McDonald MB, Liu JC, Byrd TJ, et al: Central photorefractive keratectomy for myopia. Partially sighted and normally sighted eyes. *Ophthalmology* 98:1327-1337, 1991.
11. Brancato R, Tavola A, Carones F, et al: Excimer laser photorefractive keratectomy for myopia: results in 1165 eyes, *Refract Corneal Surg* 9:95-104, 1993.
12. Pepose JS, Laycock KA, Miller JK, et al: Reactivation of latent herpes simplex virus by excimer laser photokeratectomy, *Am J Ophthalmol* 114:45-50, 1992.
13. Serdahl CL, Mannis MJ, et al: Infiltrative keratitis associated with disposable soft contact lenses, *Arch Ophthalmol* 107:332-333, 1989.
14. Nesburn AB, Maguen E, Caroline PC: A method for sterile insertion of soft contact lenses, *Contact Lens Spectrum,* March 1992.
15. Wilson LA: Tight lens syndrome in contact lenses. In Dabezies O Jr, editors: *Contact lenses: the CLAO guide to basic and clinical practice,* New York, 1984, Grune & Stratton.
16. Malley DS, Steinert RF, Puliafito CA, et al: Immunofluorescence study of corneal wound healing after excimer laser anterior keratectomy in the monkey eye, *Arch Ophthalmol* 108:1316-1322, 1990.
17. Hanna KD, Pouliquen Y, Waring GO, et al: Corneal stromal wound healing in rabbits after 193 nm excimer laser surface ablation, *Arch Ophthalmol* 107:895-901, 1989.
18. Fantes FE, Hanna KD, Waring GO, et al: Wound healing after

excimer laser keratomileusis (photorefractive keratectomy) in monkeys, *Arch Ophthalmol* 108:665-675, 1990.

19. Marhsall J, Trokel SL, Rothery S, et al: Long term healing of the central cornea after photorefractive keratectomy using an excimer laser, *Ophthalmology* 95:1411-1421, 1988.

20. Waring GO, Rodrigues MM, Laibson PR: Corneal dystrophies. I. Dystrophies of the epithelium, Bowman's layer and stroma, *Surv Ophthalmol* 23:71-122, 1978.

21. Kim JH, Hahn TW, Lee YC: Photorefractive keratectomy in 202 myopic eyes, 1-year results, *Refract Corneal Surg* 9(suppl):S11-S15, 1993.

22. Machat JJ, Tayfour F: Photorefractive keratectomy for myopia, preliminary results in 147 eyes, *Refract Corneal Surg* 9(suppl):S16-S18, 1993.

23. Roberts CW, Koester CJ: Optical zone diameters for photorefractive corneal surgery, *Invest Ophthalmol Vis Sci* 34:2275-2281, 1993.

24. Maloney RK: Corneal topography and optical zone location in photorefractive keratectomy, *Refract Corneal Surg* 6:363-371, 1990.

25. Maguire LJ, Zabel RW, Parker P, et al: Topography and raytracing analysis of patients with excellent visual acuity 3 months after excimer laser photorefractive keratectomy for myopia, *Refract Corneal Surg* 7:122-128, 1991.

26. Taylor HR, Guest CS, Kelly P, et al: Comparison of excimer laser treatment of astigmatism and myopia, *Arch Ophthalmol* 111:1621-1626, 1993.

27. Lin DTC, Sutton HF, Berman M: Corneal topography following excimer photorefractive keratectomy for myopia, *J Cataract Refract Surg* 19(suppl):149-154, 1993.

28. Parker PJ, Klyce SD, Ryan BL, et al: Central topographic islands following photorefractive keratectomy, *Invest Ophthalmol Vis Sci* 34(suppl):803, 1993.

29. Krueger RR, McDonnell PJ, Wang XW, et al: Corneal surface morphology following excimer laser ablation with humidified gases, *Arch Ophthalmol* 111:1131-1137, 1993.

30. Seiler T, Wollensak J: Myopic photorefractive keratectomy with the excimer laser, *Ophthalmology* 98:1156-1163, 1991.

31. Pallikaris IG, Tsilimbaris MK, Papatzanaki ME, et al: Paraformaldehyde-induced keratitis after photorefractive keratectomy, *Am J Ophthalmol* 114:339-344, 1992.

32. Kim JH, Hahn TW, Lee YC: Clinical experience of two-step photorefractive keratectomy in 19 eyes with high myopia, *Refract Corneal Surg* 9(suppl):S44-S47, 1992.

33. Hersh PS, Jordan AJ, Mayers M: Corneal graft rejection episode after excimer laser phototherapeutic keratectomy, *Arch Ophthamol* 111:735-736, 1993.

11

Reoperations

Daniel Epstein, Björn Tengroth, Per Fagerholm, Helen Hamberg-Nystrom

Regression of effect is a well-documented phenomenon in photorefractive keratectomy (PRK) performed with the early (small-diameter) Summit technology units. In eyes with preoperative refractions ranging from −2.00 D to −6.00 D, 10% to 15% regress back to a myopia greater than 1.00 D by 12 months after surgery.

Eyes displaying regression of effect can be treated with topical corticosteroids such as fluoromethalone and dexamethasone. Such treatment promptly reverses regression in most eyes, even to the extent of, e.g., converting a myopic shift of −1.50 D to a hyperopia of +1.00 D (Fig. 11-1).

However, not all eyes with regression respond to topical corticosteroid treatment. When failure to respond is established (usually a therapeutic trial of 2-4 weeks with a twice-daily to thrice-daily schedule is sufficient to determine response), and when stability of (myopic) refraction for at least 6 months has been documented, re-treatment with the excimer laser may be considered.

PATIENTS AND METHODS

We report on 47 eyes (45 patients) that had previously undergone PRK for myopia and were re-treated with excimer laser PRK because of regression to varying degrees of myopia. Re-treatment was performed between 12 and 29 months (mean 20.1 ±5.1 months) after initial PRK, and minimum follow-up was 6 months.

The 26 males and 19 females had a mean age of 32.2 ±5.4 years (range, 22-47 years). Their mean refraction prior to the first PRK was −5.13 ±1.22 D (range, −2.60−−7.50 D), and their mean myopia prior to re-treatment was −2.28 ±0.98 D (range, −1.00−−5.00 D) (Fig. 11-2).

In the majority of cases, regression of effect developed during the first 6 months after the initial procedure. In accordance with our standard protocol, all of these eyes were first treated conservatively with topical dexamethasone (1 mg/mL) once regression to a myopia of −0.50 D or greater was noted. If they failed to respond to this strategy, treatment was discontinued and follow-ups were scheduled to establish stability of refraction prior to re-treatment. Failure to respond ranged from no significant refractive change (<0.50 D) to only partial reversal of the myopic shift, with a significant residual postoperative myopia (≥1.00 D).

All eyes had a pre-re-treatment visual acuity correctable to 20/20 or better with spectacles. Pre-re-treatment stability of refraction was established by repeated evaluations of manifest refractions. Re-treatment was performed only when refraction remained stable for at least 6 months. The mean time interval between the first and second PRK procedures was 20.1 ±5.1 months (range, 12-29 months).

Pre-re-treatment subepithelial corneal haze ranged from trace to 2+ on a clinical scale graded from 0 (completely clear cornea) to 4+ (severely dense opacity that obscures completely the details of intraocular structures).

All eyes had originally undergone PRK with an ExciMed UV-200 LA excimer laser (Summit Technology, Waltham, Mass.). This argon fluoride laser, with spectral emission at 193 nm, has a pulse frequency fixed at 10 Hz. The pulse energy resulted in a radiant exposure of 180 mJ/cm^2. The original ablated central optical zones had diameters of 4.1 mm, 4.3 mm, or 4.5 mm, depending on the original preoperative refraction.

Eight of the 47 retreatments were performed with the same Summit machine. The only parameter which

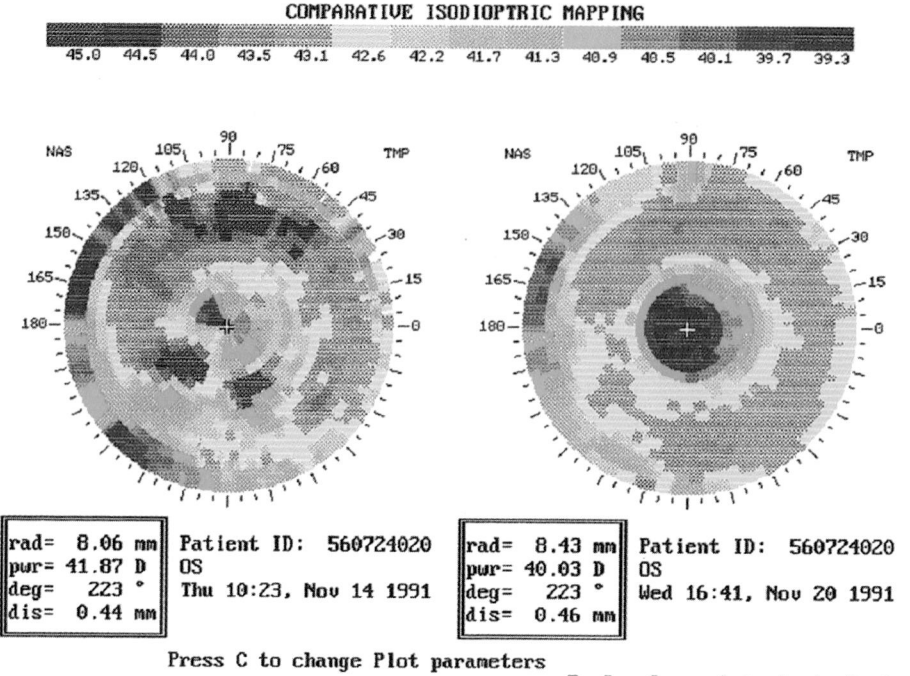

Fig. 11-1. Videokeratographs of a post-PRK eye before and 6 days after restarting topical dexamethasone therapy because of regression of effect. There was a +3.00 D change in refractive spherical equivalent within these 6 days.

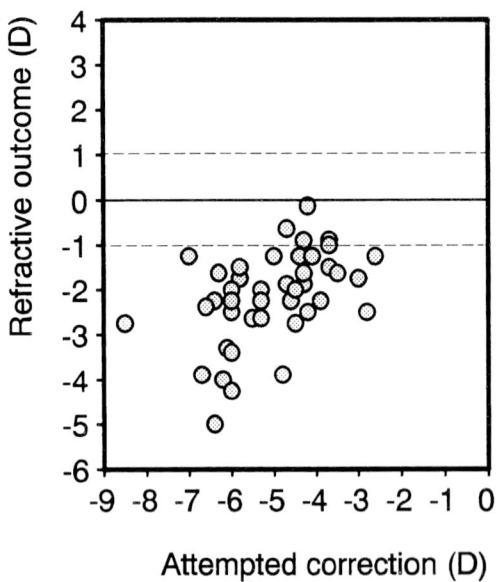

Fig. 11-2. Scattergram shows attempted correction (spherical equivalent) at first PRK and refractive outcome after that first procedure.

had been changed was the optical zone, now 5.0 mm for all patients re-treated with the Summit unit.

The remaining 39 retreatments were performed with the VISX Twenty-Twenty excimer laser (VISX Inc., Santa Clara, Calif.). Emitting 193-nm light at a repetition rate of 5 Hz and a fluence of 160 mJ/cm².

This laser offers the option of either a 5.0-mm or a 6.0-mm optical zone. It also has the capacity of correcting astigmatism. Twenty-nine of the eyes in the VISX group were treated with 6.0-mm ablations, 10 with 5.0-mm central zones. In 12 of the 39 eyes retreatment included astigmatism correction, a mode not available at the time of the original surgery.

The surgical procedure was identical in all eyes. PRK was preceded by topical anesthesia with tetracaine 0.5%, and the removal of the epithelium with a Beaver blade (Becton Dickinson AcuteCare, Franklin Lakes, N.J.). Once the epithelium has been removed, the original ablation zone (whose precise borders are often only faintly discernible at the slit lamp, especially when haze is graded as trace) becomes clearly visible. With the patient fixating on a target within the laser, PRK was performed, the surgeon centering on the original ablation area (which in turn had been centered on the entrance pupil). The attempted correction matched the manifest refraction.

Postoperative treatment consisted of cincainum-bibrocatholum ointment (a combination of a topical anesthetic and an antiseptic component in a paraffin–petroleum jelly base), and patching overnight. Standard post-PRK topical corticosteroid (dexamethasone 1 mg/mL) therapy was started on the first postoperative day. The eyes were treated for 3 months (five times daily for 1 month, three times daily for 1 month, and once daily for 1 month).

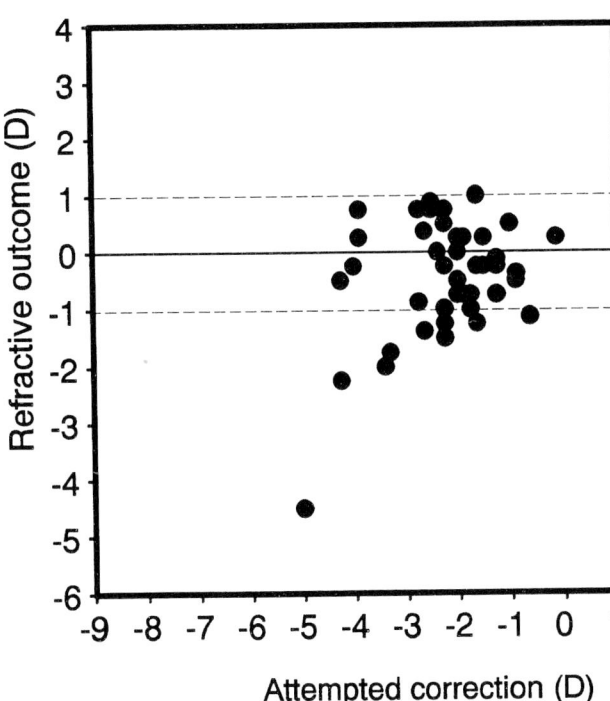

Fig. 11-3. Scattergram shows refraction (spherical equivalent) 6 months following re-treatment with the excimer laser.

Table 11-1. Mean refraction after retreatment (D)

6 months post-retreatment	12 months post-retreatment
−0.41 ±1.07 (+1.00 to −4.50)	−0.56 ±1.33 (+0.50 to −5.50)

Mean refraction after retreatment. There was no statistically significant difference between the refractive outcomes at 6 and 12 months post-retreatment.

Table 11-2. Subgroup mean refraction after retreatment (D)

	6 months post-retreatment	12 months post-retreatment
Eyes within 1.00 D of emmetropia	−0.02 ±0.57	−0.11 ±0.47
Eyes outside of 1.00 D of emmetropia	−1.81 ±1.13	−3.42 ±2.01

Mean refraction after retreatment, presented in subgroups (within or outside of 1.00 D of emmetropia). There was no statistically significant difference between the 6- and 12-month results in either of the subgroups.

Patients were seen for follow-up examinations 1, 3, 6, and 12 months after surgery. Visual acuity, refraction, autorefraction, autokeratometry, tonometry, and slit-lamp examinations of the cornea and anterior segment were performed at each visit.

Mean follow-up time was 8.9 ±2.9 months (range, 6-17 months). No patient was lost to follow-up.

RESULTS

Mean refraction 6 months after re-treatment was −0.41 ±1.07 (range, +1.00-−4.50 D) (Fig. 11-3, Table 11-1). There was a statistically significant difference ($P < .01$) between this postreablation mean and the group's mean refraction (−2.28 ±0.98 D) prior to the reoperation. Twelve months after reablation, mean refraction was −0.56 ±1.33 D (range, +0.50-−5.50 D), also significantly different ($P < .01$) from the mean prereoperation refraction. There was, however, no significant difference between the mean refractions 6 and 12 months after reoperation.

Six months after re-treatment, 80.9% of the eyes had a refraction between −1.00 D and +1.00 D. At 12 months, the equivalent figure was 86.9%. While the vast majority of the eyes had been re-treated with the VISX unit, there was no apparent difference between the refractive results of the Summit and VISX lasers at 6 or 12 months post re-treatment.

The eyes whose refraction after reoperation was within 1.00 D of emmetropia had a mean refraction of −0.02 ±0.57 D at 6 months and a mean of −0.11

±0.47 D at 12 months post re-treatment. The eyes that displayed refractions outside of 1.00 D of emmetropia (in effect, myopia greater than −1.00 D) had a mean myopia of −1.81 ±1.13 D at 6 months and a mean of −3.42 ±2.01 D 12 months after reoperation (Table 11-2). There was no statistically significant difference between the mean refractions at 6 and 12 months of the eyes with refractions within 1.00 D of emmetropia. Also the mean refractions of eyes with myopia greater than −1.00 D were not significantly different at these two post-re-treatment stages.

The mean pre-re-treatment refraction of the eyes that were within 1.00 D of emmetropia at 6 months was −2.14 ±0.92 D, and the mean pre-re-treatment refraction of the eyes displaying a myopia greater than −1.00 D at 6 months was −2.84 ±1.43 D. There was no statistically significant difference between these two means.

For the eyes that were within 1.00 D of emmetropia at 12 months post re-treatment, mean pre-re-treatment refraction was −2.62 ±0.98 D. The eyes that had a myopia greater than −1.00 D at 12 months had a mean pre-re-treatment refraction of −3.25 ±1.41 D. There was no significant difference between the two means.

Thirty-four percent of the eyes showed a post-re-treatment hyperopia of at least 0.25 D at 6 months. These eyes had a mean refraction of +0.56 ±0.26 D (range, +0.25-+1.00 D). At 12 months, 34.8% of the eyes displayed a hyperopia of at least 0.25 D, with a mean refraction of +0.36 ±0.12 D (range, +0.25-+0.50

D). There was a statistically significant difference between these two means.

For both 6- and 12-month refractive outcomes, there was no statistically significant difference between the pre-re-treatment refraction means of eyes that displayed a hyperopia of at least 0.25 D after retreatment, and the pre-re-treatment refraction means of eyes with a post-re-treatment myopia greater than -1.00 D.

Similarly, there was no significant difference between the original (preinitial PRK) refraction means of the eyes that showed a post-re-treatment hyperopia of at least 0.25 D and the original refraction means of eyes that developed a myopia greater than -1.00 D. This was true for both 6 and 12 months post retreatment.

At 6 months after reoperation, 38 (80.9%) of the eyes had an uncorrected visual acuity greater than or equal to 20/40. At 12 months, the equivalent figure was 73.9%. Forty-four eyes (93.6%) were correctable to 20/20 or better after re-treatment. Of the remaining three eyes, two showed a loss of one Snellen line at 6 months, the third a loss of two lines. None of these three eyes had reached the 12-month follow-up point.

Before re-treatment, 43 (91.5%) of the eyes had a subepithelial corneal haze less than or equal to 1+. At 6 months after re-treatment, 43 (91.5%) of the eyes displayed a haze less than or equal to 1+, and at 12 months 44 (93.6%) showed such a haze.* Thirteen eyes (27.7%) showed a slight increase in haze after retreatment. Five of these 13 eyes belonged to the group which developed a myopia greater than -1.00 D after reablation. Thirteen eyes (27.7%) showed a slight decrease in haze after re-treatment. None of these eyes had a post-re-treatment myopia greater than -1.00 D.

DISCUSSION

It is well established that following PRK, a regression of effect (i.e., a myopic shift) occurs in a variable number of patients. The incidence of regression appears to be associated with the preoperative refraction. The higher the preoperative myopia, the more common is regression of effect.

We have previously shown that the highest myopes (-5.00 to -7.50 D) in our patient population had a mean refraction at 12 months after PRK which was significantly more myopic than the mean refractions of lower myopes (-1.25 to -4.90 D). We have also shown that at 12 and 15 months postoperatively, practically

all regressions to greater than -1.00 D developed in eyes with a preoperative myopia greater than 4.00 D.

Such regressions after PRK can be reversed in most eyes through treatment with topical corticosteroids. It has not been established how topical corticosteroids reverse regression in the human eye. But it has been shown that topical dexamethasone treatment significantly decreased hyaluronic acid concentration in rabbit corneas which had undergone excimer laser keratectomy. Since hyaluronic acid is a large molecule that can bind considerable amounts of water, these rabbit studies suggest the possibility that corneal hydration after excimer ablation may be influenced by topical corticosteroids.

The 47 eyes reported here had failed to respond to topical dexamethasone therapy and were therefore retreated with excimer laser PRK (Figs. 11-4 and 11-5). With mean refraction 6 months following re-treatment at -0.41 ± 1.07 D, the result is admittedly not quite as good as that obtained in eyes which required only one PRK procedure. In single-procedure eyes in our patient population, mean refraction at 6 months was $+0.21 \pm 0.90$ D. It is interesting to note that Seiler and co-workers, in a report on re-treatments, obtained a result similar to ours, with a mean myopia 6 months after reablation of -0.29 D. However, the standard deviation in the Seiler material was considerably higher (± 2.37 D).

At 6 months after re-treatment, 80.9% of the eyes were within 1.00 D of emmetropia. Again, this was a slightly poorer result than in eyes which underwent only one PRK. Eighty-six percent of our singletreatment eyes were within 1.00 D of emmetropia 12 months postoperatively. In the study of Seiler and coworkers, only 63% had a manifest refraction between -1.00 D and $+1.00$ D 6 months after re-treatment.

Uncorrected visual acuity greater than or equal to 20/40 was documented in 80.9% of the eyes 6 months after reablation. By comparison, in single-PRK eyes in our patient material, 91% had a visual acuity greater than or equal to 20/40 12 months postoperatively. Seiler and co-workers did not report uncorrected visual acuity results.

Interestingly, neither the original (preinitial PRK) refraction nor the pre-re-treatment refraction served as an indicator of potential successful refractive outcome after reoperation. For these two variables, there was no statistically significant difference between the eyes that displayed a post-re-treatment myopia greater than -1.00 D (i.e., that regressed again) and the eyes that showed a postreablation refraction greater than or equal to 0.25 D.

These observations suggest that even eyes with preinitial PRK myopias as high as -7.50 D can ultimately obtain excellent refractive results. While such eyes run a greater risk of regression, re-treatment ap-

---

*A haze less than or equal to 1+ (on a clinical scale graded from 0 [completely clear cornea] to 4+ [severely dense opacity that obscures completely the details of intraocular structures]) is of a mild intensity which has not been shown to adversely affect visual acuity.

pears to be a means of bringing the refractive outcome of these eyes in line with that of eyes with lower preoperative myopia.

Although three eyes showed a loss of one or two Snellen lines at the 6-month follow-up examination, the loss may not be permanent. In our experience of some 3000 PRK procedures for myopia, some eyes exhibit an apparent Snellen line loss as late as 6 to 9 months postoperatively, and then recover to their preoperative visual acuity. The most common cause of the temporary line loss has been transient irregular astigmatism. The three eyes with line loss in this patient group also showed slightly irregular corneal surfaces.

We have refrained from extrapolating, on the basis of our material, the incidence of reoperations to be expected in a given population of PRK eyes. It is, after all, not certain that all excimer lasers currently being used produce the same percentage of regressions.

Unlike Seller and co-workers, we have had no patients where corneal scarring was the indication for reoperation. For the group as a whole, subepithelial corneal haze as such did not appear to increase after retreatment. While 27.7% of the eyes showed a slight increase in haze after reoperation, an equal percentage displayed a slight decrease. Consequently, it may be reasonable to state that reablation does not necessarily lead to increased scarring.

A further interesting observation with regard to haze was that only 5 of the 13 eyes which showed a slight increase in haze after re-treatment belonged to the group that had developed a myopia greater than 1.00 D after reablation. While it has previously been reported that intensity of haze and regression are correlated, we have shown in an earlier study that only haze in the 3+ to 4+ range always correlated with regression to myopia. In this patient group there were no eyes with haze graded at 3+ or 4+, and, accordingly, no convincing correlation between increase in haze and regression after re-treatment.

Because most of the re-treatments were performed with the VISX excimer, it was not possible to perform a matched analysis comparing the results of the VISX and Summit units. However, there was no apparent difference in post-re-treatment refractive outcome between the two lasers.

Our results show that eyes that regress to myopia after excimer laser PRK can be successfully re-treated, with reablation performed in the same manner as the original PRK. At 6 and 12 months after re-treatment, refractive results and uncorrected visual acuity improved in the majority of the eyes. If these refractive results remain stable over the long term, re-treatment may offer a modality for improving the overall success rate of PRK.

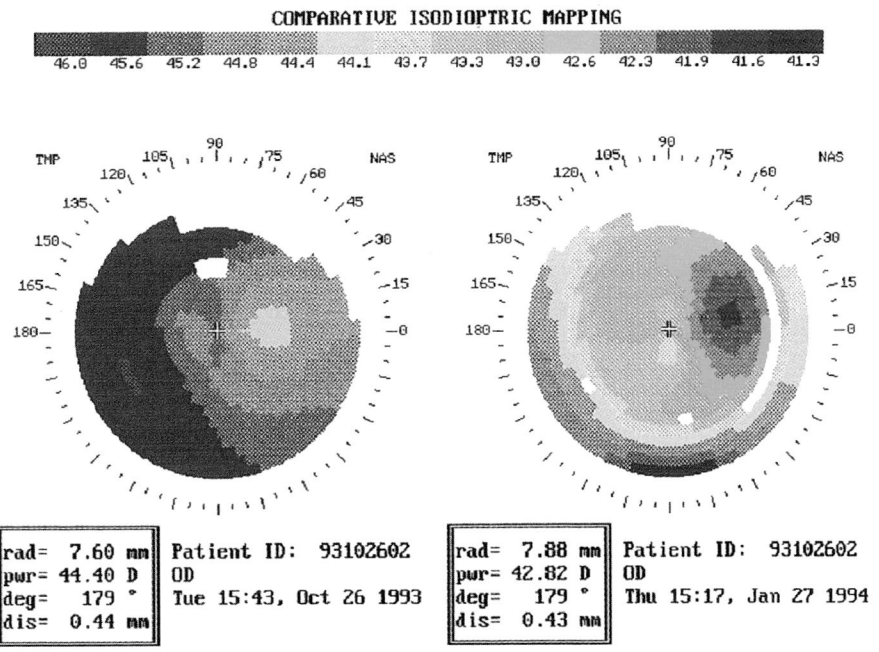

Fig. 11-4. Videokeratographs of an eye which originally underwent PRK for a myopia of 3.50 D. After initial emmetropia, regression stabilized at −1.25 D following failure to reverse it with topical dexamethasone. The *left* videokeratograph shows the corneal topography 2 months prior to re-treatment. The *right* videokeratograph was taken 1 month after re-treatment, with refraction at +0.25 D.

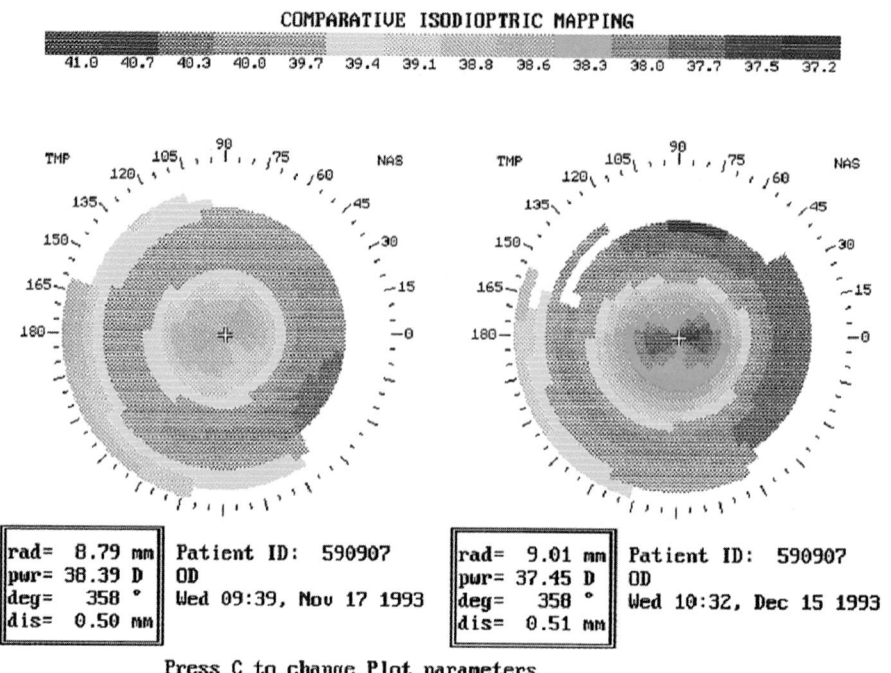

Fig. 11-5. Videokeratographs of an eye which originally underwent PRK for a myopia of 5.30 D. After initial emmetropia, regression stabilized at −1.00 D, following failure to reverse it with topical dexamethasone. The *left* videokeratograph shows the corneal topography immediately prior to re-treatment. The right videokeratograph was taken 1 month after re-treatment, with refraction at +0.50 D.

Admittedly, mean refraction after re-treatment showed a little over 0.50 D more myopia than was seen in eyes requiring only one procedure, and the percentage of eyes within 1.00 D of emmetropia as well as those with uncorrected visual acuity greater than or equal to 20/40 was slightly lower than in eyes that did not require re-treatment. But the improvement in refraction and uncorrected visual acuity after re-treatment overshadowed the slightly poorer results as compared to single-PRK eyes.

Since corneal haze has always been a central issue in photorefractive surgery, it is also interesting to note that our results indicate that re-treatment need not lead to a substantial increase of postoperative subepithelial corneal haze.

12

Radial Keratotomy and Excimer Laser Photoablation for the Correction of Myopia*

Perry S. Binder, James J. Salz

The current era of refractive surgery began with the introduction of radial keratotomy (RK).[1] Since then, numerous procedures to correct myopia, astigmatism, and hyperopia have been developed and tested.[2] Many subsequently lost favor because they were unpredictable, had an unsatisfactory complication rate, or were not efficacious (Table 12-1), although some procedures have survived owing to improved technology, e.g., myopic keratomileusis. RK currently enjoys the position as the most widely employed refractive surgical procedure because the unwanted and unexpected complications associated with the early procedures have been eliminated.[3,4]

Excimer laser photorefractive keratectomy (PRK) has stimulated renewed interest in correcting refractive errors because of its potential to minimize surgeon error, while theoretically having the capability of providing more predictable results compared to RK.[5,6] Both PRK and RK attract candidates with similar clinical indications (Table 12-2). However, the expense of delivering these procedures is significantly different. Therefore, because of current patient and physician interest in refractive surgery it is important to determine which procedure is better suited for the correction of myopia.

In the last few years, researchers have presented experimental[7-15] and preliminary clinical results[16-28] of excimer laser PRK. In order to make a decision whether or not this technology is to be recommended over RK (or any other surgical procedure for myopia correction), we need a basis for evaluating and comparing current and future technology to RK, which has been accepted as the standard refractive surgical procedure for correcting low to moderate myopia of less than 6 to 8 D. Based upon our 13 years of RK and 3-year excimer laser experience,[2,3,29-49,29-61] in this chapter we compare both procedures, while placing the risks and benefits of each into proper perspective.

EFFICACY AND PREDICTABILITY

Radial keratotomy has been used to correct 2 to 8 D of myopia, while the excimer laser has been used to correct 1 to 20 D of myopia (see Table 12-2). Most published results of excimer PRK have excluded candidates with naturally occurring astigmatism greater than 1 D. Candidates with more astigmatism can undergo incisional keratotomy (simultaneous radial and astigmatic surgery), incisional correction of the astigmatic refractive error, and later excimer laser photoablation for the residual myopic refractive error, or they can undergo combined astigmatic and myopic PRK currently under investigation in the United States. Successful clinical results of 16-,[1,62,63] 8-,[50,51,64-70] and 4-incision RK procedures[44,50,52,71,72] have been published.

The Prospective Evaluation of Radial Keratotomy (PERK) study, which was designed in 1980-1981, has been considered the benchmark against which refractive surgical procedures are compared.[51,68,54-60] The PERK study used instrumentation that was consid-

*Portions of this chapter have previously appeared in J Refract Corneal Surg Jul/Aug 1994.

Table 12-1. History of refractive surgical procedures*

Procedure	Year began	Error corrected	Problems	Current status
Keratotomy	1977	M,Ast	S,P	M,Ast
Keratophakia	1979	A	LBCVA,P,$	Disuse
Keratomileusis	1980	A,M,H	LBCVA,W,$,P	In situ
Epikeratoplasy	1980	A,M,H,KC	P,S,W	A,KC
Polysulphone	1980	M,H	LBCVA,P,S,W	Disuse
Electrosurgical kerato-plasty	1981	H,KC	P,S,W	Disuse
Excimer laser photoblation	1985	M,Ast	S,$	M,Ast
Phakic IOL	1986	M	W	M
Radiothermal kerato-plasty Ho:YAG	1987	H,M	P,S,W	Disuse
Collagen shrinkage Myopic hydrogel	1988	M,Ast,H	S,$	H,M,Ast
Intracorneal implants	1988	M,A,H	P,S,W	Disuse

M = myopia; A = aphakia; Ast = astigmatism; H = hyperopia; KC = keratoconus; P = predictability; LBCVA = loss best corrected visual acuity; S = stability; W = wound-healing problems; $ = expense; IOL = intraocular lens; Ho:YAG = holmium:yttrium-aluminum-garnet laser.

Table 12-2. Indications and inclusion criteria for myopia surgery

	Radial keratotomy	Excimer laser photorefractive keratectomy
Myopia (D)	−2--8*	−2--20†
Patient age	>18 yr	>18 yr
Previous corneal surgery	No	No
External ocular disease	No	No
Keratoconus	No	Yes‡
Astigmatism (D)	0-6	<1§
Corneal thickness limits	No	No
Corneal power limits (D)	<40.00	Unknown‖

*Age dependent.
†Under phase II Food and Drug Administration (FDA) study.
‡Apical scarring only.
§Under phase II FDA study.
‖Theoretically no limits.

ered state of the art at that time. By today's standards it would be considered marginal; the surgical algorithm used is out of date because age was not considered and reoperations (enhancement procedures) were not performed. Multiple surgeons with varying surgical experience performed eight-incision RKs with only three optical zones at multiple sites. The surgical protocol was appropriately limited to allow statistical assessment of surgical and patient variables. Additional procedures for undercorrections were discouraged to aid understanding the predictability of the procedure and patient age was ignored in surgical planning. The

results of this elegant study have been reported with 5 years of follow-up with a 10-year study now underway. There is no doubt that the PERK study has provided excellent information about an evolving procedure, but because of the limitations imposed by the study and the era in which it was performed, the clinical and refractive results (summarized by Waring and Lindstrom[73]) cannot be expected to be representative of contemporary RK surgical results that use three, four, six, or eight incisions, newer instruments, and secondary enhancement procedures.[53,74-76]

Predictability of refractive error and postoperative unaided visual acuity begin to decrease with more than 4 D of preoperative myopia, depending on patient selection and preexisting astigmatism. Werblin[75] recently presented a series of 205 eyes from his initial personal RK cases 1 year after surgery using contemporary surgical instrumentation and enhancement procedures. Including enhancement procedures for both over- and undercorrections and wound repairs performed in 31% of eyes, 99% of all eyes in his series had 20/40 or better acuity without correction. Robin et al.[76] recently summarized the results from a contemporary retrospective series which demonstrated over 98% of eyes to be 20/40 or better without correction and 55% to be within 0.5 D of emmetropia after 35% of the eyes had enhancement procedures.

Predictability can be described in terms of the number of eyes achieving refractive errors within 1 D or 0.5 D of emmetropia.[77] The percentage of eyes within this range after RK is dependent on patient age and preoperative refractive error; the surgeon selects the number and length of incisions to achieve the proper correction. Repeat operations (enhancement procedures) are employed to improve the refractive results. Since one goal of refractive surgery is to provide patients with driver's license vision without correction, most studies have reported the postoperative percentage of eyes with 20/40 or better uncorrected visual acuity (summarized by Waring and Lindstrom[73]). Because accommodation can confound results after refractive surgery and because 20/40 unaided acuity is not a predictable result, a more realistic goal would be to eliminate spectacles completely; a recent retrospective review of the patients in the PERK study has suggested that 20/20 uncorrected acuity is necessary to achieve this goal (G.O. Waring III, personal communication, Oct. 10, 1993). With increasing preoperative myopia and patient age, the distribution of refractive errors following surgery widens. With RK, certain predictive parameters have been determined, such as preoperative myopia, patient age, number and depth of incisions, and incision length,[56] whereas the only currently identified predictive parameter identified with the excimer laser is ablation depth contour.

The results following PRK have been similar to those for RK in the low myopia groups, but the early preliminary results of eyes with greater than 4 to 6 D of myopia suggest a tighter distribution of results compared to RK.* However, it must be stressed that the RK data have accumulated over 12 years compared to less than 3 years for the PRK data and that RK studies generally report results after multiple procedures for many eyes while early PRK reports are based on one procedure per eye.

One of us (J.J.S.) has recently retrospectively compared his personal results of RK and PRK on patients who had either procedure performed on one or both of their eyes during the past 3 years. The PRK patients represent all patients who underwent PRK and have at least 6 months of follow-up. The RK patients include only those patients who had at least 1 month of follow-up and so does not represent a consecutive series with the RK patients. The endpoint for this comparison was the uncorrected visual acuity and refraction as of their last examination, which was from 1 month to 3 years for the RK patients (1-month results generally predict 1-year RK results; see Williams, Chen, Lindstrom: *ARVO Abstracts* 148-149, 1990) and from 6 months to 3 years for PRK patients. Tables 12-3 and 12-4 summarize the results of this retrospective comparison of the two procedures by one surgeon.

Analysis of Tables 12-3 and 12-4 shows that although both procedures were equally effective (94% of eyes had 20/40 or better uncorrected visual acuity) in correcting up to 3 D of myopia, PRK achieved a higher percentage (83%) of eyes corrected to within 0.5 D of emmetropia than RK (68%). However, these ex-

*References 16, 17, 21, 22, 24-28, 49, 61, 78-87.

Table 12-3. Radial keratotomy data analysis*

	34 eyes −1.13--3.00	53 eyes† −3.1--6.0	26 eyes‡ − 6.1--9.00
20/20	41%	31%	
20/25-20/40	53%	59%	23%
20/40 or better	*94%*	*92%*	*77%*
±0.50 D	68%	65%	8%
±0.51-1.0 D	26%	28%	46%
>−1.0 D	3%	7%	23%
>+1.0 D	3%	0%	0%
±1.0 D	*94%*	*94%*	*77%*
Reoperations visual activity	17%	22%	27% (two eyes had three reoperations)
Loss of best reoperations visual acuity two lines or more			3% (one eye)

*Analysis comprises 113 eyes of 86 patients with preoperative myopia of −1.13 to −9.0 D with up to 4.0 D of astigmatism, followed for 1 month to 3 years (data as of last examination).
†Six eyes targeted for monovision are excluded from data analysis.
‡Four eyes targeted for monovision are excluded from data analysis.

Table 12-4. Photorefractive keratectomy (PRK) Data Analysis*

	36 eyes −1.00--3.00	55 eyes† −3.10--6.00	8 eyes −6.1--7.62
20/20	55%	36%	12%
20/25-20/40	42%	42%	50%
20/40 or better	*94%*	*78%*	*62%*
<20/40	3%	22%	37%
±0.5 D	83%	47%	37%
±0.51-1.0 D	17%	35%	37%
±1.0 D	*100%*	*80%*	*75%*
>+1.0 D	0	2%	0
>−1.0 D	0	18%	25%
Reoperations	0	2%	0
Loss of best corrected visual acuity two lines or more	0	2% (one eye)	0

*Analysis comprises 99 eyes of 75 patients with preoperative myopia of −1.50 to −7.52 D with up to 2.0 D of astigmatism followed for 6 months to 3 years (data as of last examination). Eight eyes underwent combined myopia plus astigmatic PRK.
†Two eyes targeted for monovision are excluded from analysis.

cellent results for low myopia were achieved with a single procedure with PRK but required additional surgery in 17% of the RK patients.

For eyes between 3.1 and 6.0 D of preoperative myopia, the RK results are superior with greater than 90% of the eyes obtaining 20/40 or better uncorrected visual acuity and corrected to within 1 D of emmetropia compared to about 80% with PRK. But the

RK eyes required additional surgery in 22% of the eyes while the PRK results were accomplished with one procedure. When these two groups are combined (−1-−6 D), 92% of the RK eyes obtained an uncorrected visual acuity of 20/40 or better with a 20% reoperation rate compared to 86% of the PRK eyes that underwent single procedure.

Above 6.1 D, the 77% of RK eyes achieved an uncorrected visual acuity of 20/40 or better. However, these patients were carefully selected because many of them were over the age of 40 years and it is well known that older patients obtain more effect from RK, and an undercorrection of 1 or 2 D allows them to read without glasses. This group required a second or third surgery in 27% of the eyes; the PRK group (albeit only eight eyes) achieved similar results with a single procedure.

Virtually all of the PRK patients that did not achieve a satisfactory outcome were undercorrected. Therefore, a second procedure in these eyes would most likely significantly improve the results. Also, since these patients were treated with the initial PRK algorithms it is probable that a new algorithm delivering more pulses to eyes above −3 D should reduce the undercorrections for future patients undergoing PRK.

El Maghraby and colleagues (presented to the American Academy of Ophthalmology, Dallas, Nov. 11, 1992) reported a 1-year comparison of RK in one eye and PRK in the opposite mate eye of 26 consecutive patients. At 1 year, 86% of the RK eyes and 92% of the PRK eyes had 20/40 or better uncorrected visual acuity; 90% of RK eyes and 82% of PRK eyes were within 1 D of emmetropia. The PRK eyes were undergoing a regression of refractive effect from month 6 to month 12, whereas the refractive error in the RK eyes appeared to be stable. The differences between the two procedures were not statistically significant at 1 year. We have performed similar procedures in fewer patients and have obtained similar results (Table 12-5).

The patient in case 11, Table 12-5, had a poor response to RK despite excellent incision depth achieved by an experienced surgeon who appropriately referred her for PRK in her other eye. She has obtained an excellent result in her PRK eye. Younger patients with more than 6 D of myopia may be more appropriate candidates for PRK. Fig. 12-1 is a slit-lamp photograph of the RK eye from case 10 and Fig. 12-2 is a photograph of the PRK eye. This 48-year-old patient, underwent a four-incision 3.0-mm optical zone procedure for −6.62 D with the expectation of an undercorrection (−1.25 D) for near vision in her nondominant eye. The PRK eye was targeted for full correction. Although it is impressive to see a four-incision RK correct over 5.0 D of

Table 12-5. Results of radial keratotomy (RK) in one eye and photorefractive keratectomy (PRK) in the mate eye

Patient data*	RK eyes	PRK eyes†
Case 1		
Uncorrected vision	20/40	20/40
PreOp SphEq (D)	−7.87	−6.50
PostOp SphEq (D)	−0.87	−1.25
Time to 20/20 BCVA	14 days	30 days
Mean corneal power	41.62	44.00
Follow-up (mo)	15	18
No. of procedures	1	1
Case 2		
Uncorrected vision	20/30	20/20
PreOp SphEq (D)	−5.62	−5.50
PostOp SphEq (D)	−0.37	−0.75
Time to 20/20 BCVA	7 days	28 days
Mean corneal power	41.50	44.00
Follow-up (mo)	8	13
No. of procedures	1	1
Case 3		
Uncorrected vision	20/40	20/30
PreOp SphEq (D)	−6.37	−5.37
PostOp SphEq (D)	−0.25	−0.75
Time to 20/20 BCVA	7 days	30 days
Mean corneal power	38.75	41.37
Follow-up (mo)	14	13
No. of procedures	1	1
Case 4		
Uncorrected vision	20/40	20/40
PreOp SphEq (D)	−7.12	−7.75
PostOp SphEq (D)	−1.50	−0.37
Time to 20/20 BCVA	9 days	15 days
Mean corneal power	40.25	38.32
Follow-up (mo)	9	6
No. of procedures	1	1
Case 5		
Uncorrected vision	20/50	20/40
PreOp SphEq (D)	−6.50	−10.00
PostOp SphEq (D)	+1.62	−4.62
Time to 20/20 BCVA	7 days	30 days
Mean corneal power	38.68	42.00
Follow-up (mo)	17	9
No. of procedures	1	1
Case 6		
Uncorrected vision	20/20	20/20
PreOp SphEq (D)	−7.50	−8.75
PostOp SphEq (D)	−3.87	0.00
Time to 20/20 BCVA	90 days	30 days
Mean corneal power	42.50	38.92
Follow-up (mo)	7	6
No. of procedures	2	1

*PreOp/PostOp SphEq = preoperative/postoperative spherical equivalent refractions; BCVA = best corrected visual acuity.
†Two eyes underwent astigmatic keratectomy (AK).

Table 12-5. Results of radial keratotomy (RK) in one eye and photorefractive keratectomy (PRK) in the mate eye—cont'd.

Patient data*	RK eyes	PRK eyes†
Case 7		
Uncorrected vision	20/25	20/50
PreOp SphEq (D)	−7.37	−8.75
PostOp SphEq (D)	−0.37	−0.25
Time to 20/20 BCVA	14 days	30 days
Mean corneal power	39.37	38.32
Follow-up (mo)	13	6
No. of procedures	1	1
Case 8		
Uncorrected vision	20/30	20/25
PreOp SphEq (D)	−6.00	−5.87
PostOp SphEq (D)	−0.87	−0.37
Time to 20/20 BCVA	5 days	120 days
Mean corneal power	40.50	41.00
Follow-up	5 yr	2.5 yr PRK
		2 mo AK
No. of procedures	2 RKs	1 PRK, 2 AK
Case 9		
Uncorrected vision	20/20	20/25
PreOp SphEq (D)	−2.62	−2.50
PostOp SphEq (D)	−0.25	−0.37
Time to 20/20 BCVA	7 days	30 days
Mean corneal power	39.62	40.12
Follow-up (mo)	62	25
No. of procedures	1	1
Case 10		
Uncorrected vision	20/100	20/32
	(monovision)	
PreOp SphEq (D)	−6.62	−7.37
PostOp SphEq (D)	−1.25	−0.50
	(monovision)	
Time to 20/20 BCVA	7 days	3 mo
Mean corneal power	38.75	39.50
Follow-up (mo)	14	12
No. of procedures	1	1
Case 11		
Uncorrected vision	20/200	20/30
PreOp SphEq (D)	−6.50	−6.00
PostOp SphEq (D)	−3.00	−0.37
Time to 20/20 BCVA	5 mo	3 mo
Mean corneal power	43.25	36.50
Follow-up (mo)	18	6
No. of procedures	1	1
Case 12		
Uncorrected vision	20/25	20/32
PreOp SphEq (D)	−2.75	−3.25
PostOp SphEq (D)	+0.63	−0.62
Time to 20/20 BCVA	1 day	1 mo
Mean corneal power	41.00	41.75
Follow-up (mo)	26	18
No. of procedures	3	1

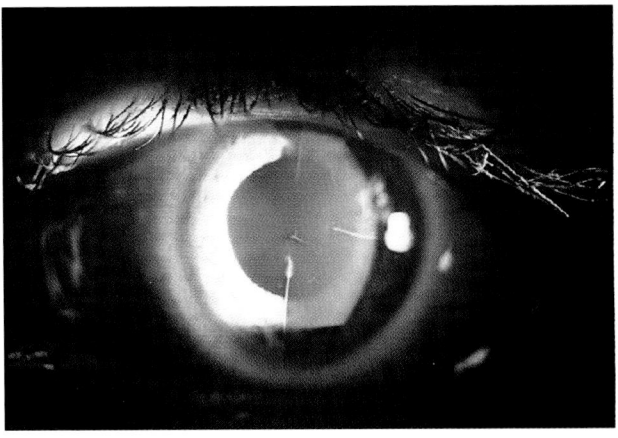

Fig. 12-1. Slit-lamp photograph of a four-incision RK, 3.0-mm optical zone, left eye, in a 48-year-old patient targeted for near vision in this eye. Preoperative spherical equivalent was −6.62 D; postoperative spherical equivalent was −1.25 D 1 year after surgery (see Table 12-5, case 10).

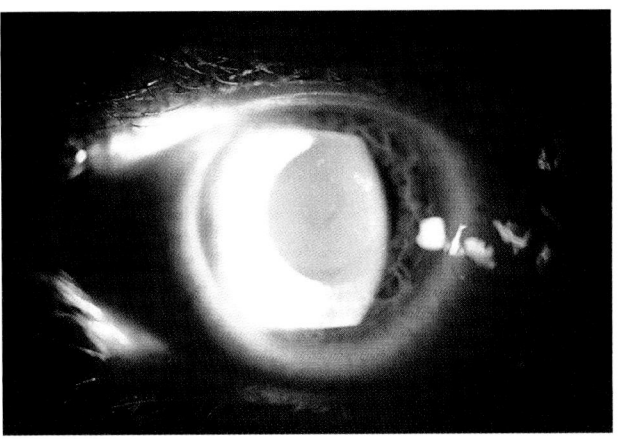

Fig. 12-2. Slit-lamp photograph of the right eye of the patient described in Fig. 12-1 6 months following PRK, 6.0-mm ablation zone, 95-μm ablation depth, targeted for distance vision. Preoperative spherical equivalent was −7.37 D; postoperative spherical equivalent was −0.50 D at 1 year; uncorrected visual acuity was 20/30 (see Table 12-5, case 10).

myopia (see Fig. 12-1), it is even more impressive to see a perfectly clear cornea following a PRK correction of 6.75 D of myopia (Fig. 12-2).

Predictability can be defined in terms of symmetry of refraction when the goal of surgery is emmetropia in both eyes (symmetry of refraction in cases of intended undercorrection for monovision in presbyopic patients is not considered). In the PERK study[68] 92% of mate eyes had spherical equivalent refractions within 3 D of each other. We currently do not have published information on bilateral PRK patients, but one of us (J.J.S.) analyzed 27 bilateral PRK patients for symmetry of outcome. In 19 patients (76%) the eyes were corrected to within 0.5 D of each other; 25 patients (93%) achieved corrections within 1 D of fellow

Table 12-6. Comparison of theoretical tissue excision after photorefractive keratectomy with postoperative ultrasonic central corneal pachymetry*

Case no.	Preoperative spherical equivalents (D)	Postoperative spherical equivalents (D)	Theoretical excision (μm)	Ultrasonically measured (μm)
1	−5.50	−0.50	46.20	46.00
2	−5.75	−0.37	46.62	47.00
3	−4.25	+1.12	36.25	25.00
4	−2.63	+3.00	40.30	40.00
5	−5.50	−0.25	26.64	21.00
6	−4.50	+1.00	38.06	22.00
7	−6.50	+0.12	44.70	51.00
8	−6.25	0.00	50.00	46.00
9	−6.38	+0.62	50.60	61.00
10	−5.13	+1.62	42.63	52.00
11	−6.13	−0.75	50.20	38.00
12	−3.00	−0.62	32.00	15.00
13	−5.63	−1.00	47.00	47.00
14	−2.62	0.00	30.00	50.00
15	−2.63	+0.75	29.00	35.00
16	−6.13	0.00	76.00	88.00
17	−4.50	0.00	47.00	78.00
18	−5.62	−1.00	47.00	47.00
19	−5.12	−0.25	43.00	57.00
20	−4.50	0.00	42.63	40.00

*Measurement with ultrasonic pachymetry at 1 month post operation to avoid the impact of epithelial hyperplasia and stromal wound healing.

eyes and in all patients both eyes were corrected to within 2 D of each other.

Predictability may be assessed by the change in corneal curvature for a given number of incisions performed with a specific optical clear zone diameter utilized during RK. With the excimer laser, the percentage of eyes within 1 D of emmetropia, the percentage of eyes with 20/40 or better uncorrected vision, and the amount of corneal tissue removed to achieve those results can be measured. However, it is not clear at this time if the thickness of corneal tissue excised is predictive of refractive outcome. Based on the PRK results of one of us (P.S.B.), at 1 month the predicted amount of resected corneal stroma was within 10% of the ultrasonically measured removed tissue from the central cornea in most eyes (Table 12-6). Because epithelial hyperplasia and new collagen production will increase corneal thickness, data taken less than 1 month following surgery will closely approximate the amount of tissue excised, whereas readings taken after 3 months will reflect the wound healing response.

RK surgeons use nomograms for determining a surgical plan to correct myopia and astigmatism. Some nomograms use patient age and the preoperative spherical equivalent (measured at the spectacles plane) as the only parameters that determine the surgical procedure, whereas others use patient sex and corneal power in addition to age and refractive error to determine the proper surgical procedure. Nomograms are based on one surgeon's experience and are usually determined retrospectively. These nomograms arbitrarily divide surgical categories into 3- to 5-year groups such as patients aged 21 to 25 years, 26 to 30 years, etc. Analysis of these nomograms reveals inconsistencies as one reads from one age group across to another. For example, reading from age 25 in one column to age 26 in another suggests less surgery should be performed for a different myopic error as soon as one has a birthday.

Since nomograms are based on the experience of one surgeon, it is difficult for most surgeons to duplicate the subtle nuances of incision production that led to the nomogram and consequently surgeons who religiously follow the nomogram may have undercorrected cases. In contrast, experienced RK surgeons might overcorrect cases using these nomograms because they achieve significantly greater effect with their incisions compared to novice RK surgeons. Nomograms that suggest a given effect can be achieved for enhancement procedures if a given surgical protocol is followed must be viewed with caution. Individual refractive and wound-healing responses simply make the predictability of enhancement procedures poor. The art of RK definitely comes into play for enhancement procedures. Recognizing the difficulties encountered when one follows a nomogram, some surgeons prefer to perform four incision procedures on many primary cases to determine the individual's response to the surgery and then either lengthen the initial incisions to a smaller optical zone or add four additional incisions, or do both in a combined procedure, if necessary. This approach minimizes the risk of overcorrection. One of us (J.J.S.) favors this approach while the other (P.S.B.) attempts to correct the refractive error with one operation based on his own surgical experience, but with a bias toward undercorrecting.

The only nomogram for PRK is built into the computer software. It only uses the refractive spherical equivalent (corrected to the corneal plane) as the major determinant for the surgical parameters.[88] The nomogram was based on the determination of ablation rates in animal and human eye bank eyes and the wound-healing effects. As experience increased, the programs have permitted increasing single ablation diameters from 4.5 mm to 7.0 mm and the use of multiple ablation diameters to produce aspherical ablations. The early clinical results after PRK suggest that the nomogram is surprisingly predictable for many surgeons, especially for eyes with less than 4 D of myopia. This should prove to be an advantage for PRK compared to RK as novice surgeons should be able to achieve results comparable to experienced PRK surgeons.

We need to carefully assess the refractive, topographic, and pachymetric data after PRK to improve the predictability of these nomograms. Above 4 D of myopia (see Table 12-4), most of the published results reveal a tendency toward undercorrection. These results could theoretically be improved by adjusting the PRK algorithm above 4 D to deliver more laser pulses for future patients or by performing a second PRK on undercorrected patients, or by both.

TIME TO RECOVER BEST CORRECTED SPECTACLE VISUAL ACUITY

For some patients, the time to recover best corrected spectacles visual acuity (BCVA) may be an important factor in making the decision as to which procedure to undertake. Published results suggest that eyes achieve their best level of uncorrected acuity in days after RK[51,89] compared to weeks after PRK.[22,28,82] This difference may be artificial because the protocol for PRK does not require that the patient return until 1 month after the epithelium has healed over the ablation. Eyes may recover BCVA earlier than 1 month, but acuity will not be measured until that visit. We believe that the majority of PRK patients are within one line of their BCVA within 2 to 4 weeks.

SAFETY

Before we can recommend a refractive surgical procedure for our patients (or even ourselves), we need to know how safe a specific technique is, the primary concern of safety being the risk of loss of BCVA. The risk of losing BCVA after RK was primarily related to

surgical technique with older instrumentation and lack of experience with the procedure. In the PERK study,[51,56] 3% of eyes lost two or more lines of BCVA at 5 years after surgery. All but three eyes maintained better than corrected visual acuity 20/20 line; two eyes lost one line of BCVA to 20/25 and one eye lost two lines from 20/20 to 20/30. Current RK technique rarely produces loss of more than two lines of BCVA. Causes of loss of BCVA are ocular trauma producing rupture of the globe,[36,90,91] delayed bacterial keratitis,[92-100] incisions within the central clear zone, decentered optical clear zones, and multifocal aspherical topography (irregular astigmatism).

Some of the preliminary studies following PRK have demonstrated a small percentage of eyes that have lost more than one line of BCVA.* The 1-year analysis of 521 eyes for the VISX phase III study for up to 6 D of myopia revealed loss of more than 1.6 lines of BCVA in eight eyes (1.5%). Two of these eyes lost from 20/12.5 to 20/20 and three eyes regained the lost visual acuity by 18 months. It should be noted that 54% of these 521 eyes underwent PRK without nitrogen flow across the cornea and none of these eyes lost more than 1.6 lines of BCVA.

The cause for this loss of BCVA has been assumed to be scarring of the cornea, but no specific study, to our knowledge, has correlated corneal scarring with loss of BCVA; decentered ablations have also been suggested as potential cause of vision loss. Fig. 12-3 illustrates the greatest amount of corneal scarring we encountered following PRK at 1 year. This eye was retreated with an initial improvement in visual acuity and haze. However, 3 months after the second PRK, the haze again increased despite aggressive topical corticosteroid treatment. Fig. 12-4 represents the slit-lamp appearance of this eye at 18 months after the retreatment when BCVA was 20/50, representing a two-line loss for this patient. Several studies after PRK have documented an improvement in BCVA, possibly based on increased magnification associated with elimination of myopic refractive errors, or other as yet undefined factors.

Another way of assessing the safety of a refractive surgical procedure is the number of eyes requiring reoperation or additional surgical procedures since reoperation increases the risks associated with any procedure. Reoperation is fairly common following RK because many surgeons prefer to perform an initial four-incision RK procedure and wait to assess the refractive results before performing additional surgery because of the concern of the risk of overcorrection. Reoperation is more common following astigmatic keratotomy[74,75,102-104] because of the less predictable results associated with astigmatism surgery.

---

*References 22, 23, 27, 28, 82, 83, 87, 101.

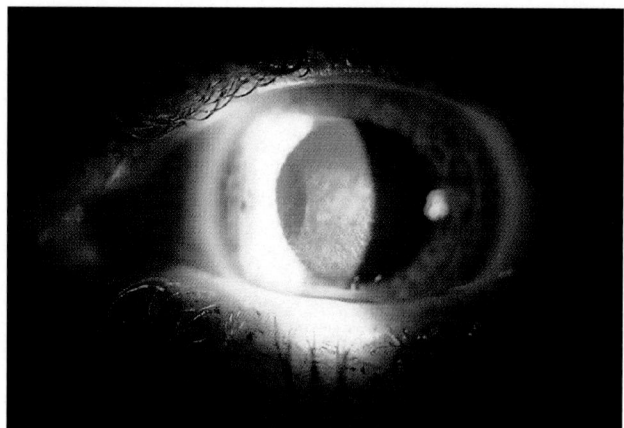

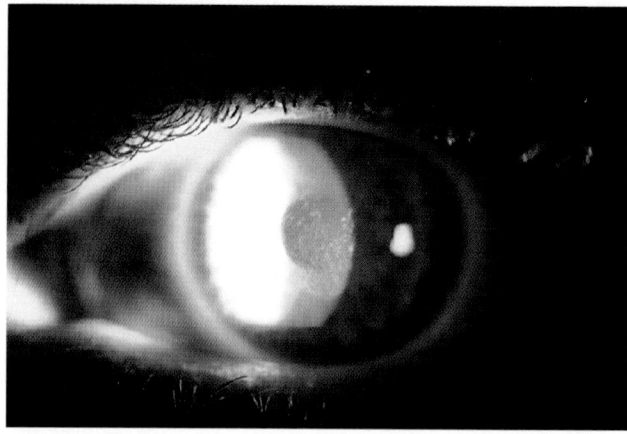

Fig. 12-3. Slit lamp photograph of a patient with grade 2.5 corneal haze 1 year after PRK (with nitrogen flow) for −5.75 D of myopia. Refraction is −3.5 −0.50 × 120 = 20/40.

Fig. 12-4. Slit-lamp photograph of the same eye shown in Figure 12-3, 18 months after second PRK. Although haze is improved, the patient is still symptomatic with glare and halos at night. Refraction is −3.75 −2.00 × 40 = 20/50.

Reoperations are less common following PRK compared to RK. In the phase III VISX study for up to 6 D of myopia, 10.4% of 691 eyes have been re-treated for undercorrection (two eyes were retreated for excessive haze and undercorrection). Twenty-nine of these eyes now have a 6-month follow-up and 80% have an uncorrected visual acuity of 20/40 or better. This would seem to indicate that re-treatment following PRK will significantly improve the results since the majority of eyes that have not achieved a satisfactory outcome following PRK are undercorrected.

In a series of 30 reoperations reported by Seiler et al.[27] for undercorrection of refractive error or reoperations for corneal scarring after PRK, or both, all but six eyes were within one line of their preoperative (preexcimer laser) BCVA. Two eyes lost four lines of BCVA to 20/50, one eye to 20/60, and three eyes lost BCVA from 20/20 to 20/33. These re-treatments were generally successful since 19 (63%) of these 30 eyes had sperical equivalent refraction between −1.00 and +1.00 D at 6 months (see Chapter 11).

The number of eyes undergoing penetrating keratoplasty following RK have been relatively few, with the main indications being irregular astigmatism and severe light sensitivity.[94,105] Recently, Colin (personal communication, Sept. 8, 1992) reported a series of corneal transplants performed after refractive surgical procedures. He documented eight corneal transplants that were performed following excimer laser photoablation. The indications for the primary laser procedures were for corneal scarring (five cases), undercorrected myopic epikeratoplasty (two cases), and a corneal perforation in one case of rheumatoid arthritis. In a separate manuscript, one of us (P.S.B.) reported the morphologic results of a study of 12 corneas following phototherapeutic excimer laser photoablation.[48] The main reason these eyes required kerato-

plasty was failure to remove the primary abnormality.

Studies of glare and photophobia following RK have documented that less than 5% of eyes have severe light-scattering complications.[106,107] Glare and photophobia may be associated with light scatter across the scars to produce the starburst symptoms or induced irregular astigmatism. Symptoms are usually more frequent at night as the pupil dilates beyond the optical clear zone. Although some RK nomograms use optical clear zone diameters of 2.75 mm, most RK surgeons prefer to limit the clear zone diameter to 3.00 mm; when given a choice of a 3.00-mm-diameter optical clear zone with four incisions or a 4.00-mm optical clear zone with eight incisions, many RK surgeons will choose the larger optical clear zone diameter provided all other surgical indications are equal.

The severity and frequency of similar complications following PRK have been associated with ablation diameters less than 5.0 mm, and transient induced optical aberrations such as multifocal corneas and decentered optics due to the superficial corneal wound-healing response.[108-112] Unlike RK patients, PRK patients are more likely to complain of a halo effect instead of a starburst. The recent elimination of ablation diameters less than 6.0 mm appears to have reduced light scatter symptoms. The light scatter symptoms following PRK are more frequent in the first few months following surgery, but can persist beyond 1 year. Long-term studies will define the time course of these symptoms.

The use of corneal topography to assess irregular astigmatism and wound healing following refractive surgery is in its infancy.[113-120] Topographic mapping of eyes following RK and PRK produces similar features with a gentle sloping pattern to the corneal power profile. The diameter of these profile changes are surprisingly similar, but some differences can be detected when one inspects the corneal power profile image. The finding of similar profile changes with these different procedures suggests that the part of the cornea forming the optical image is similar for these procedures even though PRK uses 5- to 6-mm-diameter ablations and RK uses optical clear zones of 3 to 4 mm (Fig. 12-5). To our knowledge, no study has quantified the differences in any induced, irregular astigmatism between RK and PRK. However, the multifocal pattern is more common after RK.[118] Until we have a quantitative means of interpreting the topographic maps, we will be unable to determine what patterns are consistent with loss of BCVA or light scatter complications.[118,121-123]

An early concern with RK was the risk of endothelial cell loss. Specular microscopic studies have demonstrated a small, nonprogressive cell loss after RK.[124,125] The excimer laser has produced endothelial cell loss in animal models when the laser was used to create radial excisions.[126] Recently, Beldavs and co-workers[127] reported a 17% central cell loss 1 month after PRK in 15 eyes which decreased to 9.1% at 1 year and to approximately 4.0% at 18 months. The authors have concluded that there was no significant cell loss when all eyes operated on at their center were studied (K. Thompson, M.D., personal communication, Oct. 22, 1993). Other clinical studies have failed to document significant cell loss for an entire study population, although individual cases have been found to have significant cell loss.[128] The national VISX phase III study for up to 6 D of myopia documents a 5% endothelial cell loss at 1 year.

Previous acute studies of the endothelium under an ablation site have not demonstrated cell damage or loss. Studies performed 1 to 3 weeks after PRK in rabbits and monkeys have documented fibrillar changes in Descemet's membrane without documenting any endothelial changes.[9,10] If we assume the findings of Beldavs and co-workers were not artifactitious, how can we explain the mechanism of endothelial cell loss?

In a preliminary laboratory study by one of us (P.S.B.) the mate human donor eye was ablated using the contralateral eye as a control, and both corneal-scleral rims were placed in an air-liquid organ culture model[129] for 7 days and quantitative endothelial cell counts performed. Twenty percent to 33% cell loss was found in the corneas ablated with a phototherapeutic keratectomy (PTK) profile at 150 μm depth. Acoustic damage from the laser shock wave, focal intraocular inflammation, release of chemical mediators of inflammation from the remaining epithelium or from the stroma, focal stromal edema, secondary irradiation,[130] or endothelial toxicity of topical drugs applied to the eye during reepithelialization in the absence of an epithelial barrier are possible contributors to cell loss.

Since the preliminary study of Beldavs and co-workers[127] and our laboratory findings are the first to document endothelial loss after PRK, we do not know the degree or duration of cell loss or if it is related to the model tested or to laser energy or to the mechanical technique of epithelial removal. A recent study has demonstrated keratocyte loss following simple epithelial debridement without evidence of endothelial damage.[131] Previous studies following bending of the cornea during intracapsular extraction have demonstrated that simple mechanical trauma could be one factor responsible for endothelial cell loss. Will we detect endothelial cell loss after repeat excimer laser procedures that repeat epithelial debridement and irradiation?

RK weakens the structural integrity of the cornea. Indeed, several articles have documented traumatic corneal rupture after RK,[36,90] but other articles have reported no corneal rupture after severe facial trauma in patients that had previously undergone RK.[91,132,133] There is no evidence of increased risk of corneal rupture after PRK. Other sight-threatening complications have been reported after RK,* but most had been associated with early techniques and poor instrumentation. In our opinion, the risks of the complications associated with microperforations and late-onset bacterial keratitis remain with current incisional keratotomy procedures, although the risk is apparently no greater than that of infectious keratitis following extended wear of contact lenses.[136,137] The recent interest in performing RK with centripetal incisions may increase the optical light-scattering complications with invasion of the optical clear zone. Night glare and photophobia have been reported following RK.[55,138,139] Optical clear zone diameters of less than 3.00 mm, decentered optical clear zones, incisions within the optical clear zone, and excessive wound scarring near the optical clear zone are the major factors responsible for these symptoms because they produce spherical and optical aberrations. Early PRK protocols utilized ablation diameters as small as 4.0 mm. These small ablation zones produced complaints of glare and photophobia due to the optical aberrations at the edge of the ablation zones. Some surgeons are now reablating these patients with intended ablation diameters of 6 or 7 mm to increase the diameter of the functional optical zone, but no studies of these procedures have been published.

STABILITY

The final refractive effect of RK and PRK is dependent on wound healing of the cornea. There have been no definitive studies that demonstrate a clinical benefit of using topical corticosteroids following RK; most

---

*References 3, 38, 99, 100, 134, 135.

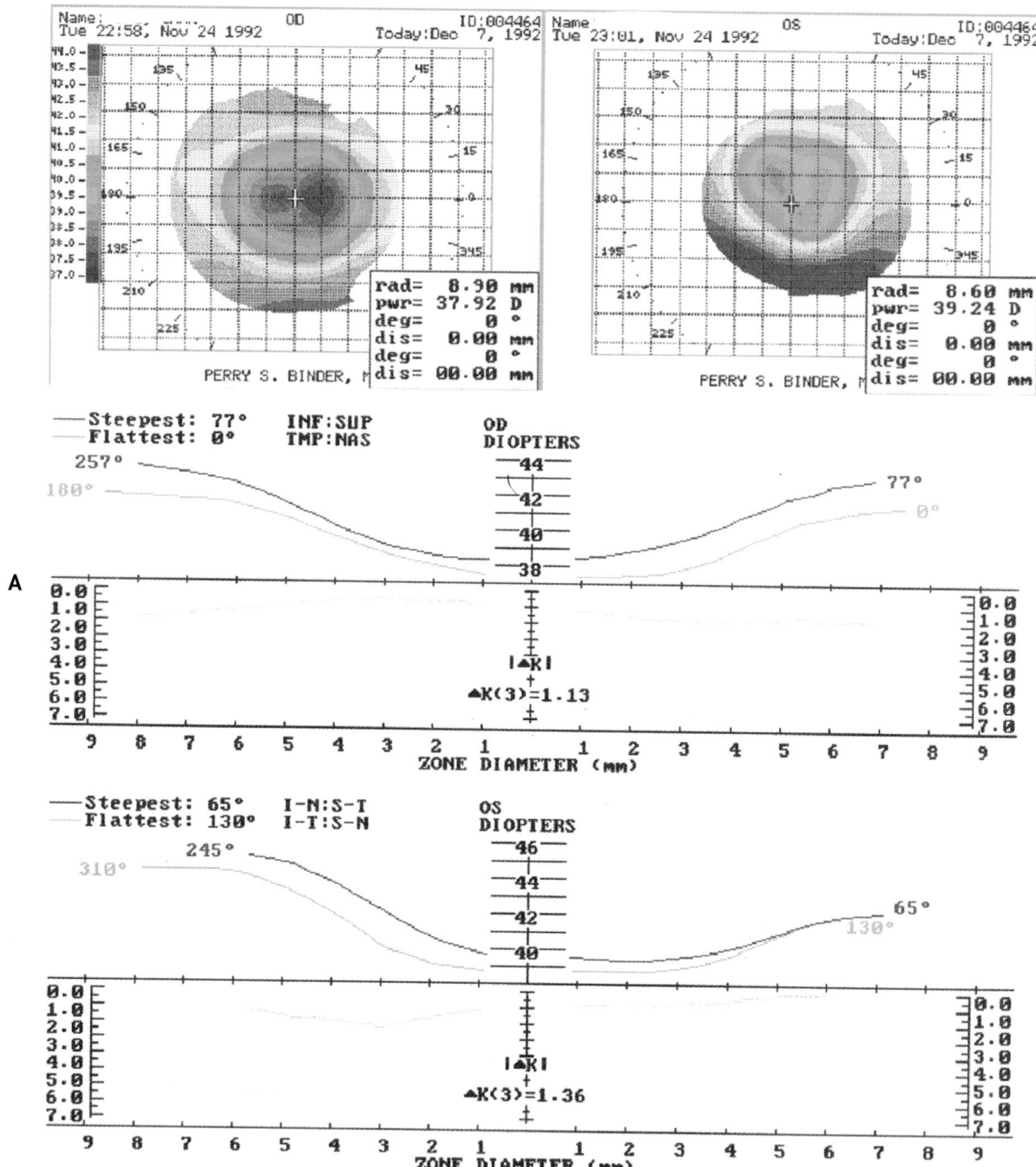

Fig. 12-5. Topographic maps of three cases listed in Table 12-5. **A,** *Case 1:* The centration and diameter of the PRK *(OD)* and RK *(OS)* procedures are similar, whereas the difference power map suggests that the left eye has a steeper inferior topography. The power profile map demonstrates a more gentle wound profile with PRK. *Case 2:* The central cornea is flatter following PRK *(OD)* compared with the RK *(OS)* eye. The RK topography is steeper compared to the PRK eye. The power profile map demonstrates asymmetric ablation after PRK *(top)* whereas the RK profile appears symmetric. *Case 3:* The PRK eye *(OD)* has a more irregular topography and an apparently decentered ablation zone compared to the RK eye *(OS)*. The power profile is smoother in the RK eye *(bottom)*. Such topographic comparisons suggest that similar diameters of corneal flattening produce similar refractive results (see Table 12-5) even though different ablation zones and optical clear zones are utilized.

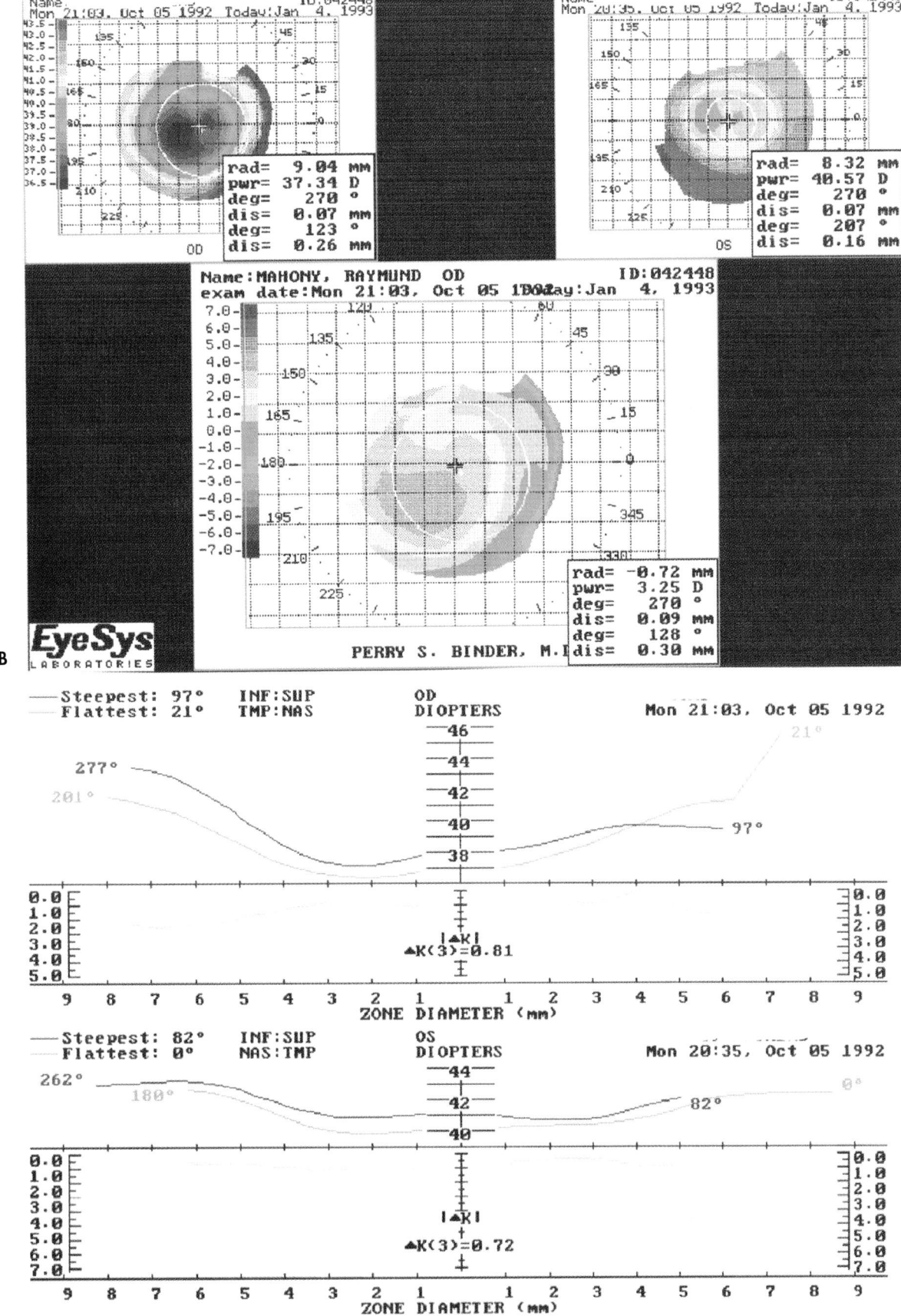

Fig. 12-5. For legend see p. 174.

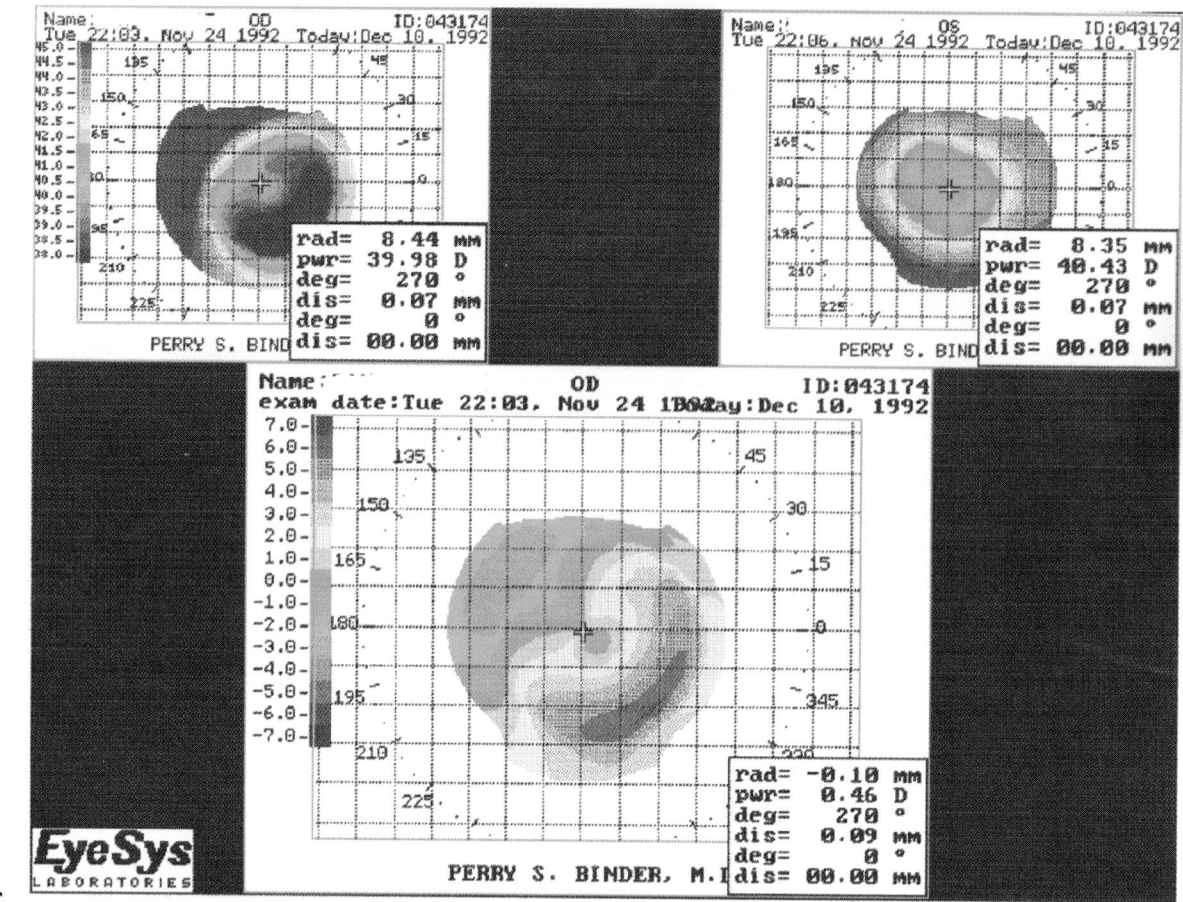

C

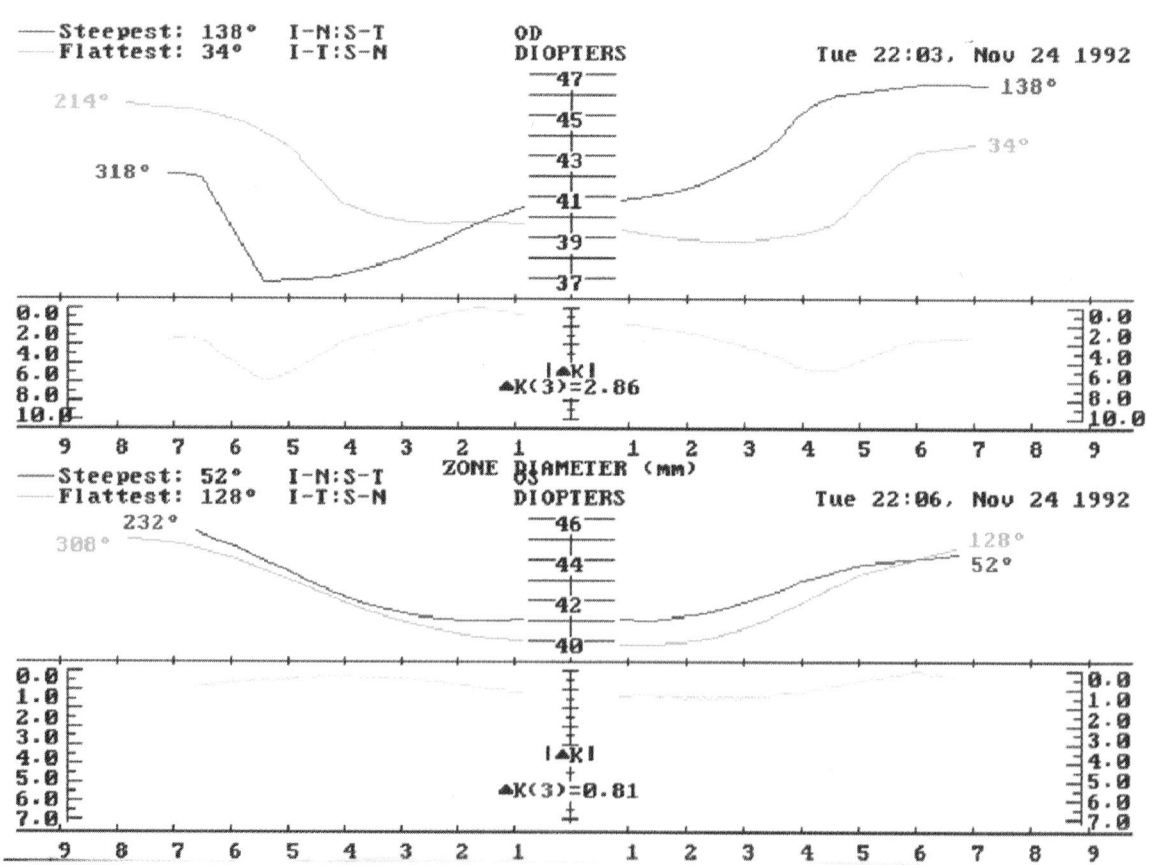

Fig. 12-5. For legend see p. 174.

surgical protocols for PRK require the use of topical steroids for at least 1 month to as long as 6 months after surgery. Up to 12% or more of eyes have developed steroid-induced ocular hypertension after PRK.[21,22,27,84] The incidence of steroid-induced cataract formation after PRK has not been determined. Whether steroids play a role in the reduction of wound healing, whether they have an effect on regression, or whether they provide better clinical results is controversial.[28,81,82,84,140] Gartry and co-workers[141] and others[142] have found no benefit on final refractive outcome with corticosteroid use. In contrast, Tengroth et al.[143,144] believe corticosteroids are beneficial for refractive outcome. At present, it is difficult to reach a conclusion about the beneficial effects of corticosteroids because too many variables are involved. For example, the duration, concentration, and type of corticosteroid used varies across studies. At the same time, surgeons used different ablation diameters, fluences, and ablation rates as different excimer lasers were used. Variable preoperative spherical equivalents were present; if deeper excisions are required for greater preoperative myopia, one might expect to achieve less effect the greater the power of the diopters to be corrected. To date no study has been able to isolate these factors to assess the effect of corticosteroids.

Diurnal Fluctuation in Visual Acuity

Refractive surgical procedures need to be assessed on the basis of the stability of refraction and visual acuity following the operation. In the early years of RK, excessive numbers of incisions (16-32) were associated with diurnal fluctuation in uncorrected vision and refractive error. Today, with four-, six-, and eight-incision procedures, fluctuation in vision from morning to night usually stabilizes in most cases within the first few months following surgery; by 1 year, few of the eyes have such optical variability.[51,55,58] In eyes with vision fluctuation that has lasted for years, only eyeglasses are used for night driving owing to undercorrection, night myopia, and diurnal increases in myopia.[145] With PRK, once the refractive error has stabilized, vision usually remains stable unless regression occurs.

Long-Term Effects

The instability of RK and the regression of effect after PRK are no doubt influenced by corneal wound healing. The major long-term complication following RK is progression of effect (hyperopic shift). Unfortunately, no surgical or patient parameter has been definitively demonstrated to determine which eye is going to develop this complication.* Deitz et al.[146] have suggested that the primary incision depth was corre-

lated with progression of effect while the PERK study[147] correlated clear zone diameter with progression of effect. Several studies performed in the early 1980s have documented a progression of effect in the hyperopic direction in 13% to 31% of eyes that has exceeded 1 D over a 3- to 5-year period. Recently, Dietz (personal communication, Nov. 13, 1993) reported that 20 (48%) of 42 of the initial 225 eyes (19% follow-up) that he first reported between 1979 and 1983 to have "progressive hyperopia" continued to have more than 1 D of progression of refractive effect between 7 and 12 years after surgery. Lindstrom (personal communication, Nov. 7, 1992) reported that 21% of eyes that had four incisions had developed more than 1 D of progression of refractive effect up to 8.5 years after surgery. The PERK study suggests 60% to 80% of eyes stabilize refractive errors between 12 and 18 months.[147]

PRK procedures tend to produce initial overcorrections (as do most RK procedures), most likely because of planned overcorrection in the computer algorithms. This overcorrection response may vary between instruments since they use different computer programs, energy delivery, and fluences.

In contrast to RK, eyes tend to lose effect following PRK, i.e., they undergo a refractive regression over time.* The cause of regression is thought to be a combination of epithelial hyperplasia and corneal wound healing (described as "remodeling"), which could represent collagen deposition, proteoglycan production, or changes in corneal hydration. Durrie (personal communication, Nov. 7, 1992) has suggested there may be three types of wound-healing response following PRK: (1) eyes that do not heal and whose corneas remain clear with hyperopic refractive errors; (2) eyes that heal "normally" producing transient haze; and (3) eyes that heal with excessive haze and undergo significant regression of refractive effect. We do not yet know if the regression effect progresses peripherally to centrally within the area of the ablation, or if it occurs first in the central cornea.

Fig. 12-6 displays a serial topographic study of an eye with a stable refractive error after PRK. In comparison, Fig. 12-7 is a serial study of an eye that developed a regression of effect between 3 and 6 months after surgery. Although the diameters of the ablation effect are similar, the corneal power profiles are significantly different reflecting a steepening of the previously flattened central cornea. This change could represent epithelial hyperplasia or increasing corneal thickness produced by the wound-healing response, but in this particular eye there was no significant increase in ultrasonic central corneal thickness, which suggests only subtle changes had occurred in epithelial or stromal thickness.

---

*References 60, 64, 65, 70, 146, 147.

*References 25, 61, 79, 81, 82, 87.

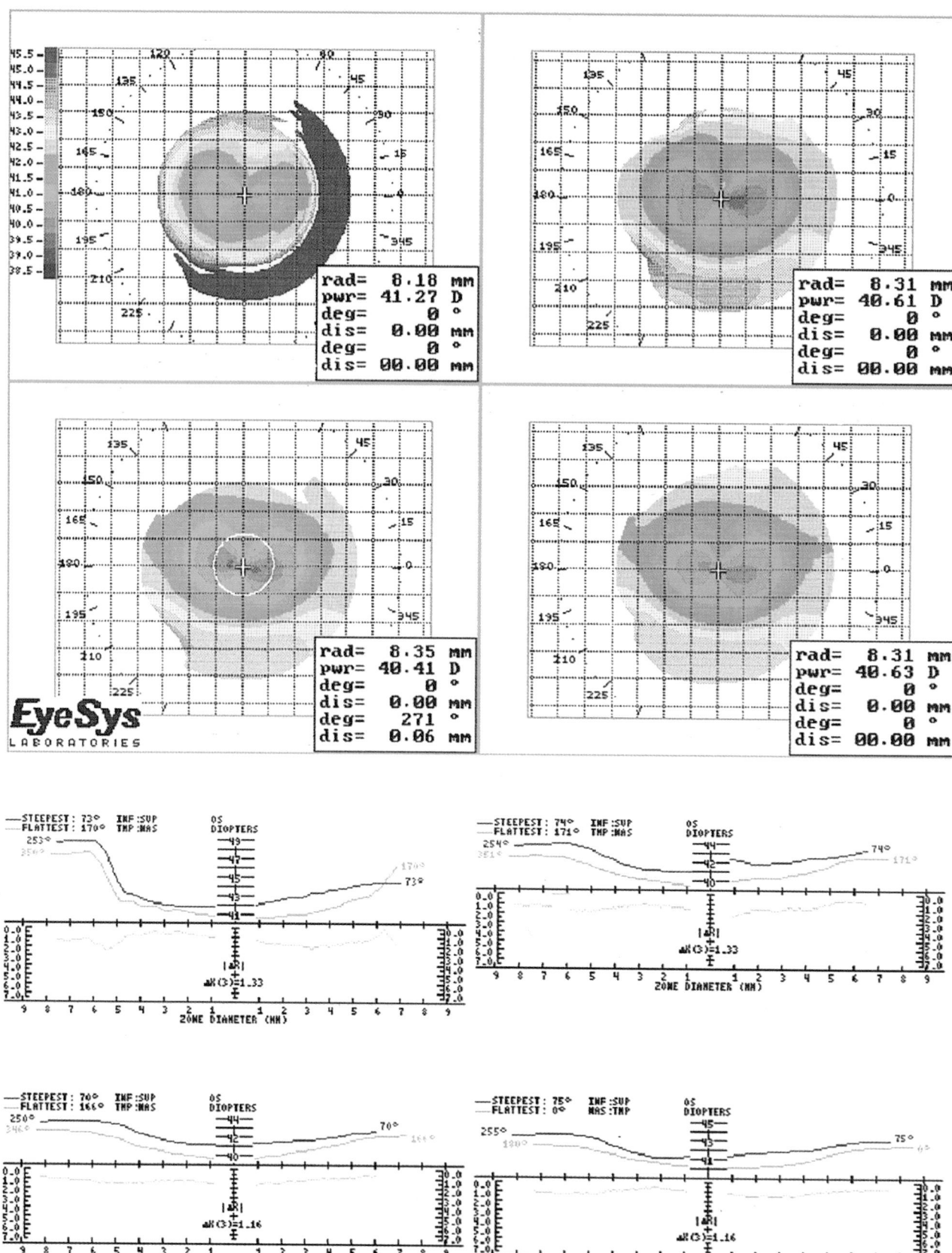

Fig. 12-6. *Top:* Topographic study of one eye that underwent PRK in June 1991 and was studied at 3 months *(top left)*, 6 months *(top right)*, 12 months *(bottom left)*, and 15 months *(bottom right)*. The diameter and shape of the ablation profile remain stable during the study period. *Bottom:* Serial power profile map at the same time periods of study. Note the change in profile from month 3 compared to the other time periods, which probably reflects epithelial hyperplasia at the ablation edges. The overall shape of the ablation profile, however, remains constant, as did the uncorrected acuity and refractive error.

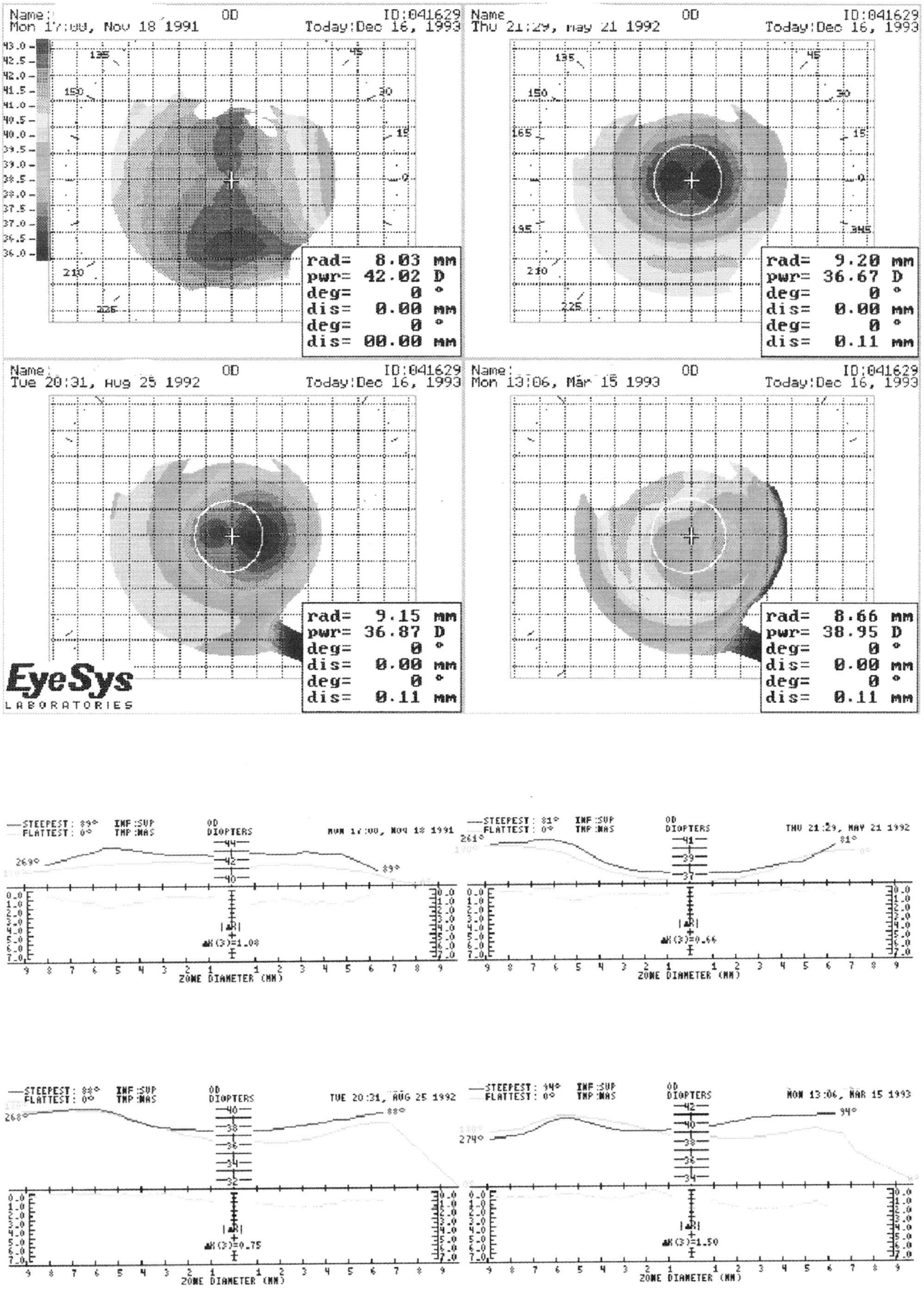

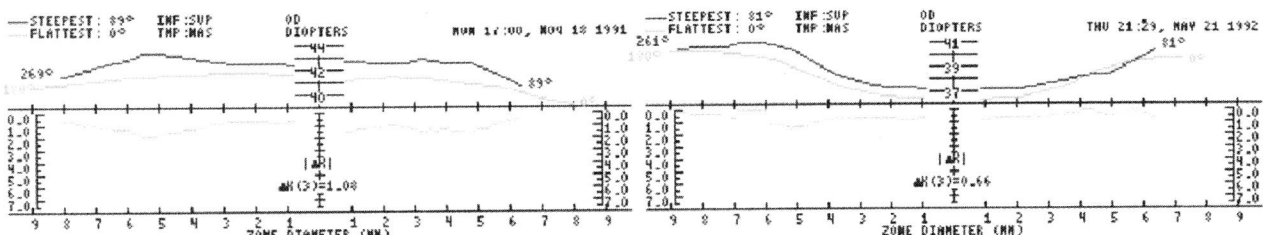

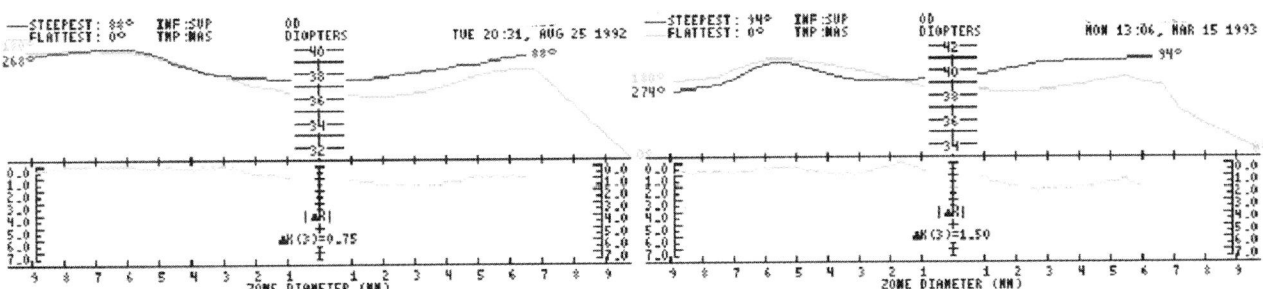

Fig. 12-7. *Top:* Topographic study of a case of refractive regression after PRK. *Top left:* 1 month after surgery. The uncorrected acuity was 20/25, the spherical equivalent was −0.50 D, and the mean corneal power was 39.78 D. *Right:* 6 months after surgery the uncorrected acuity was 20/70, the spherical equivalent was −1.75 D and the mean corneal power was 41.77 D. The ablation diameter has decreased during this time period. *Bottom:* Power profile map at 1 month post operation *(top)* and at 6 months *(bottom)*. Note the change in the contour of the power profile and the steepening of the corneal power.

These subtle changes are not unexpected. For example, after an RK procedure designed to correct 5 D of myopia, the corneal power has been documented to decrease from 45 D (7.5 mm radius) to 41 D (8.23 mm) (there is usually more refractive change than the keratometry-measured change after refractive surgery), which represents a reduction of curvature of 73 μm.[148] Applying this analysis to PRK, a reduction of 1 D of refractive effect would represent 20% of the curvature change (5 D to 4 D of achieved correction), or 14 μm. This subtle change in corneal thickness cannot be accurately detected with current technology. Although such an analysis is logical, the use of keratometry to analyze refractive benefit may not be meaningful.[149] Nevertheless, topography is useful in assessing the effects of refractive surgery.

Refractive progression after RK may shed light on the mechanism of regression after PRK. Histologic examination of eyes after RK[35] has failed to demonstrate epithelial hyperplasia over the central cornea unoperated on. However, histologic examination of animal[7,8] and human eyes[48] after PRK clearly demonstrates epithelial hyperplasia in almost every specimen. Since the reduction in corneal power is roughly similar for the same amount of myopia reduction for RK and PRK, we can conclude that the epithelial response is stimulated differently between these two procedures.

Examination of topographic maps after RK and PRK suggests there is a more gradual change in the corneal power from the central to the peripheral cornea, i.e., the transition from the unablated area to the ablated area is more rapid (steep) after PRK. This finding suggests that a gradual taper of the ablation profile might alter epithelial hyperplasia, but in our recent study of high myopia corrected with a three-zone ablation profile,[49] the regression effect was unaltered. Perhaps a larger (>6.0 mm) single-zone ablation diameter or larger or more complex ablation profiles may influence the epithelial fill-in response.

The effect of a hyperopic shift after RK can be to improve the visual and refractive results of an eye that had been undercorrected, but to worsen the results of eyes that were corrected to emmetropia or were overcorrected immediately after the RK surgery. Of greater concern is the fact that no study has demonstrated the progression of effect to cease. If progression of effect is truly procedural-independent, i.e., if it occurs with equal frequency after four incision procedures performed with currently available thin-profile diamond blades compared to previously performed RK procedures that used eight or more incisions, then refractive surgeons may need to carefully consider performing RK. Lindstrom has recently proposed the concept of "mini RK" (where centrifugal incisions stop or centripetal incisions start at a 7.0- to 8.0-mm optical zone) as a possible technique to reduce the incidence of hyperopic drift. It will take 3 to 4 years to establish whether the mini-RK technique results in a more stable outcome. Since we do not have the ability at present to improve the wound-healing response after any corneal surgical procedure, and since we do not have an operation that can predictably correct the hyperopia that occurs with progression of effect after RK, refractive surgeons should strongly consider undercorrecting each case to allow for the unpredictable percentage of eyes that will develop a progression of effect.

The regression of effect after PRK is a different concern. Most cases of refractive regression occur early (months), whereas progression of effect after RK persists for years. Regression of effect will tend to reduce the refractive and visual benefits of all eyes that were initially overcorrected. Significant regressions are treated with reoperations which carry the risk of loss of BCVA.[27] Alternatively, undercorrected cases (and cases that have suffered a regression) could receive a secondary RK procedure. No data have yet been published on the effect of performing RK after PRK, but we are aware of one case in which a −19.50- D preoperative spherical equivalent was reduced to −7.00 D after a primary PRK procedure. Six months later, an eight-incision RK procedure was performed (L.T. Nordan, personal communication, May 8, 1993). After a delay of 3 months, the refractive error decreased and the uncorrected visual acuity improved from 20/800 (pre-RK) to 20/50. Clearly, RK has the problem of long-term progression of effect and PRK has the problem of short-term regression of effect. The severity and incidence of these respective complications will most likely determine which procedure will continue to be utilized or if some newer technique will replace both procedures.

ADJUSTABILITY

Because many refractive surgical procedures do not provide the desired result after a single operation, repeat operations (enhancement procedures) may be necessary. In order for a procedure to be widely accepted, therefore, it must be able to undergo repeat surgery; i.e., it must be an adjustable procedure.

At the present time, radial and astigmatic keratotomy can be used to adjust undercorrected PRK eyes or eyes with excessive post-PRK astigmatism. Fig. 12-8 is a slit-lamp photograph of a patient (see Table 12-5, case 8) who underwent arcuate incisions to correct 2 D of PRK-induced astigmatism which improved his uncorrected visual acuity from 20/60 to 20/30. How often do repeat operations result in improved uncorrected vision, and in the percentage of eyes closer to emmetropia? Werblin[75] recently reported a series of 205 consecutive RK procedures. After one operation in 139 eyes, 71% of eyes had 20/40 or better visual

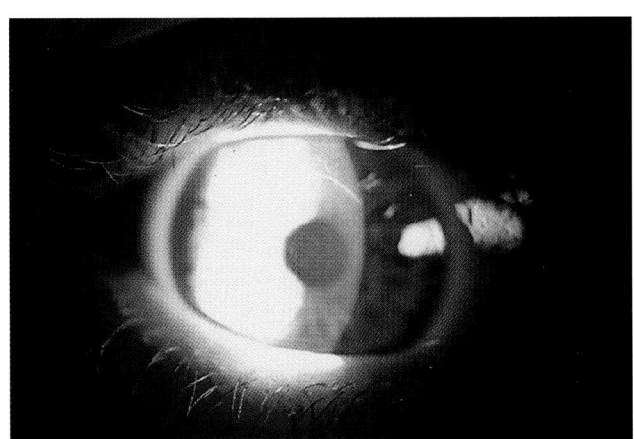

Fig. 12-8. Slit-lamp photograph of a patient who underwent astigmatic keratotomy 18 months after PRK for reduction of PRK-induced astigmatism (see Table 12-3, case 8). Preoperative uncorrected visual acuity was 20/60, refraction plano was −2.75 × 170. Postastigmatic keratotomy uncorrected visual acuity was 20/30 at 3 months; refraction plano was −0.50 × 170.

acuity without correction; after incisional enhancement procedures for undercorrection and induced astigmatism and suturing procedures for overcorrections, 99% had 20/40 or better uncorrected acuity, although many eyes had to undergo three or more procedures. In a recent retrospective series of 393 eyes operated on by one surgeon, 56% of eyes achieved 20/40 unaided visual acuity with one operation, 29% underwent one enhancement procedure, 12% underwent two enhancements, and 3% had three enhancement procedures to achieve a final result of 20/40 or better in 98% of the eyes.[89] Most RK surgeons believe enhancement procedures are extremely useful for treating undercorrected cases, in contrast to performing aggressive primary surgery which carries the risk of an overcorrection and the subsequent necessity of performing a highly unpredictable suturing procedure.

In comparison to RK, between 70% and 92% of eyes with less than 6 D of preoperative myopia have been reported to have 20/40 or better uncorrected acuity after a single PRK procedure. Recently, Seiler and co-workers[27] demonstrated that reoperation for cases of corneal scarring achieves similar refractive and visual goals as those cases that have undergone reoperation for undercorrection. Sixty-three percent of the spherical equivalent refractive errors were between +1.00 and −1.00 D at 6 months. Six of 298 eyes lost two lines of BCVA (compared to their pre-primary laser surgery) following reoperation (see Chapter 11).

We do not know at this time what laser variables should be utilized for the repeat excimer laser operations. What previous history of RK and clinical findings are predictors of results for PRK following RK?

What topographic and clinical findings following PRK are predictive of results following a repeat PRK? Since RK and PRK can be applied to pseudophakic eyes and eyes that have undergone corneal transplant, we also need to determine the predictors of clinical results in such cases.

The percentage of eyes that are refitted with contact lenses is relatively low for RK and has yet to be reported for PRK. In most cases, contact lens wear does appear to restore BCVA after RK. Spectacles, on the other hand, are more commonly used following refractive surgical procedures to provide BCVA, but they cannot correct irregular astigmatism. Recently, there have been anecdotal reports of increasing myopia following repeat PRK which has been thought to be due to structural weakening (and concomitant anterior bulging) of the cornea produced by excessive tissue removal. Other reports of poor refractive results following RK have been suggested to be due to operations performed on undiagnosed cases of early keratoconus (JJ Scragoussi, personal communication, Nov. 13, 1993).

We have to determine if the cause of significant undercorrection is truly due to weakening of the cornea's structure, thereby negating the refractive result, or if the loss of effect was simply due to the wound-healing factors that produce regression of effect, or if contact lens–induced corneal molding (orthokeratology) had been present prior to surgery and the surgeon performed surgery for the amount of myopia that had not been reduced by the contact lens wear. One of us (P.S.B.) has treated two such RK cases after orthokeratology, not recognizing that the target correction represented residual refractive error that had not been treated by the orthokeratology. Following RK for the residual refractive error, the cornea returned to its pre-orthokeratology topography, negating the refractive benefit of the RK procedure.

REVERSIBILITY

The ideal refractive surgical procedure should restore the eye to its preoperative condition. Unfortunately, neither RK nor PRK is reversible. The difficulties encountered in trying to surgically correct an overcorrected RK procedure emphasizes the impossibility of "erasing" surgical incisions.[150-153] The only potentially reversible procedures that are currently being studied are synthetic epikeratoplasty procedures that do not violate Bowman's layer,[154] the intrastromal ring,[155] and phakic intraocular lens implants for correction of myopia.[156]

COSTS

The current surgical technique for RK utilizes radial markers to assist incision orientation and length; globe fixation devices; calibration microscopes for predictably extending crystalline blades; and new thinner, single- or double-edged or square diamond blades to produce more predictable incision width and depth. Blade extension is based on ultrasonic pachymetry. The surgical procedure is determined by individual surgeon nomograms. The cost of equipment can be as low as $5000 to as high as $50,000. If one adds corneal topography (which we think is extremely important in understanding refractive surgical procedures), and an operating microscope, then the cost increases another $35,000 to $45,000. The procedure takes 5 to 15 minutes to perform, and the patient achieves his or her approximate final refractive error within 1 month following surgery. The cost to the patient may vary between $1000 and $2000 per eye in the United States. These procedures are usually performed in a surgical suite within the surgeon's office without a facility fee, or in an ambulatory surgical center. One surgical fee usually covers all surgical procedures and expenses, including reoperations performed within a fixed period of time following the primary procedure. The second eye is usually operated on at the same time or within 1 week to 3 months of the first eye. No study has yet demonstrated if the final refractive results are better with separate procedures than with simultaneous procedures.

In contrast to RK, PRK requires a minimal surgical instrument expense consisting of a lid speculum, a blade or spatula to remove epithelium, and an optical clear zone marker, amounting in all to about $250, but a huge initial expense of over $450,000 for the laser, with an additional ongoing expense of at least one part-time technician and the annual upkeep of the machine, which can approximate $40,000. This upfront expense is significantly less if the laser is leased or otherwise financed.

The surgical fee to the patient is shared between the facility and the surgeon (assuming the two are different). The typical cost to the patient for both surgeon and facility varies between $2000 and $3000 per eye. One surgical fee is charged by the surgeon, but if additional procedures are needed, an additional facility fee may be charged to compensate for the upkeep expense. Once the procedure is approved by the Food and Drug Administration (FDA) the second eye will be operated on within 1 to 4 weeks of the first (or simultaneously), whereas under the current FDA protocol, 6 months must elapse between surgical procedures in the same patient. Until it is demonstrated that there is no significant difference in the final refractive and visual result when both eyes are operated on simultaneously with PRK vs. separate operations, we recommend that only one eye undergo PRK at one surgical setting.

CONCLUSIONS

Radial keratotomy has been performed clinically for over 14 years in the United States. In addition to the usual surgeon learning curve, which is required with any new surgical procedure, we learned later about the common incidence of progression of effect and the rare risk of bacterial keratitis following RK. It is therefore not surprising that we are also undergoing a learning curve with the excimer laser, with many questions still remaining unanswered. The surgical technique with the excimer laser is highly variable from surgical center to surgical center. The technique of epithelial removal (mechanically by blade or with the laser), whether the ablation is performed under a dry, semidry, or moist condition, and whether patient ocular fixation is achieved with external instrumentation or tracking devices are some of the variables. Although currently available lasers use different techniques of placing an ablation profile on the cornea (rotating ring vs. scanning slit vs. contracting iris diaphragm), no one laser has produced results superior to another (Trokel S: presented at the American Academy of Ophthalmology Annual Convention, Dallas, Nov. 8, 1992). Whether the direction of the diaphragm expansion or closure[157] plays a final role in regression or stability has yet to be clinically documented. Similarly, ablation profiles using a single or multiple ablation zones are being studied; it is not clear whether one has an advantage over the other, although multiple ablation zones can provide the same refractive change with removal of less corneal tissue compared to single ablation profiles. The parameters chosen in the software are based on theoretical assumptions which are being modified by clinical results.

Considering how early we are in the evaluation of a new surgical procedure, the results of excimer laser photoablation have been superior to those that were obtained with RK 4 years after RK was introduced into the United States. Unfortunately, we are not going to be able to improve the clinical results after PRK until we become more consistent in reporting the results of our procedures. Basic information has to be published in a concise and digestible fashion with minimal standards for reporting the results, as suggested by Waring.[77] We need to adhere to surgical protocols so that we can understand exactly what we have done, and then be able to intelligently modify the procedure; when protocols are changed in the middle of an experiment, it is difficult to interpret clinical results.

A recent survey performed by the American Society for Cataract and Refractive Surgery found a doubling of their members performing RK from 1992 to 1993 (*Ocular Surgery News*, May 12, 1993). One has to ask that if the socioeconomic conditions that were present in America in 1984 were existing in 1993, how

Table 12-7. Comparison of radial keratotomy (RK) and photorefractive keratectomy (PRK) based on current clinical results

	RK	PRK
Efficacy	1-8 D	1-16 D
Age-dependent	Yes	No
Predictability	Similar	Similar
Safety	Keratitis	Scar formation
	Wound rupture	Endothelial loss?
	Loss of ≥2 lines of BCVA* (3%)	Loss of BCVA* ?%
Stability	Progression 13%-31%	Regression ?%
Adjustable	Yes	No
Reversible	No	No
Costs	Low	Very expensive
Reoperation	Common	10%
Years of experience	14	4
Vision recovery	Days	Weeks
Fluctuation acuity	5%	No
Glare	5%	Not established
Upkeep expense	Minimal	Significant
Astigmatism limits	6 D	Not established

*BCVA = best corrected visual acuity.

interested would the ophthalmologist be in spending over half a million dollars for excimer laser technology or $50,000 to perform RK? Newer lasers, some solid-state, are being studied for their ability to modify refractive errors. Whether these new modalities and their approaches are going to compete with excimer PRK and RK remains to be demonstrated.

RECOMMENDATIONS

Once the facts about new refractive procedures are known and the risks and benefits established, one is able to compare a new technology with existing procedures. Only when the new procedure is either equally efficacious at a lesser cost or is more efficacious without increased risk can it be recommended to replace the current procedure. Based on what is currently known about RK and PRK in 1993, the two procedures have equal pros and cons while being equally able to correct myopia (Table 12-7). If PRK produces equivalent, more stable results at a greater expense, but in a single operation, then it may replace RK. Currently, the two procedures are not mutually exclusive. Undercorrected RK cases can undergo subsequent PRK and perhaps the reverse procedure can be done. For cases with excessive naturally occurring astigmatism and myopia, the astigmatic component can be performed with crystalline blades either before or after the myopic component is corrected with the exci-

mer laser. Until PRK can be demonstrated to provide results superior to RK, the incisional procedures will remain in vogue. If a new technology such as the intracorneal ring or the holmium:yttrium-aluminum-garnet laser or an intrastromal solid-state laser can correct myopia to a more predictable degree compared to RK and PRK, then these current popular procedures may become obsolete.

REFERENCES

1. Fyodorov SN, Durnev VV: Operation of dosage dissection of corneal circular ligament in cases of myopia of mild degree, *Ann Ophthalmol* 11:1885-1890, 1979.
2. Binder PS: What we have learned about corneal wound healing from refractive surgery, *J Refract Corneal Surg* 5:98-120, 1989.
3. Binder PS: Optical problems following refractive surgery, *Ophthalmol* 93:739-740, 1986.
4. Waring GO III: *Refractive keratotomy for myopia and astigmatism,* St Louis, 1991, Mosby-Year Book.
5. Waring GO III: Development of a system for excimer laser corneal surgery, *Trans Am Ophthalmol Soc* 87:855-983, 1989.
6. Trokel SL: Evolution of excimer laser corneal surgery, *J Cataract Refract Surg* 15:373-383, 1989.
7. Fantes FE, Hanna KD, Waring GO III, et al: Photorefractive keratectomy in monkeys, *Arch Ophthalmol* 108:665-675, 1990.
8. SundarRaj N, Geiss MJ III, Fantes F, et al: Healing of excimer laser ablated monkey corneas: an immunohistochemical evaluation, *Arch Ophthalmol* 108:1604-1610, 1990.
9. Gaster RN, Binder PS, Coalwell K, et al: Corneal surface ablation by 193 nm excimer laser and wound healing in rabbits, *Invest Ophthalmol Vis Sci* 30:90-98, 1989.
10. Hanna K, Pouliquen Y, Waring GO III: Corneal stromal wound healing in rabbits after 193 nm excimer laser surface ablation, *Arch Ophthalmol* 107:895-901, 1989.
11. Malley DS, Steinert RF, Puliafito CA, et al: Immunofluorescence study of corneal wound healing after excimer laser anterior keratectomy in the monkey eye, *Arch Ophthalmol* 108:1316-1322, 1990.
12. Gipson I, Spurr-Michaud S, Tisdale A, et al: Reassembly of the anchoring structures of the corneal epithelium during wound repair in the rabbit, *Invest Ophthalmol Vis Sci* 30:425-434, 1989.
13. Hanna K, Pouliquen Y, Savoldelli M, et al: Corneal wound healing in monkeys 18 months after excimer laser photorefractive keratectomy, *Refract Corneal Surg* 6:340-345, 1990.
14. Hanna K, Pouliquen Y, Fantes F, et al: Long term corneal wound healing in monkeys after initial and repeated excimer laser keratomileusis, *Invest Ophthalmol Vis Sci* 31(suppl):478, 1990.
15. Hanna K, Pouliquin Y, Waring GI, et al: Corneal wound healing in monkeys after repeated excimer laser photorefractive keratectomy, *Arch Ophthalmol* 110:1286-1291, 1992.
16. McDonald MB, Frantz JM, Klyce SD, et al: One-year refractive results of central photorefractive keratectomy for myopia in the nonhuman primate cornea, *Arch Ophthalmol* 108:40-47, 1990.
17. Zabel RW, Sher NA, Ostrov CS, et al: Myopic excimer laser keratectomy: a preliminary report, *Refract Corneal Surg* 6:329-334, 1990.
18. Taylor DM, L'Esperance FA Jr, Del Pero RA, et al: Human excimer laser lamellar keratectomy, *Ophthalmology* 96(5):654-664, 1989.
19. L'Esperance FA, Warner JW, Telfair WB: Excimer laser instrumention and technique for human corneal surgery, *Arch Ophthalmol* 107:131-139, 1989.

20. McDonald MB, Frantz JM, Klyce SD, et al: Central photorefractive keratectomy for myopia: the blind eye study, *Arch Ophthalmol* 108:799-808, 1990.

21. Seiler T, Kahle G, Kriegerowski M: Excimer laser (193 nm) myopic keratomileusis in sighted and blind human eyes, *Refract Corneal Surg* 6:165-173, 1990.

22. Seiler T, Wollensak J: Myopic photorefractive keratectomy with the excimer laser. One year follow-up, *Ophthalmol* 98:1156-1163, 1991.

23. McDonald MB, Liu JC, Byrd TJ, et al: Central photorefractive keratectomy for myopia. Partially sighted and normally sighted eyes, *Ophthalmology* 98:1327-1337, 1991.

24. Eiferman RA, O'Neill KP, Forgey DR, et al: Excimer laser photorefractive keratectomy for myopia: six-month results, *Refract Corneal Surg* 7:344-347, 1991.

25. Sher NA, Barak M, DeMarchi J, et al: Excimer laser photorefractive keratectomy in high myopia. A multicenter study. Presented at ASCRS Conference, 1992.

26. Lohmann CP, Gartry DS, Kerr Muir M, et al: Corneal haze after excimer laser refractive surgery: objective measurements and functional implications, *Eur J Ophthalmol* 1:173-180, 1991.

27. Seiler T, Derse M, Pham T: Repeated excimer laser treatment after photorefractive keratectomy, *Arch Ophthalmol* 110:1230-1233, 1992.

28. Gartry D, Kerr Muir M, Lohmann C, et al: The effect of topical corticosteroids on refractive outcome and corneal haze after photorefractive keratectomy, *Arch Ophthalmol* 110:944-952, 1992.

29. Stainer GA, Shaw EL, Binder PS, et al: Histopathology of a case of radial keratotomy, *Arch Ophthalmol* 100:1473-1477, 1982.

30. Binder PS, Barraquer JI, Villasenor RA, et al: *The histopathology of human refractive keratoplasty. International Congress of Ophthalmology, Acta XXIV*, Philadelphia, 1982, JB Lippincott.

31. Deg J, Zavala E, Binder P: Delayed corneal wound healing following radial keratotomy, *Ophthalmology* 92:734-740, 1985.

32. Baumgartner SD, Binder PS: Refractive keratoplasty. Histopathology of clinical specimens, *Ophthalmology* 92:1606-1615, 1985.

33. Binder PS, Nayak SK, Deg JK, et al: An ultrastructural and histochemical study of long-term wound healing after radial keratotomy, *Am J Ophthalmol* 103:432-440, 1987.

34. Binder PS: Pathologic findings in cases of refractive corneal surgery. In *Transactions of the New Orleans Academy of Ophthalmology*. New York, 1987, Raven Press.

35. Deg JK, Binder PS: Wound healing after astigmatic keratotomy in human eyes, *Ophthalmology* 94:1290-1298, 1987.

36. Binder PS, Waring GOI, Arrowsmith PR, et al: Histopathology of traumatic corneal rupture after radial keratotomy, *Arch Ophthalmol* 106:1584-1590, 1988.

37. Melles G, Binder PS: A comparison of wound healing in sutured and unsutured wounds, *Arch Ophthalmol* 108:1460-1469, 1990.

38. Binder P: Presumed epithelial ingrowth after radial keratotomy, *CLAO J* 12:247-250, 1986.

39. Melles G, Binder PS: The effect of radial keratotomy incision direction on wound depth, *Refract Corneal Surg* 6:394-403, 1990.

40. Binder PS, Stainer GA, Zavala EY, et al: Acute morphologic features of radial keratotomy, *Arch Ophthalmol* 101:1113-1116, 1983.

41. Waring GO III, Binder PS: Atlas of astigmatic keratotomy. In Waring GO III, editor: *Radial keratotomy*, St Louis, 1991, Mosby-Year Book.

42. Binder PS, Waring GO III: Keratotomy procedures for astigmatism correction. In Waring GO III, editor: *Radial keratotomy*, St Louis, 1991, Mosby-Year Book.

43. Melles GRJ, Wijdh RHJ, Cost B, et al: Keratotomy incision direction. Effect of blade configuration, knife action and intraocular pressure on incision depth and shape, *Cornea* 12:299-309, 1993.

44. Melles G, Attie T, Go M, et al: Three versus four radial keratotomy incisions, *J Cataract Refract Surg* 18:27-36, 1992.

45. Gaster RN, Berns MW, Binder PS, et al: Corneal shield design for 193 nm excimer laser surgery of the cornea, *Invest Ophthalmol Vis Sci* 28(suppl):109, 1987.

46. Burstein N, Gaster R, Binder P: Corneal healing after excimer surface ablation, *SPIE Proc* 908:57-64, 1988.

47. Binder PS: Excimer laser photoablation. Clinical results and treatment of complications in 1992, *Arch Ophthalmol* 110:1221-1222, 1992.

48. Binder P, Anderson J, Rock M, et al: The morphologic features of human excimer laser photoablation (abstract), *Ophthalmology* 99:142, 1992.

49. Heitzman J, Binder P, Kassar B, et al: The correction of high myopia with the excimer laser, *Arch Ophthalmol* 1993, in press.

50. Salz JJ, Salz MS: Results of four and eight incision radial keratotomy for 6 to 12 diopters of myopia, *J Refract Surg* 4:46-50, 1988.

51. Waring G III, Lynn M, Gelender H, et al: Results of the Prospective Evaluation of Radial Keratotomy (PERK) study one year after surgery, *Ophthalmology* 92:177-198, 1985.

52. Salz JJ, Villasenor RA, Elander R, et al: Four incision radial keratotomy for low to moderate myopia, *Ophthalmology* 93:727-733, 1986.

53. Salz JJ, Salz JM, Salz M, et al: Ten years experience with a conservative approach to radial keratotomy, *Refract Corneal Surg* 7:12-22, 1991.

54. Bourque LB, Rubenstein R, Cosand B, et al: Psychosocial characteristics of candidates for the Prospective Evaluation of Radial Keratotomy (PERK) study, *Arch Ophthalmol* 102:1187-1192, 1984.

55. Bourque LB, Cosand BB, Drews C, et al: Reported patient satisfaction, fluctuation of vision, and glare among patients one year after surgery in the PERK study, *Arch Ophthalmol* 104:356-363, 1986.

56. Lynn MJ, Waring GO III, Sperduto RD, et al: Factors affecting outcome and predictability of radial keratotomy in the PERK study, *Arch Ophthalmol* 105:42-51, 1987.

57. Waring GO III, Moffitt SD, Gelender H, et al: Rationale for and design of the National Eye Institute Prospective Evaluation of Radial Keratotomy (PERK) study, *Ophthalmology* 90:40-58, 1983.

58. Waring GO III, Lynn MJ, Fielding B, et al: Results of the Prospective Evaluation of Radial Keratotomy (PERK) study four years after surgery for myopia, *JAMA* 263:1083-1091, 1990.

59. Waring GO III, Lynn MJ, Nizam A, et al: Results of the Prospective Evaluation of Radial Keratotomy (PERK) study five years after surgery, *Ophthalmology* 98:1164-1176, 1991.

60. Waring GO III, Lynn MJ, Strahlman ER, et al: Stability of refraction during four years after radial keratotomy in the Prospective Evaluation of Radial Keratotomy (PERK) study, *Am J Ophthalmol* 111:133-144, 1991.

61. Salz J, Maguen E, Macy J, et al: Results of photorefractive keratectomy (PRK) at Cedars-Sinai Medical Center (abstract), *Ophthalmololy* 99:106, 1992.

62. Dietz M, Sanders D, Marks R: Radial keratotomy: an overview of the Kansas City study, *Ophthalmology* 91:467-478, 1984.

63. Arrowsmith PN, Sanders DR, Marks RG: Visual, refractive and keratometric results of radial keratotomy, *Arch Ophthalmol* 101:873-881, 1983.

64. Arrowsmith P, Marks R: Visual, refractive and keratometric results of radial keratotomy, *Arch Ophthalmol* 107:506-511, 1989.

65. Dietz M, Sanders D, Raanan M: A consecutive series (1982-1985) of radial keratotomies performed with the diamond blade, *Am J Ophthalmol* 103:417-422, 1987.

66. Kremer FB, Marks RG: Radial keratotomy: prospective evaluation of safety and efficacy, *Ophthalmic Surg* 14:925-930, 1984.

67. Lavery FL: Comparative results of 200 consecutive radial keratotomy cases using three different nomograms, *J Refract Surg* 3:88-91, 1987.

68. Lynn MJ, Waring GO III, Nizam A, et al: Symmetry of refractive and visual acuity outcome in Prospective Evaluation of Radial Keratotomy (PERK) study, *Refract Corneal Surg* 5:75-81, 1989.

69. Neumann AC, Osher RH, Fenzl RE: Radial keratotomy: a comprehensive evaluation, *Doc Ophthalmol* 56:275-301, 1984.

70. Sawelson H, Marks R: Five-year results of radial keratotomy, *Refract Corneal Surg* 5:8-20, 1989.

71. Spigelman AV, Williams PA, Nichols BD, et al: Four incision radial keraotomy, *J Cataract Refract Surg* 14:125-128, 1988.

72. Spigelman AV, Williams PA, Lindstrom RL: Further studies of four incision radial keratotomy, *Refract Corneal Surg* 5:292-295, 1989.

73. Waring G III, Lindstrom KL Results of refractive keratotomy. In Waring GO III, editor: *Refractive keratotomy for myopia and astigmatism*, St Louis, 1991, Mosby-Year Book.

74. Schneider D, Draghic T, and Murthy R: Combined myopia and astigmatism surgery. Review of 350 cases, *J Cataract Refract Surg* 18:370-374, 1992.

75. Werblin, T: Radial keratotomy in the US: an evolving procedure (abstract), *Ophthalmology* 99:107, 1992.

76. Robin S, Rubenstein J, Epstein R, et al: Casebeer-system refractive keratotomy: a multi-surgeon retrospective evaluation, *Invest Ophthalmol Vis Sci* 34:1243, 1993.

77. Waring GO III: Standardized data collection and reporting for refractive surgery, *Refract Corneal Surg* 7(suppl):3-45, 1992.

78. Lohmann C, Gartry D, Kerr Muir M, et al: "Haze" in photorefractive keratectomy: its origins and consequences, *Laser Light Ophthalmol* 4:15-34, 1991.

79. Gartry D, Kerr Muir M, Marshall J:, Excimer laser photorefractive keratectomy, *Ophthalmology* 99:1209-1219, 1992.

80. McDonald M, Leach D, Ahmed S, et al: Photorefractive keratectomy (PRK) phase III (abstract), *Ophthalmology* 99:106, 1992.

81. Gartry D, Muir M, Marshall J, et al: The effect of topical corticosteroids on refraction and corneal haze following excimer laser treatment of myopia (abstract), *Ophthalmology* 99:106, 1992.

82. Piebenga L, Deitz M, Irvine J, et al: The effectiveness of excimer photorefractive keratectomy for myopia (abstract), *Ophthalmology* 99:106, 1992.

83. Waring G III, Maloney R, Hagen K, et al: Refractive and visual results of a multicenter trial of excimer laser photorefractive keratectomy (abstract), *Ophthalmology* 99:106, 1992.

84. Seiler T, Wollensak J, Jean B: Complications of myopic photorefractive keratectomy (PRK) with the excimer laser (abstract), *Ophthalmology* 99:107, 1992.

85. Weinstock S, Weinstock J: Excimer laser keratectomy for the correction of myopia, *CLAO J* 19:133-136, 1992.

86. Weinstock J: The results of excimer laser keratectomy (laser K) in higher myopes (abstract), *Ophthalmology* 99:127, 1992.

87. Flicker L, Steele A, Kirkness C, et al: Excimer laser photorefractive keratoplasty for myopia (abstract), *Ophthalmology* 99:127, 1992.

88. Munnerlyn R, Kooms SJ, Marshall J: Photorefractive keratectomy: a technique for laser refractive surgery, *J Cataract Refract Surg* 14:46-52, 1988.

89. Gordon J, Casebeer J, Lee P, et al: Retrospective clinical study of the Casebeer system for incisional keratorefractive surgery, *Invest Ophthalmol Vis Sci* 34:1243, 1993.

90. Bloom HR, Sands J, Schneider D: Corneal rupture from blunt trauma 22 months after radial keratotomy, *Refract Corneal Surg* 6:197-199, 1990.

91. Spivack L: Case report: radial keratotomy incisions remain intact despite facial trauma from plane crash, *J Refract Surg* 3:59-60, 1987.

92. Insler MS, Semple HC: Delayed microbial keratitis following radial keratotomy, *CLAO J* 14:163-164, 1988.

93. Geggel HS: Delayed sterile keratitis following radial keratotomy requiring corneal transplantation for visual rehabilitation, *Refrac Corneal Surg* 6:55-58, 1990.

94. Karr DJ, Grutzmacher RD, Reel MJ: Radial keratotomy complicated by sterile keratitis and corneal perforation: histopathologic case report and review of complications, *Ophthalmology* 92:1244-1248, 1985.

95. Mandelbaum S, Waring GO III, K, F.R., Culbertson WW, et al: Late development of ulcerative keratitis in radial keratotomy scars, *Arch Ophthalmol* 104:1156-1160, 1986.

96. Shivitz IA, Arrowsmith PN: Delayed keratitis after radial keratotomy, *Arch Ophthalmol* 104:1153-1155, 1986.

97. Gelender H, Flynn HW, Mandelbaum SH: Bacterial endophthalmitis resulting from radial keratotomy, *Am J Ophthalmol* 93:323-326, 1982.

98. Mackman G: Delayed sterile keratitis following radial keratotomy successfully treated with conjunctival flap, *Refract Corneal Surg* 8:122-124, 1992.

99. Les Jardins S, Bertrand I, Massin M: Intraoperative and early postoperative complications in 466 radial keratotomies, *Refract Corneal Surg* 8:215-216, 1992.

100. Durand L, Monnot J-P, Burillon C, et al: Complications of radial keratotomy: eyes with keratoconus and late wound dehiscence, *Refract and Corneal Surg* 8:311-314, 1992.

101. Sher N, Chen V, Bowers R, et al: The use of the 193-nm excimer laser for myopic photorefractive keratectomy in sighted eyes. A multicenter study, *Arch Ophthalmol* 109:1525-1530, 1991.

102. Villasenor RA, Cox KC: Radial keratotomy: reoperations, *J Refract Surg* 1:35-57, 1985.

103. Hofmann RF: Reoperations after radial and astigmatic keratotomy, *J Refract Surg*, 3:119-128, 1987.

104. Sawelson H, Marks RG: Two year results of re-operations for radial keratotomy, *Arch Ophthalmol* 106:497-501, 1988.

105. Hersh PS, Kalevar V, Kenyon KR: Penetrating keratoplasty for severe complications of radial keratotomy, *Cornea* 10:170-174, 1991.

106. Ginsburg AP, Waring GO III, Steinberg EB, et al: Contrast sensitivity under photopic conditions in the Prospective Evaluation of Radial Keratotomy (PERK) study, *Am J Ophthalmol* 6:82-91, 1990.

107. Santos VR, Waring GO III, Lynn MJ, et al: Morning-to-evening change in refraction corneal curvature, and visual acuity two to four years after radial keratotomy: the Prospective Evaluation of Radial Keratotomy (PERK) Study, *Ophthalmology* 95:1487-1493, 1988.

108. Klyce S, Wilson S, McDonald M, et al: Corneal topography after excimer laser keratectomy, *Invest Ophthalmol Vis Sci* 32 (suppl):721, 1991.

109. Wilson SE, Klyce SD, McDonald MB, et al: Changes in corneal topography after excimer laser photorefractive keratectomy for myopia, *Ophthalmology* 98:1338-1347, 1991.

110. Klyce SD, Smolek MK: Corneal topography of excimer laser photorefractive keratectomy, 19(suppl):122-130, 1993.

111. Lohman CP, Timberlake GT, Fitzke FW, et al: Corneal light scattering after excimer laser photorefractive keratectomy: the objective measurements of haze, *Refract Corneal Surg* 8:114-121, 1993.

112. Lohman CP, Fitzke F, O'Bart D, et al: Corneal light scattering and visual performance in myopic individuals with spectacles, contact lens, or excimer laser photorefractive keratectomy, *Am J Ophthalmol* 115:444-453, 1993.

113. McDonnell PJ, McClusky DJ, Garbus JJ: Corneal topography and fluctuating visual acuity after radial keratotomy, *Ophthalmology* 98:665-670, 1989.

114. Bogan SJ, Maloney RK, Drews CD, et al: Computer-assisted videokeratography of corneal topography after radial keratotomy, *Arch Ophthalmol* 109:834-841, 1991.

115. McDonnell PJ, Garbus J, Lopez PF: Topographic analysis and visual acuity after radial keratotomy, *Am J Ophthalmol* 106:692-695, 1988.

116. Lopez PF, Maloney RK, Goodman GL, et al: Topography of the corneal optical zone after radial keratotomy, *Invest Ophthalmol Vis Sci* 29(suppl):389, 1988.

117. McDonnell PJ, Garbus J: Corneal topographic changes after radial keratotomy, *Ophthalmology* 96:45-49, 1989.

118. Maguire LJ, Bourne WM: A multifocal lens effect as a complication of radial keratotomy, *Refract Corneal Surg* 5:394-399, 1989.

119. Rowsey JJ, Waring GO III, Monlux R, et al: Corneal topography as a predictor of refractive change in the Prospective Evaluation of Radial Keratotomy (PERK) study, *Ophthalmic Surg* 22:370-380, 1991.

120. Kwitko S, Gritz DC, Garbus JJ, et al: Diurnal variation of corneal topography after radial keratotomy, *Arch Ophthalmol* 110:351-356, 1992.

121. Maguire LJ, Zabel RW, Parker P, et al: Topography and raytracing analysis of patient with excellent visual acuity 3 months after excimer laser photorefractive keratectomy for myopia, *Refract Corneal Surg* 7:122-128, 1991.

122. Maguire LJ: Corneal topography of patients with excellent Snellen visual acuity after epikeratophakia for aphakia, *Am J Ophthalmol* 109:162-167, 1990.

123. Weston BC, Camp J, Maguire LJ: A method to evaluate the reproducibility of topography systems (abstract), *Invest Ophthalmol Vis Sci* 33(suppl):696, 1992.

124. Chiba K, Oak SS, Tsubota K, et al: Morphometric analysis of corneal endothelium following radial keratotomy, *J Cataract Refract Surg* 13:263-267, 1987.

125. McRae SM, Matsuda M, Rich LF: The effect of radial keratotomy on the corneal endothelium, *Am J Ophthalmol* 100:538-542, 1985.

126. Dehm EJ, Puliafito CA, Adler CM, et al: Corneal endothelial injury in rabbits following excimer laser ablation at 193 and 248 nm, *Arch Ophthalmol* 104:1364-1368, 1986.

127. Beldavs R, Thompson K, Waring G III, et al: Quantitative specular microscopy after PRK, (abstract), *Ophthalmology* 99:125, 1992.

128. Carones F, Brancato R, Venturi E, et al: The corneal endothelium after myopic excimer laser photorefractive keratectomy, (abstract), *Invest Ophthalmol Vis Sci* 34:804, 1993.

129. Richard NR, Anderson JA, Weiss JL, et al: Air/liquid corneal organ culture: a light microscopic study, *Curr Eye Res* 10:739-749, 1991.

130. Krueger R, Sliney D, and Trokel S: Photokeratitis from subablative 193-nanometer excimer laser radiation, *Refract Corneal Surg* 8:274-279, 1992.

131. Szerenyi K, Campos M, Raman S, et al: Keratocyte loss after corneal de-epithelialization in primates and rabbits, *Invest Ophthalmol Vis Sci* 34:802, 1993.

132. Feldman RM, Crapotta JA, Feldman ST, et al: Retinal detachment following radial and astigmatic keratotomy, *Refract Corneal Surg* 7:252-253, 1991.

133. John ME, Schmitt TE: Traumatic hyphema after radial keratotomy, *Ann Ophthalmol* 15:930-932, 1983.

134. Koch DD, Liu JF, Hyde LL, et al: Refractive complications of cataract surgery after radial keratotomy, *Am J Ophthalmol* 108:676-682, 1989.

135. Damiano RE, Forstot SL: Extreme corneal flattening after radial keratotomy, *Am J Ophthalmology* 112:738, 1991.

136. Buehler P, Schein O, Stamler J, et al: The increased risk of ulcerative keratitis among disposable soft contact lens users, *Arch Ophthalmol* 110:1555-1558, 1992.

137. Matthews T, Frazer D, Minassian D, et al: Risks of keratitis and patterns of use with disposable contact lenses, *Arch Ophthalmol* 110:1559-1562, 1992.

138. Veraart HGN, Vandenberg TJTP, Ijspeert, et al: Stray light in radial keratotomy and the influence of pupil size and stray-light angle, *Am J Ophthalmol* 114, 1992.

139. Vandenberg TJTP: On the relation between glare and straylight, *Doc Ophthalomol* 78:177-181, 1991.

140. Talamo JH, Gollamudi S, Green WR, et al: Modulation of corneal wound healing after excimer laser keratomileusis using topical mitomycin C and steroids, *Arch Ophthalmol* 109:1141-1146, 1991.

141. Gartry DS, Kerr-Muir MD, Lohmann CP, et al: The effect of topical corticosteriods on refractive outcome and corneal haze after photorefractive keratectomy, *Arch Ophthalmol* 110:944-952, 1992.

142. Piebengna LW, Deitz MR, Irvine JW, et al: The effectiveness of excimer photorefractive keratectomy for myopia (abstract), *Opthalmology* 99:106, 1992.

143. Tengroth B, Fagerhorm P, Soderberg H, et al: Effects of corticosteroids in postoperative care following photorefractive keratectomies, *Refract Corneal Surg* 9:61-64, 1992.

144. Tengroth B, Epstein D, Fagerholm P, et al: Excimer laser photorefractive keratectomy for myopia. Clinical results in sighted eyes, *Ophthalmology* 100:739-746, 1993.

145. Bourque LB, Lynn MJ, Waring GO III, et al: Spectacle and contact lens wearing six years after radial keratotomy in the PERK study, *Ophthalmology* in press.

146. Dietz M, Sanders D, Raanan M: Progressive hyperopia in radial keratotomy, *Ophthalmology* 93:1284-1288, 1986.

147. Waring G III, Lynn M, Kutner M: Stability of refraction after refractive keratotomy. In Waring GO III, editor: *Refractive keratotomy for myopia and astigmatism*, St Louis, 1991, Mosby-Year Book.

148. Colliac JP, Shammas H: Optics for photorefractive keratectomy, *J Cataract Refract Surg* 19:356-363, 1993.

149. Holliday JT, Waring GO III: Optics and topography of radial keratotomy. In Waring GO III, editor: *Refractive keratotomy for myopia and astigmatism*, St Louis, 1992, Mosby-Year Book.

150. Starling JC, Hoffmann RF: A new surgical technique for the correction of hyperopia after radial keratotomy: an experimental model, *J Refract Surg* 2:9-14, 1986.

151. Lindquist TD, Williams PA, Lindstrom RL: Surgical treatment of overcorrection following radial keratotomy: evaluation of clinical effectiveness, *Ophthalmic Surg* 22:12-15, 1991.

152. Damiano RE, Forstot SL, Dukes DK: Surgical correction of hyperopia following radial keratotomy, *Refract Corneal Surg* 8:75-79, 1992.

153. Lyle WA, Jin J-C: Circular and interrupted suture technique for correction of hyperopia following radial keratotomy, *Refract Corneal Surg* 8:80-83, 1992.

154. Thompson K, Gipson I, Waring G, et al: Synthetic epikeratoplasty in rhesus monkeys with human type IV collagen, 12:35-45, 1993.

155. Fouraker B, Shanzlin D, Assil K: Evaluation of the intrastromal corneal ring in non-sighted eyes (abstract), *Ophthalmology* 99:124, 1992.

156. Colin J, Mimouni F, Robinet A, et al: The surgical treatment of high myopia: comparison of epikeratoplasty, keratomileusis and minus power anterior chamber lenses, *Refract Corneal Surg* 6:245-251, 1990.

157. Campos M, Cuevas K, Shieh E, et al: Corneal wound healing after excimer laser ablation in rabbits: expanding versus contracting aperatures, *Refract Corneal Surg* 8:378-381, 1992.

13

Excimer Laser Keratomileusis

Part I

Tarek Salah, George O. Waring III,
Akef El-Maghraby

Part II

Stephen Slade, Stephen Brint, Luis Ruiz, Stephen Updegraff

Part III

Craig Kliger, Robert K. Maloney

This chapter is divided into three sections each having been contributed by a separate group of authors. The first section discusses the results of excimer laser keratomileusis (ELK) in the corneal bed under a hinged flap from the El-Maghraby Eye Hospital in Saudi Arabia and was contributed by Drs. Tarek Salah, George O. Waring III, and Akef El-Maghraby. The second section contributed by Drs. Stephen Slade, Stephen Brint, Stephen Updegraff, and Luis Ruiz gives ELK results from Bogota, Columbia, and the U.S. Clinical Trials with the Summit Laser. The third section discuss Elk results of the Jules Stein Eye Institute and is presented by Drs. Craig Klinger and Robert K. Maloney.

Excimer Laser Keratomileusis in the Corneal Bed Under a Hinged Flap: Results in Saudi Arabia at the El-Maghraby Eye Hospital

Tarek Salah, George O. Waring III,
Akef El-Maghraby

A broad spectrum of ophthalmic techniques is now available for correction of refractive errors.[1,2] From a clinical perspective, these operations are often presented as different techniques used for different amounts of myopia. For example, radial keratotomy and photorefractive keratectomy (PRK) are considered most effective from approximately 1.50 D to 6.00 D of myopia, keratomileusis on the back of the disk is often selected for myopia between 7 D and 15 D, and keratomileusis in situ for approximately 12 D to 30 D of myopia. Minus-power intraocular lenses may be implanted in phakic eyes to correct approximately 10 D to 25 D.

It would be ideal to find a procedure that could correct the full range of myopia, including compound myopic astigmatism and, indeed, hyperopia. We think that keratomileusis in situ performed with an excimer laser in the corneal bed beneath a hinged flap or anterior cornea may be such a procedure.

DEVELOPMENT OF KERATOMILEUSIS

The history and development of techniques of keratomileusis span some 40 years of innovation and improvements[3-6] (Table 13-1).

The technology has evolved continuously. Microkeratomes have changed from those that are manually advanced with blades of varying quality to those that are mechanically advanced using blades of uniform quality. Current models include one-piece instruments with a turbine drive instead of a motor drive. Techniques of making the refractive cut have evolved from the use of the complex cyrolathe, with its resulting tissue damage, through the use of microkeratomes advanced manually or mechanically to make the refractive cut on the back of the button or in the corneal bed, to the current use of the excimer laser with its micron accuracy. The suction rings with their dovetail guides have advanced from a large set of rings with individual heights for cutting different diameters of the disk, through adjustable rings where a single ring can

Table 13-1. The history and development of keratomileusis

	Clinical publications (yr)	Location and shape of stromal refractive cut	Approx thickness of disk (μ)	Disk tissue injury	Sutures	Complexity of equipment*	Complexity of surg procedure*
Cryolathe on disk	Barraquer[7] (1964)	Disk,	300	Freeze	Yes	++++	++++
Planar, non freeze on disk	Krumeich[8] (1987)	Disk, concave	300	Mechanical dessication	Yes	+++	+++
In situ†; manual and automated microkeratome	Ruiz & Rowsey[9] (1986)‡	Bed, plane	160	Dessication	Yes or no	++	++
In situ; flap technique	Barraquer[10] (1980)	Bed, plane	160	Minimal	No	++	++
Excimer laser on disk	Buratto & Ferarri[11] (1992)	Disk, concave	300	Dessication	Yes	++++	+++
In situ, excimer laser	Pallikaris et al.[12] (1990)	Bed, concave	160	Mild	No	++++	+++
In situ, excimer laser flap	Slade (1992)§	Bed, concave	160	Minimal	No	++++	++

*+ = minimal; ++ = mild; +++ = moderate; ++++ = severe (author's grading).
†Automated lamellar keratoplasty.
‡Presented at American Academy of Ophthalmology, New Orleans, LA, November 1986.
§Oral communication, September/October 1993.

cut all desired diameters, and now to the use of a single ring for the creation of a simple flap. Positioning the corneal tissue after the refractive cut has evolved from standard edge to two-edge suturing through the use of antitorque sutures and the resurrection of the old overlay sutures, to the current technique of no sutures, particularly with the use of a hinged flap.

We think that excimer laser keratomileusis in situ with a flap represents the most advanced combination of this long process of development.

DEVELOPMENT OF KERATOMILEUSIS IN SITU

The concept of creating a corneal flap and removing central flap and removing central tissue from the bed was first described by Pureskin[13] in 1966, who demonstrated that the smaller the diameter of the resected disk, the larger the refractive change, an operation he referred to as "stromectomy." Pureskin used a trephine to manually resect the stroma in the bed. For example, in a series of 93 eyes, he demonstrated that an 8.00-mm-diameter disk could induce 2.50 D of corneal flattening, whereas a 4.00-mm-diameter disc could induce approximately 12 D of corneal flattening.

José Barraquer[3] created a corneal flap and used a microkeratome to resect a disc of stromal tissue from the bed, but abandoned the technique in favor of cryolathe keratomileusis on the disk.

In the late 1980s, Ruiz[9] working in Bogota, Colombia, with Barraquer, revised the idea of keratomileusis in situ, using the planar resection principles of Krumeich, and called the technique in situ keratomileusis. He first removed a plano corneal disk with the microkeratome, and then used a suction ring with a different height to resect a plano disk from the exposed stromal bed. The anterior disc was sutured back in place, and the effect of the procedure was to create a flattening of the central cornea.[9] Ruiz never published a series of cases, and the technique underwent a number of changes, including changing preoperative nomograms, and was plagued with poor predictability and mild irregular astigmatism.[14,15]

One of the most significant advances by Ruiz in the growth of keratomileusis in situ was the conversion from the use of a manually advanced microkeratome to the use of a mechanically advanced microkeratome. However, the variable quality of individual instruments was responsible for some of the variable clinical results.

In the late 1980s, Chiron Ophthalmic procured the rights to the mechanically advanced microkeratome, known as the Corneal Shaper, improved the quality of manufacture, and launched an international campaign that combined the talents of surgeons and marketers. They renamed keratomileusis in situ "automated lamellar keratoplasty (ALK)" with the appropriate modifier "for myopia." The marketing campaign was aimed at ophthalmologists who wanted to be on the cutting edge of refractive surgery, and who were stymied by the slow regulatory investigation of excimer laser PRK in the United States. In spite of the heavy promotion, the procedure remained intrinsically restricted by the fact that the refractive cut was not truly "refractive," but the resection of a plano disc from the stromal bed.

DEVELOPMENT OF EXCIMER LASER KERATOMILEUSIS IN SITU

The use of the excimer laser to create the refractive cut in keratomileusis has developed along two lines. The first is that described originally by Buratto in Milan, Italy,[16,17] in which a 300-µm-thick disk of cornea is removed, inverted, and the excimer laser used to perform the refractive ablation on the back of the disc. Buratto called this photokeratomileusis (PKM), and considered it a logical extension of Krumeich's planar nonfreeze keratomileusis.[11,16,17]

The second direction is excimer laser keratomileusis in situ, initially developed by Pallikaris in Keraklion, Crete.[12] In 1988, Pallikaris and colleagues carried out their initial study in rabbit eyes which demonstrated a slight postoperative lamellar haze which gradually decreased over 1 month. Histologically, the epithelium appeared normal; there was a slight increase in keratocytes at the interface. The corollary of this was the absence of postoperative clinically significant haze as compared to PRK, which the authors attributed to lack of disruption of the epithelium and epithelial-stromal interaction. In 1989, Pallikaris carried out the procedure in a blind human eye, and began studies on sighted human eyes in 1991. He has carried out comparative studies on PRK and excimer laser keratomileusis in situ. Pallikaris suggested the name laser in situ keratomileusis (LASIK) for this procedure, including the flap. Pallikaris used a manually advanced microkeratome of his own design.[5,12,18-20]

The combination of a mechanically advanced microkeratome and excimer laser keratomileusis in situ technique under a flap was first done by Slade in Houston, Texas, in 1993, as an extension and combination of the microkeratome keratomileusis in situ (ALK) and excimer laser keratomileusis on the disk. He colloquially dubbed the technique "flap and zap." Further developments of the technique have been carried out by Brint in New Orleans, Ruiz in Bogota, and by our group in Jeddah, Saudi Arabia.

Since November 1993, our group has performed over 200 excimer laser keratomileusis in situ proce-

dures under a corneal flap. We have not only enrolled patients in a prospective consecutive series but are enrolling patients in a prospective randomized trial that compares PRK for myopia in one eye with excimer laser keratomileusis in the bed under a flap for myopia in the other, using the same laser and ablation diameter.

EXCIMER LASER KERATOMILEUSIS IN SITU
Advantages

1. The procedure can be performed in an outpatient setting under topical anesthesia without postoperative patching. Thus, it is user-friendly for the patient. The procedure takes 5 to 15 minutes, depending on the skill of the surgeon and the team, and the procedure obviates the discomfort and potential complications of intraorbital anesthesia.

2. As outlined above, the ophthalmic community has over 30 years of clinical experience with keratomileusis of various types, so the overall feasibility of the technique is well established. What is missing are refinements to enhance the predictability of the refractive outcome and to decrease irregular postoperative astigmatism. There is thus little chance of unexpected long-term complications such as marked regression or progression of the refractive change, late scarring in the stromal bed, progressive development of irregular astigmatism, or long-term structural changes in the corneal disc.

3. The procedure is extraocular, increasing its overall safety when compared to intraocular lens implantation with or without clear lens extraction. There has been no reported damage to the corneal endothelium, but further detailed studies are necessary in this regard. Theoretically, the procedure can correct all ametropias. Currently, a full range of myopia can be corrected, from approximately 2 D to 30 D, depending on technique and parameters. Compound myopic astigmatism has been corrected but further refinements are necessary. When excimer laser techniques to correct hyperopia are developed, they should be able to be used in situ under a corneal flap. Thus, the procedure has the potential to be "one-technique-fits-all." The procedure utilizes a mechanically advancing microkeratome, which ensures a constant rate of cutting and constant pressure on the eye, decreasing the chance of an irregular cut with irregular astigmatism. It is highly likely that design and technique improvements in automated microkeratomes will come a long in the future, together with better quality control in instrument manufacture and finer blade quality.

4. The procedure uses an argon fluoride 193-nm ex-

cimer laser, which essentially functions as a computerized robot to remove corneal tissue. The extensive worldwide experience in excimer laser PRK can be easily transferred to excimer laser in situ techniques.

5. The entire procedure can be performed under the excimer laser if it has the proper mechanical configuration, obviating the need for an operating microscope and for moving the patient from one instrument to another.

6. The use a hinged corneal flap is an enormous advantage because it speeds surgery and minimizes the exposure time of the stroma so that there are fewer particles in the bed. Most important, it allows good realignment when it is replaced, and does not require suturing, so there is less chance of inducing irregular astigmatism by misalignment or suture distortion.

7. The dimensions of the corneal flap do not have to be exact. A diameter of 7 to 9 mm and a thickness of 100 to 200 μm are adequate. Thus, neither the instrument manufacturer nor the surgeon is under pressure to achieve an exact diameter or thickness, as is necessary when one is performing the refractive cut with the microkeratome. In addition, the corneal disk is thinner (approximately 150 μm) than the disk used for standard keratomileusis (300 μm). This helps to maintain the mechanical integrity of the globe and decreases the chance of gradual long-term ectasia of the cornea.

8. The refractive cut performed by the excimer laser is spherocylindrical, a considerable advantage toward obtaining a predictable refractive outcome when compared to ALK with its plano refractive resection.

9. There is very little pain after surgery, presumably because the epithelium is minimally disrupted. This is particularly noticeable when compared to the pain after radial keratotomy or PRK. Most patients do not require topical, nonsteroidal anti-inflammatory agents or oral analgesics.

10. The mechanical structure of the cornea is preserved, because a thin anterior disk is removed and replaced. This eliminates the chance of traumatic rupture of the globe or progression of refraction in the hyperopic direction as found after radial keratotomy.

11. The structure of the anterior cornea is preserved with no disruption of central Bowman's layer. This increases the chance of having a smooth corneal surface and reduces the chance of irregular astigmatism. Most important, it eliminates the specter of subepithelial stromal wound healing, as seen in PRK.

12. Recovery of vision after surgery is rapid, because the central anterior surface is minimally disrupted and there is little stromal edema and no postoperative cicatricial haze.

13. Corneal wound healing has minimal effect on the refractive outcome. This is exceedingly important because it greatly reduces the individual variability in corneal wound healing that characterizes radial keratotomy and PRK. Apparently, the stromal keratocytes are quite happy in their lamellar bed, and if they do not receive cytokine messages, they undergo little reactive fibroplasia. Topical corticosteroids are not necessary after surgery, which decreases the chance of induced rises in intraocular pressure, of cataract caused by the misuse of steroids, and the variable wound healing that results from the steroids.

14. Theoretically, the predictability of refractive outcome should be good, but this awaits clinical confirmation.

15. Postoperative modification of the refractive outcome is still possible, using reablation of the bed after simple dissection and elevation of the flap, or with refractive keratotomy. This makes the procedure somewhat adjustable.

16. Long-term stability should be good based on past experience with keratomileusis, especially since there is no cryogenic injury or removal of the disk.

Disadvantages

There is no perfect surgical procedure and there are numerous drawbacks with the flap-and-zap technique.

1. The equipment is expensive. An excimer laser with its attendant support systems costs approximately $500,000 and the Corneal Shaper adds another $40,000.

2. Both instruments are technically complex. A talented and well-trained operating room staff is necessary to maintain the Corneal Shaper in good working condition. The surgeon must double-check the instrument at the beginning of every case and assemble it himself. A technician or engineer must be available to troubleshoot the excimer laser when it has problems, a job that is beyond the ability of medically trained personnel.

3. The surgeon does not have the ability to monitor and modulate the procedure intraoperatively. Once the microkeratome begins advancing across the cornea, the surgeon can stop it, but he or she cannot observe the bed or the flap as they are being cut. Similarly, during the excimer laser ablation, the laser beam is invisible and the configuration of the ablation on the stroma cannot be detected by visual inspection. Thus, the surgeon is at the mercy of the technology, an uncomfortable position for most surgeons.

4. The surgical algorithms continue to change, and the

technique is clearly in a phase of rapid change and development. This requires that the surgeon remain abreast of changes in the procedure—and even contribute to them.

5. The instrumentation continues to change. Many new designs of excimer lasers are being created, some of which can accommodate the microkeratome and some of which cannot. Changes in microkeratome design and use are also occurring. Changes in excimer laser technology include smaller lasers with scanning slits, improved algorithms for better contours and edge tapers, and more fail-safe mechanisms to decrease downtime. Changes in microkeratome technology include the use of an automatic stopper to help create a fixed-sized hinge on the flap and a single-sized smaller suction ring that fits more easily onto the surface of the eye.

Surgical Technique

As with any developing new technique, variations abound. We detail the technique that we currently find useful as of mid-1994.

Surgery is performed in an outpatient operating suite. The surgeon performs a normal preoperative scrub. The patient's lids are prepared with betadine solution. A fenestrated plastic adhesive is draped so that the lashes are folded back over the lid margins. A wire Barraquer lid speculum is used. A topical anesthetic is applied. Preoperatively, topical pilocarpine 1% is instilled to constrict the pupil.

We currently use a Summit OmniMed I laser (Summit Technology, Waltham, Mass.) with the capability of a 6.5-mm-diameter spot and a coaxial microscope. We use the following variables: wavelength, 193 nm; fluence, 180 mJ/cm^2; repetition rate, 10 Hz; ablation diameter, 6.0 mm; ablation algorithm, Summit PRK or myopic keratomileusis (MKM). A dilating diaphragm is used.

Prior to use we calibrate the instrument according to the manufacturer's instructions by ablating a 100-μm-thick Wratten filter, noting the number of pulses necessary. We ablate a Polaroid film to observe the uniformity of the energy distribution of the beam. Periodically, we ablate a plastic disk, which is scanned by the manufacturer. The Summit laser is not adjustable and if the calibration procedures are inexact, a trained engineer must adjust the laser.

We use the Automated Corneal Shaper (Chiron Ophthalmic, Irvine, Calif) (Fig. 13-1). Suction is set a 25 mm Hg. The suction ring is set to full diameter, which creates a corneal disk between 7.2 and 7.6 mm. A new microkeratome blade is used for each patient. Base plate no. 160 that is designated to cut a 160-μm-thick corneal flap is used. The microkeratome is assembled and undergoes multiple steps of testing pre-

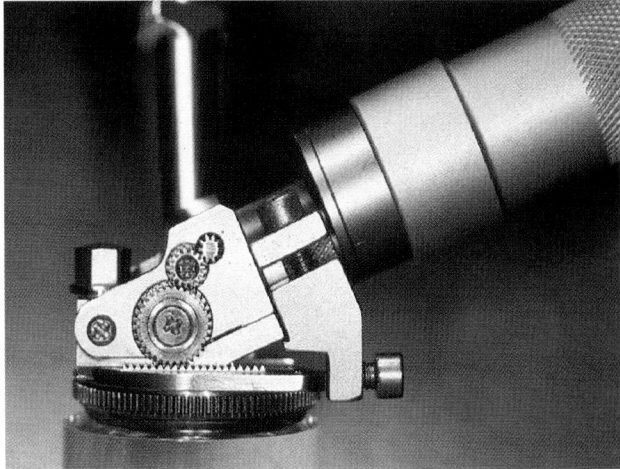

Fig. 13-1. The automatic corneal shaper with the Hansa stopper in position. (Courtesy of Stephen Slade.)

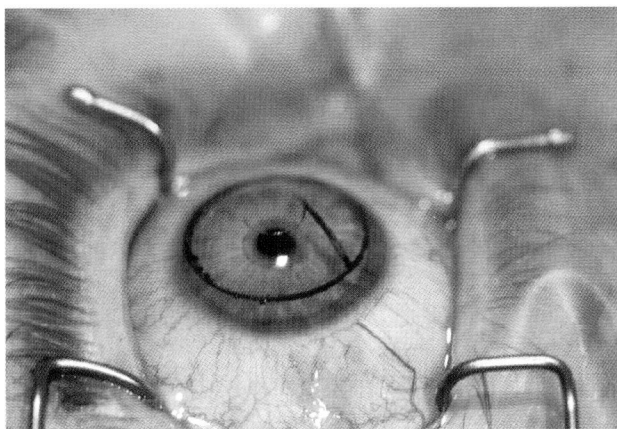

Fig. 13-2. The eye after being marked with a Ruiz concentric marker showing the positioning marks. (Courtesy of Stephen Slade.)

operatively to ensure proper movement of the gears, proper sliding of the blade without binding, proper suction of the ring, and proper advancement of the microkeratome through the dovetail of the suction ring. We mark the center of the pupil and use a Ruiz concentric marker, which has an outer ring diameter of 11 mm, to assist in centering the suction ring (Fig. 13-2). Two semiradial lines of gentian violet are used, which helps to reposition the corneal flap.

The suction ring is inserted between the lid speculum (it is best to use a speculum with open blades) and the globe is centered in the suction ring by digital manipulation (Fig. 13-3). Suction is applied and a Barraquer applanation tonometer is used to verify that the intraocular pressure is greater than 65 mm Hg. An applanation lens is used to verify that the diameter of the disk is 7.2 mm or greater.

The surface of the globe and suction ring are moistened and the microkeratome is inserted into the dove-

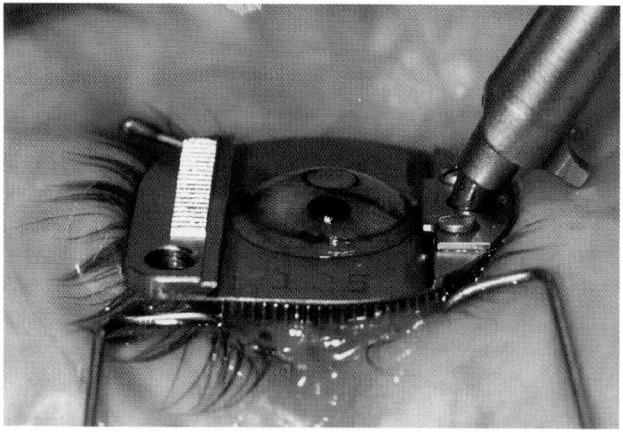

Fig. 13-3. The suction ring in place between the blades of the lid speculum. (Courtesy of Stephen Slade.)

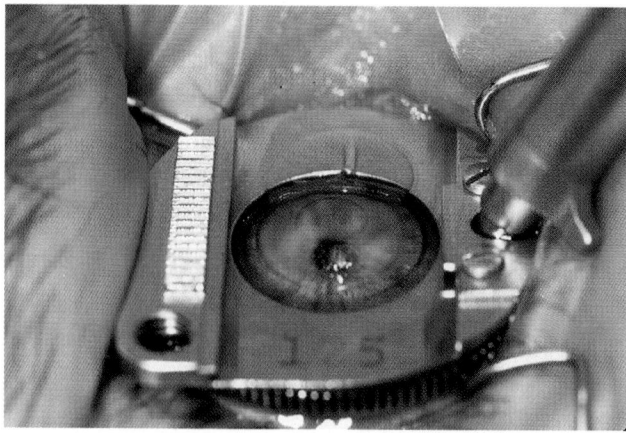

Fig. 13-5. The 160-μm corneal flap is folded back onto the surface of the suction ring. (Courtesy of Stephen Slade.)

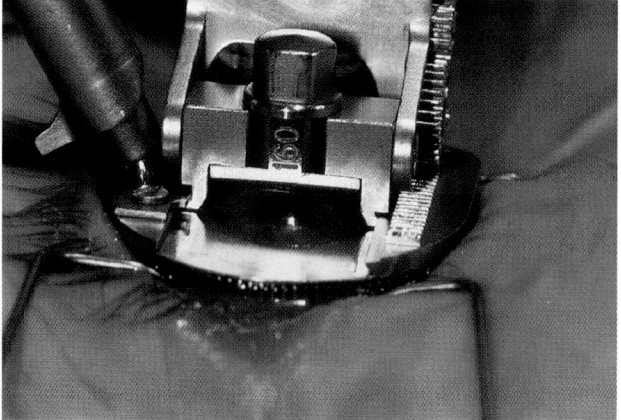

Fig. 13-4. The microkeratome in position to cut the corneal flap. (Courtesy of Stephen Slade.)

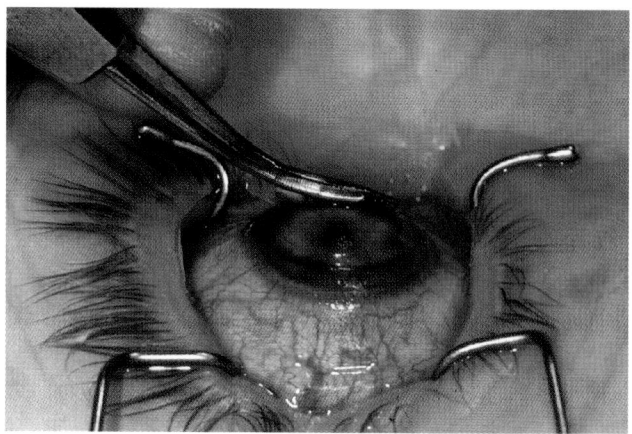

Fig. 13-6. The curved tying forceps are used to gently reposition the flap onto the bed. (Courtesy of Stephen Slade.)

tail of the ring and advanced to the edge of the toothed gear track. The surgeon steadies the microkeratome by the wire leading to the motor and activates the foot pedal. The microkeratome advances mechanically and stops 0.50 mm short of a complete resection (Fig. 13-4). The method of stopping is either the mechanical "stopper" or the lifting of the surgeon's foot when the leading edge of the blade reaches the second screw on the suction ring. The microkeratome is then reversed by pressing on the other end of the pedal and removed from the eye, leaving the disc in place. The suction is turned off, but the ring is left on the eye to aid in control and centration.

The excimer laser is centered, with the patient being instructed to view the fixation light. The two helium-neon beams are focused on the surface of the cornea, and are then observed to be present at 3 and 9 o'clock on the pupil, insuring centration on the pupil. An angled tying forceps is then slid into the corneal bed and the flap is folded back briskly onto the surface of the suction ring (Figs. 13-5 and 13-6). The laser is

again focused onto the surface of the stromal bed, and centered. During these manipulations the technician has programmed the laser, calling out the variables to the surgeon as a double-check. The surgeon activates the laser with the foot pedal, and the dilating diaphragm completes the ablation. If the patient's eye moves more than what is expected by microsaccades, the surgeon stops the ablation, recenters the eye, and completes the ablation.

One drop of balanced salt solution (BSS) is placed on the stromal bed, and a long cannula is inserted beneath the epithelial surface of the flap (Fig. 13-7). The flap is reapplied to the surface of the cornea with a brisk maneuver and the fluid on the surface allows the disk to settle gently. There is no irrigation or washing of the bed. The surgeon removes the suction ring from the surface of the eye.

Two cellulose microsponges are used to gently manipulate the cornea until the two semiradial alignment lines are properly oriented. The edge of the flap is then dried, bottled oxygen flows through a millipore fil-

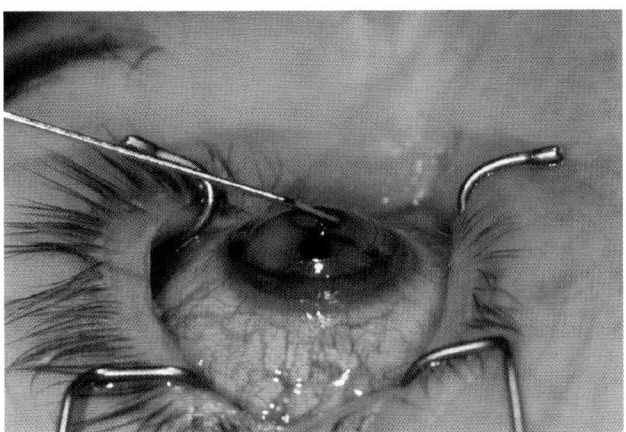

Fig. 13-7. Balanced salt solution is used to keep the surface epithelium wet. (Courtesy of Stephen Slade.)

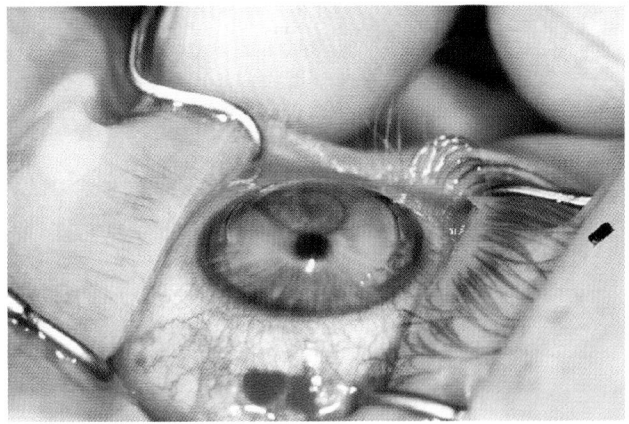

Fig. 13-8. The cornea is inspected for proper positioning of the flap and proper adhesion. (Courtesy of Stephen Slade.)

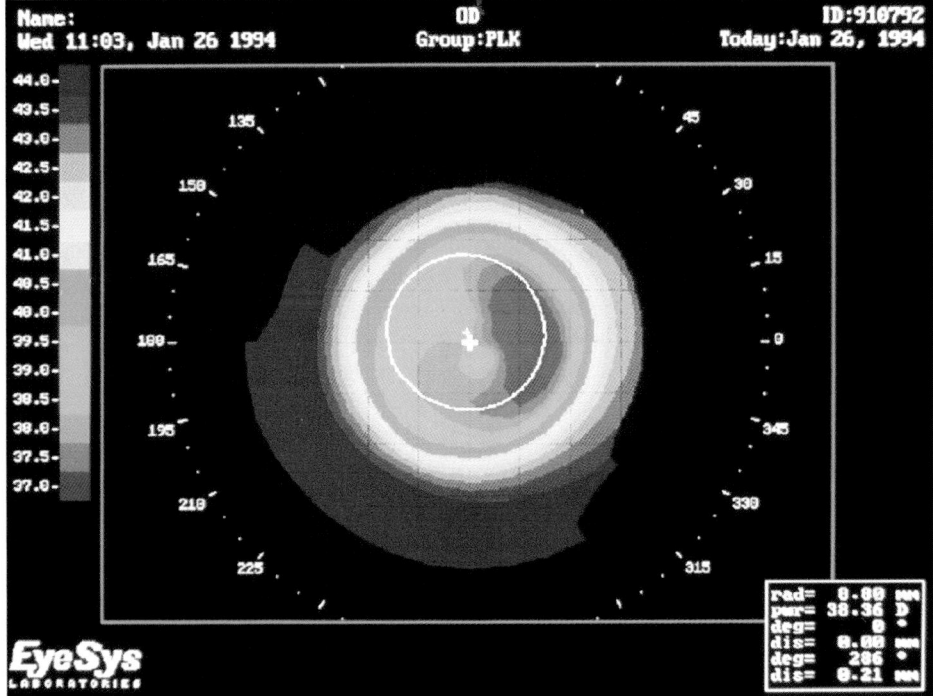

Fig. 13-9. Videokeratography showing central flattening with moderate tapering of the edges. (Courtesy of Stephen Slade.)

ter and a cannula at 4 L/min and is used to dry the flap, which helps it to adhere in place. Proper adherence of the flap can be seen with depression of the peripheral cornea, which creates radiating lines that extend into the disk indicating that the disk is adherent to the bed.

Topical gentamicin is applied. All drapes and hardware are removed, and a mild patch is applied. The patient is helped to the recovery area.

Fifteen to 30 minutes after the procedure, the patch is removed and the cornea is inspected for proper positioning of the flap (Fig. 13-8). If the flap is in any

way misaligned, the patient is taken back under the operating microscope and the flap is lifted and repositioned. However, this is an undesirable event because it increases the chance of seeding epithelium into the stromal bed.

Postoperatively, no topical corticosteroids are used. Topical antibiotics are used four times daily for 4 days. In general, systemic analgesics are not necessary.

Results of Pilot Study

The first 59 eyes of 34 patients done at the El Maghraby Eye Hospital in Jeddah, Saudi Arabia, were en-

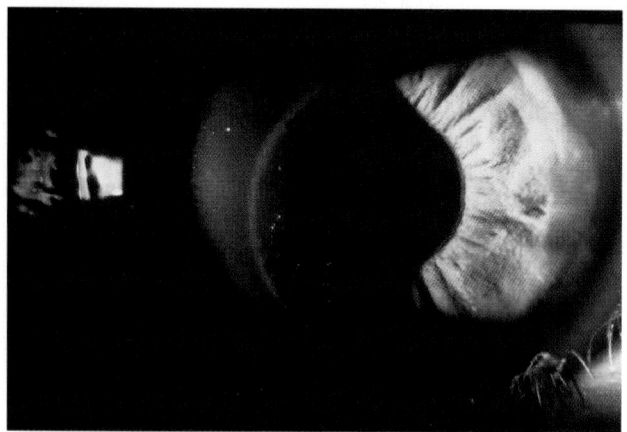

Fig. 13-10. A faint circular scar was present around the edge of the flap in most eyes. (Courtesy of Stephen Slade.)

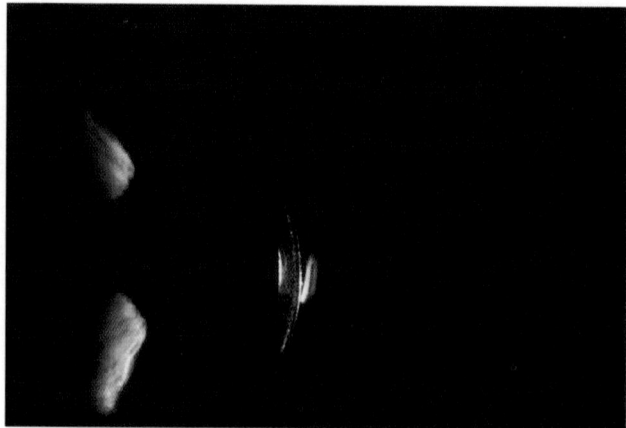

Fig. 13-11. A slit-lamp view at day 1 shows a very clear, thin corneal flap over the clear stromal bed where the ablation has been laid down. (Courtesy of Stephen Slade.)

tered into a prospective trial. Sixty-two percent of the patients were male. The mean age was 29.9 years (range, 18-45 years). The procedures were done in November and December 1993. The technique used is described above.

Follow-up is currently short, with a mean of 8 weeks. Eighty percent of the eyes were followed at least 1 month. In general, both eyes of the patient were treated in one sitting.

Preoperatively, the mean spherical equivalent refraction was −9.36 D. Postoperatively, the mean spherical equivalent refraction was −0.87 D. Keratometric power changed from a mean of 44.38 D preoperatively to a mean of 33.38 D postoperatively.

Of 44 eyes with complete information at the last follow-up examination, 32 (73%) were within 1 D of emmetropia. Only 1 eye was overcorrected by +0.75 D. The remaining 12 (26%) eyes were undercorrected, 14% less than 2.0 D, 9% with 2.0 to 2.9 D, and 4% with 3.0 D or more.

Preoperatively, all eyes had uncorrected visual acuity of 20/200 or worse. Postoperatively, 76% saw 20/40 or better without correction, and 44% saw 20/20 or better without correction. Change in best spectacles visual acuity was one line or less in 82% of eyes, 10% of eyes losing two lines, and 8% gaining two to four lines.

Videokeratography was done on all eyes, and generally showed a symmetric flattening of the central cornea with moderate tapering of the edges (Fig. 13-9). Two eyes showed what we interpreted as clinically meaningful decentration, with multiple corneal powers over the pupil.

Complications included small epithelial plaques in the stromal bed in 5% of eyes, none showing significant progression and none requiring scraping or removal. There were fine particles in the bed, but considerably less than we were used to seeing after other

techniques of keratomileusis. There was no subepithelial haze and trace haze to 1+ in the stromal bed, which was transient. After a few weeks, it was very difficult to tell where the stromal bed was; however, a circular faint scar was present around the edge of the flap in most eyes (Fig. 13-10).

In two eyes, the width of the flap was too great and the ablation overlapped the flap itself onto the back of the disk, but this did not seem to create identifiable clinical problems (Fig. 13-11).

Obviously, the results on this series of eyes are fragmentary and short term and are presented in this chapter only to give an indication of the general direction and level of success of the procedure. A complete follow-up of the series over a longer time will be necessary to draw firm conclusions about the outcome of this technique.

REFERENCES

1. Thompson K, Waring G: *Classification of refractive surgery*, Philadelphia, 1992, WB Saunders.
2. Waring G: Making sense of keratospeak IV—classification of refractive surgery, 1992, *Arch Ophthalmol* 110:1385-1391, 1992.
3. Barraquer J: *Cirugia refractiva de la cornea*, Bogota, Colombia, 1989, Instituto Barraquer de America.
4. Maxwell W, Nordan L: Myopic keratomileusis. In Thompson F, editor: *Myopia surgery*, New York, 1990: Macmillan.
5. Price F: Keratomileusis. In Nordan L, Maxwell A, Davison J, editors: *The surgical rehabilitation of vision*, New York, 1992, Gower.
6. Price F: Keratomileusis. In Thompson K, Waring G, editors: *Contemporary refractive surgery, ophthalmology clinics of* North America, Philadelphia, 1992, WB Saunders.
7. Barraquer J: Queratomileusis para la correccion de la miopia, *Arch Soc Am Oftalmol Optom* 5:27-48, 1964.
8. Krumeich J, Swinger C: Non-freeze epikeratophakia for the correction of myopia, *Am J Ophthalmol* 103:397-403, 1987.
9. Ruiz L, Rowsey J: In situ keratomileusis, *Invest Ophthalmol Vis Sci* 29(suppl):392, 1988.
10. Barraquer J: *Queratomileusis y queratofaquia*, Bogota, Colombia, 1980, Instituto Barraquer de America.
11. Buratto L, Ferrari M, Rama P: Excimer laser intrastromal keratomileusis, *Am J Ophthalmol* 113:291-295, 1992.

12. Pallikaris I, Papatsanaki M, Stathi E, et al: Laser in situ kerato-mileusis, *Lasers Surg Med* 10:463-468, 1990.

13. Pureskin N: Weakening ocular refraction by means of partial stromectomy of cornea under experimental conditions, *Vestnik Oftalmologii* 80:1, 1967.

14. Arenas-Archila E, Sanchez-Thorin J, Naranjo-Uribe J, et al: Myopic keratomileusis in situ: a preliminary report, *J Cataract Refract Surg* 17:424-435, 1991.

15. Bas M, Nano H: In situ keratomileusis results in 30 eyes at 15 months, *Refract Corneal Surg* 7:223-231, 1991.

16. Buratto L, Ferarri M: Excimer laser intrastromal keratomileusis. In Buratto L, editor: *Chirurgia della myopia assile mediante cheratomileusi,* Milan, 1993, CAMO.

17. Buratto L, Ferrari M: Excimer laser intrastromal keratomileusis: case reports, *J Cataract Refract Surg* 18:37-41, 1992.

18. Siganos D, Pallikaris I: Laser in situ keratomileusis in partially sighted eyes, *Invest Ophthalmol Vis Sci* 34:800, 1993.

19. Pallikaris I, Papatzanaki M, Siganos D, et al: A corneal flap technique for laser in situ keratomileusis. Human studies, *Arch Ophthalmol* 145:1699-1702, 1991.

20. Pallikaris I, Papatzanaki M, Siganos D, et al: Technica de colgajo corneal para la queratomileusis in situ mediana laser estudios en humanos, *Arch Ophthalmol* 3:127-130, 1992.

Excimer Myopic Keratomileusis: Bogota Experience

Luis Ruiz, Stephen G. Slade, Stephen A. Updegraff

The first cases with the excimer MKM technique in Bogota were began on August 8, 1993. These patients were done with Luis Ruiz as the medical monitor, working with Stephen Slade and Stephen Updegraff. While all the patients were treated in Bogota with this study, all follow-up was done as a collaborative effort with physicians from Houston working with the staff of the Clinico Centro Ophthalmico in Bogota. In this initial group of patients, 119 eyes were treated. Sixty-five percent of these patients were female. The mean age was 32 years. The study design divided the patients into five groups with their eyes bilaterally randomized. Excimer ALK on the bed, the flap technique (group I) (Fig. 13-12); ALK excimer on the cap, the Buratto technique (group II); standard ALK with the flap (group III); ALK with a free cap (group IV); and standard PRK (group V). The excimer ALK with the flap technique with an automated keratome was first done by Slade based on the work of Pallikaris in Greece who first performed it with a manual keratome. Preoperatively, the refractions for the Bogota groups ranged from −5.92 D with the Buratto technique to −7.32 D with the standard ALK flap technique. The PRK patients used as a control averaged −3.3 D. The lamellar refractive patients had a rapid return of best corrected visual acuity of 20/40 or better by day 1. Of the excimer ALK flap technique patients, 82.9% were 20/40 or better on day 1, which improved to 94.8% by 6 months. The range for the lamellar groups were

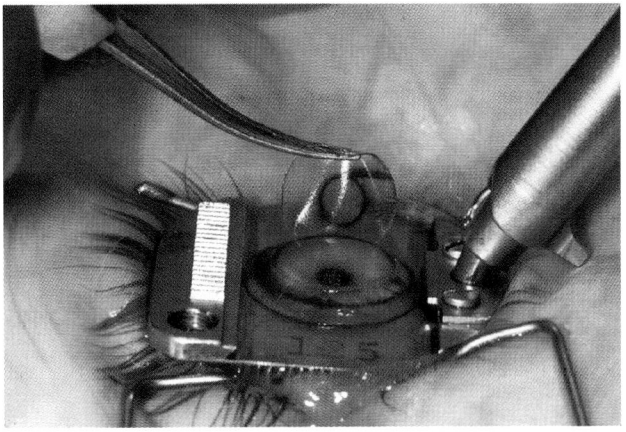

Fig. 13-12. The 160-μm corneal flap being reflected back just before the ablation is laid down for the excimer automated lamellar keratoplasty flap technique.

from 73.9% with the standard ALK flap to 91.3% with the ALK excimer cap. The PRK group showed a reduced best corrected visual acuity at day 1 of 25%, but rapidly returned to 100% of patients by 6 months. At day 1 65.5% of the patients with excimer ALK on the bed beneath the flap showed 20/40 or better uncorrected visual acuity, compared with 56.5% of the patients with excimer on the cap with the Buratto technique, 43% of the patients with standard ALK with the flap, 60% of the patients with standard ALK with the cap, and 60% of the patients with ALK with the cap. By 6 months there was marked regression in the excimer ALK patients with the cap, although some regression was noted in all cases. At 6 months, the uncorrected visual acuity of the PRK patients was the best, with 75% of these patients seeing 20/40 or better. The second best group was 63.4% at 6 months. No eyes lost more than two lines of best corrected visual acuity at 6 months. The surgery was fairly astigmatism-neutral with mean cylinder changes being very small, from 0.08 to 0.28%. The conclusion of the study was that for the higher myopes, the ALK excimer flap technique was the most effective method, while the PRK had the best results for moderate myopes (Fig. 13-13).

Excimer Laser Myopic Keratomileusis: United States Experience

Stephen G. Slade, Stephen F. Brint, Stephen A. Updegraff

On June 22, 1991, the Summit phase I excimer myopic keratomileusis protocol began under the direction of Stephen Brint, medical monitor. The first patients were done in New Orleans with Brint and Stephen Slade, and later cases were added by Slade in Hous-

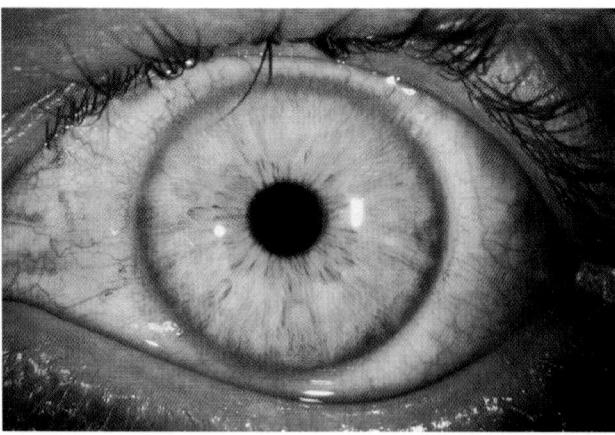

Fig. 13-13. Typically appearance 1 day postoperatively with a clear cornea and only slight hyperemia of the conjunctiva.

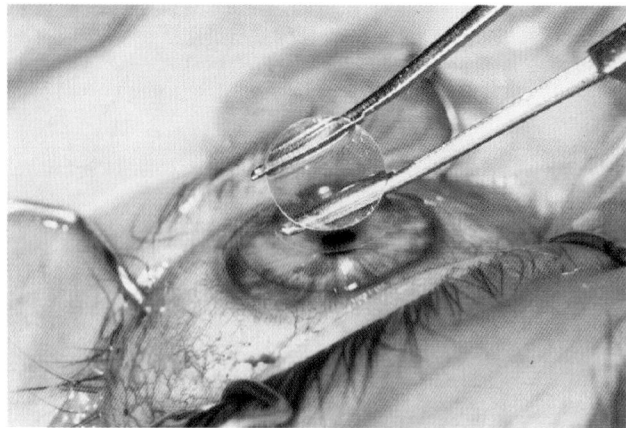

Fig. 13-14. The 300-μm corneal disk after being removed with the microkeratome ready to be placed into the antidesiccation chamber and ablated.

ton, Robert Maloney in Los Angeles, and George Waring, Doyle Stulting, Keith Thompson, and Robert Epstein in Atlanta. The original Summit excimer MKM technique was based on the work of Lucio Buratto. In this technique a thick 300-μm disk of tissue is removed with a microkeratome and placed stromal side up in an antidesiccation chamber (Fig. 13-14). The corneal disk is then positioned beneath the excimer laser and the stromal surface is ablated. The tissue lens was sutured in place in the early cases; later, the surgery was done sutureless. Four cases in the original 57 eyes under the Summit study were done with an in situ technique. In the Summit study a 5-mm optical zone was used in the majority of cases. Attempted corrections ranged from 6.0 to −19.00 D. Mean ablation depth was 90.7 μm with a range from 61 to 167 μm. Of the 30 eyes followed in Houston, postoperative visual acuities at day 1 were good with 16 of the 30 seeing 20/40 or better uncorrected. In general, these patients were more comfortable than other refractive patients at day 1. The patients' uncorrected visual acuity continued to improve with 13 out of the first 17 eyes done in Houston seeing 20/40 or better at 1 month. At 6 months in the overall series, 31 of 47 eyes (66%) 20/40 or better uncorrected. At 6 months, in this group, 71.7% of eyes fell within 2 D of their target refraction, and 47.8% fell within 1 D. Only three eyes, or 6.4%, lost greater than two lines of best corrected visual acuity. The accuracy of the attempted vs. the achieved refraction is indicated in the scattergram Figure 13-15.

There were complications noted in the study, including patient complaints of foreign body sensation, discomfort, glare, and halos. However, these were all reported as trace or mild with only one eye reporting moderate glare. There was trace haze seen in several eyes, along with iron lines. Two eyes were eliminated from the study because they required homoplastic grafts to replace the excimer laser–ablated tissue. Two

patients that were done sutureless also required sutures postoperatively after the lenses were judged not to be properly attached on day 1.

This study represents the earliest United States experience and has the longest-term follow-up. With other trials beginning and further work within the Summit study as it begins phase II, more information will be gathered as to the value of this technique.

Excimer Laser Myopic Keratomileusis at the Jules Stein Eye Institute, Los Angeles
Craig H. Kliger, Robert K. Maloney

LAMELLAR SURGERY—AN OVERVIEW

In 1964 José Barraquer[1] reported a surgical treatment for high myopia which he termed *keratomileusis* (corneal chiseling or sculpting). Using this "in-button" technique, a lamellar corneal button of uniform thickness was removed with a microkeratome. It was frozen and reshaped on a cryolathe to reduce its central thickness, thus achieving the required corneal flattening when the button was replaced on the residual stromal bed. Hyperopic corrections could also be achieved by concentrically thinning the peripheral aspect of the button, permitting the central portion to steepen when the button was replaced, although this was not widely performed because of technical difficulty.

Unfortunately, the freezing necessary to permit controlled removal of stromal tissue from the lenticle with the cryolathe proved to be a major disadvantage, as this produced tissue changes that could limit the corneal clarity and the predictability of the outcome. Swinger et al.[2] in an attempt to improve on this technique, described an alternative method for removal of the required tissue from the posterior surface of the lenticle that did not require freezing. For myopic cor-

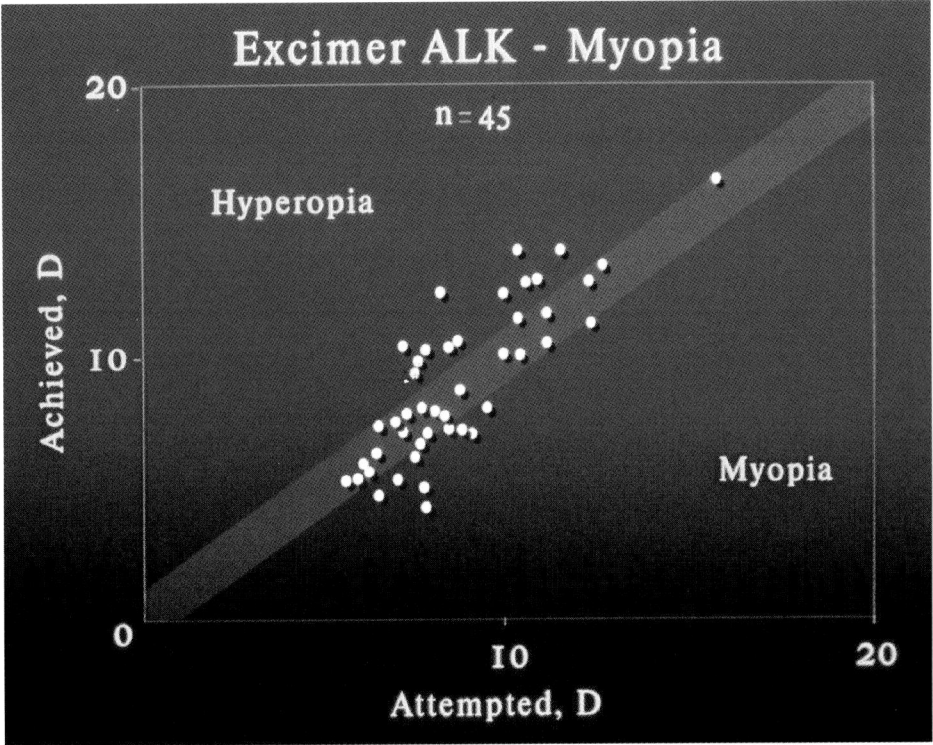

Fig. 13-15. Scattergram of the Summit (United States) results showing achieved vs. attempted dioptic correction.

rection, the lenticle was placed epithelium side down over a rigid convex template and held in place with vacuum suction while a keratome was passed in a planar fashion across the button to remove the necessary tissue.

In 1991, Arenas-Arehila et al.[3] described a different in situ technique to achieve correction of myopia, in which the second (refractive) cut is performed on the residual stromal bed rather than the lenticle. As in the Swinger et al. method, excision of central tissue achieves the flattening to yield the refractive change.

Several innovations have generally enhanced reproducibility and reduced complications of lamellar surgery in recent years. The most important of these is the automation of the microkeratome pass. Also of note is the development of the flap technique[4] in which the lenticle remains attached by a hinge created by stopping the microkeratome just before it emerges from the stromal bed. The flap technique is suitable for in situ keratomileusis. It eliminates the possibility of lenticle loss postoperatively and obviates the need for suturing.

Because radial keratotomy and PRK have been very successful in the predictable treatment of low to moderate levels of myopia (−1-−6 D), keratomileusis is normally reserved for candidate eyes exceeding −6 D, up to approximately −25 D. The upper range of cor-

rection is limited by the amount of tissue that can be safely removed from the corneal thickness. If the postoperative cornea is less than 300 μm thick, iatrogenic keratoconus may result.

LASER KERATOMILEUSIS

The excimer laser offers another method for the controlled removal of tissue for myopic keratomileusis. This technology permits myopic excision of tissue either from the lenticle itself (in-button) or from the stromal bed (in situ). Figure 13-16 schematically demonstrates laser myopic keratomileusis in-button and in situ, and compares them to mechanical in situ treatment.

The excimer laser offers several theoretical advantages over mechanical techniques. Because placement of the laser treatment is largely independent of the centration of the initial lenticle, one can better control the location of actual tissue removal, and thus centration of the refractive effect, with respect to the entrance pupil. This is most helpful when using the in-button techniques because the center of the entrance pupil can be marked preoperatively and the mark is still visible on the epithelial surface of the button during ablation.

Mechanical failure during the refractive cut is one of the feared complications of mechanical keratomileusis because it can produce a step in the stromal bed

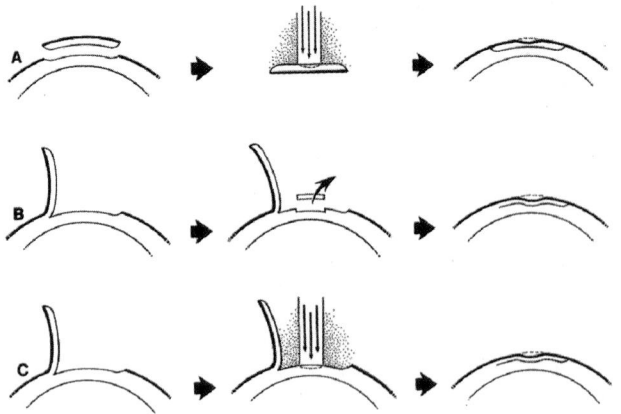

Fig. 13-16. Comparison of methods: **A,** Excimer laser myopic keratomileusis in-button. **B,** Mechanical myopic keratomileusis. **C,** Excimer laser myopic keratomileusis in situ. Compare the constant stromal thickness in **A** to the constant lenticle thickness in **B** and **C.** For graphical emphasis, myopic cuts are shown such that they would produce a concave final corneal surface, when in reality this surface is less convex.

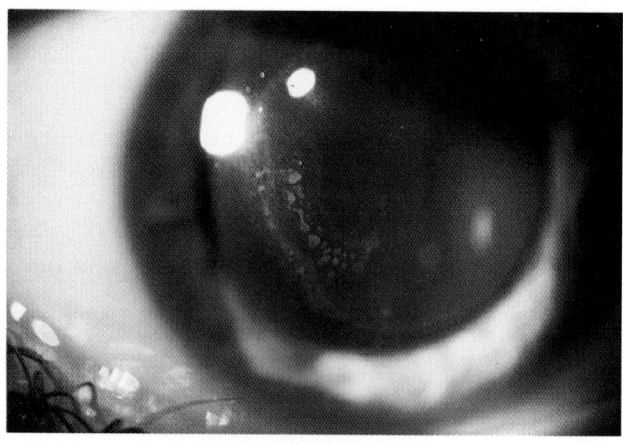

Fig. 13-17. Epithelialization of the lenticle-stromal bed interface. Similar to epithelial downgrowth in a cataract wound, epithelialization of the interface results in light scattering and regression of the effect of surgery by filling in the void created by ablation, possibly in an irregular fashion. It is treated by peeling back the lenticle, replacing it after careful scraping of the encroaching epithelial tissue.

and cause severe irregular astigmatism. Failure of the excimer laser while making the refractive ablation should produce simple undercorrection, since tissue removal is symmetric over the area of ablation. Of course, mechanical failure during the primary keratectomy is a possibility in all lamellar surgery.

Another potential advantage of the laser technique is that the laser leaves a true myopic ablation zone that is deeper centrally and shallower peripherally. The refractive cut with the microkeratome is actually planar, removing a uniform depth of tissue. Myopic correction results from draping of the lenticle over the edge of the cut. This might lead to more spherical aberration.

In-Button or In Situ?

Laser MKM can be performed in-button or in situ. Each technique has its advantages. The in-button technique avoids possible endothelial damage secondary to shock waves transmitted to deeper tissues by laser energy. If significant irregular astigmatism develops due to an irregular in-button ablation, a donor homograft lenticle can be substituted for the damaged host tissue. Either complication using in situ techniques will likely require penetrating keratoplasty to correct.

In situ laser MKM allows the use of the flap technique, eliminating the need for suturing of the button. However, if a retrobulbar injection is used, the patient cannot fixate during ablation, so centration can be more difficult with this technique. Because of its better safety, we generally prefer the in-button technique.

Excimer Laser Myopic Keratomileusis (In-Button)

Familiarity with conventional keratomileusis is essential, as is adequate training in the use of the excimer laser device.

Corneal markings and anesthesia. After the patient is brought into the surgical suite and placed in the supine position, the center of the entrance pupil is identified and marked with a surgical marking pen while the patient fixates coaxially with the surgeon's eye. At the surgeon's option, the patient can then be given a retrobulbar or peribulbar injection of lidocaine.

Once anesthesia (and akinesia, if desired) is obtained, asymmetric corneal markings are placed to allow proper reorientation of the lenticle after laser treatment.

Laser parameters. The laser is tested, programmed, and armed prior to the primary keratectomy. The amount of myopic correction is the same as for myopic PRK. To ensure that the lenticle created in subsequent steps is not perforated by laser treatment, the surgeon should determine the number of pulses needed to achieve the desired myopic correction at the chosen ablation zone diameter, usually 5 mm. To calculate the ablation depth, the number of pulses is multiplied by the depth of ablation per pulse, which depends on the fluence of the laser. An approximate value is 0.4 μm per pulse at a fluence of 180 mJ/cm^2. It should be noted that the ablation depth per pulse given with many laser systems *underestimates* the amount of tissue removal because it represents resultant tissue removal *after* wound healing has occurred.

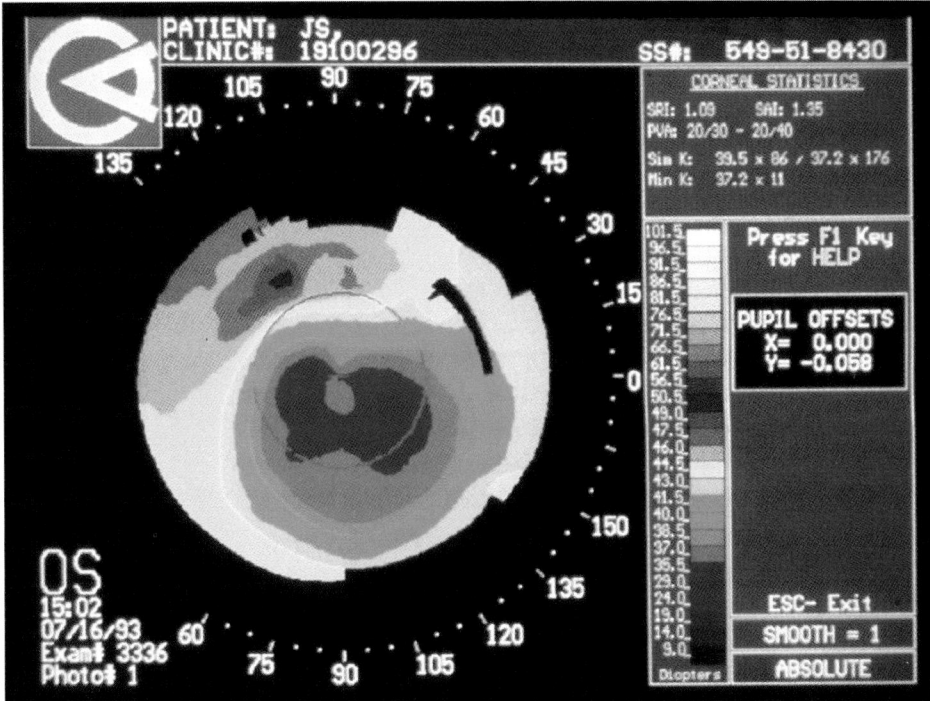

Fig. 13-18. Decentration of the ablation zone. Corneal topography showing location of laser ablation inferior to the entrance pupil, resulting in complaints of glare and halos. Decentration is unusual with the in-button technique because of the ease of centration of the detached button. If this occurs when the in-button technique is used, this problem can be treated with a lenticle homograft. In situ treatment will likely require penetrating keratoplasty.

The surgeon should plan to leave a minimum thickness of 100 μm centrally after ablation. Usually a 300-μm-thick primary lenticle will allow sufficient residual thickness.

Lenticle excision, hydration, and ablation. The suction ring is then centered on the entrance pupil, and a lenticle of sufficient stromal thickness, again usually 300 μm, is then excised and its thickness verified. If the button is too thin for the calculated ablation depth, either in situ ablation can be performed, or the ablation diameter reduced (which reduces the depth of ablation).

In addition to creating a lenticle of adequate depth, maintaining adequate hydration is essential, as dehydration can itself lead to overcorrection.[5] We use an antidesiccation chamber to transfer the tissue to the laser device. Once settings are confirmed, ablation is performed on the stromal side, centered on the epithelial entrance pupil mark.

Replacing the lenticle. The lenticle and bed are then irrigated with BSS to remove particulate debris and antibiotic, and the lenticle replaced using the asymmetric markings to restore it to its original ori-

entation. After approximately 5 minutes, the edge of the lenticle is tested to ensure tight adherence.

Usually no suture is necessary. However, for added safety, a suture can be placed. A running 10-0 nylon suture can be used as in the traditional technique. Alternatively a single 10-0 nylon interrupted suture tied very loosely at the 12-o'clock position is effective, and may result in less irregular astigmatism than a running suture. If the latter option is chosen, it is important to keep in mind that this suture is not intended to physically maintain the orientation of the lenticle, but rather to prevent its loss should it become dislodged. Therefore, excess tightening may result in undesired interface striae and possible irregular astigmatism.

EXPERIENCE AND RESULTS

As of this writing, laser MKM is an investigational procedure in the United States undergoing an Food and Drug Administration (FDA)–supervised multicenter clinical trial. Eleven patients who have undergone this surgery at the Jules Stein Eye Institute in Los Angeles had a mean preoperative spherical equivalent of -11.6 ± 2.6 D (mean $\pm$SD). On average, they experienced an undercorrection compared to attempted correction of 0.6 ±1.9 D at 3 months, 1.3 ±2.6D at 6 months, and 1.0 ±2.8 D at 1 year.

Four of the 11 patients completing 3 months of follow-up experienced a two-line loss of best corrected visual acuity. For those completing 6 months of follow-up, 2 of 9 patients, and for 1 year of follow-up, 1 of 5, had a two-line loss. As combined data from the various centers become available, the efficacy of this procedure as compared to mechanical MKM should become apparent.

COMPLICATIONS

The complications of excimer laser MKM can be divided into those related lamellar surgery in general and those unique to the use of the excimer laser.

The most common complication that affects lamellar surgery is irregular astigmatism. Loss of the lenticle is possible if a sutureless technique is used. Epithelialization of the lenticle-bed interface (Fig. 13-17) can also occur, but can be minimized by limiting the handling of the lenticle.

The complication almost unique to the laser is perforation of the lenticle (Fig. 13-18), which can be prevented by carefully following the above-described procedure. Decentration of the ablation zone (Fig. 13-19) can occur even with the in-button technique, resulting in unpredictable optical aberrations.

As with any surgical procedure, familiarity with the sources, and active avoidance, of potential complications can eliminate their occurrence.

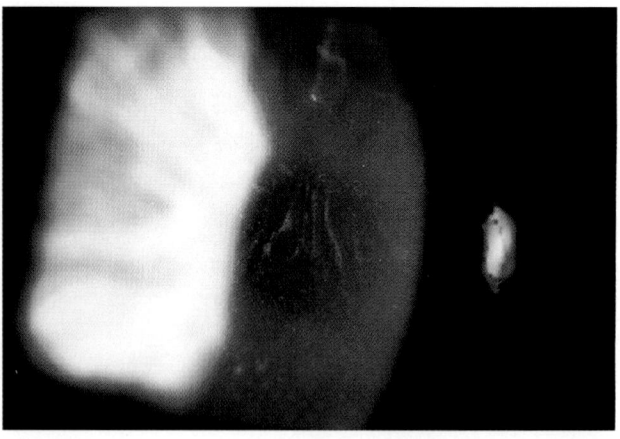

Fig. 13-19. Near perforation of the lenticle after in-button ablation. Folds in Bowman's layer are present centrally owing to the extreme thinness of the button. Uncorrected vision was still 20/20.

REFERENCES

1. Barraquer JI: Keratomileusis for the correction of myopia, *Arch Soc Am Oftal Optom* 5:27-48, 1964.
2. Swinger CA, Krumeich J, Cassiday D: Planar lamellar refractive keratoplasty, *J Refract Surg* 2:17-24, 1986.
3. Arenas-Archila E, Sanches-Thorin JC, Haranjo-Uribe GP, et al: Myopic keratomileusis in situ: a preliminary report, *J Cataract Refract Surg* 109:1699-1702, 1991.
4. Pallikaris IG, Papatzanaki ME, Sigamos DS, et al: A corneal flap technique for laser in situ keratomileusis, *Arch Ophthalmol* 145:1699-1702, 1991.
5. Dougherty PJ, Wellish KL, Maloney RK: Excimer laser ablation rate and corneal hydration (abstract), *Invest Ophthalmol Vis Sci* 34(suppl):801, 1993.

14

A Comparison of the Summit and VISX Excimer Lasers: Clinical Experience at the Gimbel Eye Centre

John A. van Westenbrugge, Howard V. Gimbel

This discussion is limited to our comparison of the Summit and VISX excimer lasers from a clinical perspective. It is our objective to enable the reader to have a more complete knowledge of the relative strengths and weaknesses of these two major excimer laser systems. Although based on the information in this chapter, certain refractive surgeons may decide that one laser or the other is more suitable for their specific purposes, we would have our readers complete the chapter with increased knowledge of both lasers but with no definite commitment to one or the other.

Although the new Summit OmniMed has an associated holmium laser as an option, we do not address the holmium laser as we have no significant experience with either its glaucoma or refractive applications.

The conclusions in this chapter are largely based on our own work, but we wish to acknowledge the contributions of our co-workers: (1) Dr. Harold Johnson in Edmonton, who has done extensive work with the ExciMed 200 LA laser, and more recently has done the majority of the work with the Summit OmniMed laser; and (2) Drs. Jacinthe Kassab and Robert Beldavs in Calgary. J.A.V. is the principle author of this chapter and he accepts full responsibility for any errors or omissions. The chapter is written from his perspective.

IMPARTIALITY

The value of a chapter such as this is only as good as the impartiality of the author(s). We have no proprietary interest in either Summit or VISX and have not served as consultants for either company. We currently have one VISX laser at our Calgary office and one Summit laser each at our Edmonton (Alberta) and Saskatoon (Saskatchewan) satellites. We are presently considering the purchase of a third Summit excimer laser for an additional satellite office. The argument might be made that we would be inclined to take a position of neutrality with regard to the Summit and VISX lasers, maintaining that they are equal because we have invested money in both of them. However, in the 5½ years that we have been working with excimer lasers, we have had opportunities to purchase both and in fact would have been in a position to get rid of one laser in favor of the other if we had been so inclined. The present higher proportion of Summit lasers is simply a reflection of economics and opportunity in laser purchase rather than an indication of favoring the Summit over the VISX excimer laser.

HISTORY OF REFRACTIVE SURGERY AT THE GIMBEL EYE CENTRE

The history of the refractive surgery at the Gimbel Eye Centre in Calgary gives readers the context of the situation in which our judgments were made and a better sense of our credentials as refractive surgeons.

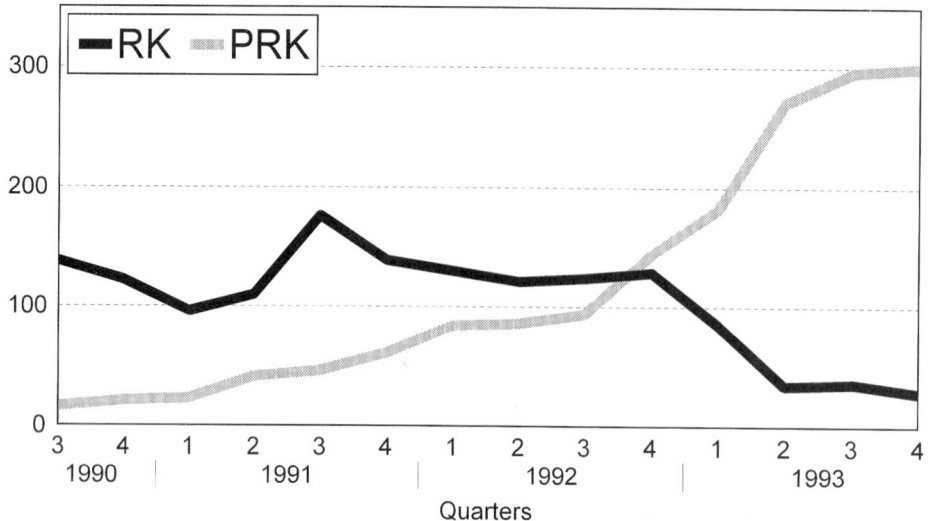

Fig. 14-1. Number of cases of RK and PRK 1990-1994 (GEC Calgary).

H.V.G. began radial keratotomy (RK) at the Gimbel Eye Centre in August 1984, after several years of consideration and after having taken a number of courses taught by various leaders in the field. We were one of the few centers offering refractive surgery in western Canada. As a result, the RK practice grew steadily during the 1980s to a volume of approximately 400 to 500 cases per year prior to starting photorefractive keratectomy (PRK) in June 1990. J.A.V. did not do RK because he was aware of the significant learning curve and had become aware of the possibility of laser refractive surgery becoming available in the next few years. Both of us were involved in the preoperative assessment, preoperative counseling, and postoperative follow-up of RK patients and were able to obtain a good knowledge base of the expectations and unique characteristics of a refractive surgery practice.

We followed with interest the early development of both VISX and Summit. We followed more closely the development of the Summit excimer laser because at that time the Summit laser cost significantly less than the VISX. Because we were uncertain as to the role of the excimer laser and its ultimate usefulness we wished to reduce our initial financial risk. Also, the smaller size and simpler requirements of the Summit system appealed to us at that time. Although we were aware of the differences between the two laser systems we felt that we did not have any information significantly favoring one system over the other and therefore elected first to purchase a Summit ExciMed laser which we first had in place in our clinic in December 1988. At that time, we used the excimer laser for only limited phototherapeutic keratectomy (PTK) applications and for partial external trabeculectomy procedures which had been pioneered for the Summit laser by Dr. Theo Seiler.

Our first procedure in December 1988 was in fact a partial external trabeculectomy (PET) which was effective in controlling eye pressure for a patient who had undergone previous multiple glaucoma procedures. Ultimately, the PET procedure proved to have similar problems to standard trabeculectomy with regard to maintaining an adequate bleb and because there was therefore no demonstrated advantage over standard trabeculectomy, the procedure was discontinued. We did obtain valuable experience, however, in becoming familiar with the characteristics of the excimer beam and the functioning of the machine.

From December 1988 until we began PRK in June 1990 we did a limited number of further PET procedures and PTK procedures with favorable results, but we shall not detail our PET and PTK experience here. On June 12, 1990 we performed the first PRK procedure in Canada and we cautiously began to do several cases per week following this.

The Transition of Photorefractive Keratectomy

The graph in Fig. 14-1 shows the relative numbers of RK and PRK patients done from mid-1990 to the end of 1993. We would have expected a more symmetric inverse relationship between numbers of RK and PRK but we believe that, as observed by others, the advent of PRK aroused great interest in the population in refractive surgery in general. Once patients had been motivated to enquire into refractive surgery, many chose to opt for the more established RK procedure. During this time we took great care to give as balanced a presentation as possible of the two procedures to every potential refractive surgery candidate.

Table 14-1 gives the absolute numbers of both cases done for each quarter starting from mid-1990 and also gives the ratio of PRK to RK cases. It is interesting to

Table 14-1. Ratio of cases of PRK to RK: 1990-1993

Year	Quarter	Ratio	RK	PRK
1990	3	1:9	138	16
	4	1:6	122	21
1991	1	1:4	96	23
	2	1:3	110	41
	3	1:3	176	46
	4	1:2	139	61
1992	1	1:1.5	130	84
	2	1:1.4	121	86
	3	1:1.3	124	94
	4	1:1.1	129	144
1993	1	2:1	85	182
	2	8:1	34	271
	3	8:1	36	296
	4	11:1	28	300

Table 14-2. Myopic PRK cases: June 1990 to January 1994

Place of study	Laser	No. of cases
Calgary	Summit	461
Edmonton	Summit	820
Calgary	VISX	1506
Total		2787

Table 14-3. Technical parameters of the Summit OmniMed and VISX Twenty/Twenty excimer lasers

	Summit OmniMed	VISX Twenty/Twenty
Ablation rate (μ/pulse)	0.25	0.25
Ablation zone (mm)	6.5	6
Pulses/sec	10	6
Gas	ArF	ArF
Beam wavelength (nm)	193	193
Energy (ml)	150	240
Fluence (mj/cm^2)	180	160

observe that while we still offer RK, the ratios have almost exactly reversed over these 3½ years. We now perform RK primarily for patients under 3 D.

Initial PRK with the Summit laser, starting on June 12, 1990, used a 4.5-mm optical zone. On June 26, 1991 we began to use a 5.0-mm optical zone. Primarily because of our interest in doing astigmatic correction, we purchased a VISX laser which we began to use in October 1992. Our Summit laser at that time was moved to our Edmonton satellite with any patients requiring significant astigmatic correction being referred to our Calgary center.

The total number of myopic PRK cases done at the Gimbel Eye Centre as of the end of January 1994 was 2787. The breakdown in the numbers is shown in Table 14-2. In September 1993 the Summit laser in our Edmonton office was upgraded to a Summit OmniMed laser with a 6.5-mm optical zone.

COMPARISON OF THE SUMMIT AND VISX LASERS
Challenges

The major challenge present in comparing the two excimer lasers is the rapid evolution of the lasers. Any statistical data of significance relate to a model of laser at least 1 or 2 years old and either manufacturer might challenge any differences presented statistically by indicating that changes have been made to improve upon any deficiencies which might seem apparent. Therefore, any comparison between the two lasers must of necessity be somewhat historical.

Similarities

Both the Summit and VISX excimer lasers are broad area ablation lasers with an iris diaphragm regulating

basic spherical correction. Basic physical parameters are listed in Table 14-3.

Convergent Evolution

It is interesting to observe how these two competitors in the excimer laser field have shown certain features of convergent evolution which have reduced the differences between them.

1. Fixation of the eye: The Summit laser uses patient fixation only, without the use of any suction ring or other stabilizing device used by the surgeon. VISX began with the use of a suction ring handpiece and has now moved to patient fixation.

2. Clearing of photoablated material: The Summit laser has never used a device for clearing of the gaseous photoablated material, whereas the VISX began with nitrogen gas flow over the cornea. This was discontinued by VISX because of indications that the drying caused increased haze.

3. Direction of iris diaphragm movement: The Summit uses a pattern that starts with the smallest-diameter ablation first and expanding out to the largest ablation diameter. VISX began by using a pattern that started with the largest-diameter ablation first, contracting into the smallest-diameter ablation, but VISX has now gone to the same "in-to-out" pattern as Summit.

4. Optical zone size: VISX began with a 6.0-mm optical zone as compared to the 4.5-mm optical zone used by Summit. Summit moved to increase their optical zone to 5.0 mm and has now increased it to 6.5 mm.

5. Astigmatism correction: VISX has led in astigmatic correction using an expanding slit superimposed as required on the circular iris diaphragm pattern. Summit plans to have available in the near future (as of the time of this writing in April 1994), an ablatable mask with a pattern of astigmatism correction that can be placed in the optical rail. To this point the ablatable mask has had to be handheld over the cornea.
6. Surgeon's view: The VISX began with a "coaxial" (more about this later) viewing microscope system, whereas the Summit view was an off-axis view. The Summit has since adopted a more similar coaxial view.

Shared Strengths and Weaknesses

The relatively well-established VISX and Summit excimer lasers are now being challenged by a number of additional manufacturers and claims are being made for second-generation lasers (see Appendix).

One of the advantages claimed by the newer laser manufacturers is a larger optical zone than either the VISX 6.0-mm or the Summit OmniMed 6.5-mm optical zone. From our personal experience to date, we do not believe that there would be a great advantage to an optical zone significantly larger than 6.0 mm, although a blend zone at the margins of the optical zone may be of benefit.

The other major innovation being introduced is that of a scanning slit or circle pattern with claims that greater homogeneity of the beam pattern can be obtained. However, some of the scanning patterns do require associated eye-tracking technology, technology which remains unproven to date, and adds another level of complexity to the apparatus.

Strongly in favor of both the Summit and VISX lasers is that they have the most extensive track records, both within the United States Food and Drug Administration (FDA) trials and at centers outside of the United States. They both have a large database of patients with extensive follow-up. Despite claims made on a theoretical basis by any new manufacturer, the new systems remain unproven by comparison with the VISX and Summit excimer lasers.

Physical Structure

The VISX laser is a larger machine than the Summit, requiring a larger physical space and higher voltage as well as access to a liquid nitrogen supply. These are relative disadvantages for the VISX but we do not think that this would be a significant factor in differentiating between the two machines for most users.

Chair

The VISX has a Dexta chair that is connected directly to the laser structure and swivels on a base allowing easy positioning of the patient under the laser. Controls for patient movement are hand-controlled just below the eyepieces and are easy to understand and use, but this does have the disadvantage of occupying one hand during the procedure. The movements include an initial slow fine movement and then a faster movement if the control pressure is maintained.

The Summit Dexta chair is not directly connected to its smaller laser structure and therefore must be carefully positioned initially. Because of the lack of a swivel base, it is slightly more awkward to position the patient under the laser. Once the patient is positioned, a foot control is used for final adjustment. It has x, y, and z controls as three separate foot switches beside one another on the same control box. The foot control is less intuitive than the VISX hand control but does leave both hands free. The positioning control movements are significantly coarser than for the VISX.

Parameters

We are not qualified to comment on the specific engineering aspects of the optics, fluence, repetition rate, and similar parameters and there are arguments for and against the various ranges and elements of these parameters. Often there are tradeoffs and balances between elements that make it impossible to say that one particular level of fluence, repetition rate, or certain elements of optics are superior to another and one must view the system as a whole. We believe that the actual demonstrated patient results need to be the ultimate test by which the system is judged and we address this later in the chapter.

The repetition rate deserves some comment. The VISX operates at six pulses per second and the Summit at ten pulses per second. For the novice photorefractive surgeon, the slower rate of the VISX is comforting in that one has a better sense of control over the procedure and is better able to monitor what is happening, and act upon it if patient movement or other factors make it desirable to stop the procedure. The higher repetition rate of the Summit is more desirable in terms of decreased time required for patient fixation. Ultimately, with more experience and confidence, one appreciates the more rapid ablation times. When doing phototherapeutic procedures some of which may involve using methylcellulose as a smoothing agent, numerous pulses may be required and it is nicer to have these delivered at a faster rate.

The foot control of the Summit, which allows one to have both hands free to manipulate the patient's head and eye position, as well as the higher repetition rate, tends to make the Summit more efficient and comfortable to use for PTK procedures.

Surgeon View and Centering System

The microscope and centering device for both the VISX and Summit are interlinked and should be discussed together. Neither laser gives a true coaxial view, i.e., where one or both eyepieces would see directly along the same line as the excimer laser beam. If the viewer was restricted to one such eyepiece or if both eyepieces were truly coaxial with the excimer beam, this would not allow stereopsis. The VISX has always had the line of sight for the two eyepieces on either side of the laser beam, with one eyepiece having a crosshair plus concentric ring pattern to which the excimer beam can be aligned. The VISX has a continuous hand-operated zoom and focus located next to the x or y chair movement button, both of which are located just below the eyepieces of the microscope.

The original Summit suffered for some time under the disadvantage of having an off-axis alignment of the line of sight, but this has now been addressed with the OmniMed, in which, as in the VISX, the line of sight for the two eyepieces is on either side of the excimer laser beam. The Summit does not have a continuous zoom magnification. It has a stepped magnification, but this offers an adequate range of magnifications. As indicated earlier the x or y and z (focus) controls are all located on a foot control. The centering device for the Summit consists of two helium-neon beams which come in from either side at the 3- and 9-o'clock position and cross over at the desired plane of laser action.

X and Y Positioning

This discussion of x and y positioning of the eye assumes that the ablation should be centered over the entrance pupil. For the VISX one centers the crosshair and concentric ring over the center of the entrance pupil and with the fine controls of the VISX chair this is easy to do. Because one calibrates the position of the excimer beam to the crosshair and concentric rings of the one eyepiece only, we advise using this eyepiece only to ensure accurate centration of the excimer beam over the entrance pupil.

For the Summit one uses the dual helium-neon beam to center over the entrance pupil. The standard procedure with the Summit is to use pilocarpine to constrict the pupil so that the beam is not lost in the pupil but shows up distinctly on the iris on either side of the pupil at 3 and 9 o'clock with the two beams crossing over and meeting at the corneal plane precisely over the pupil center. We have some concern that the use of pilocarpine may slightly alter the pupil center from its normal physiologic resting center but we have had no evidence in our experience that this has significantly affected the result for any patient. For the Summit OmniMed laser the quality of the helium-neon aiming beams is much improved over those used with the ExciMed and we personally believe that one could obtain an accurate sense of centration without necessarily using pilocarpine to constrict the pupil. We believe that if the pupil were too large to have the helium-neon beam shining on the iris itself, one could still adequately center the pupil with the aid of the fused spot of the two helium-neon beams seen at the corneal surface. This spot becomes easier to see on the dry corneal surface or dry Bowman's membrane than on the clear untouched tear film.

With the Summit, one uses the coarser control of the chair to bring the eye very close to the final position and then one tends to use small adjustments of the patient's head position to reach the final positioning point, and this does work quite well.

Illumination

We digress briefly to discuss illumination here because it has some bearing on the z axis or focal plane control to be discussed next.

The illumination for the VISX comes from a bright continuous ring of light around the microscope objective (and main laser axis) and is seen on the clear tear film as a clear ring image. Illumination for the Summit OmniMed laser comes from a number of separate lights in a circle pattern around the microscope objective (and main laser axis). As well, Summit has a flexible gooseneck light that can be brought in at various angles. This can be useful in providing a somewhat different angle of illumination, especially when the main illumination lights are turned down. Therefore, the Summit has somewhat more flexibility in lighting angle and direction compared to the VISX.

Z-Axis Control

The two helium-neon beams of the Summit give not only centering position but also an absolute point in space at which the eye can be positioned in the z axis. One must therefore adjust the eyepieces to ensure that one's optimal focal plane coincides with this point in space determined by the beams.

With the VISX, it is somewhat more difficult to be certain of determining an absolute constant fixed point on the z axis. The ring light, when initially seen reflected from a clear corneal surface, has an image that is below the actual corneal surface owing to the properties of a convex mirror. When one then dries the cornea and removes the epithelium exposing Bowman's membrane, one no longer has a clear image below the corneal surface to focus on, but rather one tends to use the z-axis control to move the eye down slightly to focus more precisely on the corneal plane. Because there is potential for patient movement up or down after one has made the initial focus or because adjustments may need to be made for other reasons, one must depend on this focus point at the corneal plane, which is different from the original focal plane on the image of the ring light. Since one is depending on a clear focus of the corneal plane to determine the patient's eye position on the z axis, if one is not bilaterally emmetropic, one must also make sure that one's eyepiece adjustment is properly set prior to positioning of the patient's eye under the laser. We would emphasize that the difference between these two focal planes is quite small and therefore not likely to be of clinical significance, but it is somewhat less precisely determined than the point in space determined by the two helium-neon beams of the Summit.

CALIBRATION

The Summit and VISX lasers use quite different techniques for calibration by the end user and this deserves some description.

Centration

Assuring appropriate centration is straightforward for both machines. For the Summit one simply fires an ablation pattern onto a piece of photo paper and ensures that the two helium-neon beams are precisely centered at their crossover point relative to the ablation pattern. If perfect centration is not observed, adjustments are made to the two beams so that they coincide with the path of the excimer laser beam.

For the VISX, one fires on thermal-sensitive paper (fax or calculator) which gives a distinct pattern, and this is viewed with just the eyepiece that has the crosshair and concentric rings, to ensure that it is centered. If it is not centered one is able to make x and y adjustments of the excimer laser beam to make it coincide with the center of the crosshair.

Calibration of Excimer Output

Calibration of exact output of the laser as determined by the end user is quite different for the two lasers. Laser output determined by the company is similar in that one makes a cut in plastic according to certain parameters and this is sent in and analyzed by the company which then gives feedback on what the performance of the individual laser is at a given time. However, this does not give reassurance immediately prior to the procedure to the physician using the device, and this must be done by different means:

1. For the Summit, ablation is done through a gelatin filter of standard thickness and the number of pulses required to penetrate the gel is recorded and compared against a standard. One may also get an impression of beam uniformity and homogeneity by the points at which the excimer beam first penetrates the gel.
2. For the VISX, a cut is made in plastic according to specified parameters and one is then able to read

the refractive result in a lensometer and adjust the output for the patient by using a calibration table based on this result. The reading in the lensometer is not perfectly clear but with some practice one can obtain a good level of consistency in reading this pattern.

By comparison with the Summit, the calibration technique for the VISX certainly provides a similar modality in the form of the lensometer reading. But the ultimate effectiveness of the calibration technique and thus the consistency of laser output is still probably best judged by overall consistency of end results as shown by analysis of patient data. Another important difference is that VISX recommends that a calibration be done immediately before every patient, whereas Summit only requires a calibration with each new gas fill. This means that patient turnover is faster with the Summit because 10 to 15 patients may be done with a single gas fill. The VISX can do a similar number of patients on a single gas fill, but the recommended calibration between patients increases turnover time.

Although one does not have the reassurance of a calibration between patients with the Summit, we have no reason to believe from our results that the laser shows significant variation in output during a gas fill. The VISX shows good consistency from calibration to calibration and one could probably increase the number of patients done per calibration if this was allowed by the company.

Beam Homogeneity and Contour

Fig. 14-2 shows a light microscopy magnification of the peripheral portion of cuts from the Summit, VISX, and Nidek, one of the new scanning mode excimer lasers. The Summit and VISX show similar fine, step-like patterns. The Summit shows an overlying fine, wavy pattern that is more prominent on the right-hand side of the picture. In contrast with both the Summit and VISX, the Nidek shows a somewhat greater, overall smoothness but is quite markedly different from the Summit and VISX in that it uses fewer and larger steps for the same 1.0 D cut. When comparing the Summit and VISX excimer beams pattern in plastic there is a definite difference in appearance. The Summit beam shows noticeably more waviness and point-to-point variation within the beam than does the VISX. This is the reason why it is difficult, even in the lower ranges, to obtain a direct lensometer reading from a Summit cut in plastic and virtually impossible in higher diopter ranges. Although the irregularities are quite apparent on looking at the plastic, the actual difference in depth from point to point is very small–well below the size of the epithelial cells that will cover the area. Whether these point-to-point variations in the Summit give rise to stronger healing

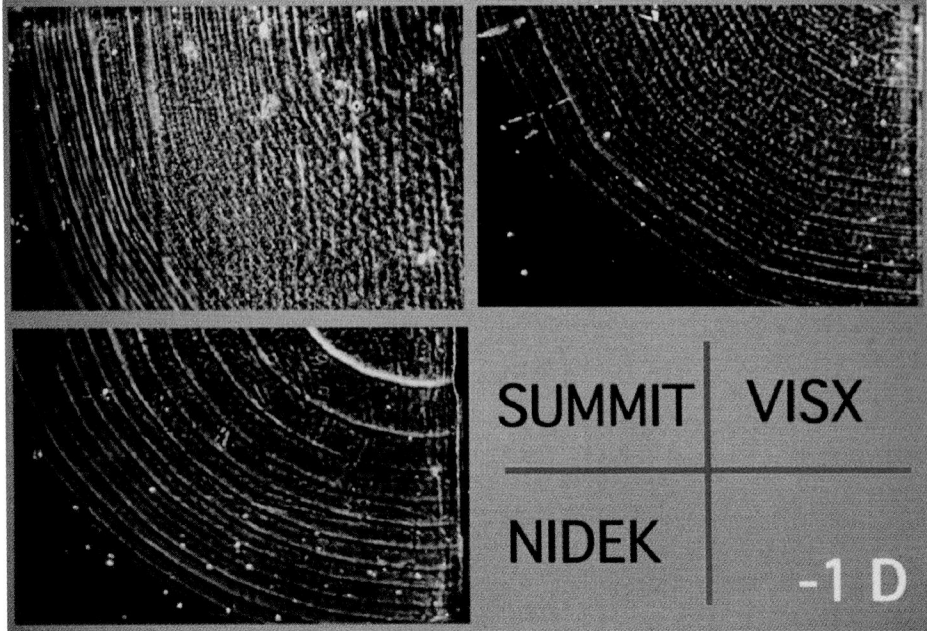

Fig. 14-2. Composite of high magnification photos of excimer ablation patterns.

responses or more haze can probably be best judged by reviewing the overall clinical results. We feel that they do not.

Probably of greater significance is the character of the overall beam contour. The main issue currently related to the question of beam contour is that of the central island. This issue is addressed in more detail in the discussion in Chapter 10 by Drs. Maguen and Machat. Promoters of the Summit laser have maintained that this is a beam configuration problem and limited to the VISX (recent reports seem to indicate that it is also present in the Technolas). Others maintain that it is a factor related to larger optical zone size. Our own limited experience appears to suggest that there is an element of truth to both positions.

VISX Central Island

We were not aware of the central island phenomenon when we initially began to use the VISX laser. Therefore we can only make a rough estimate of our incidence of central island for the following reasons: (1) While we do corneal mapping for all patients as a baseline prior to surgery, we tend to only use it postoperatively if we are suspicious of some particular problem. (2) Because of the wide geographic distribution of our patients in western Canada, our follow-up by patients at our own facility is less than it might be in other centers and therefore we may not have corneal maps on all patients affected.

We estimate that 20% to 25% of our patients show some element of central island but that only 2% to 3% have significant persisting effects from this which

would require a later, separate central island treatment. For some time, we did do a separate central island treatment as a preventive measure (as part of the initial refractive surgery) but found that an occasional patient would still present with a central island. It was also our impression that we obtained a higher number of overcorrections using this technique and there was more variability in response with the use of this separate central island treatment.

We have recently had an opportunity to test a software modification for central island which has reduced the incidence of any significant central island to approximately 10% and those central islands that do occur tend to be of lower magnitude, many of them clearing by 3 month's time. We only began using the Summit OmniMed laser in September 1993, but we have been doing corneal maps at 1 month on all patients who return to our office for follow-up, regardless of whether they had any subjective complaints. Out of 94 Summit OmniMed cases checked at 1 month postoperatively, we have noted two central islands. We have not been able to determine any common factors that would indicate patients prone to central island, but the presence of the central island with the Summit OmniMed system, even though at a very low incidence, suggests that at least some of the theories regarding certain corneal qualities, hydration patterns, ablation dynamics, and so forth, may well be true.

Astigmatism Correction

The VISX laser has certainly led the way in astigmatism correction and this ability to do astigmatism

Table 14-4. 41 Case study of elliptical pattern astigmatic correction

Mean preop cyl	−1.49 D
Mean p/o cyl	−0.77 D
Mean reduction of astigmatism	−0.73 D (48.6%)
p value	0.007

Elliptical Pattern (n = 41) 6 months postop.

Table 14-5. Myopic PRK refractive results of VISX and summit excimer lasers*

	OZ	Mean S.E. (D)(s.d.)	Range
Summit	5	Preop −5.89 (±2.12)	−2.00 to −11.50
(n = 169)		Postop −0.72 (±1.76)	3.75 to −10.50
VISX	6	Preop −5.90 (±2.14)	−2.00 to −11.38
(n = 169)		Postop −0.27 (± 1.87)	6.38 to −8.25

*Retrospective match-controlled review: Summit versus VISX at 6 months postop.

correction was one of the primary reasons why we decided to add it to our practice despite satisfactory performance by the Summit excimer laser in spherical correction. The VISX laser uses a slit superimposed on the iris diaphragm pattern to give varying amounts of astigmatic correction combined with spherical correction. Cylinder correction can also be performed even when there is no spherical component.

We found after an initial small internal study that we were obtaining approximately 25% to 75% correction of the astigmatism with the original VISX algorithm (average, 50%). We therefore elected to consistently add 30% to the astigmatic correction, reasoning that even those patients currently obtaining 75% correction would be unlikely to have astigmatism correction. This has indeed improved the overall performance of the astigmatism correction from an average of 50% to 60%. Because we are adding an additional 30% to the astigmatism we elected to reduce the associated spherical correction by an amount equivalent to 15% of the original cylinder so as to reduce the chances of obtaining overall overcorrection as a result of our adjustment.

The Summit laser has for some time had available the erodible or ablatable mask for astigmatic correction. To this point, however, the mask has had to be handheld above the eye and we found that, especially with the coarser controls of the Summit chair, it was very difficult and time-consuming to accurately and consistently position this mask. This raised questions as to whether one might inadvertently introduce some significant decentration with its use, or dehdyration of the cornea, while taking time to position the mask.

Of the handful of cases that we have done, we found an approximate 50% reduction in cylinder (similar to the VISX) but we await the introduction of a mask that can be inserted into the optical rail before rendering any judgment on its accuracy and effectiveness in astigmatism correction.

In an analysis of 41 cases of elliptic pattern astigmatic correction with the VISX excimer laser, we obtained an almost 50% reduction in the cylinder (Table 14-4). (This was without our 30% correction factor.) The VISX astigmatic correction offers two modes called elliptic and sequential. In the elliptic pattern there is a more physiologic tapering of the astigmatic pattern along both axes, whereas the sequential pattern makes essentially a cylindrical cut from the corneal surface leaving a definite stepped edge at either end of the long axis of the astigmatic correction. The elliptic pattern can be used where the sphere is equal to or greater than the cylinder correction (e.g., −3.00, −3.00 × 180 or −3.00 −1.50 × 180). The sequential pattern must be used where the cylinder correction exceeds the amount of sphere (e.g., −3.00 −3.25 × 180 or −1.00 −3.00 × 180). Although we have done most cases with the elliptic correction, we have found similar results with the two patterns, but generally prefer using the elliptic pattern as much as possible because of its seemingly more physiologic recontouring of the cornea.

Clinical Comparison

We compared the two lasers retrospectively for the purpose of this chapter. We had not contemplated doing a prospective comparison of the two lasers up to this point because we felt that the difference between the 5-mm optical zone for the Summit and the 6-mm optical zone for the VISX would probably invalidate such a comparison in the opinion of most outside observers. This then remains a significant difference in this retrospective study.

We matched spherical corrections (1.00 D or less of astigmatism) to within 0.25 D, with the range for the Summit being −2.0 D to −11.50 D and for the VISX from −2.0 D to −11.38 D (Table 14-5). The cases were compared at the 6-month postoperative interval. This limited the number of cases available from the VISX group because we had only used the VISX for a little over 1 year. Additionally, for many of the VISX cases with 1.00 D of astigmatism, we had chosen to use astigmatic correction which would make them ineligible for comparison. The Summit group resulted in a postoperative spherical equivalent of −0.72 (+1.76), while the VISX group was −0.17 D (±1.87).

Medications

The majority of the Summit cases used dexamethasone 1.0% (Maxidex) four times daily for the first month, followed by fluoromethalone (FML) in a taper-

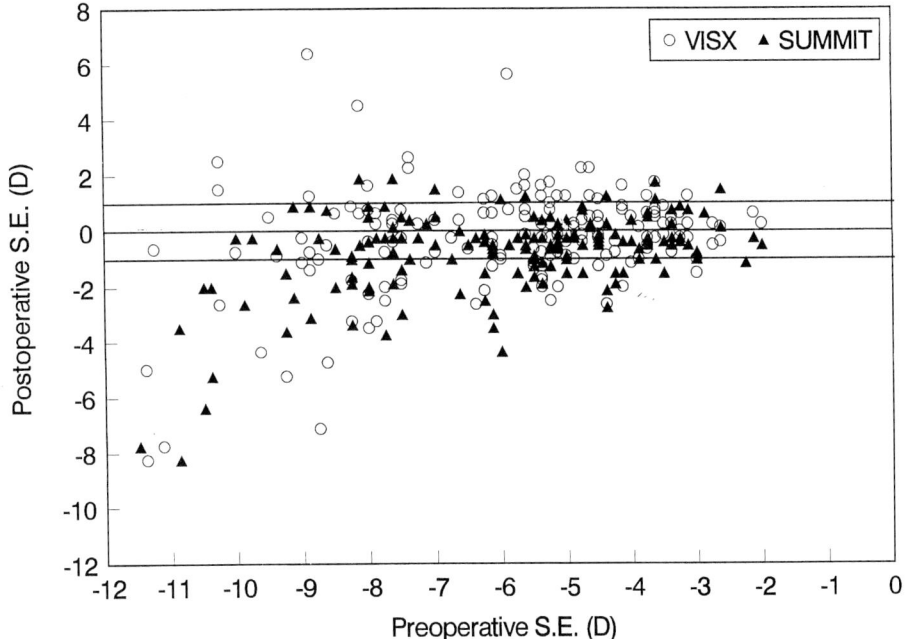

Fig. 14-3. Scattergram of pre and post-op S.E. comparing VISX and Summit lasers.

ing dose over the following 2 to 3 months. The majority of VISX cases used fluoromethalone 0.1% and ketorolac 0.5% (Acular) on a tapering pattern for 3 to 4 months postoperatively starting at four times daily for the first month. We have noted more recently that for patients showing strong haze and regression effects (type III response), enhancement (excimer retreatment) followed by application of fluoromethalone and ketorolac for an extended period of time postoperatively has reduced the recurrence rate of haze and regression. Because we are now using this routinely for all our VISX patients, one might expect that this would reduce the incidence and severity of haze for VISX patients as compared to Summit patients. On the other hand, the larger optical zone used for the VISX would mean deeper ablation depths for the VISX patients of the same level of correction and we would expect this to give rise to more haze. This may have some bearing on the incidence of haze reported in comparing the Summit and VISX groups, but these two factors, one in favor of the VISX and the other in favor of the Summit, may be canceling each other out.

Refractive Results

Table 14-6 summarizes the results over the entire range of correction for both lasers. The two lasers show no significant difference between them of eyes achieving 20/20 or better, 20/40 or better, or spherical equivalents within ±1.0 D of emmetropia. Figure 14-3 shows the correlation between preoperative and 6 months postoperative spherical equivalents for the two lasers. In observing the significant outliers, one

Table 14-6. Visual acuity results of VISX and Summit excimer lasers

	Summit		VISX
VAsc 20/20 or better	53.8%	p = 0.2	46.1%
VAsc 20/40 or better	80.5%	p = 0.9	79.1%
Achieved SE* ±1.00 D	65%	p = 0.7	62%

*Achieved spherical equivalent ± 1 D emmetropia.

should be aware that even after 6 months, most of the hyperopic corrections will tend to decrease and most of the major undercorrections would not as yet have had enhancement. Figure 14-4 shows preoperative myopic uncorrected visual acuity at 6 months by preoperative spherical equivalent. Of the 46 matched eyes with preoperative myopia of −2.0 to −4.0 D, 73.9% achieved a visual acuity of 20/20 or better in the VISX group compared with 71.7% in the Summit group. For 55 eyes per laser group with preoperative myopia of between 4.0 D and 6.0 D (58.2% and 60.0%) achieved 20/20 or better. For eyes with preoperative myopia greater than 6.0 D, 38.2% and 41.2% achieved an uncorrected visual acuity of 20/20 or better in the VISX and Summit groups, respectively.

Postoperative Spherical Equivalents Over Time

The question has often been raised as to whether one laser or the other shows greater overcorrection initially. As shown in Figure 14-5 there is little difference in the postoperative pattern in our comparison group.

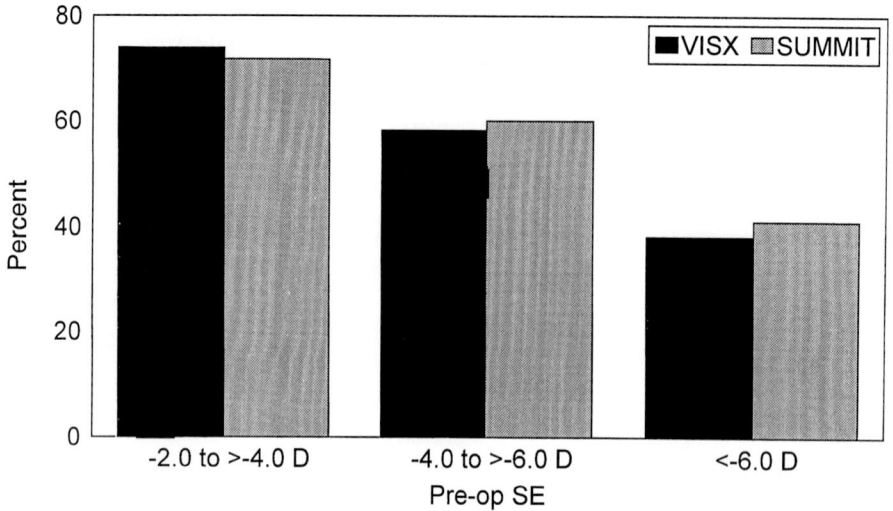

Fig. 14-4. Uncorrected visual acuities of 20/20 or better achieved by the VISX and Summit excimer lasers. Grouped according to preoperative spherical equivalent (SE).

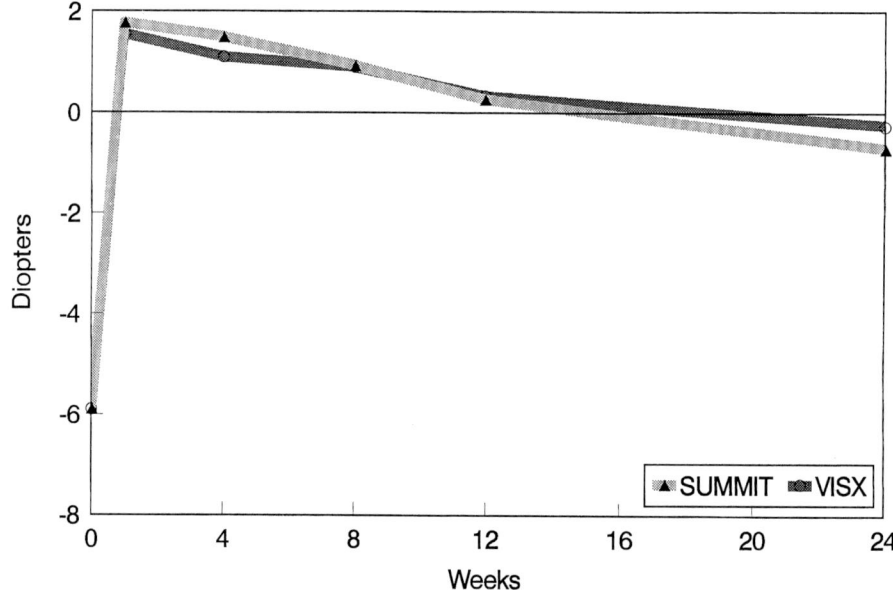

Fig. 14-5. A comparison of the Summit and VISX S.E. over time.

Both lasers still show some apparent regression at 24 weeks postoperatively, primarily because the higher corrections in our group still tended to show some regression, thus bringing down the average, even at 6 months and somewhat beyond.

Corneal Haze

The prevalence of haze at 6 months postoperatively at the various levels is noted in Table 14-7. For the majority of patients the cornea is rated as clear at 6 months. The Summit laser shows somewhat more patients at the trace and moderate level, whereas the

Table 14-7. Haze results of VISX and Summit lasers.*

	Summit (n = 169)		VISX (n = 169)
Clear	98 (58%)	p = 0.57	104 (62.7%)
Trace	49 (29%)	p = 0.13	36 (21.3%)
Mild	13 (7.7%)	p = 0.08	24 (14.2%)
Moderate	7 (4.1%)	p = 0.17	2 (1.2%)
Marked	2 (1.2%)	p = 0.98	3 (1.8%)

*Retrospective match-controlled review: Prevalence of haze at 6 months postop.

Table 14-8. BCVA loss in two or more lines at 6 months postop in VISX and summit lasers

	Patient	BCVA	Haze	Ref at 6 mo.	Preop Ref
Summit (n = 169)	1	20/30	Trace-mild	$-0.25\ -0.75 \times 05$	$-5.00\ -0.25 \times 08$
	2	20/40	Moderate	$-0.25\ -1.75 \times 34$	$-9.00\ -0.75$
	3	20/25	Moderate	$-3.0\ -1.25 \times 155$	$-8.00\ -1.00$
	4	20/30	Mild	$+0.50\ -1.25 \times 60$	$-6.00\ -0.50 \times 78$
VISX (n = 169)	1	20/30	Moderate	-2.50	$-7.25\ -1.00 \times 154$
	2	20/25	Mild	$-1.75\ -0.50 \times 150$	$-7.50\ -1.25 \times 101$
	3	20/50	Marked	$-7.00\ -1.00 \times 180$	$-10.75\ -0.75 \times 160$
	4	20/30	Marked	-7.00	$-10.00\ -0.75 \times 150$
	5	20/40	Marked	$+2.50\ -1.75 \times 55$	$-6.00\ -1.00 \times 90$

VISX laser shows more patients at the mild level. Overall there does not appear to be any statistically significant difference between the prevalence of haze at 6 months postoperatively. Most cases of haze would continue to improve after 6 months and most cases showing moderate or marked haze would also be associated with regression and in most cases would be re-treated.

Best Corrected Visual Acuity Loss

Of our total population of 169 patients in each group, there were only nine patients demonstrating two or more lines of loss of best corrected visual acuity at 6 months: four for the Summit and five for the VISX. These results are summarized in Table 14-8.

No patient had worse than 20/50 vision. All patients were at least 5 D and six of the nine patients had moderate to marked haze. Four of these six cases also showed significant regression and would be retreated with the excimer laser likely clearing most, if not all, of the haze with re-treatment. There was no significant difference in the incidence of loss of best corrected visual acuity.

CONCLUSION

In our experience the VISX and Summit lasers have performed in a satisfactory manner with no statisti-

cally significant difference between their corrections of simple spherical myopia. The difference in optical zone size is significant in terms of patient satisfaction for night vision situations, but this is now irrelevant in view of the fact that both lasers have ablation diameters of at least 6 mm. We summarize the main differences between the two lasers as follows:

1. The VISX has better astigmatism correction capability.
2. The Summit shows minimal central island effect.
3. The Summit allows treatment of more patients within a given period.
4. The Summit is simpler and somewhat less expensive to operate.
5. The VISX is more comfortable to use in regard to patient positioning and surgeon position and function.

For patients with any significant degree of astigmatism (greater than 1 D) we prefer the VISX laser, and for simple spherical corrections, primarily because of the central island concern, we prefer the Summit. We recommend both the VISX and Summit lasers at present over any new lasers, but recommend keeping an open mind with regard to new developments.

Phototherapeutic Keratectomy: The VISX Experience

Dimitri T. Azar, Sandeep Jain, Kristin Woods, Walter Stark,
Donald R. Sanders, Shigeru Kinoshita

EXCIMER LASER

The VISX excimer laser is an argon fluoride laser that emits high-energy ultraviolet radiation of 193-nm wavelength. It is capable of ablating the cornea with submicron precision without significant injury to adjacent nonablated tissue. It can be used for the controlled removal of corneal tissue in creating a new corneal curvature or in reconstructive superficial keratectomy.

PHOTOTHERAPEUTIC KERATECTOMY

Phototherapeutic keratectomy (PTK) is the removal of anterior layers of a diseased cornea using the excimer laser. Excimer laser ablation has great potential for excising corneal opacities and smoothing corneal surface irregularities.

PTK is currently undergoing Food and Drug Administration (FDA)–sponsored multicentric trials to assess its safety and therapeutic effectiveness in humans. In 1983, Trokel et al.[1] introduced the excimer laser as a prospective tool in corneal surgery, but not until 1988 was it used in investigational protocols involving humans.[2] The far-ultraviolet light, which is emitted in pulses, ablates corneal tissue with unprecedented precision.[2-4] The photochemical laser-tissue interaction, termed *ablative photodecomposition*, allows accurate removal of tissue.[1,5] It removes surface molecules by disrupting and breaking organic molecular bonds, but does not cause optical breakdown.[1,4]

The depth and shape of excimer laser ablative photodecomposition can be accurately controlled to within several microns.[1,4,6] Compared with mechanical methods, this allows for a more exact removal of the stroma and, in turn, provides a relatively smooth base for better reepithelialization and re-formation of basement membrane complexes, and produces minimal corneal scarring.[2,4,6] Use of the excimer laser in corneal surgery also reduces the risks involved in handling donor buttons.[6]

Safety

The 193-nm laser radiation is considered to be within the limits of safety for ultraviolet light used in corneal surgery. In contrast to the erosions and irregular and diffuse tissue damage caused by the 248-nm krypton excimer laser, the argon laser produces a focused smooth-edge incision with relatively no adjacent tissue damage. Incisions made with diamond and steel blades also produce irregular and diffuse tissue damage, whereas the excimer laser produces incisions with sealed surfaces and smooth lamellar sections.[6,7] Adjacent tissues undergo minimal distortion and suffer no apparent thermal damage. The stromal lamellae show no evidence of distant disorganization.[1,2,4,6] There is evidence of endothelial cell loss, which may be due to shock waves; however, as long as the unablated stromal thickness is more than 40 μm, the endothelium remains intact.[6] The only cells affected by the radiation or wound-healing process are generally those that are actually exposed to the laser energy.[8,9] The possibility of DNA damage and thermal side effects in the surrounding tissue is a controversial issue; the 193-nm radiation is less potentially mutagenic than that of longer wavelengths.[3,8]

Precision

Wound healing following PTK differs from that of classic surgery, in that there is a very clear boundary between the tissue involved in wound healing and the adjacent cellular structures.[8] Reepithelialization and complete wound healing begin quickly and are associated with a small degree of tissue reorganization.[6] The laser provides corneal surgeons with an excellent cutting instrument for the management of anterior stromal opacities, one which no other current form of surgical intervention can provide.[6] Successfully treated patients can postpone or avoid more invasive surgical procedures, such as penetrating or lamellar keratoplasty.[2]

PHOTOTHERAPEUTIC KERATECTOMY PROTOCOL

Inclusion Criteria

All patients entering the FDA-sponsored PTK trials have significant functional impairment and are candidates for conventional invasive surgery. In accordance with FDA regulations, patients must meet the eligibility criteria defined by the individual Institutional Review Boards and VISX.

Visual impairment due to opacities in the anterior third of the cornea. The opacities may result from surgical or nonsurgical trauma, corneal inflammations, dystrophies, and degenerations. Therapeutic excimer laser ablations have been used to successfully treat posttraumatic and postinfectious leukoma; herpetic scars; Reis-Buckler's, granular, and lattice stromal dystrophy; corneal nodule; and recurrent band keratopathy.

Visual impairment due to fine corneal surface irregularities. The irregularities may result from epithelial dystrophies, Reis-Buckler's dystrophy, band keratopathy, and peripheral corneal degenerations, or may arise from surgical procedures such as lamellar keratectomy.

Superficial infectious keratitis resistant to medical treatment. Therapeutic excimer laser ablations have been used in the successful sterilization of microorganism cultures, experimental microbial keratitis, and a case of infectious crystalline keratopathy.[10-13] This indication for surgery has not often been employed because of the risk of spreading of microorganisms during treatment.[14]

In a review of 271 consecutive PTK cases at 17 centers in the United States, Sanders[15] observed that 55% of patients had corneal scars or leukomas, 39% had corneal dystrophies, and 5% had corneal surface irregularities.

Significant functional impairment due to pathologic or postsurgical refractive abnormalities of the eye. The abnormalities include significant anisometropia, symptomatic anisokonia, and residual refractive error following refractive corneal surgery, intraocular lens implantation, keratoplasty, or trauma.

Exclusion Criteria

Patients who are immunocompromised and those having uncontrolled uveitis, severe blepharitis, lagophthalmos, or dry eye do not qualify as candidates for PTK under the VISX protocol. One third of total corneal thickness is the maximum amount of corneal tissue that can be removed with PTK. The pretreatment corneal thickness must be such that the immediate posttreatment corneal thickness will not be less than 250 μm. In patients with similar pathologic changes in both eyes, the nondominant eye is treated first. The minimum time period between two treatments, whether second eye treatment or same eye retreatment, is set at 6 months.

Relative Contraindications

Phototherapeutic keratectomy may induce significant hyperopia in many patients. Patients who are near plano correction, or who are already hyperopic, may not qualify as candidates for PTK.

PREOPERATIVE EVALUATION

Preoperative evaluations are performed within 90 days of the procedure. Visual acuity is evaluated without correction and with manifest refraction. Visual potential is evaluated with pinhole, hard contact lens, and potential acuity meter. Pupil size is recorded in normal room light and near-dark illumination. Anterior segment examination, slit-lamp biomicroscopy, and dilated fundus examination are performed, as well as measurement of ocular pressure, keratometry, and ultrasonic pachymetry. External, slit-lamp photographs and computerized topographic analysis of the cornea are also obtained. The depth of the intended treatment is measured using an optical pachymeter.

Patients are informed of the investigational nature of the laser procedure, and a signed informed consent document is obtained prior to surgery.

PREOPERATIVE PREPARATION

Patients receive preoperative systemic medications (analgesic-sedatives). Unless contraindicated, 30 mg of codeine and 10 mg of diazepam are administered orally. The patient is placed in the operating chair and positioned under the microscope. The use of a Vac-Pac headrest minimizes head movements. The eye is draped and prepared for surgery. The patient fixates on the blinking red light of the microscope.

Currently, all procedures are performed under topical anesthesia with 0.5% proparacaine drops. Before treatment, the plane of the corneal surface is determined by focusing the microscope at high magnification (×18). The magnification is then decreased to the normal level (×12) for final centering on the entrance pupil. Poor centration of laser treatment may result in a suboptimal outcome.

The laser is calibrated before each treatment to ensure optimal performance. The overall operation of the laser is confirmed by ablating a standard lens (−4D) into a polymethylmethacrylate (PMMA) test block using photorefractive keratectomy (PRK) software. The lens is read by a lensometer, and when it has the predetermined optical power, the appropriate value for the corneal ablation rate is determined using the nomograms, and entered into the computer program.

VISX LASER TREATMENT
Parameters

Table 15-1 summarizes the laser parameters that are ordinarily adopted for PTK using the VISX laser. Initiation and termination of ablation are achieved using foot pedal control. Nitrogen gas flow, used during the

Table 15-1. Typical laser parameters for phototherapeutic keratectomy

Fluence	160 ±10 mJ/cm^2
Repetition rate	5 Hz
Ablation rate	0.20-0.35 μm per pulse
Ablation diameter	5.5-6.0 mm including 0.5-mm transition zone
Ablation depths	
Epithelium	40 μm (default value) or as determined by pachymetry
Stroma	Depth of scar or opacity (postoperative corneal thickness should be ≥250 μm)

PMMA calibration, is not used intraoperatively because of potential desiccation of the cornea.

Epithelial Removal: Manual vs. Laser

Ablation through the epithelium is performed with straight walled cuts. The decision whether to ablate using the laser or to remove the epithelium manually is based on the smoothness of the epithelium relative to the envisioned smoothness of Bowman's layer. When the anterior stromal surface is irregular, the epithelium, in situ, acts as a smoothing agent and is ablated with the laser. If the anterior surface of the stroma is judged to be smooth, the epithelium may be removed manually with a Bard-Parker blade.

Masking Agents

Following epithelial removal, a masking fluid (surface modulator) may be applied to help achieve a regular and smooth stromal surface by masking the deeper tissues (valleys) while exposing the protruding irregularities (peaks). The fluid in valleys prevents ablation of underlying tissue, while the exposed peaks are ablated. A highly viscous fluid does not cover an irregular surface uniformly, resists leveling, and tends to partially cover peaks as well as valleys. A fluid of low viscosity tends to run off quickly, exposing both peaks and valleys. Kornmehl et al.[16] have reported good results using Tears Naturale II, a solution of moderate viscosity and high absorbance at 193 nm. Gartry et al.[17] have reported 1% HPMC to be a more suitable masking agent than 2% HPMC and polyvinyl alcohol. Stark et al.[2] have used a 1:2 combination of 1% methylcellulose and Tears Naturale II. Fasano et al.[18] suggest using relatively low repetition rates, as this allows time for the applied fluid to flow over the corneal surface, filling relatively deep depressions in the cornea, and also allows the operator to make intraoperative adjustments. In addition to creating a smooth corneal surface, masking agents may reduce the amount of induced hyperopia. Table 15-2 shows masking agents used in previous studies.

Table 15-2. Masking agents used in phototherapeutic keratectomy

Study (yr)	Best masking	Moderate masking	Poor masking
Fitzsimmons & Fager-holm[19] (1991)	0.5% tetracaine	Healon yellow	2% HPMC
Fasano et al.[18] (1991)	0.3% HPMC at 2 Hz	0.3% HPMC at 10 Hz	
Kornmehl et al.[16] (1991)	Tears Naturale II	Carboxymethylcellulose sodium (Cellu-visc), Unisol	
Englanoff et al.[20] (1992)	Collagen gel		

Stromal Ablation

During stromal ablation, a transition zone 0.5 mm in width is created between the normal stromal surface and the final depth of ablation as a default setting. The slope of the S-shaped transition zone gradually increases at the top of the ablation, and gradually decreases at the bottom of ablation. The transition zone is intended to allow smooth and uniform reepithelialization over the ablation bed. This procedure is referred to as "standard taper" ablation. Stark et al.[2] have described a "modified taper" technique, wherein the surgeon attempts to decrease central flattening by moving the eye under the laser in a circular fashion, and treating the circumference of the ablation zone with a 20-μm-deep, 2-mm-diameter spot size. This edge modification creates a ring-shaped ablation pattern at the periphery of the PTK, and the resultant corneal contour simulates a convex (plus) lens. A positive trend in reducing the hyperopic shift has been reported with this technique (Fig. 15-1). Sher et al.[21] used a "smoothing" technique in their early cases, wherein the eye was moved in a circular manner under the laser beam, which was of varying aperture size. This technique was later abandoned as it was impossible to predict the achieved ablation depth. When corneal opacities or irregularities are associated with myopic refractive errors, a combination of PTK and PRK should be considered. After allowing for approximately 1 D of hyperopic shift for every 20 μm of stromal ablation, the residual refractive error can be treated with PRK.

POSTOPERATIVE TREATMENT AND EVALUATION

Postoperative medications include prophylactic antibiotics and anti-inflammatory steroids. Sub-Tenon's injection of 20 mg of gentamicin and 1 mg of dexamethasone is given immediately postoperatively. After topical application of antibiotic ointment (bacitracin and erythromycin) and instillation of a cycloplegic agent (homatropine), the eye is patched. Since the patient may experience severe pain in the first 24 hours, systemic sedative-analgesics (meperidine [Demerol] or acetaminophen [Tylenol] with codeine) are prescribed as needed. One percent prednisolone acetate or 0.1% fluoromethalone drops are used four times daily for 1 week, then tapered to once daily by 1 month. The steroid drops are continued once daily for 6 months if no steroid responsiveness occurs.

Patients are examined every 24 to 48 hours until reepithelialization, and then at 1 month, 3 months, 6 months, 12 months, and 24 months. Reepithelialization occurs within 1 week in most patients. Following reepithelialization, the postoperative examination at each visit includes symptomatic evaluation, a detailed anterior segment examination, and slit-lamp biomicroscopy. In addition, all measurements (visual acuity, ocular pressure, etc.) taken during the preoperative evaluation are repeated.

Corneal haze is monitored during the slit-lamp examination and subjectively graded as follows: 0 = clear; 0.5 = barely detectable; 1.0 = mild, not affecting refraction; 1.5 = mildly affecting refraction; 2.0 =

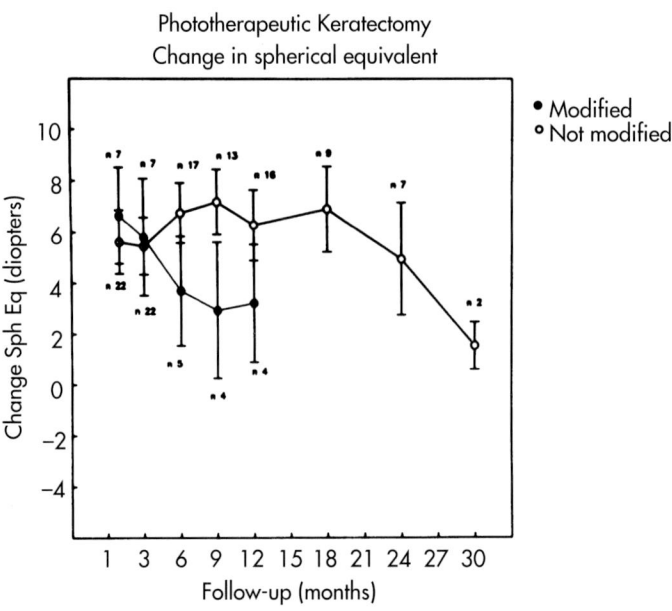

Fig. 15-1. Relationship between the induced refractive change and the time following PTK. In those patients with modified treatment, the refractive change stabilizes at a level of reduced hyperopia *(full circles)* when compared with the standard treatment *(empty circles).*

moderate, refraction possible but difficult; 3.0 = opacity preventing refraction, anterior chamber easily viewed; 4.0 = impaired view of anterior chamber; and 5.0 = inability to see the anterior chamber. The cornea is divided into five hypothetical layers (superficial and deep epithelium, anterior and posterior stroma, and endothelium), and each layer is graded separately.

Subjective methods of grading corneal haze are not accurate and reproducible, and suffer from interobserver variability and bias. Objective methods assess the magnitude of haze by measuring corneal light scattering. In collaboration with Dr. Russell McCally of the Applied Physics Laboratory at Johns Hopkins, we have developed an instrument for the objective measurement of haze. The "scatterometer" is a modified slit-lamp microscope that measures backscattered light from a defined region of the cornea under standardized illumination conditions. Corneal light scattering is related to the degree of stromal scarring following excimer laser ablations. This instrument has been tested on laboratory animals and humans and found to yield reproducible results.[22] Both objective and subjective postoperative corneal clarity scores are usually lower than preoperative scores after PTK.

RESULTS

Representative postoperative results published in previous reports are summarized in Table 15-3. Sher and colleagues[21] reported that 15% of their patients lost two or more lines of best corrected spectacles vi-sual acuity (BCVA) following PTK. Chamon et al.[22] reported a 3% loss of one line of functional visual acuity, defined as the acuity achieved with the visual aid that a patient is wearing, either contact lenses or spectacles. The mean preoperative visual acuity (logarithmic) was 20/92, and the mean postoperative visual acuity was 20/47 using manifest refraction. In 80% of patients, BCVA had improved one line or more at the most recent follow-up visit. Four patients became contact lens–tolerant after PTK.[23] The data comparing preoperative to postoperative BCVA accumulated by Sanders[15] from the 17 U.S. centers are shown in Figure 15-2, A and B. The average improvement in BCVA was 1.8 lines ($P < .001$). Ten percent (10%) of patients lost two or more lines of BCVA, while 45% gained two or more lines. Seven percent (7%) of the patients lost three or more lines, while 36% gained that much. Analysis of the reasons for decreases in BCVA showed corneal surface irregularity induced by PTK accounting for only 3% of cases. Two or more lines of improvement of uncorrected visual acuity were seen in 42% to 44% of patients, as opposed to reduction in 18% to 19% (Fig. 15-3).

The success rate of PRK depends on the attempted refractive change, and thus on the depth of ablation. Gartry et al.[25] presented data on a series of 120 eyes undergoing PRK with at least 1 year of follow-up. The success rate ranged from 95% for 2.0-D corrections to 20% for 7.0-D corrections. A similar unpredictability of refractive outcome may also accompany PTK. Eyes treated with the standard 0.5-μm taper had an average of 5.11 and 5.28 D of induced hyperopia at 3 and

Table 15-3. Initial results from three major studies

	Study		
	Sher et al.[21] (1991)	Chamon et al.[23] (1993)	Campos et al.[24] (1993)
Laser	Taunton LV 2000	VISX Twenty-Twenty	VISX Twenty-Twenty
Ablation technique	Myopic	Standard taper	Uniform depth (disk ablation)
	Combined smoothing	Modified taper	
Visual acuity			
Better	48%	74%	61%
Unchanged	36%	16%	28%
Worse	15%	10%	11%
Hyperopic shift	50%	—	56%
Best results (>75% success)	Keratoconus (apical scar)	Corneal dystrophies (lattice, granular, Reis-Buckler's); Salsman's degeneration	Corneal dystrophies (lattice, map dot, granular)
Moderate results (50%-75% success)	Corneal dystrophies; postinfectious and posttraumatic scar; Salzmann's degeneration	Corneal scars; surgically induced myopia	
Poor results (<25% success)	Recurrent erosions; herpetic scars; granular dystrophy; band keratopathy	Band keratopathy; untreated recurrent erosions	Postinfectious and posttraumatic scar; calcification; band keratopathy

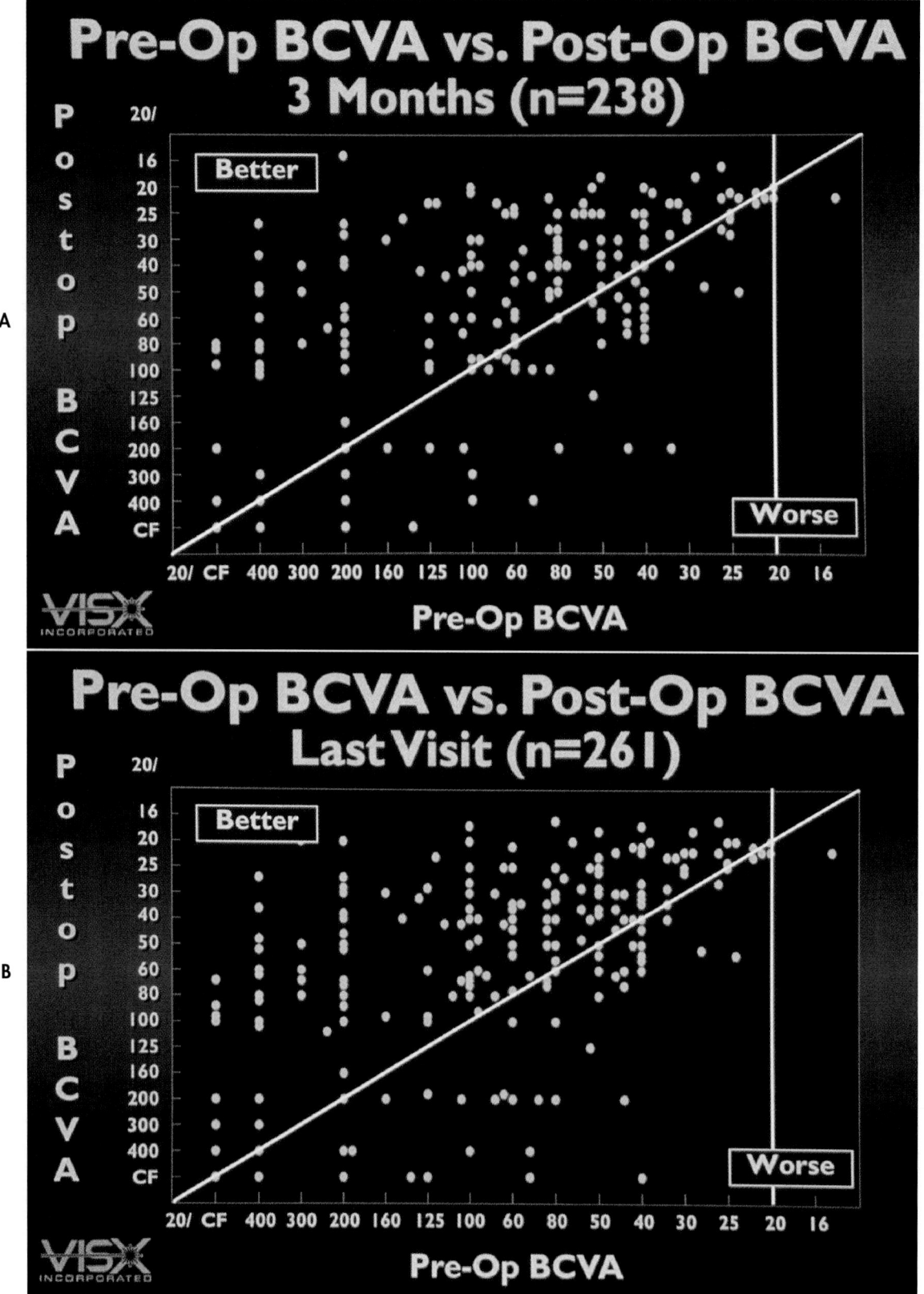

Fig. 15-2.   A, Scatterplot of pre vs. 3-month posttreatment best corrected visual acuity (BCVA). Cases above the diagonal line had an improvement in BCVA and cases below were made worse. **B,** Comparison of pretreatment vs. last-visit BCVA (1-42 months; average, 9 months).

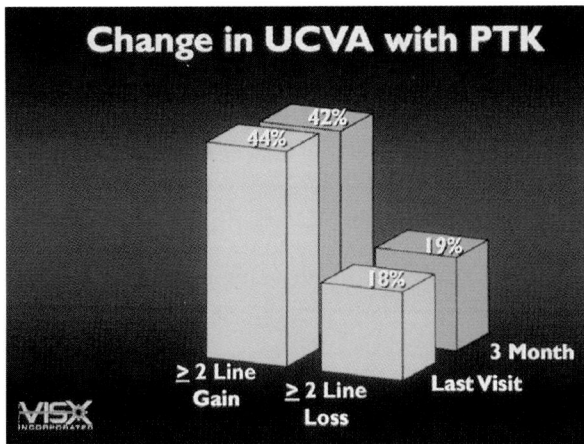

Fig. 15-3. Improvement in uncorrected visual acuity, while not a defining goal, was achieved: 42% to 44% of patients had a gain of two or more lines of uncorrected acuity, and only 18% to 19% had an equivalent loss.

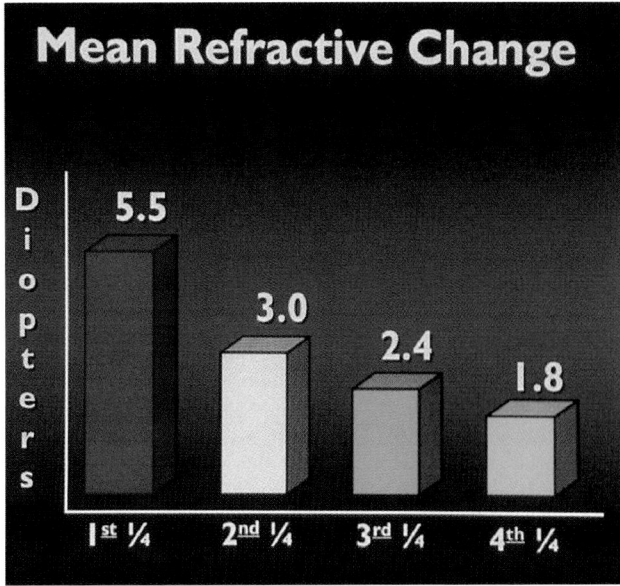

Fig. 15-4. Patients were divided into four groups or quartiles based on the date of treatment. The group or quartile that was treated initially had a change in spherical equivalent of 5.5 D. By the second quartile, the mean had been decreased by almost 50% to 3.2 D. The last series demonstrated less than 2.0 D of refractive effect. Thus, it appears that marked hyperopic shifts are no longer a problem.

36 months, respectively. Eyes treated with the modified taper showed a trend toward a decreasing amount of induced hyperopia.[23] Chamon et al.[23] observed a positive correlation between depth of stromal ablation and amount of induced hyperopia.

Campos et al.[24] performed PTK on 18 eyes. The follow-up ranged from 2 to 18 months, with a mean of 8 months. Corneal clarity improved in 77.7% of the patients, while 22.2% did not experience any improvement. In 61.1% of the patients, uncorrected visual acuity improved. An induced flattening was observed in all patients, and a hyperopic shift was observed in 55.5%. This induced hyperopia was observed to decreased by the 6-month and 1-year follow-ups. Patients with band keratopathy and corneal calcification who underwent PTK did not experience any visual improvement. As there was no recurrence of disease or surface problems in the successfully treated patients during follow-up, PTK appears to be a safe and effective way to avoid more invasive procedures for patients with selected stromal opacities.[24] Based on the dates of treatment, Sanders[15] divided the 271 patients treated at U.S. VISX centers into quartiles. He found that the first quartile had an average of 5.5 D

of hyperopic effect and the last quartile had less than 2.0 D of hyperopia (Fig. 15-4).

In addition to these studies, independent investigators have also reported results of PTK. McDonnell and Seiler[26] reported the successful management of Reis-Buckler's corneal dystrophy in two patients. Forster et al.[27] described the successful management of posttraumatic recurrent corneal erosions in all nine of their patients.

Ablation of definite corneal proturberances has produced good clinical results. Steinert and Puliafito[28] reported increased contact lens tolerance following laser ablation of a recurrent fibroblastic nodule at the apex of a longstanding keratoconic cornea. Brancato et al.[29] reported successful ablation of a posttraumatic superficial corneal nodule.

Talamo et al.[30] have described clinical treatment

Table 15-4. Strategies for successful phototherapeutic keratectomy in superficial corneal abnormalities*

Pathologic lesion	Epithelial removal	Ablation technique	Masking fluid
Elevated, focal	No	Small spot size	Preoperatively, to adjacent normal epithelium
Extensive, evenly distributed	No	Large spot size; smoothing head rotation	Intraoperatively, if irregularities are increasing
Multiple, unevenly distributed	Yes	Varying spot size	Repeated focal application

*Data from Talamo JH, Steinert RF, Puliafito CA: *Refract Corneal Surg* 8:319-324, 1992.

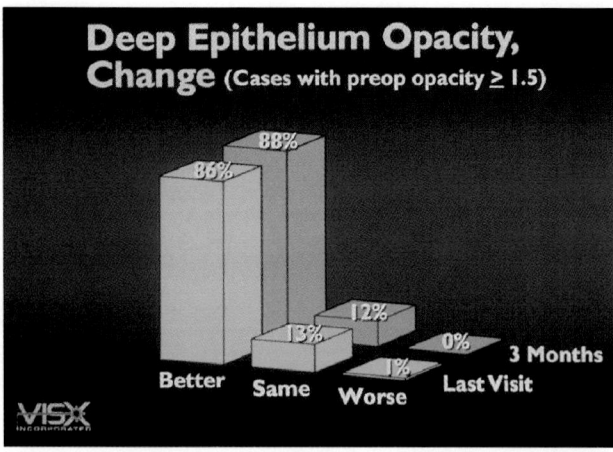

Fig. 15-5. Pre- and posttreatment changes in deep epithelial opacity scores: 86% to 88% of patients improved posttreatment and only 0% to 1% were worse. The cases improved by a statistically significant average of 3.3 categories.

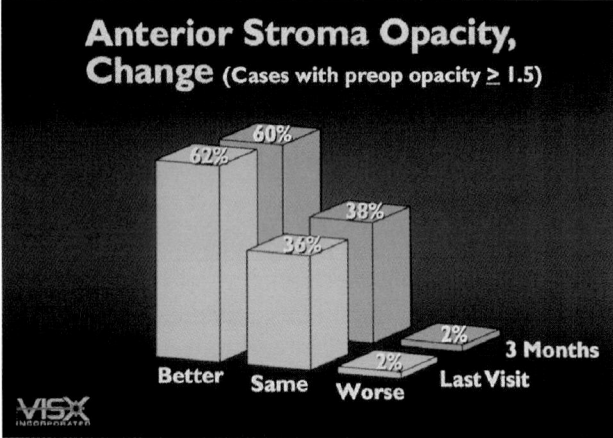

Fig. 15-6. Anterior stromal opacity change: 60% to 62% of patients improved posttreatment and 2% were worse. The cases improved by a statistically significant average of 2.0 categories.

strategies for optimizing the successful application of PTK to treatment of superficial corneal abnormalities. Table 15-4 summarizes this approach.

A study of the effect of PTK on patients with moderate to severe epithelial corneal opacities shows that 86% to 88% of patients improved following treatment, and in only 1% did the condition worsen (Fig. 15-5). Sixty percent to 62% of patients with anterior stromal opacities improved after treatment, and 2% worsened (Fig. 15-6).

The percentages of patients in Sanders' review[15] who experienced moderate to severe levels of pain and tearing before treatment were 10% and 8%, respectively. Of these patients, only one experienced postoperative tearing; the rest were improved. Similarly, there was no significant worsening of photophobia, redness, or foreign body sensation.

DISCUSSION

Patients with recurrent granular or lattice dystrophy in a graft have relatively superficial lesions (Figs. 15-7, 15-8, and 15-9). The success rate in these cases is very high and is similar to that for primary Reis-Buckler's dystrophy, in which the deposits are limited to Bowman's layer[2] (Fig. 15-10). The results of PTK in granular dystrophy are also encouraging, even when there are residual hyaline deposits, probably because most of the diffuse haze between the granular deposits is ablated (Figs. 15-11 and 15-12). A particularly dramatic example of PTK for granular dystrophy is illustrated in Figures 15-13 and 15-14 from a case treated by Professor Kinoshita at Kyoto Medical School, Japan.

Most patients with recurrent corneal erosions respond well to 5% sodium chloride, manual epithelial debridement, or anterior stromal puncture, singly or in combination. Recalcitrant cases may benefit from

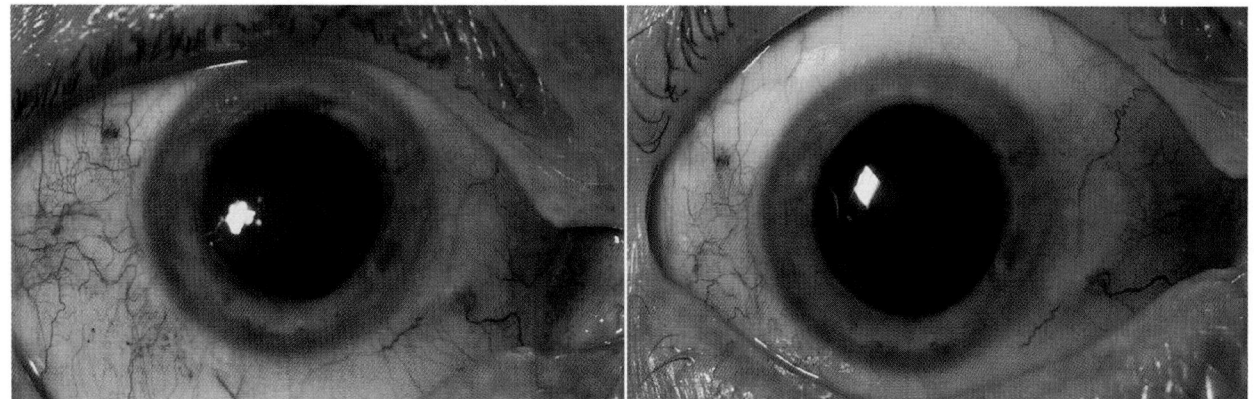

Fig. 15-7. A 47-year-old man who had undergone penetrating keratoplasty in the right eye for corneal lattice dystrophy 8 years previously presented with recurrent superficial dystrophy in the graft. **A,** clinical appearance prior to superficial laser ablation. **B,** 3 months postoperatively.

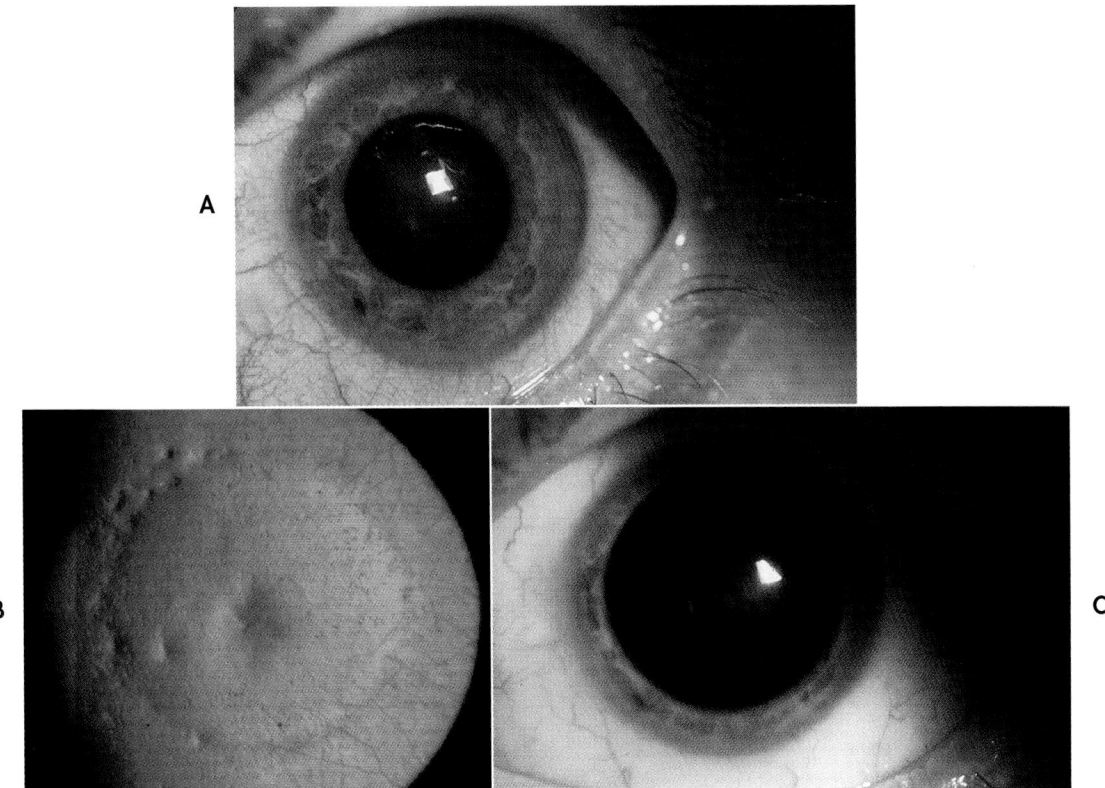

Fig. 15-8. A 31-year-old man with a history of corneal lattice dystrophy underwent PTK. Preoperative BCVA was 20/200. **A,** 75 μm stromal depth after epithelial ablation. **B,** appearance of cornea by retroillumination 3 months after PTK. **C,** marked improvement is seen 24 months postoperatively.

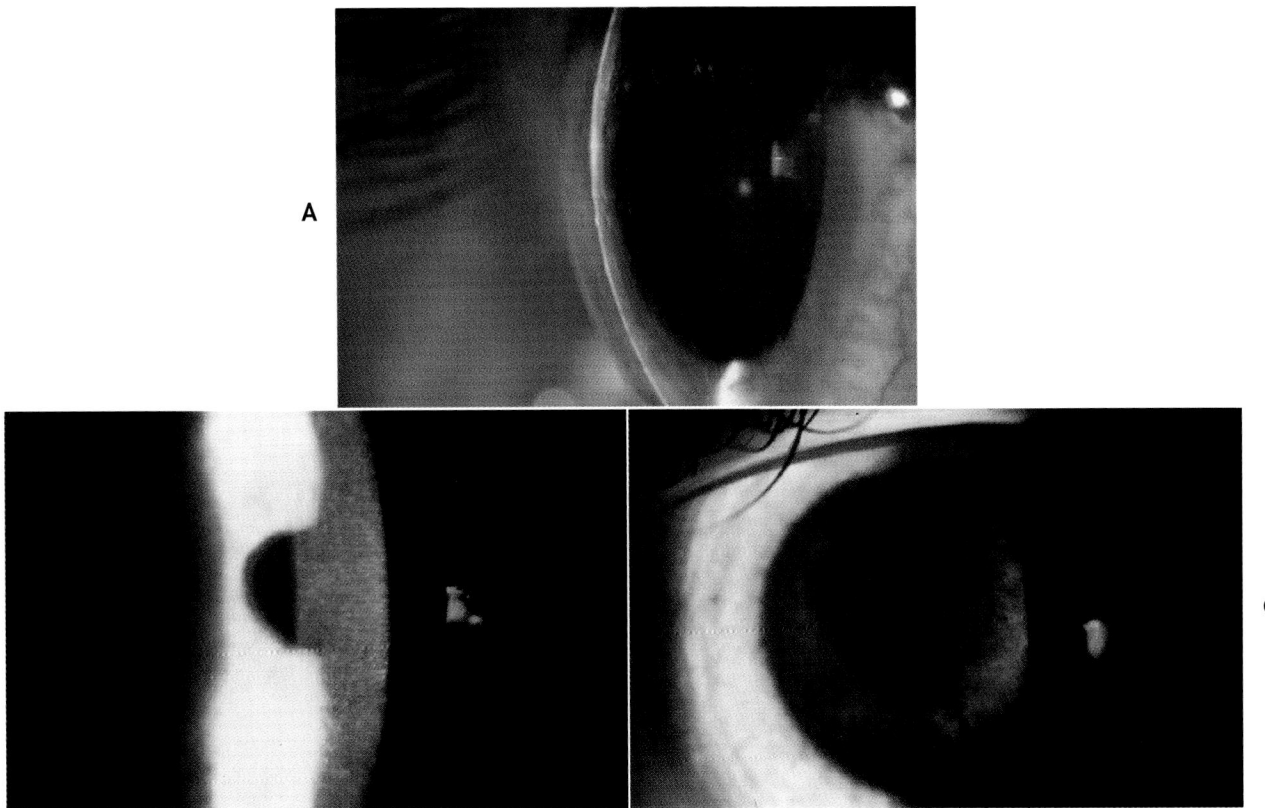

Fig. 15-9. Lattice dystrophy. **A,** preoperative appearance. **B,** 3 months post PTK. **C,** 9 months post PTK.

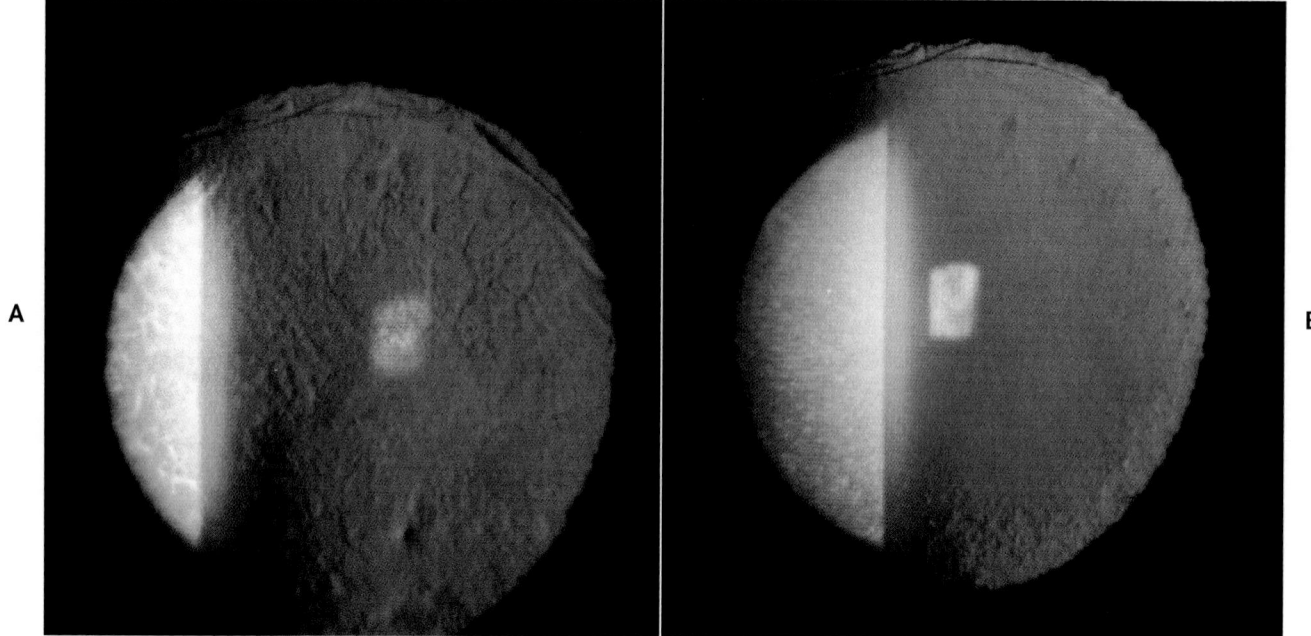

Fig. 15-10. Reis-Buckler's dystrophy. **A,** Pre-PTK. **B,** 3 months postoperatively. (From Chamon W, Azar DT, Stark WJ, et al: *Ophthalmol Clin North Am* 6:399-413, 1993. Used by permission.)

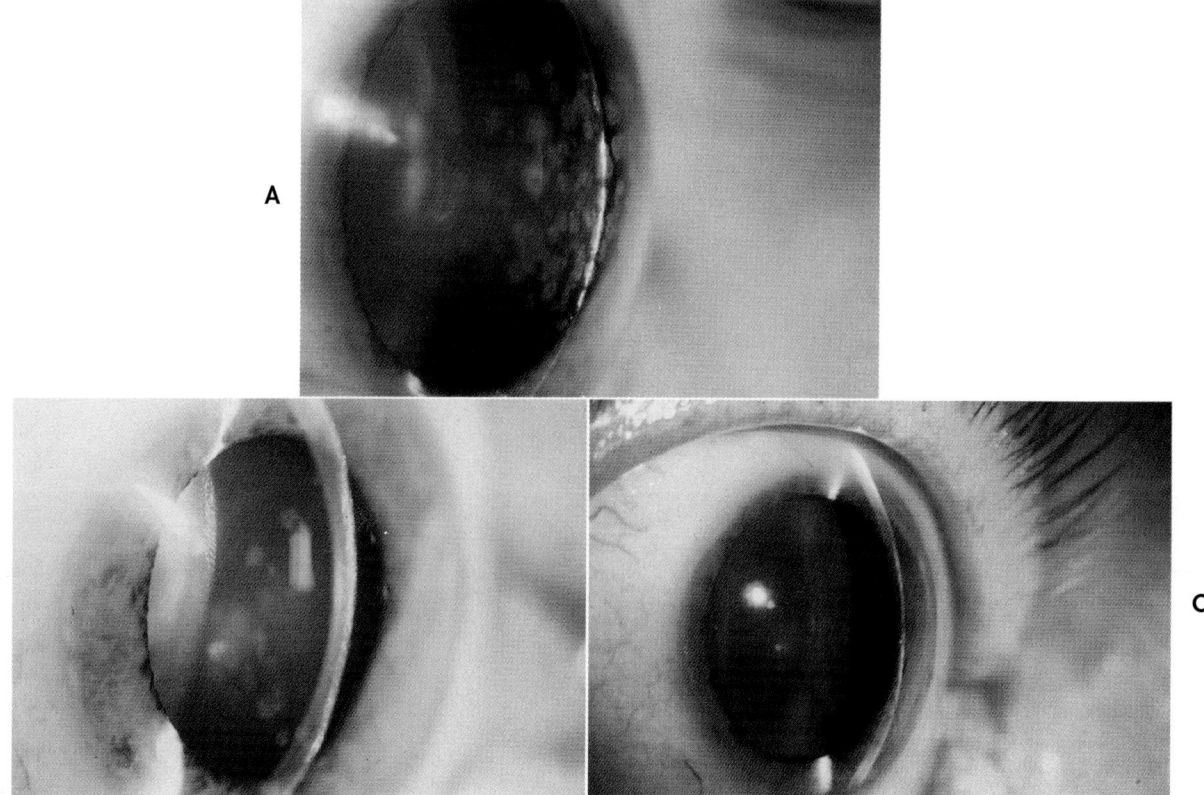

Fig. 15-11. A 73-year-old woman with a history of a granular dystrophy. The right eye received 100 μm of central ablation. **A,** Clinical appearance of granular dystrophy preoperatively, **B,** at 3 months, and **C,** at 9 months postoperatively.

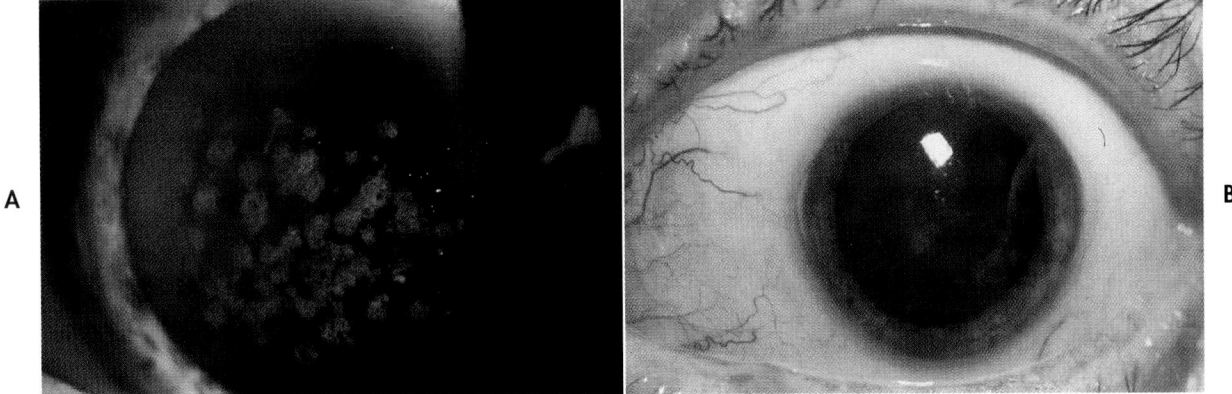

Fig. 15-12. Left eye of patient in Figure 15-11 treated with 40 μm of stromal ablation combined with a modified tapering procedure. **A,** preoperative clinical appearance of granular dystrophy. **B,** 9 months postoperatively.

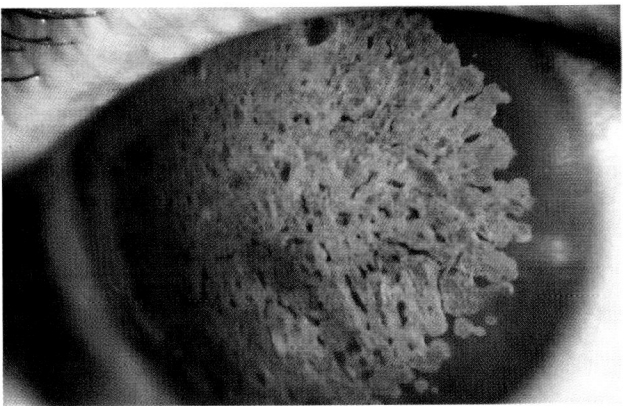

Fig. 15-13. Preoperative appearance of a patient with granular dystrophy. Visual acuity of hand motion. (Courtesy of Professor Kinoshita Kyota Medical School, Japan.)

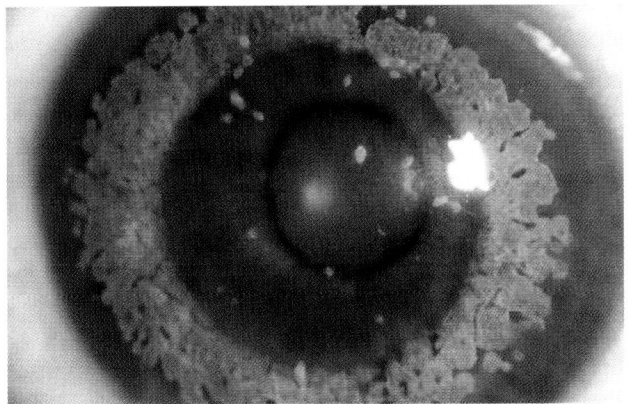

Fig. 15-14. Postoperative appearance of the patient in Figure 15-13 3 months following 195-μm ablation; 6.0-mm optical zone. Visual acuity improved to 20/400. (Courtesy of Professor Kinoshita, Kyoto Medical School, Japan.)

the use of excimer PTK to ablate the most superficial 5 to 10 μm of Bowman's layer. The depth of the treatment in this situation is relatively minimal. The ablation remains within Bowman's layer and thus, theoretically, the wound healing will differ from that following deeper PTK ablations. Additionally, the minimal depth of ablation is not associated with significant hyperopic shift. Forster et al.[27] reported successful treatment of all nine of their patients, while Sher et al.[20] report successful treatment in one of two patients that underwent PTK for traumatic recurrent erosions.

Treatment of corneal scars limited to the superficial stroma produced significant improvement of visual function in four of seven patients.[2] Campos et al.[24] reported significant visual improvement in only two of six patients with postinfectious scar, while none of the three patients with posttraumatic scar improved. Sher et al.[21] reported significant visual improvement in three of five patients with postinfectious scar while

five of the eight posttraumatic scar patients improved. These studies report a moderate success rate (33% to 62%) for the treatment of superficial corneal scars with PTK. This may be due to either the possibility that the scar ablates at a different rate than the adjacent normal stroma, or to the fact that the adjacent corneal stroma is normal and does not benefit from laser ablation (as opposed to that in corneal dystrophies). Differences in the rates of ablation for normal stroma and longstanding scar tissue, and the presence of calcified or cartilaginous tissue, may render PTK unsuccessful or may produce irregular astigmatism postoperatively.

For the most part, well-chosen PTK candidates heal relatively quickly with few but manageable complications.[2] Some patients complain of moderate to severe pain following surgery, and some have a delayed wound-healing process.[2,3] In one study, a patient with a history of heavy alcohol intake took 4 weeks to achieve corneal reepithelialization, compared to 1 week for the rest of the group. Within the same study, the cornea of a patient with Salzmann's nodular degeneration took 3 weeks to reepithelialize.[2] There is evidence of minimal corneal haze following PTK, but the principal undesired effect is the central flattening of the cornea.[2] Other postoperative complications include induced hyperopia, recurrent erosions, loss of endothelial cells, corneal ulcers, continuous epithelial defects, and infections.[2,7]

Postoperative pain may be severe during the first 24 to 48 hours. It is significantly diminished after 36 hours and is usually relieved by the time the epithelium heals. The use of cycloplegics, ice packs, peribulbar or retrobulbar anesthesia, narcotics, and disposable soft contact lenses may be required in addition to patient counseling.

According to Krueger et al.[31] the shorter penetration depth of direct 193-nm excimer laser radiation, along with the minimal fluorescent emission of longer ultraviolet wavelengths for energy exposures used in clinical applications, makes the potential side effects and risks of PTK very limited and remote. However, according to Seiler et al.,[32] DNA damage can result from clinical use of 193-nm radiation, and some regard thermal loading a major side effect. The limits of fluence and repetition rate should be defined in order to avoid thermal hazards.[33-34] Another result of ultraviolet radiation is photochemical injury, or photokeratitis; however, photokeratitis due to PTK could be caused only by irradiation with subablative laser light over a wide range of total energy exposures.[31]

If there are many complications or if the eyes do not improve significantly after PTK, the patient may need to undergo more invasive treatment such as corneal transplantation.[2]

Hyperopia appears to be the principal side effect of PTK. It may mandate the use of contact lens visual rehabilitation. Hyperopia is induced as a result of the corneal flattening that follows tissue removal, indicating that differential ablation akin to myopic PRK has occurred. Gartry et al.[17] have postulated four potential mechanisms for the hyperopic shift in some patients: (1) Constant irradiation from the laser may result in greater ablation centrally if the corneal abnormality thins progressively toward the visual axis; (2) removal of the central portions of corneal lamellae can lead to a centrifugal differential contraction and central flattening; (3) the centrifugal spray of ablation products (the plume) might provide progressively greater shielding of the stroma toward the edge of the ablated zone; (4) the increasingly oblique angle of incident radiation falling on more peripheral cornea may result in a relative decrease in energy density as the edge of the ablation zone is approached.

Various strategies have been suggested to minimize the amount of induced hyperopia, such as the modified taper technique of Stark et al.[2] Sher et al.[21] compensated for induced hyperopia by preprogramming the Taunton laser system to cut a secondary hyperopic correction ("combined" ablation). The Taunton laser system has a series of wheels for myopia, hyperopia, and astigmatism, each with 15 apertures of different diameter or shape. After the initial corneal scar is removed with a wide aperture or myopia series of apertures, a secondary set of pulses is delivered to steepen the peripheral portion of the central cornea. The use of appropriate masking agents may also minimize the hyperopic shift.

McDonnell et al.[35] have reported a case of long-standing posttraumatic superficial stromal scar that proved resistant to ablation. This complication may be minimized by the smoothing technique. Gentle rotation of the head under the laser beam blends the edges of the irregularities, much as a rough surface is smoothed with sandpaper. The treatment surface is maintained meticulously clear of debris and cellular remnants to avoid further irregularities.

Involvement of the stroma in most microorganism infections extends deeper than the clinically observable lesion. As the tissue penetration depth of 193-nm radiation is no more than 1 μm, deep stromal infiltration may limit the effectiveness of treatment of infectious keratitis with excimer laser. Reactivation of latent herpes simplex virus has been reported following excimer PTK.

HISTOPATHOLOGY

Precise removal of superficial corneal stroma results in a smooth surface, minimal scarring, reformation of basement membrane complexes, and reestablishment of the basement membrane.[2,6] After the excimer laser surgery, the eyes undergo two rapid stages of healing. The first stage of reepithelialization, and this mostly occurs within the first week.[1-6,9,36] The second stage is anchorage of the new epithelium to the underlying stroma. Hemidesmosomes and basal lamina re-form within a week.[4]

Stromal wound healing will occur only after formation of new corneal epithelium. Almost immediately after surgery, a pseudomembrane forms. Acting as a protective barrier, the pseudomembrane directs new, hyperplastic migrating epithelial cells to fill in the wound and create a smooth epithelial surface.[4,9] Epithelial hyperplasia enables new migrating epithelial cells to cover the wound, and this, along with the deposition of new stromal collagen, restores the original corneal surface contour of shallow wounds.[2,5,9] Generally, hyperplasia takes place when there are apparent irregularities in the stroma; the deeper the incision, the thicker the epithelium becomes in order to fill in and smooth out the wound surface.[36]

After reepithelialization, a hypercellular zone develops beneath the epithelium, and connective tissue is synthesized.[5] The number of keratocytes evident at the wound margins and within the anterior stroma increases, returning to normal over a few weeks.[4,36] Tissue disorganization is minimal and the number of fibrocytes increases.[2]

Deep keratectomy incisions may take longer to heal, and the re-formation may be incomplete. A residual depression may persist for 6 months or longer.[5]

Scar tissue becomes transparent after several months, but following surgery the cornea may remain hazy. Wound healing is considered to contribute to haze. Haze may result from the deposition of new collagen fibers, which scatter light entering the eye.[3,5,6,9] Postoperative treatment with steroids notably reduces the thickness of the subepithelial layer of collagen and the concentration of haze, and in effect, delays wound healing.[5] Haze usually decreases within the months following surgery.[5,36]

When ablations are closer than 40 μm to Descemet's membrane, there is a loss of endothelial cells.[6,7] Endothelial vacuolization, a reduction in density, and the displacement of endothelial cell material into Descemet's membrane are evident.[4] Even when Descemet's membrane is not cut, endothelial cell loss occurs.[7] The loss of endothelial cells may be related to a number of factors, such as fluorescence and scattering, high-pulse energy; resonance induced in the posterior border of the cornea, acoustic waves; or shock waves.[4,7,34] It is certain that endothelial cell loss is a concern in surgical applications. There is no evidence of endothelial cell loss or displacement if the ablations stay 40 μm above Descemet's membrane; however, repetition rates higher than 40 Hz may cause irreversible damage to the cornea, endothelium, and Descemet's membrane.[6,33,34]

REFERENCES

1. Trokel SL, Srinivasan R, Braren B: Excimer laser surgery of the cornea, *Am J Ophthalmol* 96:720-715, 1983.
2. Stark WJ, Chamon W, Kamp MT, et al: Clinical follow-up of 193-nm ArF excimer laser photokeratectomy, *Ophthalmology* 99:805-811, 1992.
3. Salz JJ, Maguen E, Macy JI, et al: One-year results of excimer laser photorefractive keratectomy for myopia, *Refract Corneal Surg* 8:270-273, 1992.
4. Gaster RN, Binder PS, Coalwell K, et al: Corneal surface ablation by 193 nm excimer laser and wound healing in rabbits, *Invest Ophthalmol Vis Sci* 30:90-97, 1989.
5. Tuft SJ, Zabel RW, Marshall J: Corneal repair following keratectomy, *Invest Ophthalmol Vis Sci* 30:1769-1777, 1989.
6. Marshall J, Trokel S, Rothery S, et al: Photoablative reprofiling of the cornea using an excimer laser: photorefractive keratectomy, *Lasers Ophthalmol* 1:23-44, 1986.
7. Marshall J, Trokel S, Rothery S, et al: A comparative study of corneal incisions induced by diamond and steel knives and two ultraviolet radiations from an excimer laser, *Br J Ophthalmol* 70:482-500, 1986.
8. van Setten GB, Koch JW, Tervo K, et al: Expression of tenascin and fibronectin in the rabbit cornea after excimer laser surgery, *Graefes Arch Clin Exp Ophthalmol* 320:178-182, 1982.
9. Courant D, Fritsch P, Azema A, et al: Corneal wound healing after photo-keratomileusis treatment on the primate eye, *Laser Light Ophthalmol* 3:189-195, 1990.
10. Keates RH, Drago PC, Rothchild EJ: Effect of excimer laser on microbiological organisms, *Ophthalmic Surg* 19:715-718, 1988.
11. Gottsch JD, Gilbert ML, Goodman DF, et al: Excimer laser ablative treatment of microbial keratitis, *Ophthalmology* 98:146-149, 1991.
12. Serdarevic O, Darrell RW, Krueger RR, et al: Excimer laser therapy for experimental candida keratitis, *Am J Ophthalmol* 99:534-538, 1985.
13. Eiferman RA, Forgey DR, Cook YD: Excimer laser ablation of infectious crystalline keratopathy, *Arch Ophthalmol* 110:18, 1992.
14. Pepose JS, Laycock KA, Miller JK, et al: Reactivation of latent herpes simplex virus by excimer laser photokeratectomy, *Am J Ophthalmol* 114:45-50, 1992.
15. Sanders D: Clinical evaluation of phototherapeutic keratectomy—VISX Twenty/Twenty excimer laser, written communication, Feb 7, 1994.
16. Kornmehl EW, Steinert RF, Puliafito CA: A comparative study of masking fluids for excimer laser phototherapeutic keratectomy, *Arch Ophthalmol* 109:860-863, 1991.
17. Gartry D, Muir MK, Marshall J: Excimer laser treatment of corneal surface pathology: a laboratory and clinical study, *Br J Ophthalmol* 75:258-269, 1991.
18. Fasano AP, Moreira H, McDonnell PJ, et al: Excimer laser smoothing of a reproducible model of anterior corneal surface irregularity, *Ophthalmology* 98:1782-1785, 1991.
19. Fitzsimmons TD, Fagerholm P: Superficial keratectomy with the 193 excimer laser: a reproducible model of corneal surface irregularities, *Acta Ophthalmol* 69:641-644, 1991.
20. Englanoff JS, Kolahdouz-Isfahani AH, Moreira H, et al: In situ collagen gel mold as an aid in excimer laser superficial keratectomy, *Ophthalmology* 99:1201-1208, 1992.
21. Sher NA, Bowers RA, Zabel RW, et al: Clinical use of 193-nm excimer laser in the treatment of corneal scars, *Arch Ophthalmol* 109:491-498, 1991.
22. McCally RL, Hochheimer BF, Chamon W, et al. A simple device for objective measurement of haze following excimer ablation of cornea, *SPIE* 1877:20-25, 1993.
23. Chamon W, Azar DT, Stark JW et al: Phototherapeutic keratectomy, *Ophthalmol Clin North Am* 6:399-413, 1993.
24. Campos M, Nielsen S, Szerenyi K, et al: Clinical follow-up of phototherapeutic keratectomy for treatment of corneal opacities, *Am J Ophthalmol* 115:433-440, 1993.
25. Gartry D, Kerr Muir M, Marshall J: Excimer laser photorefractive keratectomy: 18 months follow-up, *Ophthalmology* 99:1209-1219, 1992.
26. McDonnell PJ, Seiler T: Phototherapeutic keratectomy with excimer laser for Reis-Buckler's corneal dystrophy, *Refract Corneal Surg* 8:306-310, 1992
27. Forster W, Grewe S, Atzler U, et al: Phototherapeutic keratectomy in corneal diseases, *Refract Corneal Surg* 9:S85-90, 1993.
28. Steinert RF, Puliafito CA: Excimer laser phototherapeutic keratectomy for a corneal nodule, *Refract Corneal Surg* 6:352, 1990.

29. Brancatto R, Scialdone A, Carones F, et al: Excimer laser ablation of a corneal proturberance, *J Cataract Refract Surg* 18:111, 1992.

30. Talamo JH, Steinert RF, Puliafito CA: Clinical strategies for excimer laser therapeutic keratectomy, *Refract Corneal Surg* 8:319-324, 1992.

31. Krueger RR, Sliney DH, Trokel SL: Photokeratitus from subablative 193-nanometer excimer laser radiation, *Refract Corneal Surg* 8:274-279, 1992.

32. Seiler T, Bende T, Winckler K, et al: Side effects in excimer corneal surgery: DNA damage as a result of 193 nm excimer laser radiation, *Graefes Arch Clin Exp Ophthalmol* 226:276, 1988.

33. Ozler SA, Liaw LL, Neev J, et al: Acute ultrastructural changes of cornea after excimer laser ablation, *Invest Ophthalmol Vis Sci* 33:540, 1992.

34. Bende T, Seiler T, Wollensak J: Side effects in excimer corneal surgery: corneal thermal gradients, *Graefes Arch Clin Exp Ophthalmol* 226:277-280, 1988.

35. McDonnell JM, Garbus JJ, McDonnell PJ: Unsuccessful excimer laser phototherapeutic keratectomy, clinicopathologic correlation, *Arch Ophthalmol* 110:977-979, 1992.

36. Hanan KD, Pouliquen Y, Waring GO III, et al: Corneal stroma wound healing in rabbits after 193-nm excimer laser surface ablation, *Arch Ophthalmol* 107:899-900, 1989.

16

Phototherapeutic Keratectomy: the Summit Experience

Daniel S. Durrie, D. James Schumer, Timothy Cavanaugh

Phototherapeutic keratectomy is the term given to the treatment of corneal disorders with the excimer laser. Because the excimer laser can remove precise amounts of tissue (0.25 μm per pulse) over a range of areas (0.5-7.0 mm), it provides a unique way to treat superficial corneal disease. Techniques are being developed to facilitate the use of the excimer laser in the therapeutic realm.

Three distinct PTK treatment groups were categorized within the U.S. FDA clinical trial for the Summit excimer laser.[1] They consisted of: (1) corneal opacity, (2) irregular corneal surface, and (3) recurrent epithelial breakdown.

The goal in the corneal opacity group was to improve visual acuity by increasing corneal transparency. This group included patients with corneal dystrophies and scars that were significant enough to reduce the transmission of light through the cornea, thus affecting visual acuity (Fig. 16-1).

The second group included patients with corneal surface irregularities that were optically significant. The goal in this group was to improve visual acuity through smoothing the corneal refractive surface. These patients were also expected to show improvement on topographic analysis (Figs. 16-2 and 16-3).

The goal in the third group was to improve comfort by reducing recurrent epithelial breakdown. These patients had idiopathic recurrent erosion syndrome or, secondary to trauma, infectious ulcers or irregular corneal surfaces, as seen with band keratopathy and corneal dystrophies. Through smoothing and polishing the epithelial basement membrane, anterior Bowman's membrane and by removing the lesions,

the patients were made more comfortable. Figure 16-4 shows the relationships of these treatment groups and how they can overlap and interrelate.

The best patients for PTK are those that have the majority of the pathologic changes limited to the anterior 100 μm of the cornea. Ideal patients for this procedure have either elevated corneal scars or homogeneous anterior stromal scars or dystrophy limited to the anterior 100 μm (Fig. 16-5). The abnormalities in these patients are readily removed with current PTK techniques, leaving the postoperative corneal surface optically improved.[2]

Patients that are considered acceptable, but not ideal for PTK are those with minimal loss of tissue or combinations of elevated lesions and superficial corneal scarring (Fig. 16-6). These patients, with careful surgical technique, can also have excellent results with an optimal, smooth corneal surface postoperatively.

Patients considered unacceptable for PTK are those with significant loss of corneal tissue secondary to their disease as well as those with deep scars (Fig. 16-7). The position and size of the changes preclude their removal while still maintaining a refractive surface.

It is important in patient selection to be aware of the patient's preoperative refractive error. When a lesion is removed from the corneal surface it can have a significant impact on the patient's refraction. If a patient has a corneal abnormality which upon removal will significantly flatten the central cornea, a hyperopic shift in the refraction will occur (Fig. 16-8, *A*). Likewise, a paracentral lesion potentially may induce large amounts of astigmatism. A myopic shift or steep-

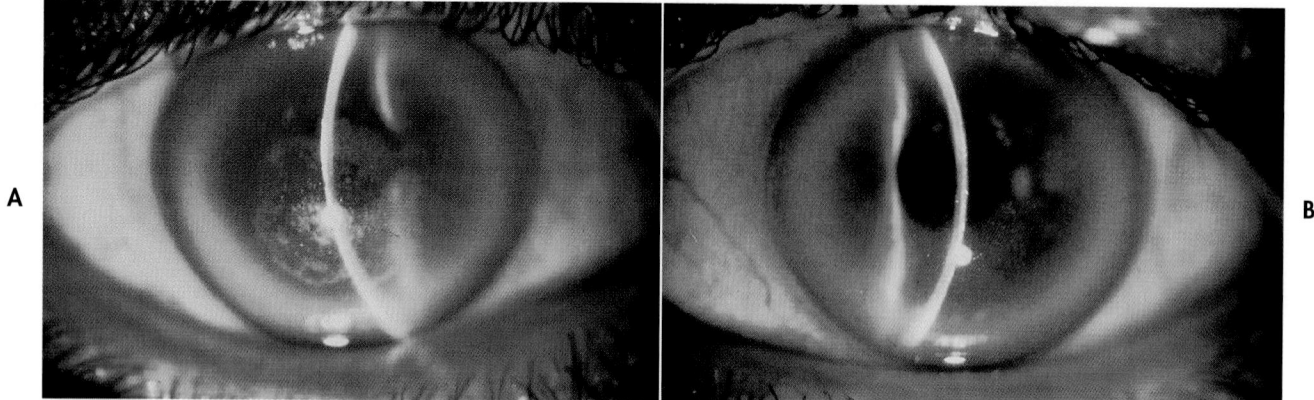

Fig. 16-1. **A** and **B,** A 58-year-old woman with central crystalline dystrophy had BCVA at plano of 20/40. One month after PTK the BCVA at +2.50 −2.00 × 90 was 20/20.

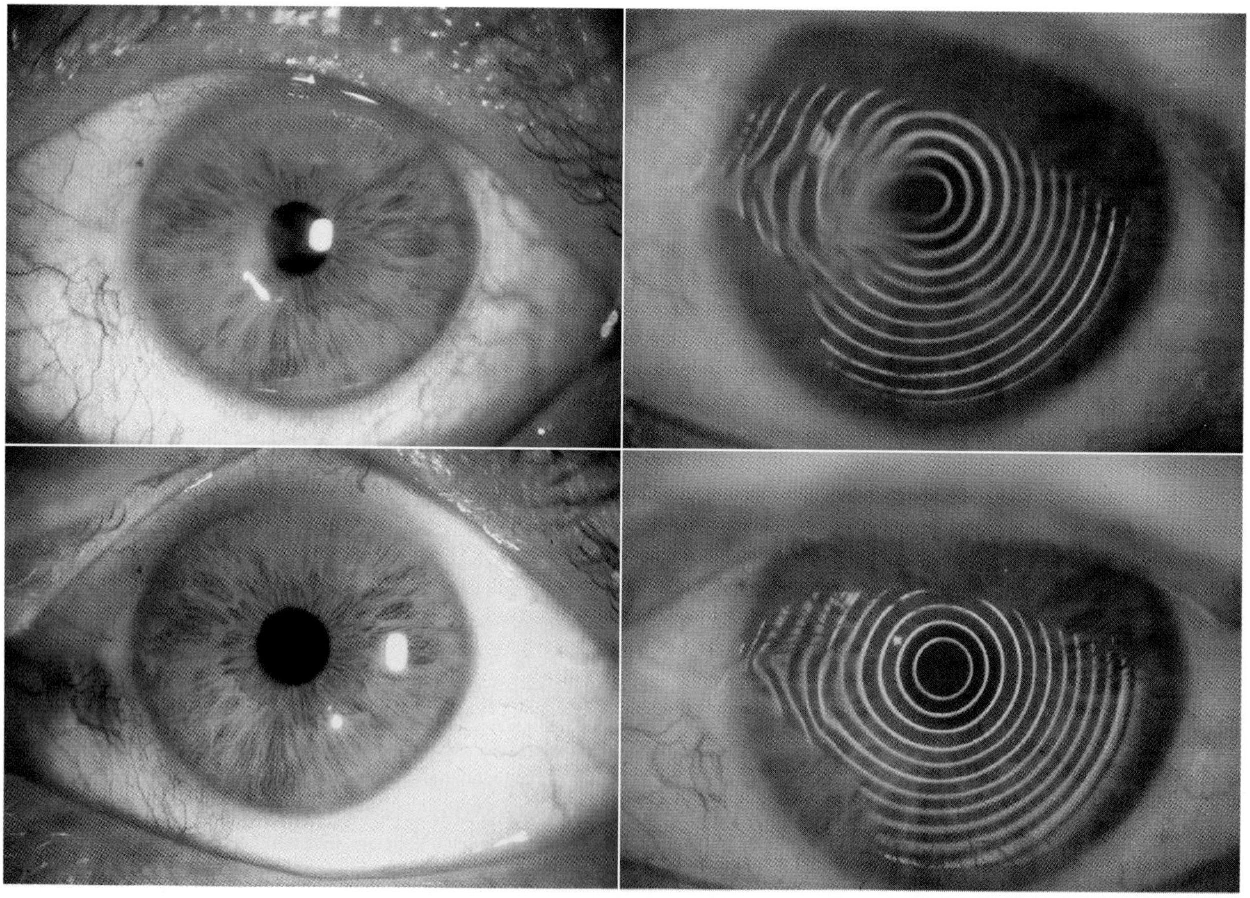

Fig. 16-2. **A** and **B,** Slit-lamp and corneoscope photograph of a superficial corneal scar status post pterygium removal. BCVA with +2.00 −3.25 at 20 was 20/40. **C** and **D,** slit-lamp and corneoscope photographs 1 year following PTK. BCVA at +2.25 −1.25 × 43 was 20/20.

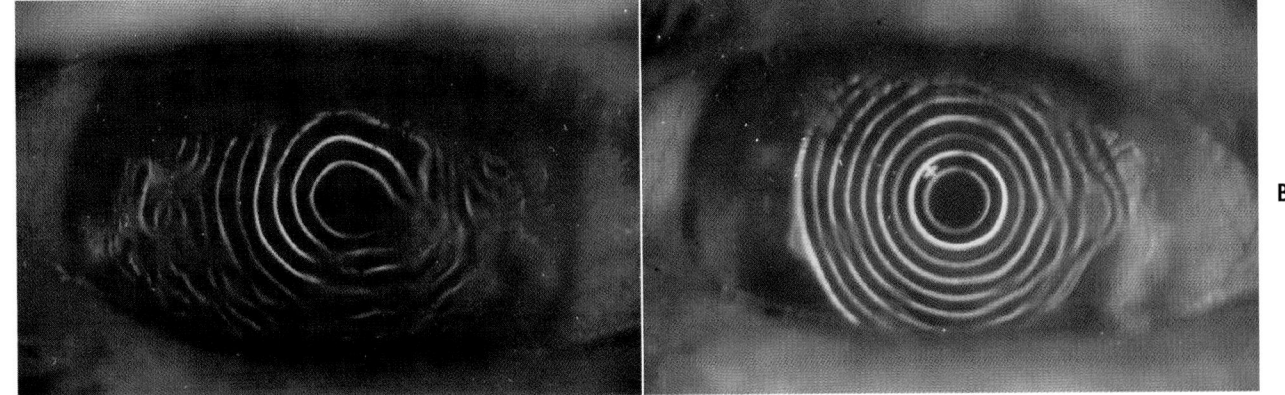

Fig. 16-3. **A,** Corneoscope photograph of a patient with Salzmann's nodular degeneration. BCVA at $-3.00 + 4.25 \times 140$ was 20/60. **B,** Corneoscope photograph 6 months following PTK. BCVA was 20/25+ with $-1.00 -0.75 \times 60$.

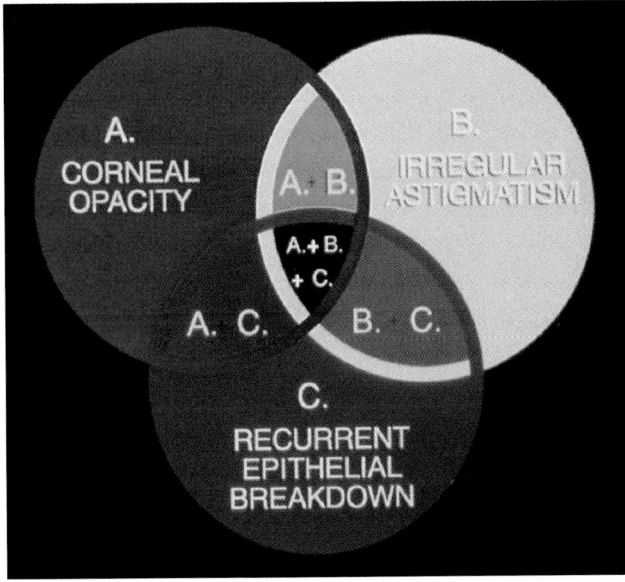

Fig. 16-4. The three groups for which PTK is efficacious. The categories are not strict and a single eye can have multiple reasons for the use of PTK.

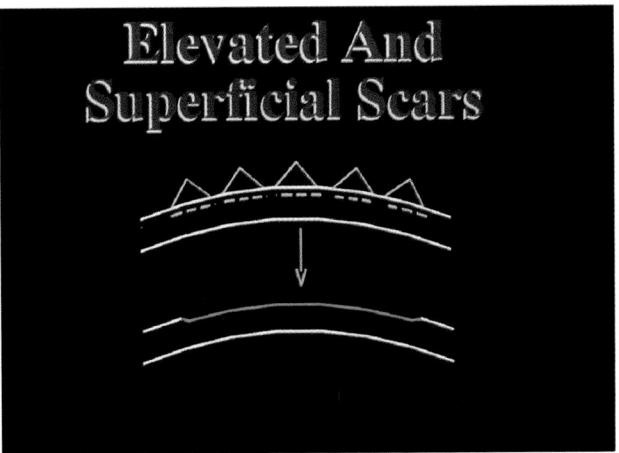

Fig. 16-5. An ideal candidate for PTK is a cornea that has either an elevated lesion or superficial stromal pathologic changes within the first 100 μm of the cornea. Current techniques can leave this patient with a smooth refractive surface.

ening of the central cornea could also result from ablation of peripheral abnormalities (Fig. 16-8, *B*). If such treatment would adversely affect the patient's uncorrected vision or induce anisometropia, the patient may not be a good candidate for PTK, despite the location or degree of the pathologic changes.

SURGICAL TECHNIQUE

The initial PTK technique described by several investigators with different laser systems can be described as the "point-and-shoot" technique.[3] The original theory was to measure the depth of the corneal opacity, dystrophy, or scar and calculate the expected number of laser pulses required to remove it. The laser was then aligned and the disk of tissue re-

moved. Early clinical results showed unacceptable levels of corneal scarring and unwanted refractive errors secondary to this technique.[3] The reason for this appears to be twofold. First of all, the disk ablation left an abrupt edge between the ablated and unablated tissue. The epithelium will hypertrophy when it approaches an edge or drop-off in the corneal surface. Studies have also shown that there can be stromal remodeling at the edge of an abrupt junction of excimer ablation to a normal corneal structure. The result is increased corneal fibrosis and epithelial hypertrophy that can increase the corneal opacity and induce a hyperopic shift[4] (Fig. 16-9). A second reason for hyperopic shift with this type of ablation is explained by the variance of energy across the laser beam. The ideal laser beam would be diagramatically represented as a top hat. The actual excimer beam has a slight drop-

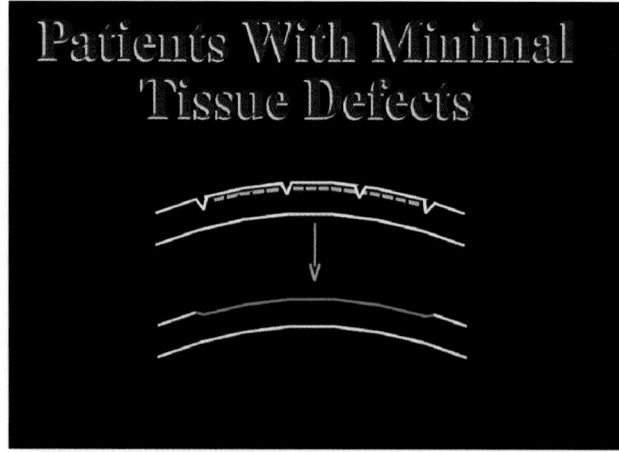

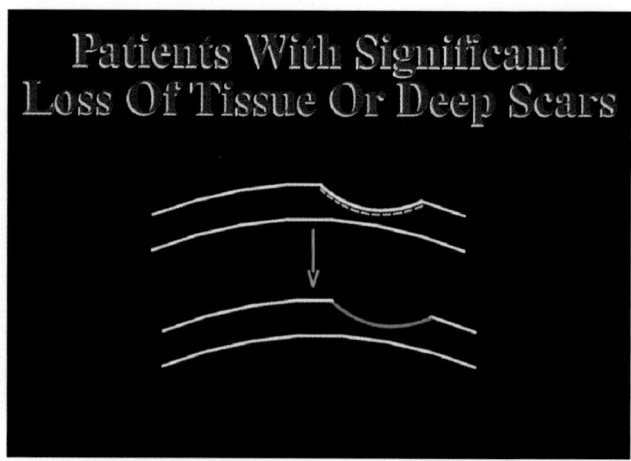

Fig. 16-6. A patient with minimal tissue loss alone or in combination with superficial corneal scarring can also be a good candidate for PTK. Through proper technique, PTK can leave the cornea with a smooth refractive surface.

Fig. 16-7. Unacceptable patients for PTK are those with large tissue defects or deep stromal pathologic changes. Upon removing these abnormalities, the cornea is left with an unacceptable refractive surface.

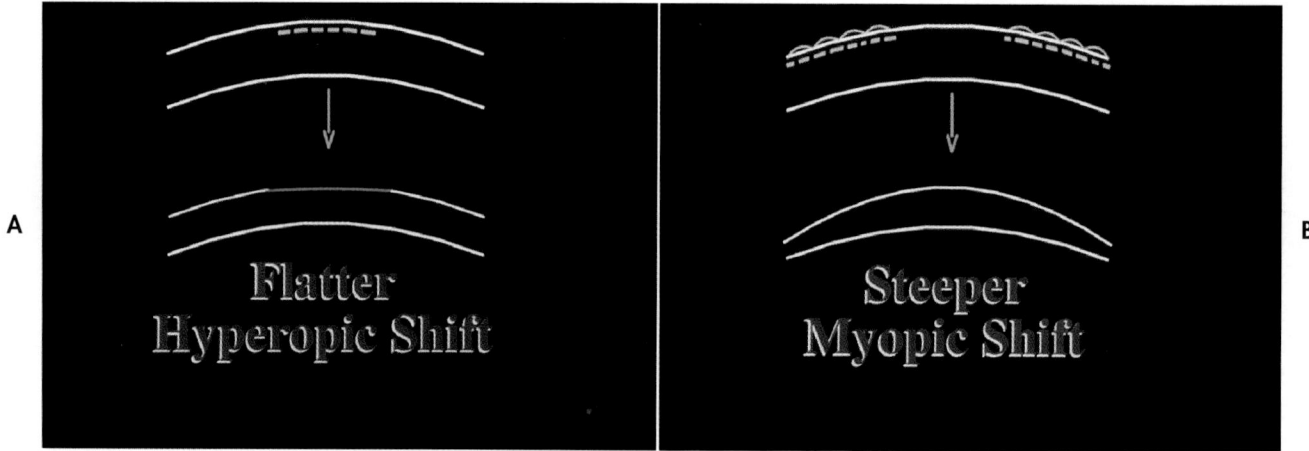

A   B

Fig. 16-8. A, Removal of a central corneal lesion can result in a flatter postoperative cornea resulting in a hyperopic shift. B, Removing a peripheral corneal lesion can lead to central steepening which will produce a myopic shift in the refraction.

off in power at the edges, leaving a beam configuration shaped more like a derby. When applied to the corneal surface in a disk-type ablation, this results in a contour that would cause a hyperopic shift (Fig. 16-10). In addition, since corneal scars, dystrophies, and deposits all have different ablation rates, the point-and-shoot technique results in an uneven final corneal surface (Fig. 16-11).

Because of these theoretical concerns a "polish technique" was devised for use in the clinical trials for PTK. Fundamental to this technique is the placement of the surgeon's hands on either side of the patient's head. As the laser treatment is performed the surgeon moves the head in a brisk controlled circular manner which allows the beam to "polish" the corneal surface. This prevents the ablation from producing an abrupt transition to the untreated cornea, as well as counter-

acting variances in laser beam energy across the beam. In the future, advanced laser delivery systems will allow the surgeon to accurately move the laser beam rather than the patient's head.

Methylcellulose will absorb excimer laser energy and is used as a polishing agent during PTK. The ideal polishing agent would be nontoxic, easy to apply, and allow for a smooth ablative surface. Methylcellulose 0.5%, uniformly painted on the cornea, will fill in very small defects allowing for a smooth corneal surface after ablation. Methylcellulose 1.0% or 2.0% is ideal to protect areas of the cornea from unwanted ablation. A combination of methylcellulose and the polishing technique can remove corneal disease while either preserving or producing an optically acceptable corneal surface (Fig. 16-12).

Figure 16-13 depicts how a PTK of an irregular cor-

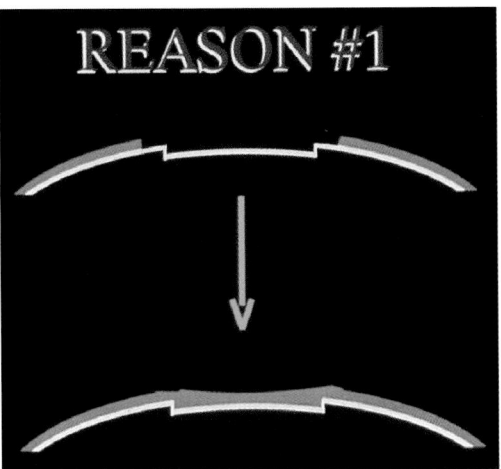

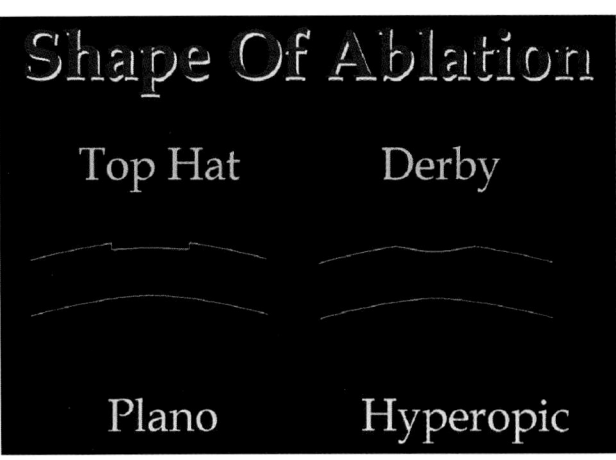

Fig. 16-9. A plano disk ablation will result in epithelial hypertrophy and corneal fibrosis, particularly at the junction between the ablated and normal cornea. A marked hyperopic shift also results.

Fig. 16-10. The ideal excimer laser beam would have a homogeneous ablation pattern creating a top-hat configuration in the cornea. The actual excimer laser beam has less energy at the periphery, creating an ablation shaped like a derby. This results in a hyperopic refractive shift.

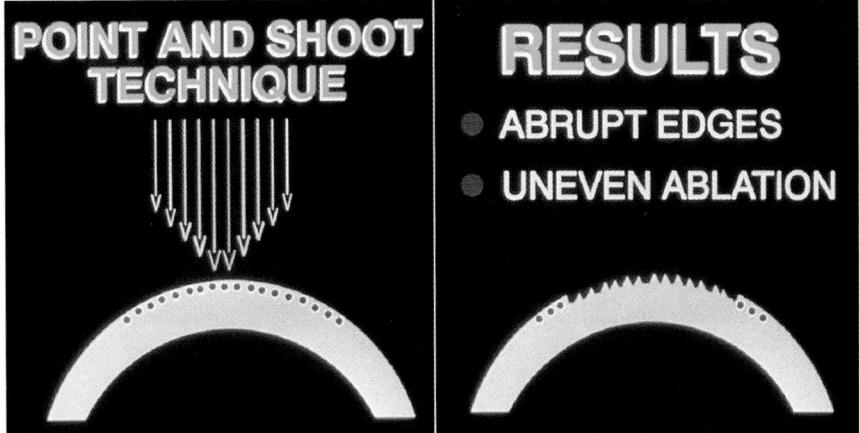

Fig. 16-11. Superficial corneal lesions can ablate at a different rate than normal cornea tissue. The resultant ablation can leave abrupt edges and an uneven pattern.

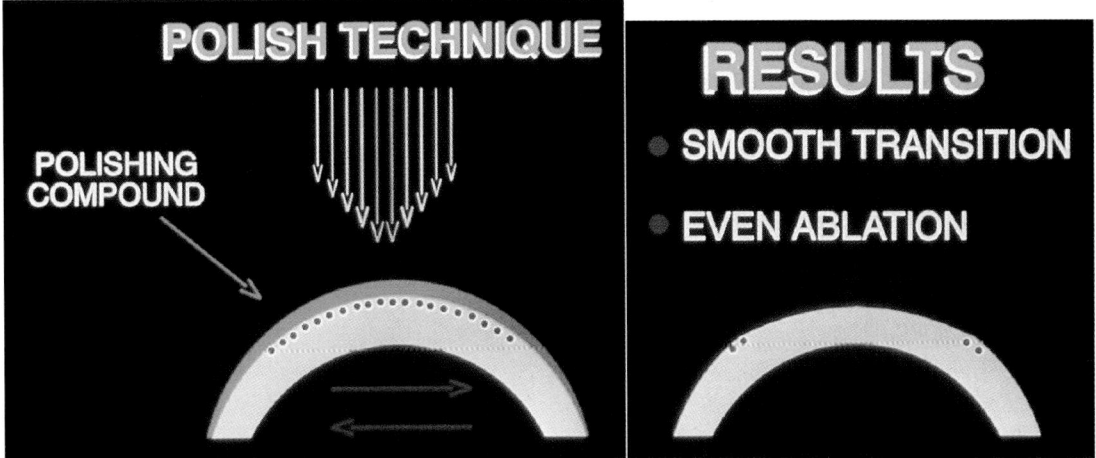

Fig. 16-12. The polish technique uses a combination of methylcellulose as a polishing compound and a circular movement of the patient's head to obtain a smooth, even ablation.

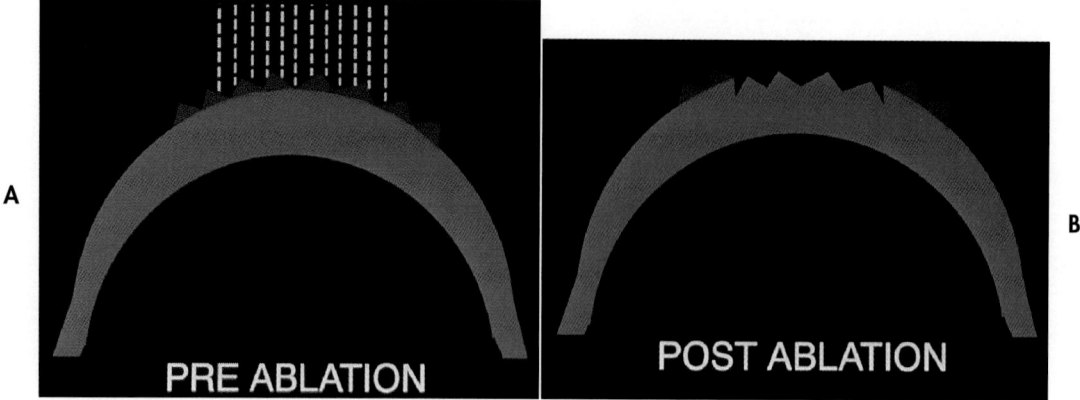

Fig. 16-13. An elevated corneal lesion ablated without the use of methylcellulose will leave an uneven corneal surface in a pattern similar to the elevated lesion.

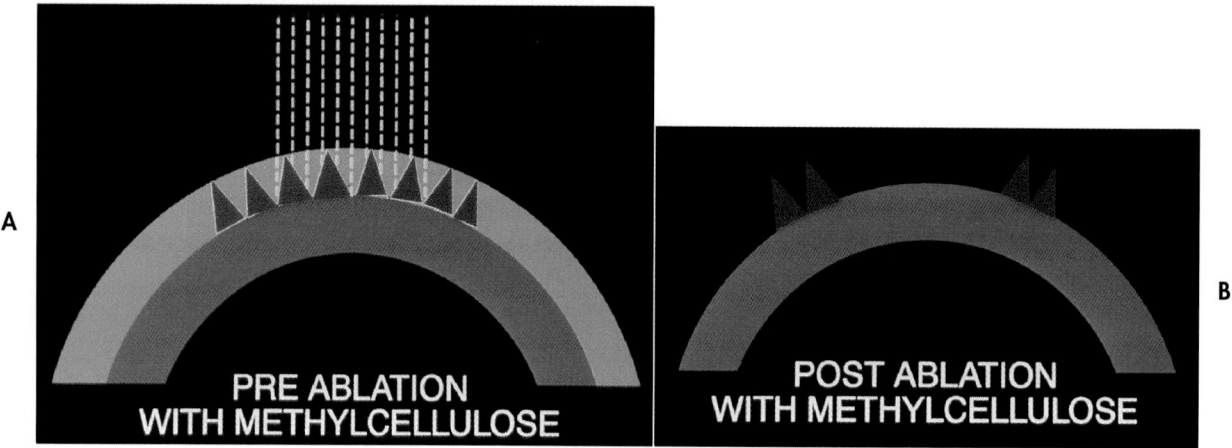

Fig. 16-14. Methylcellulose fills in the defects between elevated corneal lesions allowing for a smooth corneal surface postablation.

neal surface without methylcellulose can leave this pattern of irregularity in the cornea after ablation. The use of methylcellulose as a blocking agent to fill in the valleys produces a uniform surface after ablation (Fig. 16-14).

Using the analogy of removing rust from a chrome ball can help conceptualize the philosophy of PTK. If the goal was to maintain a spherical shape, you would not push the ball against a grinding wheel at the site where the rust spots are present. Instead, large areas of rust should be removed mechanically with either a chisel or very rough sandpaper before performing a fine finishing polish to buff the surface. In patients with large elevated scars, such as Salzmann's nodules or post–pterygium removal scars, PTK is improved by mechanically removing the bulk of the scar prior to the finishing polish with the laser. Certainly, large elevated scars can be removed with the excimer laser, but PTK is best reserved for the final steps of smoothing and polishing.

One of the learned skills in PTK is deciding when

enough laser treatment has been performed. A slit-lamp in the treatment room can be very valuable in determining the depth of treatment and whether further treatment is necessary. In addition to serial slit-lamp examinations, identifying corneal abnormalities at a level consistent with maximal treatment can be a useful tool in judging treatment depth. It is much better to err on the conservative side and undertreat patients, because repeating PTK is not difficult. Obviously, it is impossible to replace corneal tissue that has been removed in excess.

Before attempting PTK for recurrent erosions, patients should be unresponsive to traditional medical and therapeutic options such as hyperosmotic agents, bandage lenses, and patching. Prior to performing PTK, all loose epithelium surrounding the area to be treated is removed. A Weck cell sponge can be used to identify the loose epithelium and a surgical scalpel used to remove it. A 4.5- to 5.0-mm spot size is chosen and 10 to 20 pulses of the laser are applied to the surface. This removes less than 4 μm of corneal sur-

Table 16-1. The diagnoses for each treatment group in the U.S. Food and Drug Administration phototherapeutic keratectomy clinical trial

Corneal opacity group	
Lattice dystrophy	7
Corneal scar	7
Band keratopathy	5
Schnyder's crystalline dystrophy	2
Reis-Buckler's dystrophy	1
Total	22
Irregular surface group	
Salzmann's nodule	10
Anterior membrane dystrophy	6
Post–pterygium removal scars	9
Corneal scar	9
Total	34
Epithelial breakdown group	
Recurrent erosion	6
Band keratopathy	4
Corneal scar	1
Total	11

Table 16-2. Uncorrected visual acuity in the three treatment groups

	Uncorrected vision*		
	Improved	Unchanged	Decreased
Corneal opacity	64%	14%	22%
Irregular surface	69%	8%	23%
Epithelial breakdown	64%	27%	9%

*Improved or decreased represents at least one line of vision.

Table 16-3. Best crrected visual activity in the three treatment groups

	Best corrected visual acuity*		
	Improved	Unchanged	Decreased
Corneal opacity	77%	5%	18%
Irregular surface	70%	8%	22%
Epithelial breakdown	36%	46%	18%

*Improved or decreased represents at least one line of vision.

face and can be best described as microsuperficial keratectomy. This technique removes any residual basement membrane and the anterior portion of Bowman's membrane. Theoretically, this is similar to early scarification procedures as with trichloracetic acid or iodine used in the treatment of recurrent erosion. The problem with these procedures was the resultant corneal haze left in the treatment zone. PTK is one of the most successful treatments that have been developed for recalcitrant, recurrent erosion.

RESULTS

The following data are from phase II and phase III Summit ExciMed™ excimer laser clinical trials for PTK. There were a total of 67 procedures performed. Of these, 22 eyes were in the corneal opacity group, 27 eyes in the irregular surface group, and 11 eyes in the recurrent erosion group. Table 16-1 gives the diagnosis for each treatment group. The average length of follow-up is 8.2 months with a range of 3 to 21 months. Uncorrected visual acuity improved in 64% to 69% of three treatment groups (Table 16-2). This represents an improvement of at least one line of vision. Up to 23% had a loss of at least one line of vision. BCVA (best corrected visual acuity) improved in 77% of the corneal opacity group (17/22), in 70% of the irregular surface group (19/27), and in 36% (4/11) of the recurrent ero-

sion group (Table 16-3). Between 18% and 22% of eyes lost at least one line of BCVA in the three groups.

The change in the patients' spherical equivalent from preoperatively to the last postoperative visit is reported in Figure 16-15. It is obvious that a significant refractive change can be induced by PTK. Figure 16-8 depicts how either a hyperopic or myopic shift can result. In the corneal opacity group there was on average a myopic shift (preoperative average, +0.75 D; postoperative average, −0.92 D). However, there was a range of patients that had a measurable flattening and steepening (preoperative range, −9.62-+7.62, D postoperative range, −10.25-+3.00 D). Analyzing the induced refractive change in the irregular surface group, the average change was not significant (preoperative average, +0.37 D, postoperative average, +0.39 D), but again there was a range (preoperative range, −9.75-+5.12 D; postoperative range, −5.75-+5.00 D). Owing to the minimal treatment used in the recurrent epithelial breakdown group, only minimal refractive changes were seen (preoperative average, −1.59 D; postoperative average, −0.94 D).

In all three treatment groups there was an average reduction of corneal cylinder postoperatively (Table 16-4; Fig. 16-16). The corneal opacity group had almost an equal distribution of patients who had either increased or decreased cylinder postoperatively. This effect depended primarily on the site of the tissue that was removed. If the corneal lesions were elevated as seen in Figure 16-17, the astigmatism would be expected to improve. On the other hand, a lesion located below the surface may produce astigmatism as a re-

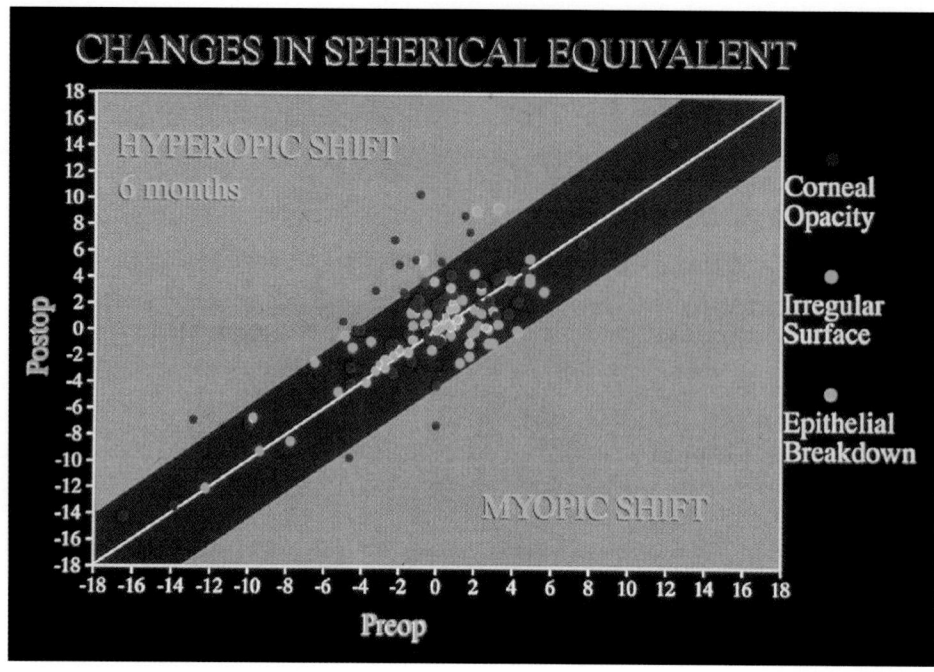

Fig. 16-15. Change in spherical equivalent for all patients in each treatment group.

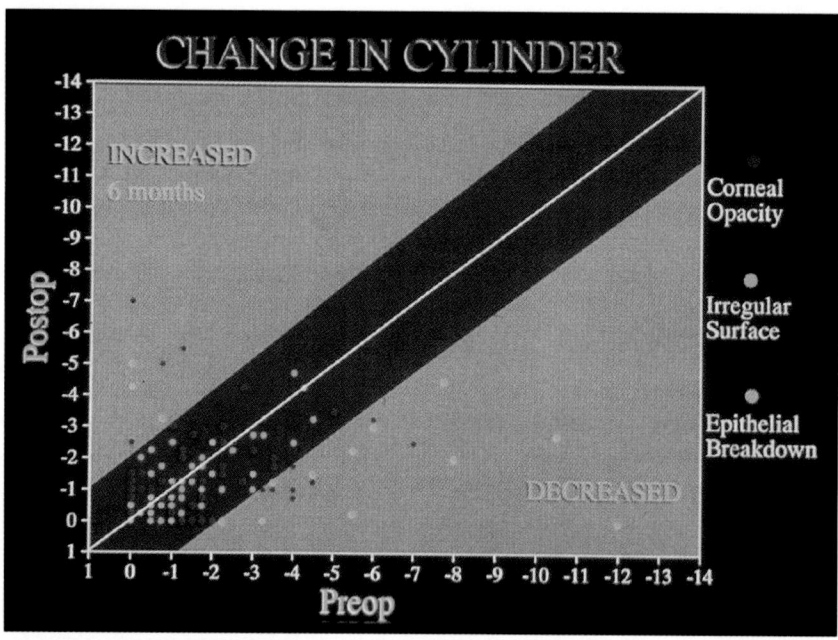

Fig. 16-16. Change in cylinder for all patients in each treatment group.

sult. These factors need to be considered in the patient selection process to make sure that the patient is a good candidate for this treatment.

Most patients demonstrate improved uncorrected vision with removal of the abnormality, and the refractive errors were not significant enough in most cases to reduce their uncorrected vision. With careful patient selection and adherence to good surgical technique, the number of patients who had a decrease in uncorrected vision postoperatively will increase in the future.

Previous reports by investigators regarding other PTK techniques have reported significant refractive error changes.[3] These results led to questioning the usefulness of PTK. The significant change from the early surgical techniques to the polishing technique used in this study, combined with good patient selection, can result in positive visual outcomes.

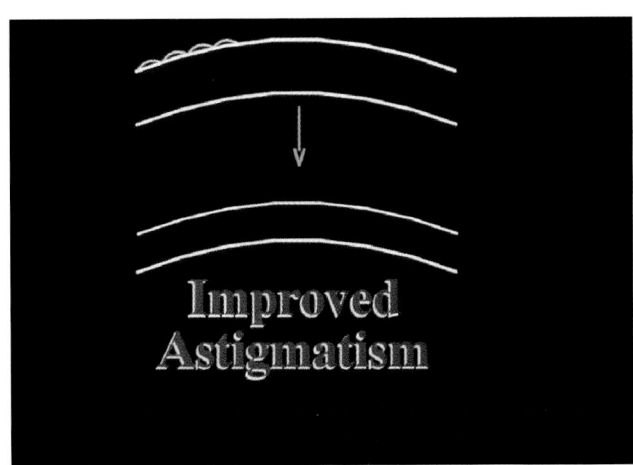

Fig. 16-17. Astigmatism produced by elevated corneal lesions can be improved by PTK.

Table 16-4. Change in cylinder after phototherapeutic keratectomy

	Preoperative average (D)	Postoperative average (D)
Corneal opacity	2.55	1.93
Irregular surface	2.12	1.17
Epithelial breakdown	1.27	1.12

CONCLUSION

Photorefractive keratectomy is an effective new treatment for superficial corneal disease. The vast majority of patients in this study have avoided more traditional surgical corrections such as lamellar or penetrating keratoplasties. For those who had failed on traditional techniques to correct recurrent erosion, a marked improvement in quality of life occurred after PTK. The PTK technique can remove a significant amount of pathologic changes from the corneal surface and provide a smoother underlying surface for reepithelialization than either a surgical scalpel or a diamond burr.

PTK has the potential to decrease morbidity for the patient as well as provide cost-effective treatment. If the excimer laser can help to prevent corneal transplantations, either lamellar or penetrating, morbidity and cost will decrease. Corneal transplantation has a significant cost for the facility, surgeon, and tissue. These procedures are also performed under either general or retrobulbar anesthesia. Replacing this with a 15- to 20-minute procedure under topical anesthesia with less potential for morbidity can bring a significant improvement in the delivery of eye care. It is our hope that the FDA will approve the excimer laser for PTK in the near future. This will have a significant impact on our ability to treat patients with corneal disease.

REFERENCES

1. *Phototherapeutic keratectomy, phase III, IRB clinical investigation protocol no. ID G880234.* Waltham, Mass, Summit Technology, 1993.
2. Thompson V, Durrie DS, Cavanavgh TB: Philosophy and technique for excimer laser phototherapeutic keratectomy, *J Refract Corneal Surg* 2:S81-S95, 1993.
3. Stark WJ, Chamon W, Azar D, et al: Phototherapeutic keratectomy: corneal opacities. In Thompson FB, McDonnell PJ, Eds. *Excimer laser surgery of the cornea*, Tokyo, 1983, Igaku-Shoin.
4. Marshall J, Trokel S, Rothery S, et al: Longterm healing of central cornea after photorefractive keratectomy using an excimer laser, *Ophthalmology* 95:1411-1421, 1988.

Laser Correction of Hyperopia

Aesculap-Meditec Results from Germany
Dieter Dausch, Monika Landesz

Sunrise Holmium Laser Results
Douglas D. Koch, Michael J. Berry, Arthur Vassiliadis, Adrian A. Abarca, Rogelio Villarreal, Elizabeth A. Haft

Summit Holmium Thermal Keratoplasty Results
Vance Thompson

VISX Blind Eye Study United States Results
Jonathan I. Macy, Anthony B. Nesburn, James J. Salz

The four sections of this chapter discuss laser techniques for the correction of hyperopia from the standpoint of both surface ablation with the excimer laser and intrastromal holmium collagen shrinkage approaches. The sections of this chapter are as follows:
1. The Aesculap-Meditec Excimer Laser: Results from Germany
2. Noncontact Holmium:YAG Laser Thermal Keratoplasty
3. Holmium:YAG Laser Themokeptoplasty Utilizing the Summit System
4. Excimer Laser Studies: Results from the United States

The surgical correction of hyperopia has proved to be much more difficult than correction of myopia. This appears to be true of incisional approaches, lamellar techniques, and more recently with various forms of laser energy.

Incisional surgery (radial keratotomy) has been quite successful in correcting myopia. Incisional surgery for hyperopia (hexagonal keratotomy) has remained controversial, primarily because of its limited efficacy, (about 2-3 D) and the frequent induction of irregular astigmatism. Lamellar surgery for the correction of hyperopia (keratophakia and hyperopic keratomileusis) is capable of correcting moderate and high hyperopia. These are demanding procedures requiring expensive instrumentation and highly skilled technicians and surgeons. Predictability is not ideal and irregular astigmatism can also be a problem. Although there is a renewed interest in lamellar techniques for the correction of hyperopia with the advent of the automated lamellar keratoplasty (ALK) technique developed by Luis Ruiz, there is very little published information about safety, efficacy, and stability.

The Aesculap-Meditec Excimer Laser: Results from Germany
Dieter Dausch, Monika Landesz

Photorefractive keratectomy (PRK) for myopia has been described in several animal and human studies with satisfactory results.[1-6] It was a logical step to extend the applications of PRK to include the correction of hyperopia. In contrast to the flattening of the central corneal portion in myopic photoablation, PRK in hyperopia is used to steepen the central cornea.

To achieve a steepening of the cornea the peripheral portion must be ablated. This necessitates a large-diameter laser beam. The excimer laser manufactured by Aesculap-Meditec, Heroldsberg, Germany, is capable of emitting a beam 7 mm in diameter. The mask used in correcting myopia[7,8] had to be altered so that only the peripheral cornea would be ablated. This modification proved to be difficult so the initiation of hyperopic PRK was delayed. The details of the hyperopic technique are described below. We think that this new technique is promising because of the relatively precise ablation that can be obtained, contrary to other lamellar procedures.

In 1990 we started a prospective study on a small group of patients to investigate the efficacy, stability, and safety of PRK for hyperopia. No previous study of this nature had been described in the literature.

SURGICAL TECHNIQUES FOR THE CORRECTION OF HYPEROPIA

Keratophakia and keratomileusis were developed by José Barraquer.[9] These techniques are lamellar keratoplasty procedures that alter the refractive state of the cornea. Both procedures involve the reshaping of parallel-faced corneal disks to produce tissue lenses capable of correcting myopia and hyperopia, including aphakia.

Keratophakia

Keratophakia is restricted to the correction of hyperopia and aphakia. A donor cornea undergoes a lamellar keratectomy, and is reshaped with a cryolathe to produce a stromal tissue lens. The stromal lens is thickest in the center and is capable of correctional hyperopia and aphakia. A lamellar keratectomy with a microkeratome is performed on the patient's cornea, the lens is placed intrastromally, and the anterior cap is sutured in place. The shape of the stromal lens creates a steepening of the cornea, thus increasing the refractive power. Corrections of up to 15 D have been achieved,[10] with 18.5% to 25% of the eyes corrected to within 3 D of emmetropia.[11,12]

Keratomileusis

Keratomileusis is a procedure that may correct either myopia or hyperopia. The patient's resected corneal disk or a corneal disk obtained from a donor eye is reshaped with a cryolathe, or modified using a microkeratome. A hyperopic correction requires removal of relatively more tissue from the peripheral part of the disk resulting in a secondary steepening of the cornea, thereby increasing the refractive power. The lenticule is sutured on the patient's lamellar keratectomy bed and corrections of 49% of eyes within 3 D of emmetropia have been described.[13]

Thermokeratoplasty

Hyperopic thermokeratoplasty was developed in the former Soviet Union and uses a probe tip preset to penetrate the corneal stroma to 90%. The needle is electrically heated and induces a coagulation of the stromal tissue resulting in shrinkage. The coagulations are applied radially in the periphery to correct hyperopia. Neumann et al.[14] describe an initial refractive change of 6 D and an undercorrection in 83% of cases at 12 months. The change in refraction increases when the optical zone decreases.

Holmium Laser

The same stromal shrinkage can be obtained by using a holium-yttrium-aluminum-garnet (Ho:YAG) laser. An in-vitro study[15] showed a keratometric change in refractive power of 5.5 to 1.0 D, depending on the diameter of the optical zone.

Excimer Laser

With the 193-nm argon fluoride (ArF) excimer laser, photoablation of the superficial corneal tissue is obtained. Unlike myopic photoablation, the central corneal portion is left untreated. To steepen the central cornea, only the periphery is ablated. The peripheral ablation technique with the excimer laser is described next.

TECHNICAL PROCEDURE FOR HYPEROPIC PHOTOREFRACTIVE KERATECTOMY
Scanning Principle

The excimer laser manufactured by Aesculap-Meditecc emits a 193-nm laser light. The exposures for large area photoablation were performed with a repetition rate of 0.5 Hz. Each complete exposure was accomplished not by a single illumination but by a scanning process. To this end, the 7 × 1-mm slit profile is moved uniformly in such a way that laser light is applied to a rectangular area measuring 7 x 10 mm. Circular areas up to 7 mm in diameter thus can be treated. The scan return points must be outside this area. The principle is illustrated in Fig. 17-1. The energy density of the individual laser beam was 250 mJ/cm², re-

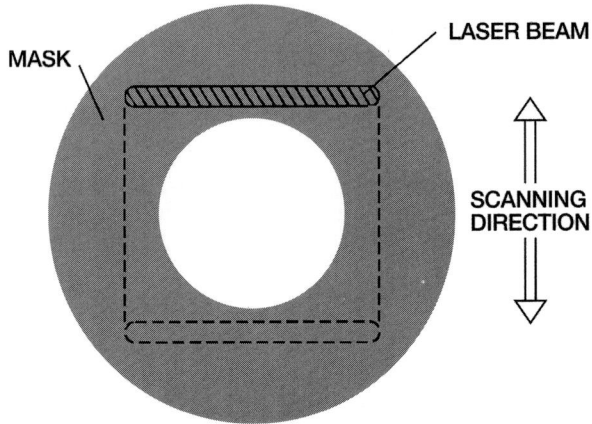

Fig. 17-1. Scanning technique for ablation of large areas.

sulting in a corneal ablation depth of 0.5 μm per pulse. However, at a repetition rate of 20 Hz the scanning process is adjusted so that there is considerable overlap of adjacent laser shots. The total effect of one scanning process is therefore an ablation of 1 μm. This overlapping method also ensures that the ablation procedure produces a smooth surface.

Technique of the Rotating Mask

The ablation profile required to correct hyperopia is presented in Fig. 17-2. The ablation profile is not created with an adjustable mechanical iris; instead, a mask with a spiral aperture is used (Fig. 17-3). The mask has to be inserted into a suction ring, which is first adjusted and fixed to the patient's eye (Fig. 17-4). The mask can be rotated over 360 degrees and is turned by a fixed angle of 4 degrees between individual laser exposures. The ablation process is completed when the mask reaches a total rotation of 360 degrees. Only then is the ablation profile rotationally symmetric. However, since a steep excision border is not permissible, a transition zone is required which extends beyond the area corrected (see Fig. 17-2). The parameters we use are as follows: the diameter of the central corrected zone is 4 mm; the overall diameter is 7 mm; there is a 1.5-mm transition zone ring around the central zone.

CLINICAL STUDIES

Two studies have investigated the correction of hyperopia with PRK.

The Study of Dausch, Klein, and Schröder

Patients. In the study of Dausch et al.[7] the patients were divided in two groups. Group I comprised 15 patients (8 females, 7 males) who underwent unilateral PRK between July and August 1990. The mean age was 36.6 ±12.9 years. The preoperative refraction ranged from +2.0 to +7.5 D. One eye was amblyopic. Emmetropia was aimed for in all cases.

Group II, comprised of eight treated aphakic eyes of eight patients, underwent therapy between July and August 1990. Their mean age was 49.5 ±10.3 years. Preoperative refraction in this group varied between +11.0 and +16.0 D. Three eyes were partially sighted, with visual acuity of less than 20/33. The surgical technique was identical in both groups.

The technical procedure applied in these patients is described above. Gentamicin ointment was used postoperatively in both groups until the epithelial defect

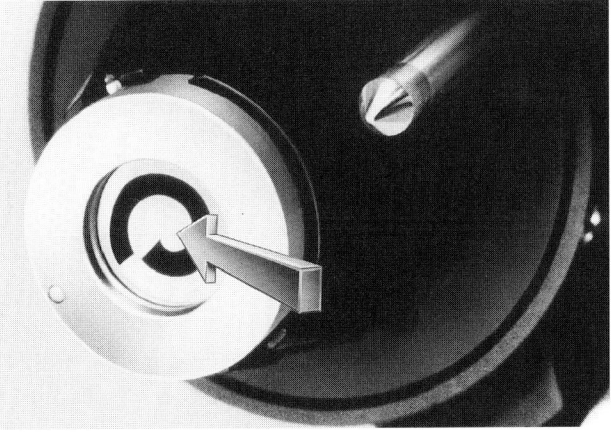

Fig. 17-3. Eye mask with spiral-shaped aperture for correction of hyperopia.

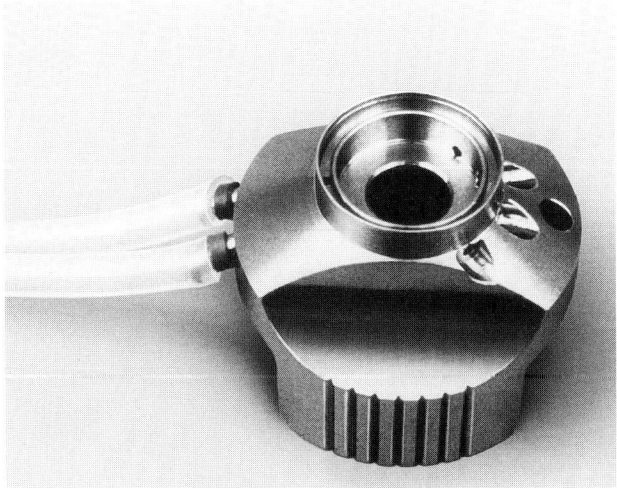

Fig. 17-4. Suction ring which has to be placed on the eye first. The mask shown in Fig. 17-3 is inserted into this ring.

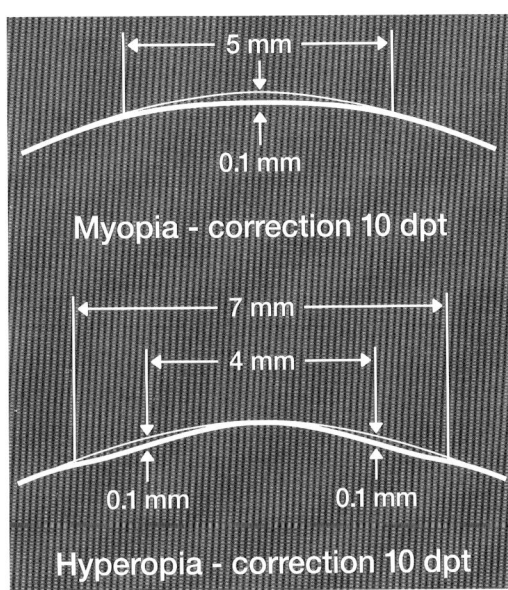

Fig. 17-2. Ablation principle for the correction of myopia and hyperopia. Cross section of ablation profile for correction of −10.00 D of myopia (*above*) and +10.0 D of hyperopia (*below*).

had healed. Fluorometholone eye drops were instilled five times a day the first month. Further medication with fluorometholone was not according to a standardized schedule, but was adapted to haze intensity and refraction.

Simultaneously, all patients received therapeutic contact lenses for a period of 3 months beginning 2 days after the epithelium was completely closed. These lenses were removed and cleaned every 4 weeks. The follow-up of both groups was 12 months.

Inclusion criteria stipulated that patients be at least 18 years old and have a stable hyperopic spherical equivalent of +2.0 D or more. Candidates with a corneal cylinder of more than 1.5 D were excluded. Patients with corneal scarring or disease, severe dry eye symptoms, blepharitis, or lagophthalmos were excluded from the study, except for long-term contact lens wearers with secondary micropannus and mild lenticular changes consistent with the patient's age. Patients with altered wound healing associated with systemic disease were excluded. The patients were given full written and oral informed consent.

Results

Refraction. The time course of the refraction in all 23 eyes is represented in Figs. 17-5 and 17-6.

Group I (+2.00-+7.50 D): The mean preoperative refraction was +4.7 (±1.6 D); at 1 month this value averaged −0.17 ±1.2 D; at 6 months, +0.33 ±1.0 D; and at 9 months, +0.53 ±1.2 D. The mean change from 1 to 9 months was 0.7 D. After 12 months, 12 eyes (80%) were within 1.0 D of emmetropia. Three eyes were outside this range (+3.5 D, +1.5 D, and +3.0 D, respectively).

Group II (+11.00-16.00 D): The mean preoperative refraction was +13.1 ±2.0 D; at 1 month this value averaged −0.5 ±1.6D; at 6 months, +1.5 ±1.3 D; and at 9 months, +2.5 ±2.1 D. Thus, the mean change in this group from 1 to 9 months was +3.0 D. Only three

of the eight eyes (37%) in group II were within 1.0 of emmetropia at 12 months.

The mean preoperative astigmatism (0.6 D; range, 0-1.25 D) was not significantly changed after 1 year (0.65 D; range, 0-1.5 D). None of the patients had an increase in astigmatism of more than 0.5 D 1 year postoperatively.

The changes in keratometer readings were significantly less marked than the changes in manifest refraction, and were of limited value. Also, the autorefractor measurement readings showed persistent hyperopia and were inconsistent with the manifest refraction.

Visual acuity. Group I (+2.00-+7.50 D): Best corrected visual acuity (BCVA) ranged preoperatively from 20/100 (amblyopic eye) to 20/20 (mean, 20/25), decreasing slightly to a mean of 20/30 (range, 20/100-20/20) at 1 month. At 12 months, only 1 eye had lost two lines, while 14 eyes showed no change or had improved. The eyes with no change or an improvement in BCVA displayed relatively good centration of the clear zone (Fig. 17-7A). A videokeratograph of one of these eyes after treatment is shown in Fig. 17-7B. The ablated zone of this eye was decentered approximately 1.3 mm inferotemporally relative to the vertex normal and this eye lost 2 lines of BCVA.

Group II (+11.00-+16.00 D): BCVA ranged preoperatively from 20/50 to 20/20 (mean, 20/35), decreasing to a mean of 20/57 (range, 20/100-20/40) at 1 month. At 12 months, two eyes displayed a decrease in BCVA compared with the preoperative value. Six eyes were unchanged or had improved.

In order to evaluate the efficacy of PRK for hyperopia, it is important to measure uncorrected visual acuity. In group I, mean uncorrected visual acuity improved from 20/60 preoperatively to 20/30 at 12 months. In group II, uncorrected visual acuity improved from less than 20/200 preoperatively to 20/80 at 12 months. Eighty percent of the eyes treated in group I, and 25% of those in group II had a visual

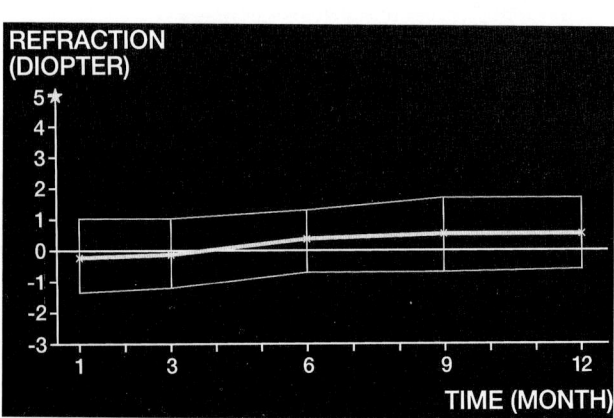

Fig. 17-5. Diagram of spherical equivalent of manifest refraction vs. time after PRK in hyperopia in group I (15 eyes with hyperopia from +2.0 to +7.50 D).

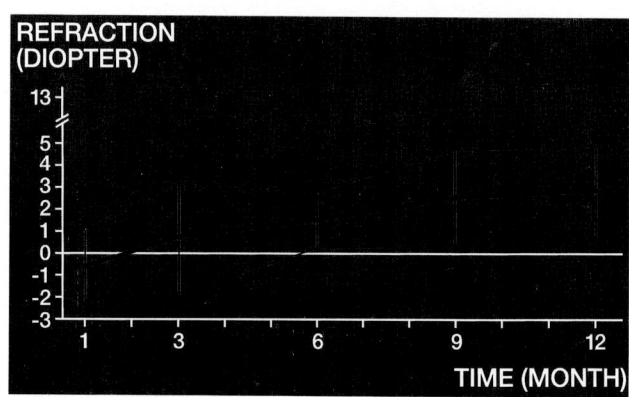

Fig. 17-6. Diagram of spherical equivalent of manifest refraction vs. time after PRK in hyperopia in group II (eight eyes with hyperopia from +11.0 to +16.0 D).

acuity of 20/40 or better, and 40% in group I and none in group II had a visual acuity of 20/20 or better without correction. However, In group I one eye was amblyopic, and in group II three partially sighted eyes did not have a preoperative potential of 20/40 or better.

Mean preoperative visual acuity under glare conditions was 20/40 in group I and 20/100 in group II. The best acuity measured with our glare tester was 0.8 (equivalent to 20/25).

At 12 months, glare visual acuity was 20/50 in group I and less than 20/200 in group II. One patient in group I lost two lines of BCVA and all eyes in group II lost more than one line.

Haze. The typical course of healing in groups I and II was as follows: After 3 to 4 weeks a ring of haze was seen (Fig. 17-8). In group I, this haze decreased or disappeared in the months that followed (Fig. 17-9). In group II, the haze was more severe from the outset, and there was practically no remission in the course of the 12-month follow-up period.

The severity of postoperative subepithelial haze was graded according to the classification devised by Dausch et al. (Table 17-1). One month after surgery, a

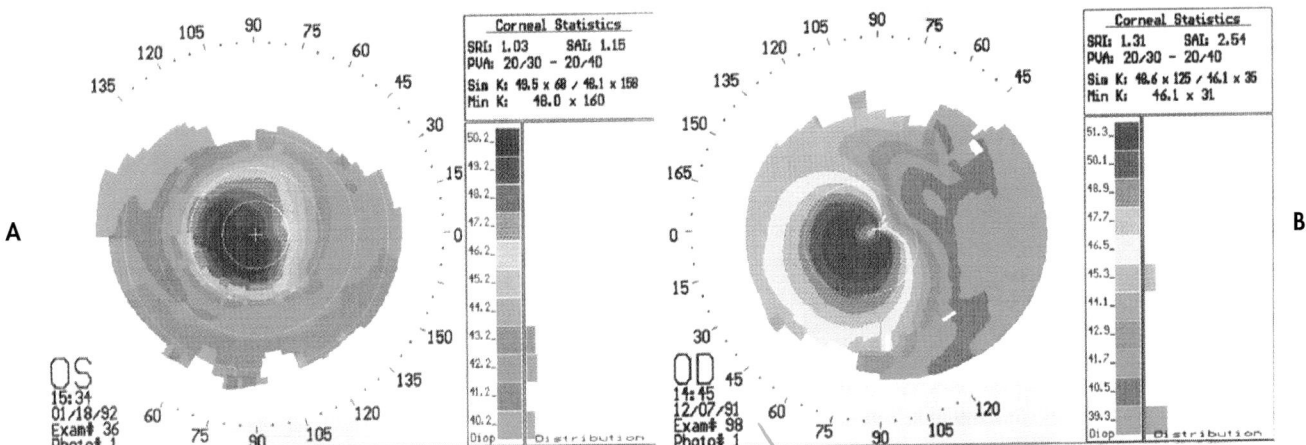

Fig. 17-7. A, Videokeratograph of an eye in which correction of +7.5 D was attempted. Uncorrected visual acuity was 20/200; best corrected spectacles visual acuity prior to surgery was 20/20. The videokeratograph shows the condition 18 months after PRK. The newly created clear zone, including the transition zone, is visible as *red, yellow,* and *green* areas. Uncorrected visual acuity 12 months after treatment was 20/20. **B,** Videokeratograph of an eye in which correction of +3.5 D was attempted. Uncorrected visual acuity was 20/20 and best corrected spectacles visual acuity (BCVA) was 20/20 prior to surgery. The videokeratograph shows the condition at 18 months after PRK. The clear zone is decentered approximately 1.3 mm inferotemporally relative to the vertex normal. Uncorrected visual acuity 12 months after treatment was 15/25; BCVA was 20/25.

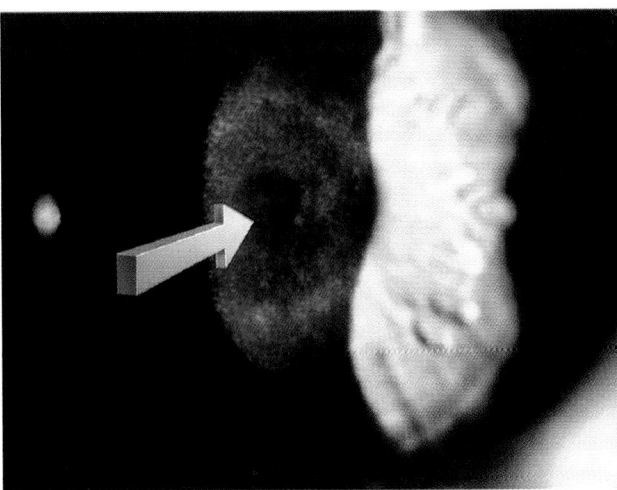

Fig. 17-8. Ring of subepithelial haze 6 weeks postoperatively. The untreated central cornea is clear.

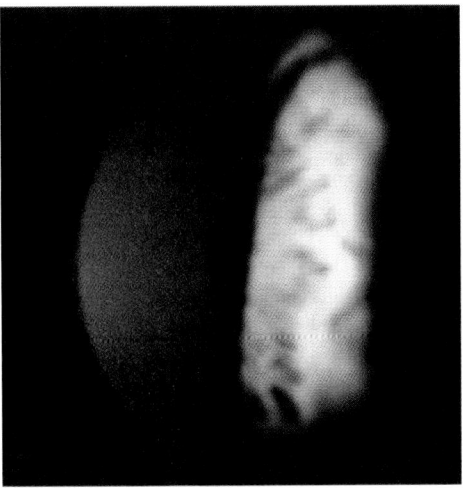

Fig. 17-9. Corneal subepithelial haze has disappeared after 6 months, leaving a clear zone.

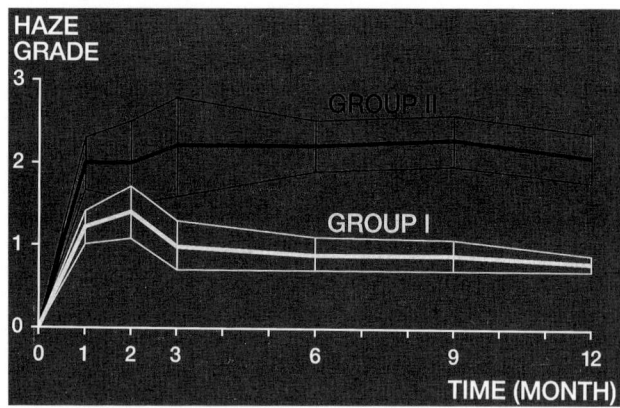

Fig. 17-10. Haze distribution: mean values with standard deviation for groups I and II. The overall mean haze score was higher in group II.

Table 15-1. Classification of haze

Grade	Corneal aspect	Postoperative best corrected visual acuity
O	Clear	No change
I	Traces of minimal reticular or spotlike haze	No change
II	Clearly visible reticular or punctate subepithelial structures	No change
III	Confluent subepithelial structures causing haze	Reduced

subepithelial ring of haze was detectable in all eyes; at that point in time, the mean haze intensity was 1.25 in group I and 2.0 in group II. The untreated corneal center, i.e., the small central area where Bowman's layer was not ablated, was clear. The intensity of the haze increased over the following 2 months. At 4 weeks, the mean haze intensity in group I was 1.25, increasing in the second month to a mean maximum of 1.4. Thereafter, it gradually but steadily decreased to 0.8 in the 12th month postoperatively (Fig. 17-10).

The mean haze intensity in group II was higher at all times, attaining 2.0 as early as 1 month postoperatively. It increased continuously until the ninth month postoperatively, thereafter decreasing slightly to 2.1 by the twelfth postoperative month.

The cornea of one eye in group II developed a ring of dense haze between 1 and 3 months postoperatively, which grew so that at 6 months the untreated central corneal region was involved. This severe haze then gradually decreased to grade II at 12 months (Fig. 17-11).

Epithelial disorders. In all cases, the epithelial defect healed within 3 days, at which time a soft contact

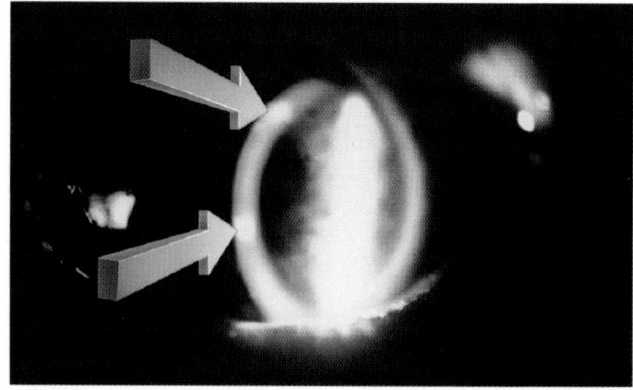

Fig. 17-11. Distinct ring-shaped haze 12 months after PRK in an aphakic eye. Attempted correction was +12.0 D. Best corrected visual acuity was 20/35 preoperatively and did not change 12 months postoperatively. The remaining refractive error was +1.0 D.

lens was applied for 3 months. All 15 eyes in group I healed without complications. However, three patients in group II displayed persistent epithelial defects. These defects, located paracentrally at the edge of the treated area, did not occur until 6 to 8 weeks after surgery. The eyes affected took 3 to 4 weeks to heal.

Subjective symptoms. All patients suffered from eye pain during the first 24 hours following surgery. After the first week and during the first month, three patients in group I and four in group II reported sporadic foreign body sensations. Almost all patients complained of halos, albeit of diminished intensity, when driving at night. At 12 months, none of the patients in group I noticed persistent halos, but all eight patients in group II considered them a problem.

One month after surgery, four patients in group I and all eight patients in group II complained of glare. After 1 year, only one patient in group I and seven in group II reported this side effect.

The Study of Anschütz and Dietzen

The hyperopic PRK study of Anschütz and Dietzen was initiated in late 1990. They used the same excimer laser of Aesculap-Meditec and the same technique with the rotating mask as described in the previous study of Dausch et al. In this study 81 hyperopic eyes were treated. In group I, 49 eyes had a manifest refraction between +2.0 D and +5.75 D. In group II, comprising 32 eyes, refraction ranged between +6.0 D and +10.0 D. The results of this study have not yet been published, but have been presented at the International Society of Refractive Keratoplasty meeting, Chicago, November 1993, and elsewhere. The main results are summarized in Figs. 17-12 and 17-13. They show the time course of the manifest refraction with a 1-year follow-up. The results are similar to those of Dausch et al.

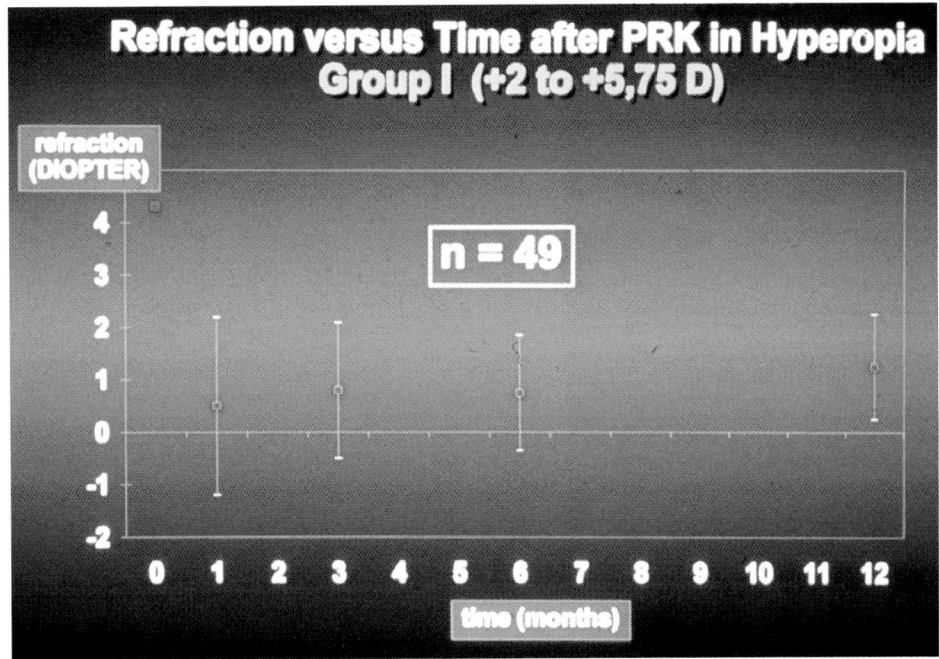

Fig. 17-12. Study of a hyperopic PRK (Anschütz and Dietzen): time course of the manifest refraction in group I (+2.0-+5.75 D).

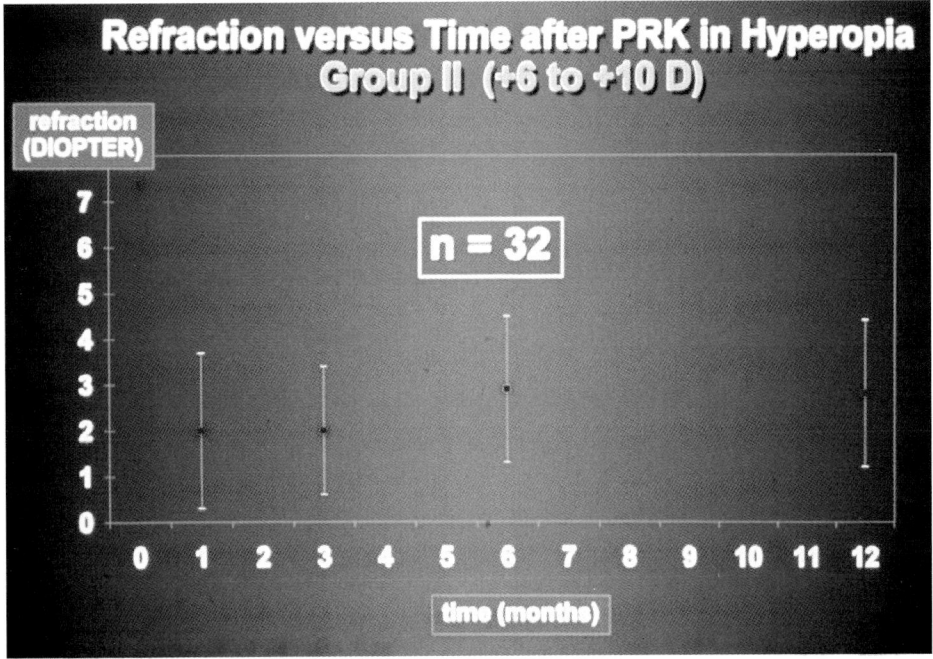

Fig. 17-13. Study of a hyperopic PRK (Anschütz and Dietzen): time course of the manifest refraction in group II (+6.0-+10.0 D).

Hyperopic Photorefractive Keratectomy in the Correction of Hyperopic and Mixed Astigmatism

With the technique of a rotating mask cylindrical ablation profiles can be realized. For this purpose the angular steps of the rotation are varied so that the angular distances are not equidistant. In this way the ab-

lation depth can be increased in one meridian. This results in a profile that has a hyperopic and cylindrical component (Fig. 17-14).

To correct mixed astigmatism, the cylindrical component is corrected as a myopic cylinder with, in addition, a spherical hyperopic component. For this pur-

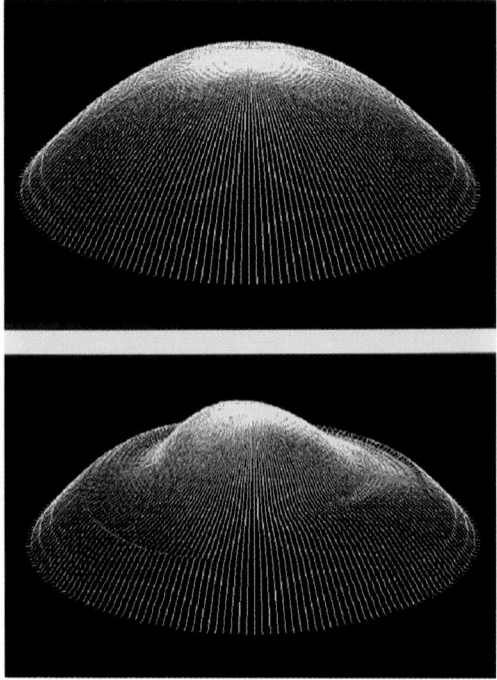

Fig. 17-14. Computer simulation of correction of a compound hyperopic astigmatism before *(top)* and after *(bottom)* treatment.

pose the mask has to be changed during the treatment sessions. The suction ring remains in place at all times. These complicated ablation profiles can be realized with a perfect superimposition of both parts of the treatment procedure.

CASE STUDIES
COMPOUND HYPEROPIC ASTIGMATISM

Patient 1 was a 55-year-old woman with naturally occurring compound hyperopic astigmatism. Her preoperative examination revealed a manifest refraction of +7.25 −3.75 × 55 degrees, keratometric readings of 47.30/44.1 at 51 degrees, uncorrected visual acuity of 20/200, and BCVA of 20/40. Preoperative corneal topography revealed a symmetric bow-tie astigmatism with a steepening of the 141-degree meridian (Fig. 17-15, *bottom left*). Ten weeks after excimer laser PRK the uncorrected visual acuity was 20/50 (0.4); the manifest refraction was +0.5 D. The keratometer readings were 54.6 at 53 degrees and 51.30 at 143 degrees. BCVA was 20/25 (0.63). Corneal topography revealed an overall steepening of the cornea (Fig. 17-15, *top left*). The difference image (Fig. 17-15, *right*) shows the ring-shaped flattened zone in the corneal periphery *(blue)* and the steepened corneal center *(red)*.

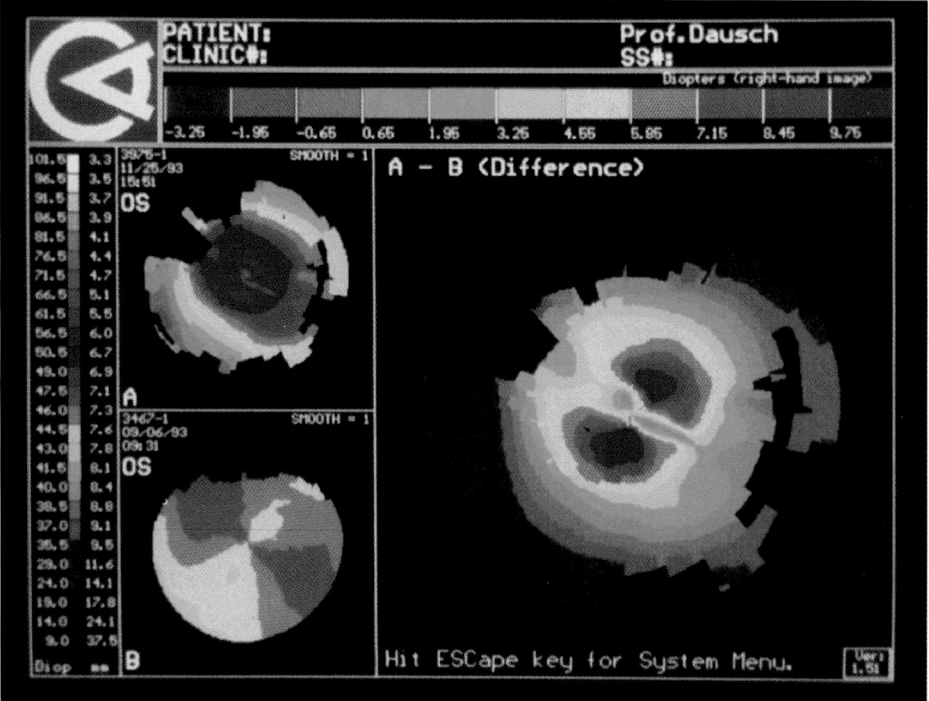

Fig. 17-15. Color-coded keratographs of patient 1 before (**B**, *Bottom left*) and 10 weeks after (**A**, *Top left*) toric ablation to correct a refractive error of +7.25 −3.75 × 55 degrees (compound hyperopic astigmatism). Postoperative keratograph shows an oval steepening of the cornea. The longer axis of this oval is aligned with the preoperative steeper axis. The difference image *(right)* shows the ring-shaped flattened zone in the corneal periphery *(blue)* and the steepened corneal center *(red, yellow, and green)*. The meridian in the axis of 53 degrees is more steepened than the meridian in the axis of 143 degrees.

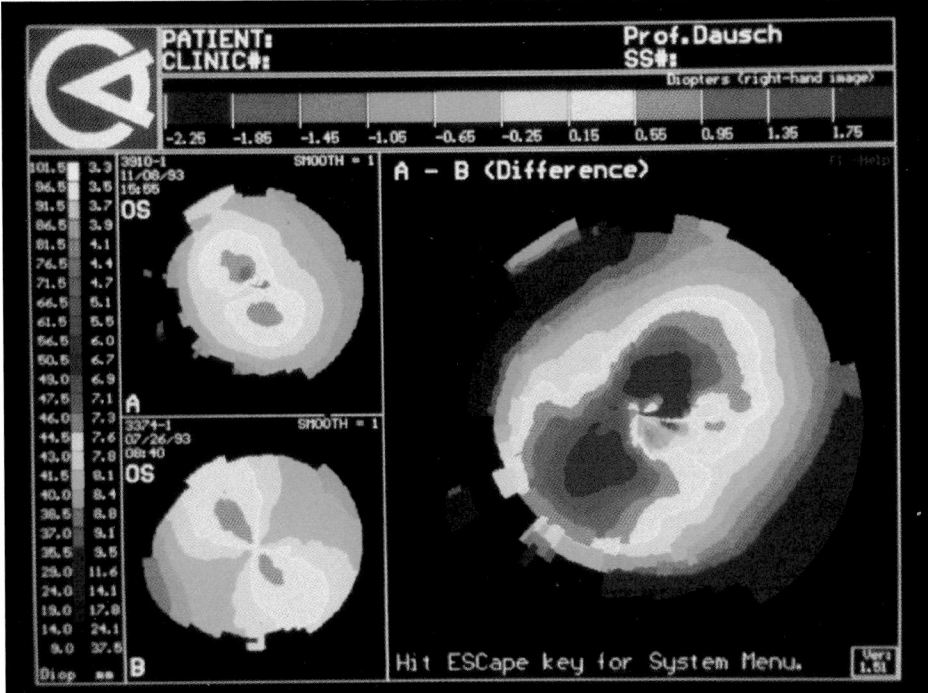

Fig. 17-16. Color-coded keratographs of patient 2 before (**B**, *bottom left*) and 2 months after (**A**, *top left*) PRK to correct a refractive error of +1.50 −4.25 × 33 degrees (mixed astigmatism). In the difference image *(right)* the ring-shaped flattening in the corneal periphery is visible *(blue)*, necessary for steepening of the corneal center. The preoperatively flatter meridian in the axis of 38 degrees is steepened for the correction of hyperopia *(red)*, and the preoperatively steeper meridian in the axis of 128 degrees is flattened for the astigmatic correction *(yellow* and *green)*.

Mixed astigmatism

Patient 2 was a 35 year-old woman with naturally occurring mixed astigmatism who was contact lens–intolerant. This patient had a preoperative manifest refraction of +1.50 −4.25 × 33 degrees, keratometric readings of 45.80 at 128 degrees and 41.70 at 38 degrees, uncorrected visual acuity of 20/100 (0.1), and BCVA of 20/20. Corneal topography revealed a typical symmetric bow-tie astigmatism with the steeper portion in the 128-degree meridian (Fig. 17-16, *bottom left*). Two months after excimer laser PRK the manifest refraction was plano, and uncorrected visual acuity was 20/20. Corneal topography revealed for the correction of hyperopia a steepening of the cornea in the preoperatively flatter meridian of 38 degrees and for the astigmatic correction a flattening in the 128 degree meridian. Biomicroscopy revealed a barely detectable haze.

SUMMARY

The previous studies on PRK in hyperopia showed a postoperative regression which was more marked in the eyes in which higher corrections had been attempted. This is in accordance with the results of PRK in myopia. Correction of higher hyperopia by PRK

also requires a deeper stromal excision and a more abrupt change in corneal curvature at the edge of the ablation, with a more marked wound-healing response.

There are important considerations about the location of haze following PRK for hyperopia. In this procedure the center of the cornea, including Bowman's layer, remains intact. The haze is therefore ring-shaped. The stromal haze is at its densest at the border of the ablated zone. Owing to this localization, the haze that develops after PRK for hyperopia does not play the same role as that following PRK for myopia.

The fact that the haze intensity after PRK for hyperopia does not affect visual acuity as much as in correcting myopia is easily explained: the center is left intact. It was found that eyes that sustained a loss of BCVA 12 months after surgery had clear central corneas. We believe that this loss of BCVA is due to a decentration of more than 1 mm relative to the vertex normal, since the videokeratograph showed the decentration to be the greatest (1.0-1.3 mm) in these eyes.

Under normal lighting conditions visual acuity had not deteriorated. However, glare tests demonstrated that visual acuity decreased under glare conditions. As in PRK for myopia, we assume that haze is not the

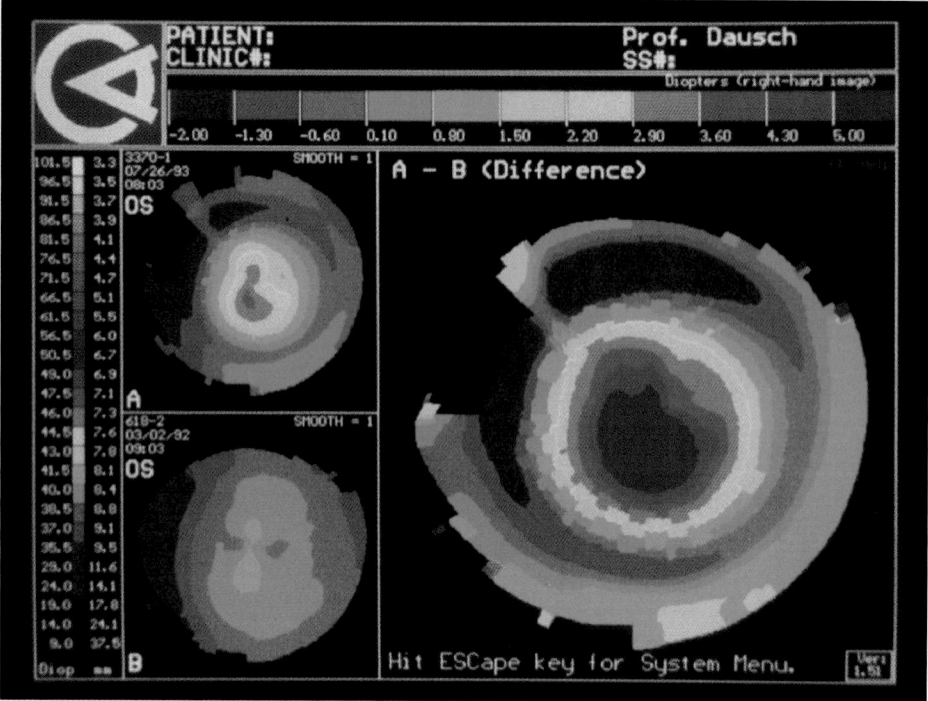

Fig. 17-17. Color-coded keratographs of an hyperopic eye before (**B**, *bottom left*) and 1.5 years after PRK (**A**, *top left*) to correct a refractive error of +8.50 −0.75 × 155 degrees. Note the large well-centered optical zone, created with a new mask with an increased outer diameter of 9-mm spiral-shaped aperture. The difference image *(right)* shows a wide ring-shaped ablation zone in the corneal periphery *(blue)* and a steepened corneal center *(red)*.

only reason for the reduced visual acuity under glare but may also occur because the central clear zone is smaller than the dilated pupil.

This difference between the pupil and the size of the treated zone may also lead to halo and glare problems. We observed a decrease in intensity of the complaints about halos and glare within 12 months.

Loss of BCVA and vision-threatening complications are important factors to investigate. Decentration of the clear zone causes a decrease in BCVA. Since we saw this problem most often in the higher hyperopic eyes we decided to abstain from PRK for hyperopia over 7.5 D. In these cases even a small error of centration leads to a marked deterioration in BCVA.

FUTURE CONSIDERATIONS

To diminish the problem of centration a new mask has been designed. The inner diameter of the spiral-shaped aperture is increased fom 4 to 6 mm; the outer diameter, including the transition zone, is increased from 7 to 9 mm. The videokeratograph in Fig. 17-17 shows the ablation zone after PRK with this new mask. This enlargement of the treated area causes fewer problems postoperatively if decentration occurs. Our experience with myopic PRK is that larger

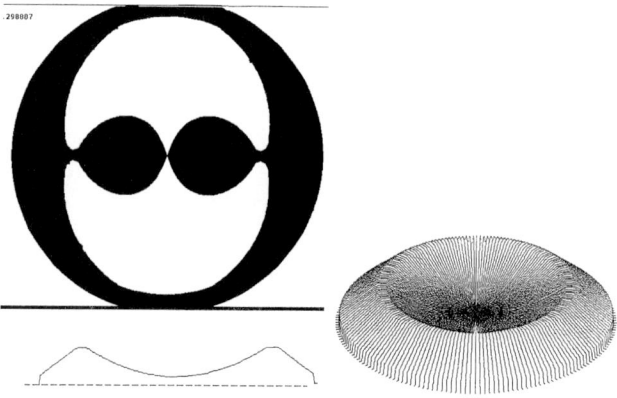

Fig. 17-18. Computer simulation of hyperopic PRK with an aspheric profile. *Top left:* Shape of the template. *Bottom left:* Cross section of the ablation profile. *Bottom right:* Three-dimensional profile of the cornea after hyperopic PRK.

zones show less regression. This could also be the case in hyperopia.

Another concept involves the idea of aspherical ablation profiles. One has to take into account that the ablation rate of Bowman's layer is higher than that of the anterior stroma, an even greater difference than the ablation rate of midstromal tissue. Bearing these facts in mind, the design of the mask should be such that an aspherical ablation profile can be achieved (Fig. 17-18). This may also improve future hyperopic PRK.

REFERENCES

1. McDonald MB, Beuerman R, Falzoni, et al: Refractive surgery with the excimer laser, *Am J Opthalmol* 103:469, 1987.
2. McDonald MB, Frantz JM, Klyce SD, et al: One year refractive results of central photorefractive keratectomy for myopia in the nonhuman primate cornea, *Arch Ophthalmol* 108:40-47, 1990.
3. DelPero RA, Gigstad JRE, Roberts AD, et al: A refractive and histopathologic study of excimer laser in primates, *Am J Ophthalmol* 109:419-429, 1990.
4. McDonald MB, Frantz JM, Klyce,SD, et al: Central photorefractive keratectomy for myopia. The blind eye study, *Arch Ophthalmol* 108:799-808, 1990.
5. Seiler T, Kahle G, Kriegerowski M: Excimer laser (193 nm) myopic keratomileusis in sighted and blind eyes, *Refract Corneal Surg* 6:165-173, 1990.
6. Seiler T, Wollensak J: Myopic photorefractive keratectomy with the excimer laser. One year follow-up, *Ophthalmology* 98:1156-1163, 1991.
7. Dausch D, Klein R, Schröder E: Photoablative, refraktive Keratektomie (PRK) zur Behandlung der Myopie. Eine Fallstudie an 134 myopen Augen mit 6-monatiger Nachbeobachtungszeit, *Fortschr Ophthalmol* 88:770-776, 1991.
8. Barraquer JI: El microqueratomo en chirurgia corneal, *Arch Soc AM Oftalmol Optom* 88:709-715, 1967.
9. Swinger CA, Barraquer JI: Keratophakia and keratomileusis. Clinical results, *Ophthalmology* 88:709-715, 1981.
10. Troutman RC, Swinger C, Goldstein M: Keratophakia update, *Ophthalmology* 88:36-38, 1981.
11. Friedlander MH, Herblin TP, Kaufman HE, et al. Clinical results of keratophakia and keratomileusis, *Ophthalmology* 88:716-720, 1981.
12. Barraquer JI: Results of hypermetropic keratomileusis *Int Opthalmol Clin* 23:25-44, 1983.
13. Neumann AC, Sanders D, Raanan M, et al: Hyperopic thermokeratoplasty: clinical evaluation, *J Cataract Refract Surg* 17:830-838, 1991.
14. Seiler T, Matallana M, Bende T: Laserkoagulation der Hornhaut mit einem Holmium:YAG Laser zur Hyperopiekorrektur, *Fortschr Ophthalmol* 88:121-124, 1991.

NonContact Holmium:YAG Laser Thermal Keratoplasty

Douglas D. Koch, Michael J. Berry, Arthur Vassiliadis, Adrian A. Abarca, Rogelio Villarreal, Elizabeth A. Haft

Thermal keratoplasty is the use of heat to alter the properties and structure of corneal stromal collagen in order to modify anterior corneal curvature. Laser thermal keratoplasty (LTK) uses laser light that is absorbed by the cornea to produce the desired temperature elevation. Thermal keratoplasty has a long and admittedly troubled history. Fortunately, new advances in laser technology and better understanding of corneal properties and of corneal topography have led to the development of safe and effective LTK procedures.

HISTORY

Lans[1] in 1898 first reported that cautery could be used to reduce astigmatism. He compared this to tissue resections and found cautery to be more effective but less stable and predictable. In isolated case reports, Wray[2] in 1914 and O'Connor[3] in 1933 each described the successful use of cautery to treat astigmatism. The literature is devoid of other clinical reports until thermal keratoplasty was reintroduced in the early 1970s as a treatment for keratoconus.

The modern era of keratoplasty was initiated by Stringer and Parr,[4] who in 1964 reported that the thermal shrinkage temperature of corneal collagen was 55° to 58° C. In the early and mid-1970s, extensive work was done in evaluating thermal keratoplasty for the treatment of keratoconus.[5-7] Thermal keratoplasty was reported to be effective in flattening the cone, eliminating the need for keratoplasty in patients who were spectacles- and contact lens–intolerant. Successful treatment of hydrops was also reported.[8] Unfortunately, treatments were complicated by poor predictability and stability and by corneal scarring, vascularization, aseptic stromal necrosis, and bullous keratopathy, as well as fibrinous iritis with hypopyon.[9] Although work with this method was abandoned in the United States, Itoi[10] in 1981 reported treatment of 750 keratoconus patients with thermal keratoplasty and stated that only 7% needed penetrating keratoplasty. Because of the shortage of donor tissue in Japan, he advocated that, in Japan, thermal keratoplasty be performed prior to penetrating keratoplasty.

In 1980, Rowsey and colleagues[11,12] reported the use of a radiofrequency probe to perform thermal keratoplasty in a more controlled fashion. Rowsey[13] abandoned this work because of problems with predictability and stability.

RECENT ADVANCES

Contemporary approaches to thermal keratoplasty began with the work of Fyodorov,[14] who developed a thermal probe consisting of a 34-gauge wire that is heated to 600° C. Treatment patterns for correction of hyperopia and astigmatism were developed. Clinical trials have demonstrated high initial corrections but with moderate regression the first few months following treatment.[15] The burns produce prominent scars that gradually fade but are still clearly apparent by 1 year postoperatively. Long-term stability is still uncertain.[16]

A critical advance in thermal keratoplasty has been the use of lasers to deliver exquisitely controllable and measurable amounts of energy to the corneal stroma. In 1990 Bruce Sand was granted a patent for performing infrared LTK, and his work led to the development of the laser discussed here. Fyodorov[17] studied the use of the carbon dioxide and erbium:glass lasers for performing thermal keratoplasty. With the latter, treating at a wavelength of 1.54 μm, Kanoda and Sorokin[18] reported correction of over 3 D of hyperopia with ongoing low-grade regression at 12 months following treatment. Other important laboratory and clinical work has been performed by Seiler, Durrie, and Thompson and their colleagues and this is reported in the following section of this chapter.

MECHANISM

Heating corneal collagen to the proper temperature can result in shrinkage to one third of its original length (Fig. 17-19). Thermal processing of collagen produces dissociation of hydrogen bonds, partial unwinding of the triple helix, cross-linking between amino acid moieties, and changes in hydration.[19-21] The amount of shrinkage is dependent upon the mechanical properties of the surrounding tissue.

There are at least three critical parameters that will determine the ultimate success of thermal keratoplasty:

1. *Collagen shrinkage temperatures.* Collagen shrinkage occurs within a relatively narrow temperature range. Allain and colleagues[22] demonstrated that relaxation of shrunken collagen begins as low as 78° C and that this temperature increases with increasing tissue age. As tissue ages, there is an increase in the number of thermally stable cross-linking bonds, resulting in a higher temperature threshold for thermally induced collagen relaxation.

2. *Keratocyte response.* We hypothesize that an important determinant of long-term stability is the avoidance of a corneal wound-healing response.

This wound-healing response would consist of keratocyte proliferation with deposition of new collagen, collagen remodeling, and production of new and abnormal glycosaminoglycans. McCalley and colleagues[23] found that keratocyte injury occurs when stromal collagen is heated to approximately 79° C. At this time we are unaware of the keratocyte response to thermal injury, and we are in the process of investigating the wound-healing response to LTK.

3. *Stability of corneal collagen.* Stability of a refractive change from LTK is presumably dependent on a long half-life of the thermally processed collagen. There is evidence that collagen turnover in the cornea may occur very slowly, perhaps with a half-life exceeding 10 or more years.[24] Lass and colleagues[25] used proline radiolabeling to study collagen turnover in corneal transplants performed in young New Zealand white rabbits. They found a moderately high turnover in collagen in the graft periphery within the first 20 days postoperatively with no significant change thereafter. They also found that little change occurred centrally. These results appear to confirm the concept that the turnover of corneal collagen is extremely slow.

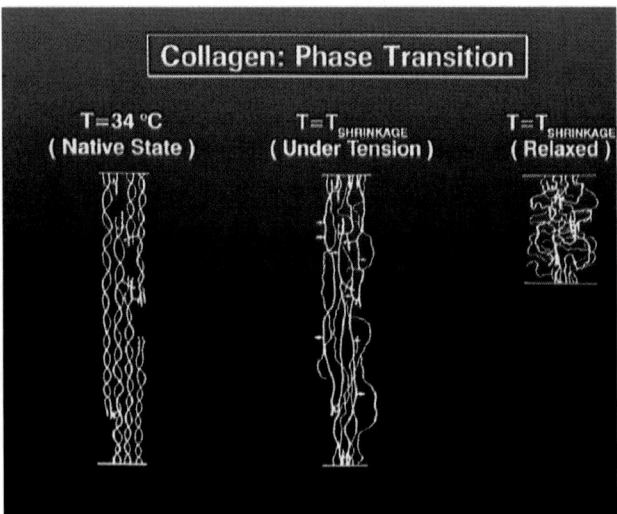

Fig. 17-19. Heating collagen above 58° C results in breakdown of the triple helix and, depending upon the surrounding tissue resistance, shrinkage to as short as one third of its original length.

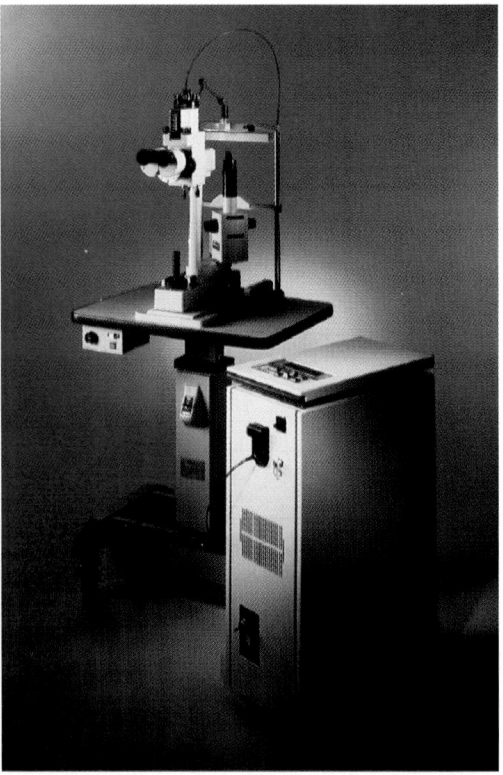

Fig. 17-20. The Ho:YAG laser (Sunrise Technologies, Fremont, Calif.). The laser is contained in the floor unit to the *right*. Laser light is delivered by a fiberoptic cable to the slit-lamp delivery system on the *left*.

NONCONTACT LASER THERMOKERATOPLASTY
Background

Laser thermokeratoplasty has been investigated with a number of different lasers, including carbon dioxide,[26] cobalt:magnesium fluoride,[27] hydrogen fluoride,[28-30] erbium:glass,[17] and holmium:YAG. All of these devices achieve their effect by delivering laser light to the cornea either with an optical delivery system or a contact probe. The light is absorbed and converted to heat, and collagen shrinkage occurs. Depending upon a large number of variables, corneal topography is thereby modified.

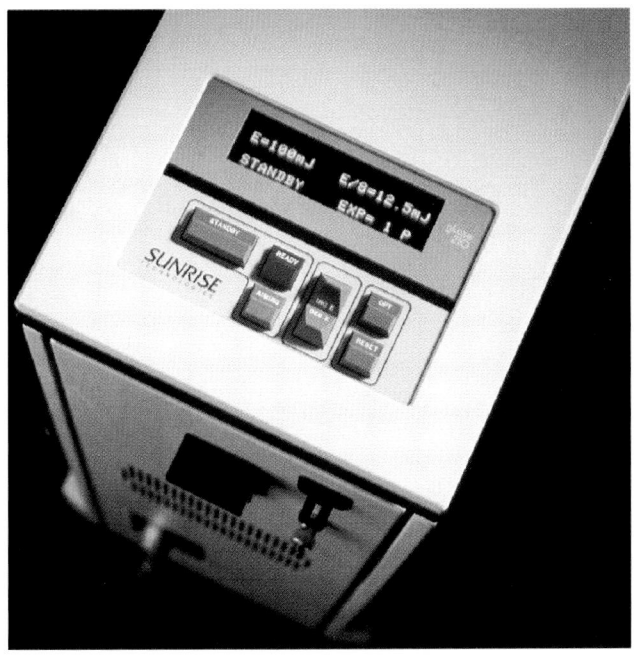

Fig. 17-21. Control panel of the Ho:YAG laser.

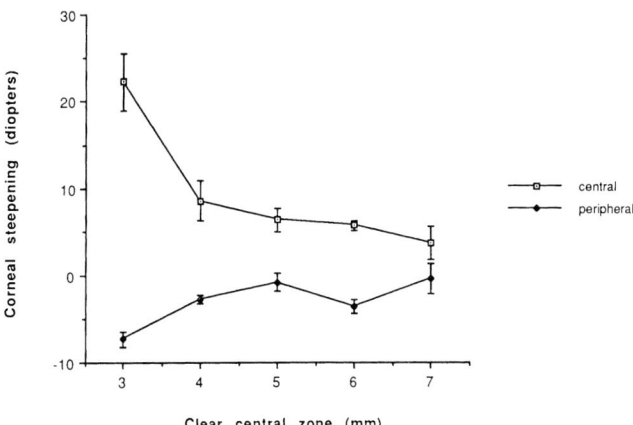

Fig. 17-23. Graph of central and peripheral corneal dioptric changes after laser thermokeratoplasty in human eye bank eyes.

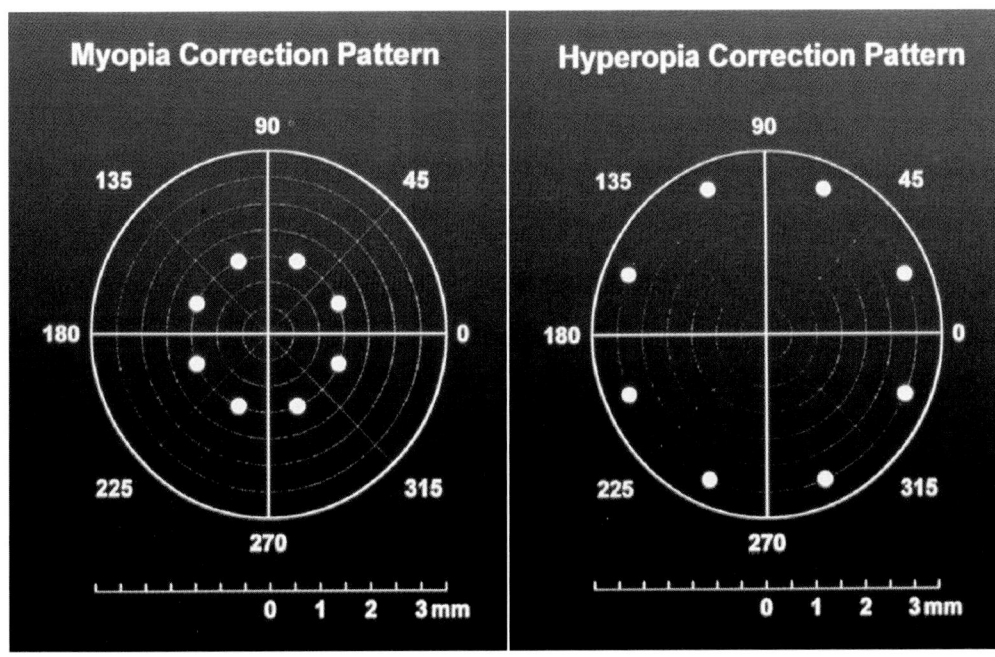

Fig. 17-22. Studies with swine and human cadaver eyes have shown that treatment at the 3.0- to 3.5-mm zones produces central corneal flattening *(left)*, whereas treatment at or beyond the 5.0-mm zone results in central corneal steepening *(right)*.

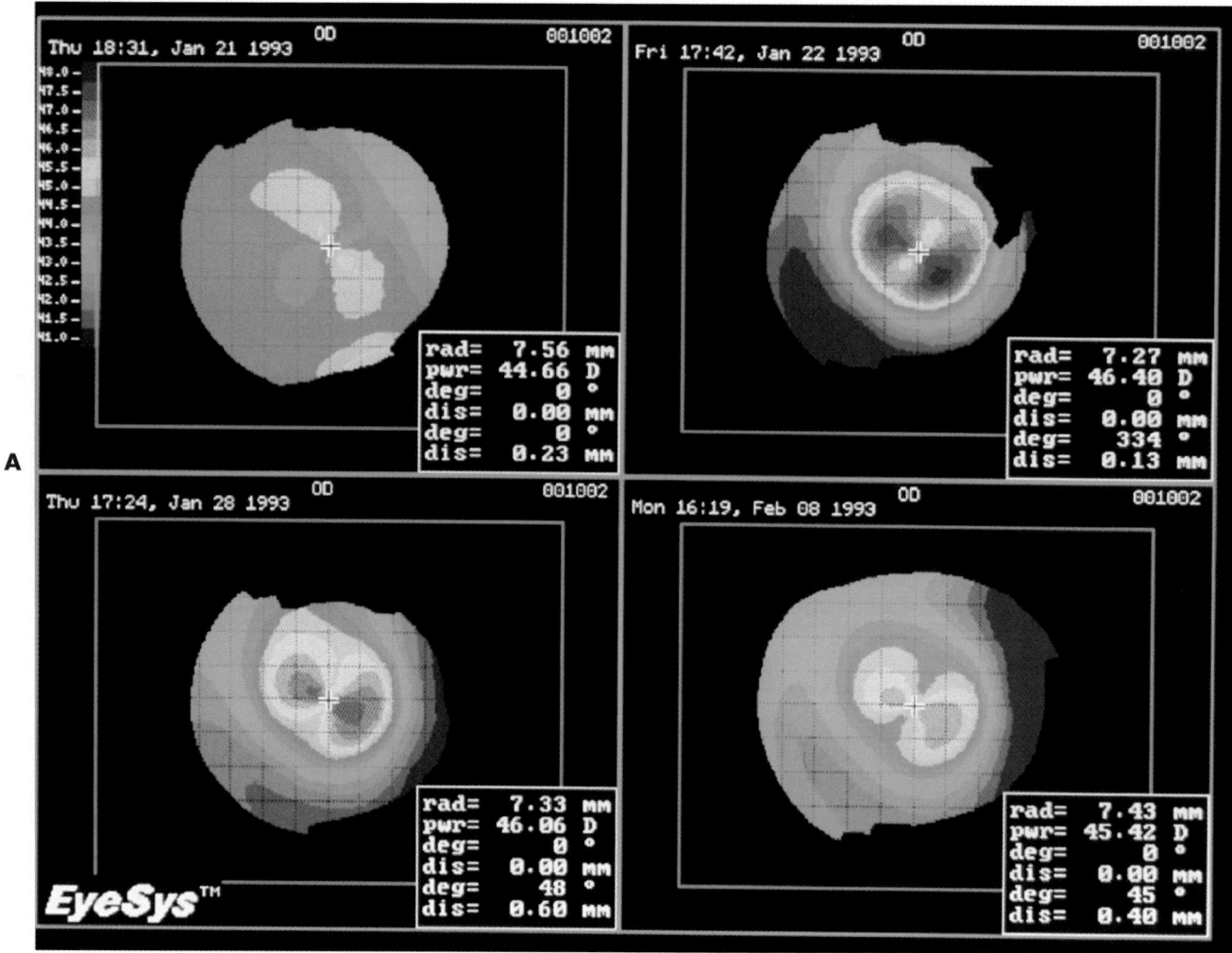

Fig. 17-24. Corneal topographic maps **A,** preoperatively *(upper left)*, and postoperatively 1 day *(upper right)*, 1 week *(lower left)*, 2 weeks *(lower right)*. **B,** 1 month *(upper left)*, 3 months *(upper right)*, and 6 months *(lower left)* following Ho:YAG laser thermal keratoplasty.

The laser device used in the studies to be described below is the Sunrise Technologies Ho:YAG laser (Sunrise Technologies, Fremont, Calif.) (Figs. 17-20 and 17-21). It is a compact, solid-state laser that operates at a wavelength of 2.13 μm, with a 250-μs pulse duration and a 5-Hz pulse repetition frequency. It utilizes a fiberoptic slit-lamp delivery system for noncontact delivery of the laser energy in one to eight spots with 500- to 600-μm spot diameter. A number of investigators have studied the potential for modifying corneal topography by performing LTK with the Sunrise device.

We performed in vitro experiments using fresh swine eyes.[31] Corneas were thinned to 0.65 mm or less by soaking them in 10% dextran, and intraocular pressure was controlled at 15 to 20 mm Hg. The epithelium was surgically removed with a blunt blade. Treatment consisted of four to eight spots with ten pulses

per spot. The range of pulse energy densities was 8 to 11 J/cm². We varied the diameter of the treatment zone and assessed corneal topographic changes with the EyeSys Corneal Analysis System (EyeSys Technologies, Inc., Houston, Tex.). We found that, at treatment zones of 3.0 and 3.5 mm, central corneal flattening of up to 9 D was produced (Fig. 17-22, *left*). A null zone in which no effect was achieved occurred in the 4.0- 4.5-mm region. At zones of 5 mm or greater, central corneal steepening of over 4 D was produced (Fig. 17-22, *right*). This latter effect could be magnified both by increasing the number of spots to 16 and by adding 16 additional spots in a second more peripheral annulus. Increased curvature change could be achieved by increasing pulse number and energy density.

Moreira et al.[32] evaluated the Sunrise device by performing LTK in 40 human cadaver eyes. Treatment pa-

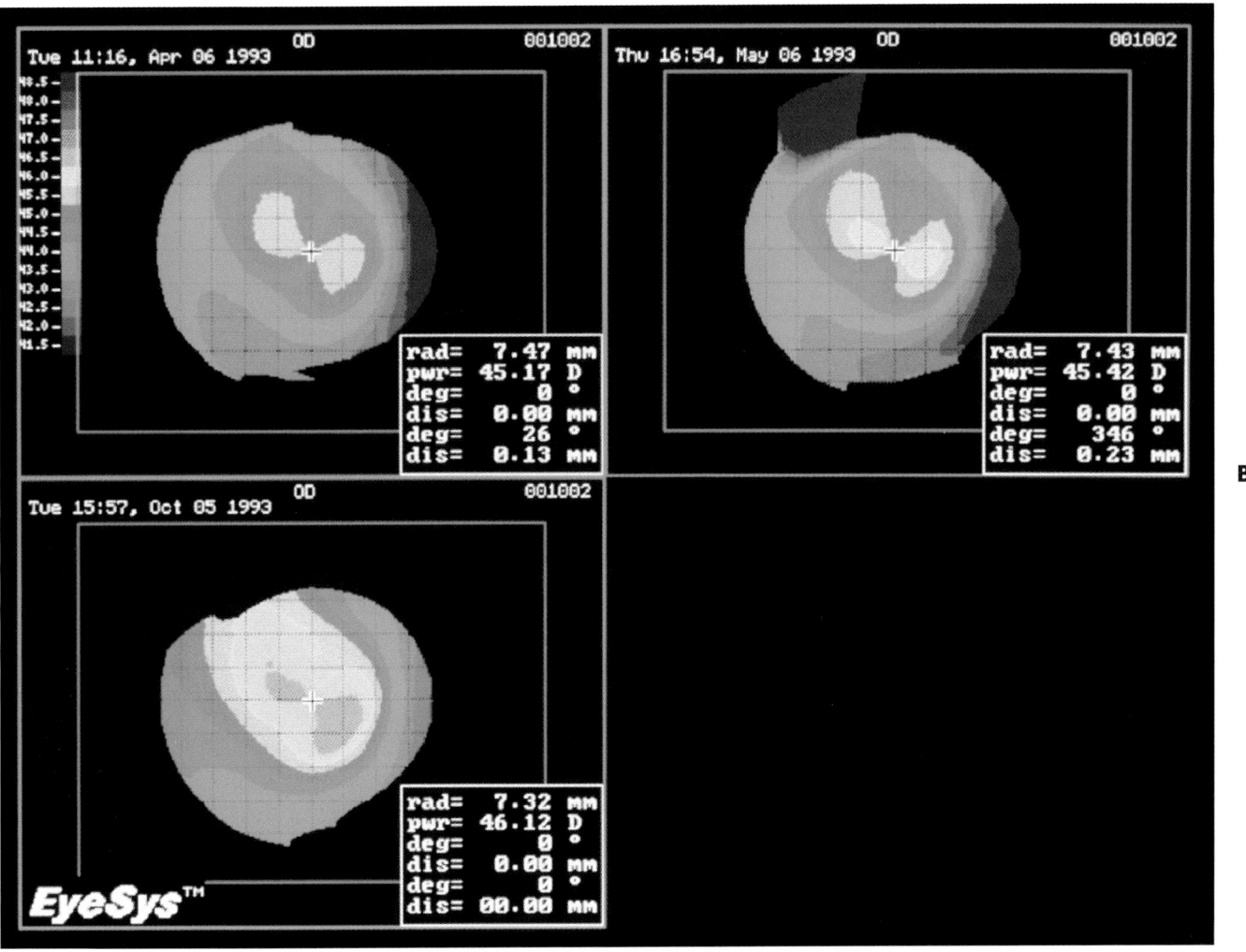

B

Fig. 17-24, cont'd. For legend see opposite page.

rameters were 32 spots, spot diameter of 300 μm, energy density of 9 J/cm^2, and treatment diameters ranging from 3 to 7 mm in 1-mm increments. They found that the laser treatment produced central corneal steepening at all treatment diameters, with the amount of induced central steepening decreasing as ring diameter increased (Fig. 17-23). Comparing the data from Moreira et al. and our studies, it is apparent that at smaller treatment zones the induced change in central corneal curvature is highly dependent upon the number of spots, spot diameter, and pulse energy density.

Moreira et al.[32] also studied histopathologic changes in rabbit corneas. At 4 weeks post treatment they noted a wedge-shaped area of altered stromal architecture extending to approximately 80% depth. At suprathreshold energies exceeding 15 J/cm^2, keratocyte nuclei became pyknotic. Minor endothelial changes were noted at 8 J/cm^2. At extremely high energies in excess of 20 J/cm^2, maximum endothelial loss was estimated to be approximately 1.2%. They

concluded that LTK with this device appeared to be safe.

First Clinical Studies

McDonnell and colleagues performed a phase I Food and Drug Administration (FDA) trial to test the safety of the Sunrise laser in nonsighted eyes (Peter J. McDonnell, a personal communication, 1994). A total of ten blind eyes were treated. Some patients experienced mild discomfort in the first 24 hours following treatment. A wedge- or bowl-shaped opacity in the anterior 30% to 50% of the cornea was noted in the treated eyes. This diminished but was still evident with the slit-lamp biomicroscopy 6 months following treatment. The intensity of the opacity was grade 1 or less in all patients. There were no complications.

Clinical Trials

Clinical trials with Sunrise Ho:YAG laser were begun outside of the United States in 1993. Initial studies were performed for the correction of hyperopia. Reported here are the treatment results of the first 16 eyes using the eight-spot pattern. Patient entry criteria were refractive hyperopia of 1 to 5 D. Mean age was 54.7 years; 3 of the 16 patients were female. Follow-up in all eyes was 6 months or greater.

The treatment protocol included the administration of proparacaine drops two or three times prior to treatment. Lids were held open with a fixation ring. Each patient received eight spots with ten pulses per spot for a total treatment duration of 2 seconds.

The laser has a central fixation light and eight helium-neon target lights that are coincident with the eight laser spots. To center the treatment, the patient fixates on the central target, and the surgeon centers

the eight spots around the patient's entrance pupil. A focusing aid has subsequently been added to ensure that the laser is focused on the anterior corneal surface, but this was not available for the initial studies. Three treatment diameters were used: 5.0 mm (2 eyes), 5.5 mm (2 eyes), and 6.0 mm (12 eyes).

Treatments at the 5.0- and 5.5-mm zones produced initial central corneal steepening, but little change persisted beyond 1 week. In the patients receiving eight spots with a 6.0-mm treatment zone, the spherical equivalent of the manifest refraction improved from +1.6 D preoperatively to +0.7 D at 6 months. Refractive change was stable from 3 months to 6 months and indeed showed only 0.4 D of regression between 1 day and 6 months. Mean uncorrected distance acuity im-

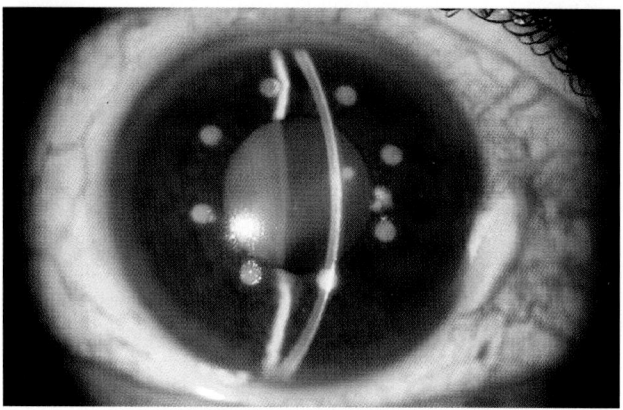

Fig. 17-25. Human cornea immediately following Ho:YAG laser thermal keratoplasty, showing moderate opacification, primarily due to epithelial opacification.

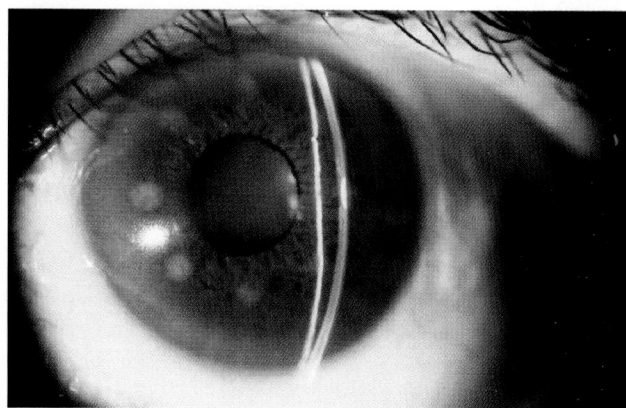

Fig. 17-26. Human cornea 6 months following laser thermal keratoplasty; the haze at the treatment sites was still evident by slit-lamp microscopy.

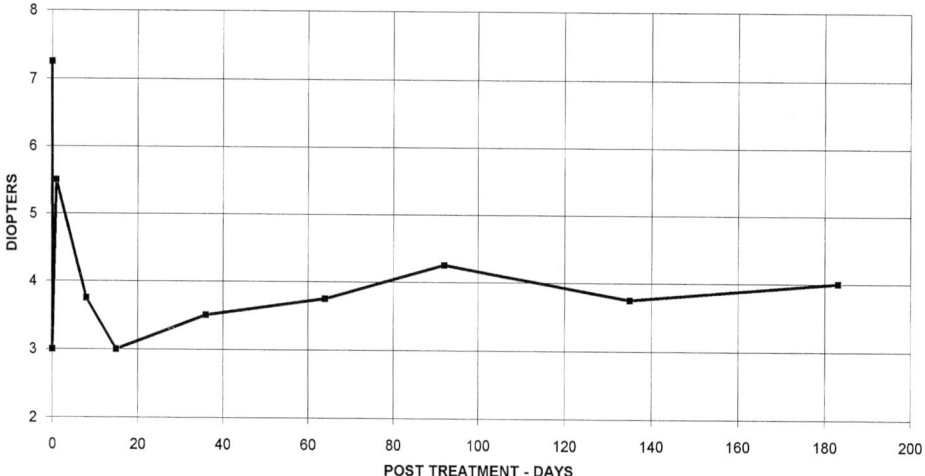

SUBJECTIVE MANIFEST (E.S.)

Fig. 17-27. Graph of manifest refraction of the left eye of a 33-year-old woman who underwent Ho:YAG laser thermal keratoplasty with the application of eight spots at 6-mm diameter, ten pulses per spot, and energy density of 8.85 J/cm². There is only 0.25 D more hyperopia at 6 months compared to 1 week following treatment.

proved from 20/80 preoperatively to 20/37 at 6 months, and the percentage of patients seeing 20/40 or better uncorrected improved from 25% to 75%. Likewise, the percentage of patients with uncorrected acuity of 20/25 or better improved from 0% to 25% at 6 months. Topographic changes closely matched the refractive changes and showed remarkably good stability by 1 week following the treatment (Fig. 17-24).

Complications included epithelial defects or staining for the first 1 to 3 days postoperatively. Haze was produced at all treatment sites. This was moderately opaque immediately following treatment, primarily due to epithelial opacification (Fig. 17-25). By 1 week, the intensity of the haze was Grade 1, and the haze continued to diminish (Fig. 17-26) but was still evident by slit-lamp microscopy at 6 months following treatment. Mean keratometric astigmatism increased from 0.5 D to 0.7 D; the maximum increase was 1.5 D (one patient). None of the patients lost BCVA, and testing with the Regan Contrast Acuity Charts (96%, 50%, 25%, 11%) (Paragon Services, Nova Scotia, Canada) showed no loss of two or more lines on any chart in all patients by 1 month following treatment.

Subsequently, other treatments have been initiated using higher energy levels and a greater number of spots. Hyperopic corrections of 3 D or greater have been achieved, again with good stability within 1 week following treatment (Fig. 17-27).

CONCLUSIONS

We believe that the preclinical and early clinical studies demonstrate that LTK is a promising treatment for correction of low to moderate hyperopia. The treatment appears to be safe and extremely well tolerated. The laser device itself has the advantages of safety, ease of use, and low cost. An important advantage of LTK is that treatments are likely to be repeatable, permitting either titration or later "touchup" of the induced change.

Extensive work is continuing to explore the potential applications of this treatment modality. We are continuing with follow-up of the treated patients to assess long-term stability. Phase II studies have begun in the United States. Additional investigations are being done to assess the effect of age, sex, previous surgery, and medications on the induced refractive change. We are studying modifications in treatment parameters to increase the effect, improve predictability, and enhance stability. We believe that noncontact LTK will be an important new addition to the refractive surgical armamentarium.

REFERENCES

1. Lans LJ: Experimentelle Untersuchungen über die Entstehung von Astigmatismus durch nicht-perforierende Corneawunden, *Graefes Arch Clin Exp Ophthalmol* 45:117-152, 1898.
2. Wray C: Case of 6 D of hypermetropic astigmatism cured by the cautery, *Trans Ophthalmol Soc U K* 34:109-110, 1914.
3. O'Connor R: Corneal cautery for high myopic astigmatism, *Am J Ophthalmol* 16:337, 1933.
4. Stringer H, Parr J: Shrinkage temperature of eye collagen, *Nature* 204:1307, 1964.
5. Gasset AR, et al: Thermokeratoplasty, *Trans Am Acad Ophthalmol Otolaryngol* 77:441-454, 1973.
6. Shaw EL, Gasset AR: Thermokeratoplasty (TKP) temperature profile, *Invest Ophthalmol Vis Sci* 13:181-186, 1974.
7. Gasset AR, Kaufman HE: Thermokeratoplasty in the treatment of keratoconus, *Am J Ophthalmol* 79:226-232, 1975.
8. Aquavella JV, Buxton JN, Shaw EL: Thermokeratoplasty in the treatment of persistent corneal hydrops, *Arch Ophthalmol* 95:81-84, 1977.
9. Aquavella JV, Smith RS, Shaw EL: Alterations in corneal morphology following thermokeratoplasty, *Arch Ophthalmol* 94:2082-2085, 1976.
10. Itoi M: Computer photokeratometry changes following thermokeratoplasty. In Schachar RA, Levy NS, Schachar L, editors: *Refractive modulation of the cornea*, Denison, Tex, 1981, LAL Publishers.
11. Rowsey JJ, Gaylor JR, Dahlstrom R, et al: Los Alamos keratoplasty techniques, *Contact Intraocular Lens Med J* 6:1-12, 1980.
12. Rowsey JJ, Doss JD: Preliminary report of Los Alamos keratoplasty techniques, *Ophthalmology* 88:755-760, 1981.
13. Rowsey JJ: Electrosurgical keratoplasty: update and retraction, *Invest Ophthalmol Vis Sci* 28:224, 1987.
14. Fyodorov SN: A new technique for the treatment of hyperopia. In Schachar RA, Levy NS, Schachar L, editors: *Keratorefractive surgery*, Denison, Tex, 1989, LAL Publishing.
15. Neumann AC: Thermokeratoplasty for hyperopia, *Contemp Refract Surg* 5:753-772, 1992.
16. Feldman ST, Ellis W, Frucht-Pery J, et al: Regression of effect following radial thermokeratoplasty in humans, *Refract Corneal Surg* 5:288-291, 1989.
17. Fyodorov SN, Semonov AD: Author's certificate no. 822407, 1980.
18. Kanoda AN, Sorokin AS: Laser correction of hypermetropic refraction. In Fyodorov SN, editor: *Microsurgery of the eye: main aspects*, Moscow, 1987, MIR Publishers.
19. Flory PJ, Garrett RR: Phase transitions in collagen and gelatin systems, *J Am Chem Soc* 80:4836-4845, 1958.
20. Deak G, Romhanyi G: The thermal shrinkage process of collagen fibres as revealed by polarization optical analysis of topooptical staining reactions, *Acta Morphol Hung* 15:195-208, 1967.
21. Verzar F, Zs-Nagy I: Electronmicroscopic analysis of thermal collagen denaturation in rat tail tendons, *Gerontolgia* 16:77-82, 1970.
22. Allain JC, Bazin S, Lelous M, et al: Isometric tensions developed during the hydrothermal swelling of rat skin, *Connect Tissue Res* 7:127-133, 1980.
23. McCally RL, et al: Stromal damage in rabbit corneas exposed to CO_2 laser radiation, *Exp Eye Res* 37:543-550, 1983.
24. Smelser GK, Polack FM, Ozanics V: Persistence of donor collagen in corneal transplants, *Exp Eye Res* 4:349-354, 1965.
25. Lass JH, et al: Collagen degradation and synthesis in experimental corneal grafts, *Exp Eye Res* 42:201-210, 1986.
26. Householder J, Horwitz LS, Murillo A, et al: Laser induced thermal keratoplasty, *SPIE Proc* 1066:18-23, 1989.
27. Horn G, Spears KG, Lopez O, et al: New refractive method for laser thermal keratoplasty with the Co:MgF_2 laser, *J Cataract Refract Surg* 16:611-616, 1990.
28. Berry MJ, Fredlin LG, Valderrama GL, et al: Temperature distributions in laser-irradiated corneas, *Invest Ophthalmol Vis Sci* 32(suppl):994, 1991.

29. Koch DD, et al: HF chemical laser photothermal keratoplasty, *Invest Ophthalmol Vis Sci* 32(suppl):994, 1991.
30. Koch DD, Padrick TD, Menefee RF, et al: Laser photothermal keratoplasty: nonhuman primate results, *Invest Ophthalmol Vis Sci* 33(suppl):768, 1992.
31. Koch DD, Abaca A, Menefee RF, et al: HO:YAG laser thermal keratoplasty: *in vitro* experiments, *Invest Ophthalmol Vis Sci* 34(suppl):1246, 1993.
32. Moreira H, Campos M, Sawusch M, et al: Holmium laser keratoplasty, *Ophthalmology* 100:752-761, 1993.
33. Ren Q, Simon G, Parel JM: Laser photo thermo keratoplasty (LPTK), *Invest Ophthalmol Vis Sci* 33(suppl):770, 1992.

HOLMIUM:YAG LASER THERMOKERATOPLASTY UTILIZING THE SUMMIT SYSTEM

Vance Thompson

Lans[1] was the first to suggest that localized heating of the cornea induced corneal power changes. Terrien[2] also published early reports on the use of cauterization to correct advanced astigmatism secondary to Terrien's disease. Since then, various modalities have been investigated to heat corneal collagen to induce corneal curvature changes. The most popular technique for shrinking collagen to date has been the Fyodorov technique of radial thermokeratoplasty.[3] Various problems, including a lack of predictability and a high incidence of regression have accompanied this procedure.[4] It is believed that Hol:YAG LTK represents an advancement in the technology of corneal collagen shrinkage.[5]

COLLAGE, HEAT, AND SHRINKAGE

Mammalian collagen contracts sharply upon application of the appropriate amount of heat. Collagen fibers can shrink to one third of their initial length with proper temperature elevations.[6] The exact temperature at which this occurs has been called the *shrinkage temperature (Ts).* The Ts for human corneal collagen is approximately 55° to 60° C. These temperatures allow collagen shrinkage without destroying the collagen fibrils. It has been shown that as soon as the temperature of collagen is increased above 65° to 70° C it starts to relax again.[7] Even higher temperatures will begin to cause necrosis of the collagen fibrils. If collagen shrinkage is performed in the periphery of the cornea, a flattening of the corneal curvature will occur at the treatment site accompanied by relative steepening in the central and midperipheral cornea (Fig. 17-28).

In the Fyodorov technique of radial thermokeratoplasty a nichrome wire probe is penetrated to 90% of the corneal depth and heated to 600° C. The coagulations are made in a radial fashion with a typical procedure consisting of eight rows of three or four applications each. I believe that one of the primary reasons for the lack of predictable results in radial thermok-

eratoplasty may be the dynamics occurring in the coagulation zone. In the central portion of the coagulation zone the collagen is exposed to temperatures as high as 600° C, which will cause necrosis of the surrounding collagen. Outside of this zone there will be collagen exposed to temperatures greater than 70° C which will lead to collagen relaxation. In the peripheral aspect of the coagulation zone temperatures in the 55° to 60° C window will be achieved with collagen shrinkage occurring mainly in this location. This rather extreme variation in heat exposure to the corneal collagen may be one of the problems associated with radial thermokeratoplasty. Reports of significant regression and lack of predictability in radial thermokeratoplasty have prompted researchers to evaluate other technologies for collagen shrinkage.[4]

THE SUMMIT TECHNOLOGY HOLMIUM:YAG LASER

I use Summit Technology's Ho:YAG laser for collagen shrinkage procedures. This is a solid-state laser which emits radiation in the infrared region (2.06 μm) of the electromagnetic spectrum. At this wavelength the cornea exhibits efficient absorption characteristics capable of increasing the temperature of water which in turn causes heat-induced shrinkage of collagen fibrils. This wavelength is ideal because the penetration depth of 2.1-μm infrared radiation is comparable to the corneal thickness, which is ideal for achieving deep, consistent collagen shrinkage zones in a controlled fashion.[8,9]

The Ho:YAG laser energy is delivered along a 600-μm core low–OH quartz fiberoptic handpiece and then focused with a specially designed sapphire tip with a cone angle of 120 degrees (Fig. 17-29). This tip

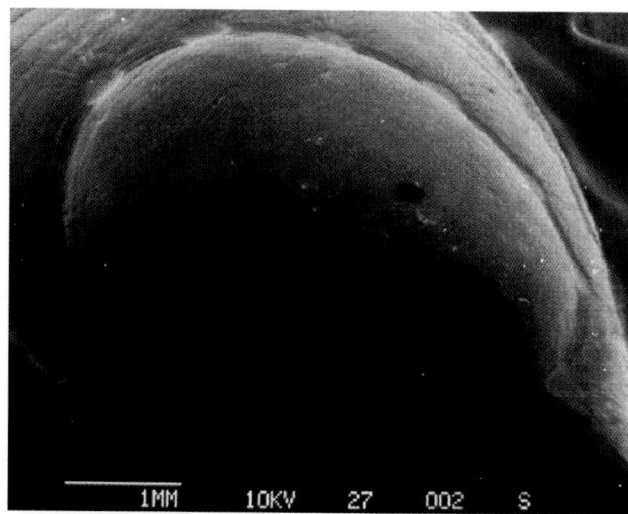

Fig. 17-28. Ho:YAG laser thermal keratoplasty scanning electron micrograph showing peripheral flattening and central steepening. (Courtesy of Theo Seiler, M.D., Ph.D., Dresden, Germany.)

is applied to the corneal surface and precisely focuses the laser energy to form a wedge-shaped (wedge angle, approximately 90 degrees) collagen shrinkage zone (Fig. 17-30). The diameter of the cone at the cornea surface is approximately 700 μm, and the apex is approximately 450 μm in depth, which maintains a safe distance from the corneal endothelium.

The Ho:YAG laser operates in a pulsed mode. Because of the short laser pulse length (0.35 ms) and relatively long thermal diffusion time of laser energy in stroma (approximately 300 ms), the volume of tissue heated during each pulse is essentially equal to the volume of tissue irradiated by the pulse. The repetition rate is 15 Hz and the energy delivered per pulse is approximately 19 mJ. Subsequent pulses arrive before heat from the previous pulse can dissi-

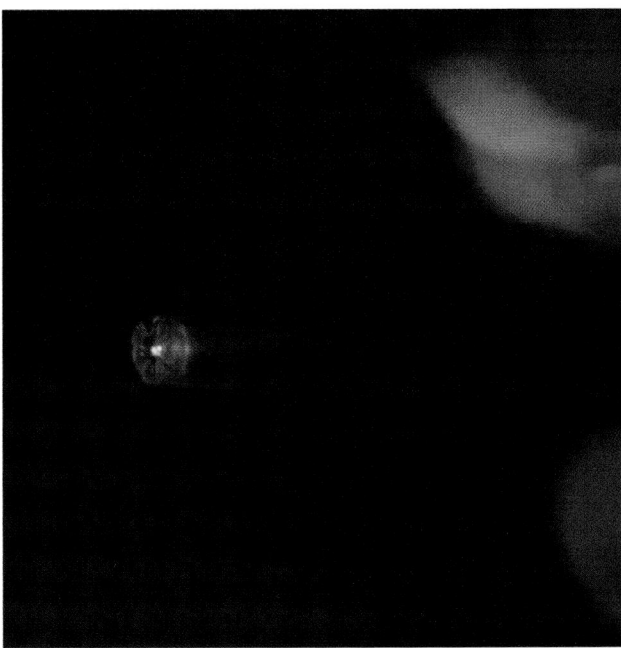

Fig. 17-29. Sapphire tip to focus holmium energy.

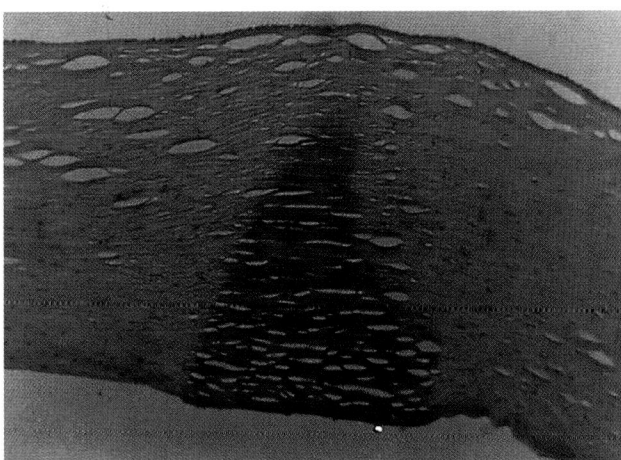

Fig. 17-30. Wedge-shaped coagulation zone achieved with sapphire focusing tip.

pate, with each treatment location receiving 25 pulses is applied to the corneal surface and precisely focuses leading to a temperature increase which raises the temperature of the collagen in that location to a maximum of approximately 60° C and effectively shrinks the collagen in that location. This system minimizes any collagen relaxation phenomenon or stromal necrosis by preventing higher temperatures from being achieved.

SURGICAL TECHNIQUE

Preoperatively, the patient receives a topical anesthetic and an antibiotic. The patient is positioned under the laser and a lid speculum is placed. With the patient fixating on the fixation light in the laser, the central cornea is marked with a 3.0-mm optical zone marker. For a hyperopic procedure one or two rings of eight treatment locations are placed at a variable optical zone, depending on the amount of treatment desired. After the marks have been placed the contact focusing tip, which has been attached to the laser handpiece, is placed in contact with the cornea at the marked treatment site. The foot pedal is pressed and the laser energy is delivered over approximately a 2-second period. During the treatment the surgeon concentrates on keeping the handpiece perpendicular to the corneal surface with a slight amount of pressure. The contact tip has friction built into it and with slight pressure the chance of a mild tremor moving the tip is minimal. After all the treatment spots have been placed the epithelium is noted to be coagulated and is subsequently removed with a cotton-tipped applicator. Antibiotic ointment is instilled, the eye is patched, and the patient is sent home with instructions to use the antibiotic ointment three times a day. The vast majority of patients are reepithelialized by day 1. Pain is typically minimal. Pain medications are not routinely prescribed.

For patients with hyperopic astigmatism the only difference in technique is the marker utilized. After marking the flat axis of astigmatism with a Mendez ruler the astigmatic marker is positioned. Marks are placed in the flat axis of astigmatism and the treatment spots are placed. It is of note that in addition to steepening the flat axis there is an overall myopic shift in the spherical equivalent so that the patients who are ideal for this treatment are those who have a hyperopic spherical equivalent that is approximately half the amount of their astigmatic correction.[5,10]

CLINICAL RESULTS

In a study on four human blind eyes, Seiler et al.[9] demonstrated that LTK successfully steepened the corneal curvature. The authors demonstrated that the amount of steepening was related to the optical zone size in a linear fashion.

Table 17-2. Phase II hyperopic laser thermal keratoplasty: six month results (n = 23)

n	Optical zone (mm)	Hyperopic correction (D)
3	7.5	1.79
11	7.0	1.32
1	6.5	1.75
4	7.0-9.0	3.03
4	6.5-9.0	3.03

Table 17-3. Phase II hyperopic laser thermal keratoplasty: one-year results (n = 18)

n	Optical zone (mm)	Hyperopic correction (D)
3	7.5	1.33
8	7.0	1.01
4	7.0-9.0	1.75
3	6.5-9.0	2.23

More recently, Durrie et al.[8] reported their results of two separate clinical studies on the correction of hyperopia in sighted human eyes using Ho:YAG LTK. In the 15 patients in the Seiler et al. study an average initial corneal steepening of 6 D was achieved. The steepening effect underwent partial regression over the first 4 months and was thought to have stabilized around 6 months. Durrie et al. then treated 10 patients in Summit Technology's FDA-monitored phase I hyperopia clinical trial and purposely overcorrected their hyperopia to allow for the regression effect. They also noted a stability of the refractive error at about 6 months and improved uncorrected vision in all 10 patients.

Twenty-five patients were entered into Summit Technology's phase II hyperopia clinical trials beginning over 1 year ago. The 6-month postoperative visit had been achieved in 23 patients at the time of this writing and the amount of hyperopia correction is shown in Table 17-2. The results of the 18 patients who had made their 1-year visit at the time of this writing are shown in Table 17-3. Note that in this study the maximum effect was achieved with eight coagulations at an inner optical zone of 6.5 mm and an additional eight coagulations placed at an outer optical zone of 9.0 mm. This double-ring treatment regressed from an average correction of 3.03 D at 6 months to 2.23 D at 1 year. One patient lost two lines of BCVA and the rest showed no change in BCVA or a slight improvement. There were no reports of infectious keratitis, recurrent erosion, corneal edema, persistent epithelial defect, or any other complication.

Observations made thus far include an increased hyperopic correction and less degree of regression with increasing age. This corresponds with the age in life (i.e., near-presbyopia) when many hyperopes become more bothered by their uncorrected visual acuity.

CONCLUSION

Ho:YAG LTK appears to show promise for the treatment of low hyperopia in the range of 3 D and under. With improved case selection, such as treating patients near presbyopic age, the results should improve. The procedure appears to be a safe form of corneal steepening with a low incidence of complications and preservation of BCVA. Further studies are concentrating on nomogram improvement and further refinement of technique.

REFERENCES

1. Lans LJ: Experimentelle Untersuchungen über Entstehung von Astigmatisumus durch nicht-perforierende Corneawunden, *Graefes Arch Clin Exp Ophthalmol* 44:117-152, 1889.
2. Terrien F: Dystrophie marginale symétrique des deux cornées avec astigmatisme régulier. Conservtif et guérison par la cautérisation ignée, *Arch Ophthalmol* 20:12, 1900.
3. Neumann AC, Fyodorov S, Sanders DR: Radial thermokeratoplasty for the correction of hyperopia, *Refract Corneal Surg* 6:404-412, 1990.
4. Feldman ST, Ellis W, Frucht-Perry J, et al: Regression of effect following radial thermokeratoplasty in humans, *Refract Corneal Surg* 5:288-291, 1989.
5. Thompson VM, Seiler T, Durrie DS, et al: Holmium:YAG laser thermokeratoplasty for hyperopia and astigmatism: an overview, *Refract Corneal Surg* 9(suppl):S134-S137, 1993.
6. Stringer AR, Shaw EL, Kaufmann HE, et al: Thermokeratoplasty, *Trans Am Acad Ophthalmol Otolaryngol* 77:441, 1973.
7. Allain JC, Lous LE, Cohen-Solal: Isometric tensions developed during the hydrothermal swelling of rat skin, *Connect Tissue Res* 7:127-133, 1980.
8. Durrie DS, Seiler T, King MC, et al: Application of the holmium:YAG laser for refractive surgery, *SPIE Proc* 1644:56-60, 1992.
9. Seiler T, Matallana M, Bende T: Laser thermokeratoplasty by means of a pulsed holmium:YAG laser for hyperopic correction, *Refract Corneal Surg* 6:335-339, 1990.
10. Thompson VM, Durrie DS, Hunkeler JD: Application of the holmium:YAG laser for refractive surgery: an update of clinical progress, *SPIE Proc* 1877:52-56, 1993.

EXCIMER LASER STUDIES: RESULTS FROM THE UNITED STATES

Jonathan I. Macy, Anthony B. Nesburn, James J. Salz

Excimer laser PRK has been increasingly investigated for a variety of refractive errors through remodeling the corneal surface. Extensive studies, under an investigational device exemption (IDE) by the FDA have evaluated myopia, astigmatism, and therapeutic applications. Laser use for hyperopic correction has been investigated much less thoroughly in the United States.

ANIMAL STUDIES
The Study of Del Pero et al.

Del Pero and associates[1] reported on six cynomolgus monkeys treated with a 193-nm excimer laser for hyperopia. The intended correction was 6 D in five monkeys and 1 D in one monkey. The beam was directed through a wheel with a series of annular apertures of decreasing width. Under computer control, the wheel was driven with a stepper motor through the different apertures. Different ablation depths and curvatures were etched onto the surface of the cornea as the laser delivered a series of pulses at each aperture setting. The intended 6-D corrections achieved a mean correction of 5.2 D at 1 year.

The Study of Keates et al.

In January 1992, Keates and colleagues[2] reported their experience with three rabbits and six cats treated with the VISX 2015 excimer laser under a protocol to treat hyperopia. They used an optical zone of 6.3 or 6.0 mm and a transition zone of 1.3 or 1.2 mm. A corrected zone of 5.0 or 4.8 mm remained. As a result of these treatments, three rabbits achieved 2.28 D of a planned 3.0-D correction. Three cats achieved 3.13 D of a planned 3.0-D correction, and the other three cats achieved 2.54 D of an intended 6.0-D correction.

CLINICAL STUDIES

As a result of these preliminary efforts, a new protocol was designed to treat human subjects for low to moderate degrees of hyperopia.[3] For treatment of hyperopia, an add-on option module has been designed by VISX to treat the profile shown in Fig. 17-31. This sculpts the central 5 mm to the new desired curvature. It also shapes an outer annulus to make the transition back to the original surface large and gradual, which appears to be necessary to prevent significant regression. This technique helps to avoid the excessive regression which has occurred when smaller transition zones are employed. Along with a larger total ablation zone, this method also allows for a larger corrected central zone, which increases the overall safety of the procedure by leaving an optically significant portion of the central cornea only slightly ablated. The technique produces an extremely smooth surface. In fact, the plastic calibration lenses are clearer and easier to read in a lensometer than the standard VISX myopia calibration lenses.

This is accomplished through the use of a variably eccentric lens used in connection with the current VISX optical delivery system. The previous method involved a total area ablation which was approximately 6.0 to 6.5 mm in diameter with a 4.8- to 5.0-mm corrected refractive correction zone leaving a 0.6- to 0.65-mm transition zone. The present approach uses a

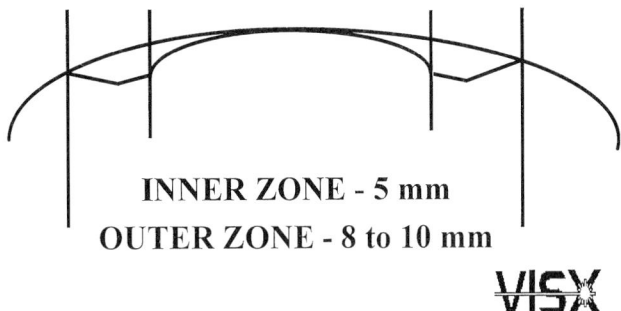

Fig. 17-31. Hyperopia treatment technique.

total ablation area of up to 9.0 mm with a 5.0-mm refractive correction zone allowing a 2.0-mm edge transition zone.

With the new H-PRK module, Ramirez-Flores and co-workers[4] treated two eyes of pigmented rabbits. They intended a +4.00-D correction over an optical zone of 5 mm. One cornea was treated over a total diameter of 8 mm and the other was treated over 10 mm. Histopathologic changes were evaluated after 12 weeks. Steepening, as measured by corneal topography with difficult fixation, was determined to be 3.3 D and 6.5 D, respectively, at that time. Using corneal topography, the authors concluded that the refractive regression that has limited earlier hyperopic procedures may be overcome with larger treatment areas. The refractive results and successful healing support the extension of H-PRK studies to blind human subjects.

In the summer of 1993, the VISX H-PRK study of the treatment of mild to moderate hyperopia began. Ten eyes were treated at three sites in the United States. At the time of this writing, 3-month follow-up is available on these eyes. A +4.00-D correction was attempted in all cases (Fig. 17-32). One eye has been excluded from the data analysis. Preoperatively, this 93-year-old woman had countfingers vision even with corrected aphakia, due to myopic maculopathy associated with an optic nerve staphyloma. After treatment, not only was it difficult to achieve reliable fixation for valid measurements but the cornea developed nodular epithelial lesions, as well as epithelial filaments.

The technique was similar to that described previously for the treatment of myopia.[5] Briefly, all eyes were screened for corneal abnormalities. Otherwise, lenticular, retinal, sensory, or neurologic causes of visual acuity below 20/200 were accepted. Refraction, corneal topography, intraocular pressure, and complete anterior and posterior segment examinations were followed by the completion of a detailed informed consent. At the modified VISX Twenty-Twenty Excimer Laser, the patient was positioned under the

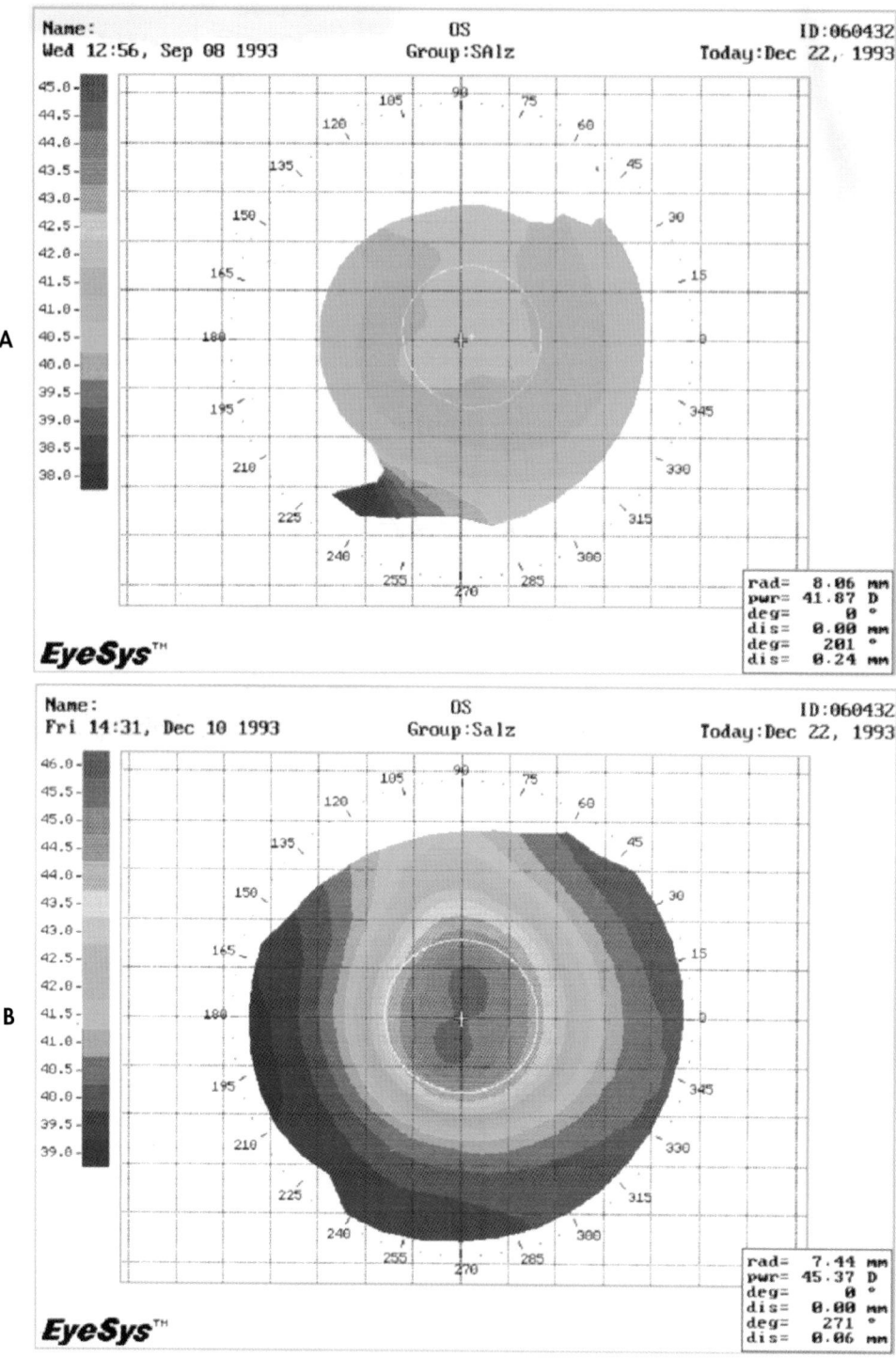

Fig. 17-32. Color-coded computer-assisted topographic maps. **A,** Preoperative corneal map, preoperative refraction +0.75 −0.25 × 85 degrees. **B,** Postoperative corneal map, postoperative refraction −2.75 −1.00 × 180 degrees.

operating microscope after the instillation of topical anesthetic eye drops. The center of the pupil was marked with an intraocular lens positioning hook and a 9- or 10-mm optical zone marker delineated the area for epithelium removal. The optical zone area was then debrided of epithelium and the surface

moistened, while the vacuum nozzle was positioned. Ablation was then completed using a Thornton ring for fixation and centering or voluntary patient fixation.

At the conclusion of treatment, topical ciprofloxacin (Ciloxan), diclofenac (Voltaren), and a disposable

Table 17-4. Refraction after VISX H-PRK treatments

Patient	Preoperative	Postoperative (3 mo)	Spherical equivalent change (D) 1 mo	3 mo	Preoperative BCVA*
LE	$+10.00 -5.00 \times \quad 5°$	$+7.00 -6.00 \times 180°$	3.62	3.50	20/200
LA	$-12.75 -1.25 \times \quad 10°$	$-17.50 -0.75 \times \quad 90°$	5.12	4.50	20/400
RA	$+0.50 -0.75 \times \quad 55°$	$-0.25 -1.50 \times \quad 45°$	4.25	1.12	HM
AM	$+7.75 -0.75 \times 105°$	$+4.50 -0.25 \times \quad 80°$	3.88	3.00	20/400
EP	$+1.75 -1.50 \times \quad 30°$	$-1.00 -2.25 \times \quad 15°$	3.75	3.12	20/400
ME	$+11.25 -1.25 \times \quad 2°$	$+9.00 -2.00 \times 175°$	0.88	2.62	CF
HN	$+7.75 -1.50 \times \quad 80°$	$+4.00 -1.00 \times \quad 90°$	3.12	3.50	20/200
GS	$+0.75 -0.25 \times \quad 85°$	$-2.75 -1.00 \times 180°$	5.12	3.88	20/400
NK	$+12.00 -1.00 \times \quad 15°$	$+7.75 -1.50 \times \quad 30°$	4.00	4.50	CF
			3.75	3.30	

*BCVA = best corrected visual acuity; HM = hand motion; CF = count fingers.

Table 17-5. Mean keratometry (D) after (VISX) H-PRK treatments

Patient	Preoperative	Postoperative 1 mo	3 mo	Change 1 mo	3 mo
LE	41.46	45.00	43.93	3.54	2.47
LA	43.38	48.06	46.50	4.68	3.12
RA	43.88	46.75	45.50	2.87	1.62
AM	41.24	45.24	43.74	4.00	2.50
EP	43.00	48.25	45.25	5.25	2.25
ME	43.50	44.25	46.75	0.75	3.25
HN	42.75	46.38	45.67	3.63	2.92
GS	42.38	46.38	45.75	4.00	3.37
NK	42.25	46.50	44.12	4.25	1.87
				3.67	2.60

soft contact lens (Acuvue) were placed on the eye. The patients used ciprofloxacin and diclofenac four times a day and were followed daily until epithelialization occurred. Then the contact lens and these drops were discontinued. Topical fluoromethalone (FML) was begun four times a day and further evaluations were done as needed until the required 1- and 3-month protocol appointments.

Results

Tables 17-4 and 17-5 detail the results of these treatments. Since preoperative visual acuity ranged from 20/200 to hand motion, the reliability and validity of the data measurements are limited. All patients achieved hyperopic corrections lasting 3 months. Mean keratometry (by ophthalmometry or computer-assisted corneal topography) steepened in all eyes. The amount of keratometric change ranged from 1.62 to 3.25 D with a mean of 2.60 D after 3 months. The amount of refractive correction at 1 month ranged from 0.88 D to 5.12 D of the intended 4.00 D. The mean correction was 3.75 D. At 3 months, correction ranged from 1.12 to 4.50 D, with a mean of 3.30 D.

Within the limitations of accurate measurement noted earlier, the corrections were quite stable over time. There was small regression of effect between 1 and 3 months in six of nine eyes. The amount of refractive regression ranged from 0.12 D to 3.12 D with a mean of 0.74 D. Three eyes showed an increased hyperopic effect from 1 to 3 months ranging from 0.38 to 1.75 D. The regression using the 8-mm ablation zone (patients RA, EP, ME, NK) was 0.88 and 3.12 D in the two eyes showing regression. The other two 8-mm eyes progressed 0.50 and 1.75 D. Four of five eyes treated with a 9-mm zone (patients LE, LA, AM, HN, GS) regressed between 1 and 3 months. Similar regression was seen in eight of nine eyes by mean keratometry between 1 and 3 months (see Table 17-5). Regression ranged from 0.62 to 3.00 D with a mean of 1.51 D.

CONCLUSIONS

One can conclude that PRK for the treatment of hyperopia appears safe and effective in the short term. In this preliminary study, a mean correction of 3.30 D of an intended 4.0-D correction has been achieved after 3 months. These data are early in the course of healing, and there must be concern about the regression between 1 and 3 months. The mean correction at 1 month was a more accurate 3.75 D. Evaluation of more eyes with longer follow-up should provide a clearer answer in the near future. It should be mentioned that there is difficulty in establishing a reproducible endpoint for keratometry and especially refractive error in "blind" eyes with poor fixation. This should be carefully considered in detailed evaluations of the numeric results rather than observations of patterns of effect. More accurate analyses await the sighted eye trials.

REFERENCES

1. Del Pero RA, Gigstad JE, Roberts AD, et al: A refractive and histopathologic study of excimer laser keratectomy in primates, *Am J Ophthalmol* 109:419-429, 1990.
2. Keates R, Martines E, Merkley K: Report of hyperopia correction on cats and New Zealand rabbits using the Excimer 2015 System, Unpublished report, January 1992.
3. Sharp SM: IDE application PRK for hyperopia VISX Twenty-Twenty Excimer Laser System for photorefractive keratectomy, Unpublished report, February 1993.
4. Ramirez-Flores S, Koons SJ, Shimmick JK, et al: Correction of hyperopia with excimer laser PRK, ARVO Abstract, submitted November 1993.
5. Salz JJ, Maguen E, Nesburn AB, et al: A two year experience with excimer laser photorefractive keratectomy for myopia, *Ophthalmology* 100:873-883, 1993.

18

Solid-State Photoablative Decomposition—The Novatec Laser

Casimir A. Swinger, Shui T. Lai

There is little question that photorefractive keratectomy (PRK) has been a major advance in corneal refractive surgery in recent years. Until now, ablation of the anterior corneal surface to produce a new surface curvature for refractive purposes, or for removal of tissue for therapeutic purposes, has been accomplished using excimer laser technology—specifically, the 193-nm wavelength systems.[1-3] Results to date clearly demonstrate that the human cornea can be reprofiled to a new curvature and, following an induced wound-healing response, produce a new corneal surface that is both optically clear and regular.

To date, the excimer laser has been used successfully to achieve correction of low to moderate myopia.[4] Correction of high myopia has been somewhat more difficult and is sometimes accompanied by instability secondary to an unpredictable wound-healing response characterized by deposition of new collagen, to a variable degree, on the ablated surface.[5] In addition, until recently, the correction of hyperopia had not been achieved. More recent developments using a larger optical zone diameter show promise, however. The correction of astigmatism has provided mixed results. It appears that regular astigmatism is correctable, but the final algorithms remain to be determined. Lastly, although the excimer laser has been able to provide a lamellar keratectomy for therapeutic purposes, the refractive power of the eye following surgery may be altered undesirably. Specifically, significant degrees of induced hyperopia sometimes accompany phototherapeutic keratectomy (PTK).[6,7]

BACKGROUND

Some of the limitations of the excimer laser when used for PRK or PTK derive from the laser system itself. Excimer lasers use a gaseous lasing medium. For this, and other reasons, the beam of the excimer laser tends to be nonhomogeneous, being characterized by occasional hot spots of varying intensity. Beam manipulation and conditioning can reduce this problem but not eliminate it. Most current excimer lasers employ a wide-beam technology that produces considerable acoustic shock when laser energy is delivered to the cornea, as the fluence is distributed over a wide surface area. This acoustic shock has been questioned as possibly playing a role in the development of corneal haze. Also, the corneal reprofiling achievable with a wide beam is limited. Customized ablations, such as for irregular astigmatism and complicated peripheral profiles, are not currently achievable with wide-beam technology. Also, to date some excimer lasers have been characterized by a relatively small optical zone, which can present problems. But increasing the optical zone while maintaining the same energy density requires greater laser size and capacity, which is a disadvantage, small optical zones are in part responsible for the regression following high myopic ablations and for the induced hyperopia following PTK.

We have developed a new laser technology that ad-

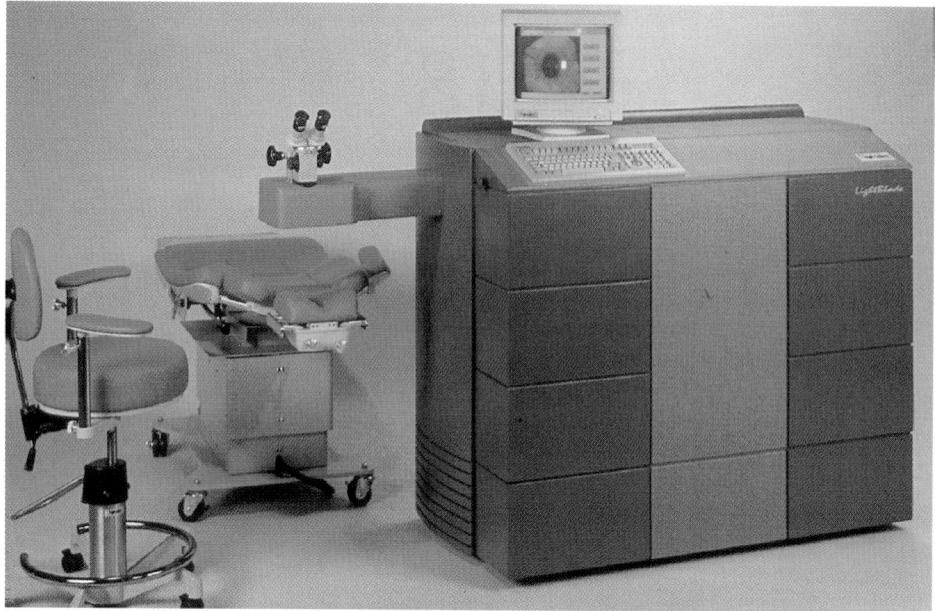

Fig. 18-1. Novatec Lightblade solid-state laser system.

dresses the current limitations of excimer laser technology.[8,9] The Novatec laser system (LightBlade model; Fig. 18-1) is designed as a potentially complete ophthalmic laser system, not only for surface ablation but also for intracorneal ablation and intraocular applications such as glaucoma, laser phaco, and vitreous surgery.

LASER SYSTEM
Solid-State Technology

The Novatec laser employs a proprietary technology, and the lasing media are solid-state laser crystals. Solid-state technology addresses current limitations of excimer lasers by providing increased reliability, ease of use, portability, and elimination of skilled technical assistance. The current operating parameters, when used for surface ablation, are approximately as follows:
- Wavelength: 0.2 μm
- Fluence: 100 mJ/cm^2
- Delivery system: scanning, computer-directed
- Spot size: 10-500 μm
- Optical zone: up to 10 mm

The Novatec laser operates in a single fundamental mode with good pulse-to-pulse stability. The surgical beam is collimated, thereby eliminating the exact requirement of microscope focusing on the surface of the patient's eye during surgery to maintain the desired fluence.

Delivery System

The system uses a computerized scanning delivery system. To truly provide flexibility in the development of surface ablation and to provide customized ablations for specific indications such as asymmetric or irregular astigmatism, a scanning delivery system is required. The Novatec workstation is capable of rapidly delivering a constant fluence with a variable spot size of up to 500 μm to anywhere on the corneal surface. Currently, optic zones up to 10 mm have been evaluated, though this can be increased if desired. The scanning pattern is concentric-circular but programmable to any desired pattern. Complex algorithms can be programmed to provide customized reprofiling. We envision that a computerized topographic map of the cornea may be inputted into the system and energy delivered under computer control with eye tracking to achieve customized ablation.

Using a scanning beam technology and a fluence lower than that of commercially available excimer lasers, the amount of energy applied to the cornea at any instant is dramatically reduced, thereby reducing acoustic shock. In practice, this is demonstrable during surgery as the procedure is almost without perceptible sound, unlike excimer surface ablation which produces a sonic component.

Coaxial Fixation

The Novatec laser employs surgical and patient fixation beams that are colinear. When aligned with the patient's visual axis, they eliminate parallax error and should improve centration of the procedure.[10]

Eye Tracker

The Novatec system is the only surface ablation laser with an eye tracker. Eye tracking is important in improving the centration of the ablation and in accomodating customized ablations. Decentration can result in edge flare, glare, or various types of subjective symptoms in addition to reduced acuity and induced astigmatism. The eye tracker, which has a rapid response time, is coupled to the computerized delivery system and allows energy to be delivered to the appropriate site despite random eye movements. Should eye movement be gross, the firing of the laser is aborted through activation of a shutter until the eye once again is relatively fixated on the target and the laser reactivated by the surgeon. In conjunction with corneal topography, it is anticipated that the eye tracker will play a critical role in ensuring that laser energy is indeed being delivered to appropriate locations on the cornea as the ablation is executed.

Multiple Modalities and Modular Design

There are currently two avenues of corneal laser development—surface ablation and intrastromal ablation. It may well be that a combination of these two modalities may be indicated, either as primary and secondary procedures, or even as a combined ablation. For example, it may be that a laser microkeratome resection may be combined with ablation of the bed in a combined intrastromal surgery, using a penetrating wavelength, followed by photoablative decomposition using an ultraviolet (UV) wavelength. To this end, the Novatec system is being developed to accommodate both modalities and to allow surgeons to evaluate the relative efficacy of both approaches. Certainly, delivery of both UV and penetrating wavelengths would demand separate delivery systems. In addition, the penetrating wavelength may also be used within the eye for performance of iridotomy, trabeculectomy, capsulectomy, capsulorhexis, laser phaco, or vitreous photodisruption.

Surgical Microscope

The workstation is designed with an integrated ophthalmic grade surgical microscope that can also be used to perform nonlaser refractive surgery such as radial keratotomy or keratomileusis. In addition, video imaging equipment can be coupled to the microscope for teaching and documentation.

PRELIMINARY INVESTIGATIONS

Preclinical studies with the laser system have been performed using both the UV surface modality and the intrastromal modality with a penetrating wavelength, though the former is emphasized here.

Human Eye Bank Eye Studies

The Novatec LightBlade surgical system was evaluated in a series of human eye bank eyes and results indicated that the scanning delivery system is capable of providing a surface quality which is comparable or superior to that provided by current excimer laser technology. An example of the fine surface quality produced by the scanning delivery system, obtained by scanning electron microscopy, is demonstrated in Fig. 18-2. In addition, light and electron microscopy were also performed on sections of the eye bank eyes. Transmission electron microscopy demonstrated a very thin pseudomembrane, approximately 1 μm thick, overlying the ablated surface, with maintenance of normal corneal structure beneath the ablated area (Fig. 18-3).

Animal Studies

Several in vivo studies have been performed, both in rabbits and in nonhuman primates.[9,11,12] Initially, optical zones were 5 mm. The epithelium was removed by a plano laser ablation to a depth of 40 μm. All evaluations were performed by highly experienced refractive surgeons with extensive excimer laser experience, and impartial outside observers were enlisted.

The first study was performed in albino rabbits and consisted of either a 3-D or a 6-D myopic ablation.[9] There were no operative or postoperative complications. Epithelial healing was normal, and all defects healed by the third day. Pachymetric measurements confirmed the corneal thinning following ablation observed on slit-lamp examination. The average thinning at 4 weeks follow-up in the 3-D eyes was 40 μm, and for the 6-D group it was 60 μm. Corneal topography showed corneal flattening with good regular-

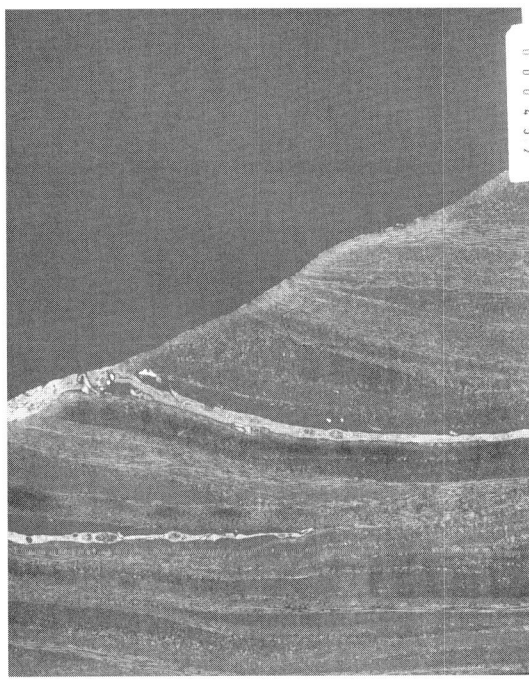

Fig. 18-2. Scanning electron microscopy (×30) of the corneal surface of a human eye bank eye following 6-D myopic PRK.

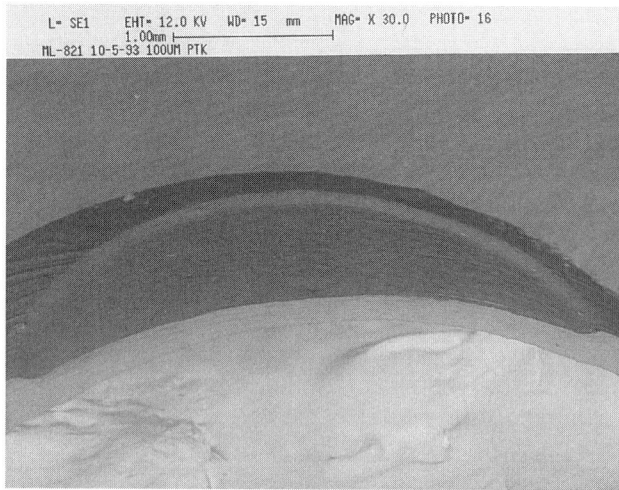

```
L= SE1    EHT= 12.0 KV   WD= 15   mm    MAG= X 30.0   PHOTO= 16
                          1.00mm
ML-821 10-5-93 100UM PTK
```

Fig. 18-3. Transmission electron microscopy (×10,500) of the anterior cornea of an eye bank eye following 6-D myopic PRK.

ity. At 4 weeks postoperatively, haze was minimal with means of 0.56 for the 3-D group and 0.5 for the 6-D group. No eye had haze of 1.0 or greater.

A second series, a randomized prospective study in albino rabbits, compared the results of myopic PRK obtained with the Novatec laser to those using the VISX Twenty-Twenty excimer laser.[11] One eye of each rabbit was randomly assigned to Novatec and the fellow eye to VISX. Ablations were either for 3 D or 6 D, and optical zones were 5 mm.

There were no operative or postoperative complications in either group. Epithelial healing was normal in all eyes and completed by day 3.5. Quantitative analysis of epithelial closure was performed on a ×160 enlargement of the slit-lamp photograph. There was no statistically significant difference ($P > .20$) in the rate of closure or epithelial defect sizes between the Novatec- and VISX-treated eyes. A comparison between the pachymetric data for 3-D and 6-D ablations for each laser was made. The data indicated that the mean ablated depths were not statistically different for the two lasers when measured at intervals of 4 to 6 weeks. Evaluation of haze showed no statistically significant difference ($P = .09-.40$) between the two lasers at any time point up to 3 months for either the 3-D or the 6-D groups. Maximum haze for any eye in the study was 1.5.

The conclusion of the study was that rabbit corneas ablated by either the VISX Twenty-Twenty or the Novatec lasers for myopic corrections of 3 D or 6 D are indistinguishable from one another over the short term on the basis of clinical appearance, epithelialization, pachymetry, or amount or pattern of haze.

A further study evaluated the Novatec laser prospectively in a nonhuman primate model (owl mon-

key) to ensure both satisfactory ablation of the primate eye, which possesses Bowman's membrane, and safety.[12] Initially, 3-D and 5-D myopic ablations with a 5-mm optical zone were performed. Later, multizonal high myopic ablations of 10 D or 20 D with 8-mm optical zones were performed. In addition, four hyperopic ablations of 5 D with an 8-mm optical zone were evaluated.

There were no operative or postoperative complications in any eye. Clinically, epithelialization proceeded normally. The rate of epithelialization in the low myopia group was not significantly different from the rabbit eyes for 5-mm optical zone ablations ($P > .20$). Ablations with 8-mm optical zones took slightly longer (average of 4 days) to epithelialize, as the ablated defect is more than 2.5 times larger than a 5-mm defect. Nevertheless, the defects closed without complication.

Clinical examination at the time of surgery demonstrated corneal thinning with good surface quality. Pachymetry showed the mean control preoperative corneal thickness to be 398 μm, and this was reduced to 332 μm and 289 μm respectively in the 10-D and 20-D ablations at 1 month. Corneal topography was performed on several eyes, and one example (Fig. 18-4) demonstrated a 14-D correction at 1 month.

Evaluation of haze indicated a greater degree of haze in the nonhuman primates than in the rabbit eyes. Rapid wound healing with a robust wound-healing response is well documented in the nonhuman primate eye, and was expected.[13] There was, however, no eye with scarring or haze greater than 3/5 at any time up to 6 months, even in the 20-D group. For myopic PRK of 3 to 20 D, mean haze for all eyes (N=12) was 1.19 (range, 0.5-2.0) at 5 weeks and trace haze at 6 months (all eyes clear or trace except one eye with 1.0). For four eyes that underwent a 5-D hyperopic PRK, mean haze was 1.0 (range, 0.75-1.25) at 1 month and clear in three eyes and 1.0 in the fourth eye at 6 months.

Initial evaluation of hyperopic ablations in primates was carried out for 5-D corrections using an 8-mm optical zone. Topography indicated that hyperopic correction was achievable. Fig. 18-5, a topographic map of an ablated bank eye, demonstrates both a hyperopic correction and the fact that the surface quality at time 0 following ablation allows topography to be performed.

In conclusion, the Novatec laser is capable of ablating the primate cornea while producing a clinically regular surface. The primate cornea, following Novatec PRK, undergoes normal epithelialization. Haze develops, as in human corneas, and its magnitude appears acceptable. The Novatec laser exhibited no safety problems in these limited series of studies.

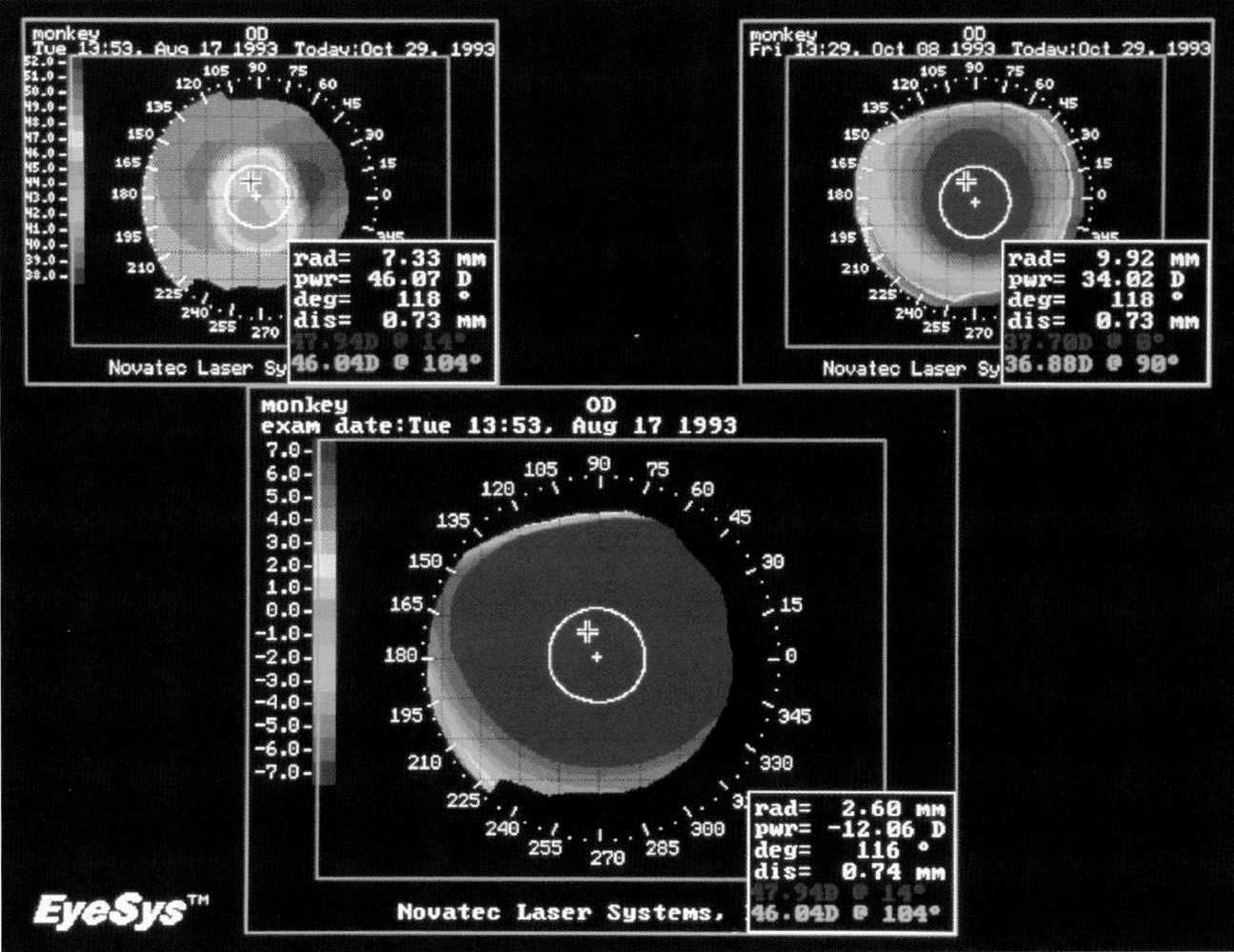

Fig. 18-4. Corneal topography demonstrates 14 D of central flattening in an owl monkey 1 month following myopic PRK.

OTHER APPLICATIONS

As mentioned earlier, the Novatec laser can operate either with a UV (photoablative decomposition) or a penetrating wavelength (photodisruption). Using the penetrating wavelength and a newly developed delivery system, we have been able to perform intrastromal ablation with good precision. We have performed arcuate and radial keratectomy, where the incision length, spacing, and depth are accurately controlled; intrastromal cavitation (Fig. 18-6); and excision for penetrating keratoplasty. The use of laser technology promises to increase the safety and accuracy of these procedures. In addition, we are investigating the possibility of performing a lamellar keratectomy by laser (laser microkeratome). This would allow the performance of keratomileusis-like surgery without any mechanical cutting devices. An example of a keratectomized bed following removal of an intact lamellar cap is shown in Fig. 18-7.

We have also used the laser to perform iridotomy, to create a smooth capsulorhexis, and to ablate the lens. In addition, vitreous abnormalities may be treatable using this modality.

SUMMARY

The Novatec solid-state laser is a second-generation corneal laser. It embodies features such as eye tracking and a scanning delivery system that will allow more sophisticated development of corneal refractive surgical procedures not currently achievable with current laser technology. Its solid-state technology promises portability, ease of use, and reduced maintenance considerations.

Preclinical evaluation of the Novatec laser has demonstrated efficacy in the correction of low to moderate myopia, and clinical results appear, even at this early stage of development, comparable to those obtainable with current excimer lasers. Its large optical zone capability and scanning delivery system may well provide improved correction of high myopia, hy-

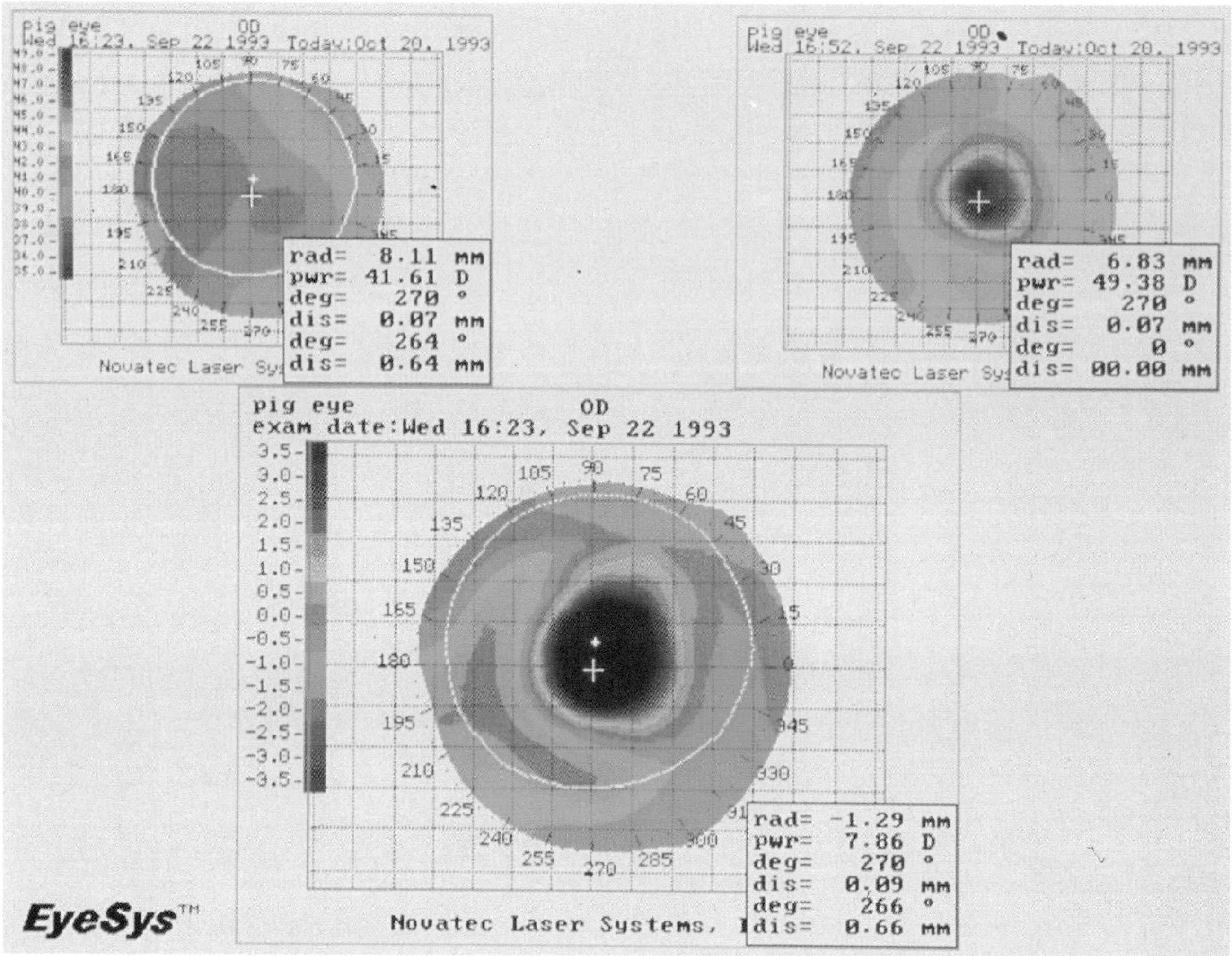

pig eye OD
Wed 16:23, Sep 22 1993 Today:Oct 20, 1993
rad= 8.11 mm
pwr= 41.61 D
deg= 270 °
dis= 0.07 mm
deg= 264 °
dis= 0.64 mm
Novatec Laser Sy
pig eye OD
Wed 16:52, Sep 22 1993 Today:Oct 20, 1993
rad= 6.83 mm
pwr= 49.38 D
deg= 270 °
dis= 0.07 mm
deg= 0 °
dis= 00.00 mm
Novatec Laser Sy
pig eye OD
exam date:Wed 16:23, Sep 22 1993
3.5-
3.0-
2.5-
2.0-
1.5-
1.0-
0.5-
0.0-
-0.5-
-1.0-
-1.5-
-2.0-
-2.5-
-3.0-
-3.5-
rad= -1.29 mm
pwr= 7.86 D
deg= 270 °
dis= 0.09 mm
deg= 266 °
dis= 0.66 mm
Novatec Laser Systems,
EyeSys™

Fig. 18-5. Corneal topography demonstrates central corneal steepening following 5-D hyperopic PRK.

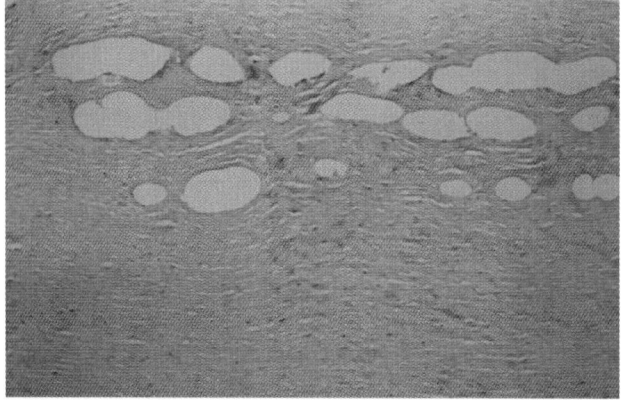

Fig. 18-6. Three layers of cavities (intrastromal ablation), evenly spaced, demonstrate the ability of the LightBlade to photodisrupt corneal stroma in a controlled manner.

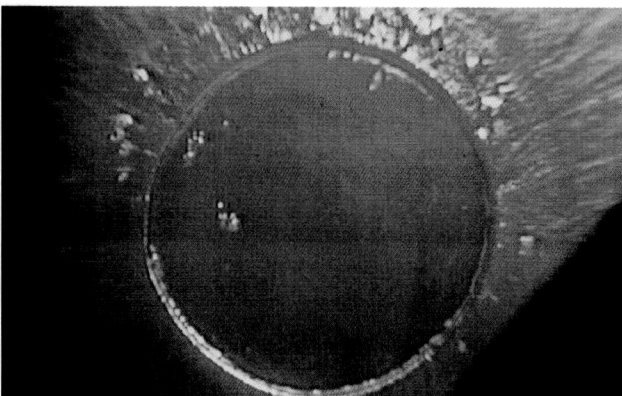

Fig. 18-7. Corneal stromal bed following removal of an intact lamellar disk of tissue by the Novatec laser microkeratome.

peropia, and varieties of astigmatism. Preliminary evaluation of the intrastromal-intraocular mode confirmed the performance of a wide range of procedures not possible with excimer laser technology.

An investigational device exemption (IDE) is currently pending for correction of low to moderate myopia by surface ablation, and human trials are expected to commence shortly.

REFERENCES

1. Trokel SL, Srinivasan R, Braren B: Excimer laser surgery of the cornea, *Am J Ophthalmol* 96:710-715, 1983.
2. Del Pero RA, Gigstad JE, Roberts AD, et al: A refractive and histopathologic study of excimer laser keratectomy in primates, *Am J Ophthalmol* 109:419-429, 1990.
3. Taylor DM, L'Esperance FA, Del Pero RA, et al: Human excimer laser lamellar keratectomy: a clinical study, *Ophthalmology* 96:654-664, 1989.
4. Salz JJ, Maguen E, Nesburn AB, et al: A two-year experience with excimer laser photorefractive keratectomy for myopia, *Ophthalmology* 100:873-882, 1993.
5. Lindstrom RL, Sher NA, Barak M, et al: Excimer laser photorefractive keratectomy in high myopia: a multicenter study, *Trans Am Ophthalmol Soc* 90:277-296, 1992.
6. Sher NA, Bowers RA, Zabel RW, et al: Clinical use of the 193-nm excimer laser in the treatment of corneal scars, *Arch Ophthalmol* 109:491-498, 1991.
7. Stark WJ, Chamon W, Kamp MT, et al: Clinical follow-up of 193 nm ArF excimer laser photokeratectomy, *Ophthalmology* 99:805-812, 1992.
8. Swinger CA, Lai ST: A new solid state laser for corneal surgery Presented at the International Society of Refractive Keratoplasty meeting, Dallas, Nov 7, 1992.
9. Swinger CA, Lai ST, Lai M, et al: Myopic photorefractive keratectomy using a scanning delivery system. In preparation.
10. Klyce SD, Smolek MK: Corneal topography of excimer laser photorefractive keratectomy, *J Cataract Refract Surg* 19:122-130, 1993.
11. Swinger CA, Lai ST, Salz JJ, et al.: A comparison of two photorefractive lasers for correction of myopia by surface ablation in a rabbit model. In preparation.
12. Swinger CA, Lai ST, Binder PS, et al: Myopic photorefractive keratectomy using the Novatec laser in non-human primates. In preparation.
13. Melles GR, Binder PS: Effect of wound location, orientation, direction, and postoperative time on unsutured corneal wound healing morphology in monkeys, *Refract Corneal Surg* 8:427-38, 1992.

19

Alternative Lasers and Strategies for Corneal Modification

Section I
J. James Rowsey, Scott X. Stevens, Bradley D. Fouraker

Section II
Douglas D. Koch, Michael J. Berry, Arthur Vassiliadis, Elizabeth A. Haft

This chapter is divided into two sections. The first section on the design and application of Intrastromal Lasers is discussed by J. James Rowsey, Scott X. Stevens and Bradley D. Fouraker. The second section on the application of laser thermal keratoplasty (LTK) to the cornea for correction of astigmatism and myopia is discussed by Douglas D. Koch, Michael J. Berry, Arthur Vassiliadis, and Elizabeth A. Haft.

Intrastromal Lasers

Scott X. Stevens, Bradley D. Fouraker, J. James Rowsey

Several methods have been used to change the refractive power of the cornea to treat myopia, hyperopia, and astigmatism. Radial keratotomy, astigmatic keratotomy, radial keratectomy, phototherapeutic keratectomy, in situ keratomileusis (also known as anterior lamellar keratectomy), and epikeratoplasty are just a few of the methods utilized and being developed. In situ keratomileusis often provides the clearest central cornea because tissue is removed from within the corneal stroma and is therefore not dependent upon superficial wound healing. Lasers are currently being developed which similarly remove intrastromal corneal tissue without corneal cap removal. Intrastromal corneal laser plasma-mediated ablation provides potential for the future treatment of myopia, hyperopia, and astigmatism.

LASER DESIGN

Intrastromal laser surgery is accomplished with solid-state lasers. Solid-state lasers are potentially more reliable and require less maintenance than gas laser systems, like the excimer. These lasers allow for a wide range of applications but require an excellent aiming mechanism.

Two solid-state lasers currently accomplish intrastromal corneal ablation: the neodymium:yttrium-aluminum-garnet (Nd:YAG) and the neodymium:yttrium-lithium fluoride (Nd:YLF) lasers.

PHOTODISRUPTION

The Nd:YAG laser utilizes an yttrium-aluminum-garnet (YAG) crystal doped with neodymium ions as the active laser medium. In short-pulse operation, a closed shutter in the laser cavity increases energy storage in the YAG crystal prior to lasing action. Opening the shutter produces very short light pulses of very high power. Power is defined as energy/time, just as acceleration is velocity/time.[1] Typical *Q-switched* Nd:YAG systems produce light pulses in the range of 2- to 30-ns (2-30 $\times$ 10^{-9} second) duration whereas *mode-locked* systems produce a group of light pulses in the range of 20- to 40 ps (20-40 $\times$ 10^{-12} second) duration. The typical wavelength of an Nd:YAG laser is 1064 nm. Therefore solid-state lasers are effective at disrupting even transparent tissue because a tremendous amount of power is delivered to a small focal spot. The term used to describe this laser-tissue interaction is *photodisruption* or *plasma-mediated ablation*.[2] Photodisruption occurs secondary to a microscopic and localized temperature increase from 37° to 15,000° C (The sun surface temperature is approximately 5000° C.). The term utilized to quantify the amount of power delivered to a focal area is *irradiance,* or less properly, *power density.* The high concentration of power in such a small focal spot results in ionization of the target tissue in a small volume of space at the laser beam focus resulting in the formation of "plasma." The small amount of plasma created by the ophthalmic photodisruptors has been termed *microplasma.*[3] Plasma is considered to be the "fourth state of matter."[4] It is a gaseous state, formed when electrons are stripped from atoms in a gas, liquid, or solid. Plasma has the mechanical properties of a gas and the electrical properties of a metal.[4] Plasma itself, when created, has some unique properties: (1) it expands rapidly outward, creating shock and acoustic (pressure) waves that mechanically disrupt tissue adjacent to the disintegrated area and (2) the plasma formation absorbs or scatters radiation arriving later within the laser pulse.[5-7]

OPTICAL BREAKDOWN

The amount of irradiance required to produce plasma in a substance is known as its *optical breakdown threshold.* The optical breakdown threshold that can be obtained varies with numerous parameters that affect clinical applications and photodisruptor design. In general, with homogeneous substances, one can reduce the threshold of optical breakdown by (1) increasing the laser pulse duration, (2) increasing the spot size, or (3) increasing the wavelength of incident laser light. Increasing the laser pulse duration or spot size increases the yield of low-level excited starting electrons. With increased pulse duration, greater thermal and acoustic damage occur. Increasing the wavelength increases photon capture in the ionization growth stage of laser beam formation. Breakdown threshold is also strongly influenced by the properties of the target material. In general, threshold is lowered by the presence of microscopic impurities (i.e., keratocytes) that act as sites for focal heating and starting electrons.[1]

LASER CORE DESIGN

The current intrastromal lasers are Q-switched photodisruptors alone or in combination with a mode-locked function and use a solid-state crystal laser sources. In a crystal laser, a flashlamp excites a significant fraction of active atoms in the crystal rod (i.e., ND ions) to create a "population inversion". Population inversion is a condition in which more atoms are in their excited state than in their ground state. Placement of mirrors at the ends of the rod creates an optical cavity in which "stimulated emission" occurs preferentially along the axis of the rod, producing a light beam (laser beam) which is

highly monochromatic and spatially coherent. Now, if one places an opaque switch ("Q-switch") within the cavity, laser emission can be retarded until a very high level of population inversion is achieved. The switch is then suddenly opened and a "giant" pulse of light escapes from the cavity. The Q-switch commonly used in photodisruptors today is a electro-optic device that remains opaque until an electrical signal switches it into a transparent condition. This electro-optic device is called a "Pockels cell."[1,8]

FUNDAMENTAL MODE

A laser beam is also influenced by the geometry of the laser cavity. The transverse mode structure influences the distribution of energy across the laser beam. The distribution of energy is determined by the boundary conditions of the laser cavity, characterized by transverse electromagnetic modes (TEMs), which arise from cavity resonances. Placement of an aperture in the cavity to limit the laser beam output to only the fundamental mode (TEM^{00}) reduces the total energy produced, but results in a gaussian distribution of energy across the laser beam which permits better focusing of the beam resulting in a smaller spot size with higher irradiance.[1]

MODE-LOCKING

Mode-locking allows photons to travel a prescribed number of trips between the ends of the laser cavity before leaving the cavity. Separation of these longitudinal modes by mode-locking provides a beam with a train of brief spikes. The peak power of the individual spikes is considerably higher than power levels achieved with Q-switched laser pulses. The relative power of the individual mode-locked spikes tends to follow the shape of the Q-switched pulse, and the total duration of the mode-locked laser pulse is the same as the Q-switched pulse.[1]

Clinical laser systems consist of: (1) a high-power, short-pulse laser source; (2) a low-power aiming or focusing laser source such as a continuous-wave, helium-neon laser that produces a red light of 632.8 nm; (3) an attachment that connects the laser source to a slit-lamp delivery system; (4) a lens system that focuses the solid-state laser beam into a small spot at the working distance of the slit lamp; and (5) a slit-lamp biomicroscope. Intrastromal corneal photodisruption requires precise axial focus. For this reason the solid-state lasers have been equipped with computer-controlled tracking devices.

CONE ANGLE

In addition to the laser system itself, high irradiance can be accomplished by adjusting the converging lens within the laser delivery system, known as the *cone angle.* The size of the spot is directly proportional to

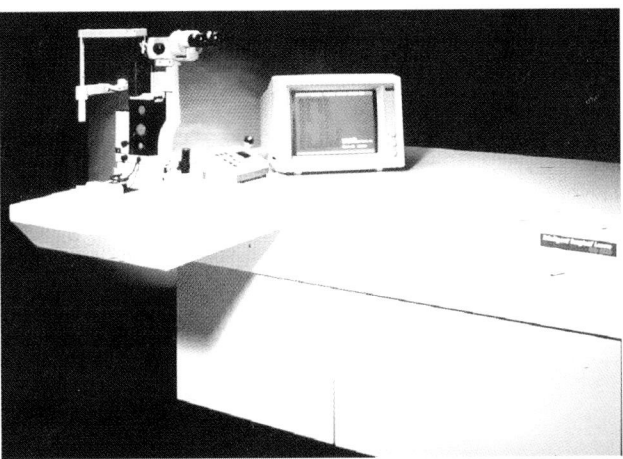

Fig. 19-1. Displays the ISL Q-switched mode-locking Nd:YLF laser with a wavelength of 1053 nm.

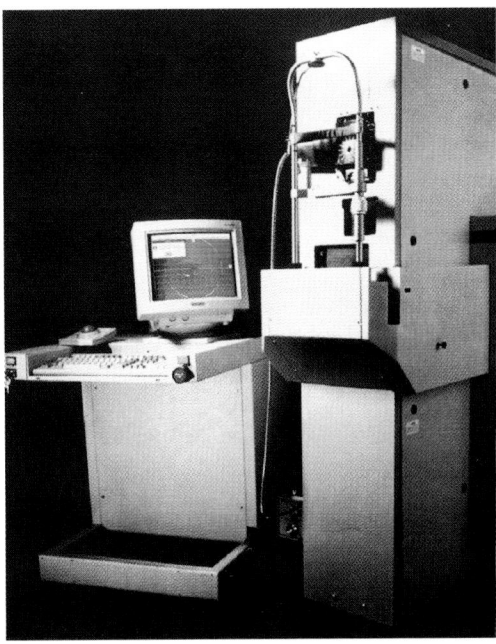

Fig. 19-2. Displays the Phoenix doubled frequency pulsed Q-switched Nd:YAG laser with a wavelength of 532 nm.

the focal length of the converging lens. Therefore a short focal length lens provides a smaller beam waist and a larger cone angle. A larger cone angle will cause the beam to diverge rapidly after leaving the focal point, resulting in lower irradiance posterior to the focal point. A long focal length lens will provide a smaller cone angle, producing a larger spot size that has lower irradiance in the focal plane and higher irradiance posterior to the focal point. Most solid-state systems use a cone angle of around 16 degrees for standard YAG capsulotomy. Intrastromal corneal lasers have increased the cone angle to between 22 and 32 degrees to ensure high target irradiance and low posterior irradiance.

Understanding the fundamental terms of solid-state laser technology which influence optical breakdown threshold is important. There are currently two companies manufacturing solid-state lasers for corneal intrastromal ablation. These companies are Phoenix Lasers, Inc. and Intelligent Surgical Lasers, Inc. (ISL).

ISL utilizes a Q-switched mode-locking Nd:YLF laser with a wavelength of 1053 nm, a repetition rate of 10 to 1000 pulses per second, pulse energy of 20 to 350 μJ, and a pulse width of 45 ps. These laser parameters in combination with a cone angle of 32 degrees creates a spot size of 7 μm. The maximal diameter of pattern disruption is 6.0 mm. The laser delivery system is a modified Moeller-Wedel Variflex operating microscope. The laser tracking device incorporated within the laser separates laser spots by 10 to 15 μm (Fig. 19-1).

Phoenix has developed a doubled-frequency-pulsed Q-switched Nd:YAG laser with a wavelength of 532 nm, repetition rate of 10 to 200 pulses per second, a pulse energy of 20 to 550 μJ, and a pulse width less than 10 ns. These laser parameters in combination with a cone angle of 22.5 degrees create a spot size of

15 μm. The laser tracking device incorporated within the laser separates laser applications by 20 μm. The maximal diameter of pattern disruption is 12 mm. The laser delivery system is based on computer tracking after head stabilization (Fig. 19-2).

One of the major differences between the two lasers is the length of the laser pulse width. The ISL uses a pulse width 200 times shorter than the Phoenix system. The shorter pulse width is possible because ISL utilizes a solid-state optical gain medium, Nd:YLF, closely related to Nd:YAG but without several of its undesirable features. Nd:YLF is only weakly affected by thermal birefrigence which allows a simpler laser cavity design and inherently allows a higher ratio of TEM^{00} to multimode average power.[9] Purely TEM^{00} mode beams can be focused to spot sizes smaller than multimode beams. In addition, Nd:YLF has a relatively large fluorescence line width compared to Nd:YAG, which allows the generation of shorter-duration pulses.[10] Nd:YLF also has a longer upper-level fluorescence lifetime compared to Nd:YAG, which allows greater energy storage and thus higher peak pulse powers under Q-switched or mode-locked operation.[3] Original studies compared Nd:YLF Q-switched picosecond photodisruptors with Nd:-YAG multimode nanosecond photodisruptors. Multimode Nd:YAG lasers suffered from poor beam quality and were unable to achieve the small focal spot size required to achieve the requisite peak powers for photodisruption. Therefore, more energy had to be deposited into the treatment site, resulting in a larger zone of effect and more propensity to damage downstream structures owing to thermal and acoustic effects.[2,5,6,11] The Phoenix system is able to produce a spot size 10 to 20 μm in diameter, resulting in peak powers greater than 10 W/cm^2 for pulse durations of less than 8 ns with energies of 80 to 150 μJ. Spot size actually may be a more important parameter affecting photodisruption than pulse duration.

SPOT SIZE

Spot size appears to be an important parameter, but precise measurement of spot size in tissue is difficult. Another important parameter is spot separation or the distance between individual laser applications. Spots placed too close together will overlap and the cavitation bubbles produced will tend to absorb laser energy intended for adjacent tissue resulting in inadequate photodisruption.[11] If the spots are placed too far apart, the cornea remains pocked or "Swiss-cheesed," resulting in irregular or variable corneal topography.

Optimal laser energy for intrastromal ablation appears to be in the range of 20 to 40 μJ with the picosecond Nd:YLF laser. Utilizing laser energies greater than 40 μJ is associated with more corneal scarring and greater risk of endothelial damage secondary to acoustic and thermal side effects. Corneal haze resolves with topical corticosteroid therapy.

The ultimate key to successful intrastromal corneal laser photodisruption is the precise placement of a focal laser pulse within the corneal stroma. ISL and Phoenix both have corneal tracking devices employed in the laser delivery system to accomplish precise placement of the laser pulses within the corneal stroma along x, y, and z coordinates.

Preliminary animal studies have been accomplished with both systems. Ablation threshold for human epithelium, Bowman's layer, and stroma is 6.1 ± 1.8 J/cm^2, 21.0 ±5.1 J/cm^2, and 10.4 ±1.8 J/cm^2 respectively for the Nd:YLF laser.[3] The authors of this study recorded threshold energy when a visible "spark" was produced. Preliminary work with the Phoenix system revealed that the ablation threshold for corneal stroma is 11.3 J/cm^2 and was documented with histopathologic evidence of tissue fragmentation, not just the presence of a "spark." The ablation threshold for human epithelium, Bowman's layer, and stroma may be greater when based on histopathology and not on visible optical breakdown.

Transmission and scanning electron microscopy of treated rabbit corneas support theories put forth in previous discussions on the formation of plasma. Once plasma is formed, shock waves in tissue are thought to be generated by several mechanisms alone or in combination: rapid expansion of plasma; photon scattering within the plasma; absorption of laser energy by a nonthermal method; radiation pressure; thermal expansion caused by focal heating; or phase

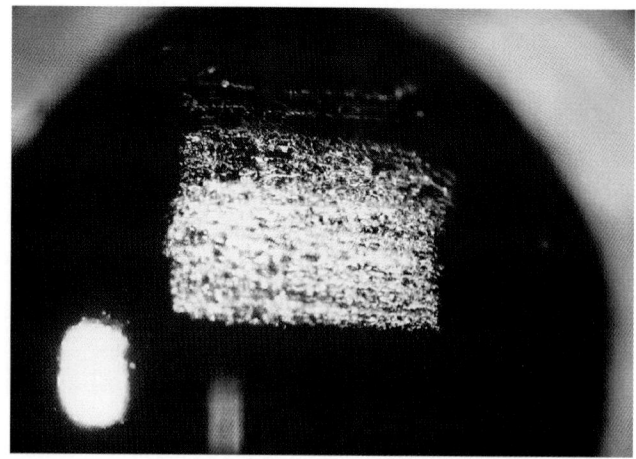

Fig. 19-3. Demonstrates the cavitation bubbles present in a cat cornea after intrastromal laser ablation.

changes within the tissue plasma.[1] Transmission electron microscopy demonstrates fragmentation of collagen fibrils and evidence of thermal damage at the plasma-tissue interface. Collagen fibril fragmentation appears secondary to the initial high-energy shock waves. Adjacent areas show disruption of normal collagen orientation and may represent evidence of a shock wave–acoustic wave gradient effect. This effect is visible 20 to 30 μm from the treatment site. The acoustic effect is secondary to the supersonic velocity of the plasma formation. The velocity of the acoustic wave travels outward approximately 100 μm in about 50 μs and then rapidly diminishes.[11] Therefore, within a distance of 100 μm from the center of the emission, the acoustic disturbance is nonlinear and has shock wave properties. Laser spots placed within 100 to 150 μm of the rabbit corneal endothelium result in acute loss of endothelium. The loss of the corneal endothelium is secondary to the acoustic effect of the laser impulse. Placement of intrastromal laser spots 330 μm deep in the cat cornea (within 200 μm of the cat corneal endothelium) by the Phoenix system results in loss of the corneal endothelium underlying the treatment site. Current algorithms place the intrastromal treatment within the anterior 150 μm of the cornea.[12,13] Immediately following the laser procedure, the cornea is opalescent because of the presence of intrastromal cavitation bubbles (Fig. 19-3). These bubbles resolve spontaneously over 6 hours. Associated corneal edema typically resolves over the subsequent 48 to 72 hours and corneal topography begins to shift as the cornea thins and collapses over the treatment sites. Intracorneal haze dissipates over the following 2 to 3 weeks.

ISL has developed pattern configurations for the treatment of myopia, hyperopia, and astigmatism. A myopic ablation is accomplished by treating the central cornea in three to four layers in a stepwise fash-

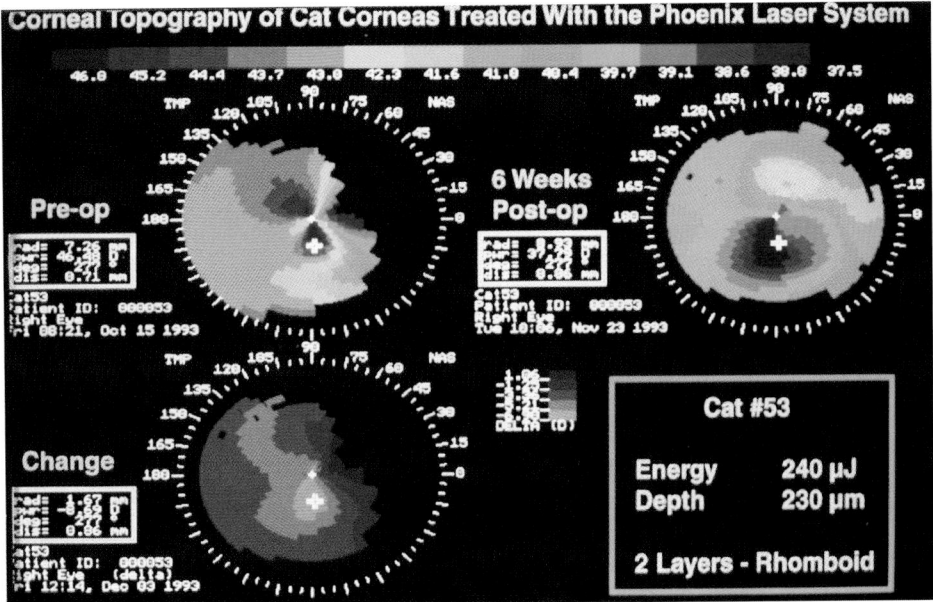

Fig. 19-4. EyeSys corneal topography of a cat eye six weeks after receiving a rhomboid treatment shows 9 D of flattening directly over the treatment site with an adjacent 5 D of steepening.

ion. The layers range from 3 to 6 mm in diameter. The most posterior stromal layer is 3 mm in diameter. The laser moves in a spiral-circumferential pattern from the cornea center to the periphery. Upon completion of the 3-mm layer the laser moves just anterior to this treatment layer and ablates a 4-mm zone in a similar fashion. Once the 4-mm zone is completed, the laser moves anterior and ablates a 5-mm optical zone followed by a 6-mm ablation zone. Completion of the treatment leaves a bowl-like configuration within the anterior one third of the corneal stroma. The intrastromal ionized plasma is absorbed, and the cornea collapses resulting in central corneal flattening. In limited human European studies, 2 to 3 D of correction have been achieved with this algorithm. Mark Speaker and his colleague Micheal Nissen, recently developed an algorithm in which the laser ablates ten spiral layers, 6 mm in diameter, starting 120 μm deep in the rabbit cornea. The rabbits achieved 15 to 20 D of flattening in the immediate postoperative period. No long-term data on stability or regression are available. Initial animal studies with the Phoenix system where we placed two thomboid patterns above and below the visual axis indicate that we can obtain up to 9 D of flattening over the treatment sites with an adjacent 5 D of central steepening (Fig. 19-4).

The pattern configuration for the treatment of hyperopia entails the removal of an intrastromal ring of tissue. Laser treatment is initiated 150 μm deep in the corneal stroma and three to four layers of tissue are removed extending from the 2.0-mm to the 6.0-mm optical zone. The central 2.0 mm is not treated. The plasma is absorbed and the midperipheral cornea collapses resulting in a hyperopic shift in topography.

Several laser parameters must be satisfied before widespread clinical use is possible. Centration of the treatment zone is critical as well as stabilizing the eye during treatment. The cornea becomes distorted in the process of treatment secondary to the intrastromal cavitation bubbles. The corneal distortion displaces the applanation system which is important for beam-tracking. Other parameters which also need to be determined for adequate dose-response curves include optimal laser energy, optimal spot size, spot separation, and layer separation.

REFERENCES

1. Mainster MA, Sliney DH, Belcher CD III, et al: Laser photodisruptors: damage mechanisms, instrument design and safety, *Ophthalmology* 90:973–991, 1983.
2. Stern D, Puliafito CA, Dobi ET, et al: Corneal ablation by nanosecond, picosecond and femtosecond lasers at 532nm and 625nm, *Arch Ophthalmol* 107:587–592, 1989.
3. Niemz MH, Klancnik EG, Bille JF: Plasma-mediated ablation of corneal tissue at 1053nm using a Nd:YLF oscillator/regenerative amplifier laser, *Lasers Med Sci* 11:426–431, 1991.
4. Boulnois JL: Photophysical processes in recent medical laser developments: a review, *Lasers Med Sci* 1:47–66, 1986.
5. Steinert RF, Puliafito CA, Kittrell C: Plasma shielding by Q-switched and mode-locked Nd-YAG lasers, *Ophthalmology* 90:1003–1006, 1983.
6. Steinert RF, Puliafito CA, Trokel S: Plasma formation and shielding by three ophthalmic Nd:YAG lasers, *Am J Ophthalmol* 96:427-434, 1983.
7. Vogel A, Hentschel W, Holzfuss J, et al: Cavitation bubble dynamics and acoustic transient generation in ocular surgery with

pulsed neodymium:YAG lasers, *Ophthalmology* 93:1259-1269, 1986.

8. L'Esperance FA: *Ophthalmic lasers,* vol I, ed 3, St Louis, 1989, Mosby-Year Book.

9. Murray JE: Pulsed gain and thermal lensing of Nd:LiYF$_4$, *IEEE J Quantum Electron* 4:488-491, 1983.

10. Pollak TM, Wing WF, Grasso RJ, C et al: Laser operation of Nd:YLF, *IEEE J Quantum Electron* 2:159-162, 1982.

11. Fujimoto JG, Lin WZ, Ippen EP, et al: Time-resolved studies of Nd:YAG laser-induced breakdown, *Invest Ophthalmol Vis Sci* 26:1771-1777, 1985.

12. Remmel RM, Dardenne CM, Bille JF: Intrastromal tissue removal using an infrared picosecond Nd:YLF ophthalmic laser operating at 1053nm. *Lasers Light Ophthalmol* 4:169-173, 1992.

13. Frueh BE, Bille JF, Brown SI: Intrastromal relaxing excisions in rabbits with a picosecond infrared laser, *Laser Light Ophthalmol* 4:165-168, 1992.

Laser Thermal Keratoplasty for Correction of Astigmatism and Myopia

Douglas D. Koch, Michael J. Berry, Arthur Vassiliadis, Elizabeth A. Haft

The background and principles of laser thermal keratoplasty (LTK) and its application for the correction of hyperopia have been described in Chapter 15. By applying thermal energy to the appropriate regions of the cornea, corrections of astigmatism and myopia can also be effected.

Laboratory Studies

Some of the important in vitro and in vivo studies of LTK for correction of myopia were performed by Berry et al using the hydrogen fluoride chemical laser, which is a continuous-wave gas laser.[1-3] A wavelength of 2.61 μm, with a treatment annulus of approximately 500 μm width, was used in a series of 12 juvenile rabbits. Treatment zones were 4 to 5 mm, and 200 to 400 mJ of energy were delivered. One eye was treated and the other eye followed as a control; follow-up was up to 6 months. Corneal topographic changes were monitored using the Corneascope (KERA Corp., Santa Clara, Calif.), comparing the average curvatures of the first three rings to the fellow eye at all intervals.

In 4 of the 12 rabbits, persistent central corneal flattening of up to 3 D was noted for up to 6 months. In the two rabbits with 6-month follow-up, the effect stabilized by 1 month posttreatment. Moderate haze was noted at the treatment site immediately following irradiation, but the opacity was barely detectable with the slit lamp at 1 week and was undetectable by 3 months postoperatively (Fig. 19-5).

Arcuate treatments were also attempted in one rabbit. Eight diopters of net steepening was induced along the treated meridian and 2 D were present at 2

months (at which point the animal died of unrelated causes).

As previously noted, the Sunrise holmium:YAG laser (Sunrise Technologies, Fremont, Calif.) has been extensively studied using swine eyes in vitro.[4] In these studies, central corneal flattening could be achieved by treating with eight spots at the 3.0- and 3.5-mm diameter zones. Astigmatic corrections were achieved by treating with two pairs of spots applied along the flat corneal meridian. The net change in corneal curvature (i.e., overall flattening or steepening) depends on the diameter of the treatment zone. These parameters follow those that were noted for the spherical corrections: astigmatic treatments at the 3.0- and 3.5-mm zones flatten the central cornea, whereas treatments at 5.0 mm and above steepen the central cornea.

Clinical Studies

Clinical studies of LTK for correction of myopia will commence once treatment patterns are developed that will not produce clinically significant long-lasting corneal haze at the treatment sites. In patients undergoing LTK for correction of hyperopia, the laser-induced opacities in the midperipheral cornea appear to have absolutely no deleterious effect on vision, but similar treatments near the center of the cornea to correct myopia could produce problems with glare or decreased contrast sensitivity. Fortunately, it is likely that lower energy densities will be required to correct myopia. At given energy densities, central treatments at 3.0- and 3.5-mm zones produced over twice the change (flattening) achieved by the hyperopic treatments at the larger treatment zones. This is presumably because localized flattening is required to produce central corneal flattening, whereas the belt-tightening effect that produces hyperopic corrections requires local corneal flattening in the region of treat-

Table 19-1. Holmium:YAG laser thermal keratoplasty for correction of astigmatism in the partially amblyopic left eye of a 54-year-old female.

Day	Uncorrected VA	Best corrected VA	Manifest refraction
Pre	20/300	20/50	+2.25-4.5×24
Post 1	20/60	—	—
8	20/60	20/60	plano
24	20/30	20/30	plano
45	20/25	20/25	plano
71	20/50	20/50	+0.5-0.75×15

Two pairs of spots were delivered along the 24-degree meridian at the 6-mm optical zone. The energy density was 8.44 J/cm². By refraction (and also by keratometry), 3.75 D of astigmatism have been corrected two months postoperatively.

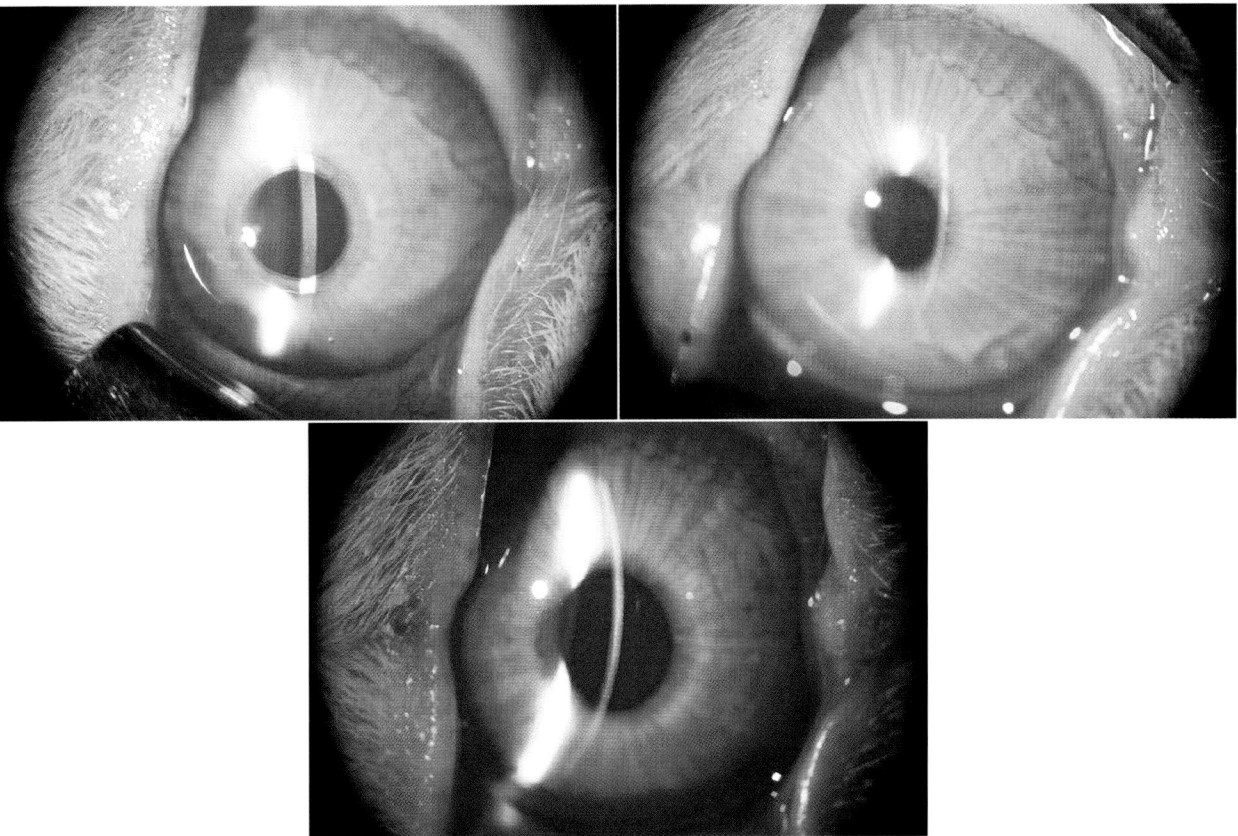

Fig. 19-5. Rabbit cornea following hydrogen fluoride laser thermal keratoplasty to produce central corneal flattening. Moderate haze was present at the treatment site immediately following irradiation (*left*), but the opacity was barely detectable with the slit lamp at one week (*right*) and was undetectable by three months postoperatively (*bottom*).

Hyperopic Astigmatism Correction Pattern   Myopic Astigmatism Correction Pattern

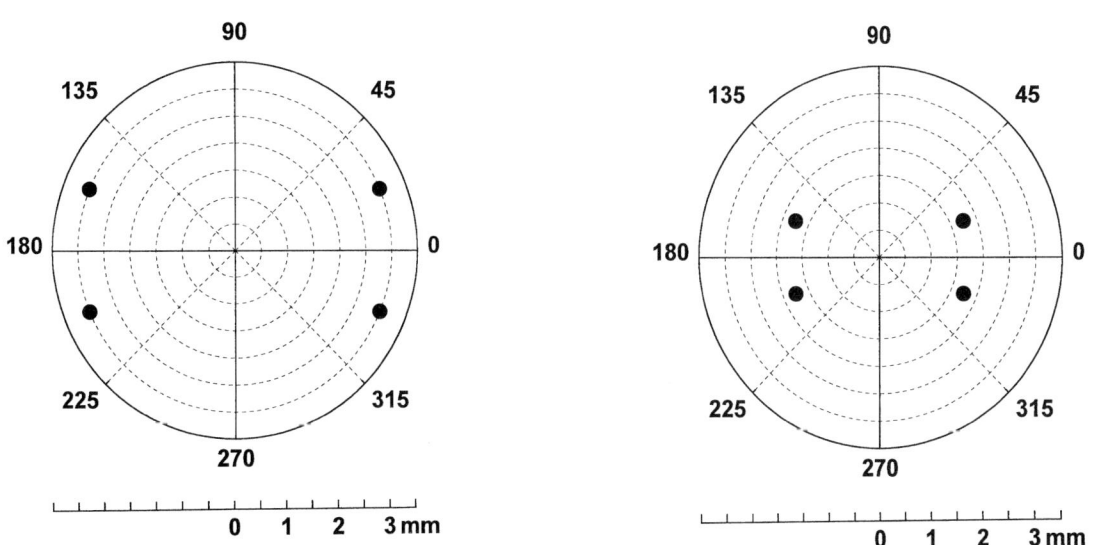

Fig. 19-6. Treatment patterns for correction of hyperopic (*left*) and myopic (*right*) astigmatism as determined in studies with swine and human cadaver eyes.

ment with the central corneal steepening occurring as a secondary effect.

Trials for correction of astigmatism have begun outside the United States. Treatments have consisted of two pairs of spots applied along the flat meridian at the 6.0- or 7.0-mm optical zones (Fig. 19-6). Astigmatic corrections of up to 4 D have been achieved (Table 19-1). Maximum follow-up is 6 months, and studies are ongoing.

CONCLUSION

Laser thermal keratoplasty is a promising treatment for correction of astigmatism and may also prove to be a useful therapy for the correction of myopia. Studies are proceeding to better understand the effects of treatment parameters (e.g., number of spots, spot size, energy density, number of pulses, treatment pattern, and pharmacologic modulation) and patient-response characteristics (as a function of age, sex, corneal thick-

ness, intraocular pressure, and other factors yet to be determined). The advantages of noncontact Ho:YAG LTK—speed, ease for surgeon and patient, low cost, high instrument reliability, and the ability to titrate and to re-treat—warrant continued investigation of this modality of laser refractive surgery for correction of astigmatism and myopia.

REFERENCES

1. Berry MJ, Fredin LG, Valderrama GL, et al: Temperature distributions in laser-irradiated corneas, *Invest Ophthalmol Vis Sci* 32(suppl):994, 1991.
2. Koch DD, Padrick TD, Halligan DT, et al: HF chemical laser photothermal keratoplasty, *Invest Ophthalmol Vis Sci* 32(suppl):94, 1991.
3. Koch DD, Padrick TD, Menefee RF, et al: Laser photothermal keratoplasty: nonhuman primate results, *Invest Ophthalmol Vis Sci* 33(suppl):768, 1992.
4. Koch DD, Abaraca A, Menefee RF, et al: Ho:YAG laser thermal keratoplasty: *in vitro* experiments, *Invest Ophthalmol Vis Sci* 34(suppl):1246, 1993.

Appendix

A. Comparison of Commercially Available Excimer Lasers
B. Sample Informed Consent for Excimer Laser Photorefractive
Keratectomy for Phase III FDA Trial (Courtesy
of VISX Corporation, Sunnyvale, California)

Ronald R. Krueger, M.D.

Appendix A: Internationally available excimer lasers for corneal surgery: Clinical, technical and economic features

Manufacturer model/name	VISX 20/20 B	VISX 20/20 C (under develop.)	Summit Omni Med	Technolas Keracor 116
Distributor	Alcon Surgical (Ft. Worth, TX)	Alcon Surgical (Ft. Worth, TX)	Summit Tech., Inc., (Waltham, MA)	Chiron Vision Corp. (Irvine, CA)
Installation consideration				
Dimension (cm) L × W. H	274 × 84 × 147	200 × 92 × 122	99 × 71 × 165	220 × 130 × 200
Weight (Kg)	955	630	635	600
Electrical requirements	220 v, 3 phase, 20 amp	220 v, 1 phase, 20 amp	110 or 220 v, 1 phase, 15 or 10 amp	220 v, 1 phase, 16 amp
Gas cylinder requirements	3 cylinders, ArF pre-mix, He, liquid N_2	2 cylinders ArF pre-mix, He	2 cylinders ArF pre-mix, N_2	1 cylinder ArF pre-mix
Instrumentation				
Laser cooling system	Air-cooled	Internal water-cooled	Internal water-cooled	Internal water-cooled
Computer system	IBM PC: external	IBM PC: imbedded	Fixed microchip	IBM PC
Delivery system	Operating microscope	Operating microscope	Operating microscope	Operating microscope
Laser beam homogenization	Rotating prism plus integrator	Rotating prism plus integrator	None	Optical integrator
Beam shaping	Iris and slit	Iris and slit	Iris and ablatable mask	Iris with beam scanning
Evacuation system	Vacuum nozzle (optional nitrogen gas blower)	Vacuum nozzle aspirator	None	Evacuation nozzle
Patient fixation system	Single coaxial LED	Single coaxial LED	Coaxial LED within circle	Single coaxial LED
Tracking system	None	Under development	None	Optional "active" tracking system
Preparation				
Gas fill	Every 1-2 days	Every 2-3 days	Every day	Every 5-10 patients
Energy calibration	Internal joulemeter	Internal joulemeter plus ablation depth	Internal joulemeter, optional gelatin film ablation	Fluence plate
Homogeneity check	Calibration card ablation quality	Calibration card quality plus (BIP)*	PMMA profilometry	Special foil
Refractive check	Ablation of calibration card lens	Ablation of calibration card lens	None	None
Operator adjustment	Adjustment based on lens ablation reading	Auto adjustment by program	None	Reprogramming based on number of pulses through foil
Procedure				
Eye fixation	Patient or mechanical fixation	Patient or mechanical fixation	Patient self-fixation	Patient or mechanical fixation
Surgeon alignment	Optical reticule align	Heads up display	2 HeNe laser spots on either side of pupil	2 HeNe laser spots alignment on cornea

Modified from Krueger RR: Excimer laser: A step-up in complexity and responsibility for the ophthalmic laser surgeon; *J Refract Corneal Surg* 10:83-89, 1994; and Moretti M: International ophthalmic excimer lasers. *Medical Laser Insight* (newsletter) Jan 1994.
*(BIP) = beam intensity profilometer

Appendix A: Internationally available excimer lasers for corneal surgery: Clinical, technical and economic features—cont'd

Schwind Keratom	Nidek EC-5000	Meditec MEL 60	Laser Sight Compak − 200
Coherent Medical, Inc. (Palo Alto, CA)	Nidek, Inc. (Freemont, CA)	Aesculap-Meditec (Herolds-berg, Germany)	Laser Sight, Inc. (Orlando, FL)
$160 \times 80 \times 65$	$136 \times 75 \times 147$	$175 \times 65 \times 160$	$46 \times 67 \times 107$
900	650	450	135
230 v, 1 phase, 16 amp	220 v, 1 phase, 20 amp	220 v, 1 phase, 20 amp	110 v, 1 phase, 16 amp
2 cylinder Ar N_2 (Self-contained halogen generator)	3 cylinders ArF pre-mix, N_2, He	1 cylinder ArF pre-mix, N_2	2 cylinders ArF pre-mix, H_2 or N_2
Air-cooled	Air-cooled	Air-cooled	Air-cooled
IBM PC	IBM PC	N/A	IBM PC
Operating microscope	Operating microscope	Operating microscope	Operating microscope
Prismatic integrator	Scanning and rotating broad band	Scanning slit	Scanning spot
Band with "fractile mask" apertures, telescopic zoom	Iris and slit	Rotating mask	None
Circumferential laminar flow vacuum	Aspiratory within optional suction cup	Vacuum aspiration in mask	Air blowing
Blinking co-axial HeNe laser	Single co-axial LED	Single coaxial filament	Single coaxial LED
"Passive" eye tracking	None	None	None
Once a week	Every 2 days	Every day	Every day
Fluence sensor, gelatin film ablation	Internal joulemeter	Internal joulemeter with electronic adjustment	External power meter
Gelatin film ablation	None	Photo paper ablation	None
None	Ablation PMMA lens	None	None
Reprogramming based on pulses for perforation of film	Reprogramming based on lens ablation reading	Change aspiration flow (internal adjustment)	System gas refill when energy too low
Patient self-fixation	Patient or mechanical	Mechanical only	Patient self-fixation
3 HeNe laser spot alignment on cornea	2 slit & 1 HeNe spot alignment on cornea	2 HeNe laser spot alignment on cornea	2 HeNe laser spots alignment on cornea
20 seconds	23 seconds	100 seconds	30-50 seconds

Continued

Appendix A: Internationally available excimer lasers for corneal surgery: Clinical, technical and economic features—cont'd

Manufacturer model/name	VISX 20/20 B	VISX 20/20 C (under develop.)	Summit Omni Med	Technolas Keracor 116
Procedure (cont'd)				
Ablation time (-5D correction)	40 seconds	25 seconds	25 seconds	19 seconds
Treatment parameters				
Spot size (Max)	6.0 mm	6.5 mm	6.5 mm	7.0 mm
Energy density ("Fluence")	160 mJ/cm^2	160 mJ/cm^2	180 mJ/cm^2	120-200 mJ/cm^2
Ablation pulse rate	6 Hz	10 Hz	10 Hz	10 Hz
Transition zone	None	Under development	None	Aspheric up to 7.0 mm
Cost				
System purchase	N/A	N/A	$425K	$450K
Annual service contract	$35K	N/A	$35K	$45K
Treatment capability (US trial status)				
Myopic PRK	Expanding iris (phase III)	Expanding iris (equivalency tests underway)	Expanding iris (phase III)	Expanding iris (Phase IIb)
Astigmatic PRK	Expanding iris & slit (phase III)	Expanding iris and slit (equivalency tests underway)	Ablatable mask (Phase IIb)	Expanding iris with meridional scanning beam (application for IDE)
Hyperopic PRK	Variable rotating slit with eccentric lens (Phase IIa)	Variable rotating slit with eccentric lens (equivalency tests underway)	Ablatable mask (phase II)	Expanding iris with annular scanning beam (application for IDE)
PTK	Open iris and/or slit, 0.6 to 6.0 mm circle or slit for smoothing (panel recommended for approval)	Open iris and/or slit. 0.6 to 6.0 mm circle or slit for smoothing	Open iris, 1.0 to 6.5 mm circle for smoothing (advisory panel approval for use)	Open iris, 0.8 to 3.5 mm circle with joystick for smoothing (phase IIb)

Appendix A: Internationally available excimer lasers for corneal surgery: Clinical, technical and economic features—cont'd

Schwind Keratom	Nidek EC-5000	Meditec MEL 60	Laser Sight Compak − 200
8.0 mm	6.5 mm achieved by 7 × 2 mm band	7.0 to 8.0 mm achieved by 10 × 1.5 mm slit	3.0 to 9.0 mm achieved by 0.8-1.2 mm spot
<250 mJ/cm^2	130 mJ/cm^2	250 mJ/cm^2	160-300 mJ/cm^2
10 Hz (1-30 Hz programmable)	5 scans/sec (50 Hz)	20 Hz	80-100 Hz
9.0 mm	9.0 mm	9.0 mm	None
$390-520 K	$440K	$400-440K	$300-350
$30K	$35K	$40K	$15-20K
Series of circular masks (IDE application pending)	Expanding iris with scanning and rotating beam (application for IDE)	Rotating hourglass mask aperture (none)	Scanning spot (phase I)
Series of elliptical masks (IDE application pending)	Expanding iris & slit with scanning and rotating beam (application for IDE)	Variably rotating hourglass mask aperture (none)	Scanning spot along meridian (none)
Series of annular masks (IDE application pending)	None	Rotating inverse "hourglass" mask aperture (none)	Scanning spot in annular pattern (none)
Large diameter mask, 0.6 to 6.0 mm circle for smoothing (IDE application pending)	Open iris or rectangle, 0.5 to 6.5 mm spot for smoothing (application for IDE)	Large diameter scanning, methylcellulose for smoothing (none)	Scanning spot (none)

APPENDIX B: SAMPLE CONSENT FORM
EXCIMER LASER FOR PHOTOREFRACTIVE KERATECTOMY
PHASE III

_____
(Name of Institution)

INVESTIGATOR(S):   _____

_____

PHONE: _____

INTRODUCTION:

My doctor has described to me a research program involving an investigational laser sponsored by VISX, Incorporated. This laser is used to reshape the front of the cornea by a procedure called photorefractive keratectomy (PRK), thereby possibly reducing or eliminating the need for glasses or contact lenses in the case of nearsightedness (myopia). I understand that the correction obtained may not be completely adequate, and that additional correction with glasses or contact lenses may be needed. I have been told that the purpose of the research is to determine the safety and effectiveness of this laser.

I understand that, while Phases I, IIa, and IIb of this study have been performed on partially sighted and sighted humans, and the procedure has been found to be effective and has produced no ill effects to date, the beneficial results of this treatment are not completely known. My participation will be in Phase III of this study, which will involve 700 patients and will start when permission has been received from the Food and Drug Administration.

INCLUSIONS:

Included will be patients 18 years or older, of either sex and any race, who are nearsighted in both eyes, and who will be available for follow-up for the duration of the study.

EXCLUSIONS:

Excluded will be anyone with residual, recurrent, or active ocular disease or abnormality except for myopia in either eye, or with active or residual disease(s) likely to affect wound healing capability.

TREATMENT:

If I agree to participate in this study, the following procedure will be used:

The eye being treated will receive either a topical or local anesthetic, and there should be little or no discomfort during the procedure. Because patients often experience pain in the hours following treatment, pain relieving medication will be prescribed by the physician.

I will be lying on my back under the laser. The doctor will control treatment pulses with a footswitch. Because of the laser energy, I may see a flash of light and hear a "ticking" sound. The laser will remove a minute amount of the front of my cornea in an attempt to reshape the front surface of my eye such that my need for glasses will be decreased or eliminated. This method may be much less traumatic than conventional radial keratotomy or other corneal surgery.

BENEFITS:

It is felt that PRK with the excimer laser may offer benefits that are not available with surgical radial keratotomy. These benefits may include a higher rate of successful treatment, less operative trauma, and fewer risks than associated with conventional treatment. The benefits of excimer laser therapy cannot be guaranteed. My participation in this study may be of no benefit and is not guaranteed not to be harmful.

RISKS:

I understand that, similar to alternative treatments, it is possible this laser surgery may make my vision worse. Complications may include corneal perforations; corneal scarring; glare; changes in the epithelium or recurrent erosions; damage to the inside of the cornea; cataract formation; corneal infection; infection inside the eye. Although these conditions are rare, it is possible that if significant reduction in vision is produced as a result of these complications, my cornea may have to be removed and replaced with a clear cornea (corneal transplant).

ALTERNATIVE TREATMENTS:

I understand that I may decide not to have this operation at all. If I decide not to have this operation for the correction of nearsightedness, I understand that there are other methods of restoring useful vision in myopia without surgery, including glasses, contact lenses, or radial keratotomy.

PERIODIC TESTS AND FOLLOW-UP:

Because of the need to monitor my progress during and after treatment, I understand that I will have certain tests on a regular basis. These include vision examinations and numerous ophthalmologic examinations. My doctor has explained these tests to me and has told me they will be performed every 24 to 48 hours until the outer layer (epithelium) of my cornea has grown back, and then at one month, three months, six months, one year, eighteen months, and two years. I also understand that I may be required to return more frequently if my doctor feels this is necessary.

FINANCIAL RESPONSIBILITY:

I understand that I will not be paid to participate in this study and that I am financially responsible for all physician fees, laboratory costs, and other procedures required for my treatment and follow-up. These costs may or may not be covered by my medical insurance.

I understand that participation in this study will not result in any extra charges above and beyond those routinely incurred by patients with similar illnesses. The costs of unforeseen complications must be met by me.

LIABILITY:

My participation in this research project does not waive any of my legal rights nor can the Investigator, the Institution, or the study Sponsor (instrument manufacturer) be released from any liability for injuries arising out of this procedure should they occur.

WITHDRAWAL:

I understand that I am not required to enter this program. If I agree to participate, it will be a voluntary decision. I understand that I am free to withdraw from this study at any time, and that my refusal to continue in the research Protocol will not jeopardize or prevent my continued medical care in this institution now or in the future. If I wish to withdraw, I understand that it is important to notify my doctor so that he/she can plan for my continuing medical care.

I also understand that my physician, after consulting with me, can withdraw me from this study if, in his/her best medical judgment, continuing the treatment will not be in my best interest.

CONFIDENTIALITY:

I understand that the results of this study will be released to the Food and Drug Administration. I also understand that the results of this study may be published. However, my privacy will be protected and my name will not be used in any manner whatsoever.

VOLUNTARY CONSENT:

I certify that other alternative surgical procedures have been explained to me, and I have rejected them. I certify that I have read the preceding, that I understand its contents, and that any questions I have pertaining to the preceding have been answered by my physician(s) and that my permission is freely given. A copy of this consent form has been given to me.

_____   _____
Patient's Signature and Date   Type or Print Patient's Name

I was present during the explanation referred to above, as well as the patient's opportunity for questions, and hereby witness his/her consent.

_____   _____
Witness' Signature and Date   Type or Print Witness' Name

INDEX